ADULT NURSING

A NURSING PROCESS

APPROACH

ADULT NURSING
A NURSING PROCESS APPROACH

Edited by

Barbara C. Long

MSN, RN
*Associate Professor Emeritus of Medical–Surgical Nursing,
Frances Payne Bolton School of Nursing,
Case Western Reserve University,
Cleveland, Ohio*

Wilma J. Phipps

PhD, RN, FAAN
*Professor Emeritus of Medical–Surgical Nursing,
Frances Payne Bolton School of Nursing,
Case Western Reserve University,
Cleveland, Ohio*

Virginia L. Cassmeyer

PhD, RN, CS
*Associate Professor,
School of Nursing,
University of Kansas,
Kansas City, Kansas*

With UK Editors

Christine Brooker, BSc, RN, RM, RNT
Formerly Senior Lecturer, Nursing Studies, South Bank University
Valerie El Gamel, DN(e), RGN, Dip Counselling, Dip. Prof. Studies
in Nursing
With Prakash Gotecha, BSc, MRPharmS

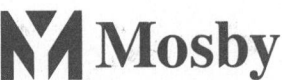 Mosby

Copyright © 1995 Times Mirror International Publishers Limited.

Published in 1995 by Mosby, an imprint of Times Mirror International Publishers Limited.

Typeset by Techset Composition Limited

Printed by Vincenzo Bona s.r.l., Turin

ISBN 0 7234 2004 1

For full details of all Mosby titles please write to Times Mirror International Publishers Ltd, Lynton House, 7-12 Tavistock Square, London WC1H 9LB, England.

A CIP catalogue record for this book is available from the British Library.

This book should not be used as a prime source for prescribing and dispensing drugs. The publisher, editors, and contributors have undertaken reasonable endeavours to check dosage and nursing content for accuracy. We recommend that the reader should always check the manufacturer's product information for changes in dosage or administration before administering any medication.

Developmental Editor:	Amy Salter
Cover Designer:	Lara Last
Production:	Joseph Lynch
Cover Illustration:	Ian Hands
Cover Photograph:	Cover photograph © 1994 Bruce Bailey/Select Photos, London
Indexer:	Nina Boyd
Publisher:	Griselda Campbell

Contents

Preface

Adult nursing encompasses the nursing care of adults who are at risk for, or who are experiencing, pathophysiological disorders. The study of adult nursing, therefore, includes knowledge of pathophysiological disorders (including medical therapy), methods of prevention, and nursing activities to assist people to achieve their optimal health. To facilitate learning, the authors of this text have chosen to focus on the essential information required by students specializing in adult nursing.

The Nursing Process approach is used in this text, particularly in the latter units that discuss pathophysiological disorders. To facilitate student learning, emphasis is placed on correlating the content of the implementation stage with the assessment stage and the nursing analysis/nursing problems stage.

Specific features of this text include:
- specific content on the care of the elderly including assessment, interventions, and common complications in elderly people, which are summarized in highlighted boxes throughout the text
- aetiologies of specific disorders, which are discussed fully throughout the text, and content on pathophysiology which includes the bases of observed symptoms
- rationales for nursing interventions, including activities that promote achievement of therapeutic goals and activities directed specifically towards achievement of patient outcomes. These are included to help students understand the difference between interdependent and independent nursing actions.

This book has been adapted from the third edition of the successful US textbook, *Medical–Surgical Nursing: A Nursing Process Approach*, with the generous permission of Barbara Long, Wilma Phipps, and Virginia Cassmeyer. The editors of the UK edition are qualified British nurses who have combined teaching nursing with clinical work. Although the basic information from the US text remains unchanged, it has been adapted, where appropriate, to include specific information relevant to UK statistics, units of measurement, nursing terminology, philosophy of care, and organization/operation of health care in the United Kingdom.

Throughout the book, the recipients of nursing care are referred to as patients rather than clients. Although client is widely used in the nursing community, the article "Complexities and Clarity in Nurse–Client and Nurse–Patient Relationships" by L. Nowakowski, which appeared in the July–August 1985 issue of the *Journal of Professional Nursing*, makes a real distinction between who is a client and who is a patient. Using her framework, the authors decided that patient was a better term to use in this book.

THE STRUCTURE OF THE BOOK

Unit 1: Introduces students to the nature of adult medical-surgical nursing and the importance of quality management in nursing.

Unit 2: Focuses on health promotion including special needs of the elderly and the role nutrition and stress management play in maintaining wellness.

Unit 3: Describes the nature of and care required for people experiencing common problems encountered in medical-surgical practice.

Unit 4: Concentrates on infection control and provides the underlying theory on HIV infection and AIDS.

Unit 5: Provides information on the care of patients undergoing surgery.

Units 6–11: Discuss specific problems of functional areas and form the main part of this text concentrating on gas transport problems, metabolic and endocrine problems, problems with digestion or elimination, sexual and reproductive problems, problems of cognition, sensation and motion, and problems of defence and protection.

THE FORMAT OF THE CHAPTERS
The overall organization of the chapters in the specific health problems are structured as follows:

Review of anatomy and physiology
Prevention and health education
Major Health Problems
Aetiology/Epidemiology
Pathophysiology
Nursing Process
  Assessment
  Nursing analysis
  Planning: expected patient outcomes
  Implementation
    Assisting with achievement of therapeutic goals
    Interventions to achieve patient outcomes
  Evaluation

The chapters are designed to aid effective student learning and to assist readers in quickly finding particular subjects. Each chapters contains:

Chapter outline — the chapter content at a glance.

Learning outcomes — the main concepts which can be learned from the chapter.

Boxed highlights — to emphasize important issues relevant to the chapter, such as cultural diversity, or varying priorities around the UK.

Nursing process stages — to present clearly the nurse's role in assessing, planning, implementing and evaluating care.

Illustrations — there are clear diagrams and photographs to illustrate the text.

Chapter summary — to provide an overview of the topics discussed in the chapter.

Study questions — to encourage reflection on practical situations, and to assess critically understanding of the content.

References and selected readings — to give full citations of the literature and research on which the chapter is based.

Further reading - recommendations for further resources, which will assist in understanding the needs of particular patients.

SUPPLEMENTARY TEACHING MATERIALS

Transparency Acetates — over 100 high quality transparencies of the images taken directly from the original American textbook are available. This set of acetates provides an ideal teaching supplement for both you and your students.
Computerised Test Bank — comprising an easy-access set of multiple choice questions this text bank is available in both MAC and IBM format.

ALSO AVAILABLE FOR QUALIFIED ADOPTERS:

Mosby's Nursing Skills Video Series — combining a well-developed coverage of clinical procedures with high quality video presentation, this series of videos engages the student in learning the skills most fundamental to nursing practice. Each skill is demonstrated by a nurse, explaining the procedure, related equipment and interaction with the patient. This is backed up with an accompanying manual providing objectives, skills, checklists and revision worksheets for each video.
Mosby's Medical Assistant Video Series — this set of seven videos provides an excellent medium for teaching core clinical–medical assisting skills. Each video covers specific skills and procedures, with clear demonstrations in hospital settings, backed up by graphic screens which highlight key points. The videos are supported by an instructor's guide which outlines the objectives and materials covered in each programme.

Acknowledgements

The editors and publisher gratefully acknowledge the following people for their assistance with this book:

Jane Appleton; Lynda Archer; Steve Cavanagh; Mavis Cox; Andrea Ford; Martin Gisby; Georgina Massy; Vidar Melby; Mrs S O'Shea; Mrs A E Stalker; Hannah Tudge.

Contributors to US edition:

Terri Abraham, MSN, RN, CCRN; Martha L Allen, MSN, RN; Dorothy R Blevins, MSN, RN; Mary Jo Boehnlein, MSN, RN, CNA; Frances R Chester, BSN, RN, MPA, CPQA; Elizabeth Cameron Eckstein, MSN, RN; H Fred Farley, MSN, RN; Sally M Featherstone, MN, RN, CS; Diane E Fritsch, MSN, RN, CCRN; Greer Glazer, PhD, RN; Rosemarie Hogan, MSN, RN; Maura A Hopkins, MSN, RN; Donald D Kautz, MSN, RN, CS, CRRN; Deborah Goldenberg Klein, MSN, RN, CS, CCRN; Denise M Kresevic, MSN, RN, CS; Mary Kay Lehman, MSN, RN; Ruth A Lincoln, MSN, RN, RNC; Gail Osterfield, MSN, RN; Carol G Phipps, MSN, RN; Dora A Rice, MSN, RN, CIC; Rebecca Anne Roberts, MSN, RN, ET; Grace A Rotter, MSN, RN, CIC; Elizabeth Anne Schenk, MSN, RN; Susan Moeller Schneider, MSN, RN; Barbara J Sibley, MA, MS, ND, RN, RNC; Carol E Smith, PhD, RN; Roberta A Stokes, MSN, RN, CHN, CNN, CS; Kathryn Sabo Thompson, MSN, RN; M Eileen Walsh, MSN, RN; Judith H Watt-Watson, MScN, RN; E Ronald Wright, PhD; Nancy Fugate Woods, PhD, RN, FAAN; Mary A (Sandy) Wyper, PhD, RN; Lynne C Yurko, BSN, RN.

Adult Nursing Practice

Perspectives of Adult Nursing

Barbara C. Long

After studying this chapter, the learner should be able to:

- Differentiate the practice of adult nursing from other nursing disciplines.
- Differentiate health promotion and prevention of illness, and the three levels of prevention.
- Identify stages of disease development.
- Differentiate independent and interdependent nursing functions.
- Describe five steps of nursing process.
- Identify ethical issues that may occur in the practice of adult nursing.

SCOPE OF ADULT NURSING

Adult nursing practice encompasses the nursing care of adults who are at risk for or who are experiencing pathophysiological disorders. In most health care centres children are separated from adults because of their different needs, and the specialty practice of paediatric nursing has developed with the focus on the nursing care of children. Thus adult nursing practice has developed primarily as the nursing care of people (1) who have attained physical/developmental maturity, (2) who are at risk for or who have expressed variations in their personal norms of physical functioning, and (3) who may require therapeutic medical or surgical intervention.

In the past *medical care* was the general term for the care given to sick people by professionals; the term is now used to denote the care given by members of the medical profession. The trend in British society is towards a health orientation; therefore, *health care* is the more acceptable term for the care provided by all health care professionals. The term *health care* is broader in that it includes assisting people to stay well in addition to providing care when they are ill. The care of the sick remains a primary responsibility of health care professionals, and this care is still provided primarily in health care institutions such as acute hospitals or long-term care centres. There is an increased use, however, of day care and primary care, as well as other types of health care services, in part because it is more economic to keep people well than to provide care when they are sick.[33]

Nurses are one group of health care professionals. In addition to participating in health promotion, nurses are actively involved in prevention of disease and health education for people who are at high risk for acquiring specific diseases. Health promotion, disease prevention, and care of people with specific pathophysiological disorders require a knowledge base of the following:

1. Health and illness
2. Factors influencing the occurrence and course of specific disorders
3. Common responses to the disorders
4. Nursing interventions that assist people to achieve optimal health or to die with maximum comfort and dignity

HEALTH AND ILLNESS

Health and illness are complex concepts, and they are interpreted in different ways by different individuals or groups. Both health and illness are multidimensional concepts; that is, there are multiple aspects to be considered and multiple factors that may be of influence.

Definitions of Health

During the early centuries, health was defined in terms of that which was normal or natural. Therefore, anything abnormal or against nature was considered not healthy and to be avoided; for example, lepers were called "unclean". Treatment of diseases consisted of amulets or spells to drive out the evil or unnatural spirits causing the abnormality.

"Leeching" was a popular treatment and consisted of applying leeches (blood-sucking worms) to suck out the tainted blood. Wounds were treated by cautery to burn out the evil forces that would prevent healing. Even in more modern times, "tonics", which often included a laxative, were taken frequently by people to stay healthy.

In later years health was defined primarily as freedom from disease. During the middle of the 20th century the concept of *mental health* was introduced, meaning the ability of the individual to cope successfully with stress in a functional manner. In 1974 the World Health Organization (WHO) defined health more broadly: complete physical, mental, and social well-being and not merely the absence of disease and infirmity. This definition introduced the concept of the subjective as well as the objective physical or behavioural responses.

The various views about health usually contain one or more of the following perspectives:

Biological or clinical: absence of pathological condition

Psychological: well-being and self-actualization

Sociological: ability to meet social responsibilities and role functions

Adaptive: adaptation to a changing environment

Patients and health care providers may have different views of health and may therefore be working towards different goals that may or may not be in conflict. For example, people who "feel well" and who hold the view that health is a sense of well-being may not be willing to follow-up on screening tests even when a disease may be suspected by the clinician.

Health is a dynamic, ever-changing state. It reflects the person's level of functioning in various physiological, psychological, and sociocultural dimensions. People can simultaneously be functioning at a high level in one aspect, such as nutrition, but at a low level in another aspect, such as oxygenation or self-esteem. Nursing is concerned with holistic health, the effect of functioning of the subcomponents on total functioning. Thus each patient is assessed in various dimensions, with consideration given for the person's overall functioning and sense of well-being. Each person has different genetic factors and is exposed to different environmental factors. There is therefore *no one* nursing approach for all people who are at risk for or who have a specific illness, disease, or injury. The approach used by nurses to provide care to a specific patient depends on the pertinent factors unique to that patient.

Health Promotion and Illness Prevention

The goal of nursing is to assist people to achieve optimal health, the highest level of functioning that is achievable for each person. This includes activities that promote health and prevent illness.

Health promotion

Health promotion refers to activities directed towards helping people maintain or achieve a high level of functioning and feeling of well-being. The nursing activities include teaching, counselling, and motivating people to develop life-styles that include adequate nutrition, exercise, and rest or relaxation. People functioning at a high level have an increased capacity to withstand physical and emotional stressors. (See Chapter 4 for further information on health promotion.)

Health promotion activities are carried out whenever the opportunities occur. Thus health teaching and counselling are instituted not only with well people but also when people are hospitalized. For example, teaching about adequate nutrition can be done while assisting a patient to select items from a hospital menu.

Illness Prevention

Prevention refers to activities directed towards protecting people from potential or actual threats to health and the subsequent consequences.[27] In other words, prevention means inhibiting the development of disease, slowing down the progression of disease, and protecting the body from further harmful effects. There are three different levels of protection: primary, secondary, and tertiary.

Primary prevention

Primary prevention includes specific protective measures against disease or trauma, such as immunizations against diphtheria or measles, environmental sanitation, and protection against occupational hazards (for example, wearing safety glasses to prevent eye injuries). Early successes in primary prevention have been the result of activities directed at preventing the occurrence of infectious diseases such as polio or smallpox through immunization and typhoid fever through purification of water. More recently dental caries have been reduced by fluoridation of water supplies.

The major health problems today are chronic diseases and accidental injuries and their sequelae, both of which require modification of deeply rooted behaviours such as use of alcohol, tobacco and drugs, and poor nutritional and exercise patterns. Health promotion activities are considered a form of primary prevention.

Secondary prevention

Secondary prevention includes early detection and prompt intervention to stop the disease at an early stage, decrease the intensity, or prevent complications. This is accomplished by screening for diseases such as diabetes, carcinoma in situ, tuberculosis, or glaucoma. The purpose is to detect early symptoms about which the patient is unaware or lacks knowledge, so that prompt intervention is effective for control or cure. Screening for contacts of people with sexually transmitted diseases and treating the infected person to prevent spread of the disease are other examples of secondary prevention.

Tertiary prevention

Tertiary prevention consists of activities that prevent or limit disabilities and help restore the person with a disability to an optimal level of functioning (for example, rehabilitation). Tertiary prevention begins in the early period of recovery from an illness and includes activities such as moving and turning immobile patients to prevent respiratory complications or decubiti, encouraging leg exercises to prevent muscle weakness, and encouraging or assisting with limb exercises to prevent contractures.

Rehabilitation programmes for people with cardiac disease or with disabilities resulting from a cerebral vascular accident (stroke) are initiated before the patient is discharged from the hospital. Chapter 10 discusses the concept of rehabilitation in more detail. Preventive measures for specific disorders are described in the appropriate chapters of this text.

At Risk Status

Some people are considered to have a greater possibility of becoming ill or acquiring a specific disease because of the presence of certain factors. These people are considered to be *at risk* and the specific factors are termed *risk factors*. For example, a woman over age 35 with a family history of breast cancer who had her first menstrual period before age 12 and who has never had a child would be considered at high risk for developing breast cancer because several of the known risk factors for breast cancer are present. This woman may not develop breast cancer; however, a greater than normal probability exists that she might.

Some risk factors, such as age and genetic factors, cannot be altered, whereas other factors, such as smoking or diet, are under the control of the person. To alter the risk factor, people need to receive information related to the specific health threats. People frequently test the validity of health information by asking laypeople and professionals about the specific risks. Knowing about the risks does not always result in altered behaviour, since some people receive satisfaction from the risk behaviours and deny the risk for themselves, even in the presence of contradictory information, saying, in effect, "It won't happen to me." Frequently there is no direct causal relationship, therefore the behaviours are easy for some people to dismiss. There are also no immediate tangible rewards for engaging in the desired behaviours. Some people therefore deliberately choose to continue engaging in the risk behaviours.

To promote health behaviours that decrease the at risk status, people first have to receive the information. Then positive reinforcement for altering behaviour is more effective than negative comments about the at risk behaviours. Group sessions (such as weight loss groups or smokers groups) may be helpful when participants reinforce each other's positive behaviours. Finally, health care professionals should be *role models*, demonstrating the desired health behaviours.

Illness

Although the terms *illness* and *disease* are sometimes used interchangeably, the terms do not relate to the same concepts. A person with a chronic disease such as diabetes may say, "I feel well." Illness is a more abstract term than disease and is essentially the opposite of wellness. Both illness and wellness have a strong subjective component, that of feeling ill or that of feeling well. Illness implies malfunctioning, a lower level of functioning.

Humans are constantly responding and adapting to changes in the external and internal (body) environments. A variety of chemical, physical, biological, and psychosocial factors in the external environment can influence a person's

Table 1-1 Environmental factors affecting health

Type	Examples	Possible effects
Chemical	Lead, arsenic	Poisoning
	Cholesterol	Myocardial infarction
Physical	Motor vehicles	Accidents
	High noise level	Deafness
	Heat	Burns, heatstroke
	Cold	Frostbite, hypothermia
	Radiation	Cancer
Biological	Bacteria, virus, fungi	Infections
Psychosocial	Stress	Ulcers, hypertension

functioning (Table 1-1, p.6). Defence mechanisms, either biological (Chapter 33) or psychological (Chapter 5), serve to protect the person from environmental factors that may cause harm. Illness results when defence mechanisms become inadequate or inappropriate.

A relatively stable internal environment is necessary for cellular growth and functioning. The process of maintaining this relatively constant environment is the process of *homeostasis* or *dynamic equilibrium*. The term *dynamic equilibrium* is more descriptive, because it implies fluctuations within a normal range rather than a static condition. Maintaining a dynamic equilibrium involves an adequate exchange of oxygen and carbon dioxide through respiration, an adequate nutrient supply to meet basal metabolic needs, and a normal balance of fluids and electrolytes. Variations above or below normal ranges lead to illness and disease.

Disease

Diseases are specific pathological conditions with characteristic signs and symptoms. Diseases may involve a specific organ or body part or may affect the body as a whole. Functioning of the part or body system may be impaired. The body has many integrated defence mechanisms and compensatory responses that maintain functioning for a period of time when a threat to the system occurs, but if the causative factors or stressors persist, altered structure or functioning results. Terms commonly used when discussing specific diseases are listed in Table 1-2.

Diseases have a natural life history, usually progressing through stages. The time factor varies; acute diseases have a sudden onset and are usually of short duration, whereas chronic diseases often have a gradual or indefinite onset and have a longer duration. In the first stage of development of a disease, the *presymptomatic* or *subclinical stage*, pathogenic changes have started to occur but no detectable signs or symptoms are apparent. Examples of this stage are the formation of atheromatous plaques in the coronary vessel or early malignant growth.[20] The second stage, the *clinical stage*, is characterized by the presence of signs and symptoms. It is at this stage that the person may seek help. The third stage, the *rehabilitation stage*, occurs with chronic diseases and is characterized by residual disabilities. During this stage the person must learn how to adapt to changes in life-style that result from the disability and learn how to prevent further disability.

Illness Behaviour and Sick Role

When people perceive that they are ill, they may take action for relief of symptoms; they may decide to take no action; or they may vacillate between action and no action. People who decide to take action may seek help from a friend or family member, from a "folk-specialist" (someone of their cultural group who is frequently consulted about illness), from a professional such as a minister, or from a health care professional. Nonhealth care people may either deal with the problems themselves or refer the patient to someone else. Often these people act as gatekeeper in helping make the decision when and from whom the sick person should seek help. People who perceive they are ill but take no action do so for a variety of reasons (Box 1-1). Low income people are more apt to seek assistance when they are ill if the health care provider or agency is within the community and easily accessible. Some people know they should take action but some reason holds them back and thus they vacillate between action and no action.

Some people are labelled as "noncompliant" because they do not follow the directions of the health care provider. Noncompliance may be defined as the failure of the person to participate in carrying out the plan of care after initially indicating the intention to comply or because of the presence of factors that prevent action.[14] Failure to carry out an action may result from some of the same reasons as failure to seek health care rather than a deliberate action of noncompliance.

When illness becomes legitimized by the doctor during the clinical stage, the patient assumes the *sick role* and is exempted from normal social roles and responsibilities as required by the type and severity of the illnes . The social expectation is that the sick person seeks help and wants to get well. The sick role permits the patient to assume a dependent relationship that facilitates receiving the required health care. Many people find the sick role undesirable and have difficulty with the enforced dependency, although they see it as necessary to achieve the desired end, that is, wellness. They find it helpful if they are kept informed and allowed to make decisions if they are able and desire to do so. The patientis expected to relinquish the sick role and assume increasing independence during the recovery and rehabilitation stage.

ADULT NURSING PRACTICE
Types of Nursing Practice

Nursing actions can be divided into two types—independent and interdependent. *Independent* nursing actions are those which the nurse takes after analysis of data pertaining to those aspects of the patient's health that are amenable to nursing intervention. Providing quality care for people at risk for or experiencing pathophysiological disorders requires a systematic approach. In recent years the term *nursing process* has become synonymous with the systematic approach used in providing nursing care.

Interdependent nursing practice consists of activities carried out in collaboration with other health care professionals, such as doctors, dietitians, and physiotherapists.

Table 1-2   Terminology used with diseases

Catergory	Term	Definition
Duration	Acute	Disease with sudden onset and short duration
	Chronic	Disease of long duration; onset may be insidious or may follow an acute disorder
Characteristics	Incidence	Frequency of occurrence of a disease
	Onset	Beginning of a disease
	Course	Pattern of development and resolution
	Duration	Length of time disease is present
	Prognosis	Ultimate outcome
Factors	Epidemiology	Rate and influencing factors of disease occurring in given populations
	Aetiology	Cause of disease
	Pathophysiology	Physiological mechanisms and effects of disease processes
Phenomena	Signs	Observable changes in body function (objective)
	Symptoms	Indication of disease perceived by the patient (subjective)
	Syndrome	Cluster of signs and symptoms that collectively indicate altered functioning
Results	Spontaneous resolution	Healing that occurs with little or no treatment
	Therapeutic intervention	Treatment directed towards a cure or alleviation of signs and symptoms
Statistics	Morbidity	Number of people having the disease in a given population
	Mortality	Number of people who die from the disease

Nurses participate in team planning with other health care professionals. Nurses are the health care professionals who have the greatest patient contact. They are therefore in a position to assist other professionals by providing additional data through monitoring and by carrying out prescribed treatments patients are unable to do for themselves, sometimes termed a *dependent* function. As patients are able to assume greater responsibility for their own care, *self-care activities* are promoted.

Knowledge Base

The ability to plan and implement nursing care, monitor the patient's condition, and carry out treatments effectively requires a sound knowledge base not only about people and factors pertaining to their health but also about the pathophysiological disorders per se. The following types of knowledge about diseases can be useful in planning and providing patient care: epidemiology and aetiology, pathophysiology, signs and symptoms of disease, and medical therapy.

Knowledge of epidemiological and aetiological factors helps to identify the populations at risk. *Epidemiology* is the study of the incidence, distribution, and determinants of diseases and injuries in human populations. In other words, epidemiology is concerned with the extent of specific diseases or injuries in specific groups of people and the factors that influence that distribution.[20] *Aetiology* refers to the specific causes of a disease. Most diseases have *multiple causality*; that is, multiple factors are working and interacting together that lead to disease occurrence. This is an important point when teaching about prevention of disease, since avoidance of only one factor may not prevent disease occurrence.

Pathophysiology is the study of the effect of disease (pathology) on body organs and systems and on total body functioning. A *pathophysiological* disorder is one in which there is altered physiological functioning, as differentiated

---

1-1

Selected reasons for not seeking health care

Denial that symptoms are present
Symptoms not viewed as important
Fear of consequences (for example, pain, cancer, death)
Fear of health care professionals or health care agencies
Lack of knowledge concerning which symptoms require medical care
Lack of availability of transportation
Lack of money for transportation
Disabilities that hinder getting to health care agency

---

from a *pathopsychological* disorder in which there is altered mental functioning. Knowledge of the physiological effects of pathology and the nature of the compensatory or adaptive responses facilitates understanding of patient responses for the purposes of monitoring the patient's status for maladaptive responses and teaching the patient about the disease.

Knowledge of the signs and symptoms and medical therapies of common diseases facilitates monitoring for presence and course of diseases, supporting and teaching the patient, and carrying out therapies patients cannot do for themselves.

Frameworks for Nursing Practice

The focus of nursing practice depends on the nurse's philosophical framework. In earlier years of professional nursing, the medical model was the primary approach. Thus when a systematic approach to data collection was first initiated, *body systems* was a framework that was commonly used. For example, data that pertained specifically to the respiratory system were collected, then analysed to identify respiratory problems.

Another framework that has been used in the practice of adult nursing is *human needs*. Maslow describes a hierarchy of needs in which physiological needs are the most basic, followed by safety, love and belonging, self-esteem, and self-actualization. The needs are ranked in ascending order from the needs that are basic to survival to those that focus on development of self (growth-motivated needs). In principle, the more basic needs are satisfied first. For example, a person who is having difficulty breathing (physiological need for oxygen) attends to that need before dealing with a feeling of loss of worth as a person (self-esteem). In most situations, however, the needs in the hierarchy exist simultaneously to different extents. Lower level needs have to be met, at least partially, before seeking gratification of higher order needs. For example, a person may omit a meal to carry out an activity that increases self-esteem. New needs usually emerge gradually except when danger is present or when the person is acutely ill.

The use of human needs as a framework for nursing care consists of collecting and analysing data that pertain to each of the need categories. The concept of hierarchy of needs is useful during planning of care by helping to set priorities; for example, survival needs would usually take priority over growth needs.

Several theoretical frameworks have been developed specifically for nursing practice and serve as a reference to guide nurses in assessment and implementation of nursing care. The concepts are abstract to allow for broad application. All the frameworks are applicable to the care of patients with medical-surgical disorders. In the United Kingdom the model developed by Roper, Logan and Tierney is widely used. Other commonly used frameworks include Rogers' Life Process model, Roy's Adaptation model, Orem's Self-care Agency model, and Johnson's Behavioural Systems model. The manner in which data are organized and used differs with the conceptual framework, but the underlying process used by the nurse is the same.

NURSING PROCESS

The systematic approach used to carry out nursing's independent functions is frequently termed *nursing process*. It is a way of thinking and acting based on the scientific method rather than on intuition. It provides organization and direction of nursing activities, a means for predicting outcomes and evaluating results, and a method for establishing standards of nursing care.

Nursing process provides a framework for (1) identification of health care needs amenable to nursing care, (2) determination of patient goals (outcomes) and nursing actions, (3) implementation of nursing actions, and (4) evaluation of results of nursing actions. This systematic process is usually divided into either four or five steps; the overall process is the same regardless of the number of steps. The five-step process is as follows:

1. Assessment: collecting patient data of pertinence to nursing
2. Nursing analysis: using the collected data to identify the patient's health care needs or problems that can be influenced by nursing care (nursing diagnoses, a term used in the United States)
3. Planning: determining priorities, expected patient outcomes, and specific nursing actions
4. Implementation: carrying out the planned nursing actions necessary to accomplish the defined goals
5. Evaluation: determining the extent to which the goals have been achieved

Nurses who use a four-step approach include nursing analysis as part of assessment; thus the four steps become assessment, planning, implementation, and evaluation.

Nursing process is discussed in great detail in fundamentals of nursing texts and in some books devoted to the topic; thus only a brief summary is presented here.

Assessment

An initial assessment is made when the person first enters the hospital or health care agency. However, since health is a dynamic, ever-changing state, assessment must be a continuous, ongoing process.

Data may be collected from a primary source (patient) or from secondary sources (family, friends, patient records, health team members). The data may be subjective or objective (Table 1-3). The differentiation is important. *Subjective* data are necessary for providing understanding of the patient's experience and sense of illness or well-being, but since these data cannot be validated, they are subject to wide interpretation. For example, one person may describe a specific pain intensity as "severe," whereas another person may describe the same pain intensity as "mild." *Objective* data are verifiable and measurable; for example, each person palpating the same lymph node can describe it as 2 × 3 cm in size, oval shaped, and freely movable. Subjective data are collected either by a nursing history or during patient/family interactions. Objective data are obtained by means of a head-to-toe physical examination or by physical inspection carried on during nursing care activities. Data specific to patients with medical-surgical disorders are described in later chapters of the text. Differentiation is made between subjective and objective data.

Nursing Analysis (needs or problems)

The second step of nursing process is making conclusions from the collected data. The process of data analysis may be referred to as nursing analysis or *diagnosis*.

Some form of organizing framework for the data is required to facilitate data analysis. Nurses who practise in the United Kingdom will find the taxonomy developed for *nursing diagnoses*, by the North American Nursing Diagnosis Association (NANDA), most interesting. The NANDA nursing diagnoses are grouped under the nine headings of exchanging, communicating, relating, valuing, choosing, moving, perceiving, knowing, and feeling. The practice of nursing in the United Kingdom is undergoing rapid changes and it is always useful to study the experience of others before initiating fundamental alterations in practice.

Table 1-3 Types of data

Type	Definition	Methods	Examples
Subjective	Statements by the person concerning thoughts or feelings (psychological, physical) that cannot be validated	Interview, interaction	Statements about pain, nausea, itching Statements about fears, desires, beliefs, attitudes, values
Objective	Data perceptible by the external senses that can be validated by others	Inspection, auscultation, palpation, percussion, olfaction	Vomiting, scratching, auditory breath sounds, palpable lymph nodes, breath odour

General conclusions

Four general conclusions can be drawn from the nurse's analysis of patient data:

1. Data is insufficient; more data must be gathered before conclusions can be made
2. The person or family is functioning at optimal level and is not at high risk; no interventions are required
3. The person or family is functioning well, but health risk factors are high; a high risk for dysfunction is present, such as "Infection, high risk for"
4. The person or family is functioning inadequately and actions are desirable

When dysfunctions are identified, one of three approaches may be taken. First, the person or family may have already identified the dysfunction and may have taken appropriate actions; therefore no further help is needed. Second, action is needed that is better carried out by another health professional; the nurse makes the appropriate referral. In the third option, nursing interventions are indicated and the nurse then determines the problem.

Problems (nursing diagnosis)

Although problems have been defined in various ways, most definitions include the following characteristics:

1. A statement or conclusion
2. An actual or high-risk health problem
3. Identified from a nursing assessment
4. The legal and educational domain of nursing

Some nursing actions, however, do *not* ensue from nurse-identified problems. Recall that nursing actions may be of two types, independent and interdependent or collaborative. Identifying a specific problem and carrying out actions appropriate for the problem are nursing's independent actions. Monitoring activities to collect data for the doctor (collaborative action) is not an action that ensues from nursing analysis.

Statements about a specific problem are not limited to dysfunction (patient problems). The goal of nursing is optimal health of the person/family; support and assistance may be needed to help people *maintain* certain health practices. For example, one woman sought assistance from a nurse to help her work through her feelings about caring for her dying mother. The woman was coping satisfactorily but needed support from the nurse to maintain coping.

Planning

Planning nursing care involves several steps:

1. Setting priorities when several problems have been identified
2. Determining goals (outcomes) of care for each problem
3. Selecting specific nursing actions

Setting priorities

When several problems have been identified, it must be determined which problems take priority. One approach is the basic needs approach. Problems that pertain to physiological and safety needs usually take precedence over love and belonging or self-esteem needs.

Priorities can also be determined by considering threats to the integrity of the individual. The following priority system can be used:

First Immediate life-threatening problems (for example, lack of oxygen)

Second Threats to physiological or psychological integrity for which the person is at *high risk*

Third Threats to physiological or psychological integrity for which the person is at *low risk* (but which may occur if action is not taken)

Fourth Health maintenance

This system does not deny the importance of health maintenance but emphasizes that when health problems are present, these problems are attended to first.

Setting of priorities does not mean numbering each problem from 1 to N in order of importance. It means that when a large number of problems have been identified, the most important problems are selected to be principally addressed.

Goal setting

The next step in planning is to determine the goals or desired patient outcomes to be achieved. *Mutual nurse-patient goal setting* is implemented whenever possible so that there is congruency between what both the nurse and the patient expect as a result of nursing interventions. The role of the nurse is to facilitate the patient's recovery and future health maintenance; thus both must be moving towards the same goals.

Goals (expected patient outcomes) are stated as *observable patient behaviours:* behaviour (or signs) that is observed in the patient if the goal is met. For example, the statement "prevent skin breakdown" is a poor goal, since it indicates nursing action and does not indicate a patient outcome to be met. The same idea stated in observable patient-outcome terms is "skin on sacral area remains intact, no redness is observed." To evaluate whether this goal had been met, the sacral area is inspected for signs of redness or breakdown in skin integrity.

Patient outcomes are written according to the following criteria: have measurable verbs, be specific in content and time, and be attainable.[5] Examples of verbs that are *not* measurable are "understands," "knows," or "appreciates." Time is included when appropriate; for example, "Walks around room 24/6, to nurses' station 25/6, and to lounge 26/6." The more specifically the expected outcomes are written, the easier is the evaluation. The expected patient outcomes serve as the criteria for evaluation.

Health care agencies participate in quality assurance review (see Chapter 2). During the process of quality assurance review, *standards* are developed and outcome criteria are identified. Some of these outcome criteria are useful guidelines in determining expected patient outcomes.

Goals are derived primarily from the first part (the pattern of functioning) of the problem statement.

Example:

Problem	Activity intolerance: decreased muscle strength (legs) related to decreased activity
Long-term goal	Leg muscles test at full baseline strength
Short-term goal	Patient raises legs 2 inches above bed against resistance within 3 days

Long-term goals describe what patient behaviours are expected for resolution of the problem. Short-term goals describe expected patient behaviours indicating that action is headed in the right direction towards resolution, that is, they are short steps to be achieved towards reaching the long-term goal.

Selection of nursing actions

Usually several alternative actions can be chosen to reach a desired outcome or goal. Selection of actions is usually guided by the second part (aetiological factors) of the problem. For example, different nursing actions are selected for a problem of "Sleep pattern disturbance: insomnia related to fear of surgery" than are selected for a problem of "Sleep pattern disturbance: insomnia related to persistent cough."

The action alternatives are identified and choices are made depending on the specific patient situation. Patient input is sought when feasible. When a nurse follows a preset plan of action for any given problem, patient care is not individualized and there is less potential for accomplishment of the desired outcomes. The determination of action alternatives is based on knowledge from experts, suggestions from the patient, observations of actions of others, suggestions from other health care providers, and the nurse's own creativity. Actions are based on scientific principles.

Selection of action is based on the following guidelines:
The greatest possibility of success
The least risk
The least discomfort
The least intrusiveness for the patient

Once the course of action has been selected, the *frequency* of action must also be determined. For example, the frequency of deep breathing and coughing exercises selected as an activity would be planned at different intervals for different patients based on risk factors such as obesity and smoking habits identified through analysis of the data.

Implementation

Nursing interventions for people who are at risk for or who have pathophysiological disorders are directed towards *restoring* optimal health and *maintaining* optimal health (see Box 1-2). Although the major focus of the care of the person who is ill may be health restoration, health maintenance interventions may be carried out concurrently to help the person maintain optimal functioning wherever possible. The interventions selected for a specific patient will be determined by the identified problems and the specific pathophysiological disorders present or for which the person is at risk. Possible nursing interventions are described in appropriate chapters in this text.

Because the goal of nursing care is the patient's optimal health, self-care is stressed to the extent possible; the patient is usually ultimately responsible for ongoing health maintenance. Thus teaching, supporting, and motivating are major nursing strategies. If self-care is impossible or inappropriate, the nurse then compensates for the patient's inability by performing the actions. Monitoring is an ongoing strategy; the type and degree usually depend on the illness or disease.

Recording (documentation)

Actions that have been taken and the patient's response to the actions need to be documented. Responses to monitoring activities are most easily recorded on *flow sheets*. The flow sheets provide a means of quick comparison of a specific monitoring parameter over time. Data such as vital signs, fluid intake and output, activity, and urine tests are recorded as they are gathered. In some institutions these sheets subsequently become part of the patient's permanent record. In others the data are recopied onto other sheets in the permanent record. Flow sheets are used extensively in special care areas such as intensive care units, where continual monitoring of several parameters is necessary.

Different formats may be used to record nursing interventions and patient responses. Forms or narrative notes may be used for charting significant data pertaining to each problem. The important point is that, regardless of the format used by the health care agency, activities that were carried out must be documented to clarify the nursing care provided and to serve as a data base for evaluation of the effectiveness of the care provided.

Evaluation

The last step of nursing process consists of determining whether the desired outcomes are met, analysing the effectiveness of nursing interventions, and planning for subsequent care. The method of evaluation consists of

Guidelines for Care

1-2

Patients at risk for or who have a pathophysiological disorder

Health restoration

Assisting with achievement of therapeutic goals
   Monitoring for signs of healing or complications
   Carrying out prescribed medical therapies that the patient is unable to do for self
Promoting functioning of those mechanisms necessary for optimal health, for example, oxygenation, nutrition, elimination
Promoting comfort and activities of daily living (ADL)
Modifying the environment to enhance healing and wellness
Counselling and teaching
   Promoting coping and adaptation to changes in health care
   Teaching the patient to care for self

Health maintenance

Monitoring for changes in health status
Teaching the patient and family or friends
   The nature of the illness or disease
   Signs and symptoms indicating presence of disease or complications to be reported to doctor
   Health promotion activities (nutrition, activity, etc.)
   Specific preventive measures
   Rationale for medical therapies
   Name, dosage, actions, and side effects of prescribed medications
   Availability of community resources
   Need for continual monitoring or follow-up care, as necessary

1-3

Possible reasons for not achieving patient goals

Database	Incomplete; changes in data
Problems	Inaccurate data analysis; inaccurate statement
Goals	Unrelated to problem; nonspecific; unrealistic
Nursing actions	Unrelated to problem or goal(s); nonspecific, therefore poorly implemented; inadequate in degree of action taken

collecting data from the patient based on the criteria established as patient goals (outcomes). Thus the more specifically the goals are stated in observable patient behaviours, the easier the task of evaluation. For example, a problem of "Constipation, related to inadequate fluid intake" could have a goal of "Stool soft and formed." Evaluation then consists of inspecting the stool. If it is soft and formed, the goal is achieved and the patient's constipation is corrected.

Some of the reasons why goals are not achieved are listed in Box 1-3.

Once the possible reason for the lack of goal achievement is identified, revisions are made and the process is repeated. As can be noted, nursing care is an ongoing and dynamic process that requires constant assessment and evaluation.

ETHICAL DILEMMAS IN ADULT NURSING

An ethical dilemma arises when, based on moral considerations, one of two opposing actions can be taken and the person perceives the possibility of either response. Evidence can be presented to support either action, but the evidence on both sides is inconclusive.[8]

Numerous ethical dilemmas arise in medical-surgical nursing practice. The dilemmas are not solely the domain of medical-surgical nursing but occur to a large extent during the care of these patients. These dilemmas may include, but are not limited to, the following:

1. Withholding information from the patient
2. Providing informed consent
3. Use of invasive techniques
4. Selection of patients for scarce therapies (such as organ transplantation)
5. Withholding or withdrawing treatment/nourishment
6. Quality of life versus prolongation of life
7. Right to commit suicide with terminal illness
8. Euthanasia
9. Definitions of death

Nursing students have an opportunity to discuss the ethical issues and to obtain feedback and support from lecturers, tutors, mentors and fellow students. Because ethical dilemmas are complex and do not have one conclusive action, the professional nurse may be frequently faced with unresolved issues. Mechanisms have been developed to assist nurses to cope with conflicts that ensue. Team conferences may be held under the leadership of a nurse ethicist who has advanced preparation in ethics. Interdisciplinary conferences may also be instituted. Support may be given on an individual basis with the nurse ethicist or counsellor.

Some ethical issues are discussed in appropriate chapters of this text. The reference list for this chapter includes some resources from the literature that may be helpful.

SUMMARY

1. Adult nursing focuses on the care of adults who are at risk for or who have medical-surgical disorders.
2. Health promotion refers to activities directed towards helping people to maintain or achieve a high level of functioning and feeling of well-being.
3. Prevention refers to activities directed towards protecting people from potential or actual threats to health and the subsequent consequences.
4. Primary prevention includes protective measures against disease or trauma. Secondary prevention includes early detection and treatment to decrease the intensity or to prevent complications. Tertiary prevention con-

sists of activities that prevent or limit disabilities and help promote rehabilitation.

5. People at risk are those considered to have a greater possibility of becoming ill or acquiring a certain disease. Factors that place the person at risk are termed risk factors.

6. Illness can be considered the opposite of wellness and implies a lower level of functioning. Disease is a pathological process having a characteristic set of signs and symptoms. Diseases may be acute or chronic.

7. The stages of disease progression are (1) presymptomatic or subclinical stage in which changes are occurring but no signs or symptoms are present; (2) the clinical stage, characterized by signs and symptoms; and (3) the rehabilitation stage (in chronic diseases), characterized by residual disabilities.

8. The sick role exempts the person from normal social roles and responsibilities and permits the person to assume a dependent relationship that facilitates receiving the required medical care.

9. Independent nursing actions are those which the nurse takes after analysis of data pertaining to those aspects of the person's health that are amenable to nursing intervention. Interdependent or collaborative nursing actions are those taken by the nurse in assisting other health care professionals.

10. Epidemiology is the study of the incidence, distribution, and determinants of diseases and injuries in human populations. Aetiology refers to the study of specific causes of diseases.

11. Pathophysiology is the study of the effect of disease on body organs and systems and on total body functioning.

12. Signs are objective evidence and symptoms are subjective evidence of disease or dysfunction.

13. The five steps of nursing process are assessment nursing, data analysis, planning, implementation, and evaluation.

14. Numerous ethical dilemmas occur in adult nursing practice, including withholding of information or therapies, use of invasive techiques, and issues associated with death.

15. Nurse ethicists can practice nurses to cope with conflicts resulting from ethical dilemmas.

STUDY QUESTIONS

- What are some practices you follow that promote health or prevent disease? What practices do you follow that are deterrents to health? How difficult would it be for you to change your behaviour?
- How do the three levels of prevention differ?
- What theoretical framework do you use in the practice of nursing? Can you correlate Gordon's functional health patterns with your framework for data analysis?
- How do the different parts of a problem statement assist you in planning nursing care?
- Read some of the chapter references that cite specific ethical dilemmas. To what extent do you think these dilemmas might provide conflicts to you in the care of these patients?

REFERENCES AND SELECTED READING

1. Alfaro R: *Application of nursing process: a step-by-step guide*, Philadelphia, 1986, JB Lippincott.
2. Allen CV: *Comprehending the nursing process: a workbook approach*, Norwalk, CT, 1991, Appleton & Lange.
3. American Nurses' Association: *Ethics in nursing*, Kansas City, MO, 1988, The Association.
4. American Nurses Association Committee on Ethics: *Guidelines on withholding or withdrawing food and fluids*, Kansas City, MO, 1988, The Association.
5. Carpenito LJ: *Handbook of nursing diagnosis*, ed 4, Hagerstown, MD, 1991, JB Lippincott.
6.* Carpenito LJ: *Nursing care plans and documentation: nursing diagnoses and collaborative problems*, Hagerstown, MD, 1991, JB Lippincott Co.
7.* Cassells J, Redman B: Preparing students to be moral agents in clinical nursing practice, *Nurs Clin North Am* 24:463-473, 1989.
8. Davis AJ, Aroskar MA: *Ethical dilemmas and nursing practice*, ed 3, Norwalk, CT, 1991, Appleton & Lange.
9. Edelman C, Mandle CL: *Health promotion throughout the life span*, St Louis, 1986, Mosby–Year Book.
10. Fowler MD, Levine-Ariff J: *Ethics at the bedside: a source book for the critical care nurse*, Hagerstown, MD, 1987, JB Lippincott.
11. Friedman E, editor: *Making choices: ethics issues for health care professionals*, Chicago, 1986, American Hospital Association.
12. Gillick MR: Common-sense models of health and disease, *N Engl J Med* 313(11):700-703, 1985.
13. Gordon M: *Manual of nursing diagnosis 1991-1992*, St Louis, 1991, Mosby–Year Book.
14.* Gordon M: *Nursing diagnosis: process and application*, ed 2, St Louis, 1987, Mosby–Year Book.
15. Greenberg JS: Health and wellness: a conceptual differentiation, *J Sch Health* 55:403-406, 1985.
16. Griffith-Kenney JW, Christensen PJ: *Nursing process, application of theories, frameworks and models*, ed 2, St Louis, 1986, Mosby–Year Book.
17.* Iwerson E: Dilemmas in practice: life at what cost? *Am J Nurs* 88:639-640, 1988.
18.* Iyer P, Camp N: *Nursing documentation: a nursing process approach*, St Louis, 1991, Mosby–Year Book.
19. Kim MJ, McFarland GK, McLane AM: *Pocket guide to nursing diagnoses*, ed 4, St Louis, 1991, Mosby–Year Book.
20. Mausner JS, Kramer S: *Epidemiology: an introductory text*, ed 2, Philadelphia, 1985, WB Saunders.
21. McFarland GK, McFarlane EA: *Nursing diagnosis and intervention: planning for patient care*, St Louis, 1989, Mosby–Year Book.
22.* Mitchell C: Dilemmas in practice: steadying the hand that feeds, *Am J Nurs* 87:293-296, 1987.
23.* Mumma CM: Withholding nutrition: a nursing perspective, *Nurs Adm Q* 10(3):31-38, 1986.
24.* Muyskens JL: Dilemmas in practice: acting alone, *Am J Nurs* 87:1141-1146, 1987.
25.* Otte DM, Allen KS: Ethical principles in the nursing care of terminally ill adults, *Oncol Nurs Forum* 14(5):87-91, 1987.
26.* Pauly-O'Neill S: Dilemmas in practice: questioning the use of invasive technology, *AJN* 91(1):19-20, 1991.
27. Pender NJ: *Health promotion in nursing practice*, ed 3, Norwalk, Ct, 1987, Appleton & Lange.
28. Prohaska TR, et al: Health practices and illness cognition in young, middle aged, and elderly adults, *J Gerontol* 40:569-578, 1985.
29. Silva M: *Ethical decision making in nursing*, Norwalk, CT, 1989, Appleton & Lange.
30.* Thomasma DC: Ethics and professional practice in oncology, *Sem Oncol Nurs* 5(2):89-94, 1989.
31. Thomasma DC: The range of euthanasia, *Am Coll Surg Bull* 73(8):3-13, 1988.
32. Webster JA: The wellness mode: feeling good about you, *AORN J* 41:713-718, 1985.
33. American Nurses Association: *Nursing: a social policy statement*, No. NP-63, Kansas City, MO, 1980, The Association.
34. Maudinger MO, Jauron GD: Developing a nursing diagnosis, *Nurs Outlook* 23:94-98, 1975.

*Recommended for student reading.

FURTHER READING

Aggleton P, Chalmers H: *Nursing Models and the Nursing Process,* London, 1986, Macmillan Press Limited.

Cavanagh S: *Orem's Model in Action,* London, 1991, Macmillan Press Limited.

Chapman CM: *Theory of Nursing: Practical Application*, London, 1985, Harper and Row Publishers.

Kershaw B, Price B: *The Riehl Interaction Model in Action,* London, 1993, Macmillan Press Limited.

Open University: *A Systematic Approach to Nursing Care,* Milton Keynes, 1984, Open University.

Pearson A, Vaughan B: *Nursing Models for Practice,* London, 1986, Heinemann.

Roper N, Logan WW, and Tierney AJ: *Using a Model for Nursing,* Edinburgh, 1983, Churchill Livingstone.

Teasdale K: Partnership With Patients? *The Professional Nurse,* 2(12):397-399, 1987.

Wilson-Barnett J, Macleod-Clark J: *Research in Health Promotion and Nursing,* London, 1993, Macmillan Press Limited.

Yassin T, Watkins S: What influences care planning? Nurses' attitudes towards care plans, *Professional Nurse* 8(9):572-577, 1993.

2

Quality Management in Nursing

Frances R. Chester
Mary Lou Monahan

Edited by Kevin Teasdale

After studying this chapter, the learner should be able to:
- Define quality management.
- Identify three reasons why quality management is an important aspect of the practice of *modern* nursing.
- Describe the steps of the model for quality assurance.
- State the difference between standards and criteria.
- Name five mechanisms involved in implementing quality management *programmes.*
- Describe the use of quality indicators as one means for monitoring quality of care.

IMPETUS FOR QUALITY MANAGEMENT

Nursing is committed to professional excellence in providing the highest quality of care possible. Implicit in this commitment is the responsibility to evaluate the quality and appropriateness of that care. However, it has only been in the last 21 years that attempts have been made to develop an extrinsic, systematic approach to monitor and improve care. The impetus for this change has come from a variety of sources: (1) legislation and government policy initiatives; (2) economic factors; (3) the nursing profession itself. Until recently this process was known as quality assurance; it is now called quality management.

Legislation and Government Policy Initiatives

The National Health Service (NHS) and Community Care Act of 1990[8d] has divided the management structure of the NHS into organizations responsible for *purchasing* health care on behalf of their local population (District Health Authorities, Family Health Services Authorities and GP Fundholders), and organizations responsible for *providing* health care (NHS Trusts and General Practices). Each year, these purchasers and providers seek to agree contracts which specify not only activity levels and financial support, but which also specify the quality of the services to be delivered. This change in the structure of the health service has linked quality with funding and has therefore placed a high premium on quality management in all services.

The introduction of the Patients' Charter[8b] has publicized ten key rights for all who use the NHS and has specified nine standards of service which the NHS will be aiming to provide. The Charter is a product of the consumer movement of the 1970s and 1980s which awakened the general public to the fact that they could reasonably question the quality of the services which they were offered in hospital and in the community.

In 1992 the British government published the White Paper *The Health of the Nation*[8a] which set out targets for promoting health and reducing illness in five main areas: coronary heart disease and strokes; cancers; mental illness; HIV/AIDS and sexual health; and accidents. NHS purchasers are reviewing public health policy in the light of these targets and are introducing quality standards linked to the targets into funding agreements with local providers. The Chief Nursing Officer at the Department of Health has published a handbook[8c] emphasizing the key role which nurses must play in the achievement of *The Health of the Nation* targets.

Economic Factors

Because health care costs have assumed an increasing share of the gross national product in the past two decades, the government and the NHS management executive have increased scrutiny of the cost effectiveness of services. At the level of service provision, this has led to requirements that all parts of the NHS demonstrate annual efficiency savings. However, at the level of public health planning, reviewing the cost of illness raises *even more* vital questions about the relation of quality of care to cost. For example, the principle of "high cost/low benefit" is defined by poor quality of healthcare in terms of overdiagnosis or overtreatment, which can lead to excessive health care expenditures even in the absence of any iatrogenic or untoward consequences. Poor quality in the form of misdiagnosis, mistreatment, or inadequate nursing care can increase mortality or morbidity, length of hospital stay, and loss of earnings, and, therefore, this poor quality can increase the costs of health care to individuals and to society.

The current economic situation where health care costs appear to be growing steadily as a proportion of the gross national product has clear implications for nursing, since it is the largest health care profession and therefore the one which consumes the largest slice of the overall NHS budget. More than ever before, the nursing profession must demonstrate the value and benefits of its service if it wishes to retain government and consumer support.

Professional Standards

Last but certainly not least, the nursing profession itself places as its highest goal the delivery of quality health care. The United Kingdom Central Council for Nursing, Midwifery and Health Visiting (UKCC) has devised and published a Code of Professional Conduct[24] (Box 2-1) and has supplemented this with additional guidance papers in areas such as the scope of professional practice, standards for records and record keeping, standards for the administration of medicines, and a framework for the exercise of accountability in professional practice. The aim is to help individual nurses understand their specific responsibility and accountability for the delivery of nursing care. The code of conduct and associated guidelines and standards identify the elements of nursing care that must be met to ensure that quality care is delivered, and to provide a baseline for measuring quality.

The UKCC is the governing body of Nursing in the United Kingdom. Some of its members are appointed by the government, but others are directly elected by the

---

2-1

Extracts from the UKCC Code of Professional Conduct

'Each registered nurse, midwife and health visitor shall act, at all times, in such a manner as to:

- Safeguard and promote the interests of individual patients and clients;
- Serve the interests of society;
  -justify public trust and confidence and
  -uphold and enhance the good standing and reputation of the professions.'

The Code specifies sixteen actions which professionals must take in order to exercise personal accountability for their practice, consistent with four aims stated above.

From United Kingdom Central Council for Nursing, Midwifery and Health Visiting (3rd edition: June 1992), Code of Professional Conduct. UKCC, 23 Portland Place, London W1N 3AF.

profession. The UKCC has established a live register of all practising nurses, with a regular requirement for periodic re-registration. Midwives already have to demonstrate that they have maintained and updated the quality of their professional practice before they re-register. It has been proposed that a similar requirement should be established for nurses: thus formally linking the concept of demonstration of competence and continuing education with eligibility for continued membership of the profession. The UKCC also holds regular hearings into the professional conduct of individuals and has the authority to remove nurses from the register if necessary. Thus the nursing profession in the United Kingdom has established its own framework for professional practice together with a structure for monitoring and controlling practice which dovetails well with the legislative and economic pressures for quality management.

In addition to the formal professional code and structures of the UKCC, the Nursing profession, through the Royal College of Nursing (RCN), has published guidance on how detailed quality standards may be developed in each clinical area.[2a] The RCN committee argued that:

"Statements related to nursing care can be valid only if set by those familiar with the values, objectives and practice of nursing care and it is the responsibility of the nursing profession alone to agree an acceptable level of excellence."[19a]

The committee stated that individualized patient care was a particularly important area of nursing responsibility and suggested three general standards consistent with this:

"The nursing care of each patient should be individually planned, the plan being based on an assessment of individual needs. The care given should be systematically recorded and subsequently reviewed to see how far the goals have been reached.

The individual nurse should accept accountability for her individual nursing action."[18a,19b]

Although these RCN statements do not identify every area where clinical standards need to be developed and monitored, they do help nurses to identify situations on which their attention could be most productively focused.

DEFINITION OF QUALITY MANAGEMENT

Quality management can be described on two levels. In its strictest sense, it is a set of techniques for assuring the maintenance and improvement of standards and the efficiency and effectiveness of nursing care; more broadly, it is an effort to control nursing practice. As such, it involves relationships between nurses and consumers and between nurses and governmental bodies.

Quality management can be defined as a process that involves evaluating the degree of excellence of the observable and measurable characteristics of delivered nursing care. The purpose of quality management is always twofold. *First*, it determines the extent to which predetermined standards are being met by a particular nursing programme. *Second*, these findings are used to make decisions about changes that are to be implemented by people carrying out the programme of care. *Both* must be in place if nursing is to ensure its accountability to the consumer. Although the specific target of each evaluation may differ

depending on the information about quality that is desired, the purpose of the evaluation is always the same.

Nurses who are engaged in the delivery of health services cannot escape inclusion of quality management reviews in their practice responsibilities. Indeed, some proficiency in evaluation must be part of the modern nurse's basic repertoire.

The quality management process is not mysterious. Most nurses are well on their way to expertise in this area by virtue of their basic education and experience. Nurses who are expert in the care of specific patient populations (for example, patients with cardiac disease) possess the knowledge necessary to determine desired health processes and outcomes for that population. These nurses are well acquainted with nursing interventions to be used in assisting patients towards health and wellness. They are also aware of the observable changes that will occur at certain intervals in the course of healing.

Most nurses are not expert, however, in the methods used to conduct these evaluations. The following section describes the steps in the quality management review process.

QUALITY MANAGEMENT PROCESS

A variety of techniques have been proposed to perform the quality management review. Presented here is a widely-used problem-solving model. Its eight steps include the following:

1. Identify values or basic philosophy/beliefs
2. Identify standards and criteria
3. Measure degree of attainment of standards and criteria
4. Interpret strengths and weaknesses
5. Identify possible courses of action
6. Select a course of action
7. Take action
8. Reevaluate

The model is best understood as a cycle or control loop, as illustrated in Fig. 2.1.

Topics for quality management reviews are generally placed in some order of priority based on their frequency of occurrence and their real or potential impact on patient care. Impact is usually gauged by whether efficiency or effectiveness of patient care is affected. Efficiency is generally defined in terms of accomplishing a task with a minimum of resources (time, money, staff); effectiveness is defined in terms of accomplishment of predetermined goals. The focus for evaluation may be the nurse, the ward, department or directorate, or Unit/Trust as a whole.

If the focus of the evaluation is the nurse, it can include the actions of a single nurse or of all the nurses in a department, and any area of nursing activity can be examined. For example, is the ward manager satisfied with the primary nursing programme instituted 3 months ago? What criteria do the nursing staff use to determine the frequency of vital sign monitoring in the immediate postoperative period? Are the nursing standards for administration of intravenous therapy being adhered to?

If the Unit or Trust is the focus of the quality management review, it might examine the administrative structure,

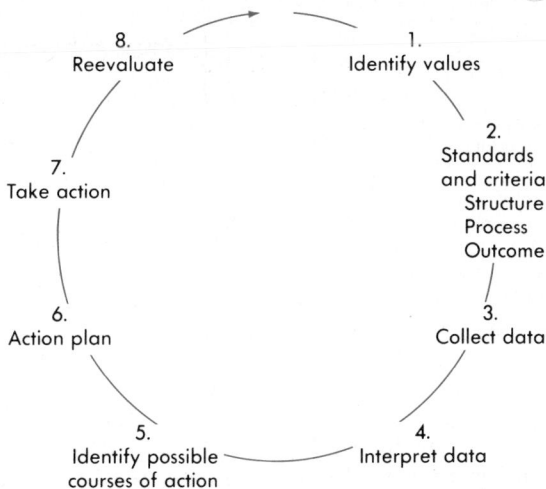

Fig. 2-1   Model for quality assurance review. (From American Nurses' Association: *Quality assurance for nursing care,* Kansas City, Mo, 1976, The Association. Reprinted by permission of the American Nurses' Association.)

the physical environment and equipment, or staffing. For example, a review could be implemented to determine whether regular appraisal or performance reviews are taking place for nursing staff and whether these are used as a basis for planning continuing education. Or a review could be undertaken with the risk management adviser to determine whether lifting and handling practices and equipment are safe and conform with current Health and Safety legislation.

When nursing care or a nursing care problem is the focus of the review, it is generally best to limit the scope to a certain population (for example, patients with certain diagnoses, surgical procedures, nursing care problems, or degree of illness) so that the project is manageable in terms of all the variables that are to be considered.

It is critical to remember the perspective of the patient must be considered in any evaluation. In selected instances, such as using patient outcomes or in attempting to validate patient care plans, direct input from the patients themselves is essential.

Steps in a Quality Management Review

Step 1: Identify values or beliefs

Before the implementation of the quality management model there must be an examination of the societal, professional, and individual values and beliefs that guide health care in the respective clinical area, directorate or Trust. The very word quality implies that someone somewhere has determined that certain outcomes have more value than others. As applied to nursing care, the individual nurse, nursing team, directorate, Trust, and community *interact* to influence the development of the criteria to be used in the review process.

To cite some obvious examples, in an intensive care unit a high value is placed on technical interventions designed to save life, whereas in a hospice the philosophy is more likely to value palliative interventions which promote quality of life or a peaceful death. Whatever the setting, the set of values must be identified and understood if the quality

assurance review is to be fair and accurate.

Step 2: Identify structure, process, outcome, standards, and criteria

A *standard* is the desirable or achievable level or range of performance of a certain criterion, or a framework against which performance is compared. An example of a standard is, "Every patient will have an admission assessment by a registered nurse." A *criterion measure* is that variable believed to be the indicator of the quality of care, for example, "The assessment form will be completed by the admitting nurse within 8 hours of admission."

The *standards for nursing practice* are generally developed by *clinical nursing leaders* in the institution, *using their professional expertise* as well as *professional research and literature.* The standards are made operational by construction of the criterion elements. These criteria, which are the actual evaluation criteria, are generally developed by a quality assurance committee, the nursing practice committee, or some similar group.

The actual criteria that are developed can be of three types: structure, process, and outcome (Box 2-2). *Structure criteria describe the environment elements, setting, and conditions within which the nurse-patient relationship occurs.* It includes the philosophy and objectives of the institution; its fiscal resources, equipment, physical facilities, management structure, accreditation, and licensure; and the quality and characteristics of the professional and technical employees. Examples of structure criteria include, "Hospital beds must be 3 feet apart." "All patients must sign the required consent form before any invasive or surgical procedure." "The current PIN number of each registered nurse must be on file in the main nursing office."

Process criteria describe the nature and sequence of nursing care activities. For example, process criteria might describe the nursing plan for a patient who demands pain medication every $1\frac{1}{2}$ hours, although he or she has made a contract with his or her primary nurse that he or she will not do so. A teaching plan for a diabetic patient is another example.

2-2	**Example of standards and outcomes**

Patient goal Adequate pain medication to enable mobilization and pulmonary hygiene.

Structure	Pain medication is available and ordered by physician.
Process	Nursing staff assess patient at least every 4 hours for discomfort.
Outcome	Patient has adequate pain control, and is able to ambulate, cough, and deep breathe.

2-3	**Outcome criteria for the person with a colostomy or ileostomy**

The patient or significant other can do the following:
1. Demonstrate how to measure the stoma for an appliance. (The stoma shrinks as healing occurs. Measure the stoma before purchasing more appliances.)
2. Demonstrate proper application of the appliance. (Application includes appliance removal, skin care, and reapplying an appliance.)
3. State plans for follow-up care.
4. State community resources available for obtaining permanent appliances, and list support groups.
5. State need to observe stoma and skin around it for redness, bleeding, or excoriation.
6 Patient or significant other has information packet, which has been reviewed with the nurse.

Outcome criteria focus on the results of the processes of health care. Many experts consider them the ultimate indicators of the quality of patient care. For the patient the outcome is measurable in terms of change in health, knowledge, or functional status. Examples of outcome criteria for the person with an ostomy are listed in Box 2-3.

After the criteria are written, they are validated, generally by "consensus among peers." The rationale for this validation step is to ensure that all criteria are correct and relevant and reflect nursing practice at the particular institution. Usually, nurses most expert in the selected clinical area are chosen to do the review.

The final step in the criteria writing process is the establishment, by the quality management committee and the "nurse experts," of a specific and observable level of performance for each criterion measure. For example, for the outcome criterion, "Patient or significant other is able to demonstrate proper technique in insulin administration," at least 90% compliance might be expected. However, for the outcome criterion, "Patient is able to apply own stoma appliance," the committee may decide that 80% compliance is appropriate, because many of the patients are elderly, are not completely independent in activities of daily living by the time of discharge, and are frequently discharged to nursing homes.

Step 3: Measure degree of attainment of standards and criteria

Many methods are available to collect data to assess the attainment of the standards and criteria. The degree to which the actual practice exceeds, meets, or falls below the validated criteria provides the data necessary to evaluate the strengths and weaknesses of the nursing care programme. Data collection methods might include *questionnaires, staff interviews, patient interviews, self-assessment questionnaires, performance evaluations, utilization reviews, patient care audits, patient or staff complaints*, and *direct observation*. Whatever the method selected, the data should be easily accessible, and questions of efficiency and accuracy should be considered.

Specific questions that the quality management review committee needs to answer at this point include:

1. Who will collect the data?
2. What will be the source of the data?
3. Where will the data be collected?
4. When will the data be collected?
5. How will the data be collected?

The answers to these questions will assist the committee in deciding whether the review can be accomplished as planned given the inherent requirements for efficiency and accuracy. As a final check, the committee should be certain that each criterion measure is written so that a decision can be easily made as to whether or not the standard has been met.

Once the data is collected, the results are tabulated, and it is determined whether the percentage of yes and no answers corresponds to the previously established level of performance (for example, percentage of compliance) for each criterion. If the level of performance does not achieve the expectations, the criterion for this evaluation item has not been met.

Table 2-1, overleaf, illustrates one method for keeping track of a multicriterion evaluation process.

Step 4: Interpret strengths and weaknesses

The degree to which the levels of performance have been met serves as the basis for describing the strengths and weaknesses of the nursing care programme. However, it is essential that certain subtle factors are not overlooked before final judgments are made. Consider the following: One *outcome criteria for a patient with a pacemaker is, "The patient or significant other is able to take a pulse."* A retrospective nursing audit was performed on patients with pacemakers to determine whether the outcome was being met. On nursing unit A, 95% of the patients could take their pulse, whereas on nursing unit C, only 65% of the patients could. Careful inspection of the patient data revealed that, in general, patients on unit C were older, had fewer significant others, and were frequently discharged to extended care facilities. Comparing the two units using this

Table 2-1

Outcome criteria for person with colostomy	Level of performance (percentage of compliance)*	Identified problems, strengths, and weaknesses
Patient or significant others can do the following:		
Demonstrate how to measure the stoma for an appliance.	85%	One patient was blind; no documentation on two patients.
Demonstrate proper application of the appliance.	85%	Two patients stated it would have been helpful to have a mirror provided; one patient was blind.
State plans for follow-up care.	60%	Forty per cent of patients were being transferred to an extended care facility
State community resources available and support groups.	80%	Twenty per cent of charts audited had one of these components missing.
State need to observe stoma and skin around it for redness and excoriation.	75%	No documentation of this being done on 25% of charts.
Patient or significant other has stoma care informational booklet, which has been reviewed with nurse.	100%	

*Expected compliance in these areas is 100%.

information provided insights into reasons for the differences in the units that would have been missed if the evaluator had not questioned why the figures from the two units were so different.

Step 5: Identify possible courses of action

After identifying the strengths and weaknesses, possible courses of action to correct the weaknesses are developed. The goal of the action plan is elimination of the weaknesses and reinforcement of the strengths of the existing programme. Consideration should be given to how best to motivate the nursing staff to implement the desired changes. Generally the best results are obtained when those staff most affected by the quality management review are involved in the planning of subsequent courses of action.

Solutions to the identified problems can be numerous and can include administrative changes, further clinical research into the problem, continuing education, changes in practice, environmental changes, a reward system for improved compliance, or even the organization of peer pressure. Each of the possible solutions has advantages and disadvantages, and the peer group has to weigh each one.

Step 6: Select a course of action

After examining the alternatives, the peer group selects the course of action, based on such considerations as the identified problem, available resources, and organizational structure. How the course of action is implemented varies among institutions. Different institutions make varying decisions about how the plan for change is presented to the administration and how the change is to be implemented. In the case of a nursing practice change, at one institution the director of nursing may wish to make the final decision and at another institution the director of nursing may only wish to be informed of the findings, delegating to the committee responsibility to make appropriate changes.

Step 7: Take action

Improving the quality of nursing care implies change, and sooner or later some action must be taken. Implementation of selected action generally includes time frames, people responsible for overseeing each step of the plan, and selection of a date for reevaluation. This action step is critical to the success of the quality management review.

Step 8: Reevaluate the process

We have added this step to the original ANA model. The rationale for its addition is to illustrate that *once a corrective action or other type of action is taken, the action is monitored to ascertain if it is effective in solving the problem.* Therefore, once an action is taken, the cycle begins over again. See Box 2-4 for a clinical example of a quality management review.

MONITORING ACTIVITIES AND INSTRUMENTS

In addition to problem-focused quality management reviews, a variety of methods have been devised for ongoing assessment of the nursing care programme. Some of the more frequently used methods are described here.

Incident Reports

Whenever an accident or untoward event occurs involving a patient, nurse or visitor, an incident report must be completed. Complaints received and investigated also generate detailed reports. It is important that these are seen as valuable sources of information which must be used in quality management. Increases in certain types of incidents, such as medication errors or patient falls, are signals to the quality assurance team that a review of either of these two areas may be indicated.

Quality Indicators

Quality indicators are those items that a purchasing organization believes are important indicators of quality patient care. The annual service agreement between an NHS Trust and a District Health Authority will contain a detailed range of quality indicators.[22a] For example, "No patient should wait more than six weeks for an initial non-urgent out-patient appointment"; or "all care should be provided in as homely and caring a setting as possible, upholding the

2-4

Quality management review topic: learning needs of the patient with a colostomy or ileostomy

Step 1: Identify values
Patient and family education and patient involvement in care are high priorities at this institution. Nurses on the surgical units were concerned that stoma care patients, in particular, were not receiving adequate discharge information.

Step 2: Identify criteria
The outcome criteria (revised in 1990) for the person with a colostomy or ileostomy were selected as the evaluation criteria (see Box 2-3).

Step 3: Collect data
Charts of 30 patients with the discharge diagnosis of some types of stoma were selected at random from patients discharged in the previous 6 months. Review of patients' records using the outcome criteria for the person with a colostomy or ileostomy revealed incomplete teaching plans and no record of the patients having received any type of information booklets. (The rule is, "If it isn't documented, it hasn't been done.")

Step 4: Interpret data
The quality management committee was certain that the patients had received more information than was documented in the record. But where was such documentation to be found? It was also apparent to the committee that some of the criterion elements required updating.

Step 5: Identify possible courses of action
It was observed that the documentation system for discharge planning for these patients needed to be more efficient, yet more thorough. The surgical nursing staff suggested that the outcome criteria sheet be printed on a Nurse's Note Sheet. Another suggestion was to use a large stamp containing elements of the teaching plan, which could be checked off as completed. A group of experienced nurses was formed, who, with the assistance of the clinical nurse specialist, rewrote and assisted in the validation process for the outcome criteria.

Step 6: Write the action plan
The quality management committee met with the surgical nursing staff and concluded that the best choice was to have the outcome criteria overprinted on the Nurse's Note Sheet. The appropriate administrative approval was obtained.

Step 7: Implement the action plan
One member of the quality management committee was assigned to oversee the production of the new forms. After they were obtained, the unit nursing staff took the responsibility for introducing them and explaining their purpose to the other staff members. An evaluation was planned for 4 months later.

Step 8: Reevaluate
Four months after the implementation, the surgical nursing staff conducted a repeat review. There was 100% compliance with each criterion element.

---

dignity, privacy, and individual choice of the patient at all times"; "waiting time in out-patient clinics should not exceed 30 minutes before the patient is seen by a member of medical staff"; "a nursing care plan, based on a model of nursing, should be developed after an assessment of the patient by a registered nurse." It is vital that the clinical team in each area is aware of the quality indicators agreed with purchasers and takes active measures to apply a model for quality assurance in pursuit of each indicator.

Standard Instruments

There are several standard instruments commercially available for measuring quality of care. "Monitor"[10a] has been widely used in the United Kingdom. It assesses four aspects of nursing care: assessment and planning, physical care, non-physical care, and evaluation of care. It is an adaptation for the UK of the Rush Medicus Nursing Process Methodology. It contains four patient-based questionnaires, relating to different levels of dependency. Specially trained assessors visit the clinical area to administer the questionnaires, with two assessors on a 25-bed ward, the process will take approximately two days.[10b] The outcome is a set of scores for each aspect of nursing care and each dependency level. Norms are available to assist interpretation, but detailed follow-up work is required to clarify the reasons for low scores in particular areas and to plan remedial action. "QUALPACS"[25] is a rival scale designed to measure the quality of nursing care. It focuses on the following aspects of care: Actions designed to meet the psychosocial needs of individual patients and of groups;

actions to meet physical needs; communication on behalf of the patient; general actions; and an assessment of professional expectations concerning patient care. The items on the scale are assessed primarily by observation, with two assessors using a seven-point scale. The process will yield a general mean score and sub-section scores. As with "Monitor", the instrument does not complete the control cycle, since further action must be taken to investigate the meaning of particular scores and to determine any improvements required.

The advantage of these and similar instruments is that they contain specific, measurable standards and give clear and practical guidance on how those standards can be evaluated in an objective way. A further advantage is that if several clinical areas are using the same instrument, their performance may be compared. The disadvantage of standard instruments is that they are "top-down" they impose standards on nursing staff, instead of allowing them to develop standards for themselves. The commitment which comes from devising one's own standards may therefore be lost. Linked with this, experienced staff may question the relevance and appropriateness of some of the prescribed standards to their particular clinical area. These instruments introduce a systematic approach to the measuring aspect of quality management, but they do not provide a complete answer to the question of how to maintain a genuine and continuing commitment to quality from the staff who are delivering the care.

Nursing Audit

Nursing Audit is best seen as the process of evaluating the quality of specific aspects of nursing care and taking action to produce defined improvements. The NHS Management Executive[15a] stated that: "It incorporates the systematic and critical analysis by nurses, midwives and health visitors, in conjunction with other staff, of the planning, delivery and evaluation of Nursing and Midwifery care, in terms of their use of resources and outcomes for patients and clients and introduces appropriate change in response to that analysis." Thus it embraces issues relating not only to clinical care, but to workload management, deployment, personnel management, organizational arrangements and the environment of care.[21a]

This process of nursing audit may be divided into two types: retrospective and concurrent. A retrospective audit is a critical examination of nursing actions, with a view to improvement in practice. A retrospective review is performed after the patient has been discharged. The reviewer has the advantage of using data from the patient's entire stay, from admission to discharge, and of evaluating the results for a large number of comparable patients. One advantage of a retrospective audit is that sometimes practitioners gain impressions from single cases in which they are personally involved. These impressions, however, may not be borne out by later systematic study of a large number of cases.

A concurrent audit is a critical examination of the patient's progress towards a desired health status (outcome) and patient care management activities (processes) while the care is in progress. Patient questionnaires, interviews, and observation of care as it is being given, and review of the patient record are possible sources of data for a concurrent review. Concurrent review has the advantage of providing opportunities for making changes in the ongoing care of individual patients and of groups. Retrospective and concurrent audits each have their own advantages and may be used singly or together in a quality management review.

Peer Review

Nursing peer review occurs when *practising* nurses establish standards and criteria and evaluate the quality of each other's patient care. The peer review process may be performed within a single unit or by specialty. It may be a highly formalized process, but is also a feature of all specialist consultancy and advice given by one nurse to another. At its worst it is a form of professional game in which practitioners spend time mutually congratulating each other. At its best it is an initiative which springs from the desire of secure and confident practitioners to develop the quality of their care through mutual critical evaluation.

Patient Satisfaction Surveys

A patient satisfaction questionnaire is generally used when written data concerning a patient's perception of his or her care is needed. This can be particularly helpful when standard quality measurement instruments are used, since these generally omit the patients' view of nursing care. However, obtaining an objective measure is difficult, since patients tend to report high levels of satisfaction and it is difficult to bring them to differentiate between aspects of care.[5a] The construction of the questionnaire or interview protocol needs particularly careful attention.[13a] Many Units/Trusts routinely distribute questionnaires to all patients and request that they complete them; others invite the Community Health Council or similar independent bodies to conduct patient satisfaction surveys.

Staff Satisfaction Surveys

Staff satisfaction surveys, either questionnaires or interviews, are less frequently used in the UK to assess general employee satisfaction or to elicit responses to proposed or recently-introduced changes in care delivery and staff deployment. They can be used as a way of motivating staff by allowing them to see how their views can shape the overall process of service delivery.

Infection Control Reports

Because nurses are involved in the direct care of patients, they are likely also to be involved in infection surveillance and control programmes, in support of a designated infection control nurse. Clearly this is an area where audit by one profession alone will be unsatisfactory and where the move towards multidisciplinary clinical audit is gaining momentum — including projects which collect data from both primary and secondary care practitioners.

ETHICAL ISSUES

Several other issues are being raised as part of the quality management process. These issues relate to confidentiality of patient information and ethical problems encountered as part of the quality management process. Both of these are discussed below.

Confidentiality and the Quality Management Process

Confidentiality of data is an issue frequently associated with quality management. The availability and use of evaluative data about a patient or groups of patients has always been of concern to health professionals. The increasing use of *computerized data* about patients has generated enormous concern for potential *threats to privacy*. Most quality management studies can be conducted without the recording of patients' names and are reported in terms of *aggregate data*. Review of care provided to an individual patient requires constant vigilance to ensure protection of the patient's identity.

Ethics and Quality Management

Ethical problems can and do influence the quality management concerns of nurses. Certainly there are traditional areas of mutual interest: patient education, informed consent, and unnecessary surgery or procedures. But ethical problems probably occur much more frequently than is apparent through patient care evaluation, particularly because quality management has focused largely on technical aspects of care — whether appropriate tests are ordered, whether surgical complications were prevented or managed, and whether patient records list the steps taken in treatment.

For several reasons, quality management will need to focus more on *ethical decision making* in the future.

First, the rapidly increasing opportunities in patient care will provide more options for patients and providers. A heart transplant for one patient, for example, may mean that a heart must be sacrificed in a "brain dead" patient who is on a ventilator. *Balancing individual rights* with *social good* will become more *frequent* and more difficult in the future.

Second, as resources continue to diminish, problems of *distributive justice* will arise. It is possible that in the future some type of health care *rationing* could exist. Who should receive this service? How much service should they receive? Who should pay? As public policymakers attempt to reduce all care choices to cost-benefit analyses, nurses must be aware of the limitations of these calculations and the inability of accounting for human pain and suffering mathematically.

Third, nurses as well as other health professionals must participate in these ethical decisions or risk losing their unique influence entirely. For example, in cases of the comatose, terminally ill patient, peer review would focus not only on the clinical aspects of death but also on the human dimension. Were the wishes of the patient or significant others followed? Did the health care provider confer with the patient and/or family to keep them totally informed? Were the providers guided by the wishes of the patient and family? Did the provider seek competent, objective, and relevant third-party opinions?

None of the decisions can be made irrespective of the law. But there are questions of quality that lie within the realm of quality management activity. In addition to questions of nontreatment, other *ethical dilemmas* must be recognized, analyzed, and resolved within a quality assurance framework. One approach suggests that decisions themselves are less important than the approach taken by the participants. In analyzing problems did they use accurate and necessary information? Was the reasoning logical? Did the decision-maker account for the values and rights of the individual? Use of the systematic quality assurance process has much to offer in this area in the future.

FUTURE TRENDS

The application of *total quality management* (TQM) concepts and the principles of *continuous quality improvement* (CQI) are becoming important and successful strategies in health care organizations as they cope with the changes in the industry. TQM is a conceptual approach different from quality management. It calls for continuous improvement in the total process that provides care, not simply in the improved actions of the individual nurse. Improvement is based upon both outcome and process.

TQM demands that the change be based on the needs of the patient, not the values of the providers. It requires the meaningful participation of all health care personnel that a patient may come in contact with and a rapid and thoughtful response from top management to suggestions made by participating personnel. An example of TQM is a product utilized for the patient's colostomy causing a skin reaction. Follow-up would include determining if other patients are also having skin reactions and if the vendor supplying the product has received other reports of reactions. Top management may then make the decision to have the product discontinued for patient care based on the nurse's findings and a report from the vendor.

CQI does not replace *quality management* but complements and enhances existing efforts. The efforts range from improved patient care, employee morale, patient satisfaction, and outcomes to decrease costs and duplication of services.

SUMMARY

1. Nursing's commitment to professional excellence in cludes monitoring the quality of care given.
2. Three factors have influenced quality management in nursing. These are (1) legislation and government policy initiatives, (2) economic factors, and (3) professional standards.
3. The UKCC Code of Professional Conduct and the work of RCN Standards of Care Project provide the framework within which detailed standards of nursing care can be developed.
4. A basic control-loop model of quality assurance consists of 8 steps.
   a. Identify values or basic philosophy/beliefs.
   b. Identify standards and criteria for structure, pro cess and outcomes.
   c. Measure the degree of attainment of standards and criteria.
   d. Interpret strengths and weaknesses.
   e. Identify possible courses of action.
   f. Select a course of action.
   g. Take action.
   h. Reevaluate.
5. Quality management is an ongoing process in which

the results of the evaluation of patient care are interpreted so that improvements may be introduced.

6. The introduction of the purchaser-provider agreements has led to the specification of quality indicators which providers must meet if they are to retain funding.

7. Standard measuring instruments are commercially available but need to be used with care as part of a wider quality management programme.

8. Nursing audit is the process of investigating key areas of nursing care, using retrospective and/or concurrent data.

9. Peer review works best when it springs from an initiative led by the staff themselves.

10. Patient satisfaction surveys are difficult to carry out but are a vital element in the quality management process.

11. Staff satisfaction surveys offer a way of empowering nurses and may yield valuable suggestions for improving the quality of the working environment.

12. Quality management demands attention to ethical issues arising from the process of data collection and from the resulting analysis of outcomes.

13. Total quality management and continuous quality improvement is an ongoing process that places primary emphasis on improving collaborative practice approaches and requiring evaluation of the interdependent outcomes of these combined efforts.

STUDY QUESTIONS

• Find and review the purchaser quality standards which apply to your Unit/Trust and clinical area.

• Identify four nursing process standards for the care of patients in your specialty.

• Identify one clinical problem and the steps you would use to assess it using the model of quality assurance.

• Identify one ethical issue arising from the process of quality management in your clinical area. Discuss the issue with your colleagues.

REFERENCES AND SUGGESTED READINGS

1. American Nurses' Association: Task force on nursing practice standards and guidelines: working paper, *J Nurs Qual Assur* 5(3):1–17, 1991.

2. Andrews SL: QA vs. QI: the changing role of quality in health care, *JQA* 13(1):14–15, 38, 1991.

3. Arikian MA, Kingery C, Beall K, Abbott R: Education and QA: a model for continuous improvement in skin integrity, *J Nurs Qual Assur* 5(1):1–7, 1990.

4.* Batslden PB: Building knowledge for quality improvement in healthcare: an introductory glossary, *JQA* 13(5):8–12, 1991.

5. Bliersbach C: Quality improvement: one-third of the quality equation, *JQA* 13(5):58f–61, 1991.

5a. Bond S, Thomas LH: Measuring patients' satisfaction with nursing care, *J Adv Nurs* 17(1):52–63, 1992.

6. Brannon D: Quality assurance feedback as a nursing management strategy, *Hospital Health Services Adm* 34(4):547–555, 1989.

7. Conningon ME, Dupuis P: *Unit-based nursing quality assurance*, Rockville, Md, 1990, Aspen Publishers.

8.* Crockett D, Sutcliffe S: Staff participation in nursing quality assurance, *Nurs Manage* 17(10):41–42, 1986.

8a. Department of Health: *The health of the nation: A strategy for health in England*, HMSO, London, 1992.

8b. Department of Health: *The patient's charter*, HMSO, London, 1991.

8c. Department of Health: *Targeting practice: the contribution of nurses, midwives and health visitors*, HMSO, London, 1993.

8d. Department of Health: *Working for patients*, HMSO, London, 1990.

9.* Fralic MF, Kowalski PM, Llewellyn FA: The staff nurse as quality monitors, *Amer J Nurs* 91(4):41–42, 1991.

10. Goldmann RC: Nursing process components as a framework for monitoring and evaluation activities, *J Nurs Qual Assur* 4(4):17–25, 1990.

10a. Goldstone LA, Ball JA, Collier MM: *Monitor: an index of the quality of nursing care for acute medical and surgical wards*, Newcastle upon Tyne Polytechnic Products Limited, Newcastle upon Tyne, 1983.

10b. Goldstone LA: Monitor, in Pearson A, (ed), *Nursing quality measurement*, John Wiley and Sons, Chichester, 1987.

11. Joint Commission on Accreditation of Healthcare Organizations: *Accreditation manual for hospitals*, Chicago, 1991, The Commission.

12. Jones KR: Maintaining quality in a changing environment, *Nurs Econ* 9(3):159–164, 1991.

12a. Kitson A: *Standards of care: a framework for quality*, Scutari Press, Middlesex, 1989.

13. Kravlovec OJ, Huttner CA, Dixon MD: The application of total quality management concepts in a service-line cardiovascular program, *Nurs Admin Q* 15(2):1–8, 1991.

13a. Locker D, Dunt D: Theoretical and methodological issues in sociological studies of consumer satisfaction with medical care, *Social Science and Medicine*, 12:283–292, 1978.

14. Lynn ML, Osborn DP: Deming's quality principles: a health care application, *Hospital Health Services Adm* 36(1):111–120, 1991.

15. McLaughlin CP, Kaluzny AD: Total quality management in health: making it work, *Health Care Manage Rev* 15(3):7–14, 1990.

15a. NHS Management Executive: *Framework of audit for nursing services*, HMSO, London, 1991.

16. Omachonu VK: Quality of care: new criteria for evaluation, *Health Care Manage Rev* 15(4):43–50, 1990.

17.* Osinski EG: Developing patient outcomes as a quality measure of nursing care, *Nurs Manage* 18(10):28–29, 1987.

18. Ott MJ: Quality assurance: monitoring individual compliance with standards of nursing care, *Nurs Manage* 18(5):57–64, 1987.

18a. Pearson A: Nursing and quality, in Pearson, A (ed), *Nursing quality measurement*, John Wiley and Sons, Chichester, 1987.

19. Redfern SJ: Measuring the quality of nursing care: a consideration of different approaches, *J Adv Nurs* 15(11):1260–71, 1990.

19a. Royal College of Nursing: *Standards of nursing care*, RCN, London, 1980.

19b. Royal College of Nursing: *Towards standards*, RCN, London, 1981.

20. Sinioris ME: TQM: the new frontier for quality and productivity improvement in health care, *JQA* 12(4):14–17, 1990.

21. Slee VN: Quality management nee quality assurance, *JONA* 21(5):9–12, 1991.

21a. Snowley GD, Nicklin PJ, Birch JA: *Objectives for care*, Wolfe Publishing Limited, London, 1992.

22.* Taylor AG, Hudson K, Keeling A: Quality nursing care: the consumers' perspective revisited, *J Nurs Qual Assur* 5(2):23–31, 1991.

22a. Teasdale K: *Managing the changes in health care*, Wolfe Publishing Limited, London, 1992.

23. Tucker SM, Canobbio MM, Paquette EV, Wells MF: *Patient care standards: nursing process, diagnosis, and outcome*, ed. 5, St Louis, 1992, Mosby-Year Book.

24. United Kingdom Central Council: *Code of professional conduct for the nurse, midwife and health visitor*, ed. 2, UKCC, London, 1984.

25. Wandelt M, Ager J: *Quality patient care scale*, Appleton-Century Crofts, New York, 1974.

*Recommended for student reading.

Health Promotion and Illness Prevention

3

Promotion of Health in the Elderly

Ruth Lincoln

After studying this chapter, the learner should be able to:

- Distinguish between primary and secondary changes of ageing.
- Describe psychosocial aspects of ageing.
- Compare health concerns of elderly adults with those of younger adults.
- Describe health promotion strategies for the older adult.
- Describe special precautions for the hospitalized elderly.

This chapter discusses the characteristics of the elderly from a health perspective. Major health needs of the elderly and the role of the nurse in assisting the elderly with health promotion and health problems are addressed. The chapter focuses on assisting elderly people to improve the quality of their lives.

The number of people over the age of 65 in the United Kingdom is increasing dramatically. The elderly population, at 10,522,000 in 1990, is predicted to be at 11,667,000 by 2011 and 14,615,000 by 2030. In the United Kingdom between 1989 and 2030, the total population is projected to rise by 7%, whilst the population between 60 and 74 years is projected to rise by 36%, and that of 75 years and over by 44%. The largest growth is occurring amongst those over 85 years.[40,41]

The elderly account for the highest proportion of those with chronic illness and functional disability. Improving the quality of life, rather than searching for means to increase longevity, becomes of utmost importance.

CONCEPTS OF AGEING

Although 65 years of age is usually considered the beginning of late adulthood, tremendous individual variation exists. Age is more a sociocultural concept than a physiological or chronological one.

Theories of Ageing

Biological ageing theory focuses on cellular ageing; changes in replicating cells, loss of or injury to cells, and changes in noncellular materials or regulatory systems that "programme" ageing. One cellular theory postulates that a limited number of cell divisions occur under the influence of a biological clock or programme. Another explanation maintains that ageing is a random chemical process, influenced by damage from free radicals. Radiation "hits" lead to cellular mutations, which cause ageing as they accumulate over the years.

Physiological theories of ageing relate the ageing process to a decline in the immune system. Either the immune system succumbs as ageing progresses or an autoimmunity develops. As immune competence decreases, the incidence of infections, cancer, and autoimmune diseases rises.

Another physiological theory maintains that "crosslinking" occurs in collagen cells. As the cross-linkages accumulate, organs deteriorate from impaired function.[11]

None of these theories has been accepted as the final truth about ageing. Researchers continue to seek the answer to the question: What causes the body to age?

Physiological Ageing

In late adulthood, physiological function does not correlate with chronological age. Adult years are not characterized by specific events at particular ages, with the exception of menopause. Some biological variables remain constant throughout the lifespan (for example, fasting blood sugar, blood pH). However, the normal range for some electrolytes and enzymes is different for the elderly than for younger adults. Other body functions begin a gradual decline after age 30, continuing into the late decades.

Certain generalizations can be made, however:
1. The older the age group, the greater the variability among individuals.
2. The rate of decline varies among body functions.
3. Changes previously thought to be associated with ageing have been shown to result from lack of physical conditioning or from disease.

Primary and Secondary Ageing

Primary ageing refers to biological changes that are universal, gradual, intrinsic, and inevitable. Greying hair and wrinkles are examples of primary ageing changes. *Secondary ageing* refers to pathophysiological conditions. These may be more prevalent in the elderly but are not universal. More importantly, secondary changes are treatable and sometimes reversible. In the past, many conditions that were attributed to old age have been proven to be pathological. Some of these are senility, arthritis, loss of hearing, muscle weakness, and incontinence. The 93-year-old man who complained to his doctor about his gimpy right leg is an example of primary versus secondary ageing. The doctor said, "You're old; you have to put up with aches and pains." The old man retorted, "Tell that to my left leg."

The nurse working with the elderly must know the common ageing changes. Assessment should include baseline function, prediction of functional changes, and discrimination between primary and secondary ageing. Because the elderly often believe the myths regarding what they "must put up with," they need to be encouraged to seek medical treatment for their chronic and acute conditions. Some symptoms, such as weakness and fatigue, are helped by diet and exercise.

Sexuality

Both men and women maintain interest in sexual activity into the late adulthood years. More women cease having sexual activity after age 65 than do men. The primary reasons for the cessation are lack of acceptable sexual partner for widows or an ailing husband for married women (rather than lack of interest).[31]

Cultural attitudes toward the elderly influence both sexes. Older men and women are frequently thought of as sexually unattractive and lacking in ability to engage in sex. However, Masters and Johnson[36] have found that, although sexual responses are slower, the elderly still have the same phases of excitement, plateau, orgasm, and resolution as younger people. Men, in particular, can expect adequate sexual performance up to and beyond the eighth decade (see Chapter 26).

Sexual problems occur more frequently for the elderly. Women may have dyspareunia as a result of vaginal thinning and decreased lubrication. These factors are caused by postmenopausal steroid starvation. Men tend to be affected by secondary impotence related to performance anxiety and low self-esteem. Diabetes, alcohol, and medications for hypertension are other prominent causes of impotence.

Masters and Johnson report a condition known as "widower's syndrome."[36] Following an extended period of sexual inactivity, a man cannot achieve or maintain an erection. An equivalent condition occurs in women: the vagina constricts and undergoes atrophic changes. The conclusion is that those who do not engage in sexual activity lose the ability.

Sexuality is more than the physical act of intercourse. Elderly people continue to need human companionship and the sharing of love and affection. Nurses need to be aware of the components of sexuality and how the elderly may be affected by chronic illness, loss of a partner, and need for touch. Being sensitive to family dynamics is just as important for a newly married couple in their seventies as for a young couple.[31] Through counselling the nurse can explain ageing changes, suggesting vaginal lubrication for women and extra physical stimulation for men. Changes in sexual position and styles of lovemaking are appropriate for those with disabling diseases. Nurses have a vital role in enabling elderly people to express their need for love and affection.

Unfortunately, the elderly are susceptible to sexually transmitted disease, though not in the same numbers as younger adults. Acquired immune deficiency syndrome (AIDS) is becoming increasingly prevalent in the elderly as the epidemic spreads among all age groups. The "at risk" categories differ for elderly (for example, not as many are intravenous drug abusers).[29] However, other risk factors are present: the decline in the ability of the immune system to ward off infections makes them more susceptible to organisms from sexually transmitted diseases. Women in particular are more vulnerable because of the friable vaginal lining that occurs with ageing. "Safe sex" education and counselling for those at risk should not be overlooked just because the person is over 65 years of age.[29]

Psychosocial Ageing

Ageing has long been associated with deterioration in function rather than an expansion of abilities. New evidence is accumulating to support multifactor systems theories to account for the richness and variety encountered among older adults.

Reed proposes the view that adult development is a progressive, not a decremental, phenomenon.[38] She emphasizes the role of person–environment interactions in successful ageing, and views ageing, behaviour not as decremental, but as "trade-offs." Important concepts are that adults:

1. Have a clearer perception of themselves and others not clouded by the context of the situation
2. Are better equipped to engage in complex and meaningful interactions with others
3. Conceptualize problems better and delegate less complex details to others
4. Are better able to predict future consequences
5. Develop more realistic solutions to problems
6. Are increasingly capable of transforming conflicts into meaningful experiences.

The "trade-offs" for the older adult are a decreased intellectual dexterity, decreased flexibility in thinking, and loss of ability to remember details. These may appear as deficiencies to young adults, but actually help the elderly provide a stabilizing force for society.

A positive outlook on ageing is crucial to the nurse's capacity to evaluate the abilities of the elderly in any setting.

An 84-year-old woman admitted to the hospital from a nursing home is not the equivalent of a regressed child. She should be regarded as an experienced adult, integrally related to the environment, no matter what her functional level.

Nurses are challenged to facilitate wellbeing among adults who have developed useful modes of functioning as they age. Strategies are not appropriate if they are based on physical strength, deftness of function, and speed of recall. The developmental tasks of late adulthood are summarized in Box 3-1. Box 3-2 discusses research on the effect of restricted activity in the elderly.

Intellectual Function

Intellectual function curves stay relatively stable throughout a person's lifespan. Research has shown that many components of cognitive function remain intact in the elderly. Problem solving, verbal ability, recognition, and memory span are examples of areas in which normal elderly people scored well.[33] Only when the tests were timed and speed was important did results decline.

The implications for the nurse are clear when devising teaching strategies for the elderly. Older adults are capable of learning. They retain content best when it is related to something familiar, is sequenced, and plenty of time is allowed to learn each facet.

3-1

Tasks of late adulthood

Adjusting to declining physical strength and health
Adjusting to retirement and change in financial status
Accepting reorganized family patterns
Adjusting to new pattern of social and civic responsibilities
Adjusting to death of significant others
Establishing affiliation with one's age group
Maintaining satisfactory living arrangements
Developing point of view about death

3-2

Nursing Research

Sholes D, *et al*: **Tracking progress toward national health objectives in the elderly: What do restricted activity days signify?** *Am J Public Health* 81(4):485-588, 1991.

This study evaluated restricted activity days (RAD) as an outcome measure in a random study of 2300 health maintenance organization enrollees. RAD is the measure by which health objectives in 1990 were evaluated for prevention of functional disability in older adults. RAD was more correlated with physical disability measures than with mental, social, and global self-perceived health.

Health Problems

Chronic diseases are a major health problem and are much more common among the elderly population (see Box 3-3). Estimates show that 85% of the elderly have one or more chronic diseases. Heart disease and hypertension are the most prevalent, with 50% of people over the age of 65 years having observable signs of heart disease. Gastrointestinal disorders, rheumatism, and arthritis affect large numbers of the elderly. Visual problems, atherosclerosis, lung disease, and hypertension appear to be associated with lower socioeconomic status.

The figures on prevalence of health problems may be misleading. The important issues are: what is normal functioning and how disabling are the chronic conditions?

Despite chronic disease, 83% of people over the age of 65 have little difficulty carrying out activities of daily living. Only 5% live in nursing homes, although 35% will be in a nursing home at one time or another. Another 5% are homebound.

The following factors are important to remember when evaluating the physical capacities of the elderly:

1. Organ systems have a great compensatory ability, despite loss of cells and tissue through ageing (such as in the brain, kidney, heart, and liver).
2. Compensatory mechanisms may fail when the organism is stressed through illness and disease (for example, renal failure can occur with urinary tract infection).
3. The body takes a longer time to return to normal following a stressful event.
4. Once a stressful event has occurred, the individual may not return to baseline function.
5. The immune system is decreasingly effective as the individual ages, causing increased susceptibility to infection. The elderly are much more prone to pneumonia, skin infections, urinary tract infection, and sepsis.
6. The symptomatology of a particular disease is often atypical in the elderly (for example, a myocardial infarction without severe crushing chest pain, an infection without a fever, a gastrointestinal haemorrhage without severe stomach pain).
7. The most typical sign that an individual has had a change in physical wellbeing is sudden onset of confusion.

Stress situations may produce more pronounced reactions in the elderly and require a longer period of readjustment (Box 3-4).

PREVENTION AND HEALTH EDUCATION
Primary Prevention

The goal of health care for the elderly is to keep people functioning at the optimal level for their age. Health promotion is just as important for the elderly person as for the young person. Nurses in any health care setting have an ideal opportunity to assist elderly people with health promotion.

Even in the acute care setting where the focus is on illness, the nurse should identify priority needs and introduce an educational programme designed to enhance the person's lifestyle after hospitalization.

The four main areas the nurse should address are *health habits* (smoking and drinking), *exercise*, *nutrition*, and *immunizations*. This section also addresses general principles in teaching the elderly.

Health habits

Nursing assessment in any setting should include questions regarding smoking and alcohol use. Smoking cessation can have positive health benefits for a person at any age. Reduced incidence of respiratory infections and improved ventilatory capacity are two of these. A smoking history should tell not only packs per day, but also the meaning of smoking to the individual, habits connected with smoking (for example, eating and drinking, reading, answering the phone) and attempts made to stop in the past. The nurse can help the elder to analyse his or her smoking behaviour to find ways to cut down or quit. Encourage the use of stop smoking programmes, such as those led by G.P. or practice nurses.

Alcohol abuse is a largely unrecognized problem among the elderly. The signs and symptoms are similar to other

---

3-3

Major health problems of late adulthood

Heart disease
Hypertension
Cancer
Renal disease
Chronic obstructive pulmonary disease
Acute pulmonary disease (pneumonia, pulmonary oedema)
Vascular disease (cerebrovascular accident, peripheral vascular disease)
Arthritis
Skin disorders
Accidents
Alcoholism

3-4

Stressful life changes for the elderly

Loss of driver's licence
Multiple relocations
Hemiplegia
Sensory deficits
Hospitalization
Institutionalization
Mechanical speech difficulties
Loss of children and friends
Dispersal of significant belongings
Incompetency proceedings
Inheritance conflicts
Birth of grandchildren
Moving to a nursing home
Inadequate health insurance coverage

secondary ageing processes; tremors, sleep difficulties, gait abnormalities, depression, and malnutrition. The elderly person and his or her family may deny the seriousness of the problem, and health professionals may neglect to assess the individual for alcohol abuse.

Elderly people have a decreased tolerance for alcohol because of a declining ability of the liver to detoxify and metabolize it. Loneliness and depression may intensify the feelings that lead to drinking. Heavy drinking contributes to confusion, injuries from falls, self-neglect, and malnutrition.[8]

The nurse should always be alert to symptoms that hint of alcohol abuse and ask questions regarding drinking habits. Teach patients about ageing changes that aggravate the effect of alcohol and inform them about community agencies that are available to assist with alcohol problems. Many of these agencies have chapters of Alcoholics Anonymous.

Exercise

An exercise programme has many benefits for the older person, whether or not they have engaged in exercise in the past. Exercise increases endurance, strengthens the muscles, and enhances the cardiovascular system. Table 3-1 shows the benefits to the body systems.

A variety of exercise programmes are recommended depending on the interests of the older person. The best and simplest is a walking programme. Walking 30 to 60 minutes three times a week can improve fitness quickly and easily.

Other forms of exercise that may appeal to the older person are swimming, water exercise, cycling, gardening, dancing, and many other sports. Whatever the type of programme, the following guidelines are important:

1. Seek the advice of a doctor before starting a strenuous exercise programme.
2. Do not exercise to the point of dyspnoea or pain.
3. Stop if signs of activity intolerance appear; dizziness, nausea, palpitations, or fatigue.[26]

When advising elderly people about an exercise programme, the nurse should instruct them in taking their pulse rate and teach them to aim for 75% to 85% of the maximum heart rate.[26] Aerobic exercise, which increases oxygen uptake and strengthens the cardiovascular system, should be performed three or more times weekly for maximum benefit.

Nutrition

Nutritional requirements of elderly people differ from those of younger adults. The physical changes associated with ageing, changes in the gastrointestinal tract, the digestive enzymes, and metabolism all affect nutritional status. Social factors may have as much impact on the individual's nutrition as physical changes. Some of these are loneliness, difficulty obtaining food, difficulty in preparing food, and social isolation. Malnutrition is common (see Box 3-5).

Immunizations

The elderly should be advised to have yearly immunizations against influenza and a one time immunization against pneumonia, particularly if they are at high risk (see Box 3-6). As the immunological system ages, the elderly person becomes more susceptible to acute communicable diseases. The reserve capacity to recover from stress declines as well. High-risk individuals are those with chronic disorders of the pulmonary and cardiovascular systems. Immunizations for influenza change annually as different strains of the influenza virus are identified. The best advice is to have patients check with their doctors.

Health education

The elderly adult learner presents an interesting challenge to the nurse in any setting. The same teaching–learning principles apply to the older person as to a younger adult, with some additional guidelines. As with any adult learner, the environment must be comfortable and familiar, so as

Table 3-1 Benefits of exercise

System	Benefit
Cardiovascular	Increased maximum oxygen consumption
	Increased cardiac output
	Reduced mean blood pressure
Pulmonary	Reduced loss of Vo_2 maximum
Musculoskeletal	Increased bone mineral content
	Decreased loss of calcium
	Preservation of lean muscle mass
Regulatory system	Increased basal metabolic care
	Increased haemoregulation
Nervous system	Decreased sleeplessness
	Decreased anxiety

From Schilke J: Slowing the aging process with physical activity, *J Gerontol Nurs* 17(5):5-9, 1991

3-5

Causes of malnutrition in the elderly

Acute and chronic illness
Limited financial resources
Psychological factors such as boredom and lack of companionship while eating
Loss of teeth
Faulty eating patterns
Fads and notions regarding certain foods
Lack of energy to prepare foods
Lack of knowledge of appropriate nutrition
Decreased digestive enzymes

3-6

Immunizations for the elderly

Pneumococcal 23-valent vaccine; given one time
Influenza vaccine; given annually in the autumn
Tetanus vaccine, for penetrating injuries, or booster; given every 10 years.[26]

not to distract from the learning process. For the elderly person, this means the nurse must take particular care to ensure that the patient is warm, relaxed, and free from pain and other discomforts. The older adult may have a hearing or vision impairment that inhibits the learning process, and the nurse must take these into consideration when planning teaching methods.

The nurse should teach the content of any teaching plan in several short sessions. Focus on single elements of the topic, reinforcing previous learning. This is especially true if the person has a short attention span or is distracted by the treatments and equipment in the environment.

One problem the nurse may overlook in the elderly patient is low literacy.[16] When a patient has cognitive and sensory impairments, the lack of good reading and vocabulary skills may hamper well-intentioned educational efforts. Low literacy provokes several reactions. The person may say she or he understands the teaching, when in fact he or she did not, resulting in withdrawal from the situation or disregarding complicated instructions. The following are hints for teaching patients with low literacy:

1. Use simple one- or two-syllable words.
2. Use large print materials.
3. Use pictures with colours and symbols.
4. Divide teaching sessions into segments.
5. Reinforce previous learning.
6. Give positive rewards for mastering content (for example, praise, attention, touch).
7. Involve other family members in the teaching process.[16]

Secondary Prevention

Health screening

Health screening is as important for the elderly as for the younger adult. The elderly person should have an annual physical examination.

Medications

The elderly use a highly disproportionate amount of medications compared with the younger adult. Most elderly take three or more therapeutic agents, and drug reactions and interactions are far more prevalent.

Four problems affect the elderly as they take medications: drug interactions, adverse reactions, drug and food interactions, and medication errors. Each category is detailed in the following discussion.

Drug interactions

Some medications interact with others, causing harmful effects. Table 3-2 shows some of the possible combinations that are problems for the elderly.

Adverse reactions

Medications that cause no problems for middle-aged adults may be harmful for the elderly because of the physiological changes mentioned previously.

Beta blockers can be particularly problematic for elders because these commonly prescribed agents depress cardiac contractility, leading to lethargy and dyspnoea. Elderly people are more prone to orthostatic hypotension, hypo-

Table 3-2 Drug interactions and their potential results

Drug A	Drug B	Potential results
Digoxin	Frusemide	Reduced potassium produced by B could increase risk of arrhythmia produced by A
Warfarin	Aspirin	Protein displacement of A by B could increase risk of bleeding
Tetracycline	Antacid	Absorption impairment of A by B could reduce the antibiotic efficacy of A

From Hershey L, Whitney C: *Drugs and the elderly*. In Kart C, Metress E, Metress S, editors: *Aging, health, and society*, Boston, 1988, Jones & Bartlett.

glycaemia, reduced peripheral circulation, and depression, all of which are possible side effects of beta blockers.[23]

Drug and food interactions

Some foods may inhibit or change the effect of a particular medication more dramatically in elderly than middle-aged people. Levodopa, taken by patients with Parkinson's disease, has a reduced effect if taken with a high-protein meal. The antidepressants in the monoamine oxidase inhibitor (MAO) group are affected by tyramine in red wine, blue cheese, and herring, causing severe hypertension.[17]

Medication errors

Medication errors are common among the elderly. Some of the typical ones, when the person is taking own medication, are omitting prescribed drugs, taking drugs at the wrong times, and taking medications without fully knowing why they are prescribed. *In studies of medication errors, the people most likely to err were those who took the most medications, those who lived alone, and those who were relatively less well-educated.*[17]

Facilitating learning about medications

First, the nurse should make a detailed and thorough assessment whenever he or she comes in contact with the elderly.

Education is based on the strengths and weaknesses found in the medication history. If the patient does not know the name of the drug, but remembers the pink "heart" pill, the nurse emphasizes the pink propranolel pill for the heart when discussing the medication. When administering medications in the acute care setting, the nurse is obligated to repeat the name, dose, and desired effect of the drugs. Through repetition, even people with cognitive and learning impairments start to gain name recognition for their medications.

Whenever possible, patients should be allowed to take their own medications in the hospital setting. Self-medication allows the nurse to assess the patient's understanding of the drugs and the timing of them. It also provides an opportunity to observe side effects, such as lethargy or hypotension.

When teaching the patient how to take medications at home, the nurse must allow sufficient time for adequate learning. The following hints assist the nurse:

1. Teach in several short sessions spread over 1 to 2 days rather than one crammed session as the patient is being discharged.
2. Simplify medication schedules; for example, use coloured stickers for different bottles.
3. Use large print instructions.
4. Coordinate times for medications with the person's daily schedule, for example with meals, when reading the paper, before or after brushing the teeth.
5. Use pictures for a person who cannot read well, for example, use a drawing of a clock with hands showing the medication time.
6. Use compliance aids if necessary; these are available from the pharmacy and designed to contain a week's supply of medicines in daily compartments, further divided into times of day.
7. Emphasize important reminders; take with food, take all the medication.
8. Remind the patients to carry a list of medications with them and show it to any doctor, at any clinic, or when coming to the hospital.[34]

MAJOR HEALTH PROBLEMS OF THE ELDERLY

Although many elderly people maintain indepedant life-styles, they are usually affected by one or more health problems. The number of problems increases proportionately as the person ages. This section addresses the systems most likely to show effects of primary and secondry ageing. The nursing prosses is the framework for each system.

COGNITIVE PERCEPTUAL PROBLEMS

The elderly differ from their younger counterparts in several aspects of cognitive and perceptual function. *The most dramatic changes occur in the central nervous system; the peripheral motor neurons and the autonomic nervous system remain relatively constant throughout the lifespan.*

The changes listed in Box 3-7 affect complex processes such as learning, memory, language, and mentation. Although loss of memory is not considered a primary ageing change, many older people have progressively increasing

---

3-7

Ageing changes

Decreased brain weight
Diminished enzyme activity
Slowed reflexes
Decreased sensory receptors for temperature, pain, and tactile discrimination
Weakening of interneuron connections
Increased response time
Chronic hypoxia

---

problems with short-term memory. Pain and temperature, taste, and touch are all dulled to some extent as one ages. Hearing and vision become less acute as the elder experiences *presbyopia* and *presbycusis* (see Chapter 30). Long-distance vision is less acute, as is night vision, and tolerance for glare decreases. The older person has more difficulty hearing high tones and discriminating speech in noisy situations.

Nursing Process
Assessment
Subjective data

Orientation: obtain information about long- and short-term memory, judgment, abstract thinking, insight, loss of vision and hearing, changes in ability to recognize hot and cold, and pain.

Objective data

Determine the patient's ability to discriminate between hot and cold objects, and hearing and visual losses.

Although delirium (temporary) is the more common form of confusion, the nurse should be aware that *chronic dementia* may be present. The most common dementia is *Alzheimer's disease*, which afflicts 50% to 60% of those who have organic brain disease (see Chapter 29). This devastating condition progressively affects the memory until the patient no longer remembers how to eat, dress, or toilet and is unable to recognize loved ones' faces. *The patient and family need great support and encouragement when the patient with Alzheimer's disease is hospitalized for an acute illness.*

Using a modified mental status examination (Box 3-8), the nurse can efficiently determine the amount of orientation and judgment the elder retains.

Nursing analysis

Nursing analyses are determined from assessment of patient data. Possible problems for people with cognitive perceptual difficulties may include, but are not limited to, the following:

Problem	Possible aetiologies
Thought processes, altered	Acute confusional states, chronic dementia (Alzheimer's disease), stress,
Sensory/perceptual alteration	CVA, dementia, diabetes, neuromuscular diseases

Planning: expected patient outcomes

Expected patient outcomes for the person with a cognitive perceptual problem may include, but are not limited to, the following:

1. Maintains orientation
2. States that he or she understands procedures and routines
3. Remains free from harm during hospitalization

Implementation
Interventions to achieve patient outcomes
Promoting orientation

Give patients detailed, repeated explanations of where they are and what is being done to them. Place glasses and hearing aid on the patient while he or she is awake.

3-8

Mental status examination

Orientation
What day is it?
What season is it?
What is the holiday closest to today? (past or future)

Long-term memory
How old are you?
What is your birth date?
What happened at Pearl Harbour? *or,* What happened to President Kennedy?

Short-term memory
What was the last meal you ate?

Abstract thinking
What is 2 plus 2? 5 minus 3?

Insight
What do you think is wrong with you?

Judgement
What would you do if you spilled your tray on the floor? *or,* What would you do if you had to go to the bathroom?

From Lincoln R: University Hospitals of Cleveland, 1986.

Maintaining adequate hydration and pain control is often sufficient to clear a confused state. *A friend or relative staying through the night could eliminate the need for restraints, and an antihistamine that causes drowsiness is preferable to a sedative for sleep*[39].

When caring for confused patients, the nurse should endeavour to maintain as structured an environment as possible. Fitting the patient's usual routine to that of the hospital may be difficult, but any adaptations that can be made help maintain the elder's orientation. Competing stimuli should be kept to a minimum. The following general guidelines may prove helpful when caring for a confused or demented patient:

1. Use the first name of the patient and ask the patient to call you by your first name.
2. Give simple one-step directions, repeat as necessary.
3. Encourage any remaining social skills.
4. Promote reminiscence and life review.
5. Use distraction for negative behaviour (never scold or argue).
6. Decrease physical stressors such as pain or full bladder.
7. Allow rest or "time-out" periods that alternate with physically active periods.
8. Speak slowly and distinctly in one- or two-syllable words.
9. Avoid tranquilizers and sedatives as much as possible.
10. Reduce extraneous stimuli such as TV, radio, or large groups of people.[7]

Promoting communication

The ability to communicate is often impaired in patients with cognitive deficits. *Those who know what the nurse is asking but have trouble following directions need physical guidance, such as laying out the articles for the bath. People who have difficulty understanding what is being said need verbal prompts and someone to show them the desired behaviour. When attention disorders are present, the nurse may need to prompt the patient frequently.*[12]

Reducing agitation

Agitation in an elderly demented patient can be one of the most difficult behaviours for the nurse to manage. Agitated patients may pull out intravenous lines, disrupt dressings, remove catheters, fall out of bed, wander about, and generally create problems. Helpful strategies for the agitated elder may also be useful in preventing agitation. Looking for the possible meaning of the behaviour gives clues to interventions. Removal of clothing may indicate a need for toileting. Respond to kicking and biting by removing as much stimuli as possible, including other people in the environment. If the person is agitated at bath time, the nurse should leave and return when the patient is less agitated. The same advice is true for giving medications. A minimum of physical and chemical restraints should be used.[27]

Using touch

Touch is of great value in caring for confused patients.[32] Even the most demented person, who has lost the ability to understand verbal communication, can recognize the tender healing touch of a compassionate nurse. Elderly people who have been alone or institutionalized may suffer most from lack of physical contact. The nurse who uses touch for comfort, protection, and affection finds this an important part of the care of all elderly.

Maintaining sensory function

The eyes of older people adjust more slowly to changes in light. Bright lights or sunlight may be almost unbearable; therefore, blinds may need to be partially drawn. Many elderly people see poorly in the dark; night lights are used to reduce confusion and to prevent accidents among those who get up during the night. Many older people require glasses or contact lenses. These visual aids must be protected from damage or loss and need to be kept clean for best use.

The major changes that affect the hearing of elderly adults are difficulties with speech discrimination, loss of ability to hear high-pitched tones, and problems with background noises. Nurses should make certain that any hearing aids are functioning correctly and are used when the patient is awake.

Pocket talkers are available for the hearing impaired. When speaking, talk slowly and face the patient with good lighting so the patient can see your face as you talk.

Evaluation

Questions to consider include the following:
1. Has the patient regained or maintained orientation to the surroundings?
2. Can the patient state understanding of treatment regime?

3. Has the patient remained free from injury during hospitalizations?
4. Is the patient able to hear and see well enough to communicate with others?

MUSCULOSKELETAL PROBLEMS

One of the most common problems of secondary ageing is joint and muscle disease (see Box 3-9). *Osteoarthritis, rheumatism, and osteoporosis are prevalent among the elderly.* As joints stiffen and muscle tone decreases, the individual may develop an awkward, halting gait. The ability to rise from a chair or to get in and out of cars or buses becomes difficult. Impaired gait, cardiovascular changes, sensory deficits, and osteoporosis make the elderly susceptible to falls. The factors contributing to falls are listed in Box 3-10. Falls account for 23% of deaths and injuries in people over the age of 65.

Nursing Process
Assessment

Subjective data

Obtain information from the patient about limitations of joint and muscle movement, ability to walk, turn, and go up stairs. Learn about problems the patient has with bathing, dressing, toileting, grooming, eating, and carrying out household tasks.

Objective data

Check patient for muscle tone and strength, joint flexibility, range-of-motion, and gait, and whether the patient uses aids such as a walking stick, walking frame, or crutches.

Nursing analysis

Nursing analyses are determined from assessment of patient data. Possible problems for the person with

---

3-9	Ageing changes of musculoskeletal system

Decreased lean muscle mass
Increased body fat
Decreased muscle strength
Demineralization of bones
Decreased joint mobility

3-10	Factors associated with falls

Intrinsic	**Extrinsic**
Limited mobility	Poor lighting
Decreased vision	Unfamiliar environment
Confused mental state	Loose slippers
Orthostatic hypotension	Cluttered equipment
Decreased ability to maintain equilibrium	and furniture

---

musculoskeletal difficulties may include, but are not limited to, the following:

Problem	**Possible aetiologies**
Mobility, impaired physical	Arthritis, osteoporosis, neuro-muscular diseases, stroke
Self-care deficit	Same as above

Planning: expected patient outcomes

Expected patient outcomes for the person with musculoskeletal problems may include, but are not limited to, the following:
1. Walks in the hall with assistance at least three times daily.
2. Transfers from the bed to the chair with one assistant.
3. Washes own face, hands, and trunk.
4. Feeds oneself after tray is set up.
5. Transfers independently to the bedside commode, using quad cane.
6. Is safe from harm and injury.

Implementation

Assisting with achievement of therapeutic goals

Physiotherapists and occupational therapists are involved early in the hospitalization to arrange a programme of care that maintains as much independence for the patient as possible. Sometimes providing a cane or walking frame and raising a toilet seat are all that are necessary to maintain functional independence. In other cases, devices, such as long-handled spoons and reachers, may help patients to dress and feed themselves.

Interventions to achieve patient outcomes
Promoting mobility

The elderly often have fragile bones and joints from osteoarthritis and osteoporosis. Use caution when working with the person. Do not lift an elderly person under the armpits when assisting to move, stand, walk, or transfer from one surface to another. Support the person's trunk and joints as the person is moved. Transfer and lifting sheets are helpful and may allow one caregiver to move or transfer the patient without additional help.

Active and passive range-of-motion exercises are as important for the elderly person as for the younger adult. Because elders may have more limitations of joint motion, great care must be taken not to move the joint past the point of resistance or pain.

Progressive activity, such as getting the patient out of bed soon after admission, and progressive ambulation are essential aspects of nursing care that help maintain independence and function. The term *dysfunctional syndrome* as applied to the elderly *refers to a loss of function through imposed bedrest and altered nutrition patterns during hospitalization.*[19] This decline occurs despite improved medical health and is attributable to a lack of aggressive measures designed to maintain the person's baseline function.

Prevention of dysfunctional syndrome includes early

ambulation, arrangements for independence in toileting, dining in a central location in a social situation, and encouraging independence in bathing, grooming, and dressing. Fulfilling the goal of functional independence necessitates ingenuity and patience on the part of the nurse. It involves spending more time allowing the elder to do for herself or himself instead of doing it for them. This may require increased staffing.

Preventing orthostatic hypotension

Orthostatic hypotension is a special problem of some elderly that increases the risk of falling. This condition is caused by an inadequate baroreceptor response to sudden changes of position or changes during the digestive process. When the person gets out of bed, rises from a hot bath, or eats a large meal, blood pressure may drop precipitously, causing the patient to become faint and fall.

The nurse should *teach the following measures to prevent orthostatic hypotension:*

1. Sleep with the head of bed elevated 8 to 12 inches.
2. Get up slowly from lying position in three stages: sit up, dangle feet over side of bed, then stand up.
3. Do not bend all the way to the floor or stand up quickly.
4. Postpone grooming activities, such as shaving and bathing, to 1 hour after arising.
5. Wear support hose at night.
6. Get out of a hot bath slowly.
7. Wait for an hour or so after a meal to engage in strenuous activity.
8. Be cautious with position changes 1 hour after taking antihypertensive medications.
9. Use a rocking chair to increase circulation.
10. Avoid the Valsalva manoeuvre.[1]

Evaluation

Questions to consider include the following:
1. Is the patient able to transfer independently?
2. Is the patient walking further each day?
3. Is the patient able to feed self, dress self, bathe self, toilet self?
4. Is joint mobility maintained?
5. Is patient safety maintained?

CARDIOPULMONARY PROBLEMS

One of the most pronounced changes that occurs as a person ages is the decline in pulmonary function. Although the changes in the cardiovascular system are not as dramatic, some differences exist between the older and the younger adult (see Box 3-11).

Nursing Process
Assessment

Subjective data

Seek information from the patient about fatigue, especially with normal routines, breathlessness, palpitations, swollen ankles, need to sleep with several pillows, persistent cough, falls with dizziness, chest pain, confusion, and medication history.

3-11 | **Ageing changes of respiratory and cardiovascular systems**

Respiratory system
Decreased elasticity of lungs and chest wall
Decreased recoil of lungs
Increased residual lung volume
Decreased forced expiratory volume
Decreased oxygen pressure (Po_2) (Po_2 decreases about 4 mm Hg/decade)

Cardiovascular system
Decreased elasticity of blood vessels
Decreased cardiac output
Possible blocking of blood vessels by fatty deposits (atherosclerosis)
Increased peripheral vascular resistance leading to increased blood pressure
Slowed circulation
Decreased efficiency of valves in veins of lower extremities

Objective data

Check the patient's vital signs, orthostatic blood pressure, oedema, use of accessory breathing muscles, condition of legs and feet, capillary refill, temperature of hands and feet, and peripheral pulses.

Nursing analysis

Nursing analyses are determined from assessment of patient data. Possible nursing problems for the person with cardiopulmonary problems may include, but are not limited to, the following:

Problem	Possible aetiologies
Breathing pattern, ineffective	Chronic obstructive pulmonary disease (COPD), sedentary lifestyle, bronchitis, pneumonia
Cardiac output, decreased	Congestive heart failure (CHF), stress
Activity intolerance	Sedentary lifestyle, immobility

Planning: expected patient outcomes

Expected patient outcomes for the person with cardiopulmonary changes may include, but are not limited to, the following:
1. Walks the length of the room without dyspnoea.
2. Maintains normal respiratory rate.
3. Accomplishes own Activities of Daily Living (ADL) with a minimum of fatigue.

Implementation

Interventions to achieve patient outcome
Decreasing fatigue

The primary focus of the nurse in caring for the patient with an ineffective breathing pattern or activity intolerance is coping with the residual effects of fatigue. Energy-saving techniques are valuable for the patient who becomes breathless with exertion or who has chronic fatigue.

1. Sit rather than stand for grooming or household chores.
2. Take frequent rest periods between activities.
3. Avoid extremes of temperature.
4. Wear loose clothing and use long-handled reachers.
5. Have friends or family help with household chores.
6. Plan meals in advance and organize cooking activities.
7. Sit down while preparing meals.
8. Practise relaxation exercises.
9. Remove self from stressful situations.

Facilitating learning

Smoking and exposure to secondary passive smoke are the biggest risk factors in developing pulmonary disease at any age. The nurse can promote a smoke-free environment by encourageing smokers to stop smoking and referring them to smoking cessation programmes. Even the elderly patient can enjoy improved health with the cessation of smoking.[17]

The nurse should teach the patient to report any unusual signs or symptoms. Cardiopulmonary disease often has an atypical presentation in the elderly. Therefore symptoms that seem insignificant may indicate a serious problem. Some *symptoms to watch for are chronic indigestion, heartburn, confusion, tingling or numbness in the extremities, shortness of breath, and oedema not alleviated by elevating the feet.* Frequent blood pressure checks are important. Other tips are to avoid tight garters and crossing legs and to engage in a suitable exercise programme (see primary prevention on p. 30).

Medications should be reviewed frequently, because the elderly are more prone to side effects and drug interactions, especially when taking heart medications.

Evaluation

Questions to consider include the following:
1. Can the patient walk a prescribed distance without dyspnoea?
2. Is normal respiratory rate maintained?
3. Can ADL be accomplished successfully with a minimum of fatigue?

GASTROINTESTINAL PROBLEMS

The changes in the gastrointestinal system can affect the mouth, teeth, and gums; the oesophagus and stomach; and the large and small intestines (see Box 3-12).

Nursing Process
Assessment
Subjective data

Inquire about the patient's appetite, dysphagia, choking, condition of teeth and gums, types of foods and liquids taken, symptoms following meals, problems with constipation, indigestion, and bowel habits.

3-12	Ageing changes of gastrointestinal systems	
	Decreased motility	Decreased salivation
	Decreased enzymal activity	Decreased taste
	Atrophied musculature	Decreased sphincter tone
	Decreased absorption	Decreased metabolism

Objective data

Assess the condition of the patient's mouth and mucous membranes, presence of gag reflex, and chewing and swallowing ability. Perform an abdominal assessment.

Nursing analysis

Nursing analyses are determined from assessment of patient data. Possible nursing problems for the patient with gastrointestinal problems may include, but are not limited to, the following:

Planning: expected patient outcomes

Expected patient outcomes for the patient with gastrointestinal problems may include, but are not limited to, the following:
1. Maintains/regains weight.
2. States satisfaction with diet.
3. Has normal bowel movements and patterns.

Implementation
Interventions to achieve patient outcomes
Maintaining/regaining weight

For the person who tends to choke, check the fit of dentures, suggest slower eating with smaller bites, and alternating liquids with solids.

If the patient has a poor appetite, determine high-protein, high-calorie foods that appeal to him or her; offer small frequent meals. People with a hiatal hernia and/or oesophageal reflux can be helped by avoiding cold liquids, sitting up for 1 to 2 hours after meals, and taking small doses of antacids and H_2 antagonists such as cimetidine or ranitidine. Teach the patient to keep the head raised during sleep by elevating the head of the bed on 3-inch blocks.[6]

Preventing aspiration

To prevent aspiration in a patient with decreased sensation in the mouth and throat, try giving soft foods such as custard, gelatin, and apple sauce rather than liquids. Give small bites and wait between mouthfuls. Ask the patient to keep the head bent forward. Put the utensil in the patient's hand, giving verbal directions, to promote independence. If patient needs help, sit beside him or her and tell him/her each food that will be fed.[17]

Promoting alternative feeding methods

For patients who are unable to chew or swallow, two main feeding alternatives are available. The easiest and least complicated is the percutaneous enterostomal gastrostomy (PEG) (see Chapter 23). Under local anaesthesia, a small tube is placed directly into the stomach through the abdominal wall and stitched in place. After 24 hours, the tube is used to give enriched formula feedings either continuously or in several bolus feedings. Another alternative is a nasogastric tube placed through the nose into the stomach through which feedings can be given. Patients must be observed closely for the possibility of aspiration, the head is kept elevated during feeding, and small amounts are given at first to test tolerance. One complication of tube feedings is diarrhoea. This can be managed by slowing down the feeding and giving high-fibre formulas. The dietitian or nutritionist can be consulted about the type of tube feeding.[6]

Relieving constipation

A very wide range of constipation remedies exist, and a large number of elderly people use laxatives regularly. In many cases, the use of laxatives may contribute to constipation. Laxatives hinder the absorption of vitamins and may upset the patient's electrolyte balance.

Teaching should focus on developing or maintaining normal habits. Because of decreased sphincter control, removing laxatives from the patient's routine may be difficult, but normal patterns can be resumed with use of stool softeners and bulk-forming agents, such as ispaghula. Patients should be advised to use natural substances to aid elimination, such as prunes and prune juice. Adding bran to cereal or other foods is sometimes helpful. The elderly often neglect to drink enough fluids for fear of incontinence or because limited mobility creates problems getting to the toilet. Sometimes by merely increasing the intake of water, the person can relieve constipation.

When trying to regain normal bowel habits, the patient should go to the bathroom after breakfast and other meals to take advantage of the gastrocolic reflex. Sometimes using a glycerin suppository may stimulate the bowels. The elderly people should be encouraged to keep trying to regain normal habits; sometimes the process takes several weeks, after years of laxative use. Use enemas only as a last resort. If the stool is very hard and impacted, use an oil retention enema before the cleansing enema to soften the stool. Use greater caution when giving cleansing enemas to the elderly than to younger adults. The rectal mucosa may be very friable and easily traumatized. The elderly are much more prone to electrolyte imbalances and can become very weak and hypokalaemic following administration of multiple enemas.

Evaluation

Questions to consider include the following:
1. Is the patient's weight being maintained or increasing?
2. Is the patient stating satisfaction with diet?
3. Are the bowel patterns more normal?
4. Does the patient state satisfaction with amount and frequency of bowel movements?

INTEGUMENTARY PROBLEMS

The primary ageing changes that occur in the integumentary system are the ones most noticeable to the lay person and are commonly associated with "growing old" (see Box 3-13).

The skin changes occur as the basal membrane flattens and epidermal turnover rate diminishes. These changes cause a decrease in the barrier function of the skin, making it more susceptible to irritants and allergens. As the hair follicles decrease and melanocytes become less active, the hair becomes grey and thin. Decreased sweat production and decreased subcutaneous fat lead to altered thermoregulation, making the elderly more prone to hypothermia in the winter and heat exhaustion in the summer. Wrinkling is due to loss of elasticity and decreased subcu-

3-13	**Ageing changes of the integumentary system**
Greying hair	Decreased elasticity of skin
Loss of connective tissue	Loss of subcutaneous fat
Decreased vascularity	
Liver spots	Decreased skin turgor
Senile purpura	Tooth loss
Decreased seborrhoeic secretions	Malodorous breath
Seborrhoeic keratoses	Receding gums
Decreased venous circulation	Hardened nails
	Corns, calluses

taneous fat. Fingernails and toenails become brittle and thick, with many deformities resulting from trauma and circulatory impairment.[17]

Nursing Process
Assessment
Subjective data

Obtain information from the patient about dry skin, pruritus, skin and nail infections, tooth loss and decay, gum disease, bathing patterns, use of emollients, skin-care habits, mouth-care habits, and foot problems.

Objective data

Assess the patient for dryness of skin, skin turgor (test over sternum, not on forearm), rashes and skin lesions, condition of hair, nails, gums, and mouth, and capillary refill.

Nursing analysis

Nursing analyses are determined from assesment of patient data. Possible nursing problems for the person with integumentary system problems may include, but are not limited to, the following:

Problem	Possible aetiologies
Skin integrity, impaired	Dehydration, immobility, shearing, poor venous circulation, incontinence
Oral mucous membranes, altered	Gingivitis, stomatitis, tooth loss

Planning: expected patient outcomes

Expected patient outcomes for the person with integumentary problems may include, but are not limited to, the following:

1. Skin and mucous membranes remain intact.
2. No signs of infection are present.
3. Feet remain healthy.

Implementation
Interventions to achieve patient outcomes
Maintaining skin integrity

Dryness and itching. The elderly are especially prone to very dry, itching skin, called "senile pruritus." The best treatment is frequent use of creams and emollients. Elderly people do not need daily baths, but they should include more sponge baths in their routine and decrease the use of soap. Liquid cleansers made for sensitive skin are often recommended in place of soap. Hot showers or baths should be avoided, and skin should be patted instead of rubbed dry. Perfumed creams and perfumes containing alcohol can be drying and irritating to already compromised skin texture.

Skin tumours. Both benign and malignant skin tumours are common in the elderly, especially those individuals who have prolonged exposure to the sun. Elderly people should be advised to see a doctor if they have any changes in their skin, especially changes in moles or pigmented areas. The major concern is that a skin lesion might be a *malignant melanoma*. If found early these tumours can be removed with no further complications. Teaching should include daily inspection of skin, wearing protective clothing for work or leisure activities out-of-doors, and avoiding exposure to the ultraviolet rays of the sun. When out in the sun, the elderly should wear a sunscreen lotion with a skin protection factor of at least 15.

Preventing pressure sores and shearing lesions

Elderly patients who are bed bound for all or part of the day are especially susceptible to *pressure sores* and *shearing lesions*. Pressure sores are ischaemic areas of breakdown that occur when fragile tissue is compressed between a bony prominence (sacrum, heels, scapulae) and a firm surface such as a mattress or a chair. Shearing lesions arise from loss of outer layers of skin, resulting from friction when a person is moved or turned in bed. Treatment of deep pressure sores can cost thousands of pounds. Nurses can help prevent this serious complication.

Prevention requires meticulous attention to relief of pressure through turning schedules and pressure-reducing devices. Maintaining clear, dry skin, adequate hydration (up to 2400 ml/day) and supplemental nutrition for the malnourished is equally critical to prevention of pressure sores.

Promoting proper foot care

Elderly people have more corns, calluses, bunions, hammer toes, and horny toenails than younger people. They are taught to wear protective footwear, clean and inspect feet daily, and guard against frostbite and burns. For difficult toenails or other foot problems, a chiropodist should be consulted. Diabetic patients should never cut their own toenails but should have a professional attend to foot care.[24]

Preventing intravenous therapy injury

Elderly people create special problems for the phlebotomist and intravenous therapist. Their veins are fragile and inelastic, making it difficult to enlarge them with a tourniquet. Haematomas form quickly. Sometimes anatomic markings are not in the usual places. When choosing a vein, use the network on the back of the forearm, the cephalic vein on the thumb side of the hand, and the basilar vein on the posterior arm.[10]

Select as small a cannula as possible, protect the skin with proper skin preparation, and use the indirect method of entering the vein. Maintain traction on the skin during insertion. Always remove the needle gently so as not to damage the vein.[10]

Maintaining mucous membranes and dental health

Tooth decay is not a serious problem among the elderly; they are much more afflicted by peridontal disease. Peridontal disease is responsible for most tooth loss after age 35.[2] Gingivitis (gum disease) and periodontitis (bone disease) occur when plaque develops in gum crevices, then the bacterial growth causes receding gums and invasion of the bone.[17]

For sore receding gums, broken teeth, ill-fitting dentures, or malodorous breath, the nurse should refer the patient to a dentist or oral health clinic. Other helpful measures include:

1. Frequent mouth care for patients who are using oxygen, are taking nothing by mouth, or are immunosuppressed.
2. Use of emollients to lips and nares for patients who are using oxygen or nasogastric tubes.
3. Frequent suctioning of secretions for those who cannot handle secretions themselves.
4. Treatment of yeast (thrush) infections.

Evaluation
Questions to consider include the following:
1. Is skin integrity maintained?
2. Are there any signs of infection or pressure sores?
3. Is skin on the feet intact?
4. Are the mucous membranes intact?
5. Does the patient have access to regular dental care?

URINARY PROBLEMS

Although ageing leads to decreased kidney function, most elderly can maintain normal voiding. Incontinence is always a result of pathological process and not of primary ageing, (see Box 3-14).

Nursing Process
Assessment
Subjective data

Obtain information from the patient about usual urinary patterns, any changes in habits, pain, hesitancy, burning, urgency, and loss of control. If incontinence exists, assess amount, frequency, type of management, and loss of control with sneezing, coughing, or movement.

3-14	**Ageing changes of urinary system** Reduced renal blood flow Decreased glomerular filtration rate Decreased bladder muscle tone

Objective data

Observe the patient's urine for colour, consistency, amount, and presence of blood. If cloudy, or if sediment is present, send urine for culture and sensitivity.

Nursing analysis

Nursing analyses are determined from assessment of patient data. Possible nursing problems for the person with urinary problems may include, but are not limited to, the following:

Problem	Possible aetiologies
Incontinence, functional	Altered environment, sensory, cognitive, or mobility deficits

Planning: expected patient outcomes

Expected patient outcomes for the person with urinary elimination problems may include, but are not limited to, the following:
1. Increased time between voidings.
2. Decreased number of incontinent episodes.

Implementation
Interventions to achieve patient outcomes
Minimizing functional incontinence

Elderly people are especially susceptible to functional incontinence. Factors affecting this condition are urinary infections, inability to get to the bathroom, and altered fluid intake caused by illness and hospitalization. Use of restraints and attachment of multiple tubes often hinder the ability of the person to accomplish independent toileting. The presence of cognitive impairment and limited mobility complicates the situation.

The nurse can assist the patient getting to the bathroom independently through modification of the environment. This may involve moving furniture and equipment to clear a path to the bathroom or arranging for a bedside commode to be placed near enough to the patient's bed for easy use. Sometimes providing a cane or walking frame is all that is necessary, as well as giving the patient some privacy. If special equipment presents a hindrance, the nurse can teach the patient how to manipulate intravenous tubing or machinery or urge the patient to call for assistance.

It is important for the nurse to remember that incontinence is embarrassing and shameful for the patient. The patient should be treated in a kind, unflustered manner, never scolded, and helped to avoid future incidents. The nurse may tell the patient that urinary control in the hospital is much more difficult where the surroundings are unfamiliar and assure the patient that when he or she returns home, continence may be regained or improved.

Continuous intravenous fluids, having nothing orally because of diagnostic studies, and altered eating schedules may interfere with voiding patterns. Whenever possible, fluids should be encouraged, up to 2 L/day, with the bulk of the liquids given between 8 AM and 7 PM. Limiting the fluids at night helps prevent incontinent episodes during sleeping hours. If the patient is restrained or hindered by intravenous or other tubings, he or she should be offered opportunities to void before and after meals and at bedtime. Urinary tract infections are common and should be treated with the appropriate antibiotics.

Some elderly men can only void when standing. Others may have urinary frequency and hesitancy because of an enlarged prostate, which is common in older men. Assistance should be provided as necessary to handle these difficult problems. Maintaining as much independence as possible is important in keeping the elderly person from losing functional capacity.

Promoting urinary elimination

Foley catheters may be placed in some patients to monitor and accurately record urinary output. After the catheter is removed, the elderly patient may have trouble regaining bladder control, especially if mild incontinence was present previously.

The best approach for urinary retention following catheter removal is to do a straight catheterization every 6 to 8 hours until the person is able to void voluntarily. This is much preferable to reinserting the indwelling catheter. For the person who is incontinent, teaching Kegel strengthening exercises may help tone the pelvic floor muscles. The patient should be reassured that most incontinence ceases after a routine of fluids and voiding has been re-established.

For any elderly person who has problems with incontinence, it is important for the nurse to determine what type of incontinence is present. In many cases, stress and urge incontinence are exaggerated by functional incontinence. *Urinary incontinence is never a normal part of ageing.* The nurse may be the first person to discover the patient's problem, and referrals for incontinence studies can be a vital part of the nursing care.

Evaluation

Questions to consider include the following:
1. Have the number of incontinent episodes decreased?
2. Is the patient able to toilet independently?
3. Does the patient state that control of incontinent episodes is to his or her satisfaction?

OTHER PHYSIOLOGICAL PROBLEMS

DEHYDRATION

Dehydration is a common problem among the elderly and is a frequent cause of admission to the hospital.

Nursing Process
Assessment

Subjective data

Seek information from the patient about usual fluid intake, types of fluids preferred, thirst, ability to handle fluid containers, swallowing ability, usual pattern of consumption, changes in intake related to illness, and medications that affect intake and output (diuretics, laxatives).

Objective data

Assess the patient for skin turgor, texture, fragility, and temperature; condition of mucous membranes; weakness, and orientation.

Nursing analysis

Nursing analyses are determined from assessment of patient data. Possible problems for the patient with dehydration may include, but are not limited to, the following:

Problem	Possible aetiologies
Fluid volume deficit or Fluid volume deficit, high risk for	Dysphagia, congestive heart failure, medications, dementia, depression, stroke, hypertension, use of diuretics, inability to obtain fluids, fear of incontinence, fever, diarrhoea, renal, failure

Planning: expected patient outcomes

Expected patient outcomes for the person with dehydration may include, but are not limited to, the following:
1. Takes 2000 ml of fluid in 24 hours.
2. Intake is greater than output for 48 hours.
3. Skin and mucous membranes are intact and moist.
4. Urine is light amber colour and is clear.

Implementation

Interventions to achieve patient outcomes

Promoting hydration

The nurse can take several steps to promote hydration: encourage fluid intake of 7 to 8 glasses a day; offer a variety of fluids, especially juices; weigh the patient daily; keep accurate intake and output records; and provide cups and jugs that the people can handle.

Facilitating learning

Instruct the patient in the importance of maintaining adequate fluid intake. Teach which fluids are best: soups and fruit juices may have high sodium content; milk increases phlegm; alcohol depresses the CNS; coffee, tea, and colas contain caffeine, which is a stimulant; soft drinks and gelatins are high in sugar.[18]

Evaluation

Questions to consider include the following:
1. Is the volume of fluids adequate?
2. Is the intake greater than the output?
3. Are skin and mucous membranes moist, pink, and intact?
4. What are the colour and consistency of urine?

PAIN

Nursing Process
Assessment

Assessment of pain in the elderly person is more complex than in the younger adult. Pain may appear in atypical forms. Conditions that normally cause pain in young people may not do so in the elderly.

The nurse assesses for location, quality, intensity, onset, duration, and physical manifestations of pain in the same manner as for any patient. In addition, the nurse must attend to the impact of pain on activities of daily living, gait, and behaviour.

Factors that affect pain in the elderly are different than those affecting younger people. Impaired vision and hearing, problems expressing oneself, ability to concentrate, and cognitive changes may interfere with assessment. More attention must be paid to nonverbal expressions, as well as soliciting comments from family members.[14]

The belief system of the elderly person affects his or her expression of pain. Some believe that pain is a normal part of the ageing process and must be endured stoically. If the person fears loss of autonomy, she or he may deny having pain. A fear of serious illness may lead to denial of pain. Some ethnic groups believe showing pain is not acceptable, whereas others may be more vocal when they experience pain.

An atypical presentation of pain is much more common in the elderly. For example, one half of patients with myocardial infarctions have no pain. Diseases usually associated with severe pain, such as peptic ulcer, appendicitis, and pneumonia, may only provoke mild pain in older people. Some abdominal emergencies present as chest pain at first. Depression masks pain and pain may be difficult to assess, especially if the patient is also cognitively impaired.

Taking all these factors into consideration, the nurse must establish rapport with the elderly person by taking plenty of time and phrasing questions in several different ways. For the aphasic patient, a pain chart with a drawing of a body to which the patient may point may be helpful. Patients may be asked to rate their pain using a pain scale numbered 1 to 10, with 10 being the most severe pain ever felt and 1 for the least severe pain (see Chapter 8 for more information). Showing concern for the patient and his or her suffering rather than dismissing the pain as "part of growing old" assists immeasurably in gathering accurate data.

Nursing analysis

Nursing analyses are determined from assessment of patient data. Possible nursing problems for the person with pain may include, but are not limited to, the following:

Problem	Possible aetiologies
Pain	Pathophysiological changes, trauma/diagnos-tic tests, immobility, improper positioning, disability

Planning: expected patient outcomes

Expected patient outcomes for the person with pain may include, but are not limited to, the following:

1. States pain is decreased.
2. Exhibits fewer nonverbal signs of pain.
3. Is more independent in ADL.

Implementation

Interventions to achieve patient outcomes
Alleviating/minimizing pain

Problem	Possible aetiologies
Nutrition, less than body requirements	Poorly fitting dentures, tooth loss, lack of sensation, hiatal hernia, loss of taste or smell, anorexia
Constipation	Lack of muscle tone, reliance on use of laxatives/enemas, lack of bulk in diet, low fluid intake

In the care of the elderly, the nurse should consider a variety of modifications in managing pain that differ from those used with the younger adult. Elderly people are more prone to mild arthritis and fibrositis. The incidence of osteoporosis, especially involving the spine and femur, is very high in elderly women. Great care must be taken to protect the joints, back, and shoulders when transferring, moving, and turning. Where one nurse could handle a younger adult, two people may be needed to move the older patient in bed or to help him or her walk.

Protective adipose tissue under the skin disappears with age, and the volume of circulating blood, particularly to the small outer arteries, may be diminished. This affects the ability to withstand cold without discomfort. Several layers of light-weight clothing are warmer than fewer heavy layers when the person is cold. Many elderly people wish to wear socks and additional clothing in bed. Provision must be made to prevent drafts in the room while maintaining good air circulation.

Elderly patients may tolerate smaller doses of pain medications than younger adults (see secondary prevention, p. 53). *Bizarre reactions to pain medications may occur, such as hallucinations, delirium, aggravated pain, and agitation.* Great caution should be used in starting and/or changing dosages of narcotics to prevent reactions and interactions. The nonsteroidal antiinflammatory medications are used for treating pain from arthritis and neuralgias. These drugs create fewer side effects, and elderly patients tolerate them better (see Chapter 32 for more information about these medications).

Evaluation

Questions to consider include the following:

1. Does the patient show less evidence of pain?
2. Does the patient rate pain between 2 and 3?
3. Is the patient able to do ADL more independently?

SPECIAL CONSIDERATIONS

SLEEP PATTERN DISTURBANCE

Elderly people have less Stage 4 (deep) sleep and more periods of wakefulness than younger adults. Rapid eye movement (REM) sleep is often interrupted, causing sleepiness and a pattern of napping throughout the day. The nurse should recognize that elderly people do not necessarily need more sleep than younger adults, but that the sleep is obtained in shorter periods throughout the day rather than just at night.

A variety of measures are helpful for sleeplessness. A glass of warm milk at bedtime and a soothing back rub, as well as following usual nighttime routines, help prepare the patient for sleep. Keep a low nightlight on, lower the bed, and provide adequate supervision at night to prevent accidents. If the person is likely to get up for toileting, place a bedside commode next to the bed and teach the person how to use it safely. A short-acting hypnotic may be given for a few days, although with care because daytime drowsiness, confusion and ataxia may occur.

DIAGNOSTIC TESTS

Diagnostic tests should be judiciously spaced to prevent overtaxing the elderly individual. Routine preparations for tests may need to be modified to prevent exhaustion or dehydration. Elderly people may become weak or dizzy from test preparations such as multiple enemas or the withholding of food. Do not leave weak patients unattended on a treatment table. Advise people who are dizzy to sit up slowly and to remain sitting on the edge of the table for a few moments before standing. The dizziness is caused by the slow compensation of inelastic blood vessels.

Place pads under the normal curves of the back and under bony prominences in elderly patients who must lie on treatment or operating room tables for lengthy periods because they develop pressure sores rapidly. If the patient is placed in the lithotomy position, place both legs in (and remove both from) the stirrups at the same time to prevent pull on unresilient muscles.

ANAESTHESIA AND SURGERY

For the patient who is undergoing surgery, age in itself is not a risk factor. The risk factors for the elderly are the presence and severity of any underlying disease, such as congestive heart failure, renal disease, ischaemic heart problems, or chronic obstructive lung disease.[11] The surgeon and anaesthetist study the patient carefully to determine how much risk is involved. Their recommendations are made according to the type of surgery and concerns about cardiopulmonary function.

During the preoperative period, the nurse assists the patient in restoring fluids that have been lost through dehydration, bowel disease, or blood loss. In addition, the nurse provides basic preoperative teaching. Teaching is particularly important for an elderly person with cognitive deficits and who may need extra time and patience to understand the procedures that have been planned. Family members may be concerned that the person's age makes him or her a poor risk. They need careful detailed explanations of the surgery and the intraoperative procedures.

When choosing anaesthesia for the elderly, the anaesthetist is most likely to use a regional anaesthetic. If general anaesthesia is necessary, then shorter-acting anaesthetic agents are best. With underlying cardiopulmonary disease, the risks are greater for aspiration, shock, pulmonary oedema, and myocardial infarction.[11]

Postoperatively the elderly are more prone to confusion and sleepiness. Other problems are *hypothermia, respiratory depression, fluctuations in blood pressure, and renal failure.*

Postoperative nursing care focuses careful attention to vital signs, being alert to early signs of shock or hypertension. Warm blankets are even more important for the elderly than for the younger adult. Monitor urinary output, BUN, and creatinine carefully. The people who is confused may require frequent reorientation and repetition of instructions. Having a familiar family member at the bedside helps the elderly patient who is frightened and confused. Although they should be used as little as possible, restraints may be necessary in the early postoperative period to keep the person from tugging at intravenous lines, nasogastric tubes, and oxygen tubes. Attendance by a significant other may eliminate the need for restraints.

The postoperative course may be longer for the elderly patient. As the functional reserve capacity is decreased, the individual may be more susceptible to urinary and pulmonary infections. Return to baseline function requires more effort on the part of both the nurse and the patient. If the patient is discharged while still below his or her normal function level, relatives or home nursing services will be needed to meet the patient's needs until full recuperation is accomplished.

DIABETES

Elderly people are more susceptible to abnormalities in glucoregulation than are younger people. In the elderly, the presenting signs are not an elevated blood sugar but microvascular changes that go undetected until signs and symptoms of complications, such as neuropathy, nephropathy, or retinopathy, occur. The fasting blood sugar may be normal; a glucose-tolerance test is needed for a definite diagnosis. Factors that lead to a decline in glucose tolerance in the elderly are obesity, deconditioning, decreased muscle mass, poor diet, coexisting diseases, and medications.[11]

The diagnosis is often made when the patient is under care for some other condition such as an infection, workup for surgery, or other complicating illness. Noninsulin-dependent diabetes is seen most often in obese patients over 50 years of age who have had significant glucose intolerance for several years before being detected.

The goal of medicine is not vigorous treatment of the hyperglycaemia but rather adequate control in the hope of minimizing organ complications. About half of elderly diabetics need sulphonylurea drugs and fewer than half require insulin.[11] The nurse teaches the patient the significance of weight loss (80% of elderly diabetics are overweight), aerobic exercise, and good foot and skin care. See Chapter 20 for more information about diabetes.

PSYCHOSOCIAL CHANGES
General Care

In dealing with psychosocial changes the nurse assesses the physiological changes, the diseases present, and the person's emotional makeup and apparent adjustment to the particular situation. Older people frequently talk at length about their families and the past; their conversations may give clues to interests that should be encouraged and to problems confronting them. Plans should be made to help them maintain as much independence as possible despite their limitations. Community resources are available to assist older people maintain independence and meet their social needs (see Box 3-15).

Elderly patients are often lonely and appreciate just talking with others. Volunteers may provide a service by visiting with the elderly. Many patients appreciate visits with a member of the clergy. When visiting with elderly people, it should be remembered that, although they commonly talk about events and activities in their own past, they usually are interested in the activities of younger people and of the world around them.

The need to be useful is important to all patients. There are many tasks in which even the elderly person who is ill may be able to participate. At home, the elderly may be able to help with the dishes or with meal preparation. They may be interested in crafts or making useful items. The older person may be quite slow, and great care must be taken not to show impatience, which may discourage further participation.

Depression is not uncommon in the elderly, and the elderly may be suicidal. Nurses need to be alert to signs of depression and thoughts of suicide, especially in older people who are lonely and may not have a social support system. Box 3-16 describes a recent study of suicide in the elderly and makes several recommendations of which nurses should be aware.

3-16

Nursing Research

Frierson R: Suicide attempts by the old and very old, *Arch Intern Med* 151(1):141–144, 1991.

A study of suicide attempts was made among 95 elderly patients in the U.S. (age 60 to 90) and evaluated by a consult service after a suicide attempt. The subjects differed significantly when compared with younger age groups who attempted suicide, but the younger age groups were similar to the elderly who successfully committed suicide. Recommendations are increased detection and treatment of depression and alcoholism, early psychiatric referral, limited access to firearms, and strategies to decrease social isolation.

3-15	Community Support services for older people	
	Senior citizen centres	Social, nutritional, educational, and counselling services
	Geriatric day care centres	Assistive daytime nursing care, and social, nutritional, and rehabilitative services may be available
	Nursing homes	Care in private home for the older person who is unable to live alone
	Meals on Wheels	Meals delivered to the person's home
	Home help services	Household chores, shopping, and so on
	Transportation service	Arranged pickup by public transportation system
	District nursing service	Skilled home nursing care
	Legal services	Will, settlement of estate
	Respite care	Short-term care to support primary carer, provided by hospitals, extended care facilities, or community nursing service
	Counselling services	Private governmental, public services for patient and carers
	Support groups	Private, nonprofit groups related to specific diagnosis
	Rehabilitation services	Physiotherapy and occupational therapy in home or hospital

Elderly people are usually aware of death as an imminent possibility and sometimes see it as a welcome event. The issue should not be avoided. If the patient shows genuine concern about impending death, the nurse can encourage discussion of feelings (Chapter 11). The family may also need opportunities to discuss their feelings about death.

Discharge Planning

Following hospitalization the younger adult most frequently returns home to an independent lifestyle, whereas the older adult must be evaluated for ability and resources to manage at home. Some of the factors to consider are:

1. Has patient been functioning independently before hospitalization?
2. If patient is independent, has function returned to baseline?
3. Are appropriate care or support people at home?
4. Are other dependent disabled people in the home?
5. What is the health of the primary care?
6. How capable are the carers emotionally, physically, mentally?
7. What financial resources are available for home care, such as supplies and equipment?

The patient who has declining function and requires increasing amounts of assistance with activities of daily living usually has three choices for discharge placement:

1. Home, with family care
2. Home with family and/or professional nursing services or other assistance
3. Nursing home or extended care facility

The nurse often becomes the coordinator for the discharge planning for the elderly patient who needs assistance after discharge. For the patient returning home, the nurse must ensure that the patient understands the transfer techniques taught by the physiotherapist, physical care, use of special equipment, and knowledge of medications. If the patient needs home nursing services, the nurse makes the appropriate referral, listing all the patient's needs. Social work services are necessary for the patient who must be transferred to an extended care facility or needs financial assistance.

In the case of the patient who may need institutional care, the nurse has a key role. First, the patient's functional abilities must be delineated thoroughly to determine if placement is really necessary. Then the nurse and social worker help the family choose the appropriate facility by giving them a list of available places and teaching them how to evaluate each one. This is frequently a difficult task for family members, who may feel guilty about removing the patient from the home. The nurse gives emotional support during the decision-making process to both the family and the patient, who may view the decision negatively because he or she is losing autonomy.

The nurse may be caught in a controversy between the patient's wishes to return home and the wishes of the family and doctor to institutionalize the patient. It is not unusual for the patient to deny the amount of care needed. In such a situation, ethical principles must be carefully considered.

Patient autonomy may need to be weighed against the greatest good for the greatest number (the family). The process involves listing alternatives, predicting consequences, and selecting the solution based on those consequences. For example, a positive consequence results if a patient with declining physical function is returned home. However, harm could occur from a fall, and continued physical decline might result (negative consequence). Therefore the protected environment of the nursing home would be a positive consequence, and the family would be relieved from the burden of care.[15]

Each case must be decided individually with as much input from all parties as possible. The nurse is obligated to support the process and the chosen solution, no matter what her or his peopleal values. In many cases the options are limited, and the solution brings sadness to all involved.

Terminating Treatment

The nurse is frequently involved in decisions about initiating or withholding treatments for the elderly person who is terminally ill. No simple legislated answers exist to the questions, "Who should have treatment?" or "Is withholding fluids and food a form of passive euthanasia?" Some countries have legal provision for a *living will*, but even this document does not guarantee that the patient's wishes will be followed in the event he or she is incompetent or unable to make known his or her desires.

Some experts recommend that *a durable power of attorney for health care* be obtained while the person is mentally competent. Then when the patient becomes ill or incapacitated, the person with the durable power of attorney can act on the patient's behalf and assure that the patient's wishes are carried out.

When a patient has no living will or durable power of attorney, the health team must consider the following factors when making decisions regarding withholding of treatments:

1. Did the patient express any wishes when competent?
2. What are the wishes of the family?
3. Does the giving of treatment represent a disproportionate burden to others?
4. What is the quality of life for the individual?[15]

The nurse can act as advocate for the patient by interviewing family members, supporting the decision-making process, and encouraging the parties involved to make the decisions without haste. Wishes the patient expresses while competent should be carefully documented in the patient's record.

Living Wills

In September, 1992, the Terrence Higgins Trust and the Centre of Medical Law and Ethics at Kings College, London, published a form for a living will, which enables patients to appoint a health care proxy to make medical decisions if the patient is permanently unconscious or mentally incapacitated, and to name the person who should be contacted if death is imminent.[17a] In the United States, many states have passed laws giving such documents legal authority. In addition, the Patient Self-Determination Act, a US federal law instituted in 1990, requires hospitals admitting patients to inform the patient of his or her right to make an advance directive.

In Britain, living wills currently have no legislatire backing and their effects have yet to be tested in the courts. However, in a case concerning administration of a blood transfusion to a Jehovah's Witness, Lord Donaldson, Master of the Rolls, ruled that a form could be used to register a valid refusal, provided the patient understood its significance.[5a] In this case, the court made it clear that any refusal to consent to life-saving treatment could be considered legally binding only if the following four criteria are met:

1. The patient is capable of making the decision (is not mentally impaired and is free from the influence of drug treatment)
2. The patient's will has not been overborne by the influence of a third party
3. The patient understands the nature and effect of the treatment which he or she is refusing or consenting to
4. The refusal of treatment covers the actual situation in which the treatment is needed.[17a]

Although the form is designed for people with HIV infection or AIDS, it is also suitable for general use. It provides for choices about medical treatment in the event of a terminal illness, permanent severe mental impairment with physical illness, or permanent unconsciousness.

The Voluntary Euthanasia Society (formerly Exit) is supporting a private member's bill aimed at giving legal force to living wills.

THE RIGHTS OF OLDER PEOPLE

The RCN's Association for the Care of Elderly People (ACE), and Focus on Older People, Nursing and Mental health (FOCUS) 42 belive that older people should:

- Have equal rights and responsibilities to all other citit zens.
- Have equal access to health care.
- Receive regular, skilled and comprehensive assesment of their health needs, including mental health.
- Receive care tailored to their individual needs.
- Be able to make decisions about the kinds of care they recive.
- Recive a high standard of care.
- Be able to maitain their dignity and independance of choice
- Be able to choose where they want to be cared for — whether in their own home or in a residential nursing home.
- Be cared for in a homely enviroment, wherever it may be
- Have easy access to a general practitioner and to the full range of mult-professional health and social suport whether they are in residential care or living in their own homes.

SUMMARY

1. People in late adulthood focus on life accomplishments and look toward life's end, while maintaining autonomy and dignity.
2. Elderly adults often have more than one chronic illness, with the incidence increasing with age.

3. Nursing care must be tailored according to the specific physical, psychological, sexual, and social effects of any disease or illness on the individual.
4. Nurses need to be cognizant of the differences between primary and secondary ageing changes in elderly.
5. Nursing care should be predicated on the belief that late adulthood is a time of diversity, richness, and increasing complexity.
6. Health promotion is as important for older age groups as for younger people in maintaining a high quality of life.
7. The strengths of the older person should be given the same consideration as their disabilities when devising health care strategies.
8. Many conditions have the initial symptom of confusion in the elderly.
9. The elderly are more susceptible to falls, but restraints are not an adequate intervention.
10. The elderly are often malnourished because of physiological and social ageing changes.
11. Constipation is a secondary ageing change and can be controlled with diet and habit training.
12. Urinary incontinence is a secondary ageing change. The most common form is functional incontinence.
13. Hearing and vision defects affect the ability of the elderly to communicate adequately.
14. The elderly experience many minor discomforts, but some do not have pain as a typical symptom of disease.
15. Dehydration is diagnosed for many elderly when admitted to the acute-care setting.
16. Helping the elderly with discharge planning is a major nursing role.
17. Supporting decision-making in an ethical context is a challenge for the nurse who works with aged people.
18. The purpose of the Patient Self-Determination Act (PSDA) that went into effect in the United States on December 1, 1991, is to ensure that the patient's wishes about prolongation of life be respected.
19. Geriatric nursing standards provide a context of car for the nurse.

STUDY QUESTIONS

- Talk with and observe people over 65 years of age. How do you and they differ in terms of physical development and major concerns in your lives?
- Review the eating patterns of an elderly person of your acquaintance; compare his or her food intake with your understanding of an adequate diet. If there are inadequacies, what are some possible reasons?
- From what you have read in newspapers and heard discussed, what would you select as major problems of elderly people in your community?
- What services are available for the elderly in your community?
- Compare your grandparents or other elderly relatives with other elderly acquaintances for differentiation in primary and secondary ageing.

REFERENCES AND SELECTED READINGS

1.* Aronson L, Carlson-Wolfe N, and Schoener S: Pressures that fall on rising, *Geriatr Nurs* 12:(2)58-60, 1991.
2.* Berg R, Cassells J: *The second fifty years*, Washington, DC, 1990, NationalAcademy Press.
3.* Blakeslee J, et al: Making the transition to restraint-free care, *J Gerontol Nurs* 17(2):4-8, 1991.
4.* Bosek MSD, Fitzpatrick J: Legally speaking—finding the right words, *RN* 54(11):66-67, 1991.
5. Brower T: Alternatives to restraints, *J Gerontol Nurs* 17(2): 18-20, 1991.
5a. Dyer C: Living will allows choice of medical care, *Br Med J* 305:602–603,
6. Esberger K: Guide to gastrointestinal problems of elders, *Geriatr Nurs* 12(2):74-75, 1991.
7. Gilmore G, Whitehouse P, Wykle M: *Memory, aging, and dementia*, New York, 1987, Springer Publishing.
8. Gray M: Polypharmacy in the elderly, *Orthop Nurs* 9(6):49, 1990.
9. Greve P: Legally speaking—Advance directives—what the new law means to you, *RN* 54(11):63-66, 1991.
10.* Hadaway L: Intravenous tips, *Geriatr Nurs* 12(2):78, 1991.
11. Hazzard W, et al: *Principles of geriatric medicine*, New York, 1990, McGraw-Hill.
12. Heacock P, et al: Caring for the cognitivity impaired, *J Gerontol Nurs* 17(3):22-26, 1991.
13. US Dept of Health and Human Services: *Healthy People 2000: National health promotion and disease preventions: 1991 objectives*, Washington, DC, 1990, US Government Printing Office.
14. Herr K, Mowby P: Pain assessment in the elderly, *J Gerontol Nurs* 17(4):13-19, 1991.
15.* Hogstel M: Safety or autonomy, *J Gerontol Nurs* 17(3): 5-10, 1991.
16. Hussey L: Overcoming the clinical barriers of low literacy and medication noncompliance among elderly, *J Gerontol Nurs* 17(3):27-29, 1991.
17. Kart C, Metress E, Metress S: *Aging, health, and society*, Boston, 1988, Jones & Bartlett Publishers.
17a. Korgaonkar G, Tribe D: Living wills and the law, *Br J Hosp Med* 49(8):576-578, 1993.
18.* Kositzke J: A question of balance: dehydration in the elderly, *J Gerontol Nurs* 16(4):7-9, 1990.
19. Landefeld S, Palmer R, Kresevic D: Dysfunctional syn-drome, *GAS Abstracts*, 1990.
20. Lang N, et al: *Quality of health care for older people in America*, Kansas City, Mo, 1990, American Nurses' Associa-tion.
21. McCaffery M, Beebe A: *Pain: clinical manual for nursing practice*, St. Louis, 1989, Mosby-Yearbook.
22. Melers C: Antibiotics: Old drugs, new information, *Geriatr Nurs* 12(2):61-63, 1991.
23. Newbern V: Beta blockers, *Geriatric Nurs* 12(2):119-121, 1991.
24. Osterman H, Stuck R: The aging foot, *Orthop Nurs* 9(6):43, 1990.
25. Palmore E, et al: *Normal aging III*, Durham, NC, 1985, Duke University Press.
26. Pastorino C, Dickey T: Health promotion for the elderly, *Orthop Nurs* 9(60):36, 1990.
27. Roper J, Shapiro J, Chang B: Agitation in the demented patient, *J Gerontol Nurs* 17(3):17, 1991.
28.* Schilke J: Slowing the aging process with physical activity, *J Gerontol Nurs* 17(6):5-9, 1991.
29. Scura K, Whipple B: Older adults as an HIV positive risk group, *J Gerontol Nurs* 16(1):6-10, 1990.
30. Talashek M, Tichy A, Epping H: Sexually trans-mitted disease in elderly, *J Gerontol Nurs* 16(4):33,1990.
31. Travis S: Older adults' sexuality and remarriage, *J Gerontol Nurs* 13:9, 1987.
32.* Vortherms R: Clinically improving communication through touch, *J Gerontol Nurs* 17(5):6-9, 1991.
33. Birren J, Schale K: *Handbook of the psychology of aging*, New York, 1977, Van Nostrand Reinhold.
34. Boyce M: *Guidelines for printed materials for older adults*, Battle Creek, Mich, 1981, Michigan Health Council.
35. Butler R: *Why survive? Being old in America*, New York, 1975, Harper & Row.

36. Masters W, Johnson V: *Human sexual response,* Boston, 1966, Little, Brown, & Co.

37. Murray R, Zentner J: *Nursing assessment and health promo-tion through the lifespan,* Englewood Cliffs, NJ, 1979, Prentice-Hall.

38. Reed P: Implications of the life-span developmental frame-work for wellbeing in adulthood and aging, *Adv Nurs Sci* 6(1):18-25, 1983.

39. Wolanin MO, Phillips L: *Confusion: Prevention and care,* St Louis, 1981, Mosby-Yearbook.

40. Age Concern: *Older people in the United Kingdom: Some basic facts,* London, 1993.

41. Office of Population Censuses and Surveys: U.K. *National population projections* based on the 1989 population census: 15, 16, 34.

*Recommended for student reading.

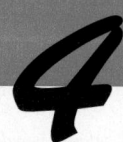

4

Health Promotion: Nutrition and Exercise

Barbara C. Long

After studying this chapter, the learner should be able to:

- Describe factors affecting health-promoting behaviours and approaches to facilitate health promotion.
- Differentiate nutrient standards, food guides, and dietary guidelines in terms of purpose.
- Describe the dietary guidelines recommended by Department of Health and those recommended in the United States
- Differentiate between saturated, monounsaturated, and polyunsaturated fats, and cholesterol in terms of definition and recommendations for health.
- Use the daily food guide to evaluate adequacy of nutrient intake.
- Explain approaches to facilitate weight loss and weight gain.

| | |

Box 4-1

Health Strategies: Areas for action

Coronary Heart Disease (CHD) and Stroke
Diet
Smoking
Hypertension
Lack of exercise
Excess alcohol

Cancer
Smoking
Screening
Sunlight

Mental Illness
Improve services

HIV/AIDS and Sexual Health (great risks)
Sexual health
Family planning

Accidents (often avoidable)
An important cause of morbidity and mortality
in the young and very old

From Secretary of State for Health: *The Health of the Nation: A Strategy for Health in England,* London, HMSO, 1992.

Health promotion and disease prevention have become major aspects of health care in the United Kingdom. During 1992, the Secretary of State for Health presented a paper entitled *The Health of the Nation: A Strategy for Health in England.* The paper identified key areas for action (Box 4-1) during the period up to 2010 and set out a number of targets:

1. A reduction in deaths from coronary heart disease (CHD) and stroke.
2. A reduction in deaths from breast cancer in women invited for screening, and in the incidence of invasive cancer of the cervix.
3. A fall in lung cancer deaths, and prevention of an annual increase in skin cancer.
4. A significant improvement in the health and social functioning of the mentally ill.
5. A reduction in suicide rates, both overall and in people with severe mental illness.
6. A fall in the incidence of gonorrhoea (indicator of HIV/AIDS infection).
7. A reduction in the conception rates in women under 16 years of age.
8. A decline in the number of deaths caused by accidents in several age groups.

Because the goal of nursing is to assist people to achieve optimal health (Chapter 1), nurses are among the leaders of health professionals working towards meeting the national health targets. Recently introduced Project 2000 Diploma courses in nursing have placed new emphasis on health promotion, health teaching, and self-care. Nurses are well prepared as health teachers and health advocates.

Therefore health promotion is one aspect of medical–surgical nursing.

HEALTH PROMOTION IN ADULT NURSING PRACTICE

Health promotion can be defined as activities directed towards helping people maintain or achieve a high level of functioning and wellbeing. Health promotion is an integral part of nursing care for all types of patients and clients in all types of environments of care. In day care centres, health promotion assumes a major focus. In acute care centres the major focus is assisting patients to regain their health (illness care). However, health care must also be considered; that which is healthy must be promoted or maintained.

Health promotion strengthens the person's capacity to withstand physical and emotional stress. Thus the person who is in an excellent nutritional state, has good physical endurance, and copes well with stress, is at less risk of developing a pathophysiological disorder, and has resources to use in regaining optimal functioning more quickly if illness or disease does occur.

Factors Affecting Health-Promoting Behaviours

Why do some people take actions that promote a high level of functioning, whereas others do not? Pender[26] has identified factors that (1) affect the individual's perceptions, (2) modify behaviours, and (3) influence the likelihood of health-promoting actions (Figure 4-1).

Individual perceptions

Motivation to participate in health-promoting behaviours is influenced by the person's perceptions about health and perceptions about self:

1. Perceptions about health
   a. Value placed on health by the person
   b. Desire for the highest achievable health level versus that for maintaining status quo
   c. Evaluation of present health status
   d. Perceived benefits of the health-promoting behaviours
2. Perceptions about self
   a. Perceived control over own behaviour (internal versus external control)
   b. Desire for mastery of the environment
   c. Self-concept
   d. Self-esteem

Thus people who do not value health or see a need to improve their health status, who are not self-motivated, or who have a poor self-concept are less likely to engage in health-promoting behaviours. Nursing approaches in these situations include helping these people identify their values and explore feelings about themselves with emphasis placed on identifying strengths. Helping these people set their own goals (thus exerting internal control) greatly increases the likelihood of achieving desired behaviours.

Modifying factors

Pender[26] has identified categories of modifying factors: demographic (age, sex, ethnicity, education, income),

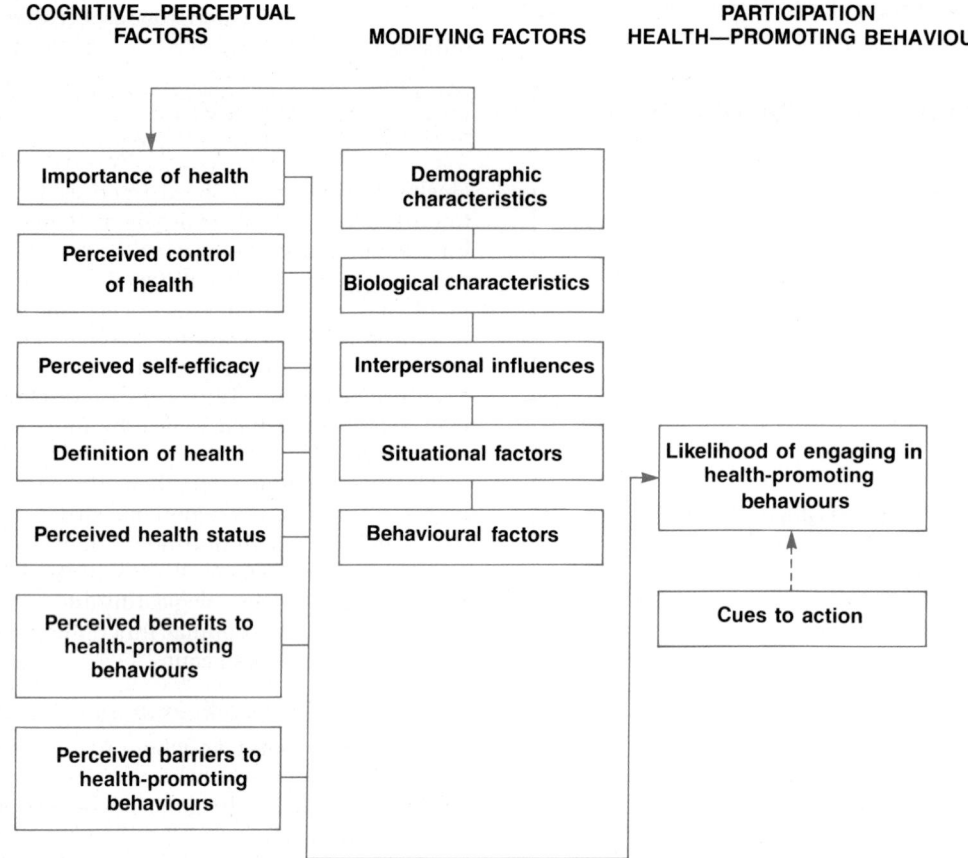

Fig. 4-1   Pender's health promotion model. (From Pender NJ: *Health promotion in nursing practice,* ed 2, East Norwalk, Ct, 1987, Appleton & Lange.)

biological, interpersonal, situational, and behavioural variables. The specific effect of demographic variables on health-promoting behaviours is not clearly established and requires further research.

The major interpersonal factors influencing health-promoting behaviours are the *influence of family or friends* and the *family patterns of health care.* People more likely to participate are those who have support for the health-promoting behaviours from family or friends and who have been raised in a family in which health-promoting behaviours are valued. Health teaching is enhanced when the patient's support people are included in the teaching.

Situational factors include the availability of opportunities to engage in health-promoting behaviours. For example, facilitation of a nutritionally balanced weight control programme is enhanced by the availability of fruits and vegetables rather than vending machines with sweets and crisps. Nurses can assist patients in exploring alternative ways of achieving their goals.

Health-promoting actions

The probability that a person will engage in health-promoting actions is influenced by actual or perceived barriers to action, such as cost, time, or ability, and the presence of cues to action.[26] Nursing approaches include assisting the person in differentiating between perceived and actual

barriers and promoting behaviours directed towards overcoming actual barriers.

Cues to action include hearing about activities that promote health either in interactions with others or through the mass media. Nursing strategies include health teaching of patients or encouraging patients to read, to listen to radio, or to watch television programmes that emphasize health promotion. Nurses also need to be instrumental in the development of these health-teaching tools.

Additional strategies that may be used to motivate people and help them develop positive health behaviours include modelling, self-confrontation, and behaviour modification. The nurse who carries out positive health behaviours, such as exercising regularly, serves as a *model* that others may emulate. Modelling positive health behaviours is an important nursing role function that, unfortunately, is not carried out to the degree that it should if health promotion is truly valued. *Self-confrontation* includes helping people identify inconsistencies in health beliefs, values, or behaviours; dissatisfaction with these inconsistencies that follow the awareness may lead to behavioural changes.[26]

Behaviour modification, or operant conditioning, consists of changing the behaviour by means of a cognitive plan that is made by the person with the health care professional and rewards positive behaviours. Positive reinforcement of desired behaviours increases the likelihood of desirable behaviour repetitions. The person is involved throughout the process. Behaviour modification is accomplished over a period of time by the following self-actions:

1. Setting own goals
2. Self-monitoring
3. Developing a personal reward system
4. Obtaining positive feedback
5. Developing a new self-concept
6. Developing and implementing an activity programme

Behaviour modification has been useful in weight reduction programmes (p. 58). (See Pender[26] for in-depth discussion of these and other methods that facilitate health promotion.)

Health promotion includes eating a well-balanced diet with emphasis on weight control, regular exercise, and reduction of stress. Stress management is discussed in Chapter 6. Health promotion also includes practices that decrease the risk of disease, such as not smoking, and eating a low-fat, low-salt, high-fibre diet. Specific aspects of health promotion are also discussed in various chapters, such as those for cancer and for respiratory and cardiovascular disorders. The following discussion focuses on nutrition and exercise.

NUTRITION

Food excesses and imbalances of certain food components are of as much concern in the United Kingdom as nutrient deficiencies. Dietary factors are associated with the leading causes of death in British and American adults: cancer, heart disease and stroke. *The Health of the Nation* report (1992)[7b] identifies the following risk-factor targets for diet and nutrition:

1. Reduce, by at least 12%, the average percentage of energy obtained from total fat intake (35% of energy or less).
2. Reduce, by at least 35%, the average percentage of energy obtained from saturated fatty acids (11% of energy or less).
3. Reduce, by 25% and 35% respectively, the proportion of obese men and women (6% of men and 8% of women or less).
4. Reduce, by 30%, the proportion of people who exceed the recommended intake of alcohol — men 21 units/week and women 14 units/week (men 18% and women 7%).

These topics are discussed in the following pages.

Nutritional Guidelines

There are three types of nutritional guidelines for health promotion: nutrient standards, food guides, and dietary guidelines.

Nutrient standards

Dietary standards are designed for the maintenance of good nutrition of practically all healthy people in the United Kingdom. *Dietary reference values* (DRVs), which include the *reference nutrient intake* (RNI), *estimated average requirement* (EAR), *lower reference nutrient intake* (LRNI), and *safe intake* (listed in Appendix C), are the accepted nutrient standards for proteins, energy, vitamins, and

minerals. These recently introduced DRVs (Department of Health 1991) which replace *recommended daily amounts* (RDAs), differ for age groups of children, men, and women based on weight and height. Labels found on many food products still include comparisons of the product with the RDAs. Because the food labels are listed as percentages of the total RDAs, people can easily make a rough estimate for their own use to determine if they are receiving the desired quantity of the nutrients.

Food guides

Food guides provide a *practical* approach for organizing food intake to ensure the needed variety and balance of required nutrients. Two examples of food guides are the *Basic Four daily food guide* (p. 56) and *food exchange lists* commonly used with dietary control of diabetes mellitus (Chapter 20).

Dietary guidelines

Dietary guidelines are general statements to provide people with direction towards a healthy diet. The guidelines are directed not only towards general health promotion, but also towards reducing risk of disease. Therefore they reflect the current emphases on prevention of the major diseases, such as heart disease and cancer. The dietary guidelines for the American public developed by the Department of Health and Human Services (DHHS) and the nutrition section of the U.S. Department of Agriculture[33] are a good example and can be compared with the guidelines adapted from those produced by the National Advisory Committee on Nutrition Education (NACNE) in 1983:

United States guidelines	NACNE guidelines
1. Eat a variety of foods	
2. Maintain ideal weight	Reduce body weight to normal
3. Avoid too much fat, saturated fat and cholesterol	Reduce the amount of energy obtained from fat (38% to 30%)
	Reduce the amount of saturated fats
	Replace saturated fats with polyunsaturated fats
4. Eat foods with adequate starch and fibre	Increase intake of unrefined carbohydrates–fibre (20% to 30%)
5. Avoid too much sugar	Reduce refined carbohydrate intake (sugar)
6. Avoid too much sodium	Reduce salt intake
7. Drink alcohol in moderation	Alcohol should provide no more than 4% of the total energy intake

The seven guidelines for the United States are presented in the following discussion.

Eat a variety of foods

The greater the variety of foods ingested, the more likely the person is to receive the required nutrients. Good nutritional status exists when the necessary nutrients (protein, fat, carbohydrate, minerals, vitamins, and water) are consumed in sufficient amounts and are used appropriately

Table 4-1 Height and weight tables for adults with desirable weights for people aged 25 and over

Men*					Women*†			
Height		Small frame (lb)	Medium frame (lb)	Large frame (lb)	Height		Small frame (lb)	Medium frame (lb)	Large frame (lb)
ft	in				ft	in			
5	2	112-120	118-129	126-141	4	10	92-98	96-107	104-119
5	3	115-123	121-133	129-144	4	11	94-101	98-110	106-122
5	4	118-126	124-136	132-148	5	0	96-104	101-113	109-125
5	5	121-129	127-139	135-152	5	1	99-107	104-116	112-128
5	6	124-133	130-143	138-156	5	2	102-110	107-119	115-131
5	7	128-137	134-147	142-161	5	3	105-113	110-122	118-134
5	8	132-141	138-152	147-166	5	4	108-116	113-126	121-138
5	9	136-145	142-156	151-170	5	5	111-119	116-130	125-142
5	10	140-150	146-160	155-174	5	6	114-123	120-135	129-146
5	11	144-154	150-165	159-179	5	7	118-127	124-139	133-150
6	0	148-158	154-170	164-184	5	8	122-131	128-143	137-154
6	1	152-162	158-175	168-189	5	9	126-135	132-147	141-158
6	2	156-167	162-180	173-194	5	10	130-140	136-151	145-163
6	3	160-171	167-185	178-199	5	11	134-144	140-155	149-168
6	4	164-175	172-190	182-204	6	0	138-148	144-159	153-173

From Metropolitan Life Insurance Co., New York.
*Height for men with shoes with 1-in heels; height for women with shoes with 2-in heels.
†For women 18-25 years old, subtract 1 lb for each year under 25.

by the body to meet needs. All people need the same nutrients throughout life.

All nutrients are equally important, although they are not required in equal amounts. The nutrients providing energy (protein, fats, carbohydrates) and water are required in much larger quantities than vitamins that regulate body processes. The differences in the quantities of various nutrients required by an individual are much greater than the change in amounts of any one nutrient over the life cycle. Growth, basal metabolic needs, and physical activity are the major factors responsible for changing nutrient needs. Disease, trauma, variations in metabolism (normal and or abnormal), medications, and treatments can also affect needs. The major effects of good nutrition include the following:

Growth and development of tissues/organs

Source of energy for metabolic processes and physical activity

Tissue healing and repair

Resistance to infection

One method to ensure a good variety of foods is to follow the guidelines of the Basic Four food groups: dairy products, meat/protein, vegetables/fruits, and bread/cereal (see p. 56).

Maintain ideal weight

Weight control is a major concern of many people; at least one out of every four adults is following a weight-reducing diet at any given time.[36] *Ideal body weight* (IBW) is difficult to identify because of individual variations, such as sex, age, genetic framework, and metabolic needs. Two men of the same age may weigh the same, but one may be an athlete and have large amounts of muscle with little fat, whereas the other may have considerable fat. However, height and weight tables are practical guides for determin-

ing a *general* weight range (Table 4-1). The height and weight table must be used with caution because it is based on "averages" and the "average person" does not exist.

The terms *overweight* and *obesity* must be differentiated and may be described in different ways. However, *overweight* generally refers to weight between the high point and 20% above IBW established by height and weight standards. *Obesity* is described as *more than* 20% above the height and weight standards. *Massive obesity* places the person at a high risk for numerous disorders; this condition is discussed in Chapter 23. Overweight, as contrasted to massive obesity, has not yet been demonstrated as placing the person at risk for disease.[36] Many people, however, do not feel at their optimal level of fitness and self-esteem when they are overweight. Thus, health promotion usually includes helping people maintain their IBW by restricting energy input (high-calorie foods) while increasing energy output (physical activity) (see p.59).

Underweight is described as 20% below the accepted weight and height standards. Unplanned weight loss may be an early sign of a medical disorder and medical evaluation should be sought. Some weight loss may be due to inadequate calorie intake or failure to increase calorie intake when physical activity is increased. Undernutrition leads to nutritional deficits that affect growth and development, metabolism, and the body's protective mechanisms. *Hospitalized patients are at risk for malnutrition* for several reasons. First, stress and increased metabolic rates from certain disorders deplete nutrient stores. Secondly, the patient is less active and may be relatively immobile. Thirdly, the patient may not be ingesting the required nutrients because of anorexia, nausea/vomiting, missed meals because of tests or surgery, or prescribed restrictive diets. Ongoing assessment of the patient's nutrient status is important. Protein–calorie malnutrition, a severe form of

---

4-2 | **Definition of terms pertaining to fats and cholesterol**

Lipids A group of fatty substances that are insoluble in water.

Triglycerides Simple lipids that are composed of one molecule of glycerol linked to three molecules of fatty acids.

Saturated fats Fatty acids that have no double bonds in the carbon chains: the fatty acid is filled (saturated) with hydrogen atoms; usually of animal origin.

Monounsaturated fats Fatty acids that have one double bond (one less hydrogen atom); of plant origin (for example, olive oil).

Polyunsaturated fats Fatty acids that have two or more double bonds (fewer hydrogen atoms; of plant origin (for example, vegetable oils).

Lipoproteins The form in which fats are carried in the blood stream: the unsoluble fat is wrapped in a water-soluble protein; may be low or high density.

Cholesterol A steroid that is found in animal fats and body tissues; most cholesterol is synthesized in the body; carried in blood stream attached primarily to low-density lipoproteins; of animal origin only.

4-3 | **Foods high in sodium**

Salt-preserved foods: ham, bacon, sausage, hot dogs, cold meat
Salted or smoked fish
Salted snacks: crackers, popcorn, pretzels, crisps, nuts
Spices/condiments: meat tenderizer, stock cubes, celery salt, garlic salt, monosodium glutamate, pickles, olives, Worcestershire sauce, soy sauce
Cheese

---

undernutrition can occur in hospital (Dickerson 1986) and is discussed in Chapter 23.

Avoid too much fat, saturated fat, and cholesterol

We need fat in our foods, particularly to supply essential fatty acids, especially linoleic acid that cannot be synthesized in the body. The body synthesizes fats from amino acids, but food provides an additional supply. Excess fats that the body cannot use are deposited in the tissue, adding to body weight. In addition, research strongly supports a relationship between dietary fat and the incidence of cancer, especially cancer of the breast, colon and rectum, and prostate.[2]

The public is becoming better informed about the effects of high levels of serum cholesterol as a risk factor for coronary heart disease. High serum triglycerides are additional risk factors (Chapter 17). A 1990 survey in the U.S. found that 65% of adults reported having had their cholesterol levels tested; however, only 24% stated that they were trying to lower their cholesterol levels through dietary means.[1] In the U.S. the following guidelines exist for adults:

1. Have cholesterol level measured every 5 years
2. Know your cholesterol level
3. Take steps to lower the cholesterol level, if elevated

In the United Kingdom, the Department of Health has identified a cholesterol of above 5.2mmol/l as undesirable because of the increased risk for coronary heart disease.[7a]

The phrase "avoid too much fat, saturated fat, and cholesterol" is vague; therefore more direction is needed. The health-risk factor targets identified in *The Health of the Nation* report (1992) include some concerned with fat intake. These targets cover both overall fat intake and, more specifically, the consumption of saturated fatty acids in terms of the percentage of energy obtained from fat in the diet (see page 51).

The different types of fats are defined in Box 4-2. Note that the more hydrogen is found in the fatty acid, the more it is saturated. Although saturated fats are usually of animal origin, unsaturated oils can be hardened commercially by injection of hydrogen gas to saturate them, producing margarines. About 40% of fats are visible in foods; the remainder is hidden, especially in red meats. Note also that cholesterol is not a fat but is related in that it is carried in the serum attached to fatty acids. Cholesterol is essential as a precursor to body steroids, for the development of bile acids, and as a component of cell membranes. Excess serum cholesterol not excreted contributes to the formation of atheromatous plaques in linings of blood vessels, especially the coronary arteries. This leads to blocking of the blood vessels. For some individuals with a higher than normal serum cholesterol level the use of low cholesterol diets, as part of a general reduction in the intake of saturated fatty acids, may favourably influence the risk of coronary heart disease. Recommended foods with lower cholesterol are listed on p. 58.

Eat foods with adequate starch and fibre

Starch is a polysaccharide (complex carbohydrate) found primarily in cereal grains, legumes, and vegetables (especially potatoes). It is the most important source of carbohydrate because it contains more nutrients than sugars. Carbohydrates are a vital energy source for the body. The suggested recommendations include increasing the daily intake for grain products and legumes to 6 *or more daily servings*.

Dietary fibre contains cellulose and some noncellulose polysaccharides. Cellulose is not digestible; therefore it remains in the gastrointestinal tract, providing bulk to help stimulate peristalsis in the intestines. The noncellulose polysaccharides absorb water to add to the bulk. Noncellulose substances also bind dietary cholesterol, preventing its absorption. Dietary fibre, therefore, is important to promote normal bowel elimination and to decrease dietary cholesterol absorption. In addition dietary fibre has been shown to have an inverse association with colon cancer; that is, a high intake of dietary fibre decreases the risk for colon cancer.[2] Sources of dietary fibre include whole grains (wheat, rye, oats) used in cereals and breads, bran, fruits, and vegetables.

4-4	Effect of some drugs on nutritional status	
Antacids	Iron: decreased absorption	
	Thiamine: reduced absorption	
Aspirin	Vitamin C: lower plasma levels	
	Vitamin K: reduced absorption	
Isoniazid	Nicotinic acid: antagonism	
	Vitamin B-6: antagonism	
Liquid paraffin	Vitamin A and D: reduced absorption	
Methotrexate	Folic acid: antagonism	
	Vitamin B-12: reduced absorption	
Neomycin	Nutrients: reduced absorption	
Oral contra- ceptives	Altered lipid profile	
	Folic acid: antagonism (rare)	
	Vitamin A: increased plasma levels	
	Vitamin B-6: antagonism	
	Vitamin C: lower plasma levels	
	Vitamin B-12: lower plasma levels	
Penicillins	Potassium: increased excretion	
Phenytoin	Folic acid: antagonism	
Tetracyclines	Vitamin C: lower plasma levels	
	Iron: decreased absorption	
Thiazides	Potassium: increased excretion	
	Zinc: increased excretion	
	Magnesium: increased excretion	
Trimethoprim	Folic acid: antagonism	

4-5	Medications to be taken with food	
Allopurinol		Nitrofurantoin
Aminophylline		NSAIDs
Cefuroxime		Phenytoin
Ferrous sulphate		Pivampicillin
Griseofulvin		Prednisolone
Labetolol		Theophylline
Metronidazole		Tinidazole
Nifedipine		Triamterene

The current intake of dietary fibres in the U.K. is about 10 to 13 g daily. The Department of Health recommends *increasing daily fibre intake to* an average of 18 g/d with an upper limit of 32 g to avoid adverse effects. Suggestions for increasing overall intake include consuming up to five portions of fruit or vegetables and up to six portions of grain/legumes daily. These suggested amounts would provide an adequate fibre intake for most people.

Avoid too much sugar

Excess amounts of sugar add to caloric intake without supplying nutrients; they also contribute to formation of dental caries. In general, sugars in British adult diets average about 18% of daily calories. People who diet by cutting out sugar but continue to consume fats, deceive themselves because fats provide almost double the amount of calories. Use of artificial sweeteners does not necessarily reduce calories because the artificial sweeteners do not relieve the desire for "something sweet", and the person then may turn to fats to achieve the feeling of satiety.[36] Substituting complex carbohydrates for some of the sugars provides for greater intake of essential nutrients and feelings of satiety.

Avoid too much sodium

Sodium, a major body electrolyte (Chapter 6), can affect blood pressure levels. Although the cause of hypertension is unknown, a decreased sodium intake can help decrease blood pressure in people with hypertension. Sodium in the form of salt-cured or salt-pickled foods has been associated with the increased incidence of gastric cancer.[2] Foods that are high in sodium are listed in Box 4-3. Many British diets are high in sodium, and dietary recommendations suggest that sodium intake be decreased to promote health. Suggestions for reducing sodium intake include the following:

- Increase the proportion of households that purchase foods low in sodium
- Prepare foods without adding salt
- Do not add salt at the table.

Drink alcohol in moderation

Alcohol is high in calories but low in nutrients. Excess alcohol intake leads to medical disorders and possible alcohol abuse. People who drink excessively often do not eat balanced meals and therefore experience malnutrition. A large percentage of motor vehicle accidents (a major public health problem) are caused by people who have been drinking alcohol. All health guidelines suggest that if you drink alcohol, you should do so in moderation (no more than 14 units for non-pregnant women and 21 units for men in one week).

Food–Drug Interactions

Some medications may affect nutritional status if taken over a period of time (see Box 4-4). Conversely, food can reduce or enhance absorption of oral medications.

Drugs are absorbed more readily if the stomach is free of food. Drugs taken with water when the stomach is empty move rapidly into the small intestines, where much drug absorption takes place. Fatty foods delay gastric emptying; therefore, drugs that are absorbed in the small intestine have delayed absorption if taken with a meal high in fats. Food adversely affects absorption of antimicrobial drugs, particularly the tetracyclines, some penicillins, and the sulphonamides. Some antimicrobials, such as ampicillin, cloxacillin, and tetracycline, are unstable in acid and should be taken half an hour before food; acid food, such as lemon juice, may also inactivate these drugs. Medications are taken with food as absorption is enhanced or they have a gastric irritant effect (see Box 4-5).

Drugs that are slightly acidic, such as aspirin, ionize and are absorbed in the stomach. If the stomach pH increases, such as by the ingestion of milk or antacids, the rate and extent of absorption of these drugs decrease. Increase in stomach acidity may also break down the protective coating of spansules or enteric-coated tablets, resulting in the premature release of contents.

Food components can interact with oral medication by the chemical or physical binding of one substance on another, thus interfering with absorption of either the food component or the drug. Tetracycline binds to calcium, aluminum, or magnesium ions when taken with milk or antacids. This decreases absorption of tetracycline. Foods containing tyramine (cheeses, wines) may interact with monoamine oxidase (MAO) inhibitors, such as phenelzine or tranylcypromine, which are antidepressants, causing hypertensive reactions.

Nursing Process
Assessment

To assess nutritional status (see Goodinson 1987, 13a.b.c.d), it is necessary to determine the supply of available nutrients, the sources available for metabolic processes, body size, and physical signs. Data are obtained primarily by patient interview, by observing the patient's general appearance, and by physical examination (N.B. biochemical methods will be used by the medical staff).

Subjective data

Data to be collected to determine nutritional status include the following:
Food intake
    Typical day food/fluid pattern (type, amount)
    Recent changes in amount and type of intake
    Recent changes in appetite
Eating ability
    Dentures (fit, comfort)
    Problems with chewing or swallowing
Weight
    Usual and current weight
    Patient's perception of weight level
    If overweight/underweight: lifetime patterns, feelings about weight, reasons for recent change
Food supplements, medications, drugs (types, duration)

Food intake

When collecting data about nutrition, it is especially important to phrase the questions so that patients describe what they typically eat rather than what they think they should. For example, the question, "Do you usually drink orange juice for breakfast?" implies (1) that breakfast is a desirable or expected behaviour and (2) that orange juice is essential. Thus the patient may answer. "Yes," believing that is the expected answer, when in fact neither orange juice nor breakfast is usually consumed. A better approach is to say, "Tell me what you typically eat and drink in a day. What do you usually eat or drink first?" Questioning should elicit a picture of total food consumption for a day including all snacks. Designation by meals or snacks is not really necessary and may bias answers by implying value judgments.[24]

Identification of amount consumed is as important as the type of food. Often people find this difficult to estimate. Those familiar with cooking may be able to estimate in terms of weight, tablespoons or cups. For the hospitalized patient the equipment or portions on the plate tray can be used as a basis for comparison.

Table 4-2 Estimating body frame from height/wrist ratio

Sex	Frame size		
	Small	Medium	Large
Male	r > 10.4	r = 9.6 to 10.4	r < 9.6
Female	r > 10.9	r = 9.9 to 10.9	r < 9.9

Changes in appetite or in the amount or type of food or fluids ingested may be the result of illness (for example, anorexia, nausea, vomiting, or pain), self-imposed dietary regimens, or emotional or physical stress.

Additional data

If nutritional intake is identified as inadequate, additional data facilitates analysis and planning:
1. Food and fluid likes and dislikes
2. Financial resources
3. Facilities and ability for purchasing, storing, and preparing food
4. Problems with prescribed diets

Objective data
Height and weight

Height and weight are easily measured and are important data to obtain and use. The most reliable weight measurement is in the morning after voiding and before eating or drinking fluids. The patient's weight and height are compared with a table of recommended values (see Table 4-1, p. 52). Interpretation of the table requires knowing frame size, which is determined by comparing height with wrist circumference. Measure the wrist distal to the styloid process on the right hand.[7] The height/wrist ratio (r) formula is as follows:

$$r = \frac{\text{Height (cm)}}{\text{Wrist circumference (cm)}}$$

Compare the ratio (r) with Table 4-2 to determine frame size.

Physical examination data

The time elapsing between the lack of nutrient supply and the actual appearance of clinical signs that are obvious on physical examination can be as little as a week or as long as several years. Data from a head-to-toe physical examination that suggest malnutrition may include the following:
Hair: lack of shine, thin and sparse, easily plucked
Eyes: pale conjunctiva, fissures at corner of eyelids
Lips: redness, dry, scaly, oedema, fissures at corners of lips
Tongue: swollen, smooth, raw, scaly, enlarged papillae
Teeth: cavities, loose or missing teeth
Gums: bleed easily, spongy
Skin: lack of subcutaneous fat, dryness, petechiae
Nails: brittle, ridged, spoon-shaped
Muscles: decreased muscle tone, tenderness, difficulty walking

Table 4-3 Daily food guide for adults

Food group (serving/day)	Amount/serving	Nutrients supplied
Dairy 2 or more	(1 cup = 225ml approx.) 1 c milk 40 g (1 ½ oz) cheese 1 ¾ c ice cream 1 c yogurt	Protein, calcium, phosphorus, ribo-flavin, other vitamins and minerals (except iron and vitamin C)
Meat protein or alternative 2 or more	60 to 75 g lean meat, poultry, fish 2 eggs (egg intake should be limited) 1 c cooked beans, peas, lentils 4 Tbsp peanut butter	Protein, fat, B complex vitamins, plant products lack vitamin B_{12})
Vegetables/fruits 4 or more total 1 dark green or deep yellow at least every other day	½ c broccoli, kale, carrots, spinach, sweet potatoes, turnip or greens, apricots, melon, pumpkin	Vitamin A
1/day (vitamin C sources)	½ c citrus fruits/juices, cabbage, broccoli, brussels sprouts, peppers, strawberries, tomatoes	Vitamin C
2 to 3/day (other)	½ c medium potato or apple, other vegetables or fruits	All fruits/vegetables: vitamins, minerals (low sodium), fibre
Bread/cereal 4 or more (whole grain or enriched)	1 slice bread 30 g dry cereal ½ to ¾ c cooked cereal, rice, pasta	Complex carbohydrates, protein, iron, thiamin, riboflavin, niacin

Body mass index

A relative index of body fatness can be determined by calculating the body mass index (BMI) using the following formula:

$$BMI = \frac{Weight\ (kg)}{Height\ (m)^2}$$

Divide the number of pounds by 2.2 to determine weight in kg. Divide the number of inches by 39.37 to determine height in metres; then multiply this number by itself to square it. For example, the BMI calculation of a person who weighs 125 lbs and is 5 ft 3 in tall is as follows:

$$125 \div 2.2 = 56.8\ kg$$

$$5\ ft\ 3\ in = 63\ in;\ 63 \div 39.37 = 1.6;\ 1.6 \times 1.6 = 2.56$$

Therefore, the BMI would be $56.8 \div 2.56 = 22.18\ kg/m^2$

For health maintenance, the BMI range for adults is 20 to 25 kg/m².[36] A person above that range, especially above 30 kg/m², is at risk. The person in the sample calculation is not at a health risk for overweight at the present time.

Skinfold measurement

Body fat can be estimated by skinfold measurements. Calipers are used to measure skinfolds by compressing the skin and subcutaneous fat, not muscle, into a fold at specific body sites (for example, biceps, triceps, subcapsular, and suprailiac areas).

Data analysis: health care needs influenced by nursing care

Analysis of food intake

Food guides developed to help people choose the kinds and amounts of food to eat for health can be used for rapid evaluation of adequacy of the diet eaten at home or food intake in the hospital. Many different food guides are available, since to be effective they must be devised for a specific country or culture and feature the foods readily available and acceptable to the people being evaluated.

An example of a daily food guide is shown in Table 4-3. The guide groups staple food items rich in protein, vitamins, and minerals into four major classes according to their major nutrient contributions. Recommendations are made for the number and size of servings to be selected from each food group. To evaluate a diet quickly, check to see if the recommended types of food and servings are included in the usual dietary pattern.

Because foods are mixtures of nutrients, the protein, vitamin, and mineral requirements are substantially met when the daily intake includes the recommended servings from each group. The calorie level of the basic diet is low, but it is approximately sufficient for adult basal metabolism. Adequacy of energy intake is best judged by evaluation of body weight. In this method of evaluation, fats, oils, and sweets are not tabulated because they provide primarily energy.

Each food group contributes particular nutrients to the total diet. The absence of any one food group from the diet

4-6	Types of diet modifications	
	Protein	Increased with losses from tissue catabolism, bleeding, exudates
		Decreased for chronic renal failure or hepatic coma
		Elimination of specific proteins (for example, allergies or malabsorption of gluten)
	Fats	Increased to provide essential calories in concentrated form
		Decreased for pain with gallbladder disease
		Modified for disorders of digestion or absorption, lipid metabolism, or to alter serum lipid levels
	Carbohy-drates	Increased for weight gain
		Decreased for weight loss or diabetes mellitus
		Changed from simple to complex carbohydrates in diabetes mellitus
		Elimination of specific carbohydrates with disorders of carbohydrate intolerance (for example, lactase deficiency)
	Vitamins	Increased for vitamin deficiency
		Provided in an alternate form to enhance absorption or use
	Minerals	Sodium restriction with hypertension, fluid retention, kidney disease
		Potassium and calcium increased or decreased for lack or excess
		Provided by prescription for deficiency
	Liquid, soft, pureed	Postoperative, diseases of gastrointestinal tract, difficulty with chewing or swallowing
	Elimination diets	Food allergies

or particular types of food should alert the nurse that the person has a potential nutrition problem.

The daily food guide can also be used for evaluating vegetarian diets. Many people are vegetarians and their reasons vary (for example, religion, food cost, philosophy). The diets vary as well. Generally, the lacto-ovovegetarian (includes milk products and eggs) diet is nutritionally sound when a variety of foods is included. People on more restricted vegetarian (vegan) diets should be considered at nutritional risk and candidates for more detailed study (refer to dietitian). One potential problem with the vegan diet is vitamin B_{12} insufficiency unless fortified cereal or a dietary supplement is taken. The young adult who has changed to a vegan diet may use body stores of B_{12} for a time (a 5-year store is possible), but is at potential risk, especially if intake of folacin in vegetables is high, masking the signs of megaloblastic anaemia.

Health Care Needs influenced by nursing

Nursing diagnoses are determined from analysis of patient data. Possible health care needs for the person with a nutritional imbalance include the following:

Problem	Possible aetiologies
Knowledge deficit	Lack of information
Nutrition, altered: high risk for more than body requirements	Dysfunctional eating behaviours
Nutrition, altered: more than body requirements	Dysfunctional eating behaviours, lack of exercise
Nutrition, altered: less than body requirements	Dysfunctional eating behaviours, anorexia, decreased intake because of tests or surgery

Planning: expected patient outcomes

Expected patient outcomes to promote good nutritional status may include, but are not limited to, the following:

1. Describes desired servings for each food group to meet basic nutritional needs.
2. Maintains weight within desired weight ranges.
3. Describes modifications in dietary intake to correct existing or potential nutritional deficits or excesses.

Implementation

Interventions to achieve patient outcomes
Facilitating patient teaching

Good nutrition can be promoted by giving positive reinforcement for selection of balanced meals from hospital menus. Teaching patients with specific knowledge deficits includes identification of the patient's motivation to learn. Patients with extensive lack of knowledge about food preparation, particularly with ways of preparing nutritionally balanced meals at low cost, may profit from the services of a dietitian.

The daily food guide (Table 4-3) is a useful tool for teaching people a method of evaluating their own food intake. The dietitian may be helpful in developing a specific food guide for people whose cultural patterns or personal preferences (for example, vegetarians) do not fit the standard food guides.

People who have been prescribed a dietary modification may need interpretation of the rationale for the diet and assistance in planning acceptable meals using the prescribed dietary plan (see Box 4-6). The dietitian usually initiates the discussion of a new diet to be used at home, but the nurse serves as interpreter to the patient by providing explanations about the diet and feedback on how to make changes in current dietary patterns to meet the dietary prescription. Because the patients are the ones who must implement the dietary changes, they need to internalize the need for a behaviour change. This takes active participation in all phases of the learning process. The person who does the cooking and shopping (if not the patient) also needs to

Table 4-4 Guidelines for decreasing dietry fats and cholesterol

Food groups	Use	Decrease
Meat	Fish, skinned poultry, lean cuts of meat	Fatty meats, sausages, hot dogs, cold meats, e.g. ham
Milk prod-ucts	Skimmed or 1% milk, low-fat cheeses, and yogurt	Whole milk, whole milk yogurt, natural cheeses, sour cream
	Egg whites	Egg yolks
Fruits	All fruits	
Vegetables	All vegetables	Butter or sauces added to vegetables
Bread/cereal	Low-fat crackers and biscuits, homemade baked goods with limited unsaturated fats	High fat crackers and biscuits, commercially baked goods, foods made with saturated fats
	Whole grain breads/cereals; rice pasta	Breads/cereals without whole grain: egg noodles
Fats/oils	Corn, safflower, sesame, soybean, and sun-flower oils	Coconut and palm kernel oil; butter, saturated fat, bacon fat
	Seeds and nuts	Coconut

From Expert Panel: Report of the National Cholesterol Education Program Expert Panel on detection, evaluation, and treatment of high blood cholesterol in adults, *Arch Intern Med* 148:36-69, 1988.

be involved in the learning process. Dietary changes are more likely to be implemented if the changes can be easily adjusted to the family's usual meal plans.

Facilitating weight loss

Diet. Diet is the most important method of weight reduction. Weight loss for some people may be achieved by eating three regular, balanced meals a day that include the four basic food groups and avoiding fried foods, sugars, and between-meal snacks. Other people achieve better results with planned, frequent small meals. Some obese people omit breakfast but then snack frequently and thus ingest more calories and fewer required nutrients. Therefore, *changes in eating patterns* are usually required for permanent weight loss.

People consuming high levels of calories before weight-reduction diets are likely to be successful in achieving rapid weight loss, because the calorie deficit between need and the recommended diet is large. There is a difference in weight loss patterns between men and women. If both a man and a woman are instructed to adhere to a 1000-calorie intake, the man should lose at a faster rate, not because he is more cooperative but because his calorie deficit is greater.[24]

Rapid weight loss is usually the result of loss of fluid rather than fat. Thus after an initial successful loss of weight on a weight-control diet, a plateau is reached when weight appears to remain constant or decrease only slightly. This can be discouraging to the person who is following the prescribed approach. Reinforcement to continue the regimen is usually needed at this point.

Diets are planned on an individual basis, with the caloric intake set at a level below the person's caloric need for maintaining weight. The calorie intake should come from complex carbohydrates and proteins. A protein intake of about 1 g/kg of ideal body weight should be maintained. Fats must be decreased. Salt-free diets are of no long-term value for weight reduction, because the weight loss relates to water loss, and the weight returns when salt is added to the diet. *Fasting* diets are controversial. Rapid weight loss may be necessary in some instances; however, weight gain follow-

ing the fasting period is a common occurrence. Most fasting programmes use a high-protein liquid; some commercial products use hydrolyzed collagen that is low in nutritional value. Close medical supervision is imperative for fasting diets because risks (such as ketosis, metabolic acidosis, hypokalaemia, hepatic impairment, renal insufficiency, and death) are high.

Fad diets should generally be avoided, although they usually induce rapid weight loss in a relatively easy way. However, nutrients will be lost (marked protein catabolism with losses of nitrogen, phosphorus, calcium, potassium, sodium, and water). Weight then returns to the original level after termination of the diet, because the person's general pattern of eating has not been changed.

Exercise. Exercise is an essential component of any weight control programme. It promotes expenditure of energy and makes body appearance more pleasing to the person and thus desirable to maintain. Although the actual number of calories used are few, the combination of diet and exercise promotes loss of fat rather than lean tissue. It is important that the exercise programme be agreeable to the person so that it becomes a pattern of behaviour to be continued throughout life (see p. 59).

Behaviour modification for weight control. Behaviour modification (p. 50) for weight control consists of changing the pattern of eating and exercising. Without changes in eating behaviours and exercise participation, overweight people usually return to their original weight after dieting.

Self-control is important in learning to change eating habits to facilitate weight loss and to maintain desirable body weight. Setting one's own goals and developing a personal reward system can facilitate motivation to participate in the desirable behaviours. Self-monitoring by means of planning the menus and keeping food diaries increases the person's awareness of the foods consumed. (Many people are unaware of the number of calories consumed, especially by "nibbling".)

Reinforcement from others is a major factor in the success of a weight control programme. The effectiveness of weight control groups, such as Weight Watchers, is based on this concept.

Facilitating weight gain

People who are underweight or have inadequate nutritional stores need encouragement to eat the right nutrients and calories. Motivating someone with anorexia to eat can be a challenge. Interventions that can correct the cause lead to improved appetite. Determining the person's likes and dislikes, providing an environment conducive to eating, and providing several small meals rather than three large meals a day may facilitate an adequate nutritional intake.

If the patient can eat, a high-calorie, high-protein diet is indicated to provide energy and amino acids for tissue building. The diet is essentially a normal one with added protein and supplementary high-caloric feedings. High-protein diets are contraindicated if a patient has liver disease because protein catabolism takes place in the liver. For those with protein-calorie malnutrition, enteral and parenteral feedings are frequently necessary (see Chapter 23).

Facilitating control of dietary fats and cholesterol

As cited previously (p. 53), adults should know their cholesterol levels and should take measures to decrease the level if it is greater than 5.2mmol/l. The usual diet is 10% to 15% of kcal *higher* in total fats (10% higher in saturated fats, 5% higher in monounsaturated fats, and slightly higher in polyunsaturated fats) than the recommended levels. The cholesterol levels of average diets in the U.S. are higher than 300 mg/d[11], but dietary intake of cholesterol appears to have little influence on the serum cholesterol level if saturated fatty acids provide only a small amount of total energy.[7a] Therefore, it is necessary for all people to modify these intakes to the recommended levels (p. 76). Guidelines for decreasing fats and cholesterol are listed in Table 4-4.

Maintaining a low-saturated fat, low-cholesterol diet is not always easy because it involves deleting some well-liked foods, such as high-fat cheeses and cold meat. Learning to eat a diet that is lower in saturated fats and cholesterol, as with other types of permanent diet changes, requires a change in eating behaviour patterns (behaviour modification, p. 50). People need to know the differences among the types of fats, cholesterol and fat content of foods, and how to read food labels.[21] For example, many producers of plant-based products advertise that their product has zero cholesterol; this is in fact true, but one must remember that cholesterol comes only from animal products. The advertised product may be high in saturated fats, which the body can then use to produce cholesterol.

EXERCISE

Regular physical activity can help individuals feel well, cope with stress, enhance normal body functioning, and decrease risk factors for some diseases. Lack of exercise is cited in connection with the incidence of coronary heart disease and stroke.[7b] It has been found that the actual number of adults who participate in moderate daily activity or in vigorous exercise at least 3 times a week is far below the desired levels.[27] Much health teaching and active promotion of exercise and fitness are necessary. In the U.S. the following objectives for the Year 2000[35] have been set:

- Increase to more than 30% the proportion of people older than age 6 who engage regularly, preferably daily, in light to moderate activity for at least 30 minutes per day.
- Increase to more than 20% the proportion of people older than age 18 who engage in vigorous physical activity for more than 20 minutes, 3 or more days a week.

Although a positive trend has developed towards increased exercise in recent years, many adults live a sedentary lifestyle. People are aware that activity or mobility is necessary for health but many still do not take the effort to increase their activity level. Those who do not value exercise as a means of maintaining optimal health often find excuses for not participating in a planned exercise programme on an on-going basis. Exercise does imply effort; if exercise is not valued, the effort is not made.

Benefits of Exercise

A programme of regular exercise can have both psychological and physiological benefits. a physically fit person also generally has greater endurance and faster recovery time (return to resting rate), which can contribute to more rapid recovery from illness.

Exercise is important *regardless of age*. Some elderly people believe they are too old to begin an active fitness programme, but these programmes are possible even for those with chronic illness. The fitness programme is individually planned and based on the person's interests, capabilities, and limitations.

Physically, exercise enhances cardiovascular fitness, endurance, muscle strength, flexibility, and weight control. It has positive effects on the musculoskeletal, neurosensory, circulatory, respiratory, gastrointestinal, and urinary systems.

Exercise Programmes
Classification of exercise

Activity or exercise should be incorporated into one's lifestyle, e.g. using the stairs not the lift, attaining the same importance as eating or sleeping. Physical activity performed on a regular basis gives a sense of wellbeing that is part of feeling healthy. And feeling healthy contributes to longer life.

SUMMARY

1. Factors influencing health-promoting behaviours include perceptions about health and self, demo graphic factors, influence of family or friends, family patterns of health care, availability of opportunities to engage in health-promoting behaviours, and actual or perceived barriers to health-promoting actions.
2. Health-promoting strategies include health teaching, modelling, self-confrontation, and behaviour modification.
3. Three types of nutritional guidelines are nutrient standards (dietary reference values), food guides (the Basic Four and food exchange lists), and dietary guidelines.
4. A recommended dietary guideline includes (1) eating a variety of foods; (2) maintaining ideal weight; (3)

avoidingtoo much fat, saturated fat, and cholesterol; (4) eating foods with adequate starch and fibre; (5) avoidingtoo much sugar; (6) avoidingtoo much sodium; and (7) consuming alcohol in moderation.

5. Overweight refers to weight between ideal body weight and 20% above ideal body weight (IBW). Obesity is more than 20% above the height–weight standards. Underweight is 20% below the height–weight standards.

6. Guidelines for cholesterol awareness and actions include having cholesterol measured every 5 years, knowing your cholesterol level, and taking steps to lower the elevated cholesterol level. A reduction in dietary intake of cholesterol is recommended.

7. Dietary fibre provides bulk to help stimulate intestinal peristalsis, binds dietary cholesterol to prevent absorption, and is a factor in reducing risk for cancer of the colon. An average intake of 18 g/d of dietary fibre with a maximum of 32 g/d is recommended.

8. Recommendations for decreasing sodium intake include eating foods low in sodium, preparing foods without adding salt, and not adding salt at the table.

9. Medications may affect nutritional status; food can, in turn, affect absorption of oral medications.

10. The dietary food guide is useful for a quick dietary assessment and for use in health teaching.

11. Methods of weight reduction include diet, exercise, and behaviour modification.

12. Exercise enhances cardiovascular fitness, endurance, muscle strength, flexibility, weight control, sense of wellbeing, sleep, and ability to cope with stress. Exercise also has a positive effect on the body systems, decreases risk factors of coronary artery disease, provides better control of hypertension, and assists in reducing addictive behaviours.

STUDY QUESTIONS

- Select a health behaviour that you do not follow. How does this behaviour relate to your definition of health? What factors can you identify that may be barriers to the desired behaviours?
- In what ways do your eating behaviours differ from the recommended dietary guidelines? What measures could you take to meet or maintain each of the guidelines?
- Why would it be ineffective to tell an overweight person he/she should lose weight?
- How often do you engage in 15 minutes or more of aerobic activities each week? What changes, if any, could you make to meet recommendations for health promotion?

REFERENCES AND SELECTED READINGS

1. *Americans aware of cholesterol dangers*, April 10, 1991, Cleveland, The Plain Dealer.
2. Butrum RR, Clifford CK, Lanza E: NCI dietary guidelines: rationale, *Am J Clin Nutr* 48:888-895, 1988.
3.* Cerato PL: How safe are modified fasts, *RN* 52(11):79-81, 1989.
4. Clark JB, Queener SF, Karb VB: *Pharmacologic basis of nursing practice,* ed 3, St Louis, 1990, Mosby–Year Book.
5.* Clark SR: Compliance and health behavior, *Top Clin Nurs* 7(4):39-46, 1986.
6. Cornacchia HJ, Barrett S: *Consumer health: a guide to intelligent decisions,* ed 4, St Louis, 1989, Mosby–Year Book.
7.* Curtas S, Chapman G, Meguid MM: Evaluation of nutritional status, *Nurs Clin North Am* 24:301-312, 1989.
7a. Department of Health, *Dietary Reference Values for Food Energy and Nutrients for the United Kingdom,* Report on Health and Social Subjects, no.
41. Report of the Panel on Dietary Reference Values of the Committee on Medical Aspects of Food Policy. London, HMSO, 1991.
7b. Department of Health, *The Health of the Nation: A Strategy for Health in England,* Presented to Parliament by the Secretary of State for Health. London, HMSO, 1992.
7c. Dickerson JWT, and Booth EM, *Clinical Nutrition for Nurses, Dietitians and Other Health Professionals.* London, Faber and Faber, 1985.
7d. Dickerson JWT, and Booth EM, Hospital Induced Malnutrition: a cause for concern, *The Professional Nurse,* 1, (11), 293-296, 1986.
8. Dychtwald K, Flower J: *Age wave: the challenges and opportunities of an aging America,* Los Angeles, 1989, Jeremy P Tarcher.
9. Dychtwald K, MacLean J: *Wellness and health promotion for the elderly,* Rockville, Md, 1986, Aspen Systems.
10. Ebersole P, Hess P: *Toward healthy aging: human needs and nursing response,* ed 3, St Louis, 1989, Mosby–Year Book.
10a. Ewles L, Simnett I, *Promoting Health. A Practical Guide,* ed 2. London, Scutari Press, 1992.
11. Expert Panel: Report of the National Cholesterol EducationProgramme Expert Panel on detection, evaluation, and treatment of high blood cholesterol in adults, *Arch Intern Med* 148:36-69, 1988.
12. Factors related to cholesterol screening and cholesterol level awareness, *MMWR* 39(37):633-637, 1990.
13. Getchell B: *Fit: a personal guide,* ed 2, Indianapolis, 1986, Benchmark Press.
13a. Goodinson SM, Assessment of nutritional status, *The Professional Nurse,* 2, (11), 367-369, 1987a.
13b. Goodinson SM, Anthropometric assessment of nutritional status, *The Professional Nurse,* 2, (12), 338-393, 1987b.
13c. Goodinson SM, Biochemical assessment of nutritional status, *The Professional Nurse,* 3, (2), 8-12, 1987c.
13d. Goodinson SM, Assessing nutritional status: Subjective methods, *The Professional Nurse,* 3, (2), 48-51, 1987d.
14. Haskell WL, Montoye HJ, Orenstein D: Physical activity and exercise to achieve health-related physical fitness components, *Public Health Rep* 100(2):202-210, 1985.
15. Hospital malnutrition still abounds, *Nutr Rev* 46:315-317, 1988.
16. Johnson C, Greenland P: Effects of exercise, dietary cholesterol, and dietary fat on blood lipids, *Arch Intern Med* 150:137-140, 1990.
17. Krause MV, Mahan LK: *Food, nutrition, and diet therapy,* ed 8, Philadelphia, 1991, WB Saunders.
18. Marwick C: Changes brewing for food labels as national concern about diet and health continues to grow, *JAMA* 262:752-755, 1989.
19.* Massachusetts Medical Society Committee on Nutrition: Fast-food fare: consumer guidelines, *New Eng J Med* 321:752-753, 1989.
20. McCain GH: Sources of health information for consumers and health practitioners, *Fam Community Health* 9(2):46-50, 1986.
21.* McCann BS: Promoting adherence to low-fat, low-cholesterol diets: review and recommendations, *J Am Dietetic Assoc* 90:1408-1414, 1990.
22. Molloy D: Now is the time to advocate wellness, *Am Nurse* April 4, 1991.
22a. National Advisory Committee on Nutritional Education (NACNE), *Proposals for Nutritional Guidelines for Health Education in Britain.* London, Health Education Council, 1983.
23. National Research Council: *Recommended dietary allow-ances,* ed 10, National Academy Press, Washington, DC, 1989, The Council.
24. Neville J: *Assessment of nutritional status and dietary counseling.* In Phipps WJ, et al, editors: *Medical–surgical nursing: concepts and clinical practice,* ed 4, St Louis, 1991, Mosby–Year Book.
25. Nowak RK, Schultz KO: A comparison of two methods for determination of body frame size, *J Am Dietetic Assoc* 87:339-341, 1987.
26.* Pender NJ: *Health promotion in nursing practice,* ed 2, Norwalk, Ct, 1987, Appleton & Lange.
27. Progress toward achieving the 1990 national objectives for physical fitness and exercise, *MMWR* 38(26):449-453, 1989.
28. Public Health Service: *Promoting health-preventing disease: Year 2000 objectives for the nation, draft for public review and comment,* Washington, DC, 1989, US Dept of Health and Human Services.

29. Public Health Service: *Healthy people 2000: nationalhealth promotion and disease prevention objectives*, Washington, DC, 1990, US Dept of Health and Human Services.

30. Schectman G, et al: Dietary intake of American reporting adherence to low-cholesterol diet (NHANES II), *Am J Public Health* 80:698-703, 1990.

31. Stoto MA, Behrens R, Rosemont C, editors: *Healthy people 2000: citizens chart the course*, Washington, DC, 1990, National Academy Press.

32. *Surgeon General's report on nutrition and health*, Washington, DC, 1988, US Dept of Health and Human Services.

32a. Taylor S, Goodinson-MacLaren S, *Nutritional Support: A Team Approach*, London, Mosby–Year Book Europe Limited, 1992.

33. US Dept of Agriculture, Human Nutrition Information Service: *Nutrition and your health: dietary guidelines for Americans; eat a variety of foods*, Washington DC, 1986, US Superintendent of Documents.

34. US Dept of Agriculture and the US Dept of Health and Human Services: *Nutrition and your health: dietary guidelines for Americans*, ed 2, Washington, DC, 1985, US Superintendent of Documents.

35. US Dept of Health and Human Services and Public Health Service: *Healthy People 2000: national health promotion and disease prevention objectives*, 1991, Washington, DC, US Government Printing Office.

36. Williams SR: *Essentials of nutrition and diet therapy*, ed 5, St Louis, 1990, Mosby–Year Book.

37. Year 2000 national health objectives, *MMWR* 38(37): 629-633, 1989.

37a. Wilson-Barnet J, Macleod-Clark J, Editors *Research in Health Promotion and Nursing*. London, Macmillan Press Limited, 1993.

38. Cantu RC: *Toward fitness: guided exercise for those with health problems*, New York, 1980, Human Sciences Press.

39. Cantu RC: Health maintenance through physical conditioning, Littleton, Mass, 1981, PSG Publishing.

40. Cooper KH: *The aerobics way*, New York, 1977, M Evans & Co. Inc.

41. Stefee P: Malnutrition in hospitalized patients, *JAMA* 244:2630-2635, 1980.

*Recommended for student reading.

5

Stressors, Stress, and Stress Management

Virginia L. Cassmeyer
Barbara C. Long
May Wykle

After studying this chapter, the learner should be able to:

- Define adaptation.
- Differentiate between stressors and stress response.
- Explain the relationship of dealing with stressors to optimal functioning and growth.
- Describe the neuroendocrine response to stressors.
- Describe behavioural responses to stressors.
- Define coping.
- Describe types of coping strategies.
- Identify assessment parameters of anxiety.
- Describe interventions for persons with anxiety.

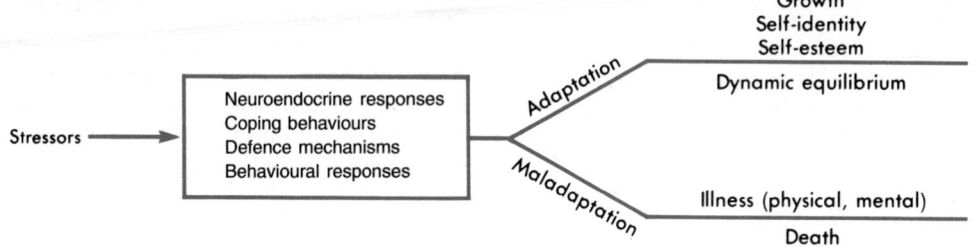

Fig. 5-1 Responses to stressors may lead to adaptation or maladaptation.

Promotion of health involves activities that facilitate a sense of wellbeing. This implies a feeling of "ease," which is accomplished in part by coping effectively with internal or external stressors. Nurses can help patients learn how to cope with stressors in positive ways and thus prevent or diminish the effects of the stressors and the stress response. This chapter discusses various concepts of adaptation, stressors, stress response, and stress management.

ADAPTATION

Humans can be conceptualized as open systems that respond to stimuli from the internal and external environments. This process of interaction can be termed *adaptation*. In this context, adaptation has neither positive nor negative values. However, many prefer to use the term in a positive sense, to mean the process of interaction with the environment that promotes homeostasis or dynamic equilibrium and growth. The process that leads to inadequate functioning is then termed *maladaptation*.

Human beings adapt biologically, psychologically, emotionally, and socially. The goal of biological adaptation is survival or stability of internal processes. When the ability to maintain this equilibrium is lost, pathophysiological disorders result. Psychological and emotional adaptation is directed towards preservation of self-identity and self-esteem. The person adapting in these modes is mentally healthy, whereas maladaptation leads to mental illness. Social adaptation depends on the sociocultural expectations of the society of which the person is a member. A maladaptive or socially deviant behaviour in one society may be acceptable in another.

Although any changing environmental stimuli can initiate the need for adaptation, stressors create major adaptive demands for individuals. As shown in Figure 5-1, the neuroendocrine responses, coping behaviours, defence mechanisms, and behavioural responses are major strategies available for meeting adaptive demands associated with stressors. Nurses work with people in adaptation at many levels including:

1. Helping to identify and remove stressors requiring adaptive demands.
2. Supporting healthy strategies that help to meet the adaptive demands of stressors.
3. Helping people use higher level defence mechanisms.

4. Helping people deal with the psychological responses to stressors.
5. Helping people develop alternative coping behaviours or behavioural responses to stressors.
6. Helping people deal with the illnesses that result if adaptation is not effective.

STRESSORS/STRESS AS CONCEPTS

The ability of the human body to initiate and sustain a response to stressors is one of the major protective mechanisms that allows individuals to exist in a hostile environment. Both the healthy and ill—those in the hospital, in extended care facilities, or in their own homes—are exposed to stressors. Because stressors are so ubiquitous, the individual must possess mechanisms to deal with them.

Stressors

Before exploring the responses to stressors, the concept of stressors will be discussed. A *stressor* can be defined as a noxious or threatening stimulus that can elicit a stress response. A stressor may be actual or potential, biophysical–chemical, or psychosocial–cultural. Although most of the stressors that are experienced by patients in the hospital are negative stimuli and severe in nature, stressors can be positive stimuli, such as marriage, physical exercise, or the birth of a child. Stressors also can be nonsevere, everyday hassles. Important in the definition of stressors is that, although some of the more severe stimuli would probably be perceived as a stressor for anyone, individuals differ as to which stimuli are stressors.

Many different studies have shown that stressors can be biological, physical, chemical, social, developmental, cultural, or psychological stimuli.[28,32,40] Stressors can range from the daily hassles of an alarm clock that does not go off on time, to an approaching deadline, to the onset of the common cold in a relatively healthy person, to major burns over 50% of the body. The stressors that the nurse deals with vary depending on the patient population. The nurse in an outpatient setting, in home health care, or in discharge planning may focus more on daily hassles and primary health care problems. The nurse working with patients during the acute or critical stages of illness may deal with more severe stressors.

Stress

The term *stress* has been used for many years to denote mental strain, for example, "He's under stress." Every person has some definition for the word stress. For the purpose of this chapter *stress* is defined as:

> An integrated body response, including intellectual, behavioural, emotional, and physiological components, to a stimuli that is perceived on a conscious or unconscious level as noxious or threatening. The response serves as a protective mechanism. It is elicited to allow the individual to adapt to or adjust to noxious or threatening stimuli and is graded. The response varies depending on the type, strength, and duration of the stimuli and is modified by characteristics of the person.

The response to stressors may have either negative or positive results or both. For example, a person may experience pain (a stressor). The pain may cause anorexia, which may lead to nutrient imbalance and inactivity, which may lead to the side effects of immobility. These are negative results. On the other hand, the presence of pain may guide the person to seek medical intervention. This may lead to removal of the underlying condition causing the pain and a positive result occurs.

Stress is not necessarily something to be avoided, and in fact a certain amount of normal stress (*eustress*) is considered necessary for adaptation. For example, microorganisms can upset cellular function, leading to disequilibrium and death. However, exposure to microorganisms in limited numbers or of decreased strength can help the body develop mechanisms to defend against subsequent exposures. Similarly, exposure to daily hassles helps develop useful coping methods that facilitate dealing with new stressors. Coping with biological or psychosocial stressors in an adaptive manner aids optimal functioning and growth. Maladaptation leads to dysfunction and pathophysiological or psychopathological disorders.

RESPONSES TO STRESSORS
Integrated Psychobiological Response

People respond to stressors as a *unified whole*, that is, compensatory or defence mechanisms are initiated to help the individual cope with the stressor biologically and psychologically. Some of the evoked responses are biological, others are behavioural, and both frequently occur simultaneously. For example, anxiety can cause sweaty palms, pale skin, and frequent voiding, as well as decreased attention span, decreased ability to follow directions, or immobility. For the purpose of learning, however, it is easier to separate physiological responses from behavioural responses.

The scientist with whom the concepts of stress and stressor are most closely associated is Hans Selye. When he was a medical student, Selye observed in diverse people with various diseases similar signs and symptoms that he labelled as the *syndrome of just being sick*.[67] When he first observed this syndrome, he questioned whether the underlying mechanism could be identified. Years later, while involved in experimental studies designed to discover a new hormone, he noted that injections of a tissue extract, which supposedly contained the hormone, resulted in enlarge-

ment of the adrenal cortex, ulcers of the gastrointestinal tract, and atrophy of the lymph nodes and thymus gland.[65] Although Selye[67] at first ascribed these changes to the hypothetical hormone supposedly in the tissue extract, he later found that injections of any extracts, as well as other stimuli, such as cold and X-rays, caused the same response.

General Adaptation Syndrome

Selye labelled this nonspecific response to various agents the general adaptation syndrome (GAS).[65,67] GAS became known as the stress syndrome and was viewed as having three stages: alarm reaction, resistance, and exhaustion. The first two stages are repeated continuously throughout life as people encounter stressors. The exhaustion stage occurs when resistance cannot be sustained, and altered functioning then results.

Alarm reaction stage. During the initial alarm stage (shock), the "fight or flight" response is initiated. The individual prepares to counteract the stressor or remove himself or herself from the stressor. If the shock is too severe, a "freeze" response occurs; the person is overwhelmed by the stressor and cannot fight or flee. During the alarm reaction stage, the neuroendocrine mechanisms are activated. If the compensatory mechanisms are sufficient to deal with the stressor, the individual returns to the prestressed level.

Resistance stage. Continual and prolonged application of the stressor leads to the resistance stage. During this stage, continued adrenocortical activity facilitates adaptation. Energy is required to maintain a high level of resistance. If the stressor is maintained a sufficient time, stress-related pathophysiological disorders may result. If adaptation is successful and the stressor removed, the person may return to the prestressed level.

Exhaustion stage. If the original stressor is so damaging that defence mechanisms are ineffective or if the stressor is not removed and energy to maintain resistance is depleted, the exhaustion stage occurs. Examples of extreme stressors are arterial bleeding, pressure on the hypothalamus, overwhelming infection, blockage of a major branch of the coronary artery, or sudden death of a spouse. Unless the primary biological condition can be controlled promptly, death may ensue.

The meaning of the stressor for the individual is one of the major factors influencing the stress response. Stressors creating a change that is viewed negatively have a high probability of an increased stress response. For example, a woman who places great value on her body as a means of personal and sexual gratification will likely experience a greater response to removal of a breast than a woman who places less significance on her bodily appearance.

The individual's *perception* of the stressor (and hence the meaning that is interpreted) is influenced by cognitive ability, verbal skills, past experiences, interpersonal relationships, significant others' responses, and feelings of control. A sense of control over the stressor helps to decrease the response. For example, patients who know in advance some measures to decrease postoperative pain (that is, have control over the pain) usually adapt more effectively in the postoperative period. People who have developed a repertoire of coping skills can select one that facilitates adaptation to a new stressor. Thus people who have had to cope with numerous intense stressors in the past are often able to cope effectively when crises occur.

When health status is poor, less energy is available to deal with environmental stimuli, and responses to stressors may be affected. Nutritional deficits especially place the person at higher risk of maladaptive responses (see Chapter 4).

Another important factor in relation to psychological and emotional influences on physiological stressors is that in some experiments[60,61] where physical stressors were induced while controlling or minimizing the discomfort, suddenness, or unpleasantness of the stimuli, the GAS was not elicited. This may mean that all stressor stimuli must have a psychosocial–cultural component.

One criticism of Selye's work relates to his description of the stress response as nonspecific. This characteristic meant that the same response occurred regardless of the stressor. Current data do not support this assumption. In animal studies,[59] different hormonal and neurochemical responses occur in response to different stressors. Despite these criticisms, Selye's work still provides the basis of the physiological response that can be elicited by stressors and an appreciation of the various stimuli that may serve as stressors in many people.

Neuroendocrine Response to Stressors

The physiological components involved in the stress response include the central nervous system, the hypothalamus, the sympathetic nervous system, the anterior and posterior pituitary gland, and the adrenal cortex and medulla. These physiological components and their secretions (hormones and catecholamines) are responsible for the neuroendocrine response to stressors. As discussed earlier in this chapter, not all of these components are necessarily involved in the response to every stressor; but to provide holistic nursing care, the nurse must know the effects of response to stressors of each of these components of the neuroendocrine response.

The physiological components of the neuroendocrine stress response are shown in Figure 5-2. Stressors, either perceived at the level of the *central nervous system* or on an unconscious level by *baroreceptors, chemoreceptors*, or *glucoreceptors*, which transfer information to the *medulla oblongata*, serve as the *afferent input*. This information is eventually forwarded to the *hypothalamus*, which coordinates the response. The hypothalamus activates the *sympathetic nervous system* and the *anterior* and *posterior pituitary glands*. The *adrenal medulla* is activated when the sympathetic nervous system is stimulated.

The hypothalamus stimulates the anterior pituitary gland by releasing hormones such as corticotropin-releasing hormone (CRH), growth hormone-releasing hormone (GHRH), or prolactin-releasing hormone (PRH) or by inhibiting its secretion of inhibiting hormones. For example, dopamine acts as a prolactin-inhibiting hormone (PIH), and thus prolactin secretion is increased when dopamine secretion is decreased.

Adrenocorticotropin hormone (ACTH), which is released from the anterior pituitary gland, stimulates the release of cortisol from the adrenal cortex. The adrenal cortex also releases the hormone aldosterone in response to ACTH secretion. However, the major controller of aldosterone secretion is the renin–angiotensin system, which is shown in Figure 5-3.

Another endocrine gland activated by the hypothalamus is the posterior pituitary gland. The posterior pituitary gland, when stimulated, releases antidiuretic hormone (ADH) or vasopressin. The effects of stimulation of the sympathetic nervous system, anterior and posterior pituitary glands, and adrenal cortex and medulla are mediated by the catecholamines and hormones released by the nervous system or the glands.

Catecholamines

The catecholamines, adrenaline and noradrenaline, act by stimulating receptors unique for them. The receptors are located on various cells throughout the body. The catecholamine receptors are divided into two major classes, alpha (α) and beta (β), with two subclasses of each major class. The activation of these receptors by endogenous or exogenous catecholamines results in selected physiological actions.

Stimulation of α_1 receptors is primarily associated with excitation or stimulation, and stimulation of α_2 receptors is primarily associated with relaxation or inhibition. Stimulation of β_1 receptors is primarily associated with stimulation of cardiac activity, and stimulation of β_2 receptors is associated with all other effects associated with beta receptors such as bronchial dilation.

During the neuroendocrine response to stressors, both noradrenaline and adrenaline are released. Noradrenaline binds primarily to α receptors, whereas adrenaline activates both α and β receptors. The effects of catecholamines during the stress response then are due to a combination of the actions of both catecholamines and activation of several different receptors. The effects seen with the release of catecholamines during the stress response are summarized in Table 5-1 on p. 68.

Cortisol

Cortisol is released from the adrenal cortex under the control of CRH and ACTH. Cortisol has major effects on metabolism and fluid and electrolyte balance and has antiinflammatory and immunosuppressant effects. It enhances the activity of other hormones. Detailed information of the effects of cortisol on the body are presented in Box 5-1 on p. 69.

Aldosterone

Aldosterone is released from the adrenal cortex primarily in response to activation of the renin–angiotensin system as diagrammed in Figure 5-3 on p. 67. Some aldosterone is released in response to ACTH from the anterior pituitary gland. Aldosterone acts on the distal kidney tubule cells and causes reabsorption of sodium and water and excretion of potassium and hydrogen ions. Aldosterone helps to maintain vascular volume and blood pressure.

Stressors

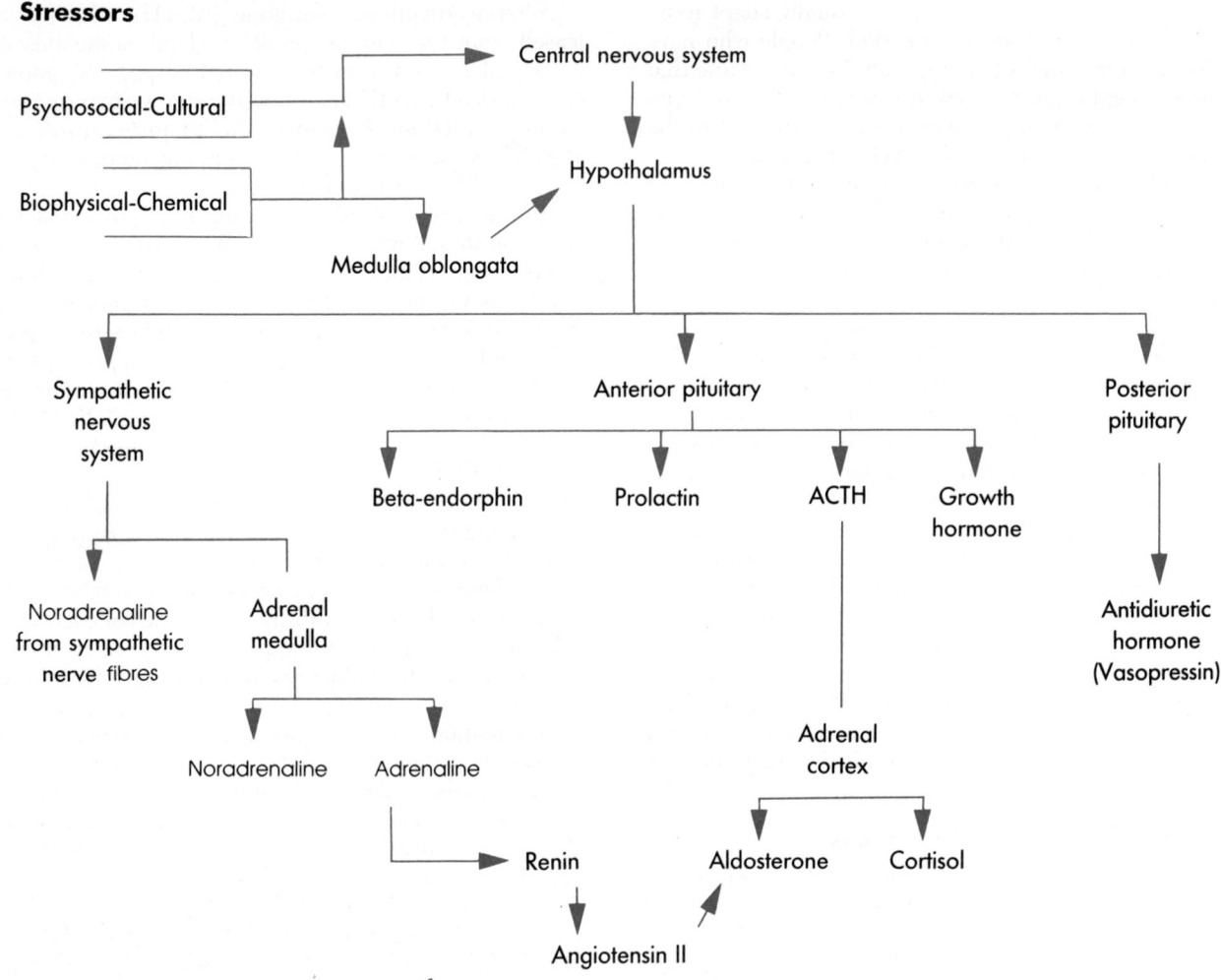

Fig. 5-2 Physiological components involved in the neuroendocrine response to stressors.

Antidiuretic hormone

Antidiuretic hormone (ADH) or vasopressin is released during the neuroendocrine response to stressors. ADH acts on the kidneys to increase water reabsorption. Water is reabsorbed in response to the osmotic gradient established by the difference in osmolality of the tubular fluid and the medullary interstitial fluid. ADH controls the osmolality of body fluid. ADH in high concentration can result in arteriole vasoconstriction and can help to increase blood pressure.

Other pituitary hormones

Endogenous opiates (β-endorphins) are released as part of the neuroendocrine response to stressors. Release of endogenous opiates in stressful situations may account for the analgesic effect experienced by trauma patients.

Growth hormone is released from the anterior pituitary during the neuroendocrine response to stressors. Hypoglycaemia and strenuous exercise are two stressors associated with an increase in growth hormone. Growth hormone helps to provide nutrients for the energy needs during the stress response. It helps to maintain the blood glucose level, and increases lipolysis, free fatty acid levels, and ketone formation, which provide nutrients for various tissues, such as skeletal and cardiac muscles.

Prolactin[24] is released in the presence of certain stressors. The function of prolactin in relation to dealing with stressors is unknown.

The overall effects of the release of the hormones and catecholamines during a neuroendocrine response to stressors, if the response is effective, are summarized in Box 5-2 on p. 69.

Coping

Coping refers to processes or skills that individuals use to deal with events, circumstances, or situations that are out of the ordinary and thus become stressors. Coping strategies are overall plans of action for overcoming stressors.[2] Thus coping is a general behavioural response to stressors.

People cope with stressors in one or more ways (see Table 5-2 on p. 68). Actions to cope with stressors may be adaptive or maladaptive, depending on the achieved level of

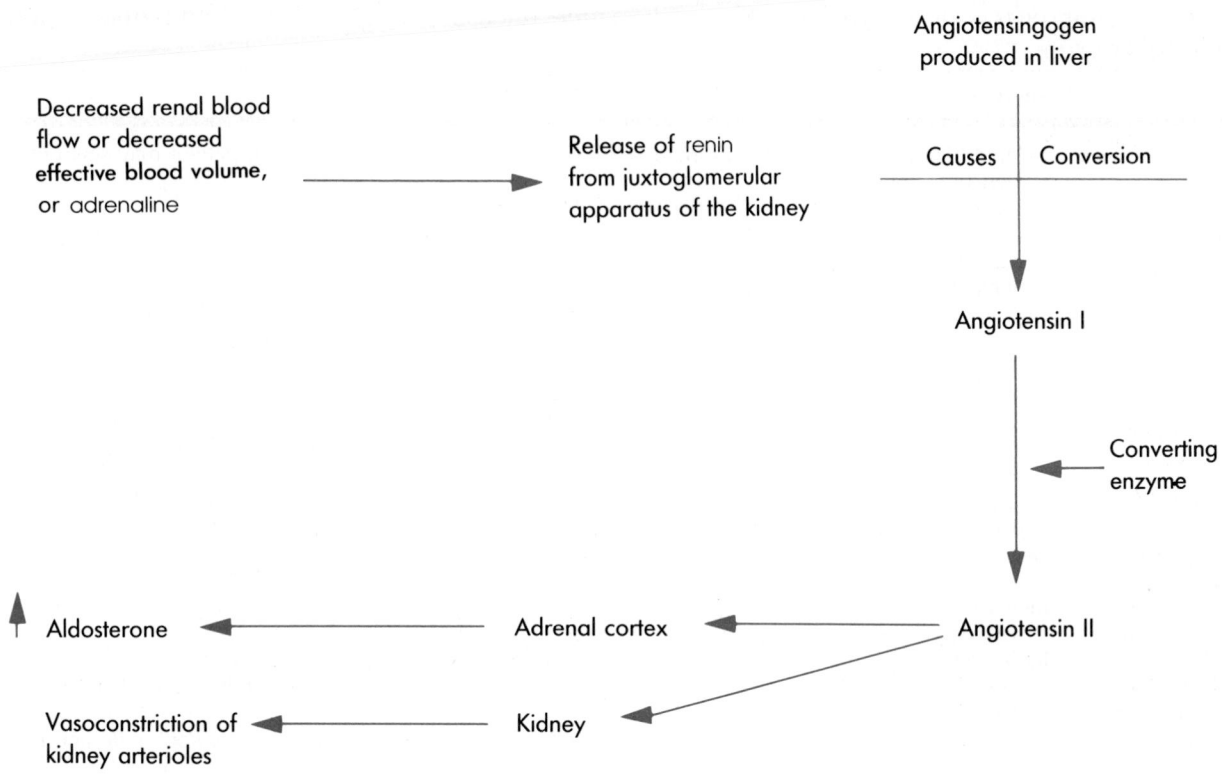

Fig. 5-3   Renin–angiotensin–aldosterone system.

functioning. Some people respond to most stressors in one characteristic mode; however, this limits their ability for adaptation when new stressors occur that interfere with this coping mode. For example, people who generally respond to stressors by physical activity are severely hampered when an illness (stressor) occurs that decreases physical mobility. People who have developed several coping strategies are better able to cope effectively with new stressors.

Defence Mechanisms

Defence mechanisms are unconscious processes used by individuals in adjustment to life stressors. They evolve during personality development and serve to protect the personality, satisfy emotional needs, maintain harmony between conflicting tendencies, and reduce tension or anxiety by modifying reality to make it more acceptable. Defence mechanisms are compromise solutions.

There are two levels of defence mechanisms: those that are considered more primitive and those that are of a higher level. Defence mechanisms are used by mentally healthy people as well as by those who are neurotic or psychotic. In the mentally healthy, defence mechanisms are used less frequently, and those mechanisms of a more primitive kind are avoided. Defence mechanisms become pathological when they are overused.

A defence mechanism is effective when it succeeds in easing intrapsychic tensions. When lower level defence mechanisms fail, a more pathological process evolves, and

the person exhibits psychiatric symptoms. All defence mechanisms are unconscious with the exception of suppression. Two defence mechanisms, denial and repression, are frequently manifested by the hospitalized patient and are discussed in more detail in the following section.

Denial

One of the defence mechanisms used frequently in dealing with illness is denial. This mechanism occurs during the early stages of crisis after the initial stressful impact. Denial of the illness helps the person deal with increased tension by protecting the ego (self) from reality. The pattern used by the person is similar to games played by children when they close their eyes and believe no one can see them. "It's not there because I don't see it." That which cannot be perceived is therefore not painful.

During denial intolerable thoughts are disowned. The ego gets rid of unwelcome facts (such as an illness) while still retaining its faculty for reality testing. The person manifests denial by disowning any body changes. For example, patients with coronary disease may deny they have had heart attacks and blame their discomfort on indigestion. Patients may even deny the severity of the pain and act as though the pain were not present.

Denial works well for the person who has been independent and has a self-image of a strong, self-made individual or who views sickness as a sign of weakness. Denial can be complete or partial and includes a "splitting"

Table 5-1 Systemic effects of adrenaline and noradrenaline release during the neuroendocrine response to stressors

Organ	Effects
Brain	Dilated blood vessels resulting in increased blood flow; increased metabolism; patient may seem more alert or restless
Eyes	Pupil dilation; patient appears startled
Heart	Dilated coronary blood vessels with increased blood flow; increased heart rate and contractility; patient's cardiac output and stroke volume may increase if the heart is able to keep up with icreased demand
Peripheral vascular system	Constriction of arterioles to skin, mucosa, renal, and abdominal, viscera, with decreased blood flow; increased constriction of veins with increased venous return; skin is cool and pale; urine output may be decreased; ischaemia with resultant tissue death and failure of kidneys and abdominal viscera may occur; toe temperature may be decreased
Lungs	Dilation of pulmonary vascular bed; bronchodilation; increased rate and depth of respiration; oxygen uptake and excretion of CO_2 increases; and the patient may show respiratory alkalosis ($\downarrow$ pCO_2 and $\uparrow$ pH)
Gastrointestinal tract (GI)	Decreased motility and secretion; production of mucus is decreased and with decreased blood flow patient may have irritation of GI tract and GI bleeding
Exocrine pancreas	Decreased secretions
Endocrine pancreas	Decreased insulin secretion
Liver	Increased gluconeogenesis and glycogenolysis; decreased glycogen synthesis; these processes along with decreased insulin and decreased glucose uptake may result in hyperglycaemia
Adipose tissue	Increased lipolysis and fatty acid production; serum may show increased triglycerides or cholesterol
Skeletal muscle	Increased muscle glucogenolysis; decreased glucose uptake, increased contractility; generalized muscle tension may be evident
Skin, sweat glands	Decreased blood flow, increased localized secretion of sweat; piloerection; skin is cool, pale and moist; goose bumps may be evident

From Phipps WJ, *et al*: *Medical-surgical nursing: concepts and clinical practice,* ed 4, St Louis, 1991, Mosby–Year Book.

of thoughts, feelings, and actions; for example, the patient may own the thoughts but deny the feelings.

Approaches that may be useful when working with the person exhibiting denial include the following:

1. Explore fears and anxieties underlying the denial.
2. Avoid direct confrontation of denial.
3. Assist person in controlling selected aspects of care.
4. Provide reassurance of the person's worth as a human being despite being in a dependent state.
5. Reinforce behaviours indicating reality acceptance.
6. Set limits kindly but firmly when denial behaviour interferes with treatment.

Regression

Regression is a defence mechanism often seen in people who are ill, because regression facilitates acceptance of the patient role. Regression makes a dependency relationship possible because of the individual's reversion to behaviour patterns of an earlier level of development. Illness necessitates patients placing themselves in the hands of competent others. They often become self-centered and concerned only with their own needs and interests. These interests focus on what is happening to the person and on their acceptance or rejection by caregivers. Often regression helps patients promote conservation of energy.

Approaches that may be useful when working with the person exhibiting regression include the following:

1. Explore the observable behaviour with the patient.
2. Discuss the patient's goals.
3. Discuss the patient's unreadiness to attain goals and revise as appropriate.

Table 5-2 Types of coping strategies

Category	Examples
Action	Taking walks, washing floors, gardening
Cognitive	Problem solving
Intrapsychic	Religion, activities to search for meaning of stress
Interpersonal	Use of support people, talking it over with someone
Emotional	Use of defence mechanisms, such as denial

Specific Behavioural Responses

Stressors and the stress response lead to behaviours that are either adaptive or maladaptive. People who display adaptive behaviour are those who make appropriate use of their coping mechanisms and do not exhibit symptoms of psychological disturbance. Those with maladaptive behaviour are at the end of the spectrum (Fig. 5-4 on p. 70); their psychiatric symptoms are a way of dealing with the increased stress. (For further information on maladaptive behaviour consult a psychiatric–mental health text.) Anxiety and other common behaviours resulting from the stress of illness are discussed in the following section.

Anxiety

Anxiety is a psychological response to stressors with both physiological and psychological components. It is a feeling of dread or uneasiness from an unrecognized source. Anxiety results when a person perceives a threat to the self

---

5-1

Systemic effects of cortisol release during the neuroendocrine response to stressors

Metabolic effects

Maintains blood glucose by:
  Increasing gluconeogenesis
  Decreasing glucose uptake by many body cells, particularly muscle
Increases protein catabolism, which provides substrate for glucose formation
Promotes lipolysis to provide alternative nutrient sources

Fluid and electrolyte effects

Promotes sodium and water retention
Promotes potassium excretion

Antiinflammatory/immunosuppressive effects

Decreases eosinophils, basophils, monocytes, and lymphocytes in the circulation
Increases neutrophil (polymorphonuclear leukocytes) by movement from bone marrow and circulatory pools
Decreases leukocyte accumulation at infalmmatory sites
Inhibits release of inflammatory substances (kinins, prostaglandins, leukotrienes)
Degrades collagen
Decreases scar tissue formation
Decreases lymphoid tissue mass, participation of T-lymphocytes in cellular-mediated immunity, and production of interleukin 1 and 2

Miscellaneous effects

Maintains emotional stability
Increases red blood cell formation
Possibly increases platelet formation
Increases gastric acid and pepsin production
Is permissive for other hormones and catecholamines (cortisol is necessary for the full functioning of some other hormones and catecholamines), particularly in relation to blood pressure control, cardiac output, and metabolic effects of adrenaline and noradrenaline.

From Phipps WJ, et al: *Medical-surgical nursing: co ncepts and clinical practice,* ed 4, St Louis, 1991, Mosby–Year Book.

5-2

Overall effects of an effective stress response

Increased glucose and fatty acids for energy
Increased oxygen uptake
Increased excretion of CO_2
Maintenance of blood volume and cardiac output
Increased muscle activity
Increased mental alertness

---

anxiousness manifested by behavioural changes is communicated interpersonally. Highly anxious people can transmit the sense of anxiousness to others; for example, a very anxious patient can heighten a family member's anxiety and vice versa.

Although the ego attempts to deal with anxiety through the use of defence mechanisms, certain degrees of anxiety are reflected in behaviours resulting from a discharge of energy necessary to restore equilibrium. These responses range from behaviour that is adaptive to behaviour that is considered, by our social standards, maladaptive (see Fig. 5-4, overleaf). The types of behavioural reactions that occur are influenced by psychosociocultural factors, basic personality development, past experiences, values, and economic status. Because anxiety is so common, assessment criteria, nursing diagnoses, outcomes, and interventions are discussed in detail in the Nursing Process section of this chapter.

Aggressive behaviour

Whenever self-concept is threatened, individuals may respond by aggression, a way that makes them feel less helpless and more powerful. Aggression is one way of handling anxiety. People are often angry at the loss of health status and question what is happening to them. They become irritable and uncooperative and may project their anger on others and become demanding. Expression of anger in socially acceptable ways prevents anger from being turned inward, causing depression.

Approaches that prove to be useful when working with a person exhibiting aggressive behaviour include the following:

1. Provide opportunities for the person to express feelings and the reasons for the feelings.
2. Accept expressions of hostility without retaliation or making the person feel guilty.
3. Anticipate the demands of the patient.
4. Maintain eye contact with the patient.
5. Approach patient in calm, direct manner without any signs of aggression.
6. Decrease environmental stimuli.
7. Set limits.
8. Provide outlets, if possible, for increased psychomotor activity within the confines of the hospital unit.
9. Chemical or physical restraints are used only if all other measures fail and the person becomes harmful to others or to self.

either physically or psychologically (such as to self-esteem, body image, or identity).

Anxiety is manifested in different levels ranging from mild to severe.[62] In Box 5-3, overleaf, note the changes in the way the person relates to the environment associated with the different levels of anxiety. Awareness, which is heightened with mild anxiety, begins to decrease until the panic stage, in which perceptions of the environment become distorted. People can vacillate among the several levels of anxiety. The level of anxiety engendered and its manifestations depend on the person's maturity, understanding of need, level of self-esteem, and coping mechanisms.

Anxiety is a psychological response that cannot be seen; it is only implied by the individual's actions. The state of

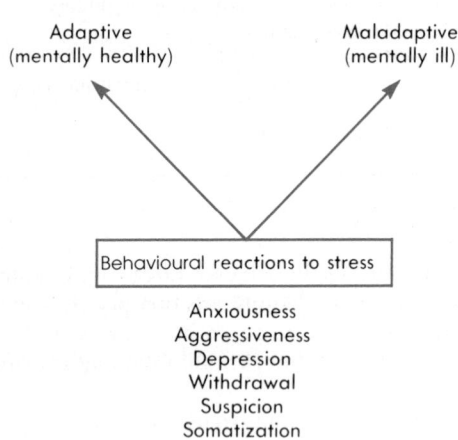

Fig. 5-4 Behavioural responses of persons experiencing anxiety from stress, such as illness, range from adaptive to maladaptive behaviour.

5-3	Levels of anxiety	
	Level	**Behaviour patterns**
	Mild anxiety	Increased alertness
		Quick eye movements
		Increased hearing ability
		Increased awareness
	Moderate anxiety	Decreased awareness of environmental details
		Focus on selected aspects of self (or illness)
	Severe anxiety	Disturbances in thought patterns
		Incongruency of thoughts, feelings, and actions
		Perceptual field greatly decreased
	Panic	Distorted perceptions of environment
		Inability to see or understand situation
		Unpredictable responses
		Random motor activity

Depressed behaviour

Depression is a normal response to illness, once the illness has been accepted. The person may describe feelings of sadness or unhappiness. Some common signs of depressed behaviour include the following:

1. Decreased interaction with others.
2. Lack of interest in activities or environment.
3. Voiced concern about illness and amount of care required.
4. Expressed wish for or concerns about dying.
5. Dependent behaviour.
6. Decreased activity.
7. Complaints of fatigue or inability to sleep.
8. Crying spells.

Any expressions about suicide should be taken seriously and the person referred for immediate counselling.

Approaches useful when working with a person exhibiting depressed behaviour include the following:

1. Approach the patient in a serious mood.
2. Convey by action and communication an understanding of what the person must be feeling.
3. Help the person express feelings.
4. Convey acceptance of the right to feel sad.
5. Listen to the person so that the anger can be turned outward.

Withdrawn behaviour

Withdrawal is commonly noted during illness. It permits the person to conserve mental and physical energy needed to deal with stressors and to promote repair and restoration. Withdrawn patients usually do not pose many problems and are apt to be labelled "good" patients. They demand little from others and thus may be overlooked. Withdrawn patients regress more easily to earlier levels of behaviour at which they can accept the patient role. They may have feelings of low self-worth.

Approaches that may be useful when working with the withdrawn person may include the following:

1. Spend time with the person, even if you are both silent, to increase the person's self-worth.
2. Provide gentle encouragement to talk, express feelings, and relate to others.

Suspicious behaviour

A sense of powerlessness or lack of control as a result of stressors and the stress response and anxiety may lead to suspicious behaviour. Suspicious patients have difficulty with trust and may have had previous experiences in which they learned to distrust others. They are often suspicious of the health care staff, the health care routines, the medicine, and the procedures. Whispered conversations by others within the person's hearing may reinforce feelings of suspiciousness that others are talking about the person.

Approaches that may be useful when working with people exhibiting suspicious behaviour may include the following:

1. Let the person talk about concerns but do not insist.
2. Keep promises made to the person to promote trust.
3. Avoid an overzealous approach, which may make the person more suspicious.
4. Provide explanations of procedures and routines so the person knows what to expect.
5. Avoid whispering or talking about the person within his or her hearing.

Somatic behaviour

A familiar reaction to illness is one that can be called *flight into illness*. Patients somaticize their concerns; that is, they have learned to express anxiety through complaints about a variety of physical symptoms. They may be preoccupied with body functions and feelings of pain. Vague complaints of backache, headache, or fatigue are expressed to legitimize the *attention needed*. Staff often become angry at patients who use somatic behaviour because of the frequent vague symptomatic complaints. Staff members feel "caught" if they minimize the symptoms, because there is always the possibility that the complaints are truly connected with an illness. Guilt on the part of staff prevails for some time if a complaining patient who was ignored is diagnosed as having a physical illness.

Approaches that may be useful for the person exhibiting somatic behaviour may include the following:

1. Accept all symptoms and report them.
2. Spend time with the person and listen to physical complaints with some limit setting.
3. Use a saturation technique to provide needed attention.

Nursing Process
Assessment

The conclusion that a person is demonstrating anxious behaviour can be made when several signs of anxiety are present. With mild anxiety the signs are fewer and less prominent. Signs of anxiety are more overt in people who are experiencing severe anxiety or panic.

Subjective data

Subjective data may include the following[12,21]:

1. States feeling apprehensive, uncertain, fearful, out of control, helpless, or anxious
2. States fears of unspecific consequences
3. States feeling overexcited, rattled, distressed, or jittery
4. States feeling tired and having difficulty sleeping

Data from the initial nursing history and the situation (such as proposed surgery, diagnostic tests) may provide clues to possible aetiologies.

The physiological signs of anxiety result from the stimulation of the sympathetic nervous system and the adrenal medulla. Restlessness and an increased awareness of the environment are early signs of anxiety. The person focuses more on the self as anxiety increases. Physiological signs usually begin with moderate anxiety and are more prevalent and intense during severe anxiety and panic.

Nursing analysis

The nursing analysis of *anxiety* is best qualified whenever possible by citing the anxiety level (mild, moderate, severe, or panic, as noted in Box 5-3). Possible *aetiologies* include the following[21]:

Threat to self-concept
Threat of death
Threat to or change in health status, socioeconomic status, role functioning, environment, or interaction patterns
Situational and maturational crises
Interpersonal transmission and contagion
Unmet needs

Planning: expected patient outcomes

The expected patient outcomes depend on the behaviours demonstrated by the anxious person; the outcomes indicate a decrease in the exhibited behaviours. Expected patient outcomes for the anxious person may include, but are not limited to, the following:

1. The person states feeling more relaxed and less anxious.
2. The person states sleep is improved.
3. Vital signs return to usual norms.
4. Elimination is regular.
5. Diaphoresis is decreased.
6. Muscles are relaxed and the person rests quietly.
7. The person demonstrates increased ability to follow directions.
8. The person demonstrates effective coping skills.

Implementation

Interventions for the person experiencing stressors and the stress response may include general interventions to reduce the effects of the stressor and the stress response, crises intervention for panic, specific support approaches, and additional stress management therapies.

General interventions to achieve patient outcomes

Nursing actions support the body's mechanisms for handling stressors and provide an environment that permits the person to mobilize defences.

Supporting protective mechanisms

Rest is absolutely essential with severe stressors and the stress response to maintain energy supply for metabolic functions essential for life. The person is kept comfortably warm but never overly warm, because overheating causes vasodilation and counteracts the arteriolar constriction necessary to ensure an adequate blood supply to vital organs.

Even a minor stress response can cause annoying discomforts such as backache, generalized muscle tension, and headache. These discomforts can act as additional stressors, and comfort measures such as back rubs, position changes, and back support to relax the muscles are indicated. Pain should be alleviated as much as possible, and noise and disturbance should be kept to a minimum. During a severe stress response, oral food and fluids may need to be withheld until nausea subsides and gastrointestinal tract activity returns to normal.

Providing structure

Structure decreases anxiety and is helpful for the person experiencing mild or moderate anxiety. Explanations are one method of providing structure. Each new experience should be explained to patients and, if possible, related to familiar experiences. The higher the level of anxiety, the more simple should be the explanations.

If patients are to have treatments or tests, they need to be given some idea of what will be done, the preparation involved, and the reasons why the procedure is necessary. To remove water jugs and inform patients that they cannot have any more water until after X-ray examinations can generate many anxious thoughts: "What X-ray examination?" "I wonder when it is?" "What will it be like?" "It must be something special if I can't have any water." Lack of knowledge as a cause of anxiety reflects the nurse's lack of consideration for patients' rights.

Explanations should be given in the patient's own terms, at appropriate times, and repeated as necessary. If the patient is very anxious, repeated explanation may be necessary, since extreme anxiety reduces intellectual function. It is useless to give explanations to patients who are severely anxious or sedated or to those who have high temperatures or severe pain. Repetition is often required for older people and children because they may have short attention spans or poor recent memory.

Time spent in giving explanations to relatives is not wasted. Not only does it relieve their anxieties, which may be transmitted to the patient, but it also saves having to untangle misinformation. Often the family is helpful in interpreting necessary instructions to the patient in a manner that the patient understands and accepts.

Promoting exploration of feelings

In most instances a large part of the nurse's work is to encourage patients to express anxieties, to help patients see the fear in their situations, to help them seek outlets for their fears and tensions, and to allay these negative feelings whenever possible. Nurses provide opportunities for the patient to talk, but they should not probe. There is a difference between prying into a patient's thoughts and beliefs and eliciting information that aids in the understanding of behaviour and in planning for care. Without seeming unduly curious, one can usually find some topic of personal interest to the patient that provides an opening. A picture on the bedside table may create such an example. Nurses who listen with sincere interest and without making judgments about the patient may begin to gain insight into the patient as a person. More important, the patient may begin to speak about personal fears.

As soon as the patient begins to talk about feelings, the nurse should proceed with conversation, taking cues from what the patient offers. The nurse who feels inadequate or anxious may cut off the conversation. For instance, if a patient says, "You know, I don't think I'll ever get to see my little boy again," a common response is, "Oh, don't say that, certainly you will; you're going to be all right," when the patient may very well not be all right. Would it not be better to respond, "What makes you feel this way?" Such a response helps the patient explore the subject and leaves opportunity for the patient to examine this concern. The nurse who is willing to listen to patients, to be guided by their reactions, and to work with them rather than to make decisions for them will give them needed emotional support. Solving patient's problems, even if it were possible, is not the aim of nursing. Indeed, it would tend to make patients less healthy psychologically.

The art of meaningful communication involves more than just listening; it includes moving the conversation so that the patient's attempts to communicate are assisted. Observing the patient for facial changes and general body movements provides opportunities for the nurse to discover from the individual the full meaning of the situation. For example, consider the patient who sucks in air while talking. The mouth becomes drier and drier as the tongue seems to stick in the mouth. These patients are not at ease and show anxiety even though their words may be quite innocuous. A simple statement such as, "Your mouth seems very dry. Would a glass of water help?" allows the nurse to clarify observations. Such an approach gives the patient a chance to tell what is being felt and to gain understanding by talking about it.

The nurse helps patients examine those problems that they are able to bring into awareness. Underlying problems should be handled by people trained in psychotherapy. A nurse needs to recognize normal anxiety reactions and to report exaggerated reactions that may indicate the need for psychiatric referral.

When any patient's anxiety increases to a high level, the nurse may need to sit with the patient. The nurse's presence is often reassuring. If possible, the patient is helped to recognize the anxiety by the nurse asking, "Are you uncomfortable?" or "What are you feeling?" In severe anxiety and panic, being there is most important, and touch may be used as a means of reassurance. Some severely anxious people, however, view touching as an intrusion of their personal boundary, and the nurse needs to keep this in mind. When the patient is able to talk, the nurse helps the patient to describe what is happening, what has happened, and what is expected to happen.

Supporting coping mechanisms

There is no one specific or best way to cope with any given situation. What is useful to one individual may be inappropriate for another. The nature of the stressor, the developmental level of the individual, the social and cultural environment, and the physical and interpersonal resources available all influence the style and effectiveness of coping strategies.

It is most useful to help a person to cope in ways that are congruent with previously established styles. Data must therefore be collected to identify the person's usual coping strategies. One method is by asking the question, "What do you usually do when things get tough?" Weisman suggests seven simple questions that may obtain a great deal of information about coping strategies[70]:

1. What problems, if any, do you see this illness creating?
2. How do you plan to deal with them?
3. When faced with a problem you must do something about, what do you do?
4. How does it usually work out?
5. To whom do you turn when you need help?
6. What has happened in the past when you have asked for help?
7. What kinds of problems usually tend to upset you or get you down?

These questions establish perception of the current problems, present and usual ways of dealing with problems, sources and responses to help, and recurrent problems that affect coping.

Stress management includes reinforcing appropriate coping mechanisms and helping the person explore alternative strategies if existing coping mechanisms are inappropriate.

Facilitating problem solving

Some people solve problems in a haphazard manner while others are very structured in their approach to problem solving. Problem solving can be a means for coping with stressors and the stress response and is more effective if the problem-solving steps are consciously followed. The steps include the following:

1. Gathering data
2. Identifying the problem (or effect of stressor)
3. Identifying factors affecting the problem or stressor
4. Determining goals
5. Exploring alternative ways and consequences to achieve the goals
6. Implementing actions
7. Evaluating effectiveness of actions

If the stressor has been identified, the nurse first assists the patient in exploring feelings and reactions associated with the stressor. Often people are not consciously aware of what they are feeling and therefore may select inappropriate actions. People vary in their ability to identify problems and in their desire to discuss personal feelings, although it is widely accepted that talking does help. If the patient is urged indiscriminately to talk about problems, the relationship becomes superficial and mechanical. The identification of the consequences of actions is often omitted but is an important component if problem solving is to be effective.

Problem solving reduces ambiguity and feelings of loss of control. People who do not generally employ conscious problem solving as a means of coping with stressors may benefit from learning about problem solving as a strategy for coping with stress.

Teaching relaxation techniques

Relaxation exercises are developed from the concept that the stress response with anxiety does not and cannot exist when the muscles of the body are relaxed. Relaxation exercises do not "cure" the stressors or the stress response but do help to minimize effects of the stress response and give the person a sense of control. A daily programme of relaxation exercises has an effect on physiological responses to stressors (for example, lowering of elevated blood pressure or elevated blood sugars) and in psychological responses to stressors (for example, decreased level of anxiety) (See Research Box 5-4). They are also helpful on a short-term basis when anxiety is present.

There are four basic components of relaxation techniques:

1. *Quiet environment*: deleting all possible noise and distractions
2. *Comfortable position*: sitting with no undue muscle tension
3. *Passive attitude*: emptying all thoughts from the conscious mind
4. *Mental device*: focusing on a sound, word, phrase, mental image, object, or breathing pattern to shift the mind from logical, externally oriented thoughts

The important factor is that the person empties the mind

Nursing Research 5-4

Monro BH, et al: Effect of relaxation therapy on post-myocardial infarction patient's rehabilitation, *Nurs Res* 37:231-235, 1988.

This experimental study involved 57 subjects (27 experimental, 30 control) who were participants in a U.S. cardiac rehabilitation programme. The study was designed to measure whether practising Benson's relaxation techniques resulted in improvement in psychosocial functioning as measured by Sickness Impact Profile, aerobic conditioning level (MET level), systolic and diastolic blood pressure, or heart rate. The study also explored the influence of behavioural style on the outcome measures.

The major finding was that diastolic blood pressure was reduced and maintained over a 3-month period. Systolic blood pressure was also reduced, but the reduction was not statistically significant. Subjects in this study showed improvement in psychosocial functioning, aerobic conditioning, and heart rates, but the practice of the relaxation techniques did not enhance these improvements. Behavioural style was not related to outcome measures.

The lack of significant findings for some of the outcome measures may have been related to the nonspecificity of the measures. For example, the measure of behaviour style did not contain many items regarding hostility and anger, which may be the most important factors of personality type related to coronary risk. The measure used to evaluate psychosocial functioning focused on illness rather than overall psychosocial functioning.

of all thoughts and concentrates on the mental device. It is natural for the mind to wander. When this occurs, the person simply redirects the mind back to the mental device. Each relaxation session should take approximately 20 minutes. One method is the progressive relaxation method (Box 5-5, overleaf).

Providing antianxiety medications

In some instances, the patient may be prescribed an antianxiety medication to reduce the anxiety symptoms. The antianxiety agents may be divided into two groups, the benzodiazepines and the nonbenzodiazepines (Table 5-3, overleaf). Note that the dosage is less for elderly people who metabolize the drugs slowly, resulting in a prolonged depressant effect. Dosage should also be reduced for people with impaired liver or kidney function.

The benzodiazepines are the most frequently prescribed antianxiety agents. These drugs act by inhibiting transmission of stimuli from the limbic system of the brain (septum, amygdala, and hippocampus). Side effects include drowsiness, dizziness, and weakness which are potentiated by other CNS depressants such as alcohol; ability to drive or operate machinery may be impaired.

Antianxiety agents produce muscle relaxation and a sense of wellbeing. The drugs are prescribed for short-term relief of anxiety but not for anxiety from daily stressors. Long-term therapy leads to increased tolerance and de-

5-5

Progressive relaxation

1. Assume a comfortable position in a quiet room
2. Begin by focusing on easy breathing
3. Tense specific muscle groups (see step 5) for 5 to 7 seconds, then relax quickly
4. Concentrate for 10 seconds on the sensations of the relaxed muscles
5. Follow a sequence, repeating each muscle group, tensing two or three times:
    a. Hand and arm: clench fist, pull elbow tightly, wrinkle nose, purse lips, smile with teeth tightly clenched
    b. Face: wrinkle forehead, close eyes tightly, wrinkle nose, purse lips, smile with teeth tightly clenched
    c. Neck: pull chin to chest
    d. Trunk: pull shoulder blades together, tighten stomach and buttocks
    e. Leg and foot: push down with leg, point toes upward (dorsiflexion) dominant leg first
6. Repeat process in any areas in which increased tension has been identified

pendence; larger doses are then needed to produce the desired effects.

The Committee on Safety of Medicines (CSM) has advised that benzodiazepines are indicated only for 2-4 weeks treatment if anxiety is severe and disabling; treatment for "mild" anxiety is not recommended.

SUMMARY

1. Adaptation is a process of interaction with the environment that promotes homeostasis and growth. Maladaptation leads to inadequate functioning.
2. Responses to stressors include neuroendocrine response, coping behaviours, defence mechanisms, and specific behavioural responses.
3. Response to stressors is influenced by the type of stimuli, the meaning of the stressor, perception of stressor, sense of control, coping resources, and health status.
4. The general adaptation syndrome consists of three stages: alarm reaction, resistance, and exhaustion. The first two stages occur frequently throughout life; death may ensue from exhaustion.
5. The physiological stress response consists of stimulation of the sympathetic nervous system, adrenal medulla, anterior and posterior pituitary glands, and the adrenal cortex.
6. The neuroendocrine response to stress is integrated by the hypothalamus.
7. Noradrenaline released by the sympathetic nervous system and the adrenal medulla primarily causes vasoconstriction of blood vessels of the skin, mucous membrane, and abdominal and pelvic organs, thus shifting blood to blood vessels of the heart, lung, and brain, which have been dilated by the action of adrenaline.
8. In addition to dilating selected blood vessels, adrenaline increases cardiac function, dilates bronchial smooth muscles, and alters metabolism to provide substrates for energy needs.
9. Cortisol, acting in concert with catecholamines, growth hormone, and glucagon, helps to mobilize substrates for energy.

10. Cortisol may also serve a major function by its antiinflammatory and immunosuppressive actions by dampening the stress response to prevent overactivity.
11. Water and sodium balance, osmolality, and blood volume are protected by the action of aldosterone and ADH, which are released during the neuroendocrine response to stressors.
12. Types of coping strategies include action, cognitive, intrapsychic, interpersonal, or emotional strategies.
13. Defence mechanisms are unconscious mechanisms used by individuals in adjustment to life stressors. Mentally healthy people use defence mechanisms occasionally, avoiding more primitive mechanisms.
14. Some specific behavioural responses to stressors include anxiety, aggressive behaviour, depressed behaviour, withdrawn behaviour, suspicious behaviour, and somatic behaviour.
15. Anxiety results when a person perceives a threat to the self, either physically or psychologically.
16. Anxiety may be mild, moderate, severe, or a state of panic. When anxiety increases, awareness of the environment decreases and physiological signs increase.
17. Rest and relief of discomfort conserve energy for coping with stressors and the stress response; providing explanations provides structure, which helps to decrease anxiety. Exploration of feelings helps to relieve tension associated with the stress response, and problem solving reduces feelings of loss of control associated with the stress response.
18. Relaxation is the opposite of the tension associated with the stress response; it also gives the person a sense of control. Basic components of relaxation techniques are quiet environment, comfortable position, passive attitude, and a mental device to remove externally oriented thoughts.
19. The most frequently prescribed antianxiety agents are the benzodiazepines. Alcohol or other CNS depressants should be avoided when taking antianxiety agents.

STUDY QUESTIONS

• Should you try to lead a life that is free from stressors? Explain.

Table 5-3 Antianxiety agents

Generic name	Usual adult dosage	Usual elderly dosage
Benzodiazepines		
Alprazolam	0.25-0.5 mg tid	0.25 mg bid/tid
Bromazepam	3-18 mg daily	1.5-9 mg daily
Chlordiazepoxide	10 mg tid	5 mg tid
Clobazam	20-30 mg daily	10-20 mg daily
Clorazepate	7.5-22.5 mg daily	7.5-15 mg daily
Diazepam	2-10 mg tid	2 mg tid
Lorazepam	1-4 mg daily	0.5-2 mg daily
Medazepam	15-30 mg daily	5-15 mg daily
Oxazepam	15-30 mg tid/qid	10-20 mg tid/qid
Nonbenzodiazepines		
Buspirone HCI	15-30 mg daily	Same as adult dosage
Chlormezanone	200mg tid/qid	100 mg tid/qid
Hydroxyzine HCI	50-100 mg qid	25-50 mg qid
Meprobamate	400 mg tid/qid	200 mg tid/qid

- Think back over several situations when you were experiencing the stress response. What type of physical symptoms did you experience? What is the physiological reason for each symptom that you experienced? Were the symptoms always the same? If not, state why.
- In what way(s) do you cope with stressors? What other coping strategies might be useful for you?
- Try the relaxation technique described in this chapter. Describe the sensations experienced during relaxation. How did you feel after completing the exercise? What types of difficulties did you have in carrying out the relaxation exercises? Identify a patient situation from your experience where you think relaxation exer-cises might have been a useful nursing intervention.

REFERENCES AND SELECTED READINGS

1.* Agras S: Panic: facing fears, phobias, and anxiety, New York, 1985, WH Freeman.

2.* Aguilera DC: Crisis intervention: theory and methodology, ed 6, St Louis 1989, Mosby–Year Book.

3. Beck C, Rawlins R, Williams S: Mental health—psychiatric nursing: a holistic life-cycle, ed 2, St Louis, 1987, Mosby–Year Book.

4.* Benner P, Wrubel J: The primacy of caring: stress and coping in health and illness, Menlo Park, Calif, 1989, Addison Wesley.

5. Berne RM, Levy MN: Physiology, ed 2, St Louis, 1988, Mosby–Year Book.

6.* Billings CV: Come here, nurse! Am J Nurs 86:915-916, 1986.

7.* Crockett MS: How a disabled, depressed patient learned to break an unhappy cycle, Am J Nurs 86:294-297, 1986.

8.* Dossey B: Awakening the inner healer, Am J Nurs 91:30-34, 1991.

9. Ebersole R, Hess R: Toward healthy aging: human needs and nursing response, ed 3, St Louis, 1990, Mosby–Year Book.

10. Gaillard RC, Al-DamLeiji S: Stress and the pituitary adrenal axis, Baillieres Clin Endocrinol Metab 1:319-354, 1987.

11.* Glod C: Psychopharmacology and clinical practice, Nurs Clin North Am 26:375-399, 1991.

12. Gordon M: Manual of nursing diagnosis 1991-1992, St Louis, 1991, Mosby–Year Book.

13. Granner D: Hormones of the adrenal medulla. In Murray RK, et al, editors: Harper's biochemistry, 21, New York, 1988, Lange Medical Books.

14. Groer MW, Shekleton ME: Basic pathophysiology: a holistic approach, ed 3, St Louis, 1989, Mosby–Year Book.

15. Guzzetta C: Effect of relaxation and music therapy on patients in a coronary care unit with presumptive acute myocardial infarction, Heart Lung 18:609-616, 1989.

16.* Harris B: Drugs and depression, Am J Nurs 86:292-293, 1986.

17.* Hillhouse J, Adler C: Stress, health, and immunity: a review of the literature and implications for the nursing profession, Holistic Nursing Practice 1991:5(4):22-31.

18.* Hornberger CA: Perceived stressors, perceived stress response, and level of cardiac reactivity in wellness sample, University of Kansas School of Nursing, Kansas City, 1989(unpublished master's thesis).

19. Johnson D: Metabolic and endocrine alterations in the multiple injured patient, Crit Care Nurs Q 11(2):35-41, 1988.

20. Karb V, Queener SF, Freeman JB: Handbook of drugs for nursing practice, St Louis, 1989, Mosby–Year Book.

21. Kim MJ, McFarland GK, McLane AM: Pocket guide to nursing diagnosis, ed 3, St Louis, 1989, Mosby–Year Book.

22. Kuhn MM: Pharmacotherapeutics: a nursing process approach, ed 2, Philadelphia, 1991, FA Davis.

23.* Lindsay AM, Carrieri VK: Stress response, In Lindsay AM, Carrieri VK, West CM, editors: Pathophysiological phenomenon in nursing: human responses to illness, Philadelphia, 1986, WB Saunders.

24. McCance K, Huether SE: Pathophysiology: the biologic base for disease in adults and children, St Louis, 1990, Mosby–Year Book.

25. McEwen B, Brinton RE: Neuroendocrine aspects of adaptation, Prog Brain Res 72:11-26, 1987.

26. McKenry LM, Salerno E: Mosby's pharmacology in nursing, ed 17, St Louis, 1989, Mosby–Year Book.

27. Mellion MB: Exercise therapy for anxiety and depression:what are the specific considerations for clinical application? Postgrad Med 77(3):91-95, 1985.

28. Meyer D: Development of an instrument to measure perceived environmental stressors of surgical intensive care patients, University of Kansas, Kansas City, 1985 (unpublished master's thesis).

29.* Minot SR: Depression: what does it mean? Am J Nurs 86:283-287, 1986.

30. Moos R: Coping with physical illness, ed 2, New York, 1985, Plenum Publishing.

31. Munro BH, et al: Effect of relaxation therapy on post-myocardial infarction patient's rehabilitation, Nurs Res 37, 231-235, 1988.

32.* Owen PL: A dozen tasks vie for your attention at the same time, with no respite in sight—what can you do to keep stress at bay? Am J Nurs 86:52-53, 1986.

33. Pender NJ: Effects of progressive muscle relaxation training on anxiety and health locus of control among hypertensive adults, Res Nurs Health 8(1):67-72, 1985.

34.* Roberts J, et al: Coping revisited: the relation between appraised seriousness of an event, coping responses and adjustment to illness, Nurs Pap 19:45-54, 1987.

35. Robinson L: Stress and anxiety, *Nurs Clin North Am* 25:935-943, 1990.

36. Shoemaker W, et al, editors: *Textbook of critical care*, ed 2, Philadelphia, 1989, WB Saunders.

37. Stevens K: Patients' perception of music during surgery, *J Adv Nurs* 15:1045-1051, 1990.

38. Symposium on anxiety disorders, *Psychiatr Clin North Am* 8(1):1-179, 1985.

39. Axelrod J, Reisine T: Stress hormones: their interaction and regulation, *Science* 224:452-453, 1984.

40. Ballard KS: *Identification of environmental stress for patients in the surgical intensive care unit*, University of Kansas, Kansas City, 1979 (unpublished master's thesis).

41. Benson H: *The relaxation response*, New York, 1975, William Morrow.

42. Cannon WD: Stresses and strains of homeostasis, *Am J Med Sci* 189:1-14, 1935.

43. Cannon WB: *The wisdom of the body*, New York, 1963, WW Norton.

44. Caplan G: *Principles of preventative psychiatry*, New York, 1964, Basic Books.

45. Carlson CE, editor: *Behavioral concepts and nursing interventions*, ed 2, Philadelphia, 1978, WB Saunders.

46.* Clarke M: Stress and coping: constructs for nursing, *J Adv Nurs*, 9:3-13, 1984.

47. Cox T: *Stress*, New York, 1978, Macmillan Press.

48. Curtis J, Detert R: *How to relax*, Palo Alto, Calif, 1981, Mayfield Publishing.

49. Danskin D, Crow M: *Biofeedback: an introduction and guide*, Palo Alto, Calif, 1981, Mayfield Publishing.

50. Hetzel BS, et al: Changes in urinary 17-hydroxy-corticosteroid excretion during stressful life situations in man, *J Clin Endocrinol* 15:1057-1068, 1955.

51. Hoff LA: *People in crisis: understanding and helping*, Menlo Park, Calif, 1984, Addison-Wesley.

52. Hyman RB, Woog P: Stressful life events and illness onset: a review of crucial variables, *Res Nurs Health* 5:155-163, 1982.

53.* Jasmin SA, Hill L, Smith N: Keeping your delicate balance: the art of managing stress, *Nurs 81* 11(6)52-57, 1981.

54.* Jupp H, et al: Group cognitive/anxiety management, *J Adv Nurs* 9:573-580, 1984.

55. Kogan HN, Betrus P: Self-management: a nursing mode of therapeutic influence, *Adv Nurs Sci* 6:55-73, 1984.

56. Lazarus R: *Patterns of adjustment*, New York, 1976, McGraw Hill.

57. Lazarus R: *Psychological stress and the coping process*, New York, 1966, McGraw Hill.

58. Lazarus RS, Folkman S: *Stress, appraisal and coping*, New York, 1984, Springer Publishing.

59. Lenox RH, et al: Specific hormonal and neurochemical responses to different stressors, *Neuroendocrinology* 30: 300-308, 1980.

60. Mason JW: A re-evaluation of the concept of nonspecificity in stress theory, *J Psychiatric Res* 8:323-333, 1971.

61. Mason J: *Specificity in the organization of neuroendocrine response profiles*. In Seeman P, Brown GM, editors: *Frontiers in neurology and neuroscience research*, First International Symposium of the Neuroscience Institute, University of Toronto, 1974.

62. Peplau H: *A working definition of anxiety*. In Burd S, Marshall M, editors: *Some clinical approaches to psychiatric nursing*, New York, 1963, Macmillan Publishing.

63.* Selye H: *Stress in health and disease*, Sevenoaks, 1976, Butterworth.

64.* Selye H: *Stress without distress*, New York, 1975, New American Library.

65. Selye H: The general adaptation syndrome and the diseases of adaptation. *J Clin Endocrinol* 6:117-230, 1946.

66. Selye H: *The stress of life*, rev ed, New York, 1976, McGraw-Hill.

67. Selye H: The stress syndrome, *Am J Nurs* 65:97-99, 1965.

68. Shontz F: *The psychological aspects of physical illness and disability*, New York, 1975, Macmillan Publishing.

69.* Sutterley DC: Stress and health: a survey of self-regulation modalities, *Top Clini Nurs* 1(1): 1-29, 1979.

70.* Weisman A: *Coping with cancer*, New York, 1979, McGraw-Hill.

*Recommended for student reading.

Common Problems Encountered in Adult Nursing

6

Fluid and Electrolyte Imbalances

Mary Kay Lehman
Barbara Soltis

After studying this chapter, the learner should be able to:

- Describe the mechanisms for maintaining fluid and electrolyte balance.
- Describe the effects of fluid deficit and excess.
- Describe the mechanisms and effects of deficits and excesses of sodium, potassium, calcium, and magnesium.
- Describe the mechanisms that maintain acid–base balance.
- Describe the causes and effects of metabolic and respiratory acidosis and alkalosis.
- Identify data indicating fluid or electrolyte imbalances.
- Develop a nursing care plan for a patient with a fluid and electrolyte imbalance.

The *internal environment* is a term used to describe body water and the constituent electrolytes and other dissolved substances that sustain all the physiological processes that maintain life. The amount and distribution of water in the various body compartments, as well as the type and amount of electrolytes and nonelectrolytes dissolved in the water, are kept in an extremely delicate balance by a number of control mechanisms. These mechanisms are so effective that normal values have been established for all constituents of the internal environment in healthy individuals. Knowledge of these normal values is used for detection and correction of imbalances that occur during illness.

The assessment and maintenance of a patient's fluid and electrolyte balance is a major nursing responsibility. This chapter describes some basic information about water and electrolytes in the body and the causes and effects of common fluid and electrolyte imbalances. The last part of the chapter discusses nursing measures employed to prevent, identify, and alleviate these imbalances and to relieve discomfort.

BASIC MECHANISMS OF FLUID AND ELECTROLYTE BALANCE

Body Water

A large percentage of body weight is composed of water containing dissolved particles of organic and inorganic substances vital to life. A newborn infant's weight is approximately 75% water, whereas a young adult male's is about 60% and a female's 50%. The percentage of body weight that is water gradually declines with age. Because fat contains little water, the more obese an individual is, the smaller the percentage of weight that is water. Both obese and aged persons have increased risk of morbidity and mortality in situations involving fluid loss because they have less fluid reserve on which to draw.

Fluid distribution

Fluid and electrolytes are found in the body either within the cell (*intracellular*) or outside the cell (*extracellular*). The extracellular fluid (ECF) is contained in two compartments: the *interstitial* fluid (fluid between the cells) and *intravascular* fluid (fluid in the blood vessels). The largest percentage of body water is located in the billions of individual body cells.

Fluid balance

Body fluid is constantly being lost and must be replaced for normal processes to continue. With an average daily intake of food and liquids, the healthy body easily maintains compartmental balance. The body receives water from ingested food and fluids and through metabolism of both foodstuffs and body tissues. Solid foods, such as meat and vegetables, contain 60% to 90% water. The normal daily replacement of water equals the normal daily loss. Easily measurable intake (liquid) and easily measurable output (urine) tend to be approximately equal, emphasizing the great need for recording patient fluid intake and output accurately.

Two vital processes demand continual expenditure of water: the removal of body heat by vaporization of water through the skin and lungs, and the excretion of urea and other metabolic wastes by the kidneys. The volume of water used in these processes varies greatly with external influences such as temperature and humidity.

Body Electrolyte Component

Types of body electrolytes

All body fluids contain chemical compounds. Chemical compounds in solution may be classified as electrolytes or nonelectrolytes on the basis of their ability to conduct an electric current in solution. *Electrolytes in solution break up into charged particles called ions.* Sodium chloride in solution exists as positively charged sodium ions, Na^+, and negatively charged chloride ions, Cl^-. *Positively charged ions are called cations. Negatively charged ions are called anions.* Proteins are special types of charged molecules. They have a charge that depends on the pH of the body fluids. At normal plasma pH (7.4) the proteins exist with a net negative charge. Nonelectrolytes such as urea, dextrose, and creatine remain molecularly intact and are essentially uncharged.

Each electrolyte has specific functions. *The general functions of all electrolytes are to (1) promote neuromuscular irritability, (2) maintain body fluid volume and osmolality, (3) distribute body water between fluid compartments, and (4) regulate acid-base balance.*

Distribution of body electrolytes

The three fluid compartments contain similar electrolytes, but the concentration of the electrolytes in each compartment varies greatly. Electrolytes move between compartments, but most of the exchange occurs between *interstitial* and *intravascular* fluids.

Differences in individual ion concentrations occur in various *extracellular* fluids. For instance, gastric secretion is acid; hence the concentration of hydrogen ions is high. Pancreatic secretion, on the other hand, is more alkaline than plasma and contains a high concentration of hydrogen carbonate. Gastric and pancreatic secretions and bile all contain high concentrations of sodium ions. Knowing the common electrolytes found in various body fluids is helpful in preventing depletion of necessary substances and in noting early signs of imbalance.

Electrolyte balance

In health the ratio of cations to anions in each of the body fluids and the concentration of the various ions in these fluids are relatively constant. Dietary intake and, in some instances, intravenous infusions are the routes by which an individual obtains a supply of electrolytes to replace daily losses and to keep the body in electrolyte balance. Electrolyte loss is mainly through the kidneys, with smaller losses through the skin and lungs and relatively minimal losses through the bowel. The kidneys selectively excrete certain electrolytes, retaining those needed for normal body fluid composition. Hormonal influences affect the kidneys' selective function. For example, the adrenocortical hormone aldosterone favours sodium reabsorption and the excretion of potassium.

Mechanisms for Fluid and Electrolyte Movement

Fluids, electrolytes, gases, and small molecules move freely through the semipermeable membranes that separate compartments. This movement occurs constantly as oxygen and nutrients are carried to cells and wastes are removed from cells by the blood. In spite of the constant movement of water and dissolved particles (*solutes*) back and forth, the actual amount of water and concentration of solutes in each compartment remain relatively unchanged when the body is functioning normally. *The mechanisms by which water and solutes move are osmosis, diffusion, and filtration.*

Osmosis

Osmosis is the movement of a solvent (water) through a semipermeable membrane from an area of lower concentration of solute to an area of higher concentration. The water moves to dilute the more highly concentrated solution until an equilibrium is reached on both sides of the semipermeable membrane. *The concentration of solute in any one compartment is called osmotic pressure or osmolality and is determined by* the *total number* of *dissolved particles per unit of solvent.*

Because of their large size, *protein molecules* normally have *little movement between compartments.* Their presence, especially in the intravascular fluid, creates a pressure called *colloid osmotic* or *oncotic* pressure, which *functions to hold water within the compartment.*

Diffusion

Diffusion is the movement of a solute from an area of greater concentration to an area of lesser concentration. This is known as *movement down a concentration gradient.* Diffusion includes dispersion of solute throughout the fluid within a compartment, as well as movement of the solute through a membrane that separates two compartments until its concentration is equal on both sides of the membrane. The semipermeable walls of blood vessels and cells contain tiny pores through which small molecules and electrolytes diffuse freely.

Large molecules such as glucose are too large to pass through membrane pores and are assisted in crossing the membrane by *carrier substances*; this process is known as *facilitated diffusion.*

Filtration

Filtration pressure is another means by which water and diffusible particles are moved through a membrane. Movement occurs because the weight or pressure of the fluid is greater on one side of the membrane than on the other. Filtration pressure is discussed later in this chapter in relation to normal exchange of water and solutes across capillary membranes.

Hormonal Control

Three hormones play a particularly vital role in maintaining fluid and electrolyte balance as follows:
1. *Antidiuretic hormone* (ADH)
   a. Is produced in the hypothalamus and stored and released from the posterior pituitary gland
   b. Acts on the renal tubules to retain water and to decrease urinary output
2. *Aldosterone*
   a. Is secreted by the adrenal cortex
   b. Acts on the renal tubules to reabsorb sodium and to excrete potassium
   c. Increases circulatory volume by reabsorbing water along with sodium
3. *Parathormone*
   a. Produced by the parathyroid glands
   b. Promotes absorption of calcium from the intestine
   c. Promotes release of calcium from bone
   d. Increases the excretion of phosphate ions by the kidneys

FLUID AND ELECTROLYTE IMBALANCE

Almost all medical–surgical conditions threaten fluid and electrolyte balance. There may be deficits or excesses of water or of any electrolyte. Actually, several imbalances occur simultaneously because of the interrelationship of body fluids and their electrolytes. For clarity, *imbalances of body fluid and of each ion are considered separately.*

Fluid Imbalances

Osmolality is determined by the total number of particles dissolved in a unit of solvent. The osmolality of body fluid is measured in milliosmols or thousandths of an osmol because the number of particles in solution is relatively small. Normal osmolality of body fluids is approximately 300 mOsm/L. Solutions relate to normal osmolality in the following ways:
1. *Isosmolar*: same osmolality as body fluids
2. *Hyposmolar*: less osmolality than body fluids
3. *Hyperosmolar*: greater osmolality than body fluids

When the body gains or loses fluid in excess of normal fluid balance, the intercompartmental fluid movement that occurs depends on whether the extracellular fluid becomes hyperosmolar or hyposmolar,[2] or remains isosmolar. The effects of different types of fluid imbalances are illustrated in Table 6-1.

Fluid loss

There are a number of ways in which body fluids and electrolytes contained therein are lost or made unavailable for normal fluid and electrolyte balance, as summarized in the list below.

Losses of fluid and electrolytes

Skin: diaphoresis, oozing from severe wounds or burns
GI tract: profuse salivation, vomiting, diarrhoea, GI drainage, enemas
Kidneys: diuretics, polyuria
Haemorrhage
Trapping of fluids: wound swelling, oedema, ascites, intestinal obstruction

Electrolyte Imbalances

Clinically, serum electrolytes are measured in millimoles per litre (mmol/l), but for an indication of the chemical combining activity of an electrolyte the unit milliequivalents per litre (mEq/l) is more useful. For example, 1 mEq of the cation sodium is available to combine with 1mEq of an

Table 6-1 Fluid imbalances

Pathophysiology		Signs and symptoms	Therapy
Isosmolar fluid deficit	Decreased body water and electrolytes; extracellular fluid remains isosmolar but volume decreases	Hypotension, increased pulse and respirations, cool skin, delayed vein filling, shock, decreased urinary output	Replacement of water sodium: oral intake of salty fluids; IV of normal saline
Hyperosmolar fluid deficit	Decreased body water more than decreased electrolytes; water moves out of cells to dilute extracellular fluid (cellular dehydration)	Thirst; skin flushed, dry, poor turgor; dry coated tongue; increased body temperature; increased haemoglobin and haematocrit levels; apprehension, restlessness	Water taken orally, if possible; IV of 5% dextrose in water; additional water given with tube feedings
Hyposmolar fluid excess (water intoxication)	Excess body water without excess electrolytes; water moves into cells, causing cells to swell	Behaviour changes, confusion, incoordination; sudden weight gain; warm moist skin; lethargy, convulsions	Water restriction; for severe signs, 3% to 5% sodium chloride IV
Isosmolar fluid excess (oedema)	Excess body water and sodium; excess fluid moves into extracellular spaces	Oedema of dependent body parts: pitting oedema over bony prominences; swollen, tight, shiny skin Pulmonary oedema: dyspnoea; wheezing cough with frothy sputum; cyanosis	Elevation of dependent part; treatment of underlying condition; diuretics, reduced salt intake; treatment of pulmonary oedema

anion such as chloride or hydrogen carbonate. The concentration of cations in blood serum or plasma is the same as the concentration of anions when expressed in terms of milliequivalents. This is a useful measurement of electrolytes as it gives information about the relationship between cations and anions. *No single electrolyte can be out of balance without causing some others to be out of balance.*

Sodium, potassium, and *calcium* are all *essential* for the *passage of nerve impulses.* Whenever the concentrations of any of these cations are increased or decreased in body fluids, the increase or decrease is reflected in the stimulation of muscles by nerves. The muscles may become weak and atonic because of inadequate stimulation, or they may become somewhat spastic because of excess stimulation. For example, a decrease in calcium concentration in body fluids causes the stimulus to be increased and results in muscle spasms. GI and cardiac symptoms, so often produced by electrolyte imbalances, result in part from changes in neural stimulation on the muscles of these systems.

With *cation imbalances,* the *distribution of body fluids* is *frequently upset.* Abnormal collections of fluid probably cause some of the GI symptoms such as nausea, vomiting, and diarrhoea. Decreased amounts may cause anorexia, dyspepsia, and constipation. It is thought that oedema of cerebral tissues may be responsible for headache, convulsions, and coma.

Sodium

Sodium deficit (hyponatraemia)

The normal concentration of sodium in the blood is 138 to 145 mmol/l. A low sodium level in the blood (*hyponatraemia*) can indicate either a deficit of sodium or an excess of water. Whenever sodium is lost from the body fluids, *the osmotic pressure of the ECF decreases and water diffuses into the cell, where there is greater osmotic pressure.*

The *plasma volume is then decreased,* and *symptoms of hypovolaemia may be present.* In response to this reduction of the sodium concentration in the extracellular fluid, potassium moves out of the intracellular fluid. Therefore, the patient with sodium imbalance is also likely to have a potassium imbalance.

Sodium depletion results most often from the loss of GI secretions. It can also occur from losses through the skin and in the shifting of body fluids so that the sodium is not accessible for use.

Anyone who is perspiring profusely because of environmental conditions, exercise, or fever is losing large amounts of both sodium and water. If salt is not replaced with water, such as by drinking salty fluids, water intoxication occurs. The ability of the cells to depolarize and repolarize normally is impaired in sodium deficit.

Treatment of shock, if present, is the first concern. Saline solution, usually 0.9% sodium chloride, *is given intravenously* at a *rapid* rate. Plasma expanders may also be infused.

If other electrolytes (potassium, calcium, hydrogen carbonate) have been depleted, these also need to be replaced. Treatment that alleviates the underlying cause will prevent further sodium loss. Salt or salty foods are added to the diet for sodium depletion, which develops slowly or follows profuse perspiration (diaphoresis) or vomiting.

Safety measures, such as the use of cot sides on the bed, supervision of ambulation, and frequent observation, are necessary if the patient becomes weak or confused or experiences marked hypotension.

Sodium excess (hypernatraemia)

A serum sodium level greater than 145 mmol/l is known as *hypernatraemia.* There are actually *two kinds of sodium excess, oedema* and *hypernatraemia.* When there is a *sodium* and *water excess, oedema exists*; when there is an *excess of sodium in relation to water* in the *extracellular compartment, hypernatraemia exists*.

Hypernatraemia does not necessarily indicate an excess of total body sodium.

If fluids are greatly limited or if excess salt is taken into the body and retained because of poor renal function, sodium may be concentrated in body fluids. Excess intravascular sodium causes fluid to be withdrawn from interstitial spaces. Extracellular fluids become hyperosmolar and draw water from the cells, causing cellular dehydration. If fluids are not given to dilute the sodium and if excretion of sodium is not increased, severe fluid and electrolyte disturbances occur, causing manic excitement, tachycardia, and eventual death.

Water alone is given to treat sodium excess. If cardiac and renal function is normal, a liberal amount of water is administered orally, or 5% dextrose in water is given intravenously. In the absence of normal cardiac and renal function, hydration must be carried out with caution to prevent fluid overloading in the patient.

Diuretics are of *value* in *removing sodium*. *If sodium excess is severe*, with or without excess water retention, and *does not respond to other treatment, renal dialysis may be necessary.*

Potassium

Potassium is the major cation of the cells. During the *formation of new tissue (anabolism)* or *when glucose is converted to glycogen, potassium enters the cell.* With *tissue breakdown (catabolism), potassium leaves the cell.* This occurs with trauma, dehydration, or starvation. The normal serum level of potassium is 3.5 to 5.0 mmol/l.

Potassium deficit (hypokalaemia)

A serum potassium level below 3.5 mmol/l is known as hypokalaemia. The body's mechanism for conserving potassium is not as effective as that for conserving sodium, and the kidneys may excrete potassium even when the body needs it. *Whenever sodium is being retained in the body through reabsorption by the kidney tubules, potassium is excreted.* Thus *whenever aldosterone secretion is increased,* such as in *stress, potassium is excreted. Potassium depletion,* therefore, *is common* in *many diseases* and *injuries* and *during therapy such as surgery. Potassium* may also be *lost through the urine* as a *result of certain diuretics* such as the thiazides and frusemide.

The patient who has a balanced diet withheld for several days, is dehydrated, or is given large amounts of parenteral fluids with no replacement of potassium develops potassium depletion. Dilution of extracellular potassium by the administration of 5% dextrose without potassium supplements and potassium loss caused by catabolism of body proteins account for many electrolyte imbalances in the postoperative patient.

The practice of giving multiple enemas is becoming less common because it is now known that some of the enema fluid is absorbed and dilutes the potassium in the interstitial compartment, upsetting the balance between compartments. Solutions for hyperosmolar enemas may damage cells in the bowel mucosa, causing potassium loss.

Potassium has *a direct effect on cardiac and skeletal muscle function.* The patient with *potassium deficit* shows *characteristic electrocardiographic changes* of *flattened or inverted T waves with a prolonged Q-T interval* (see Chapter 16). The most *striking symptom of hypokalaemia is muscle weakness.* Digitalis toxicity can occur in patients taking cardiac glycosides if they develop hypokalaemia. With severe hypokalaemia, the patient may die unless potassium is administered promptly.

The *safest way to administer potassium is orally.* Fresh fruits (especially oranges and bananas) or foods high in protein are good sources of potassium. A potassium salt may be prescribed orally; if given in liquid form, it should be given in fruit or vegetable juice or chilled to increase palatability. When potassium is given intraven-ously, it must be diluted, and the rate of flow must be monitored closely to prevent hyperkalaemia and atrial arrest. The usual rate of infusion should not exceed 20 MMol of potassium per hour. Potassium is never given in a bolus or IV push.

Potassium excess (hyperkalaemia)

A serum potassium level greater than 5.0 mmol/l is termed hyperkalaemia. This condition does not occur as frequently as hypokalaemia, especially if renal function is normal.

As previously stated, *whenever there is severe tissue damage, potassium is released from the cells into the extracellular fluids.* Because shock usually accompanies this damage, renal function is reduced, and a high blood potassium level results. There is great danger in giving extra potassium to any patient with poor renal function. If the patient is dehydrated or has lost vascular fluid, glucose and water or plasma expanders usually are given until renal function returns. Untreated adrenal insufficiency also is a contraindication for giving potassium.

The *patient with hyperkalaemia develops spasticity of muscles* because of their overstimulation by nerve impulses. The patient *complains of nausea, colic, diarrhoea, and skeletal muscle spasms.* The muscles later become weak because the overstimulation produces an accumulation of lactic acid and because potassium is lost from the muscle cells.

If the condition is not controlled, overstimulation of the cardiac muscle causes the heartbeat to become irregular and eventually stop. ECG evidence of potassium elevation includes tall, peaked, symmetric, or tented T waves with a short Q-T interval. As the blood potassium level increases further, the QRS spreads and atrial arrest occurs.

If the patient who has hyperkalaemia needs a blood transfusion, *fresh* blood must be used. Cells in blood that has been stored for several days tend to release potassium during storage. A transfusion of stored blood may further increase the patient's serum potassium level.

When hyperkalaemia occurs, the patient is allowed nothing orally, and infusion of 10% glucose with 50 units of insulin is often given to induce transfer of potassium from the serum to the intracellular fluid. If the patient is in a state of acidosis (p. 89), correction of the situation results in movement of potassium back to the cell.

Sodium polystyrene sulphonate, a cation exchange resin, can be given orally or rectally. It results in the release of sodium and binding of potassium, with the potassium then excreted in the stool. If the patient is in renal failure or if the serum potassium is dangerously high, haemodialysis is necessary. The patient is placed on absolute bed rest until the potassium blood level is returned to normal.

Calcium

There is a considerable amount of calcium in the human body, most of it located in the bony skeleton and a small amount dissolved in body fluids. Serum calcium level must be maintained at a level of 2.1 to 2.6 MMol/L to maintain vital functions of neuromuscular irritability and blood clotting. Calcium is present in the blood in two forms: free ionized calcium and calcium bound to protein. Only ionized calcium is physiologically active. Both *parathyroid hormone* and *vitamin* D are necessary for normal absorption of calcium from the GI tract, for reabsorption of calcium from bone to maintain the normal serum calcium level, and for prevention of excess calcium loss in urine.

Calcium deficit (hypocalcaemia)

A *decrease in serum calcium level below 2.1 mmol/l is termed hypocalcaemia.* Some conditions lead to excessive calcium binding, such as the infusion of large amounts of blood containing citrate (citrate is a blood preservative and binds calcium) and alkalosis (more calcium is bound in an alkaline medium). When these conditions are present, the patient begins to show signs of calcium deficit, because, although the total amount of blood calcium is not changed, there is less physiologically active (unbound, ionized) calcium available.

Patients with pancreatic disease or disease of the small intestine may fail to absorb calcium from the GI tract, and they may excrete abnormally large amounts of calcium in the faeces, thus reducing the blood level of calcium. *Hypocalcaemia* may also occur during the diuretic phase of acute renal failure as calcium is excreted.

The *patient with a calcium deficiency* usually *first complains of numbness and tingling of the nose, ears, fingers, and toes.* If calcium is not given at that time, painful muscular spasms, especially of the feet and hands (carpopedal spasm), muscle twitching, and convulsions may follow (*tetany*).

The specific treatment for a low blood level of calcium is the administration of calcium salts orally or intravenously.

Calcium excess (hypercalcaemia)

A *serum calcium level above 2.6 mmol/l is called hypercalcaemia.* It may be caused by calcium leaving the bone and concentrating in the ECF (as seen in bone diseases such as cancer or with prolonged immobilization) or by increased intake and absorption of calcium.

Normal retention of calcium in the bones is believed to be caused by the pressure exerted on bones by active movement or exercise. When a large amount of calcium accumulates in the extracellular fluid and passes through the kidneys, calcium can precipitate and form stones (calculi), a not infrequent complication of immobilization. Calcium precipitates more readily in alkaline solution. This can be a problem in a urinary tract infection, which increases the alkalinity of the urine.

Treatment for hypercalcaemia is removal of the cause. Intravenous saline and a diuretic (frusemide) may be given to promote renal excretion of the calcium. Oral or intravenous phosphate may also be given because calcium is excreted when phosphorus serum levels are increased. Plicamycin, a potent antitumour drug, has been used successfully to reduce serum calcium. If the hypercalcaemia is caused by multiple myeloma or other cancers, glucocorticoids may be effective in reducing hypercalcaemia, either because they decrease the size of the tumour or because the effect of the tumour on bone is reduced.

Because persons with marked hypercalcaemia often are losing calcium from their bones or have malignant involvement of bone, special care should be taken to prevent pathological fractures. Great care must also be taken with any physical nursing activity, e.g. massage, and active or passive movements.

Careful *attention* must be *directed* to the *prevention of calcium stone formation in the kidneys.* Acid-ash fruit juices, cranberry and prune juice, or ascorbic acid can be given to promote urinary acidification and discourage stone formation. Urinary tract infections must be avoided. Good perineal care and meticulous technique in caring for indwelling catheters are mandatory.

Unless they are *contraindicated, people* with *hypercalcaemia are encouraged to drink 3000 to 4000 ml of fluids* per *day* to reduce the possibility of renal calculi and to overcome the thirst that accompanies hypercalcaemia.

Magnesium

The normal serum magnesium level is within the range of 0.75 to 1.0 mmol/l. About 50% of magnesium is located in bones, 5% in ECF, and the remaining 45% within the cells. It functions in the activation of enzymatic reactions, especially in carbohydrate metabolism. Magnesium has a sedative effect on the CNS similar to that of calcium. High serum levels result in vasodilation and lowering of blood pressure; this is a rare occurrence except with kidney failure.

Metabolically, magnesium is closely interrelated with both calcium and potassium. In the presence of a large amount of calcium in the GI tract, calcium is absorbed in preference to magnesium, and the magnesium is excreted. Conversely, low calcium levels increase magnesium absorption. The kidneys effectively conserve magnesium when intake is low.

Magnesium deficit (hypomagnesaemia)

Hypomagnesaemia is a serum magnesium level below 0.75 mmol/l. It may be caused by impaired absorption from the GI tract, excess loss through the kidneys, or prolonged malnutrition.

A low serum magnesium level leads to increased neuromuscular irritability. Hypomagnesaemia is usually manifested by behavioural and neurological symptoms such as confusion, hallucination, convulsions, increased reflexes, muscle spasms, and paraesthesias.

Nursing responsibilities for the patient with hypomagnesaemia include the following:
1. Encouraging foods high in magnesium (fruit, green vegetables, whole grain cereals, milk, meat, and nuts)

2. Careful observation and supervision of the patient who is confused or hallucinating
3. Providing for patient safety if convulsions occur

Magnesium excess (hypermagnesaemia)

Hypermagnesaemia is a serum magnesium level greater than 1.0 mmol/l. The action of magnesium is on the neuromuscular junction where a high magnesium level blocks acetylcholine release, decreasing the excitability of the muscle cells. Hypermagnesaemia rarely develops unless there is renal failure, although it has been identified in diabetic ketoacidosis where there is severe water loss. In people with renal failure, frequent use of magnesium-containing antacids or cathartics can cause toxicity. The vasodilating effect of magnesium is accentuated in hypermagnesaemia and can lead to hypotension. There may be loss of deep tendon reflexes, respiratory depression, and cardiac arrest.

Correction of the underlying cause corrects magnesium excess. If renal failure is present, dialysis is necessary. Intravenous calcium gluconate may be a useful temporary treatment, because calcium has an antagonistic effect on magnesium.

ACID–BASE BALANCE AND IMBALANCE
Regulation of Acid–Base Balance

Cells are sensitive to changes in the pH (hydrogen ion concentration) of body fluids. The maintenance of a stable pH of body fluids is essential to life. Normal body fluid is slightly alkaline (pH 7.35 to 7.45). A pH reading less than 7.35 is present in acidosis, and a reading greater than 7.45 is present in alkalosis. Limits of pH compatible with life are 7.0 to 7.8. The pH is kept relatively constant by the buffer systems in the body. Mechanisms that regulate acid–base balance include chemical buffer systems, the respiratory system, and the kidneys (Table 6-2, overleaf).

Buffer system

A *buffer is a substance that can act as a chemical sponge,* either soaking up or releasing hydrogen ions so that the pH remains relatively stable. The main buffer systems of the body are the carbonic acid–hydrogen carbonate system, the phosphate system, and protein. The carbonic acid–hydrogen carbonate system is the most important clinically. If this buffer system is stable, the other buffer systems are stable.

Two types of carbonate are present in body fluids—carbonic acid (H_2CO_3) and hydrogen carbonate (HCO_3^-). The ability of the body to keep the pH of body fluids within normal limits relies essentially on main-tenance of the normal ratio of *one part of carbonic acid to 20 parts of hydrogen carbonate* (Fig. 6-1).

Carbonic acid concentration is controlled by the lungs, because if carbon dioxide is retained in large amounts, more is available to combine with water to form carbonic acid in the following chemical reaction:

$$CO_2 + H_2O \rightleftarrows H_2CO_3$$

The amount of carbon dioxide expelled is varied by the rate and depth of respiration.

Hydrogen carbonate concentration is controlled by the kidneys, which selectively retain or excrete hydrogen carbonate, depending on body needs.

Respiratory control of pH

The respiratory control centre in the brain responds to increases of carbon dioxide and hydrogen ions in body fluids. Rate and depth of respiration are in turn controlled by the respiratory control of pH as follows: (1) when pH decreases (more acid), respiratory rate and depth are increased, and there is greater excretion of carbon dioxide through the lungs; thus less carbon dioxide is present to produce carbonic acid by the reaction: $CO_2 + H_2O \rightleftarrows H_2CO_3$, and the pH increases towards alkalinity; and (2) when pH rises above the normal range (more alkaline), the respiratory centre is depressed, rate and depth of respiration decrease, carbon dioxide is retained, and more carbonic acid is formed, moving the pH towards acidity.

Because carbon dioxide is constantly being formed as a product of metabolism, the concentration of carbon dioxide in the body must be continuously balanced between the rate of metabolism and the rate of pulmonary excretion. *The buffering capacity of the respiratory system is more than double that of all the chemical buffers combined.*

Renal regulation of pH

Both chemical buffers and respiratory regulation have limited ability to make complete adjustments in pH, and it remains for the kidneys to make permanent adjustments in the pH of body fluids. The renal regulation of pH is effected by control of the retention or excretion of hydrogen carbonate and hydrogen ions. The kidneys usually excrete an acid urine because of the excess of acid metabolic products (non-volatile acids), which must be eliminated by the renal route. Normally, almost all of the hydrogen carbonate formed by the kidneys is retained.

Hydrogen ions secreted by kidney tubule cells and hydrogen carbonate filtered into the glomerular filtrate combine in the kidney tubules to form carbon dioxide and water, which are excreted through exhalation (CO_2) and in urine (H_2O). In acidosis, excess hydrogen ions are secreted

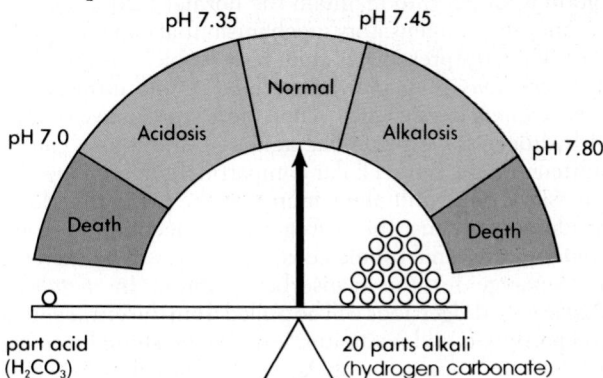

Fig. 6-1   Note that the relationship of 1 part carbonic acid to 20 parts hydrogen carbonate maintains hydrogen ion concentration (pH) within normal limits. Increase in H_2CO_3 or decrease in HCO_3^- causes acidosis; similarly, decrease in H_2CO_3 or increase in HCO_3^- causes alkalosis. (Redrawn from Abbott Laboratories: *Fluid and electrolytes*, North Chicago, 1970, Abbott Laboratories.)

Table 6-2 Mechanisms regulating acid–base balance

	Action time	Effect
Chemical buffers in cells and body	Instantaneous	Combine with acids or bases added to the system to prevent marked changes in pH
Respiratory system	Minutes to hours	Controls CO_2 concentration in ECF by changes in rate and depth of respiration
Kidneys	Hours to days	Increases or decreases quantity of $NaHCO_3$ in ECF
		Combines HCO_3^- or H^+ with other substances and excretes them in urine

into the kidney tubules, where they combine with buffers and are excreted in the urine. In alkalosis, hydrogen carbonate ions enter the tubules, where there is a lack of the hydrogen ions with which they normally combine to form carbonic acid; the hydrogen carbonate ions combine instead with sodium or other cations and are excreted in the urine. Hydrogen ions can be exchanged for sodium and potassium ions in the kidney tubules; therefore excretion or conservation of hydrogen ions can result in imbalances of sodium and potassium.

Compensation

Carbonic acid (H_2CO_3) excess or deficit is referred to as *respiratory* acidosis or alkalosis, whereas base hydrogen carbonate change is called *metabolic* acidosis or alkalosis.

Maintenance of the 1:20 ratio of carbonic acid to hydrogen carbonate is crucial to keeping serum pH within the normal range. Actual amounts of both hydrogen carbonate and carbonic acid may vary, but the pH remains normal as long as the 1:20 ratio exists. For example, if the P_{CO_2} indicator of carbonic acid rises, the hydrogen carbonate rises to keep the normal ratio between these two substances intact. This effort of the body to maintain normal pH when acidosis or alkalosis occurs is known as *compensation*.

In compensation, the kidneys attempt to compensate for changes in blood CO_2 by making a corresponding change in blood *hydrogen carbonate*, and the lungs attempt to compensate for abnormal changes in blood hydrogen carbonate by making corresponding changes in blood CO_2. Compensation is an effort to maintain the normal 1:20 ratio.

Another compensatory mechanism that can be used by the body in the presence of acid–base problems is *shifting of hydrogen ions from the extracellular to the intracellular compartment or vice versa*. When there is an increased level of hydrogen ions (metabolic acidosis), these ions can be shifted into the intracellular compartment in exchange for *potassium*. This shift alone increases the pH in the blood. In addition, because the hydrogen ion concentration is now higher in the renal tubule cells, hydrogen will be excreted in exchange for the reabsorbed sodium. In *metabolic alkalosis*, hydrogen ions will be pulled from the intracellular compartment, and potassium ions will be shifted into the intracellular compartment. Again, this shift alone will help to lower the pH. Also, because potassium ion concentration is now higher in the renal tubule cells, potassium will be excreted for the conserved sodium, and hydrogen ions will also be conserved. These *compensatory mechanisms can lead to hyperkalaemia when metabolic acidosis is present and hypokalaemia when metabolic alkalosis is present*.

It must be remembered that the buffer systems and the compensatory mechanisms provide for only temporary adjustment, and the underlying cause of the disturbance must be identified and corrected. However, the kidney can make permanent adjustments as seen in people who have respiratory acidosis as a result of chronic obstructive pulmonary disease (see Chapter 16).

Types of Acid–Base Disturbances

There are two types of acidosis (respiratory and metabolic) and two types of alkalosis (respiratory and metabolic). Table 6-3 shows the four types that occur and their compensatory mechanisms. The *major effect of acidosis is depression of the CNS* as evidenced by *disorientation* followed by *coma. Alkalosis is characterized by overexcitability of the nervous system,* and *the muscles may go into a state of tetany and convulsions.* Acid–base imbalances always produce an imbalance of the body's electrolytes as well; therefore symptoms of these imbalances also occur.

Laboratory tests

Information about a patient's acid–base status is obtained by testing a sample of arterial blood (arterial blood gas) for the following values:

1. pH (normal 7.35-7.45): measure of hydrogen ion concentration.
2. P_{CO_2} (normal 5.3 kPa or 40 mmHg): partial pressure of carbon dioxide.
3. Hydrogen carbonate (normal 27 mmol/l): sometimes reported as carbon dioxide content, which is a measure of all carbon dioxide dissolved in the blood as carbonic acid and hydrogen carbonate.

The P_{O_2}, partial pressure of oxygen, is also measured and indicates how well the patient is obtaining oxygen, but does not indicate the acid–base status.

Carbonic acid excess (respiratory acidosis)

Any condition that decreases the rate of pulmonary ventilation increases the concentration of dissolved carbon dioxide and hydrogen ions and results in a build-up of carbonic acid known as respiratory acidosis. The *excess of carbon dioxide (hypercapnia) can cause carbon dioxide narcosis.* In this condition *carbon dioxide levels are so high that they no longer stimulate the respiratory centre* (medulla) *but depress it.* Associated with the decreased respiratory rate are lack of oxygen and hypoxia. *During respiratory acidosis, potassium moves out of the cells,* producing hyperkalaemia. *Ventricular fibrillation may occur if the blood potassium level is greatly increased.*

Treatment is aimed at increasing the alveolar ventilation rate to improve the exchange of carbon dioxide and oxygen.

Table 6-3 Types of acid–base disturbances and compensatory mechanisms

Disturbance	Physiological causes	Method of compensation
Respiratory acidosis	Carbonic acid excess: lungs not removing sufficient CO_2 (hypoventilation)	Hydrogen carbonate production by kidneys increased; hydrogen carbonate retained and chloride excreted instead by kidneys; secretion and excretion of hydrogen ions in urine increased
Respiratory alkalosis	Carbonic acid deficit; lungs removing too much CO_2 (hyperventilation)	Kidneys increase excretion of hydrogen carbonate ions
Metabolic acidosis	Hydrogen carbonate deficit; retention of acid metabolites, diabetic ketoacidosis, excess acid intake (salicylate poisoning), loss of hydrogen carbonate, hyperkalaemia	Increased rate and depth of respiration cause increased excretion of CO_2 by lungs; formation of hydrogen carbonate ions in the kidneys increased
Metabolic alkalosis	Hydrogen carbonate excess: excess intake (sodium hydrogen carbonate, carbonated drinks) or retention of hydrogen carbonate Potassium depletion	Rate and depth of respiration decreased; lungs retain more CO_2; kidneys excrete hydrogen carbonate Loss of acid

This objective is accomplished with bronchodilators, and by physiotherapy in patients with obstruction of respiratory passages. Because the respiratory centre is narcotized by increased amounts of carbon dioxide, the lowered oxygen tension of the blood maintains respiration. If a patient whose respiratory drive is dependent on a low P_{O_2} is given large amounts of oxygen, the stimulus for breathing is removed, and respirations will cease. For this reason, oxygen is never given to patients with carbon dioxide narcosis. Low concentration oxygen, e.g. 24% via a *venturi effect* mask (where the oxygen is diluted with room air drawn into the mask), is given to a patient with chronic obstructive pulmonary disease who maintains a chronically high P_{CO_2}. Respiratory treatments are usually given using compressed air or room air instead of oxygen in these situations.

The major nursing responsibility is to recognize patients who have the potential for developing respiratory acidosis because of conditions that interfere with normal respiratory gas exchange. A patient whose airway is compromised by the presence of secretions must be encouraged to cough frequently or may need to have nasopharyngeal or tracheal suctioning.

Carbonic acid deficit (respiratory alkalosis)

Excessive pulmonary ventilation decreases hydrogen ion concentration and the formation of carbonic acid, leading to respiratory alkalosis. A common cause of respiratory alkalosis is *hyperventilation.* A person who hyperventilates blows off large amounts of carbon dioxide.

Respiratory alkalosis can be prevented in a person who is hyperventilating by administering a few whiffs of carbon dioxide or by having the person breathe into a paper bag and then rebreathe the exhaled carbon dioxide. Care should be taken in adjusting mechanical respirators so that the patient is not being forced to breathe too deeply or too rapidly.

The *patient may complain of lightheadedness and numb-*

ness or tingling of the fingers and toes. If the alkalosis becomes more severe, tetany and convulsions may be present. Serum potassium levels will decrease because potassium moves into the cells as hydrogen ions move out in an attempt to correct the alkalosis.

Treating the underlying condition usually effectively resolves respiratory alkalosis. Respiratory alkalosis becomes especially dangerous when it leads to cardiac dysrhythmias caused partly by a decreased serum potassium level. If a patient who is receiving assisted ventilation complains of dizziness or shows any signs of muscle irritability, it is likely that the depth of respiration is too great, and the respiratory rate of the machine should be decreased. If tetany is present, calcium gluconate is given intravenously. Renal function must be maintained to promote renal compensation of the alkalosis.

Hydrogen carbonate deficit (metabolic acidosis)

When acid production or addition of acid by ingestion exceeds acid loss, hydrogen carbonate attempts to buffer the acid load; however, the *hydrogen carbonate supply* soon *becomes depleted* and a *hydrogen carbonate deficit, metabolic acidosis, results* (see Table 6-3). Hydrogen carbonate may also become depleted by losses of large amounts of alkaline secretions, such as intestinal secretions.

Increased acid production occurs during the development of ketoacidosis, uraemic acidosis, or lactic acidosis. In *ketoacidosis,* glucose either cannot be used or is not available for oxidation. The body compensates for this by using body fat for energy, thus producing abnormal amounts of ketone bodies, which are fatty acids. Ketoacidosis also develops in anyone who does not eat sufficient food to meet daily needs and in whom body fat must be burned for energy. It is the reason why extremely low-carbohydrate or high-protein-zero-carbohydrate reduction diets are criticized by nutrition experts.

Lactic acidosis results when lactic acid is produced in large quantities such as in prolonged strenuous muscle exercise or when oxidation takes place in cells without adequate oxygen such as occurs in heart failure and shock. Uraemic acidosis results from the *inability of the failing kidney to excrete the acid end products of metabolism.*

Hyperkalaemia may result during metabolic acidosis; as the hydrogen ion concentration of the extracellular fluid increases, hydrogen moves into the cell and potassium moves out into the bloodstream.

The *patient in acidosis becomes hyperpnoeic and has deep, periodic breathing. Hyperventilation* represents an attempt to blow off carbon dioxide and to lower the P_{CO_2}, thus compensating for the acidosis. If the *condition is untreated, disorientation, stupor, coma, and death occur.*

Metabolic acidosis is controlled by giving an intravenous solution of sodium hydrogen carbonate or sodium lactate. Sodium hydrogen carbonate sometimes is given orally if it can be retained. Treatment of the condition precipitating the acidosis is then instituted.

Hydrogen carbonate excess (metabolic alkalosis)

When acid loss is greater than acid production, hydrogen ions are lost from body fluids and hydrogen carbonate excess (*metabolic alkalosis*) *exists.* An excess may also occur with an excessive intake of sodium hydrogen carbonate or other alkaline salt, especially if renal function is impaired.

Loss of potassium can also *lead to metabolic alkalosis.* When potassium is lost from the body, hydrogen ions move into the cells to replace the lost potassium, leaving a decreased hydrogen ion concentration in the extracellular fluid, that is, metabolic alkalosis (see Table 6-3).

In *metabolic alkalosis, breathing becomes depressed in an effort to conserve carbon dioxide for combination with hydrogen ions in the blood to raise the blood level of carbonic acid* (see Table 6-3).

Treatment consists of administration of sodium chloride or ammonium chloride. If the condition is associated with a loss of sodium chloride, potassium must be restored because it is lost with the sodium.

The nurse assists in maintenance of good respiratory function so that compensation can take place through this mechanism. *Careful monitoring of the patient for adequate renal function and safety precautions are important in the nursing care of patients with metabolic alkalosis.* Because convulsions may occur, precautions are taken for the patient's protection.

People must be cautioned against the excessive use of sodium hydrogen carbonate to alleviate indigestion. Controlling the conditions that can cause metabolic alkalosis can prevent this imbalance from developing. If drug therapy is causing the alkalosis, these drugs should be discontinued, and others substituted where possible.

ASSESSMENT OF FLUID AND ELECTROLYTE BALANCE

Patient Data

The nurse should be familiar with signs and symptoms of fluid and electrolyte disturbances. Because these *symptoms* are *frequently subtle*, it is necessary to have a high degree of sensitivity to the possibility of occurrence in certain people, as in the following:

1. Has an illness of a type that usually disrupts fluid and electrolyte balance.
2. Has medical or surgical treatments that result in imbalances.
3. Has considerable limitation of food and fluids intake.
4. Sustains significant loss of body fluids.

By knowing of conditions that put an individual at risk and making careful ongoing assessments, the nurse can prevent or detect imbalances before they become severe.

Subjective data include *thirst, headache, pain, nausea, dyspnoea,* and *orthopnoea.* The time of origin and a description of symptoms are noted. *Objective data,* as noted in Table 6-4, *can be compared to the baseline assessment* obtained at the time of the patient's initial contact with health care providers.

Laboratory Values

Laboratory determinations of serum levels of the specific electrolytes help in making decisions concerning electrolyte excesses or deficits. When electrolyte disturbances develop slowly, symptoms may not be pronounced, and the problem may be detected only by a determination of the electrolyte concentration in the patient's blood. When there is *excess water, haemodilution occurs* and the *haemoglobin* and *haematocrit levels decrease.* With excessive fluid loss, there is haemoconcentration and the haematocrit and blood urea levels increase.

Additional Data

Important data to be considered in assessing fluid balances are comparison of fluid intake to output and changes in patient weight. Acutely ill medical patients and patients undergoing major surgery need to have their fluid intake and output and daily weight closely monitored. The practice of totalling the fluid intake and output every shift or every 24 hours provides additional data for determining whether or not the patient has a fluid imbalance.

Fluid intake

The intake record should show the type and amount of all fluids the patient has received and the route by which these were administered. This includes fluids given orally, parenterally, rectally, or fluids administered by tubes and retained by the patient. Foods that are eaten in a semisolid state but are basically liquid, such as ice cream, are recorded as fluids. To record the fluid intake of ice chips, the amount of ice chips is divided by two (60 ml of ice chips equals 30 ml water). Patients may receive considerable amounts of fluid through the frequent sucking of ice chips.

Fluid output

Urinary output

Urinary output is recorded as to time and amount of each voiding to help evaluate renal function. If renal function is a major concern, such as in the patient with

Table 6-4 Data supporting fluid and electrolyte imbalances

	Signs and symptoms	Imbalance
Change in mental status	Irritable, restless	Sodium or potassium excess
	Confusion, lethargy	Sodium or calcium excess or deficit
		Hyposmolar fluid excess
		Isosmolar fluid deficit
Head/neck	Dry, sticky mucous membranes	Sodium excess
	Facial puffiness (oedema)	Isosmolar fluid excess
	Distended neck veins (raised JVP)	Isosmolar fluid excess
	Thirst, dry mucous membranes, longitudinal furrows on tongue	Isosmolar fluid deficit
	Flat neck veins in supine position	Isosmolar fluid deficit
Temperature	Increase	Water loss, sodium excess
	Decrease	Fluid excess
GI	Absent bowel sounds (ileus)	Potassium deficit
	Anorexia, nausea, vomiting	Fluid excess or deficit
		Potassium excess or deficit
		Calcium excess
Circulation	Increased blood pressure	Increased circulatory volume
		Magnesium deficit
	Decreased blood pressure	Decreased circulatory volume
		Magnesium excess
	Increased pulse, slow vein filling	Potassium excess or deficit
		Isosmolar fluid deficit
	Bounding pulse	Increased circulating volume
		Potassium excess or deficit
		Sodium excess
	Weak, irregular pulse	Potassium excess or deficit
	Cardiac dysrhythmias	Potassium excess or deficit
Respiration	Dyspnoea, orthopnoea, moist breath sounds	Isosmolar fluid excess
	Decreased rate	Magnesium excess
Skin	Pale, cool extremities (without oedema)	Decreased circulating volume
	Pitting oedema	Isosmolar fluid excess
	Poor turgor (test over sternum)	Fluid deficit, sodium excess
	Dryness in groin, axillae	Isosmolar fluid deficit
	Flushed dry skin	Sodium excess
Neuromuscular	Numbness, tingling around mouth, fingers, toes	Calcium deficit
	Increased irritability, muscle spasms	Calcium deficit
	Muscle weakness, paralysis	Potassium deficit
	Decreased muscle tone, decreased deep tendon reflexes	Magnesium deficit
	Abdominal cramps	Potassium excess

shock, an indwelling catheter is used so the amount of urine can be recorded every hour and fluid intake regulated accordingly.

Wound drainage

Any drainage from a tube/drain draining a wound is measured and the amount and character of the drainage is recorded. If there is excessive drainage on dressings, it may be necessary to weigh the dressings. Fluid loss equals the difference between the wet weight and dry weight of the dressing.

GI drainage

Electrolytes are lost in large amounts with vomiting, diarrhoea, and gastric and intestinal drainage. The amount and kind vary according to the type of GI fluid lost. For determination of the amount and type of fluid replacement, vomitus, GI drainage, and liquid stools are measured as accurately as possible and are described as to consistency, colour, and odour (Table 6-5). Fluid used to irrigate nasogastric tubes is subtracted from total drainage before the amount of drainage is recorded.

Other output

Fluid aspirated from any body cavity, such as the abdomen or pleural spaces, must be measured. This fluid contains not only electrolytes but also proteins.

Diaphoresis is difficult to measure. If the clothing and linen become saturated, there may be as much as 1000 ml of fluid lost in perspiration. Dry and wet weights may be taken to get a more accurate measure of the amount of fluid loss.

Daily weight

The *daily weight record* is *the best way to determine the onset of dehydration or the accumulation of fluid* either as general-

Table 6-5 GI output

Type of fluid	Consistency	Colour	Odour
Gastric	Watery	Pale yellow-green	Sour Fruity odour with metabolic acidosis
Biliary	Thicker than gastric	Bright yellow to dark green	Acrid odour and bitter taste
Intestinal	Thick	Dark green to brown	Faecal

ized oedema or as "hidden" fluid in body cavities. *An increase of 1 kg in weight is equal to the retention of 1 L of fluid.* If the weight record is to be useful, the *patient must be weighed* on the *same scale* and at the *same hour* each day and must be *wearing the same amount of clothing.* Usually weights are taken in the early morning before the patient has eaten or defaecated but after voiding.

Urine specific gravity

The specific gravity of urine is a measure of the density (amount of solutes) in a sample of urine compared with the density of pure water (which is 1.000). Normal range for urine specific gravity is approximately 1.003 to 1.030. A person with renal impairment excretes a small amount of dilute urine (low specific gravity) because of the inability of the kidneys to concentrate solutes in the urine. The relationship between specific gravity and fluid deficit or excess is summarized as follows:

Fluid deficit: small urine volume with high specific gravity
Fluid excess: large urine volume with low specific gravity

INTERVENTIONS FOR PATIENTS WITH FLUID AND ELECTROLYTE IMBALANCE

Important nursing functions include prevention of fluid and electrolyte imbalance, assessment of patients to recognize and report early signs of imbalance, planning and carrying out actions related to therapy to correct the condition, and relief of symptoms.

Prevention of Fluid and Electrolyte Imbalance

Unless preventive measures are employed, many medical–surgical conditions and therapies may lead to fluid and electrolyte imbalance. In some frequently encountered situations, attention to preventive aspects may lessen the possibility of the development of serious fluid and electrolyte imbalance.

Prevention of inadequate fluid intake

Any patient who is unable to ask for fluids, to identify a need for fluid, or to swallow easily may develop a fluid deficit. The fluid intake of these patients is monitored, and specific plans are made to offer fluids at regular intervals. Some conditions placing patients at risk for fluid deficit are as follows: aphasia, catatonia, confusion, disorientation, dysphagia, weakness, and tube feedings.

Prevention of imbalances from GI fluid loss

Vomiting and diarrhoea

Vomiting and diarrhoea are common symptoms of many illnesses. Sodium and some potassium are lost in vomiting and diarrhoea, whereas chloride is lost only from vomitus. As soon as fluids are tolerated, the patient may be served salty broth and tea or another fluid high in potassium to replace the losses. Dry salty crackers are often tolerated when fluids are not and can be used to replace sodium. These measures keep the patient from feeling weak and exhausted.

Draining fistulas

A patient with a *draining fistula* from any portion of the GI tract loses *sodium, calcium,* and some *potassium,* and dietary supplements are needed. Extra milk can replace all the losses if tolerated by the patient. The vitamin D in the milk enables the body to use the calcium in the milk. Patients with a permanent fistulous opening, such as an ileostomy, need to be especially careful to supplement their sodium and potassium intake when vomiting, diarrhoea, or fever adds to the already unusually large loss of electrolytes.

Nasogastric drainage

Routine *intravenous replacement usually is adequate to compensate* for *losses through nasogastric drainage, unless* the *patient* has *been sucking many ice chips or the tube has been irrigated frequently with water.* Both of these practices, although they seem to be harmless because the fluid is removed immediately through the aspiration apparatus, stimulate the secretion of gastric juices. Aspiration of gastric juices of the stomach at rest may lead to loss of electrolytes and fluid. If irrigation of the tube is necessary, physiologically normal saline is used.

Enemas

Repeated enemas may result in water intoxication and potassium loss. If there is a prescription for enemas until the returns are clear, it is best not to give more than three enemas at one time without consulting the doctor. If an elderly person living at home complains of pronounced weakness without apparent cause, the person is asked whether cathartics or enemas are being taken. If so, stopping this practice, eating foods with high potassium content, and increasing fluid intake may relieve the symptoms. Methods to combat constipation without taking laxatives or frequent enemas are then taught.

The Elderly with Fluid and Electrolyte Imbalances

Assessment

Obtain careful medication history: diuretics and laxatives (frequently taken by elderly—see Gupta 1980) may promote dehydration.

Monitor fluid intake and output. Confusion or apathy may lead to decreased fluid intake.

Monitor dietary intake; decreased intake leads to decreased fluids (found in foods) and decreased electrolyte intake that can affect electrolyte balance. Decreased food intake may result from lack of teeth, poorly fitting dentures, decreased taste sensation from loss of taste buds, or inability to purchase or cook foods at home.

Assess for signs of **dehydration** because of decreased ability to concentrate urine. Dehydration may occur more frequently and more rapidly in elderly than in younger adults.

> Monitor urine specific gravity; this is usually lower in the elderly (1.026).
> Watch for symptoms of dehydration that may include mental status changes, such as apathy, dulled mentation, confusion, irritability, and weakness.
> Monitor for signs of volume depletion such as brown furry tongue, dry mucous membranes, decreased saliva pool under tongue; skin turgor is *not* a good indicator of dehydration in the elderly because of loss of skin elasticity with age.
> Blood urea is normally increased in elderly.

Monitor carefully IV fluid rate and assess patient for signs of pulmonary oedema (coughing, dyspnoea, moist breath sounds). **Fluid overload** may occur more readily because of decreased cardiac reserves, decreased vasomotor response, or decreased urinary function.

Interventions

Facilitate fluid intake of at least 1500 ml/day.

> Smaller more frequent amounts of fluid are better tolerated.
> Extra free water is essential when giving tube feedings to promote excretion of high-solute loads (up to 1000 ml daily).
> Use measures to encourage a balanced dietary intake (within prescribed restrictions); small frequent meals may be better tolerated than 3 large meals per day.
> Report and record early signs of dehydration (especially mental changes) or of IV fluid overload.
> Teach patient the need for adequate hydration, control of sodium (as pertinent), and foods high in potassium (if taking diuretics).

Common disorders in elderly

Dehydration
IV fluid overload
Sodium excess
Potassium excess

Prevention of excessive fluid loss from skin, lungs, or kidneys

Diaphoresis

Diaphoresis may result from heat, strenuous exercise, or fever. Even the healthy person who is perspiring profusely needs extra salt in the diet and should drink extra fluids. Some salty fluids are needed by the patient with a fever. Patients on salt-restricted diets and those with draining fistulas are especially likely to suffer from sodium depletion and should increase their salt intake slightly when perspiring profusely.

Diuretics

Diuretics are administered to encourage excretion of sodium and water in excess of body needs. However, potassium, which may not be in excess, is also lost with the increased urinary output. The patient receiving diuretics is encouraged to eat foods that are *high in potassium but low in sodium.* Good sources are bananas and other fresh fruit.

Diuretics such as the thiazides may eventually cause sodium depletion; therefore the patient receiving extensive diuretic treatment is taught to observe for symptoms indicating sodium depletion and to report these symptoms to the doctor.

Renal or circulatory impairments

Any patient with renal or circulatory impairment, as may occur in *shock, cardiac failure, renal insufficiency,* or *constriction of blood vessels* because of disease, *may develop a fluid and electrolyte imbalance.* Common imbalances include the following:

1. Oedema from sodium and water retention
2. Hyperkalaemia
3. Hyponatraemia
4. Acidosis from inadequate tissue oxygenation
5. Overhydration

Patients with the above conditions are instructed to avoid taking too much food containing sodium, potassium, or hydrogen carbonate. They should not drink carbonated beverages. The nurse must be especially aware of overhydration whenever intravenous fluids are being given to patients with renal or circulatory impairment.

Respiratory impairments

Patients with diseases such as emphysema that limit lung excursion and therefore limit exchange of O_2 and CO_2 should *not take carbonated beverages or bicarbonate of soda.* These substances tend to make the blood more alkaline than normal, and respiration is depressed in an effort to correct this imbalance. Depression of respiration is highly undesirable for patients with obstructive lung diseases. Early recognition and treatment of these lung diseases may help prevent acid-base imbalances.

Replacement Therapy

Fluids may be replaced by various routes as follows: orally (preferred route), by intravenous infusion, or by tube feedings (see Chapter 4).

Spacing of fluids

Fluids given by any route should be spaced throughout a 24-hour period. Not only does this practice help to maintain normal body fluid levels, but it also provides for better regulation of the electrolyte balance by the kidneys and prevents the end products of metabolism and toxic materials from being excreted in concentrated form. In this way the danger of renal damage, formation of calculi, and irradiation of the lower urinary tract is reduced. In addition, fluid spacing prevents overloading of the circulation.

Concentration of fluids

Infusing *concentrated solutions* rapidly and in *large amounts into the alimentary tract causes the blood volume to drop because large amounts of fluid are needed to dilute the substance. If the circulating volume becomes considerably depleted, irreversible shock can result.* The "dumping syndrome," which sometimes occurs after gastric resection, is caused by this abnormal shift of fluid. Concentrated solutions sometimes are given intentionally to reduce cerebral oedema.

Concentrated intravenous solutions of sugar or protein should also be given slowly in small amounts because they require fluid for dilution. *Hypertonic saline solution may cause fluid to diffuse from the tissues to equalize the concentration of salt in the intravascular compartment.* The superior vena cava is the preferred site for infusions of hypertonic solutions, such as parenteral hyperalimentation, because of the rapid dilution by the larger amount of blood at this site. *If any of these concentrated solutions flows too rapidly into the vascular system, pulmonary oedema can develop.*

Oral intake

Adults who have no circulatory or renal malfunction usually need between 1500 and 3000 ml/day of fluid, depending on the amount of food consumed. Patients who have anorexia and are not eating well require more fluid to maintain a fluid balance. Medical prescriptions for fluid restriction are usually given for patients who have fluid excess (oedema or water intoxication) or whose kidneys are not functioning well.

A medical prescription may be given to the patient to "push fluids" or the nurse may make the decision that a large intake of fluids is desirable, such as for prevention of urinary stasis with its subsequent complications. No standard amount can be stated because the amount required depends on the following:
1. Size of the patient
2. Patient's circulatory and renal status
3. Amount of food intake
4. Amount of fluid loss (if appropriate)

It must be remembered that people with small or inelastic vascular systems become overhydrated easily. If the patient has had a large portion of the body such as a limb removed either by surgery or trauma, overall physical size is thereby decreased. If there is a question concerning the amount of fluids a patient should be encouraged to drink, the doctor is consulted.

Parenteral fluids

Type of fluid

The nurse needs to know the common solutions used parenterally (Table 6-6). Some of the reasons for giving the more common intravenous solutions are listed in Box 6-1. Potassium chloride may be added to maintain normal intake of potassium and to replace losses. Ascorbic acid and vitamin B may be added for nutritional purposes.

Whole blood, plasma-reduced blood, plasma, concentrated albumin, or plasma volume expanders can be given to substitute for blood protein loss and are used to establish normal blood volume and prevent shock. *Dextran is the most generally accepted plasma volume expander.* It increases the oncotic pressure of the blood, thus increasing the reabsorption of fluid from interstitial spaces. This creates an increase in plasma volume. *Low-molecular dextran decreases the viscosity of the blood, allowing greater blood flow through the capillaries; thus it is useful in treating cardiogenic, haemorrhagic, or septic shock.* It may cause prolonged bleeding time and should not be used if renal disease with severe oliguria or anuria is present. The patient is monitored for signs of anaphylactic reaction (apprehension, dyspnoea, wheezing, respirations, tightness of chest, itching, hypotension) when dextran is being given.

Intravenous fluids containing electrolytes should be run slowly to allow the body to regulate their use. The patient is monitored for signs of intoxication (excess of fluids or electrolytes) and satisfactory urinary output. *Increased serum potassium (hyperkalaemia) can be particularly dangerous, because it may cause cardiac arrest.* Renal failure and untreated adrenal insufficiency are contraindications for the use of potassium. Many doctors do not start intravenous therapy until serum electrolyte levels have been reported for the day.

6-1

Uses of common intravenous solutions

Solution	Use
Dextrose	
5% in water	Maintenance therapy when sodium not desirable
5% in saline (0.9%, 0.18%)	Maintenance therapy depending on desired amount of sodium
Sodium chloride (0.9%)	For large losses of sodium, as in loss of GI fluids, burns
M/6 molar lactate	Replacement of sodium but not chloride
Ringer's lactate	Balanced solution containing Na^+, K^+, Ca^{++}, Cl^-

Table 6-6 Solutions for intravenous use

Type of solution	Contents of solutions								
	Cations (mmol/l)					Anions (mmol/l)			Glucose (g/l)
	Na⁺	K⁺	Ca⁺⁺	Mg⁺⁺	NH⁺₄	Cl⁻	HCO₃ lactate	PO₄⁻	
Dextrose in water						50			
10% Dextrose in water									100
Normal saline (0.9%)	150					150			
3% Saline	500					500			
Ringer's solution	147	4	2			156			
5% Dextrose in Ringer's lactate	131	5	2			111	29		50
Ringer's lactate	131	5	2			111	29		
Sodium lactate M/6	167						167		
4% Dextrose in 0.18% saline	30					30			40

Amount and rate of administration

The administration rate of fluids usually is ordered by the doctor and depends on the patient's illness, the kind of fluid given, and the patient's size and age. Approximately 30 ml/kg body weight is needed to meet daily fluid requirements. Fever increases water needs by about 15% for each 1 degree Celsius rise in a patient's body temperature.[11] If there has been an acute illness resulting in a significant fluid deficit, fluid is replaced at the rate of 1000 ml/kg loss in weight. The doctor calculates water needs based on the amount needed to replace losses and the amount required to meet daily needs.

The usual rate for replacement of fluid loss is 3 ml/min; it is rarely run at a rate faster than 4 ml/min. If fluids are given continuously or if they are given when there is impaired renal or cardiac function, they are rarely run faster than 2 ml/min. Intravenous infusions that are run at too rapid a rate (sometimes seen when an infusion is "speeded up" to complete the treatment at a specified time) may result in overloading of the circulatory system and pulmonary oedema. At the first signs of increased blood volume in any patient receiving an intravenous infusion, the rate of flow is reduced and the doctor notified.

Relief of Thirst

Thirst, the first and most insistent sign of dehydration, sometimes causes the patient more misery than surgery or the symptoms of a disease. It may develop even when fluids have been withheld for only a number of hours. If fluid is being withheld intentionally, thirst often is made more bearable by explaining to patients why fluid is withheld and when they can expect to receive some.

Thirst usually is relieved rather readily by taking fluids. If fluids cannot be taken orally, the administration of fluids parenterally usually gives relief. It is often helpful to explain to the patient who is receiving an infusion that the procedure will soon provide some relief from thirst.

Mouth care allays some of the discomfort from thirst and may need to be repeated every hour. If patients can be trusted not to swallow, they may be given ice chips, which are held in the mouth and then spat out. Hard sweets, e.g. fruit-flavoured, often give relief, even though they also must be expelled. The chewing of gum may help to relieve dry mouth.

Pronounced and continued thirst, despite the administration of fluids, is not normal and is reported. In the patient recently returned from surgery, this kind of thirst may indicate internal haemorrhage, elevation of temperature, or some other untoward development. Thirst may also be an indication of hypercalcaemia or the onset of diabetes mellitus.

SUMMARY

1. Losses of fluid and electrolytes occur through the skin by diaphoresis and oozing from severe wounds or burns; from GI drainage and enemas; from the kidneys because of diuretic use and polyuria; from haemorrhage; and through the trapping of fluids by wound swelling, oedema, ascites, and intestinal obstruction.

2. A low sodium level in the blood can indicate either a deficit of sodium or an excess of water.

3. Muscle weakness, anorexia, nausea or vomiting, diminished deep tendon reflexes, lethargy, cardiac arrhythmias, and ECG changes are symptoms of hypokalaemia.

4. Nursing responsibilities for patients with hypercalcaemia include active exercises for immobilized persons, increased fluid intake, prevention of urinary tract infections, and gentle handling to prevent pathological fractures

5. Mechanisms that regulate acid–base balance include chemical buffer systems, the respiratory system, and the kidneys.

6. The respiratory control centre in the medulla oblongata responds to increases of carbon dioxide and hydrogen ions in body fluids by changing the rate and depth of respiration.

7. The renal regulation of pH is effected by control of the retention or excretion of hydrogen carbonate and hydro-gen ions.

8. The major effect of acidosis is depression of the central nervous system as evidenced by disorientation followed by coma.

9. Alkalosis is characterized by overexcitability of the nervous system, and the muscles may go into a state of tetany and convulsions.

10. Any factor that decreases the rate of pulmonary ventilation increases the concentration of dissolved carbon dioxide, carbonic acid, and hydrogen ions and results in respiratory acidosis.

11. Excess pulmonary ventilation will decrease hydrogen ion concentration and thus cause respiratory alkalosis.

12. When excess organic acids are added to the body fluids or when hydrogen carbonate is lost, a metabolic acidosis results.

13. When excessive amounts of organic acid substance and hydrogen ions are lost from the body, or when large amounts of hydrogen carbonate or lactate are added, the result is an imbalance in which there is an excess of base elements, resulting in metabolic alkalosis.

14. Monitoring fluid and electrolyte balance is particularly important in patients with an illness of the type that disrupts fluid and electrolyte balance, with medical–surgical treatments that result in imbalances, with considerable limitation of food and fluid intake, and in people who have sustained significant loss of body fluids.

15. Assessment of fluid and electrolyte balance includes the monitoring of laboratory values, fluid intake, fluid out-put (urinary output, wound drainage, GI drainage, fluid from any body cavity, diaphoresis), daily weight, and urine specific gravity.

STUDY QUESTIONS

- What would you recommend to young women to prevent osteoporosis?
- How would you explain a low potassium diet to an elderly patient with a hearing deficit?
- Explaine one common method of preventing respiratory alkalosis.
- Why are the elderly at particular risk for dehydration?
- What is the best method to administer water, electrolytes, and nutrients? Why?

REFERENCES AND SELECTED READINGS

1. Ashby D: Balancing fluids and electrolytes in the PACU, *J Post Anesth Nurs* 2(2):114-116, 1987.
2.* Barta M: Correcting electrolyte imbalances, *RN* 50(2): 30-34, 1987.
3.* Bowman M, et al: Effect of tube-feeding osmolality on serum sodium levels, *Crit Care Nurse* 9(1):22-28, 1989.
4. Brocklehurst JC, Allen S: *Geriatric medicine for students*, ed 3, New York, 1987, Churchill Livingstone.
5.* Calloway C: When the problem involves magnesium, calcium, or phosphate, *RN* 50(5):30-36, 1987.
6.* Felver L, Pendarvis J: Electrolyte imbalances: intraoperative risk factors, *AORN J* 49(4):992-1008, 1989.
7. Foss M: Acid-Base Balance, *The Professional Nurse* 3(12):509, 511-513,1988.
8.* Gasparis L, Murray EB, Ursomanno P: IV solutions: which one is right for your patient? *Nurs 89* 19(4):62-64, 1989.
9.* Gershan JA, et al: Fluid volume deficit: validating the indicators, *Heart Lung* 19(2):152-156, 1990.
10. Goldberger E: *A primer of water, electrolyte, and acid-base syndromes*, ed 7, Philadelphia, 1986, Lea & Febiger.
11. Goodinson SM: Good practice ensures minimum risk factors. Complications of peripheral venous cannulation and infusion therapy, *Professional Nurse* 6(3):175-177, 1990.
12. Groer M, Shekelton ME: *Basic pathophysiology: a conceptual approach*, St. Louis, 1989, Mosby–Year Book.
13. Gupta K: Constipation, *Geriatric Medicine*, 10(12):45, 1980.
14. Guyton A: *Textbook of medical physiology*, ed 7, Philadelphia, 1986, WB Saunders.
15. Innerarity SA: Electrolyte emergencies in the critically ill renal patient, *Crit Care Nurs Clin North Am* 2(1):89-99, 1990.
16* Janusek LW: Metabolic alkalosis: pathophysiology and the resulting signs and symptoms, *Nurs 90* 20(6):52-53, 1990.
17* Janusek LW: Metabolic acidosis: pathophysiology and the resuling signs and symptoms, *Nurs 90* 20(7):52-53, 1990.
18.* Kee JL: *Fluid and electrolytes with clinical applications (programmed approach)*, ed 4, New York, 1986, John Wiley & Sons.
19.* Mathewson M: Intravenous therapy, *Crit Care Nurs* 9(2):21-23, 26-28, 30-36, 1989.
20* Mathewson M, Mathewson R: Establishing acid–base balance, *Crit care Nurs* 7(5):77-86, 1987.
21. McVicar A, Clancy J: Which infusate do I need? Physio-logical basis of fluid therapy, *Professional Nurse* 7(9):586-591, 1992.
22. Methany NM: *Fluid and electrolyte balance: nursing considerations*, ed 3, Philadelphia, 1987, Lippincott.
23. Miller JA: Intravenous therapy in fluid and electrolyte balance, *The Professional Nurse* 4(5): 237-241, 1989.
24. Miller L, Holloway N: Water intoxication: psychogenic hyperdipsia, *Crit Care Nurse* 9(7):74-78, 1989.
25. Plumer AL: *Principles and practice of intravenous therapy*, ed 4, Boston, 1987, Little, Brown.
26.* Rinardi G: Water intoxication, *Am J Nurs* 89(12):1635-1638, 1989.
27. Robinson JR: *Fundiamentals of Acid–Base Regulation*, ed 5 Oxford, 1979, Blackwell Scientific Publications.
28. Sabiston DC (editor): *Textbook of surgery*, ed 13, Philadelphia, 1986, WB Saunders.
29. Smith LH, Wyngaarden JB: *Cecil review of general internal medicine*, ed 4, Philadelphia, 1989, WB Saunders.
30.* Sommers M: Rapid fluid resuscitation: how to correct dangerous deficits, *Nurs 90* 20(1):52-59, 1990.
31.* Symposium on fluid, electrolytes, and acid-base balance, *Nurs Clin North Am* 22(4):749-872, 1987.
32. Taylor DL: Respiratory alkalosis: pathophysiology, signs, and symptoms, *Nurs 90* 20(8):60-61, 1990.
33.* Taylor DL: Respiratory acidosis: pathophysiology, signs, and symptoms, *Nurs 90* 20(9):52-53, 1990.
34. Thompson AD, Cotton RE: *Lecture Notes on Pathology*, ed 3, Oxford, 1983, Blackwell Scientific Publication.
35.* Valle G, Lemberg L: Electrolyte imbalances in cardiovascular disease: the forgotten factor, *Heart Lung* 17(3):324-329, 1988.
36. Vander AJ, Luciano DS: *Human physiology: mechanisms of body functioning*, ed 5, New York, 1989, McGraw-Hill Book Co.
37.* Weldy NJ: *Body fluids and electrolytes (programed presentation)*, ed 6, St. Louis, 1991, Mosby–Year Book.
38. Willatts SM: *Lecture Notes on Fluid and Electrolyte Balance*, Oxford, 1982, Blackwell Scientific Publications.
39. Woodward W, Woodward T: Management of dehydrating diarrhoea, *Hosp Pract* 21(3):60, 63, 67-68, 1986.
40.* Yarnell RP, Craig MP: Detecting hypomagnesia: the most overlooked electrolyte imbalance, *Nurs 91* 54(7):55-57, 1991.
41.* Young M, Flynn K: Third spacing: when the body conceals fluid loss, *RN* 51:46-48, 1988.

*Recommended for student reading.

7

Shock

Martha L. Allen
Gail Osterfield

After studying this chapter, the learner should be able to:

- Contrast three major types of shock.
- Describe early and late pathophysiological changes that occur with shock.
- Describe organ damage that may occur with shock.
- Describe different methods of monitoring for shock.
- Describe the principles of treating shock.

7-1	**Types of shock**	
	Hypovolaemic	From loss of fluid from vascular system (through blood loss or fluid loss)
	Cardiogenic	From inability of heart to pump blood to tissues (decreased cardiac output)
	Vasogenic	From massive vasodilation (from interference with sympathetic nervous system or effects of histamine or toxins)

Shock is a syndrome characterized by hypoperfusion of body tissues. Any condition that prevents cells from receiving an adequate blood supply can interfere with their metabolism and produce shock.

Blood flow depends on pressure changes within the vascular compartment. Blood flows from areas of greater pressure to areas of lesser pressure. In the systemic circulation, the mean pressure is highest in the aorta, where the blood leaves the left ventricle, and lowest in the right atrium. In order for the necessary pressure gradients to exist so that blood can flow, the following three factors are necessary:

1. An adequate amount of blood for the heart to pump around the body
2. Ability of the heart to pump blood
3. Blood vessels with good tone, able to constrict and dilate to maintain normal pressure

Shock results from the disruption of one or more of these factors.

AETIOLOGY/EPIDEMIOLOGY

Shock may be classified as hypovolaemic, cardiogenic, or vasogenic (see Box 7-1).

Hypovolaemic Shock

Hypovolaemic shock is the most common type of shock. *Any condition that reduces the volume within the vascular compartment by 15% to 25% can result in hypovolaemic shock.* Common causes include the following:

1. Excessive blood loss: trauma (most common cause), gastrointestinal bleeding, coagulation disorders, surgery
2. Loss of body fluids other than blood: excessive diuresis (diabetic ketoacidosis or other hyperosmolar states), plasma loss from burns, fluid loss from excessive vomiting or diarrhoea
3. Movement of fluid into another body space (third space), for example, bowel obstruction (up to 5 or 10 L may collect in bowel) or peritonitis (4 to 6 L may collect in peritoneal cavity within 24 hours)

Characteristically, the signs and symptoms of hypovolaemic shock progress in direct proportion to the percentage of blood loss (see Table 7-1, overleaf).

Cardiogenic Shock

Cardiogenic shock results from the inability of the heart to pump blood sufficiently to perfuse the cells of the body. When stroke volume falls initially, cardiac output may be maintained by an increase in heart rate (Chapter 17); however, an increase in the heart rate may further damage the heart. As the heart rate increases, the period of diastole shortens and the period of systole remains relatively constant. Because the coronary arteries fill during diastole, their filling time is reduced. The heart works for longer periods and requires more oxygen and nutrients. Thus tachycardia can both increase the oxygen need of the heart and decrease its oxygen supply.

Although cardiogenic shock may be caused by various cardiac conditions including cardiac tamponade, restrictive pericarditis, pulmonary embolism, severe valvular disease, or dysrhythmias, the most common cause by far is myocardial infarction. Studies have shown that in most patients who die from cardiogenic shock, at least 40% of the left ventricle was damaged by a recent infarction or by a recent infarction plus a previous scar. In spite of improvements in managing cardiogenic shock, the mortality still remains above 80%. (Additional information on cardiogenic shock is given in Chapter 17.)

Vasogenic Shock

Vasogenic shock is caused by massive dilation of the blood vessels, resulting in disproportion between the size of the vascular space and the amount of blood contained. As arterial blood pressure falls, the difference between arterial and venous pressures decreases. Because blood flow depends on pressure differences, blood flow decreases. Blood pools in the blood vessels, resulting in decreased venous return to the heart. Cardiac output falls, and blood pressure decreases even further.

Initially in vasogenic shock, the extremities are warm because of vasodilation. However, as cardiac output decreases and tissue perfusion is reduced, *compensatory vasoconstriction occurs.*

Loss of vascular tone may result from a number of conditions. *Neurogenic shock results from interference with the sympathetic nervous system, which helps maintain vasomotor tone.* Spinal cord injury, spinal anaesthesia, and, rarely, brain damage are among the causes. *Anaphylactic shock occurs when there is massive dilation of the blood vessels from the direct effect on the vessels of a substance such as histamine.* Histamine, released by mast cells and basophils, has a powerful dilating effect on blood vessels, particularly capillaries. The endothelial cells that line the capillaries separate and expose the basement membrane, which is permeable to fluid and plasma proteins, resulting in hypovolaemia.[11]

Septic shock, another form of vasogenic shock, may result from various infections, including those caused by both Gram-positive and Gram-negative bacteria, viruses, and fungi, although it most commonly results from Gram-negative bacterial infections. The primary sites of infection are usually the urinary tract, respiratory tract, or blood. Organisms that ordinarily dwell in the gastrointestinal tract may cause sepsis and shock if they enter the bloodstream.

Septic shock is commonly seen in hospitals. Approxi-

Table 7-1 Clinical manifestations of hypovolaemic shock

Parameter (for a 70 kg male)	Class I early	Class II moderate	Class III major or progressive	Class IV severe or profound
Approximate blood volume loss (ml)	Up to 750	750-1500	1500-2000	2000 or more
% of blood volume	Up to 15%	15-30%	30-40%	40% or more
Neurological/behavioural status	Slightly anxious	Mildly anxious, restless; muscle fatigue and weakness evident	Agitated, confused; progressive decrease in activity; progressive thirst evident	Stuporous, lethergic, unconscious; dilated pupils may be evident
Heart rate	<100	>100 Mild tachycardia	>120 Tachycardia	140 or higher Irregular pulse, decreased pulse amplitude
Blood pressure	Normal	Normal	Decreased	Severe hypotension
Pulse pressure (mm Hg)	Normal or increased	Decreased	Decreased	Decreased
Respirations	14-20, normal	20-30, normal	30-40, hyperpnoea	>35, shallow, irregular
Urine output (ml/h)	30 or more	20-30	5-15	Negligible
Capillary blanch test	Normal	Slight delay	Defined delay	No refilling observed
Skin	Pale pink, slightly cool	Slightly cold, pale	Cold and moist	Cold and cyanotic, mottled

From McQuillan KA and Wiles CE: Initial management of traumatic shock. In Cardona DV and others: *Trauma nursing from resuscitation through rehabilitation.* Philadelphia, 1988, WB Saunders.

mately one in every 100 patients in hospitals will develop sepsis, and of these 40 will develop septic shock.[40] Conditions that predispose to septic shock include the following:

1. Age, both the very young and the very elderly
2. Malnutrition
3. General debilitation
4. Immunosuppressive and steroid therapy
5. Chronic disease of the immune system (for example, AIDS)
6. Any surgery (for example, urological or gastrointestinal surgery)
7. All forms of instrumentation (for example, intravenous lines, indwelling catheters, and diagnostic procedures)

Elderly men are particularly susceptible to septic shock because of the high incidence of prostatic hypertrophy in this group. They are more likely to develop urinary tract infections and to have urological surgical procedures.

The mechanism by which septic shock occurs is not completely understood. Some believe that early in sepsis, fluid leaks out of the vascular system, and the resultant shock is simply a form of hypovolaemic shock.[29] Others see the primary cause as faulty cellular metabolism from the direct effect of the toxin.[50] *Although the early pathophysiology of septic shock is not completely understood, it is known that when some organisms enter the bloodstream, they are destroyed by the immune system and a toxin is released.* This toxin, in some way, causes the characteristic symptoms of early septic shock (increased cardiac output, peripheral vasodilation, skin flushing, hyperthermia, increased renal output, and respiratory alkalosis).[40] As septic shock progresses and cardiac output decreases, it resembles other types of shock, with low urinary output, vasoconstriction, and cool moist skin.

PATHOPHYSIOLOGY
Early Stage

In the early stage of shock the body responds to hypoperfusion as it would to any other stressor. Many of the changes that occur are mediated through the sympathetic nervous system. *Stimulation of the sympathetic nervous system results in secretion of adrenaline and noradrenaline by the adrenal medulla.* Both alpha- and beta-adrenergic receptors are stimulated throughout the body. *Alpha receptors respond by causing vasoconstriction,* and *beta receptors respond by causing vasodilation (beta 1)* and *increased rate and strength of contraction of the heart (beta 2).* The skin and the abdominal organs, which are rich in alpha receptors, receive a decreased blood supply because of vasoconstriction. The heart and skeletal muscles, which are rich in beta receptors, receive an increased blood supply because of vasodilation. The heart beats more rapidly and more forcefully and the respiratory rate increases in response to beta stimulation, thereby increasing oxygen delivery to the tissues. All of the compensatory responses that are mediated through the sympathetic nervous system occur rapidly.

Another compensatory response, mediated through the renin–angiotensin system, occurs more slowly. As cardiac output decreases, the blood supply to the kidneys also decreases. The juxtaglomerular cells respond by secreting *renin,* which *acts upon a plasma protein, converting it to angiotensin I.* This is converted to *angiotensin II,* which has *two major effects:* it *causes vasoconstriction* and it causes the *adrenal cortex to secrete aldosterone. Aldosterone* causes the kidneys to *retain sodium and water,* and *secrete potassium,* resulting in an *increased blood volume.* The secretion of potassium may result in hypokalaemia during this stage of shock. *Decreased cardiac output* results in *decreased hydrostatic pressure in the capillaries,* causing *fluid to shift from the interstitial space into the capillaries.* This also improves blood volume.

For a short period of time the compensatory mechanisms have a beneficial effect. The most vital organs, the heart and the brain, receive an adequate blood supply at the expense of the less vital organs, such as the kidneys and other abdominal organs. This allows time for the underlying cause of shock to be corrected. However, if the underlying problem is not or cannot be corrected, the compensatory mechanisms will not be able to continue to supply sufficient blood to vital organs and the compensatory mechanisms themselves will have a deleterious effect on the body. Shock will then progress to a later stage.

Late Stage

As shock progresses, blood flow to all body tissues becomes impaired. Cells in vasoconstricted organs receive *insufficient oxygen*, and aerobic metabolism is replaced by *anaerobic metabolism*. Energy, in the form of adenosine triphosphate (ATP), is produced very inefficiently. *Lactic acid cannot be metabolized* in the *absence of oxygen*, so it accumulates in the body, resulting in *metabolic acidosis. With insufficient ATP, the sodium–potassium pump fails; potassium leaves the cells and sodium and water enter them.* Organelles within the cells are damaged. Rupture of the cell wall of the lysosomes is particularly dangerous. They normally have an important role in phagocytosis and contain digestive enzymes. When their cell walls are destroyed, the digestive enzymes are released into the cell and autodigestion of the cell occurs.[21] This process can spread from cell to cell, resulting in organ death.

Acid metabolites cause dilation at the arteriole end of the capillaries (precapillary sphincter) and constriction at the venule end of the capillary (postcapillary sphincter), increasing *intracapillary hydrostatic pressure.* This results in *a fluid shift out of the capillary, further decreasing blood* volume. Increased capillary permeability may occur, particularly in septic shock, as large amounts of *histamine* and *serotonin* are *released in response to Gram-negative toxins.* As proteins leak out of the capillaries, fluid follows and the blood volume is even further reduced. As the *blood supply to the kidneys is decreased, oliguria* or *anuria* occurs. The *blood urea nitrogen* (BUN) and *serum creatinine* levels rise. *Cellular damage releases potassium* into the blood, and the impaired kidneys are unable to excrete it. *Hyperkalaemia, which results, depresses the contractility and conduction in the heart.*

Vasoconstriction of the splanchnic vessels in response to sympathetic stimulation *causes ischaemia of the abdominal organs.* Of *particular importance* is the *pancreas.* In response to hypoxaemia the pancreas produces and secretes a substance called myocardial depressant factor (MDF), which depresses contractility of the heart. As compensatory mechanisms fail, blood supply to the heart decreases and electrical and mechanical activity are impaired.

Box 7-2 summarizes the pathophysiological changes in early and late shock.

7-2

Major pathophysiological changes in shock

Change	Effect
Early stage (compensatory stage)	
Increased adrenaline and noradrenaline	Increased cardiac output to send more blood to tissues
Alpha and beta receptors stimulated	
Alpha effects	
Skin	Vasoconstriction and decreased blood supply
Beta effects	
Heart and skeletal muscles	Vasodilatation and increased blood supply and heart rate
Renin–angiotensin response	Vasoconstriction and secretion of aldosterone; sodium and water retention and potassium loss
Increased glucocorticoids and mineralocorticoids	Sodium and fluid retention to increase intravascular volume
	Potassium loss
Hypoxaemia (↓ Pa_{O_2})	Hyperventilation; provides more oxygen to tissues; may cause respiratory alkalosis
Decreased hydrostatic fluid pressure	Fluid shifts from interstitial space to capillaries to increase vascular volume
Late stage (noncompensatory stage)	
Decreased blood flow to heart	Impaired cardiac pumping ability (decreased cardiac ouput); blood pressure decreases
Anaerobic metabolism	Acidosis; decreased adenosine trisphosphate (ATP); failure of cellular N^+–K^+ pump (K^+ leaves cell, Na^+ and water enter cell); cellular damage
Arteriolar dilation and venule constriction	Fluid shift from intravascular to interstitial space
Decreased blood flow to kidney	Decreased kidney function (oliguria or anuria, retention of nitrogenous waste products)
Decreased blood flow to pancreas	Production of myocardial depressant factor (MDF)

Shock is a dynamic process with shock itself causing shock[15] as is depicted in Fig. 7-1. At some point a cycle begins that cannot be interrupted, and an *irreversible stage of shock* ensues. *Even if the primary problem that caused the shock is corrected and good supportive care is given, the patient will die.* However, the exact point at which shock becomes irreversible cannot be determined. Regardless of the patient's symptoms, all efforts should be made to reverse the progression of shock.

ORGAN DAMAGE
Kidneys

The kidneys contain about 2,400,000 nephrons, each of which is capable of forming urine. Each nephron is composed of a glomerulus, made up of capillaries and the collecting tubules (Chapter 25). Under normal conditions the pressure within the glomerulus is sufficiently high to force fluid out of the capillaries into the collecting chamber. *When the systolic pressure falls below 70 mm Hg, glomerular filtration ceases and the body is unable to rid itself of fluid and nitrogenous wastes.*

The tubules, which are perfused by the peritubular capillaries, suffer from the lack of oxygen and nutrients. *Acute tubular necrosis* develops. The tubular epithelial cells slough and block the tubules, causing loss of function of the nephron and resulting in *acute* renal failure.

The kidneys often are affected in the early stage of shock, even before systolic blood pressure falls, because the renal vessels respond to sympathetic stimulation by constricting. *A decrease in urinary output is often an early sign of shock.*

Brain

The brain is not affected early in shock. Because it does not contain alpha-adrenergic receptors, its vessels do not constrict in response to the increased levels of adrenaline and noradrenaline, and blood is shunted to the brain (and heart) at the expense of the other organs. As shock progresses and compensatory mechanisms fail, the brain does suffer inadequate perfusion. *As cerebral hypoxia occurs, restlessness and anxiety, followed by lethargy and coma, may be seen.* Cerebral function may also be *altered* by the *increasing acidosis* and the *accumulation of toxic substances.*

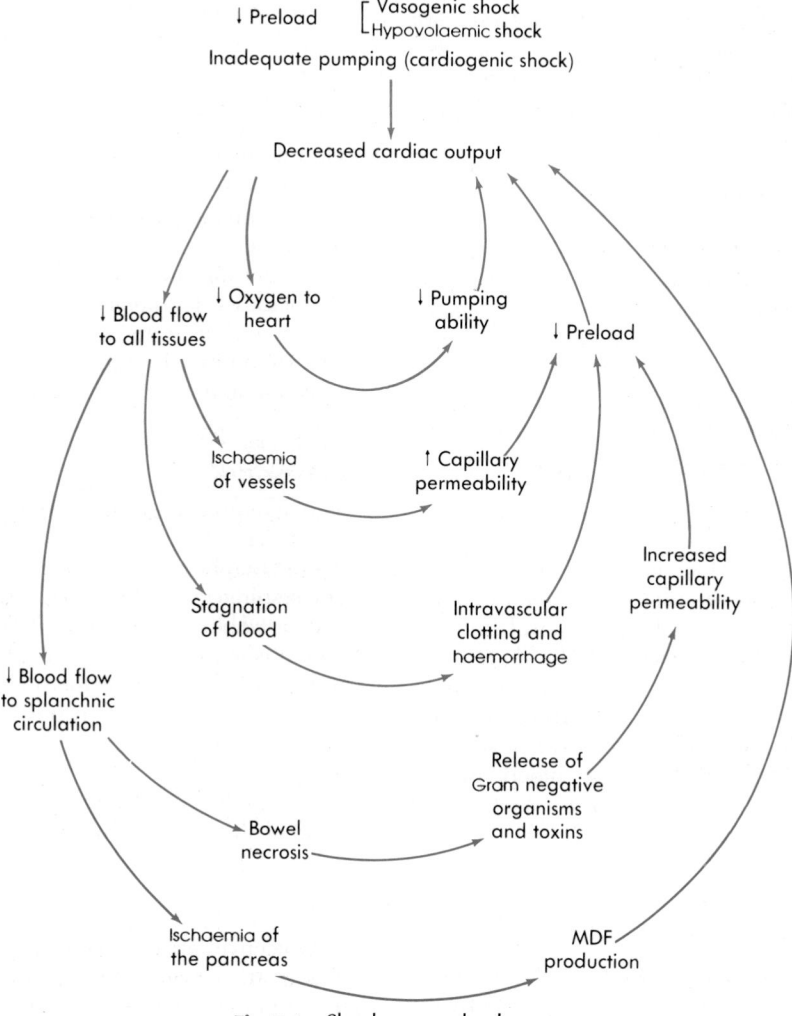

Fig. 7-1 Shock causes shock.

Heart

Although deterioration of cardiac function is a primary problem only in cardiogenic shock, the heart eventually is affected in all types of shock. As cited earlier, in the early stage of shock the heart is spared. *As shock increases, the pumping ability of the heart is affected and cardiac output decreases* (p. 142). As the heart muscle becomes increasingly hypoxic, it begins to show *disturbances of electrical activity.* Most *dysrhythmias have a detrimental effect on cardiac output,* and *some may be fatal.* In the *later stages* of shock, *deterioration of myocardial function* is probably the *most important factor* in the *further progression of shock.*[15]

Lungs

The effect of shock on the lungs has only been recently determined. During the Vietnam War, many victims of traumatic shock survived the early complications because of the use of massive blood transfusions and renal dialysis. The effect of shock on the lungs surfaced as a later complication. The pulmonary condition that results from hypoperfusion of the lungs has been known by a number of names, including shock-lung, white lung, and Da Nang lung. It is now known as adult respiratory distress syndrome (ARDS) (Chapter 16).

ARDS can result from any condition that causes hypoperfusion of the lungs, but is seen most commonly with traumatic or septic shock.[36] It is characterized by *increased permeability of the pulmonary capillaries* to *proteins* and *water,* resulting in *noncardiac pulmonary oedema. Type 2 pneumocytes are destroyed,* impairing the *production of surfactant* that normally prevents collapse of the alveoli. *Alveoli either become filled with fluid or collapse,* and lungs *become stiff.*

In the early stages, *hypoxaemia* results from impaired gas exchange and *hyperventilation* occurs, resulting in *hypocapnoea* and *respiratory alkalosis.* Platelet aggregation in the pulmonary capillaries further damages the lungs. Hypoxaemia persists despite administration of increasing amounts of oxygen. *As shock progresses, ventilation is impaired and carbon dioxide is retained. Respiratory acidosis* results. As hypoxaemia increases, platelet aggregation increases, and a destructive cycle is initiated.

Gastrointestinal Tract

Sympathetic stimulation, which occurs early in shock, causes vasoconstriction and thus decreased blood supply to the organs of the gastrointestinal tract. Bowel function decreases, and *paralytic ileus* may result. If the *blood supply is severely impaired for a length of time, necrosis of the intestinal mucosa may occur. Microorganisms* normally *found in the bowel lyse* and release *endotoxins* when they are attacked by the leukocytes in the blood. *Shock,* from whatever cause, will now also have a septic component. The *gastric mucosa commonly ulcerates* when it *becomes ischaemic, which may result in occult bleeding or massive haemorrhage.*

Liver

Sympathetic stimulation causes vasoconstriction in the liver. In the early stages of shock this can be beneficial. Normally the liver is capable of storing large amounts of blood in its veins. With *vasoconstriction it can release* up to 350 ml *blood into the general circulation,* resulting in *improved cardiac output.*

With *continued sympathetic stimulation* and *decreased blood flow,* liver tissue is affected. In *septic shock* there is an *increase in oxygen uptake* and a *decrease in energy production* in the *liver.* All types of *shock affect the metabolic functions of the liver including the excretion of bile and cholesterol, gluconeogenesis, detoxification, and protein synthesis.*[23]

The sinusoids of the liver are lined with Kupffer cells, which are part of the reticuloendothelial system (RES). These cells are very powerful phagocytes and destroy the many bacteria from the colon that reach the liver by way of the portal system. *Normally, very few bacteria get past the RES. With the destruction of the RES, bacteria enter the general circulation and produce toxins,* which under normal circumstances would be detoxified by the liver. The liver can no longer perform this function, and *overwhelming infection and toxicity result.*

Blood

Disseminated intravascular coagulation (DIC) (Chapter 19) can be a cause or a result of shock. It is characterized by *intravascular clotting,* resulting in the *formation of microthrombi in the capillaries.* Some of the *factors that* activate *clotting factors in the blood* are *acidosis, stagnation,* and *procoagulant substances* such as *bacterial toxins.*[40] *Acidosis* and *stagnation of blood are present in all types of shock,* and bacterial toxins are found in septic shock. As clotting occurs in the capillaries, clotting factors in the rest of the body become depleted. Haemorrhage may then occur from incisions, punctures, the gastrointestinal tract, and other sites. A vicious circle ensues. Intravascular clotting results in even further decrease in tissue perfusion and acidosis. The *haemorrhage caused by DIC decreases* the *cardiac output* even *further* and *worsens tissue perfusion.* The mortality in patients with DIC in association with infection and shock is very high.

Nursing Process
Assessment

The signs and symptoms of shock are summarized in Table 7-2. There are few observable signs in the early stage; the patient may be restless and complain of feeling weak. Pulse and respiratory rates may be increased. Cool, clammy skin, decreased blood pressure, and lethargy or unconsciousness are signs of the later stage. The status of patients in shock is monitored by various methods. The parameters used in assessing shock appear in Box 7-3.

Haemodynamic assessment

Haemodynamic alterations are often the first sign of the onset of shock. The patient's haemodynamic status can be assessed at various levels (Fig. 7-2).

Vital signs

Objective data that are always indicators of physiological change are the vital signs. Any incremental change (e.g., 10 points or more in blood pressure or pulse) should be a clue to increase the frequency of monitoring of these clinical

Table 7-2 Comparison of signs and symptoms in early and late shock by body system

Body system	Early shock	Late shock
Respiratory system	Hyperventilation; ↑ minute volume; ↓ P_{CO_2}; normal P_{O_2}	Respirations shallow; breath sounds may suggest congestion; ↑ P_{CO_2}; ↓ P_{O_2}
Cardiovascular system	Blood pressure normal to slightly lowered; ↑ diastolic pressure; ↓ pulse pressure; cardiac output normal; tachycardia; mild vasoconstriction in hypovolaemic and cardiogenic shock	↓ Blood pressure; ↓ cardiac output; tachycardia continues; vasoconstriction worsens in hypovolaemic, cardiogenic, and septic shock
Renal system	Normal to slightly depressed urine output; ↑ urine osmolality; ↓ urine sodium concentration. Hypokalaemia	Oliguria or complete renal shutdown; buildup of waste products. Hyperglycaemia
Acid–base balance	Respiratory alkalosis	Metabolic acidosis; respiratory acidosis
Vascular compartment	Fluids shift from interstitial space to vascular compartment; thirst	Fluids shift from vascular space to interstitial and intracellular space, causing oedema
Skin	Minimal to no changes in hypovolaemic and cardiogenic shock; warm, flushed skin in vasogenic shock	Cool, clammy skin in hypovolaemic, cardiogenic, and septic shock; cool and mottled skin in other types of shock
Haematologic system	Release of red blood cells from bone marrow to increase vascular volume; platelet aggregation	Disseminated intravascular coagulation
Mental–neurologic system	Restlessness; alertness; confusion	Lethargy; unconsciousness
Gastrointestinal–hepatic system	No obvious changes	Perfusion decreases and bowel sounds may be diminished. MDF production by hypoxic pancreas. Liver dysfunction. Possible bowel necrosis

---

7-3

Parameters for assessing status of patient in shock

Haemodynamic monitoring
Blood pressure (cuff and/or intraarterial)
Pulse
Central venous pressure
Pulmonary artery pressure
Pulmonary wedge pressure
Cardiac output
Electrocardiogram
Mixed venous O_2 saturation

Respiratory monitoring
Respiratory rate, depth
Breath sounds
Blood gases
  pH
  P_{O_2}
  P_{CO_2}
Per cent O_2 saturation
Pulse oximetry

Fluid and electrolyte monitoring
Serum electrolytes
Blood lactate and pyruvate levels
Intake
  By mouth
  Intravenous
  Nasogastric
  Irrigation solutions
  Solution in medications
Output
  Urinary
  Gastrointestinal tract
  Sweating
  Dressings
Weight
Serum creatinine level
Blood urea nitrogen level
Serum and urinary osmolality
Urinary specific gravity

Neurological monitoring
Alertness
Orientation
Mental acuity

Haematological monitoring
Erythrocytes
Haematocrit and haemoglobin levels
Leukocytes
Platelets
Prothrombin and partial thromboplastin times
Clotting time
Fibrin degradation products

Other monitoring
Bowel sounds
Skin temperature

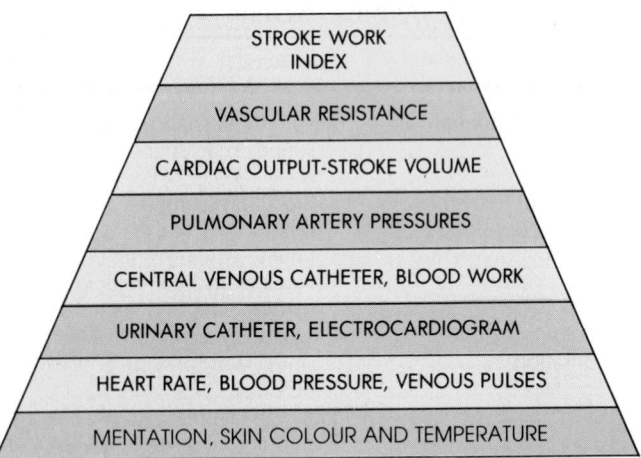

Fig. 7-2   Levels of haemodynamic monitoring. (From Ellerbe S: *Fluid and blood component therapy in the critically ill and injured,* New York, 1981, Churchill Livingstone.)

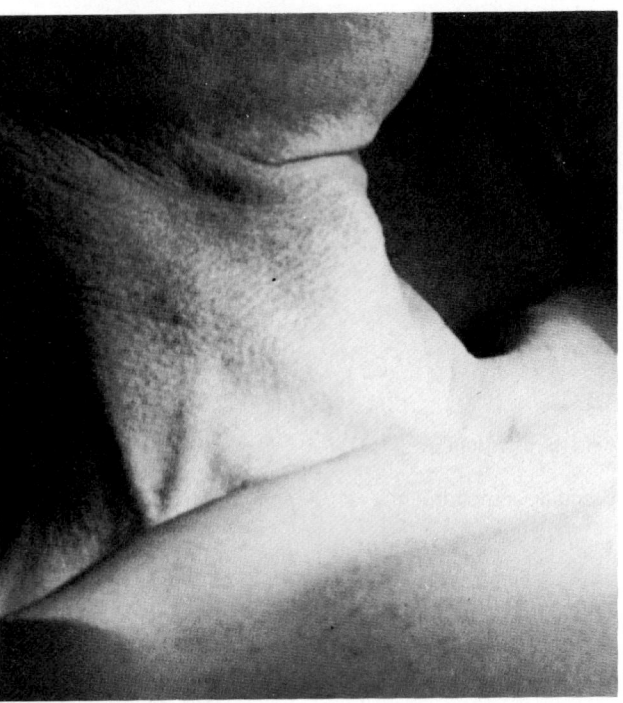

Fig. 7-3   Distended external jugular neck vein of a patient with right-sided heart failure. (From Daily EK, Schroeder J: *Techniques in bedside hemodynamic monitoring,* ed 4, St Louis, 1989, Mosby–Year Book.)

parameters. As shock progresses, the pulse becomes quite rapid and in the latter stages of shock becomes difficult to palpate. Irregularities in the pulse may develop as cardiac dysrhythmias occur.

Early in shock the blood pressure may be normal or elevated because of compensatory vasoconstriction. Blood pressure can be heard without difficulty at this early stage. However, when blood pressure starts decreasing as the pulse rate is increasing, a heightened concern for clinical instability suggestive of *progressive shock* should be considered. The monitoring of vital signs at this point could be as frequent as every half hour to hour depending on the speed and magnitude of the changes being assessed. As shock progresses, the blood pressure may be difficult to auscultate, but it may be possible to obtain the systolic pressure by palpation. If intraarterial pressure monitoring is not instituted, Doppler ultrasound (Chapter 18) may be helpful in obtaining the blood pressure.

Venous pulsation in the neck is noted. Both the external and internal jugular veins should be examined. Generally, the external jugular vein is easier to see, but in some patients with heart disease the external jugular veins are occluded by fibrosis or are absent. Because of these potential problems, venous pulsation in the internal jugular vein may be a more reliable area to assess for signs of venous pulsation and right atrial pressure. Normally, *venous pulsations* are visible when the patient is lying flat but not when the head is elevated to 45 degrees (Fig. 7-3). Flat neck veins, when the patient is in a horizontal position, often indicate *hypovolaemia,* common in most types of shock.

Central venous pressure

Central venous pressure (CVP) is a more accurate means of determining the fluid status of a patient in shock. CVP measures right ventricular filling pressure, which reflects venous return to the heart. CVP monitoring is most valuable in assessing status in patients with absolute or relative hypovolaemia, including those with vasogenic, neurogenic, and hypovolaemic shock. It is *less valuable in assessment in patients with cardiogenic shock,* who may have intravascular fluid excess.

To obtain an accurate CVP reading, a catheter is inserted into a major vein and threaded through the superior vena cava into the right atrium. The catheter is attached by a three-way stopcock to an intravenous infusion and a water manometer (Fig. 7-4). The intravenous solution (usually 5% glucose in water) is allowed to drip slowly into the vein to keep the vein open. When a reading is to be taken, the stopcock is opened to the manometer and the manometer is filled with the intravenous solution. The stopcock is then turned to the venous opening (the patient). The fluid level in the manometer should fluctuate with each respiration. The fluid is allowed to stabilize before a reading is taken, and the highest level of the fluid fluctuating in the column is used for the CVP reading. As soon as the reading is taken, the stopcock is turned to the solution position, and the infusion is continued.

For the CVP reading to be accurate, the patient must be relaxed, and the zero point of the manometer must always be at the level of the right atrium, which in most people is level with the midaxillary line. If the patient cannot be flat in bed, the zero point on the manometer is adjusted to the level of the right atrium in a sitting position. Any change in the patient's position requires that the zero point be reset. *The initial CVP reading and the position that the patient was in when it was taken should be recorded, because these will serve as a baseline for comparison with subsequent readings.* The patient should be placed in the same position for each reading, since even a slight change in position alters the CVP.

The normal values for CVP will vary with the use of different equipment; however, a range of 5 cm to 15 cm

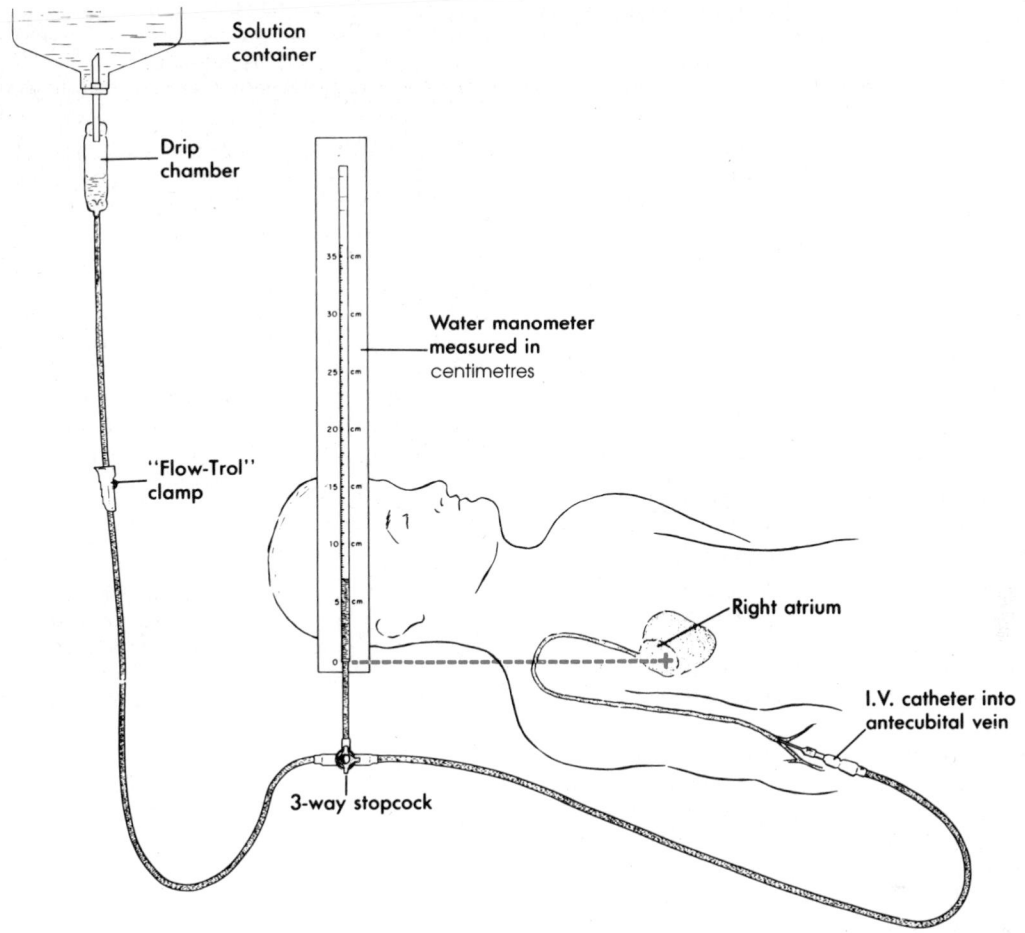

Fig. 7-4 Measurement of central venous pressure (CVP) using water manometer. Zero point on manometer is at level of midright atrium, and CVP reading is 7 cm of water.

water is acceptable. It is important to note that a change or a trend in the CVP is more important than the actual numeric value.

Central venous catheters can also be used to obtain blood samples, to assess venous oxygen saturation determinations, and to administer fluids. The catheter insertion site should be kept scrupulously clean to minimize the possibility of phlebitis. Patient movement is not restricted as long as the catheter and tubing are secured adequately and intravenous flow is maintained.

Pulmonary artery pressures

The status of the left side of the heart can best be evaluated by the measurement of pulmonary artery pressure (PAP) *and pulmonary capillary wedge resection* (PCWP). A mean PAP of less than 10 mm Hg may indicate decreased blood volume resulting in decreased preload in the left ventricle. A mean PAP of more than 20 mm Hg may indicate poor myocardial contractility and left ventricular overload. These pressures are measured with a special triple-lumen balloon-tipped (Swan-Ganz) catheter (Fig. 7-5). The catheter is inserted into a vein, usually the *subclavian*, and advanced to the *right atrium*. The balloon is inflated and carried to the right ventricle and then to the pulmonary artery by the

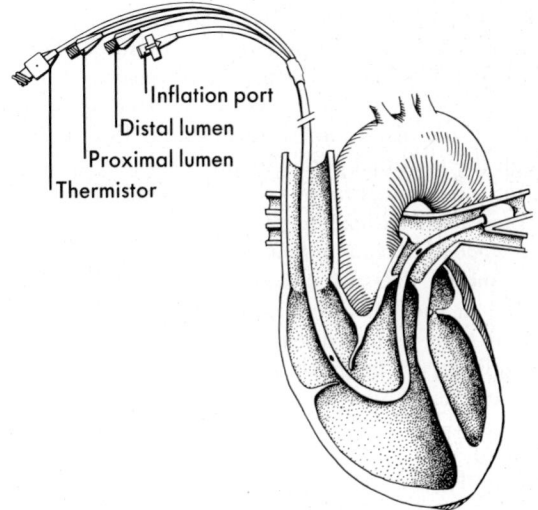

Fig. 7-5 Placement of Swan-Ganz catheter.

Table 7-3 Complications of pulmonary artery pressure monitoring

Complication	Indications	Interventions
Infection	Chills Headache Malaise Generalized aching Flushed face Warm skin Elevated temperature	1. Notify doctor immediately. 2. Prepare for removal of catheter. 3. Administer antibiotics as ordered. 4. Provide symptomatic relief.
Ventricular arrhythmias: premature ventricular contractions, or short runs of ventricular tachycardia	"Skipped heart beats" Irregular pulse PVC's noted on cardiac monitor	1. Notify doctor immediately. 2. Prepare for repositioning of catheter. 3. Administer antiarrhythmic drugs if problem persists after repositioning.
Sustained ventricular tachycardia, or ventricular fibrillation	Lightheadedness, progressing to loss of consciousness Loss of consciousness Pulselessness Dysrhythmia noted on cardiac monitor Respiratory arrest	1. Notify doctor immediately. 2. Prepare for repositioning catheter. 3. Defibrillate.
Pulmonary infarction	Chest pain Haemoptysis Fever Friction rub Elevated LDH Area of opacity on chest X-ray film Decreased Pao_2	1. Notify doctor immediately. 2. Administer oxygen. 3. Prepare for repositioning or removal of catheter. 4. Provide symptomatic relief.
Valvular damage	Depends on extent of damage Patient may be asymptomatic, or may develop symptoms of congestive heart failure or new murmur	1. Notify doctor of development of new murmur or new symptoms.

Modified from Asheervath J and Blevins D: *Handbook of clinical nursing practice*, Norwalk, Conn, 1986, Appleton-Century-Crofts.

blood flow. The balloon is then deflated and the tip of the catheter is left in the *pulmonary artery*. The opening at the tip of the catheter communicates with the distal port. The lumen from the proximal port opens into the right atrium. The distal port is connected to a transducer, which converts the pressure it senses through the catheter to an electrical signal, which is then displayed on a monitor. Thus the pressure in the pulmonary artery can be measured continuously. A continuous flush system is used to maintain patency of the distal lumen. Intravenous fluid is infused through the proximal port. The proximal port can also be used for the administration of medications.

In individuals without lung or pulmonary vascular disease, PAP is a good indicator of how well the left side of the heart is functioning. Pressure changes in the left ventricle are reflected in the left atrium and back to the pulmonary artery. If there is any disease in the lungs, however, as frequently occurs in shock, the PAP does not accurately reflect left ventricular pressure. In this case, the PCWP should be obtained. By inflating the balloon, which is near the tip of the catheter, the pulmonary artery can be occluded. This blocks communication between the pressure in the pulmonary artery and the lumen of the catheter, allowing for pressure that is ahead of the occluded artery to be transmitted through the catheter. The PCWP is identical to the left atrial pressure.

The nurse caring for the patient with pulmonary artery pressure monitoring must be aware of the common complications that can occur with this type of invasive monitoring (Table 7-3). The appearance of either a *right ventricular* or *PCWP waveform* on the monitor can have serious consequences for the patient. Dislodgement of the tip of the catheter from the pulmonary artery into the right ventricle can result in the occurrence of *premature ventricular beats* or even *ventricular tachycardia*. Progression of the catheter into a small vessel in the pulmonary vasculature can occlude the vessel and result in *pulmonary infarction*. Prolonged inflation of the balloon can have the same effect. The nurse must be able to distinguish the normal PAP waveform from both right ventricular and PCWP waveforms (Fig. 7-6). It is essential that sterile technique be maintained during the insertion of the PAP catheter and during dressing changes.

Intraarterial assessment

Intraarterial monitoring is usually instituted along with PAP monitoring. A catheter is inserted into a radial, brachial, or femoral artery and attached to a transducer in much the same way as the pulmonary artery catheter (Fig. 7-7). Because this is a high-pressure system, haemorrhage is a possible complication, and the insertion and connections in the system must be monitored frequently. The

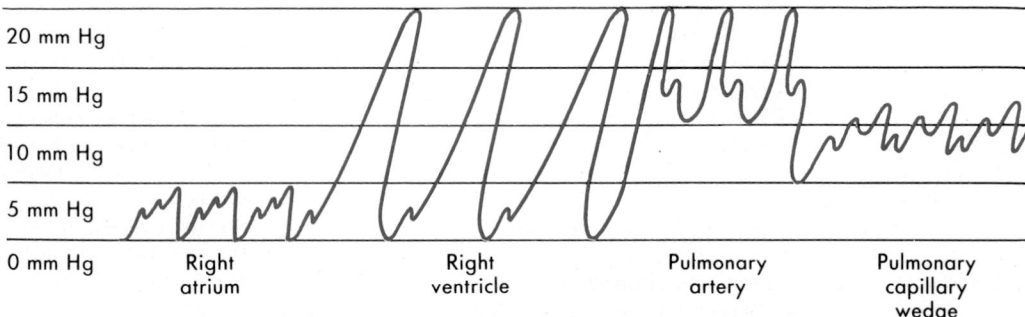

20 mm Hg				
15 mm Hg				
10 mm Hg				
5 mm Hg				
0 mm Hg	Right atrium	Right ventricle	Pulmonary artery	Pulmonary capillary wedge

Fig. 7-6 Characteristic waveforms of pulmonary artery pressure monitoring. (From Asheervath J, Blevins D: *Handbook of clinical nursing practice,* 1986, Norwalk, Ct, Appleton-Century-Crofts.)

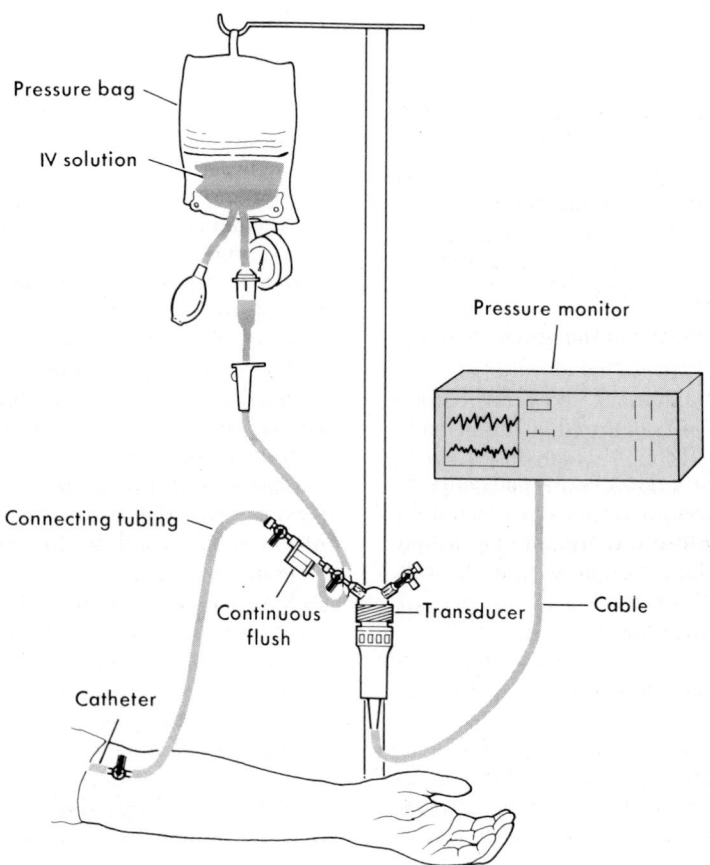

Pressure bag

IV solution

Pressure monitor

Connecting tubing

Continuous flush

Transducer

Cable

Catheter

Fig. 7-7 Connections between intraarterial catheter, transducer, monitor, and fluid. (From Daily EK, Schroeder J: *Techniques in bedside hemodynamic monitoring,* ed 4, St Louis, 1989, Mosby–Year Book.)

Table 7-4 Complications of intraarterial pressure monitoring

Complication	Indications	Intervention

Haemorrhage	Obvious excessive bleeding
	Tachycardia
	Hypotension
	Pallor
	Diaphoresis
	Tachypnoea
	Restlessness
	Dizziness
	Headache
		1. Control bleeding
		  a. If bleeding is occurring at the puncture site, apply pressure.
		  b. If part of the system has become disconnected, immediately turn the stopcocks to stop bleeding.
		2. Attach a syringe containing sterile saline until contaminated parts of the system are replaced with sterile parts.
		3. Notify the doctor if a large amount of blood has been lost.
		4. Prepare the patient for blood replacement if loss has been large.

Thrombus or embolus	Pallor, loss of pulse, and coolness of skin distal to the site of the thrombus Pain	1. Notify the doctor immediately. 2. Instruct patient to lie quietly. 3. Prepare to administer O_2.
Infection of catheter site	Redness and warmth at the site Possible fever	1. Notify the doctor 2. Prepare for removal of the catheter. 3. Send the catheter tip for culture.
Bacteraemia	High fever Chills	1. Notify the doctor. 2. Prepare for removal of the catheter.

Modified from Asheervath J and Blevins D: *Handbook of clinical nursing practice*, Norwalk, Conn, 1986, Appleton-Century-Crofts.

extremity distal to the insertion site must be monitored for signs of arterial occlusion (colour, temperature, movement, presence or absence of pulses, and pain) (Table 7-4). It is essential that sterile technique be maintained during insertion of the catheter and during dressing changes. A patient who is ill enough to require haemodynamic monitoring has little reserve to fight infection.

Cardiac output, cardiac index, and mixed venous return assessment

Some pulmonary artery catheters allow for cardiac output and cardiac index to be monitored at the bedside. Such catheters have a port through which fluid can be injected into the right atrium. *A thermistor is located at the tip of the catheter and attached to a wire that runs through the catheter and is attached to a cardiac output computer.* Saline, either iced or at room temperature, is injected into the right atrium. The solution travels with the blood into the pulmonary artery. The thermistor senses the extent of temperature change, and from these data the computer is able to calculate cardiac output. The normal cardiac index is 2.5 to 3.5 L/min/m².

Another version of the pulmonary artery catheter called the fiberoptic flow directed pulmonary artery catheter allows for continuous evaluation of the balance between supply of oxygen to the tissues and consumption of oxygen by the tissues, i.e. mixed venous oxygen saturation. Values that reflect a normal balance between supply of oxygen and oxygen consumption are 0.68 to 0.77. High values (greater than 0.77) are associated with conditions of reduced oxygen consumption in the tissues (e.g., septic shock, hypothermia, deep coma). Low values (less than 0.68) may be seen

in states of high oxygen consumption (e.g., major surgery, aggressive exercise).

Respiratory assessment

As cited earlier, hypoperfusion of the lungs, common in shock, may result in adult respiratory distress syndrome (ARDS). This may be suspected very early in the course of the disease from changes in the patient's mentation. There may be minor changes in orientation, unusual interpersonal exchanges, and mood changes. The patient is observed for *cough* and *dyspnoea*, which develop as ARDS progresses. *Changes in respiratory rate* and in the *colour of the mucous membranes and skin are important indicators of pulmonary status.* Breath sounds are auscultated. Early in the course of the disease the lungs may be clear, but as ARDS progresses, *rales and rhonchi may be heard.*

If the patient is receiving mechanical ventilation, the amount of pressure required to deliver a specific tidal volume is noted. As the *lungs* become *increasingly* stiff, the *pressure required to deliver the volume increases.* With ARDS, the pulmonary artery pressure may rise, although the pulmonary capillary wedge pressure remains normal.[36] Arterial blood gases may provide valuable information and are monitored as indicated depending on the patient's condition. Characteristically with ARDS, the Pao_2 falls, in spite of ventilation with increasing amounts of oxygen, because of *physiological shunting* of blood through the lungs to the left side of the heart. Shunting occurs because many alveoli are either collapsed or filled with fluid, and diffusion cannot occur. In the earlier stages of ARDS, when a sufficient number of alveoli are functioning, the $Paco_2$ is usually normal or more likely low because of the rapid diffusion of CO_2 and of hyperventilation that results from hypoxia. However, as the number of functioning alveoli decreases, the $Paco_2$ increases.

Arterial blood gas determinations are also used to assess the *acid–base balance* of the patient in shock. In the early stages of shock, mild *respiratory alkalosis* is common from *hyperventilation* that is part of the stress response. As shock progresses and tissues become progressively hypoxaemic, *anaerobic metabolism* takes place and *metabolic acidosis* occurs. In the *advanced stages of shock*, when *respirations decrease* and *ARDS becomes progressively worse, respiratory acidosis may also develop.*

Fluid and electrolyte assessment

The urinary output and the CVP most accurately reflect fluid status. An indwelling urinary catheter is usually inserted, and the urine output is measured hourly. Other output, such as gastrointestinal drainage, wound drainage, or perspiration, is measured or estimated as accurately as possible. *Body weight* often gives a more accurate assessment of fluid changes than the measurement of intake and output; however, this can be an inaccurate determinant of intravascular volume when "third spacing" of fluid occurs. *Noting* the presence of *oedema, auscultating* the *chest* for the *presence of fluid,* and *measuring* the *abdominal girth* for the development of *ascites are means of assessing fluid collection in the third spaces.*

In the early stages of shock, the serum potassium concentration may be abnormally low as a result of increased levels of aldosterone in response to stress. However, as shock progresses, the serum K^+ level may become abnormally high as damaged cells release K^+. As urinary output falls, the body is unable to eliminate the excess amounts of K^+ that are accumulating in the serum. If K^+ is administered in the early stage of shock, it is extremely important that the urinary output and serum electrolytes be monitored frequently so that *hyperkalaemia* can be *prevented* or *treated early* should it occur.

The concentration of other serum electrolytes may be abnormal as a result of acid–base abnormalities, altered renal function, or fluid therapy. Serum enzymes may be elevated because of ischaemia and damage to the heart, liver, and pancreas.

Neurological assessment

In shock, the brain may be adversely affected by hypoxia, acid–base imbalance, or toxins. Often, *subtle changes in mentation are the earliest signs of cerebral hypoxia.* The patient is observed for *increasing restlessness.* Sedation should not be given until the patient's status has been assessed further and it has been determined that the restlessness does not have an organic cause. In the *late stages, when perfusion of the brain is severely impaired, loss of consciousness* occurs. Vital signs and arterial blood gas determinations can aid in assessing the cause of subtle neurological changes.

Haematological assessment

The *haemoglobin* and *haematocrit* levels are valuable tools for assessing blood loss in *hypovolaemic shock secondary to haemorrhage.* It must be remembered, however, that the *haemoglobin and haematocrit levels do not drop immediately with loss of an excessive amount of blood,* because *plasma is lost along with the blood cells. The blood that remains in the intravascular compartment initially will have a normal concentration of red blood cells in less plasma and the haematocrit will be increased.* Because the kidneys retain water in response to blood loss, the blood becomes more dilute and there is a decrease in the haemoglobin and haematocrit concentrations.

Patients in shock are assessed for the development of DIC. The nurse may be the first to observe that the patient is bleeding for an excessively long time after a venipuncture or that blood is oozing from an incision. If DIC is suspected, laboratory studies are initiated, then clotting factors (including fibrinogen and platelet counts) are decreased, prothrombin time and partial thromboplastin time (aPTT) are prolonged, and fibrin degradation products are increased.

Other assessment

Abdominal assessment is important in the patient in shock. Decreased blood flow to the intestines may result in decreased peristalsis or paralytic ileus (Chapter 23). *Decreased or absent bowel sounds are noted. Gastric drainage and stools are assessed for occult blood because of the high incidence of gastrointestinal tract bleeding with shock.*

Nursing analysis

Nursing problems are determined from assessment of patient data. Possible nursing diagnoses for the person with shock include, but are not limited to, the following:

Problem	Possible aetiologies
Cardiac output, decreased	Myocardial hypoxia, myocardial depressant factor
Fluid volume deficit	Blood loss, increased capillary permeability, vasodilation
Gas exchange, impaired	Decreased lung compliance, interstitial oedema
Tissue perfusion, altered cardiopulmonary	Hypovolaemia, decreased cardiac output, redistribution of blood
Breathing pattern, ineffective	Inadequate perfusion of respiratory muscles
Airway clearance, ineffective	Decreased energy, endotracheal intubation
Anxiety	Threat of death
Oral mucous membrane, altered	Endotracheal intubation
Infection, high risk for	Invasive monitoring, Foley catheterization, decreased immune response
Sleep pattern disturbance	Intensity of nursing care
Activity intolerance	Imbalance between oxygen supply and demand

Planning: expected patient outcomes

Expected patient outcomes for the person with shock may include, but are not limited to, the following:

1. Cardiac output determination using thermodilution techniques confirms that the cardiac output is normal.
2. Intravascular volume (haemoglobin and haematocrit) returns to normal; urinary output and specific gravity are within normal limits.
3. Arterial blood gases (Po_2 and Pco_2) are within normal limits.
4. Vital signs (blood pressure, pulse) indicate normal tissue perfusion.
5. Respiratory rate and tidal volume are within normal limits.
6. Airway remains free from secretions.
7. Patient and significant others remain free of avoid able anxiety.
8. Oral mucous membrane remains moist and intact.
9. Patient is free from infection.
10. Patient sleeps for undisturbed periods of time.
11. Patient tolerates activity involved in care without an increase in pulse rate of more than 20 per minute.

Implementation

Assisting with achievement of therapeutic goals

Treatment of shock will vary to some extent, depending on the cause of the shock, the organ systems affected, and the preexisting condition of the patient. *In the early, acute phase of shock, the major role of the nurse is continuous assessment of the patient's clinical status and assisting with administration of therapies necessary to stabilize the patient's condition.*

Fundamentally, the same priorities that exist for treating any life-threatening emergency hold true for shock. The priorities for shock management are as follows:

1. Airway: A patent airway must be maintained to maximize oxygen uptake and carbon dioxide removal. To accomplish this, a nasal or oral airway may be inserted. When respiratory failure is a high potential, the airway is secured with an endotracheal tube.
2. Breathing: Oxygen is administered immediately at the level ordered. This may include preparations to ventilate the patient by mechanical ventilation. These measures support breathing and enhance ventilation and gas exchange between the airways and the circulation.
3. Circulation: The pump (the heart) is supported by the administration of fluids including blood to increase blood volume, improve cardiac output, and maximize oxygen transport to the cells. Vasoactive and cardiogenic drugs may also be prescribed to enhance cardiovascular functioning and oxygen transport to the cells.
4. Diagnosis: Shock can be treated most effectively if the underlying cause can be determined and treated. For example, if the cause of shock is hypovolaemia secondary to massive bleeding, efforts will be made to find the site of the bleeding and stop it, if possible. Blood and fluids will be used to improve intervascular

volume and cardiac output. This will then improve exchange of oxygen and carbon dioxide at the cellular level. If the cause of shock is sepsis, antibiotics will be administered intravenously, and if the cause is anaphylaxis, adrenaline is given.

Evaluation

Evaluation is based on expected patient outcomes, and questions used to measure them include the following:

1. Patient will be able to tolerate activity involved in care. Did pulse increase no more than 10 beats per minute? Did skin remain warm and dry? Did respiratory rate remain the same?
2. Patient's airway will remain free from secretions. Are lung sounds clear? Can suction catheter be inserted into airway easily?
3. Patient and significant others will remain free of avoidable anxiety. Are they able to verbalize fears? Are they free of signs of anxiety?
4. Patient will have a respiratory rate and tidal volume within normal limits. Are respirations regular? Is the respiratory rate between 16 and 22 per minute? Is the tidal volume normal for the patient's size?
5. Cardiac output will be within normal limits. Is the mean arterial blood pressure greater than 80 mm Hg? Is the pulse rate between 60 and 100 beats per minute? Is the cardiac index 2.5 to 3.5 L/min/m²? Is the PCWP between 10 and 20 mm Hg?
6. Patient will make his or her needs understood by verbal or alternate means of communication. Is the patient able to make his or her needs known? Is the patient free from anxiety when trying to communicate?
7. Intravascular volume will return to normal. Is the CVP between 6 and 15 cm water? Is the pulse volume normal? Is the pulse rate between 60 and 100 per minute?
8. Blood gases will be within normal limits. Are the blood gases within the following range? Po_2 80 to 100 mm Hg; Pco_2 35 to 45 mm Hg; HCO_3 22 to 26 mmol/L; pH 7.35 to 7.45.
9. Patient will be free from infection. Is the patient's temperature within normal range? Is the leukocyte count between 4500 and 11,000/mm? Are the catheter insertion sites free from redness, swelling, and drainage?
10. Oral mucous membrane will remain moist and intact. Is mucous membrane pink and moist? Are lips free from cracks? Is mouth free of excessn mucus?
11. Patient will have adequate rest. Does patient appear rested? Has care been planned to allow for periods of undisturbed sleep?
12. Patient will have normal tissue perfusion. Is the urinary output greater than 30 ml/h? Is the BUN between 8 and 25 mg/dl? Is the serum creatinine

between 0.6 and 1.2 mg/dl? Is the lactic acid level less than 1.9 mmol/L? Is the serum potassium level between 3.8 and 5.0 mmol/L? Is the serum sodium level between 136 and 142 mmol/L? Is the patient's skin warm, dry, and pink? Is capillary refill less than 3 seconds? Is the patient's mental status the same as before the onset of shock?

13. Patient will remain free of injury. Is the patient free from nosocomial infections? Is the patient free of abrasions? Is the patient free of complications of immobility?

SUMMARY

1. Shock is a syndrome characterized by hypoperfusion of body tissues.
2. The major classifications of shock are hypovolaemic, cardiogenic, and vasogenic shock.
3. Shock results in a derangement of cellular metabolism, and if not treated in the early stages, it can affect all body systems.
4. The early stage of shock is characterized by a stress response.
5. At some point in the progress of untreated shock, the process becomes irreversible and no treatment can save the patient.

STUDY QUESTIONS

- How would you define shock?
- What are the differences between the neurogenic form and the septic form of vasogenic shock?
- Metabolic acidosis and respiratory acidosis are typically signs of what stage of shock?
- Is fluid volume deficit a potential nursing assessment in all types of shock?

REFERENCES AND SELECTED READINGS

1. Asheervath J, Blevins D: *Handbook of clinical nursing practice*, Norwalk, Conn, 1986, Appleton-Century-Crofts.
2. Barone JE: Treatment strategies in shock: use of oxygen transport measurements, *Heart Lung* 20(1):81-86, 1991.
3. Biharri DJ, Tinker J: The therapeutic value of vasodilator prostaglandins in multiple organ failure associated with sepsis, *Intens Care* 15(1):2-7, 1988.
4. Bonato J: Blood transfusions: are they safe? *Crit Care Nurse* 9(7):40-46, 1989.
5. Bone RC: A critical evaluation of new agents for the treatment of sepsis, *JAMA* 266(12):1686-1691, 1991.
6. Brandsetter RD: The adult respiratory distress syndrome-11986, *Heart Lung* 15(2):155-164, 1986.
7. Bulle TM, Rogers WJ: Cardiogenic shock. In Hardway RM: *Shock: the reversible stage of dying*, Littleton, Mass, 1986, PSG Publishing.
8. Calandra T, et al: Treatment of gram-negative shock with human IgF antibody to Escherichia coli J5: a prospective, double blind, randomized trial, *J Infect Dis* 58(2):312-319, 1988.
9. Clowes GHA Jr: *Trauma sepsis and shock: the physiological basis of therapy*, New York, 1988, Marcel Dekker.
10. Danner RL, Parrillo JF: The role of endotoxins in human septic shock: therapeutic potential of lipid A analogs, *Prog Clin Biol Res* 286:183-200, 1989, Alan R Liss, Inc.
11. Dickerson M: Anaphylaxis and anaphylactic shock, *Crit Care Nurs Q* 11(1):674-678, 1988.
12. Dislet L, et al: Cardiogenic shock in evolving myocardial infarction, *Heart Lung* 16:649-651, 1987.
13. Dunham CM, Cowley RA: *Shock trauma/critical care handbook*, Rockville, Md, 1986, Aspen Systems.
    13a. Goldberg RJ et al: Cardiogenic shock after acute myocardial infarction, *N Engl J Med* 325(16):1117-1122, 1991.
14. Gorelick K, et al: Randomized placebo-controlled study of E5 monoclonal antiendotoxin antibody. In Larrick J, Borrebaeck C, eds: *Therapeutic monoclonal antibodies*, New York, 1990, Stockton Press.
15. Guyton AC: *Textbook of medical physiology*, ed 7, Philadelphia, 1986, WB Saunders.
16. Halfman-Franey M: Current trends in haemodynamic monitoring of patients in shock, *Crit Care Nurs Q* 11(1):9-18, 1988.
17. Hammerschmidt DE, Vercellotti GM: Granulocytes of mediators of tissue injury in shock: therapeutic implications, *Prog Clin Biol Res* 236A:19-32, 1987, Alan R. Liss.
18.* Hancock BG, Eberhard NK: The pharmacological management of shock, *Crit Care Nurs Q* 11(1):19-29, 1988.
19. Hardway RM: *Shock: the reversible stage of dying*, Littleton, Mass, 1986, PSG Publishing.
20. Hesselvik JF, Brodin B: Low dose noradrenaline in patients with septic shock and oliguria: effects on afterload, urine flow, and oxygen transport, *Crit Care Med* 17(2):179-180, 1989.
21.* Houston MC: Pathophysiology of shock, *Crit Care Nurs Clin North Am* 2(2):143-149, 1990.
22. Jefferies PR, Whelan SK: Cardiogenic shock: current management, *Crit Care Nurs Q* 11(1):48-56, 1988.
23. Jurkovich GJ, Moore EE, Eisman B: The liver in shock. In Hardaway RM: *Shock: the reversible stage of dying*, Littleton, Mass, 1986, PSG Publishing.
24.* Lancaster LE, Rice V: Nursing care: planning overview and application to the patient in shock, *Crit Care Nurs Clin North Am* 2(2):279-286, 1990.
25. Lefer AM, Hock CE: Vascular mediators in circulatory shock. In Hardaway RM: *Shock: the reversible stage of dying*, Littleton, Mass, 1986, PSG Publishing.
26. Littleton MT: Pathophysiology and assessment of sepsis and septic shock, *Crit Care Nurs Q* 11(1):30-47, 1988.
27. Littleton MT: Prostaglandins and leukotrienes as mediators of shock and trauma, *Crit Care Nurs Q* 11(2):11-20, 1988.
28. MacLean LD: Shock, *Br Med Bull* 44(2):437-452, 1988.
29. Martin E, et al: Autotransfusion systems, *Crit Care Nurs* 9(7):65-72, 1989.
30.* McMorrow ME, Daniello MC: When to suspect septic shock, *RN* 54(10):32-37, October 1991.
31.* McQuillan KA, Wiles CE: Initial management of traumatic shock. In Cardona DV, et al: *Trauma nursing from resuscitation through rehabilitation*, Philadelphia, 1988, WB Saunders.
32. McSwam NE: Pneumatic anti-shock garment: state of the art, 1988, *Ann Emerg Med* 17(5):506-526, 1988.
33. Millar S: *AACN procedure manual for critical care*, Philadelphia, 1985, WB Saunders.
34. Nagy S: Cardiodepressant and cardiostimulant factors in shock, *Prog Clin Biol Res* 236A:599-610, 1987, Alan R Liss.
35. Parrillo JE: The cardiovascular pathophysiology of sepsis, *Ann Rev Med* 49:469-485, 1989.
36. Perry AG: Shock complications: recognition and management, *Crit Care Nurs Q* 11(1):1-8, 1988.
37. Rackow RC, Astiz ME: Pathophysiology and treatment of septic shock, *JAMA* 266(4):548-554, 1991.
38. Rackow RC, Astiz ME, Weil MH: Cellular oxygen metabolism during sepsis and shock, *JAMA* 259(13):1989-1993, 1988.
39. Rice V: *Shock: a clinical syndrome, the clinical continuum of septic shock, shock management*, Secaucus, NJ, 1985, Critical Care Nurse/Hospital Publications.
40.* Rice V: Shock, a clinical syndrome: an update. Part 1, an overview of shock, *Crit Care Nurs* 11(4):20-27, 1991.
41. Rice V: Shock, a clinical syndrome: an update. Part 3, therapeutic management, *Crit Care Nurs* 11(6):41-43, 1991.
42. Schedel I: New aspects in the treatment of gram-negative bacteremia and septic shock, *Infection* 16(1):4-7, 1988.
43. Schumer W: Corticosteroids in the treatment of shock, *Prog Clin Biol Res* 236B:249-259, 1987, Alan R Liss.
44. Shoemaker WC, et al: Therapy of shock based on pathophysiology, monitoring and outcome prediction, *Crit Care Med* 18(1):19-25, 1990.
45. Soulioti AM: Naloxone for septic shock, *Lancet* 2(8620):1133-1134, 1988.
46. Strange JM, editor: *Shock trauma care plans*, Springhouse, Penn, 1987, Springhouse.

47. Stroud M, Swindell B, Bernard GR: Cellular humoral mediators of sepsis syndrome, *Nurs Clin North Am* 2(2):150-160, 1990.

48. Summers G: The clinical and haemodynamic presentation of the shock patient, *Nurs Clin North Am* 2(2):161-166, 1990.

49. Tilkian SM, Conover MB, Tilkian AG: *Clinical implications of laboratory tests,* ed 4, St Louis, 1987, Mosby–Year Book.

50. Weil MH, Rackow EC: Colloidal osmotic pressure and its implication for the fluid management of patients in shock. In Hardway RM: *Shock: the reversible stage of dying,* Littleton, Mass, 1986, PGS Publishing.

51. Flower NO: Examination of the heart: inspection and palpation of venous and arterial pulses, New York, 1978, American Heart Association.

52. Perry AG, Potter PA: Shock: comprehensive nursing management, St Louis, 1983, Mosby–Year Book.

*Recommended for student reading.

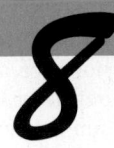

Pain

Judith H. Watt-Watson
Barbara C. Long

After studying this chapter, the learner should be able to:

- Describe some common misbeliefs about pain management.
- Describe the physiology of pain and related theories of pain transmission.
- Compare factors that influence perception and response to pain.
- Differentiate between acute and chronic pain assessment.
- Describe some assessment tools to use in clinical practice.
- Describe pharmacological and nonpharmacological approaches for pain management.
- Identify nursing implications for pain management.
- Explain the purpose and methods of the team approach for chronic pain management.

Pain is experienced by everyone to some degree. It is, however, a very individualized experience and is difficult to define or understand. It is an unpleasant feeling, entirely subjective, that only the person experiencing it can describe or evaluate. It can be evoked by a multiplicity of stimuli, but the reaction to it cannot be measured objectively. Pain is a learned experience that is influenced by the entire life situation of each individual.

Pain accompanies many disorders, as well as some therapies. It is a sensation that is frequently feared by people undergoing surgery. Although many people with cancer do *not* experience it, pain is one of the major concerns people have about cancer.

Relief of pain and discomfort is a major nursing intervention and one that requires skill in both the art and science of nursing. It requires knowledge about concepts related to pain, data collection, and useful therapies. It also requires sensitivity and empathy—an effort on the part of the nurse to understand what the patient is experiencing and to communicate understanding and caring. It requires that the nurse use a systematic approach (nursing process) with the patient in pain. Too often when a patient states that he or she has pain, medication is given without valid assessment and evaluation, resulting in undermedication, overmedication, or medication when other interventions would be more effective.

PHYSIOLOGY OF PAIN
Pain Receptors and Stimuli

Pain receptors, called *nociceptors*, are free nerve endings of unmyelinated or lightly myelinated afferent neurons. Nociceptors are located extensively in the skin and mucosa and less frequently in selected deeper structures, such as viscera, joints, arterial walls, and bile ducts. Nociceptors respond to harmful or potentially harmful stimuli that may be chemical, thermal, or mechanical.[12] Chemical stimuli for pain include histamines, bradykinin, prostaglandins, and acids, some of which are released by damaged tissues. Anoxic tissue also releases chemicals that lead to pain. Tissue swelling may cause pain by creating pressure (mechanical stimulation) on nociceptors in adjoining tissues.

After tissue injury and in some pathological conditions, pain receptors do not adapt to repeated stimulation and may become more sensitive.[10] As a result, pain sensitivity to a normally painful stimulus may be increased (*hyperalgesia*) or a normally nonpainful stimulus, such as touch, may be painful (*allodynia*).

Pain Transmission

Pain impulses are transmitted to the spinal cord by two types of fibres: thinly myelinated faster-conducting A-delta fibres and slower-conducting unmyelinated C fibres. Pain that may be described as "sharp" or "pricking" and that can be easily localized results from impulses transmitted by the A-*delta fibres*. An example of this type of pain is that felt by a needle prick. Pain that may be described as "burning," "dull," or "aching," and that is more diffuse, results from impulses transmitted by the C *fibres*. Impulses transmitted on the larger diameter myelinated A-beta and A-alpha fibres have an inhibitory effect on those transmitted over A-delta and C fibres.

The afferent nerve fibres enter the spinal cord through the dorsal root and synapse in the *dorsal horn* (Fig. 8-1). The dorsal horn consists of several layers (laminae) with interconnections. Lamina II comprises an area called *substantia gelatinosa* (SG). Substance P is released at synapses in the SG and is thought to be a major neurotransmitter of the pain impulses.

The pain impulses cross the spinal cord over interneurons and connect with *ascending spinal pathways*. The most important ascending pathways for nociceptive impulses located in the ventral half of the spinal cord are the spinothalamic tract (STT) and the spinoreticular tract (SRT). The STT is a discriminative system and conveys information about the nature and location of the stimulus to the thalamus and then to the cortex for interpretation. Impulses transmitted over the SRT (which goes to the brainstem and part of the thalamus) activate the autonomic and limbic (motivational-affective) responses.

Pain Modulation

Discovery of receptors in the brain to which opiate compounds bind led to the discovery of two naturally occurring endogenous morphine-like pentapeptides (5-amino acid compounds), met-enkephalin and leu-enkephalin. These enkephalins are classified as *endorphins* (from the terms endogenous and morphine). Other endorphins, such as beta-endorphin, have also been identified. The endorphins are thought to suppress pain by (1) acting presynaptically to *inhibit release* of the neurotransmitter substance P or (2) acting postsynaptically to *inhibit conduction* of pain impulses.[14] The endorphins are found in high concentration in the basal ganglia of the brain, thalamus, midbrain, and dorsal horn of the spinal cord.

Descending spinal pathways, from the thalamus through the midbrain and medulla to the dorsal horns of the spinal cord, conduct nociceptive *inhibitory* impulses. Serotonin is one neurotransmitter that supports these inhibitory impulses. The endogenous descending pain suppressive system is more effectively activated by nociceptive stimuli transmitted by A-delta fibres. Electrical stimulation by means of transcutaneous electrical nerve stimulation (TENS, p. 174) using low frequency and high intensity activates opiate analgesia. Acupuncture is also thought to use the opiate pathways.[14,52]

Theories of Pain Transmission

Various theories of pain transmission have been proposed[53] (Table 8-1). The affect specificity and pattern theories were early theories that led to the development of the gate control theory. Although the *gate control theory* does not fully explain pain transmission, it serves as a basis for understanding pain transmission.

The gate control theory was proposed by Melzack and Wall[58] in 1965. The theory proposes that the substantia gelatinosa (SG) in the spinal cord acts as a gating mechanism to permit or inhibit passage of pain impulses. The "gate" can be "closed" (so that the contact is not made, thus interrupting the pain impulse) by nerve impulses from the large non-nociceptive A-beta and A-alpha fibres or from the

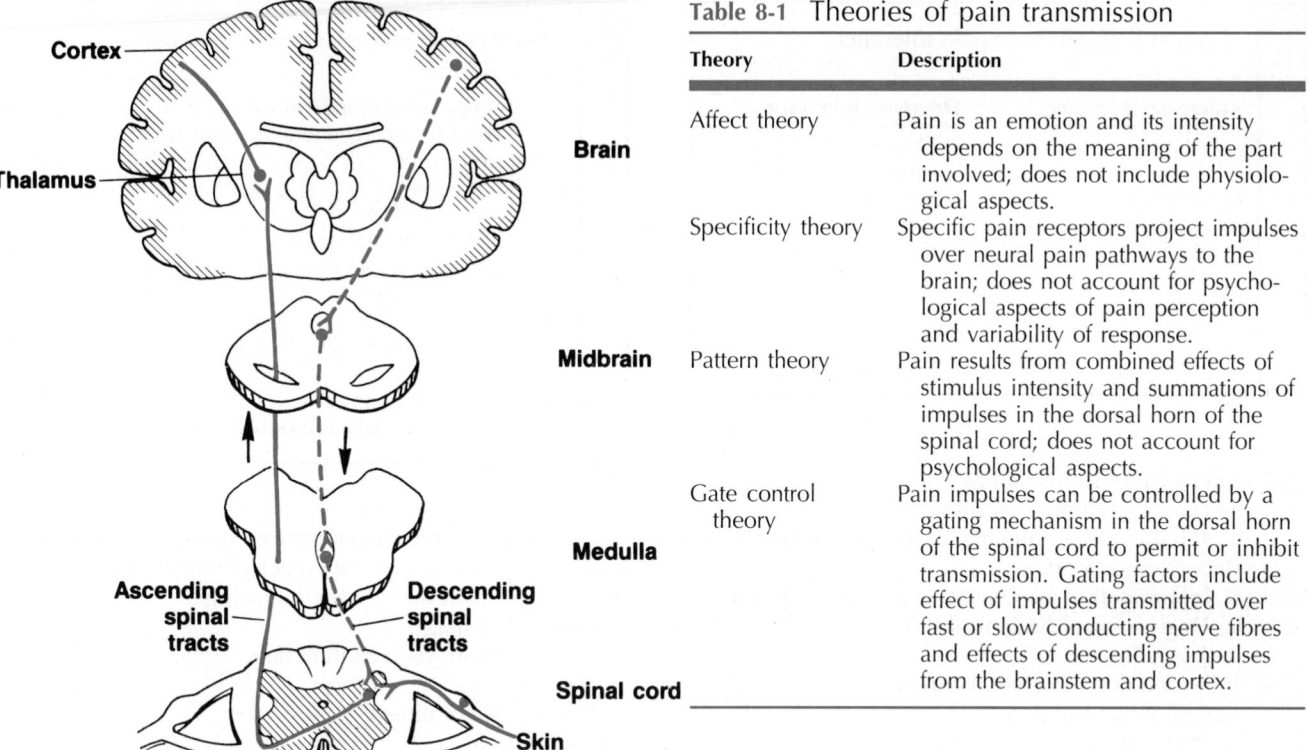

Table 8-1 Theories of pain transmission

Theory	Description
Affect theory	Pain is an emotion and its intensity depends on the meaning of the part involved; does not include physiological aspects.
Specificity theory	Specific pain receptors project impulses over neural pain pathways to the brain; does not account for psychological aspects of pain perception and variability of response.
Pattern theory	Pain results from combined effects of stimulus intensity and summations of impulses in the dorsal horn of the spinal cord; does not account for psychological aspects.
Gate control theory	Pain impulses can be controlled by a gating mechanism in the dorsal horn of the spinal cord to permit or inhibit transmission. Gating factors include effect of impulses transmitted over fast or slow conducting nerve fibres and effects of descending impulses from the brainstem and cortex.

Fig. 8-1 Pathways of pain transmission to and from cortex.

Table 8-2 Factors affecting pain transmission based on the gate control theory

Site	Close gate (block transmission)	Open gate (permit transmission)
Fibres	Impulses transmitted by large fast myelinated A-beta and A-alpha fibres	Impulses transmitted by slow small A-delta and C fibres
	Stimulation of unaffected skin areas (for example, massage)	Stimulation of affected skin areas (for example, sunburned skin)
Brainstem (descending pathway)	Endorphin effect	No endorphin effect
	Sufficient or maximum sensory input (for example, distraction)	Insufficient sensory input (for example, monotony)
Cortex	Past experiences	Past experiences
	Feelings of pain control	Anxiety

descending pathways. Impulses conducted over large fibres not only close the gate but also are sent immediately to the cortex for rapid identification, evaluation, and modification of the sensory inputs.[59] Impulses sent to the brainstem, the centre for motivational-affective and sensory-discriminative actions, can influence cognition or evaluation in the cortex. Impulses are then sent from the cortex back to the SG via corticospinal pathways to inhibit or permit passage of pain impulses. Note in Table 8-2 the various factors that can open or close the gate.

PAIN EXPERIENCE

The pain experience of every individual includes the perception of the pain sensation and the response to this perception. Tolerance to the noxious stimulus will influence both of these components.

Pain Perception

Perception of pain takes place in the cortex (cognitive–evaluative function) as a result of the stimuli transmitted up the spinothalamic and thalamic–cortical tracts. This thinking–feeling component of pain is subjective, highly complex, and individual; it is influenced by factors affecting stimulation of the nociceptors and transmission of the nociceptive impulse, as well as by cortical receptivity and interpretation:

1. Stimulation of nociceptors
   a. Increased number of stimuli
   b. Increased duration of the stimulus

8-1 | **Factors that influence pain tolerance**

Increase tolerance	Decrease tolerance
Alcohol	Fatigue
Drugs	Anger
Hypnosis	Boredom
Warmth	Anxiety
Rubbing	Persistent pain
Distraction	
Faith	
Strong beliefs	

8-2 | **Factors that influence reaction to pain**

Meaning of pain to individual
Degree of pain perception
Past experience
Cultural values
Social expectations
Physical and mental health
Parental attitudes towards pain
Setting in which pain occurs
Fear, anxiety
Usual way of responding to stressors
Age
Preparation for pain context
Health professionals' responses

2. Alteration of transmission
   a. Damage to nerve endings
   b. Inflammation, tumours, or injuries to spinal cord
3. Receptivity of cortex
   a. Inflammation, degenerative changes of brain
   b. Depression of brain function
   c. Anaesthesia
4. Interpretation in cerebral cortex
   a. Childhood training
   b. Past experience with pain
   c. Cultural values
   d. Religious beliefs
   e. Physical and mental health
   f. Knowledge and understanding
   g. Attention and distraction
   h. Fear, anxiety, tension
   i. Fatigue
   j. State of consciousness

Pain perception, therefore, can be altered by usual activities, such as reading or socialization, as well as by abnormal conditions. Damaged nerve endings may not transmit pain sensation, such as from a severe burn, and the patient may not perceive a usually painful stimuli as such.

The intensity at which the noxious stimulus is subjectively judged as painful is called the *pain detection threshold*.[12] This sensory discrimination is relatively consistent within an individual and between different individuals, relative to the location and type of stimulus.

In contrast, *pain tolerance*, which is the maximum degree of pain intensity a person is willing to experience, is highly variable.[12] Numerous factors can increase or decrease pain tolerance (Box 8-1). Tolerance can vary between different individuals in the same situation and in the same individual in differing situations. For example, a woman with a tender breast lump may complain of more pain if her mother died of breast cancer. Individuals can respond in many ways to any level of pain intensity, and pain tolerance is influenced by the meaning of the pain to the individual. It is important to remember that there is no right or wrong way to experience pain and pain is whatever and whenever the patient says it is.[26]

Meaning of Pain

Pain has different meanings for each person, which may differ for the same person at different times. In general,

most people view pain as a negative experience, although it may also have some positive aspects. Some examples of the meanings of pain include the following:
   Harm or damage
   Complication, such as infection
   New illness
   Recurrence of illness
   Fatal disease
   Increasing disability
   Loss of mobility
   Ageing
   Healing
   Necessary for cure
   Punishment for sins
   Challenge
   Appreciation for suffering of others
   Something to be tolerated
   Release from unwanted responsibilities

Numerous factors influence the meaning of pain for an individual, including age, sex, sociocultural background, environment, and past or present experiences. For example, two women may be experiencing pain from a fractured leg. To the 75-year-old woman living alone with few social contacts, pain may be interpreted on the basis of fear of ageing and inability to maintain her independent living status. The 28-year-old lawyer might interpret the pain as an expected nuisance, with the realization that healing will occur and she can get back to work soon.

Response to Pain

People respond to pain in different ways depending on their perception of the pain, including what it means to them. Some may be fearful, apprehensive, and anxious, whereas others are tolerant and optimistic. Some weep, moan, scream, beg for relief or help, threaten to destroy themselves, thrash about in bed, or move about aimlessly when in severe pain; others lie quietly in bed and may only close their eyes, grit their teeth, bite their lips, clench their hands, or perspire profusely when experiencing pain.

Some people, based on their cultural beliefs, are taught to endure severe pain without reacting outwardly, while others are very expressive about experiencing any degree of pain. People whose health beliefs and education em-

Table 8-3 Comparison of acute and chronic pain

Characteristic	Acute pain	Chronic pain
Onset	Usually sudden	May be sudden or developed insidiously
Duration	Transient (up to 3 months)	Prolonged (months to years)
Pain localization	Pain vs. nonpain areas generally well identified	Pain vs. nonpain areas less easily differentiated; intensity becomes more difficult to evaluate (change in sensations)
Clinical signs	Signs of sympathetic overactivity (such as increased blood pressure)	Usually lacks changes in vital signs (adaptation)
Purpose	Warning that something is wrong	Meaningless; no purpose
Pattern	Self-limiting or readily corrected	Continuous or intermittent; intensity may vary or remain constant
Prognosis	Likelihood of eventual complete relief	Complete relief usually not possible

phasize prevention, tend to accept pain as a warning to seek help, and expect that the cause of pain will be found and cured.

Numerous factors influence response to pain (Box 8-2). One cannot predict how any given person will respond, and value judgments should not be made concerning how a patient responds. It is very important for health professionals to recognize misbeliefs about expected pain response that prevent effective pain management (p. 119).

TYPES OF PAIN
General Types of Pain

There are two types of pain syndromes: acute and chronic. Unfortunately, a number of health care professionals provide care for the person experiencing chronic pain as though it were acute pain. There are many differences between acute and chronic pain (Table 8-3), and the approaches to pain relief are usually different, although some of the same techniques may be used.

Acute pain

Acute pain lasts no longer than 3 months. It is essentially a transient episode and informs the person that something is wrong. There is usually sudden onset from a perceived cause, and the painful areas can generally be well identified.

Sudden severe pain activates the autonomic nervous system, which may produce signs of sympathetic overactivity. These signs include tachycardia, increased blood pressure, pupillary dilation, diaphoresis, and stimulation of adrenal medullary secretion. In some situations, such as with severe visceral pain of sudden onset, vasodilation may occur with a subsequent fall in blood pressure and shock. Continuous painful stimulation can produce a steadily maintained reflex contraction of adjacent or distant muscles, such as abdominal rigidity, in people with intraabdominal pain.

Acute pain is commonly accompanied by increased muscle tension and anxiety, both of which may contribute to increased perception of pain (Fig. 8-2). If the pain is moderate or severe, overt physiological and behavioural signs facilitate assessment of the pain. The person usually seeks pain relief.

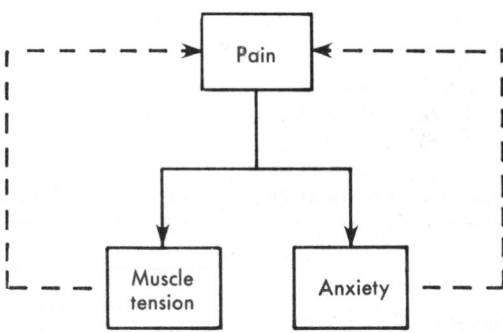

Fig. 8-2 Acute pain.

Chronic pain

Pain that persists longer than 3 months is usually classified as chronic pain. Either the source of pain is unknown or the pain cannot be eliminated. The pain sensation often becomes more diffuse, so that it is difficult for the person to identify a specific pain site. The pain may have originally been acute pain but persisted (for example, third-degree burns), or the onset may be so insidious that the person cannot state specifically when it was first experienced.

There are different types of chronic pain. *Intermittent* chronic pain occurs only at specific periods; at other times the person is pain free (migraine headaches). *Persistent* pain is always present, although there may be periods when pain is more or less intense (as seen with low back pain). One form of persistent pain may increase in frequency because of the pathological condition (pain from incurable cancer). (Cancer pain is discussed in Chapter 9.)

Chronic pain is characterized by irritability (often compounded by insomnia), which leads to decreasing interests and isolation from friends and family. Added to that is the centring of the person's life on the pain experience, with increasing feelings of helplessness and hopelessness as the pain persists. Ultimately the person withdraws from social interactions (Fig. 8-3).

The patient's world centres on ways to modify the pain experience. Patients experience tremendous disruptions in many aspects of their usual activities, including work, family roles, socialization, sleep, and leisure.[45] Some patients go from one doctor to another seeking pain relief,

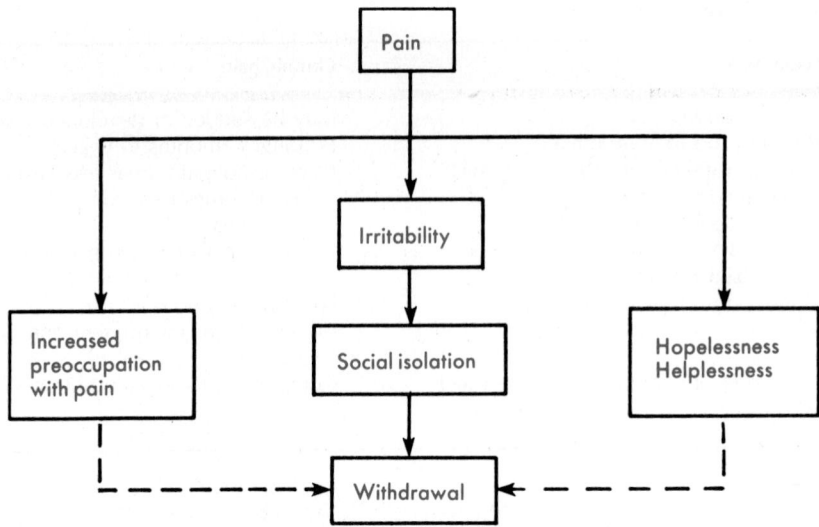

Fig. 8-3   Chronic pain.

Table 8-4   Comparison of somatic and visceral pain

| | Type of pain | | |
| | Somatic | | |
Characteristic	Superficial	Deep	Visceral
Quality	Sharp, pricking, burning	Sharp or dull and aching	Sharp, dull and aching, cramping
Localization	Good	Poor	Poor
Referred pain	No	No	Yes
Provoking stimuli	Cut, abrasion, excessive heat or cold, chemicals	Cut, pressure, heat, ischaemia, displacement (bone)	Distention, ischaemia, spasms, chemical irritants (no cutting)
Autonomic reactions	No	Yes	Yes
Reflex muscle contractions	No	Yes	Yes

which takes time, effort, and money. Even as they seek relief, they often lose faith in the ability of anyone to help them. The lack of continuity of care augments the problems. Doctors themselves may feel helpless when the patient continues to complain of pain. The development of pain clinics and inpatient teams has led to successful control of chronic pain for some (but not all) people with chronic pain.

As a means of differentiating the acute and chronic types of pain, Crue (1983) has developed a taxonomy of pain, beginning with acute pain of short duration and ending with continuous intractable pain (unrelieved by therapeutic measures)[49]:

1. *Acute*: lasts a few days, is caused by tissue injury, and can be expected to end when source is removed
2. *Subacute*: similar to acute but persists days to weeks
3. *Recurrent acute pain*: exacerbations of chronic pain
4. *Ongoing cancer pain*: caused by progressive pathology
5. *Intractable benign pain* (adequate coping): pain is continu-

ous but individual is able to live productive life
6. *Intractable benign pain* (inadequate coping): person is completely disabled by the continuous pain

Specific Types of Pain
Somatic versus visceral pain

Pain may originate in the skin and subcutaneous tissue (superficial), in the muscles and bones (deep somatic pain), or in the body organs (visceral pain). Somatic and visceral pain differ in their characteristics, particularly in the quality of pain, localization, causes, and accompanying symptoms (Table 8-4).

Referred pain

Referred pain is felt in areas other than those stimulated. It may occur when stimulation is not perceived in the primary areas. For example, somebody having a heart attack may complain only of pain radiating down the left arm when in fact the tissue damage is occurring in the myocardium.

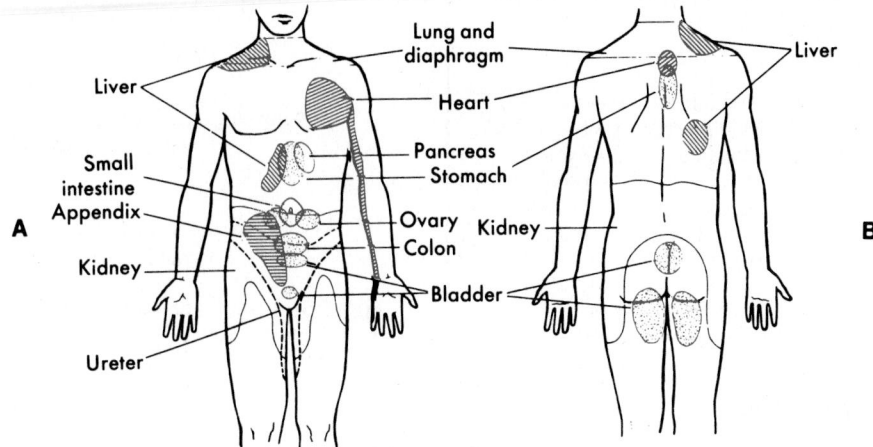

Fig. 8-4   Referred pain. **A,** Front. **B,** Back.

Referred pain occurs most often with damage or injury to visceral organs, and the pain is referred to cutaneous surfaces (Fig. 8-4). The origin of referred pain is complex and not clearly understood but may relate to one or more of the following[14]:

1. Referred pain usually occurs in structures that developed from the same embryonic dermatome.
2. Visceral and somatic nerves enter the nervous system at the same spinal level and share the same spinothalamic tracts.
3. Somatic pain is more common and the person has "learned" to interpret signals conducted on certain pathways as being somatic in origin.

The cutaneous pattern of various referred pains is fairly constant and frequently seen in practice. The nurse should be able to recognize the possibility of visceral organ disease in patients who have appropriate complaints of cutaneous pain.

Psychogenic pain

The term "psychogenic" has been used to describe pain where no physical pathology has been found or where the pain appears to have a greater psychological basis than a physical one.[39] A caution here is that diagnostic tests are not definitive measures and may not be sophisticated enough to detect pathophysiological changes. Distinguishing between physical and emotional components of pain is difficult and it is important to remember that *all pain is real*.

Neurological pain

Pain in the neurological system occurs in different forms. *Neuralgia* is sharp, spasmlike pain along the course of one or more nerves. Two common areas of neuralgia are the trigeminal nerve in the face and the sciatic nerve in the lower trunk. *Causalgia*, a form of neuralgia, is severe burning pain associated with injury to a peripheral nerve in the extremities. The patient may go to great lengths to protect against irritating stimuli (which may be something as simple as the noise of a plane overhead).

Phantom limb pain is pain or discomfort perceived by the individual to be occurring in an extremity that has been amputated. It is more likely to develop in people who had pain before amputation and may persist long after healing has occurred. The phenomenon of phantom limb pain is poorly understood, and therefore treatment is not very effective.

Nursing Process
Assessment
Acute pain

When a patient reports having pain or asks for pain medication, it is important to make a rapid assessment, collecting both subjective and objective data before taking any actions. Omission of assessment may lead to inadequate pain relief. For example, a young woman after pelvic surgery was crying loudly and demanding pain medication, which was given to her without assessment of the pain. No relief was obtained from the medication. When an assessment was finally made, it was discovered that she had a full bladder of which she was unaware. After she voided, the pain disappeared. Unfortunately, many patients continue to have pain postoperatively,[8] and many will not ask for help.[33] Use a rating scale to validate with patients the pain they are experiencing. This patient rating of pain intensity is assessed and recorded both before and 1 hour after giving any analgesic. If the pain intensity does not decrease after the analgesic, assess the adequacy and timing of the dose and necessity of change.

Subjective data

Data that are useful to obtain *before* pain is anticipated are the patient's expectations for pain relief from health caregivers. Many people are unaware of their expected role in speaking out when they have pain or discomfort. Some patients think they will be considered "complainers" or "bad patients" if they state that they are experiencing discomfort. In this situation, an explanation is given of the subjective nature of pain and the need for patient input to facilitate selection of effective pain relief measures.

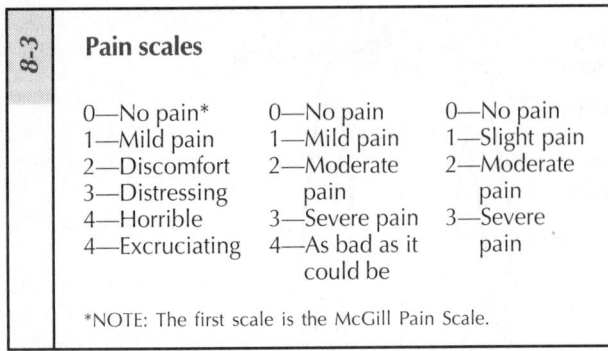

8-3

Pain scales

0—No pain*	0—No pain	0—No pain
1—Mild pain	1—Mild pain	1—Slight pain
2—Discomfort	2—Moderate	2—Moderate
3—Distressing	pain	pain
4—Horrible	3—Severe pain	3—Severe
4—Excruciating	4—As bad as it	pain
	could be	

*NOTE: The first scale is the McGill Pain Scale.

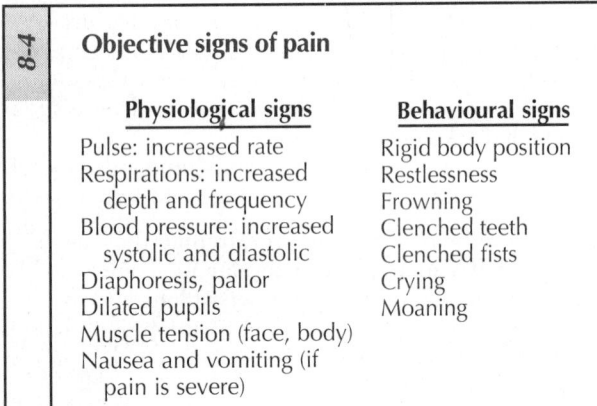

8-4

Objective signs of pain

Physiological signs	Behavioural signs
Pulse: increased rate	Rigid body position
Respirations: increased	Restlessness
depth and frequency	Frowning
Blood pressure: increased	Clenched teeth
systolic and diastolic	Clenched fists
Diaphoresis, pallor	Crying
Dilated pupils	Moaning
Muscle tension (face, body)	
Nausea and vomiting (if	
pain is severe)	

The best assessment of pain is the patient's own evaluation. Data need to be gathered about the nature of the acute pain; that is, the location, intensity, quality, timing (onset, duration, frequency, cause), and provoking and palliative factors. One approach for evaluating these characteristics is the use of the mnemonic PQRST[38]:

P Provoking factors: what makes the pain worse or relieves it
Q Quality: dull, sharp, crushing
R Region or radiation: site and radiation to other areas
S Severity or intensity
T Time: onset, duration, frequency, cause

Pain *intensity* can be determined by various means. One way is to ask the patient to describe the pain or discomfort, including a numerical rating between 0 (no pain) and 10 (worst pain possible). Other scales to assess pain intensity are outlined in Box 8-3. The obtained data are recorded. The pain scale score can also be recorded on a flow chart to provide ongoing assessment of progression of the pain. A third approach is to ask the patient to mark an X on a visual analogue scale (Fig. 8-5). Pain intensity should be assessed *at least once a shift* or more often if the patient is receiving interventions for pain (such as analgesics, relaxation exercises, or TENS). When acute pain has subsided, further data can be collected about the *meaning* of pain for the patient.

Objective data

Objective data assist the nurse in identifying possible pain or discomfort in a person who has not reported pain and in helping to clarify the subjective response.

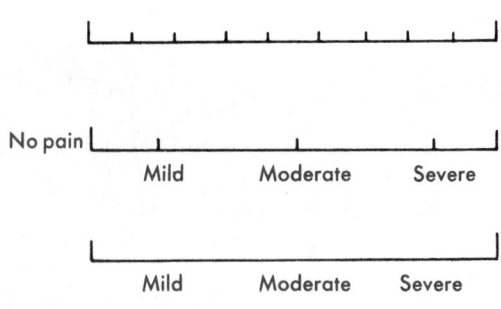

Fig. 8-5 Visual analogue pain scales. Patient marks line describing intensity of pain.

Objective signs of pain are of two types: physiological and behavioural. Remember that *physiological* signs of pain result from activation of the sympathetic nervous system (see Box 8-4). With very severe acute pain, neurogenic shock may result from the stressful insult to the system. *The behavioural* signs are not specific to pain; therefore, if the observable data suggest that pain may be present, subjective data must be elicited to validate the assumption.

Specific objective data to be collected, therefore, include the following:
1. Appearance
2. Motor behaviour
3. Affective and verbal responses
4. Vital signs
5. Skin: moisture, colour
6. Inspection and gentle palpation of painful area; identify trigger points that initiate pain, if present

Sometimes the patient's subjective response differs from the objective signs. For example, the patient may request an analgesic, a back rub, or other measure to relieve pain, but when the nurse arrives to carry out the request, the patient is found to be asleep. The patient may be exhausted from the pain and thus falls asleep. The patient who is sleeping or quiet is not necessarily pain-free. It is important to reiterate that pain is what the patient says it is, and although objective data may assist in confirming the existence of pain, the diagnosis must include both subjective and objective data.

Chronic pain
Subjective data

Long-term pain requires a much more in-depth assessment of the pain syndrome. Hospitals or pain clinics that use a team approach in providing care to the person with chronic pain often develop their own pain history form or questionnaire (see references 26, 43, and 57 for examples). This history may be collected by one or more health team members. Types of data collected may include the following:
1. Demographic data
2. Sociocultural data
3. History of the pain pattern from time of onset
4. Factors perceived to increase or decrease the pain
5. Effects of the pain on the patient's lifestyle
6. Meaning of the pain for the patient

7. Effects of the patient's pain on other family members or friends
8. Measures used in the past and present for relief of pain

Objective data

Physiological signs of pain may be absent in the person with chronic pain because of the body's compensatory mechanisms. Although there is adaptation to the pain stimuli, the pain persists. The absence of physiological signs, therefore, does not indicate absence of pain. Prolonged pain, however, may create changes in the person's appearance over time, perhaps as a result of decreased appetite or lack of interest in appearance because of fatigue or depression.

Behavioural responses to chronic pain are varied and unique to the individual. Here, also, there may be few overt signs to indicate the presence of pain. Changes usually occur in daily patterns related to sleeping, eating, socialization, and libido. If the person is extremely depressed because of the ongoing pain, withdrawal behaviour may be noted.

Nursing analysis: problems

If pain is present for which specific nursing interventions may be effective, a nursing diagnosis is made of *Pain* (specify location). Possible aetiologies may include but are not limited to: physiological (specify), trauma, diagnostic tests, immobility, improper positioning, overactivity, or pressure points.

Pain may also be an aetiological factor for other nursing diagnoses, such as the following:

Anxiety related to increasing or threatened pain
Ineffective breathing pattern: related to pain in chest or abdomen
Impaired physical mobility: related to pain
Self-care deficit (describe) related to pain
Sexual dysfunction related to pain
Sleep pattern disturbance related to pain

Planning: expected patient outcomes

Expected patient outcomes for the person experiencing pain may include, but are not limited to, the following:

1. Patient states pain is relieved or reduced to a mild level.
2. Pain-related behaviour or signs (specify) are decreased or absent.
3. If pain is present when patient is discharged, patient or significant other can
   a. Describe general measures for pain relief (such as exercises, heat, ice)
   b. Explain prescribed medications (actions, dosages, frequency, side effects)
   c. Describe when to seek medical assistance if pain is not relieved as expected
4. Patient with chronic pain can
   a. State plans to participate in ongoing therapies
   b. State plans for increasing independence in activities of daily living
   c. Identify supports for encouragement and help

The need to assess the patient with pain is ongoing, yet the nurse must begin to plan an approach with the individual in pain. Family members should be included when possible. The nurse is able to function independently with many interventions, but careful planning with other members of the health care team should ensure that all have the same patient outcomes or goals in mind.

One aspect of the treatment plan that is often forgotten or omitted is the incorporation of measures the patient thinks may help relieve the pain, even if these measures are different from those usually carried out in that institution. Without encouragement, the patient may hesitate to mention these possible remedies: for example, nonprescription liniments, special applications of heat and cold, unusual positioning, or favourite homemade foods or drinks. If there are no contraindications to the remedy the patient wishes to try, the health care team may consider using it before trying other relief measures.

The patient should be involved in planning the use of pain relief measures. For example, he or she may wish to receive parenteral analgesics at bedtime to improve sleep and to receive a less potent medication that causes less drowsiness before family members visit.

Planning for the same health care team members to care for the patient regularly should result in a more consistent approach and plan of care. Between the small group of health care team members and the patient, a plan of care can be developed in which the patient's decisions are honoured, and a daily routine can be devised that will reduce anxiety and frustration about constant changes. This plan should include, if appropriate, such items as specified hours for analgesic administration before uncomfortable procedures, specified blocks of time for rest or napping, and coordination between various departments, such as physical therapy and occupational therapy. For some patients fatigue is a great problem, so regular visits to off-unit departments should be interspersed with rest periods; for other patients the most beneficial plan includes ensuring that they go directly from one department to the next so that time is not wasted getting in and out of bed or performing other painful manoeuvres.

Implementation

Misbeliefs about pain and their effect on management

Ineffective pain management of both adults and children in a variety of settings has, unfortunately, been clearly documented.[9,33,37] There are some commonly held misbeliefs or incorrect beliefs that guide our practice and that may contribute to this ineffective pain management.[42]

Minimal or no pain should be the goal of pain management. A hospital admission should not automatically mean a pain experience for *any* patient, including elders, children, and infants. Patterns of pain intensity vary, and the diagnosis and/or type of surgery is *not* an effective primary basis for determining the amount of pain the person is experiencing or the analgesic required. Although not all pain can be removed, the use of multiple modalities can usually decrease it to at least the minimal range.

All pain tends to be assessed as acute pain. However, chronic pain differs from acute pain and needs to be assessed using different parameters (p. 118). It is important

Table 8-5 Equianalgesic* doses of commonly used opioids for moderate or severe pain

Generic name	IM/SC dose (mg)	Oral dose (mg)	Duration of action (hours)
Morphine	10	20-30†	4
Morphine, modified release	—	20-30	8-12
Pethidine	80-100	300	2-3
Codeine	120	200	3-4
Methadone	8-10	20	3-5

* When given parenterally or orally, the drug produces approximately the same analgesic effect as 10 mg morphine (IM/SC).
† Oral to parenteral ratio for morphine, modified release differs: 1 : 6, single dose for acute pain; 1 : 2 or 1 : 3, repeated doses for chronic pain. (Adapted from Tuttle CB: Drug management of pain in cancer patients, *Can Med Assoc J* 12:121-134, 1985.)

to believe that all pain is real and that malingerers (people who deliberately lie about their pain) are rare. Patients in pain will not necessarily ask for help until they are in severe pain,[33] and they may use words such as "pressure" or "soreness" instead of "pain."

Pain is a complex experience, and multiple strategies rather than only one approach are likely to be more successful. Incorrect beliefs about analgesic administration, particularly opioids, result in undermedication for patients.[48] Analgesics need to be given round the clock and titrated (regulated) so the pain levels are zero to mild. The fear of addiction should not prevent effective opioid doses as addiction rarely occurs.

It is difficult to understand and recognize another person's pain. Therefore it is crucial to gain as much information about the patient as possible instead of making assumptions about what may be happening. Recognizing misbeliefs (incorrect beliefs) is an important step to more effective pain management.

Pharmacological approaches to pain management
Analgesics

Two groups of analgesics as well as adjuvant medications are important components of effective pain management. Opioid analgesics (also called narcotics), such as morphine, act mainly on the central nervous system to alter the perception of pain. Nonopioids, such as aspirin, block impulses mainly in the periphery and decrease inflammatory related pain by inhibiting the synthesis of prostaglandins. For some types of pain, such as with bone cancer, analgesics from both groups are necessary. Adjuvant medications relieve pain, such as muscle spasms, or decrease the side effects associated with some analgesics, particularly opioids.

Nurses need to know the equianalgesic doses for both opioid and nonopioid analgesics. This means knowing the dose of any opioid that has the same strength (potency) as parenteral morphine 10 mg (Table 8-5).

Opioid analgesics. Opioids are the most effective analgesics for relief of moderate to severe pain. They must be

given round the clock to reach and maintain the steady blood levels necessary for pain relief. Side effects of opioids vary with the physiological state of the patient. Constipation is the most common side effect, and laxatives should be given to any patient receiving opioids on a regular basis. Nausea and vomiting are experienced by some; these patients usually respond well to antiemetics. Sedation and drowsiness may occur for the first 48 to 72 hours, but one needs to consider that the patient may be catching up on sleep lost because of pain. Respiratory depression is rarely a problem with standardized doses and careful titration (slowly increasing the dose). Narcan will reverse any depressive effect.

The oral route is preferred unless the patient is vomiting, unable or not permitted to swallow, or is in acute pain. Routes other than intramuscular or subcutaneous injection are rectal, intravenous, transdermal, or epidural (see Chapter 14).[17,34] Slow release preparations, such as MS Contin, are given every 8 to 12 hours, allowing less focus on the pain and better control with fewer side effects.

Concern for addiction. Patients receiving opioids for pain relief very rarely develop addiction. The incidence of opioid addiction in hospitalized patients is less than 1%.[61] Patients are taking opioids for pain relief and not for the psychological effect. Unfortunately, health professionals are overly concerned about addiction, and opioids are underprescribed by doctors and underadministered by nurses.[48]

It is important to differentiate between tolerance, dependence, and addiction, which are summarized below:

Tolerance	Larger doses are needed to produce desired effects
Dependence	Need to continue use of drug to prevent symptoms
Addiction	Behavioural pattern of compulsive drug use; drug used for psychological effect

Drug tolerance occurs with some patients and with some conditions, usually when the patient's pain is first being controlled and/or when the pain increases. This is a physiological response and requires increasing the dose until pain relief is reached. There is no ceiling or maximum amount of opioid that can be given. *Physical dependency*, appearance of physiological withdrawal symptoms, *rarely happens* because as pain decreases the dosage is gradually tapered, and no symptoms are experienced. Physical dependency and drug tolerance are involuntary behaviour.

Patient-controlled analgesia. One method of providing more adequate pain control with opioids is the system of patient-controlled analgesia (PCA). The system consists of a syringe-type infusion pump that is filled with the prescribed opioid and is attached to an intravenous injection port. PCA is activated when the patient pushes a button to release a set amount of opioid by bolus. A refractory time prevents delivery of another bolus before a preset time interval. The device also records the patient's attempts to receive the opioid in a given time period. The doctor determines the opioid dosage and the refractory

Table 8-6 NSAIDs commonly used for mild to moderate pain

Generic name	Dosage range
Diclofenac sodium	200 to 600 mg daily in divided doses
Fenoprofen	200 to 600 mg tid or qid
Ibuprofen	1.2 to 1.8 g daily in divided doses
Mefenamic acid	500 mg tid
Naproxen sodium	550 mg Bd.

time interval.

Experience has demonstrated that people using PCA tend to take less than those receiving the standard method of intramuscular injections.[21,63] PCA has been used for postoperative pain, for other types of acute pain such as sickle cell crisis, and for cancer pain.[20,36] Nursing activities related to PCA include maintaining the system, recording the number of times the patient activates the system, and monitoring the patient's pain. The patient should be the only person who activates the PCA (presses the button); this serves as a safeguard to prevent oversedation.

Nonopioid analgesics. Mild to moderate pain can generally be controlled by nonopioid analgesics, most commonly nonsteroidal anti-inflammatory agents (NSAIDs), such as aspirin, and by acetaminophen.

Paracetamol is comparable to aspirin for analgesic effects but is not anti-inflammatory. It causes less alteration in prothrombin level and has fewer side effects but can cause severe liver damage. It is useful for people who are allergic to aspirin and for whom aspirin is contraindicated.

Nonsteroidal anti-inflammatory drugs. The nonsteroidal anti-inflammatory drugs (NSAIDs) act primarily by inhibition of prostaglandin synthesis. In lower doses, these drugs have analgesic properties; in higher doses there is anti-inflammatory action in addition to analgesia. The principal uses of NSAIDs are control of moderate pain of dysmenorrhoea, arthritis and other musculoskeletal disorders, postoperative pain, and migraine. NSAIDs commonly used to control pain are listed in Table 8-6.

NSAIDs inhibit platelet aggregation with resulting increased bleeding time. Common side effects include gastrointestinal disturbances, dizziness, tinnitus, and headache. People who are hypersensitive to aspirin may also be hypersensitive to NSAIDs. Concurrent use of an NSAID with aspirin may lead to increased side effects.

Phenylbutazone is an NSAID with potent anti-inflammatory properties given for short-term therapy for moderately severe arthritis, gout, or bursitis. Although the drug has analgesic activity, it is not used as a general analgesic for moderate pain because it is poorly tolerated by many people and has numerous side effects, including haematological changes, gastric irritation, and fluid and electrolyte disturbances.

Aspirin. Acetylsalicylic acid (aspirin) is the most widely used analgesic for mild to moderate pain. Salicylates produce analgesia by blocking pain impulses peripherally

or centrally, possibly in the hypothalamus, and by inhibiting synthesis of prostaglandins. Aspirin is therefore also an anti-inflammatory agent. It has an onset of 15 to 20 minutes, peak of 1 to 2 hours, and duration of 3 to 4 hours.

Aspirin is a platelet aggregation inhibitor and a weak vitamin K antagonist. It produces an increased bleeding time and prolonged prothrombin time when given in large doses. Therefore, it is contraindicated for those receiving anticoagulant drugs.

Irritation of the gastric mucosa is a common side effect of aspirin; therefore it should not be taken on an empty stomach. Aspirin is best taken after meals or with a snack such as a glass of milk. People with a history of peptic ulcer should avoid taking aspirin. Aspirin should also be avoided by anyone taking phenylbutazone and spironolactone because of drug interaction, and by children because of risk of Reye's syndrome.

Other drugs for pain relief. Smooth muscle relaxants may be given for pain from muscle spasms and include propantheline bromide and drugs of the belladonna group, such as atropine. Antispasmodics, such as hyoscine butylbromide, may be given for GI pain.

Sedatives and antianxiety agents are sometimes prescribed for patients in pain. These drugs do *not* have an analgesic effect but may permit relaxation and decrease anxiety and thus prevent potentiation of pain. The drugs may permit the person to sleep and thus be better able to cope with the pain. In some people sedatives and antianxiety agents may lead to disorientation and agitation, which can increase the pain and decrease the ability to cope. Treating pain with analgesics is the more effective and preferred method.

Tricyclic antidepressants, such as amitriptyline, produce analgesia at doses lower than those used for depression. These drugs are useful in nerve injury pain, such as with postherpetic neuralgia (shingles).

Counterirritant drugs relieve local pain by producing counterirritation (stimulation of the large A-beta fibres). Examples of counterirritants include ointments containing methyl salicylate (oil of wintergreen) or ethyl aminobenzoate and oil of cloves (for toothaches).

Nonpharmacological approaches to pain management

Nonpharmacological approaches should be considered along with analgesics for effective pain management. This type of intervention can alter pain transmission, modify the response to pain, and modify the pain stimulus.

Alter pain transmission

Electrical stimulators. The purpose of electrical stimulators is to modify the pain stimulus by blocking or changing the painful stimulus with stimulation perceived as less painful. The success of this approach is thought to be explained by the gate control theory of pain transmission; that is, blockage of pain stimulus by stimulation of the large sensory fibres. Selected forms of electrical stimulation may activate the opiate or nonopiate descending pathways (see Box 8-5).

<table>
<tr><td>8-5</td><td colspan="2">**Methods of electrical stimulation for pain control**</td></tr>
</table>

Transcutaneous electrical nerve stimulator (TENS)	Manually controlled stimulation of specific pain areas through externally placed electrodes
Percutaneous implanted spinal cord epidural stimulator (PISCES)	Stimulation by an external transistorized receiver through leads inserted percutaneously in epidural space of spinal column
Dorsal column stimulator	Stimulation by transistorized receiver, implanted surgically in an infraclavicular or abdominal skin pouch, through electrodes surgically implanted on dorsum of spinal cord

Transcutaneous electrical nerve stimulator. The transcutaneous electrical nerve stimulator (TENS) is a battery-powered stimulator worn externally. It is a convenient, nonintrusive, nonaddictive type of pain therapy that can be learned easily by the patient. Success is variable, and it is usually used along with other pain therapies.

A number of TENS devices are on the market; all consist of a battery-powered portable pulse generator about the size of a pocket paging device. Control knobs on the generator permit adjustment of the impulse. The generator is connected by a pair of cables to electrically conductive tape electrodes placed at appropriate sites on the skin. The TENS delivers a balanced biphasic potential in a waveform.

TENS appears to be more useful for postoperative pain, posttraumatic pain, phantom limb pain, peripheral neuralgias, low back pain, and muscle and bone pain. It is less effective with cancer pain, inflammatory arthritis, trigeminal neuralgia, or with anxious or depressed people.[67]

TENS electrodes should not be placed over hair, irritated skin, sutures, carotid sinus (may produce bradycardia), laryngeal or pharyngeal muscles (may trigger spasms), or a pregnant uterus.[11] A cardiac pacemaker may interfere with TENS effects. Suggested electrode placement may include (1) directly over the painful area, (2) at trigger points along the nerve pathways, or (3) at trigger points in the same dermatome as the pain.[62]

Routine skin care at the electrode sites includes the following:

1. Remove and clean electrodes at least once a day.
2. Wash skin with soap and water.
3. Allow skin to air dry.
4. Wipe skin with a prep pad before reapplying conductor pad.

If the skin becomes irritated, it may be cleaned with milk of magnesia, rinsed well, then air dried.[62]

Spinal cord stimulators. Spinal cord stimulators are similar to the TENS except that they are intrusive procedures. Instead of electrode placement on the skin, the electrodes are placed on or near the spinal cord. This is done either surgically over the ventral surface of the spinal cord or percutaneously through the back into the epidural space. Because percutaneous placement of electrodes (PISCES) can be performed under local anaesthesia, it is preferred over surgical placement of the dorsal column stimulator electrodes. Postoperative care after dorsal column stimulator implantation includes the same care that follows

laminectomy, with monitoring for infection and leakage of cerebrospinal fluid (Chapter 29).

Neurosurgical procedures. Constant relentless chronic pain that cannot be controlled by analgesics (*intractable pain*) may be reduced or eliminated by one of various neurosurgical procedures. Other forms of pain control are usually attempted before neurosurgical procedures.

Neurosurgical procedures do not play a major role in management of chronic pain. Major limitations include short duration of relief, occurrence of dysaesthesia (pain induced by gentle touch of the skin), central pain syndrome (burning sensations in skin areas lacking sensation from surgical afferent interruptions), and possible further neurological dysfunction.[64]

Neurectomy has limitations in that peripheral nerves may regenerate. Both rhizotomy and anterolateral cordotomy require laminectomy. A more commonly used procedure is percutaneous cordotomy, a closed stereotactic procedure in which the lesion is first located by using three-dimensional coordinates. The anterospinothalamic tracts are destroyed by electrodes inserted percutaneously. The patient is awake to provide feedback, thus providing more accurate site location and better pain relief. The effect usually lasts 18 to 24 months.[64]

Rhizotomy interferes with the ability to perceive heat and cold; therefore, protection from extremes in temperatures is important for prevention of injury. The advantages of cordotomy include a wide sense of analgesia below the surgical site while preserving other sensory and motor functions. After surgery there may be temporary leg weakness and loss of bowel and bladder control from oedema of the spinal cord; these usually disappear within 2 weeks. If quadriceps setting exercises are begun in the early postoperative period, walking will be less difficult.

Pain pathways in the brain may also be interrupted by stereotactic techniques (tractotomy, thalamotomy, lobotomy). These surgical procedures are usually reserved as a final solution for patients with intractable pain, usually from malignant invasion of cranial or facial structures. Lobotomy usually results in a change in personality.

Nerve block. A nerve block involves the injection of substances such as local anaesthetics or neurolytic agents (for example, alcohol or phenol) close to nerves to block the conduction of impulses over the nerves. Nerve blocks are frequently used for the symptomatic relief of pain. They are used to treat chronic pain associated with peripheral vascular disease, trigeminal neuralgia, causalgia, and cancer.

A nerve block may be unsuccessful because of difficulty in locating the correct nerve fibre or because of the complexity of the pain. Because the nerve fibres, ganglia, and roots contain fibres other than those for pain, and because some of the injected agents may leak out of the injection site and affect other nerves, the nerve block usually produces some other type of neurological deficit.

Acupuncture. Acupuncture is an ancient form of disease treatment that can be used for pain relief. Only recently has the method been used in Western countries. Small needles are skilfully inserted and manipulated at specific body points, depending on the type and location of pain. The gate control theory provides the best explanation for the success of acupuncture: the local stimulation of large-diameter fibres by the needles "closes the gate" to pain. It is not known to what extent the psyche and the power of suggestion contribute to the effectiveness of this therapy. Nursing intervention includes careful client assessment and teaching.

Modify pain response

Behaviour modification. Behaviour modification consists of a planned change in the way a person behaves by means of rewarding desired behaviour and ignoring undesirable behaviour. Forms of behaviour modification are used unconsciously all the time: a young boy "throwing a tantrum" may be ignored, but as his behaviour becomes more appropriate his mother may reward him with her time and attention.

Behaviour modification may be useful for people with chronic pain. For example, one protocol for patients with chronic low back pain is to set a limit of 10 minutes daily for discussion of their pain experiences (with the exception of data-gathering interviews). Pain medications are given on a regular schedule to dissociate the feelings of pain with inappropriate use (reward) of analgesics or other unhealthy behaviour.

In using behavioural methods to alter pain-associated behaviour or to encourage patient activities, success will occur only with a consistent approach on the part of the health care team. Although patients should always be praised for their efforts to comply or assist with treatment regimens, a true behaviour modification programme requires careful analysis of patient behaviour and the development of a specific and comprehensive treatment plan.

Biofeedback and autogenic training. Some people are able to alter their body functions through mental concentration. In biofeedback training a machine that monitors brain wave activity (electroencephalograph [EEG]) is used. The individual concentrates on slowing his or her brain wave activity to rates at which pain and distress are unlikely to cause discomfort (that is, complete relaxation). It may take many months of regular practice to achieve the desired level of control. The nurse should encourage and praise the patient's efforts.

In autogenic training the same type of self-regulation is used to alter various autonomic nervous system functions, such as pulse, blood pressure, and muscle tension. Practised use of transcendental meditation and other methods of concentration and self-control may achieve the same degree of autoregulation without the use of sophisticated physiological monitoring equipment.

Hypnosis. Hypnosis may be used in the treatment of various conditions, particularly when these conditions are aggravated by tension and stress. Individuals are helped to alter their perception of pain through the acceptance of positive suggestions made to the subconscious. Many people are able to learn self-hypnosis. Individuals vary in their suggestibility and readiness to try this approach. The nurse's most helpful role may be to support the patient's desire to make hypnotism work.

Explanation of the problem. As a result of nursing assessment, it may become clear that the patient's response to pain is really the manifestation of a lack of knowledge about the cause of pain. Sometimes a simple explanation about what is causing the pain and how long it will last is all that is necessary. Understanding that pain or discomfort is to be expected may relieve anxiety or help the patient to alter expectations and be better prepared for what will happen. In all cases, an explanation that includes information about pain is given before each diagnostic test.

Decreasing anxiety. Because anxiety increases pain, measures taken to decrease anxiety may help to decrease pain (see Chapter 5 for a discussion of anxiety). Interventions for the patient and family with pain include the following:
1. Maintain a calm, quiet manner.
2. Help the patient explore concerns related to the pain (meaning of pain for the patient).
3. Respect the patient's response to pain, even if it differs considerably from what the nurse expects.
4. Hold the patient's hand, if appropriate.
5. Arrange for someone to be with the patient if the patient fears being alone.
6. Talk with family or close friends and help them to allay their anxieties so these are not transmitted to the patient.
7. Teach the family and close friends ways in which they can help the patient, such as massage, encouraging the patient to use distraction or relaxation techniques, or supporting painful parts when moving. People often feel helpless when observing a loved one in pain and may need help themselves to cope.

Modify the pain stimulus

Cutaneous stimulation Cutaneous stimulation innervates the large A-delta fibres to block the pain stimuli across the small C fibres. Methods of cutaneous stimulation include the following:
1. Lightly rubbing the affected area
2. Back rub

3. Application of heat or cold
4. Whirlpool massage

Reducing additional physical stimuli. Although in many instances pain cannot be prevented, it is often possible to avoid additional pain when pain is already present. For example, when moving the body or an extremity, supporting the trunk or extremity will prevent increasing the pain by unilateral pulling on muscles, joints, and ligaments. Interventions include the following list:

1. Use a turning sheet for patients with severe neck, back, or general trunk pain
2. Place a pillow under a painful joint when helping a patient change position
3. Support limbs at the joints rather than the muscle bellies when handling an extremity
4. Use special beds (Stryker frame, Egerton turning and tilting bed, profiling bed[16a]) for patients with severe general or trunk pain
5. Avoid bumping or moving the bed suddenly

Reducing auditory and visual stimuli. The patient may experience sensory overload with subsequent potentiation of pain stimuli. If nurses could stand still for 5 minutes in the patient's environment and watch and listen, they might understand that some patients are simply bombarded with noise and visual stimulation. If these are problems, it may be possible to change the environment. Changes include the following:

1. Move the patient to a quieter room away from the centre of activity.
2. Dim any bright lights; pull shades if sunlight is intense.
3. Keep verbal interactions at a minimum when pain is severe.
4. Keep television or radio at a reasonable level but not loud.
5. Control the number of people entering the patient's room according to patient's wishes.

Reducing social isolation. When external stimuli are decreased too much, the patient may lack distraction from the pain stimuli; thus pain perception is increased. Social isolation may occur for a variety of reasons: the serious nature of a patient's disease may necessitate being in a private room for an extended period; hospitalization far away from home may mean few family members and friends can visit; extended periods of hospitalization may result in friends losing interest in visiting; or the patient may complain so much that no one cares to visit to hear the monologue repeated.

Each of these causes of isolation may have a different solution. In any event, careful assessment may indicate that social isolation is a problem for the patient. Before determining the plan for addressing this problem, the patient should be consulted about the desire and need to alter the present situation. Possible nursing interventions include the following:

1. Place the patient with a compatible roommate
2. Plan frequent contacts with health team members
3. Facilitate visits by family and friends
4. Help patient to be as comfortable as possible during visits by family or friends

Therapeutic touch. A less traditional therapy, that of therapeutic touch, may be helpful to patients in pain. The rationale for the success of therapeutic touch is not clearly understood. The nurse undergoes a brief period of meditation before coming in contact with the patient. During this period the nurse quiets his or her internal energy levels and then touches the patient and transmits the healing energies. Few nurses are trained in the use of therapeutic touch as described. It does seem to be helpful for some patients and some kinds of pain.

Distraction and relaxation exercises. Patients can be taught to modify their sensory input to control pain by activities that promote distraction or relaxation.

Distraction. Distraction interferes with the pain stimulus, thereby modifying the awareness of the pain. Mild or moderate pain can be modified by focusing on activity in the environment. A very quiet environment providing little or no sensory input can actually intensify the pain experience because the individual has nothing to focus on but the painful stimulus.

Severe pain requires more active participation by the individual in an effort to block out the painful stimulus. This can be enhanced by involving two or more sensory modalities, such as vision, hearing, touch, or movement. The distractors must be powerful enough to involve the individual's total interest without resulting in fatigue. Pain of long duration requires a variety of meaningful distracters. Methods of distraction include the following:

1. Playing games, watching television
2. Talking with someone
3. Listening to favourite music
4. Rhythmic breathing
5. Focusing on an object

Waking-imagined analgesia. Waking-imagined analgesia is defined as imagining a pleasant situation when a noxious stimulus is applied. This intervention is similar to distraction except that the person concentrates on trying to relive the sensations that occurred during a previous pleasant experience rather than on enumerating the events that took place. Only a small percentage of the population in pain can use this method of analgesia; more can derive benefit from distraction alone.

Relaxation. Full relaxation decreases muscle tension and fatigue that usually accompanies pain. It also helps to decrease anxiety, thereby preventing augmentation of the pain stimulus. Carrying out relaxation techniques also serves as a form of distraction.

Not all persons with severe pain are able to achieve sufficient relaxation to have an effect on decreasing the pain sensation. Relaxation exercises may be especially beneficial for persons with chronic pain to help reduce stress that exacerbates the pain and to help the person achieve a sense of control, of being better able to cope with the pain. There are numerous forms of relaxation techniques (see Chapter 5). Success with a relaxation technique requires practice and encouragement.

Specific nursing implications for pain control

Specific nursing interventions for pain relief include those related to preventing pain, modifying the stimulus, and modifying the response to pain as previously described. General guidelines for pain relief are listed here.

Guidelines for pain relief measures
1. *Preparation for painful experiences*
   Prepare patients for what to expect in terms of discomfort and measures of pain control *before* pain occurs, whenever possible (such as before painful tests or treatments). Intensity and duration of pain are decreased because of decreased anxiety and the patient's sense of control.
2. *Preventive approach*
   Use pain relief measures *before* pain becomes moderate or severe. The more severe the pain the less the possibility of relief.
3. *Placebo response*
   Use methods that employ a placebo response, that is, some relief from discomfort not related specifically to the applied pain relief method. If the person expects relief from the pain, anxiety and muscle tension will decrease, and decreased pain is experienced. This can be accomplished by suggestion ("This should help you feel better") or by using methods the patient believes will work.
4. *Patient's ability or will to participate*
   Consider the patient's ability or will to be active or passive in using pain relief measures. Decreased ability results from severe pain, fatigue, sedation, or unconsciousness. Decreased will occurs with some people with chronic pain who have experienced numerous failures in pain relief.
5. *Varying pain relief measures*
   Use more than one type of pain relief measure when appropriate. For example, give an analgesic, rub the patient's back, and then offer some distraction, or combine an analgesic with relaxation response.
6. *Introducing new pain relief measures*
   Introduce a new method in combination with known effective methods. Some measures, such as distraction or relaxation, require practice; do not discard the new method until after several tries.
7. *Giving analgesics*
   a. Assess and record the effectiveness of analgesics given.
   b. Ask the patient for a pain rating (0 to 10) on each shift, before, and 1 hour after each analgesic given.
   c. Give analgesics to prevent or minimize pain.
   d. Give opioids on a regular basis rather than as needed when acute pain is anticipated, such as after some general surgical procedures.
   e. If the medications will be given "as needed," instruct patient to report the presence of developing or recurrent pain, and ask regularly for pain ratings.
   f. Determine which patients are at high risk for developing pain and assess them frequently for presence of increasing pain.
   g. Use the oral route, when possible, where patient is not in acute pain, can swallow, and is not nauseated.
   h. Use the parenteral route in acute intermittent pain to provide immediate, short-term relief.

Team approach for chronic pain control

In recent years knowledge of the nature of chronic pain and the need for coordinated efforts of different health care professionals have resulted in the establishment of pain clinics and inpatient pain teams for control of chronic pain.

Pain clinics. Most pain clinics use a team approach that may include doctors (medical and surgical), anaesthetist, nurse, physiotherapist, occupational therapist, social worker, psychologist, counsellor, and chaplin. Each pain clinic is organized differently and places greater emphasis on different aspects of pain relief. Usual approaches to pain relief include the following:
1. Behaviour modification (with patient's approval)
2. Medications: opioids, NSAIDs, laxatives, tricyclics
3. Exercise and activity prescriptions
4. Family training to support planned goals/activities.

The responsibility of the nurse varies depending on the available team members and may include patient assessment, documentation of observations, creating and maintaining a therapeutic milieu, providing emotional support for patient and family, and patient teaching. Nurses who work in pain clinics must be skilled in nurse–client interactions, be knowledgeable about the mechanisms of pain and the effectiveness of various treatment modalities, and possess patience and understanding as they assist patients in reaching their goals.

Inpatient chronic pain teams. People with chronic persistent pain are sometimes admitted to a hospital for evaluation or initiation of treatment by a multidisciplinary health team similar to that in a pain clinic. One example is a team for evaluation and treatment of chronic back pain. Each team member participates in the evaluation individually and collectively and in team conferences to develop a specific treatment plan. The culmination of the hospitalization is a discharge conference with the patient and family members in which future treatment plans and recommendations are presented and discussed.

Protocols are developed for the approach to be used in control of the chronic pain; all those providing patient care during the hospitalization need to become familiar with the protocols so that a consistent approach is used for pain control. For example, protocols for control of chronic back pain in one large American medical centre include an initial immobilization phase in which patients are placed in pelvic traction and instructed to move as little as possible (for example, eat in side-lying position). This phase is followed by a mobilization phase in which the patients are encouraged to be active (for example, walk to physical therapy and to the cafeteria for meals and make their own beds). The type of nursing care is therefore different depending on which phase is being implemented.

Nursing responsibilities include patient assessment, documenting observations, carrying out phase-related activities, carrying out designated behaviour modification modalities, and patient teaching.

Evaluation

Evaluation is an important component that is often forgotten in the care of the patient with pain. Evaluation is vital so that the effectiveness of the interventions continues, or that the interventions be modified, replaced with another intervention, or discontinued. The essential questions to consider in regard to *acute* pain are as follows.

Does the patient still have pain?
If so, how does it compare with the pain experienced before the intervention?
If it is better but still present, should the same intervention(s) be continued unchanged or modified?
Should new interventions be added?
If it is not better, were sufficient data obtained in the initial assessment to determine the cause of pain?
Are there new data to indicate a different diagnosis?
What are the patient's thoughts about the continuing pain and the modes of intervention?

The essential questions to consider in regard to *chronic* pain are as follows:

To what extent is the patient participating in the planned therapeutic programme?
What is the patient's assessment of present pain?
Pain teams often have special evaluation guidelines specific to their patient population and treatment goals.

SUMMARY

1. Pain is a complex universal, yet individualized, experience.
2. Nociceptors are pain receptors that respond to chemical, thermal, electrical, or mechanical stimuli. Chemical stimuli released by damaged tissues include histamines, bradykinins, prostaglandins, and acids.
3. The gate control theory proposes that the substantia gelatinosa is a gating mechanism that may modify the pain experience by 'opening' or 'closing' the gate to pain impulse transmission. The gating mechanism is influenced by impulses from A-delta and C fibres and from descending pathways from the brainstem and cortex.
4. The pain experience is influenced by the individual's pain perception and response.
5. Pain perception is subjective, highly complex, and individual. It is influenced by characteristics of the pain stimuli and transmission and by receptivity and interpretation in the cerebral cortex.
6. Pain detection threshold is the intensity of the stimulus necessary for the individual to perceive pain.
7. Pain tolerance is the maximum degree of pain intensity that someone is willing to endure before seeking relief. Pain tolerance may be increased by drugs, warmth,

counterirritation, distraction, and strong beliefs; it may be decreased by fatigue, anxiety, boredom, continuous pain, or illness.

8. Pain response is influenced by the degree of pain perception, past experiences, sociocultural values, health status, anxiety, and age.
9. Acute pain is a sudden short-term event, usually with a known source and self-limiting or readily corrected. The typical clinical signs are usually present and pain areas generally well identified. It leads to action to relieve pain with likelihood of eventual relief. Acute pain is characterized by anxiety and muscle tension.
10. Chronic pain is a prolonged situation, often with no purpose. Pain areas are less easily defined. Pain may be continuous or intermittent and with few typical clinical signs. It leads to actions to modify the pain experience. Chronic pain is characterized by increased preoccupation with pain, hopelessness, and irritability, all leading to withdrawal.
11. Superficial somatic pain is sharp and pricking, well localized, and usually not accompanied by autonomic reactions. Deep somatic and visceral pains are sharp or dull and aching, poorly localized, and usually accompanied by autonomic reactions.
12. Referred pain is felt in areas other than those stimulated; it is usually visceral in origin.
13. Pain intensity can be determined by the use of pain scales or visual analogue scales in addition to asking the patient to describe the pain.
14. Subjective data for pain include the location, intensity, quality, timing (onset, duration, frequency, cause), and provoking or palliative factors.
15. Objective data include appearance, motor behaviour, affective and verbal response, vital signs, skin colour and moisture, and inspection and palpation of painful areas.
16. Opioids provide relief of moderate to severe pain. Those with severe pain rarely develop opioid addiction. Smaller, more frequent dosages of opioids are more effective for severe acute pain, whereas larger, less frequent dosages are more effective for severe cancer pain.
17. Patient-controlled analgesia is a system of self-administration by an intravenous set-up whereby a prescribed preset bolus of opioid may be taken but not repeated until a prescribed refractory time has occurred.
18. Paracetamol and NSAIDs (such as aspirin) provide relief of mild to moderate pain.
19. Electrical stimulators include TENS and spinal cord stimulators. TENS is a nonintrusive system, easily learned by the patient and useful for postoperative, posttraumatic, peripheral neuralgia, and muscle and bone pain.
20. General nursing interventions for pain relief include preparing patients for painful experiences, using pain relief measures before pain becomes severe, varying pain relief measures, trying new approaches, and giving analgesics as effectively as possible.

STUDY QUESTIONS

- How does the assessment of acute pain differ from that of chronic pain? Think about two patients for whom you have provided care, one with acute pain and one with chronic pain. In what ways did their responses to pain differ, and how did these responses influence different management approaches?
- What misbeliefs are most prevalent in your areas of practice, and how have you tried to change them in relation to your practice and others?
- What are the equianalgesic doses and the duration of action for the most frequently administered analgesics?
- How do the following terms differ: *Pain tolerance* and *pain threshold? Pain tolerance* and *drug tolerance? Drug dependence* and *drug addiction?*
- Interview three or four patients who are using a nonpharmacological pain intervention. Compare and contrast the method, frequency of use, patient satisfaction, and effectiveness for pain relief. Were several modalities used (including drugs), and was the combination of approaches successful?

REFERENCES AND SELECTED READINGS

1.* Amadio P, Cummings D, Amadio P: Pain in the elderly: management techniques, *Pain Manag* 6(12):33-41, 1987.

2.* Baquire ML: What matters most in chronic pain management, *RN* 52(3):46-50, 1989.

3. Barkas G, Duafala ME: Advances in cancer pain management: a review of patient controlled analgesia, *J Pain Sympt Manag* 3(3):150-160, 1988.

4.* Bast C, Hayes P: PCA, a new way to spell pain relief: patient controlled analgesia, *RN* 49(8):18-20, 1986.

5.* Copp LA, editor: *Recent advances in nursing, perspectives and pain,* New York, 1985, Churchill Livingstone.

6.* Coyle N: Analgesics and pain, *Nurs Clin North Am* 22(3): 727-741, 1987.

7.* Dernham P: Phantom limb pain, *Geriatr Nurs* 7:34-37, 1986.

8.* Donovan M: Acute pain relief, *Nurs Clin North Am* 25(4):851-861, 1990.

9. Donovan M, Dillon P, McGuire L: The incidence and characteristics of pain in a sample of medical–surgical inpatients, *Pain* 30:69-78, 1987.

10. Dostrovsky J: Pathways of pain: update, *Persp Pain Manag* 1(1):4-8, 1991.

11. Driscoll CE: Pain management, *Prim Care* 14(2):337-352, 1987.

12.* Fields H: *Pain,* Toronto, 1987, McGraw-Hill Book Co.

13.* Fordham M: Psychophysiological pain theories, *Nursing* (London) 3:360-364, 1986.

14. Ganong WF: *Review of medical physiology,* ed 15, Norwalk, Conn, 1991, Appleton & Lange.

15. Gorman ES, Warfield CA: The use of opioids in the management of pain, *Hosp Pract* 21(6):48A-48H, 1986.

16.* Grainger S: No cause, no cure—but he's still in pain, *RN* 50(2):43-45, 1987.

16a. Grundy D, Russell J, Swain A: ABC of spinal cord injury, *BMJ,* 1986.

17. Haight K: What you should know about epidural analgesia, *Nurs 87* 17(9):58-59, 1987.

18.* Harrison M, Contanch PH: Pain: advances and issues in critical care, *Nurs Clin North Am* 22(3):691-697, 1987.

19.* Jacobs MK: Patient-controlled analgesia: who really benefits? *J Post Anesth Nurs* 3:404-407, 1988.

20. Kane N, et al: Use of patient-controlled analgesia in surgical oncology patients, *Oncol Nurs Forum* 15:29-32, 1988.

21.* Kleiman RL, et al: PCA vs regular IM injections for severe postop pain, *Am J Nurs* 87:1491-1492, 1987.

22. Lamb S, Barbaro NM: Neurosurgical approaches to the management of chronic pain syndromes, *Orthop Nurs* 6(1): 23-29, 1987.

23. Lasagna L: Pain and its management, *Hosp Pract* 21(10): 92C-92Y, 1986.

24.* Lisson EL: Ethical issues related to pain control, *Nurs Clin North Am* 22(3):649-659, 1987.

25.* McCaffery M: Giving meperidine for pain: should it be so mechanical? *Nurs 87* 17(4):61-64, 1987.

25a.* McCaffery M, Beebe A; Latham J, ed: *Pain: clinical manual for nursing practice, UK adaptation,* London, 1994, Mosby–Year Book Europe Ltd.

26.* McCaffery M, Beebe A: *Pain: clinical manual for nursing practice,* St Louis, 1988, Mosby–Year Book Co.

27.* McCaffery M, Ferrell B: Do you know a narcotic when you see one? *Nurs 90* 20(6):62-63, 1990.

28. McGuire DB, editor: Cancer pain seminar. *Semin Oncol Nurs* 1:81-150, 1987.

29.* McGuire L: Administering analgesics: which drugs are right for your patient? *Nurs 90* 20(4):34-41, 1990.

30.* McGuire L: The power of non-narcotic pain relievers, *RN* 53(4):28-35, 1990.

31.* Oberle K: Pain, anxiety and analgesics: a comparative studyb of elderly and younger surgical patients, *Can J Aging* 9(1):13-22, 1990.

32.* Olsson G, Parker G: A model approach to pain assessment, *Nurs 87* 17(5):52-57, 1987.

33.* Owen H, McMillan V, Rogowski D: Postoperative pain therapy: a survey of patients' expectations and their experiences, *Pain* 41(3):303-308, 1990.

34.* Paice JA: New delivery systems in pain management, *Nurs Clin North Am* 22(3):715-725, 1987.

35. Pearson BD: Pain control: an experiment in imagery, *Geriatr Nurs* 8:28-30, 1987.

36. Royburn W, et al: Patient-controlled analgesia for postcesarean section pain, *Obstet Gynecol* 72:136-139, 1988.

37. Schecter M, Allen D, Hanson K: The status of pediatric pain control: comparison of hospital analgesic usages in children and adults, *Pediatrics* 77:11-15, 1986.

38. Sheehy SB, Barber J: *Emergency nursing: principles and practice,* ed 2, St Louis, 1985, Mosby–Year Book.

39. Sternbach RA: *The psychology of pain,* ed 2, New York, 1986, Raven Press.

40. Tuttle CB: Drug management of pain in cancer patients, *Can Med Assoc J* 12:121-134, 1985.

41.* Walker M, Wong DL: A battle plan for patients in pain, *Am J Nurs* 91(6):33-36, 1991.

42.* Watt-Watson J: Misbeliefs about pain. In Watt-Watson J, Donvan M, editors: *Pain management: nursing perspective,* St Louis, 1992, Mosby–Year Book.

43. Watt-Watson J: Neurological patient with chronic pain. In Baumann A, Dewis M, editors: *Decision making in neuroscience nursing,* St Louis, 1992, Mosby–Year Book.

44.* Watt-Watson J: Nurses' knowledge of pain issues: a survey, *J Pain Sympt Manag* 2(4):207-211, 1987.

45. Watt-Watson J, Evans R, Watson CP: Relationships among coping responses and perceptions of pain intensity, depression and family functioning, *Clin J Pain* 4(2):101-106, 1988.

45a. Wild L, Coyne C: Epidural analgesia: the basics and beyond, *Am J Nurs* 92(4):26-36, 1992.

46.* Wright S: The use of therapeutic touch in the management of pain, *Nurse Clin North Am* 22(3):705-714, 1987.

47. Alberico JB: Breaking the chronic pain cycle, *Am J Nurs* 84:1222-1225, 1984.

48. Angell M: The quality of mercy, *N Engl J Med* 306(2): 98-99, 1982.

49. Crue BL: The neurophysiology and taxonomy of pain. In Brena SF, Chapman SL (editors): *Management of patients with chronic pain,* New York, 1983, SP Medical and Scientific Books.

50.* Donovan MI: Relaxation with guided imagery: a useful technique, *Cancer Nurs* 3:27-32, 1980.

51.* Friedman FB: PRN analgesics: controlling the pain or controlling the patient? *RN* 46(3):67, 1983.

52. Huhman M: Endogenous opiates and pain, *ANS* 4(4):62-71, 1982.

53.* Kim S: Pain: theory, research and nursing practice, *ANS* 2:43-59, 1980.

54.* McCaffery M: When your patient's still in pain, don't just do something, sit there, *Nurs 81* 11(6):58-61, 1981.

55.* McCaffery M: Should you administer placebos for pain? *Nurs 82* 12(2):80-85, 1982.

56.* McGuire L, Wright A: Continuous narcotic infusion, *Nurs 84* 14(12):52-57, 1982.

57.* Meissner JE: McGill-Melzak pain questionnaire, *Nurs 80* 10(1):50-51, 1980.

58.* Melzack R, Wall PD: Pain mechanisms: new theory, *Science* 150:971-979, 1965.

59. Melzack R, Wall PD: *The challenge of pain,* New York, 1983, Basic Books.

60.* Moore DE, Blacker HM: How effective is TENS for chronic pain? *Am J Nurs* 83:1175-1177, 1983.

61. Porter J, Jick H: Addiction rare in patients treated with narcotics, *N Engl J Med* 303(2):123, 1980.

62. Rudy EF: *Advanced neurological and neurosurgical nursing,* St Louis, 1984, Mosby–Year Book.

63. Tamsen A, et al: Patient-controlled analgesic therapy: clinical experience, *Acta Anaesth Scand* 74(Suppl): 157-160, 1982.

64. Warfield CA, Stein JM: Pain relief by electrical stimulation, *Hosp Pract* 18:207-218, 1983.

* Recommended for student reading

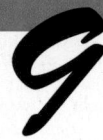

Cancer

Susan Moeller Schneider
Rosemarie M. Hogan

After studying this chapter, the learner should be able to:

- Discuss the epidemiological variables related to cancer and the nurse's role in cancer epidemiology.
- List several factors that contribute to carcinogenesis.
- Outline the pathophysiology of malignant tumours, focusing on the concepts of tumour growth and metastasis.
- Describe the nurse's role in cancer prevention and health education.
- Conduct a holistic assessment of the oncology patient.
- Identify appropriate nursing diagnoses.
- Discuss the rationale for four categories of cancer therapy and nursing interventions for patients receiving those therapies.
- Formulate a plan of care for the patient with advanced cancer.

Cancer was recognized in ancient times by skilled observers who gave it its name (from the Latin *cancri*, crab) because it stretched out in many directions like the legs of a crab. It would be preferable if the image of the crab, suggested by Hippocrates for superficial cancer in the advanced stages, could be dropped, because it maintains a legend of incurability. Forms of cancer are found in plants and in humans and other animals. The term is somewhat general and is used interchangeably with *malignant tumour* and *malignant neoplasm*.[27]

One of the least understood facts about cancer is that the name designates more than 200 diseases that have in common the production of abnormal cells that do not obey the laws of normal tissue growth.[41] Therefore cancer should never be looked on as a disease entity but only as a traditional term that describes a neoplastic process.

DEFINITION OF TERMS

The term *neoplasm* comes from the Greek word meaning "new growth" or "new formation." Normally, cell division is an orderly process with the distinct purpose of organism development or replacement of destroyed or injured cells. When cells divide without such a distinct purpose, they form neoplasms, sometimes referred to as *tumours*. Strictly speaking, a tumour is a swelling caused by any number of conditions; for example, inflammation or trauma. However, the terms *neoplasm* and *tumour* often are used interchangeably.

Oncology, a term used in association with the treatment and study of cancer, is the study of tumours (from the Greek *onkos*, mass). Neoplasms are classified broadly by distinguishing between those that are "benign" and those that are "malignant." A *malignant* neoplasm (that is, a cancer) will cause death if it is not controlled. A *benign* neoplasm usually will not cause death unless its location interferes with vital functions.[27]

ATTITUDES TOWARDS CANCER

Cancer has become one of the more curable chronic diseases. Progress is evidenced by people's knowledge about the disease and the means to prevent it, more sophisticated diagnostic techniques revealing more cancers in the early curable stages, and improved methods of treatment, particularly with radiotherapy and chemotherapy.

More effective management of the side effects of therapy has improved survival rates. Advances in antimicrobial treatments and transfusion technology have helped to combat the life-threatening complications of sepsis and haemorrhage. Despite this progress, few diseases cause greater feelings of anxiety and apprehension. A diagnosis of cancer still may carry wtih it a social stigma. The myths surrounding malignant disease, often focusing on incurability, help foster feelings of hopelessness and dread.

Nurses may also have the same negative attitudes that exist in society. For this reason it is extremely important that all nurses examine their own feelings about cancer and try to work them through, both by increasing their knowledge of the diseases and treatments and by discussing feelings openly with members of the health team. Nurses who have worked through their feelings are more able to be of assistance to patients and their families than nurses who have not done so.

The nurse's role in helping cancer patients is broad in scope and area of influence. The nurse must have correct knowledge of prevention, control, and treatment of cancer and be able to apply this information in a variety of settings. Teaching about cancer is not limited to the hospital or clinic setting but takes place in industry, at community organization meetings, and at other public forums. In addition to teaching about prevention, the nurse has an active role in treatment and control programmes in all settings in which clients are found. Clients and their families look to the nurse for assistance and guidance in all phases of illness from primary prevention to terminal care.

To be effective as a helping person, the nurse must be aware of the emotional impact that the diagnosis of cancer has on the patient and family, because this emotional response affects every aspect of nursing care. Cancer nursing is a challenge to the creativity, skill, and commitment of the nurse.

EPIDEMIOLOGY

Cancer is a disease that is universal in scope. It has existed since the beginning of history and affects humans wherever they live and whatever their race, colour, level of culture, and material progress.[4]

Cancer ranks second to heart disease as the cause of death in the United Kingdom, but significant progress has been made in prevention and treatment. In the early 1900s few cancer patients had any hope of long-term survival. In the U.S., by the 1960s, 1 in 3 was alive at least 5 years after treatment. Today about 1 out of 2 cancer patients in the United States will be saved.[5] This success can be attributed to the following:

1. Diagnosis of more cancers in the early, localized stage
2. Treatment of more patients soon after diagnosis
3. Development of new diagnostic and treatment modalities, especially chemotherapy

Cancer accounts for one in four deaths (25%) in the U.K., considerable morbidity, and huge quantities of scarce National Health Service resources.[8] The incidence of cancer and the number of deaths resulting compare unfavourably with other European countries and the U.S. For example, breast cancer in the U.K., with 60+ deaths per 100,000 females, "tops the league table," whereas countries such as Greece have only half that number. The major causes of death remain lung, breast and colorectal cancers. The pattern of cancer incidence is changing—some cancers, e.g. of the lung (male), oesophagus and stomach, are now showing a decrease,[5b] but others, such as skin cancer, are increasing.

Epidemiological Variables for Cancer

Although in general cancer shows no respect for economic or social status, there are some variations with regard to sex, site, age, race, and geographic location.

Sex and site

The average incidence of cancer is similar in both sexes. Overall survival rates (proportion of people alive 5 years

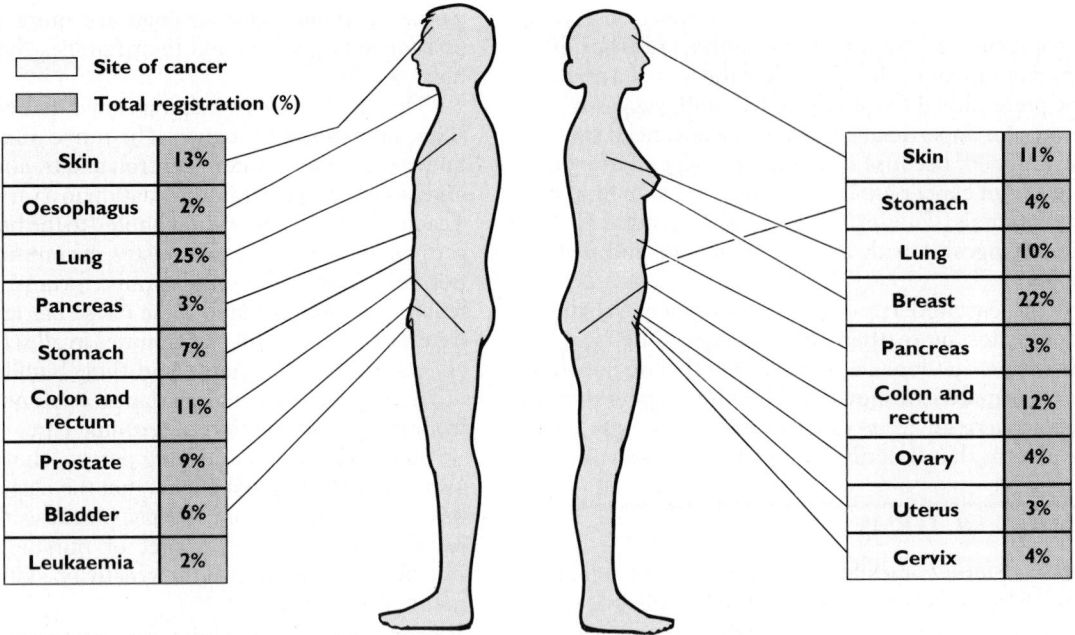

Fig. 9-1 Comparison of cancer incidence by site and sex. (Figures, 1981, taken from The Department of Health: The Health of the Nation. A Consultative Document for the Health of England, London, 1991, HMSO, and Health Education Authority: Can you avoid Cancer?, London, 1989, Health Education Authority.)

after diagnosis) for some cancers have increased, such as those for cervical cancer. Rates for most other cancers have levelled off in the past 25 years. The average cancer mortality in developed countries is higher for men than for women.

Trends in the incidence and mortality of cancers (1991) suggest the following:
1. For both sexes
   a. Steady decrease in cancer of the oesophagus and stomach
   b. Steady increase in cancer of the pancreas
   c. Slight decrease in rectal cancer deaths and a slight increase in colon cancer deaths
   d. Skin cancer increase
2. For males
   a. Increase in prostate and bladder cancer
   b. Decrease in deaths from lung cancer
3. For females
   a. Steady decrease in cancer of the uterus
   b. Increase in cancer of the cervix in younger women
   c. Deaths from breast cancer are constant in the age group 35 to 54 years but increasing in women aged 55 to 64
   d. Increase in deaths from lung cancer

Fig. 9-1 compares cancer registrations by site and sex.

Age

Although more than three-quarters of the deaths from cancer occur in people over 55 years of age,[12] cancer affects more women than men in the younger age groups, but more men are affected after the age of 60, and more children aged 3 to 13 years die of cancer than of any other disease.

However, mortality among children with cancer has declined.

Race

Cancer incidence and mortality rates in the U.S. are higher for blacks than for whites. Statistics indicate that blacks have significantly lower survival rates for cancer of the breast, colorectum, and prostate.[4,5] Oesophageal cancer has declined in whites but has risen rapidly in blacks of both sexes. Although incidence of invasive cervical cancer has declined in women of both races, the survival rate for white women is significantly higher than for black women.

Most differences in the cancer rates of black and white populations are attributed to environmental and social factors rather than to inherent biological characteristics. One study showed that urban blacks tend to be less knowledgeable about warning signals and are less likely to seek medical care if symptoms do occur. These blacks also tended to underestimate the prevalence of cancer and the choices of cure.[25] Increased risk of exposure to industrial carcinogens and limited educational opportunities among those in the lower socioeconomic group may also be contributing factors, because a higher percentage of blacks are in the lower socioeconomic group.[4] These findings will be of interest to nurses providing health care for multiracial groups and in areas where communities may be disadvantaged in terms of education, employment, income, and health care facilities.

Geographic factors

Differences occur in the geographic distribution of cancer. For example, stomach cancer is common in Japan, Latin

Table 9-1 Risk and epidemiology for five major cancer sites

Site	% cancer registration	Deaths per 100,000 (standardized mortality rates) in 1991	Risk factors	Comments
Breast females	22% (female)	50 per 100,000	Over age 50, personal or family history of breast cancer, never had children, first child after age 30	Leading cause of death from cancer in women
Colorectum males	11%	30 per 100,000	Personal or family history of colon and rectum cancer, personal or family history of polyps in colon or rectum, ulcerative colitis, diet high in beef and/or deficient in fibre content	Considered a highly curable disease when digital and proctoscopic examinations are included in routine check-ups
Lung males females	25% 10%	90 per 100,000 42 per 100,000	Heavy cigarette smoking, history of smoking 20 or more years, exposure to certain industrial substances such as asbestos, particularly for those who smoke	Leading cause of cancer among men, and rising mortality among women
Stomach males females	7% 4%	20 per 100,000 11 per 100,000	Ingestion of smoked food, history of pernicious anaemia; males affected twice as often as females	Less prevalent now, in the U.K.
Uterus—cervix females	4%	7 per 100,000	Cervical cancer: early age at first intercourse, multiple sex partners	Cervical cancer mortality has declined during past 40 years with wider use of cervical smear

America, and Eastern Europe but uncommon in Australia, New Zealand, the United States and the United Kingdom. Breast cancer is more common in Western countries but is rare in Japan. Cancer of the liver occurs frequently in parts of Africa and Asia but rarely in the United Kingdom.

Genetic differences between populations may contribute to international variations. However, observations of what happens to cancer incidence when people migrate from one country to another show that environmental (for example, air pollution) and clinical (for example, diet) factors play a more important role than genetic differences in the rate that changes occur.[7]

Nurse's Role in Cancer Epidemiology

Cancer is not only a threat to life, but its cost in loss of income and disruption of the lives of families cannot be estimated. Nurses must be in the forefront of the thousands of health professionals who are working to eradicate the disease. Cancer epidemiological research has contributed to cancer prevention and control by identifying epidemiological trends that can be used to determine individuals and groups at high risk for cancer. Nurses can play a vital role in cancer prevention by assessing people's cancer risks and teaching them about environmental and personal carcinogenic risk factors, including recommendations for prevention and early detection. Table 9-1 summarizes important epidemiological aspects and risk factors for the six major cancer sites.

AETIOLOGY: CARCINOGENESIS

The factors that contribute to the development of cancer are many and at present are not fully understood; however, certain health practices are known to decrease the possibility that cancer may occur. Because cancer is not a single disease entity, it is not likely that there is a single cause.

Cancer probably occurs as the result of the interaction of many risk factors or because of long-term exposure to a single carcinogenic agent. Factors involved in carcinogenesis include host susceptibility, environmental carcinogens, habits and customs, and viruses.

Host Susceptibility
Genetic factors

Studies of genetic factors have focused on specific cancer sites and the disease in general. Chromosomes have been studied to find evidence of the genetic origin of cancer. Chromosomal abnormalities associated with neoplasia may consist of extra or missing chromosomes or the presence of abnormal chromosomes. The question is whether these changes are the cause or the effect of cancer.[16]

A second indication of genetic origin is that cancer cells are a population of cells descendant from a single cell of origin (clones). Future generations of cancer cells are always malignant; they inherit and pass on the trait. Finally, there is a possibility that cancer arises from an innate genetic inability, possibly a defect in mitotic regulation.

Familial polyposis of the colon, a precursor of cancer, is indisputably hereditary. There is also a high incidence of breast cancer in a vertical line of descent, such as from mother to daughter.[6] Risk of breast cancer in the first-degree relative of a patient is five times that of the general population. Heredity in some way seems to be connected with bronchogenic cancer. It seems to interact with cigarette smoking to cause a synergistic effect.[4]

In general, inherited cancers are a direct expression of an inherited defect, but these syndromes are rare and account for only a small percentage of familial cancer.[4] Studies have shown that the pattern of inheritance is not usually that of single mendelian gene, and it is still not known whether the incidences of many specific cancers are a result of a combination of genetic and environmental factors.[6]

Hormonal factors

Hormones do not appear to be primary carcinogens, but rather they seem to influence carcinogenesis in the following three ways:
1. By a preparative action on the target tissues, making them susceptible to the carcinogenic agent
2. By a "permissive" influence of carcinogenesis allowing the process to progress
3. By a conditioning effect on the tumour

Hormones are capable of restraining or enhancing the growth of tumours that have developed. Hormone therapy and some surgical therapies (hypophysectomy and oophorectomy) are based on this fact.

Evidence exists that tissues that are endocrine responsive (for example, breasts, endometrium, and prostate) do not develop cancer unless they are stimulated by their growth-promoting hormones. Oestrogens have been associated with cancers such as adenocarcinoma of the vagina, hepatic tumours, breast tumours, and uterine cancer.

In addition to tissue stimulation by the hormone, carcinogenesis may be determined by the length of time of the hormonal effect. The longer the preparative influence of the hormone, the greater the chance of cancer development.

Precancerous lesions

Certain benign lesions and tumours have a tendency towards malignant change. These cancers are preventable if minor precursor conditions are treated carefully. Precancerous lesions are a large and heterogenous group. In some, cancer is inevitable, whereas in others the risk is so low that medical management disregards the cancer risk. Two examples of precancerous lesions are actinic keratoses, which appear as rough, scaly, erythematous areas on skin that has usually been exposed to sun; and leukoplakia, which are white patches of the mucous membranes[12] (see Chapter 34).

Chronic irritation

It is also known that cancer may follow chronic irritation of any part of the body. There are many ways to prevent irritation that may lead to cancer. Effort is being made in industry to protect workers from coal-tar products known to contain carcinogens. Masks and gloves are recommended in some instances, and workers are urged to wash their hands and arms thoroughly to remove all irritating substances at the end of the day's work. Occupational health nurses participate in intensive educational programmes to help workers understand the need for carrying out company safety policy that may help prevent cancer.

Immunological factors

It may be possible that failure of the normal immune mechanism may predispose to certain cancers. The change from normal to malignant cells is relatively common. These new cells are antigenically different and are recognized as such by the body's immune system. If the immune response is initiated, the malignant cell will be destroyed. That a kind of immune surveillance system may exist is suggested by the following evidence:

1. The two peaks of high incidence of tumours in humans are in early childhood and old age.[12]
2. Individuals with rare immunodeficiency disease in which there is a defect in cellular immunity have increased evidence of tumour development.
3. Individuals receiving immunosuppressive drugs to prevent organ transplant rejection have an increased evidence of neoplasia.[6]

Cancer itself appears to suppress the immune response early in the disease, as well as late in its progression. It has not been definitely established that cancer develops because of failure in immune surveillance, and at present there is not enough data to make a strong case. (The role of the immune systems and cancer therapy is discussed later in this chapter and in Chapter 18.)

Environmental Factors

In the United States it has been estimated that 70% to 90% of human cancers result from environmental factors. The view of the United Kingdom Department of Health is that, potentially, about 85% of cancer deaths in England could be avoided.[8] Occupational and environmental factors, e.g. pollution and ionizing radiation, cause a very small percentage (1% to 2%) of human cancers, but many chemical substances, *excluding* pharmaceutical and food additives in common use, are known to be carcinogenic.[42]

There are several types of chemical and physical carcinogens (cancer-producing substances). Various carcinogens may have an additive or enhancing effect on one another, and even small amounts of these substances may constitute a hazard. Carcinogens act on different organs depending on the portal of entry and the distribution in the body.[7]

Chemical pollutants

Air pollution has been blamed for the rising cancer incidence in the twentieth century. Ten polycyclic aromatic hydrocarbons have been recognized as carcinogenic. Tar and pitch and their derivatives and mineral oils containing aromatic hydrocarbons were discovered to be carcinogenic many years ago. Bladder cancer from aromatic amines is an occupational disease of workers in the rubber industry.[2] The risk of contracting lung cancer is 15 to 30 times greater among those exposed to chromium compounds. Other common occupational cancers are respiratory cancers from asbestos and leukaemia resulting from long-term inhalation of benzine.

Chemotherapeutic agents used to treat cancer are also considered carcinogens. Because these agents alter the ability of cells to replicate, they are capable of affecting healthy cells as well as tumour cells. Although data are inconclusive regarding how much risk is involved with handling antineoplastic agents, many groups e.g. Health and Safety Executive (1983) recommend using protective gowns, gloves, and masks.[31] These medications should be prepared under a vertical laminar air flow hood. Nurses should be familiar with the policies and procedures of the institution where they are employed.[26]

Health Practices
Tobacco use

There is now no question that the rate of lung cancer during the past 70 years can be attributed to the use of cigarettes. Some estimates suggest that cigarette smoking is responsible for 83% of lung cancer cases among men and 43% among women—more than 75% overall. The incidence of lung cancer in those who smoke on a regular basis is up to 40 times greater than in nonsmokers. In the past, more men than women smoked, and men smoked more heavily; however, the gap has been narrowing. The rise in the number of women smokers has captured the attention of cigarette manufacturers, who have increased their advertising efforts to the point of designing cigarettes expressly for women.

Tobacco use accounts for about 30% of all deaths from cancers (some examples are mouth, pharynx, larynx, oesophagus, pancreas, and bladder) and is also linked to heart disease, gastric ulcers, chronic bronchitis, and emphysema.[2] It is estimated that some 100,000 deaths per annum in the U.K. are linked to smoking. If smoking is discontinued, even after a habit of 30 years, there is a decrease in the evidence of lung cancer. Not smoking for 10 years reduces the risk of cancer to equal that of a person who has never smoked.[11]

There has been a steady decline in the proportion of adult smokers in the U.K. That the percentage of smokers within the population has fallen is supported by a corresponding reduction in cigarette sales during the last decade. Adults who have stopped smoking are in excess of one million and non-smokers now outnumber smokers by two to one in the U.K. However, a worrying trend is the number of young people, especially young women, who have started to smoke. The vast majority of people stop smoking on their own, without the aid of any organized programme. However, for smokers who need more intensive assistance and group support, smoking cessation clinics are available in most communities.

The Health Education Authority and various anti-smoking organizations, e.g. Action on Smoking and Health (ASH), provide information about smoking, its effects and advice on "giving up". Several of these participating organizations have produced films, videos, and other educational materials that are available to schools, organizations, and individuals. This educational material can be obtained from local health promotion units and anti-smoking organizations. One of the main concerns is how to convince young people not to start smoking. In the United States, educational and smoking control programmes have been effective in college graduates, in whom smoking prevalence has decreased by 50%. In the government paper, *Health of the Nation* (1992), the following risk factor targets are set out for the U.K.: a reduction in cigarette smoking to 20% or less of the population (male and female); a reduction in smoking in the group 11 to 15 years by 33%; that 33% of women who smoke stop at the start of their pregnancy; and that cigarette use in general be reduced by 40% or more.

The question of hazards for nonsmokers who breathe the smoke of others' cigarettes is not resolved, but recent studies have aroused concern. Two studies have shown increased risk of lung cancer among wives of cigarette smokers; however, another study found little, if any, risk for "passive smokers."[1]

Nurses have a responsibility, both as well-informed citizens and as professional people, to be aware of the most recent antismoking programmes and to interpret them to the public. One of the best ways for nurses to do this would be to stop smoking themselves. Many nurses still smoke and unfortunately do so in public places, which may result in confusing health messages for lay people.[14]

Nutrition

Nutritional habits are increasingly being investigated and implicated in the aetiology of cancer. A high incidence of cancer of the colon occurs in populations whose diet is high in refined food and low in nonabsorbable cellulose "roughage" or fibre. Evidence indicates that the incidence of colonic carcinoma is low among those who eat a largely vegetarian diet (i.e. with relatively few animal products[4]) and which is especially low in fats. Breast cancer appears to be associated with a diet high in animal fat, but the precise relationship has not been identified.[2]

Other factors in the daily diet may be responsible for cancer. These are not only specific carcinogenic agents but also certain nutritional deficiencies. Ingestion of smoked foods, which contain benzopyrene, has been correlated with an increased incidence of stomach cancer. Some epidemiological and experimental evidence suggests that high caloric intake may lead to cancer and calorie deprivation may prevent it. Obesity may increase the risk of breast, colon, gallbladder, prostate, and uterine cancer.[6]

Some foods may protect against cancer. The food additives butylated hydroxyanisole (BHA) and butylated hydroxytoluene (BHT) seem to inhibit cancer. Although reports are conflicting, some investigators believe vitamins A, B, C, and E actually have anticancer effects.[2] High-fibre foods such as fruits, vegetables, and whole grain cereals may decrease the incidence of cancer.[6]

Many food substances contain additives, contaminants, and naturally appearing substances such as aflatoxin, which may be carcinogenic. Food additives being studied include food dyes, flavouring agents, and antimicrobial preservatives such as sodium and potassium nitrite and nitrate. Although some potential carcinogens are present in the diet, the time trends do not indicate that additives now in use are significant in the aetiology of cancer. The present government policy is to keep the levels of potential carcinogenic agents in food as low as feasible, recognizing that it is almost impossible to state with absolute certainty that any ingested chemical is safe. The problem is that effects from ingesting carcinogenic agents may not be seen for decades because of the long latency periods. Childhood exposure, particularly, may provide the time for cancer to appear.

Alcohol

There is a significant association between alcohol intake and cancer of the mouth, pharynx, larynx, and oesophagus.[6] However, alcohol misuse is often associated with smoking and with vitamin and dietary deficiencies, whose roles in the aetiology of cancer are not known. It is speculated that alcohol and nutritional deficiencies enhance carcinogenesis by increasing the metabolic activities of specific tobacco carcinogens.[2] Tumours of the involved sites occur with greater frequency in men, lower socioeconomic groups, increasingly urbanized societies, and the elderly.[7]

Sexual practices

Carcinoma of the uterine cervix is less common in virgins than in sexually active women. It is higher in those who have first coitus at an early age, who have an early first marriage, and who have had multiple sex partners. Cervical cancer is more frequent in women who have had multiple pregnancies, but this factor decreases in importance when the groups of women compared started their sex life at the same age. The development of cancer seems to be connected with coitus rather than pregnancy.[6]

Carcinoma of the penis is virtually unknown among circumcised men. The means by which circumcision provides protection is not clear, but it is probably related to better hygiene. There is also a lower incidence of cancer of the uterine cervix in women whose sexual partner has been circumcised and in cultures in which the men, even though not circumcised, have a high standard of genital hygiene. Increased risk of testicular cancer is associated with undescended testicles.[6]

The correlation with sexual experience and breast cancer is the reverse of that for the uterine cervix. Breast cancer patients have usually been married and become pregnant later in life.[6] Lactation may provide some protection against breast cancer, since women who have breast-fed their infants show a lower incidence of breast malignancy. Cancer of the breast is reported to be unknown among Eskimo women and to be relatively rare among Japanese women; both cultures practise breast-feeding.

Psychosocial Factors

Stressors such as life changes, loss of a significant other, and personality variables have been suggested as aetiological factors in the development of cancer. Some researchers believe that stress alters the body's immune system, making a person more susceptible to cancer. Depression has also been linked to cancer deaths by causing changes in immune mechanisms.

Social support in the form of institutions, family, and friends may also be an important variable. The individual with low social support and high need may be at a higher risk for developing cancer. In addition, lack of social support may adversely affect coping responses to therapy and to the illness. At the present time, however, how one defines the nature of social support and the degree to which it is present or lacking is unclear.[16]

Conclusions

Carcinogenesis is a dynamic process that is influenced by many independent and poorly defined variables. The initial molecular changes are irreversible, but they may not be expressed when cooperative conditions are absent. Changes in these conditions may alter the carcinogenic process, resulting in either acceleration, inhibition, or even reversal of the process. Aetiological agents may be co-carcinogens. A genetic predisposition for a "weak" immune system along with a viral infection may lead to cancer, or oncogenic viruses may act as suppressants of the immune system. Chemical carcinogens may activate latent viral genes or inhibit the immune system's effectiveness in destroying cancer cells.

Nurses have a vital role to play in communicating to the public the factors involved in carcinogenesis. They can clarify misconceptions as well as do health teaching so that known carcinogenic practices may be eliminated. They can also set an example of good health practices for the general public, perhaps a more difficult role. As knowledgeable and concerned citizens, nurses must be initiators and supporters of efforts to have carcinogens removed from the environment.

PATHOPHYSIOLOGY

Characteristics of Malignant Cells

Normal tissue is composed of mature cells of uniform size and shape. Within each cell is a nucleus, which contains the chromosomes, a specific number for every species, and within each chromosome is deoxyribonucleic acid (DNA). DNA is a giant molecule whose chemical composition controls the characteristics of ribonucleic acid (RNA), which is found both in the nucleoli of cells and in the cytoplasm of the cell itself and which regulates cell growth and function. When ovum and sperm unite, the DNA and RNA within the chromosomes of each will govern the differentiation and future course of the trillions of cells that finally develop to form the adult organism. In the development of various organs and parts of the body, cells undergo differentiation in size, appearance, and arrangement; thus the histologist or the pathologist can look at a piece of prepared tissue through a microscope and know the portion of the body from which it came.

There are two categories of alterations in cell growth: benign and malignant. Benign neoplasms involve cellular proliferation of adult or mature cells growing slowly in an orderly manner in a capsule. These tumours do not invade surrounding tissue but may cause harm through pressure on vital structures. Benign tumours remain localized, do not metastasize (spread), and do not recur after they are completely removed (see Table 9-2).

A malignant cell is one in which the basic structure and activity have become deranged in a manner that is abnormal; the cause or causes are still poorly understood. It is believed, however, that the basic process involves a disturbance in the regulatory functions of DNA. It is known that the DNA molecule is affected by radiation in certain instances, and it is speculated that it may be affected by other factors as well.

In the neoplastic cell, normal restraints on growth are defective. It is believed that malignant neoplasms occur as the result of faulty mechanisms inside the cell nucleus.[27]

DNA, the permanent genetic material in nuclear chromosomes, contains information necessary for cell replication, the chemical code for cell growth and development To convey this information, RNA serves as a messenger.

Table 9-2 Characteristics of benign and malignant neoplasms

Characteristics	Benign	Malignant
Cell characteristics	Cells resemble normal cells of the tissue from which the tumour originated	Cells often bear little resemblance to the normal cells of the tissue from which they arose; there is both anaplasia and pleomorphism (assumption of two or more different forms)
Mode of growth	Tumour grows by expansion and does not infiltrate the surrounding tissues; encapsulated	Grows at the periphery and sends out processes that infiltrate and destroy the surrounding tissues
Rate of growth	Rate of growth is usually slow	Rate of growth is usually relatively rapid and is dependent upon level of differentiation; the more anaplastic the tumour the more rapid the rate of growth
Metastasis	Does not spread by metastasis	Gains access to the blood and lymph channels and metastasizes to other areas of the body
Recurrence	Does not recur when removed	Tends to recur when removed
General effects	Is usually a localized phenomenon that does not cause generalized effects unless by location it interferes with vital functions	Often causes generalized effects such as anaemia, weakness, and weight loss
Destruction of tissue	Does not usually cause tissue damage unless location interferes with blood flow	Often causes extensive tissue damage as the tumour outgrows its blood supply or encroaches on blood flow to the area; may also produce substances that cause cell damage
Ability to cause death	Does not usually cause death unless its location interferes with vital functions	Will usually cause death unless growth can be controlled

From Porth C: *Pathophysiology: concepts of altered health states*, ed 3, Philadelphia, 1990, JB Lippincott.

Any small change in DNA (mutation) causes a distortion of biological information, which may result in the affected cells running wild. The result is a malignant neoplasm.[2] The malignant cells lose the normal specialized function of the normal cell or may take on new characteristics and functions.

A characteristic of malignant cells that can be observed through a microscope is *loss of differentiation*, or loss of likeness to the original cell (parent tissue) from which the tumour growth originated.[15] This loss of differentiation is called *anaplasia*, and its extent is a determining factor in the degree of malignancy of the tumour.

Anaplasia is characterized by alterations in intracellular macromolecular synthesis and intercellular relationships and associations. Two types of anaplasia have been identified. In positional or organizational anaplasia, the usual distinct histological patterns in tissues are altered. In cytological anaplasia, there is increased or altered nucleic acid synthesis in growing tissues.[7] Anaplasia is one of the most reliable indicators of malignancy. It is seen only in cancers and does not appear in benign neoplasms.

Other characteristics of malignant cells that can be seen through a microscope are the presence of nuclei of various sizes, many of which contain unusually large amounts of chromatin, and the presence of mitotic figures (cells in the process of division), which denotes rapid and disorderly division of cells. The proportion of cells actively proliferating in malignant tumours is generally greater than that of normal cells.

Malignant tumours have no enclosing capsule; thus they invade adjacent or surrounding tissue, including lymph and blood vessels, through which they may spread to distant parts of the body to set up new tumours (*metastases*). Unless completely removed or destroyed, they tend to recur after treatment, and their continued presence causes death by replacing normal cells and by other means not fully understood.

Growth of malignant neoplasms

The term *neoplasm* has been defined as a relatively autonomous growth of tissues, the term *autonomy* meaning that a malignant tumour is not subject to the "rules and regulations" that govern cells and cell interaction of the healthy individual. This autonomy is relative in that the tumour is not completely independent of the tissue from which it arose.

There are considerable differences in the rate of growth of malignant tumours. The growth rate is often referred to in terms of tumour *doubling time*. Different types of tumours often have varying doubling times.[23] For example, lymphomas generally have a faster doubling time than cancers of the bone. It is also possible for tumours of the same tissue type to have different doubling times. A breast cancer may spread rapidly in one individual, whereas the growth in another individual could be extremely slow for a period of time and then could later accelerate. In general, it is has been calculated that a tumour mass will double in size 30 times before it is 1 cm in size, when there is a chance for it to be clinically detected. Occasionally, a tumour grows so slowly that it can be removed completely after a long period of time. This characteristic probably accounts for the good results obtained in a few circumstances even when treatment has been delayed. No doctor, however, ever relies on this possibility to justify delay in treatment. Occasionally, a malignant tumour grows slowly for a long time and then undergoes change, and the rate of growth increases enormously.

Spread of cancer

The rate of growth of a malignant neoplasm determines its capacity to spread. Cancer may spread by direct extension, by gravitational metastasis, or by metastatic spread.

Direct extension or invasion

Direct extension or invasion of neighbouring tissue produces the typical local effects of ulcerating, bulky, haemorrhagic masses or indurative, fibrosing lesions with tissue fixation, distortion of the structure, and the pitting of the skin seen in some breast cancer. Infection may accompany this local infiltration. Because of local spread, any cancer excision must include a margin of surrounding tissues to ensure removal of all malignant cells.

Gravitational metastasis and seeding

Gravitational metastasis involves the erosion of cancer cells into body cavities and their dropping onto the serous membrane lining the cavity. The pathway is determined by gravity or movements of the body.[16] A tumour may penetrate the wall of the stomach and its cells implant on the surface of the peritoneal cavity. In the peritoneal cavity, cells tend to gravitate to the pelvis. Cells from neoplasm of the pleura of the thoracic cavity may "drop" to the diaphragm. Cancer cells can also be implanted by the surgeon into the operative area, causing metastatic lesions (mechanical transplantation).

Metastatic spread

Metastatic spread occurs when cancer cells invade vascular or lymphatic channels and travel to distant parts of the body where implantation occurs. Lymph node metastasis is present in approximately half of all fatal cancers. In *lymph vessels*, cells may detach and become emboli, which lodge in the regional lymph nodes that receive their drainage from the tumour site. Spread continues to the next group of nodes and into the other organs. Cells also may gain access to the blood stream by way of the thoracic duct.[16]

Vascular embolism of malignant cells may occur through the veins or arteries to various parts of the body depending on the vascular drainage of the organs involved. The liver is a common metastatic site for cancers originating in the gastrointestinal tract, pancreas, and spleen because of routing through the hepatic portal vein before entering the general circulation. Because venous blood travels through the lungs, this is another common site for secondary growth via the venous system. Cancer cells in the arterial system frequently form secondary neoplasms in the bone and the brain, especially if the primary site is in the lungs, where cancer cells can gain direct access to the left heart and systemic circulation.

In metastatic spread, there is almost always a high degree of histological, cytological, and functional similarity between the primary cancer and these metastases. Consequently, the type of cell and the probable site of the primary tumour can be identified from the morphology of the metastasis. In addition, metastases usually mimic the primary tumour in the formation of cell products and secretions.

Naming and Classifying Neoplasms

Tumours derive their names from the parent tissue or the tissue type from which the growth originated (Table 9-3). This is often called the tissue of origin. In general, the names of benign tumours carry the suffix *-oma* following the name of the parent tissue, for example, *neuroma* or *fibroma*. Malignant tumours generally are of two types, those of epithelial and those of mesenchymal (connective tissue) origin. The term *carcinoma* denotes a malignant tumour of epithelial cells, and the term *sarcoma* denotes a malignant tumour of connective tissue cells.[16] Haematopoietic or blood-forming tissues are involved in malignant processes that are disseminated from the beginning, in contrast to solid tumours that initially are confined to a specific tissue or organ.

Tumours containing embryonic elements of all three primary germ layers, such as hair, teeth, and so on, are called *teratomas*. These are usually benign and often are found in the ovaries.

Some malignant tumours are known by the names of the scientists who first described them, for example, Hodgkin's disease and Wilm's tumour. Other types of malignant neoplasms occur with a wide variety of seemingly unrelated names. The diversity in naming malignant neoplasms reflects the complexities involved in identifying and classifying the many forms of cancer. However, a consistent, universal system of naming and classifying tumours is necessary to facilitate communication among researchers and health professionals.

There are two major methods for classifying cancers: *grading* according to histological criteria and *staging* according to the extent of the spread of the disease. Tumours may be *graded* by roman or arabic numerals into four grades; the higher the grade, the worse the prognosis.[15]

Histological grading

G1	Well-differentiated
G2	Moderately well-differentiated
G3, G4	Poorly to very poorly differentiated

Remember that normal cells of one organ or tissue are well differentiated from cells of another organ or tissue (p. 135). Thus, a grade 1 tumour is the most differentiated (more like the parent tissue) and, therefore, the least malignant; grade 4 is the least differentiated (more unlike the parent tissue) and has a high degree of malignancy. These classifications are useful to the doctor when determining whether the tumour may be expected to respond to radiation treatment, as well as in planning all other aspects of the patient's treatment. Usually, malignant tissue is slightly more sensitive to irradiation than normal tissue.

Determination of the extent of the spread of cancer (*staging*) and the site of the original tumour is vital for planning therapy. The International Union Against Cancer has devised the TNM system of classification: *T*, tumour; *N*, regional lymph nodes; *M*, distant metastases. Adding a number to the letters (for example, T1, T2, N1, N2) indicates the extent of the malignancy. This system provides a type of shorthand notation to describe the particular tumour (Box 9-1). The purpose of the TNM system is to

Table 9-3 Names of neoplasms

Tissue type	Benign	Malignant
Epithelium		
Skin and mucous membrane	Papilloma	Squamous cell carcinoma
Glands	Adenoma	Adenocarcinoma
Connective tissue		
Fibrous	Fibroma	Fibrosarcoma
Adipose	Lipoma	Liposarcoma
Cartilage	Chondroma	Chondrosarcoma
Bone	Osteoma	Osteosarcoma
Blood vessels	Haemangioma	Haemangiosarcoma
Lymph vessels	Lymphangioma	Lymphangiosarcoma
Muscle tissue		
Smooth muscle	Leiomyoma	Leiomyosarcoma
Striated muscle	Rhabdomyoma	Rhabdomyosarcoma
Nerve tissue		
Nerve fibre and sheath	Neuroma	Neurogenic sarcoma
Ganglion cells	Ganglioneuroma	Neuroblastoma
Glia cells	Astrocytoma	Glioblastoma multiforme
Hamatopoietic tissue		
Plasma cells		Multiple myeloma
Lymphoid		Lymphatic leukaemia
Miscellaneous		
Placenta	Hydatiform mole	Chorioepithelioma (choriocarcinoma)

define categories for all cases and also allow subsequent and more detailed information to be added. A TNM classification has been identified for major cancer sites, and the choice of treatment depends on the clinical TNM stage, both for the primary tumour and the lymph nodes.[2]

Different staging systems exist for some specific types of cancer. Two examples of this are the Dukes classification system for adenocarcinoma of the colon (Chapter 23). and the Ann Arbor system of staging for Hodgkin's lymphoma. Most authorities now advocate use of the TNM system because it can be easily understood and applied to all tumour types. The consistent terminology of the TNM system facilitates communication among health care providers.[15]

Physiological Changes with Ageing

The incidence of cancer is higher in the elderly population than in any other age group, and the chances of developing cancer increase with each decade after an individual reaches the age of 60. While a variety of physiological changes occur with the ageing process that makes the host more vulnerable to malignant growth (see later chapters for specific changes), perhaps the most significant change is the exhaustion of the immune system. Antibody functioning becomes impaired and normal cells are subject to attack when the immune system falsely identifies them as foreign substances. The compromised immune system leaves the host more vulnerable to the development of malignancies

and less capable of combating those malignancies when they do occur.[40]

Another theory regarding the increase of cancer incidence in the elderly is that a lifetime of exposure to carcinogens eventually leads to the development of cancer. The physiological changes of ageing do not naturally result in tumour formation, but it is the result of prolonged exposure to cancer-causing agents. Regardless of the cause of cancer in the elderly population, nurses need to remember to assess the patient thoroughly for the signs and symptoms of cancer.[4]

Because many older adults have chronic illnesses, early warning symptoms of malignancy are often attributed to other health conditions or are overlooked as part of the ageing process.[39] As a result, many elderly patients are seen initially with advanced malignancies that are less amenable to treatment.

PREVENTION AND HEALTH EDUCATION
Primary Prevention

The British public is more widely read and informed about health problems than ever before. Health-seeking behaviour and a desire to be more knowledgeable about health problems are indicated by the frequency of articles on topics such as cancer in the lay press. The topic of cancer is also discussed more openly than ever before. Nurses have a major responsibility in the prevention of cancer. Because

---

9-1

TNM staging classification system

Tumour

T0	No evidence of primary tumour
TIS	Carcinoma *in situ*
T1, T2, T3, T4	Ascending degrees of tumour size and involvement

Nodes

N0	No regional nodes demonstrably abnormal
N1a, N2a	Demonstrable regional lymph nodes, metastasis not suspected
N1b, N2b, N3	Demonstrable regional lymph nodes; metastasis suspected
Nx	Regional nodes cannot be assessed clinically

Metastasis

M0	No evidence of distant metastasis
M1, M2, M3	Ascending degrees of metastatic involvement of the host including distant nodes

---

9-2

Dietary guidelines for cancer prevention

Reduce the intake of total fats to 35% of total calories.

Increase intake of high fibre foods; include fruits, vegetables, and whole grain cereals. Eat fruits that are high in vitamin C, vegetables (such as broccoli, cabbage, cauliflower), and vegetables that contain carotene (dark green and dark yellow-orange), e.g. carrots, peppers.

Avoid high doses of dietary supplements.

Minimize consumption of cured, pickled, and smoked foods, and alcohol.

---

of their knowledge about the disease and their opportunity for contact with the public in the inpatient and outpatient setting, nurses have the opportunity to teach about cancer and to help motivate patients to seek treatment.

Self-care practices for primary prevention of cancer include (1) limiting sun exposure, (2) maintaining a healthy weight, (3) limiting alcohol consumption, (4) avoiding cigarettes and cigarette smoke, and (5) good hygiene. The nurse can be involved in primary prevention by educating individuals about the importance of these self-care practices, informing the public about the importance of screening examinations, and promoting the creation of a safe environment in which there is minimal exposure to carcinogens.[35]

Dietary modifications can also prevent the development of cancer. The Department of Health recommends a prudent diet that limits the intake of fats, alcohol, and processed foods. Foods high in fibre are encouraged (Box 9-2).

Secondary Prevention

The approach to early detection of cancer is worldwide. General criteria for cancer screening and testing programmes in the U.K., have been drawn up by the epidemiology section of the Department of Health. Multiphasic screening and a periodic health examination are being accepted by the public. In some cases diagnosis can be made months before the development of symptoms causes the person to seek care.

Cancer detection is expensive. Education of the public often includes convincing them that a periodic health examination is worthwhile. A great deal of cancer screening

e.g. mammography, is provided free of charge by the National Health Service. In addition, there are various private healthcare companies which offer health checks and screening which include a complete physical examination including chest radiograph, Papanicolaou smear, breast examination, urinalysis, and blood count all performed for a moderate fee. Nurses should be aware of clinics in their area where people needing such resources may be referred.

The cancer screening programmes offered by the National Health Service are under constant review. Publication of the Forrest Report (1986), which suggested that women over 50 would benefit from regular screening, led to the setting up of a national mammography programme. Cervical screening call and recall are now fully computerized with payments for family doctors who reach targets for women screened. It is worth noting that most women who die from cancer of the cervix have never had a smear test!. Cancer related checkups should also involve health counselling including information about personal cancer risk factors.[2] Women should request that the cervical smear test (Papanicolaou stain) be done if it was inadvertently overlooked by the health care provider. The cervical smear test still is one of the best means of preventing death from cervical cancer.

Early detection of cancer can decrease mortality. The guidelines for screening have been developed for people *without* symptoms; however, those who have any signs or symptoms suggestive of cancer should report them immediately to a doctor. The nurse must know and be able to explain the significance of the early warning signals (Box 9-3) and safeguards (Box 9-4). Any of these signs should be investigated medically, but their occurrence does not necessarily mean that the person has cancer.

All people should know the most common sites of cancer. In women these are the breast, uterus (cervix), lung, and colorectum (Fig. 9-1). Women should be taught to examine their breasts each month immediately after the menstrual period or, for postmenopausal women, on a designated day each month. Such self-examination and, more importantly, being "breast aware" are vital in detecting early breast cancer. Women of all ages should know the importance of reporting abnormal vaginal bleeding or other discharge between menstrual periods or after menopause. (Further information about cancer of specific organs can be found in appropriate chapters of this text.)

Table 9-4 Guidelines for cancer-related checkups

Test or examination	Sex	Age (yr)	Recommendation
Cervical smear (Papanicolaou test)	Female	Over 20; under 20 if sexually active. Repeated until age 64	Currently, at least every 5 years (20 to 64). Many doctors repeat every 3 years or more often
Pelvic examination	Female	Over 20	With cervical smear
* Endometrial tissue sample	Female	At menopause if high risk	High risk: history of infertility, obesity, failure of ovulation, abnormal uterine bleeding, prolonged oestrogen therapy
Breast self-examination	Female	Adult	Be breast aware
Breast physical examination	Female	Adult	Every 3 years
		Over 40	Yearly
Testicular self-examination	Male	At least up to 45 years	On a regular basis, e.g. monthly
Mammogram	Female	50-64	Every 3 years †
* Stool guaiac slide test	Male and Female	Over 50	Yearly
Digital rectal examination	Male and Female	Over 40	Yearly
* Sigmoidoscopic examination	Male and Female	Over 50	Every 3–5 years after two initial negative examinations 1 year apart

* Not standard screening in the U.K.
† Available to women over 64 and to those with a suspicious breast lump

---

9-3

Cancer early warning signals

Change in bowel or bladder habits
A sore that does not heal
Unusual bleeding or discharge
Thickening or lump in breast or elsewhere
Indigestion or difficulty in swallowing
Obvious change in wart or mole
Nagging cough or hoarseness

9-4

Cancer safeguards

Lung: Don't smoke cigarettes.
Colorectum: Have a proctoscopic exam as part of a regular checkup after age 40.
Breast: Practise breast awareness and self-examination.
Cervix: Have a smear test as part of a regular checkup.
Skin: Avoid overexposure to the sun.
Oral: Have a regular mouth examination by dentist.
Testes: Perform regular self-examination.
Complete body: Have an overall physical checkup annually or at 3-year intervals, depending on age.

Testicular cancer accounts for only 1% of all male cancer, but it is the commonest carcinoma in the 15- to 35-year-old age group.[5] Men, especially those in this young population, should be taught testicular self-examination (see Chapter 27). Testicular cancer, if diagnosed early, has an excellent chance for cure if treated with surgery and/or radiation therapy.

Two common misconceptions that lead people to ignore symptoms should be corrected. The first is a belief that a disease as serious as cancer must be accompanied by weight loss. Weight loss is usually a late symptom of cancer, yet a person often remarks, "I wasn't losing weight so I thought nothing serious could be wrong." Another reason for neglect of cancer is that it may not cause pain, and again the person believes the absence of pain means that the indisposition is minor. It must be repeatedly emphasised to the public that pain is not an early sign of cancer and that cancer often is far advanced before pain occurs.

Nurses also have a role in prevention and early detection of genetic cancer. They systematically obtain family cancer histories, teach about health maintenance, and do genetic counselling.[35] They may be involved in centralized familial cancer registries analogous to the monitoring of communicable diseases by health departments. Familial cancer registries would be helpful in pooling data on suspected cancer-prone families, as well as in disseminating current methods of surveillance and management of the conditions.

In addition to being knowledgeable about measures for prevention and early detection of cancer, nurses must be aware of current therapeutic modalities and their rationales. Because of lack of information, misinformation, or fear of the effects of treatment, people may put off seeking help. Clearly presented information about therapy will help to allay anxiety and confusion.

Organizations that can help meet the needs of cancer patients are listed in Box 9-5 on p. 141. Those such as the Ileostomy Association and the Breast Care and Mastectomy Association help individuals cope with body image changes and the return to a healthy state of physical functioning following cancer surgery. Cancer Link, which helps with all aspects of cancer, also provides valuable assistance for the various locally based self-help groups. Even though patients are cured of cancer, they may still have many psychosocial and physical problems.

Organizations Involved in Cancer Research, Education, Detection, and Rehabilitation

Since its inception, the National Health Service has been concerned with all aspects of cancer care. Most people obtain cancer screening, treatment and rehabilitation through National Health Service establish-men—although some private facilities do exist.

The Health Education Authority and many voluntary organizations are vital in educating the public about cancer and producing a vast amount of educational material for the use of nurses and other professional health care workers.

Actual research into causes and treatments for cancer is funded both by government and by cancer charities, the latter relying heavily upon public donations for their funding. A great deal of this research is funded by charities such as the Cancer Research Campaign, and the Imperial Cancer Research Fund which carries out research at its own facilities and funds projects in universities and medical schools.

Various charities, e.g. Marie Curie Cancer Care, Cancer Relief Macmillan Fund, and British Red Cross, help people with advanced cancer by providing funds, equipment, practical assistance, and specialist nursing.

Nurses can be articulate speakers for the cause of cancer care and cure because they are intimately aware of the effects of cancer in threat to life and financial cost, disrupted lives, and human suffering. Nurses must assertively express to their representatives in government the importance of a combined effort to eradicate cancer.

Nursing Process
Assessment
Subjective data

The doctor obtains a careful medical history inquiring into family history to determine those with a familial tendency for cancer, social history, marital and sex history, habits, occupation, and past medical history, since all may provide valuable clues to the presence of cancer.

It is especially important that the nurse obtain baseline data in relation to the cancer patient's health and health habits, since the treatment of cancer often involves complex changes in the patient's ability to meet psychological, physiological, and sociological health care. By careful collection of data the nurse can plan and carry out the complex nursing care that may be needed by the patient with cancer.

Knowledge of diagnosis

Some initial data are needed to plan care. The first important question to be answered is *whether the patient knows the diagnosis*. This information should be recorded on the nursing care plan and discussed with other health team members. This will ensure that the patient does not receive different answers to the same questions from the health care providers. Some hospitals have partially over-

come this problem by having regular meetings of all the members of the professional staff at which the information given to each patient is reviewed. If meetings of this type are not being held, nurses should take the initiative in planning such a meeting.

The nurse should also elicit from both the patient and the doctor *what the patient has been told*. Because of anxiety and the need for denial to protect the ego, the patient may have heard only part of the information given by the doctor or have misinterpreted the information. The nurse can identify any discrepancies to plan care on the basis of the patient's perceptions of the illness.

Members of the medical profession differ in their opinions regarding whether the patient with cancer should be told the diagnosis. The decision may be made by the doctor after consultation with the patient's family. The present trend is towards telling patients if they have cancer. When patients are not informed, the reasons seem to be related much more to the doctor's own attitudes and emotional reactions than to concern about the patient's reactions. The nurse may help by discussing with the doctor the reactions of the patient and the feelings expressed. It is the nurse's responsibility and sometimes a challenge to work effectively for the ultimate benefit of the patient within the seeming limitation it may impose.

Many spiritual advisors recommend telling the truth. Some people, however, may not want to know the diagnosis and may ask and then answer their own questions negatively. Some do not ask for the diagnosis because they do not wish to have confirmed what they already suspect. Some insist on knowing the diagnosis and are preoccupied with every detail of their progress and treatment in a detached but completely abnormal fashion. Finally, there are some who wish to know the facts and who can accept them in a realistic way when given an opportunity to discuss their feelings with others. Some doctors prepare the patient over a period of time and tell the complete truth when they feel the patient is ready to accept it.

It is also important to determine *how long the patient has known the diagnosis*. The patient who has just been told may be going through the initial grief reactions. The person who has known for many years may have made a realistic adaptation and may see cancer as a chronic disease and not as a death sentence. The nurse should ascertain from the doctor whether the cancer has already metastasized and, if so, whether the patient is aware of this fact. Responses of the patient with metastatic cancer will be different from those of the patient who can be more hopeful of a cure.

Coping skills

Coping skills should be identified, because the diagnosis of cancer is an enormous test of the person's inner resources, as well as those of friends and family. Some people cope by directly verbalizing fears and seeking support from others, whereas others are less direct. Some deal with problems with a problem-solving approach; others try to avoid dealing with the problem.

The patient's and family's interpersonal, physical, and financial resources must be determined. What kind of support can be expected from the family? The financial burden, e.g. through loss of income, the patient anticipates because of the therapy may affect the reaction to the disease.

9-5

Selection of organizations offering services to the cancer patient and the family

Organization	General description
Breast Care and Mastectomy Association 15–19 Britten St. London SW3 3TZ Tel. 0171 867 1103 (helpline)	Support and advice about breast cancer and surgery. Produces useful literature.
British Association of Cancer United Patients and their Families (BACUP) 121–123 Charterhouse St. London EC1M 6AA Tel. 0171 608 1661, Freeline 0800-181199 (outside London)	Advice, information and support by letter or phone for patients, family and friends. Many free publications.
British Red Cross 9 Grosvenor Cres. London SW1X 7EJ Tel. 0171 235 5454	Provides care and equipment for people in need.
Cancer Link 17 Britannia St. London WC1X 9JN Tel. 0171 833 2451	Support and information by letter or phone for patients, family, friends and health care workers. Acts as resource for nationwide network of self-help and cancer support groups.
Cancer Relief Macmillan Fund Anchor House, 15–19 Britten St. London SW3 3TZ Tel. 0171 351 7811	Provides specialist nurses for home care and hospital support posts, e.g. breast care. Also offers in-patient and day care in Macmillan Cancer Care Units. Grants in cases of need. Pain relief education for doctors and nurses.
Tenovus Cancer Information Centre 142 Whitechurch Rd. Cardiff CF4 3NA Tel. 01222 619846	Promotes wider understanding of cancer, including prevention and early detection. Provides speakers, information, counselling. Mobile screening unit in Wales.
The Leukaemia Resurch Fund 43 Great Ormond St. London WC1N 3JJ Tel. 0171 405 0101	Provides information about leukaemia and other diseases. Funds research and educates health care workers.
Women's National Cancer Control Campaign (WNCCC) 1 South Audley St. London W1Y 5DQ Tel. 0171 499 7532	Promotes prevention and early detection of cancers affecting women. Provides information, literature, speakers, and mobile screening units.

Psychological response to cancer

Once the diagnosis of cancer has been made, the patient and family may be overwhelmed and immobilized. As one patient stated, "I cried all day Saturday, Sunday, and Monday. My daughter and my husband wanted to help but they didn't know what to do or say. I know my daughter was scared that she'd get cancer, too." Not all patients can openly express their feelings. Consequently, the nurse may have difficulty gathering data in order to assess and plan intervention. Some individuals are stoic, feeling it is a sign of weakness to display their psychological devastation in public. The nurse must be alert for subtle cues that may indicate that intervention is needed.

Grief. The general psychological responses to a diagnosis of cancer are those accompanying the grieving process (see Chapter 11). The patient and family may go through a period of denial, during which there may be a delay in beginning therapy. Anxiety, depression, regressive behaviour, and anger may all be manifested (see Chapter 5).

To many the diagnosis of cancer signifies the end of life itself, the ultimate loss. Nurses must be careful that they do not communicate any negative reactions to cancer. Newly qualified practitioners must look at their own attitudes towards the disease.

Guilt. Guilt is also a frequent psychological response. Cancer patients may feel that the disease is punishment for actions in their life. They may also feel guilty if they have delayed seeking treatment.

Sense of isolation. Perhaps one of the most prevalent reactions described by patients with cancer is a sense of isolation, of being cut off from those people and things that are important to them. Patients with cancer may report that there is a gradual break in relationships. In some cases the isolation is patient-initiated, in others it may result from actions of significant others because of their negative attitude towards the disease. Perhaps the most profound isolation is psychological isolation, an inability to relate to and derive comfort from others, the feeling of being alone in a crowd.

Sexual disequilibrium. Nurses must be comfortable with their own sexuality and sensitive to the patient's responses, which may indicate that sexual tension is present.

Cancer is particularly destructive to the sexual relationship. It may so occupy the patient's life that all energy is directed to the illness. Sexual roles change. There may be fear that sexual activity may cause the cancer to spread or that the well partner may "catch" it. Treatment modalities that affect the genital organs may cause sexual dysfunction, and the psychological responses of anxiety, anger, depression, and body image changes may disrupt the sexual relationship[17] (see Chapter 26).

Fantasies of death and dying. Some patients report that they are overwhelmed with fantasies of death and dying. Most patients are more concerned about the process of dying, fearing pain, mutilation, and deterioration in both their physiological and psychological status, than with death itself. They may be open about their fantasizing, but are more apt to communicate this in less obvious ways. Patients may focus their attention and discussion on the suffering and pain of others. They may express concern about the future of their families and may speculate on what will happen to their loved ones. The nurse must be alert to these signs that patients need to talk about their view of their future.

Objective data
Local effects

Benign tumours cause serious problems if they obstruct the lumen of tubular structures such as the ureter, trachea, or intestinal tract. Intraspinal and intracranial tumours cause problems because of the pressure they exert in a closed space. Tumours may also degenerate or by the pressure they exert cause atrophy and ulceration of overlying epithelium.

Malignant tumours may produce the same problems as benign tumours. In addition, because of their size and ability to infiltrate and destroy surrounding tissue, there is a danger of obstruction, haemorrhage, ulceration, and secondary infection.

Systemic effects

The term *paraneoplastic syndrome* is used to describe the systemic effects of cancer. These can be divided into the following categories: (1) haematological, immunological, and vascular abnormalities; (2) hormonal and endocrine effects; (3) neuromyopathies; (4) skin and connective tissue disorders; (5) gastrointestinal disorders; and (6) general and metabolic disorders.[4]

Anaemia, leucopenia, and platelet deficiency may result from replacement of bone marrow by cancer cells. Patients with cancer of the gastrointestinal tract often develop anaemia secondary to chronic blood loss and malabsorption. Tumours of the endocrine glands usually cause an increase in secretion from the glands, resulting in various syndromes such as Cushing's syndrome or hyperthyroidism. In addition, some malignant tumours of the lung secrete trophic hormones, which can result in conditions resembling Cushing's syndrome.[8]

When there is a metastatic implant in the peritoneal or pleural cavity, this causes an increased production of serous fluid, and the patient develops either pleural effusion or ascites (peritoneal).

Degenerative changes can occur in the central nervous system of patients with advanced cancer, even in the absence of metastases to the area. The patient may show signs of cerebellar disease and peripheral neuritis.[4] There may be severe muscle weakness or dermatomyositis, and haemorrhage may occur if blood vessels are eroded by the growing tumour.

There is destruction of muscle protein, impaired cellular respiration (often a complication of anaemia), and neuromyopathies followed by failure of important muscle masses, such as intercostal and abdominal muscle. This results in poor pulmonary ventilation, stasis of secretions, and pneumonia. Smooth muscle failure in the urinary bladder wall and the intestinal tract results in urinary tract infection or constipation.

Cachexia is almost universal at some point in the development of malignant disease and is usually a sign of advanced cancer. It is characterized by anorexia, hypermetabolism, excess of energy consumption over nutritional supply, and wasting as a result of negative protein and fat balance in the body. Weight loss may be gradual or rapid.

The following five factors are involved in the aetiology of cachexia[3]:

1. It is possibly caused by inhibition of the hypothalamic appetite centre. Appetite may fail to increase in the face of the increased nutrient needs of the tumour.
2. There is altered gastrointestinal function, malabsorption of nutrients, especially in the small intestine, and exudation of protein and electrolytes.
3. There is increased use of nutrients by some tumours that require more amino acids and vitamins than do normal tissues. There may also be insufficient use of available nutrients.
4. There is increased secretion of nutrients such as urinary excretion of electrolytes and metabolic products.
5. The disease process, and often the chemotherapy or radiation treatment, alter the patient's sense of taste and smell. Food is no longer appetizing.

In addition, other factors that may be implicated include immobilization, drugs, and reactive depression that may accompany metastatic cancer. Along with this may be insomnia and a feeling of hopelessness, which also may contribute to anorexia and cachexia. There is an increased susceptibility to infection. Therapy for the cachectic state is rarely successful unless the underlying cancer is treated.

Pain does not always occur with cancer; when it does occur, it is usually a late sign. Cancer pain is described later in this chapter (p. 148).

The paraneoplastic syndrome often results in devastating effects on the individual host; many of these effects are similar to the side effects of antineoplastic therapy. A common myth held by some general health care consumers is that the treatment for cancer is worse than the disease itself. It is important to remember that cancer, if left untreated, will eventually result in death. All health care professionals have an obligation to inform the public about the importance of early detection and treatment.

Table 9-5 Cancer diagnostic tests

Diagnostic test	Description
Physical examination	External and internal physical assessment to evaluate clinical signs and symptoms related to local or distant effects of cancer growth and development; internal assessment done through pelvic exam and/or rectal examination.
Biopsy	Histological testing (frozen or permanent section) to confirm malignancy and to determine type of cancerous cell and degree of cellular aplasia/differentiation (that is, grading).
Incisional biopsy	Surgical removal of section of neoplasm.
Excisional biopsy	Removal of entire growth if tumour is small.
Aspiration needle biopsy	Removal of small plug of tumour by use of needle and syringe.
Cytology	Collection and slide preparation of exfoliated cells without the tissue framework provided in biopsy; the cervical smear to determine abnormal or cancerous cells is the most familiar example.
Clinical laboratory tests	Include routine blood and urine studies as well as other biochemical and chromosomal analyses (for example, measurement of the enzyme acid phosphatase for cancer of the prostate).
Body imaging X-ray examinations	Provide good visualization of chest and bone (contrast to surrounding tissue); mammography (to detect breast cancer) differs from ordinary chest X-ray examination in that it uses very slow, nonpenetrating radiation and very sensitive film.
Xerography	Uses a specially charged plate of selenium-coated metal, resulting in a detailed picture of soft tissue.
Computed Tomography (CT scan)	Uses an X-ray beam in conjunction with a computer, permitting detailed study of small parts deep in the body without the necessity of invasive procedures.
Magnetic Resonance Imaging (MRI)	Uses a very strong magnet combined with radio frequency waves and a computer to produce X-ray-like images of body chemistry in heart, brain, and other organs; no radiation is present.
Contrast examination	Addition of contrast material for X-ray examination via swallowing of a liquid (for example, barium for gastrointestinal visualization) or injection of a dye into blood or lymph vessels (for example, lymphangiography).
Nuclear scans (radioactive isotopes)	Introduction of radioactive substance into body to detect primary or metastatic cancer; the isotopes concentrate in the tumour (hot spot) or in the normal tissue surrounding the tumour (cold spot) and create an image on a scintillation detector or on photographic film.
Ultrasound (echography)	An electronic instrument detects and records echoes of sound when they are reflected at junction of tissues with different densities; not useful, at present, for lungs or stomach.
Endoscopy	Uses a telescope-like optical instrument to look at the internal organs; X-ray examination or biopsy may be done simultaneously; instruments are named for the organs they visualize: • Bronchoscope: abdomen • Laparoscope: abdomen • Cytoscope: bladder • Gastroscope: stomach • Sigmoidoscope: lower colon • Proctoscope: rectum

Diagnostic studies

The nurse needs to be able to give a simple description of various diagnostic procedures to patients and families. The tests may involve the use of complex equipment as well as the injection or ingestion of various substances. The patient's anxiety may be high, and the nurse's ability to give factual information often will help to decrease this anxiety. Specific procedures before, during, and after diagnostic testing may vary slightly from institution to institution, requiring that the nurse be knowledgeable about the common as well as the possible unique characteristics of a diagnostic test. Table 9-5 lists and describes briefly the most common diagnostic procedures when the patient presents with signs and symptoms suggestive of malignancy.

Nursing intervention during assessment phase

The emotional climate produced during the period of diagnostic examination and initial treatment is very important in determining whether patients will continue diagnostic examination, treatment, or repeated follow-up care after discharge. The care they receive in the hospital may shape their attitudes towards the disease and may determine whether they can return home and either care for themselves or be cared for by the family. An important nursing function in the care of patients with cancer is building up faith in the team involved with their care. The patient needs to feel certain that everything possible is being done and that new measures will be tried if there is any promise whatsoever of their being helpful.

Many patients may undergo extensive diagnostic examinations and surgery in large hospitals a long distance from their homes. Some patients have reported that, although they were confident that they were in "good medical hands," such confidence did not make up for the feelings that they were not always known as individuals. They needed desperately to feel that at least one person knew and understood them. Some patients experience near panic at the thought of their loved ones coming to visit and being unable to locate them. In most instances it is best for the patient to be accompanied by a relative or a close friend. It should also be recognized that even a patient in familiar surroundings may feel very much alone when awaiting diagnostic tests or surgical treatment for known or suspected cancer.

Both patient and family need something to help pass the time during the period of diagnostic tests and treatment and between steps of treatment such as surgery or X-ray therapy. Psychological relief may sometimes come from keeping occupied with usual daily activities. Anxious relatives also receive satisfaction from doing things that the patient would do, if possible, thus preserving parts of cherished routines.

Members of the family often need direction in their activity when they have just learned that a loved one has cancer. They may need to talk over immediate and long-term plans with someone not close to the family situation. The nurse can sometimes be this listening person. At other times the family can best be served by a social worker, who will help them talk through and think through a course of action.

Data analysis and planning

A sound personal philosophy and an objective, positive attitude towards the disease based on knowledge will help the nurse who is caring for the patient with cancer. The nurse should be able to give support and hope to the patient and family or friends.

Following an assessment that includes subjective and objective data, the nurse analyses the information and formulates health care needs influenced by nursing care. Because cancer is a chronic illness that often involves numerous body systems, the list of pertinent health needs can be extensive. It is often a challenge for the nurse to identify all of the pertinent health needs that will require nursing interventions for a specific patient.

The following four principles should be considered by the nurse when planning nursing interventions that are patient centred:
1. People have a right to be part of the treatment team.
2. People have the right to choose the desired degree of privacy or communication.
3. The nurse must respect the coping mechanisms of patients who are trying to maintain themselves through a difficult illness.
4. The nurse must remember not to give the appearance of hurrying, thus blocking communications.

The plan of care that a nurse develops for a patient with cancer needs to be individualized to reflect problems unique to a particular disease, treatment regimen, or the personality and life situation of the patient. The following

section will detail the nursing interventions for the patient experiencing one or more of the four treatment modalities and for the patient with chronic pain and cancer that is terminal.

Implementation

Often several doctors are involved in determining the appropriate treatment for cancer. The medical team decides on the choice of treatment on the basis of the biological characteristic of the tumour, its clinical stage (p. 195), and the condition of the patient. The histological type of the tumour is particularly important in determining the treatment to be used.

Therapy may be curative (removal of all traces of the disease from the body) or palliative (directed towards relieving symptoms only). At the present time there are four major forms of treatment: surgery, radiotherapy, chemotherapy, and immunotherapy. The latter is the newest form of treatment for cancer. Combinations of the four treatment modalities are often employed to achieve the best result for each patient.

Surgery

Surgery, the oldest method of treating cancer, may be either curative or palliative. The best treatment for cancer at present is complete surgical removal of all malignant tissues before metastasis occurs. Surgery must often be extensive and may require adjustments beyond those needed in many other conditions. There may not be time to accustom oneself gradually to the idea of surgery and the effect it can have on one's body and lifestyle. The individual often faces the prospect of mutilating surgery with only the hope that it will cure the cancer and be lifesaving. Concern about what will happen to the family may be upmost in the patient's mind. Obviously, the patient and family need empathy and understanding as they attempt to accept the recommendation for immediate surgery.

The operative procedures used to treat various types of cancer are discussed in the appropriate chapters of this book.

Radiotherapy

Radiotherapy, or the use of radiation in the treatment of disease, has been used in the treatment of cancer for about 90 years. It is estimated that approximately 60% of all cancer patients will receive radiotherapy.[4] The principal radiation agents are: (1) X-ray which consists of electromagnetic radiation produced by waves of electrical energy travelling at a very high speed; (2) radium, which is a radioactive isotope occurring freely in nature; and (3) the artificially induced radioactive isotopes produced by bombarding the isotopes of elements with highly energized particles in a cyclotron. Radiation can be delivered externally (teletherapy) or internally (brachytherapy).

Radiotherapy is effective in curing cancer in some instances; in other instances it controls the growth of cancer cells for a time. Because it may deter the growth of cancer cells, it may relieve pain even when extension of the disease is such that cure is impossible.

Radiation delivered externally (including X-rays) can harm people working with the patient *only during* the time that the patient is being treated. This is true also of the radiation from some radioactive substances used for other methods of treatment. Patients with internal radiation who emit γ-rays, however, may expose others to radiation for varying periods of time, and the time one can be exposed safely to the patient is important in planning care. The time interval required for the radioactive substance to be half dissipated is called its *half-life*. This period varies extremely widely, but as the end of the half-life is reached, danger from exposure decreases.

Exposure to radiation can be controlled three ways: *time*, *distance*, and *shielding*. All emanations are subject to the physical law of inverse-square. For example, a person who stands 2 metres away from the source of radiation receives only one-fourth as much exposure as when standing only 1 metre away. At 4 metres, only one-sixteenth of the exposure will be received. Therefore, increasing the distance from the emanations decreases the exposure. When a patient such as an infant must be held for X-ray treatment, the nurse or person who holds the patient must be careful to keep at arm's length or as far away as possible and to avoid having any body part in the direct path of the rays. *Lead-lined gloves and a lead apron, which act as a shield to reduce exposure, should be worn by anyone who attends patients during X-ray treatment or during examination by fluoroscopy.*

When the nurse knows the kind of substance used, the kind and amount of rays it emits, its half-life, and its exact location in the patient and considers these facts in relation to control of exposure, safe and adequate care for the patient can be planned.

Nurses wishing to know about radioactive substances can obtain information from the International Commission on Radiological Protection, the Health and Safety Executive and the current codes of practice produced by the Department of Health. In cities with a large hospital providing radiotherapy, a radiation physicist or the Radiation Safety Committee may be consulted.

Teletherapy

Preparation of patient. Teaching the patient and family is an important aspect of care. Orientation programmes, information booklets, and weekly group sessions for patients and families are useful methods of communicating information.

Patients who are to receive radiation therapy should know that they will be attended by radiotherapists who will be stationed outside the treatment room and who will observe the treatment and be in communication at all times. The patient must often lie absolutely still for a period of time, a very tiring experience. There is no pain associated with radiation therapy.

Early reaction. When radiation therapy is used, some degree of radiation reaction may occur. Early reactions include blanching or erythema of the skin and mucous membranes, possibly progressing to dry or moist desquamation. If the mucosa of the mouth, pharynx, bladder, or rectum is affected, there may be pain, inhibition of the normal secretions, and impairment of functions.[32]

When treatment is directed towards abdominal organs or any deep tissues there is almost always some skin reaction. There may be itching, tingling, burning, oozing, or sloughing of the skin. The term *burn* should never be used in referring to this reaction, since it implies incorrect dosage. Reddening may occur on or about the tenth day, and the skin may turn a dark plum colour after about 3 weeks. The skin may also become dry and inelastic and may crack easily.

Gastrointestinal reactions to radiation therapy are more common when treatment includes some part of the gastrointestinal tract or when the ports lie over this system. The patient may suffer nausea, vomiting, anorexia, malaise, and/or diarrhoea. Gastric emptying is slowed during the treatment phase, but usually returns to normal levels. Gastric reactions are extremely common, and almost all patients who receive moderate or large doses of radiation have these symptoms in varying degrees.

Radiation therapy also causes depression of the haematopoietic system and in turn a low white blood cell count, predisposing the patient to infection. Sloughing of tissue and subsequent haemorrhages are complications that must be considered when radiation is used in any form. Ambulatory patients are told that they should call the doctor at once should any sloughing of tissue occur.

Late reaction. Effects of radiation may be apparent months or years after therapy. Genital tissue, muscles, and kidneys may be affected, resulting in painful radionecrosis. Radiation causes destruction of fine vasculature, and the skin may show signs of atrophy (thinning and blanching), pigmentation, and telangiectasis. If there is severe vascular damage or if there are other complications that require further surgery, the irradiated tissues may fail to heal.[32]

Nursing care of patients receiving external radiation. Nursing care is directed towards preventing skin breakdown, decreasing gastrointestinal upset, and preventing infection (Box 9-6). The area to be treated is usually outlined by the radiologist at the time of the first treatment. Occasionally, a small tattoo mark is used instead of the conspicuous skin markings when treatment is given to exposed parts of the body. Marks must not be washed off until the treatment is completed because they are important guides to the radiologist. Medicated substances that may contain heavy metals such as zinc are not permitted on the skin until the series of treatments is completed, because such substances may increase the radiation dosage.

If the radiation dosage has been high and blanching or discoloration of the skin has resulted, the patient may be advised to avoid exposure to temperature changes for several years. The patient may have to take much cooler baths or showers than formerly and may have to avoid sunbathing or any other extreme of temperature. Corn starch can be applied to dry, irritated skin.[32] If X-ray treatments have been given to a woman's face, she must be cautioned regarding the use of cosmetics to cover discoloured skin. They may contain heavy, irritating oils and should not be used until consultation with the doctor.

When treatment must be given to any part of the head, patients may ask about the possibility of loss of hair. Whether hair will return after falling out depends on the amount of radiation received. Attractive scarves and wigs are useful for patients with alopecia or when returning hair is too thin.

Brachytherapy

Internal radiation may be delivered by sealed or unsealed methods. In either type special precautions may be necessary, depending on the amount of radioactive material used, its location, and the kind of rays being emitted. Special precautions may be taken if more than a tracer diagnostic dose has been given. Most hospitals have printed instruction sheets stating the precautions to be followed for each substance used. Personnel should be fully acquainted with all precautions and should be supervised in carrying them out. Generally, the patient will be placed in a single room or in a double room with another patient who is also receiving radiation therapy. A radiation precaution sign should be placed on the door to the patient's room, and visitors should be restricted.

Nursing care of patients receiving internal radiotherapy. Nursing interventions consist of the following:
1. Teach routine and reasons for precautions
2. Decrease isolation by providing radio or television for outside contact and encouraging permissible interaction with nursing staff
3. Plan trips into room to include several tasks
4. Promote comfort: complete bath before treatment, clean bed linens, turn sheet, position pillow

The patient should know that isolation is temporary, that the restrictions will be removed on a certain day, and that members of the nursing staff will be available but that they will work quickly and will remain in the room only long enough to carry out essential activities. The patient can assist in notifying family and friends about the restriction on visitors and how long it will last. The patient should also know how the radioactive substance is eliminated to lessen worry about being a danger to others, particularly after therapy is concluded.

Trips made in haste into the patient's room are disturbing psychologically, because they imply that the patient is not acceptable to others. The nurse who plans thoughtfully might deliver a letter, fresh water, and the newspaper and make pertinent observations in less time than one who plans less well and must make several trips to the patients room.

Chemotherapy

Advances in knowledge of cancer growth and chemotherapeutic agents have led to concomitant advances in cancer treatment. Improvement in overall survival and longer disease-free intervals can be directly ascribed to the use of chemotherapeutic agents, particularly in combination chemotherapy regimens and as adjuvant therapy.

Guidelines for Care | **9-6**

Patients receiving external radiation

1. *Preventing skin breakdown*
   Skin preparation: cleansing.
   Care must be taken *not* to remove skin markings used to guide radiologist.
   Vegetable fat/or oil may be ordered to protect the affected skin.
   Medicated solutions, ointments, or powders that may contain heavy metals such as zinc are *not* permitted on the skin.
   Consult radiologist about skin care for local radiation reactions; do *not* remove crusts.
   Keep dressings loose; use nonirritating tape and avoid pulling on affected skin.
   Teach patient to avoid constricting clothing or friction of any kind on exposed skin.
   Teach patient to avoid excesses of heat and cold to affected skin surfaces.
   Teach patient not to expose treatment area to the sun (sunburn).
2. *Decreasing gastrointestinal upset*
   Advise resting before and after meals to control nausea and vomiting.
   Breakfast is usually the best tolerated meal of the day.
   Suggest small frequent meals during the day.
   Sour beverages and effervescent liquids may relieve nausea.
   Suggest high-protein, high-carbohydrate, fat-free, low-residue diet to prevent nausea and vomiting; low-fibre diet for diarrhoea.
   Administer palliative medications, as ordered.
3. *Preventing infection*
   Advise patient to avoid people with upper respiratory infections.
   Use protective isolation if white blood count is low.
   Administer antibiotic drugs, as ordered.

Benefits of chemotherapy

Chemotherapy is potentially curative in gestational choriocarcinoma, acute lymphocytic leukaemia (ALL), Ewing's sarcoma, advanced Hodgkin's disease, diffuse histiocytic lymphoma, Burkitt's lymphoma, testicular cancer, and ovarian cancer. Prolonged disease-free or controlled intervals may be achieved by chemotherapy in the treatment of several non-Hodgkin's lymphomas, multiple myeloma, breast cancer, and oat cell carcinoma of the lung. In other advanced malignancies, such as colorectal carcinoma, chemotherapy rarely produces a complete response and only a few such patients experience an increased survival time. In the treatment of chronic myelogenous leukaemia (CML) and chronic lymphocytic leukaemia (CLL), although the duration of life may not be prolonged, the quality of life may be enhanced by chemotherapy because of control of symptoms. Patients and families may be told that incurable does not mean untreatable or uncontrollable.

In the care of an individual patient with cancer, the expected benefit of chemotherapy (cure, control, or palliation) should be known by the doctor, nurse, and patient. This allows for realistic goal setting by the caregivers, patients, and family. Such background also provides a perspective from which to view side effects. The potential for cure, prolonged disease-free survival, or reduction of symptoms is a benefit that most often outweighs the risk and discomfort of short-term toxicity and side effects. Conditions in which risk may outweigh benefits include overt or occult infections, bleeding dyscrasias, bone marrow depression, severe metabolic disturbances, renal or liver dysfunction, and pregnancy.

Adjuvant chemotherapy refers to chemotherapy administered after surgical removal of all known cancer present in the body. It is aimed at the destruction of micrometastases thought likely to be present but too small to be detected by current diagnostic techniques. Left untreated, the micrometastases have a high potential for tumour growth and cancer recurrence. With the use of chemotherapy at a time when the malignant cell population is small and likely to be susceptible, complete tumour cell eradication is possible. The goal is cure. (Table 9.6 indicates agents used in cancer chemotherapy.)

Adjuvant chemotherapy is now generally considered to be indicated after mastectomy in all women with involved axillary lymph nodes at the time of surgery and it has demonstrated a significant decrease in recurrence rates and prolonged disease-free intervals. Adjuvant chemotherapy also appears to be beneficial in osteogenic sarcoma and Wilms' tumour. Evidence is currently equivocal regarding its benefit in other malignancies, such as colon cancer and malignant melanoma. The precise role of adjuvant chemotherapy will be more clearly delineated during the next decade, but it is already established as one of the major developments in health care.

A feeling of wellbeing and knowledge that all diagnostic tests are negative for cancer understandably may cause the patient to question the need for adjuvant therapy. This is emphasized when side effects are experienced. A sensitivity to these feelings, coupled with the knowledge of the expected benefit of therapy, is the basis for both patient teaching and the supportive encouragement often needed for continued therapy.

Despite an intellectual understanding of the benefits of chemotherapy, it is sometimes difficult for a nurse to maintain an appropriately optimistic and realistic outlook if all one sees are those patients who did not respond to or are no longer responsive to therapy, manifest severe toxicity, or are dying. The practitioner must take into account the setting in which patients are seen. Hospital-based nurses tend to see patients at the time of diagnosis, when they are critically ill, or during the final days of life. The community nurse may see the patient at comparable points of illness while providing nursing care in the home. Discussion between the nurse and primary doctor, contact with the outpatient clinic, and readmission to the same nursing unit are useful ways of acquiring a more complete picture of an individual's response to treatment. Such positive experiences are a means of nurturing one's own faith in therapy so that a realistic and at times very optimistic approach to caring for, supporting, and teaching the chemotherapy patient exists.

Combination chemotherapy

Increased knowledge of how specific cytotoxic drugs exert their effect and of the potential for the emergence of tumour cells resistant to a specific therapy, similar to antibiotic resistance, has led to the use of combination chemotherapy. Combination chemotherapy demonstrates a therapeutic effect superior to single-agent therapy for many cancers. Drugs considered for combination chemotherapy are those that (1) are active when used alone, (2) have different mechanisms of action, (3) have a biochemical basis for possible synergism, (4) do not produce toxicity in the same organs, and (5) produce toxicity at different times after administration.[27] Repeated brief courses of drug therapy are given to reduce immunosuppressive effects.

Side effects and nursing intervention

Some degree of injury to normal cells often occurs with treatment by chemotherapeutic agents. The basis for normal cells being affected is their rate of proliferation. Many normal tissues have a high proliferation capacity, in some instances exceeding that of malignant disease. It is these rapidly proliferating tissues (the bone marrow, gastrointestinal epithelium, and hair follicles) that bear the brunt of the toxic effects of many of the cytotoxic drugs. Nursing care of patients receiving chemotherapy is summarized in Box 9-7.

Biological response modifier therapy (immunotherapy)

The role of biological response modifier (BRM) therapy in the prevention and treatment of cancer is being studied. The term BRM actually applies to the broad category of biological agents that have the potential to control the growth and metastasis of neoplasms. Immunotherapy is a subcategory of BRM therapies.[33]

Many scientists believe cancer occurs in the body more frequently than once in a lifetime; however, in most cases clinical evidence of the disease is not apparent. It is postulated that there is a natural immunity against the development of the disease and that cancer cells are destroyed almost as quickly as they develop.[16] Studies of cancer show that when the normal cell becomes malignant, it often undergoes biochemical changes resulting in formation of new cellular antigens that cause an immune response. Clinical malignancy may occur as a result of failure in the immunological surveillance system of the body.

At the present time, the immune response can handle only a limited number of tumour cells, up to 10 million. After a growth to 100 million cells, the immune response is not capable of preventing further growth. Once the cancer is large, it cannot be totally controlled by the immune system, so immunotherapy cannot be the primary mode of cancer therapy at the present time. It is used after surgery, radiotherapy, and chemotherapy have removed the bulk of the tumour.

Much is yet to be learned about the immunology of cancers. The number of cancers once thought to be immunogenical and responsive to immunotherapy is less than originally supposed. If cancer vaccines are developed, they will be effective in tumours caused by viruses, and these are probably limited in number. Even if a cancer-

Table 9-6 Agents used in cancer chemotherapy

Agent	Mechanism of action[27]	Major toxic manifestation
Alkylating Busulphan Carboplatin Carmustine Chlorambucil Cisplatin Cyclophosphamide Estramustine Ifosfamide Lomustine Melphalan Mustine Thiotepa Treosulphan	Interfere with DNA replication by attacking DNA synthesis throughout cell cycle (cell cycle nonspecific)	Bone marrow depression with thrombocytopenia and bleeding; pulmonary fibrosis; renal failure may occur
Antimetabolites Cytarabine Fluorouracil Mercaptopurine Methotrexate Thioguanine	Interfere with synthesis of essential metabolites (cell cycle specific)	Bone marrow depression; oral and gastrointestinal ulceration
Antibiotics Aclarubicin Bleomycin Dactinomycin Doxorubicin Epirubicin Idarubicin Mitomycin Mitozantrone Plicamycin	Interfere with DNA or RNA synthesis, varying with the drug (cell cycle nonspecific)	Bone marrow depression (except for bleomycin); pulmonary fibrosis with bleomycin or mitomycin; renal failure with mitomycin; cardiac toxicity with doxorubicin
Plant alkaloids Vinblastine (Velban) Vincristine (Oncovin) Vindesine	Interfere with mitosis	Bone marrow depression; areflexia Neurotroxicity with ataxia and impaired fine motor skills, paralytic ileus
Steroid hormones Adrenocorticosteroids (Prednisolone) Androgens (testosterone proprionate) Antioestrogens (tamoxifen) Oestrogens (ethinyloestradiol) Progestogens (medroxyprogesterone)	Alter the host environment for cell growth (cell cycle nonspecific)	Specific for the actions of the hormone

carrying virus is isolated, it must be attenuated so it can be given safely.

Management of cancer pain

Pain is one of the most feared effects of cancer although, contrary to popular belief, it is frequently the last symptom to appear. Even in terminal stages, 60% of people with cancer will experience mild or no pain. The aetiology of cancer pain is complex because it has physical, psychological, social, cultural and spiritual aspects.

Stages of cancer pain

Three stages of cancer pain have been described: early, intermediate, and late. Early pain usually occurs after initial surgery for diagnosis or treatment and usually subsides after the third day; thus, this pain is an acute episode: that is, it is short term and temporary.

Intermediate-stage pain results from postoperative contraction of scars and nerve entrapment or from cancer recurrence or metastasis. This pain may subside or may be controlled by palliative therapy such as radiation, chemo-

9-7

Guidelines for Care

Patients receiving chemotherapy

Bone marrow suppression or infection

*Check blood counts

Assess infection-prone areas daily to identify early signs of infection

Maintain medical asepsis through careful hand-washing

Maintain intact skin and mucous membranes

Teach avoidance of injury and breaking skin

Maintain aseptic technique during IV infusion and dressing changes

Keep fingernails short

Teach good perineal hygiene

Teach avoidance of excessive friction and importance of vaginal lubrication

Teach avoidance of anal intercourse

No enemas, rectal medications, or rectal thermometers

Encourage fastidious oral hygiene with a soft toothbrush

Inspect mouth daily for ulcers and white patches

Use lubricants to prevent drying and cracking of lips

Maintain optimal respiratory function

Assess for early signs of respiratory infection

Ask family/friends not to visit if they have colds

Maintain reverse isolation if ordered

Gastrointestinal effects: stomatitis, nausea, vomiting

Administer oral nystatin, as ordered

Use a mouthwash and lignocaine before meals to lubricate and provide an analgesic effect

Use a cleansing mouthwash of plain water or normal saline after meals

Administer antiemetic as ordered

Determine from patient best time for food and fluid intake in relation to treatment

Teach relaxation techniques and imagery, if appropriate

Alopecia

Explain that drug-induced alopecia is not permanent

Allow expression of feelings about hair loss

Scalp tourniquets or scalp hypothermia via ice pack may be ordered for patients with solid tumours to minimize hair loss with some agents (for example, vincristine)

Encourage use of wigs, hats, and scarves

Effects on skin

Inspect administration site for signs of infiltration or extravasation

Organ toxicities

Assess signs and symptoms of liver dysfunction (see Chapter 26)

Monitor cardiac status (dysrhythmias, congestive heart failure) (see Chapter 21)

Assess signs and symptoms of pulmonary toxicity (see Chapter 20)

Urinary effects: haemorrhagic cystitis, renal toxicity

Maintain hydration by encouraging drinking of large amounts of fluid (if receiving cyclophosphamide)

Monitor renal function*: check serum creatinine or creatinine clearance* (with cisplatin), urea and electrolytes, and fluid balance

Sterility

Assess knowledge of known possible effects on fertility

Provide birth control and reproductive counselling, as appropriate

* Nurses may order some routine tests in specialist units

---

therapy, neurosurgery, and analgesics. Therapy itself may initiate the pain.

Late-stage pain occurs in terminal cancer when therapy no longer controls the disease. This pain is chronic, may slowly increase in intensity, and at times may be intractable. Severe chronic pain occurs in only about 25% of patients who die from cancer.[11]

Pathophysiology

Malignant neoplasms cause pain by five physiological changes: bone destruction, obstruction of lumens (viscera or vessels), peripheral nerve involvement, pressure of growing tumours causing ischaemia or distention, and inflammation, infection, or necrosis of the tissue.

Bone destruction with infraction (fractures without displacement) is the most frequent cause of pain, usually resulting from metastatic lesions. Bone destruction may cause increased sensitivity over the area or sharp, continuous pain.

Obstruction of a viscus, such as in the gastrointestinal or genitourinary tract, causes severe, colicky, crampy-type pain. Visceral pain is dull, diffuse, and poorly localized. Obstruction of an artery, vein, or lymphatic vessel may initiate arterial ischaemia, venous engorgement, or oedema. This pain is dull, diffuse, and aching.

Infiltration or compression of peripheral nerves or nerve plexuses causes continuous, sharp, or stabbing pain sometimes accompanied by hyperaesthesia or paraesthesia.

Infiltration or distention of the integument, fascia, or tissue initiates a severe localized pain that is dull and aching, increasing in intensity as tumour size increases. An example of this is the pain resulting from distention of the abdomen by ascites or the stretching of the skin by carcinoma of the neck.

Finally, inflammation, infection, and necrosis of the tissue itself may cause pain by producing either pressure or ischaemia. Chemical mediators of pain are present during inflammation and necrosis.

Psychosocial aspects

The psychological component of cancer pain is associated with the patient's perception of the threat and stress of cancer and varies from individual to individual. Three categories of stressors have been identified: injury or threat of injury as a result of the cancer, loss or threat of loss (body part or death), and frustration of drives as a result of disabilities from the cancer *per se* or from the effect of therapies. Patients may respond with depression, decreased self-esteem, hostility, and irritability.

The sociological effects include decreased interaction and participation in activities of daily living. There is decreased productivity characterized by absenteeism from work, economic problems, and deterioration in family relationships. The spiritual effects of pain are evidenced by loss of hope and trust and an overwhelming feeling of despair, rejection, and sense of isolation.

Side effects of cancer pain include fatigue, sleeplessness, anorexia, and decreased movement followed by the complications of immobility, namely, muscle weakness, decubiti, contractures, and respiratory dysfunction.[31]

Intervention

Medical therapy in early-stage pain focuses on therapy directed at the cancer *per se*. Late-stage pain is treated symptomatically by analgesia, neurosurgery, and nerve blocks.

Cancer pain, like other types of severe pain, may occupy the patient's entire attention and, unless treated vigorously, may demoralize the patient and interfere with eating, resting, or sleeping. Interventions are directed towards helping the patient live as normal a life as possible and cope with the pain. Pain tolerance is increased when the patient's energy is preserved for enjoyable activities. General comfort measures to promote rest and sleep, good body positioning, and nutrition may do much to increase the patient's pain tolerance. Teaching patients conscious muscle relaxation during which they systematically contract and relax muscle groups throughout the body may decrease pain resulting from muscle tenseness as well as anxiety associated with the pain (see Chapter 8).

Diversionary activities help decrease the patient's perception of the pain by distraction. These activities may be physical (work, walking, rocking, swimming), social, or mental (watching television, reading, crafts). Some patients find imagery (waking-imagined analgesia) helpful. Others may try to separate the pain from their bodies thereby "quieting the mind by letting the body drop away".[31]

Medications. Drugs may be the one significant method that alleviates the pain of cancer. Aspirin is the most effective single analgesic for mild to moderate pain.[11] There is an additive and perhaps synergistic effect between aspirin and codeine; therefore, combinations of these drugs are useful in moderate acute pain and in chronic aching pain.

In severe chronic cancer pain the narcotics, with the exception of codeine, are the most effective. Although there are no significant differences among the various drugs in potency or side effects, there are significant differences in the duration of action. Those with long duration of action

Nursing Research   9-8

Ferrell B *et al.*: Effects of controlled-release morphine on quality of life for cancer pain, *Oncol Nurs Forum* 16(4):521-526, 1989.

As the title indicates, the purpose of this study was to determine the effects of controlled-release morphine on the overall quality of life for patients with cancer. Data was collected from 83 subjects in a repeated-measure design every 2 weeks for 6 weeks, using five instruments to assess quality of life, pain, and functional status. Findings indicated improved pain management with improved quality of life as measured in the study. The study concludes that nurses can greatly enhance quality of life for the patient with cancer by providing appropriate pain therapies.

are preferred for relief of chronic cancer pain.[10] Tolerance and dependence related to these drugs is not an issue. Repeated studies show that, in general, patients with chronic physiological pain do not become addicted to narcotic analgesics.[11]

There are three important principles in the administration of narcotics. The first is that the optimal dose must be determined, and initial pain control may require seemingly large doses of the narcotics. The second principle is to start with a dose that is too high rather than one that is too low because the patient may become anxious if there is no analgesia despite analgesic administration. This anxiety may exacerbate the pain. The third and most important principle is that the narcotic must be *administered regularly*, not prn. Each dose must be given before the previous dose loses effect. Prevention of pain recurrence usually requires less analgesia than treatment of pain after it has recurred (Box 9-8).

Oral administration is preferred. Parenteral therapy produces higher initial serum and tissue levels of the narcotic, but the oral doses are as effective as parenteral doses in maintaining drug levels in the body. Intramuscular and subcutaneous injections are more difficult to administer and are painful to patients with marked muscle wasting. In addition, parenteral administration may make the patient dependent on others for drug administration.[10]

Phenothiazines are the principal adjunct drug given to control severe chronic cancer pain. They are effective as antiemetics and also have an antianxiety effect.

Nurses provide the psychological and social support necessary to help the cancer patient cope with severe pain. Administration of analgesics over the 24-hour period and explanations of the physiological and pharmacological effects of the drugs can be very helpful to patients and their families (see Chapter 8).

Psychological support of patient and family

Cancer nursing demands not only caring *for* the patient but also caring *about* the patient, who may be angry, depressed, and perhaps physically unattractive because of the effects of the disease or its treatment. Communication is vital in meeting the needs of the cancer patient and the family. Validating assumptions and assisting patients in describing, clarifying, and identifying reasons for feelings are important to promote communications. In addition, the nurse must try to make explanations clear and uncomplicated. Getting feedback from the patient is one way to ensure that the message has been received.

Nursing interventions to help patient cope

Because the threat to life and the potential for other losses are great for patients with cancer, they need especially to have their existing coping mechanisms supported or to receive support if coping mechanisms are inadequate to meet their needs.

Each patient's reaction to cancer is unique, so there can be no easy formula for care. The nurse must be able to work with and accept patients' behaviour and coping style. Avoidance of false reassurance and pat answers that block communication will contribute to patient comfort. Openness, honesty, and creativity of the nurse are essential. The nurse reinforces patients' hope but is careful to avoid giving false hope, which can be more devastating than none at all. At times patients may need to deny their illness, while at other times they may want to talk about it.

Trusting patients' resilience and their will to try and helping them live as fully as possible are all appropriate interventions. When patients complain, perhaps the best response is, "Tell me how you feel. Perhaps we can do something about it." Self-esteem is maintained by fostering patients' independence, even if this involves only taking part in decision making about the care to be given.

Those working with these patients must have confidence in themselves and the ability to suspend their own concerns, needs, and desires to concentrate on patients' problems. To do this one must be able to tolerate a high level of anxiety and to look at problems on both a feeling (affective) and a thinking (cognitive) level.

Listening carefully and attentively to concerns of patients helps to calm fears. In addition, nurses who are knowledgeable about cancer, who can answer questions and clear up misconceptions, help to promote the patient's psychological wellbeing.

Nursing interventions to help family cope

The interventions that help the patient cope are also important in helping the family cope. The nurse must get to know them and their reactions. They may feel guilty, helpless, and angry, just as the patient does. Letting them know that their feelings are normal may increase their comfort. Families should not be pushed into responsibilities that they cannot handle. Some want to participate in care, others are overwhelmed by the disease and are afraid to or may not want to help. Their feelings need to be respected.

Teaching the family is a major responsibility. They should be reminded not to cut the patient off from family activities and concerns. If possible, the patient should be included in family decision making and planning. In their desire to help their loved ones, families may unintentionally contribute to the patient's sense of isolation by shielding him or her from family concerns.[29]

9-9	**Health care needs, which may be influenced by nursing, for the patient with terminal cancer**

Airway clearance, ineffective
Constipation
Family processes, altered
Fatigue
Fear (specify)
Grieving: anticipatory, dysfunctional
Nutrition, altered: less than body requirements
Oral mucous membrane, altered
Pain
Powerlessness
Self-care deficit, bathing/hygiene
Skin integrity, impaired: high risk for
Social isolation

Interdisciplinary approach to care

The skills of many members of the health team may be required to meet the needs of the cancer patient. Clear, concise communication of ideas about care and the planned interventions is essential for coordination, continuity, and integration of care. Team conferences help establish goals and promote the sharing of expertise. The social worker, occupational therapist, minister, and psychologist may all be needed to contribute to the patient's wellbeing. The nurse, who spends the most time with the patient, may be the first person to recognize that the patient and family could benefit from the services of health team members.

Rehabilitation of the cancer patient to an optimal level of functioning through the efforts of many health team members results in a more satisfying life for the patient and the family. Often the community nurse is called on to give care, teach, counsel, and support the patient and family after discharge.

Supportive care of the patient with terminal cancer
Planning care

When all possible therapies have failed to control the spread of cancer, the patient and family have many special problems. They need encouragement and help in living as normally as possible, in planning for the late stages of the patient's illness, and in adjusting to death and its implications for the family.

Before nurses can help the patient and family, they must have developed a mature philosophy that allows acceptance of death as an eventual reality for everyone. This philosophy is not acquired overnight. The nurse needs the opportunity to discuss feelings about caring for the patient whose death is imminent because the nurse's attitude towards death and suffering will affect the ability to plan and give care to the patient with advanced cancer. (See Chapter 11 for a discussion of death and dying.)

No one can say with certainty when death will come. The patient may ask about the length of time remaining, but no absolute answer can be given. Doctors may have made a statement to the patient about life expectancy. The nursing staff should know what the patient has been told because the patient's willingness to participate in self-care and attitude towards the illness may be influenced by his or her perception of life expectancy.

Planning, doing, and achieving are the best way to prevent the hopelessness and despair that may overwhelm the patient. Every effort must be put forth to meet the patient's physiological needs so that higher-order psychological needs may be expressed. The patient who is in pain or feels "dirty" will probably have difficulty expressing concerns and fears.

Other factors to consider in planning care are the personality of the patient, feelings about death and illness, and the reactions of those significant others whose opinion the patient values. The goal of nursing care should be to relieve physical, mental, and spiritual distress. The most common health care needs for the patient with cancer that is terminal are listed in Box 9-9.

Planning home care. At least half of all deaths from cancer occur in the patients' home. Planning for home care of the patient without completely disrupting the rest of the family takes the concerted efforts of many people. Patients must always be consulted, and their wishes should be respected in the early stages of the disease. In the final stages they may be too ill to be bothered or concerned with making decisions. The doctor, the social worker, and the nurse must work together with the local home hospice and agencies, such as Marie Curie Cancer Care, to ensure continuity of care from the hospital to the home. The principles governing suitability for home care are similar to those for any patient receiving home care, although the patient with cancer may not live as long as many others with chronic long-term illnesses. Medical and nursing supervision must be available; it must be possible for required care to be given; both patient and family must want the patient home; and home facilities must be suitable. Rehabilitation teams may also be sent into the home to help the patient and family.

The growth of the *hospice* concept, a place where patients may come for short or long periods for nursing care and then return to their homes as their condition warrants, is exciting. The hospice tries to maintain a homelike setting while relieving the family of the emotional and physical burden of constant care. Hospice programmes provide medical, social, and psychological support for patients and their families so that dying can be truly dignified.

The hospice concept may also be implemented as home care for the patient with the inpatient facility as a backup for home care. If a family wishes to go away on a trip, for example, the patient may request to stay in the hospice. The ultimate goal of the hospice is for the family to develop its ability to give care; thus the relationship of the hospice to the family becomes primarily one of consultation and referral. The family is aided in remaining the patient's primary support system.

Hospice staff are multidisciplinary and are employed and evaluated based on their interests and abilities to care for the terminally ill person. The focus of activities is care rather than cure, with an emphasis on symptom control. Actions are identified to help the patient and family deal with their chief concerns.[29]

Nursing interventions during advanced cancer stages

Counselling and guidance

Avoiding false hope. Occasionally, there is a mistake in diagnosis or the disease is in some way arrested for a long time. If the patient assumes that one of these occurrences may take place, the nurse should not suggest facing probable reality. The nurse must, however, avoid encouraging false hope. Many patients accept their prognosis philosophically, with the hope that a cure for cancer will be found before their disease is far advanced. Some patients are better able to accept the situation if their religious faith can be strengthened. Some patients and their families find it helpful to live each day as fully as possible without looking too far ahead. Sometimes patients with cancer have few symptoms and are able to carry on quite well until shortly before death.

Nurses also must be careful that they do not experience false hope. The inability to fulfill the hope to sustain life may make it more difficult for nurses to accept the patient's death and they may see themselves as having failed.[29]

Encouraging social and vocational activities. Patients with advanced cancer should resume their regular work if they can possibly do so, for work makes them feel as though they are still an active part of their group and worthy of the approval of others. It was said many centuries ago that employment is a person's best doctor, and this concept applies particularly to those whose existence is seriously threatened by cancer. Social activities and all experiences associated with normal family life should be continued whenever possible. There is probably no greater service the nurse can give to patients with uncontrollable cancer than to help them continue their everyday lives in any way possible. Family members often need guidance in seeing the patient's need to live as normally as possible.

Decreasing fear of helplessness. Patients may be haunted by fear of brain involvement, loss of mental faculties, and the possibility that they may become completely helpless and dependent on others. By these fears they express a basic human wish: the wish to leave the world with as much dignity as possible. The nurse should urge the patient and family to discuss such fears with the doctor. The patient may feel that the doctor is too busy and that questions are too trivial to justify the use of the doctor's time. Some questions, however, are not trivial at all, and a satisfactory answer to them adds tremendously to the patient's peace of mind. Metastasis to the brain in patients who have other metastases is somewhat rare, and some patients suffer more from fear of damage to the brain than is justified. The patient should know that good general hygiene, good nutrition, being up and about for part of each day, and doing deep-breathing exercises with attention to posture all help to prevent helplessness. A positive approach to all problems certainly shortens the time of helplessness and makes the patient more content.

Facilitating activities of daily living.

Promoting comfort. Giving good nursing care to the patient in an advanced stage of cancer is challenging. Promoting the patient's comfort should be high on the list of goals. Nursing measures that increase rest and sleep and reduce pain (p. 150) will help maintain the patient's physical and psychological wellbeing.

Maintaining nutrition. Cachexia is a frequent problem. Anorexia may accompany therapy, and the increased protein needs of the body resulting from tumour growth may be difficult to meet. Mealtimes should be incorporated with family visiting, or patients can eat together if possible. A high-protein diet enhances the response from therapy, and an adequate intake of calories spares protein for cell building. Because chewing may be difficult, food should be cut in small pieces and creamed or combined with cooked vegetables, rice, or noodles. Meat may also be minced or used as a base for soups or stews. Fish, cottage cheese, and eggs are also good sources of protein.

Total parenteral nutrition (TPN) may be used as an adjunct to therapy. TPN has not been found to stimulate tumour growth and it may result in a return of immune system competence, a decrease in sepsis, wound healing, and an increase in response to chemotherapy.

Maintaining elimination. Diarrhoea may be a problem, but constipation is more likely. If the patient is receiving narcotics, especially opium derivatives, peristalsis is decreased.[10] Patients receiving the plant alkaloid vincristine (Oncovin) may develop neurotoxicity, causing a high faecal impaction. Increasing the intake of fibre and fluids in the diet, maintaining activity, and using stool softeners may be helpful. Enemas and laxatives may be necessary.

Maintaining personal hygiene. Careful and meticulous hygiene is essential. Careful bathing and attention to skin, hair, and clothing will all promote self-esteem in the patient. Odours from body exudates, draining wounds, and incontinence may occur. Soiled dressings and bed linen are changed immediately. Judicious use of deodorizers is helpful, but deodorizers do not take the place of good hygiene.

Preventing effects of immobility. Pressure sores may be a severe problem. The combination of inactivity, poor nutrition, and incontinence seen in patients with advanced cancer predisposes them to skin breakdown. Maintaining the patient's activity by getting him or her out of bed as much as possible will prevent pressure and also promote the patient's joint mobility and muscle strength.

Teaching patient and family. The nurse is involved in teaching during most interactions with the patient and family. Careful explanations about care and sensitivity to what the patient thinks and feels about the disease contribute to the nurse's effectiveness in promoting change in the patient's behaviour. When possible, self-care activities should be emphasized. Maintaining the patient's independence whenever possible should be the goal while recognizing that the time may come when dependence is necessary.

Evaluation

Because of the diversity and complexity of cancer, evaluation of care is especially dependent on the expected patient outcomes that have been identified. Care is based on the patient's level of physical and psychosocial capacities and value systems. Questions to consider include the following:

1. Have identified learning needs been met with patient teaching?
2. Have the patient and significant others had opportunities to express feelings and concerns?
3. Has the patient participated in decision-making as desired?
4. Has hope been maintained, without giving false hope?
5. Is the patient as comfortable as possible?
6. Are good ventilation, nutrition, and elimination being maintained?
7. Are usual activities of daily living being carried out, with assistance given as needed?
8. Is the patient active within existing limits?
9. Have coping methods been supported and support services been identified?

SUMMARY

1. The term *cancer* refers to more than 200 diseases that have in common the production of abnormal cells that do not obey the laws of normal tissue growth.
2. Early diagnosis and new treatment advances have increased the survival rate so that today one out of every two people with cancer can survive.
3. Malignant cells are characterized by larger irregular nuclei, increased rates of mitosis, atypical appearance, loss of contact inhibition, and increased concentration of RNA.
4. Cancer spread occurs by three routes: direct extension or invasion, gravitational metastasis or seeding, and metastasis via blood or lymph vessels.
5. The chance of developing cancer increases with each decade after an individual reaches age 60. This may result from an exhaustion of the immune system or from a lifelong exposure to environmental carcinogens.
6. Environmental factors, host susceptibility, health practices, and psychosocial factors all contribute to carcinogenesis.
7. Common sites of cancer in women are the breast, colorectum, lung, ovary and uterus (cervix).
8. Common sites of cancer in males are the prostate, lung, and colorectum.
9. Psychological responses to cancer can range from stoicism to extreme anger. Loneliness, depression, denial, anxiety, and guilt are common reactions.
10. The term *paraneoplastic syndrome* is used to describe the systemic effects of cancer.
11. Surgery is the oldest treatment for cancer and involves removal of the tumour for cure or palliation.
12. Radiotherapy uses radiation to destroy or delay the growth of the rapidly reproducing malignant cells.
13. Chemotherapeutic drugs bring about changes in the cell cycle phases and interrupt cell growth and replication.
14. Biological response modifier therapies are therapeutic agents that alter the interaction between the tumour

and the host by influencing the host's biological response to cancer cells.

15. Malignant neoplasms cause pain by five physiological changes: bone destruction, obstruction of lumens, peripheral nerve involvement, pressure of growing tumours, and inflammation, infection, and necrosis of tissue.

16. Even in terminal stages, 60% of people with cancer will experience mild or no pain.

STUDY QUESTIONS

* Look at Fig. 11-1. What are the three most common cancers for men and for women? What preventive measures can be taken for each of the common cancers?
* The doctor's report states that the patient's tumour is staged as T1, N1, M0. What does this mean? What nursing implications does this have?
* What organizations in your community provide services to patients with cancer?
* What are the benefits and disadvantages of the four treatment modalities for cancer? What is the nurse's role in each of these modalities?
* What nursing care services are provided by hospices?

REFERENCES AND SELECTED READINGS

1. American Cancer Society: *Cancer facts and figures 1991*, New York, 1991, The Society.
2. American Cancer Society: *Cancer manual*, ed 8, Boston, 1989, The Society.
3. Averette HE, Boike GM, Jarrell MA: Effects of cancer chemotherapy on gonadal function and reproductive capacity, *CA* 40(4):199-209, 1990.
4. Baird SB, McCorkle R, Grant M: *Cancer nursing: a comprehensive textbook*, Philadelphia, 1991, WB Saunders.
5. Boring CC, Squires TS, Tong T: Cancer statistics, *CA* 41(1):19-36, 1991.
5a. Burkitt DP, Walker ARP, Painter NS: Effect of dietary fibre on stools and transit times and its role in the causation of disease, *Lancet*, ii:1408-1412, 1972.
5b. Central Statistical Office, Editor Rose P: *Social Trends 23*, London, 1993, HMSO.
5c. Clayson ME: Breast awareness may reduce mortality. A health education opportunity for women admitted to hospital. *Professional Nurse* 7(7):442-446, 1992.
6. Crowley MJ: *Risk factors*. In Ziegfeld CR, editor: *Core curriculum for oncology nursing*, Philadelphia, 1987, WB Saunders.
7.* D'Agostino NS: Managing nutrition problems in advanced cancer, *Am J Nurs* 89:50-56, 1989.
8. Department of Health: The Health of the Nation: A Consultative Document for Health in England. Presented to Parliament by the Secretary of State for Health, London, 1991, HMSO.
8a. Department of Health: The Health of the Nation: A strategy for Health in England. Presented to Parliament by the Secretary of State for Health. London, 1992, HMSO.
8b. DeVita V Jr, Hellman S, Rosenberg SA: *Cancer principles and practice of oncology*, ed 3, Philadelphia, 1989, JB Lippincott.
8c. Doll R, Peto R: *The causes of cancer*, Oxford, 1981, Oxford University Press.
8d.* Dudjak LA, Fleck AE: BRMs: new drug therapy comes of age, *RN* 54(10):42-47, 1991.
9.* Ferrell BR, Schneider C: Experience and management of cancer pain at home, *Cancer Nurs* 11:84-90, 1988.
10. Ferrell B et al: Effects of controlled-release morphine on quality of life for cancer pain, *Oncol Nurs Forum* 16(4):521-526, 1989.
11.* Foley KM: The treatment of pain in the patient with cancer, *CA* 36(4):195-215, 1987.
11a. Forrest P: Breast Cancer Screening Report, London, 1986, HMSO.
12. Frank-Strombert M: The role of the nurse in early detection of cancer: population sixty-six years of age and older, *Oncol Nurs Forum* 13(3):66-74, 1986.

12a. Gammon J: Which way out of the crisis? Coping strategies for dealing with cancer, *Professional Nurse*, 8(8):488-493, 1993.
13. Garfinkel L, Silverberg E: Lung cancer and smoking trends in the United States over the past 25 years, *CA* 41(3):137-145, 1991.
14. Garfinkel MA, Stellman SD: Cigarette smoking among doctors, dentists, and nurses, *CA* 36(1):2-8, 1986.
15. Gordon D: *Staging: a classification system for cancer*. In Ziegfeld CR, editor: *Core curriculum for oncology nursing*, Philadelphia, 1987, WB Saunders.
15a. Graves D, Nash A: A friendship that inspires hope. A study of Macmillan nurses' working patterns, *Professional Nurse*, 7(7):478-485, 1992.
15b. Greener M: Cancer self-help groups: a vital support link. *Professional Nurse*, 6(11):662-664, 1991.
16. Groenwald SL: Cancer nursing: principles and practice, ed 2, Boston, 1990, Jones & Bartlett.
16a. Health and Safety Executive: Precautions for the safe handling of cytotoxic drugs. Guidance Note MS 21, London, 1983, HMSO.
16b. Health Education Authority: Can you avoid cancer? A guide to reducing your risks, London, 1988, Health Education Authority.
17. Hogan R: Human sexuality: a nursing perspective, ed 2, New York, 1985, Appleton-Century Crofts.
17a. Holmes S: Support can boost the body's defences. Nutrition in cancer care, *Professional Nurse*, 7(2):83-89, 1991.
18.* Jarvis W: Helping your patients deal with questionable cancer treatments, *CA* 36(5):293-301, 1986.
19.* Jassak PF, Stricklin LA: Interleukin-2: an overview, *Oncol Nurs Forum* 13(6):17-22, 1986.
20. Kane NE et al: Use of patient-controlled analgesia in surgical oncology patients, *Oncol Nurs Forum* 15:29-37, 1988.
20a. Kelsey S: Can we care to the end? Do nurses have the skills for terminal care? *Professional Nurse*, 7(4):216-219, 1992.
21.* Lewandowski W, Jones SL: The family with cancer: nursing interventions throughout the course of living with cancer, *Cancer Nurs* 11:313-321, 1988.
22.* Lewis F, Levita M: Understanding radiotherapy, *Cancer Nurs* 11:174-185, 1988.
23. Lovejoy N: *Alterations in cell biology*. In Ziegfeld CR, editor: *Core curriculum for oncology nursing*, Philadelphia, 1987, WB Saunders.
23a. McVey L: A direct assault on abdominal cancer, *RN* 55(2):46-52, 1992.
24.* Melone L et al.: A teaching booklet for patients receiving GM-CSF therapy, *Oncol Nurs Forum* 18(3):593-597, 1991.
25. Million-Underwood S, Sanders E: Factors contributing to health promotion behaviours among African-American men, *Oncol Nurs Forum* 17(5):707-712, 1990.
26. Oncology Nursing Society: *Cancer chemotherapy guidelines for nursing education and practice*, Pittsburgh, 1984, The Society.
26a. Ponder MA: Can cancers be inherited? *Professional Nurse*, 6(10):593-597, 1991.
27. Porth C: Pathophysiology: concepts of altered health states, ed 3, Philadelphia, 1990, JB Lippincott.
28. Rose MA: Health promotion and risk prevention: applications for cancer survivors, *Oncol Nurs Forum* 16:335-340, 1989.
29.* Scanlon C: Creating a vision of hope: the challenge of palliative care, *Oncol Nurs Forum* 16(4):527-541, 1989.
30.* Schneider SM, Distelhorst CW: Chemotherapy-induced emergencies, *Semin Oncol* 16(6):572-578, 1989.
31.* Sprass J: Cancer pain and suffering: clinical lessons from life, literature, and legend, *Oncol Nurs Forum* 12(14):23-31, 1985.
32.* Strohl RA: The nursing role in radiation oncology: symptom management of acute and chronic reactions, *Oncol Nurs Forum* 15(4):429-434, 1988.
33. Suppers VJ, McClamrock EA: Biologicals in cancer treatment: future effects on nursing practice, *Oncol Nurs Forum* 12(3):27-32, 1985.
34. Taylor KM et al.: Recombinant human granulocyte colonstimulating factor recovery after high-dose chemotherapy and autologous bone marrow transplantation in Hodgkin's disease, *J Clin Oncol* 7(12):1791-1799, 1989.
35. Valentine A: Early detection measures. In Ziegfeld CR: *Core curriculum for oncology nursing*, Philadelphia, 1987, WB Saunders.
36. Varricchio CG: Cultural and ethnic dimensions of cancer nursing care: introduction, *Oncol Nurs Forum* 14(3):57-58, 1987.
37.* Walters P: Chemotherapy: a nurse's guide to action, administration, and side effects, *RN* 53(2):52-68, 1990.
38. American Cancer Society: *Public attitudes toward cancer and cancer tests*, New York, 1980, The Society.
38.* Goodman SG, Wickham R: Venous access devices: an overview, *Oncol Nurs Forum* 11(5):16-23, 1984.
40.* McIntire SM, Cioppa AL: Cancer nursing: a developmental approach, New York, 1984, John Wiley & Sons.
41. Rosenbaum EH: Living with cancer, St Louis, 1982, Mosby–Year Book.
42. Schottenfeld D, Haas JF: Carcinogens in the workplace, *CA* 29:173-183, 1977.

*Recommended for student reading.

10

Chronic Illness

Wilma J. Phipps

After studying this chapter, the learner should be able to:

- Differentiate between acute and chronic illness.
- Describe factors that influence chronic illness.
- Identify areas of assessment for the chronically ill person.
- Describe physical and psychosocial interventions for the person with a chronic illness.
- Define rehabilitation and the roles of team members and of the patient.
- Describe different patterns and facilities for continuing care.
- Identify major health goals related to chronic health problems to be achieved by the year 2000.
- Discuss strategies for promoting health.

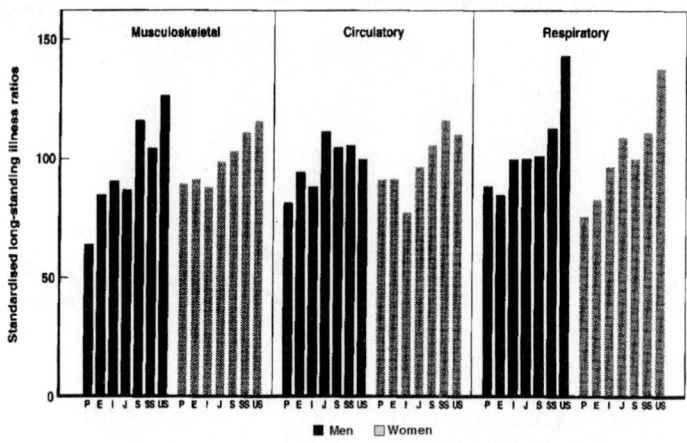

Fig. 10-1   Standardized long-standing illness ratios for men and women in different socio-economic groups, Great Britain, 1988/89. (From *On the state of Public Health*, Office of Population Census and Surveys, 1990. Used with permission)

There is increasing awareness in Britain of great pockets of unmet needs among people with long-term health problems. These individuals have needs that extend beyond the strictly medical. Their problems demand the use of multiple sources of help and care. In many cases the coping capacities of chronically ill individuals are reduced because of advancing age, serious functional impairment and disability, and limited personal, social, and financial resources.

Chronic disease is not an entity in itself but an umbrella term that encompasses long-lasting diseases, which are often associated with some degree of disability. According to the 1989 General Household Survey (GHS), an annual survey of 20,000 adults and 5,000 children, 32% of those surveyed reported having a long-standing illness, 18% reported having a long-standing illness which limited their activities, and 13% reported having had restricted activity in the previous two weeks, due to illness.[11a] Each chronic illness is unique and has a different impact on the individual, family, and community. Nevertheless, common problems and complications that accompany the various chronic health problems can be studied in general to help the nurse understand and care for individuals with specific long-term illnesses.

The incidence and prevalence of chronic diseases have increased since the beginning of the twentieth century. *Incidence* refers to the number of cases of illness that had their onset during a specified period of time. Commonly, health statistics report the number of new cases for a calendar year. *Prevalence* refers to the total number of cases at a given point in time. Thus, prevalence rates are higher than incidence rates because they include all people (cases) with a specified condition (old cases) and those who acquired the condition during a specified period of time (new cases).

The reason that both the incidence and prevalence are increased for *chronic diseases* is because fewer people are dying from *acute diseases*. There is decreased mortality from infectious diseases such as whooping cough and chickenpox in children and tuberculosis and pneumonia in people

of all ages. Improved sanitation, the introduction of effective vaccines and mass immunizations, and the discovery of antibiotics have all contributed to this decrease in deaths from infectious diseases. In Britain, the proportion of infants immunized against diphtheria, poliomyelitis and tetanus increased from 73% to 92% between 1976 and 1990. Although the rates of immunization for whooping cough dropped due to safety concerns during the 1970s, rates of immunization had again increased by 1990-1991.[8a]

Using type of employment as an indicator of socioeconomic status, Figure 10-1 illustrates that, from 1988 to 1989, more "unskilled" men and women suffered from musculoskeletal, circulatory and respiratory illnesses than "professional" men and women. This seems to indicate that people from higher income levels may be better educated about preventive health measures and they are able to afford better diet, better housing, and have medical care. In general, people in manual occupations (social classes IIIM, IV and V) have higher rates of illness and death than those in non-manual groups (social classes I, II and IIIN). In addition, death rates from the leading causes of death are generally higher in manual groups. There are, however, variations in death rates within these groups, which may be partly due to differences in risk behaviours. People in manual groups, for example, are more likely to smoke, drink larger amounts of alcohol, and to consume foods containing less vitamin C and ß-carotene.[24a]

Disability refers to any long- or short-term *reduction of activity* as the result of an acute or chronic condition. *Limitation of activity* is used to describe a *long-term reduction* in a person's ability to perform the kind or amount of activity associated with a particular age group. *Restriction of activity* is generally used to refer to a relatively short-term reduction in a person's activity below his or her normal capacity.

Heart disease is the leading cause of death in Britain today. Other leading causes of death are circulatory diseases, including stroke (46%); cancers (25%); and respiratory diseases (11%)(Fig 10-2). All the leading causes of death have risk factors associated with life-style and many of these diseases may be prevented by effective control of smoking, blood pressure, diet, and alcohol consumption.

Death rates from other causes have also been increasing. The cumulative total of deaths due to AIDS reported in England by March, 1992, was 3,336. In 1992, 15,133 cases of HIV infection had been reported in England, but the actual number of people who have been infected (many of them unaware) is certainly higher.[24a]

DEFINITION OF ACUTE AND CHRONIC ILLNESS

An *acute illness* is one caused by a disease that produces symptoms and signs soon after exposure to the cause, that runs a short course, and from which there is usually a full recovery or an abrupt termination in death. An acute illness may become chronic. For example, a common cold may develop into chronic sinusitis. A *chronic illness* is one caused by disease that produces symptoms and signs within a variable period of time, that runs a long course, and from which there is only partial recovery. The National Health Survey conducted in the U.S. defines chronic conditions as follows: (1) the conditions were first noticed 3 months or more before the date of the interview, or (2) they belong to a group of conditions (including heart disease, diabetes, and others) that are considered chronic regardless of when they began.[41] This follows the pattern of the U.S. *Commission on Chronic Illness*, which in 1949 *defined chronic illness as any impairment or deviation from normal that has one or more of the following characteristics.*

1. The illness or impairment is permanent.
2. The illness or impairment leaves residual disability.
3. The illness or impairment is caused by nonreversible pathological alteration.
4. The illness or impairment requires a long period of supervision, observation, or care.

This definition is still in use more than 40 years later.

The symptoms and general reactions caused by chronic disease may subside with proper treatment and care. The period during which the disease is controlled and symptoms are not obvious is known as *remission*. However, at a future time the disease may become active again with recurrence of pronounced symptoms. This is known as an *exacerbation* of the disease.

Exacerbations of chronic disease often cause the patient to seek medical attention and may lead to hospitalization. The needs of a patient who has an acute illness may be very different from those of the patient with an acute exacerbation of a chronic disease. For example, a young person may enter the hospital with complaints of fever, chest pain, shortness of breath, fatigue, and a productive cough. If the diagnosis is pneumonia, the patient usually can be assured of recovery after a period of rest and a course of antibiotic treatment. However, if the diagnosis is rheumatic heart disease and if the patient is being admitted to the hospital for the third, fourth, or fifth time, the reassurance needed will not be so definite, clear-cut, or easy to give. In such a case it is necessary to begin planning care that will extend beyond the period of hospitalization, taking into consideration many aspects

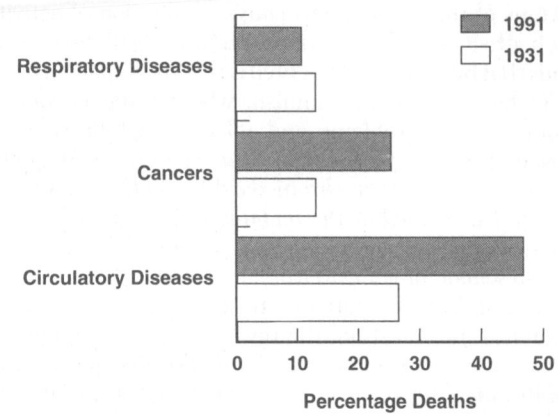

Fig. 10-2 Major causes of death 1931 and 1991, England and Wales. (From Registrar General's Statisitical Review 1931 and OPCS 1991, from *The Health of the Nation*, HMSO, 1992.)

of the patient's total life situation. The concerns of the patient who has repeated attacks of illness will be very different from the concerns of the one who has a short-term illness.

Further, the needs of patients who are admitted to the hospital with an acute illness but who also have an underlying chronic condition must not be overlooked. For example, elderly patients who enter the hospital with pneumonia may receive treatment for the pneumonia and recover from their illness. However, they may still be hampered by the arteriosclerotic heart disease and arthritis that they have had for years. Also these two chronic conditions may have been aggravated by the acute infection, or the return to former activity may be hindered by joint stiffness resulting from bed rest and inactivity. Consideration of a patient's several diagnoses can help in preventing new problems associated with the chronic illness.

Strauss,[44] a well-known medical sociologist, has described the following problems experienced by people with chronic illness:

1. Preventing and managing medical crises
2. Controlling symptoms
3. Following prescribed regimen
4. Maintaining normal interactions with others
5. Adjusting to recurrent patterns in the course of the disease
6. Arranging payment for treatment

The emotional, social, and economic implication of chronic illnesses are discussed later in this chapter.

IMPACT OF CHRONIC ILLNESS ON SOCIETY

The U.S. National Health Survey of 1989 classified chronic conditions in the following categories: (1) *selected skin and musculoskeletal conditions*, (2) *impairments (visual, hearing, speech, paralysis, deformity, or orthopaedic impairment)*, (3) *selected digestive conditions*, (4) *selected conditions of the genitourinary, nervous, endocrine, metabolic, and blood and blood-forming systems*, (5) *selected circulatory conditions*, and (6) *selected respiratory conditions*.[42]

Many of these conditions cause a limitation of activity, which affects the life-style of the chronically ill. One of the trends that has been documented is that the impact of acute illness has seemed to diminish, whereas the burden of chronic health problems and related disability has increased. *Limitation of activity is a measure of long-term disability resulting from chronic health problems or impairment and is defined as the inability to carry on the major activity for one's age group, such as cooking, keeping house, going to school, or going to work.*

Some activity limitations are associated with mental disabilities, but most are the result of physical handicaps caused by heart conditions and arthritis. *Because chronic disability increases in direct proportion to age, people over 65 years of age are most prone to severe chronic disability.*

As the population of the U.K. ages, the number of people with chronic illness will continue to increase. The inability to work or to move about influences greatly the kind of medical treatment and health supervision needed by people who have a chronic illness. Some people only need periodic medical examination and perhaps continuing treatment with medications; others may require complete physical care. Some have a disease that progresses very slowly without remissions, whereas others may have episodes of acute illness and then seem comparatively well for a time. Each person requires a thorough assessment to determine the stage of the illness, the course the illness is likely to take, the type of care needed, and the method by which that care will be delivered if the individual is to be helped appropriately.

Factors That Influence Chronic Illness
Age

Different age groups have different kinds of experience with acute and chronic diseases. The young are more likely to experience short, intense, acute conditions that are quickly over. The elderly are more likely to have long, drawn-out chronic diseases; nevertheless, it is true that anyone can have either an acute or a chronic disease at any age. Chronic illness and disability may date from birth (for example, spina bifida with neurological damage), or it may originate in childhood, adolescence, or early adult life (for example, multiple sclerosis, rheumatoid arthritis). *The major chronic illnesses among those 65 years and over identified in the National Health Survey conducted in the United States, were arthritis, diabetes, heart disease, and hypertension.*

Because of strides made in paediatric medicine, children who 30 years ago would have died from diseases such as cystic fibrosis are living longer. The reduction in death rates among the younger age groups has allowed a higher percentage of the population to reach the age of greatest risk from chronic diseases. Cancer develops far more frequently in older people.

Much remains to be learned about interactions of the normal, pathological, and physiological changes of ageing with various diseases. A common question that is asked is "When does ageing end and illness begin?" Differences found in age groups or changes found in individuals as they age represent normal ageing; that is, a universal, intrinsic process of growth and development that is inevitable, irreversible, unpreventable, but ultimately detrimental. Even though ageing, a normal process, is distinct from chronic disease, a pathological process, *chronic illness often accompanies ageing.* The problems of ageing and chronic disease are influenced in major ways by each other; for example, the social problems confronting the aged are strongly influenced by the presence and severity of chronic disabilities. Remissions and exacerbations are possibilities with chronic illness; they are not with ageing.

Although many people now live into their 80s, it is not likely that all those years will be active and independent ones. Thus, improving the functional independence and not just the length of later life is an important element in promoting the health of this group.

One measure of health that considers quality as well as the length of life is the years of healthy life. Whereas people aged 65 and older have 16.4 years of life remaining on average, it is estimated that they have about 12 years of healthy life remaining. *Thus quality of life is determined by the individual's ability to perform activities of daily living so that he or she can be independent.*

Race and ethnicity

Race or ethnic group membership is a factor that influences chronic health problems. Race-specific rates measure the association between disease occurrence and race. Data on specific conditions indicate not only that some problems are more prevalent among nonwhites (for example, blacks and Asians) but also that many nonwhites fail to receive necessary care. Rates of ill health and death also differ among various ethnic minorities. In Britain, for example, death rates for coronary heart disease are higher in people from the Indian subcontinent than in the white population, but lower in Indians than in Afro-Caribbeans.[24a] In the US, *nonwhites are more than three times more likely to die of hypertension than whites of the same age group.*[41] *The findings of the US Task Force on Black and Minority Health, which were released late in 1985, found that 60,000 excess deaths occur each year in minority populations.*[30]

The excess number of preventable deaths is derived by calculating the difference between the number of deaths in the black population and the number that would have been expected to occur by applying the average annual age-specific rates of the white population to the mid-period black population (as of 1983).[24] *This means that there would be no excess black deaths if the mortality rates of blacks and whites were the same.*

Cultural values

Western culture tends to be cure oriented, therefore, health care for acute conditions is often more valued than is health care for the chronically ill. In contrast to the exciting aspects of sophisticated and mechanical technology, caring for chronically ill people is often considered boring. The continued struggle to cope with day-to-day living soon becomes tedious for ill people, their families, and health professionals. *The rewards of treating chronic illness cannot be measured by a cure but by the prevention of complications and by helping individuals function at their optimal level.*

The cultural context has many symbolic meanings, beliefs, and values that health professionals need to understand to meet individuals' health needs. Some individuals may view their chronic disease as a form of punishment from God. Thus they may experience a sense of guilt. Individuals who view their chronic disease as a "leper phenomenon" may experience a sense of social rejection. Others may see their chronic illness as a destructive force without meaning or simply as a physical response of their body. Appreciation of the person's beliefs and behaviour in the context of his or her cultural heritage rather than denial of the cultural influence increases understanding between the health professional and the chronically ill person. Differences need not imply deviance. It is possible to introduce health practices in a manner congruent with the individual's cultural values.

Cost of Disability

Chronically ill people and their families are subjected to great personal and emotional losses that must be dealt with—loss of self-esteem, loss of status within the family, loss of independence, feelings of rejection, and feelings of helplessness are only a few. These can be more devastating than economic deprivation, which is a constant problem.

The economic cost to patients, families and government for providing health care and social care for people with chronic illnesses is considerable. Under Section 21 of the National Assistance Act, 1948, local authorities have a statutory duty to provide residential accommodation for people who, because of age or infirmity, are in need of care and attention.[8a] The concept of "priority groups" in health and social care services can be traced back to a 1976 consultative document issued by the Department of Health and Social Security (now the Department of Health). This was the first time government had attempted to establish priorities within health and social services.[11b] A survey published by the Office of Population Census and Surveys in 1988 indicated that six million adults in Britain had some physical, mental or sensory disability. More than four million of these people are 65 years old or older.[19a]

The cost of medications to control or maintain a patient's health status may require a major portion of the family budget. Additional expenses may include special diets and equipment, home modifications (for example, ramps or widening of doors for wheelchairs) and transportation.

The ability of the individual family to pay its own way is determined in part by which member of the family becomes disabled. Older studies showed that the family suffered less economic deprivation if the wife was disabled. In those studies, three quarters of the chronically ill people unable to carry out their jobs were men. Today, however, more and more households are headed by women who are single parents and are the only wage earners for the family. Women who head households will need additional help and support and nurses should be sensitive to their needs.

Some financial assistance is provided by the Department of Health and Social Security. Social Security benefits are the second most important source of income in Britain, after wages and salaries. Social Security is the largest single public expenditure programme and accounted for one-third of all general government spending in 1991-1992.[20b]

People with chronic illnesses may have considerable difficulty in paying for prescribed therapy. It is not uncommon for the person with limited resources to weigh whether to purchase medications or food because there is not enough money to do both.

In considering the cost of disability to the community, it must be realized that most individuals who are unable to work must be supported by others, either from private or from public funds. In 1991, sickness and invalidity benefits were claimed by the following age groups: 2.12% of 20–29-year-olds, 0.182% of 30–39-year-olds, 0.300% of 40–49-year-olds, 0.559% of 50–59-year-olds and 0.558% of over 60-year-olds also claimed sickness or invalidity benefit.[20b]

CHRONICALLY ILL PEOPLE AND THEIR FAMILIES

The effects of chronic illness on individuals and their families are numerous and varied. The first impact of the disability may nearly immobilize them. Time must be provided them to talk through their concerns and fears before they can be expected to begin coping with their new situation.

Marked changes often take place, and are often required to take place, in family living as a result of chronic illness. Some families may find themselves drawn closer together. Other families may drift apart, the individual members being incapable of helping one another. At times, chronic illness may threaten an individual's basic emotional stability, and the whole situation may be unbearable to others. Sometimes the individual's emotional needs may not have been apparent to the family early in the illness, but when such needs grow obvious, relatives feel inadequate to cope with the situation. *The length of illness, periodical hospitalizations, and increased financial, emotional, and social burdens are stressors that threaten the family's integrity.*

Many people struggle on their own to assume the full financial burden of the illness and consequently expose other members of the family to lower standards of nutrition, housing, and care. Many times relatives move in with one another, arguments develop, and family ties are strained or broken. Public assistance may be acceptable to some families, whereas others find it impossible to accept.

Chronic illness imposes additional problems of learning how to cope with restrictions on activities of daily living, how to prevent or identify medical crises that occur, and how to carry out treatment regimens as delineated by the health care provider. Family members also need to learn about the restrictions, not only to be of assistance to the chronically ill person, but also because their own activity patterns may be disrupted by the person's activities.

Because chronic illness may have periods of exacerbation when symptoms become more acute and medical crises may occur, patients and family members need to know which symptoms must be reported to the doctor as well as the time interval for reporting these symptoms. They also need to know how to contact the doctor and what measures to take if a medical crisis occurs. For example, the person who has a history of myocardial infarction and that person's family members must know what to do if the person experiences severe chest pain. Should the person be taken immediately to a hospital or should the doctor be contacted first? Patient and family should plan in advance the sequence of actions to take during a medical crisis, depending on the nature and extent of the presenting symptoms.

Compliance and Noncompliance

People with chronic illness are often labelled as "compliant" or "noncompliant" in carrying out regimens prescribed for them. There are many factors that influence the person's ability or motivation to carry out the prescribed regimen. If the person does not carry out the regimen (noncompliant), it does not necessarily mean that the individual is refusing to do so deliberately, although this may sometimes occur.

Before the nursing diagnosis of noncompliance is made, the nurse needs to assess the situation to determine the reasons that the patient is not complying with therapeutic recommendations. The aetiology of noncompliance includes the patient's value system (health beliefs, cultural influence, spiritual values).[37] The following are some possible reasons for nonadherence to a prescribed therapy:

1. Failure to understand or internalize the reason for the recommendations
2. Procedures that are difficult to learn and carry out
3. Time required to carry out therapy
4. Side effects of therapy (medications, exercises, etc.)
5. Being embarrassed when carrying out regimen in front of others
6. Social isolation and lack of support and positive reinforcement

Conflicts occur within the family structure when one family member recognizes the importance of carrying out the prescribed regimen but another does not. For example, a wife may see the need for continuing checkups and medication for her husband's hypertension, whereas he may perceive this as needless because he feels well and has no symptoms. People vary from time to time in the extent of compliance. Individuals who are not hospitalized are their own health care agents and they (or their partners) determine the actions that are taken.

Coping mechanisms that have been developed should not be tampered with unless, based on a thorough understanding of the situation, viable and more appropriate alternatives can be proposed. If the goal of maintaining the chronically ill person in the optimal state of health is being interfered with by the individual's or the family's attitudes or capacities, a change in those attitudes or capacities is necessary, but it must be a change that is mutually acceptable.

Prevention of Chronic Illness

Because chronic disease evolves over time and pathological changes may become irreversible, the goal is to detect risk factors as early as possible.

Generally, prevention means inhibiting the development of a disease before it occurs. The term includes several levels of prevention to interrupt or slow the progression of disease (see Box 10-1).

Chronically ill people and their families require long-term care. The nursing profession has been concerned with chronic health problems and the challenge involved in providing long-term nursing care to chronically ill individuals and their families.

The American Academy of Nursing has made the following statement regarding long-term care:

> Long-term care is the provision of that range of services—physical, psychological, spiritual, and social, including socioeconomic—needed to help people attain, maintain, or regain their optimal level of functioning. It includes health maintenance throughout the life span as well as care during acute and protracted illness and disability. Such care is the legitimate province of nurses who now are making social contributions through health teaching and promotion, prevention of illness, and rehabilitation.[33]

In the past nursing has followed the general pattern of providing health services by placing the emphasis on acute and episodic care rather than on health promotion and health maintenance. However, there is an emerging consensus among the health community that the health strategy must be changed dramatically to emphasize the prevention of disease. In the same vein, Health of the Nation report proposed that "nursing assume major responsibility for health promotion, maintenance, and teaching within the context of its definition of long-term care."[33]

Another way of looking at prevention has been identified by Albee. He has developed a "prevention equation" for preventing dysfunction:

$$\text{Incidence of dysfunction} = \frac{\text{Stress} + \text{Constitutional vulnerabilities}}{\text{Social supports} + \text{Coping skills} + \text{Competence}}$$

The two major strategies for preventing dysfunction are decreasing the values in the numerator (that is, decreasing stressors or constitutional vulnerabilities) and increasing the values in the denominator (that is, increasing social supports, coping skills, and competence). It is more difficult to have an impact on the numerator of the prevention equation because stressors in our lives cannot always be controlled; however, creative ways to decrease individual and societal stressors must continually be sought. It is easier to affect the denominator by strengthening social supports, coping skills, and competence. For more information see Chapter 5 for a discussion of stressors, stress, and stress management.

One valuable tool that has been developed to assist people to identify their own risk factors and change their life-styles is the health hazard appraisal (HHA).[36] The HHA is a screening process that includes a comprehensive questionnaire and the taking of certain physical measurements. Based on probability tables, a risk assessment is then calculated from each person's profile along with goals that would result in risk reduction. Counselling and follow-up are provided to reinforce the data.

Levels of prevention

Primary
Health promotion
Specific protection against diseases (vaccines)

Secondary
Early detection of disease
Prompt intervention to halt progression of disease

Tertiary
Rehabilitation (appropriate to the stage of disability)
Prevention of further complications
Restoration of optimal functioning to highest possible level

Nursing Process
Assessment of the person with a chronic illness

Before a plan of care can be devised for the chronically ill person, a thorough assessment of needs and capabilities must be carried out. Included in such an assessment are the individual's *physical, psychological, social, and financial status.*

Physical status

Because medical diagnoses do not accurately reflect the physical status and functioning of the chronically ill person, the use of a profile system or assessment tool may be instituted as a guide for those working with the patient. One such tool[39] provides a guide for grading the patient in six different categories: (1) physical condition including cardiovascular, pulmonary, gastrointestinal (GI), genitourinary, endocrine, or cerebrovascular disorders; (2) upper extremities, structure and function, including the shoulder girdle and cervical and upper dorsal spine; (3) lower extremities, structure and function, including the pelvis and lower dorsal and lumbar sacral spine; (4) sensory components relating to speech, vision, and hearing; (5) excretory function, including the bowels and bladder; and (6) mental and emotional status. The ability of the person to carry out activities of daily living (for example, dressing, feeding, bathing, brushing teeth, combing hair, toileting, and moving from place to place) specifically need to be assessed. The completed assessment should indicate in what areas the patient has difficulty and the extent of that difficulty. Such a guide can be used in planning goals for care, both immediate and long term, and will be useful in assisting the individual and the family to make realistic plans for care. Because a chronic condition is not static, reassessment should be carried out at regular intervals whether there is improvement or regression.

The impact of chronic illness on the person's desire for or ability to participate in sexual activities should be assessed. Changes in body appearance, shortness of breath, and musculoskeletal or neurological impairments may make it seem to the person that they can no longer be sexually active. In addition, the side effects of certain medications tend to decrease sexual desire or cause impotence. The nurse should determine if concern about sexual ability is a problem for the person, and if it is, appropriate action including referral can be taken. (See Chapter 26 for more information about sexuality in health and illness.)

Psychological status

Assessment of the individual's psychological needs and capabilities includes determining attitudes and stage of adaptation to the illness, feelings concerning how illness affects the family or significant others, and the person's own goals in regard to living with an illness. For example, individuals who are almost totally helpless as a result of an accidental spinal cord injury may seem to have no interest in learning ways to help themselves. Their families may react in the same manner and be of little help to them. Both the individuals and their families need interest and support from nurses and other professionals as they learn to cope with the change in their life situations.

Feelings of anxiety, frustration, irritability, bitterness, and guilt may be expressed by some chronically ill people who face unending pain and loss of economic and social security. Some people become obsessed with their health problems, and spend much of each day thinking about what will happen and what to do. Guilt may result from being unable to work and support oneself or from the belief, as a result of a search for some purpose or reason for the affliction, that one must deserve the suffering. *Depression is common among chronically ill people, especially those who feel powerless. Powerlessness can be the result of feeling unable to control or overcome what has happened to one.*[17]

Social and financial status

Social and financial status must be considered because they relate specifically to the kind of support and resources available to the individuals in meeting their goals. It would be unrealistic, for example, to plan for a hydraulic bath chair if the patient could not afford it, family members were unavailable to help operate it, or the patient's landlord would not permit it to be installed. Alternative methods of helping the patient to take a bath would have to be explored.

The social assessment includes living arrangements, family roles, support of family, cultural and social group memberships, education, and vocational and avocational activities. The data collected through the performance of this kind of thorough assessment should make it possible to devise a *plan of care directed towards the accomplishment of attainable goals that are mutually acceptable to the patient, the family, and the carers.*

Nursing analysis

Nursing problems are determined from assessment of patient data. Possible nursing problems for the person with a chronic illness may include, but are not limited to, the following:

Problem	Possible aetiologies
Activity intolerance	Bed rest, immobility, generalized weakness, sedentary life-style
Adjustment, impaired	Disability requiring change in life-style; inadequate support systems; impaired cognition, sensory over load; altered locus of control; incomplete grieving
Anxiety	Threat to self-concept; threat of change in health status, socioeconomic status, and role functioning
Breathing pattern, ineffective	Neuromuscular impairment, pain, musculoskeletal impairment
Communication, impaired verbal	Aphasia, physical impairment
Constipation	Change in life-style, immobility, inadequate nutrition, inadequate fluid intake
Coping, ineffective family: compromised	Inadequate or incorrect information, temporary family disorganization and role changes, prolonged disability of significant person
Diversional activity deficit	Long-term hospitalization
Fear	Loss of body part, long-term illness, pain, life-style changes
Health maintenance, altered	Altered communication skills, decreased motor skills
Home maintenance management, impaired	Insufficient family resources, lack of knowledge/role modelling, inadequate support systems
Hopelessness	Prolonged activity restriction, failing physical condition, long-term stress
Incontinence, functional	Altered environment; sensory, cognitive, or mobility deficits
Incontinence, reflex	Neurological impairment
Injury, high risk for	Sensory/motor deficits, lack of awareness of environmental hazards
Knowledge deficit	Lack of exposure/recall, cognitive limitation
Mobility, impaired physical	Intolerance to activity; decreased strength/endurance; pain/discomfort; cognitive, neuromuscular, or musculoskeletal impairment; depression; severe anxiety
Nutrition, altered: less than body requirements	Chewing or swallowing difficulties, inability to obtain food
Pain	Immobility, improper positioning, pressure points
Powerlessness	Health care environment, illness-related regimen, lifestyle of helplessness
Self-care deficit, bathing/hygiene, dressing/grooming, feeding/toileting	Intolerance to activity/fatigue, pain/discomfort, perceptional/cognitive impairment, musculoskeletal impairment, depression
Self-esteem disturbance	Severe trauma, change in body appearance, change in social involvement
Sexual dysfunction	Altered body structure, physiological limitations
Skin integrity, impaired	Mechanical forces (pressure, shearing), immobility
Social interaction, impaired	Poor communication skills, self-concept disturbance, absence of supportive others, altered thought processes

Planning: expected patient outcomes

Because outcomes for specific chronic diseases are discussed in the chapters dealing with those diseases not all possible outcomes will be discussed here. However, in general it may be stated that on discharge from the hospital or other care facility, patients with chronic disease or their family members should be able to do the following:

1. Demonstrate or explain those measures that must be taken to avoid further preventable disability.
2. Demonstrate or explain those self-care activities of which they are capable.
3. Identify those activities for which help is needed.
4. Explain who will be available to help with those activities and on what basis that help will be available.
5. Recognize the effect that change in body appearance and social involvement have on self-esteem.
6. Recognize the need to work on coping skills of patient and family.
7. Explain what community resources are available and how to obtain them.
8. Discuss in reasonable detail their plans for follow-up care and reevaluation.

Implementation

Interventions to achieve patient outcomes

Limiting Disability

The first focus in intervention for the chronically ill person is on preventing and reducing disability and enabling the person to remain a socially functioning individual in every respect. Some disabilities among chronically ill people might have been prevented if prompt, aggressive, suitable medical and nursing care had been available at the onset of the illness. *Many of the difficulties that limit these individuals may not have been caused by the disease itself but may have developed because of immobility during the acute phase of the illness.*

Keeping the patient's body in good alignment, maintaining joint range and strength, and preventing decubitus ulcers are physical measures that must constantly be borne in mind. (For further information, see Chapter 34.) A careful plan of rest and activity helps preserve physical resources and makes the day purposeful. If assistance is needed, it should be given until the person can manage the activity by himself or herself or until an alternative method of management can be taught.

Promoting self-care

Asking the patient to identify what is meaningful is a primary step towards helping develop self-care. Physical needs are of paramount importance for chronically ill people. Meeting these physical needs provides a way to convey to such individuals an interest in their progress and welfare. For chronically ill people who must be hospitalized, it is important that they be allowed to perform as much of their own care as possible. People who have been independent in self-care before hospitalization should not be allowed to regress in these abilities if at all possible. Helping them to take their own baths, attend to toilet needs, and groom themselves can give some sense of accomplishment and help them maintain their self-respect. Helping them to be dressed appropriately promotes a sense of well-being. Success in performing portions of their own self-care may be stimulating enough to strengthen ill people's motivation; they and their families then may make amazing strides in thinking through and working out future problems themselves. For their planning to be realistic and ultimately functional, all health care personnel must teach chronically ill people the total physiological ramifications of their disability as well as methods of coping with those ramifications.

People who are in their homes or in substitute homes should be encouraged to dress in regular, comfortable street clothing rather than pyjamas or gowns. Visitors to the home and family members who constantly see such individuals dressed in nightclothes think of them as sick and are reminded of their illness. Seeing them dressed as usual helps to maintain normal attitudes, relationships, and expectations.

Promoting self-esteem

The care of chronically ill people requires alertness in feeling, seeing, and hearing. Continued warmth and interest are necessary to the self-esteem of any chronically ill person. Very often a relationship based on an understanding of these requirements promotes self-esteem and helps the individual to become highly motivated. It may be taxing to listen to the same questions and say the same things day after day, but the nature of chronic illness may require this attention, and the manner in which responses are given will convey warmth and interest. The world of chronically ill people, whether they are in the hospital or elsewhere, becomes narrowed and circumscribed. They treasure and are interested in those things and those people who are close to them. Their conversations may be largely about themselves, their immediate environment, a few close objects, and the people who are close to them. Although they may be confined to bed and to their room, others can keep them up to date on outside news. Depending on their level of adaptation to their illness, they may welcome hearing about outside events, or they may not be able to think beyond themselves. When they reach the stage of being able to look beyond themselves, newspapers, magazines, radio, television, or creating something with their own hands may help to keep up their interest in others and in outside events.

Supporting coping skills

Coping skills may be challenged by persistent, ongoing problems such as chronic pain, recurring medical expenses, or continuing difficulties in carrying out activities of daily living. Usual coping methods may become impossible; for example, a person who usually copes by *expending energy in physical activity* may become unable to do so. The person who *usually copes by discussing problems with family members* will need to find an alternative method if family communication patterns break down. The person can be helped to identify usual coping methods and to explore alternative approaches when necessary.

It is important to recognize that chronically ill people or their families may suffer from unresolved sadness known as *chronic grief*. Chronic grief may be defined as accumulated or prolonged grief. It extends over long periods, with permanent characteristics developing in many people, and carries with it a potential for decreased functioning. The causes are varied, and new waves of grief are constantly triggered. One example is grief caused by the losses associated with ageing: youth, dreams, jobs, hair, friends, family, health, visual acuity, social role, money, body parts, and mobility. Each loss is accompanied by grief, which builds on previous grief like bricks in creating a wall. In chronic grief the person may be faced with repeated acute episodes. These episodes may coincide with exacerbation of the condition, facing a new limitation, or meeting new indignities. Each new episode requires a renewed struggle back and forth through the various stages of grief.[43]

The nurse can assist by listening and helping the person explore feelings and the content related to these feelings. Because the grief is ongoing, family members can also be helped to identify their feelings and strengthen the communication patterns within the family structure for mutual support of its members.

Clarifying nurse–patient values

Before nurses can work effectively with chronically ill people they need to be able to distinguish between their own values, standards, and goals and those of the patient. In day-to-day contact with individuals who are making little or no progress, it is tempting to make plans for their future because of a sincere interest in helping them. This is particularly true when the patient's age is similar to one's own. There may be a feeling that something must be done to speed progress. One may become frustrated by the feeling of wanting to do something or wanting to see some marked change. However, the nurse must recognize that *management of chronically ill people requires a slow-moving, persistent pace* with *possibly little or no change for a long time*. The person's physical and mental condition must be maintained at its present level or improved, and efforts must be made to progress and encourage the family's adaptation to the patient's condition. Eagerness and readiness to progress will be determining factors for the future. *The "doing" in the care of the chronically ill person is not always a physical action with the hands. Often the maintenance of a positive approach and attitude and a demonstration of real interest are the greatest help to the patient.* Teaching patients to perform activities related to their own care independently rather than performing those activities for them may also lead to progress.

Supporting the person with a progressive disability

Health care personnel must also be prepared to provide care for patients whose disease will follow a course of progressive disability, as in multiple sclerosis or rheumatoid arthritis. In these instances, goals of care must be modified to retard the downhill progression of disability rather than to achieve maintenance or improvement of physical status. Helping the patient and family cope with progressive deterioration and in some cases eventual death is a demanding task. Those who wish additional information relating to this aspect of care are referred to the literature on this subject.[45]

People with a disability, whether obvious to others or unrecognizable, should not be viewed from the standpoint of the disability alone but for their abilities as well. Usually the greatest need is for comprehensive health services and continuing care. Comprehensive care is provided to patients according to their needs in an appropriate, continuous, and dynamic pattern. Accommodating the plan of care to the needs and goals of individual patients rather than to those of the health service is the essence of comprehensive care.

Providing community resources

There has been an increasing interest in providing programmes for chronically ill people and in assisting them and disabled people to assume a more active role in their communities. Volunteer workers may act as readers both in hospitals and in homes or may assist with other diversional activities. Institutions are required to make aids such as ramps available to individuals who are unable to climb stairs or who are in wheelchairs. With the development of structural changes that facilitate mobility, some people with physical limitations are more involved in local activities and associations. Nurses can assist by supporting the further development of these structural changes in all community buildings and by encouraging the participation of chronically ill people in community activities of interest. Various information sources may be obtained from national organizations, involved with chronic illness and disability. Many of these agencies have services available in the community (see Box 10-2). Programmes, facilities, and legislation of this nature reflect the public's increasing awareness of the difficulties faced by chronically ill and disabled people.

Evaluation

Questions to be asked about the patient with a chronic illness include the following:

1. Can the patient or family demonstrate or explain the measures necessary to avoid further preventable disability?
2. Can the patient demonstrate or explain the self-care activities of which they are capable?

3. Can the patient identify the activities for which help is needed?
4. Can the patient explain who will be available to help with the above activities and on what basis they will be available?
5. Can the patient verbalize the effect that change in body appearance and social involvement has had on his or her self-esteem?
6. Do interactions between the patient and family members give evidence that they have been working to improve their coping skills?
7. Can the patient or family explain what community resources they are using and how they obtained them?
8. Can the patient discuss plans for follow-up care and re-evaluation?

REHABILITATION

Rehabilitation is the process of assisting the individual with a disability to realize his or her particular goals, physically, mentally, socially, and economically. As such, *rehabilitation is an active concept* and *must be clearly differentiated from the concept of maintenance care.* Following a thorough assessment of patients' disabilities and capabilities, assumptions can be made regarding the potential for improving their conditions. If improvement can be made, patients are candidates for rehabilitation. If improvement cannot be made, care is directed toward maintaining the current condition, that is, preventing further disability. The process of rehabilitation can be viewed more appropriately as *patient education* rather than *patient care.* One must remember, however, that the rehabilitation of every patient will reach an end point, that is, a point at which no further progress is possible. At that time, the focus of care reverts to that of maintenance.

The purpose or extent of rehabilitation ranges from employment or reemployment for the disabled person to the more limited achievement of developing self-care abilities. This latter accomplishment can be just as important to the individual as earning money and may represent that person's greatest life achievement. This might be true, for example, for a person who was born with a severe physical disability such as cerebral palsy.

Success in learning to adjust to living with a disability depends on the *person's premorbid personality, total life experience,* and *premorbid family relationships,* as well as *the person's current behaviour and motivation.* Certainly, some rehabilitation can occur in any health agency; nevertheless, the greater the number of rehabilitation disciplines made available as needed to individuals, the greater is their chance of achieving their highest potential. The rehabilitative process, as with any form of education, is involved as deeply in the motives and purposes of the teacher as in those of the learner.

People with disabilities, whether obvious to others or unrecognizable, should not be viewed from the standpoint of their disability alone. Usually the greatest need is for comprehensive health services and continuing care. *Comprehensive care is that which is provided to patients according to their needs in an appropriate, continuous, and dynamic pattern.* Accommodating the plan of care to the needs and goals of individual patients rather than to those of the providers of care is the essence of comprehensive care.

Interdisciplinary Approach

The number of professional people required to assist the patient and family with rehabilitation will vary. *Most often the patient, the family, the doctor, and the nurse can work out a practical plan.* If a patient's problems are complex, other members may be added to the team. Typically, such a team consists of a doctor, nurse, discharge coordinator, medical social worker, vocational counsellor, psychologist, speech therapist, occupational and physical therapists, and a caseworker from the patient's social agency. Teamwork requires that members of the team be able to use their special knowledge and skill and understand the value of their contribution to the patient's care. In addition, team members need some understanding of each other's professional functions and contributions.*One of the cooperative efforts of the involved team members is to meet regularly to evaluate patients and their abilities thoroughly. Based on this assessment,each patient and the team devise a plan to foster readjustment, compensation, and the learning of new ways to manage self-care and living.*

Rehabilitation Centres

People with very complex problems of rehabilitation may need to receive care at specialized centres for rehabilitation, or they may receive care at home combined with visits to day rehabilitation centres. The variety of specialized centres includes teaching and research centres (centres located in and operated by hospitals and medical schools), community centres with facilities for inpatients, community outpatient centres, skilled nursing homes with an active rehabilitation service and staff, including physio and occupational therapists, and vocational rehabilitation centres. In addition to centres that provide multiple services for the physically disabled, specialized centres provide rehabilitation for blind, deaf, mentally ill, and mentally retarded people. Most centres offer a wide range of services that usually fall into the following three areas:

Physical area

Physical, nursing, and medical evaluation
Physiotherapy
Occupational therapy
Speech therapy
Medical and nursing supervision of
appropriate activities

Psycho-social area

Evaluation
Personal counselling
Social service
Psychiatric service
Recreational therapy

Vocational area

Work evaluation
Vocational counselling
Prevocational experience
Industrial fitness of programmes
Trial employment in sheltered workshops
Vocational training
Terminal employment in sheltered workshops
Placement

Several advantages exist for patients participating in organized programmes for rehabilitation. They have an opportunity to see and be with others who have similar or more extensive disabilities. Often they progress more rapidly when they realize that others have similar difficulties and are overcoming them. Group therapy often arouses a competitive spirit, and a formerly reluctant person may become willing and diligent. On the other hand, all personnel need to be alert to those patients who have had the opposite reaction. Patients who see others advance in activity while they either do not improve or progress very slowly may become so discouraged that they give up trying. In some cases, the person becomes very depressed and may be suicidal. The nurse should be aware of changes in the person's behaviour and be sensitive to any expression of suicidal ideas.

On a rehabilitation unit activities are scaled so that individuals can see their own progress in comparison with their beginning abilities. Patients may take an active interest in keeping their own scores. After a programme of therapy has been planned and is scheduled as to time of day, patients can help to keep themselves on the schedule by having a copy of it at the bedside. Individuals can then be assisted to gradually assume more responsibility for readying themselves for scheduled activities. In addition, a master plan of activities for all patients on the unit can be a useful device for nurses, doctors, and therapists. The plan can be kept in a central place on the unit and should list name, activity, and time of activity for each patient. This type of plan is also helpful when a patient's progress is to be re-evaluated.

Rehabilitation programmes can be organized through the health services, or through charitable and voluntary organizations. The latter two organizations are more likely to be able to assist with grants for physical or practical provisions, and most rehabilitation centres/organizations can provide technical and practical guidance.

All people of working age with a substantial job handicap resulting from either physical or mental impairment are eligible for help or assistance. The purpose of rehabilitation services is to *preserve*, *develop*, or *restore* the ability of disabled people to earn their own livings. The individual services offered are medical care, counselling and guidance, training, and job finding. The local Disablement Resettlement Officer (contact number in local phone book) will be able to provide the client and the carer with up-to-date information and guidance.

10-2

Community resources involved in chronic health problems

Various types of information may be obtained by writing to these organizations. In addition, services of the various agencies are usually available at the local level.

Alzheimer's Disease Society
158–160 Balham High Rd
London
SW12 9BN
0181-675 6557
0181-675 8040 Fax

Arthritis Care
5 Grosvenor Crescent
London
SW1X 7ER
0171-235 0902
0171-259 5330 Fax

Association of Cystic Fibrosis
(Adults UK)
5 Blyth Rd
Bromley
Kent BR1 3RD
0181-464 7211/2
0181-313 0472 Fax

Association of Retired Persons
3rd Floor
Green Coat House
Francis St
London
SW1P 1DZ
0171-828 0500
0171-834 3829 Fax

Asthma Society of Ireland
24 Anglesea St
Dublin 2
Republic of Ireland
353 (1) 716551

British Association for Service to
the Elderly
119 Hassell St
Newcastle under Lyme
Staffs ST5 1AX
01782-66037
01782-612725 Fax

British Association of Cancer
United Patients (BACUP)
121/123 Charterhouse St
London EC1M 6AA
01800-181199 Freeline
0171-608 1038 Counselling
service

British Colostomy Association
15 Station Rd
Reading RG1 1LG
01734-391537
01734-569095 Fax

British Diabetic Association
10 Queen Anne St
London
W1M 0BD
0171-323-1531
0171-637 3644 Fax

British Geriatrics Society
1 St Andrews Place
London NW1 4LB
0171-935 4004
0171-224 0454 Fax

British Institute of Mental Handicap
The Crescent
Wolverhampton Rd
Kidderminster
Hereford and Worcester
DY10 3PP
01562-850251

British Nutrition Foundation
15 Belgrave Sq
London SW1X 8PG
0171-235 4904
0171-2355336 Fax

Cancer After Care and Rehabilitation
Society
21 Zetland Rd
Bristol BS6 7AH
01272-427419

Cancer Relief Macmillan Fund
15–19 Britten St
London SW3 3TZ
0171-351 7811
0171-376 8098 Fax

Clinical Genetics Society Northern
Region Genetics
19 Claremont Pl
Newcastle-upon-Tyne
NE2 4AA
0191-232 5131

CRUSE—Bereavement Care
126 Sheen Rd
Richmond
Surrey TW9 1UR
0181-940 4818

Cystic Fibrosis Association of Ireland
24 Lower Rathmines Rd
Dublin 6
Republic of Ireland
353 (1) 962433

Cystic Fibrosis Research Trust
5 Blyth Rd
Bromley BR1 3RS
0181-464 7211
0181-313 0472 Fax

Disabled Living Foundation
380–384 Harrow Rd
London W9 2HH
0171-286 6111

Down's Syndrome Association
153–155 Mitcham Rd
London SW17 9PG
0181-682 4001

Family Heart Association
7 High St
Kidlington
Oxford
OX5 2DH
018675-70292
018675-70295 Fax

HEADWAY
National Head Injury Association Ltd
7 King Edward Court
King Edward St
Nottinghamshire NG1 1EW
0115 9240800
0115 9240432

Irish Cancer Society
5 Northumberland Rd
Dublin 4
Republic of Ireland
353 (1) 681855

Irish Diabetic Association
82–83 Lower Gardiner St
Dublin 1
Republic of Ireland
353 (1) 363022

Let's Face It
c/o Christine Piff
10 Wood End
Crowthorne
Berks RG11 6DQ
01344-774405

Leukemia Care Society
14 Kingfisher Ct
Venny Bridge
Pinhoe
Exeter EX4 8JN
01392-64848

MIND—National Association for Mental Health
22 Harley St
London W1N 2ED
0171-637 0741

Multiple Sclerosis Society of
Great Britain & Northern
Ireland
25 Effie Rd
London SW6 1EE
0171-7366267
0171-7369861 Fax

Multiple Sclerosis Society of
Ireland
2 Sandymount Green
Dublin 4
Republic of Ireland
353 (1) 2694599
353 (1) 2693746 Fax

Muscular Dystrophy Group of
Great Britain
35 Macaulay Rd
London SW4 0QP
0171-720 8055

Muscular Dystrophy Society
of Ireland Ltd
2 Sandymount Green
Dublin 4
Republic of Ireland
353 (1) 2694599
353 (1) 2693746 Fax

National Association for Mental After
Care in Residential Care
PO Box 71
Derby DE1 9HB
01332-293617
01332-32072 Fax

National Association for the Mentally
Handicapped of Ireland,
5 Fitzwilliam Place
Dublin 2
Republic of Ireland
353 (1) 766035
353 (1) 760517 Fax

National Association for the
Relief of Paget's Disease
University of Manchester
Dept of Medicine

Hope Hospital
Salford M6 8HD
0161-787 4949
0161-787 4344 Fax

National Association of Laryngectomee
Clubs
Ground Floor
6 Rickett St
Fulham
London SW6 1RU
0171-381 9993

National Asthma Campaign
Providence House
Providence Place
London N1 0NT
0171-226 2260
0171-704 0740 Fax

National Back Pain Association
31–33 Park Rd
Teddington
Middx TW11 0AB
0181-977 5474
0181-943 5318 Fax

National Federation of Kidney
Patients Association
6 Stanley St
Worksop
Nottinghamshire S81 7HX
01909-487795
01909-481723 Fax

National League of the Blind
and Disabled
2 Tenterden Rd
London N17 8BE
0181-808 6030

National League of the Blind
of Ireland
35 Gardiner Place
Dublin 1
Republic of Ireland
353 (1) 742792

National Library for the Blind
Cromwell Rd
Bredbury
Stockport SK6 2SG
0161-494 0217
0161-406 6728 Fax

National Society for Epilepsy
Chalfont Centre for Epilepsy
Chalfont St Peter
Gerrards Cross
Bucks SL9 0RJ
012407-3991
012407-71927 Fax

Oesophageal Patients' Association
16 Whitefields Crescent
Solihull
West Midlands B91 3NU
0121-704 9860

Parkinson's Disease Society
of the United Kingdom
22 Upper Woburn Place
London
WC1H 0RA
0171-383 3513
0171-383 5754 Fax

Rehabilitation Institute
Roslyn Park
Sandymount
Dublin 4
Republic of Ireland
353 (1) 2698422
353 (1) 839732

Royal Association for Disability
and Rehabilitation (RADAR)
25 Mortimer St
London W1N 8AB
0171-6375400

Sickle Cell Society
54 Station Rd
London NW10 4UA
0181-961 7795

Spastics Society
12 Park Crescent
London W1N 4EQ
0171-636 5020
01800 626216 (help line)
0171-436 2601 Fax

Stroke Association
CHSA House
Whitecross St
London EC1Y 8JJ
0171-490 7999
0171-490 2686 Fax

Role of the Patient in Rehabilitation

The most important contributions to patients' rehabilitation are made by the patients themselves. The patient, his or her family, the nurse, the doctor, the social worker, the occupational therapist, and sometimes others planning together can arrive at the best plans for the future, but the patient's attitudes, acceptance, and motivation are the most important considerations. If the patient cannot adjust to the disability, whatever it is and however extensive, attempts at rehabilitation usually are hindered. Patients must make the decisions and they change at their own pace. If they are agreeable to suggestions but make little or no effort to try them, one should question if they really have accepted them.

Self-care is encouraged within existing limitations. The patient's behaviour from day to day can be the first indication of the direction of positive motivation. For example, if the patient makes every effort to resume normal daily activities such as feeding, bathing, and dressing, one can be certain that the person has a sincere desire to be independent. As patients become ready for more advanced activities, such as ambulation and sheltered work areas, they need continuing genuine interest and support. As obstacles arise, patients may be able to accept and eventually overcome them. Patients who are truly motivated towards helping themselves never seem to give up, finding ways of accomplishing activities that professional personnel might believe impossible. Each person working with the chronically ill patient has seen that many times life has meaning for the individual even though it may not be readily apparent to others. Some patients, however, when faced with an added burden, cannot accept it and give up trying. Guidance and support for the families of such patients become tremendously important. Health care personnel who understand these attitudes and behaviours can help make life more satisfying for the chronically ill person and can positively influence the behaviours of the family, professional co-workers, and the public.

Role of the Nurse in Rehabilitation

The concepts of comprehensive nursing care and rehabilitation can be considered synonymous. Helping the patient and family to help themselves is an integral part of nursing care. Nurses who work with patients who have disabilities have two major responsibilities: (1) to ensure that disability from disease or disuse is limited as much as possible and (2) to see that a rehabilitation programme is planned and implemented.

Limiting disability

Limitation of disability is the nurse's main responsibility and requires attention to the prevention of complications, to the early recognition of symptoms of exacerbations or complications, and to the prevention of deformity. For patients with chronic illnesses, the onset of exacerbations or complications is frequently subtle, marked by minute changes in functional ability or general performance or attitude. Nurses, working closely with such patients and understanding the pathophysiology of their diseases, are frequently the first to recognize initial signs of difficulty and make provision for appropriate intervention.

To be effective in the rehabilitation process, nurses must have an understanding of the techniques used by the various therapists so that they can plan and work cooperatively with them in caring for the patient. This knowledge is also used to help the patient employ appropriate techniques in carrying out activities of daily living.

CONTINUING CARE

Traditionally, health care professionals have assumed responsibility for the patient's well-being within the hospital and little to no responsibility for the patient and family in the home setting. This dichotomy between health care in the home and hospital facility made little sense. With chronically ill individuals the dichotomy interferes with a smooth transition from hospital to home. *The major portion of health care for people with chronic illnesses occurs in the home; thus ongoing communications must exist between the patient and health professionals.* Strauss et al.[45] advocate that sick people participate more in their care within health facilities and that health care professionals play a greater role in aiding chronically sick people *and* their families to cope with their problems at home. Social forces such as shorter hospital stays have made it necessary for nurses to be more aware of home health care needs.

Self-Help Groups

Self-help groups are associated with self-care. These groups may or may not include the guidance of health care personnel. They provide social support to their members through the creation of a caring community, and they increase members' coping skills through the sharing of information, experiences, and problem solutions. Examples of self-help groups include those for women who have had mastectomies and those for individuals who have colostomies, diabetes, or obesity. There are now self-help groups or clubs for patients with a variety of conditions. Nurses should learn what groups are available to patients in their community. A telephone call to an association such as BACUP, British Heart Foundation or National League for the Blind and Disabled, can elicit information about clubs available to patients who have the specific condition served by the agency.

In some hospitals and nursing homes nurses have been instrumental in setting up support groups for families of patients with chronic health problems such as Alzheimer's disease. It can be expected that more support groups, both those for patients and those for families, will be developing in the near future. Changes in governmental health policy (care in the community) have resulted in shorter hospital stays for both acute and chronic illnesses. As a result, patients and their families need to be better prepared to care for the patient in the home because patients are sent home sooner than in the past and their needs for continuing care are greater.

Facilities for Continuing Care

It is impossible to include here all the facilities that provide continuing care. Each of the programmes mentioned has its own criteria for acceptance of patients for the services it renders. *Before application for service is made and before the programme is discussed with the patient and family, the individual patient's eligibility for that service should be determined.*

Ambulatory care

The term *ambulatory care* is used interchangeably with *outpatient care* and *refers to first-contact health care services as well as to continuing contact services in settings that do not require overnight stays.* The use of ambulatory care facilities has expanded because of the increase in chronic illness and the increase in cost of inpatient services. A good ambulatory care service constitutes one of the most important elements of the hospital's contribution to community health. There is a trend towards development of ambulatory care facilities within the community to assist disabled, aged, or disadvantaged people to obtain needed health care. An ambulatory care centre usually provides long-term follow-up care needed by the person with a chronic illness, in addition to preventive health care, diagnostic workups, and treatment of acute illnesses for which hospitalization is unnecessary.

Home care

Before World War II the home was the place where medical treatment was given. Well-to-do people rarely went to a hospital; they received the services of a private doctor in their own home, and the family or nurses employed by the family were responsible for the day-to-day care. Poor families were among the first people to use hospitals. The philosophy of home care can be traced as far back as 1796, when the Boston Dispensary provided medical care to the sick poor in their homes.

One of the most obvious reasons for the development of home care programmes was to provide care to patients with long-term illnesses who did not need the around-the-clock services of an institution and yet who were too ill to go to an outpatient centre. Caring for patients at home is often desired by the individual and family, and it also releases hospital beds for use by acutely ill patients.

Today home care is being provided for acutely ill patients discharged from the hospital earlier than in the past and has meant that many patients are being discharged while they still need skilled nursing care. As a result, many hospitals have set up home care programmes to supply nursing care and other services to their patients after discharge.

Often the issue arises as to who should pay for home health services and who should be reimbursed for health care provided. America has for many years exercised a purchaser/provider financial service, and the American Nurses Association's position is that reimbursement systems should foster care of individuals in their homes based on the following premises[4]:

1. Home health care is humane and respectful of the individual's dignity and integrity.
2. Home care or care within the community can be less costly than institutional care.
3. Nursing care is the primary element in home care.
4. Payment systems for home care should recognize

nurses as the major providers of home care, and nurses should be reimbursed on their own authority. Home care may not be possible for all patients. For those living in smaller dwellings, adequate space for the patient, necessary equipment (oxygen, intravenous fluids, and so on) and for other members of the family may be at a premium. The choice of home care, independent living centre, or institutional care depends not only on the desires of the patient and the family, but also on the ability to finance the care. Despite many inconveniences, some families wish to have the patient with them. The family's understanding of the patient and their ability to assist one another will make a great difference in choosing between home care or other living arrangements. Not only may space be inadequate, but many times it is impossible to have a family member in attendance with the patient during the day. Family members who work cannot afford to sacrifice jobs to stay with the patient. However, many families find it easier financially to have the patient at home and are able to make satisfactory arrangements even though the facilities are limited.

Many communities in Britain provide Meals-on-Wheels for homebound people. Most programmes provide one hot meal daily and food that does not need to be heated for at least one other meal. The cost differs widely and depends on the services offered, such as special diets, and on the sponsorship of the plan. Volunteer groups frequently deliver the meals. This service alone often makes it possible for a chronically ill or aged person to remain at home.

Home care services

The early discharge of patients from hospitals has increased the need for these services even more. Home care workers provide physical care to the patient after a registered nurse evaluates the home situation and the patient's need for physical personal care. They are also responsible for keeping the patient's environment clean. Ongoing supervision of the home care worker can lie between the registered nurse and social services.

Day care centres

In many communities some senior centres and nursing homes are expanding their facilities and services to include day care centres. Many chronically ill people are able to live with their families but require 24-hour attendance. Often the carer in the family has to work. Day care centres can provide a place where the chronically ill person can be looked after on a daily basis. Nursing services, physio and occupational therapy, recreational therapy, meals, and, in some instances, transportation to and from the centre are provided. This form of service may allow a person to remain at home with the family rather than having to resort to institutional care.

Respite care services

Some nursing homes and hospitals maintain a specified number of beds for respite care. As the name implies, these beds are available on a short-term basis to provide respite for families who have a chronically ill person at home. The day-to-day care of the patient, often 24 hours a day, is a very trying experience for any family. To provide the family or primary carer with a period free of this responsibility, respite care may be the answer.

Services such as Marie Curie, can be employed either privately or through the hospital to sit with a patient (with cancer) in order to give the carer a "break". Many hospice units have developed sitting services also, and can supply respite care in the patient's own home for part of a day, for 24 hours, or for extended periods depending on need.

Sheltered Accommodation

Some people with chronic illnesses may be unable to cope with the demands of maintaining a home but wish to live as independently as possible. Various options are available in some communities; these range from accommodation where people cook their meals but have the flat maintained, to accommodation where people can have their own living area but where one or more meals a day and other services are available. Sheltered accommodation is designed with such features as handrails for support in ambulation, wide doors to facilitate passage of wheelchairs, and emergency call systems.

Institutional care

Institutional care may be necessary when alternatives are not available, or the type of care needed by the patient requires close professional supervision. This includes chronic disease hospitals, skilled care facilities, convalescent homes, rest homes, homes for the aged, and nursing homes. Chelsea Pensioners Association provides services for men and women who have served in one of the British Armed forces. The patient's potential for rehabilitation, need for maintenance care, or the level of physical disability are factors that determine eligibility for placement in any of these facilities. A large or limited selection of outside facilities may be available, depending on the community.

Role of the Nurse in Continuing Health Care

A nurse may be involved in continuing health care in several ways: (1) as an independent nurse practitioner assisting the person with chronic illness to cope with problems incurred by the illness; (2) as a public health nurse or community nurse involved in a primary rehabilitative programme in the home; (3) as a supervisor of home care workers; or (4) as a nurse in a hospital concerned about the care patients will be receiving after they leave the hospital, particularly when the patient's rehabilitation programme is not completed before discharge or when rehabilitation is not possible. Any of these nurses may also be involved in research pertaining to chronic illness. Some concepts that need further study in the area of chronic disease include social stigmatization, effects of isolation, and effects of chronic illness on the family, marriage, and domestic and occupational roles. Research will make a major contribution to clarification of these general concepts by identifying their relationship to chronic health problems.

Nurses must know the community resources available to patients to inform them and their families about what resources they might obtain, the types of service from which they may benefit, and what referrals they need for obtaining those

services (see Box 10-2 for a list of community resources). The hospital nurse should clearly communicate to the continuing care agency the data pertinent to the patient's care so that continuity is ensured. Teamwork and continuity are the keys to successful rehabilitation and management services for patients, and they must be practised at all stages of care if patients are to realize their fullest potential.

FOCUS ON THE FUTURE
Priority Care Services

As mentioned earlier, the context of "priority groups" can be traced back to a 1976 consultative document. It was coined to refer to groups of people in need who had historically been neglected by the health service, that is:
- Elderly people
- Mentally ill people
- Mentally handicapped people
- Physically and sensorily handicapped people

There was an emerging consensus in the mid to late 1970s that these groups must receive greater priority. The DHSS guidance in 1977 was significantly diluted in comparison to the aspirations of the 1976 consultative document, and was to become weaker still by 1981 when the DHSS published a handbook of policies and priorities.

Implications for nursing

It is important for nurses to know about the provisions of the priority care services so that they can provide the disabled with optimum information.

Nurses working in the rehabilitation settings will be able to employ nursing interventions that will assist the disabled person to function at his or her highest possible level. The role of the nurse in rehabilitation is discussed earlier in this chapter (see p. 168).

All nurses as citizens can be advocates for the disabled and help articulate their needs to the general public. Nurses can be active in their own communities to ensure that the public accommodations and public service provisions are carried out.[32]

Health Care Goals for the Year 2000

The Health of the Nation Green Paper, published in June, 1991, stimulated extensive public debate. More than 2000 individuals and organizations contributed their views. Dozens of conferences, seminars and workshops were held. Newspaper and journal articles were written debating the issues raised on health and how it might be improved. The strategy:
- Selects five key areas for action
- Sets national objectives and targets in the key areas
- Indicates the action needed to achieve the targets
- Outlines initiatives to help implement the strategy
- Sets the framework for monitoring, development and review

Five key areas, in which substantial improvement in health can be achieved were selected (see Box 10-4), and each area has national targets. The majority of the targets relate to the year 2000, but some look further to the future.

10-3

Aims of priority care services

Elderly People

Strengthen primary and community care services to enable elderly people to live at home. (It was acknowledged that some might need the additional support of sheltered accommodation, but that this form of housing provision would be available to relatively few.)
Encourage an active approach to treatment and rehabilitation, to enable elderly people to return to the community.
Maintain capacity in the general acute sector to deal with the increasing number of elderly patients.
Maintain adequate provision for elderly people requiring long-term care.

Mentally Ill People

In keeping with a community-focused approach, it is envisaged there should be a widespread hospital closure programme, and provide a service reaching out into the community.

Mentally Handicapped

Provide a locally-based service that enables mentally handicapped people to be with their families, where possible, or in a local community setting.
Help develop the capabilities of each individual so that he or she can live as independent a life as possible.
Support those looking after mentally handicapped people at home by providing day services and short-term residential care.

Physically Disabled

Relieve pressure on carers through more short-term carers and treatment.
Improve arrangements for caring for younger disabled people separately from elderly people.
Help those with hearing impairments make best use of the improved range of aids.
Improve co-ordination between authorities to ensure visually handicapped people are aware of, and can benefit from, the services and advice available to them.

From NAHAT *NHS Handbook*, 8th edition, JMH Publishing, Kent, United Kingdom, 1993/1994.

Within the key areas, emphasis is placed on risk factors, such as smoking and dietary imbalances.

Health in England Today

Health in the U.K. is better than it has ever been. Many diseases have been brought under control and some almost eliminated. A century ago, four out of ten babies did not survive to adulthood. Life expectancy at birth was only 44 years for boys and 48 years for girls. As recently as the early 1930s, 2500 women died during pregnancy or childbirth every year. Today, infant mortality, a basic indicator of any nation's health, stands at under eight per 1000 live births.

10-4

Key areas identified by *The Health of the Nation* (1992)

Coronary heart disease and stroke
Cancers
Mental illness
HIV/AIDS and sexual health
Accidents

Life expectancy at birth is now 73 years for boys and 79 years for girls. Over the last century, death rates from infectious diseases have fallen dramatically; although immunization and the development of effective treatments have played their part, the improvement in health has essentially resulted from social and public health measures.[24a]

Health of the Nation Main Targets

Coronary Heart Disease (CHD) and Stroke
1. To reduce death rates for both CHD and stroke in people under 65 by at least 40% by the year 2000 (from 58 per 100,000 population in 1990 to no more than 35 per 100,000 for CHD, and from 12.5 per 100,000 population in 1990 to no more than 7.5 per 100,000 for stroke).
2. To reduce the death rate for CHD in people aged 65 to 74 by at least 30% by the year 2000 (from 899 per 100,000 population in 1990 to no more than 629 per 100,000)
3. To reduce the death rate for stroke in people aged 65 to 74 by at least 40% by the year 2000 (from 265 per 100,000 population in 1990 to no more than 159 per 100,000).
4. To reduce the prevalence of cigarette smoking in men and women aged 16 and over to no more than 20% by

Table 10.1	Five broad goals for the year 2000

1. To reduce the level of ill-health and death caused by coronary heart disease and stroke, and the risk factors associated with them.
2. To reduce ill-health and death caused by breast and cervical cancer, skin cancers, lung cancer and other conditions associated with them
3. To reduce ill-health and death caused by mental illness.
4. To reduce the incidence of HIV, and other sexually transmitted diseases, to reduce the number of un wanted pregnancies, and to ensure the provision of effective family planning services for those people who want them.
5. To reduce ill-health, disability and death caused by accidents.

Source: Secretary of State for Health: *The health of the nation—a strategy for health in England*, London, HMSO, 1992.

the year 2000 (a reduction of at least 35% in men and 29% in women, from a prevalence in 1990 of 31% and 28% respectively).

5. To reduce the average percentage of food energy derived by the population from saturated fatty acids by at least 35% by 2005 (from 17% in 1990 to no more than 11%).
6. To reduce the average percentage of food energy derived by the population from total fat by at least 12% by 2005 (from about 40% in 1990 to no more than 35%).
7. To reduce the percentages of men and women aged 16–64 who are obese by at least 25% for men and at least 33% for women by 2005 (from 8% for men and 12% for women in 1986/87 to no more than 6% and 8% respectively).
8. To reduce mean systolic blood pressure in the adult population by at least 5 mmHg by 2005.
9. To reduce the proportion of men drinking more than 21 units of alcohol per week from 28% in 1990 to 18% by 2005, and the proportion of women drinking more than 14 units of alcohol per week from 11% in 1990 to 7% by 2005.

Cancers

1. To reduce the death rate for breast cancer in the population invited for screening by at least 25% by the year 2000 (from 95.1/100,000 in 1990 to no more than 71.3/100,000).
2. To reduce the incidence of invasive cervical cancer by at least 20% by the year 2000 (from 15/100,000 in 1986 to no more than 12/100,000).
3. To halt the year on year increase in the incidence of skin cancer by 2005.
4. To reduce the death rate for lung cancer by at least 30% in men under 75 and 15% in women under 75 by 2010 (from 60/100,000 men and 24.1/100,000 women in 1990 to no more than 42 and 20.5 respectively).

5. To reduce the prevalence of cigarette smoking in men and women aged 16 and over to no more than 20% by the year 2000 (reduction of at least 35% in men and 29% in women from a prevalence in 1990 of 31% and 28% respectively).
6. In addition to the overall reduction in prevalence, at least a third of women smokers to stop smoking at the start of their pregnancy by the year 2000.
7. To reduce the consumption of cigarettes by at least 40% by the year 2000 (from 98 billion manufactured cigarettes per year in 1990 to 59 billion).
8. To reduce smoking prevalence among 11–15 year olds by at least 33% by 1994 (from about 8% in 1988 to less than 6%).

Mental Illness

1. To improve significantly the health and social functioning of mentally ill people.
2. To reduce the overall suicide rate by at least 15% by the year 2000 (from 11.1/100,000 in 1990 to no more than 9.4).
3. To reduce the suicide rate of severely mentally ill people by at least 33% by the year 2000 (from the estimate of 15% in 1990 to no more than 10%).

HIV/AIDS and Sexual Health

1. To reduce the incidence of gonorrhoea among men and women aged 15–64 by at last 20% by 1995 (from 61 new cases per 100,000 in 1990 to no more than 49 new cases per 100,000).
2. To reduce the rate of conceptions among the under 16 year olds by at least 50% by the year 2000 (from 9.5 per 1000 girls aged 13–15 in 1989 to no more than 4.8).
3. To reduce the percentage of injecting drug misusers who report sharing injecting equipment in the previous four weeks by at least 50% by 1997 and by at least a further 50% by the year 2000 (from 20% in 1990 to no more than 10% by 1997 and no more than 5% by the year 2000).

Accidents

1. To reduce the death rate for accidents among children aged under 15 by at least 33% by 2005 (from 6.7 per 100,000 in 1990 to no more than 4.5/100,000).
2. To reduce the death rate for accidents among young people aged 15–24 by at least 25% by 2005 (from 23.2 per 100,000 in 1990 to no more than 17.4 per 100,000).
3. To reduce the death rate for accidents among people aged 65 and over by at least 33% by 2005 (from 56.7 per 100,000 in 1990 to no more than 38 per 100,000).

Management System for People With Chronic Conditions

In looking at health care for the chronically ill, it seems obvious that some changes need to be made. One consultant to hospitals in America has suggested that hospitals need to look at their focus on acute care and give higher priority to care of the chronically ill.[14] He recommends that hospitals develop Chronic Disease Centres just as they have developed Ambulatory Surgery Centres. He points out that the present health care delivery system is oriented to intervening in the disease process and "fixing" the condition whereas people with a chronic condition are trying to minimize their chronic condition and live as normal lives as possible.

He also suggests that Chronic Disease Centres could become the primary care provider for people with chronic conditions. His suggestion will not be acceptable to all care providers including many nurses who believe that clinical nurse specialists and nurse practitioners are the ideal health care providers for these patients because much of their care involves teaching and counselling, which are central parts of the nursing role.

Burkhardt et al. describe the results of a research project using the Quality of Life Scale (QOLS) and point out what nurses might wish to keep in mind as they work with people with chronic conditions.[2]

> There is no reason to believe people with a stable chronic illness or condition cannot have as high a quality of life as those without chronic illness although care must be taken to see that the definition and measurement of *[quality of life]* be *[clearly subjective satisfaction]* and not be confounded with objective measure of health status.

SUMMARY

1. Chronic health problems are one of the major health problems in Britain.
2. The incidence and prevalence of chronic diseases have increased in this century and can be expected to increase even more as the population ages.
3. According to the GHS census, 32% of respondents indicated they had a long-standing illness; 18% a limiting long standing illness, and 13% restricted activity in the previous two weeks.
4. There are major disparities in the health of ethnic groups in Britain when compared with the white population.
5. The characteristics of chronic illnesses include one or more of the following: (1) illness or impairment that is permanent, (2) residual disability, and (3) nonreversible pathological alteration, which requires a long period of care.
6. Chronic illnesses may be present from birth or develop during childhood, adolescence, early adult life, or old age.
7. Today some children with chronic illnesses such as cystic fibrosis live into early adulthood because of more effective treatment.
8. Major chronic illnesses of adults include arthritis, diabetes, heart disease, and hypertension. The rates for arthritis and hypertension are higher in blacks than in whites.
9. Cultural values determine how both nurses and patients view chronic illness.
10. The economic costs of chronic illness are considerable and many people will require some type of financial assistance.
11. Failure to understand or internalize the reason for therapeutic recommendations, procedures that are difficult to learn and carry out, time necessary to carry out therapy, side effects of therapy, inability to pay for prescribed therapy, and social isolation and lack of support and positive reinforcement are possible reasons why a person may be noncompliant with therapeutic recommendations.
12. It is important that nurses be involved in prevention of chronic illness.
13. There are three levels of prevention: primary, secondary, and tertiary, and the nurse has an important role to play at each level.
14. Primary prevention involves health promotion and specific protection against disease (such as immunization against poliomyelitis).
15. Secondary prevention includes early detection of disease and prompt intervention to halt progression of disease.
16. Tertiary prevention includes rehabilitation appropriate to the stage of disability, prevention of further complications, and restoring optimal functioning to the highest possible level.
17. Depression is common among the chronically ill, especially those who feel powerless about controlling or overcoming what has happened to them.
18. Rehabilitation is best carried out in a setting where an intradisciplinary team of nurses, physicians, physiotherapists and occupational therapists, social workers and, when necessary, speech therapists are available to work together in planning the therapeutic regimen for the patient and in assisting and supporting the patient with the prescribed therapy.
19. The nurse should be familiar with the facilities for continuing care in his or her community and the eligibility requirements for each facility.
20. The term Priority Care Services was coined to refer to groups of people in need which had historically been neglected by the health service. The DHSS issued guidelines in 1977 in service provision for these four groups, but they were considered to be considerably diluted from the original 1976 consultative document.
21. Health for all by the year 2000 WHO initiative was the central theme on which the Health of the National document was built. This document identifies five key areas for improving health surveillance.
22. Nurses need to be aware of the plans of the state in which they reside for meeting the goals for the year 2000.

STUDY QUESTIONS

- What types of patients do you think are most in need of rehabilitation? Outline the rehabilitation needs of a patient you are now caring for or have cared for in the past.

- What proportion of the patients on the hospital unit to which you are assigned has a chronic illness as either a primary or secondary diagnosis? What proportion has more than one chronic health problem? What age group is affected most by more than one chronic health problem?

- What resources are available in your community for the care of the chronically ill? Are the facilities adequate for the number of people needing care? How are these facilities supported financially?

- From what you have learned in anatomy, outline in detail the physical movements necessary to rise from a sitting position in a chair to a standing position. Describe how you would assist a patient to stand while allowing him or her to be as independent as possible.

REFERENCES AND SELECTED READINGS

1. American Cancer Society: 1991 *Cancer facts and figures,* Atlanta, 1991, The Society.

2.* Burckhardt CS et al: Quality of life of adults with chronic illness: a psychometric study, *Res Nurs Health* 12:347–354, 1989.

3. Centers for Disease Control Report to the Secretary's task force on black and minority health, *MMWR* 35(8), 1986.

4.* Centers for Disease Control chronic disease reports, *MMWR* 38(S-1), 1989.

5.* Centers for Disease Control: Progress in chronic disease prevention, *MMWR* 38(8), 1989.

6.* Centers for Disease Control: Progress in chronic disease prevention, *MMWR* 38(12), 1989.

7.* Centers for Disease Control: Health objectives for the nation, *MMWR* 38(37), 1989.

8.* Centers for Disease Control: Chronic disease reports in the morbidity and mortality weekly report (MMWR) 38(S-1), 1989.

8a. Central Statistical Office: *Social trends—crime and justice,* London, HMSO, 1993.

9. Council on Ethical and Judicial Affairs: Black-white disparities in health care, *JAMA* 263(17):2344-2346, 1990.

10. Council on Scientific Affairs: Home care in the 1990s, *JAMA* 263(8):1241-1244, 1990.

11. DeLisa JA, Jain SS: Physical medicine and rehabilitation, *JAMA* 265(23):358-359, 1991.

11a. Department of Health: *On the state of the public health for the year 1990,* London, HMSO.

11b. Department of Health and Social Services: *Priorities for health and personal social services in England—a consultative document,* London, HMSO, 1976.

12. Dittmar S: *Rehabilitation nursing,* St Louis, 1989, Mosby–Year Book.

13.* Older Americans present a double challenge: preventing disability and providing care, *Am J Pub Health,* 81(3):287-288, March 1991 (editorial).

14. Henry WF: Chronic care needs to be a higher priority, *Hospitals* Feb 20: 68, 1991.

15. Kahn KL et al: Comparing outcomes of care before and after implementation of the DRG-based prospective payment system, *JAMA* 264(15):1984-1988, 1990.

16. Kemper P, Murtaugh CM: Lifetime use of nursing home care, *New Engl J Med* 324(9):595-600, 1991.

17.* Lambert VA, Lambert CE, editors: Adaptation to chronic illness, *Nurs Clin North Am* 22:527-644, 1987.

18.* Leidy NK: A structural model of stress, psychosocial resources, and symptomatic experiences in chronic physical illness, *Nurs Outlook* 34(4):230-236, 1990.

19. Lubkin IM: *Chronic illness: impact and interventions,* Boston, 1986, Jones & Bartlett Publishing.

19a. National Association of Health Trusts: *NHS handbook,* 8/e, Kent, United Kingdom, JMH Publishing, 1993.

20. National Center for Health Statistics: *Vital statistics of the United States, 1980,* vol 11, Mortality, part B, DHHS, Pub No (PHS) 85-1102, Washington, DC, 1985, US Government Printing Office.

20a. Office of Population Census and Surveys: *Population and vital statistics,* London, HMSO, 1990.

20b. Office of Population Census and Surveys: *Sickness and invalidity benefits,* London, HMSO, 1991.

21.* Pollock SE: Human response to chronic illness: physiologic and psychosocial adaptation, *Nurs Res* 35:90-95, 1986.

22. Primomo J, Yates BC, Woods NF: Social support for women during chronic illnesses: the relationship among sources and types to adjustment, *Res Nurs Health* 13:153-161, 1990.

23. Public Health Service: Vital and health statistics: current estimates from the National Health Interview Survey, 1989, US Department of Health, Education, and Welfare.

24.* Schwartz E, et al: Black/white comparisons of deaths preventable by medical intervention: United States and the District of Columbia 1980-1986, *Int J Epidemiol* 19(3):591-598, 1990.

24a. Secretary of State for Health: *The health of the nation—a strategy for health in England,* London, HMSO, 1992.

25. Shaughnessy PW, Kramer AM: The increased needs of patients in nursing homes and patients receiving home health care, *New Engl J Med* 322(1):21–27, 1990.

26.* Stewart Al, et·al: Functional status and well-being of patients with chronic conditions, *JAMA* 262(7):907-193, 1989.

27. US Bureau of the Census: *Statistical abstract of the United States, 1986,* annual ed 107, Washington, DC, 1987, US Government Printing Office.

28. US Department of Health and Human Services: *Healthy People 2000: national health promotion and disease prevention objectives,* Washington, DC, 1990, US Government Printing Office.

29. US Department of Health and Human Services: *Vital and health statistics: current estimates from the national health interview survey,* 1989, Washington, 1990, US Government Printing Office.

30. US Department of Health and Human Services, Secretary's task force on black and minority health, Washington, 1985, US Government Printing Office.

31.* Van Horne WA, Tonnesen TV, editors: *Ethnicity and health,* Madison, 1988, The University of Wisconsin System Institute on Race and Ethnicity.

32.* Watson PG: The Americans with Disabilities Act: More rights for people with disabilities, *Rehab Nurs* 15(6): 325-328, 1990.

33.* American Academy of Nursing: Long-term care: some issues for nursing, Kansas City, Mo, 1976, American Nurses' Association.

34.* American Nurses' Association: A national policy for health care: principles and positions, Kansas City, Mo, 1977, The Association.

35. Expectation of life in the United States at a new high, *Stat Bull* 61(4):13-15, 1980.

36.* Johnson JH, editor: Rehabilitation nursing: *Nurs Clin North Am* 15:2, 1980.

37. Leslie PM: Nursing diagnosis: use in long-term care, *Am J Nurs* 81:1012-1014, 1981.

38. Morris R, editor: Allocating health resources for the aged and disabled, Lexington, Mass, 1981, Lexington Books.

39. Moskowitz E, McCann CB: Classification of disability in the chronically ill and aging, *J Chronic Dis* 5:342-346, 1957.

40.* Olson EV: The hazards of immobility, *Am J Nurs* 67:780-797, 1967.

41. Public Health Service: *Vital and health statistics: current estimates from the Health Interview Survey (1981),* series 10, No 141, Rockville, Md, Oct 1982, US Dept of Health, Education, and Welfare.

42. Public Health Service: *Vital and health statistics: health characteristics of persons with chronic activity limitations (1979),* series 10, No 137, Rockville, Md, Dec 1981, US Dept of Health and Human Services.

43. Ryan S, Wassenberg C, editors: Community health and home care nursing, *Nurs Clin North Am* 15:2, 1980.

44.* Sorensen K, Armis DB: Understanding the world of the chronically ill, *Am J Nurs* 67:811-817, 1967.

45.* Strauss AL et al: Chronic illness and the quality of life, ed 2, St Louis, 1984, Mosby Year–Book.

46. Thom A: Home health care agencies in the 1980s, *Home Health Care Serv Q* 3:5-24, 1982.

47. US Dept of Health, Education, and Welfare: *Healthy people, Surgeon General's report on health promotion and disease prevention*, Washington, DC, 1979, US Government Printing Office.

48.* Wright BA: Value-laden beliefs and principles for rehabilitation, *Rehabil Lit* 12:266-269, 1981.

FURTHER READING

Anonymous. Honoring the personal side of chronic illness: systemic lupus erythematosus, *Nursing,* 15 (11 World Ed):52–7, Nov. 1985.

Barnes G: Asthma: latest developments in care, *Professional Nurse,* June, 3(9):364-8. 1988.

Brandt KD, Potts MK, Barton R, Sokolek C: How financial barriers can frustrate good arthritis care, *Geriatrics* May; 43(5):83-8. 1988.

Burke TR: The economic impact of alcohol abuse and alcoholism, *Public Health Report* Nov-Dec: 103(6):564-8., 1988.

Cohen FL: Narcolepsy: a review of a common, life-long sleep disorder, *Journal of Advanced Nursing* Sep; 13(5):546–56, 1988.

Cooper J: Food intolerance and joint symptoms: historical review and present day application, *Physiotherapy* 77(12):847–58 Dec. 1991.

Cottingham B: Rationing community care, *Nursing Times* March 16-22, 84(11):16-7 1988. O'Connor S, Wright M. An ongoing partnership in care: nursing innovations in a rehabilitation ward, *Professional Nurse* 7(6):266, 368-70 March 1992.

Murphy E. Government must act on community care, (editorial) *BMJ* Dec 17; 297 (6663):1558-9 1988.

Thorne SE, Robinson CA: Reciprocal trust in health care relationships, *Journal of Advanced Nursing,* Nov; 13(6):782-9 1988.

*Recommended for student reading.

11

Loss, Dying, and Death

Sally M. Featherstone

After studying this chapter, the learner should be able to:

- Describe losses to self, external losses, and factors influencing loss experiences.
- Describe the phases of life-threatening illness.
- Discuss the basis tasks of grief.
- Discuss the crisis model as an assessment tool for coping.
- Describe nursing interventions for patients/families coping with life-threatening events.
- Compare patient/family tasks associated with each phase of the dying process.
- Discuss the process and stress of nurses' grief and survival strategies when working with dying patients and bereaved families.

Nurses who work with terminally ill and bereaved people often develop a heightened empathy and identification with their patients. This occurs because the loss experience is so universal that everyone has experienced its impact. These losses can prepare us for the ultimate loss in death. Grief is the normal and universal response to loss.

Dying and death are not synonymous; they are distinct and separate events. Almost nothing can be known about death, at least on this side of parapsychology and faith. A great deal, however, can be known about dying. A pattern of dying is lived by each person in his or her lifetime. Life can be described as a migration through many little dyings, losses, and grieving for those losses. Growth, change, and maturing occur by adaptation to the losses occurring throughout one's lifetime. Nurses can learn about the "big" dying by understanding the "little" dyings.[38]

UNDERSTANDING LOSS
Basic Assumptions

When people do not do "grief work" following any significant loss, they are at risk for emotional, mental, and social problems. A review of the literature reveals many examples of increased morbidity, both physical and mental, following significant losses.[9,16,21,23,43] There is an increase in the breakup of marriages and other significant relationships following the loss of a child or when one partner suffers a loss of body part or function.[24]

Loss is defined as any change in a person's situation that reduces the probability of achieving goals or when a person is without something he/she formerly possessed. It can be anticipatory. A loss need not have occurred to stimulate a grief response. Loss is inevitable and inescapable—no one is exempt from loss. There are hardly any gains in life that have not grown out of or been accompanied by loss; for example, a person who receives a promotion gains in stature and income, but may simultaneously lose the support of his or her previous peer group. Losses accumulated without resolution lead to energy depletion and increased vulnerability to psychological stress. Loss is a complex phenomenon.

Categories of Loss

Losses can be described as related to the self or as external to the self (Box 11-1). Self losses include the loss of the psychological self, the sociocultural self, the physical self, and the spiritual self. The ultimate loss of self is the loss of self because of death. External losses include the loss of objects, possessions, loved ones, support, and environment.[25]

Self losses

Loss of the psychological self includes loss of self-esteem and personal identity. Some examples are:
1. Mrs Smith, who has been married for many years suddenly loses her husband. She not only loses her husband, but she also loses all that being Mrs Smith meant.
2. John Jones has been a Professor of English for 30 years. He recently retired and no longer has the

11-1	**Categories of loss**

Self losses
    Loss of the psychological self
    Loss of the sociocultural self
    Loss of the physical self
    Loss of the spiritual self
External losses
    Objects, possessions
    Loved ones
    Environment
    Support
Real or imagined losses
Present or anticipated losses

responsibilities that go with being a teacher. He is no longer Professor Jones, just Mr Jones.

Any loss that affects the way one perceives oneself as a competent and capable person impacts the psychological self.

Loss of the sociocultural self includes the loss of language, associations, and the meanings of one's cultural heritage. Loss of the sociocultural self occurs when a person is suddenly thrust into an alien culture or has divided loyalties to different cultures. A nurse can belong to a religious group whose beliefs are in conflict with her work assignments, as in the case of a Catholic who is assigned to work in a family planning clinic. Society's demand for conformity places much pressure on people with different values and beliefs and often causes a person to be separated from familiar and comforting surroundings and people. This can be observed in countries with a history of colonization; for example in the United Sates, the native Americans have been forced to integrate into the Anglo-Saxon way of life. When confronted with life-threatening situations, they may well worry about possible discrimination and, fearful of giving expression to their needs, remain silent.[10] This can also be seen when patients are hospitalized. They no longer have control over their surroundings. They are expected to learn how to be "good" patients. People are shaped by the cultural values of the ethnic, religious, and social segment of the society in which they are reared. When access to that network is denied, the person suffers the loss of the sociocultural self.

Losses of the physical self are more obvious, but their impact is not necessarily so clear. The extent, duration, and visibility of the loss will influence how the individual responds to the loss. Loss of one leg could be less significant than the loss of both legs. A temporary loss of body function is much more easily adapted to than a permanent loss would be. People confined to wheelchairs often report being treated as incompetent. Beland relates the story of going shopping in a wheelchair—the shop assistant asked Beland's companion what Beland wanted instead of speaking to Beland directly.[24] The meaning of the particular body part involved will also have an impact. It will make a significant difference if the people who lose the use of their legs are football players or accountants. The loss to the football player is central to his life goals and therefore is likely to have a much greater impact than the same loss might have on an accountant whose legs are not critical to success as an accountant.

Loss of the spiritual self refers to the loss of hope, values, and beliefs. Many writers have identified the critical role that maintenance of hope plays for the person with a life-threatening illness. Without hope, despair sets in and the patient gives up.*

External losses

External losses include the loss of objects, possessions, loved ones, environment, and support. These losses can be real or imagined, present or anticipated. The importance of the loss of objects or possessions is influenced by the value of the object, both monetary and sentimental, and the usefulness of the object. A lost loved one may be a family member, a friend, or an acquaintance. The loss can occur through separation, moving, promotion, or death. The loss of familiar surroundings or other supports can leave one feeling vulnerable and lonely. The impact of loss through the death of a loved one is discussed later.

Factors Influencing Loss

Loss is a complex phenomenon, influenced by many factors (Box 11-2). A review of these factors is helpful in understanding what a specific loss means to an individual. Generalizations about personal experiences and behaviour are useful only when one is committed to understanding and accepting individual variations.

Childhood experiences can impact the way one perceives and reacts to a loss. How parents handle losses can influence a child's view of loss as a challenge or something to be avoided at all costs. If parents protect a child from experiencing the grief associated with loss, the child may think that loss is something bad. A child's first experience with death is often the death of a pet, such as when a pet goldfish dies. Parents can use this as an opportunity to discuss death or they can cover it up by replacing the dead fish before the child knows what has happened. A child who is punished for losing things, as in the nursery rhyme about the three little kittens who lost their mittens, may later experience guilt as the predominant emotion related to loss.

The significance assigned to the loss can be related to the objective or subjective value of the object. An illustration of this is the story of a couple who is in the process of moving. The wife has a heavy old mantle clock that has been in the family for generations. The husband thinks the clock is ugly and it weighs a ton. The removal people lift the clock out of the removal van and drop it. The clock shatters. The wife is horrified and bursts into tears. The husband can barely contain his glee. The objective value of the clock is the same, but its subjective value to each of the people involved has a major impact on their response to the loss.

One's *physical and emotional status* at the time of a loss can have a significant influence on one's response. Nurse Nelly is getting ready for work. She woke up with a headache and she is running late; the alarm did not go off. She is anxious because her new nurse manager starts today.

---

*References 1, 3, 7, 8, 12, 15.

11-2	**Factors influencing loss experiences**

Factors influencing loss experiences

Childhood experiences
Significance assigned to the loss
Physical and emotional state
Accumulated loss experience
View of loss as crisis
Visibility
Duration and timing
Abruptness or suddenness
Financial impact
Availability of resources
Cultural factors
Personal attributes
Relationship with the lost person
Death surround

Nelly cannot find her car keys. She feels overwhelmed and dissolves into a sobbing heap on the floor. On a normal day she would have been slightly irritated and would have remembered that she has a spare set of keys and would only have lost a few minutes.

Accumulated losses can impact how a person responds to a current loss, especially if there are unresolved losses. A nurse was interviewing a family after the loss of a baby to sudden infant death syndrome. The grandparents were present. The grandmother began to sob uncontrollably. The nurse inquired about the grandmother's past experience with loss and found that she had recently lost a son in a car accident and had a history of miscarriages that she had never been able to talk about.

View of the loss as a crisis is an important factor. It can be helpful to understand how a person experiencing the loss perceives his or her ability to cope. A crisis is defined by the person experiencing the event. The balancing forces of crisis are (1) the person's view of the situation; (2) the feelings experienced and expressed; (3) previous problem-solving efforts made in this situation; and (4) the person's support system, both internal and external. If any of these balancing forces are absent or unavailable to people coping with the loss, they are likely to perceive themselves as being in crisis.

Visibility can have both a positive and negative effect on the loss. Visibility of the loss can increase the support offered, as in the example where a family loses its home in a fire and the neighbourhood offers support through donations and assistance. Visibility can have a negative effect when it brings forth nonsupportive expressions, as in the situation of a person who has experienced a facially disfiguring accident that causes people to stare in horror. Other losses may fail to call forth support because they are invisible, as in the case of the loss of a baby before term.

Duration and timing can impact a loss depending on the degree of goal disruption that results from the time spent in resolving the loss. An athlete who suffers a broken leg may only be disrupted temporarily. However, if the break occurs before a key event, it may result in the athlete not getting an opportunity to compete at that level. If the break is of short duration, and timing is not an issue, the athlete may resume

Table 11-1   Children's responses to loss and death

Age years	Developmental stage/task	Concept of death	Grief response
2–4	Egocentric. Believes world centres around self. Narcissistic. No cognitive understanding. Pre-conceptual, unable to grasp concepts.	Seen as abandonment. Seen as reversible. "Did you know my daddy died—when will he be home?"	Intense, brief. Very present-oriented. Most aware of altered pattern of care.
4–7	Gaining sense of autonomy. Exploring world outside of self. Gaining language. Fantasy. Initiative phase. Concerns of guilt.	Death still seen as reversible. Personification of death. Feels responsible, because of wishes, thoughts. "It's my fault. I was mad at her and wished she would die."	Verbalization. Great concern with process. How? Why? Repetitive questioning.
7–11	Concrete. Industry versus inferiority. Begins socialization. Developing of cognitive ability. Begins logical thinking.	Death as punishment. Fear of bodily harm, mutilation. Difficult transition period; still wants to see death as reversible, but beginning to see it as final.	Specific questions. Desire for details. Concern with how others respond. What is the right way? How should they respond? Begins to mourn.
11–18	Formal problem solving. Abstract thinking. Integration of own personality.	"Adult" approach. Conceptualizes death. Works at making sense of teachings.	Depression. Denial. Repression. Willing to talk to people outside family. Traditional mourning.

Modified from Metzgar M: Little ears, big issues: children and loss, Seattle, 1990 (pamphlet).

his or her career with little effect. However, an accident that results in permanent paralysis will have a major impact on the loss adjustment of the individual.

Abruptness or suddenness of the loss will influence how one copes with it. It is generally agreed that a sudden loss is more difficult to cope with than one that is expected and for which a person has had time to prepare.

Financial impact adds a secondary loss. The longer and more extensive the loss, the greater the expense usually involved. This is particularly significant when the primary loss results in the inability of the individual to return to work. Bereaved families have been known to express a great deal of anger and pain upon receiving a large bill incurred by a family member who died because it adds insult to injury.

Availability of resources, both internal and external, are important to the individual's ability to cope with the challenges resulting from the loss. Prior experience in successfully coping with loss can provide the internal support to deal with the current loss. However, if the loss is sufficiently different and catastrophic, such as a sudden violent death, previous coping is not likely to suffice to support the individual. External support from family, friends, acquaintances, and professional or community services is essential.[9]

Culture is the dynamic system of values that informs and influences most loss situations. Culture is an integrated system of learned patterns of behaviour, ideas, and products that are characteristic of a society. It affects the assessment of comfort needs of the dying and the kind of care provided. It influences the selection, perception, and evaluation of healthcare providers and their methods. It shapes beliefs about the cause of loss and death. It determines the disposition of the body and funeral and burial rites. It influences grief responses and bereavement roles.[47] The nurse must not rely on stereotypes because there are

variations within any group of people. Each patient and family's grief reactions will be a blend of culture, personal habits, and raw emotion.

Personal attributes that affect loss include age, sex, socioeconomic status, and education or occupation. The age at which a loss is experienced will impact the loss (Table 11-1). In their review of the literature, Stroebe and Stroebe[21] concluded that men and younger people were at greatest risk, with social support likely to be the moderating factor. Socioeconomic status and education affected the response to loss only in terms of the options for coping made available to the person experiencing the loss.

Relationship with the lost person will impact the loss according to the meaning and significance of the relationship to the survivor. It cannot be automatically assumed that one type of loss is more serious than another. It is not necessarily true that the loss of a parent will bring more grief than the loss of a grandparent. The griever may have had a more intimate relationship with the grandparent. The qualities of the relationship are more important than the relationship itself. For some people the loss of a pet may be a more significant loss than the loss of a person. The psychological nature of the relationship and the strength of the attachment will have a significant impact on the griever. For example, a relationship characterized by ambivalence is more difficult to resolve than one that is not conflicted. Those who are strongly dependent upon the lost person often have more problems than others.[47] It has been said that to lose your parents is to lose your past, to lose your child is to lose your future, and to lose your spouse is to lose your present.

The *death surround* refers to the immediate circumstance of the death or loss. It includes the location, type of loss or death, the reason for the loss, and the degree of preparation for the loss. Ideally the griever will feel that the

11-3

Beneficial ways in which death affects our perceptions of life

It helps us savour life.

It provides an opposite by which to judge being alive.

It gives us a sense of a real, individual existence.

It gives meaning to courage and integrity, allowing us to express our convictions effectively.

It provides us with the strength to make major decisions.

It reveals the importance of intimacy in our lives.

It helps us to ascribe meaning to our lives; this is especially useful to older people.

It shows us the importance of ego-transcending achievements.

It allows us to see our achievements as being significant..

From Rando TA: *Grief, dying, and death*, Champaign, Ill, 1984, Research Press.

11-4

Phases of life-threatening illness

Prediagnostic phase. Often precedes diagnosis. Here the patient recognizes symptoms or risk factors of illness. The basic ongoing process is a health-seeking one in which the patient recognizes some element of risk and selects strategies to cope with this perceived threat.

Acute phase. Centres around the crisis of diagnosis. The patient is faced with a diagnosis of life-threatening illness and now must make a series of decisions—medical, psychological, and interpersonal—on how, at least initially, to cope.

Chronic phase. The patient is struggling with the disease and its treatment. Many patients may attempt, with varying degrees of success, to live a reasonably normal life within the confines of the disease. Often this period is punctuated by a series of illness-related crises.

Terminal phase. The disease has progressed to a point in which death is inevitable. Death is no longer merely possible, it is now likely.

Data from Doka K: *The Terrible Threat,* Book in preparation, 1992.

circumstances are appropriate. To the extent the "surround" can be accepted, the grief will be more amenable to resolution.[47]

DYING AND DEATH

Dying is an integral part of life. It is as natural and predictable as being born. Death is dreaded, whereas birth is often welcomed and celebrated. Death is an issue to be avoided. Throughout history, humanity has been concerned with death. Philosophy, religion, and science have all attempted to find answers to explain and control death. In spite of technological advances, death continues to be inevitable, and this knowledge influences how we look at life.

Death affects our perceptions of life in beneficial ways, such as giving us an appreciation for living, helping us savour life, and giving us a sense of real existence (Box 11-3). It can, however, also threaten us with the negation of ourselves and all that we value. We tend to be future-oriented and the thought of no future arouses anxiety. Attitudes towards death may range from complete denial to complete and existential acceptance. The particular attitude adopted influences our lives significantly.[19,47]

One person may choose to deny the reality of death, will avoid talking about death, will not attend wakes or funerals, may postpone making a will or having a physical examination. Another person will have faith in life after death and, through religion, can believe that this life is merely a prelude to the afterlife. It is critical to understand not only how our patients view death, but also our own personal feelings about death. We can have a variety of personal gut-level responses to death, but these responses do not prevent our being effective in working with the dying and the bereaved, if we are aware of them. It is normal and natural to have less-than-positive feelings about death.[37]

There is a "living–dying" interval between the time of diagnosis and death. Pattison offers a model of the dying process that emphasizes three phases: an acute phase that centres around the issue of diagnosis, a chronic phase that emphasizes living with disease, and the terminal phase when the impending death is both certain and paramount.[46] Doka[5] has adapted this model to a model of "life-threatening illness" (Box 11-4). It is clear that throughout each phase the patient and family will be coping with different loss issues. Dying or coping with illness is not an isolated process; rather it is part of the process of life. Models are valuable because they help organize information, but they are at best generalities. Models can be helpful when they contribute to our understanding of the individual experiences, but they are destructive when they impose that reality on the patient.

Kubler-Ross's model of the five stages of dying—denial, anger, bargaining, depression, and acceptance—has been misused when nurses tried to classify the many different responses of patients into one of the five stages or to move the patient from denial to acceptance.

GRIEF, MOURNING, AND BEREAVEMENT

The terms *grief*, *mourning*, and *bereavement* have been used interchangeably and have been assigned specific meaning. In this chapter they mean the following:

Grief is the process of psychological, social, and somatic reactions to a perceived loss. It is manifested in all three areas and changes over time. It is a natural, often expected reaction, to many kinds of loss, not just death. Grief is based on the unique, individual perception of the loss by the griever.

Mourning includes a wide array of intrapsychic processes, conscious and unconscious, that are the result of

Table 11-2 Comparison of major theories of grief

Kubler-Ross stages	Lindemann stages	Parkes/Bowlby phases	Engel
Denial and isolation	Shock/disbelief	Numbness	Shock/disbelief
Anger	Acute mourning	Yearning/searching	Developing awareness
Bargaining	Resolution of grief	Disorganization and despair	Restitution
Depression		Reorganization	Resolve the loss
Acceptance			Idealization
			Final outcome

loss. It is also a response to loss that is culturally and socially influenced. Grief may be conceptualized as a transitional phase in the overarching process of mourning.

Bereavement is the state of having suffered a loss.

Basic Tasks of Grief

An understanding of the grief process requires knowledge of the basic tasks of grief. Lindemann offered his conceptualization in 1944 and his theory has been incorporated into contemporary researchers' definitions of the grief process.[22,45,47] There are three basic tasks that constitute grief work:

1. Emancipation from the bondage of the lost object.
2. Readjustment to the environment in which the lost object is missing.
3. Formation of new relationships.

Emancipation from the lost object is the task of "untying the ties that bind" the griever to the lost person or object. This does not mean that what is lost is forgotten or not loved, but rather that the griever can invest the energy previously placed in the lost person in new relationships. The relationship with the lost person remains, but in altered form, in the mind and heart of the griever. What is changed is the ongoing investment in, and attachment to, the lost person as living. The energy that previously kept that relationship alive must now be channelled elsewhere, where it can be returned.

Readjustment to the environment is the task in which the griever accommodates to a world without the lost object or person. The griever experiences many distressing feelings while struggling to bear the pain of separation and becoming accustomed to the loved one's absence.

Formation of new relationships involves the reinvestment of the emotional energy that is withdrawn from the previous relationship in someone or something else. The time it takes before a griever can reinvest will depend on a host of factors, but at some point in time the griever should be able to take the energy that had been used to keep the previous relationship alive and redirect it towards establishing and maintaining rewarding investments in others.[47]

Lindemann's term "grief work" is accurate because grief requires the expenditure of both physical and emotional energy. The work of grieving involves grieving for the actual lost person or object and for all the hopes, dreams, fantasies, and unfulfilled expectations the griever had in terms of the relationship. The loss of a child not only involves the loss of the person, but all the dreams the parents had for the child and the parents' expectation that they would outlive their child. It does not seem to matter if the child was lost before birth or at a later age. From the moment that parents become aware of the child's conception, they begin to dream.

Another complicating factor in accomplishing the grief work is that loss resurrects old issues and conflicts in the griever. The feelings reawakened by these memories can be overwhelming. Conflicts around childhood dependency, ambivalence, parent–child relationships, and security can be stirred by the experience of loss and may make the work of grief more difficult.

Many theorists have described the grief process as having stages or phases (Table 11-2). The responses described include (1) shock, disbelief, and numbness; (2) intense mourning, developing awareness and acceptance of the unwanted reality of the loss, accompanied by disorganization; and (3) reestablishment of homeostasis, recovery, restitution, and reorganization.

Engel[28] describes successful mourning as being evident in the ability to remember comfortably and realistically both the pleasures and disappointments of the lost relationship. Most theorists agree that mourning generally lasts a year or more. There is no one right way or one right time frame for grief.

More and more death educators and counsellors are looking to task theories to assist in understanding the needs of grievers. Worden[22] described four tasks of grief and mourning:

1. To accept the reality of the loss.
2. To experience the pain of the grief.
3. To adjust to an environment in which the deceased is missing.
4. To withdraw emotional energy and reinvest it in another relationship.

In describing a model bereavement programme, O'Toole[15] integrates the tasks of grieving into three phases of caring for the patient and family coping with a life-threatening illness: (1) living with the illness phase, (2) active dying phase, and (3) follow-up bereavement phase. These are discussed in the section on nursing care of the patient/family coping with life-threatening illness and death.

Complicated Mourning/Dysfunctional Grieving

There are four possible types of complicated outcomes of grief: (1) persevering, unusually intense or distorted occurrences of normal grief symptoms; (2) syndromes of expression (absence, inhibition, or delay), distortions (rooted in anger, guilt, or lack of anticipation,) or problems ending (that is, chronic grief); (3) diagnosable mental or physical disorders; and (4) suicide.[19]

11-5

Symptoms and behaviours of unresolved grief [22,41,42]

Overactivity without a sense of loss.

Acquisition of symptoms belonging to the last illness of the deceased.

Development of psychosomatic illness.

Alteration in relationships with friends and relatives.

Furious hostility against specific people somehow connected with the death.

Wooden and formal conduct masking hostile feelings.

Lasting loss of patterns of social interaction.

Actions detrimental to one's social and economic wellbeing; for example, giving away belongings.

Agitated depression with tension, agitation, insomnia, feelings of worthlessness, bitter self-accusation, obvious need for punishment, and even suicidal tendencies.

History of delayed or prolonged grief.

A feeling the death occurred yesterday, even though the loss took place months or years ago.

Unwillingness to move the possessions of the deceased after a reasonable amount of time.

Inability to discuss the deceased without crying, particularly over a year after the loss.

A relatively minor event triggering major grief reactions.

False euphoria subsequent to the death.

Overidentification with the deceased.

Phobias about illness or death.

11-6

Nursing Research

Lasker JN, LJ Toedter: Acute versus chronic grief: the case of pregnancy loss, *Am J Orthopsychiatry* 61(4):510–522, 1991.

This study considered some of the problems in measuring the extent of grief for any type of loss, but particularly "chronic" or "complicated" grief. A scale for measuring grief after pregnancy loss was tested on data from a longitudinal study of 138 women and 56 men who had experienced a perinatal loss. The results suggested that it is possible to distinguish between less severe (crying and sadness) and more severe dimensions of grief (withdrawal and despair). It was found that it may be possible to identify the long-term potential for chronic disturbed responses soon after the loss. Measures were taken at 2 months and 2 years. Scores on "Difficulty coping" and "Despair" are the best predictors, as represented by the level of one's mental health and social and marital support.

Six high risk factors make it more likely that such complications will occur: (1) sudden, unanticipated death, especially when it is traumatic, violent, mutilating, or random; (2) ambivalence or marked dependence or co-dependence in the relationship with the deceased; (3) perceived lack of social support, especially for disenfranchised grief; (4) liabilities of the mourner, including mental health problems; (5) loss of a child; and (6) perception of the death or the suffering as preventable (for example, cases in which persons take "too long" to die).[19]

Various theorists have described behaviours indicative of unresolved grief (Box 11-5). There is disagreement whether these behaviours are indicative of "dysfunctional grieving" or complicating factors influencing the manifestation of grief. Whatever the case, it is important for the nurse to recognize and refer these patients for appropriate counselling and/or treatment (Box 11-6).

Nursing Process
Assessment of patient/family experiencing loss/dying/death

It is recognized that each loss experience is different. Generalizations are made for the sake of discussion. The focus of the nursing process discussion will be primarily on the patient coping with a life-threatening illness, dying, and death. (The use of the term *family* throughout this chapter refers not only to a legally defined family, but recognizes the nontraditional relationships or significant others as family.)

Crisis assessment

The crisis model provides the nurse with an ongoing framework to help determine how much and what type of assistance is needed by the patient or family. A crisis is subjectively defined by the patient or family when they perceive the situation with which they are confronted as sufficiently different from previous experiences or so overwhelming that habitual problem-solving activities are not adequate to resolve the challenge.

There are four balancing forces to be assessed. First, the nurse needs to determine how realistic a view the patient and family have. Do they see the illness as fatal or are they able to see possible alternatives for the future? If their view of the situation is distorted, then the first challenge will be to provide them with accurate information; if it is clear that their misperception is caused by anxiety, then reducing the level of anxiety will be the necessary first step.

The second balancing force is the ability to identify and express feelings related to the situation. For example, after the loss of a child, fathers identify feeling the same emotions as mothers, but their modes of expression are often different. Fathers often chose activities for expressing feelings, whereas mothers will frequently cry and exhibit other overt expressions of sorrow. It is important not to assume that just because fathers are not showing their feelings they are not experiencing as much pain as mothers. Another example would be at the time of diagnosis of a life-threatening illness that has been described as a turning point, a time of crisis when the patient's whole orientation changes: one's worst fears may be realized and patients may recognize or perceive that they are now either in a struggle for life or an inexorable slide towards death. This confrontation with death can overwhelm the patient and family.[5]

The third balancing force is having successful problem-solving skills. Death is not as frequent an occurrence as it was in the past. It is an unfamiliar and frightening experience for many people. Confrontation with a life-threatening illness and possible death calls upon all the problem-solving skills a patient and family can muster. It would not be surprising that they would need assistance to cope with this event. The process of rendering a diagnosis is often very difficult; during this time patients undergo a multiplicity of tests and procedures and also experience a great deal of uncertainty. Despite the uncertainty of both diagnosis and prognosis, being diagnosed as having a life-threatening illness is an intense crisis filled with anxiety, affect, and a host of personal and interpersonal issues. Tensions and anxieties mount and individuals must either mobilize coping mechanisms or experience personal disorganization. Despite this crisis of uncertain nature, patients often have to make decisions that may radically affect the quality, nature, and even duration of life.[5]

The fourth balancing force is support. Coping with a life-threatening illness or loss due to a death is inevitably a family issue, for everyone's life is changed when one member of a family experiences illness or dies. The grief and emotional responses of each family member may be so intense that they are unable to give each other the support they need.

Nursing assessment is an ongoing process throughout the illness and into the dying phase. A thorough assessment includes input from the patient and significant others (Box 11-7).

Tasks of the living–dying phase

The nurse assesses the tasks confronting the patient and family at each phase of the living–dying continuum. O'Toole has described these phases and their related tasks: (1) the living with illness phase, (2) the active dying phase, (3) the time of death and (4) the follow-up bereavement phase.[15]

11-7

Nursing assessment: input from patient with life-threatening illness and significant others

General perception of each individual

Awareness of clinical diagnosis and prognosis
Philosophy of living and beliefs about dying
Expected physiological and behavioural changes
Past experiences with major illness, loss, or crisis
Concurrent life crises or losses
Financial impact of illness, loss, or death
Degree of dependence or autonomy of family members

Perceived strengths, desires, and hopes

Personal abilities and coping techniques
Personal support systems
Availability of resources
Beliefs, religious convictions, and cultural views of dying, death, and bereavement
Past experiences with loss, dying, and death
Expectations about care, use of life supports, and advanced directives
Communication patterns

The living with illness phase begins for the patient at the time when the illness is first diagnosed; for the nurse it begins with the initial assessment. The key tasks for the patient and family during this phase include:

1. The need to obtain and gain understanding and information regarding the illness process. This can include information about medical and nursing treatments, what to expect, and what patient and family need to do. It may also include having access to information regarding all treatment options available, both traditional and alternative methods. At this time it is appropriate to assess the patient and family's understanding of the grief process.

2. The need for assistance and information about limitations imposed by the illness and what resources are available to assist them.

3. A period of adjustment as family members develop new roles.

4. The patient and family's need to develop a trusting relationship with their caregivers.

5. The need for assistance in maintaining hope while dealing with the reality of the disease process and the implications of the threat to life.

6. The family's needs to develop strategies to meet the needs of the ill person which recognize the need of the ill person to retain as much control over his or her life as possible.

7. The patient and family's need to discover coping patterns that will assist in limiting their awareness of the impact of losses and conserve energy so that living can continue.

8. The need to maintain and/or restore relationships with significant people; the need to tie up loose ends.

9. The time, to some degree, to recognize and to resolve unfinished business.

10. The caregivers' need to develop a system that permits them to care for themselves and continue living as fully as possible. The focus for the patient and family is on *living*.

It would be ideal, if in every case there could be sufficient time in the phases of illness and dying to allow the patient and family adequate time to complete all their tasks. All too often the living–dying period is too short, leaving the patient and family with unfinished business. That is why familiarity with the tasks confronting the patient and family, along with a careful assessment, completed as rapidly as possible, will provide the nurse with the data needed to plan optimal care.

Patient/family tasks of the active dying phase

The active dying phase is characterized by the period of physical and mental decline that indicates that death is near. Tasks of this phase are an integral part of the grief process of the survivors, just as the tasks of the earlier phase were a preparation for this phase. Completion of the tasks of this phase are significant in how the bereaved survivors will later remember the dying experience. This phase is often seen as part of the shock or numbing experience of grief when memories are recorded, stored, and frozen in vivid and graphic forms. Patient/family tasks of the active dying phase include the following:

1. If the patient is cared for at home, the caregivers will need instruction on the care of the terminally ill.
2. The family caregiver needs to regulate emotions to attend to personal needs, the dying person's need, and the family system needs.
3. The patient and family will experience the pain of separation, as the patient may begin to withdraw.
4. The need to remain sufficiently engaged to provide care, comfort, and presence to the dying person and other family members.
5. The time for completion of significant issues of reconciliation and forgiveness.
6. As far as possible, the time to accept or recognize that earth life is ending.
7. The need for some form of acknowledgment of the bonds of the dying person to those who remain, and some formalization of the creation of memories.
8. The dying person's needs for assurance that he or she will be remembered. Fears most often associated with dying are the fear of pain, disfigurement, abandonment, helplessness, loss of self-worth, and extinction.

Tasks at the time of death

1. Assessment of the need and wish of the family to be present at the time of death.
2. The patient should not be left alone at the time of death.
3. Assessment of who the patient/family want present, such as clergy, other family members, or friends.
4. The family's needs for information about what to expect at the time of death.
5. The family's need for assistance in notifying the appropriate people about the death, such as an undertaker.
6. The family's need for permission to remain alone with the patient's body after death.

Family tasks after death

1. If the patient died at home, the family needs assistance with preparing the body.
2. They may need assistance in arranging funeral/memorial rituals meaningful to them and the deceased.
3. They may want and need encouragement to use this period to reminisce about the "good days" prior to and during the illness.
4. They may need support in experiencing the tasks of grief, described earlier, and in expressing their grief, both individually and as a group.

Not all bereaved people need or want formal intervention following the loss of a loved one. They will ultimately move through their grief work with or without intervention; however, there is evidence that suggests people move faster through the grieving process when they receive formal support. The need for support is determined through careful crisis assessment and determination of possible dysfunctional grieving.

Nursing analysis

Problems are determined from analysis of patient data. Possible problems for the person coping with loss, dying, or death may include, but are not limited to, the following:

Problems	Possible aetiologies
Anxiety	Threat to self-concept, change in health status/socioeconomic status/role functioning/environment, crisis, and threat of death
Role performance, altered	Changes in social involvement due to life-threatening illness
Hopelessness	Failing physical condition, abandonment
Denial	Threat to life
Powerlessness	Healthcare environment, interpersonal interaction, illness-related regimen
Grieving, anticipatory	Potential loss of significant person/object/body part
Social interaction, impaired	Poor communication skills, self-concept disturbance, absence of supporting others, altered thought processes
Social isolation	Alteration in physical appearance, state of wellness or altered mental status, death of a significant other
Grieving, dysfunctional	Actual or perceived loss

Planning: expected patient outcomes

Planning patient and family care is a team effort including the patient, family, doctor, nurse, social worker, and other healthcare providers, as appropriate. Successful planning incorporates the needs and goals of the family as well as the goals of the healthcare team.

Two issues that nurses may need to consider while caring for dying patients and their families are organ donation and advance directives. There are procedures, both legal and medical, where organ/tissue donation is to occur and situations where the wishes of the patient take the form of an advance directive ('living will').

In appropriate situations, the medical team caring for a patient in hospital will offer patients and families the option to donate organs and or tissue after death. It is recommended that discussion be conducted in a sensitive and caring manner. The intent of these recommendations is to ensure an adequate number of organs and tissues for those whose lives depend on transplantation of healthy organs or tissues. There remains an acute shortage of donated organs, eyes, and tissues, and there are still many thousands of people in the United Kingdom known to be awaiting life-saving transplant surgery. Another important benefit is that the option to donate may offer a sense of comfort to the grieving family of a dying loved one.[17]

Most hospitals have well-established organ donation policies and procedures based on local, regional, national, and international requirements. Usually, the medical team will make the request but there may be local variation (for example, a transplant co-ordinator may be involved). It is incumbent on nurses to know the policy in the institution where they work, as well as being knowledgeable about the basic information regarding organ donation. It is often the nurse at the bedside who has the opportunity to discuss this issue with the patient or family.

The issue of advance directives has come to the forefront in many countries within the last few years. Advance directives are signed and witnessed documents providing specific instructions for healthcare treatment in the event that a person is unable to make those decisions personally at the time they are needed. The form varies from country to country. Documents may take the form of the standard Health Care Treatment Directive, additional specific written instructions, a Values History, a written statement that provides information about the person's personal values as they relate to life and healthcare, and a Enduring Power of Attorney for Health Care Decisions. It is important to know the law related to advanced directives and your nursing responsibilities in seeing that it is not violated.

The advance directives are based on the person's right to self-determination. Every adult has the freedom to accept or refuse any recommended medical treatment. Every person who completes an advance directives should give a copy to his or her family doctor and to family or friends to ensure that it is available when necessary. Advance directives should be seen not only as protection for personal rights, but also as a guide to a person's healthcare providers.[6]

In areas of the United States where advance directives are recognized, the attending doctor and hospital must comply with the provisions of the patient's Health Care Treatment Directive or transfer the patient to another doctor, unless there is reason to doubt the validity of the Health Care Treatment Directive.

A person may revoke his or her Health Care Treatment Directive at any time and in any manner in which the person is able to communicate his or her intent.

Expected patient/family outcomes for people coping with loss, dying, or death may include, but are not limited to, the following:

1. Experience a reduced anxiety level as evidenced by: decreased tension, less apprehension, ability to discuss anxiety related to illness, the ability to identify stressors, and the ability to learn.
2. Demonstrate effective coping skills as evidenced by the ability to problem solve.
3. Engage in functional role performance as evidenced by being able to discuss role expectations and changes with each other and by using constructive strategies to cope with the changes related to the patient's deteriorating condition.
4. Maintained hope, as evidenced by the patient performing self-care activities as long as possible, by participating in diversional activities as long as possible, and by maintaining relationships. Patient and family will be able to express feelings, both verbally and nonverbally, as they choose. They will identify realistic goals.
5. Express some reduction in concerns. (Denial will be at a level that supports the patient's progress.)
6. Participate during the living-with-illness phase in constructive anticipatory grief work as evidenced by discussing thoughts and feelings related to anticipated losses, utilizing appropriate resources, meeting ongoing needs, and maintaining constructive relationships.
7. Demonstrate increased ability to cope with interpersonal encounters and social situations. They will express feelings in a constructive, socially acceptable manner.
8. Experience a reduced level of social isolation and spend time daily with trusted people.
9. Demonstrate normal grief work, acknowledging awareness of loss, verbalizing or in some comfortable manner expressing thoughts and feelings related to their losses. They will develop goals that are congruent with loss and that reflect individual values and choices.[8]

It is imperative that nurses include themselves in the assessment and planning phase. It is important to be aware of one's own loss experiences, unresolved griefs, beliefs about loss, dying, and death. Nurses who have not worked through their own grief issues are vulnerable when exposed to the loss of others. Unresolved griefs can be reactivated, preventing nurses from being able to respond to the needs of the patient or family. It colours their perceptions and ability to assess accurately and objectively. Rando[47] noted the following prerequisites for working with the dying:

1. A personal confrontation with death in the sense of having started to come to grips with one's own mortality. This can never be done completely, but the issue needs to have been addressed.
2. An understanding of the grief process and an appreciation for the total experience of the dying patient.
3. Effective listening skills and the ability to respond appropriately, nonverbally as well as verbally.
4. A commitment to giving part of oneself to the dying person and to working with families after death when appropriate.
5. A knowledge of one's own personal limits, knowing when there is a need to get away from death and how to avoid burnout.

British nurses responsible for planning patient/family care will find the "Dying Person's Bill of Rights" created at a workshop on "The Terminally Ill Patient and the Helping Person" in Lansing, Michigan in 1975 (Box 11-8) most helpful.

Implementation

Living with illness phase

Many interventions are appropriate throughout the care period. The thrust of intervention with patients and families coping with life-threatening illness is the maintenance of hope, dignity, and quality of life.

Establishing a trusting relationship is the key to all that follows. It is important that, as much as possible, the same nursing staff work with these patients and families. It is threatening to come into a foreign environment and undergo strange procedures that are often painful. Patients and families need someone they can rely on, who knows

11-8

The dying person's bill of rights

I have the right to be treated as a living human being until I die.

I have the right to maintain a sense of hopefulness however changing its focus may be.

I have the right to be cared for by those who can maintain a sense of hopefulness, however changing this might be.

I have the right to express my feeling and emotions about my approaching death in my own way.

I have the right to participate in decisions concerning my care.

I have the right to expect continuing medical and nursing attention even though "cure" goals must be changed to "comfort" goals.

I have the right not to die alone.

I have the right to be free from pain.

I have the right to have my questions answered honestly.

I have the right not to be deceived.

I have the right to have help from and for my family in accepting my death.

I have the right to die in peace and dignity.

I have the right to retain my individuality and not be judged for my decisions, which may be contrary to beliefs of others.

I have the right to discuss and enlarge my religious and/or spiritual experiences, whatever these may mean to others.

I have the right to expect that the sanctity of the human body will be respected after death.

I have the right to be cared for by caring, sensitive, knowledgeable people who will attempt to understand my needs and will be able to gain some satisfaction in helping me face my death.

This Bill of Rights was created at a workshop on "The Terminally Ill Patient and the Helping Person," in Lansing, Mich, sponsored by the Southwestern Michigan Inservice Education Council and conducted by Amelia J. Barbus, Associate Professor of Nursing, Wayne State University, Detroit, 1975.

---

them and can assist them through this frightening and anxiety-producing experience. The nurse promotes the trusting relationship by first listening to the patient and family and hearing where they are in their coping process and what they say they need, not what they should need.

Be physically and emotionally present to offer security and support. When people are feeling anxious or emotionally stressed they often respond positively to the gentle touch of a hand or the offer of a hug. However, be aware that some people are not comfortable with being touched or would not welcome it from a relative stranger. Be aware of nonverbal feedback and, if in doubt, ask permission before touching such people.

The healthcare team can then move on to assisting the family in recognizing, accepting, and using their individual and collective coping styles to meet their needs. The family will need information and assistance in meeting the physical needs of the patient. In the hospital, the nursing staff provides most of the patient's care, including the family when appropriate, and assures them of their continued importance in the patient's care. Some families want to do as much as possible for their loved one; others are not able to participate. It is important to respect the choices of the patient and family in these matters. The patient and family should be included in decisions throughout the hospitalization and preparation for discharge. Encourage the person with the illness to retain as much control as possible.

The nurse can begin to explore with the family the impact of the illness and assist them in preparing for possible role changes. This can be especially important if the relationship involves dependency of the well partner. Encourage and assist the family to maintain as high a degree of normal living as possible. Recognize special events such as birthdays and anniversaries as a way to affirm that life is still valuable and in process and to encourage reminiscences. Normalize the experience, discussing common

emotional responses and anticipatory grieving. Assist the patient and family in recognizing that they are grieving for themselves and for the other and of the naturalness of these reactions. Provide information on the grief process. As appropriate, encourage and provide opportunities for families to meet with each other to obtain information and clarification, to express feelings, to identify their needs for reconciliation, and to recognize and accept their various coping styles. Encourage patient/family support networks and assist in identifying resources, both personal and community.

When families choose to take the patient home for care, be sure that they are well prepared before discharge for what they will need to know. Teach them basic care, including feeding techniques when appropriate. Assist them in selecting foods that will be easy to chew and swallow and that are as palatable as possible. Have them assist in bathing, mouth care, and other hygiene measures so they will know how to perform these when they return home. Teach them simple transfer techniques to prevent injury to themselves and the patient. Discuss routines, including the need for rest periods. Arrange for local hospice services to assist the family if they are receptive; emphasize the importance of continuity of care and 24-hour availability for periods when the patient is experiencing an emotional or physical crisis and needs ongoing support.

Provide teaching, information, and encouragement in the use of creative outlets for expressing feelings and communicating with others. Encourage the use of taperecorded messages, drawings, writings, imagery, music, and poetry. This also assists patients and families in creating memories that can be very comforting later. Teach the patient and family relaxation techniques.

The maintenance of hope can be difficult during this time. As the patient's condition deteriorates, the challenge becomes one of assisting the patient and family in translat-

Signs and symptoms of approaching death

The arms and legs may become cool to the touch and the underside of the body may become darker in colour. These symptoms are the result of the blood circulation slowing down.

The patient will spend more and more time sleeping during the day and at times will be difficult to arouse. This results from slowing of the body's metabolism.

The patient may lose bladder or bowel control, resulting in incontinence.

Oral secretions may become more profuse and collect in the back of the throat, producing what is commonly referred to as the "death rattle". This is a result of decreased fluid intake and the patient's inability to cough up normal saliva.

The patient's vision and hearing decrease slightly, with hearing generally being the last sense to be lost.

The patient may become restless, pulling at bed linen and having visions of people or things. This is the result of decreased oxygen to the brain, as well as the decreased metabolism.

The patient will have a decreased need for food and drink.

The patient's breathing pattern will change during sleep to an irregular pace with 10- to 30-second periods of no breathing.

Signs of death include no breathing, no heartbeat, no response to shaking or shouting, loss of bladder and bowel control, eyelids slightly open with eyes fixed on one spot, and jaws relaxed and mouth slightly open.

Note: Not all these symptoms will appear at the same time and some may never appear.

---

ing their hope for a cure into realistic hopes that are focused on short-term achievable goals. This may be the hope for a comfortable and painfree life, or the desire to live long enough to participate in some important family event, like the wedding of a son. Hope can take many forms; the challenge for the nurse is to help the patient and family identify those hopes that are most important to them and that will help them cope.

Active dying phase

It is important to provide the family with realistic information about the course of the illness and the signs and symptoms of impending death. Hospices frequently give families both verbal and written information (Box 11-9) whereas in hospitals this is rarely discussed. Families have often expressed fear of what happens at the time of death and consequently may avoid being present, leaving the patient feeling alone and abandoned. When possible, encourage family members to have someone supportive be with them during this time. Ensure that they take adequate breaks and supplement their vigil if needed by people from the family support network, staff, or volunteers.

Continue to listen and to provide a supportive presence. Coach the family and model for them ways to interact with the dying patient. Speak to the patient, even if unresponsive and call him or her by name. Encourage family members to talk to the patient and assure him or her that he or she is significant to the family and will be remembered. Encourage the family to recognize that in terminal illness, dying is a process that often occurs over time and that the patient, although dying, is still alive.

It may be necessary to give the family permission to recognize that it is "okay" for them to continue to live even in the presence of death. Encourage them to bring food or beverages into the patient's room. Provide them with opportunities to express their sorrow and the pain of the loss. At the same time, demonstrate acceptance and support to family members who do not express their feelings.

When appropriate, model and coach the family in giving the patient "permission to die" and in saying "goodbye." If needed, give family members the permission to not be present during this stage; convey your acceptance of such a decision. Keep the family informed as the patient's condition changes. If the family chooses to be present, offer support, acceptance, and assurance, especially to those who fear the time of death or of being present at the time of death.

At time of death

Offer to call the clergy or other support people identified by the patient and family. Allow the family time to be alone with the body of their loved one if they wish. Model acceptance of the body, by touching and calling the dead person by name. If the family was not present at the time of death, encourage them that this is a time when they can still say anything that they will later regret not having said. Point out that we do not know how long the patient's life force is present and that there is still time to say "I love you" or whatever else they want to say. Give and model comfort and caring through shared tears, touch, listening, and acceptance. Provide a calm, reassuring, and caring presence.

Assist or prepare the body according to hospital protocol; in the home, assist the family in preparing the body for removal to the chapel of rest. If requested or needed, support the family in arranging funeral or memorial rituals that are meaningful to them. If possible, attend the wake, visit to chapel of rest, or memorial service and let the family know of your presence and that you care. A special bond often forms between the family and the nurse because of having shared one of the most important events of their lives.

Care for nurse caregiver
Process and stress of nurse's grief

Because many patients die in hospitals rather than in homes, nurses have evolved in the role of "surrogate griever." Nurses who work with the terminally ill and with bereaved people develop a heightened empathy and identification with their patients. This occurs because the loss experience is so universal that we have all experienced its impact. Dying and bereaved individuals force us to confront death and loss. Nurses take emotional risks and form bonds that demand a grief response. When this is experienced intensely in a serial fashion without adequate processing, nurses can become subject to bereavement overload.[47]

Nurses are susceptible to all the emotions of grief: frustration, sadness, guilt, anxiety, depression, helplessness, and anger. They need to do for themselves what they do for their patients to help them with their grief work. There are, however, roadblocks to nurses' grieving:

- Social negation of the loss and isolation from support: few hospitals provide opportunities for nurses to grieve lost patients formally. The nurses' families and friends often cannot understand how the death of a relative stranger can cause such intense grief. Hence the nurse is left to grieve alone or to go on as if nothing important has occurred.
- "Professionalism": Nurses are expected to be strong.
- Ambivalence and feelings of guilt towards the dead person can result when the nurse had mixed feelings about the patient. If the patient was a particularly difficult person to like or to care for, the nurse may even feel a sense of relief when death occurs. This can be incompatible with the idea that a nurse is "supposed to love everyone equally."
- Nurses often have a need to be in control, so they may not be able to show how they feel or may even suppress their feelings.
- Multiple losses can be overwhelming. It is not uncommon on some nursing units for several patients to die in a very short period of time, leaving little or no time for proper processing of the nurses' grief.
- Old, unresolved losses suffered by the nurse can be reawakened and can prevent the nurse from dealing with the current losses.

Nurses' responses to loss are subject to the same influences discussed earlier in this chapter. Other factors include unique genetic and developmental history, prior loss history, stress management, professional training, values and beliefs, the particular developmental period in the nurse's life, the number and intensity of life changes at any given period of time, the nurse's personal motivation for working with the terminally ill, and the nurse's personal level of energy and rest requirements.

Strategies for survival

It is incumbent upon the hospital or other work groups employing nurses in the care of the terminally ill to build into the organization a formalized process for recognizing and allowing the grieving process to take place. This can be done on the unit level or hospitalwide. Some hospitals have instituted regular meetings that the staff can attend to share the losses they have experienced and to talk about patients who have recently died.

Nurses have the responsibility to take steps to care for themselves:

1. Take regular breaks from the patient care area and consider rotating out of high-stress nursing areas.
2. Identify specific patients that are most difficult, so that they can be anticipated and counteracted. Ask for special assistance in working in these specific situations.
3. Acknowledge physical needs as key factors in stress reduction.
4. Integrate decompression routines into daily life. Before leaving the work area take a moment to review the day and set it aside before going home.
5. Engage in life-affirming activities, for example, spend time with lively healthy children.
6. View losses as an opportunity to reevaluate and grow.
7. Avoid the "rescuer" or "saviour" complex; recognize limits.
8. Recognize the need for support and do not hesitate to ask for it.
9. Say "I choose" rather than "I should."
10. Develop the skills of setting limits and feeling okay about saying "no."
11. Laugh and play in the face of tragedy without guilt.
12. Seek consultation on a regular basis.

Evaluation: patient/family/nurse

A review of the projected outcomes provides the evaluation criteria:

1. Did the patient or family express a positive reduction in their initial level of anxiety and an increase in positive coping skills?
2. Were patient and family able to make the necessary role adjustments while preserving the patient's self-esteem and without overwhelming the family with the new responsibilities?
3. Did the patient and family find satisfactory expression of their feelings and grief?
4. Was hope redefined as the patient's condition changed?
5. Were patient and family able to maintain an appropriate level of denial, allowing them to adjust to the patient's deteriorating condition?
6. Did the patient and family maintain social interaction throughout the illness–dying process at a level satisfactory to them?
7. Did the nurse develop useful strategies for dealing with stress related to working with loss, dying, and death?

SUMMARY

1. Dying and death are distinct and separate events that are part of the continuum of life. Grief is the normal response to any loss. It is a lifelong normative process as each new loss experience is met. Grief is an active, not a passive process; it takes work and emotional energy. When people do not do "grief work" following any significant loss, they are at risk for emotional, mental, and social problems. The role of the nurse is to assist the patient and family in making choices related to their tasks of grieving.
2. Loss is inevitable and inescapable.
3. Losses can be described as self losses or external losses.
4. Self losses include the loss of the psychological self, the sociocultural self, the physical self, and the spiritual self.
5. External losses include loss of objects, possessions, loved ones, environment, and support.

6. Losses can be real, imagined, present, or anticipated.
7. Many factors influence the way an individual responds to loss: childhood experiences, significance assigned to the loss, the physical and emotional state of the individual, accumulated loss experiences, view of loss as crisis, visibility, duration and timing, abruptness or suddeness, financial drain, availability of resources, cultural factors, personal attributes, relationship with the lost person, and the death surround.
8. Dying is an integral part of life, as natural and predictable as birth.
9. Dying can help us to appreciate and understand life.
10. Models of dying and grief are useful in conceptualizing the processes, but should never be used prescriptively.
11. The terms *grief*, *mourning*, and *bereavement* are used to describe the process and state of having suffered a loss.
12. The tasks of grief help in understanding the needs of the griever.
13. Complicated or dysfunctional grief should be identified by the nurse and referred for appropriate intervention.
14. The crisis model provides a framework for assessing patient and family perspectives on loss as a possibly overwhelming event that needs professional intervention.
15. Nursing assessment includes a review of the tasks confronting patients and families during each phase of the living–dying continuum.
16. The nurse needs to be aware of the patient's wishes with regard to organ/tissue donation and advanced directives, as well as legal and hospital regulations on these issues.
17. Nurses experience all the emotions of grief not only in response to their own losses but also in response to the deaths of their patients.
18. It is imperative that nurses care for themselves.
19. Patients and families properly supported through their early illness and final living–dying experiences will be able to make the necessary emotional adjustments to the changes in their lives so that growth and maturing are more likely to occur.

STUDY QUESTIONS

- Complete the following "Personal Loss" Inventory[39] and discuss your responses with a member of your group:
- List the three most significant losses you have personally sustained in life to date. They do not need to be in any hierarchical order and can involve people, things, hopes, beliefs, or attitudes. Be brief and concrete.
- In which of these losses have you completed your grief work? How has this promoted self-affirmation, creative living, and growth? Be specific.
- In which of the three losses noted have you not completed your grieving? In what ways is this manifest in your living today?
- How would you explain the grieving process to a patient with a newly diagnosed life-threatening illness?
- Differentiate between the dying process and death.

- Select a patient you are currently working with and review the patient's loss history. What factors influencing loss are most pertinent in planning care?
- Share with a member of your group the steps you take to manage the stress in your life.

REFERENCES AND SELECTED READINGS

1. Bruss CR: Nursing diagnosis of hopelessness, *J Psychosoc Nurs* 26(3):28-31, 1988.
2. Corr CA: A task-based approach to coping with dying. Paper presented at the ADEC conference, Duluth, Minn, April 1991.
3. DeSpelder LA, Strickland AL: *The last dance: encountering death and dying*, ed 2, Mountain View, Calif, 1987, Mayfield Publishing.
4.* Dobratz, MC: Hospice nursing: present perspective and future directives, *Cancer Nurs* 13(2):116-122, 1990.
5. Doka KJ: *The terrible threat*, Book in preparation, 1991.
6. Emanuel LL, Emanuel EJ: The medical directive, *JAMA*, 261(22):3288-3293, 1989.
7.* Grollman EA: *In sickness and in health: how to cope when your loved one is ill*, Boston, 1987, Beacon Press.
8. Kim MJ, McFarland GK, McLane AM: *Pocket guide to nursing diagnosis*, ed 3, St Louis, 1989, Mosby–Year Book.
9. Lasker JN, Toedter LJ: Acute versus chronic grief: the case of pregnancy loss, *Am J Orthopsychiatry* 61(4):510-522, 1991.
10.* Lawson LV: Culturally sensitive support for grieving parents, *MCN* 15:76-79, March/April 1990.
11. Leavitt PF, McDowell WA, Lewis SJ: *The patient who is dying*. In Lewis S et al, editors: *Manual of psychosocial nursing and interventions*, ed 3, Philadelphia, 1989, WB Saunders.
12. Longo DC, Williams RA, editors: *Clinical practice in psychosocial nursing: assessment and intervention*, ed 2, Norwalk, Conn, 1986, Appleton-Century-Crofts.
13. Metzgar M: *Little ears, big issues: children and loss*, Seattle, 1990.
14.* Mount BM: *Dealing with our losses*, *J Clin Oncol* 4(7):1127-1134, 1986.
15. O'Toole D: *Bridging the bereavement gap*, ed 2, LaPeer, Mich, 1985, The Bereavement Project.
16. Parkes CM: *Bereavement: studies of grief in adult life*, ed 2, Madison, Conn, 1987, International Universities Press.
17. Perryman JP: Providing the option to donate, *The Forum*: (Newsletter of the Association for Death Education and Counseling) 13:6, 1989.
18. Rando TA: *Loss and anticipatory grief*, Lexington, Mass, 1986, Lexington Books.
19. Rando TA: *Treatment of complicated mourning*, Book in preparation, 1992.
20. Redmond LM: *Surviving: when someone you love was murdered*, Clearwater, Fla, 1989, Psychological Consultation and Education Services.
21. Stroebe W, Stroebe MS: *Bereavement and health: the psychological and physical consequences of partner loss*, Cambridge, UK, 1987, Cambridge University Press.
22. Worden JW: *Grief counseling and grief therapy: a handbook for the mental health practitioner*, ed 2, New York, 1990, Springer Publishing.
23. Zisook S: *Biopsychosocial aspects of bereavement*, Washington, DC, 1987, American Psychiatric Press.
24. Beland-Werner JA, editor: *Grief responses to long-term illness and disability: manifestations and nursing interventions*, Reston, Va, 1980, Reston Publishing.
25. Bower F, editor: *Nursing and the concept of loss*, New York, 1980, Wiley Medical Publications.
26. Bowlby J: *Attachment and loss: loss, sadness, and depression*, vol 3, New York, 1980, Basic Books.
27. Daniel EJ: *Any other song: a plea for holistic communication*, Bowie, Md, 1980, Prentice-Hall.
28. Engel G: *Psychological development in health and disease*, Philadelphia, 1962, WB Saunders.
29. Feifel H: *New meanings of death*, New York, 1977, McGraw-Hill.
30.* Glaser BG, Strauss AL: The social loss of dying patients, *AJN* 63:119-121, 1964.
31.* Glaser GB, Strauss AL: *A time for dying*, Chicago, 1968, Aldine de Gruyter.
32. Glick IO, Weiss RS, Parkes CM: *The first year of bereavement*, New York, 1974, Wiley.
33. Harper GC: *Death: the coping mechanism of the health professional*, Greenville, SC, 1977, Southwestern University Press.

34. Jackson EN: *Understanding grief: its roots, dynamics, and treatment*, Nashville, 1957, Abingdon Press.

35. Kalish RA: *Death, grief, and caring relationships*, Monterey, Calif, 1981, Brooks/Cole.

36. Kastenbaum RJ: *Death, society and human experience*, St Louis, 1977, Mosby–Year Book.

37.* Kavanaugh R: *Facing death*, Baltimore, 1974, Penguin Books.

38.* Keleman S: *Living your dying*, New York, 1983, Bantam Books.

39. Knott JE, et al: *Thanatopics: a manual of structured learning experiences for death education*, Kingston, RI, 1982, SLE Publications.

40. Koestenbaum P: *Is there an answer to death?* Englewood Cliffs, NJ, 1976, Prentice-Hall.

41.* Kubler-Ross E: *On death and dying*, New York, 1969, Macmillan.

42. Lazare A: Unresolved grief. In Lazare A, editor: *Outpatient psychiatry: diagnosis and treatment*, Baltimore, 1979, Williams & Wilkins.

43. Lindemann E: Symptomatology and management of acute grief, *Am J Psychiatry* 101:141-148, 1944.

44. Maslach C: *Burnout—the cost of caring*, Englewood Cliffs, NJ, 1982, Prentice Hall.

45.* Parkes CM, Weiss RS: *Recovery from bereavement*, New York, 1983, Basic Books.

46. Pattison EM: The living-dying process. In Garfield CA, editor: *Psychosocial care of the dying patient*, New York, 1978, McGraw-Hill.

47. Rando TA: *Grief, dying, and death*, Champaign, Ill, 1984, Research Press.

48. Raphael B: *The anatomy of bereavement*, New York, 1983, Basic Books.

49. Simos BG: *A time to grieve: loss as a universal human experience*, New York, 1979, Family Service Association of America.

50. Vachon MLS: Motivation and stress experienced by staff working with the terminally ill, *Death Education*, 2:113-122, 1978.

FURTHER READING

Allmark P: Euthanasia, dying well and the slippery slope, *Adv Nurs* 18(8):1178-1182, 1993.

Buckman R: *How to break bad news. A guide for health care professionals*, London, 1993, Macmillan Press Ltd.

Clarke J: The day after a death, *Nurs Times* 89(12):46-47, 1993.

Claxton JW: Paving the way to acceptance. Psychological adaptation to death and dying in cancer, *Professional Nurse* 8(4): 206-211, 1993.

Crombie A: Gift of life, *Nurs Times* 89(16):25, 1993.

Department of Social Security and Central Office of Information: *What to do after a death. A guide to what you must do and the help you can get*, London, 1991, HMSO.

Ellis P: Euthanasia: the way to a peaceful end? *Professional Nurse* 7(3):157-160, 1991.

Ellison G: A private disaster, *Nurs Times* 88(52):59-60, 1992.

Ewins D, Bryant J: Relative comfort, *Nurs Times* 88(52):61-63, 1992.

Farrar A: How much do they want to know? Communicating with dying patients, *Professional Nurse* 7(9):606-610, 1992.

Farrell M: What to do after a bereavement, *Professional Nurse* 5(10):539-542, 1990.

Hollinworth H: Comfort of strangers, *Nurs Times* 88(40):38-40, 1992.

House N: Helping to reach an understanding. Palliative care for people from ethnic minority groups, *Professional Nurse* 8(5): 329-333, 1993.

Jones A: Actors in an emotional drama. Inter-related grief in terminal care, *Professional Nurse* 6(10):598-603, 1991.

Kelsey S: Can we care to the end? Do nurses have the skills for terminal care? *Professional Nurse* 7(4):216-219, 1992.

Nash A: A terminal case? Burnout in palliative care, *The Professional Nurse* 4(9):443-444, 1989.

Reynolds P et al.: Cancer and communication: information given in an oncology clinic, *Br Med J* 1:1449-1450, 1981.

Satterthwaite HJ: When right and wrong are a matter of opinion. The ethics of organ transplantation, *Professional Nurse* 5(8): 434-438, 1990.

Warren J: Match point, *Nurs Times* 89(16):29-31, 1993.

Wight C: Organ donation, *The Professional Nurse* 3(2):40-44, 1987.

*Recommended for student reading.

Infection

12

Infection Control

Grace A. Rotter
Dora Rice
Elizabeth Cameron Eckstein

After studying this chapter, the learner should be able to:

- Describe the chain of infection.
- Identify high-risk factors for infection.
- Describe white blood cell response to infection.
- Identify community approaches to infection control and describe immunization programmes.
- Define nosocomial infections and measures of prevention and control.
- Compare category-specific isolation precautions and body substance isolation, including major components of each.

The field of infection control is a challenging one, with the identification of new pathogens (for example, human immunodeficiency virus or HIV) and advances in research uncovering new information that may change current thinking and practices. Infection control nurses (ICNs) serve as a valuable resource because they interact with virtually every department in a hospital as they survey for infections and teach staff how to prevent and control infection. The ICN is an important link between personnel from various hospital departments. When there is a question or problem regarding infection control, the ICN should be called on without hesitation.

The epidemiological method used by infection control nurses now serves as a model for the study of other adverse outcomes of hospitalization: for example, falls. Quality management departments of many hospitals consult ICNs in the design and implementation of monitors and focused studies. Informing health care workers of rates of patient outcomes results in changes in practice, which ultimately improves patient outcomes.

The current epidemic of acquired immunodeficiency syndrome (AIDS), caused by the HIV, has presented infection control nurses with the challenge of developing a system of isolation that would prevent transmission of this and other frequently undiagnosed infections in health care settings and the community. Body substance isolation (BSI) is a new system developed by ICN's Jackson and Lynch.[31] This system emphasizes universal precautions when in contact with the body fluids of all patients.

This chapter presents an overview of the role of the nurse in the prevention and control of infection. For further information regarding a specific infectious disease, consult the chapter in which the site of the disease is discussed; for example, Chapter 22 for hepatitis, Chapter 16 for tuberculosis, and so on.

THE INFECTIOUS DISEASE PROCESS
Definitions

A number of definitions are useful when describing certain conditions related to the infectious disease process. These are presented in Table 12-1.

The question of whether somebody has an infection or colonization can be difficult to answer. What is important to realize is that people who are colonized, as well as those who are infected, can easily serve as a source of infection to themselves and to others who are at risk.

Chain of Infection

Essential to appropriate intervention in the prevention and control of infection is an understanding of the infectious disease process. All infectious diseases occur as a result of a sequence of events (Fig. 12-1). Often the reservoir for an agent responsible for an outbreak of an infection is not readily apparent and, in fact, may never be identified. If the process of infection is well understood, however, appropriate and effective control measures can be instituted even though the original source of the causative agent is not known.

Once the agent has left the reservoir, it needs a *mode of transmission* to a host. Modes and examples of how infection is spread by each mode are explained in Box 12-1.

Table 12-1 Selected definitions related to the infectious disease process

Term	Definition
Pathogen	Microorganism or substance capable of producing disease
Pathogenicity	Capability of pathogen to infect and produce disease; determined by ability to survive and multiply outside host, virulence, dose, host specificity, and resistance of host
Invasiveness	Injury to host as a result of presence and spread of pathogen through body tissues
Toxigenicity	Injury to host as a result of effects to host of toxins produced by pathogen
Incubation period	Period of time after pathogen enters host and before clinical symptoms of infection appear
Infection	Presence in the body of a pathogen that multiplies and produces effects injurious to the host
Apparent (symptomatic, clinical)	Clinical signs and symptoms present
Inapparent (asymptomatic, subclinical)	No perceivable signs or symptoms present
Acute	Rapid onset, immediate host response, severe symptoms, and usually short course
Chronic	Insidious onset, delayed host response, mild symptoms, and long course
Latent	Pathogen ever-present in host, symptoms present only intermittently, often in response to a stimulus; pathogen dormant at other times
Localized	Focal point of symptoms or injury
Generalized	Systemic, whole body involvement
Superinfection	New infection by a pathogen different from one that caused initial infection
Colonization	Presence of pathogenic microorganisms in or on a host that do not produce injury or incite an injurious body response
Normal flora	Presence of nonpathogenic microorganisms that normally reside in various body locations without invasion or harm (may become pathogenic if introduced into an area in which they do not normally reside)
Contamination	Presence of pathogenic microorganisms on inanimate objects or in substances

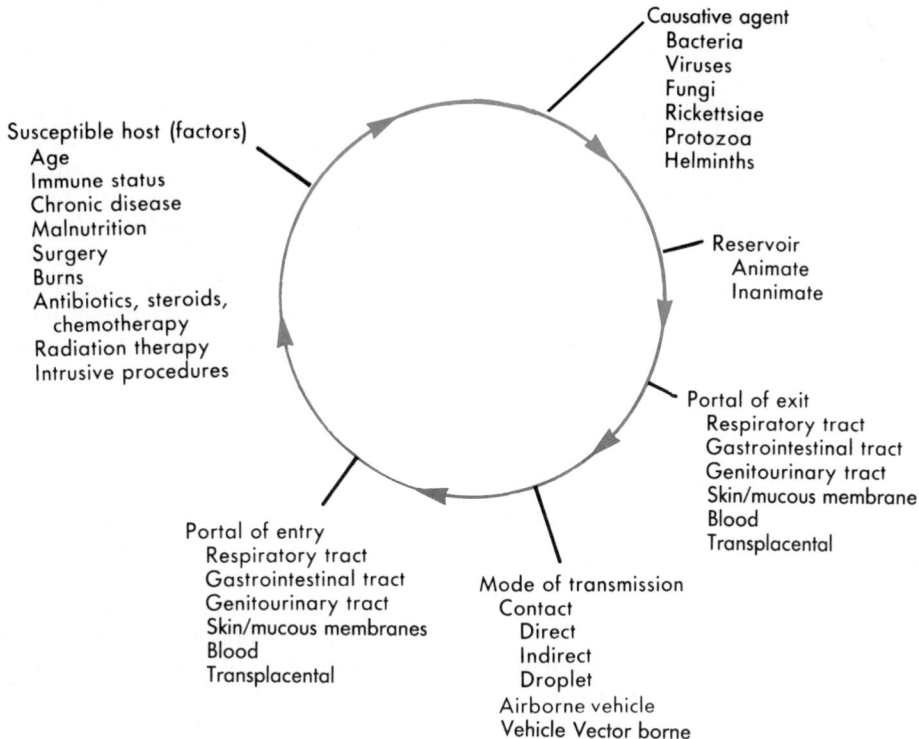

Fig. 12-1   The infectious disease process.

Entry of an infectious agent into a host does not mean that the agent will proliferate and cause infection. Infection depends on the dose and virulence of the agent and the *susceptibility of the host*. The healthy human body is extremely resistant to infection; however, when the basic biological defence mechanisms of the body are compromised, an infectious organism has a much greater chance of causing an infection. Chapter 33 deals with many of the factors of biological defence exhibited by the host to prevent infection and injury. Some of the factors that affect host susceptibility to infection are included in Box 12-2.

No one factor alone is responsible for an infection. Rather, there are a number of variables—the *agent*, the *environment*, and the *host*—that determine the outcome and towards which prevention and control measures are directed. To intervene effectively in the infectious disease process it is important that all of these concepts be understood.

Assessment

The establishment of an infection within the human body leads to a number of specific and generalized manifesta-

12-1	**Examples of modes of transmission of infection**	
	Mode	**Example**
	I. Contact	HIV infection, gonorrhoea, syphilis
	Direct: (source to host)	
	Indirect: by way of intermediate object	
	Hands	*Staphylococcus aureus* wound infection
	Fomites (e.g., hypodermic needle)	Hepatitis B, HIV infection
	Surgical instruments	*Staphylococcus aureus* wound infection
	Droplet (large particles)	Meningococcal meningitis, influenza
	Host inhales droplets expelled from reservoir	
	II. Airborne: host inhales droplet nuclei (1 to 5 micrometers) in air	Chicken pox (varicella), pulmonary tuberculosis
	III. Vehicle: ingested or administered substance	
	Food, water	Hapatitis A, salmonellosis
	Blood products	Hepatitis B, HIV infection
	IV fluids	Enterobacter bacteraemia, fungaemia
	IV. Vector: animate intermediary (usually insect)	Malaria, Rocky Mountain spotted fever, yellow fever, Lyme disease

---

12-2

Factors affecting host susceptibility to infection

Age	Young and old most susceptible
Impaired immune status	HIV infection, leukaemia, immunosuppressive drugs, radiation therapy, steroids
Chronic diseases	Diabetes, cancer, COPD, end-stage renal disease
Poor nutritional status	
Invasive devices, surgery	Intravenous catheters, chest tubes, urinary catheters, artificial airways
Impaired skin integrity	Burns, decubitus
Altered body flora	Antibiotics, antacid therapy

---

tions. The exact signs and symptoms elicited in the host depend on the agent responsible for the infection and the site of the infection. (For details on host response to specific infectious disease, see the particular chapter that discusses the disease site.) Early recognition of infection is a crucial step to initiating prompt treatment. There are some general subjective, objective, and diagnostic findings that can alert the nurse to suspect an infection, even if the causative agent is not known. These are summarized here.

The normal white blood cell (WBC) count in blood is 5000 to 10,000 WBC/mm³. With the presence of a serious infection the number of WBCs rises above 10,000/mm³ in response to the infectious inflammation. Leukocyte values between 10,000 and 20,000 are considered slightly elevated, 20,000 to 40,000 moderately elevated, and greater than 40,000 greatly elevated. In a few infectious diseases the number of WBCs in circulation actually drops, which is also a significant piece of diagnostic datum.

None of the signs and symptoms present in localized or generalized infections is diagnostic in itself. Many can be demonstrated by other disease processes. They can also serve as helpful clues in the diagnosis of a suspected infectious process.

Diagnostic Tests

Diagnostic tests are important in the diagnosis of an infection. Some of the diagnostic tests used to obtain data are the following:

  Bacterial, viral, and fungal cultures, Gram stain
  Antigen/antibody detection
  Blood counts
  Skin tests
  Radiological tests
  Gallium scans
  Ultrasound examinations
  CT scan
  MRI examinations
Specimens for microbiological testing are perhaps the most frequently ordered when an infection is suspected.

Proper collection and handling of laboratory specimens are essential to ensure accurate laboratory results. Inappropriate collection or handling of specimens may lead to unnecessary delays in test results or to inaccurate results, thus affecting the therapy given to the patient. When an infection is suspected, cultures are taken of the suspected site. If the patient has a fever and the site of infection is unknown, cultures are commonly taken of the blood, urine, sputum, and any other possible sites of infection. This may include spinal fluid cultures, aspirates of body fluid, or intravenous catheter tips. *It is imperative that these cultures be obtained before the initiation of antibiotic therapy whenever possible because antibiotics can suppress any bacteria that are present and give inaccurate or false–negative culture results.* Cultures should be obtained in a manner that avoids contamination. Aseptic preparation of the site to be cultured, observance of aseptic technique, and placing specimens in an appropriate container are crucial factors to be observed in ensuring the best sample. Once obtained, the specimen must be properly stored and transported promptly to the laboratory. Each institution should have guidelines for the proper method for collecting and handling specimens for the laboratory (Box 12-3).

Interpretation of laboratory results is sometimes difficult. Certain body sites have bacteria known as normal flora, which reside there in a commensalistic (intimate) relationship with the host. These bacteria do not cause infection in the normal host. The skin, upper respiratory tract, vagina, urethra, and bowel are examples of body sites in which normal bacterial flora can be found. The bacteria found vary from site to site, and knowing the normal flora is helpful in discerning the significance of laboratory culture results. *A Clinician's Dictionary of Bacteria and*

12-3

General guidelines for specimen collection

Objective

To obtain specimen containing infecting pathogen that is free of contamination

Method

1. Wash hands.
2. Prepare site aseptically.
3. Collect specimen using aseptic technique; wear gloves if appropriate; avoid coughing, sneezing, or talking.
4. Obtain adequate amount of specimen.
5. Collect and transport in sterile container appropriate for type of specimen.
6. Label requisition with patient's name, location, date, and time of collection, type of specimen, how obtained (for example, clean void or catheter urine), test requested, and current antibiotic therapy.
7. Store properly and transport promptly to laboratory.
8. Keep record of test

Fungi[15] is an excellent publication that lists in detail the normal flora of various sites. It must be emphasized that laboratory results alone cannot be used to make diagnostic and therapeutic decisions. Rather, they are used in conjunction with the clinical status of the patient to make appropriate diagnostic and therapeutic decisions.

Knowledge about the infectious disease process and about how to recognize or suspect an infectious process is vital to the prevention and control of infectious diseases in both community and hospital settings.

INFECTION CONTROL IN THE COMMUNITY

An infectious disease is termed a communicable disease when it is highly transmissable to other people. Smallpox is an example of a communicable disease that, through cooperative efforts worldwide, has been successfully eradicated. The methods used to eradicate smallpox throughout the world can serve as a model of how to eliminate other communicable diseases. The eradication of smallpox also demonstrates the importance of accurate reporting of communicable diseases to the proper authorities so that prevention and control measures can be instituted.

The community health nurse plays a vital role in the collection of data, surveillance activities, immunization programmes, education, and other control measures. Doctors and health care facilities have a responsibility to report communicable diseases promptly to the health department. Health agencies in the community can use the reported data to determine potential or real problems, to identify the causative agent and its source (if possible), and to identify the population at risk. A method to control the problem, care for the exposed, and protect the population at risk can then be devised and implemented.

The HIV epidemic has posed the greatest communicable disease threat in recent years. Since first identified as a communicable disease in 1981, much has been learned through epidemiological research. AIDS was first described in homosexual males and then in intravenous drug users and haemophiliacs. This discovery helped to identify the routes of transmission as sexual contact, contaminated needles, and blood transfusions. In 1983 the virus was first isolated. In Britain the virus was named human *T lymphotrophic virus III* (*HTLV III*). The French named the same virus *lymphadenopathy virus* (*LAV*). Later the virus was renamed *human immunodeficiency virus* (*HIV*). Since first recognized as a communicable disease, no new routes of transmission have been identified.

In October 1987 the screening of all blood and blood products for HIV antibody was begun in Britain. This has almost eliminated blood transfusions as a source of HIV infection. Today, those most at risk for HIV infection are people who engage in high-risk behaviour: having multiple sexual partners, sharing intravenous needles, or being a sexual partner of a person who engages in high-risk behaviour. In addition, HIV infection may be transmitted from an infected mother to fetus *in utero* from maternal circulation or during labour and delivery. Casual contact has not been identified as a means of transmission. Nonsexual cohabitants of HIV-infected people have not become infected. The risk of transmission of HIV to a health care worker from an infected patient via needle-stick has been calculated as 1:250.[21] Improved technology to decrease exposure of health care workers to needles and other sharps is needed. In 1991, the first case of transmission of HIV from health care worker to patient during an invasive procedure was reported in US.

Until a cure or vaccine is available, the only effective control measure is education. Educational programmes emphasize the routes of transmission, identify high-risk behaviour, and instruct in safer sexual practices. Nurses participate in AIDS education programmes in schools, in the media, community centres, and churches. Nurses are also engaged in HIV counselling. It is essential that the nurse be well informed and provide accurate information in a sensitive and nonjudgmental manner.

AIDS is discussed in detail in Chapter 13.

Prevention and Control Measures

One method of prevention and control of disease in the community involves environmental control measures such as sanitation techniques that ensure a pure water supply and proper disposal of sewage and other potentially infectious materials. These measures have been legislated into building codes and governmental regulations. Similarly, there are regulations regarding health practices in institutions that handle, package, and prepare foods. Another example of an environmental control measure is the spraying of a designated area to kill mosquitos, which are implicated in the spread of viral encephalitis. Spraying usually is done only after an outbreak has been identified.

Depending on the communicable disease, care of exposed people and protection of the population at risk for contracting the disease may entail prophylaxis, immunization, or careful monitoring of only new cases. Often, simple adherence to basic principles of hygiene is sufficient. Determination of additional required measures should be made by the local health department. Attempts are made to reach those at risk and inform them of the preventive measures. Education of the public is a key component of these efforts.

In the U.K., the European targets for immunization form the basis for immunization policy. In 1986, two reports to Parliament highlighted the U.K.'s poor record on immunization.[15a,34a] However, recent trends in immunization rates for the U.K. have been more encouraging. Diphtheria, polio and tetanus have all but disappeared from the mortality and disease statistics. The Department of Health set a target of 90% vaccine uptake by 1990 for measles, rubella, polio, diphtheria and tetanus, and aims to eliminate these diseases by the year 2000. The U.K. is now approaching both national and international targets for immunization uptake of rubella, measles and pertussis (whooping cough).[28a]

A more recent concern because of air travel is the elimination of the barriers of time and distance and the possibility of a person with an infectious disease being brought from a remote area of the world to a major population centre where the disease can be readily spread to a susceptible public.

The dramatic control of several infectious diseases has been caused by the development and use of a variety of

Table 12-2 Outline of the recommended vaccination programme for children

Recommended age	Vaccine(s)*	Comments
2 months	DTP	Given in 3 doses at intervals of 4 weeks
	Haemophilus influenza type B	
	Polio (oral)	
12 to 15 months	MMR	
	Haemophilus influenza type B	
School age	DT	At entry to school or nursery
	Polio (oral)	
	MMR	If not previously immunized
10 to 14 years	BCG	After tuberculin test
	Rubella	For girls only
16 years	Polio (oral)	Given when leaving school or before
	Tetanus	starting work or further education

* *DTP*, diphtheria, tetanus, pertussis; *MMR*, measles, mumps, rubella.

inactivated vaccines and live attenuated antigens. The potential for eradication of common infectious diseases brings with it major responsibilities for public health agencies, doctors, and nurses. Ways must be found not only to carry out planned programmes of immunization, but also to educate the public to the hazards of apathy and failure to maintain proper levels of immunization. Progress in control and eradication requires that all aspects of these programmes be continually evaluated.

Immunization Programmes

Immunization programmes have played and continue to play a primary role in the control of infectious disease throughout the world. The body can be stimulated to produce antibodies against some specific diseases without actually having the disease (*active artificial immunity*). Temporary protection sometimes can be provided by injecting antibodies produced by other people or animals into the bloodstream of a human being (*passive artificial immunity*).

Recommendations concerning current immunization schedules are found in *Immunisation against Infectious Diseases*, a handbook published annually by the Department of Health, Welsh Office, Scottish Office and the DHSS (Northern Ireland). The reader should refer to these resources when there are questions about proper immunization practices, prophylaxis, interruption in immunization schedules, or adverse reactions and side effects.

Active immunization

If 90% of the population is protected against organisms that required continued passage through human beings to reproduce and live, the disease caused by the organism can be virtually eliminated because there are too few susceptible hosts for organism spread. Smallpox has been eliminated from the world in this way. It is ineffectual, however, against organisms such as tetanus bacilli that can exist indefinitely (in the soil), and in this instance each individual must be immunized to be protected. If the disease is one not prevalent in the environment, such as diphtheria , or is not spread from person to person by direct contact, such as tetanus, the inoculation must be repeated at regular intervals to maintain protection. This inoculation is called a

booster dose, and usually one-tenth of the original inoculating dose is sufficient.

An inoculation often causes a local tissue response. Symptoms of inflammation (redness, tenderness, swelling, sometimes ulceration) appear at the site of the injection, and generalized symptoms of widespread tissue involvement (slight febrile reactions, general malaise, muscle aching) for 1 or 2 days are common.

Active artificial immunization against many bacilli and viruses is now available. Everybody should be encouraged to avail themselves of the protection advised by health officials in their local area. They also should be advised to keep a permanent record of the date of each immunization.

Primary immunization schedules

In the U.K. it is recommended that all children be immunized against diphtheria, pertussis, (whooping cough), tetanus (DPT); measles, mumps, and rubella (MMR); and poliomyelitis (OPV) (see Table 12-2). Children who have not been immunized as infants can be immunized at any age. All susceptible children, adolescents, and adults should be immunized unless contraindicated.

Routine vaccination against smallpox is no longer recommended because the side effects and complications of the vaccine are greater than the danger of acquiring the disease. The vaccine is indicated only for laboratory workers who are directly involved with smallpox or closely related orthopox viruses. However, the armed forces vaccinate all personnel serving overseas.

At the present time, immunization against typhoid fever is recommended only when there is exposure to a typhoid carrier in the household, when there is an outbreak of typhoid in a community, or for travellers to countries where typhoid is endemic.

Immunization to protect against other diseases is given on a selective basis; that is, groups at a high risk are immunized. Hepatitis B vaccine is an excellent example of a vaccine that is recommended only for people at high risk of acquiring the virus.

Because of the prevalence of *influenza* and its potential for causing death, immunization against influenza is recommended for all individuals at increased risk of adverse consequences from infection of the lower respiratory tract.

A vaccine is currently available that protects against 23 types of streptococcal pneumonia.

Passive immunization

Passive immunization usually is reserved for situations in which the disease would be detrimental to the individual. For example, it is rarely given to prevent a disease such as chickenpox or mumps in children because they are at an optimal age for the body to respond immunologically with minimal inflammatory response. On the other hand, an adult exposed to the same diseases often would be given antibodies because adults may have a severe pathological response. *Immunization is given to all age groups exposed to pathogens that cause serious diseases such as hepatitis, poliomyelitis, diphtheria, tetanus, or rabies.*

Products used for passive immunization may be specific to the disease. Antitoxins and immune animal and human sera are examples. These materials contain elevated levels of immune globulins, which can specifically detoxify the toxin, neutralize the virus, or inactivate the bacterium. The whole blood of a patient who has recently recovered from a disease against which antibodies are produced also may be used. Antitoxins are available for diphtheria, tetanus, botulism, gas gangrene, and the venom of snakes. *Human immune serum* is available for mumps, measles, pertussis, rabies, poliomyelitis, and tetanus.

Immune serum globulin (ISG), or gamma globulin (γ-globulin), is an antibody-rich fraction of pooled plasma from normal donors. The rationale for pooling plasma is that someone among the donors will have had the diseases and will have developed antibodies against them. The *globulin fraction* of the plasma carries the antibodies, and because it is known not to transmit the virus of hepatitis, it is considered safe to use. Because of occasional side effects, it is now recommended that the use of immune serum globulin be limited to those disorders in which its efficacy has been definitely established. These are measles prophylaxis or modification, viral hepatitis type A prophylaxis or modification, and immune deficiency diseases.

Special human immune serum globulins are derived from the sera of people previously immunized or convalescing from specific diseases. Tetanus immune globulin (human) is of value in prophylaxis and treatment of tetanus in those who have not received prior immunization. Pertussis immune globulin (human) and mumps immune globulin (human) are of uncertain or unproved value in the prevention and treatment of pertussis and mumps, respectively. Hepatitis B immune globulin (human) is available for prophylaxis after exposure to hepatitis B. Zoster immune globulin (human) is available for restricted use for prophylaxis against chickenpox.

Nursing responsibilities

Teaching

The greatest responsibility of the nurse in immunization programmes is to teach the public the advantages of immunization and encourage widespread participation in programmes recommended by the local public health officer.

In teaching it is advisable to provide the public with the following information: (1) *against what disease protection is being given*, (2) *why immunization is desirable, and* (3) *when booster doses should be obtained.* The relative safety of the immunization and the advantages of immunization early in life should be stressed.

The nurse is responsible for assessing people before immunization because there are some contraindications to receiving certain immunizing substances. Those that are prepared in chicken or duck embryos may cause an allergic reaction in those allergic to eggs. Many people are allergic to horse serum, and substances containing horse serum, such as tetanus antitoxin, should never be given unless a small amount of the substance has been injected intradermally (a sensitivity test) and after 20 minutes produces no "hive" reaction about the injection site. *Active immunological products should not be given while a person has a cold or other infection because the inflammatory reaction from the immunization will be greater than usual.*

Live attenuated virus vaccines should *not be given to people* with *alterations in their immune status* because virus replication after administration may be unchecked in these individuals. OPV viruses are excreted by the recipient of the vaccine and are communicable to other people, so individuals who live with an immunocompromised person should not receive OPV.

Before leaving the clinic, the patient and/or family members should be instructed about the expected effects of an inoculation and told to contact the doctor or to report to a hospital casualty department if any other symptoms develop. The patient is cautioned not to scratch any lesion produced by an inoculation. If a severe local reaction with redness, swelling, and tenderness occurs, the doctor may order the application of hot, wet dressings. If the lesion is open, these dressings should be sterile.

When antitoxins, antisera, or antivenims are given, the patient is kept under observation for 20 to 30 minutes. Symptoms of severe allergic response usually will appear within that period of time. The responsibility of the nurse working in employee health programmes is to educate personnel to achieve and maintain immune status and participate in screening programmes, for example, tuberculosis, varicella, and rubella.

Yearly chest X-ray examinations are no longer recommended for the routine management of people with positive tuberculin skin tests. Health care workers with negative tuberculin tests should be tested yearly. If a worker who has had a negative test turns positive, she or he should be offered prophylactic isoniazed (INH). Additionally, the source of the infection should be identified if possible. (For more information see Chapter 16.) After the initial chest X-ray examination following a skin test conversion, yearly chest X-ray examinations have not been shown to be of significant clinical value and are not cost effective in monitoring people for early disease. Health care and public safety workers who have contact with blood should maintain their immune status against hepatitis B.

Table 12-3 U.S.A. infection rates per 1000 discharges by site and hospital category, 1984

	UTI	SW1	LRI	BACT	CUT	OTH	All sites
Nonteaching hospital	9.9	3.6	4.2	1.3	1.1	2.0	22.2
Small teaching hospital	13.9	6.0	5.4	1.9	1.8	4.7	33.8
Large teaching hospital	14.2	6.6	7.7	3.9	2.6	6.4	41.4

From Centers for Disease control: CDC Surveillance Summaries, 1986; 35 (No. 1SS)
UTI, Urinary tract infection; *SWI,* Surgical wound infection; *LRI,* Lower respiratory tract infection; *BACT,* Primary bacteraemia; *CUT,* Cutaneous infection; *OTH,* Other.

Home care

People with communicable diseases are frequently cared for at home. The district nurse is often asked to teach family members how to care for the patient and how to protect family members, friends, and neighbours. The same principles apply in the home as in the hospital.

Regardless of the disease, good hand washing technique should be practised and gloves should be worn for contact with any body substance. A smock or apron can be worn to protect the clothes from soiling. A mask, if indicated, can be improvised from any closely woven absorbable material, or disposable ones can be purchased at a chemist. All liquid wastes can be flushed down a toilet. Garbage and other wastes containing body substances can be wrapped in newspaper and placed in a plastic bag before being discarded in a rubbish container. Dishes should be washed in hot, soapy water. Separate dishes are not required. Laundry should be washed in a washing machine with a detergent. Chlorine bleach or a disinfectant should be added if linen is soiled with body substances. The local health department should be consulted for full information regarding specific communicable diseases.

The special problems the nurse encounters in controlling *hospital-acquired infections* will be the focus of the remainder of this chapter.

INFECTION CONTROL IN THE HOSPITAL
Scope of the Problem

A *nosocomial* infection is one that is not present or incubating at the time a person is admitted to the hospital but which develops after admission. A *community-acquired* infection is one that is present or incubating at the time of admission to the hospital. The nurse should be aware of the problem of nosocomial infections, their effects on patient morbidity, mortality, and increased hospital costs, as well as the legal aspects concerning them. The nurse also should be knowledgeable about the types of infections seen most often, the common pathogens and how they are transmitted, factors that predispose a patient to a nosocomial infection, how to recognize those at risk of infection, and the prevention and control measures necessary to decrease the incidence of nosocomial infections.

It is estimated that 3% to 5% of all patients discharged from hospital each year develop nosocomial infections.[25] In addition to the considerable morbidity and mortality caused by these infections, their diagnoses and treatment (including additional days of hospitalization) cost more than £1 billion per year. The Department of Health requires that those institutions seeking accreditation have a programme of infection control centred around monitoring (1) patients with infections, (2) patient care practices, (3) antibiotic usage, (4) health of personnel, and (5) the environment of the institution. The Department of Health and the Communicable Disease Surveillance Centre (CDSC) have developed guidelines for the prevention and control of infectious diseases for use in patient care centres. Because of these external forces, as well as to provide the best possible care for their patients, hospitals are recognizing the need to increase infection surveillance and to upgrade programmes to prevent nosocomial infections.

As seen in Table 12-3, the incidence of nosocomial infections varies with the type of hospital, and this can be attributed to differences in the size of hospitals, the severity of illness in the patient population, the susceptibility of the patient population, and the number of personnel who have hands-on contact with the patients. The patient with the greatest risk of developing a nosocomial infection is one with a chronic illness, a prolonged hospital stay, and the most direct contact with various hospital personnel (that is, doctors, students, nurses, or therapists). These factors hold true not only for variations of infection rates from institution to institution, but also for variations in infection rates within an institution. Certain patient care areas are considered to be *high-risk areas* for developing nosocomial infections. These areas understandably are those that care for patients who have decreased host defences, are immunocompromised, or in whom invasive procedures and devices are common. Areas generally considered to be high risk are (1) intensive care units (including neonatal units), (2) burn units, (3) dialysis units, and (4) oncology units. The infection rate in these areas may be well over 20%.

Although ICU patients account for only 15% of hospital admissions, they account for 50% or more of nosocomial infections.[26]

People at Risk

The nurse needs to be able to recognize those patients who are at the greatest risk of a nosocomial infection. Some of the factors that predispose a person to infection are mentioned on p. 196. Probably the single most important factor predisposing a patient to a nosocomial infection is the severity of the patient's underlying disease.

A person admitted to the hospital with an infection may develop during the hospitalization a *superinfection* with another organism. Often this superinfection is with a more virulent or drug-resistant organism. For example, a patient admitted with a leg ulcer infected with *Staphylococcus aureus* may develop further infection (not colonization) with *Pseudomonas aeruginosa*. Furthermore, if this infection progresses to involve the bloodstream, then a *secondary bacteraemia* has occurred. Infection can occur secondary to (1) an existing infection, (2) an underlying disease process, or (3) an anatomic defect that may be causing obstruction. An example of this is the man who has benign prostate hypertrophy (BPH) and who develops a urinary tract infection secondary to the obstruction caused by the BPH.

The most common site for a nosocomial infection is the urinary tract; 75% of these infections are related to instrumentation, including in-dwelling urinary catheters, catheterizations, and urological procedures. Infected surgical wounds, followed by lower respiratory tract infections, and then bloodstream infections (some associated with the use of intravascular lines) are the next most frequently encountered types of nosocomial infections. Together these sites account for about 80% of all nosocomial infections.

Pathogens Causing Nosocomial Infections

The pathogens commonly responsible for nosocomial infections and their common sources are listed in Table 12-4. Changes in the aetiological agents of nosocomial infections occurred in the 1980s. Organisms causing these infections are now increasingly likely to be resistant to most antibiotics, which leaves fewer options for treatment.

According to National Nosocomial Infections Surveillance System (NNIS) data from 1986 to 1989, *Escherichia coli* continues to be the most common pathogen responsible for hospital-acquired infection. Other pathogens responsible for 10% or more of the total number of infections include enterococci, *Pseudomonas aeruginosa*, and *Staphylococcus aureus*. Coagulase negative staphylococcus, once considered an insignificant source of nosocomial infection, is now responsible for close to 10% of all hospital-acquired infections. These infections are primarily seen in patients with intravascular devices and are caused by the ability of the organism to adhere to the walls of the device.

Serratia marcescens is a Gram-negative organism responsible for 2% of nosocomial infections. Its ability rapidly to develop resistance to antibiotics has made it a potential source of nosocomial infection outbreaks, especially in intensive care units. Because the mode of transmission is direct or indirect contact on the hands of personnel or on contaminated articles, *good hand-washing* and *aseptic techniques are the most effective measures to prevent outbreaks.*

Candida albicans is a yeastlike fungus that can *cause infection, especially in immunocompromised patients* or in *patients receiving antibiotics.* These patients have a decrease in their normal flora, which provides a niche for *Candida* organisms to settle in and proliferate. *Candida vaginitis and oral thrush are common complications of antibiotic therapy.* Antibiotics suppress bacterial growth but do not affect fungal growth; special antifungal agents are necessary to control these infections unless the normal flora returns following discontinuance of the antibiotics.

Methicillin sodium-resistant *Staphylococcus aureus* (MRSA) is a pathogen causing increasing concern among health care workers. Methicillin sodium is one of the penicillins specifically developed to treat S. *aureus* infections. Because S. *aureus* is a common surgical wound pathogen, the concern is that MRSA infections will be more difficult and expensive to treat. Currently the antibiotic of choice for treating MRSA infection is vancomycin, which must be given intravenously and may be ototoxic and nephrotoxic. It is considerably more expensive than the methicillin-group antibiotics. Once introduced into an institution, MRSA becomes endemic, and eradication measures have been largely unsuccessful. The hands of health caregivers have been associated with cross-infections. Patients colonized with MRSA should not be transferred to another health care institution because institutions are afraid of the spread of this pathogen.

Prevention and Control Measures

In the hospital there are many potential sources of infection, including patients, personnel, visitors, equipment, and linen. Patients may become infected with organisms from either the external environment (*exogenous*) or, as is often seen in the severely immunocompromised host, from their own internal organisms (*endogenous*). Virtually any microorganism can be a potential pathogen to the immunocompromised patient. Most of the causative or-

Table 12-4   Modes of transmission of some common pathogens

Pathogen	Source
Gram-positive cocci	
Staphylococcus areus	Contaminated objects, hands, and nasal tracts of health care workers, air, self
Coagulase-negative *Staphyloccus*	Self, hands of health care workers, invasive devices
Group A *Streptococcus* organisms	Direct contact, air, hands, rarely objects
Enterococcus organisms	Self, hands of health care workers, contaminated environmental surfaces
Gram-negative rods	
Escherichia, Klebsiella, Enterobacter	Self, hands of health care workers, contaminated solutions
Proteus, Salmonella, Providencia, Serratia, Citrobacter	Contaminated food and water, hands of health care workers, self
Pseudomonas	Contaminated environment, hands, self
Anaerobic bacteria	
Clostridium, Bacteroides	Self, contaminated environment, hands
Fungal organisms	
Yeasts	Self, hands of health care workers
Fungi	Air, contaminated environment
Viruses	
Varicella	Air, direct contact
Herpes	Self, direct contact, air
Rubella	Direct contact, air
Hepatitis B	Contaminated instruments or injectables, direct contact

12-4

Prevention of, and control measures for, nosocomial infections

Control of external environment (exogenous sources of infection)
Health caregivers
1. In good health—do not care for patients when ill
2. Keep immunization current
3. Practise effective hand washing between each patient
   If skin dry, rough, or broken, seek appropriate attention
   If active herpes simplex infection of hand (herpetic whitlow), do not give direct patient care until lesion healed
4. Wear gloves when contact with any body substance is anticipated

Housekeeping and sanitation
1. Bed linens not shaken in air or thrown on floor
2. Proper disposal of wastes—solid and liquid
3. Proper cleaning and sterilization of contaminated articles
4. Proper ventilation for adequate air exchanges
   Modern hospitals—patients' rooms under negative pressure
   Negative pressure keeps air from patients' rooms from moving into hallways
5. Proper mopping and damp dusting to remove dust and other environmental resevoirs of infection

Control of internal environment (endogenous sources of infection)
1. Preventive measures aimed at increasing patient's defence mechanisms and thus reducing risk of infection
   Teach patient about good nutrition
   Teach patient about personal hygiene, especially hand washing
2. Be aware that normal flora of patient can be disrupted when patient is receiving antibiotics or chemotherapy and colonization may occur
   Give antibiotics on time as scheduled
   Teach patient about appropriate use of antibiotics and dangers of taking them when not prescribed by doctor.

ganisms are present in the external environment of the patient and are introduced into the body through direct contact or by contact with contaminated materials. In many instances nosocomial infections could be prevented by strict aseptic technique when giving care to the patient and by greater restraint in the use of invasive procedures and antibiotics. A summary of some of the prevention and control measures is presented in Box 12-4. The reader is referred to Reference 39 for greater detail.

Protection by isolation

The purpose of isolation is to protect both the health caregiver from exposure to infectious agents and the patient from cross-infection. In the U.S. in 1983 the Centers for Disease Control (CDC) published revised guidelines for isolation precautions in hospitals. Two systems were offered for use. One was based on categories of isolation, and the other listed disease-specific isolation precautions. Hospitals were advised to choose the system most appropriate for their needs. There were seven major categories of isolation: strict, contact, respiratory, tuberculosis (AFB), enteric, drainage/secretion, and blood/body fluid. Protective isolation was eliminated as a category because it has not been shown to reduce the risk of infection in the immunocompromised patient.

The current HIV epidemic has emphasized the need for health caregivers to consider the blood and body fluids of all patients as potentially infectious. Although it has been shown that the risk of HIV transmission to health caregivers is low, other pathogens such as hepatitis A virus, hepatitis B virus, hepatitis virus C, cytomegalovirus, herpes simplex virus, Epstein–Barr virus, and *Staphylococcus aureus* are more easily transmitted in health care settings. Infections with these agents are frequently undiagnosed before initial contact with the patient. Therefore, taking precautions with the body fluids of all patients will both protect the health caregiver and reduce nosocomial transmission of pathogens. In August 1987 the CDC published new recommendations for the prevention of HIV transmission in health care settings. These guidelines recommend the elimination of a separate blood/body fluid category, because these precautions are to be taken with all patients. Many hospitals have eliminated all the old isolation categories and implemented a system called *body substance isolation* (BSI). BSI protects both the health careworker and patients because it is not dependent on a diagnosis to initiate precautions. Following are explanations of (1) category-specific isolation and universal blood/body fluid precautions (Box 12-5) and (2) BSI (Box 12-6).

General principles of isolation

Some general principles apply regardless of the type of isolation. Gowns, gloves, and masks should be used only once and then discarded in an appropriate receptacle before leaving the patient's room. Supplies should be available convenient to each patient's room. Hands must be washed before and after patient contact, even when gloves are a required part of the isolation procedure. Masks become ineffective when they are moist and therefore should never be reused. They should be worn over the nose and mouth and should not hang around the neck and then be reused. Disposable used articles and other waste should be placed in an impervious bag and the bag should be securely closed before it is discarded. Mattresses and pillows should be covered with impervious plastic.

The reader can see the similarity between the CDC's universal blood/body fluid precautions and BSI. The difference is that BSI does not require the other categories except for airborne transmitted diseases because the BSI technique prevents the transmission of the diseases in the other categories. There is redundancy in the CDC's category-specific and universal blood/body fluid precaution system.

12-5

Universal blood/body fluid precautions

Because medical history and examination cannot reliably identify all patients infected with HIV or other blood-borne pathogens, blood and body fluid precautions should be consistently used for all patients.

Specifications for universal blood/body fluid precautions

1. Gloves are worn for touching blood and body fluids, mucous membranes, or nonintact skin of all patients, for handling items or surfaces soiled with blood or body fluids, and for performing venipuncture and other vascular access procedures. Gloves should be changed after contact with each patient.
2. Masks and protective eyewear or face shields should be worn during procedures that are likely to generate droplets of blood or other body fluids to prevent exposure of mucous membranes of the mouth, nose, and eyes.
3. Gowns or aprons should be worn during procedures that are likely to generate splashes of blood or other body fluids.
4. Hands and other skin surfaces should be washed immediately and thoroughly if contaminated with blood or other body fluids. Hands should be washed immediately after gloves are removed.
5. Disposable articles contaminated with body substances should be bagged and discarded according to local and state regulations.
6. Care should be taken to avoid needle-stick injuries. Used needles should not be recapped or bent; they should be placed in a designated puncture-resistant container as close to point of use as possible.
7. Blood spills should be cleaned up promptly with a solution of 5.25% sodium hypochlorite diluted 1 : 10 with water or an approved "hospital disinfectant" that is also tuberculocidal.

Universal blood and body fluid precautions protect the caregiver from blood-borne communicable diseases. Diseases recognized as being transmitted by blood include:

Acquired immunodeficiency syndrome (AIDS)
Arthropod-borne viral fevers (for example, dengue, yellow fever)
Babesiosis
Creutzfeldt–Jakob disease
Hepatitis B (including HBsAg carrier)
Hepatitis C
Leptospirosis
Malaria
Rat-bite fever
Relapsing fever
Syphilis, primary and secondary (skin and mucous membrane lesions)

12-6

Body substance isolation

All body substances are potentially infectious. Faeces, sputum, and wound drainage always contain infectious organisms, whereas blood, urine, and other body fluids sometimes contain infectious organisms. The colonized, subclinical, and diagnosed infections are all communicable. However, category-specific or disease specific isolation protects against only the diagnosed communicable infection. Therefore, protection against communicable disease transmission (health careworker and patient) can be achieved only by taking precautions with the body substances of all patients. Precautions should be determined by the anticipated interaction with a patient's body substances. Under this system, labelling patients with diagnosed infections would serve as a hindrance and support a double standard of practice. For example, a double standard exists when caregivers wear gloves when handling the urine of a patient with diagnosed *Serratia* urinary tract infection but not when handling the urine of other patients. Under BSI, the caregiver would be instructed to wear gloves for handling the urine of all patients.

Specifications for body substance isolation

1. Gloves for contact with mucous membranes, nonintact skin, and moist body substances. Gloves are changed after each patient contact.
2. Gown or plastic apron if soiling of clothing is likely.
3. Mask and eye protection if splashing of moist body substances is likely.
4. A private room is indicated if personal hygiene is poor or if body substances contaminate the environment.
5. Trash and linen bagged securely to prevent leakage.
6. Needles are disposed of uncapped and unbent at the point of use in a puncture-resistant container. Safe recapping using a one-handed or device-assisted technique is used when necessary.
7. Blood spills of all patients should be cleaned by a gloved person using a solution of 5.25% sodium hypochlorite (household bleach) diluted 1 : 10 in water or a hospital disinfectant that is tuberculocidal.
8. A sign explaining BSI technique is placed in each patient's room.
9. Patients with airborne transmitted diseases require a private room with a sign to alert staff and visitors to check with the nurse before entering the room. Special ventilation is indicated. A mask is required to enter the room of a patient with pulmonary tuberculosis or meningococcal disease. Only immune persons should enter the room of a patient with chickenpox.

From Lynch P, Jackson M: Isolation practices: How much is too much or not enough? *Asepsis: The Infection Control Forum* 8(4):2-5, 1986.

SUMMARY

1. The sequence of events in the chain of infection involves (1) a causative agent, (2) a reservoir, (3) a portal of exit, (4) a mode of transmission, (5) a portal of entry, and (6) a susceptible host.
2. Modes of transmission are (1) contact (direct, indirect, and droplet), (2) airborne, (3) vehicle, and (4) vector.
3. Whenever possible, appropriate cultures should be obtained before the initiation of antibiotic therapy.
4. The D.H.S.S. recommends that children be immunized against diphtheria, pertussis, and tetanus (DPT); measles, mumps, and rubella (MMR); and poliomyelitis (OPV).
5. Health caregivers who have frequent contact with blood and blood products should be immunized against hepatitis B virus.
6. Passive immunity is temporary, lasting a few weeks without stimulating antibody production in the recipient.
7. A nosocomial infection is one that is not present or incubating at the time a person is admitted to the hospital but which develops after admission.
8. A community-acquired infection is one that is present or is incubating at the time of admission to the hospital.
9. Hand washing is the single most important measure in preventing cross-infections.
10. Aseptic technique is an important factor in preventing nosocomial infection.
11. Two systems of isolation are (1) CDC category-specific isolation with universal blood/body fluid precautions and (2) body substance isolation (BSI).
12. Adherence to currently recommended isolation practices is the best protection that health careworkers have from occupationally acquired infection.
13. Health careworkers should direct problems concerning any aspect of infection control to the infection control nurse, the hospital epidemiologist, or the infection control committee in their institution.

REFERENCES AND SELECTED READINGS

1. Abbot Diagnostic Division: Transmission in Medical Situations, National AIDS Manual, Spring 1993.
1a. American Hospital Association: AIDS/HIV infection policy: ensuring a safe hospital environment, *AHA Report*, pp 1-27, 1987.
2. American Public Health Association: *Control of communicable disease in man*, ed 15, New York, 1990, The Association.
3. Bennett JV, Brachman PS, editors: *Hospital infections*, Boston, 1986, Little, Brown & Co.
4. Bowell B: Assessing infection risk, *Nursing (London)* 4(12): 12-23, 1990.
5. Centers for Disease Control: Nosocomial infection surveillance, 1984, *MMWR* 35(1SS):17-29, 1986.
6.* Centers for Disease Control: Recommendations for prevention of HIV transmission in health-care settings, *MMWR* 36(2S):3-17, 1987.
7.* Centers for Disease Control: Perspectives in disease prevention and health promotion: Public Health Services Guidelines for counseling and antibody testing to prevent HIV infection and AIDS, *MMWR* 36(31):509-515, 1987.
8. Centers for Disease Control: Recommendations of the Immunization Practices Committee (ACIP): Pneumococcal polysaccharide vaccine, *MMWR* 38(5):64-76, 1989.
9. Centers for Disease Control: Recommendations of the Immunization Practices Advisory Committee (ACIP): General recommendations on immunization, *MMWR* 38(13):206-227, 1989.
10.* Centers for Disease Control: Recommendations of the Immunization Practices Advisory Committee (ACIP): Protection against viral hepatitis, *MMWR* 39(RR-2):1-26, 1990.
11. Centers for Disease Control: Recommendations of the Immunization Practices Committee (ACIP): Prevention and control of influenza, *MMWR* 39(RR-7):1-15, 1990.
12. Centers for Disease Control: Guidelines for preventing the transmission of tuberculosis in health-care settings with special focus on HIV-related issues, *MMWR* 39(RR-17):1-28, 1990.
13. Centers for Disease Control: Update: Transmission of HIV infection during an invasive dental procedure—Florida, *MMWR* 40(2):21-27, 1991.
14. Centers for Disease Control: Recommendations of the Immunization Practices Advisory Committee (ACIP): Diphtheria, tetanus, and pertussis: recommendations for vaccine use and other preventive measures, *MMWR* 40(RR-10):1-28, 1991.
15. *A clinician's dictionary of bacteria and fungi*, Indianapolis, 1986, Eli Lilly.
15a. Committee of Public Accounts, House of Commons Forty-fourth Report, Session 1985-86, *Preventive Medicine*, London, HMSO 1986.
16.* Cooper D: Optimizing wound healing, *Nurs Clin North Am* 25(1):165-180, 1990.
17. Craven DE, Steger KA, Barber TW: Preventing nosocomial pneumonia: state of the art and perspectives for the 1990s, *Am J Med* 91(suppl 3B):44-53, 1991.
17a. Department of Health: Vaccination and immunisation 1980-1990/91. Summary information from forms KC50, KC50A, KC51, SM12B.
18. Friedland GH, Klein RS: Transmission of human immunodeficiency virus, *N Engl J Med* 317(18):1125-1135, 1987.
19. Garner JS, et al.: CDC definitions for nosocomial infections, *Am J Infect Control* 16:128-140, 1988.
20. Gaynes RP: The NNIS system: plans for the 1990s and beyond, *Am J Med* 91(suppl 3B):116-120, 1991.
21.* Gerberding JL: Reducing occupational risk of HIV infection, *Hosp Prac* June 15, 1991, pp 103-117.
22. Gerberding JL, Henderson DK: Design of rational infection control policies for human immunodeficiency viral infection, *J Infect Dis* 156(6):861-864, 1987.
23. Haley RW: The nationwide nosocomial infection rate: a new need for vital statistics, *Am J Epidemiol* 121(2):159-166, 1985.
24. Haley RW: Measuring the costs of nosocomial infections: methods for estimating economic burden on the hospital, *Am J Med* 91(suppl 3B):32-38, 1991.
25. Haley RW, et al.: The efficacy of infection surveillance and control programmes in preventing nosocomial infections in US hospitals, *Am J Epidemiol* 121(2):206-215, 1985.
26. Healthy people 2000: National health promotion and disease prevention objectives, US Department of Health and Human Services, Washington, DC, 1990.
27. Infection control in critical care units, *Crit Care Nurs Quart* 11(4), 1989.
28.* Jagger J, Pearson RD: Universal precautions: still missing the point on needlesticks, *Infect Control Hosp Epidemiol* 12(4):211-213, 1991.
28a. King Edward's Hospital Fund for London, *The Nation's Health: A Strategy for the 1990s*, London, Bell and Bain, Ltd. 1991.
29. Kunin C: *Detection, prevention, and management of urinary tract infections*, ed 4, Philadelphia, 1987, Lea & Febiger.
30. Larson E: Infection control, *Ann Rev Nurs Res* 7:95-113, 1989.
31. Lynch P, Jackson M: Isolation practices: how much is too much or not enough? Asepsis: the Infection Control Forum 8(4):2-5, 1986.
32.* Lynch P, et al.: Why not treat all body substances as infectious? *Am J Nurs* 15(3):1137-1139, 1987.
32a. Miller E, Waight P, Rousseau SA, Hambling MN, Rushton P, Ellis D, et al.: Congenital rubella in the Asian community in Britain. *BMJ* 1990, 301:1391.
33.* Mooney BR, Armington LC: Infection control—how to prevent nosocomial infections, *RN* 50(9):21-23, 1987.
34. Nafziger DA, Wenzel RP: Catheter-related infections: reducing the risk and the consequences, *J Crit Illness* 5(8):857-865, 1990.

34a. National Health Service, *Preventive Medicine,* London, HMSO 1986.

35. Nichols RL: Surgical wound infection, *Am J Med* 91(suppl 3B):54-64, 1991.

36. Norwood S, et al.: Catheter-related infections and associated septicemia, *Chest* 99(4)968-75, 1991.

36a. Shovein J, Young MS: MRSA: Pandora's box for hospitals, *Amer J Nurs* 92(2):48-52.

37. Stamm WE: Catheter-associated urinary tract infections: epidemiology, pathogenesis, and prevention, *Am J Med* 91(suppl 3B):65-75, 1991.

38.* Wysocki AB: Surgical wound healing, *AORN* 49(2):502-524, 1989.

39. Garner JS, Simmons BP: Guideline for isolation precautions in hospitals, *Infect Control* 4(4):245-325, 1983.

40. Larson E: Clinical microbiology and infection control, 1984, Cambridge, Mass, Blackwell Scientific Publications.

FURTHER READING

Department of Health: *Immunisation against Infectious Disease,* London, 1992, HMSO.

Communicable Disease Report, Vol 3, Review 3, Feb 1993, London, ISSN 0144-3186.

O.P.C.S., Communicable Disease Statistics England and Wales, London, 1991, HMSO.

* Recommended for student reading.

13

Management of People with HIV Infection and AIDS

Denise M. Kresevic

After studying this chapter, the learner should be able to:

- Describe three common ways by which the HIV infection is spread.
- List the infection control measures to be used when caring for a person with AIDS.
- Indentify three nursing problems and interventions for patients with HIV infection.
- Discuss the role of the nurse in addressing psychosocial, legal, and ethical issues related to the HIV epidemic.

Since the time of Florence Nightingale, nurses have provided care for individuals and families with communicable disease. One of the most dreaded communicable diseases of the twentieth century is AIDS (acquired immunodeficiency syndrome). AIDS is caused by the human immunodeficiency virus (HIV). Individuals infected with this virus suffer severe compromise of the body's ability to fight various infections and rare forms of cancer. The incidence of AIDS and HIV infection continues to increase steadily worldwide. Therefore it is crucial that nurses have an understanding of (1) epidemiology, (2) disease prevention, (3) pathophysiology, and (4) nursing care of individuals infected with HIV.

EPIDEMIOLOGY AND PREVENTION

In 1980, doctors in the U.S. began noticing a number of unusual infections, including forms of skin cancer and pneumonia among young homosexuals in New York and San Francisco. By September 1982, the U.S. Public Health Service had coined the acronym AIDS (acquired immune deficiency syndrome). All those affected were in their late 20s or early 30s, were homosexual, were from the Los Angeles area (but did not know each other) and all had developed *Pneumocysitis carinii* pneumonia, a rare illness that develops when the immune system is suppressed. Epidemiologists and researchers studying these cases concluded that the cause of the fatal pneumonias and skin cancers was an underlying immune deficiency syndrome. Research efforts continued to isolate the causative immune deficiency virus. Before 1986 different researchers attributed various names to the virus: AIDS-related virus (ARV), lymphadenopathy-associated virus (LAV), and human T-lymphotropic virus type III (HTLV III). It was not until 1986 that the virus believed to cause AIDS was defined and named HIV.

The World Health Organization (WHO) estimates that more than 600,000 people, worldwide, have AIDS (Table 13-1); another 6 to 10 million in over 152 countries are infected but asymptomatic. The numbers of infected women and elderly continue to rise. It is also estimated that by the year 2000 from 12 to 18 million people worldwide will be infected with HIV.

Virus Transmission and Risk Behaviours

A critical need exists to educate health care professionals, patients, and families about disease transmission and identified risk behaviours for HIV infection. The human immunodeficiency virus has been found in a variety of body fluids including blood, semen, cerebrospinal fluids (CSF), urine, stool, and saliva. Blood serum and CSF of infected individuals contain the highest concentrations of the virus and thus are the most likely means of transmission. Although HIV has also been found in varying concentrations in urine, stool, and saliva, no evidence exists that disease transmission has occurred via these body secretions.

There are *three major methods of HIV transmission*: (1) *intimate contact with body secretions*, including *semen* and *vaginal secretions* that occur *during sexual intercourse*, (2) *contact* with *infected blood* through *blood transfusions* or the *sharing of needles* during intravenous drug use, and (3) *maternal–infant transfer* via *placental exchange* or *breast milk*.

Although any member of the population may acquire AIDS, certain behaviours place individuals at increased risk for exposure to HIV based on disease transmission patterns. Populations at highest risk for exposure to HIV include homosexual and bisexual men, intravenous drug users, heterosexual partners of HIV-infected individuals, infants born to HIV-infected parents, and individuals who have received blood or blood products, especially before 1985 (Table 13-2).

The number of women with AIDS continues to increase with the greatest risk factor in 1990 being intravenous drug use. The incidence of AIDS in the elderly has been relatively low. Ten percent of all cases of AIDS have been reported in those aged 50 years and over. Of those cases, only 4% have occurred in those aged 70 years and older. Because of the latency period (up to 10 years) of this disease it is expected that the number of cases among the elderly will continue to increase.

Table 13-2 Number of AIDS cases in the United Kingdom by exposure category as of March 1993

Risk Group	Number of cases
Homosexual men	11,809
Heterosexual men	1,243
Heterosexual women	1,415
Male IV drug users	1,635
Female IV drug users	744
Homosexual men IV drug users	257
Male haemophiliacs	1,203
Female haemophiliacs	11
Male blood transfusion	88
Female blood transfusion	87
Mother to child	163
Male undetermined	683
Female undetermined	133

Data cited by National AIDS Helpline; Communicable Disease Department. Numbers reflect only those who have submitted themselves for testing or have been admitted for care.

Table 13-1 Cases of AIDS reported to the WHO, January 1993

Africa		Americas		Europe	
Ivory Coast	10,792	Brazil	31,364	France	21,487
Malawi	22,300	Mexico	11,034	Italy	14,483
Uganda	34,611	USA2	242,146	Spain	14,991
Tanzania	34,605	All others	28,539	All others	28,919
Zaire	18,186				
Zimbabwe	12,514				
All others	78,024				
Africa total	211,032	Americas total	313,083	Europe total	80,180
Asia	2,582	Oceania	4,082	World total	611,580

From Stewart G: Predictable and Preventable: *Nursing Times* June 30 1993, 89(26):29-32.

More than 60% of the reported cases worldwide of HIV infection and AIDS have been in homosexual and bisexual men.[13] The greatest identified risk factor for HIV transmission in this group is anal intercourse. Such intercourse may be traumatic to fragile mucous membranes, resulting in microscopic tears and possible semen–blood transmission of the virus. The appropriate and consistent use of latex condoms, nonoxynol-9 spermicide, and water-soluble lubricants may decrease the risk of trauma and disease transmission with anal intercourse in this risk group.[29]

Transmission of HIV by vaginal heterosexual intercourse is also possible. Associated risk factors for heterosexual transmission include anal intercourse, multiple sexual partners who may be infected and asymptomatic, and frequent sexual intercourse with multiple partners; these behaviours increase opportunities for exposure to infected body fluids. Studies on nonsexual household contacts, sharing of eating utensils and bathroom facilities, and close personal contact have *not* resulted in the transmission of HIV.[29,41]

Although the risk of HIV infection to health careworkers is low, it remains a potential risk for those workers exposed to body secretions such as blood, urine, and stool. The Monks report[17a] highlighted the lack of formal training for health advisers in genito-urinary medicine clinics, where the risk of possible infection transfer was considered potentially high. By June 1990, 34 cases worldwide of occupational exposures had been reported to the Centers for Disease Control. Eighty per cent of the exposures were attributed to needle-stick injuries. This represents a 0.5% risk of HIV seropositive conversion if injured with a contaminated hollow-bore needle. To address this problem, several needle and syringe manufactures have offered various anti-stick systems which may give additional protection from accidental needle-stick injuries to caregivers with accidental needle-sticks and mucous membrane exposures. *Mucous membrane exposure* occurs by *blood splashing into the mouth, nose, or open cuts on the hands.*

Clearly the most important strategies for health careworkers are good handwashing, avoidance of recapping needles, and the use of gloves whenever exposure to any patient's body secretions is likely to occur.[52]

For health care-workers infected with HIV and desiring to continue to practise, the CDC recently issued guidelines. These guidelines recommend these health workers refrain from invasive procedures, such as surgery.[14a, 22a]

Infection Control Measures

In addition to health education strategies, infection control is one of the most important areas of concern for nurses caring for patients with HIV infection, whether in the hospital or home environment. Infection control procedures based on knowledge of disease transmission are essential to dispel the many emotional fears and myths surrounding the HIV infection. *Handwashing* remains the single most important principle of infection control for all diseases.[51] Handwashing is critical to protect immunocompromised patients and caregivers; it should be performed before and after contact with each patient and after removal of gloves. *Gloves* should be used whenever there will be *contact with body secretions: during care of lesions,* when *coming into contact with blood* (such as during dressing changes or starting intravenous lines), when *cleaning incontinent patients of urine or stool,* when *changing soiled linens,* and when *performing oral care.* In addition, caregivers should *keep fingernails cleaned* and well *trimmed to prevent punctures to gloves* and *possible transmission of the virus.*

Gloves are not necessary for casual contact such as bathing (without the presence of lesions), feeding, or ambulating patients.[52]

Soiled dressings, wet linens, and respiratory equipment should be discarded in heavy plastic bags. Puncture-resistant needle disposal containers should be in close proximity to all patient care areas. Needles should be disposed of promptly, *WITHOUT RECAPPING,* because recapping is the most frequent cause of accidental needlesticks. Soap dispensers should be within close proximity of all patient care areas, and gloves should be worn for clean-up of urine, stool, or blood spills.

Standard household and institutional cleaning is important to protect all immunocompromised patients. Institutional cleaning agents used for floor and bathroom facilities are sufficient. A freshly mixed solution of bleach and water in a 1:10 parts mixture is used for home cleaning of floors, countertops, toilets, and spills. Standard laundering using bleach, and dishwashing using hot water and air drying, are sufficient to protect caregivers and family members from HIV infection. However, *personal care items* such as *razors and toothbrushes should never be shared because of possible transmission* by *blood serum.* Pet excretion may pose a unique threat to immunocompromised patients. Patients with HIV infection who desire to keep their pets may require assistance in care, especially in cleaning bird cages, cat litter boxes, or fish tanks.[52]

The infection control guidelines previously mentioned are sufficient to protect pregnant women. Clearly, use of infection control measures is essential for all patients, regardless of known HIV infection, because this is the only way to ensure protection of caregivers. Patients' family members and all members of the health care team, including dietary workers and transport personnel, need basic education about HIV infection and infection control policies.

PATHOPHYSIOLOGY
Mechanism of HIV Infection

Infection with HIV renders the immune system severely compromised (see Chapter 33). The immune system, composed of organs and cells, protects the body from infections, cell mutations, and environmental toxins. The cells of the immune system are composed of lymphocytes, macrophages, and monocytes. Lymphocytes are further differentiated as T cells or B cells. HIV attacks T cells, which are responsible for all mediated immunity and protect the body from malignant cells, viruses, and parasites. The T cells are formed in the bone marrow and develop in the thymus. Two types of T cells produced by the body are T_4 inducer or helper cells, and T_8 cytotoxic or suppressor cells.

HIV has an affinity for invasion of the T_4 helper cells, but *it may also invade other components of the immune system, including B cells, macrophages, and nerve cells, severely compromising cell-mediated immunity.*

Individuals infected with HIV usually have almost twice as many T_8 suppressor cells as T_4 helper cells. This abnormal cell ratio renders HIV-infected people immunocompromised and thus susceptible to a host of infections, malignancies, and abnormal laboratory results (Table 13-3).[18,26,40]

HIV is classified as a retrovirus. Retroviruses carry their genetic code in RNA rather than DNA material. In retroviruses an enzyme known as reverse transcriptase converts RNA to DNA, which is incorporated into the host cell's genetic material. Thus the virus invades the host cell, living within it and replicating itself (Fig. 13-1). Based on

these cellular pathologies of the HIV infection, the CDC defines AIDS as "*a disease at least moderately predictive of a cell-mediated immunity occurring in persons with no known cause for diminished resistance to that disease.*"[41]

HIV Infection Continuum and Clinical Manifestations

HIV infection may remain dormant for several years, producing no clinical symptoms.[18] This prolonged incubation period is of great concern because individuals may be asymptomatic but contagious. Others infected with the virus may experience transient acute symptoms of fever, muscle aches, rashes, diarrhoea, and gastrointestinal cramping that occur 2 to 6 weeks after exposure and then resolve (Fig. 13-2 and Table 13-4). Other patients exposed to the virus and harbouring HIV antibodies exhibit chronic symptoms of diffuse noncancerous lymph node enlargement, or *persistent generalized lymphadenopathy* (PGL), fever, chills, night sweats, and weight loss.

Patients exposed to the virus, who are harbouring HIV antibodies and who experience night sweats, fever, weight loss, fatigue, oedema, and abnormal laboratory immune values including altered T_4 and T_8 cell ratios, but who have no infections or malignancies, are diagnosed as having AIDS-related complex (ARC). ARC can be a very debilitating disease.[9] However, *acquired immunodeficiency syndrome, or AIDS, is the most severe HIV disease.* Patients with AIDS continue to experience all the same symptoms,

Table 13-3 Common laboratory abnormalities associated with HIV infection and AIDS

Disorder	Laboratory findings
Anaemia	Haematocrit <30%
Leukopenia	WBC <2500/cm³
Lymphopenia	Helper T cells 400/mm³
Decreased T_4/T_8 ratio	Ratio 1 : 2
Thrombocytopenia	Platelets <150,000

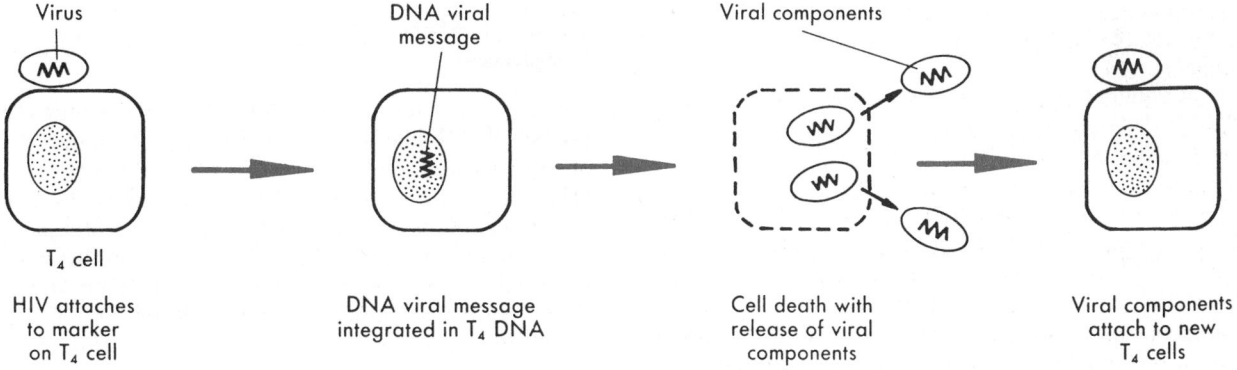

Fig. 13-1 Mechanism of HIV action.

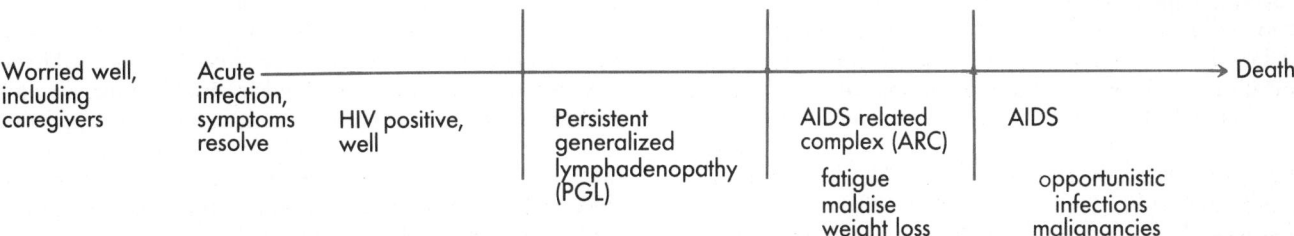

Fig. 13-2 Continuum of HIV infection; only some people proceed from infection to AIDS and death.

Table 13-4 Progression of HIV infection[11]

Group	Type	Characteristics
I	Acute infection	Fever, malaise with seroconversion
II	Asymptomatic infection	Seroconversion; no symptoms
III	Persistent generalized lymphadenopathy (PGL)	Lymphadenopathy more than 3 months in absence of explainable illness
IV	Other HIV disease	(See subgroups)
IV-1	Constitutional disease (ARC)	Diarrhoea or fever persisting more than 1 month; involuntary weight loss of greater than 10% of baseline
I	Neurological disease	HIV encephalopathy or dementia; peripheral neuropathy
IV-3	Secondary infectious diseases	*Pneumocystis carinii* pneumonia; candidiasis; extrapulmonary cryptococcosis; mycobacterial infection; CMV infection; herpes infections
IV-4	Secondary cancers	Kaposi's sarcoma, non-Hodgkin's lymphoma, primary limphoma of the brain

Modified from Centers of Disease Control: Pneumocystis pneumonia: Los Angeles, *MMWR* 30:250-252, 1981.

Table 13-5 Opportunistic infections and neoplasms associated with HIV infection

Agent	Body system affected
Infection	
Protozoal	
Pneumocystis carinii	Respiratory
Toxoplasma gondii	Neurological and disseminated
Cryptosporidium	Gastrointestinal
Bacterial	
Mycobacterium avium intracellulare	Disseminated
Mycobacterium tuberculosis	Respiratory, neurological or disseminated
Fungal	
Candida albicans	Gastrointestinal (mouth and or oesophagus) Disseminated
Cryptococcus neoformans	Neurological or disseminated
Viral	
Herpes simplex	Integumentary (mouth, genital, perianal)
Varicella-zoster	Integumentary
Cytomegalovirus	Neurological (eyes) disseminated
Neoplastic diseases	
Kaposi's sarcoma (epidemic form)	Skin and mucous membranes
Burkitt's lymphoma	Lymph system
Non-Hodgkin's lymphomas	Lymph system
Hodgkin's disease	Lymph system
Chronic lymphocytic leukaemia	White blood cells

including fatigue, weight loss, fever, diarrhoea, and oedema.[6] In addition, *opportunistic infections may be life-threatening*, and rare forms of cancers also invade the body (Table 13-5). *Opportunistic infections* prey on compromised immune systems.

Patients with AIDS, similar to patients with cancer, patients with an organ-transplant, and those receiving immunosuppressive therapy to prevent rejection, become susceptible to infections that individuals with intact immune systems are able to fight.

Nursing Process
Assessment

Some patients may be asymptomatic; others may report nonspecific "flulike" symptoms of fever, chills, night sweats, or dry, nonproductive cough. The clinical diversity of the HIV infection can make identification and assessment of infected patients difficult. Nurses may encounter patients experiencing various clinical symptoms including fatigue, fever, diarrhoea, or confusion, depending on the continuum of illness. Patients identified at risk for HIV infection either by sexual history, drug history, or flulike symptoms should be further assessed for the presence of opportunistic infections, rashes, and neoplasms (see Table 13-5).

Identification of people at risk

Health assessments of all patients should include an appraisal of potential risk factors for HIV infection. Obtaining a complete, accurate history of sexual behaviour, including past and present sexual activities, will be necessary and requires skilful interviewing techniques and a professional relationship based on trust. Nurses need to be comfortable explaining the need for information on intimate sexual activities, and phrasing questions in appropriate but comprehensible terms. The sexual health history, in addition to identifying individuals at risk for possible HIV infection, may also be an opportunity for health education and disease prevention (see Box 13-1).

Sample sexual history

1. When did you first become sexually active? With whom? For how long? Type of sexual activity practised:
   - Mutual masturbation
   - French kissing
   - Vaginal intercourse
   - Anal intercourse
   - Oral intercourse
   - Use of objects to enhance stimulation
   - Use of contraceptives
2. Are you currently sexually active? With whom? For how long? Type of sexual activity?
3. Do you currently have any concerns about your sexuality or sexual activity?
4. Do you suspect that any of your sexual partners have been infected with herpes, syphilis, gonorrhea, or AIDS? (Patients may need further explanations of specific types of infections and symptoms).

Information on the use of mood-affecting drugs such as alcohol, marijuana, heroin, cocaine, crack, barbiturates, tranquillizers, butyl nitrate, or amphetamines should also be obtained. Frequency and routes of administration including oral, smoking, sniffing, snorting, or injecting drugs should be explored. Needle exposure through the sharing of drug paraphernalia, tattoos, or acupuncture treatment should also be assessed.[39]

Individuals identified as being at risk for HIV infection should be counselled about the significance of testing and the necessity for follow-up. Patients with evidence of risk factors and any clinical symptoms should be referred for blood testing and medical evaluation of symptoms to diagnose exposure to the HIV infection.

AIDS and the elderly

Although much is still unknown about the immune function and ageing, in general ageing is associated with depressed cell-mediated immunity, impaired antibody production, and increased autoantibody production (see Chapter 33). These ageing changes often result in decreased capacity to resist infections.

The majority of elderly people with AIDS to date have been traced to blood transfusions associated with common surgical procedures such as coronary bypass and valve surgery and joint replacements. Given the long incubation period, the risk of contamination from blood transfusions, and the decreased capacity of the elderly to resist infections, the incidence of HIV in this age group is projected to rise steadily.

Recognition of the HIV infection in the elderly may be difficult for several reasons. A diagnosis of AIDS may be missed in the elderly who frequently have symptoms such as pneumonia, dementia, shortness of breath, weakness, fatigue, poor nutritional intake, and weight loss. In addition, caregivers may fail to evaluate thoroughly such risk factors as intravenous drug use and homosexuality in this age group.

The elderly with compromised immune functions or chronic illnesses such as heart and respiratory disease often have little reserve to resist or fight the multiple infections that may accompany the HIV infection. In general, this age group exhibits more side effects from aggressive antibiotic therapy used to fight infections. Increasing numbers of acutely ill elders suffering from multiple infections associated with the HIV infection poses unique clinical challenges for nurses in all settings.

Diagnostic tests: HIV seropositivity

Individuals who have been exposed to HIV and have had sufficient time for increased antibody production can be tested for infection. Two tests may be used to diagnose infection. The most common test is the enzyme-linked immunosorbent assay (ELISA). This test was originally developed as a screening tool for potential blood donors. Because the ELISA is a sensitive screening test for HIV infection, *false positive* tests are possible. Individuals who are not infected with HIV but have had multiple blood transfusions or pregnancies may have false positive results. In addition, a *false negative* ELISA test may occur during the so-called "window period." The window period is that time between exposure to the virus and the development of sufficient antibodies. The window period for HIV may be a few weeks or up to 3 months.[40] An additional confirmatory test called the *Western Blot* is usually used as a means of accurately diagnosing HIV-infected people. In general, the use of both the ELISA and Western Blot is able to provide over 99% accurate diagnosis of HIV infection.

A person with a positive test result is called HIV seropositive. This result indicates exposure to the HIV infection. Although it is not known at present how many seropositive individuals develop AIDS, it is believed that a majority die of AIDS complications.[40]

Nursing Analysis

Because of the different HIV infection categories on the HIV infection continuum and the great variety of symptoms, nursing care plans for people with HIV infection or AIDS will show a variety of nursing problems based on analysis of patient data. Some possible nursing problems for the person with HIV infection include, but are not limited to, the following:

Problem	Possible aetiologies
Knowledge deficit	Lack of exposure/recall, misinterpretation of information about HIV
Infection, high risk for	Decreased immune response
Body temperature, altered, high risk for	Infection, dehydration
Nutrition, altered: less than body requirements	Nausea, vomiting, diarrhoea, alterations in oral mucous membranes, dysphagia
Coping, ineffective individual, family	Inadequate or incorrect information or understanding, crisis, prolonged disability of significant person, societal mores
Anxiety	Threat to self-concept, threat of death, threat to/change in health status/socioeconomic status

Injury, high risk for	Confusion, dementia, weakness
Skin integrity, impaired	Pressure sores, infected lesions
Self-care deficit	Activity intolerance, dyspnoea, fatigue, depression, visual impairments, cognitive dysfunction
Social isolation	Societal biases, alteration in physical appearance or mental status, lack of knowledge about AIDS virus transmission
Grieving, anticipatory	Probable patient death

Planning: expected patient outcomes

Expected patient outcomes for the person with HIV infection or AIDS may include, but are not limited to, the following:

1. The patient and significant others verbalize an understanding of disease pathophysiology, transmission of the virus, basic infection control measures, diagnostic tests, and common treatment modalities.
2. Secondary infections do not occur or are identified early for treatment. HIV transmission to significant others and caregivers does not occur.
3. Body temperature decreases.
4. Weight loss, electrolyte imbalance, and discomfort are minimized. Patient ingests adequate fluids and a balanced diet daily.
5. Patient and significant others describe usual coping strategies and explore alternative strategies.
6. Patient demonstrates fewer signs of anxiety.
7. Patient endeavours to remain free from injury such as falls.
8. Skin and mucous membranes are moist; skin turgor is good.
9. Patient participates in ADL at optimal level of functioning.
10. Patient has opportunities to interact with others on a social basis.
11. Patient and sigificant others engage in anticipatory grieving through communication that leads to sharing of feelings, decision making, and problem resolution, as pertinent.
12. The patient and family will be able to discuss perceptions related to the meaning of their life, their suffering, and wishes for continued treatment or with holding of treatment.

Implementation

Interventions to achieve patient outcomes
Facilitating learning for people at risk

Nursing care needs vary along the illness continuum of HIV infection. Interventions are directed towards several groups of patients, including (1) "worried" well, (2) individuals with risk factors, (3) asymptomatic HIV-infected, (4) HIV-infected patients with clinical symptoms and their families; and (5) terminally ill HIV-infected individuals and their families. Nursing care of worried well individuals and family emphasizes education about HIV infection. Nurses will be required to serve as health resources for various community and institutional settings ranging from hospi-

tals, churches, and schools to occupational settings. A majority of health education about HIV infection focuses on clarifying myths and helping individuals cope with their anxiety and emotion-laden fears surrounding this epidemic. The challenge for nurses providing health education about HIV infection is to impart accurate, concise information that addresses the fears of contagion and disease transmission. Inherent in such education is a multitude of complex educational issues, including human sexuality.

Educational strategies, whether directed towards the worried well or those infected with HIV, must emphasize accurate information about disease transmission and safer sex practices. Safe sex refers to abstinence or a mutually monogamous sexual relationship with a noninfected partner. Risky sexual practices include multiple sexual partners and anal sex. The use of water-soluble lubricants and latex condoms with the spermicide nonoxynol-9 may increase the safety of vaginal and anal intercourse.

Both the worried well and those identified as being at risk for HIV infection need education and referral for antibody tests. Before testing, individuals require extensive counselling on the significance of test results and follow-up care and treatment. It is *important to stress* in counselling *that a one-time negative antibody test is meaningless if exposure to risk factors continues.* Some patients practising intravenous drug use need additional referral and treatment to eliminate the risk behaviour. One of the most difficult issues in caring for patients at high risk of contracting and transmitting the HIV infection is the balance of patient confidentiality and the caregiver's responsibility to share information regarding potential risk to the patient's sexual partners and loved ones. Education and counselling may be accomplished through individual teaching, role modelling, informal group discussions, or lectures. However, teaching requires more than spoken words. Learning should be reinforced by allowing people to express their concerns, answering questions, and using printed resources for future reference; repetition is essential. See Box 13-2 for guidelines for teaching.

The *Health of the Nation* report[36a] published by the Department of Health establishes uniform health goals in order to decrease the spread of HIV. However, setting targets for reducing risk factors is made difficult by the absence of baseline data on sexual behaviour in the general population. Estimates of sexual behaviour will become available from the national survey of sexual attitudes and lifestyles, as well as surveys of knowledge; attitudes and behaviour undertaken by the Health Education Authority.[23b] Box 13-3 gives an outline of national objectives and strategies.

Patients and families along the HIV continuum, from the worried well to those terminally ill with the virus, require much health teaching and counselling. The goal of counselling is to impart accurate information that empowers patients and families to make informed decisions and mobilize adequate mechanisms of support and adaptation for coping with multiple stressors.

Patients with HIV infection have many questions and concerns about the disease and its transmission, prognosis, and treatment. Initially, most patients are in a state of shock and disbelief. Information should be given in small segments with opportunities for repetition. Many patients

13-2

Guidelines for teaching patients with HIV and their significant others

Common risk factors for transmission of HIV infection include sharing of needles and other drug paraphernalia by IV drug abusers; anal intercourse; and blood transfusions.

Ways to prevent spread of HIV infection include limiting sexual partners and using latex condoms with nonoxynol-9 spermicide; cleaning of needles by IV drug abusers and not sharing needles with others; and autologous blood donations before elective surgery.

Symptoms of AIDS—fevers, dry cough, and night sweats.

Diagnostic tests—ELISA and Western Blot.

Healthful living practices—good nutrition, exercise, and stress reduction.

Community resources available to people with HIV infection including health clinics, support groups, community nurses, and resources for AIDS education.

13-3

Prevalance targets for the year 2000, and strategies to prevent the spread of HIV

	Prevalence/1000 population	
	Baseline	Year 2000 target
1. Male homosexuals attending GU Medical clinics in London	200	200
Outside London	50	50
2. Heterosexuals attending GU Medical clinics (non-injecting drug users) in London	7	10
Outside London	3	5
3. Injecting drug users attending services in London	20	20
Outside London	10	10

4. To reduce the incidence of gonorrhoea among men and women aged 15 to 64 years by at least 20% by 1995 (from 61 new cases per 100,000 population in 1990 to no more than 49 new cases per 100,000).

5. To reduce the rate of conceptions among the under 16s by at least 50% by the year 2000 (from 9.5 per 1,000 girls aged 13 to 15 years in 1989 to no more than 4.8).

6. To reduce the percentage of injecting drug misusers who report sharing injecting equipment in the previous 4 weeks by at least 50% by 1997, and by at least a further 50% by the year 2000 (from 20% in 1990 to no more than 10% by 1997, and no more than 5% by the year 2000).

The Secretary of State. *The Health of the Nation:* A summary. HMSO 1992.

require assistance with the decision to share the fact of their illness with significant others. All sexual partners who are potentially at risk for contracting the disease have the right to know of their own potential risk of illness.

Additional information may be obtained from the following sources: National AIDS Helpline Tel. 0800 567123; a good source for statistics and clinical drug trials is the Department of Public Health, Tel. 0181 200 4400.

Preventing infections

Normal environments can be a source of lethal infections for the immunocompromised patient. Nursing care for people with HIV infection or AIDS must stress meticulous personal hygiene, close observation of potential sources of infection, frequent handwashing, and avoidance of environmental microbes. Infection control measures (p. 208) are essential.

Patients with HIV infection are encouraged and assisted to bathe daily. Most patients will require a bed bath; tub baths should be avoided if the patient has a rash. Whenever possible, showers are recommended. Patients suffering from diarrhoea require frequent cleaning with a gentle soap and liberal application of moisture barriers to prevent skin breakdown. Special attention to oral care to prevent infection and promote adequate nutrition and comfort is important. Soft toothbrushes and nonabrasive toothpaste and rinses will decrease the chances of trauma and secondary infections. Rinses with sodium bicarbonate, saline, or lemon and hydrogen peroxide are useful before meals and at bedtime. Oral care after meals helps prevent tooth decay and infections.

Pulmonary infection occurs frequently with HIV. Thus patients are taught and coached through deep-breathing and coughing exercises at least every 4 hours while awake to promote airway clearance and prevent atelectasis.

Meticulous skin care is necessary to minimize infections and promote comfort. Patients with decreased mobility may benefit from the use of air mattresses and frequent turning schedules to prevent decubiti. Turning sheets are used when necessary to prevent friction and injury. A high-protein diet will help prevent skin breakdown by providing essential amino acids for healing. Oedematous limbs are elevated using pillows to promote circulation. Emollients can be used liberally to prevent skin drying and cracking. Skin lesions are washed separately using a clean washcloth and gloves to prevent contamination.

Biopsy sites and intravenous insertion sites can be sources of infection. Observe sites daily for redness, warmth, pain, or drainage. Sites that are suggestive of infection should have wound cultures to confirm or rule out infection. Avoid plastic occlusive dressings; they have been shown to increase the risk of infection in some immunocompromised patients. Change dressings at least every other day. Avoid sources of microbes, such as fresh plants and dietary servings of rare meat and fresh vegetables or fruits.

Attention must be paid to the patient's environment. The room should be dusted and mopped daily using damp cloths to prevent air distribution of microbes. Supplies should be neatly stocked. Dietary trays are removed after meals, and additional dietary supplements are stored outside the patient's room. In most cases, except with airborne infections such as tuberculosis, the patient's door may be kept open to minimize odours, promote adequate ventilation, and decrease feelings of isolation. Private rooms for patients with HIV infection are not usually necessary except with specific infections such as tuberculosis. Patients are not placed in a room with another patient who has an infection. The single most important factor that protects immunocompromised patients from infections is the practise of consistent good handwashing techniques by patients, caregivers, and visitors. Care of the patient with HIV infection is summarized in Box 13-4.

Modifying alterations in body temperature

Fever, a common result of HIV infection, may be caused by dehydration or multiple infections, including *P. carinii* pneumonia, cytomegalovirus, and *Mycobacterium avium intracellulare*. Fevers may also be caused by infection from intravenous lines or biopsy sites.

All patients with HIV infection should be monitored for fever and adequate fluid intake. Temperatures of hospital-ized patients are assessed every 4 hours, body temperatures greater than 37.5° C or 101.5° F are reported to the doctor for medical follow-up. Diagnostic tests for fevers may include chest X-ray examinations or blood cultures for detection of specific pathogens. Patients with fevers may require several tepid sponge baths and linen changes to promote comfort. Fever and sweating may increase fluid loss and contribute to dehydration; therefore patients should ingest at least 2500 ml of fluid per day. Accurate daily intake and output are recorded and evaluated.

Daily monitoring of intravenous sites and other wounds for possible infection is also critical. Fevers are cautiously treated with antipyretics such as paracetamol (used with zidovudine). The use of aspirin is contraindicated with HIV infection because the infection itself may alter normal blood coagulation. Intravenous therapy may be necessary to provide adequate hydration. Despite meticulous personal hygiene and nursing care, some patients with HIV infection may continue to have persistent temperature elevation with no explained cause.

Guidelines for care 13-4

The patient with HIV infection/AIDS

Prevent infection.

1. Wash hands frequently and use emollient for patient and caregiver.
2. Use a gentle liquid soap; avoid bar soaps that may irritate skin.
3. Provide for daily showering or basin bath; avoid tub bath if rashes are present.
4. Use a separate washcloth for lesions.
5. Use soft toothbrushes, nonabrasive toothpaste; and mouth rinses with sodium bicarbonate, saline, or lemon and hydrogen peroxide before meals and at bedtime.
6. Use measures to prevent skin pressure, such as turning sheets, sheepskin, or eggcrate or air mattresses.
7. Elevate and support areas of oedema.
8. Observe biopsy sites and IV insertion sites daily for signs of infection.
9. Change dressings at least every other day; avoid plastic occlusive dressings.
10. Avoid sources of microbes, such as fresh plants or ingestion of fresh fruits and vegetables.
11. Carry out measures to prevent spread of infection; use of gloves for contact with bodily secretions, double plastic bags to dispose of bodily secretions, use of bleach and water (1 : 10) for cleaning of contaminated areas.

Modify alterations in body temperature.

1. Administer prescribed antibiotics, IV fluids, or antipyretics.
2. Encourage fluid intake >2500 ml.
3. Maintain daily intake and output records.
4. Weigh daily.
5. Provide tepid sponge baths and linen changes as necessary.
6. Instruct patient in deep-breathing and coughing exercises to prevent atelectasis and additional fever.

Promote good nutrition.

1. Provide instruction for high-calorie, high-protein, high-potassium, low-residue diet.
2. Encourage high-calorie, high-potassium snacks.
3. Suggest foods that are easy to swallow (gelatin, yogurt, puddings) when dysphagia is present.
4. Avoid foods that are spicy or acidic, rare meats, and raw fruits and vegetables.
5. Provide oral care before patient eats.
6. Encourage patient to get out of bed and sit up for meals if possible.
7. Avoid odours by aerating room.
8. Make appropriate dietary consultations.

Promote self-care.

1. Assess realistic functional ability.
2. Plan, supervise, and assist with ADL as necessary.
3. Encourage patient to be as active and independent as possible.
4. Assist patient with range-of-motion exercise to prevent contractures.
5. Provide equipment aids for eating, walking, and commodes to promote patient independence.
6. Pace activities and schedule rest periods to prevent fatigue.

Provide counselling.

1. Assess and support patient coping mechanisms.
2. Explore with patient and significant others normality of grief responses.
3. Assist patient and significant others in acknowledging and planning for anticipated losses.
4. Provide information as desired and necessary, depending on the ability to perceive.
5. Suggest religious support, where appropriate.
6. Facilitate participation in support groups or individual counselling as pertinent.

Promoting optimal nutrition

Patients with HIV infection are frequently plagued by alterations in gastrointestinal function, such as dysphagia, nausea, vomiting, and diarrhoea. Infections such as *Candida* and *Cryptosporidiosis* also contribute to alterations in food and fluid intake and absorption, resulting in reduced nutrition. Depression may be manifested by changes in appetite.

Daily weight and food and fluid intake are monitored and recorded. Nutritional intake may be increased by attention to oral hygiene, positioning, socialization, and attention to individual preferences. Patients and caregivers are taught about nutritional factors that contribute to health despite the HIV infection.

Patients are encouraged to get out of bed and sit up for meals to aid digestion and decrease the possibility of aspiration. Odours should be minimized because they may contribute to nausea. Oral hygiene, including mouth rinses before meals, enhances the taste of food and stimulates digestive juices. Whenever possible, significant others can be encouraged to visit during meals and to bring home-prepared food. Patients may prefer frequent small meals or snacks spaced throughout the day to prevent indigestion and fatigue.

Adequate nutrition can be enhanced by the following:

1. Daily oral intake of 2500 ml to 3000 ml of fluids to prevent dehydration, especially with diarrhoea; suggested fluids are water, fruit juices, soups, and jelly.
2. Foods high in potassium (to replace that lost by diarrhoea) include bananas, apricots, and orange juice.
3. Textured foods that are easy to swallow and tolerate include jelly, yogurt, and pudding.
4. Foods high in protein that are easily tolerated include peanut butter, honey, and instant meal drinks.
5. Avoid foods with naturally occurring microbes (rare meat, raw fruits and vegetables) and foods that aggravate dysphagia (spicy, acidic, or raw fruits and vegetables).

Multiple medications may alter the normal taste of foods, and patients may need to be encouraged to try new or differently prepared foods. Collaboration with dieticians may be useful. At times, dietary supplements may be needed to maintain adequate caloric intake. All supplements, especially those containing lactose, should be evaluated as potentially causing diarrhoea. Dysphagia resulting from oral *Candida* may be treated with oral medications such as nystatin or lignocaine to decrease discomfort and increase nutritional intake. Patients living alone in their own homes often require assistance with shopping and meal preparation.

Some severely malnourished patients may require oral nutritional supplements or parenteral hyperalimentation (Chapter 23).

Assisting with coping

Individuals who are exposed to HIV infection, but are without symptoms or complications of infections or cancers, live with a great deal of uncertainty and anxiety interspersed with denial and hopefulness. The role of the nurse in this stage of the disease process is to provide continued education about the disease of AIDS, as well as to assist in realistic goal setting. Patients are encouraged to participate in their own care and to maintain positive relationships.

As the HIV infection progresses with clinical complications of infections and cancers, patients experience multiple losses including loss of energy, self-care deficit requiring assistance with activities of daily living, and loss of independence, employment, finances, and hope. The reality of death emerges. Nursing care focuses on a philosophy of facing life a day at a time and living each day to the fullest extent possible by resolving multiple conflicts. This may be a time for strengthening personal and spiritual relationships.

Empathic listening and the ability to help patients find meaning in life become critical nursing interventions. Assisting families and significant others, including lovers, to provide support to the terminally ill patient despite their own anger and grief is a unique nursing challenge. Such care, although emotionally draining for the nurse, can provide tremendous positive feelings of professional accomplishment.

Box 13-5 presents the results of a U.S. research study of people with HIV infection and AIDS.

The diagnosis of HIV infection, with a social stigma, poor prognosis, and lethal nature, is indeed a catastrophic event for patients and caregivers. Patients experience a variety of intense emotions that threaten self-esteem and predispose to depression and feelings of powerlessness. Anxiety is a response that pervades the entire HIV illness continuum. Anxiety and denial often accompany the initial diagnosis and intensify with physical decline and loss of independence, job, and finances. Anxiety may be incapacitating as death becomes a reality. Nursing interventions to promote effective coping focus on exploring and strengthening healthful coping strategies and maintaining sources of psychological support.

13-5

Nursing Research

Korniewicz DM, Obrien ME, Larson E: Coping with AIDS and HIV: psychosocial adaptation, *J Psychosoc Nurs Men Health Serv* 28(3):14-21, 1990.

In this study four groups of patients were interviewed: those with HIV risk factors such as homosexuality but with unknown seropositive status, HIV-infected individuals with no symptoms, HIV-infected individuals with early symptoms of AIDS such as vomiting and weight loss, and those with late symptoms of AIDS including opportunistic infections. Through patient interviews and chart reviews the investigators found that individuals infected with the HIV virus, but not yet exhibiting symptoms, experienced the greatest feelings of powerlessness. Based on these findings *the researchers recommend that nurses providing care to HIV-infected patients pay particular attention to newly diagnosed individuals rather than postpone psychosocial interventions until physical symptoms of AIDS are apparent.*

Reducing anxiety

Individuals experiencing the anxiety of HIV infection are often in a state of crisis (see Chapter 5 for further information). Continued clarification and education about the HIV infection, complications, and treatment are critical. Every effort should be made to include the patient in planning medical and nursing care. An assessment of past coping styles and support systems should be made early and continually reevaluated. Healthful patterns of coping, such as talking or relaxation and meditation, are encouraged. Relationships with family, friends, and lovers should be maintained and may be strengthened through the HIV crisis. Conversely, past conflicts, especially among family members, may persist and intensify during the HIV crisis.

Occasionally anxiety, denial, depression, and even grief may persist for extended periods, interfering with daily functioning, productive communication and relationships, and even the ability to make decisions. The nurse must be able to assess normal periods of anxiety, depression, and grief, as well as refer patients and significant others for psychological evaluation and counselling for ineffective coping patterns. Although reactions of anxiety and depression are normal, professional intervention is necessary whenever they preclude communication and daily functioning for an extended time (usually longer than 3 months). Patients with HIV infection and depression should be assessed for suicidal ideation because this phenomenon occasionally occurs in terminally ill patients who are experiencing anxiety and fear of further pain and physical decline. Early recognition of depression is critical because some cases of depression and anxiety may respond to medications and psychotherapy.

Individuals with diffuse anxiety often feel they have little control over their daily existence. A schedule of activities that patients develop with guidance from health care professionals may decrease anxiety and feelings of powerlessness. Opportunities for spiritual support and comfort should be explored. Significant others may also experience anxiety. Community support groups for patients and significant others may offer additional sources of support and contribute to healthful coping. Planned uninterrupted time with only the nurse, patient, and significant others may create a supportive environment that decreases anxiety and promotes healthful coping.

Preventing injury

Safety is a critical need for patients with HIV infection who are at increased risk for accidents and injury because of decreased physical and cognitive function. The patient's environment is assessed to ensure strategic placement of items such as call lights and urinals. Use of cot sides and restraints may be necessary to prevent injury but should never be substituted for frequent observation. Both patients and significant others should be aware of safety needs and the rationale for interventions to prevent injury. Referrals to occupational and physiotherapy may be useful in developing a coordinated plan of care to maximize safe independent functioning.

Promoting skin integrity

As the patient becomes increasingly ill and is unable to meet self-care needs, the potential for skin breakdown is high. Nursing emphasis is on frequent turning and keeping the skin clean, dry, and well lubricated with moisturizers. Special mattresses or beds may be used to minimize pressure on bony prominences. Improving the patient's nutritional intake will also help prevent skin breakdown.

Promoting self-care and safety

Many people infected with HIV suffer from fatigue, dyspnoea, depression, or cognitive impairments requiring assistance with activities of daily living. Immunocompromised patients are particularly vulnerable to environmental pathogens and require meticulous daily hygiene. A daily schedule of activity that includes turning, positioning, sitting up for meals, bathing, and toileting will minimize the risks of secondary infections and contribute to feelings of positive self-esteem.

Patients are encouraged to remain as active and as independent as possible. The use of energy conservation and pacing of activities is very effective in maintaining independence and comfort. Adaptive equipment such as assistive eating devices, walkers, or bedside commodes may also promote independence and safety. Some patients may require assistance with range-of-motion exercises to prevent contractures.

Supporting interactions to minimize social isolation

The psychosocial aspects of AIDS are devastating. Because no cure presently exists for the HIV infection, the diagnosis of HIV infection, like a diagnosis of cancer, brings potential denial, fear, depression, and anger. The social stigma of AIDS, based on associations with homosexuality, intravenous drug abuse, and sexual transmission, cannot be minimized.[49] One of the earliest issues that HIV-infected individuals face is sharing the information with significant others. Tremendous fear of family anger, rejection, or abandonment is a real concern.

Often families and friends who are struggling with their own anxieties and fears abandon the patient. When this happens, the nurse should try to assist the patient to find other sources of social support. In some cities there are support groups for patients and separate groups for significant others. HIV-infected individuals who have been exposed by contaminated blood or unknowingly through heterosexual relationships may feel unique and intense anger and hostility. These patients are usually supported by their families and friends. They can be isolated by other people who do not understand that HIV and AIDS are not spread by casual contact.

Assisting with grieving

Like patients with other terminal illnesses, patients diagnosed with the HIV infection may experience strong emotions of fear, anger, denial, or quiet depression. Some patients benefit from individual empathic listening and exploring feelings, fears, and treatment options. Other patients may benefit from support groups with patients experiencing similar feelings. Significant others, including family and lovers, experience their own feelings of fear, anger, and embarrassment. Individual counselling and support groups may be helpful for loved ones who will need to be a source of support for the patient. Practical issues such as employment disability, housing discrimination, insurance coverage, and preparation for death also need to be addressed. Referral to social workers and appropriate community agencies can alleviate many concerns that plague acutely and terminally ill patients. Continued participation in religious services and the support of fellow worshippers and clergy should not be overlooked as a source of healthy coping. Many members of the clergy are experienced in grief counselling and can be helpful to patients and significant others.

Evaluation

Evaluation is based on the expected patient outcomes. Questions to consider include the following:
1. Can the patient and significant others explain the disease pathophysiology, transmission of the virus, basic infection-control measures, diagnostic tests, and common treatment modalities?
2. Have secondary infections been avoided or identified early, and has HIV transmission to significant others and caregivers been avoided?
3. Has the patient's body temperature decreased?
4. Have weight loss, electrolyte imbalance, and discomfort been minimized, and is the patient ingesting adequate fluids and a balanced diet daily?
5. Can the patient and significant others describe usual coping strategies and have they developed alternative strategies?
6. Is the patient's anxiety reduced?
7. Has the patient remained free from injuries such as falls?
8. Are the patient's skin and mucous membranes moist, and is skin turgor good?
9. Does the patient participate in ADL at the optimal level of functioning?
10. Does the patient have opportunities to interact with others on a social basis?
11. Have the patient and significant others engaged in anticipatory grieving?
12. Can the patient and significant others discuss perceptions regarding the meaning of their lives, their suffering, and their wishes for the continuation or withholding of treatment?

DRUG THERAPY

Because there is no cure for HIV infection at present, treatment has been aimed at slowing progression of the disease, managing symptoms, and providing palliative care. Table 13-6 lists some of the current drug regimens used to treat HIV infections and malignancy. Multiple clinical trials of various drugs to slow progression of the HIV infection are now under way. In 1987 the first such drug, zidovudine was released for treatment. It acts by inhibiting the replication of the human immunodeficiency virus. In some individuals, zidovudine has been effective in reducing the number of opportunistic infections and dementia symptoms.

However, it has many side effects including malaise, headache, fever, nausea, vomiting, insomnia, and myalgia. Toxic effects occur in about 50% of patients. These include anaemia, bone marrow suppression, reduced white blood

count, and low platelet counts. Patients on zidovudine require weekly blood testing to monitor for toxic effects.[42] Some patients may require blood transfusions to counter the toxic effects of the drug.

Zidovudine therapy has also been suggested as a preventive measure in the management of occupational exposure to HIV.[14] Lower doses of it are being prescribed prophylactically for health care-workers who have had an occupational exposure.

Two other oral agents—didanosine and zalcitabine—have shown promise in slowing virus progression. These agents, like zidovudine, inhibit the enzyme, reverse transcryptase, and prevent the HIV from multiplying. Patients on didanosine are monitored for the following side effects: diarrhoea, insomnia, headache, peripheral neuropathy, and pancreatitis.

SOCIAL, ETHICAL, AND LEGAL ISSUES

The HIV epidemic has brought with it not only a dismal prognosis, but also severe social stigmatization, public fear, and a growing number of legal and ethical issues. Nurses providing care in a variety of settings will face many of these issues that may jeopardize the quality of patient care. In addition, nurses caring for patients with the HIV infection will face many personal stresses including fear of personal contamination and disease transmission to family members, and burnout related to caring for terminally ill young patients with controversial lifestyles. The professional commitment needed by nurses who provide care to HIV-infected patients requires clarification of personal values regarding the issues of homosexuality and drug use.

Inherent in nursing is a respect for life, dignity, and social justice. The United Kingdom Central Council (UKCC) Code of Conduct reaffirms that the profession of nursing provides services with respect for human dignity and the uniqueness of each client, unrestricted by social or economic status, personal attributes, or the nature of health problems.[37b]

The very nature of nurses' work constitutes a level of risk for various diseases that does not exist in other professions. In upholding the moral principle of justice, risks and withholding of care must be carefully balanced with potential benefits of care. In addition, individual nurses and institutions have a responsibility to take reasonable precautions to protect caregivers from harm while providing medical and nursing care to patients.

As long as the HIV infection remains a downhill continuum with multiple complications and eventual death, nurses caring for patients with progressive AIDS will be involved in decisions regarding the selective withholding of treatment while preserving the quality of life and human dignity. The role of nursing in the terminal phase of illness is a critical one. When no medical treatments can be offered to the patient, nursing has everything to offer, including providing physical care that makes the patient more comfortable, identifying values, exploring the meaning of life with the patient and significant others, supporting bonds between the patient and significant others, and providing

Table 13-6 Pharmacological treatment of HIV infections and malignancy

Generic name	Infection/malignancy	Side effects
doxorubicin (systemic)	Kaposi's sarcoma	Leukopenia or infection (fever, chills, sore throat); stomatitis; oesophagitis, flank stomach, or joint pain; pain at injection site; peripheral oedema; fast or irregular heartbeat; shortness of breath; gastrointestinal bleeding; thrombocytopenia (unusual bleeding or bruising); changes in skin colour; diarrhoea, nausea, vomiting; skin rash or itching; hair loss; reddish colour to urine
co-trimoxazole (systemic)	*Pneumocystis carinii* pneumonia	Skin rash or itching; Stevens–Johnson syndrome (myalgia, arthralgia, redness, blistering, peeling or loosening of the skin); extreme fatigue, dysphagia, fever, leukopenia (sore throat); Thrombocytopenia (unusual bleeding or bruising); hepatitis (dark urine, pale stools, yellow skin, and/or sclera); crystalluria, haematuria, diarrhoea, dizziness, headache; anorexia, nausea, vomiting
bleomycin (systemic)	Kaposi's sarcoma	Cough, shortness of breath, pneumonitis, fever, chills, stomatitis, confusion, syncope, sweating, changes in skin colour and texture, rashes, swelling of fingers, nausea, vomiting and anorexia, weight loss, hair loss
ganciclovir (systemic)	Cytomegalovirus (CMV) (CMV retinitis and CMV colitis)	Under investigation Leukopenia, bone marrow depression, elevation of serum liver enzymes, neutropenia, eosinophilia, decreased platelet count; oedema, nausea, myalgias, headache, anorexia, disorientation, hallucinations, rash, phlebitis
fluconazole	Candidiasis, cryptococcal meningitis	Nausea, headache
amphotericin B (systemic)	Cryptococcus	Anorexia, headache, fever, chills and rigors, convulsions, myalgia, pain at injection site, tinnitus, hypotension, atrial fibrillation, hypokalaemia, decreased renal function, anaphylactic reactions
ketoconazole	Candidiasis (oral and systemic) Histoplasmosis	Headache, dizziness Nausea, vomiting Itching, nervousness Gynaecomastia
pentamidine	*Pneumocystis carinii* pneumonia	*Parenteral*: anorexia, nausea and vomiting, leukopenia, thrombocytopenia, hypoglycaemia, hypotension, pain at injection site, hepatotoxicity, decreased renal function *Aerosol*: bronchospasm, fatigue, dizziness, burning pain in back throat, bitter metabolic aftertaste, conjuctivitis, haemoptysis
acyclovir	Herpes simplex Herpes zoster Varicella	*Oral*: change in menstrual period, skin rash, diarrhoea, dizziness, headache, myalgia, nausea and vomiting, acne, anorexia, somnolence *Parenteral*: skin rashes or hives, haematuria, lightheadedness, headaches, hypotension, sweating, confusion, tremors, abdominal pain, dyspnoea, oliguria, unusual thirst, extreme fatigue
dapsone	Dermatitis herpetiformis	Nausea and vomiting, abdominal pains, vertigo, blurred vision, tinnitus, insomnia, fever, headache, psychosis, phototoxicity, tachycardia, albuminuria, nephrotic syndrome, hypoalbuminaemia, male infertility

13-6

Nursing Research

Flaskerud JH, Lewis MA, Shin D: Changing nurses' AIDS-related knowledge and attitudes through continuing education, *J Cont Ed Nurs* 20(4):148-154, 1989.

The purpose of this study was to measure changes in nurses' knowledge and attitudes following attendance at a continuing education conference. The conference topics included epidemiology of AIDS, infection control, sexual history taking, counselling and psychosocial and institutional support for health careworkers. Using a pretest, posttest, and a 3-month follow-up structured questionnaire, the researchers found significant increases in knowledge and attitude scores.

13-7

Nursing Research

Martin DA: Effects of ethical dilemmas on stress felt by nurses providing care to AIDS patients, *Crit Care Nurs Quar* 12:53-62, 1990.

The purpose of this study was to examine the nature and prevalence of ethical dilemmas encountered by nurses who provide care to patients hospitalized with AIDS-related illnesses. Half of the nurses reported a high degree of emotional exhaustion. However, there was a correlation between overall years of nursing experience and ability to cope. *The most frequent dilemmas reported were related to issues of dying* and *"do not resuscitate" orders. The second category of dilemmas surrounded issues of pain and symptom management.* Coping strategies ranged from venting emotions to deciding to leave the nursing unit or institution.

comfort measures and support that will allow the patient to have a peaceful death.

Nurses must continually help the health care team, family, and significant others to focus on the patient's desires. This principle of autonomy is a valuable guide for many ethical decisions regarding terminally ill patients. Nurse caregivers providing such intense physical and psychological care also need support. Peer support through informal sharing or a structured support group is an effective strategy that may alleviate feelings of helplessness.

Legal issues such as confidentiality, mandatory testing, employee screening, and school attendance of children infected with HIV remain controversial. Therefore it will be important for all nurses to keep themselves informed of policy developments and to influence, whenever possible, such decisions based on the ethical principle of justice. (For further information about ethical issues, see Boxes 13-6 and 13-7.)

SUMMARY

1. The three major methods of transmission of human immunodeficiency virus (HIV) are by intimate contact with semen or vaginal secretions through sexual contact, by infected blood through blood transfusions or sharing of IV drug needles, and by mother-to-infant transfer through placenta or breast milk.

2. Risk behaviours for HIV infection include anal intercourse, frequent sexual intercourse with multiple partners, and sharing IV drug needles.

3. Populations at highest risk include homosexual and bisexual men, IV drug users, heterosexual partners of HIV-infected individuals, infants born to HIV-infected parents, and individuals and their sexual partners who received blood transfusions before 1985.

4. HIV infection is not spread by nonsexual household contacts.

5. Infection control measures include handwashing before and after patient contact and after removal of gloves; wearing gloves whenever there will be contact with body secretions; disposing of soiled dressings, wet linens, and respiratory equipment in heavy plastic bags; disposing of needles *without capping* in puncture-resistant needle disposal containers; environmental cleaning with institutional cleaning agents or a 1:10 dilution of bleach and water; and use of bleach when laundering.

6. The human immunodeficiency virus is a retrovirus that invades helper T cells, incorporates its DNA into the genetic material of the helper T cell, and replicates itself, destroying the helper T cell. The decreased number of helper T cells causes immunodeficiency.

7. People exposed to HIV may develop an acute infection (similar to mononucleosis) or may be asymptomatic, harbouring the virus for several years. The asymptomatic person may unknowingly transmit the virus to others. Some people develop a persistent generalized lymphadenopathy in the absence of explainable illness. Not all people appear to progress to AIDS-related complex (ARC) or AIDS.

8. ARC is a debilitating syndrome of fever, diarrhoea, weight loss greater than 10% of baseline, fatigue, oedema, and abnormal laboratory immune values (altered T_4/T_8 ratio, leukopenia, lymphopenia, thrombocytopenia).

9. AIDS is the most severe HIV disease. In addition to the symptoms of ARC, the AIDS patient develops opportunistic infections and/or malignancies. Death eventually ensues.

10. Opportunistic infections may be protozoal, bacterial, viral, or fungal; the most common infection is *Pneumocystis carinii* pneumonia. The most common malignancy is Kaposi's sarcoma.

11. The ELISA test, indicating the presence of HIV *antibodies*, is the most often used diagnostic test for HIV infection. If this test is positive, a Western Blot test is used to confirm the results.

12. Interventions for persons with HIV infection depend on the symptoms and presence of infections or malignancies. Nursing interventions include prevention of infection, modification of alterations in body temperature, promotion of self-care, safety, and good nutrition, counselling, assisting with coping; and patient teaching.

13. To slow progression of HIV infection, zidovudine is now being used. Zidovudine acts by inhibiting the replication of HIV. There are many toxic effects, and

patients receiving zidovudine require weekly blood tests, and may require blood transfusions to treat toxic effects. Lower doses of zidovudine may be prescribed prophylactically for people with occupational exposure. Two newer oral agents—didanosine and zalcitabine, whose action is similar to zidovudine, are being tested in patients.

14. Numerous social, ethical, and legal issues need to be considered regarding care of people with HIV infections.

STUDY QUESTIONS

- You have been assigned to care for your first HIV-infected patient. What things should you consider before providing care?
- The local school has asked you to give a presentation on AIDS. What areas of content will you include? What teaching strategies and media might be helpful?
- Several of your peers confide in you that they would never care for a patient with AIDS. What ethical principles can help you clarify your views on this issue?
- What strategies can nurse caregivers use to alleviate fear and stress while caring for terminally ill HIV-infected patients and their families?
- You are preparing a family to provide home care for their son with AIDS. What learning needs must you assess?

REFERENCES AND SELECTED READINGS

1. Ahluwalia IB: The epidemiology of AIDS. In Blanchet KD, editor: *AIDS: a health care management response*, Rockville, Md, 1988, Aspen.
2. American Nurses Association: *Code for nurses with interpretative statements*, Kansas City, Mo, 1985, The Association.
3. American Nurses Association: *Nursing and the human responses to AIDS/HIV infection*, Kansas City, Mo, 1988, The Association.
3a.* Anastasi JK: Why give corticosteroids for *Pneumocystis carinii* pneumonia? *Am J Nurs* 92(2):30-32,1992.
3b.* Anastasi JK and Riviera JL: AIDS drug update, DDI and DDC,*RN* 52(11):41-43, 1992.
3c.* Andrullis DP, et al.: Comparisons of hospital care for patients with AIDS and other HIV-related conditions, *JAMA* 267(18):2482-2486, 1992.
4.* Barrick B: Light at the end of the tunnel, *Am J Nurs* 90(11):37-40, 1990.
5.* Beckham MM, Rudy EB: Acquired immunodeficiency syndrome: impact and implication for the neurological system, *Neurosci Nurs* 18:7-10, 1986.
6. Bennett J, Gee G: History and overview of HIV infection. In Gee G and Moran TA, editors: *AIDS: concepts in nursing practice*, Baltimore, 1988, Williams & Wilkins.
7. Blanchet KD: *AIDS: a health care management response*, Rockville, Md, 1988, Aspen.
8. Carey JT: The clinical spectrum of AIDS. In Blanchet KD: *AIDS: a health care management response*, Rockville, Md, 1988, Aspen.
9. Carpenito LJ: *Nursing diagnosis: application to clinical practice*, ed 2, Philadelphia, 1987, JB Lippincott.
10. Carr G: Medical treatment of persons with AIDS/ARC. In Lewis A, editor: *Nursing care of the person with AIDS/ARC*, Rockville, Md, 1988, Aspen.
11. Centers for Disease Control: Classification system for human T-lymphotropic virus III/lymphadenopathy-associated virus infections, *MMWR* 35:334-339, 1986.
12. Centers for Disease Control: Revision of the CDC surveillance case definition for acquired immunodeficiency syndrome, *MMWR* 36:3-16, 1987.
13. Centers for Disease Control: Update: universal precautions for prevention of transmission of human immunodeficiency virus, hepatitis B virus, and other bloodborne pathogens in health care settings, *MMWR* 37:24, 1988.
14. Centers for Disease Control: Public Health Service statement on management of occupational exposure to HIV, including considerations regarding zidovudine postexposure use, *MMWR* 39(RR-1):1-14, 1990.
14a. Centers for Disease Control: Recommendations for preventing transmission of human immunodeficiency virus and hepatitis B virus to patients during exposure-prone procedures, *MMWR* 40(RR):1-9, 1991.
14b. Centers for Disease Control: *HIV-AIDS surveillance report*, January 1992, 1-22.
15. Christ GH, Weiner LS: Psychosocial issues in AIDS. In DeVita VT Jr et al., editors: *AIDS: etiology, diagnosis, treat-ment, and prevention*, Philadelphia, 1985, JB Lippincott.
16. Cohen F: Immunologic impairment, infection and AIDS in the aging patient, *Crit Care Nurs Q* 12(1):38-44; 1989.
17.* Durham J, Cohen F: *The person with AIDS: nursing perspective*, New York, 1987, Springer.
17a.Department of Health: Working group to examineworkloads in genitourinary medicineclinics,report,1988.
17b. Farthing CF, Brown SE, Straughton RCD, Cream JJ, Mühlemann M: *A Colour Atlas of AIDS*, London, 1986, Wolfe Medical Publications.
18. Fauci AS, et al.: The acquired immunodeficiency syndrome: an update, *Ann Intern Med* 102:800-813, 1985.
19.* Fillit H, et al.: AIDS in the elderly, *AIDS Patient Care* 4(1):8-12, 1990.
20.* Flaskerud JH: AIDS: the psychosocial dimension, *J Psy-chosoc Nurs* 25:4-36, 1987.
21. Flaskerud JH: Nurses call out for AIDS information, *Nurs Health Care* 8:557-562, 1987.
22.* Flaskerud JH: *AIDS/HIV infection: a reference guide for nursing professionals*, Orlando, Fla, 1989, WB Saunders.
22a. General Medical Council: HIV infection and AIDS: The Ethical considerations, Annual report of the G.M.C., June 1993.
22b. Graham MH, et al.: The effect on survival of early treatment of human immunodeficiency virus infection, *N Engl J Med* 326(16):1037-1041, 1992.
23. Hatfield S, Dunkel J: Understanding and working with the emotional reactions of staff. In Lewis A, editor: *Nursing care of the person with AIDS/ARC*, Rockville, Md, 1988, Aspen.
23a. Hayward Jones I: *The Nurse's Code*: A practical approach to the code of professional conduct for nurses, midwives and health visitors.
23b. Health Education Authority: AIDS strategic monitor: report on the survey period Nov 1987–Dec 1988, London, HEA, 1988.
24. *Healthy people 2000: National health promotion and disease prevention objectives*, Department of Health & Human Services, Public Health Service, Washington, DC, Government Printing Office, 1990.
25. Hughes AM, et al.: *AIDS home care and hospice manual*, San Francisco, 1987, AIDS Home Care and Hospice Program, UNA of San Francisco.
25a. Illman J: History Lesson, *N.T.* 89(26):26-29, June 30 1993.
26. Justice AC, Feinstein AR, Wells CK: A new prog- nostic staging system for the acquired immuno-deficiency syndrome, *New Engl J Med* 320(22):1388-1489, 1989.
27. Kaplan LD, Wofsy CB, Volberding PA: Treatment of patients with acquired immunodeficiency syndrome and associated manifestations, *JAMA* 257:1367-1374, 1987.
28.* Koenig BA: Ethical and legal issues in the AIDS epidemic. In Lewis A, editor: *Nursing care of the person with AIDS/ARC*, Rockville, Md, 1988, Aspen.
29. Koop CE: *Surgeon General's report on acquired immune deficiency syndrome*, Rockville, Md, 1986, US Dept of Health and Human Services.
30. Leads from MMWR: Acquired immune deficiency syndrome,*JAMA* 252:1298-1301, 1985.
31.* Lewis A: *Nursing care of the person with AIDS/ARC*, Rockville, Md, 1988, Aspen.
32. Masur H, et al.: Infectious complications of AIDS. In DeVita VT Jr, et al., editors: *AIDS: etiology, diagnosis, treatment, and prevention*, Philadelphia, 1985, JB Lippincott.
33. Menke EM: *HIV and AIDS: an introduction for nurses*, Columbus, Ohio, 1989, East Central AIDS Education and Training Grant.
34.* Nelson WJ: Nursing care of the acutely ill person with AIDS. In Durham JD and Cohen FL, editors: *The person with AIDS: nursing perspective*, New York, 1987, Springer.
35. Pender NJH: *Health promotion in nursing practice*, Norwalk, Conn, 1987, Appleton & Lange.
35a. Rumbold G: *Ethics in Nursing Practice*, London, 1989, Baillière Tindall.
36.* Scherer P: How AIDS attacks the brain, *Am J Nurs* 90(1):44-53, 1990.
36a. Secretary of State for Health: The Health of the Nation report, London, HMSO, 1991.
37. Smith CL: Nursing management of aerosolized penta-midine administration, *AIDS Patient Care* 4(1):13-17,1990.

37a. Stewart P: Predictable and Preventable, *N.T.* 89(26): 29-32, June 30 1993.

37b. UKCC: The code of Professional Conduct for Nurses, Midwives and Health Visitors, UKCC, London, 1983.

38. Ulrich SP, Canale SW, Wendell SA: *Nursing care planning guides: a nursing diagnosis approach*, Philadelphia, 1986, WB Saunders.

39.* Ungarvski PJ: Learning to live with AIDS, *Nurs Mirror* 160:20-22, 1985.

40. Ungarvski PJ: *Living with AIDS: a caregivers guide*, New York, 1987, National Center for Homecare Education Research.

41. Volberding PA: The clinical spectrum of the acquired immunodeficiency syndrome: implications for com-prehensive patient care, *Ann Intern Med* 103:729-733,1985.

42. Volberding PA: Kaposi's sarcoma and the acquired immunodeficiency syndrome, *Med Clin North Am* 70:665-675, 1986.

43.* Weaver K: Reversible malnutrition in AIDS, *Am J Nurs* 91(9):34-31, 1991.

44. White K: "Why weren't you just more careful?" *AIDS Patient Care* 4(3):13-16, 1990.

45. Wolfe P: Clinical manifestations and treatment. In Flaskerud JF, editor: *AIDS/HIV infection: a reference guide for nursing professionals*, Philadelphia, 1989, WB Saunders Co.

45a. Worden W: *Grief Counselling and Grief Therapy*, Cam-bridge, 1982, Tavistock/Routledge.

45b. Wright S, Mackereth P: Waking up to Reality, *N.T.* 89(26) 32-33, June 30 1993.

46. American Nurses Association: *Nursing: a social policy statement*, Kansas City, Mo, 1980, The Association.

47. Beauchamp T, Childress J: *Principles of biomedical ethics*, New York, 1979, Oxford University Press.

48. Centers for Disease Control: *Pneumocystis* pneumonia: Los Angeles, *MMWR* 30:250-252, 1981.

49. Fowler MDM: *Ethics and nursing, 1983-1984: the ideal of service, the reality of history*, Los Angeles, 1984, University of Southern California.

50. Jameton A: *Nursing practice: the ethical issues*, Englewood Cliffs, NJ, 1984, Prentice Hall.

51.* Ungvarski PJ: Acquired immune deficiency syndrome, *Nurs Mirror* 157:17-20, 1983.

52. Ungvarski PJ: Infection control in the patient with AIDS, *J Hosp Infect* 5(A):111-113, 1984.

*Recommended for student reading.

Perioperative Nursing

Unit Five

14

The Patient Undergoing Surgery

Carole G. Phipps
Barbara C. Long

After studying this chapter, the learner should be able to:

- Differentiate among ways of admitting surgical patients.
- Describe different purposes of surgery.
- Identify psychological and physiological responses to surgery.
- Identify risk factors for surgery.
- Explain the nature of informed consent and related nursing responsibilities.
- Explain the rationale for collection of physiological data for the preoperative patient.
- Explain the preoperative preparation of the patient (diet, bowel and skin preparation).
- Identify common learning needs of preoperative patients and methods for deep breathing and coughing and leg exercises.
- Identify final preparation of the patient for surgery.
- Identify nursing interventions to meet patient needs in the postanaesthetic period.
- Discuss the rationale for collection of data necessary to plan nursing care when the patient returns to the ward or unit.
- Describe the types and process of wound healing and interventions that promote wound healing.
- Explain wound dehiscence and evisceration and appropriate nursing interventions.
- Identify postoperative respiratory and circulatory problems, assessment parameters, and preventive measures.
- Describe possible postoperative problems with fluid and electrolyte balance, nutrition, elimination, and inactivity, and the assessment parameters and preventive measures.
- Describe measures to promote patients' physical and psychological comfort in the postoperative period.

Surgery is one of the major modes of medical therapy. It is a stressful experience because it involves a threat to body integrity and sometimes a threat to life itself. Pain frequently occurs. The nurse can assist the person to cope with the stressors, to seek relief from the pain, and to return to optimal functioning.

The surgical (perioperative) experience can be divided into three stages: preoperative, intraoperative, and postoperative. This chapter discusses these stages with the emphasis upon pre- and postoperative nursing care. Details of care after admission to the theatre suite are not included and readers are directed to a specialist book for further details of intraoperative care.

The primary role of the perioperative nurse is that of a patient advocate. In order to fulfil this role the perioperative nurse must possess scientific and techical knowledge and also acquire a variety of technical skills. Incorporation of this knowledge with the nursing process enables the nurse to collaborate with other team members to provide effective, safe, and efficient care for the patient undergoing surgical intervention.

ELECTIVE ADMISSION FOR SURGERY

People scheduled for elective surgery were formerly all admitted to the hospital 1 or more days before surgery for medical examination, laboratory testing, and patient teaching, the necessary elements of preoperative care. Increasingly in recent years, patients having many types of surgery are either admitted to the hospital as inpatients on the day of surgery (same-day surgery), or to a day (ambulatory) surgical centre (either hospital- or community-based).

Day (Ambulatory) Surgery

Day case patients are admitted to the day case ward on the morning of surgery, remain there for their immediate postoperative care, and are then discharged to their homes before the end of the day. The surgery itself is uncomplicated and does not require expert postoperative care.

Success in day surgery depends on several factors, including preoperative testing and teaching facilities, physical status of the patient, and home care support people.

Age, per se, is not a limiting factor, and in fact, many elderly people have increased benefits from day case surgery versus inpatient surgery, e.g. reductions in postoperative complications. Additional care requirements may be needed for elderly people, including providing time and attention needed for adjustment.

Same-Day Surgery

Surgical patients who are admitted to the hospital approximately 2 hours before surgery and who require inpatient postoperative care are classified as undergoing same-day surgery. Same-day surgery patients require their preoperative preparation before the day of surgery because of time constraints. The admission management involves the necessary medical examination and testing procedures, as well as comprehensive preoperative nursing assessment, patient education, and discharge planning.[21]

Early Hospital Admission

Patients who are admitted 1 or more days before planned surgery are those whose medical condition warrants it (such as patients with brittle diabetes) or those who require parenteral antibiotics or hydration, or bowel preparation.

All categories of admission require the necessary *preoperative preparation* (Box 14-1). The nurse in the preoperative prehospital period is in a position to perform the required comprehensive assessment to plan and initiate interventions from admission to discharge. This is of utmost importance for the day surgical patients who must have a responsible person take them home and provide any necessary care.

14-1	**Components of preoperative preparation**
	Preoperative tests (see Table 14-6)
	History and physical examination
	Anaesthesia consult
	Nursing assessment
	Preoperative eduction

TYPES OF SURGERY
Classification

Surgeries may be classified in several ways, such as by location, extent, or purpose of the surgery.

Location

Surgery may be performed externally or internally. In *external surgery* the skin or underlying tissues are readily accessible to the surgeon. *Plastic surgery* (Chapter 34) is an example of external surgery. *Internal surgery* involves penetration of the body. Surgery of major internal organs may lead to decreased function if sufficient tissue is removed.

Surgery may also be classified by location of body parts or systems, such as cardiovascular surgery, chest surgery, neurological surgery, and so on. Information specific to these types of surgery can be found elsewhere in the text.

Extent

Surgery may be classified as minor or major. *Minor surgery* is simple surgery that presents little risk to life. It may be performed in a doctor's surgery, a clinic, or an outpatient or inpatient surgical suite. Although the operation is termed "minor," it may not be viewed as minor by the patient and may evoke some fears.

Major surgery is usually performed in an inpatient surgical suite. It is more serious than minor surgery and may involve risk to life.

Purpose

There are several reasons for performing surgery (Table 14-1). The surgeon explains the method and purpose for the proposed surgery to the patient and family. Because the preoperative period is often a time of increased anxiety for the patient or family, they may not perceive or understand

Table 14-1 Purpose of surgery

Type of surgery	Reason performed	Examples
Diagnostic	Determine cause of symptoms	Biopsy, exploratory laparotomy
Curative	Removal of diseased part	Appendicectomy
Restorative	Strengthen weakened areas	Herniorrhaphy
	Correct deformities	Mitral valve replacement
	Rejoin a separated area	Bone pinning
Palliative	Relieve symptoms without curing disease	Sympathectomy
Cosmetic	Improve appearance	Rhinoplasty

the reason for the surgery and may require further clarification, which the nurse can provide.

Surgical Procedures

Most surgical procedures are given names that describe the site of the surgery and the type of surgery performed. For example, a hysterectomy is the removal of (-ectomy) the uterus (hyster-).

Common surgical suffixes

-ectomy	Removal of an organ or gland
-rrhapy	Suturing or stitching
-ostomy	Providing an opening (stoma)
-otomy	Cutting into
-plasty	Plastic repair
-scopy	Looking into

Some procedures, however, carry the name of the surgeon who developed the technique, such as the Heineke-Mikulicz procedure (widening of the pyloric opening of the stomach).

The most common method of performing surgery is cutting into the tissue and exposing the operative field. In recent years the "scope" approach has been introduced for certain types of surgery, for example, arthroscopy (knee) or laparoscopy (removal of gallbladder). It is estimated that by the year 2000 much elective surgery will be performed through a scope (see Fig. 27-10). In this method, a very small puncture incision is made to introduce the scope, which is attached to a video screen for visualization of the operative area. Two to three additional puncture incisions are made to introduce instruments. Lasers can be used (with great caution) to cut away tissue, obliterate tissue, repair tissue, or stop bleeding. The advantage of the scope method of surgery is more rapid patient recovery, with less discomfort, although there are disadvantages, such as perforation of structures.

EFFECTS OF SURGERY ON THE PATIENT

Surgery is a potential or actual threat to a person's integrity and thus may produce both physiological and psychological stress reactions. The physiological stress reaction is directly related to the extent of the surgery, that is, the more extensive the surgery, the greater the physiological response. The psychological response, however, is not directly related. A relatively minor surgical procedure, such as removal of a cyst from the face, may evoke a greater psychological response than removal of an organ

such as the spleen because of the former's potential for scarring. Removal of the uterus, however, may evoke a greater response than would removal of the spleen. This is because of the implications and values attached to the uterus.

Physiological Responses

Major surgery is a stressor to the body and evokes a neuroendocrine response. The response, which consists of sympathetic nervous system and hormonal responses (Table 14-2), serves to protect the body from the threat of injury (Fig. 14-1). (Review Chapter 5 for the neuroendocrine response to stress). When the stress to the system is severe or if blood loss is excessive, the body's compensatory mechanisms are overwhelmed, and shock is the result. Certain types of anaesthesia used may also contribute to shock formation.

Metabolic responses also occur. Carbohydrates and fats are metabolized to produce energy. Body proteins are broken down to provide a supply of the amino acids used to build new tissues. Those amino acids that are not used are broken down to nitrogen end products, such as urea, and excreted. This leads to *a negative nitrogen balance;* that is, nitrogen loss exceeds nitrogen intake. All these factors lead to weight loss after major surgery. A high protein intake is necessary for healing and for restoration of optimal functioning.

Psychological Responses

People differ in the way they perceive the meaning of surgery, and thus they respond in different ways. There are, however, some common fears and concerns. Some fears underlying preoperative anxiety are general and some more specific. Following is a list of these fears.

General	Specific
Fear of unknown	Diagnosis of malignancy
Loss of control	Anaesthesia
Loss of love from significant others	Dying
	Pain
Threat of sexuality	Disfigurement
	Permanent limitation

Fear of the unknown is the most common. If the diagnosis is uncertain, fear of malignancy is frequent, regardless of the probability of occurrence. Fears concerning anaesthesia are usually related to dying, "going to sleep and never waking up." Some people are concerned about what they will say when they are awakening from

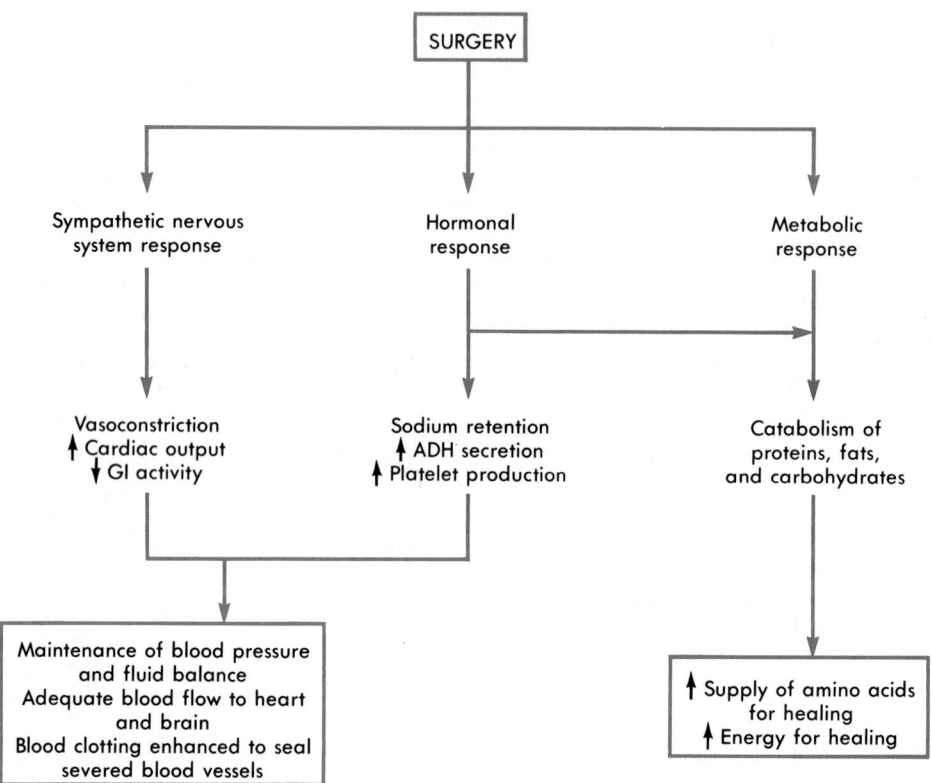

Fig. 14-1 Positive effects of the pathophysiological response to surgery.

Table 14-2 Effects of physiological responses to surgery

Response	Positive effect	Negative effect
Sympathetic nervous system		
Vasoconstriction	Maintain blood pressure, adequate blood flow to heart and brain	
Increased cardiac output	Maintain blood pressure	
Decreased GI activity		Anorexia, distention and pain, constipation
Hormonal		
Increased glucocorticoid secretion (adrenal cortex)		
Sodium retention	Increased blood volume	Potassium loss
Protein and fat catabolism	Increased energy, amino acids available for healing	Weight loss
Increased platelet production	Prevent bleeding through clotting	Possible thrombus formation
Increased ADH secretion (posterior pituitary)	Increased blood volume	Possible fluid overload

Table 14-3 Potential postoperative complications in elderly people

Dysfunction	Possible effects
Decreased circulaion	Shock, wound infection, thrombophlebitis
Decreased kidney function	Prolonged response to anaesthesia, fluid and electrolyte imbalances (especially overhydration)
Decreased respiratory function	Atelectasis, pneumonia
Decreased mobility	Atelectasis, pneumonia, thrombophlebitis, constipation, or faecal impaction

anaesthesia. Fears concerning pain, disfigurement, or permanent disability may be realistic or may be influenced by myths, lack of information, or lurid stories told by friends. The patient may also have other concerns related to hospitalization, such as job, income, and family.

People with anxiety so high that they cannot talk about and begin to cope with their anxiety before surgery frequently experience difficulty in the postoperative period. They are more apt to be angry, resentful, confused, or depressed. They are also more vulnerable to psychotic reactions than are people with lower levels of anxiety.

Lack of any emotional response to surgery may indicate denial; this precludes dealing with and coping with the anxiety before surgery. Some anxiety enables the individual to identify and begin to cope with feelings. These people usually have a smoother postoperative course.

Elderly People's Response to Surgery

The ability of the elderly patient to tolerate surgery depends on the extent of physiological changes that have occurred with the ageing process, the duration of the surgical procedure, and the presence of one or more chronic diseases. The changes that affect responses to surgery are cardiovascular, renal, pulmonary, and musculoskeletal (Table 14-3).

The greater the number of changes present, the greater the potential for the development of a postoperative complication. Heart rate changes in the elderly occur more slowly than in younger people; therefore, the pulse rate *may not* be a good index in assessment of shock, and a longer period of time may be necessary to wait for pulse stabilization after activity.

The duration of the surgical experience can affect the response of elderly people to surgery. Surgery of short duration is more easily tolerated. Presence of chronic diseases such as pulmonary, cardiac, or CNS disease limits the elderly person by prolonging recovery or by increasing the risk of mortality. Certain types of surgery present low or high risks for elderly people:

Lower risk	Higher risk
Elective	Thoracic
Away from diaphragm	Radical head and neck
Not involving infections	Closure of wound dehiscence
Permitting early mobility	Perforated ulcer
Requiring minimal narcotics	Colostomy following obstruction

RISK FACTORS FOR SURGERY

A number of variables influence physiological and psychological responses throughout the surgical experience.

Age

Surgery can be performed on people of any age, from neonates (and even on the foetus) to the very old. People at extremes of age are less able to tolerate stress such as tissue trauma (surgery) or infection.

Nutrition

Malnourished people are poorer surgical risks than the well nourished and are more likely to develop postoperative complications. *Undernourished* people already have diminished reserves of carbohydrates and fats. Body proteins will be used to provide the energy to maintain metabolic functioning of cells; thus nitrogen imbalances will be greater than normal and less protein will be available for healing. Wound healing is considerably delayed in undernourished people, and wound separation and infection may occur. Elective surgery is delayed until the patient's nutritional status is improved. Conditions predisposing the person to preoperative malnutrition include chronic inflammatory disorders, liver and renal disease, gastrointestinal cancer, and congestive heart failure.

The *obese* person presents numerous risks during the surgical experience:

Respiratory complications
Vital signs fluctuations
Wound separation and infection
Incisional hernias
Thrombophlebitis

The organs are enlarged and excessive demands are placed on the cardiovascular system. Fatty tissue has reduced circulation so wounds heal more slowly. Obese people have greater difficulty expanding their chests, moving in bed, and walking.

Neuroendocrine Response Ineffectiveness

The neuroendocrine response assists the person in coping with the stress of surgery. If this response is ineffective, postoperative complications such as shock and delayed wound healing may occur. In addition, anaesthesia may be tolerated poorly, and fluid and electrolyte imbalances are more likely to occur because of insufficient adrenocortical activity. People with diseases of the adrenal gland or the sympathetic nervous system or those who are under a great deal of stress before surgery may do less well postoperatively because of inability to retain sodium. Infants and elderly also have diminished neuroendocrine responses.

Chronic Disease

The existence of one or more chronic diseases does not necessarily increase surgical risk. The nature and extent of the diseases and the degree to which they are under control are the important variables. Surgery may be delayed until optimal condition is achieved.

Pulmonary disease, such as chronic obstructive pulmonary disease (COPD), may affect the person's response to the anaesthetic and ability to cope with respiratory problems after surgery.

Cardiovascular disease can affect the individual's response to surgery because a heart that pumps effectively and blood vessels that constrict effectively are necessary for the prevention of shock and of fluid imbalances.

Renal insufficiency can increase the risk of surgery because of difficulty in the removal of increased amounts of electrolytes, especially potassium, and waste products from catabolism. People with renal disease are prone to developing fluid overload.

The patient with *diabetes mellitus* should have the disease well controlled before surgery.

Smoking

Smoke irritates the tracheobronchial tree, resulting in increased secretions. Therefore, smokers are at higher risk for developing postoperative pulmonary complications. Most surgeons and anaesthetists prefer that people who smoke stop smoking for a period of time before surgery.

INFORMED CONSENT

Written permission must be obtained from the patient for each operation performed and is usually obtained for major diagnostic procedures, such as thoracentesis, cystoscopy, or bronchoscopy, which involve entry into the body cavity. The consent implies that the patient has been provided with the knowledge necessary to understand (1) the nature of the procedure to be performed, (2) the available options, and (3) the risks associated with each option. Signed permission protects the patient from undergoing unauthorized surgery and protects the surgeon and hospital against claims of unauthorized surgery or that the patient was unaware of the risks involved.

Legal responsibility for obtaining informed consent from the patient resides with the surgeon. Doctors will document that the necessary information has been provided for the patient. Signing of the official consent form is primarily evidence that the *consent process* has occurred— that the patient is aware of the concept of informed consent.

In the role of patient advocate, the nurse identifies that the patient has discussed with the doctor the risks and benefits of the procedure and the alternatives. The nurse uses skills of teaching and counselling to clarify any patient misconceptions and to facilitate the decision-making process by the patient. This process must occur before the patient receives any sedation. Patients may decide to refuse surgery, and it is their right to do so. Nurses have the responsibility to see that the decision is an *informed* decision.

If an adult is incapable of giving informed consent, consent must be obtained from the next of kin. A parent or legal guardian usually provides consent for a minor child. Minors over the age of 16 may sign their own consent form.

In an emergency situation, the surgeon may operate without written permission, although every effort is made to contact a family member or guardian if time permits.

Nursing Process
Assessment

Data are collected by the nurse in the preoperative period, often before admission, to identify the patient's (1) knowledge of events that will occur, (2) psychological readiness for surgery, and (3) physiological status before surgery. Specific data to be collected are listed in Box 14-2.

Patient knowledge

A major nursing strategy in the preoperative period is teaching the patient about forthcoming events and exercises that can be used in the postoperative period to decrease the potential for complications.[6] The nurse should determine existing knowledge and readiness to learn, and teach at a level appropriate to the person's understanding.

Psychological readiness for surgery

The degree of anxiety felt by the patient needs to be assessed. Patients may not be able to identify specific concerns, and further exploration may be necessary. If the nurse has identified clues from the patient's behaviour that moderate to severe anxiety is present, these complications need to be validated with the patient. If the collected data indicate that the patient is severely anxious or if the patient describes fear of dying while in surgery, report this information to the doctor for further evaluation.

Knowledge of the patient's religion can help the nurse identify a possible source of support. The effect of family or significant others on anxiety needs to be determined. Some family members or friends increase the patient's anxiety by transmitting their own anxiety. Others are calm, and it is observed that the patient's anxiety is reduced when they are present.

Table 14-4 Medications that can adversely affect anaesthesia or surgery

Medication	Effect
Antibiotics	Potentiate muscle relaxants
Anticoagulants	Increase bleeding and haemorrhage
Antihypertensives	Affect anaesthesia and compensatory ability (hypotension may occur)
Aspirin	↓ Platelet aggregation
	Potentiates effect of anticoagulants
Diuretics (thiazides)	Possible potassium imbalance
Steroids	↓ Neuroendocrine response
	Antiinflammatory effect, may delay wound healing
Tranquillizers	Potentiate effect of narcotics and barbiturates
	Hypotension

Changes in sleep patterns or frequent urination also provide clues about increased anxiety.

Signs of anxiety in the preoperative patient are no different from those in other people. Physical signs include an increased pulse rate and respiratory rate, moist palms, constant hand movements or motor-verbal activity, and restlessness.

Physiological status

Data are collected in the preoperative period concerning the patient's physiological status to obtain baseline data for comparison in the intraoperative and postoperative phases and to identify potential postoperative problems requiring preoperative intervention. Admission histories and physical examinations by the doctor and assessment by the nurse are good sources of pertinent data. The doctor may order special tests (Table 14-5) to detect the presence of diseases that may affect the perioperative course. Nurses should explain the relevance of such tests.

Ability to communicate

Data relating to the senses and language indicate the patient's ability to understand directions and to receive support in theatre. Deficits need to be communicated with the theatre staff.

Oxygenation

Respiratory data are especially important for determining the postoperative risks and the person's ability to expand their lungs and do deep breathing. Circulatory data are particularly important when the patient is elderly or is undergoing cardiovascular surgery. People with chronic lung, heart, or peripheral vascular disease may have more difficulties with tissue oxygenation in the postoperative period.

Nutrition

The height-to-weight ratio indicates whether the patient is overweight or underweight (see Chapter 4). People who are at risk for postoperative nutritional deficiency should be identified early. Inadequate dietary intake, nausea, anorexia, and poor conditions of the mouth and teeth will influence preoperative nutritional intake and may be factors to consider in the postoperative period.

Elimination

Decreased activity after surgery predisposes a patient to constipation.

Activity

Mobility and ambulation are important activities in the postoperative period for preventing postoperative compli-

---

14-2

Preoperative nursing assessment

Subjective data

Knowledge and past experiences
    Understanding of proposed surgery
        Site and type
        Information about hospitalization, postoperative limitations
        Preoperative routines and tests
        Postoperative routines
    Previous surgical experiences
Psychological readiness for surgery
    Concerns or fears about proposed surgery
    Usual coping methods
    Religion and its meanings for patient
    Living will or Advance Directives
    Cultural beliefs or practices related to surgery
        Refusal of treatment such as transfusion of blood or blood products
    Family and close friends
        Accessibility (distance)
        Perception of family and friends as source of support
        Present living situation
    Changes in sleep patterns
    Increased urinary frequency
Physiological status
    Medications (Table 14-4)
    Allergies
    Sensory difficulties
    Nutritional status
    Elimination: defaecation, urination and menstrual cycle if appropriate

Motor: difficulties with ambulation, movement of arms and legs, use of walking aids
Prosthetic devices: dentures, artificial eye or limb, contact lenses, pacemakers, broviac mediport
Comfort: ability to sleep, presence of pain or discomfort, expectations regarding relief of postoperative pain
Risk factors: smoking, alcohol, illicit drugs

Objective data

Speech patterns: repetition of themes, change of topic, avoidance of topics related to feelings (anxiety); ability to understand English
Degree of interaction with others (anxiety)
Behaviour: excessive hand movements, restlessness, withdrawal, or excessive activity (anxiety)
Height and weight
Vital signs
Sensory: ability to see, hear, and speak
Skin: turgor, presence of lesions, rashes, or bruising
Mouth: dentures, condition of teeth and mucous membranes
Motor ability: any limitation to walking, sitting, or moving in bed, coordination with ambulation

Table 14-5 Preoperative tests to establish baselines and detect presence of diseases that can affect patient responses in intraoperative or postoperative phases

System	Test	Disease or condition
Respiratory	Chest radiograph	Tuberculosis or other pulmonary disease
	Vital capacity	Tuberculosis, chronic obstructive lung disease, bronchitis, asthma
	Pulmonary function	
	Blood gas studies	
Circulatory	Electrocardiogram, echocardiogram	Cardiac dysrrhythmias, myocardial damage
	Blood studies	
	WBC and differential	Chronic infection
	RBC haemoglobin, haematocrit	Anaemia
	Electrolytes	Electrolyte imbalances
	Platelet count, bleeding and clotting times, prothrombin	Liver disease, blood dyscrasias
	Typing and crossmatching	Compatibility for transfusion
	Blood volume	Heart disease
Renal	Urine studies	
	Bacteria	Urinary tract infection
	Routine ward test	Kidney disease
	Blood studies	
	Creatine, urea, electrolytes	Kidney disease
Metabolic	Blood sugar, urine sugar, acetone	Diabetes mellitus
		Starvation

cations. The patient's ability to move and walk preoperatively will determine actions that must be taken to enhance maximum mobility.

Comfort

The pain-relieving routines need to be clarified to the patient to prevent misunderstandings. The various modalities for pain management also need to be explained. Pain modalities may include patient-controlled analgesia (PCA) or the use of an epidural catheter. Because the epidural catheter is placed before general anaesthesia is given, the anaesthetist or surgeon discusses this with the patient preoperatively.

Nursing Analysis

Problems are determined from analysis of patient data. Possible preoperative problems may include, but are not limited to, the following:

Problem	Possible aetiologies
Anxiety	Threat of death, threat to role functioning, threat of unmet needs, fear of the unknown
Fear	Anaesthesia, surgery (type), loss of body part, anticipated pain, possible lifestyle changes
Knowledge deficit (events pertaining to surgery)	Lack of exposure/recall, information misinterpretation, cognitive impairment, severe anxiety
Infection, high risk for	Lack of knowledge, decreased nutrition
Injury, high risk for	Sensory/motor deficits, lack of awareness of environmental hazards

Planning: expected patient outcomes

Expected patient outcomes for the preoperative patient may include, but are not limited to, the following:

1. Demonstrates no more than moderate anxiety.
2. Describes (if conscious) the surgery to be performed and has signed the operative consent form.
3. Describes events and physical activities expected in the early postoperative period (turning, effective deep breathing, and leg exercises).
4. Wears a legible identification band that has been checked and an allergy band (if pertinent).
5. Does not wear nail polish or acrylic nails, hairgrips or wigs, dentures, or jewellery to the theatre (articles have been stored for safekeeping).
6. Voids urine before going to theatre.
7. Receives preanaesthetic medication as ordered, if informed consent is signed.

Implementation

Assisting with achievement of therapeutic goals
Medical interventions: correction of existing deficiencies

Postoperative complications can be minimized if existing medical conditions are treated or are under good control before surgery. For example, dehydration from vomiting and diarrhoea is treated with parenteral fluids.

Patients with chronic diseases should be at their optimal health level before surgery. The undernourished patient should receive a high-protein, high-carbohydrate diet rich in vitamins B_1, C, and K. If an oral diet is poorly tolerated or poorly absorbed, total parenteral nutrition (TPN) will be initiated. The obese patient receives a weight-reducing diet. Patients with low haematocrit levels from autologous blood donation (Chapter 33) are prescribed iron-rich diets and iron supplements.

Patients with chronic obstructive pulmonary disease are frequently placed on vigorous physiotherapy to decrease postoperative respiratory complications. Smoking is restricted for all patients preoperatively and especially for patients with lung disease. Diabetes mellitus should be under good control.

Preoperative preparation

Diet. Except in bowel surgery for which patients may receive a low-residue or clear liquid diet, a normal diet is permitted on the day before surgery. Usually patients are permitted fluids up to 4-6 hours before surgery, but there may be local variations. Presence of food or fluids in the stomach increases the possibility of aspiration of gastric contents should the patient vomit while under anaesthesia. If it should be discovered that the patient has consumed food or fluids whilst "nil by mouth", the surgeon should be notified because this may necessitate delaying the surgical procedure. If a local or spinal anaesthetic is planned, it is still common practice to keep the patient nil orally.

Patients who are dehydrated will usually have parenteral fluids initiated before surgery. Patients having surgery where reduced peristalsis is anticipated, e.g. on the gastrointestinal tract, will have a nasogastric tube passed just before or during surgery.

Bowel preparation. Enemas and or washouts are usually given preoperatively only for surgery of the GI tract or the pelvic, perineal, or perianal areas. The purpose of the preoperative enema is to prevent injury to the colon, to provide better visualization of the surgical area, and to prevent constipation or faecal impaction postoperatively.

If enemas or washouts are to be given until the returns are clear, it is important to remember that fluid excess and potassium deficits can occur with repeated enemas or washouts. Bowel washouts may be given for 2-3 days prior to surgery. Repeated enemas/washouts are very tiring and may irritate rectal and bowel mucosa.

Patients may be given a glycerine suppository to use the night before surgery to clean out the lower bowel. This helps to prevent postoperative constipation when ambulation is delayed. Bowel cleansing preparations may also be prescribed.

Skin preparation. The purpose of preoperative skin preparation is to free the operative site of as many microorganisms as possible. In many instances showering well with a chlorhexidine preparation will suffice. In certain types of surgery, such as for placing orthopaedic implants, infections can lead to dysfunction so several showers are prescribed. Same-day surgery patients are given a chlorhexidine preparation and instructed to shower twice, the night before surgery and on the morning of admission.

Hair may be removed from the surgical site because microorganisms cling to the hair. Shaving or clipping of the hair may be ordered either the night before or immediately before surgery (preferred approach). The skin should not be scratched or nicked because microorganisms can harbour in broken skin surfaces. A depilatory may be used if the skin is not sensitive to the depilatory.

Shaving of hair on certain areas of the body may have a special meaning for some people. These areas include the face, head, and pubic area. If the entire head is to be shaved, it is frequently carried out after the patient has been anaesthetized. The eyebrows are not shaved. Pubic hair is shaved only when necessary; the regrowth of this hair is uncomfortable to many patients.

An area larger than the anticipated incision is shaved to permit flexibility in location and size of incision.

Interventions to achieve patient outcomes
Preparing patient psychologically for surgery

Both patient and family need opportunities to discuss their concerns and fears about the forthcoming surgery.

Providing time for patients to talk with a supportive, knowledgeable individual helps them to begin to identify the reasons for their anxiety and to marshal coping responses. It is helpful for the nurse to provide for a quiet unhurried time to sit down with the person or family and give them an opportunity to ask questions and to talk about concerns. Touch is often a helpful form of communication, sending the message, "I care". Knowing that a nurse is interested and cares helps to reduce anxiety. It is helpful for the person to know that some anxiety is "normal".

Loss of control is one of the fears associated with surgery. It is important that a patient understands the type of anaesthesia recommended. Allowing people to participate in decision making in regard to their own care, when feasible, helps them partially to keep control. Identifying and carrying out measures to help the patient meet physical needs in the preoperative phase may help provide a feeling of security about having postoperative needs met and thus allay some anxiety.

Teaching (from preparation for surgery to discharge instructions) is an important nursing function in the preoperative phase. This teaching helps to allay anxiety when the patient knows what to expect. Also, if people are to move towards self-care and independence, they need to know early the what, why, and how of activities that will help them regain an optimal level of functioning after surgery. They also need to know what to expect when they go home or go to a rehabilitation or extended-care facility. It is particularly useful to provide *written* instructions whenever possible, especially for activities the patient and family are to carry out.

Explaining events

Fear of the unknown can be decreased by an understanding of the events that will occur. The amount of information to give preoperatively depends on the individual patient. A good rule to follow is to ask patients what they would like to know about forthcoming surgery and to base responses on the types of questions asked. Simple explanations are indicated for people under considerable stress or those with severe pain. A highly anxious person may not take in and remember information given. Information helpful for preoperative patients is listed in Box 14-3.

Facilitating teaching

Effective deep breathing exercises. Some people are at high risk for developing postoperative pulmonary complications such as atelectasis or pneumonia, e.g. smokers, the elderly, those with lung disease, obesity and thoracic/upper abdominal surgery. These people need to carry out deep breathing exercises in the early postoperative period.

14-3

Helpful information for preoperative patients and families

Preoperative tests—reason, preparation
Preoperative routines; sequence of events
Special equipment needed
Transfer to theatre (time, checking procedures)
Recovery room
   Place where patient will awaken
   Frequent monitoring of vital signs
Probable postoperative therapies
   Deep breathing and leg exercises
   Anticipated treatments (for example, I.V.)
   Pain medication routines, and modalities of
      management

Coughing is *contraindicated* in intracranial surgery and surgery of the eye, ear, nose, and throat, because it either increases pressure, causing tissue damage and dislodging of sutures, or dislodges a clot.

The person needs to know how to perform diaphragmatic breathing, as this increases lung expansion by permitting the diaphragm to descend fully. With diaphragmatic breathing, the abdomen *rises with inspiration* and *falls with expiration*. If diaphragmatic breathing does not occur naturally, the person can be taught to inspire deeply while pushing the abdomen up against the hand.

The method for effective deep breathing exercises is listed as follows:
1. Upright position with knees flexed to relax abdomen and allow full chest expansion.
2. Place a hand lightly on the abdomen.
3. Breathe in slowly through nose, letting chest expand and feeling abdomen rise against hand.
4. Hold breath for 5 seconds.
5. Exhale slowly through pursed lips (abdomen contracts).
6. Inhale and exhale 7 more times.

If a thoracic or high abdominal incision is present, the person can "splint" the incision with a pillow during coughing to relieve stress or pull on the incision.

Leg exercises. Venous stasis in the postoperative period may lead to thrombophlebitis (blood clot). People at high risk include those who (1) will have decreased mobility after surgery, (2) have a history of decreased peripheral circulation, or (3) undergo cardiovascular or pelvic surgery. These patients will need to carry out exercises postoperatively to prevent venous stasis in the legs. Tightening and relaxing leg muscles helps to "pump" the blood along the veins. Valves in the veins prevent back flow of blood.

People at high risk may have sequential compression devices applied before, during, and after surgery to promote venous return. Antiembolic stockings, either thigh-high or knee-high, may also be used. People who will be restricted to bed rest for several days after surgery will need to exercise the legs to maintain muscle tone to facilitate ambulation at a later date. These people need to learn to carry out ankle pumps, quadriceps sets, and gluteal tightening exercises as taught by the physiotherapist.

Promoting mobility

Moving and turning in bed helps to prevent pulmonary and circulatory complications, prevent decubiti, stimulate peristalsis, and decrease pain. During the preoperative period, people can be taught how to move and turn in bed. They can also be taught how to sit up on the side of the bed with the least amount of pull on the incision.

Carrying out final preparation for surgery

Preventing injury. Measures taken to protect the patient from errors of identification or injury include the following:
1. Check identification band for secureness and legibility and allergy band if allergies present.
2. Remove hair grips and wigs; protect hair with a cap.
3. Remove jewellery; wedding ring may be taped to patient's finger.
4. Remove nail polish and acrylic nails (for assessment of circulation during surgery).
5. Remove contact lenses and store correctly.
6. Remove any prostheses (dentures, false eyes, and so on); store safely.
7. Leave hearing aid in place if patient is unable to hear without the aid (inform theatre nurse).
8. Apply SCDs and/or antiembolic stockings if patient is at high risk for thromboembolism or shock (elderly, marked varicosities, pelvic surgery, time-consuming surgery).
9. Ask patient to empty bladder immediately before receiving preanaesthetic medication.
10. Instruct patient to stay in bed until transported to the operating theatre.
11. Ensure patient can reach call system.

Administering preanaesthetic medication. If a patient is in the hospital the night before surgery, a sedative may be prescribed to ensure a full night's sleep.

Preanaesthetic medications, commonly referred to as *premedication*, are given about 45 to 90 minutes before surgery is anticipated. Preanaesthetic medications are given to decrease anxiety, to provide a smoother induction and maintenance of anaesthesia, to diminish undesirable reflexes during emergence from anaesthesia, to decrease secretions, and to block vagal impulses that produce bradycardia.

The effects of commonly used preanaesthetic medications are listed in Table 14-6. Adults frequently receive a combination of drugs. Dosages may be decreased in the elderly.

Any delay in giving the medication is reported to the anaesthetist. All preoperative routines are completed before the preanaesthetic medication is given. The patient should remain in bed following administration of the medication to promote maximum effect and to prevent falls from dizziness. Cot sides may be raised, the bed is placed in low position, the call signal is placed within reach, and the patient is instructed not to get out of bed.

One major effect desired before surgery is decreased anxiety. It must be reemphasized that psychological preparation is the most effective approach to help allay anxiety. The administration of preanaesthetic medication without any attempt at psychological preparation may render the patient drowsy, but it does not reduce anxiety.

Some drugs other than preanaesthetic agents, such as insulin, antihypertensive agents, and cardiac medications, may be prescribed for the day of surgery. Oral medications are given with only a small sip of water. Administration of all medications is recorded.

Recording. A check list that includes the final preparations is often used. Presence of impairments such as blindness or deafness should be noted for use by the surgical staff.

Before the patient leaves for surgery the notes are checked for completeness as to the following:
1. Skin preparation done and checked by nurse
2. Vital signs (temperature, pulse, respiration, blood pressure) charted
3. Premedications charted
4. Other medication charted
5. Weight and height recorded (for use by anaesthetist)
6. Consent signed, and attached to notes

7. All recent laboratory, radiographic, and ECG reports attached to notes
8. Previous hospital notes

Evaluation
Questions to ask may include the following:
1. Is the patient's anxiety level no more than moderate?
2. Does the patient understand the nature of the surgical procedure to be performed, and has the consent form been signed?
3. Has the patient been taught about turning, effective deep breathing, and leg exercises?
4. Is the patient wearing a legible identification band that has been checked?
5. Have all removable objects been stored for safekeeping?
6. Has nailpolish or acrylic nails been removed?
7. Has the patient voided urine just before receiving premedication?
8. Has the premedication been given and charted?
9. Are the notes complete?

Table 14-6 Commonly used preanaesthetic medications

Drug	Desired effect	Undesired effect
Benzodiazepines e.g.		
Diazepam	Reduces anxiety, promotes relaxation	Orthostatic and general hypotension; drowsiness and decreased coordination
Narcotics e.g.		
Morphine sulphate	Reduces anxiety, promotes realaxation, decreases preoperative pain, decreases amount of anaesthetic needed	Depresses respiration, circulation, and gastric motility; may cause nausea and vomiting
Pethidine hydrochloride	Same as for morphine sulphate	Same as for morphine sulphate
H₂ receptor antagonists e.g.		
Cimetidine	Decreases gastric acid and gastric volume	Rare; confusion may occur in elderly people
Antacid, nonparticulate		
Sodium citrate (Bicitra)	Increases gastric pH; less pulmonary damage with aspiration	None
Antiemetics e.g.		
Metoclopramide	Enhances gastric emptying	Restlessness, confusion
Neuroleptanalgesic agent		
Fentanyl and droperidol	General quiescence, state of indifference, decreased motor activity, analgesia, antiemetic	Respiratory depression, muscle rigidity, hypotension
Anticholinergics		
Atropine sulphate	Decreased secretions, prevention of laryngospasms and bradycardia	Excessive dryness of mouth, tachycardia, confusion, restlessness
Scopolamine hydrochloride	Decreased secretions, amnesia, state of indifference, sedation	Excessive dryness of mouth; profound confusion and restlessness in the elderly
Glycopyrronium bromide	Same as atropine sulphate	Same as atropine sulphate

Nursing Care Plan

Preoperative patient

DATA: Mrs. G. is an active 76-year-old widowed housewife with a history of osteoarthritis in her left hip. She has been experiencing difficulty ambulating and has had increased pain, especially at night. She denies any history of falls or trauma. She is scheduled for a total hip replacement.

1. Mrs. G. has been hospitalized only once before and has never had major surgery.
2. She lives alone in a two-storey house with a bathroom on the first floor.
3. She states she is worried about being anaesthetized and of the pain after surgery.
4. She expresses much anxiety about being a burden on her family and not going back to her home after surgery.
5. Mrs. G. has strong supportive family and friends.

Nursing analysis: Knowledge deficit related to lack of information regarding hip replacement surgery

Expected patient outcomes	Nursing interventions	Rationale
Mrs. G. describes the sequence of events that will occur on the morning of surgery Mrs. G. repeats preoperative expectations	Review with Mrs. G. and family what to expect in terms of activities related to the day of surgery Provide rationale for preparation for surgery and give written instructions	Knowledge of expected events helps to decrease anxiety and facilitate coping Knowing why the preoperative activities are necessary and having notes to refer to will facilitate her carrying out the instructions
Mrs. G. demonstrates effective deep breathing exercises	Teach rationale and method of effective deep breathing exercises; ask her to demonstrate and suggest she practise at home	Mrs. G. will be less mobile after surgery; she is at high risk for pulmonary complications

Nursing analysis: Anxiety, related to surgery and threat of losing independence

Expected patient outcomes	Nursing interventions	Rationale
Mrs. G. is relaxed before surgery	Clarify her understanding of anaesthesia, its administration and effects	Mrs. G. may have heard inaccurate stories about anaesthesia or may be worried about waking up. Clarification will decrease anxiety
	Explain methods of postoperative pain relief and control she may have	Knowing that pain control is possible decreases anxiety

Nursing analysis: Home maintenance management, impaired related to inadequate living situation

Expected patient outcomes	Nursing interventions	Rationale
Mrs. G. states she is comfortable about her decision to go to an extended-care facility for 4 to 5 days before going home	Call social services to arrange for placement	Mrs. G. will be unable to go home until she can climb stairs with crutches or walker
	Arrange for transportation to extended-care facility	Mrs. G. will require transportation because of her limited mobility
	Order equipment and supplies for home care after surgery	Mrs. G. will require equipment for home care; advance ordering will facilitate her return home

TRANSPORTATION TO OPERATING THEATRE

Personnel transporting the patient bring the trolley from the operating theatre and identify themselves to the nurse. The ward nurse assigned to prepare the patient for surgery checks the patient record, accompanies the transportation staff to the patient's bedside, checks the patient's identification band, and signs the patient identification form. Patients should be protected from draughts

The patient's family or close friends are provided with the following information:

1. Expected time intervals
   a. Patient is sent to theatre some time before surgery actually commences
   b. Surgery may be delayed if the previous operation took longer than anticipated
   c. Patient will be sent to a recovery room after surgery for varying periods of time
2. Method of receiving information when surgery is completed
3. Where to wait/obtain meals and beverages if staying in the hospital
4. What to expect when patient returns from surgery (condition, special equipment, etc.)

N.B. Details of specialist intraoperative care and interventions can be found in a text dealing specifically with theatre nursing. Some examples are included in the list of selected readings.

The postoperative period begins as soon as the operation is completed. If a general anaesthetic has been given, the patient is usually taken to a postanaesthesia recovery unit for the postanaesthetic phase.

POSTANAESTHETIC PHASE

The immediate postanaesthetic period is critical. The patient must be observed diligently and must receive intensive physical and psychological support until the major effects of the anaesthetic have worn off and the overall condition stabilizes. The nurse is largely responsible for the care of the patient at this time.

The patient is accompanied to the recovery unit by the anaesthetist and another member of the operating theatre professional staff. The recovery room nurse assesses the patient's status, obtains report, and begins recording the recovery unit notes.

Much of the ongoing nursing care provided in the immediate postanaesthetic period depends on the surgical procedure performed and type of anaesthetic given, and is discussed elsewhere in this text (see specific surgical care for each body system). Some outcomes, however, are the same for all patients: pulmonary ventilation, circulation, and fluid and electrolyte balance are maintained, injury is prevented, and comfort is promoted.

Nursing Process
Assessment

The initial patient assessment may be done by the recovery nurse or jointly with a member of the theatre team. Data are primarily objective because the patient is often partly asleep. Data are collected pertaining to airway patency, vital signs, pressure readings, level of consciousness,

---

14-4

Postanaesthesia assessment

Airway	Patency, presence/adequacy of artificial airway
Vital signs	Respiratory rate, depth, character
	Heart rate (pulse, pulse oximeter, or cardiac monitor)
	Blood pressure (cuff or arterial line)
	Temperature
Pressure readings (as indicated)	Pulmonary artery wedge pressure (Chapter 7), central venous pressure (Chapter 7), intracranial (Chapter 29)
Level of consciousness	
Patient position	Position to facilitate breathing, to prevent pressure on body parts or invasive lines, and to promote comfort
Tissue oxygenation	Skin: colour, temperature, moisture
	Nail beds: colour, capillary refill
	Lips/oral mucosa: colour
	Pulse oximetry
	Peripheral pulses: presence, strength (as indicated)
Dressing/suture line	Dressings: dry or minimal drainage
	Suture line (if visible): colour, approximation of wound edges
Fluid lines/tubes	Intravenous fluids: rate, amount in bag, infusion site
	Other lines: patency, connection
	Drainage tubes: patency, connection, character and amount of drainage

---

patient position, tissue oxygenation, and dressings, or suture line, fluids lines, and tubes (Box 14-4). Many recovery units use a rating scale to evaluate postanaesthesia recovery. Ongoing data is collected on these same parameters and recorded on flow sheets or nurses notes to show changes in the patient's status.

Nursing Analysis

Problems are determined from analysis of patient data. Possible problems for the postanaesthesia patient may include, but are not limited to, the following:

Problem	Possible causes
Airway clearance, ineffective	Inability to remove secretions, relaxed tongue blocking airway
Gas exchange, impaired	Anaesthetic, narcotics, incisional pain
Cardiac output, decreased	Anaesthetic, blood loss
Hypothermia	Anaesthetic, body exposure in cold operating theatre
Fluid deficit	Blood loss, fluid loss

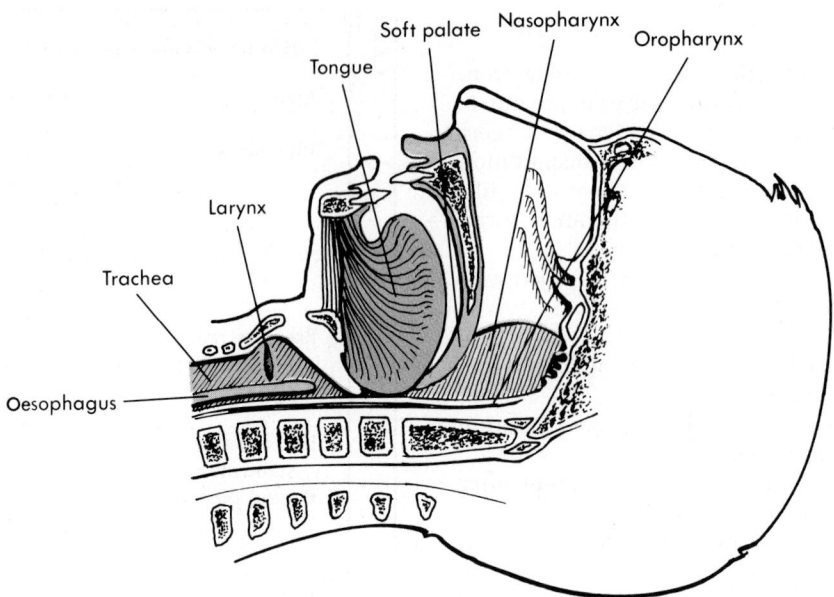

Fig. 14-2   Obstruction of airway by tongue blocking oropharynx in unconscious person lying in supine position.

Problem	Possible causes
Fluid excess	Fluid replacement in excess of body's ability to remove fluids
Injury, high risk for	Anaesthetic, immobility
Pain	Incision
Anxiety	Knowledge deficit, fear of results of surgery

Planning: expected patient outcomes

Expected patient outcomes for the postanaesthesia patient may include, but are not limited to, the following:

1. Breath sounds are clear.
2. Respiratory rate is 12 to 20 breaths per minute and regular.
3. Oxygen saturation levels are within normal levels.
4. Blood pressure returns to patient's usual level.
5. Temperature returns to patient's usual level.
6. Skin is warm and dry, pulse is regular, urinary output usually slightly less than fluid intake.
7. Pulmonary oedema does not occur.
8. Sleep is quiet and face is relaxed.

Implementation

Maintaining pulmonary ventilation

In the immediate postanaesthetic period, two of the most common causes of inadequate pulmonary exchange are airway obstruction and hypoventilation.

Airway patency

Airway obstruction most frequently occurs as a result of the tongue, which is relaxed against the pharynx (Fig. 14-2), or of secretions or other fluids collecting in the pharynx, trachea, or bronchial tree. This can be prevented by proper positioning, use of an artificial airway, or removal of secretions.

Positioning. Until protective reflexes have returned, the best position for the majority of patients is on their side or *semiprone* position with the head tilted back and the jaw supported forward. It is important to remember that aspiration can occur unless the *whole body* is turned.

Artificial airway. Some patients are admitted to the recovery unit with an *endotracheal tube* in place; however, the endotracheal tube is usually removed in the operating theatre. (Care of the patient with an endotracheal tube is described in Chapter 16.)

An oropharyngeal or nasopharyngeal airway is often left in place after administration of a general anaesthetic to keep the passage open and the tongue forward until pharyngeal reflexes have returned (Fig. 14-3). They are removed as soon as the patient begins to awaken and has regained coughing and swallowing reflexes. After this time their presence can be irritating and can stimulate vomiting or laryngospasm.

Removal of secretions. If the patient cannot cough up and expectorate secretions, they must be removed by suctioning. Pharyngeal suctioning is usually all that is necessary, although intratracheal suctioning may be indicated.

Adequate ventilation

Immediate postoperative hypoventilation can result from drugs (anaesthetics, narcotics, tranquillizers, sedatives), incisional pain, obesity, chronic lung disease, or pressure on the diaphragm. Inadequate ventilation leads to hypoxaemia. Arterial oxygen saturation (Sao_2) can be monitored either by arterial blood gas measurements or by pulse oximetry. *Pulse oximetry* is a noninvasive method providing continuous monitoring of Sao_2 for assessment of gas exchange. The system consists of a probe applied to a finger, of the patient's vital signs.

Blood pressure, pulse, and respirations are usually taken as follows: (1) every 15 minutes until stable, (2) every half hour for 2 hours, then (3) every 4 hours until ordered otherwise. More frequent monitoring may be indicated. In many hospitals, the monitoring of vital signs every 15 minutes is continued for a long as the patient is in the recovery unit and for at least 1 hour after leaving the recovery unit. The pulse rate, volume, and rhythm, and the respiratory rate and character are carefully noted and recorded. Preoperative vital signs are used as a baseline for comparison.

Cardiac output may be monitored by the thermistor of a pulmonary artery catheter if one is in place. Cardiac dysrrhythmias can be noted on a cardiac monitor.

Hypotension

Many factors can cause circulatory changes that result in lowering of blood pressure (see Box 14-5). A mild decrease in blood pressure from the normal preoperative

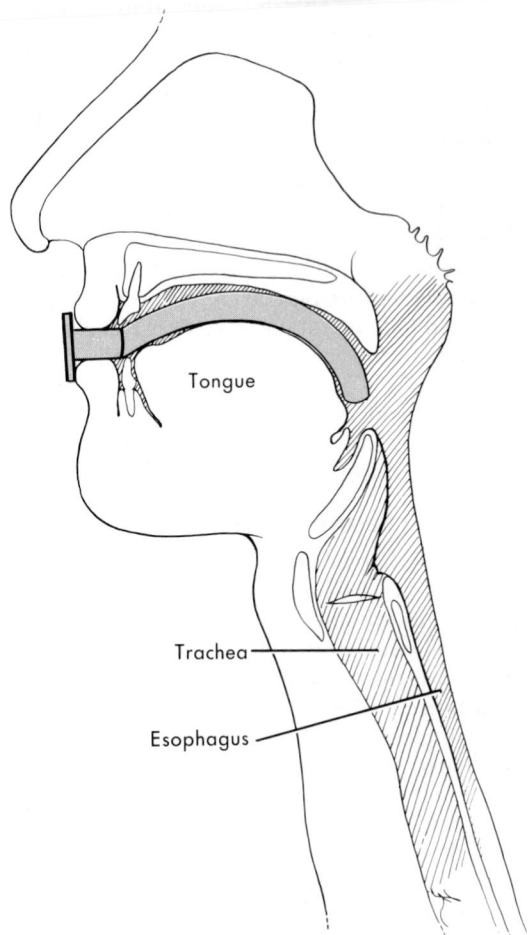

Fig. 14-3   Airway in place to prevent tongue from falling back against pharynx and blocking airway.

14-5	**Possible causes of postoperative shock**
	Moving patient from operating table to bed/trolley
	Jarring patient (bed/trolley) during transport
	Reactions to drugs and anaesthesia
	Loss of blood and other body fluids
	Cardiac dysrrhythmias
	Cardiac failure
	Inadequate ventilation
	Pain
	Residual sympathectomy from conductive anaesthesia

---

toe, earlobe, or the nose. Oxygenation and ventilation to facilitate gas exchange can be enhanced by oxygen therapy and breathing exercises.

Oxygen therapy

Oxygen is usually given postoperatively because after anaesthesia almost all patients have decreased pulmonary expansion and areas of atelectasis, both of which result in hypoxaemia. Oxygen is administered by nasal cannula, disposable face mask or shield, or endotracheal or tracheostomy tube if one is in place.

Breathing exercises

Deep-breathing exercises are started as soon as the patient is conscious and able to follow directions. If the patient is unconscious or will not breathe deeply when stimulated, the physiotherapist or nurse can hyperventilate the lungs passively by using a breathing bag and mask.

Maintaining circulation

Hypotension and cardiac dysrrhythmias are the most common cardiovascular complications in the immediate postanaesthetic period. Early recognition and management of these complications before they become serious enough to diminish cardiac output depend on frequent assessment

range is not uncommon during the early postoperative period. It is usually well tolerated in healthy patients and does not require treatment. Shock must be prevented because the brain, heart, kidneys, and other vital organs do not tolerate long periods of hypoxaemia. Measures to control shock are immediately instituted when signs of shock occur (Chapter 7).

Cardiac dysrrhythmias

Hypoxaemia and hypercapnia are common causes of postoperative cardiac dysrrhythmias, especially premature beats and sinus tachycardia. These dysrrhythmias often can be suppressed by adequate ventilation. Other common causes of postoperative cardiac dysrrhythmias include pain, hypovolaemia, gastric distention, and acidosis. Significant dysrrythmias are treated by attending to the underlying cause when possible. Antiarrhythmic drugs may be prescribed (Chapter 17).

Promoting normal temperature

Hypothermia, a core temperature of less than 36°C (96.8° F), occurs in 60% to 80% of all postoperative patients.[4] Contributing factors include body exposure in a cold theatre, the effects of cold solutions, and as a consequence of some anaesthetics. The elderly person is especially affected. The patient experiences discomfort from the cold.

Hypothermia increases the length of time spent by the patient in recovery unit unless warming methods are used. The patient is monitored for signs of continued hypothermia: persistent low temperature, shivering, and patient reports of still feeling cold even after warming methods. Warm blankets are usually applied to the body, especially around the feet, and adding warmth around the head is also helpful. A newer method is convective warming therapy in which a disposable cover inflated with warm air from a heating unit is placed over the patient; warm air passes out through the underside, providing constantly moving warm air.[4]

Maintaining fluid balance

Fluid deficit may result from inadequate replacement of body fluids lost during surgery or from continued fluid losses. *Fluid excess* may occur from large volumes of fluids replaced by intravenous fluids when kidney function is inadequate (as evidenced by oliguria). Careful monitoring of intravenous fluids and urinary output is essential to ensure adequacy of replacement and prevention of fluid overload (Chapter 6).

Preventing injury

To prevent falls after anaesthesia, cot sides on the trolley or bed are raised and left so until the patient is fully awake. The patient is placed in good body alignment to prevent nerve damage and muscle and joint strain from lying in one position for a long time. Patients who may vomit are positioned on their side to prevent aspiration.

Relieving pain

Postoperative pain management in the recovery unit is now usually under the direction of the anaesthetist. Narcotics may be given intramuscularly, intravenously, by patient-controlled analgesia (PCA), by continuous epidural infusion, or intrathecally. *PCA* is now commonly used because it affords better control of postoperative pain and requires smaller dosages of narcotics.[54]

Good postoperative pain control is also achieved by narcotics (morphine, fentanyl, alfentanil, diamorphine) given by continuous drip or by PCA in the *epidural* space. This method reduces respiratory, sympathetic, motor, and sensory disturbances as compared to parenteral administration. Epidural analgesia blocks innervation of the bladder, leading to an inability to void urine; therefore an in-dwelling catheter is necessary during therapy. Other side effects may include pruritus and nausea.

Transcutaneous electrical nerve stimulation (TENS) may also be used for pain control. Other forms of pain management are also important, such as providing information to decrease anxiety (which intensifies the pain experience), and encouraging methods to promote relaxation (Chapter 8).

Promoting psychological comfort

The immediate postanaesthetic period is often frightening for the patient. While awakening from anaesthesia, the patient needs frequent orientation to place and reassurance of not being alone. The patient also needs to know that the operation is over and that recovery from anaesthesia is satisfactory. Careful explanations of procedures being carried out are given even when it appears that the patient is not alert.

Evaluation

Evaluation is based on the identified expected patient outcomes. Questions to consider include the following:
1. Are breath sounds clear?
2. Is respiratory rate 12-20/min and regular?
3. Are oxygen saturation levels within normal levels?
4. Is blood pressure at patient's usual level?
5. Is temperature at patient's usual level?
6. Is skin warm and dry, pulse regular, and urinary output slightly less than fluid intake?
7. Has pulmonary oedema been avoided?
8. Is patient's sleep quiet and face relaxed?

Discharge from Recovery Unit

Patients are discharged from the recovery unit when the following criteria have been met:
1. Vital signs are stable and indicate adequate respiratory and circulatory function.
2. Patient is awake or easily aroused and can call for assistance if needed.
3. Postsurgical complications have been thoroughly evaluated and are under control.
4. After regional anaesthesia, motor and partial sensory functions have returned to all anaesthetized areas.

Acutely ill patients who require further close supervision are transferred to an intensive care unit. Most patients are transferred to their ward. The ward is notified to expect the patient, and all pertinent information concerning the patient's status is communicated to the nurse who will continue to provide postoperative nursing care. The recovery room nurse writes a discharge summary note before the patient leaves the recovery unit.

ADMISSION OF PATIENT TO WARD
Preparation of Ward

The patient's bed is prepared to facilitate patient transfer and monitoring (see Box 14-6).

Many surgeons visit the patient to describe briefly what was found and to provide reassurance. The family is frequently highly anxious concerning the patient's condi-

---

14-6	**Preparing for the patient's return from surgery**
	1. Make bed into pack to facilitate easy transfer of patient.
	2. Use clean linen to minimize infection risk.
	3. Provide sufficient covers (patient may feel cold).
	4. Clear a passageway to the bed.
	5. Provide necessary equipment
	a. Intravenous pole
	b. Sphygmomanometer
	c. Any special equipment as designated by recovery room nurse.

tion and may not perceive or understand all that the staff tell them. The nurse needs to know what information was given to the patient and family to be able to answer their questions.

Safety

Bed cot sides are kept raised until the patient is fully awake and responding or to prevent the heavily medicated patient from falling. The patient is instructed early regarding permissibility of ambulation and the need to call for assistance for initial attempts. The call cord should be easily accessible to the patient.

Family members

If family members are present in the room when the patient returns, they may be asked to wait outside until the patient has been transferred and assessed. Before leaving the patient, the nurse invites the family to return, explains equipment, and describes the patient's state of awareness and comfort. Family members who understand what is occurring can offer support to the patient.

Nursing Process

14-7

Patient assessment on return from recovery room

Respiratory status
Patency of airway
Respirations: depth, rate, character
Breath sounds: presence, character

Circulatory status
Pulse, blood pressure, temperature
Skin colour, temperature
Capillary filling

Neurological status
Level of consciousness, ability to move extremities

Dressing
Presence of drainage
Presence of tubes to be connected to drainage systems

Comfort
Presence of pain, nausea, vomiting
Patient positioned for comfort and to facilitate ventilation

Safety
Necessity for cot side
Call cord within reach

Equipment
Monitors connected and functioning
Intravenous fluids: rate, amount in bag, patency of tubing
Drainage systems (for example, nasogastric, chest, urinary): type, patency of tubing, connection of appropriate container, character and amount of drainage

---

Assessment
Initial assessment

As soon as the patient is positioned on the bed in the ward, the nurse makes a rapid assessment of the patient's condition. Parameters to assess include respiratory, circulatory, neurological status, dressing, patient comfort and safety, and functioning of equipment (see Box 14-7).

Subjective data

The patient is asked for symptoms of discomfort after having been transferred to the bed and positioned. This gives the nurse a quick indication of the level of alertness and symptoms of discomfort. An indirect question such as, "How do you feel?" will elicit data concerning nausea or pain without focusing on a specific area. Pain perception is frequently increased at this time because of the movement from trolley to bed. It is important to find out location, onset, and change in pain intensity and not to assume that the pain is incisional.

Nausea occurs less frequently postoperatively with the use of newer anaesthetics. There is greater possibility of nausea when the stomach has been manipulated extensively during the surgical procedure or if considerable amounts of narcotics have been administered. The vomit bowl should be easily available but not too obvious if vomiting is a possibility.

Objective data
Respiratory status

Respirations may be increased or decreased (see Table 14-7). If hypoventilation is present, oxygen may be given if a nasal cannula is in place.

Noisy respirations may be caused by airway obstruction from the tongue falling back against the pharynx or from secretions. The patient with noisy respirations is assisted in coughing and then positioned on their side if possible. Suctioning may be indicated if coughing does not clear the airway.

Deep-breathing and coughing measures are instituted immediately in all patients who have had general anaesthesia.

Circulatory status

The pulse, blood pressure, skin colour and temperature, and capillary filling are assessed (Table 14-7). Signs of shock or haemorrhage are reported immediately to the surgeon. Hypotensive changes may be related to shock, although other signs of shock usually occur before changes in blood pressure. The skin often feels cool to the touch after surgery hypovolaemia from blood loss, or vasoconstriction from stress. Restlessness is an early sign of shock.

After surgery of the extremities, local circulation is assessed by the presence and strength of peripheral pulses *distal* to the operative site or plaster cast. If the dressing is too tight, it should be loosened, if permissible, or reported at once to the surgeon.

Level of consciousness

Level of consciousness can be ascertained by asking the patient to respond to simple questions or commands. A decrease in consciousness level may indicate shock (from

Table 14-7 Some causes of vital sign changes in early postoperative phase

Vital sign	Increase	Decrease
Temperature	Stress reaction (low-grade fever)	Cold theatre and recovery unit
Pulse rate	Jarring during transfer	Cardiac glycoside overdose
	Shock, haemorrhage	Cardiac dysrhythmias
	Hypoventilation	
	Acute gastric dilation	
	Pain	
	Anxiety	
	Cardiac dysrrhythmias	
Respiratory rate	Hypoventilation: poor positioning, tight chest or upper abdominal dressing, obesity, gastric dilation	Drugs: anaesthetics, narcotics, sedatives
Blood pressure	Anxiety ($\uparrow$ systolic)	Jarring during transfer
	Pain	Severe pain
	Distended urinary bladder	Cardiac dysrythmias
		Shock: fluid loss, haemorrhage, acute gastric dilation

jarring motions during the transfer) and should be reported to the surgeon.

Dressing

The entire dressing is inspected with the bedding pulled back or the patient turned as necessary. A dressing applied to the side, such as after kidney surgery, may appear dry on the top visible area but may have excess drainage on the lower portion. Excess drainage is reported immediately.

Whenever it is anticipated that fluid may collect in a body area postoperatively, leading to delay in healing, the surgeon usually inserts a tube or drain to permit escape of the fluid. One end of the tube or drain is placed in or near the organ or cavity to be drained, and the other end is passed through the body wall, usually through a separate stab wound.

If small amounts of unexpected drainage are observed, especially bright red drainage, the areas can be outlined with a pen on the dressing so that the rate of drainage can be easily determined. Initially dressings are reinforced with dry dressings if drainage penetrates the outer layer; this prevents bacterial contamination through the wet dressings. If these additional dressings become wet, they are removed and replaced with new dressings, leaving the original dressing intact. Once the dressing has been changed, usually the day after surgery, it is renewed as often as necessary to prevent maceration of the skin and to promote patient comfort. In special circumstances the surgeon may issue specific instructions regarding dressing changes, e.g. skin grafts.

Body position

The patient is placed in a position of comfort that aids good ventilation. Except after spinal anaesthesia or in certain types of eye surgery or neurosurgery when the bed must remain flat, most patients prefer to sit upright. Pillows should *not* exert pressure on the popliteal area (behind the knee), because this leads to venous obstruction and potential thrombophlebitis.

Assessment of fluid lines

Fluids may be prescribed to be given intravenously or instilled in body cavities for irrigation, such as in the bladder (see Chapter 25). The contents of the fluid containers, the patency of the tubing, and the rate of fluid administration are checked. Fluids are usually given intravenously at rates ranging from minimal (to keep the line open) to 3 ml/min (180 ml/hr). If the rate is greater than 3 ml/min, and if the prescription sheet is not available in the wards, the rate should be slowed, the order checked immediately, and the rate adjusted appropriately. Rate of administration varies with the amount of fluid lost, size and age of the patient, and the underlying illness (Chapter 6).

Drainage from tubes can be accomplished by either gravity or suction. Each tube is connected to a separate drainage receptacle. All tubing is connected to the drainage receptacle and checked for patency. The amount of fluid in each receptacle is marked on the receptacle and recorded as baseline for future comparison. Colour and consistency of drainage are noted.

Data from patient's chart

After the patient has been assessed and positioned comfortably and safely, the nurse gathers additional data from the patient's charts and notes (Table 14-8) before planning and initiating general postoperative care.

Nursing Analysis

The collected data are recorded in the nursing admission notes and used to identify the specific needs of the patient in the postoperative period. The preoperative condition of the patient, type of surgery performed, and strengths and resources of the patient are determining factors in postoperative discomfort or complications. In planning the patient's care, the nurse uses previously collected data, present data, knowledge of factors related to specific types of surgery (as illustrated in succeeding chapters of this text), and specific postoperative needs and possible postoperative complications.

Table 14-8 Chart data useful in planning postoperative care

Data	Direction for action/interpretation
Surgeon's instructions	
Activity	Extent permissible
Fluids, food	Intravenous: type, amount, rate
	Oral: type
Medications	Type and frequency of medications to be taken as needed
	Medications to be started immediately
Other orders	Special orders to be carried out depending on type of surgery
Operation notes	
Postoperative diagnosis	Interpretation to patient/family
Type of surgery	Special nursing interventions
	Interpretations to patient/family
Anaesthetic	
Inhalant	Need for deep-breathing measures
Muscle relaxants	Assessment for respiratory distress
Spinal	Headache may occur
Estimated blood loss and fluid replacement	Potential for fluid and electrolyte imbalance or transfusion reactions
Drains	Possible drainage on dressing
Recovery unit notes	
Vital signs before transfer	Identification of changes related to transfer
Patient progress	Identification of persistent problems
Medications given	Times when drugs given and patient response
Urinary output	Status of renal function or urine retention

Problem	Possible aetiologies
Injury, high risk for: wound dehiscence	Excessive coughing, distention, dehydration, obesity
Infection, high risk for (wound)	Poor aseptic technique, malnutrition, existing infection
Breathing pattern, ineffective	Increased respiratory secretions, dry sticky secretions, decreased thorax expansion, pain, tight bandages or plasters, abdominal distention, medications
Tissue integrity, impaired, high risk for	Inactivity, shock, obesity, pressure on popliteal area, tight dressings or plaster
Fluid volume excess	Age (elderly), large fluid volume intake
Comfort, altered, nausea	Anaesthetic, narcotic, electrolyte imbalance
Pain	Incisional pain, sore throat from endotracheal tube, tissue anoxia from tight dressings/plaster, abdominal distention
Nutrition, altered: less than body requirements	Anorexia, nausea, weakness, pain
Urinary retention	Position for voiding urine, anaesthetic, narcotic, pelvic surgery
Constipation	Anaesthetic, narcotic, inactivity, inadequate nutrition, stress
Mobility, impaired physical	Pain, decreased strength and endurance, multiple tubes
Anxiety	Threat to self-concept; threat or change

Possible problems for the postoperative patient may include, but are not limited to, the following:

Problem	Possible aetiologies
	in health status, socioeconomic status, role functioning; unmet meets
Knowledge deficit	Lack of exposure or recall: routines, preventive measures, specific care requirements

Planning: expected patient outcomes

Expected patient outcomes for the postoperative patient may include, but are not limited to:

1. Incision heals well.
2. Breath sounds are clear.
3. No pain or redness of calf/thigh occur (thrombophlebitis).
4. Fluid intake is more than fluid output for first 24 to 48 hours, then becomes essentially equal.
5. States feeling comfortable.
6. Eats well from prescribed diet; weight loss is minimal or stabilized.
7. Stools return to usual pattern within 3 to 4 days after major surgery (earlier with minor surgery; longer after GI surgery).
8. Carries out activities of daily living at an optimal level, although fatigue may still be present.
9. Shows no outward signs of anxiety; identifies concerns, including sexual concerns, as pertinent.
10. Can explain at discharge:
    a. Home treatments, if pertinent

b. Home medications (name, dosage, frequency, side effects)
c. Dietary changes required by surgery
d. Activity limitations incurred by surgery and any exercise programmes to be carried out at home
e. When to go for follow-up.

Implementation

Promoting wound healing

Pathophysiology of wound healing

Understanding the pathophysiology of wound healing and the factors that influence wound healing provides the basis for some of the postoperative nursing care, particularly wound care, dietary requirements, and need for physical activity.

Result of wound healing. Wounds may heal by regeneration of the tissue or by *scar* formation. Injured cells that have the capacity to regenerate (Fig. 14-4) will do so if the underlying structure has not been destroyed. Muscle and nerve cells are usually unable to regenerate. When muscle cells are injured, satisfactory performance may result by hypertrophy of marginal cells. Nerve cells in the central nervous system do not regenerate. In the peripheral nervous system there is no regeneration if the cell body is

destroyed; however, if the axon is injured, there is partial degeneration of the axon, followed by regeneration.

In a typical surgical incision, muscle tissue is cut into. Although the epithelial cells regenerate over the scar tissue, the epithelial layer is so thin that the scar tissue is visible.

Types of wound healing. Tissue may heal by primary, secondary, or tertiary intention (Fig. 14-5). Healing by *primary intention* occurs with surgical wounds; all layers of the wound are closely approximated by suturing. If not infected, the wound heals quickly with minimum scarring. Healing by *secondary intention* occurs when a wound, such as an ulcer with edges that cannot be sutured, heals by filling in the area from the bottom. The wound is open, with increased chance of infection, and heals slowly with considerable scarring. With healing by *tertiary intention*, the wound is sutured several days after wounding. This may occur if the wound was very dirty or if a surgical wound breaks open after several days. The wound is more contaminated than with primary intention so scarring is greater, but less than with secondary intention.

Process of wound healing. Regardless of the type of wound healing, the process is the same. The difference is in the length of time for each phase of healing and the extent of granulation tissue formed. When tissue is injured (see Fig. 14-6), two major responses occur initially, the *stress response* (Chapter 5) and the *inflammatory response* (see below). The *immune response* is also activated to protect against invading microorganisms. A *generalized body response* occurs when there is a major injury to the tissue, partly as a result of the stress response and partly from inflammation.

In *phase I* of wound healing, leukocytes (white blood cells) ingest bacteria and debris. Fibrin is deposited throughout the clot that fills the wound, and new blood vessels develop across the wound using the fibrin threads as a framework. A thin layer of epithelial cells migrate across the wound and help to seal the wound.

Phase II lasts from 3 to 14 days after surgery. The leukocytes start disappearing and the space begins to fill with *collagen*, a white protein fibre. All layers of epithelial cells are completely regenerated in about 1 week. The new tissue is a highly vascular connective tissue, reddish from the numerous blood vessels, and is called *granulation tissue*.

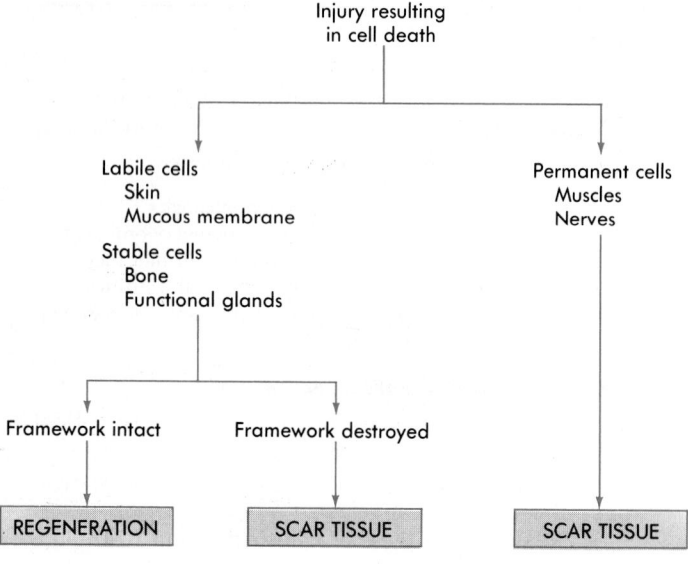

Fig. 14-4   End results of wound healing.

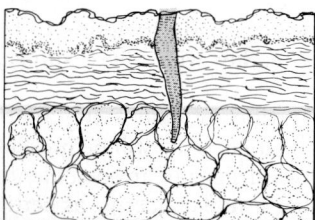 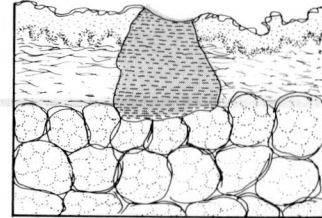 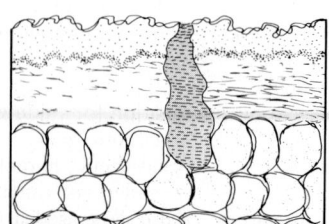

Fig. 14-5   Types of wound healing: primary, secondary, and tertiary intention.

Table 14-9 Steps of the inflammatory response

Steps	Mediators	Outcome
1. Injury	Physical, chemical, biological, immunological stimulus	Cell and tissue injury

2. Vascular response
  a. Vascular dilation
  b. Fibrin clot formation
	Histamine, plasmin, serotonin, kinins, prostaglandins released or activated by injury
	Activation of clotting mechanism
		Dilation of vessels causing stasis of blood and margination of leukocytes
		Containment of irritants

3. Fluid exudation	Histamine, kinins, prostaglandins cause opening of venule–endothelial cell junction	Fluid exudation into tissues

4. Cellular exudation
  a. Leukocyte exudation
 	
  b. Attack and engulfment of foreign materials
	Chemotactic substances released by complement activation, clot formation, and injured cells
	Neutrophils and macrophages
		Passage of leukocytes from blood to site of injury and accumulation there
		Removal and digestion of bacteria, foreign particles, and damaged tissues

5. Healing	Fibroblasts produce collagen fibres and tissue regeneration	Resolution of inflammation and formation of scar tissue

The collagen that is deposited will provide good support for the wound in 6 to 7 days. Thus skin sutures are often removed about this time, depending on the site and extent of surgery.

During *phase III*, collagen continues to be deposited. The wound now looks like a broad pinkish raised scar. During this phase, second to sixth week after surgery, the patient should avoid heavy use of the affected muscles.

The final phase, *phase IV*, lasts for several months after surgery. Although collagen continues to be deposited during this time, the wound shrinks and contracts. Because of the shrinkage the wound becomes a concave thin white line.

Interventions to promote healing

1. Promote intake of foods high in protein, zinc and vitamin C.
2. Carry out measures to increase circulation.
3. Avoid antiinflammatory drugs (such as steroids) when healing is desired; inflammation is a desired part of the healing process.
4. Prevent infection that delays healing:
   a. Change soiled wet dressings immediately.
   b. Use strict aseptic technique when changing dressings.
   c. Cover moist dressings with a dry sterile cover.

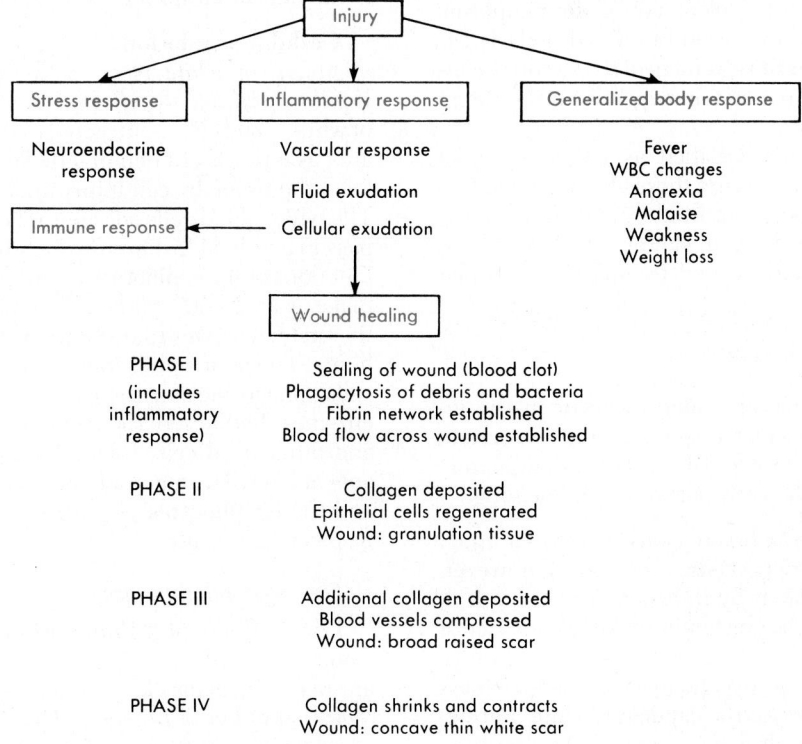

Fig. 14-6 Response of body to injury.

<table>
<tr><td>14-8</td><td colspan="2">Causes of the cardinal symptoms of inflammation</td></tr>
<tr><td></td><td>Redness</td><td>Hyperaemia from vasodilation</td></tr>
<tr><td></td><td>Heat</td><td>Vasodilation - blood vessels closer to skin surface</td></tr>
<tr><td></td><td>Swelling</td><td>Fluid exudation into tissue</td></tr>
<tr><td></td><td>Pain</td><td>Chemical (bradykinin) irritation of nerve endings and pressure of fluid in tissues</td></tr>
<tr><td></td><td>Loss of function</td><td>Tissue swelling and pain</td></tr>
</table>

14-9	Some types of inflammations	
	Cellulitis	Inflammation involving cellular and connective tissue
	Lymphadentis	Inflammation of lymph nodes
	Lymphangitis	Inflammation of lymphatic vessel
	Bacteraemia	presence of bacteria in blood
	Septicaemia	Systemic disease associated with pathogenic microorganisms and their toxins in the blood
	Abscess	Collection of pus localized by a zone of inflamed tissue
	Sinus	Suppurating channel from an abscess to the surface of the body or into a body cavity
	Peritonitis	Inflammation of the peritoneum
	Pleuritis	Inflammation of the pleura
	Empyema	Collection of pus in a body cavity, especially the pleural cavity

5. Irrigate contaminated wounds well to remove foreign substances, which delay healing.
6. Maintain suction of wound catheters. Fluid remaining in a wound space delays healing.

Inflammatory response

When injury occurs in the body, all the nonspecific and, to some degree, the specific defence mechanisms are directed towards localizing the effects of the injury, protecting against microbial invasion at the site, and preparing the site for repair. This process is called *inflammation*. When inflammation occurs at a particular site in the body, the suffix-*itis* is added to the site designation to indicate the pathological state; for example, an inflammatory response on the pericardium is termed *pericarditis*, and of the bladder, *cystitis*.

The inflammatory response can be initiated by any type of injury; for example, heat, cold, irradiation, chemicals, trauma, infection, immunological injury, or neoplasm. Whatever the stimulus, the response of the body is the same, but the extent of the involvement of the various facets of the nonspecific response system depends on the extent and severity of the injury.

Inflammations can be classified as either acute or chronic. Acute inflammations are those characterized by a sudden onset and an increased fluid exudative response. Chronic inflammations have a slower, more insidious onset, and they are characterized by increased cellular exudation (see below).

Steps of the inflammatory response.

Three major physiological responses occur in the inflammatory process: vascular response, fluid exudation, and cellular exudation (Table 14-9). The inflammatory process occurs during the early part of wound healing.

Vascular response. The first response to cellular injury is a transitory vasoconstriction (stress response); however, this is followed immediately by *vasodilation* as a result of chemical substances such as histamine or kinins released at the site of injury or invasion. The amount of blood flow to the area is thus increased (hyperaemia), causing redness and heat. Blood flow slows as the capillaries dilate. Permeability of the capillary walls is increased, facilitating fluid and cellular exudation to the injured tissue.

Fluid exudation. Fluid exudation from the capillaries into the interstitial spaces begins immediately and is most active during the first 24 hours after injury or invasion. Initially, the fluid exudate is primarily serous, but as the capillary wall becomes more permeable, protein (albumin) is lost into the interstitial spaces. Loss of large amounts of serum protein in major injuries, such as burns, leads to loss of plasma osmotic pressure. *Movement of protein into the interstitial spaces increases tissue osmotic pressure, which encourages more fluid exudation.* The *swelling from the fluid in the interstitial spaces is called oedema* (see Chapter 6).

Cellular exudation. *Cellular exudation refers to the migration of white blood cells (leukocytes) through the capillary wall into the affected tissue.* An increased number of white blood cells is attracted to the vessels in the affected area as a result of chemotactic substances being released from the tissue by cell injury and complement activation. The white blood cells adhere to the capillary wall and then pass in ameboid fashion through the widened endothelial junctions of the capillary wall. Neutrophils (PMNs), which make up about 60% of the circulating white blood cells, are the first leukocytes to respond, usually within the first few hours. The neutrophils ingest the bacteria and dead tissue cells (phagocytosis); then they die, releasing proteolytic enzymes that liquefy the dead neutrophils, dead bacteria, and other dead cells (pus). Monocytes and lymphocytes appear later. The macrophages continue the phagocytosis, and the lymphocytes play a role in the antigen–antibody response at the site.

Effects of inflammation

Local effects of inflammation. The *five local cardinal symptoms of inflammation*, identified many centuries ago, are *redness (rubor)*, *heat (calor)*, *swelling (tumour)*, *pain (dolor)*, and *loss of function*. These symptoms result from vasodilation and fluid exudation as well as irritation from chemotactic substances (Box 14-8).

The inflammatory response serves to prepare the tissue for healing and to contain the spread of bacterial invasion. To prevent the spread of bacteria, fibroblasts are attracted to the area and secrete fibrin, a threadlike substance that encircles the affected area to wall it off from healthy tissue. If there is interference with this walling-off process, bacteria can spread into the the surrounding tissue. This explains why an abscess should not be incised and drained until it has "come to a head," or untill the walling-off process is completed.

No healing will occur until inflammation has subsided and pus and dead tissue have been removed. Pus is a local accumulation of dead phagocytes, dead bacteria, and dead tissue. The bacteria most commonly causing this reaction are the staphylococci, streptococci, Neisseria, and P. aeruginosa (*pyocyanea*).

Lymph node involvement. *Bacteria may fail to be contained locally and may spread to other parts of the body by means of the lymph system* (lymphogenous) *or bloodstream* (haematogenous) (Box 14-9). If picked up by the lymph stream, the bacteria will be carried to the nearest lymph node. These nodes are located along the course of all lymph channels, and here too bacteria can be ingested and destroyed. If the bacteria are virulent enough to resist the action in the lymph nodes, leukocytes are brought in by the blood stream to attack and engulf the bacteria in the node. The node then becomes swollen and tender because of the accumulation of phagocytes, bacteria, and destroyed lymphoid tissue. This is know as lymphadenitis. Swollen lymph nodes can be palpated primarily in the neck, axilla, and groin.

Systemic effects of inflammation. Moderate to severe inflammatory responses can produce generalized systemic effects. Products from the breakdown of bacteria and white blood cells can affect the temperature-regulating centre in the hypothalamus and produce *fever*. A severe infection without accompanying fever may suggest a poor prognosis. Loss of appetite (anorexia) and fatigue may be caused by conservation of body energy needed to resist the infection. The body increases the production of white blood cells to help fight the infection, and leukocytosis (serum white blood cell levels>10,000/mm^3) may occur. With infection the *blood sedimentation rate* is also increased; that is, when an anticoagulant is added to the blood in the laboratory, the red blood cells settle to the bottom of a test tube more rapidly than normal. The increase in the sedimentation rate is believed to be caused by an increase in fibrinogen (a blood protein essential to the healing process). The sedimentation rate is elevated during the acute inflammatory stage of infection. An elevated sedimentation rate is considered to be a non-specific test because it indicates that inflammation is present, but not what is causing it. It also indicates that the body's defence mechanism for the repair of damaged tissue is operating. Because the sedimentation rate gradually returns to normal as tissues heal, it also is used to determine when physical activity can be safely resumed after an acute infection.

Resolution and healing

After the infected area is clean, new cells are produced to fill in the space left by the injury. They may be the normal structural cells, or they may be fibrotic tissue cells known as *scar tissue*. If they are fibrotic cells, they will not function as formerly but serve only to fill in the injured area. Some body cells readily regenerate; for instance, after the bowel has heald it is almost impossible to find the injured area. The respiratory tract also regenerates its tissues readily. Liver tissue has the capacity to regenerate, but over a longer period of time. Some nerve cells are always replaced with fibrous tissue. If a large amount of tissue is destroyed, structural cells may not be replaced, regardless of the type of tissue.

Care of the surgical wound

Surgical wounds, because they are aseptically created, generally heal well and quickly. For psychological reasons, and to prevent trauma until epithelialization occurs, the wound is usually covered initially by a dressing. More importantly wounds are covered to produce the warm, humid microenvironment known to enhance healing.[53]

Incisional coverings may be non-adherent gauze, semiocclusive, or occlusive dressings. Non-adherent gauze dressings permit air to reach the wound; semiocclusive dressings permit oxygen but not air to pass; occlusive dressings permit neither air nor oxygen to pass. Occlusive and semiocclusive dressings are thought to promote healing by keeping wounds moist (yet sterile) so epithelial cells can slide more easily over the surface of the wound during epithelialization.[45]

Tubes and drains are used to prevent or remove accumulation of fluid from the surgical site. Because the drain provides a passage out of tissues or body cavities, microorganisms can also travel into these areas. Aseptic technique is therefore essential in caring for tubes and drains; they are removed by the nurse, when instructed by the surgeon, usually when drainage is minimal. Tubes and drains are usually brought out of a separate incision (stab wound) to prevent infection of the operative wound. Soft drains, such as a Penrose drain (Fig. 14-9) are either stitched to the skin or have a large safety pin fastened at the distal end to prevent slippage back into the body. If an open drainage system is present, the open end of the drain should be encased in an absorbable sterile dressing or stoma bag to protect the skin; any dressing is changed frequently. Closed systems are used in preference to open drainage to reduce infection. A firm catheter, usually attached to low pressure suction such as a Hemovac, is used in place of a soft drain for closed drainage. A sump drain (Fig. 14-8) has an airflow system that facilitates fluid removal; it must be connected to constant suction.

Wound dehiscence and evisceration

Pathophysiology. Wound *dehiscence* (disruption) is partial to complete separation of the wound edges. Wound *evisceration* is protrusion of abdominal viscera through the incision (Fig. 14-10).

Wound dehiscence is rare in people under 30 but occurs in 5% of people over age 60 who are having laparotomy.

Wound separation that occurs during the first 3 postoperative days is usually a result of inadequate surgical closure. During the next 10 days, wound separation is

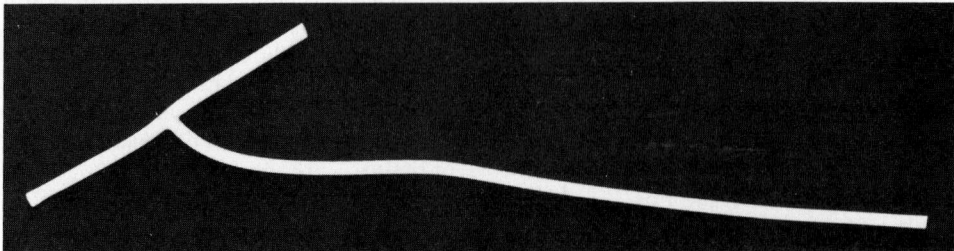

Fig. 14-7 T tube for draining common bile duct.

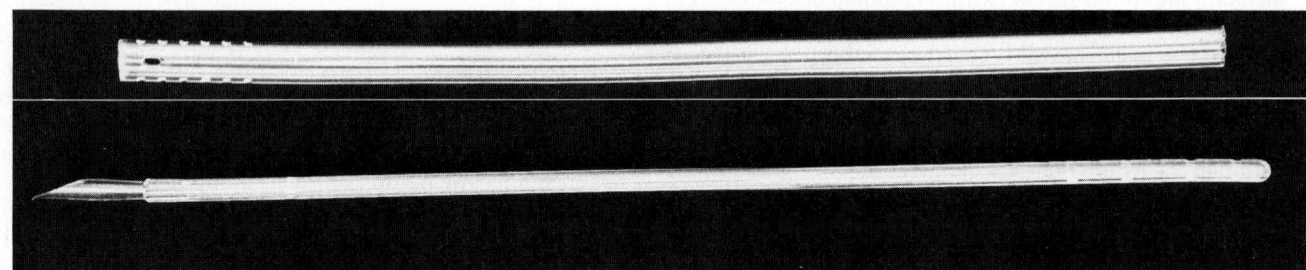

Fig. 14-8 Surgical drain tubes. *Top*, Abramson all-purpose drain has three lumens: for aspiration, irrigation, and instillation. *Bottom*, Saratoga sump drain has a tube within a tube for low-pressure suction.

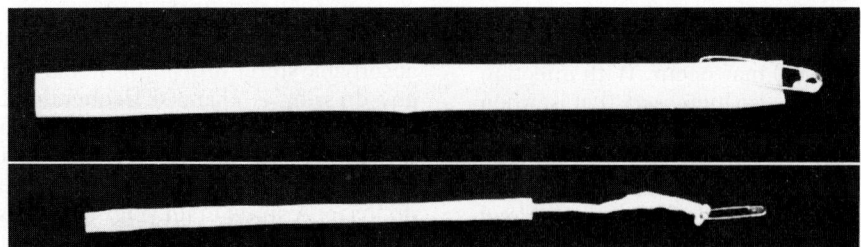

Fig. 14-9 Wound drains. *Top*, Penrose drain. *Bottom*, Cigarette drain.

usually associated with postoperative complications, such as excessive coughing or vomiting, distention, dehydration, or infection. Wound separation during phase III is usually associated with metabolic factors such as cachexia, obesity, hypoproteinaemia or avitaminosis, increased age, decreased resistance to infection, malignancy, multiple trauma, or hypothermia. These factors can also cause wound separation at an earlier time.

Assessment. The patient may complain of a "giving" sensation at the incision or a feeling of wetness with dehiscence. If evisceration has occurred and a loop of bowel is obstructed, the patient will complain of severe pain at the incision. On inspection the dressing will be found to be saturated with clear pink drainage. The wound edges may be partially or entirely separated, and loops of intestine may be visible. Signs of shock may be present.

Intervention
1. Put patient in bed in semi-recumbent position to ease strain on the incision.

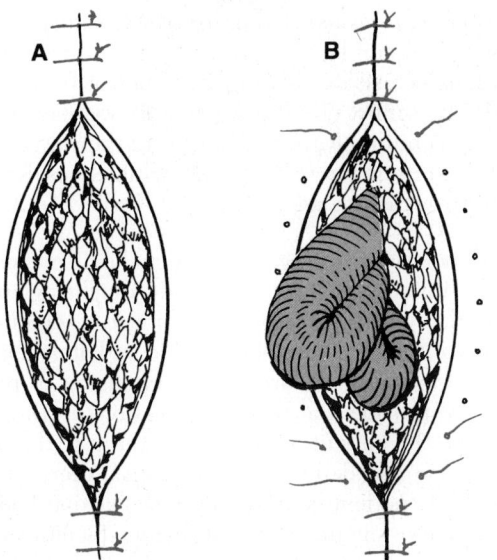

Fig. 14-10   **A,** Wound dehiscence. **B,** Wound evisceration.

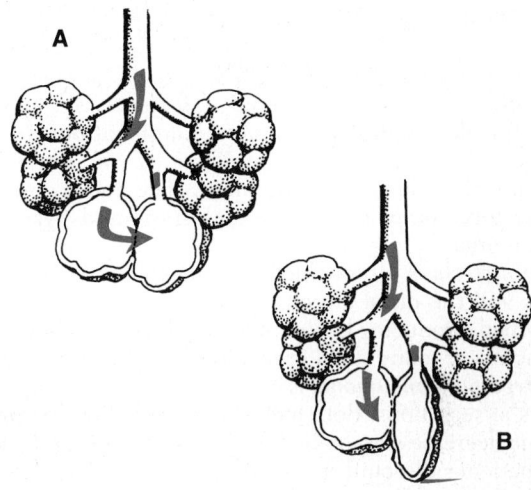

Fig. 14-11   Mucus plug blocking alveolar duct in obstructive atelectasis. **A,** Aeration of blocked alveolus through interalveolar duct with deep inspiration. **B,** Collapse of blocked alveolus with shallow inspiration.

Table 14-10   Risk factors in development of postoperative pulmonary complications

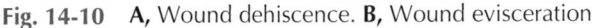

Risk factors	Effect
Increased respiratory secretions Smoking Intubation Inhalant anaesthetics Chronic lung disease Upper respiratory infection	Irritation of lining of tracheobronchial passages Decreased ciliary action to remove secretions Secretions will block bronchial passages or alveoli
Dry sticky secretions Chronic lung disease Dehydration	Difficult too cough up secretions Secretions will block bronchial passages
Decreased thorax expansion Pain (chest, upper abdomen) Obesity Age Tight dressings or plasters Skeletal abnormalities (for example, scoliosis)	Lung does not expand fully, resulting in hypoventilation of alveoli
Decreased diaphragm mobility Abdominal distention Surgery of chest or upper abdomen Muscle relaxants Neurological deficit	Decreased lung expansion, leading to hypoventilation
Depression of respiratory centre Sedatives Narcotics Acid-base imbalance	Depressed respirations result in hypoventilation
Aspiration of gastric contents Vomiting	Causes aspiration pneumonia

2. Tell patient to lie quietly and not cough, eat, or drink.
3. Cover protruding viscera with a dressing moistened with warm sterile saline solution.
4. Notify surgeon.
5. Remain with the patient until the surgeon arrives, monitor vital signs for shock.

The treatment for wound dehiscence or evisceration is immediate closure of the wound under local or general anaesthesia.

Promoting adequate respiration

Pathophysiology. Postoperative patients are at high risk for developing pulmonary complications (Table 14-10). The pulmonary complications are often preventable by nursing management. The most common respiratory complications are atelectasis and hypostatic pneumonia.

In *atelectasis* a bronchiole becomes blocked by secretions and the distal alveoli collapse as the existing air is absorbed, producing hypoventilation (Fig. 14-11). A major bronchus or many small bronchioles may be involved.

Hypostatic pneumonia is inflammation of the lung from stasis of secretions. Both atelectasis and hypostatic pneumonia decrease oxygenation, prolong recovery, and add to the patient's discomfort.

Assessment. The patient is assessed frequently during the first 24 to 48 hours after an inhalant anaesthetic. A person at high risk may need to be assessed as often as every hour. Assessment includes monitoring respirations and chest expansion, evaluating the productiveness of the cough, and observing for signs of atelectasis and pneumonia (See Box 14-10).

Intervention. After general anaesthesia most patients will need to ventilate their lungs well *at least* every 1 to 2 hours during the first postoperative day, and then every 3 to 4 hours for several days if not active.

Ventilatory measures. A number of ventilatory measures (Table 14-11) can be used in the postoperative period to prevent atelectasis by inflating the alveoli as fully as possible. The two most effective ventilatory manoeuvres that lead to maximum alveolar inflation are the yawn and the incentive spirometer (Fig. 14-13). Guidelines for using ventilatory measures are described in Table 14-12.

Positioning and turning. If the patient lies in one position with continuous pressure from body weight against the chest wall, proper ventilation and drainage of secretions on that side of the chest are not possible and atelectasis can develop (Fig. 14-14). Turning and changing of position frequently provide for better ventilation of the lungs. Encourage the patient to help in the turning; the activity will increase the depth of respirations. Alternating the height of the patient is useful: upright position facilitates diaphragm movement; low or flat position facilitates drainage and expectoration.

Maintaining circulation

Pathophysiology. Thrombophlebitis, which results from venous stasis, is a preventable postoperative complication in many situations. Platelets adhere to the venous wall, with resultant thrombus formation (Fig. 14-15). Venous stasis occurs postoperatively for a number of reasons (see Box 14-11).

Table 14-11   Common postoperative ventilatory manoeuvres

Manoeuvre	Method	Comments
Yawn	Inhale deeply with mouth open (yawn), hold breath for 3 seconds, exhale	Easy to do; good deep breath when yawn occurs
Incentive spirometer	Breath in through mouthpiece as deeply as possible, hold breath 3 seconds, exhale; work towards increasing inspiratory effort	Promotes sustained maximal inspiration; requires minimal instruction; avoid using at mealtimes (may cause nausea)
Deep breathing	Inhale deeply through nose using diaphragm (abdomen rises), exhale slowly through pursed lips	Effectiveness depends on depth of respirations; patients with chest or abdominal incisions tend to limit depth; patients need encouragement

Table 14-12   Guidelines for using ventilatory measures in postoperative patients

Nursing interventions	Rationale
Plan ventilatory measures 30 minutes after narcotic is given, if possible	Facilitates patient cooperation
Place patient in upright position, if permitted	Facilitates diaphragm and chest expansion
Suggest patient take three to five normal breaths between each deep inspiration	Prevents dizziness from hyperventilation
Splint chest or abdominal incision with towel, small pillow, or hand before cough, if necessary	Prevents additional pain and muscle strain; provides support to incision to encourage deep cough

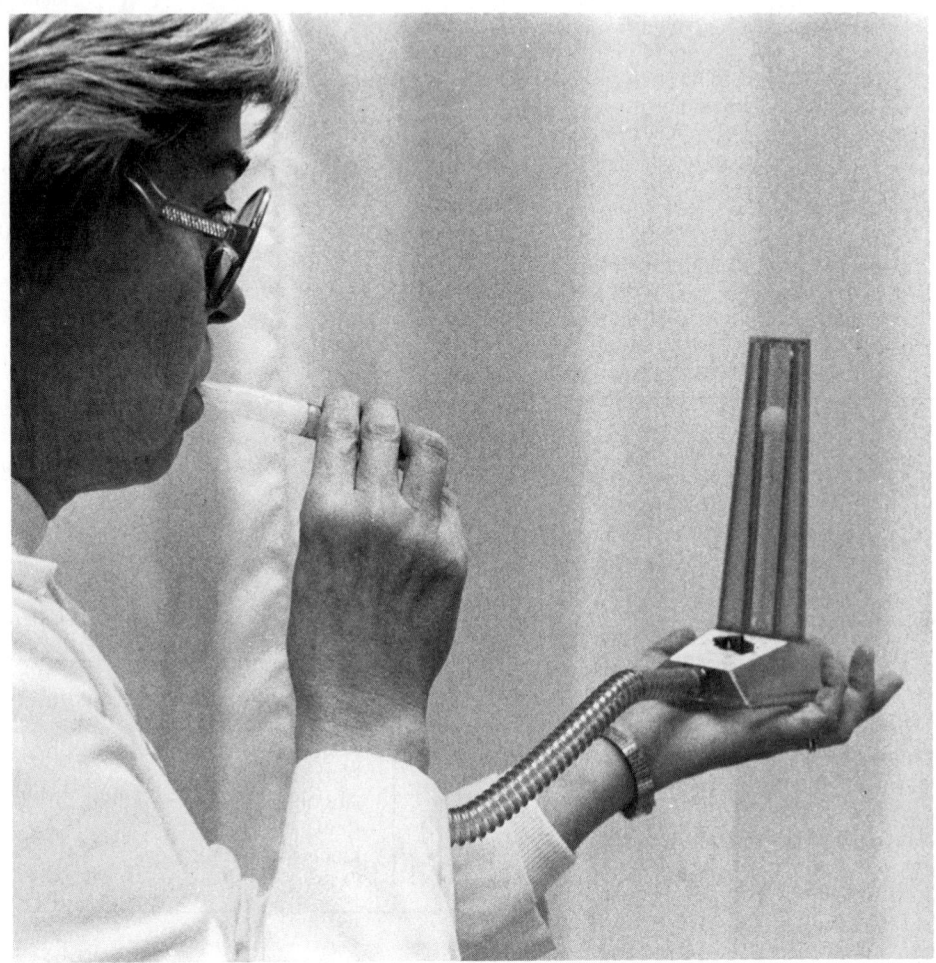

Fig. 14-12   Incentive spirometer. Ball rising with inspiration is a visual cue of deep breathing for patient.

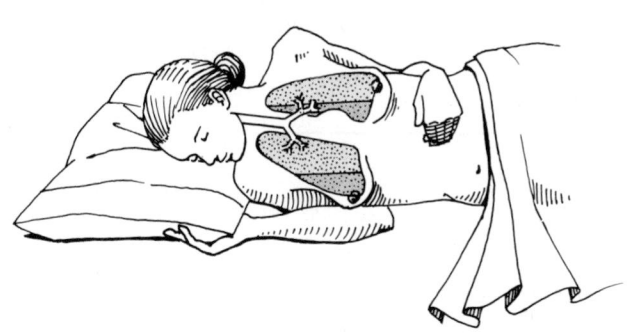

Fig. 14-13   Schematic of lungs illustrating pooling of secretions in dependent alveoli.

14-10	**Signs of postoperative pulmonary dysfunction**	
	Hypoventilation	Rapid shallow respirations
		Absent or diminished breath sounds in lower lobes
		Decreased chest expansion
	Increased secretions in airways	Rales heard on auscultation
		Nonproductive cough
	Atelectasis	Signs may be absent
		Fever, increased pulse and respirations; dyspnoea, cyanosis, and shock if a large bronchus is blocked
	Hypostatic pneumonia	Fever, dyspnoea, chest pain, cough productive of mucopurulent sputum

14-11	**Risk factors for postoperative thrombophlebitis**	
	Intrinsic factors	Older age, obesity, malnutrition, oral contraceptive use
	Pathological condition	Malignancy, congestive heart failure, history of previous deep-vein thrombosis, polycythaemia
	Types of surgery	Pelvic, abdominal, thoracic; fracture of hip or lower extremity
	Effects of surgery	Anaesthesia, shock, decreased mobility
		Prolonged sitting with legs crossed
		Pressure on popliteal area
		Tight dressings or plaster on lower extremities

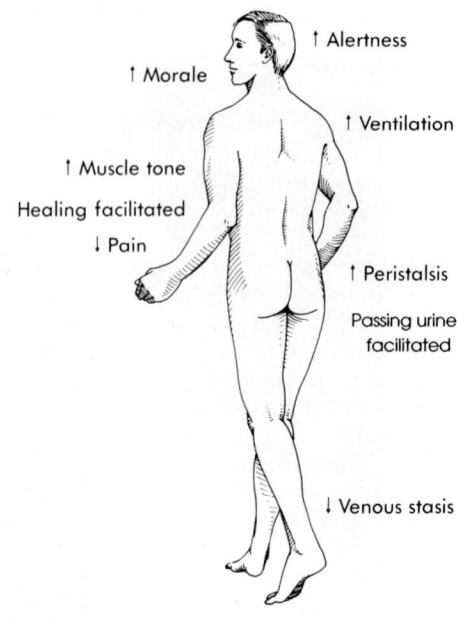

Assessment. If a patient complains of any discomfort in a leg, examine the leg (with gentle palpation) for redness and tenderness along the course of a vein if a superficial vein is involved or for tenderness and oedema if a deep vein is involved. There may be pain on dorsiflexion of the foot (Homan's signs) with deep vein thrombosis.

Prevention. *Medical* preventive measures in high-risk patients include (1) heparin prophylaxis given 2 hours preoperatively and 8 to 12 hours postoperatively, (2) aspirin in instances when heparin is contraindicated, (3) dextran, or (4) warfarin. *Intermittent external pneumatic compression* to the legs may also be prescribed. This procedure is not uncomfortable and has demonstrated marked effectiveness in high-risk patients.

Nursing preventive measures include the following:
1. Use elastic stockings.
2. Teach patient to avoid sitting for long periods (pressure on popliteal area) and to elevate feet when sitting to promote venous return.
3. Avoid any pressure on popliteal area (for example, pillow under knee) that can impede venous return.

Fig. 14-15 Benefits from early postoperative ambulation.

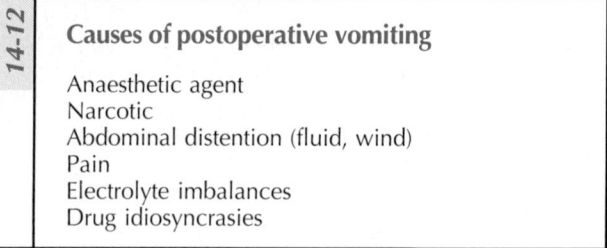

14-12	**Causes of postoperative vomiting**
	Anaesthetic agent
	Narcotic
	Abdominal distention (fluid, wind)
	Pain
	Electrolyte imbalances
	Drug idiosyncrasies

4. Teach and encourage leg exercises for the inactive patient.
5. Encourage early ambulation to facilitate venous return and thus prevent venous stasis.

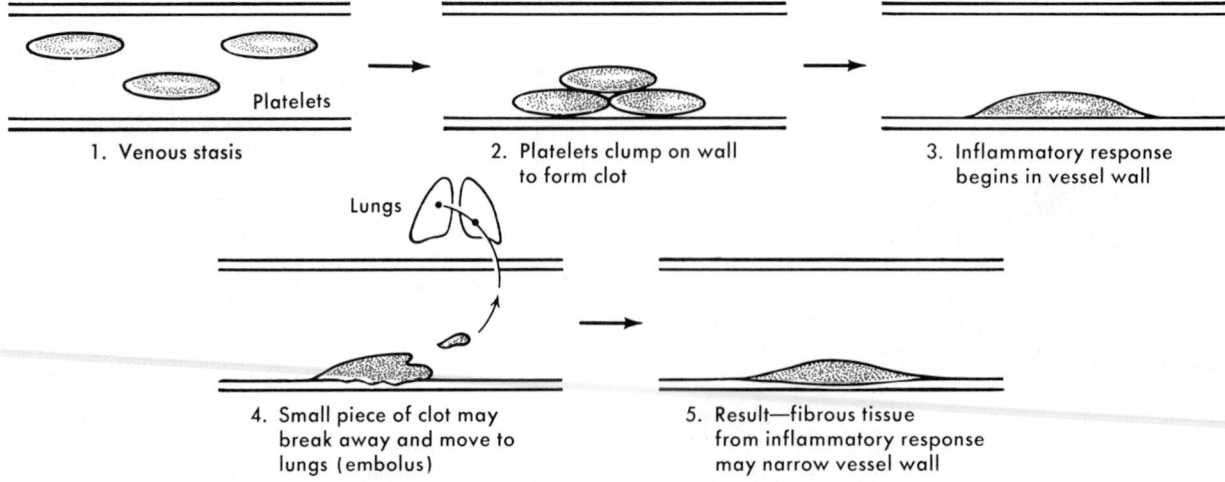

Fig. 14-14 Diagram illustrating formation of thrombus on wall of vein following venous stasis resulting in narrowing of blood vessel.

6. Deep breathing to facilitate venous return.

Intervention. The care of the patient with thrombophlebitis is discussed in Chapter 18. At the first sign of possible thrombophlebitis, ask the patient to return to bed and notify the doctor. Rest, heat, elastic bandages, and anticoagulant therapy are usually prescribed.

Maintaining fluid and electrolyte balance

Pathophysiology. Fluid is lost during surgery through blood loss and increased insensible fluid loss through the lungs and skin. During the surgical procedure the blood loss is estimated and fluids are replaced intravenously.

For at least the first 24 to 48 hours after surgery, fluids are retained by the body because of the stimulation of antidiuretic hormone (ADH), as part of the stress response to trauma and the effect of anaesthesia. During surgery there is also renal vasoconstriction and increased aldosterone activity, leading to increased sodium retention and subsequent water retention. *Overhydration* can occur with vigorous fluid replacement, especially in very small or elderly people. Both water intoxication and pulmonary oedema can occur, depending on the type and amount of fluids given. (For further information on fluid overload, see Chapter 6).

Sodium and potassium depletion can occur in the postoperative patient from the loss of blood or body fluids during surgery or the loss of gastrointestinal secretions. Potassium is also lost during catabolism (tissue breakdown), especially after severe trauma or crush injuries. Loss of gastric secretions can result in chloride loss, producing metabolic alkalosis.

Assessment. Monitor for signs of fluid overload, particularly in small sized or elderly people:
1. Behaviour: change in behaviour, confusion
2. Skin: warm, moist
3. Neck: distended neck veins
4. Respiration: dyspnoea, cough, moist breath sounds
5. Anorexia, nausea, vomiting
6. Fatigue
7. Weight gain (weigh high-risk patients)

Intervention. Intravenous administration of fluids is monitored carefully so that fluids are given evenly over the entire 24 hours. Usually 2000 to 2500 ml of 5% dextrose in normal saline or Ringer's lactate is given daily. If signs of fluid overload appear, slow the intravenous fluid to a keep-open rate and notify doctor.

Fluids are started orally as soon as peristalsis is present. Sips of water are offered first to see if fluids can be tolerated. Some people better tolerate sucking on ice chips. Ice chips must be recorded as fluid intake (two parts ice equal one part water). As soon as the patient can tolerate drinking fluids, the intravenous fluid administrations are discontinued on medical instruction.

Promoting comfort

The major discomforts after surgery are nausea and vomiting, abdominal distention and wind pains, and incisional pain. *Sore throat* may also occur from irritation of the endotracheal tube used during anaesthesia. Notify the anaesthetist if hoarseness persists longer than 24 hours, signifying possible injury to a laryngeal nerve.

Nausea and vomiting

Nausea and vomiting, which occur less frequently with the newer anaesthetic agents, may be related to a number of factors (Box 14-12). Nausea resulting from anaesthesia is self-limiting, and usually lasts only 24 to 48 hours.

Persistent postoperative vomiting is usually a symptom of pyloric obstruction, intestinal obstruction, or peritonitis. Vomiting tires the patient, puts strain on the incision, and causes excessive loss of fluids and electrolytes. Choking while vomiting may lead to aspiration pneumonia.

Interventions for the person who is experiencing vomiting include the following:
1. Lie on side to prevent aspiration
2. No food or fluids until vomiting subsides
3. Sips of fluid (ice chips, hot tea) or dry solid food (crackers) after vomiting subsides
4. Frequent oral care and chance to clean teeth
5. Prescribed antiemetics given parenterally

Abdominal distention and wind pains

Pathophysiology. Postoperative *distention* results from accumulation of nonabsorbable gas in the intestines caused by decreased intestinal activity from handling of the bowel during surgery, by swallowing of air during recovery from anaesthesia or attempts to overcome nausea, and by movement of gases from the bloodstream to the atonic portion of the bowel. Narcotics also decrease intestinal activity. Distention is experienced to some degree by most patients after abdominal and renal surgery. *Wind pains* are caused by contractions of the unaffected portions of the bowel in an attempt to move the accumulated gas through the intestinal tract.

Assessment. If the patient complains of diffuse or cramping abdominal pain, monitor the following:
1. Measurement of abdominal girth with tape measure
2. Presence of signs of shock from acute gastric dilation

Intervention. If the stomach is distended, the fluid and gas can be aspirated with a nasogastric tube. General distention or wind pains from sluggish intestinal peristalsis can be relieved by passage of flatus.

There are a number of interventions that may be helpful in moving the gas along the colon and facilitating passage:
1. Ambulation: most effective method to stimulate peristalsis and get the gas moving so it can be expelled
2. Avoidance of very hot or cold liquids: sucking ice chips does not have the same effect because the water warms before it reaches the stomach
3. Exercise to stimulate movement of the gas from right to left and prevent buildup[47]
4. Pelvic rock to stimulate peristalsis[31]
5. Abdominal massage to help push gas along colon[47]
6. Rectal tube for 20 minutes every 4 hours as necessary: tube stimulates lower colonic peristalsis and permits easy passage of the gas past the anal sphincters (rarely)

Pain

Pathophysiology. Pain is common after nearly all types of surgical procedures in which there has been cutting, pulling, or manipulation of tissues and organs. It may result from stimulation of nerve endings by chemical substances released at the time of surgery or from tissue ischaemia caused by interference of blood supply to the part, such as by pressure, muscle spasm, or oedema. After surgery other factors can add to the sensation of pain, such as infections, distention, muscle spasms surrounding the incisional area, anxiety, and tight dressings or plaster (see Box 14-13).

Postoperative pain usually lasts 24 to 48 hours but may continue longer depending on the extent of the surgery, the pain threshold of the patient, and response to pain (Chapter 8). The presence of pain can prolong convalescence because it may interfere with return to activity.

Assessment. When the patient complains of pain in the postoperative period, do not assume that the pain is incisional. Subjective data include origin, area involved, nature of the pain, and possible cause from the patient's point of view. Objective data include observation of facial expressions, body position, activity, muscle rigidity, and pulse rate.

Intervention. It is often impossible to prevent postoperative pain, but it can be minimized so that the patient is relatively comfortable. Patients with adequate preoperative instructions and confidence in the surgeon, the nurse, and the outcome of the surgery usually have less postoperative pain than apprehensive patients, because they have less tension.[26] Measures to reduce anxiety and apprehension will also help reduce pain. Relief of pain may encourage the patient to move and breathe more deeply, thus preventing postoperative complications, which cause more pain.

If the cause of pain is determined to be other than incisional, measures are taken to relieve the cause e.g. emptying a full bladder can relieve what was thought to be pain from a lower abdominal incision.

Incisional pain can be relieved by nursing measures and by analgesics.

1. Encourage patient to move in bed or to ambulate, to decrease pain from muscle tension and increase circulation to the part.
2. Move the injured part as a whole; for example, move trunk as one unit.
3. Support an injured limb during a move (a pillow is a useful support).
4. Teach relaxation and distraction techniques, if suitable (Chapter 5).
5. Give PRN medications according to the guidelines for acute pain (Chapter 8).
   a. Narcotics are usually required on a regular basis for 12 to 48 hours after major surgery. Do not hesitate to use full narcotic dosages as prescribed; narcotic addiction is unlikely.
   b. Assess the patient for pain frequently during this period. Tell patient to request medication *before* the pain becomes severe. Analgesia is less effective when pain is severe.
   c. Monitor patient receiving pethidine for signs of orthostatic hypotension (dizziness, fainting, rapid pulse) during ambulation.
   d. Nonnarcotics may provide relief after 48 to 72 hours following major surgery.

Epidural analgesia is now commonly used following major surgery; it improves pain relief with less sedation and facilitates postoperative mobility. The anaesthetist inserts a small-lumen epidural catheter that can be fitted with an injection cap or can be attached by tubing to a continuous infusion pump. Morphine sulphate is the primary analgesic of choice, although fentanyl and other narcotics may also be used. Pain relief begins in 30 to 60 minutes and lasts 6 to 12 hours.[56] Better pain relief results with a regular dose schedule than PRN. No other narcotics or CNS depressants should be given concurrently. Keep an ampoule of naloxone (0.4 mg) available (to counteract an opioid overdose).[56] Monitor the patient for decreasing level of consciousness and shallow respirations; intake and output (to distinguish between hypovolaemia and urinary retention resulting from opioid action); and signs of epidural catheter leakage, infection, or bleeding.[56]

Patient-controlled analgesia (PCA) is also commonly used for control of severe pain following major surgery. PCA is a method by which the patient can self-administer the narcotic by pressing a button to deliver (intravenously or by epidural catheter) a predetermined dose of analgesic. Controls are built into the system to prevent overdosage (see Chapter 8). Because pain is a powerful respiratory stimulant, narcotics rarely produce respiratory depression when given for postoperative pain. Patients using PCA usually have better relief of postoperative pain and use smaller dosages than narcotics given on demand (PRN).[54]

Transcutaneous electrical nerve stimulation (TENS) is an additional method for postoperative pain relief (see Chapter 8). The electrodes are applied to the skin on either side of the incision. The electrodes are then connected to a battery-powered portable pulse generator. The stimulation is patient-controlled.

14-13

Common postoperative pain syndromes

Pain with fever
Pain with vomiting and abdominal distention
Suprapubic discomfort
Pain with coldness or numbness to part
Wound infection
Gas collecting in intestinal tract
Full bladder
Decreased circulation from tight dressing or plaster or from venous stasis

---

14-14

Causes of postoperative urinary retention

Recumbent position
Nervous tension
Anaesthetic; decreased bladder sensation and ability to pass urine
Narcotic: decreased bladder sensation
Pelvic surgery: interference with innervation of bladder muscles, local oedema

For relief of postoperative pain, a *high-frequency* (80 to 100 Hz) *low-intensity* (12 to 20 mA) impulse appears to be the most effective. The intensity is determined preoperatively on a trial-and-error basis by the patient. A tingling sensation may be experienced. The patient can vary the intensity according to the pain level. The best results are obtained when the TENS is used at periodic intervals, such as for a 60-minute period, rather than continuously. It may be helpful to provide stimulation for about 30 minutes before painful activities.

Maintaining adequate nutrition

Pathophysiology. The best way to supply essential foods is orally. Weight loss usually occurs after surgery as a result of catabolism, nutrients used for healing, and inadequate caloric intake while receiving fluids intravenously. Rapid weight loss indicates *fluid* loss: rapid weight gain indicates fluid retention.

Food substances of special importance in wound healing are protein, zinc and vitamin C. During catabolism in the early postoperative period, a negative nitrogen balance occurs; more nitrogen is lost than is taken in. Protein intake is necessary to restore nitrogen balance and to provide the necessary amino acids for anabolism. Vitamin C is stored only in small amounts in the tissues, so must be supplied daily from an external source.

Peristalsis decreases temporarily after *abdominal and pelvic* surgeries because of handling of the gastrointestinal organs during surgery. Peristalsis then returns gradually in 24 to 48 hours (72 hours after colon surgery).

Assessment
1. The doctor will monitor bowel sounds until heard regularly, or patient passes flatus, indicating return of peristalsis.
2. Weigh the patient for whom weight loss may present a problem, that is, the person who is severely undernourished or receiving feedings intravenously for 1 week or longer.
3. Monitor meal trays to identify those people who are not eating foods high in protein and vitamin C.

Intervention. After abdominal or pelvic surgery, the patient usually receives intravenous fluids until bowel sounds are heard. Poorly nourished patients may require total parenteral nutrition (TPN). When peristalsis has been identified, clear liquids (water, tea, coffee, broth, juice) are permitted until they are well tolerated. Full liquids (milk products, cream soups, high-protein drinks, ice cream) are then introduced. Soft foods are then permitted, and finally a normal diet is permitted, as tolerated by the patient. The goal is to move the patient to a full balanced diet as soon as possible.

Other nursing interventions include the following:
1. Encourage and teach postoperative patients to eat foods high in protein, zinc and vitamin C.
2. Do not force food. Instead, offer frequent small amounts of food or high-protein, high-calorie liquids (such as milk shakes or special manufactured products).
3. Encourage activity to improve appetite.
4. Discuss with underweight people their plans for obtaining the desired nutrients after discharge.

Maintaining elimination
Urine elimination

Pathophysiology. A patient who is well hydrated usually passes urine within 6 to 8 hours after surgery. Although 2000 to 3000 ml solution usually is given intravenously on the day of surgery, the first voiding may be 200 ml or less, and the total urinary output for the day may be less than 1500 ml. The small amount of urinary output results from the loss of body fluid during surgery, increased insensible fluid loss, vomiting, and increased secretion of antidiuretic hormone. As body functions stabilize, fluid and electrolyte balance returns to normal in about 48 hours.

Urinary retention, or the inability to pass urine, may occur in the early postoperative period for several reasons (see Box 14-14). A full bladder may increase pressure on an incision, causing bleeding and pain. *Urinary tract infections* may occur in patients who must have prolonged bed rest after surgery, have a history of urinary tract infections, have had pelvic surgery, or have in-dwelling catheters.

14-15

Causes of postoperative constipation

Neuroendocrine response to stress (decreased gastrointestinal motility)
Anaesthetic agents
Narcotics
Inactivity
Decreased intake of high-fibre foods

14-16

Effects of early postoperative ambulation

Increased rate and depth of breathing
Prevention of atelectasis and hypostatic pneumonia
Increased mental alertness from increased oxygenation to brain

Increased circulation
Nutrients required for healing are more available to wound
Prevention of thrombophlebitis
Increased kidney function

Increased micturition
Decreased pain

Increased metabolism
Prevention of urinary retention
Prevention of loss of muscle tone
Restoration of nitrogen balance

Increased peristalsis
Promotion of expulsion of flatus
Prevention of abdominal distention and wind pains
Prevention of constipation
Prevention of paralytic ileus

Assessment

1. Monitor urinary output until output equals fluid intake.
2. If patient does not pass enough urine, especially within 6 to 8 hours, assess for urinary retention (suprapubic distention, sensation of full bladder, suprapubic discomfort).
3. If patient complains of frequency of urination with burning, check body temperature, send a clean midstream urine specimen to laboratory for microscopy, culture and sensitivity, and notify doctor.

Intervention. If urinary retention is present, carry out measures to facilitate voiding (Chapter 25). Catheterization may be delayed longer than the usual 8 hours postoperatively for patients other than those having lower abdominal or pelvic surgery, in the hope that the patient will pass urine normally. Bethanechol chloride or carbachol may be ordered by the doctor for acute postoperative urine retention; however, catheterization is the preferred method.

If the bladder must be catheterized repeatedly after surgery, an in-dwelling catheter may be inserted. Fluids are then encouraged up to 3000 ml, unless contraindicated, to prevent urinary stasis that leads to infection.

Bowel elimination

Pathophysiology. Peristalsis will be decreased for at least 24 hours after abdominal or pelvic surgery and for several days after surgery of the gastrointestinal tract. No bowel movement can occur when peristalsis is absent or significantly decreased. *Constipation* occurs frequently after major surgery for several reasons (see Box 14-15). A bowel movement may be intentionally delayed after burns of the buttocks or extensive rectal surgery to prevent additional trauma.

Assessment

1. Monitor daily for passing flatus/bowel movement.
2. After abdominal surgery, assess and record signs returning peristalsis (bowel sounds, passing flatus).
3. Examine stool for amount and consistency; small dry, hard stool indicates constipation.
4. Assess for potential constipation:
   a. Narcotics given frequently or in high doses
   b. Inactivity
   c. Fluid intake less than 1200 ml/day
   d. Previous history of constipation

Intervention

1. Institute measures to *prevent* constipation for the first 2 or 3 days after major surgery:
   a. Facilitate fluid intake of 2000 to 3000 ml/day
   b. Encourage maximal activity
   c. Provide toilet privileges as early as possible
2. If no bowel movement within 3 or 4 days after surgery:
   a. Consult doctor about a laxative order. An osmotic laxative enema may be necessary if an oral agent is ineffective
   b. Encourage intake of foods high in fibre, if permissible

Maintaining activity

Pathophysiology. Early ambulation has been a significant factor in hastening postoperative recovery and preventing postoperative complications (see Box 14-16 and Fig. 14-15). Ambulation is usually contraindicated when there is a severe infection or thrombophlebitis

Assessment. Before helping the patient to ambulate for the first few times after major surgery, an assessment is made of the patient's level of alertness to follow directions, cardiovascular status, and motor status:

1. Level of alertness
2. Cardiovascular status
   a. Assess pulse and respiratory rate and depth while supine, then after sitting
   b. Observe skin colour for pallor while sitting
   c. Note complaints of dizziness when sitting
3. Motor status
   a. Assess muscle strength of legs
   b. Assess sitting ability

It is also important to know of any limitations to ambulation present preoperatively, e.g. arthritis. The patient who used a walking frame preoperatively will need assistance for a longer time.

Intervention

1. Encourage muscle-strengthening exercises before ambulation.
2. Ask the patient sit on side of bed (legs dangling) to become accustomed to upright position before ambulating the first time. Be sure *pulse has stabilized* (returned to baseline) before ambulation.
   a. Clamp off nasogastric tube until patient has ambulated, then reconnect.
   b. Keep urinary catheter connected to drainage bag; carry bag or pin bag to inside of dressing gown.
   c. Attach intravenous bag to a mobile stand.
3. Use two people to assist a weak patient receiving intravenous fluids to ambulate.
4. Encourage patient to walk further at each ambulation.

The word *ambulate* means to move from place to place, to walk. Sitting in a chair is not considered ambulation. After ambulating, the patient may sit in a chair if permitted, but should be advised to stand and walk at intervals and to elevate the legs while sitting to prevent venous pooling.

Helping meet psychological needs

Psychological factors. Some of the concerns that were present preoperatively may continue into the postoperative period. These concerns fall into essentially three categories: concerns specific to the surgery performed, concerns over loss of a body part, and concerns about the future. Future concerns include those related to changes in sexuality, economic status, prognosis, or permanent effects. Sexuality may be threatened by enforced absence from home or by a specific surgical procedure.

Assessment. Anxieties will be expressed in many different ways. It must be remembered that expressions such as anger, resentfulness, crying, excessive joking, inappropriate laughter, or withdrawal may all be signs of anxiety and are often seen in the postoperative period.

Intervention. Sitting down and talking with surgical patients about their concerns is an important nursing action. Time must be planned for this. If a specific concern is expected, such as sexual functioning after a prostatectomy, the topic may have to be introduced by the nurse in order to let the patient know that it is permissible to talk about it.

Evaluation

Evaluation is based on the identified outcomes, which vary greatly, depending on the type of surgery performed and the patient response to surgery. Questions to consider include the following:

1. Have postoperative complications or injury been avoided?
2. Is the incision healing well?
3. Are breath sounds clear and have atelectasis and pneumonia been avoided?
4. Has thrombophlebitis been avoided?
5. Has overhydration been avoided?
6. Does the person state feeling comfortable?
7. Has weight been stabilized?
8. Have usual elimination patterns been reestablished?
9. Does the person carry out ADL at an optimal level and ambulate at prescribed levels?
10. Has the person had an opportunity to explore concerns related to surgery?
11. Does the person know the medication therapy, treatments, dietary restrictions, or activity prescription to be carried out at home and when to attend for follow-up care?

DISCHARGE PLANNING

During hospitalization the patient and family should be prepared for any care that must be given at home, and any necessary arrangements for convalescent care should be completed before discharge. Patients are helped to become as self-sufficient as possible before being discharged so they do not have to depend any more than necessary on the assistance of relatives and friends.

If dressings are needed, the patient may be given supplies to take home. The patient and family must know where in the community they can get dressings and other materials. A community nurse is a useful resource person when treatment of almost any kind is to be provided at home.

On discharge the patient may be given an appointment for a follow-up examination in the outpatient clinic. The patient should understand the importance of returning for this consultation.

Normal activities should be resumed gradually. Driving is usually permitted after the outpatient follow-up appointment for major surgery, but the patient should avoid any heavy lifting, pushing, or pulling for at least 12 weeks following surgery.

SUMMARY

1. Elective admission for surgery may be by way of day case surgery, same-day surgery, or early hospital admission. All preoperative patients require the necessary preoperative preparation.
2. Surgery may be classified by location (external, internal, or body system) or by extent (major or minor).
3. The purpose of surgery may be diagnostic, curative, restorative, palliative, or cosmetic.
4. Surgery is a stressor; therefore, it evokes neuroendocrine and metabolic responses to stress.
5. Anxiety and fear are common responses to anticipated surgery. People with severe anxiety are poor candidates for surgery.
6. Risk factors for surgery include extremes of age, malnutrition, neuroendocrine response ineffectiveness, selected chronic diseases, and smoking.
7. Patients must know about the nature and risks of the proposed surgery and available options for care before signing a consent form (informed consent). The doctor is responsible for obtaining informed consent; the nurse facilitates the process and ensures that the consent form has been signed before surgery.
8. Data are collected by the nurse in the preoperative period to identify the patient's knowledge about surgery and psychological response (for planning of preoperative care); physiological data are collected to establish a baseline for future comparison and to identify potential postoperative problems.
9. Preoperative medical care includes treatment of existing medical conditions, including nutritional status, to facilitate optimal health status (except in emergency surgery).
10. Psychological preparation of the patient for surgery includes helping the person explore concerns or fear about surgery and providing desired information about the perioperative experience.
11. Preanaesthetic medications are given to decrease anxiety; facilitate induction, maintenance, and emergence from anaesthesia; decrease secretions; and prevent bradycardia. The patient remains in bed to facilitate drug effects and to prevent falls from dizziness.
12. The most common problems encountered in the postanaesthetic phase are airway obstruction, hypoventilation, hypotension, cardiac dysrrhythmias, and pain.
13. Measures to prevent postanaesthesia pulmonary problems include lying on side, artificial airway until patient begins to awaken, suctioning secretions that patient is unable to cough up, oxygen therapy, and initiation of breathing exercises.
14. Common causes of vital sign changes in the early postoperative period include shock, pain, anxiety, hypoventilation, jarring during transfer, distended urinary bladder, and drugs.
15. Postoperative hypothermia may cause discomfort, hypertension, cardiac dysrrhythmias, and tissue hypoxia.
16. Narcotics in the recovery unit may be given intramuscularly, intravenously, intrathecally, by patient-controlled analgesia (PCA), or by continuous epidural infusion.
17. Regeneration of tissue or scarring depend on the types of injured cells and intactness of the underlying structure.

18. Healing by primary or tertiary intention involves suturing the incision, immediate or delayed; healing by secondary intention consists of healing from the bottom.
19. Responses that occur following tissue injury include stress, inflammatory, immune, and generalized body responses followed by wound healing.
20. Interventions to promote wound healing include intake of protein, zinc and vitamin C, avoidance of antiinflammatory drugs, and prevention of wound infection and of fluid build-up in wound spaces.
21. People at high risk for postoperative pulmonary complications are those with increased or dry respiratory secretions, decreased thorax expansion, decreased diaphragm mobility, depression of respiratory centre by drugs, or aspirated gastric contents.
22. Measures to prevent postoperative thrombophlebitis include providing elastic stockings for people at high risk, avoiding pressure on popliteal area or leg massage, and encouraging leg exercises and early ambulation.
23. Incisional pain can be minimized by medication in combination with movement and ambulation, teaching relaxation and distraction techniques, and supporting injured parts.

STUDY QUESTIONS

- What general reactions do you believe you would have if told you must have immediate major surgery? What questions would you want answered? Based on this, what would be important to include in your preoperative teaching?
- Using Fig. 14-1, explain in lay terms the positive effects of the pathophysiological responses to surgery.
- Examine the informed consent form of your hospital. What is your responsibility in this situation?
- Examine the charts of several patients who have had surgery. What preanaesthetic medications were given? What were the purposes of these medications?
- After the same type of major surgery, in what ways should the general postoperative care differ between a male athlete aged 25 and a man aged 75 with arthritis of hands and hips? Explain the rationale for your answer.
- Examine the charts and nursing notes of two or three postoperative patients.
- What changes in vital signs occurred during the early postoperative period as compared to the preoperative baseline? What were the possible reasons for these changes?
- What types of preventive respiratory measures were used and what was the effect? What other nursing actions could have been taken?
- Did any postoperative complications occur? If so, what risk factors were present? How could the complication have been prevented?
- How did the patients compare in their response to postoperative ambulation? Did some need more encouragement than others? What positive effects would ambulation have for each patient?

REFERENCES AND SELECTED READINGS

1. Association of Operating Room Nurses Inc: *AORN standards and recommended practices for perioperative nursing*, Denver, 1989, The Association.
2. Atkinson LJ, Kohn ML: *Berry and Kohn's introduction to operating room technique*, ed 6, New York, 1986, McGraw-Hill.
3. Atsberger DB, et al: Postoperative pain management in the PACU: nurse's challenge, *J Post Anesth Nurs* 3:399-403, 1988.
4. Augustine SD: Hypothermia therapy in the postanesthesia care unit: a review, *J Post Anesth Nurs* 5:254-265, 1990.
5. Blansett MT: The effects of rewarming hypothermic postanesthesia patients using thermadrape covering, heat lamps, and warmed cotton blankets, *J Post Anesth Nurs* 5: 80-84, 1990.
6. Boore JRP: *Prescription for recovery: The effect of pre-operative preparation of surgical patients on post-operative stress, recovery and infection*, London, 1978, Royal College of Nursing.
7. Bragg CL: Practical aspects of epidural and intrathecal narcotic analgesia in the intensive care setting. *Heart Lung* 18:599-608, 1989.
8.* Bray CA: Postoperative pain: altering the patient's experience through education, *AORN J* 43:672-683, 1986.
9.* Brozenec S: Caring for the postoperative patient with an abdominal drain, *Nursing 85* 15(4):55-57, 1985.
10.* Burge S, et al: How painful are postop incisions? *Am J Nurs* 86:1263-1265, 1986.
11.* Carroll PF: Artificial airways: real risks, *Nursing 86* 16(8): 56-59, 1986.
12.* Cerrato PL: What diet does for wound healing, *RN* 51(6): 73-77, 1988.
13.* Closs SJ: An exploratory analysis of nurses' provision of postoperative analgesic drugs, *J Adv Nurs* 15:42-49, 1990.
14. Coleman DL: Control of postoperative pain: nonnarcotic and narcotic alternatives and their effect on pulmonary functioning, *Chest* 92:520-528, 1987.
15.* Crawford FJ: Ambulatory surgery: the elderly patient, *AORN J* 41:356-369, 1985.
16.* Crocker DG: Acute postoperative pain: cause and control, *Orthop Nurs* 5(2):11-15, 1986.
17. David JA: *Wound management*, Springhouse, Penn, 1988, Springhouse.
18.* Deters GE: Managing complications after abdominal surgery, *RN* 50(3):27-32, 1987.
19. Emery P: Ambulatory surgery. In Rothrock JC: *Perioperative nursing care planning*, St Louis, 1990, Mosby–Year Book.
20.* Erhardt BS: Pulse oximetry: an easy way to check oxygen saturation, *Nursing 90* 20(3):50-54, 1990.
21. Evaluating the usefulness of routine preoperative tests, *AORN J* 45:696, 1987.
22. Fraulini KE, Borchardt AC: Guide to solving postanesthesia problems, *Nursing 88* 18(5):66-86, 1988.
23. Garibaldi RA, et al: The impact of preoperative skin disinfection on preventing wound contamination, *Infect Control Hosp Epidemiol* 9(3):109-115, 1988.
24. Hargreaves A, Lander J: Use of transcutaneous electrical nerve stimulation for postoperative pain, *Nurs Res* 38(3): 159-161, 1989.
25. Hathaway D: Effect of preoperative instruction on postoperative outcome: a meta-analysis, *Nurs Res* 35: 269-275, 1986.
26. Hayward J: *Information, a prescription against pain*, London, 1975, Royal College of Nursing.
27. Heffline MS: Exploring nursing intervention for acute pain in the postanesthesia care unit, *J Post Anesth Nurs* 5:321-328, 1990.
28.* Hogue E: What you should know about informed consent, *Nursing 86* 16(6):47-48, 1986.
29.* Jackson MF: Implications of surgery in very elderly patients, *AORN J* 50:859-866, 1989.
30. Johnston M: Preoperative emotional states and postoperative recovery, *Adv Psychosom Med* 15:1-22, 1986.
31.* Kearns PC: Exercises to ease pain after abdominal surgery, *RN* 49(7):45-48, 1986.
32. Kneedler J, Dodge G: *Perioperative patient care*, ed 2, Boston, 1987, Blackwell Scientific Publications.
33.* Kresl JS: Patient-controlled analgesia, *AORN J* 48: 481-487, 1988.
34.* Latz PA, Wyble SJ: Elderly patients: perioperative nursing implications, *AORN J* 46:238-253, 1987.

*Recommended for student reading.

35.* Leeson IL: Pain and the postoperative patient, *Nursing (Oxford)* 2:1289-1290, 1985.

36. Lemmink JA: Infection control: when a surgical wound becomes infected, *RN* 50(9):24-27, 1987.

37.* Litwack K: Administering preoperative medications, *Nursing 91* 21(8):44-47, 1991.

38.* Litwack K, Parnass S: Practical points in the management of postoperative nausea and vomiting, *J Post Anesth Nurs* 3:275-277, 1988.

39. Meeker MH, Rothrock JC: *Alexander's care of the patient in surgery*, ed 9, St Louis, 1990, Mosby–Year Book.

40.* Miracle VA: How to perform basic airway management, *Nursing 90* 20(4):55-60, 1990.

41.* Montanari J: Wound dehiscence, *Nursing 86* 16(20):33, 1986.

42. Mortenson M, McMullin C: Discharge score for surgical outpatients, *Am J Nurs* 86:1347-1348, 1986.

43. Murray SE: Patient assessment in the postanesthesia care unit: a critical care approach, *J Post Anesth Nurs* 4:232-238, 1989.

44. Musgrave SF: Acute postoperative pain: the cause and the care, *J Post Anesth Nurs* 5:329-337, 1990.

45.* Neuberger GB: Wound care: what's clear, what's not, *Nursing 87* 17(20):34-37, 1987.

46.* Neuberger GB, Richling JB: A new look at wound care, *Nursing 85* 15(2):34-41, 1985.

47.* Nichols RR: Simple remedies for postoperative gas pain, *RN* 49(2):42-44, 1986.

48. Rogers M, Reich P: Psychological intervention with surgical patients: evaluation outcomes, *Adv Psychsom Med* 15:23-50, 1986.

49. Rothrock JC: *Perioperative nursing care planning*, St Louis, 1990, Mosby–Year Book.

50.* Rowland MA: Myths and facts about postop discomfort, *Am J Nurs* (5):61-64, 1990.

51. Schoessler M: Perceptions of preoperative education in patients admitted the morning of surgery, *Patient Educ Counsel* 14(2):127-136, 1989.

52. Torrington KG, et al: Perioperative respiratory therapy (PORT): a program of preoperative risk assessment and individualized postoperative care, *Chest* 93:946-951, 1988.

53. Turner TD: Absorbents and wound dressings, *Nursing* 2(12):(supplement 1-7), 1983.

54. Way LW: *Current surgical diagnosis and treatment,* ed 9, Los Altos, Calif, 1991, Appleton & Lange.

55.* Wetchler BV: Patient selection criteria for 1987: ambulatory surgery, *AORN J* 44:30-36, 1987.

56. Wild L, Coyne C: Epidural analgesia: the basics and beyond, *Am J Nurs* 92(4):26-36, 1992.

57. Williams SR: *Essentials of nutrition and diet therapy*, ed 5, St Louis, 1990, Mosby–Year Book.

58. Worley B: Preadmission testing and teaching: more satisfaction at less cost . . . surgical admissions, *Nurs Manage* 17(12):32-33, 1986.

59.* Wound management: Update 88, *Nursing 88* 18(6):33-37, 1988.

FURTHER READING

Baldwin C: Welcome Visitor, *Nursing Times*, 89(4):44-46, 1993.

Birrell J: Managing Anxiety, *The Professional Nurse*, 3(7): 243-246, 1988.

Drug and Therapeutics Bulletin: Day case surgery, *Drugs and Therapeutics Bulletin* 26(9):23-24, 1991.

Garrett G: A new lease of life. Nursing care of elderly surgical patients, *Professional Nurse* 8(1):15-20, 1992.

Griffiths-Jones A: Wound care: can the nursing process help? Implementing a wound care policy, *Professional Nurse*, 6(4): 208-212, 1991.

Hamilton Smith: *Nil by Mouth?* London, 1972, Royal College of Nursing.

Hayward J: *Information, a prescription against pain*, London, 1975, Royal College of Nursing.

Love C: Deep vein thrombosis—threat to recovery, *Nursing Times* 86(5):40-43, 1990.

Love C: Deep vein thrombosis—methods of prevention, *Nursing Times* 86(6):52-55, 1990.

Morison M: *A colour guide to the nursing management of wounds*, London, 1992, Mosby–Year Book Europe, Limited.

Spencer KE, Bale S: A logical approach. Management of surgical wounds, *Professional Nurse* 5(6):303-308, 1990.

Wilson-Barnett J, Batehup L: *Patient problems: A research base for nursing care*, London, 1988, Scutari Press.

Gas Transport Problems

15

The Patient with Nose and Throat Problems

Wilma J. Phipps

After studying this chapter, the learner should be able to:
- Describe pathophysiological bases of upper respiratory infections and therapeutic modalities.
- Discuss the nursing care of people having nose and sinus surgery and tonsillectomy.
- Describe aetiology and symptoms of cancer of the larynx, and postoperative care following surgery.

Disorders of the nose and throat are very common, and nurses in particular are often asked to give advice about these problems. To be effective, nurses need a basic understanding of the structure and function of the organs of the upper airway, as well as knowledge of the medical and nursing regimens for problems affecting the upper airway.

ANATOMY AND PHYSIOLOGY
Nose and Sinuses

The nose is supported by the nasal bones, the nasal processes of the maxillary bones, the cartilaginous and bony parts of the septum, and the upper and lower nasal cartilages. The septum, which divides the nares, is rarely straight in adults because at some time it has been injured.

The nasal cavities are located between the roof of the mouth and the frontal, ethmoid, and sphenoid bones. Three projections, which are lined with mucous membrane and called the *turbinate bones*, are located on the lateral walls of each nasal cavity (Fig. 15-1). Their purpose is to increase the mucous membrane surface over which air passes as it travels to the nasopharynx, thus allowing for precipitation of inhaled particles and warming and moistening the inhaled air.

The mucous membrane posterior to the vestibule (anterior part) of the nose contains cilia that beat in a constant wave-like motion to carry mucus into the nasopharynx. Trapped in the mucus are bacteria, dust, and other foreign matter entering the nose. The olfactory epithelium is located in a small area superiorly and provides the end organ of smell.

There are four sets of paranasal sinuses located on either side of the head (Fig. 15-2). These sinuses are air-filled spaces in the skull that drain into the nasal cavities through openings behind the turbinates. The maxillary sinuses are the largest and most accessible. The sinuses are lined with mucous membrane continuous with that of the nose.

Upper Throat: Pharynx and Tonsils

The pharynx is the space behind the oral and nasal cavities that extends from the base of the skull to the larynx. The pharynx can be considered in three parts: the nasopharynx, the oropharynx, and the laryngopharynx (Fig. 15-3). It is lined with mucous membrane.

The opening of the eustachian tubes and the adenoids are located in the nasopharynx, the palatine tonsils anterior to the oropharynx, and the lingual tonsils in the hypopharynx. The adenoids and tonsils are lymphoid tissue that help to filter the circulating lymph of bacteria or other foreign matter that penetrate the body, especially by way of the nose or mouth.

The oral pharynx serves both the respiratory and digestive systems. In the lower regions of the laryngopharynx the *larynx* and *oesophagus* form separate passageways for air and food.

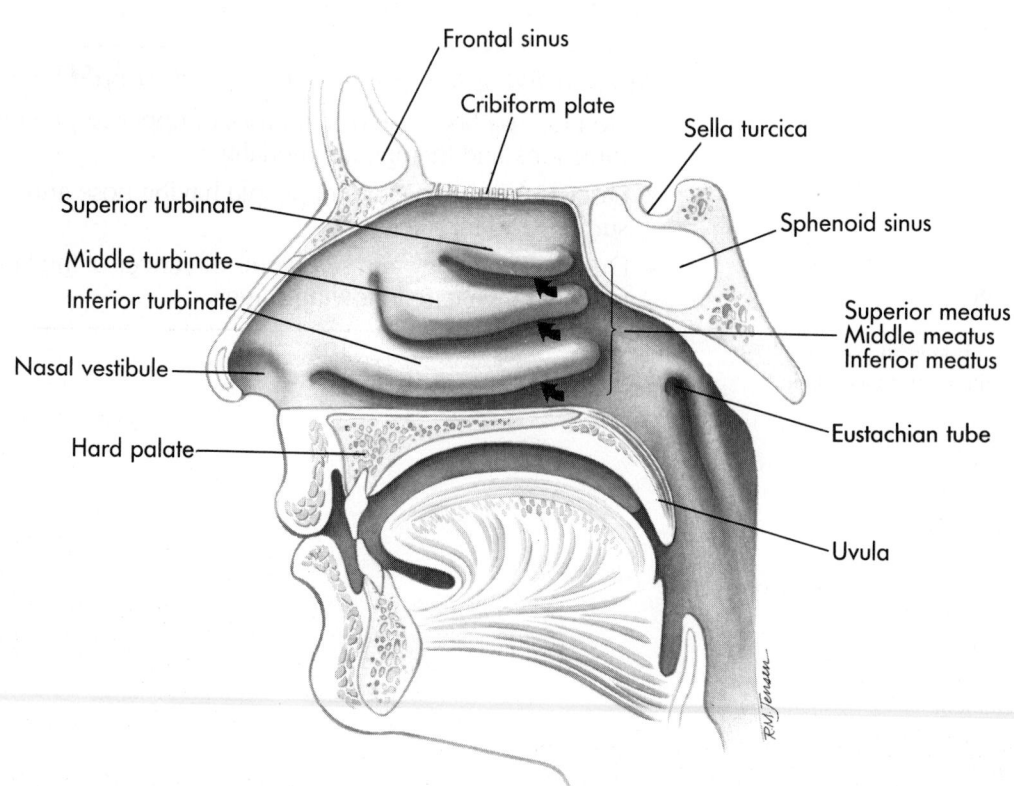

Fig. 15-1 Lateral wall of nose, showing superior, middle, and inferior turbinates. (From DeWeese DD, *et al: Otolaryngology—head and neck surgery*, ed 7, St Louis, 1988, Mosby–Year Book.)

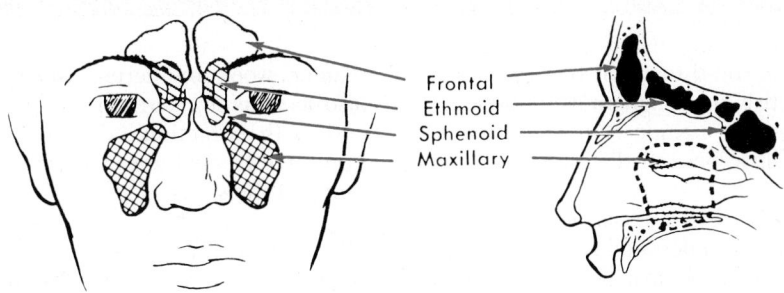

Fig. 15-2   Location of sinuses.

Frontal
Ethmoid
Sphenoid
Maxillary

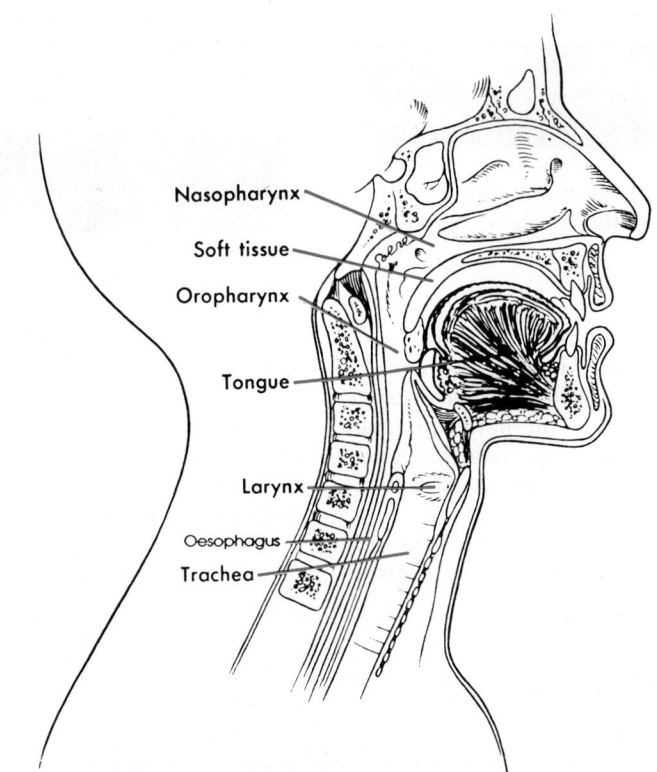

Nasopharynx
Soft tissue
Oropharynx
Tongue
Larynx
Oesophagus
Trachea

Fig. 15-3   Sagittal section of head showing pharynx and larynx.

Lower Throat: Larynx and Laryngopharynx

The larynx ("voice box") forms the upper extremity of the trachea. The framework of the larynx is made up of several cartilages held together by muscle and ligaments. The cartilaginous framework protects the vocal cords and affords a stiffness that permits an airway. The thyroid cartilage, the "Adam's apple," is the largest cartilaginous element in the larynx and protects the inner structures. The hyoid bone forms an attachment for the larynx and tongue. The larynx is lined with mucosa continuous with that of the laryngopharynx and trachea. The vagus nerve innervates the larynx.

The chief function of the larynx is to serve as an airway between the pharynx and trachea. A leaf-shaped lid of fibrocartilage (epiglottis) protects the glottis by covering the entrance to the larynx during swallowing to prevent aspiration of food or fluids. The closing of the glottis also allows for an increase of intrathoracic pressure, which is needed, for example, in coughing or lifting. This increased pressure increases the use of the muscles of the shoulder and thorax.

In addition, a most important function of the larynx is phonation. The larynx creates sounds as a result of vocal cord vibrations that are formed into speech patterns by the movement of the pharynx, palate, tongue, teeth, and lips.

Major Health Problems of the Nose and Throat

Most disorders of the nose and throat may be categorized as inflammatory, obstructive, or malignant as follows:

1. Inflammatory disorders include rhinitis, sinusitis, pharyngitis, tonsillitis, peritonsillar abscess, and laryngitis.
2. Obstructive disorders include nasal polyps, hypertrophy of the turbinates, a deviated septum, foreign bodies, and fractures (nasal, maxillary, zygomatic). Airway obstruction is discussed in Chapter 16.
3. Malignant disorders include carcinoma of the nasopharynx, of the maxillary and ethmoid sinuses, of the tonsil, and of the larynx.

Inflammations of the Nose and Sinuses

Inflammations may develop in the nose and sinuses (Table 15-1). A more detailed discussion of these conditions follows.

Aetiology

Inflammations of the upper airway structures may result from numerous viruses and bacteria. Many filtrable viruses (such as the more than 100 identified rhinoviruses, adenovirus, echovirus, influenza and parainfluenza viruses, and coxsackievirus) may serve as aetiologic agents of inflammations. Bacteria include primarily streptococci, staphylococci, and pneumococci.

Inflammations of the nose and sinuses are often an allergic reaction to pollen of grass and flowers, dust, animal dander, wool, and certain foods. Maxillary sinusitis may also occur as an extension of infection from abscessed teeth and tooth extraction, because the apices of many of the upper teeth roots are in close contact with the mucosal lining of the sinus.

Pathophysiology

Signs and symptoms seen with inflammations of the nose and throat result from the inflammatory process. Redness and oedema of the mucous membrane occur early. Discharge from the nose and sinuses include fluid exudate from the inflammatory process (which may be serous or purulent if infection is present), as well as mucous secretions. General malaise and fever are part of the systemic response to inflammation.

Infections of the Nose and Sinuses

The skin around the external nose is easily irritated during acute attacks of rhinitis or sinusitis. Furunculosis and cellulitis occasionally develop. Infections around the nose are extremely dangerous because the venous blood supply from this area drains directly into the cerebral venous sinuses. Septicaemia, therefore, can occur easily, and for this reason no pimple or lesion in the area should ever be squeezed or "picked." Hot packs may be used. If any infection in or around the nose persists or shows even a slight tendency to spread or increase in severity, a doctor should be consulted.

REVIEW

Table 15-1 Infections of the nose and sinuses

Disorder	Signs and symptoms	Medical therapy
Acute rhinitis (coryza, common cold)	Initial: dryness of mucous membranes, chills, general malaise 12–24 hours; profuse watery discharge, sneezing, tearing of eyes	Rest, fluids, moist inhalations, antihistamines and decongestants
Allergic rhinitis (hay fever)	Sneezing, nasal obstruction, watery nasal discharge, frontal headache, itching of eyes and nose	Separation of people from sensitizing allergens, desensitization, antihistamines; topical nasal steroids
Chronic rhinitis	Stuffiness and pressure in the nose; nasal discharge, which may be serous, mucopurulent or purulent; polyp formation; frontal headache; vertigo; sneezing	Antibiotics, avoidance of the offending allergens, antihistamines; polypectomy may be necessary
Sinusitis		
Acute	Constant severe headache, pain over sinuses, orbital oedema, nasal discharge, fever	Rest, analgesics, oral nasal decongestants, systemic antibiotics, local heat, topical nasal decongestants
Chronic	Chronic purulent nasal discharge, dull sinus headache, loss of ability to smell	Surgery; sinus irrigations

RHINITIS
Aetiology/Epidemiology

Rhinitis refers to inflammation of the mucous membrane of the nose. It may be acute or chronic.

Acute rhinitis (coryza, common cold) is an inflammatory condition of the mucous membranes of the nose and accessory sinuses caused by a filtrable virus. It affects almost everyone at some time and occurs most often in the winter, with additional high incidence in early autumn and spring. Some of the known causes of the common cold are more than 100 serotypes of rhinoviruses, adenoviruses, echoviruses, influenza and parainfluenza viruses, and coxsackievirus. The common cold is spread by droplet nuclei from sneezing, and the condition is contagious for the first two to three days.

Most people with colds contaminate their hands when coughing or sneezing, contaminating everything they touch. Others can become infected when touching the telephone, computer, or anything else that has been touched by the person with the cold. Also, many colds are believed to be spread when shaking hands with the person who has a cold.

Secondary invasion by bacteria may complicate the cold, possibly causing pneumonia, bronchitis, sinusitis, and otitis media.

Allergic rhinitis (hay fever) can be acute and seasonal when caused by the pollen of grass and flowers, or it may be chronic and perennial when associated with numerous allergens, such as house dust, animal dander, wool, and certain foods.

Chronic rhinitis is a chronic inflammation of the mucous membrane caused by repeated acute infections, by an allergy, or by vasomotor rhinitis. The cause of vasomotor rhinitis is unclear, but this condition may result from an instability of the autonomic nervous system caused by stress, tension, or some endocrine disorder. Often it is mistaken for nasal allergy, but the allergen cannot be identified. Formation of nasal mucus is increased, leading to a runny nose. Rhinitis can also be caused by the overuse of nose drops (*rhinitis medicamentosa*); a rebound phenomenon occurs after the immediate effect of the nose drops with the return to congestion. Discontinuing use of the nose drops usually clears up this condition within a week or two. The correct administration of nose drops is listed in Box 15-1.

In all forms of rhinitis sneezing, nasal discharge with nasal obstruction, and headache, are present, but the form of these symptoms varies with the type of rhinitis (Table 15-2). Acute rhinitis also includes signs of acute inflammation (early chilliness followed by "feverishness" and malaise). A painful throat is not always associated with a cold. However, the pharynx may feel sore because of early dryness followed by irritation from postnasal drainage. If uncomplicated, the cold is usually self-limiting and lasts for about one week.

In chronic rhinitis, acute symptoms are absent. The chief complaint is nasal obstruction accompanied by a feeling of stuffiness and pressure in the nose. Polyp formation may occur and vertigo may be present.

Interventions

No specific treatment is available for the common cold. Over-the-counter cold remedies usually contain one or more drugs, including antihistamines, sympathomimetics, and analgesics. Differences of opinion exist concerning the effectiveness of antihistamines in relieving cold symptoms. If taken during the onset of the cold, the allergic manifestations (sneezing, tearing, watery discharge) may be relieved; use during the latter stages may only cause drowsiness. Sympathomimetic drugs (such as phenylephrine [Neosynephrine] and phenyl-propanolamine) are nasal decongestants and help to relieve the nasal stuffiness. Vitamin C has no significant protective or inhib-

---

15-1

Correct administration of nose drops

1. Wash hands.
2. Assume a position that facilitates flow of medication.
   a. Sit in chair and tip head well backward, or
   b. Lie down with head extended over edge of bed, or
   c. Lie down with pillow under shoulders and head tipped backward.
3. Turn head to side that receives the drops.
4. Place no more than 3 drops of solution into each nostril at one time (unless otherwise prescribed).
5. Remain in position with head tilted backward for 5 minutes to permit solution to reach posterior nares.
6. If marked congestion is still present 10 minutes after nose drop insertion, another drop or two of solution may be administered (nasal constriction of swollen mucosa from first insertion may facilitate additional drops reaching posterior nares).

Table 15-2 Signs and symptoms of rhinitis

	Acute rhinitis	Allergic rhinitis	Chronic rhinitis
Nasal discharge	Initially watery, then mucoid	Thin, watery	Serous, mucopurulent, or purulent
Eyes	Tearing during early phase	Tearing, itching	No tearing
Tubinates	Oedematous	Pale, oedematous, mucoid	Enlarged
Nasal polyps	No	Yes	Yes
Headache	Generalized	Frontal	Frontal

itory effect on colds.[10] Antibiotics are used only for complicating secondary infections. Also see the Nursing Process section under Sinusitis.

Nose drops are sometimes recommended for infrequent use (every four hours for a few days) if there is some nasal obstruction. Many ear, nose, and throat (ENT) doctors now believe that the frequent use of nose drops results in rhinitis medicamentosa, an "addiction" of the nasal mucosa to their use.[10] Some doctors believe that the obstruction of the nose may be a protective device that prevents the spread of infection to other parts of the body.

For allergic rhinitis, the treatment consists of maintaining an allergen-free environment (see Chapter 33). Hyposensitization or desensitization (administering the allergen in gradually increasing doses to establish an "immunity") may be helpful. Antihistamines give relief to most people, but their effectiveness often decreases as the "hay fever season" continues.

For chronic rhinitis, antihistamines may give relief. When nasal obstruction persists, surgery may be necessary to remove polyps (polypectomy) or to remove tissue obstruction (septoplasty).

Nasal irrigations are now seldom used in the treatment of chronic rhinitis. Details of the procedure are described in texts on fundamentals of nursing or ENT. Care should be taken to ensure that both nostrils are open and that the pressure in the nostrils is not excessive (the irrigating container should not be higher than 30 to 38 cm above the level of the nose). Excess pressure may force infected material into the sinuses or the middle ear.

SINUSITIS
Aetiology/Epidemiology

The sinuses are air-filled cavities lined with mucous membrane. Any inflammation of the mucous membranes of the sinuses is called *sinusitis*. This is still a frequent disorder, although it is less common since the advent of antibiotics. Often patients who complain of sinusitis do not have a sinus infection but some other disorder. When an ENT doctor refers to sinusitis, a *bacterial invasion of the mucous membrane is implied*. Only about 10% of the patients who consult an ENT doctor because of "sinus trouble" are diagnosed as having sinusitis.

Sinusitis is classified as follows:
- Acute suppurative
- Subacute suppurative
- Chronic suppurative
- Allergic
- Hyperplastic.

The most common cause of *acute suppurative sinusitis* is the obstruction of the paranasal sinuses that blocks the egress of secretions from the sinuses. These secretions become infected, giving rise to acute suppurative sinusitis. The organisms most often responsible are *Streptococcus pneumoniae*, beta-haemolytic *Streptococcus*, *Haemophilus influenzae*, coagulase-positive *Staphylococcus aureus*, and *Klebsiella pneumoniae*. More than 50% of maxillary sinus infections are caused by *S. pneumoniae* and *H. influenzae*. Another 30% are caused by anaerobic bacteria, which are

often dental in origin. *Cultures are not helpful* because multiple organisms are usually found.

Acute Suppurative Sinusitis

The signs and symptoms of acute suppurative sinusitis are listed in Table 15-3. Symptoms worsen over 48 to 72 hours until there is severe localized pain and tenderness over the involved sinus (Box 15-2). The patient often believes that the pain is due to an infected tooth. Pain is localized and may be referred to another site.

In acute frontal and maxillary sinusitis, pain usually does not appear until one to two hours after awakening. It increases for three to four hours and then becomes less severe in the afternoon and evening.

There may be bloody or blood-tinged discharge from the nose in the first 24 to 48 hours. The discharge rapidly becomes purulent and copious, blocking the nose. The throat may become inflamed and sore on one side because of the purulent discharge.

On examination, the involved nasal mucosa is hyperaemic and oedematous, and the turbinates are enlarged. X-ray films show that the involved sinus is clouded, and a fluid level is visible. Usually the diagnosis is established without radiographs. If there are recurrent episodes of acute sinusitis, radiographs or computerized tomography (CT) scans are indicated to rule out underlying pathology.

Subacute Suppurative Sinusitis

The medical measures described in Table 15-3 cure more than 90% of patients with acute suppurative sinusitis; a subacute infection persists in the remaining 10%. Persistent purulent discharge is the only constant symptom. A radiograph or CT scan is indicated to determine whether one or more sinuses are involved. Because it is uncommon for acute sinusitis to persist, the causative organism may be unusual.[10] Special culture techniques may be necessary, and antibiotic sensitivity studies are essential. The most commonly isolated organisms are *H. influenzae*, *H. pneumoniae* and *Branhamella catarrhalis*. *Branhamella catarrhalis* is not sensitive to penicillins, and treatment requires systemic sulphonamide therapy or erythromycin with a sulphonamide. Pain is not severe and requires no medication. Treatment consists of vasoconstriction of nasal mucosa, heat, and irrigation of the involved sinus (Table 15-3).

Antral irrigation, in which the anterior wall of the maxillary sinus is punctured, is the preferred treatment for subacute sinusitis. Anaesthesia is obtained with an injec-

15-2	**Location of pain with sinusitis**	
	Sinus	**Pain location**
	Maxillary	Over cheek and upper teeth
	Frontal	Above the eyebrow
	Ethmoid	Medial and deep in the eye.
	Sphenoid	Deep behind the eye, over the occiput, or top of head

REVIEW

Table 15-3   Sinusitis: signs and symptoms and treatment

Type	Signs and symptoms	Medical therapy
Acute suppurative sinusitis	Stuffy nose, slowly developing pressure over involved sinus General malaise, toxicity, headache, slightly elevated or normal temperature	Antibiotics for 14 days Cefaclor, cefuroxime axetil, penicillin V, and erythromycin are effective against the three most common pathogens. Bedrest, humidity, hydration, decongestations, and expectorants. *Antihistamines should be avoided.* Relief pain may require codeine or meperidine. Wet hot packs over affected sinus continuously or for 1-2 hours four times a day
Subacute suppurative sinusitis present in about 10% of patients	Persistent purulent nasal discharge that lasts longer than 2 weeks but less than 4 weeks	Vasoconstrictors, heat and irrigation of involved sinus
Chronic suppurative sinusitis	Purulent nasal discharge, persistent nasal congestion, postnasal drip, halitosis, anosomia, and sometimes sinus headache. Persistent headache requires surgical consult	A small percentage of patients may be cured by repeated irrigation, antihistamines, and antibiotics Most patients require surgery: Caldwell-Luc surgery is the most common cal prodedure

tion of 2 to 3 ml of 1% lignocaine with 1:100,000 adrenaline under the upper lip. A 16-gauge needle (with stylet in place) is rotated through the soft tissue and bone. When proper placement of the needle is assured, saline solution is instilled to wash out the sinus. Antibiotic solutions may be used, but mechanical cleansing is more important than the solution used.[10]

It is not possible to irrigate the ethmoid sinuses directly, and *ethmoiditis* is treated with systemic antibiotics. The antibiotics should be continued for 10 to 14 days.[10] Proper treatment of subacute sinusitis is the best means of preventing *chronic suppurative sinusitis.*

Chronic Suppurative Sinusitis

When suppurative sinusitis is not treated or is inadequately treated during the acute or subacute phase, or when the mucosa is damaged from recurrent attacks, permanent change may occur. Bacteria can invade the tissue of the sinuses, become walled off, and produce chronic inflammation. With prolonged infection of soft tissue, pathological change may become irreversible and the patient has *chronic suppurative sinusitis.*[10]

The most common and sometimes only symptom is purulent nasal discharge. In a small percentage of patients, repeated irrigation, antihistamines, and antibiotics may cure the disease. However, most patients must be treated surgically. Surgical treatment is discussed below. *Anosmia* (loss of smell) or *parosmia* (a perverted sense of smell) may result from nasal blockage.

Surgery of the Sinuses

Treatment of *chronic suppurative sinusitis* involves surgery to remove all diseased soft tissue and bone, adequate postoperative drainage, and obliteration of the sinus cavity where possible. The goal of surgery is to eradicate infection and leave contiguous structures normal. Preoperative teaching is outlined in Box 15-3.

The Caldwell-Luc procedure is the generally accepted operative procedure for chronic maxillary sinusitis. It is also called a *radical antrum* operation. Local or general anaesthesia may be used.

The external approach is preferred for ethmoid surgery because it allows better visualization and reduces the risks of complications such as damage to the optic nerve and central spinal fluid leak. Ethmoidotomy is an opening made for drainage, whereas an ethmoidectomy entails removal of ethmoid tissue (Table 15-3). The incision is made in the inner half of the eyebrow downward along the side of the nose.[22,31] Ethmoidectomy is performed for correction of nasal polyps and for ethmoiditis because nasal polyps frequently originate in the ethmoid cells.

15-3

Preoperative teaching for sinus surgery

Determine what the patient understands about the surgical procedure. Clarify misconceptions and answer patient's questions. Explain that he or she:
- Will have nothing to eat or drink 6–8 hours preoperatively.
- Will receive sedative medication before surgery.
- Will feel pressure, not pain, during surgery.
- Will have a nasal pack for 24–48 hours postoperatively.
- Will have a moustache dressing postoperatively.
- Will have some ecchymosis and swelling around the nose and eyes for 1–2 weeks postoperatively.

The osteoplastic flap operation allows for complete removal of diseased mucosa of the frontal sinus and for obliteration of the sinus so that it is no longer functional or in continuum with the inner nose.

Postoperative care for sinus surgery

Care of the patient following sinus surgery is described in Box 15-4. Gauze packing is usually inserted into the nares and removed after 48 hours. The patient thus breathes through the mouth, with subsequent dryness of mouth and lips. Mouth care is required, and warm or cool vapour inhalations often are prescribed. If there is an oral incision, mouth care is carried out before meals to improve appetite and after meals to decrease danger of infection. Antibiotics may be prescribed prophylactically. For one or two weeks swelling or ecchymosis may be present around the nose and eyes. Ice compresses will constrict blood vessels, decreasing oozing and oedema, and help relieve pain.

INFECTIONS OF THE PHARYNX AND LARYNX

ACUTE PHARYNGITIS
Aetiology/Epidemiology
Acute pharyngitis is the most common throat inflammation. It may be caused by haemolytic streptococci, staphylococci, or other bacteria or viruses. There is an increased incidence of gonococcal pharyngitis caused by the Gram-negative diplococcus *Neisseria gonorrhoeae*. The disease is increasingly found in both men and women who engage in oral–genital sex. When gonorrhoea is suspected, a throat culture should be obtained.

A severe form of acute pharyngitis is often referred to as *strep throat* because of the frequency of streptococci as the causative organisms.

Symptoms usually precede or occur simultaneously with the onset of acute rhinitis or acute sinusitis. Pharyngitis can occur after the tonsils have been removed because the remaining mucous membrane can become infected. Pharyngitis is also a common manifestation of infectious mononucleosis.

Pathophysiology
Table 15-4 summarizes the signs and symptoms and therapy for infections of the pharynx and larynx. Nursing care includes the points listed in Box 15-5 and in the following discussion:

1. Give medications as prescribed. A penicillin or eryth-romycin may be prescribed prophylactically to pre-vent superimposed infections, especially in people with a history of rheumatic fever or bacterial endocarditis.
2. If the diagnosis is gonococcal pharyngitis, the patient will need instruction in how to avoid reinfection.
3. Provide moist inhalations and ice collar if ordered.
4. Provide a liquid diet with at least 2 to 3L of fluids.
5. Bedrest if temperature is elevated; otherwise, extra rest.

Guidelines for Care 15-4

Postoperative care of the patient following surgery of sinuses

1. After general anaesthesia, position patient well onto the side to prevent swelling or aspiration of bloody drainage.
2. When the patient is awake, remind him or her to expectorate secretions and not swallow them.
3. Encourage a supported sitting position when fully awake to promote drainage and decrease oedema.
4. Apply ice compresses over nose (or ice bag over maxillary or frontal sinuses) in the early postoperative period.
5. Monitor the patient for:
   a. Excessive bleeding from nose (may be evidenced by repeated swallowing).
   b. Decreased visual acuity, especially *diplopia*, indicating damage to optic nerve or muscles of globe of eye.
   c. Complaints of pain over the involved sinus, which may indicate infection or inadequate drainage.
   d. Fever—take temperature rectally.
6. Carry out frequent mouth care using a soft toothbrush. If there is an oral incision, mouth care is carried out before meals to improve appetite and after meals to decrease danger of infection.
7. Change nasal pad when it is soiled.
8. Apply ice compresses to ecchymotic areas to constrict blood vessels, to decrease oozing and oedema, and to help relieve pain.
9. Encourage liberal fluid intake. Patient may be very thirsty because of dry mouth from mouth breathing.
10. Teach patient to:
    a. Avoid blowing nose for at least 48 hours after packing is removed to prevent bleeding.
    b. Report signs of infection (fever, purulent discharge) to surgeon.
    c. Expect tarry stools from swallowed blood for a few days.
    d. Avoid constipation (Valsalva manoeuvre can cause bleeding).
    e. Expect that ecchymosis of nose and eyes will begin to change colour over next 1-2 weeks.
    f. Take prophylactic antibiotics as prescribed. Do not stop until all medication is taken.

ACUTE FOLLICULAR TONSILLITIS
Aetiology/Epidemiology

Acute follicular tonsillitis is an acute inflammation of the tonsils and their crypts. It is usually caused by the *Streptococcus* organism. It is more likely to occur when the person's resistance is low, and is very common in children. (See Table 15-4 for summary of signs and symptoms and medical therapy.)

REVIEW

Table 15-4   Infections of the pharynx and larynx

Disorder	Signs and symptoms	Medical therapy
Pharyngitis Acute	Redness and soreness of throat, difficulty in swallowing, fever Hacking cough	Warm saline gargles, ice collar, aspirin, moist inhalations, antibiotics; anaesthetic lozenges may be given

Tonsillitis
  Acute
    follicular
	Sudden onset of sore throat, dysphagia, fever, chills, malaise	Rest, fluids, warm saline gargles, ice collar, antibiotics, analgesics, tonsillectomy may be necessary when recurrent infections do not respond to antibiotics

Laryngitis Acute	From slight huskiness to total voice loss, sore throat, dry harsh cough	Symptomatic treatment, voice rest; steam inhalations; avoidance of smoking and being near those who are smoking

Patient Teaching 15-5

Teaching for the patient with an infection of the nose or throat

1. Get additional rest (hastens recovery).
2. Drink at least 2–3L of fluid every day.
3. Medications
   a. Antihistamines are effective primarily during the initial period only; care should be taken when driving or working with heavy machinery when taking antihistamines
   b. Take prescribed antibiotics for bacterial infections for the prescribed period of time
   c. If using nose drops:
      (1) Place no more than 3 drops of solution in each nostril at one time (unless otherwise prescribed)
      (2) Keep head tilted back for about 5 minutes to permit solution to reach posterior nares
      (3) Insert 1–2 additional drops after 10 minutes if marked congestion is still present
   d. If using atomizer:
      (1) Occlude opposite nostril with finger pressure to prevent entrance of air
      (2) Administer no more than 3 sprays of solution in each nostril at one time.
4. Promote throat comfort through use of the following:
   a. Warm saline gargles
   b. Ice collar
   c. Throat lozenges
   d. Moist inhalations.
5. Avoid further upper respiratory infections
   a. Avoid direct exposure to others with respiratory infections, if possible
   b. Teach all people to cover nose and mouth with tissue when coughing or sneezing
   c. Wash hands after disposing of tissues.
6. Explain rationale for prophylactic antibiotics for people with a history of rheumatic fever or bacterial endocarditis.
7. Medical attention is required for recurring symptoms (fever, excessive pain, dysphagia, expectoration of pus).

Complications of untreated tonsillitis include heart and kidney damage, chorea, and pneumonia. Incidence of these complications is decreasing with the widespread use of penicillin and early diagnosis.

Interventions

Most physicians believe that people who have recurrent attacks of tonsillitis should have a tonsillectomy. This procedure is usually performed from four to six weeks after an acute attack has subsided.

Because the person with acute tonsillitis is usually cared for at home, the nurse should help in teaching the general public the care that is needed (Box 15-5 outlines teaching priorities). The ward nurse, the clinic nurse, the occupational health nurse, the school nurse, and the community nurse have many opportunities to do this teaching.

Tonsillectomy

Tonsillectomy for the adult may be performed under local or general anaesthesia. Haemorrhage may occur postoperatively. The doctor may be able to control minor postoperative bleeding by applying a sponge soaked in a solution of adrenaline to the site. The person who is bleeding excessively often is returned to the operating room for ligation or cauterization of the bleeding vessel. If sutures must be used, the person has more pain and discomfort than following a simple tonsillectomy. The patient may not be able to take solid food for several days. Some surgeons no longer prescribe aspirin for pain after tonsillectomy, as it increases the tendency to bleed. Paracetamol is usually ordered.

A tough, yellow, fibrous membrane that forms over the operative site begins to break away between the fourth and eighth postoperative days, and haemorrhage may occur. The separation of the membrane accounts for the throat being more painful at this time. Pink granulation tissue soon becomes apparent, and by the end of the third postoperative week, the area is covered with mucous membrane of normal appearance.

Postoperative care is outlined in Box 15-6.

LARYNGITIS
Simple Acute Laryngitis

Simple acute laryngitis is an inflammation of the mucous membrane lining the larynx and is accompanied by oedema

Postoperative care of the patient following tonsillectomy

1. Side-lying position until awake, then a supported sitting.
2. Monitor for signs of haemorrhage
   a. Repeated swallowing
   b. Vomiting of bright red blood
   c. Increased pulse rate while sleeping.
3. Diet
   a. Offer fluids when vomiting has ceased
   b. Encourage patient to take large swallows (more comfortable than small sips)
   c. Avoid using a straw (suction may cause bleeding)
   d. Ice-cold fluids better tolerated.
   e. Offer bland nourishment:
      Ice cream, cold custards, cream soups, and bland juices (for example, pear) offered initially
      Refined cereal and soft-cooked egg usually better tolerated morning after surgery
      Avoid citrus juices, hot fluids, rough or highly seasoned foods for 1 week.
4. Relieve throat discomfort:
   a. Apply ice collar as desired
   b. Give prescribed analgesic (avoid aspirin, which can increase bleeding).
5. Teach patient about the following:
   a. Avoid vigorous exercise, coughing, sneezing, clearing throat, and vigorous nose blowing for 1–2 weeks
   b. Report signs of bleeding immediately to the doctor
   c. Drink fluids (2–3L/day) until mouth odour disappears
   d. Stools may be tarry for several days from swallowed blood
   e. Throat discomfort may increase slightly between 4th and 8th postoperative day (membrane separation).

of the vocal cords. It may be caused by a cold, by sudden changes in temperature, by irritating fumes, by excessive use of the voice, or by excessive smoking. Symptoms vary from a slight huskiness to complete loss of voice. The throat may be painful and feel scratchy, and a cough may be present. (See Table 15-4 for signs and symptoms and medical therapy.)

Chronic Laryngitis

Some people who use their voices excessively, who smoke a great deal, or who work continuously where there are irritating fumes develop a chronic laryngitis. Hoarseness usually is worse in the early morning and in the evening. There may be a dry, harsh cough and a persistent need to clear the throat.

Treatment may consist of removal of irritants, voice rest, correction of faulty voice habits, steam inhalations, and cough medications. The doctor may order spraying of the throat with an antiseptic spray. To carry out this procedure properly the patient must use a spray tip that turns down at the end so that the medication reaches the vocal cords and is not dissipated in the posterior pharynx. The spray tip is placed in the back of the throat with the bent portion behind the tongue. The patient should then take one or two deep breaths and spray the medication on inhalation. This procedure may cause temporary coughing and gagging. Many medications used as throat sprays are now sold in plastic squeeze bottles with tube and spray tip attached.

OBSTRUCTIVE DISORDERS OF THE NOSE

Trauma or polyps in the nose, nasal bones, turbinates, maxillary bones, and zygomatic bones may cause obstruction. Many people with obstructions of the nose may be diagnosed and treated on an ambulatory basis.

Aetiology

Obstruction may be caused by a deviated septum, either congenital or, more commonly, as a result of trauma. Allergy and chronic sinusitis may lead to the development of nasal polyps, grape-like growths of mucous membrane and loose connective tissue in the sinus mucosa. Fractures of the nasal, maxillary, and zygomatic bones may result from falls, motor vehicle accidents, and fights. Displaced fragments from the fracture obstruct passage of air. Malignant growths may also cause obstruction.

Nosebleeds may result from a number of causes (see Box 15-7). When the bleeding stops, some nasal obstruction may occur from the blood clot until the mucosa heals. In adulthood, nosebleeds are more common in men than in women.

NASAL POLYPS

Pathophysiology

Nasal polyps are grape-like growths of mucous membrane and loose connective tissue. They are usually bilateral and are usually caused by allergic rhinitis. Polyps cause *anosmia* by preventing air from reaching the olfactory mucosa high in the nose.

Common causes of nosebleeds

Local irritation of superficial blood vessel
Trauma
Chronic infection
Lack of humidity in air breathed
Violent sneezing or noseblowing
Nose picking (most common cause)

Systemic causes
Hypertension
Blood dyscrasias (for example, leukaemia)
Deficiency in vitamin K

Interventions

Because they may obstruct breathing or block sinus drainage, nasal polyps are removed surgically if they do not respond to treatment with aerosol sprays containing corticosteroids. Even when they do respond to corticosteroid sprays, polyps reappear when the steroids are discontinued.

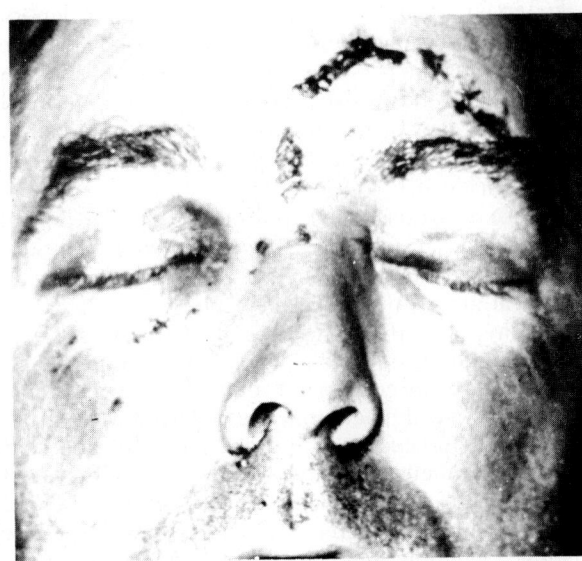

Fig. 15-4   Laterally displaced fracture of nose secondary to trauma. Pressure on convex side will restore alignment. (From Saunders WH, *et al*: *Nursing care in eye, ear, nose, and throat disorders*, ed 4, St Louis, 1979, Mosby–Year Book.)

FRACTURES OF NASAL BONES AND SEPTUM

Fractures of the nasal bones and septum commonly occur from relatively minor injuries, such as falls, or from more severe injuries, such as automobile accidents or fights. If there is no displacement of the bone, no obstruction to the airway, and no cosmetic deformity, treatment is not needed. When airway obstruction or bone displacement occurs, simple reduction is performed. Most simple nasal fractures can be reduced by applying firm pressure on the convex side of the nose (Fig 15-4). Nasal fractures should be reduced within the first 24 hours if at all possible. Local anaesthesia is used. After 24 hours reduction becomes more difficult and may require general anaesthesia.

FRACTURES OF MAXILLARY AND ZYGOMATIC BONES

Fractures of the maxillary and zygomatic bones are seen after automobile accidents and fights.[10] These fractures are generally reduced under anaesthesia. Patients may also require wiring of the teeth with all the attendant problems of that procedure.

Nursing Process
Assessment

Subjective data

Symptoms of nasal obstructions include the following:
1. Noisy, difficult breathing
2. Dry mucosa
3. Postnasal drip
4. Nasal discharge
5. Anosmia
6. Bleeding from nose.

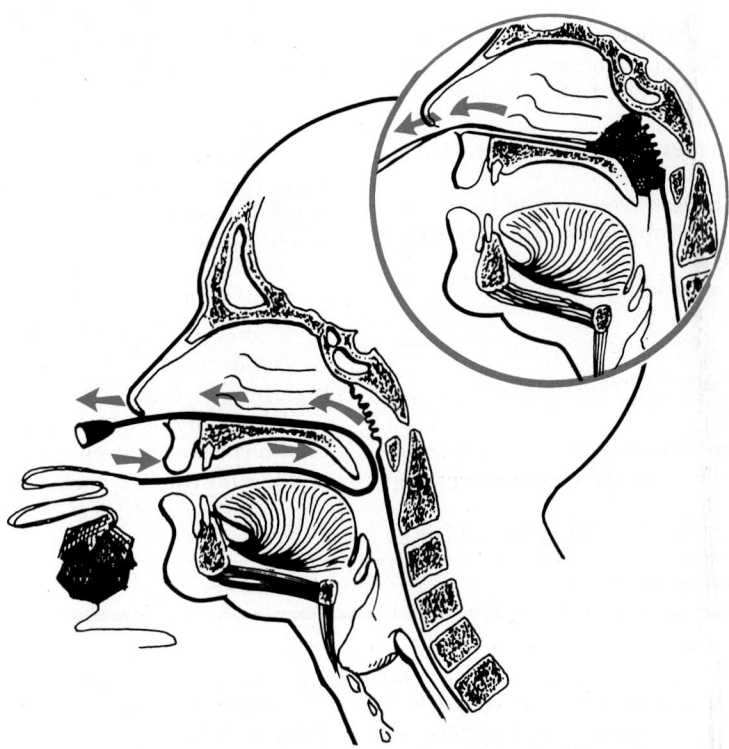

Fig. 15-5   Postnasal packing. Pack is attached to catheter then pulled through mouth to posterior nasopharynx.

If nasal trauma is present, additional symptoms include displacement of the bones, cosmetic deformity, pain, and ecchymosis around the eyes or jaw.

Objective data

1. Inspection for deformity or asymmetry.
2. Some septal deviation is common in adults and is asymptomatic.
3. Check for abnormal findings in nose
   a. Excessive redness
   b. Oedema
   c. Exudate
   d. Bleeding.

Nursing analysis

Nursing analyses are determined from an assessment of patient data. Possible nursing analyses for the person with obstruction of the nose may include, but are not limited to, the following:

Problems	Possible aetiologies
Body image disturbance	Severe trauma/disfiguring surgery
Pain	Trauma/obstruction
Knowledge deficit	Lack of exposure to information, misinterpretation of information
Sensory/perceptual alterations: olfactory	Trauma/surgery

Planning: expected patient outcomes

Expected patient outcomes for the person with an obstruction of the nose may include, but are not limited to, the following:

1. Patient maintains positive body image.
2. Patient states he or she is comfortable.
3. Patient can state care required after surgery and discharge from hospital.
4. Patient knows how to prevent nosebleeds or to treat them if they occur.
5. Patient can state signs and symptoms of complications (bleeding, drainage, and fever) that need to be reported to the surgeon.
6. Patient can breathe more easily.

Implementation

Assisting with achievement of therapeutic goals
Controlling nasal bleeding

Nosebleeds from the tiny blood vessels in the anterior part of the septum are usually controllable by compressing the soft tissue of the nose against the septum with a finger. Firm pressure should be maintained for at least 5 to 10 minutes, and it may be necessary for as long as 30 minutes. The person should breathe through the mouth during this time. Ice compresses may be applied over the nose; however, the primary benefit of the application of ice is that it requires the patient to remain still.

Bleeding may also be controlled by placing a cotton ball soaked in a topical vasoconstrictor such as phenylephrine in the nose and applying pressure. Other first-aid measures include having the person sit quietly with the head up and inclined slightly forward to prevent blood from entering the pharynx and causing gagging or swallowing of blood. The person is instructed not to blow the nose for several hours after a nosebleed.

If these measures do not control bleeding, the help of a doctor should be sought. After identifying the site of bleeding, the doctor may cauterize the bleeding vessel with a silver nitrate stick or electrode cautery.

Bleeding from the posterior part of the nasal septum is more common in elderly people and is more likely to be severe. If the bleeding point cannot be seen and cauterized, a postnasal pack may be inserted (Fig. 15-5). Because this procedure is extremely painful and sometimes causes faintness, patients may be admitted to the hospital. Pain medication, antibiotic therapy, and sedation may also be ordered for a person with posterior packing. Sedation may be ordered, because bleeding tends to be increased by apprehension and restlessness. The pack is left in place for two to five days and then gently removed.

Severe bleeding results in a drop in blood pressure, which may cause the bleeding to stop; therefore, exsanguination from the usual nosebleed is rare. To prevent recurrent haemorrhage, the person is warned not to blow the nose vigorously and to avoid dryness of the nose. This can be accomplished by using saline or nasal lubricants.

Persistent or recurrent profuse epistaxis, especially posterior epistaxis, may require surgical ligation of the external carotid artery, the ethmoid artery, or the internal maxillary artery, all of which supply blood to the nose.

Nasal surgery

When there is obstruction of the nasal passages, surgery is usually necessary. The most common surgeries are presented in Table 15-5.

Polypectomy is usually performed under local anaesthesia. Polyps are removed with a small snare or biting forcep, and the nostrils are packed for 24 hours. Because polyps

---

Table 15-5 Surgeries to relieve nasal obstruction or trauma

Procedure	Description	Comments
Nasal polypectomy	Removal of polyps from nose	Local anaesthesia given; nasal packing for 24 hours
Submucous resection	Removal of obstructive parts of cartilage and bone from nasal septum	Local anaesthesia given; both nostrils packed to provide splinting
Nasoseptoplasty	Reconstruction of nasal septum	Same as for submucous resection
Rhinoplasty	Reconstruction of external nose following trauma or for cosmetic reasons	Often combined with septoplasty following nasal trauma; nose splinted after surgery; nasal packing

and the nostrils are packed for 24 hours. Because polyps tend to recur, especially if allergy is the underlying cause, further surgery is often necessary. Ethmoidectomy and sphenoidectomy and even a Caldwell-Luc procedure may be necessary.

Nasoseptoplasty involves reconstruction of the septum and is replacing submucous resection as the operation of choice for deviated nasal septum. Reconstruction of the external nose (*rhinoplasty*) is often combined with septoplasty. It is usually performed under local anaesthesia. With rhinoplasty, the nasal bones or cartilaginous framework of the nose are altered. The nose is usually protected with a plaster-of-Paris splint, adhesive tape dressing, or plastic mould following a plastic procedure on the nasal bones. Firm healing develops on about the 10th day. Usually only the surgeon changes a rhinoplasty dressing.

Monitoring after surgery

Following nasal surgery, the patient is placed in a supported sitting position to decrease local oedema, and ice compresses are usually applied to the nose to lessen the discolouration, bleeding, and discomfort. Patients can usually apply their own ice compresses.

The patient is monitored for signs of haemorrhage Some oozing on the dressing below the nose (Fig. 15-6) is expected and this dressing may be changed as necessary. If bleeding becomes pronounced, the surgeon is notified and material for repacking the nose is prepared. This material consists of a haemostatic tray containing gauze packing, umbilical tape for posterior packing, a few small gauze sponges, small catheter (used for inserting a postnasal plug), packing forceps, tongue blades, and scissors. The surgeon may require a head mirror, good light, adrenaline 1:1000 or other vasoconstrictor, 4% topical lignocaine or 4% cocaine solution, applicators, nasal speculum, and suction.

Because packing blocks the passage of air through the nose, a partial vacuum is created during swallowing, and the person may complain of a sucking action when attempting to drink. Postnasal drainage, the presence of old blood

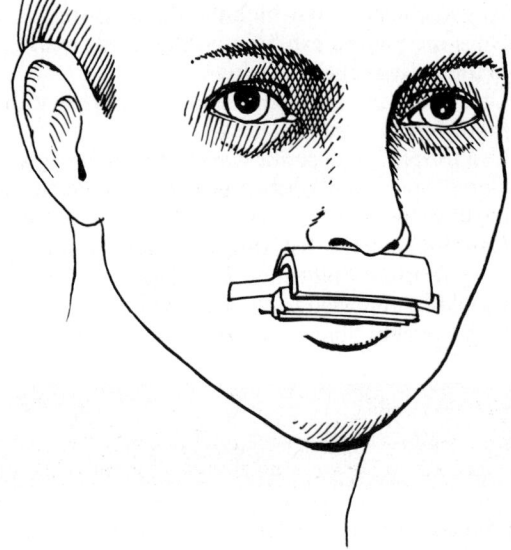

Fig. 15-6   Dressing placed under nose for nasal drainage.

in the mouth, dryness of the mouth from mouth breathing, and loss of the ability to smell often lead to anorexia. Antihistamines may be prescribed to reduce nasal secretions, and frequent mouth care is important.

Interventions to achieve patient outcomes
Facilitating learning

People with trauma to the nose should be encouraged to seek medical attention, even if obstruction is not present, because a broken nose can lead to chronic problems (for example, chronic sinusitis) if not treated. If deformities are present, the person may be disturbed about body image because of the high visibility of the face. These people need an opportunity to talk about their feelings and are encouraged to talk to the doctor about possible long-term positive changes through plastic surgery.

Evaluation

Evaluation is based on expected patient outcomes.

REVIEW

Table 15-6   Malignant disorders of nose and throat

Disorder	Description	Signs and symptoms	Medical therapy
Nasopharyngeal carcinomas	Carcinomas that obstruct nose first on one side then the other	Nasal obstruction, early metastasis to neck, bleeding	Surgery; radiation therapy
Carcinoma of maxillary and ethmoid sinuses	Relatively uncommon	Loosening of upper teeth; nasal obstruction, nosebleeds, displacement of eye, anosmia, tearing and diplopia	Chemotherapy; radiation; surgery that removes entire upper jaw (maxillectomy) and one eye (orbital enucleation)
Cancer of tonsil	May be carcinoma, lymphoepithelioma, or lymphosarcoma	Local ulceration, enlarged tonsil, pain	Surgery; radiation
Carcinoma of larynx	Squamous cell carcinoma of vocal cords and surrounding tissue	Progressive hoarseness that lasts longer than 2 weeks	Partial or total laryngectomy; radiation therapy before or after surgery

Questions to consider may include the following:

1. Does the patient exhibit a positive body image?
2. Is the patient comfortable?
3. Can the patient describe care required at home following surgery?
4. Can the patient describe ways to prevent nosebleeds?
5. Can the patient describe the expected time frame for positive cosmetic effects following rhinoplasty?
6. Can the patient list the signs and symptoms of complications (bleeding, drainage, and fever) that should be reported to the surgeon?
7. Is the patient able to breathe more easily?

MALIGNANCIES OF THE NOSE AND THROAT

Malignancies may develop in the nasopharynx, sinuses, tonsils, and larynx.

Pathophysiology

Nasopharyngeal carcinomas obstruct the nose; they metastasize early to the neck. Carcinomas of the maxillary and ethmoid sinuses may erode the adjacent nasal walls and bleed easily. Carcinoma of the maxillary sinus causes dental problems initially; other effects may include nasal obstruction, nosebleeds, and displacement of the eye. Carcinoma of the ethmoid sinus causes outward displacement of the eye, disturbance of the sense of smell, and nosebleeds. The prognosis is grave. The signs and symptoms and medical therapy of these disorders are listed in Table 15-6.

MALIGNANCY OF SINUSES

The most frequent malignancy of the nasal cavity and the paranasal sinuses is squamous cell carcinoma. The lesion is most common in the maxillary sinus. Unfortunately, there are no early symptoms to warn the patient.[10]

The diagnosis is confirmed by biopsy and CT scan, which are used to differentiate between benign and malignant lesions and to determine how far the tumour has extended.

Treatment consists of irradiation and surgery. Some surgeons prefer to irradiate the involved area before surgery, whereas other surgeons use irradation after surgery. Chemotherapeutic agents may also be prescribed in addition to surgery and radiation therapy.[10]

Maxillectomy and Orbital Enucleation

Surgery for malignancies of the sinuses consists of removal of the entire upper jaw (maxillectomy) and one eye (orbital enucleation). Split-thickness skin grafts are usually applied to the operative area. Postoperatively, the deformity of the jaw is managed with a dental prosthesis, which closes off the defect in the mouth. Several prostheses may be needed because of shrinking of the cavity as healing progresses. Radical surgery is required because of the danger of recurrence.

Postoperative care includes the following:

1. Monitor for signs of meningitis (fever, headache, neck rigidity).
2. Provide care related to nasogastric intubation (see Chapter 23).
3. Provide mouth care
   a. Use a gentle spray or oral irrigation
   b. Use saline with hydrogen peroxide, weak sodium bicarbonate, or prescribed antibiotic solution
   c. Aspiration of drainage may be necessary (care is taken to prevent trauma from suction tip).
4. Provide pain medication as needed.
5. Give prescribed prophylactic antibiotics.
6. Encourage early ambulation.
7. Provide emotional support.

People who undergo radical surgery of this type have a number of emotional adjustments to make.[25,26] The alteration in their physical appearance is readily visible; the person feels conspicuous and different. In addition to disfigurement, the person has all the normal fears of surgery and of cancer. Fear, anger, and grief are normal reactions to the situation. Fear is focused on concerns about the future, the ability to live normally, and also of being rejected. Anger and grief are common responses to the loss and the helplessness to control the loss. Oral communication also may be a problem immediately following surgery, and every effort is made to allow the person to express needs and feelings by writing if necessary. Conveying compassion and concern to the person is important.

MALIGNANCY OF TONSILS
Aetiology/Epidemiology

Malignancy of the tonsils can be one of three types: *carcinoma, lymphoepithelioma,* or *lymphosarcoma.* Carcinomas are more common in men, possibly related to the longer smoking history of some men. The carcinomas spread upward into the soft palate and usually metastasize early to the neck.

Pathophysiology

Local ulceration and otalgia (earache) are early symptoms. Lymphoepithelioma often remain small and do not ulcerate, but neck metastasis occurs early. Lymphosarcomas produce large tonsils, usually without ulceration or pain, and metastasize early to the neck.

Medical Treatment

Medical interventions for tonsillar malignancies may include radiation in conjunction with an extensive surgical procedure to remove all the malignant tissue. Chemotherapy may be used also, but it is still being tested for effectiveness. The cure rate has improved using this combined technique.[10] Recurrence often occurs locally or with distant metastasis.

MALIGNANCY OF LARYNX
Aetiology/Epidemiology

Squamous cell carcinoma of the larynx is increasing in

frequency. It is estimated that in the United States there are over 12,500 new cases and over 3,650 deaths every year.[1]

Cancer of the larynx is five times more common in men than in women, and it occurs most often in people over 60 years of age. There appears to be some relationship between cancer of the larynx and heavy smoking, alcohol use, chronic laryngitis, vocal abuse, and family predisposition to cancer. Because of the number of women who continue to be heavy smokers, the incidence of carcinoma of the larynx has increased in women. According to the American Cancer Society the percentage of deaths from laryngeal cancer in women increased 150% when figures from 1955 to 1957 and 1985 to 1987 are compared.[1]

Pathophysiology

Cancer of the larynx that is limited to the true vocal cords grows slowly because of the lymphatic supply. Elsewhere in the larynx (epiglottis, false vocal cords, and pyriform sinuses) lymphatic vessels are abundant, and cancer of these tissues often spreads rapidly and metastasizes early to the deep lymph nodes of the neck.

Any smoker who becomes progressively hoarse or is hoarse for longer than two weeks should be urged to seek medical attention at once. Hoarseness is an early symptom of cancer of the vocal cords. If treatment is given when hoarseness appears (caused by the tumour's preventing the complete approximation of the vocal cords), a cure usually is possible. Signs of metastases of cancer to other parts of the larynx include a sensation of a lump in the throat, pain in the Adam's apple that radiates to the ear, dyspnoea, dysphagia, enlarged cervical nodes, and cough). The diagnosis of cancer of the larynx is made from the patient's history, from visual examination of the larynx with indirect laryngoscopy, and from a biopsy and microscopic study of the lesion.

Diagnostic tests

A laryngeal mirror is used to visualize the larynx.

Direct laryngoscopy

When there are suspicious lesions of the larynx, a direct laryngoscopy is performed. It is usually performed with the patient under local anaesthesia with 10% cocaine or under general anaesthesia. A sedative (for example, diazepam or pethidine) and atropine sulphate (to decrease secretions) are given one hour before the examination. The person is placed in a reclining position with the head in a head holder or with the head extended over the edge of the table and manually supported by a doctor or nurse. The laryngoscope is inserted through the mouth and laryngopharynx, making the interior of the larynx easily visible. Minor surgical procedures, such as a biopsy, may be performed through the laryngoscope.

If local anaesthesia has been given, the patient should not eat or drink anything until the gag reflex returns, usually within two hours. The gag reflex can be tested by touching the back of the throat with a tongue blade or applicator. After the gag reflex returns, the patient should first try to drink water because it is the fluid least likely to cause aspiration pneumonia if it is accidentally aspirated into the trachea or lungs.

Surgery of the larynx

Treatment of carcinoma of the true vocal cord depends on the extent of the tumour involvement. If the tumour is limited to the true cord without limitation of cord movement, then radiation therapy is the best course of treatment, with cure rates of 80 to 90%. Surgical intervention is considered when extension of the tumour fixes one of the cords or extends upward or downward from the larynx. Surgery may include a partial or total laryngectomy, or radical neck dissection. Table 15-7 lists the types of laryngectomy surgery.

Partial laryngectomy

Hemilaryngectomy. In this procedure, which is also called a *vertical partial laryngectomy*, one half or more of the larynx is removed. People suitable for this procedure have malignancies involving one true vocal cord or one true vocal cord and a portion of the other. This procedure is usually well tolerated, and difficulty in swallowing is minimal. Although the quality of the voice is altered, it is adequate for communication.[10]

Supraglottic laryngectomy. When the supraglottis is invaded by cancer, a *supraglottic laryngectomy* (horizontal partial laryngectomy) is performed. The procedure usually involves the removal of endolaryngeal structures from the tip of the epiglottis down to and including the laryngeal vertical. Because the true vocal cords are preserved, the patient's voice quality is excellent. The major postoperative problem is the danger of aspiration because of difficulty in

Table 15-7 Laryngectomy surgery for cancer

Type	Description	Voice result
Partial laryngectomy		
Hemilaryngectomy	Opening into larynx through thyroid cartilage with removal of diseased false cord, arytenoid, and one side of thyroid cartilage	Hoarse voice
Supraglottic partial laryngectomy	Horizontal incision passes above true cords (left intact) with removal of epiglottis and diseased tissue	Normal voice
Total laryngectomy	Removal of epiglottis, thyroid cartilage, and 3 or 4 tracheal rings; closure of pharynx with trachea; permanent tracheostomy	No voice

swallowing. Aspiration may occur because the major reflex arc that causes closure of the larynx is initiated by sensory receptors in the supraglottic larynx, which has been removed. These patients will need special swallowing training postoperatively. Although patients take variable amounts of time to learn to swallow safely, most will be able to take feedings by mouth.

After partial laryngectomy, a temporary tracheostomy tube is inserted and removed when oedema in the surrounding tissues subsides. The person is not permitted to use the voice until the surgeon gives specific approval (usually three days postoperatively). In the past whispering was allowed, but it is now believed that whispering can further damage the voice. This problem is currently under study. The person usually adjusts quite readily to relatively minor limitations of speech. The main problems encountered by people undergoing partial laryngectomy are those of swallowing and aspiration.

Total laryngectomy

When cancer of the larynx is advanced, a total laryngectomy may be performed. This includes removal of the epiglottis, thyroid cartilage, hyoid bone, cricoid cartilage, and three or four rings of the trachea. The pharyngeal opening to the trachea is closed, the anterior wall of the laryngopharynx (hypopharynx) is closed, and the remaining trachea is brought out to the neck wound and sutured to the skin. It forms an opening (permanent tracheostomy) through which the patient breathes (Fig. 15-7). The presence of a tracheal stoma affects the sense of smell because breathing through the nose is impossible; therefore, the person does not receive olfactory sensations. The person has no voice because of removal of the larynx. The nursing care of the patient with a laryngectomy is outlined in Box 15-8.

Radical neck dissection

A radical neck dissection may be performed along with a laryngectomy in patients whose risk of metastases to the neck from carcinoma of the larynx is high. This includes *primary tumours whose size and location are known to result in metastasis and palpable cervical lymph nodes at time of surgery*. In a radical neck dissection the submandibular salivary gland, sternocleidomastoid muscle, internal jugular vein, and spinal accessory nerve are removed to assure complete removal of nodal-bearing tissue.[10] In some patients a modification of a radical neck dissection is performed. These are referred to as *modified, conservation,* or *functional* neck dissections and are used when the nodal metastatic disease is not far advanced. These procedures cause atrophy of the trapezius muscle, and the shoulder droops on the side of surgery.

Patients can be taught to do exercises with other muscles that gradually replace the function of the lost muscles. Most patients have difficulty lifting their heads. They can be taught to place both hands behind their necks with fingers interlocked when lifting the head from the pillow. The patient is more comfortable and can breathe better when placed in a supported sitting position. Pressure dressings are best avoided in radical neck dissection because they compromise the blood supply to the skin

Guidelines for Care   15-8

Postoperative care of the patient following a laryngectomy

Elevate head of bed 45°
Encourage coughing, deep breathing every 4 hours; maintain oxygen to trach collar
Incentive spirometry if ordered
Assess airway patency every shift and as required
   Vital signs
   Quality and rate of respiration
   Skin colour (pallor, cyanosis)
   Auscultation of lungs every shift and as required
Monitor hydration and ensure adequate fluid intake to maintain healthy oral mucosa; provide mouth care at least 3 times a day
   Record intake and output every shift
   Weigh daily at the same time and in same amount of clothing
Provide stoma and stoma vent care every shift and as required
Begin teaching laryngectomy care
Ambulate 3 times a day and as required
Assess anxiety level and provide emotional support
Assist patient in communicating
   Provide patient with a pen and paper
   Use questions that can be answered yes or no
   Reinforce use of artificial speech device and encourage its use
Assess suture line and stoma site every 4 hours
   Report erythema, purulent drainage, haematoma
Care for suture line and stoma site as ordered by surgeon
Monitor drain function and output
   Maintain suction to drain at level ordered
   Milk tubing every 1-2 hours for 24 hours; and then every 4 hours and as required
   Report changes in amount and colour of drainage
Administer enteral feedings per order
   Assess patient's tolerance of feedings
   Assess bowel sounds every shift and as required
   Report intolerance to feedings (nausea, fullness, inability to tolerate prescribed amount of feedings)
Record amount, consistency, and frequency of stools
Assess swallowing ability and provide support when oral diet resumes
Monitor patient's reaction to change in body image
   Be sensitive to patient's reactions to changes in appearance
   Provide time to listen to patient
   Encourage use of support groups
Prepare patient for discharge
   Monitor ability of patient or significant other to perform airway management care
   Provide patient with list of supplies necessary for home care
   Review written instructions in home-going booklet

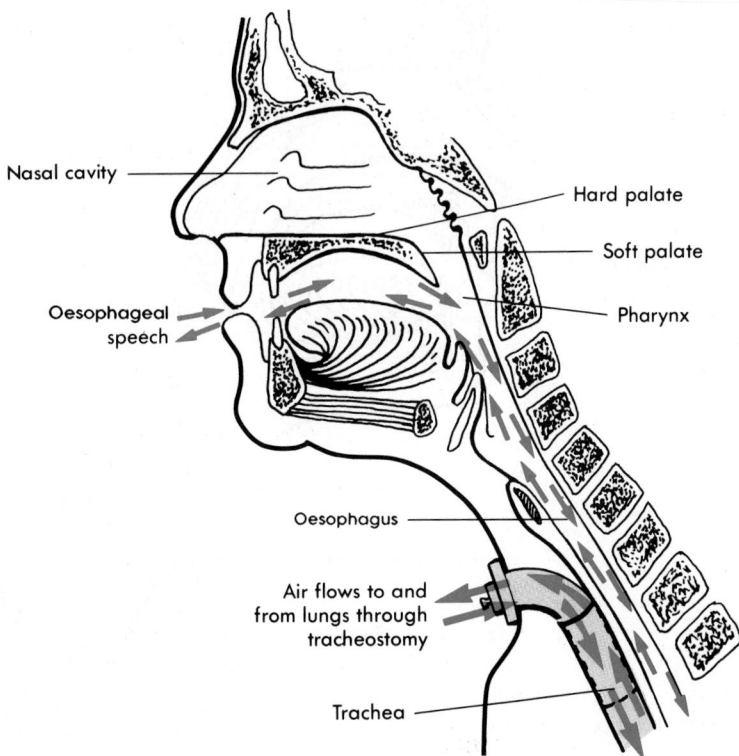

Nasal cavity

Hard palate

Soft palate

Oesophageal
speech

Pharynx

Oesophagus

Air flows to and
from lungs through
tracheostomy

Trachea

Fig. 15-7   Permanent tracheostomy: no connection exists between trachea and oesophagus.

flaps protecting the vital neck structures.

The Haemovac is one device available to keep constant drainage from the neck wound without pressure on the flaps. The Haemovac must be checked to see that it is working properly and that there is no oedema, which might indicate haematoma. The tubing is milked every one to two hours for the first 24 hours postoperatively and then every four hours and as required. Changes in the amount or colour of drainage should be reported to the surgeon.

Some alteration of appearance is readily visible, which may cause the person to feel somewhat conspicuous. Anger, grief, or denial may be part of the normal response to the change in body image. (For further information on psychological support, refer to Chapter 9.)

Radical neck dissection can be performed without laryngectomy for people whose primary malignant lesion is in the tongue, tonsil, lip, nasopharynx, or thyroid. Often the procedure accompanies other procedures and is termed a *composite resection*. Composite resections may include either radical neck dissection in addition to the removal of the mandible; removal of the mandible and resection of the floor of the mouth; or removal of the mandible, floor of the mouth, and the tongue. Emotional reactions to this type of radical surgery may be profound. Disfigurement is readily visible, and reactions to the change in body image are marked. In addition to the usual fears of surgery and cancer, the patient having a composite resection may have fears of rejection and fears concerning the future.

Preoperative care. The person who is to have a laryngectomy is told by the doctor that breathing will occur through a special opening made in the neck and that normal speech will not be possible. This is often depressing to the patient because it may threaten economic status, as well as life. In some instances, it is helpful to receive a visit from another person who has made a good recovery from laryngectomy and who has undergone rehabilitation successfully. In other instances, this visit may depress the patient further. Careful assessment must be made to determine if the person will benefit from such a visit and whether the visit should be made preoperatively, immediately after surgery, or later in the recovery period.

Often no one else can give a person reassurance that speech can be regained as well as a fellow patient. The majority of ENT units have patients who are willing to return to the ward to visit "new patients" to talk about their experience, and how they overcame specific difficulties. Great care needs to be taken, however, before these types of support agencies are used. The nurse needs to be sure of the "counselling patient", and a briefing should take place beforehand so that the nursing staff know what kind of information is going to be given out. Immediate follow-up of the patient should take place to assess his/her feelings postmeeting, and to evaluate the outcome. Further support and information in the United Kingdom can be obtained from the National Association of Laryngectomee Clubs*. The hospital speech therapist can also provide support and information to the patient and family, perhaps by teaching oesophageal speech to the family which the patient will learn.

Postoperative care. Postoperative care of the person is

---

* National Association of Laryngectomy Clubs, Ground floor, 6 Rickett Street, Fulham, London SW6 1RU.

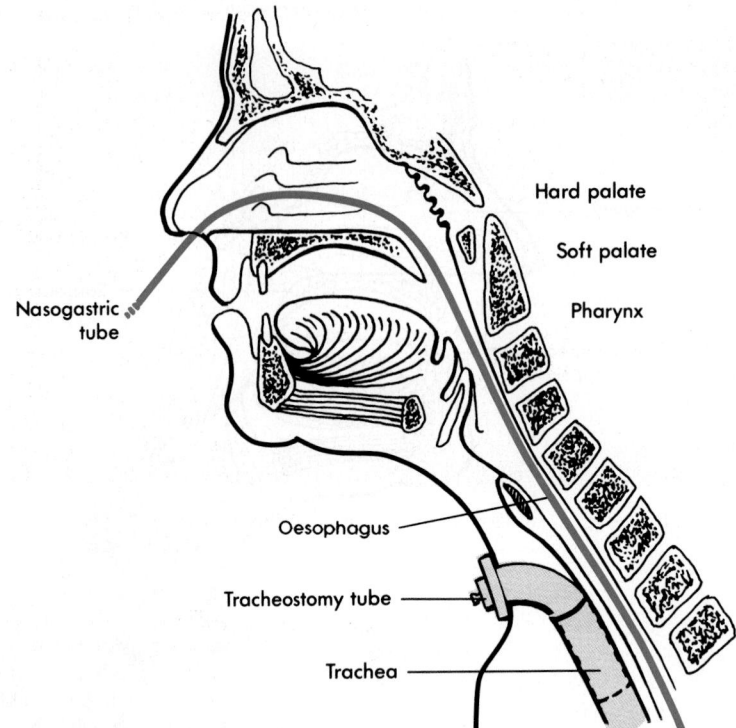

Hard palate

Soft palate

Pharynx

Nasogastric
tube

Oesophagus

Tracheostomy tube

Trachea

Fig. 15-8   Position of tracheostomy tube and nasogastric tube following total laryngectomy.

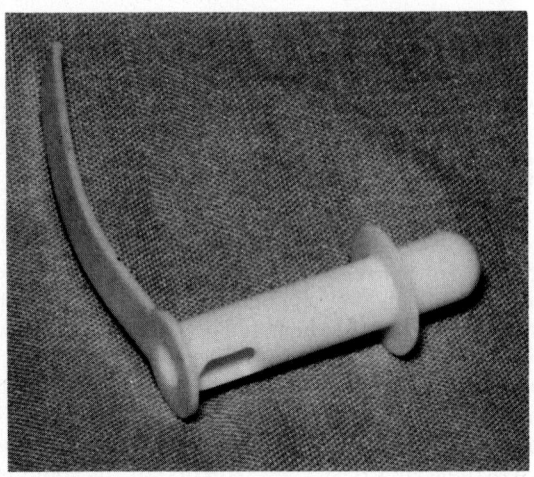

Fig. 15-9   This vocal prosthesis allows for the passage of air from the trachea into the hypopharynx but prevents the opposite flow of saliva. (From DeWeese DD, et al: *Otolaryngology—head and neck surgery*, ed 7, St Louis, 1988, Mosby–Year Book.)

essentially the same as that described for tracheostomy (Chapter 16) except that these people will have a *laryngectomy tube* in place, a tube that is shorter and wider in diameter than a tracheostomy tube. Some patients may not have a tube in the stoma after the operation because the stoma is a permanent one kept open initially by the sutures and because their surgeon believes that there is less tissue reaction and a better stoma if no tube is used. If a laryngectomy tube is used, it remains until the wound is healed and a permanent fistula has formed, usually within two to three weeks. Frequent suctioning is necessary in the early postoperative period to keep the trachea free of secretions.

A *nasogastric tube* is usually inserted during the surgical procedure for the instillation of food and fluids at regular intervals postoperatively for about 10 days (Fig. 15-8). The use of the tube to give food is thought to minimize contamination of the pharyngeal and oesophageal suture lines and to prevent fluid from leaking through the wound into the trachea before healing occurs. The nasogastric tube is removed as soon as the person can safely swallow. The person then needs careful attention in the first attempts to swallow. There may be the sensation of choking and severe coughing, which is frightening and painful. Aspiration cannot occur because the trachea no longer communicates with the oesophagus.

The sense of smell is affected after laryngectomy because breathing through the nose is impossible, therefore, the patient does not receive olfactory sensations.

Speech rehabilitation. Until recently, *oesophageal speech* was the primary speech method after laryngectomy. Although this method of speech was successful for many laryngectomees, others could never learn to use it. In addition, the increased use of radiation therapy after laryngectomy causes fibrous tissue to form, making *oesophageal speech* less possible.

For a number of years, surgeons had been working to develop other forms of speech after laryngectomy. In 1980 the first successful procedure using surgical-prosthetic voice restoration was introduced. In this procedure, a *tracheo-oesophageal puncture* (TEP) is made to create a tracheo-oesophageal fistula large enough to permit the insertion of a valve prosthesis. The TE fistula is created after the larynx has been resected and a frozen section indicates

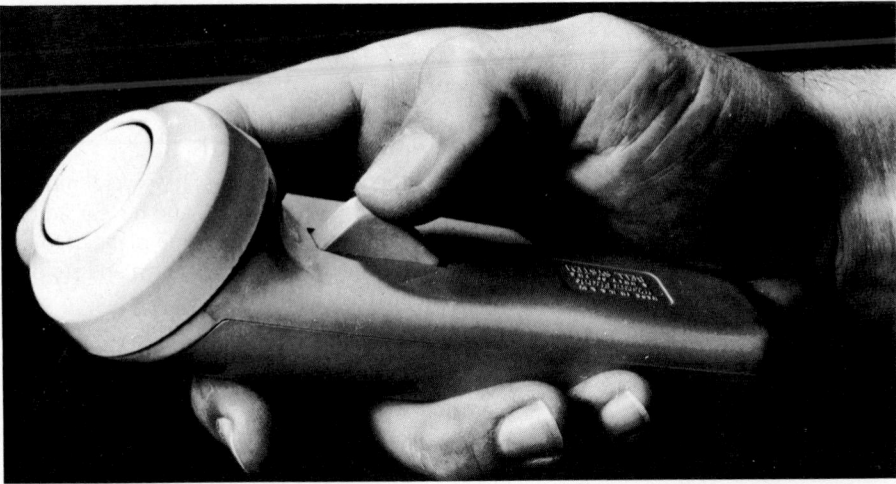

Fig. 15-10   Battery-powered electronic artificial larynx for patient who has total laryngectomy and cannot learn oesophageal speech. (Courtesy Illinois Bell Telephone Co.)

that all of the carcinoma has been removed. A red rubber catheter is pulled through the fistula into the oesophagus and sutured in place. The end of the catheter is occluded with an umbilical clamp. The patient is discharged with the catheter in place.[43] The prosthesis is a hollow tube open at the tracheal end and closed with a horizontal slit at the laryngopharyngeal end (Fig. 15-9). When the patient talks, air pressure opens the closed end, permitting air to enter the laryngopharynx. When the patient stops talking, the laryngopharyngeal end closes preventing saliva from draining into the trachea. Because air is diverted from the trachea into the oesophagus, this form of speech is referred to as *tracheo-oesophageal speech.*

The stoma must be occluded during speech, either by placing a finger over the opening or by using a special tracheostomal valve inserted after the patient has learned to use the prosthesis. The patient or family must be taught to remove, clean, and reinsert the voice prosthesis rapidly so that stenosis of the fistula does not occur. Not all patients and families are comfortable with removing and cleaning

the prosthesis, and considerable support by the speech therapist may be necessary. Ideally, the patient should be able to use the prosthesis for speaking and be able to clean and reinsert it before discharge from the hospital.

Early evidence indicates that there are several advantages of *tracheo-oesophageal speech.* These include more rapid restoration of voice, speech that is closer to normal in rate and phrasing, and speech that is more pleasing than speech with an electrolarynx. Disadvantages include reliance on a prosthesis and the rapidity with which the tracheo-oesophageal fistula may undergo stenosis.[10] For this reason, all three methods of speaking are still in use, and none are mutually exclusive. In fact, some patients find it useful to use more than one of the methods (Box 15-9).

Information about devices used to produce electronic speech can be obtained from the speech therapist, National Association of Laryngectomee Clubs, or the British Voice Association*, as can information about oesophageal speech.

Teaching the patient to use *oesophageal* speech is started as soon as the oesophageal suture line is healed. To learn

---

* British Voice Association, 77B Abbey Road, London, NW8 OAE.

15-9	Speech methods following total laryngectomy	
	Tracheo-oesophageal prosthesis	Formation of a tracheo-oesophageal fistula with insertion of a silicone prosthesis that produces a sound in the oesophagus (Fig. 15-9)
	Oesophageal speech	Speech produced by expelling swallowed air (burping) across constricted tissue in the pharyngo-oesophageal segment
	External speech aids	Mechanical devices, such as a vibrator or electronic artificial larynx, used externally (Fig. 15-10)

15-10	Patient following total laryngectomy
	1. Wear a scarf or shirt with closed collar of porous material (to warm and screen air over stoma). 2. Use caution while taking a bath or shower (to prevent aspiration of water in stoma). 3. Check with surgeon concerning swimming or boating; if swimming is permitted, use a special snorkle device designed for tracheostomees. 4. Use available community resources for support and speech rehabilitation as necessary (for example, laryngectomee clubs). 5. Seek immediate medical attention for respiratory tract infection or signs of stomal bleeding. 6. Continue medical follow-up as per doctor instructions.

Nursing Care Plan	Person with laryngectomy

DATA: Mr K, a 68-year-old man, had noted progressive hoarseness for several months. Indirect laryngoscopy and biopsy confirmed cancer of the larynx, and he was admitted for a total laryngectomy. His wife accompanied him to the hospital and planned to be with him as much as possible during his hospitalization. She was attentative and suppotive.

The following pertinent data were indentified on admission:
1. He was visibly apprehensive (pacing the floor, restless, asking repeated questions).
2. His major concerns centred on the extent of the cancer and on communication problems following the surgery.
3. His height is 175cm (5ft 10in), weight 68kg (150lb).
4. He wears glasses; near vision is poor without glasses.

Before surgery, Mr K's primary nurse spent time with him, encouraging him to express his concerns and providing information about what to expect in the postoperative period and care that would be provided. Following the interaction, Mr K's restlessness decreased and he was observed talking quietly with his wife and watching TV.

The larynx was removed during surgery; a permanent tracheostomy was performed, with insertion of a temporary laryngectomy tube. A tracheal oesophageal catheter was in place. The end of the catheter was occluded with an umbilical clamp to prevent drainage of gastric contents into the surgical wound. A nasogastric tube was inserted, to be removed after Mr K was swallowing well. During the first postoperative day, Mr K again appeared apprehensive (restlessness, pointing frequently to the tracheostomy, pulling on his wife's hand, and pointing to the call cord to call the nurse). Breath sounds in the upper lobes were clear but were absent in the lower lobes. Codeine and paracetamol were prescribed for pain.

Nursing analysis: Anxiety, related to breathing difficulties and inability to communicate

Expected patient outcomes	Nursing interventions	Rationale
Mr K rests quietly and does not call frequently for suctioning	Explain suctioning procedure and carry out regular suctioning of tracheostomy	If Mr K knows tube will be suctioned frequently, fear of possible asphyxiation should decrease
	Develop a means of communication (such as cards, with needs printed clearly, or pen and paper for writing); be sure Mr K wears his glasses	If Mr K can communicate needs, anxiety should decrease; his glasses are needed for visual communication
	After initial period and if wife is willing and able, teach her to help with suctioning tracheostomy	Participating in husband's care may assist wife in feeling she is helping, thus decreasing her anxiety (anxiety can be transmitted to patient)
	Encourage Mr K to care for own tracheostomy when feasible	Self-care enhances feeling of control of situation

Nursing analysis: Airway clearance, ineffective: related to secretions in upper airway and laryngectomy tube

Expected patient outcomes	Nursing interventions	Rationale
Respirations are effortless, quiet, and at baseline rate	Place Mr K in a supported sitting position	Position uses gravity to help expand thorax and decrease pressure on lower lobes
Breath sounds are clear at all lobes	Suction laryngectomy tube as often as needed as evidenced by noisy respirations, increased pulse and respiratory rate, and restlessness (may be as often as every 5 minutes initially)	Air blowing through secretions produces noisy respirations; pulse and respirations are increased when oxygen intake is decreased; restlessness may indicate decreased oxygen
	Provide tracheostomy care, including suctioning as needed	Keeping tube patent will facilitate air interchange
	Provide air humidification	Humidity will help keep secretions liquid for easier removal
	Encourage deep breathing and coughing	Deep breathing will help aerate lower lobes; coughing will help expel secretions

Nursing analysis: Nutrition, altered: less than body requirements related to difficulty in swallowing

Expected patient outcomes	Nursing interventions	Rationale
Weight is not more than 11kg from baseline	Give prescribed tube feedings via nasogastric tube until patient can swallow well (usually 7 days)	Tube feedings provide more nutrients than intravenous fluids; swallowing is impaired initially from postoperative oedema of lower pharynx
	When nasogastric tube is removed, give fluids only until Mr K is swallowing well	Fluids are easier to swallow than solid food until oedema subsides
	Explain anatomical changes to Mr K (no connection between oesophagus and tracheostomy)	May help to decrease Mr K's concern about choking
	Stay with Mr K during initial eating of semisolid and solid foods	Mr K may fear choking and not be willing to swallow initially; encouragement by nurse with assurance of suctioning if necessary may inspire more confidence
	Use measures to encourage eating as necessary (tray for wife so they can eat together, selection of desired foods, and a pleasant atmosphere)	Return to usual eating patterns may encourage Mr K to eat
	Encourage Mr K to monitor weight 2–3 times a week until baseline weight is regained	Participating in monitoring own weight may motivate Mr K to eat

Nursing analysis: Pain: related to surgery

Expected patient outcomes	Nursing interventions	Rationale
Mr K is relaxed and signals feeling comfortable	Give prescribed analgesic for pain	Analgesics will decrease transmission and interpretation of pain stimuli
	Encourage other pain-relieving measures such as relaxation exercises or distraction	Help to minimize pain perception
	Provide nose and mouth care while nasogastric tube is in place	Tube may irritate nose; mouth becomes dry and uncomfortable from open mouth breathing and decreased lubrication (unable to swallow fluids)

Continued.

Nursing Care Plan	Person with laryngectomy—cont'd

Nursing analysis: Knowledge deficit: related to need to care for self after discharge

Expected patient outcomes	Nursing interventions	Rationale
Mr K describes self-care	Teach Mr K description of ana-tomical changes Provide written instructions for all aspects listed below Teach Mr K care of stoma includ-ing self-suctioning Teach Mr K methods to protect stoma	Providing own care will give Mr K self-confidence; care is needed to keep the tracheostomy open for air exchange
	Advise Mr K of availability of com-munity resources and provide written list	Mr K may be interested in support groups for sharing of experiences
	Teach Mr K how to reinsert tracheo-oesophageal tube and to go to hospital if cannot reinsert	Need to maintain tracheo-oesophageal fistula so tracheo-oesophageal speech can be achieved

Nursing analysis: Communication, impaired verbal related to laryngectomy

Expected patient outcomes	Nursing interventions	Rationale
Mr K communicates with others	Encourage Mr K to communicate using system devised with him preoperatively (hand signals, writ-ing)	Absence of larynx makes speech impossible
Mr K understands need to retain tracheo-oesophageal catheter in fistula	Reinforce with Mr K preoperative teaching about tracheo-oesophageal speech and purpose of a catheter	Catheter in fistula prevents aspira-tion and maintains patency of tracheo-oesophageal fistula
Mr K understands options available to assist with speech	Review instructions about oesopha-geal and electro-oesophageal speech	Tracheo-oesophageal prosthesis will be fitted at first postoperative visit Electronic devices are available to assist him to speak as necessary
Mr K understands need for follow-up care after discharge	Reinforce need for regular follow-up with speech therapist and sur-geon after discharge	For best speech results he will be followed at least 1 year by sur-geon and speech therapist

oesophageal speech, the patient must first practise burp-ing. This provides the moving column of air needed for sound, while folds of tissue at the opening of the oesopha-gus act as the vibrating surface. The patients must learn to coordinate articulation with oesophageal vocalization made possible by aspirating air into the oesophagus. The new voice sounds are natural, although somewhat hoarse. The qualities of speech provided by the use of the nasopharynx are still present. The patient may have digestive difficulty while learning to speak; this is caused by swallowing air during practice, by unusual strain on abdominal muscles, and by nervous tension. Digestive difficulties usually abate with proficiency in speaking.

Most patients learn oesophageal speech best at a special clinic. Although some individuals may need to go to a nearby city for this instruction, they usually must remain away from home for only one or two weeks. Motivation and persistent effort are essential in learning this kind of speech; encouragement and support from the professional staff and the patient's significant others are important to the patient's morale. About 75% of all patients who have their larynx removed master some sort of speech, and the average person can return to work one or two months after leaving the hospital.

If a person is unable to learn oesophageal speech in 60 to 90 days after surgery, a *speech aid* such as a vibrator or an electronic artificial larynx (Fig. 15-10) may be pre-scribed. Various mechanical devices are available, and the new ones permit a natural type of speech, providing pitch inflections and volume control. The speech therapist can provide information about the availability and purchase of these devices.

Reconstructive surgery

Because of the extensive surgery required to treat malig-nancies of the head and neck, reconstructive surgery may be necessary. In the past, skin grafts and pedicle or rotation skin flaps were used for reconstruction. Today the *myocutaneous flap* is the major reconstructive flap used after radical neck dissection and traumatic defects of the head and neck.

Myocutaneous flaps use the axial blood supply that supplies muscle mass, as well as cutaneous and subcutaneous tissue. The inclusion of muscle with its blood supply when transferring the skin allows for a much greater range of rotation of the flap. The *pectoralis major*, the *latissimus dorsi*, the *trapezius*, and the *sternocleidomastoid muscles* can be used for *myocutaneous flaps*.

The care of these patients is complex, and there are many nursing requirements both preoperatively and postoperatively. For further information, references 29 and 38 are two excellent articles on the nursing care of these patients.

Discharge teaching

People with laryngectomies must take special precautions because of the permanent tracheostomy (Box 15-10). Usually by the time of discharge, patients with laryngectomies do not need suctioning of the tracheostomy but can cough up secretions. If suctioning is deemed necessary, patients or their families need to be told where to secure the necessary suction equipment and how to care for themselves. Suction equipment can be rented for home use or obtained in many communities through local GP services.

Nursing Process
Assessment
Subjective data

People with carcinomas of the larynx can have a variety of symptoms, which include the following:
1. Persistent hoarseness (two weeks or longer).
2. Sore throat.
3. Odynophagia (pain when swallowing).

Objective data

1. Hoarseness is obvious when speaking.
2. Patient appears restless and anxious and has many questions about impending surgery.

Nursing analysis

Nursing analyses are determined from an assessment of patient data. Possible nursing analyses for the person undergoing total laryngectomy may include, but are not

Problems	Possible aetiologies
Airway clearance, ineffective	Presence of laryngectomy tube, increased tranchobronchial secretions
Anxiety	Threat to self-concept, inability to speak, threat to socioeconomic status
Aspiration, potential for	Presence of layngectomy tube

Problems	Possible aetiologies
Body image disturbance	Disfiguring surgery
Infection, potential for	Surgical incision
Nutrition, altered; less than body requirement	Swallowing difficulty
Oral mucous membrane, altered	Surgery
Pain, postoperative	Surgery
Communication, impaired verbal	Laryngectomy

limited to, the following:

Planning: expected patient outcomes

Expected patient outcomes for the person undergoing total laryngectomy may include, but are not limited to, the following:
1. Patient maintains respiratory rate of 12 to 18 breaths per minute.
2. Respirations are quiet: breath sounds are clear in all lobes.
3. Patient does not exhibit signs of anxiety (restlessness, increased pulse and respiration).
4. Patient is able to swallow without aspirating.
5. Patient verbalizes acceptance of laryngectomy and begins to acknowledge feelings about change in body image.
6. Patient does not develop an infection in the suture line.
7. Patient's weight at time of discharge from hospital is not less than 11 kg from baseline weight.
8. Patient's oral mucous membrane is moist and pink.
9. Patient signals that he or she is feeling comfortable.
10. Patient communicates using hand signals or pen and paper.
11. Patient is a willing participant in speech rehabilitation.

Implementation
Assisting with the achievement of therapeutic goals

Nursing interventions can be found in the Nursing Care Plan on p. 282 and Box 15-8.

Evaluation

Evaluation is based on expected patient outcome. Questions to consider about a patient having a laryngectomy and TEP may include the following:
1. Does patient maintain respiratory rate of 12 to 18 breaths per minute?
2. Are respirations quiet and breath sounds clear in all lobes?
3. Does patient exhibit minimal signs of anxiety?
4. Is the patient able to swallow without aspirating?
5. Does the patient verbalize acceptance of laryngectomy?
6. Is the patient beginning to acknowledge how he or she feels about the change in body image?
7. Is the patient free of infection in the suture line?
8. Is the patient's weight within 11 kg from baseline at discharge?
9. Is patient comfortable?
10. Is the patient able to communicate using hand signals or in writing?
11. Is the patient a willing participant in speech rehabilitation?

SUMMARY

1. The major infections of the nose and sinuses are rhinitis (common cold), allergic rhinitis (hay fever), chronic rhinitis secondary to repeated infections or allergy, and sinusitis caused by bacteria or viruses.
2. Subjective assessment of the person with a nose or

sinus problem includes a careful history of infections, how they were treated and self-treatment by the person including the use of over-the-counter medications.

3. The most common throat inflammation is acute pharyngitis. Haemolytic streptococci, staphylococci, and other bacteria and viruses may be the source of infection. Pharyngitis caused by *N. gonorrhoeae* is being seen more commonly in both men and women.

4. Obstructions of the nose, such as a deviated septum, are often treated surgically by septoplasty or submucous resection (SMR); SMR is being used less frequently than in the past.

5. Postoperative care following nasal surgery includes the following:
   a. Monitor for haemorrhage.
   b. Place patient in a supported sitting position to decrease local oedema.
   c. Place ice compresses over the nose for 24 hours and as needed.
   d. Provide food and fluids as tolerated.
   e. Provide frequent oral care.
   f. Change dressing under nose as needed.
   g. Teach patient to avoid blowing nose for 48 hours after packing is removed to prevent bleeding.
   h. Teach patient to avoid constipation and vigorous coughing until healing occurs because coughing and Valsalva manoeuvre may initiate bleeding.
   i. Explain that stools may be tarry for several days.

6. Progressive or persistent hoarseness that lasts longer than two weeks requires medical evaluation for cancer of the larynx.

7. Carcinoma of the larynx is treated with a partial or total laryngectomy.

8. Partial laryngectomy may be achieved by a hemilaryngectomy, or supraglottic partial laryngectomy after which the person will be able to speak.

9. Total laryngectomy is necessary when cancer of the larynx is far advanced. People with total laryngectomy are unable to speak normally, but will be able to have some form of speech.

10. There are three major forms of speech following laryngectomy: oesophageal, tracheo-oesophageal, and external speech aide.

11. Tracheo-oesophageal speech requires the formation of a fistula after all the carcinoma has been removed. This procedure is called a TEP.

12. A radical neck dissection is commonly performed along with total laryngectomy because of the possible metastasis to the neck.
   a. Postoperatively the person will have a laryngectomy tube and a nasogastric tube in place.
   b. Communication is impaired because of the loss of ability to speak and the person will require speech rehabilitation.

REFERENCES AND SELECTED READINGS

1. American Cancer Society: *19 Cancer facts and figures*, Atlanta, 1991, The Society.

2. Baker, KH, Feldman JE: Cancers of the head and neck, *Cancer Nurs*, 10(6):293-299, 1987.

3. Brown PE, Coleman JJ: The role of radiotherapy and musculocutaneous flaps in oropharyngocutaneous fistulas, *Am J Surg* 156 and 256-260, 1988.

4. Burke RH: A simplified nasal packing, *J Oral Maxillofac Surg* 43:555, 1985.

5. Calhoun KH: Otolaryngology—head and neck surgery, *JAMA* 265(230):3152-3154, 1991.

6. Carroll PF: Laryngospasm, *Nurs 86* 16(5):33, 1986.

7. Causes of stuffy nose: external nasal deformity, *Hosp Med* 21(5):194-198, 1985.

8.* Chisholm S, et al: Duck-bill prosthesis: words of hope for the laryngectomy patient, *Nurs 86* 16(3):29-31, 1986.

9. Clark KM: *Hoarseness and laryngitis*. In Rakel RE, editors: *Conn's current therapy 1990*, Philadelphia, 1990, WB Saunders.

10. DeWeese DD, Saunders WH: *Otolaryngology, head and neck surgery*, ed 7, St Louis, 1987, Mosby–Year Book.

11. Dropkin MJ: Coping with disfigurement and dysfunction after head and neck cancer surgery: a conceptual framework, *Semin Oncol Nurs* 5(3):213-219, 1989.

12. Ebersole P, Hess P: *Toward healthy aging*, ed 3, St. Louis, 1990, Mosby–Year Book.

13. Eichel B: Ethmoiditis: pathophysiology and medical manage-ment, *Otolaryngol Clin North Am* 18(1):43-53, 1985.

14.* Feinstein D: What to teach the patient who's had a total laryngectomy, *RN* 59(4):53-57, 1987.

15. Fosso BA: Sore throat, antibiotics and rheumatic fever, *Fam Pract* 2:101-107, 1985.

16. Gantz NM: *Streptococcal pharyngitis*. In Rakel RE, editor: *Conn's current therapy 1990*, Philadelphia, 1990, WB Saunders.

17.* Grant M, Rhimer J, Padilla GV: Nutritional management in head and neck cancer patient, *Semin Oncol Nurs* 5(3):195-204, 1989.

18.* Griffin CW, et al: Learning to swallow again, *Am J Nurs* 87:314-315, 1987.

19. Harold ML: Rehabilitation of the dysphagic client following ablative surgery for laryngeal cancer, *J Soc Otorhinolaryngol Head Neck Nurses* 5(2):16-18, 1987.

20.* Harris LL, Kraege J: After T-E puncture: relearning to speak, *Am J Nurs* 86(1):55-58, 1986.

21.* Harris LL, Smith S: Chemotherapy in head and neck cancer, *Semin Oncol Nurs* 5(3):174-181, 1989.

22. Hendrickson FR: Radiation therapy treatment of larynx cancers, *Cancer* 55:2058-2061, 1985.

23. Innes AJ, Gates N: ENT surgery and disorders, with notes on nursing care and clinical management, London, 1985, Faber & Faber.

24. Jafek BW: Intranasal ethmoidectomy, *Otolaryngol Clin North Am* 18(1):61-67, 1985.

25.* Kennedy DW, et al: Endoscopic sinus surgery: ambulatory surgery, *AORN J* 42:932-936, 1985.

26. Kennedy DW, Shikhani AH: *Sinusitis*. In Rakel RE, editor: *Conn's current therapy 1990*, Philadelphia, 1990, WB Saunders.

27. Knegt PP, et al: Carcinoma of the paranasal sinuses: results of a prospective pilot study, *Cancer* 56:57-62, 1985.

28. Konda M, et al: Prognostic factors influencing relapse of squamous cell carcinoma of the maxillary sinus, *Cancer* 55:190-196, 1985.

29.* Mahon SM: Nursing interventions for the patient with a myocutaneous flap, *Cancer Nurs* 10(1):21-31, 1987.

30. Mandel JH: Pharyngeal infections: causes, findings, and management, *Postgrad Med* 77;187-193, 1985.

31. Martin LK: Management of the altered airway in the head and neck cancer patient, *Semin Oncol Nurs* 5(3):182-190, 1989.

32. Mathieson CM, Stam JH, Scott JP: Psychosocial adjustment after laryngectomy: a review of the literature, *J Otolaryngol* 19(5):331-336, 1990.

33. Minx SM, et al: Carcinoma of the parasinus: perioperative nursing responsibilities, *AORN J* 42:671-681, 1985.

34. Neal GD: External ethmoidectomy, *Otolaryngol Clin North Am* 18:55-60, 1985.

35. Panje WR: *Sinusitis*. In Rakel RE, editor: *Conn's current therapy 1991*, Philadelphia, 1991, WB Saunders.

36. Parsons JT, et al: Neck dissection after twice-a-day radio-therapy: morbidity and recurrence rates, *Head Neck* 11(5):400-404, 1989.

37.* Patry-Lahey R: Doing it better: helping a laryngectomy patient go home, *Nurs 85* 15(3):63-64, 1985.

38.* Rodzwic D, Donnard J: The use of myocutaneous flaps in reconstructive surgery for head and neck cancer, *Oncol Nurs Forum* 13(3):29-34, 1986.

39. Romm S: Cancer of the larynx: current concepts of diagnosis and treatment, *Surg Clin North Am* 66:109-118, 1986.

40.* Rook IL, Rook M: Head and neck cancer, *J Postanesth Nurs,* 4(6):363-372, 1989.

41.* Sawyer DL, Bruya MA: Care of the patient having radical neck surgery or permanent laryngostomy: a nursing diagnostic approach, *Focus Crit Care* 17(2):166-173, 1990.

42. Schleper JR: Prevention, detection, and diagnosis of head and neck cancers, *Semin Oncol Nurs* 5(3):139-149, 1989.

FURTHER READING

Allan D: Making sense of ..... tracheostomy. *Nurs Times* 83(45):36-38: 11-17, 1987.

Caruana SR: Myths and facts .... about tracheal tubes. *Nursing* 20(6): 30 June 1990.

Mapp CS: Trach care: are you aware of all the dangers? *Nursing* 18(7):34-43, 1988.

Martin LK: Management of the altered airway in the head and neck cancer patient, *Semin Oncol Nurs* 5(3): 182-190, 1989.

Roberts A: Systems and signs. Locomotor system: head, neck and shoulders, *Nurs Times* 78: Nov, 3-9, 1982.

Saunders SH: Tonsils, adenoids and grommets, *Midwife, Health Visitor and Community Nurse,* 25(12): 516-517, 1989.

Sawyer DL: Care of the patient having radical neck surgery or a permanent laryngostomy: a nursing diagnostic approach, *Focus On Critical Care* 17(2): 166-173, 1990.

* Recommended for student reading

16

The Patient with Pulmonary Problems

Wilma J. Phipps

After studying this chapter, the learner should be able to:

- Differentiate between restrictive and obstructive pulmonary disorders.
- Describe the nature of viral respiratory infections and methods of assisting effective coughing.
- Compare classic, atypical, aspiration, and haematogenous pneumonia.
- Describe measures to promote oxygenation, facilitate breathing, and provide ventilation and hydration.
- Describe incidence, preventive measures, and therapeutic approaches to tuberculosis.
- Compare fungal infections of the respiratory tract.
- Explain the pathophysiology of adult respiratory distress syndrome (ARDS).
- Describe incidence, prevention, and therapy for lung cancer.
- Describe types of chest surgery and the care of the patient undergoing chest surgery (including patients with chest drains).
- Describe the pathophysiological conditions of chest trauma (for instance, fractured ribs, penetrating wounds, and pneumothorax).
- Explain the pathophysiological conditions and interventions for chronic obstructive pulmonary disease.
- Describe the nature of respiratory insufficiency and the care of the patient with an artificial airway or mechanical ventilation.

ANATOMY AND PHYSIOLOGY OF THE RESPIRATORY TRACT

The main purpose of respiration is to provide oxygen to body cells and to remove excess carbon dioxide from them. For respiration to take place there must be a way to deliver oxygen (O_2) to the body and a circulatory system to carry it to the cells and to remove carbon dioxide (CO_2) from them. The transport of O_2 is accomplished through the upper and lower airway.

Upper Airway

The upper airway consists of the nose and sinuses, the pharynx and tonsils, and the larynx and laryngopharynx (see Chapter 15).

Lower Airway

Structure and function of the respiratory tract

The *conducting airways* (trachea, right and left main or primary bronchi, and bronchioles), which terminate into *respiratory units* (respiratory bronchioles, alveolar ducts, and alveoli), make up the lower airways (Fig. 16-1).

In addition to providing a passageway for air, the *conducting airways serve three functions: filtering, warming, and humidifying air*. Air inspired through an intact respiratory tree is cleansed of all particles larger than 2 μm in diameter before reaching the alveolus. The removal of particulate matter such as dust and bacteria preserves the sterility of the alveolus. The removal of particulate matter, such as dust and bacteria, is accomplished by the *mucociliary system, one of the lung's primary defence mechanisms*. The mucociliary system consists of cilia, which line the respiratory tract from the laryngopharynx through the terminal bronchioles, and a dual-layered *fluid lining* secreted by *goblet cells* and *subendothelial glands*. The fluid lining that lies on top of the cilia consists of a lower serous and an upper mucopolysaccharide (mucus) layer. Inhaled particles are trapped in the mucus layer and are propelled upward towards the pharynx by the continuous rapid beating of the cilia. After reaching the pharynx, mucus and particles are removed from the airways by swallowing, coughing, or sneezing. The process of particle removal by the mucociliary system is often referred to as the *mucociliary escalator.*

The warming and humidifying functions are made possible by the rich capillary blood supply in the submucosal layer of the airways. During inspiration, air is heated to body temperature, and up to 1000 ml/day of water is used to raise the humidity of the inspired air to at least 80%. On expiration, some of this water is reabsorbed, thus conserving fluid; an average of 300 ml/day is lost in normal respiration.

Within the respiratory unit, respiration occurs only in the alveoli. Alveoli, which number 300 million in adults, are minute sacs that arise from the walls of the respiratory bronchioles and alveolar ducts. *The alveolus itself is composed of a single layer of squamous epithelium and an elastic basement membrane. These two layers, together with the interstitum and the endothelial and basement layers of the adjacent capillary, form the alveolar-capillary membrane or interface.* It is across this membrane, a distance less than 1 μm, that *diffusion of carbon dioxide and oxygen occurs.* The spherical interconnected structure of the millions of alveoli provides a large (50 to 100 m) surface area for gaseous diffusion to occur.

In addition to their respiratory function, the alveoli prevent lung collapse by producing surfactant, a phospholipid that decreases surface tension and prevents interstitial fluid from traversing into the lung space. Any foreign matter that deposits in healthy alveoli is engulfed by macrophages and disposed of through the circulatory system.

Lungs and thoracic cavity

The lungs themselves are subdivided into lobes. The *right lung* has *three* lobes: *upper, middle,* and *lower.* The *left lung* has only *two* lobes: *upper* and *lower.* Air is conducted to each lobe through lobar bronchi that branch off the main bronchus. An important difference between the right and left lungs is the size of the airways leading to them. *The right bronchus is significantly wider and shorter and extends at a straighter angle from the trachea, making it the more likely lodging point of aspirated material.* The *left bronchus* is narrower and extends at more of a right angle off the trachea, making it *more difficult to suction secretions from the left lung.*

The thoracic cavity is lined with pleura. The pleura is a continuous *serous* membrane; one surface of it lines the signs and symptoms seen in anyone experiencing oxygen

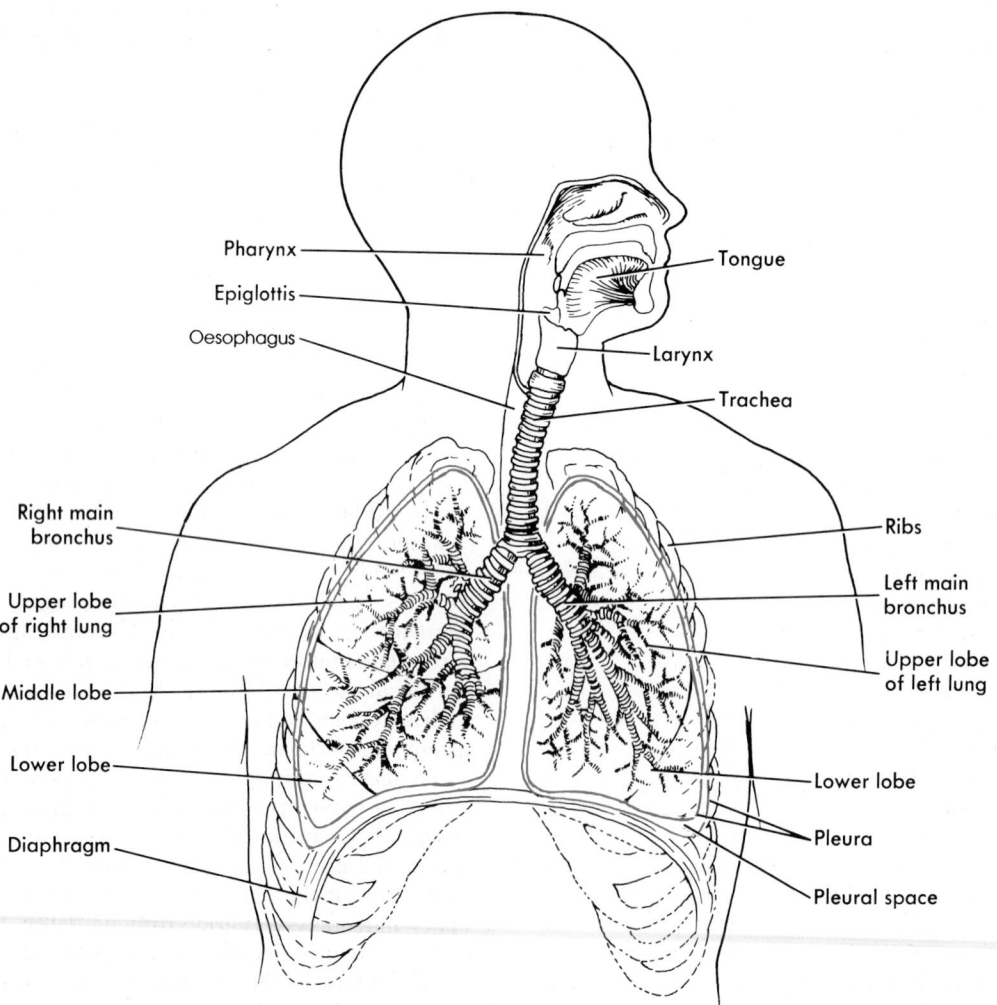

Fig. 16-1 Anatomy of the thorax and lungs.

inside of the rib cage (parietal pleura), and the other surface (visceral pleura) covers the lungs. The space between the two surfaces is known as a *potential space*. It normally contains a few millilitres of serious fluid that prevents friction rub when the two surfaces come together.

The lungs lie in and are protected by the thoracic cavity. This bony cage is composed of the sternum and ribs anteriorly and the ribs, scapulae, and vertebral column posteriorly. On the anterior surface, the apices of the lungs lie just above the clavicles and posteriorly extend to the eleventh or twelfth rib. Figure 16-1 illustrates the borders of each lobe.

Respiratory muscles

The major function of the respiratory muscles is to move air in and out of the lungs, thereby maintaining arterial blood gases within acceptable limits.[112]

The primary muscles of inspiration include the *diaphram, the external intercostals, the internal parasternal, intercostals, and the scalene muscles*. The major inspiratory muscle is the *diaphragm*, which is *innervated by the phrenic nerves*.

Altough normal quiet expiration dose not require active muscle conraction, relaxation of the abdominal muscles at the end of inspiration allows passive ascent of the diaphragm during expiration. When expiration is active, for example as a result of exercise, the *internal intercostal and abdominal muscles contract to assist expiration of air out of the lungs*.

Accessory muscles that are used when breathing is labored include the *sternocleidomastoids, pectoralis major and minor , trapezii, and laryngeal muscle*. The scalene muscles were formaly thought to be accessory muscles, but recent research has demonstrated that the contraction of these musles during inspiration is necessary for diaphragmatic descent to occur.[112]

Pulmonary ventilation

Air moves in and out of the lungs as a result of the principle of gas flow; that is, movement is from an area of greater pressure to an area of lesser pressure. At the start of inspiration, the atmospheric air pressure is greater than alveolar pressure; therefore, air moves through the respiratory passageway into the alveoli. When the alveolar pressure exceeds atmospheric pressure, expiration occurs, and air moves out of the lungs into the atmosphere.

The pressure gradient between the alveoli and the atmosphere is established by changes in the size of the thoracic cavity. *As the size of the thorax increases, pressure decreases and air flows into the lung*. Thoracic size is increased by contraction of the diaphragm and the external intercostal muscles. The diaphragm descends as it contracts and flattens, increasing the longitudinal diameter of the thorax. The external intercostals, parasternal internal intercostals, and the scalene muscles pull the ribs up and out, elevating the sternum and increasing both anteroposterior and lateral diameter of the chest.

As the thorax expands, it pulls the lungs with it because of cohesion between the moist surfaces of the lungs and chest wall. *Expiration is normally a passive process that results from the elastic recoil of the lungs and thoracic muscles*. It is this ability of the lungs to stretch and recoil that is evaluated by *pulmonary function testing* (see Table 16-6). The ability of the lungs to stretch is measured in terms of compliance. Compliance is the volume increase in lungs for every unit increase in intraalveolar pressure. This relationship is defined by the formula:

$$\text{Compliance} = \text{Change in volume} / \text{Change in pressure}$$

Thus lungs with increased (high) compliance have a larger increase in volume for each unit of pressure. *Lungs with increased compliance characterize a group of pulmonary disorders known as obstructive diseases*. Lungs with decreased (low) compliance *have a diminished volume for each unit of pressure. Decreased lung compliance characterizes lung disorders called restrictive diseases*.

The other property that affects the ability of the lungs to ventilate is *pulmonary resistance*. This property is *evaluated by measuring lung volume and airflow over time. Pulmonary resistance is made up of tissue resistance and airway resistance*. Tissue resistance results from friction created as tissues move against each other during lung expansion. Airway resistance results from friction encountered by air passing through the airways. The major factor affecting pulmonary resistance is the radius of the airways. *The following factors alter airway radius:*
(1) *bronchial innervation (for example: bronchospasm);*
(2) *external compression (for example: thoracic tumour); and*
(3) *internal obstruction (for example: mucus).*

Gas exchange (diffusion)

In the alveoli, oxygen diffuses across the alveolar-capillary membrane from the alveoli into the blood because the partial pressure of oxygen (oxygen tension, P_{O_2}) of *alveolar air* 13.3 kPa (100 mm Hg) is greater than the P_{O_2} of venous blood 5.3 kPa (40 mm Hg). Carbon dioxide diffuses in the opposite direction, because the P_{CO_2} of *venous blood* 6.1 kPa (46 mm Hg) is greater than the P_{CO_2} of alveolar air 5.3 kPa (40 mm Hg). The pulmonary diffusion capacity for carbon dioxide is much greater than the capacity for oxygen, and thus carbon dioxide diffuses more readily.

Diffusion of oxygen is decreased by the following factors: (1) *decreased atmospheric oxygen*, (2) *decreased alveolar ventilation*, (3) *decreased alveolar-capillary surface area, and* (4) *increased alveolar-capillary membrane thickness.*

Lung circulation

The lungs receive blood from the pulmonary circulation and the bronchial circulation. *Bronchial circulation* provides *blood flow* to the *tissues of the tracheobronchial tree*.

Pulmonary circulation is made up of the entire blood volume received from the right ventricle of the heart. The deoxygenated blood from the right ventricle is carried through the main pulmonary artery to successively branching vessels that follow the bronchi to the respiratory units. *Within the alveolar walls, the branching capillaries form a dense network that has been described as a sheet of blood.* Thus the circulatory system matches the vast surface created by the alveoli to provide for the rapid efficient exchange of oxygen and carbon dioxide. Newly oxygenated blood then travels via the four pulmonary veins back to the left atrium where it is circulated throughout the body via the aorta.

Ventilation-perfusion relationships

As discussed above, exchange of oxygen and carbon dioxide between alveolar air and pulmonary capillary blood occurs by gaseous *diffusion*. It is imperative that lung *ventilation (airflow) and perfusion (bloodflow)* are relatively evenly matched so that adequate oxygen and carbon dioxide exchange can occur. Both airflow to the alveoli and blood flow to the pulmonary capillaries have volumes of 4 to 6 L/min. A *normal ratio between ventilation and perfusion ranges from 0.8 to 1.2*. A low ventilation-to-perfusion ratio exists when alveoli cannot receive ambient air. Blood flowing through the capillaries in contact with the occluded alveoli would have low oxygen and high carbon dioxide levels. A clinical situation that can cause *low ventilation-to-perfusion ratios is when secretions block* bronchioles leading to alveoli. *A high ventilation-to-perfusion ratio exists when a pulmonary capillary is blocked*. In this situation oxygen and carbon dioxide levels in the alveoli remain the same as ambient air. A clinical situation that can cause high ventilation-to-perfusion ratios is pulmonary emboli.

Control of respiration

Breathing is an automatic process, but it may also be controlled voluntarily; that is, although humans do not have to think about breathing, they can breathe slower or faster at will. Voluntary control of respiration is centred in the cerebral cortex, from which impulses are sent to innervate the muscles of respiration.

Automatic control of respiration is centred in the medulla and pons. The pons is responsible for maintaining rhythmicity of respirations. The respiratory centre that is located in the medulla is controlled primarily by *central chemorecepters* that are sensitive to carbon dioxide tension (Pco_2), oxygen tension (Po_2), and acidity (pH) of arterial blood.

Peripheral chemoreceptors, located in the carotid body and aortic arch, respond to low arterial blood oxygen levels. The peripheral sensor mechanism is believed to be a built-in backup mechanism, and it does not function under normal physiological conditions.

When the central chemoreceptor is not functioning because of elevated carbon dioxide levels of more than a few days' duration CO_2 narcosis results. When this occurs it is only the person's peripheral chemoreceptor response to a decreased oxygen level that maintains respiration. Elevating the oxygen level without simultaneous lowering of the carbon dioxide level will result in apnoea and death.

Factors necessary for oxygen–carbon dioxide exchange

For breathing to take place normally, several factors are necessary: (1) an adequate supply of oxygen in the environment, (2) a patent airway, (3) a normally functioning bellows motion of the chest wall and diaphragm, (4) an adequate number of functioning alveoli and capillaries that together form a terminal respiratory unit, (5) an adequate amount of haemoglobin to carry oxygen to the cells, (6) an intact circulatory system and an effective heart pump, and (7) a functioning respiratory centre. Problems in one or more of these can result in inadequate exchange of oxygen and carbon dioxide and, if severe enough, can cause death.

Factors necessary for oxygen–carbon dioxide exchange

For breathing to take place normally, several factors are necessary: (1) an adequate supply of oxygen in the environment, (2) a patient airway, (3) a normally functioning bellows motion of functioning alveoli and capillaries that together form a terminal respiratory unit, (5) an adequate amount of haemoglobin to carry oxygen to the cells, (6) an intact circulatory system and an effective heart pump, and (7) a functioning respiratory centre. Problems in one or more of these can result in inadequate exchange of oxygen and carbon dioxide and, if severe enough, can cause death.

Maintaining an adequate supply of oxygen in the enviroment

High altitudes do not change the composition mof the air, but the oxygen pressure (Po_2) decreases.[122] People exposed to high, such as pilots, astronauts, mountian climbers, and those moving to high altitudes, have various reactions depending on the rate at which hypoxia develops, the degree of oxygen requirements as determined by physical exertion, and the duration of exposure.[122]

The initial reaction to high altitudes results in the same signs and symptoms seen in anyone experiencing oxygen lack. *Headache, dizziness, breathlessness, weakness, nausea, sweating, palpitation, dimness of vision, partial deafness, and sleeplessness occur with moderate hypoxia*.[122] With exertion, dyspnoea and other symptoms worsen. These signs and symptoms have been referred to as *mountain sickness* because they are evident as people travel to altitudes higher than those to which they have been accustomed.

These symptoms gradually disappear over days or weeks depending on the altitude, and the person is eventually able to carry out more activities without becoming short of breath. This is known as *acclimatization* and is caused in part by an increased capacity for supplying oxygen to the tissues and in part by overcoming the consequences of hypocapnia produced by excessive breathing.[122]

The *factors involved in acclimatization include:* (1) *a sustained increase in alveolar ventilation*, (2) *adjustment in the acid-base composition of the blood and other body fluids*, (3) *an increase in oxygen-carrying capacity, and* (4) *an increase in cardiac output*.[122]

People moving to higher altitudes, such as mountain climbers, are advised to allow time for their bodies to adjust to changes in various altitudes. Trained climbers, especially those ascending to very high altitudes, allow themselves weeks or even months at base camps at various altitudes in preparation for their ascent.[122]

Maintaining a patent airway

Several measures may be used to ensure a patent airway. The most basic measure involves simply positioning the person in such a way as to prevent obstruction of the airway. This is most relevant in resuscitation or in caring for an unconscious person. The position of choice is supine or on their side with the neck hyperextended. People who are unconscious may suffer airway obstruction if the tongue should fall back and cover the glottis; positioning them on their side prevents this from happening.

When a person has a mechanical obstruction of the airway and is expected to be unconscious for some time, it may be necessary to use an artificial airway (p. 363).

Maintaining bellows function of the chest wall and diaphragm

Whenever there is interference with the bellows function of the chest wall, there are changes in breathing pattern. The major cause of disruption of the bellows function is trauma to the chest involving fractures of the ribs or penetrating chest wounds. These conditions and their sequelae of paradoxical breathing and pneumothorax are discussed on p. 332.

Maintaining an adequate number of terminal respiratory units

The individual with pulmonary disease may have impaired ability to aerate alveoli. The impairment may be related to several factors. These include (1) inability to move adequate amounts of air in and out of the lungs, (2) interference with alveolar expansion secondary to an accumulation of secretions resulting in collapse of portions of the lungs (*atelectasis*), and (3) restriction of lung expansion by mechanical factors such as air in the pleural space (*pneumothorax*) or fluid or blood in the pleural space (*pleural effusion* or *haemothorax*). An increase in respiratory rate and pulse rate indicates that the body is trying to compensate for hypoxia. Patients who must make a conscious effort to breathe become very fatigued. They also become anxious because of shortness of breath and hypoxia.

Maintaining transportation of oxygen and adequate oxygenation of tissues

For oxygen to be supplied to the cells there must be (1) *an adequate amount of haemoglobin available to transport oxygen* and (2) *an effective heart pump and circulatory system to deliver the oxygen to the tissues.* The amount of oxygen delivered to body tissues each minute equals the cardiac output in litres per minute times the number of millilitres of oxygen contained in 1 L of arterial blood. In the resting state this is about 5×200, or 1000 ml O_2/min. About one fourth of this is used by the tissues, and three fourths returns to the heart in mixed venous blood. During exercise the amount of oxygen contained in 1 L of arterial blood does not increase, but the cardiac output does increase. With a cardiac output of 24 L/min, the oxygen delivered would be 24×200, or 4800 ml/min. The tissues would use three fourths of this amount, and only one fourth would be returned to the heart in mixed venous blood.[99]

An *inadequate amount of haemoglobin* (such as occurs in anaemia), *an inadequate heart pump*, or *a problem with the circulatory system can all have a deleterious effect on the delivery of oxygen.* In these situations the basic problem is treated in an attempt to increase the amount of available haemoglobin, to strengthen the heart pump and thus increase the cardiac output, or to improve the circulatory system. *Severe anaemia, carbon monoxide poisoning,*

methaemoglobinaemia, congestive heart failure, and *haemorrhage are possible interferences that must be corrected before an optimal amount of oxygen is available to the tissues.*

If *hypotension is present secondary to haemorrhage* or a *failing heart pump, there may be several sequelae.* These include (1) *anginal pain, because the coronary vessels that normally extract almost the maximal amount of oxygen* are not receiving sufficient oxygen to supply the myocardium and (2) *changes in sensorium and behaviour secondary to cerebral anoxia.* If this situation continues and there is inadequate oxygenation of tissues, respiratory or cardiac arrest may result. If an arrest occurs, cardiopulmonary resus-citation (CPR) must be instituted. CPR is discussed in detail in Chapter 17, and the reader is referred there for details.

Maintaining a functioning respiratory centre

Hypoventilation or apnoea can occur if there is *depression of the respiratory centre by general anaesthesia,* or by drugs such as morphine, heroin, barbiturates, or alcohol. Diseases of the central nervous system, such as bulbar poliomyelitis or meningitis, also depress the respiratory centre, as does an increase in intracranial pressure. In these situations the patient's respirations must be assisted until the patient is able to maintain his or her own breathing. Intubation with an endotracheal tube, supplemental oxygen, and artificial respiration with a ventilator may all be required. The conditions causing depression of the respiratory centre need to be identified and treated while the person's ventilation is being maintained by a ventilator. Details of management of patients in respiratory failure are discussed later.

Physiological Changes With Ageing

Several changes occur in the lungs and other parts of the respiratory tract with ageing.

Structural alterations in the thorax may limit lung expansion. Ribs do not move as freely because of cartilage calcification and partial contraction of respiratory muscles. Kyphosis (hunchback) secondary to osteoporosis decreases the transverse measurement of the thorax. The lungs become more rigid and less elastic. *There is a decrease in both residual volume and a decrease in vital capacity secondary to a decrease in the strength of the inspiratory and expiratory muscles.* The result is incomplete lung expansion and basilar lung collapse. These changes may *not* cause an obvious decrease in lung performance unless there is an increase in activity or stress when dyspnoea and other symptoms occur.

As a result of these changes older people are very vulnerable to respiratory problems if they develop a pulmonary infection or other illness that places stress on their already compromised respiratory system. For instance, changes in the thorax and altered muscle strength cause a decreased ability to clear the airway and cough effectively.

PHYSICAL EXAMINATION OF THE CHEST

Physical examination of the chest by the doctor provides objective data that, along with information obtained during

interview, forms the database necessary to identify problems appropriate to the individual. The pulmonary examination should be conducted with the person sitting upright on the edge of the bed, if possible. Adequate lighting and a relaxed, quiet environment are essential to obtain maximum information.

Three of the steps in the physical examination of the chest are *inspection*, *palpation*, and *percussion*.

Inspection

The patient is observed for general appearance, respiratory rate and pattern, and thoracic configuration. It is important to take adequate time to thoroughly observe the patient before moving to the "hands on" component of the examination. By observing general appearance, respiratory rate

and pattern, the presence and character of the person's cough, and sputum production, the nurse can assist the doctor to determine which components of the pulmonary examination are appro-priate for assessing the patient's current respiratory status. Table 16-1 indicates the normal and abnormal findings for each component of inspection.

Palpation

The chest is palpated to evaluate skin and chest wall status. Palpation of the chest and spinal column is a general screening technique to identify the presence of underlying abnormalities such as inflammation. The chest is also palpated for *fremitus, which are vibrations felt on the chest surface when sound passes through underlying tissue and air- or fluid-filled space.* Fremitus can be caused by secretions

Table 16-1 Possible findings by inspection in a pulmonary examination

Observe	Normal	Abnormal
General appearance	Quiet respiration Sitting or reclining without difficulty Skin translucent, appears dry Nailbeds pink Mucous membranes pink and moist* Cyanosis or pallor assessed by establishing an early individual baseline	Lips puckered when exhaling Restless and apprehensive Leans forward with hands or elbows on knees Skin: diaphoretic, dull pale, or ruddy Cyanosis: Skin or mucous membrane has bluish cast Central cyanosis: results from decreased oxygenation of blood† Peripheral cyanosis: result of local vasoconstriction or decreased output Nail clubbing: painless enlargement of terminal phalanges related to chronic tissue hypoxia
Trachea	Midline in neck	Tracheae deviation; displacement either lateral, anterior, or posterior Jugular venous distension (see Chapter 21) Cough: strong or weak, dry or wet, productive or nonproductive Sputum production: amount, colour, odour, consistency
Rate	Eupnoea: 12 to 20	Tachypnoea: rate >20 breaths/min Bradypnoea: rate <10 breaths/min
Breathing pattern	Minimal effort with inspiration: passive, quiet expiration Inspiration/expiration ratio 1 : 2 Male: diaphragmatic breathing Female: thoracic breathing	Hypernoea: increased breathing rate Accessory muscle breathing Apnoea: total absence of breathing Biots: irregular rhythm with periods of apnoea Cheyne-Stokes: cyclical deeper and shallower breaths followed by periods of apnoea Kussmaul's: deep, rapid, and regular breathing Paradoxical: portion of chest wall moves in during inhalation and out during exhalation Stridorous: audible, loud, low-pitched sound with inhalation and exhalation
Thoracic configuration	Symmetric appearance Anteroposterior diameter (AP) less than transverse diameter Spine straight Scapulae on same horizontal plane Trachea midline (centred on suprasternal notch)	Chest expands unevenly Muscular development asymmetric Barrel chest: AP diameter increased in relation to transverse diameter Kyphosis: increased thoracic curvature Scoliosis: increased lateral curvature Scapular placement *asymmetric* Trachea right or left of midline

* Dark-skinned people might have normal bluish pigmented mucous membranes.
† Central cyanosis is relevant to respiratory status. Observe nailbeds, mucous membrane, and lips.

in the large airways, a pleural friction rub, or lung consolidation. Vocal (tactile) fremitus is normally present; thus it is necessary to determine whether fremitus is increased or decreased. The chest is also palpated for symmetry and degree of lateral chest expansion from maximal exhalation to maximal inhalation. Possible normal and abnormal findings are presented in Table 16-2.

Percussion

Percussion is used to assess the lung fields and the position and movement of the diaphragm (excursion). *Percussion notes are produced from vibration created by tapping the chest wall.* The quality of the percussion note depends on the density of underlying tissue and the amount of air through which the vibration passes. Table 16-3 identifies common normal and abnormal percussion findings.

Pulmonary Auscultation

Auscultation of the lungs enables a doctor to establish baseline data for identifying current and potential lung problems that require medical and nursing interventions, such as determining the frequency for breathing exercises or the need for or effectiveness of suctioning.

Breath sounds

Breath sounds result from the movement of air through the lungs and air passages. The sounds are thought to occur as a result of two elements, the vesicular and bronchial elements. The vesicular element occurs when the walls of the alveoli are separated by air entering the alveoli from inspiration. The bronchial element is a hisslike sound resulting from air flowing past the bronchi and across the vocal chords.

The three types of breath sounds that can be heard are vesicular, bronchovesicular, and bronchial. *Vesicular breath sounds are heard over most of the lungs because of the prominence of the alveoli.* The sounds are of a low pitch and have a soft rustling or swishing quality. The sound of the inspiratory phase is longer and higher in pitch than that of the expiratory phase, which is a soft, short, low-pitched, almost inaudible sound. The relative loudness of inspiration may differ among listening sites; the sounds are usually softer at the bases of the lungs.

Bronchovesicular breath sounds are heard as one auscultates towards the main bronchi. Inspiration and expiration are loud and nearly equal in duration and intensity because of auscultating closer to the vocal chords.

Bronchial breath sounds normally are not heard over any area of lung tissue and their presence indicates consolidation such as occurs in pneumonia, or compression of lung tissue or a pleural effusion. These breath sounds are high pitched and loud; during the expiratory phase they increase in duration, pitch, and intensity.

Adventitious abnormal lung sounds

Adventitious lung sounds are abnormal sounds superimposed on breath sounds. There are essentially two kinds of abnormal sounds: (1) *crackles* or *rales* (rhymes with *pals*) caused by air flowing through moisture in the air passages

Table 16-2   Possible findings by palpation in a pulmonary examination

Palpate	Normal	Abnormal
Skin and chest wall	Skin nontender, smooth, warm, and dry	Skin moist or exceedingly dry Crepitation—"crackling" when skin palpated—due to air leak from lung into subcutaneous tissue
	Spine and ribs nontender	Localized tenderness
Fremitus*	Symmetric, mild vibrations felt on chest wall during vocalization	Increased fremitus—a result of vibrations through more solid medium such as lung tumours Decreased fremitus—a result of vibration through increased space in the chest such as pneumothorax or obesity. Asymmetric fremitus is always abnormal
Lateral chest expansion	Symmetric 3 to 8 cm expansion†	Expansion less than 3 cm, painful or assymetric†

* Normal fremitus varies from person to person. An individual's baseline must be established.
† Reduced expansion can result either from either an overexpanded chest (barrel chest) or from a restricted chest.

Table 16-3   Possible findings by percussion in a pulmonary examination

Percussion	Normal	Abnormal
Lung fields	Resonant low-pitched, hollow, easily heard sounds; equal quality bilaterally	Hyperresonant: heard with air trapping or pneumothorax Dull or flat: results from decreased air in lungs (tumour, fluid)
Diaphragm position and movement	Resting diaphragm at 10th thoracic vertebrae Each hemidiaphragm moves 3-6 cm	High position—stomach distension or phrenic nerve damage Decreased or no movement in either hemidiaphragm*

* Decreased excursion can result from hyperinflated lungs pushing down on diaphragm, diaphragmatic disorders, or loss of diaphragmatic innervation.

and (2) *wheezes* or *rhonchi* caused by air flowing through narrowed air passages (Table 16-4). A third type of sound occurs outside the lung; a *pleural friction rub* results from the rubbing of inflamed pleura between the lung and chest wall.

DIAGNOSTIC TESTS
Radiographic Examination of the Thorax and Lungs

Patients are usually familiar with X-ray examination. In recent years, there has been an increase in consumer awareness of the danger of excessive exposure to radiation. The patient should have a full explanation of the type of test to be performed and the benefits (knowledge gained) in relation to risk from radiation exposure.

Chest film studies are indicated for the following reasons:

1. Detect alterations of the lung caused by pathological processes such as tumours, inflammation, fractures, fluid or air accumulation
2. Determine appropriate therapy
3. Evaluate effectiveness of treatment
4. Determine position of tubes and catheters
5. Provide a way of following the progression of lung disease

Chest films

Chest film studies are best performed in the radiology department. However, if the patient is acutely ill, the test can be completed at the bedside with a portable X-ray machine. The X-ray camera moves from the front to the back of the body; that is, anteroposterior (AP). Standard chest x-ray films are preferably taken in the standing position, although the sitting or supine position can be used. The standard views are as follows:

1. Posteroanterior (PA)—X-rays pass through the back to the front of the body
2. Lateral—X-rays pass through the side of the body (usually left side)

Special views might be required to visualize specific parts of the chest. The special views include the following:

1. Oblique—X-ray films slanted at specific angles
2. Lordotic—X-ray films slanted at 45-degree angle from below to visualize lung apices
3. Decubitus—X-ray films taken with patient lying on either side to visualize free fluid in chest

See Box 16-1 above for details of preparation procedure.

Tomography

Tomography is a special technique that permits better visualization of a single layer or plane of the lungs. It is used to study cavities, neoplasms, and lung densities. The patient is required to lie still while an X-ray tube is rapidly moved over the lung at approximately 1-cm intervals. The procedure takes approximately 15 minutes.

Computed tomography

Computed tomography (CT) is rapidly replacing standard tomographic examination. Conventional tomography resulted in a blurred film, except for the one plane being observed. CT scanning uses computer programming to enhance and process the X-ray film "slices" to produce a clear picture of the chest cavity structures.

Table 16-4   Abnormal (adventitious) lung sounds

Type	Physiology	Auscultation	Sound	Pathology
Crackles (rales)				
Fine	Air passing through secretions in alveoli	Heard at end of inspiration	Several hairs rubbed together between fingertips	Pneumonia, heart failure (may occur normally in elderly bed-ridden people)
Medium	Air passing through secretions in bronchioles or bronchi	Heard midway during inspiration	Fizzing of carbonated drink	Later stages of pneumonia, heart failure, pulmonary oedema
Coarse	Air passing through secretions in large airways, especially trachea	Heard at beginning of inspiration	Rough gurgling	People with repressed cough reflexes, unable to clear own secretions
Wheezes (rhonchi)	Air passing through narrow passages	Heard mostly during expiration, but may also occur with inspiration	Loud musical gurgling	Obstructive lung disease
Pleural friction rub	Rubbing of inflamed pleura	May occur throughout respiratory cycle, heard best at base of lung at end of expiration	Scratching, grating, rubbing	Inflamed pleura

Preparation of patient for radiographic examination

1. Explain specific procedure.
2. Ask patient to remove all clothing above the waist and put on a gown with an opening in the back. The patient must remove metal objects above the waist because metal restricts X-ray films from passing through the body.
3. The procedure is noninvasive and should cause no discomfort.
4. Patient will probably be alone in the room, but someone is nearby and always has voice contact.
5. Patient will probably be asked to take a deep breath and hold it.
6. If it is necessary for people to be in the room with the patient while X-ray is being taken, they will wear lead aprons to protect them from radiation exposure.

Fluoroscopic examination

When dynamic information about the chest such as diaphragmatic movement, lung expansion and contraction, or cardiac action is required, fluoroscopy is the preferred examination.

Ultrasound (echogram)

In an ultrasound examination, a harmless, high-frequency sound wave is emitted and penetrates the thorax. These sound waves bounce back and are converted by a transducer to a pictorial image of the area being studied. Ultrasound of the thorax can provide information about pleural effusion or opacities in the lung.

Bronchography

A bronchogram enables the doctor to visualize the bronchial tree by X-ray film after the introduction of an iodized radiopaque liquid, which coats the bronchial mucosa. The pharynx, larynx, and major bronchi are anaesthetized with a topical anaesthetic before introduction of a metal cannula into the trachea. The radiopaque substance is then introduced, and the patient is tilted in various positions to distribute the dye to the bronchi and bronchioles. A series of X-ray films are then taken. See Box 16-2 for details.

Radiological Examination of Ventilation and Perfusion

Lung scan (pulmonary scintiphotography)

Lung scan procedures involve the use of a scanning device that records the pattern of pulmonary radioactivity after the inhalation or intravenous injection of gamma ray-emitting radionucleotides, thus providing a visual image of the distribution of ventilation or blood flow in the lungs. These studies provide valuable information about ventilation-perfusion patterns and aid in the diagnosis of parenchymal lung disease and vascular disorders such as pulmonary embolism. See Box 16-3 for preparation procedures.

In a *perfusion scan, radiopaque iodine is injected intravenously.* The lungs are then scanned, and the pattern of particle distribution in the lung vasculature is recorded. Areas of poor radionucleotide uptake are suggestive of pulmonary vascular disorders. In a *ventilation scan, the radioactive gas is inhaled, and the lungs are scanned to detect abnormal diffusion of the gas throughout the lungs.*

Pulmonary angiography

Pulmonary angiography is used to detect pulmonary emboli and a variety of congenital and acquired lesions of the pulmonary vessels. A radiopaque material is injected via a catheter into a systemic vein, the right chambers of the heart, or the pulmonary artery; and the distribution of this material is recorded on film.

Positron emission tomography (PET)

PET uses the capability of computerization to study regional pulmonary perfusion and ventilation-perfusion relationships. A radioisotope that releases positrons (positively charged particles with the same mass as an electron) is inhaled by or injected into the individual. As the short-lived radioisotope decays, it releases gamma rays that are recorded by the computerized scanner.

Preparation of patient for a bronchogram

Prebronchogram

1. Patient is instructed to do complete mouth care night and morning before procedure.
2. Patient does not eat or drink for 8 hours before procedure.
3. Dentures are removed. Document any loose teeth on preoperative sheet.
4. Shortly before the examination, patient receives a short-acting sedative and an antispasmodic.

Postbronchogram

1. Postural drainage is initiated unless contraindicated to assist in the removal of radiopaque substance.
2. Food and fluid are withheld until gag reflex returns.
3. Deep breathing, coughing, and moving about are encouraged to maintain a clear airway.

Preparation for lung scan or pulmonary angiography

Radiopaque iodine is the radionucleotide usually used for both pulmonary angiography and lung scan. Always carry out the following activities.

1. Check patient for iodine allergy.
2. Obtain a prescription to administer 10 drops of Lugol's solution several hours before the test to block thyroid uptake of radioactive iodine.

Examination of Sputum

Sputum analysis

Examinations of sputum are usually required when chest disease is suspected. The mucous membrane of the respiratory tract responds to inflammation by an increased flow of secretions that often contain causative organisms. The volume, consistency, colour, and odour of the sputum are observed and recorded (see Box 16-4).

Sputum examination includes the following tests:

1. *Gram stain* usually gives enough information about organisms and cells present to give a presumptive diagnosis.
2. *Culture* identifies specific organisms to enable making a definitive diagnosis. It should be collected before initiation of antibiotic therapy and thereafter to monitor effectiveness of antibiotic therapy.
3. *Sensitivity* serves as a guide to antimicrobial therapy by identifying antibiotics that prevent growth of the organism present in the sputum. It is collected before initiation of antibiotic therapy. Culture and sensitivity (C & S) are usually ordered together.
4. *Acid-fast bacilli* (AFB) determines the presence of mycobacterium tuberculosis which, after taking up a dye, is not decolourized by acid alcohol.
5. *Cytology* assists in identification of lung carcinoma. Sputum contains coughed cells from tracheobronchial tree; thus malignant cells might be present. Although the presence of malignant cells indicates carcinoma, the absence of cells might indicate that either there is no tumour or that the tumour is not shedding cells.
6. *Quantitative* test is the collection of sputum over a period of 24 to 72 hours.

Sputum collection

Tests to be performed on sputum are explained to the patient so that a suitable specimen will be obtained. The patient is instructed to collect only sputum that has come from deep in the lungs. When not instructed adequately, patients often expectorate saliva rather than sputum. They are likely to exhaust themselves unnecessarily by shallow, frequent coughing that yields no sputum suitable for study and that affords them little relief from discomfort. *The first sputum raised in the morning is usually the most productive of organisms.* During the night, secretions accumulate in the bronchi, and just a few deep coughs will bring them to the back of the throat. If patients do not know this fact, on awakening they may almost unconsciously cough, clear their throats, and swallow or expectorate before attempting to produce the specimen.

16-4

Sputum colour analysis

1. Colourless or clear mucoid: noninfectious process
2. Creamy yellow: staphylococcal pneumonia
3. Green: *Pseudomonas* pneumonia
4. "Currant jelly": *Klebsiella* pneumonia
5. Rusty: pneumococcal pneumonia
6. Pink frothy: pulmonary oedema

The patient should be supplied with a wide-mouthed sterile container and instructed to expectorate directly into it. Because the sight of sputum is often objectionable to the patient and to others, the outside of a glass container is covered with paper or other suitable covering. Usually 4 ml of sputum is sufficient for laboratory tests and examinations. Nursing implications for sputum collection include the following:

1. Patients who have difficulty producing sputum or who have very tenacious sputum might be dehydrated. Encourage fluid intake.
2. Collect specimen before meals to avoid possible vomiting from coughing after eating.
3. Instruct patient to rinse mouth with water before collecting specimen to decrease contamination.
4. Instruct patient to notify staff as soon as specimen is collected so that it can be sent to the laboratory as soon as possible.

Occasionally patients have difficulty producing sputum for examination. Inhalation of a hypertonic solution such as 10% saline in distilled water is used to temporarily stimulate sputum collection. Other methods to collect sputum include the following: (1) endotracheal aspiration with a suction catheter and special sputum collection container, (2) transtracheal aspiration (insertion of a needle with a catheter through the cricothyroid cartilage), and (3) fibreoptic bronchoscopy (p. 301).

Gastric washings

Gastric aspiration is occasionally used to collect gastric contents, which may contain swallowed sputum. It is usually performed when the diagnosis or suspected diagnosis is tuberculosis. Because most patients swallow sputum when coughing in the morning and during sleep, an examination of gastric contents can reveal causative organisms.

The procedure requires the following steps:

1. Breakfast is withheld before aspiration.
2. A nasogastric tube is passed into the stomach.
3. A large syringe is connected to the nasogastric tube, and a specimen of stomach contents is gently withdrawn.
4. The specimen is placed in a covered container.
5. The nasogastric tube is withdrawn.

Skin Testing

For various pulmonary disorders, the skin is tested for an antigen-antibody reaction to the proteins of the infectious agent. This cell-mediated or delayed hypersensitivity reaction is manifested by induration caused by cellular infiltration at the site of the injection in people who have been sensitized to the proteins of the infectious agent. Skin testing for *Mycobacterium* tuberculosis with either tuberculin purified protein derivative (PPD) or old tuberculin (OT) is the most common type of test. However, skin testing also can be conducted for *atypical tubercle bacilli* and for *fungal infections* resulting from *coccidioidin, histoplasmin,* and *blastomycin.* The primary purpose of skin testing is to detect individuals who are infected with the suspect organism but who do not have the disease. In this capacity, skin testing is primarily a screening device. Skin antigens can also be used for presumptive diagnosis; however, a positive skin test reaction must be substantiated with other diagnostic evidence before active disease can be confirmed. Skin testing can produce false-positive and false-negative results (usually in immunosuppressed, older, or newly infected people).

Skin test administration

Skin tests can be administered by intracutaneous injection (Mantoux method), jet gun or multiple puncture tests (Tine, mono-vacc, and Heaf-type). The *Mantoux test is the only method used for diagnosis*. The jet gun or multiple puncture methods are used *only* for pre-BCG screening tests. (See Box 16-5 for details of administration.)

Pulmonary Function Tests

Pulmonary function testing is a noninvasive method of assessing the functional capacity of the lungs. These tests cannot be used by themselves to diagnose specific diseases, but they are an integral part of the diagnostic process. Pulmonary function tests (PFTs) are used for the following purposes:

1. Screening for the presence of pulmonary disease
2. Preoperative evaluation
3. Evaluating the patient's condition for weaning from a ventilator
4. Researching pulmonary physiology
5. Documenting the progression of pulmonary disease or effects of therapy
6. Studying the effects of exercise on respiratory physiology

Assessment of lung properties

The functional ability of the lungs is assessed by measuring properties that affect ventilation and respiration.

16-5

Administration technique for the mantoux test

1. Draw up 0.1 ml of PPD, OT, atypical (tuberculin), or fungal antigen, using a tuberculin syringe and ½ inch 24- to 26-gauge needle.
2. Cleanse the site (dorsal surface of forearm).
3. Keeping skin slightly taut, insert the needle bevel upward just beneath the skin surface.
4. Inject the solution, creating a 6 to 10 mm wheal.
5. Read the test site with a millimetre ruler 48 to 72 hours after injection. The site should be lightly palpated to determine the presence or absence of induration. The largest diameter of induration should be measured and recorded in millimetres. Any erythema at the site should also be noted.
6. Interpretation of induration:
   a. 10 mm or more = highly significant for past or present infection.
   b. 5 mm to 9 mm = doubtful reaction except in persons with HIV infection.
   c. 0 to 4 mm = little or no sensitivity, however if patient's history indicates exposure, the test should be repeated.

---

1. Ventilation
   a. Static properties focus on lung distensibility; that is, on the bellows action of the thorax and lungs. Static properties are assessed through measurement of lung volumes and functional capacities.
   b. Dynamic properties are those aspects of lung mechanics that affect the resistance within the airways. These properties are assessed by pulmonary function tests that measure volume/time relationships.
2. Respiration
   a. Diffusion properties are those aspects of lung function that affect the ability of gas to move across the alveolar-capillary membrane (Table 27-8, *D*).
   b. Perfusion properties affect the supply of blood to the lungs.

Normal values for pulmonary function tests are calculated by taking into consideration the following variables for each individual being evaluated: (1) age, (2) sex, (3) height and weight, and (4) individual effort in performing each test.

Measurement of ventilation

Ventilatory studies are performed by asking the patient to breathe through a mouthpiece connected to a spirometer that measures the air moving through the apparatus. The spirometer is connected to a recording device that documents air volume, usually in litre measurements. Some measurements such as the residual volume cannot be measured directly and are calculated mathematically.

Spirometric measurement of lung *dynamic properties* are of particular clinical significance because they relate the volume of air expired to the time required for expiration. One meaningful clinical measurement is the forced expiratory volume (FEV). The FEV measures the amount of air in litres forcefully expired over 1, 2, or 3 seconds after a full inspiration. *The FEV is an accurate indicator for obstructive diseases because airway obstruction becomes worse on expiration and particularly when expiration is forceful and rapid. The FEV at 1 sec is the most clinically accurate of the three measurements and is particularly* useful when expressed as a percentage of the forced vital capacity (FVC). An FEV_1/FVC of 80% or greater is considered normal.

Measurement of respiration

It is best to measure efficiency of respiration by both PFTs and other parameters such as arterial blood gas measurements. Two variables affecting respiration that PFTs can measure are the ability of gas to diffuse across the alveolar-capillary membrane and the ratio of ventilated alveoli to perfused capillaries.

Alveolar-capillary diffusion

The ability of gas to diffuse across the alveolar-capillary membrane is measured by a test called *diffusing capacity* (D_x). The patient breathes a measured amount of carbon monoxide from a closed system. The rate of carbon monoxide removal from the closed system indicates the status of the alveolar-capillary membrane.

Ventilation-perfusion relationship

In order for the lung to perform gas exchange efficiently, the ventilation-perfusion ratio (V/Q ratio) must be balanced.

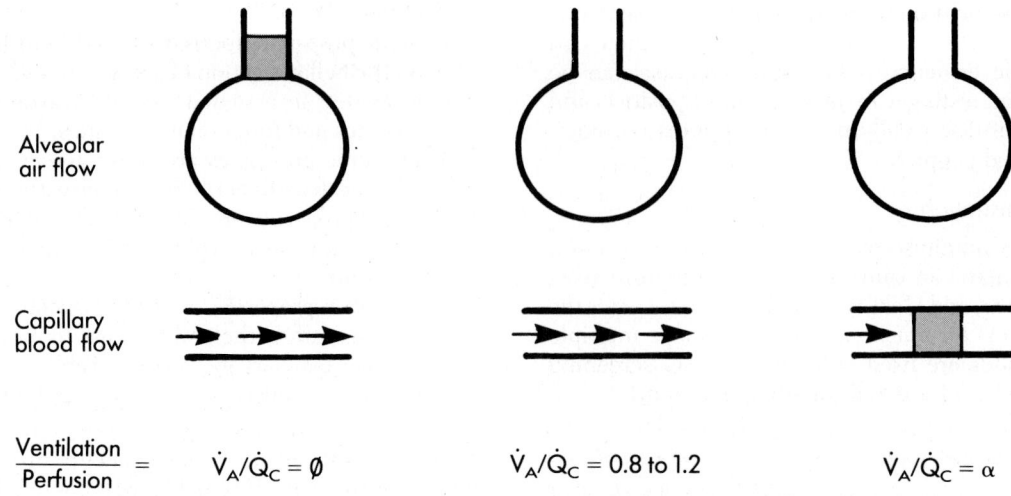

Fig. 16-2   Ventilation/perfusion relationships are as follows: *left,* bronchus blocked with secretions equals decreased ventilation, and normal perfusion equals zero gas exchange; *centre,* normal ventilation and normal perfusion is Va/Q$_c$ of 0.8 to 1.2; *right,* normal ventilation and decreased perfusion from blocked capillary as found in pulmonary emboli equals zero gas exchange. (Modified from West JB: *Ventilation, blood flow and gas exchange,* ed 3, Oxford 1977, Blackwell.)

That is, areas that receive ventilation should be well perfused with blood, and areas that receive blood flow should be capable of ventilation (Fig. 16-2). Although in the normal lung with its many millions of gas exchange units some imbalance in ventilation and perfusion exists, this has little effect on overall gas exchange function. In fact, adaptive mechanisms appear to exist that divert blood flow to the best ventilated regions of the lungs or redirect ventilation away from nonperfused areas in order to maintain a normal ratio in the range of 0.8 to 1.2. Alteration in ventilation-perfusion relationships (either overall or in circumscribed areas of lung tissue) is largely responsible for the *hypoxaemia* or *hypercapnia* seen in patients. The nitrogen washout test measures ventilation/perfusion relationships. Ambient air, and thus air in the lungs, is known to contain 80% nitrogen. The nitrogen washout test requires the patient to breathe 100% oxygen to wash out all the nitrogen from the lungs. After a measured period of time, the patient's expired air is measured for nitrogen content. Unevenly ventilated alveoli that receive less of the inspired oxygen will take longer to wash out lung nitrogen.

For pulmonary function testing, patients are required to breathe into a mouthpiece while wearing a noseclip; thus they often fear smothering or having a dyspnoeic episode. Thorough preparation for the test includes an explanation of the procedure to decrease the patient's apprehension.

Arterial Blood Gas Analysis

Arterial blood gas analysis provides objective determination of the following: (1) arterial blood oxygenation, (2) gas exchange, (3) alveolar ventilation, and (4) acid-base balance. The arterial blood gas parameters that assess function of the respiratory system are shown in Table 16-5. A blood sample is obtained from a radial, brachial, or femoral artery with a preheparinized syringe to prevent clotting. The syringe is capped after obtaining the blood sample to prevent contact with air and is placed in an ice-water container until analyzed. Pressure is maintained over the puncture site for at least 5 minutes after needle withdrawal to prevent bleeding.

Patients with blood-clotting abnormalities may require that pressure be applied to the sample site for longer than 5 minutes. Nursing implications include assessing the site periodically and applying pressure for as long as necessary to prevent haematoma formation or bruising.

Table 16-5   Arterial blood gases

Respiratory function	Measurements	Normal value
Acid base balance	pH-hydrogen ion concentration	7.35-7.45
Oxygenation	Pao$_2$: partial pressure of dissolved O$_2$ in blood	10.6-13.3 kPa (80-100 mm Hg)
	Sao$_2$: percentage of O$_2$ bound to haemoglobin	95%-98%
Ventilation	Paco$_2$: partial pressure of CO$_2$ dissolved in blood	5.0-6.0 kPa (38-45 mm Hg)

Measurement of oxygenation

Both Pao_2 and Sao_2 are used to determine the adequacy of arterial blood oxygenation. The Pao_2 measures oxygen dissolved in the blood; however, the amount of oxygen carried in the blood in this form is small. Most oxygen is transported in chemical combination with haemoglobin. The Sao_2 measures the oxyhaemoglobin saturation or that percentage of the haemoglobin that is combined with oxygen. More than 90% of the oxygen-carrying capacity of blood is accounted for by oxyhaemoglobin, with the partial pressure of oxygen acting as the driving force for this chemical combination.

The relationship of Pao_2 to Sao_2 is demonstrated in the oxyhaemoglobin dissociation curve. This relationship is not directly linear; many factors affect the affinity of the haeme molecule for oxygen. The sigmoid curve represents the saturation percentages that occur at various Pao_2 levels. As can be seen in the oxyhaemoglobin dissociation curve (Fig. 16-3), in the upper portion of the curve, haemoglobin has an increased affinity for oxygen, so that large changes in Po_2 levels can be tolerated without significantly changing the saturation. For example, at a Po_2 of 100 mm Hg, haemoglobin saturation is almost total, 97%; even if the Po_2 should fall to 70 mm Hg, the saturation would only decrease to 94%. This serves as a protective mechanism that ensures adequate tissue oxygenation even when there is mild hypoxaemia. It should be noted, however, that once the Po_2 level falls below 60 mm Hg, saturation begins to decrease sharply, thus reducing the ability of the haemoglobin to transport oxygen.

The oxygen affinity of haemoglobin is influenced by various factors. Those factors that cause the curve to shift to the left (that is, hypothermia, alkalosis, and hypocapnia) increase the affinity of oxygen but diminish the release of oxygen to the tissues. Factors that cause a shift to the right are fever, acidosis, and hypercapnia. The primary impact of a shift to the right is reduced affinity of haemoglobin for oxygen.

The Pao_2 and Sao_2 must be evaluated in relation to the amount of haemoglobin. Because Sao_2 measures saturation of haemoglobin, an anaemic person can have a normal saturation but still be inadequately oxygenated.

Assessment of ventilation

The $Paco_2$ is used as a measurement to determine the adequacy of ventilation and depends on the amount of carbon dioxide produced by the body and the ability of the lungs to eliminate it. *Hypoventilation* is shown by an elevated $Paco_2$ and *hyperventilation* is indicated by a decrease in $Paco_2$ below normal levels.

Measurement of acid-base balance

Arterial blood pH is a measurement of hydrogen ion concentration. Because pH is expressed as a negative logarithm, as the hydrogen ion concentration increases and blood becomes more acid, the pH value falls. When the hydrogen ion concentration decreases, the blood becomes more alkaline, and the pH value rises.

The lungs play an important part in maintaining normal body pH (7.35 to 7.45) by regulating $Paco_2$ through ventilation. The $Paco_2$ is related to the pH by the chemical reaction of carbon dioxide and water in the blood, which results in the formation of carbonic acid. Carbonic acid, in turn, dissociates to form hydrogen and bicarbonate ions, as illustrated in the following equation:

$$CO_2 + H_2O \rightleftarrows H_2CO_3 \rightleftarrows HCO^- + H^+$$

The maintenance of a normal pH depends on a ratio of 20 bicarbonate ions to 1 hydrogen ion. It can be seen from the equation that the presence of an elevated $Paco_2$ shifts the equilibrium equation to the right and will result in an excess of H^+ ions. When this occurs, the pH falls, and the patient is said to be in *respiratory acidosis*. Conversely, when $Paco_2$ is decreased, the equation shifts to the left, resulting in an increased pH and *respiratory alkalosis*.

Endoscopic Examination

Bronchoscopy

A bronchoscopic examination is performed by passing a bronchoscope into the trachea and bronchi (Fig. 16-4). By use of either a rigid bronchoscope or a flexible fibreoptic bronchoscope, the larynx, trachea, and bronchi can be visualized. Diagnostic bronchoscopic examination includes observation of the tracheobronchial tree for abnormalities, tissue biopsy, and aspiration of sputum for testing. Therapeutic bronchoscopic examination can be performed to remove an aspirated foreign body, to facilitate free air passage by removal of mucus plugs with suction, or to control bleeding.

Preparation for a bronchoscopy is similar to that for bronchography, except that postural drainage is less often ordered. If the patient is very apprehensive or if a sponge biopsy (abrasion of a lesion with a sponge) is to be performed or a tissue biopsy specimen is to be obtained, intravenous anaesthesia can be used.

Nursing care for patients after bronchoscopy is as follows:

1. Patient has nothing orally until gag reflex returns.
2. Patient is positioned in semi recumbent position or on either side to facilitate removal of secretions, unless doctor specifies position.

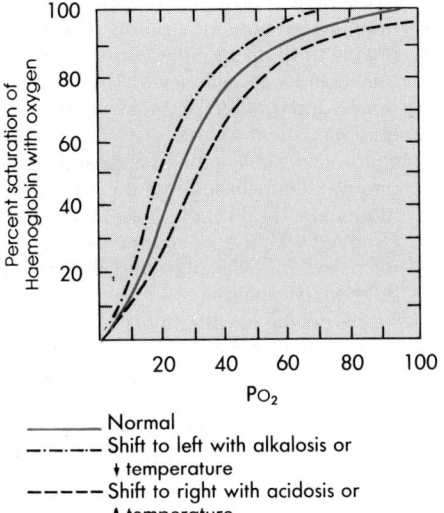

Fig. 16-3 Oxyhaemoglobin dissociation curve. (From Comroe JH Jr: *Physiology of respiration*, ed 2, St Louis, 1974, Mosby–Year Book.)

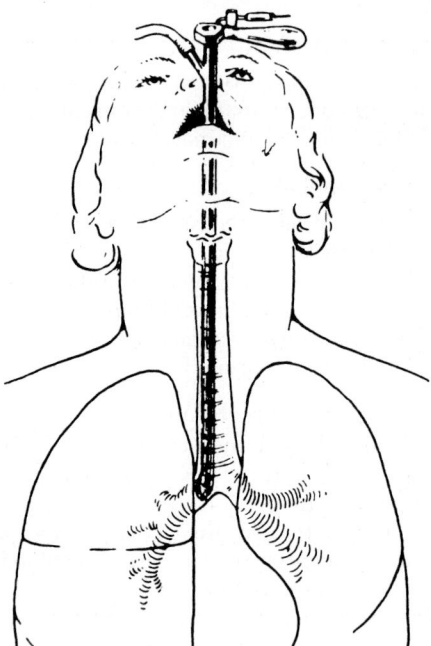

Fig. 16-4 Bronchoscope inserted through trachea into bronchus. (From DeWeese DD, Saunders WH: *Textbook of oto laryngology*, ed 7, St Louis, 1987, Mosby-Year Book.)

3. All sputum is saved for culture and cytological studies. *Note:* If bronchograms were performed, sputum cannot be used for cytological examination, because the dye impedes cell fixation.
4. Patient is monitored for signs of laryngeal oedema or laryngospasms such as stridor or increasing shortness of breath.
5. If lung tissue biopsy is taken, sputum is monitored for signs of haemorrhage. *Note:* Blood-streaked sputum can be expected for a few days after biopsy.

Mediastinoscopy

In mediastinoscopy a *mediastinoscope*, which is an instrument much like a bronchoscope, is inserted through a small incision in the suprasternal notch and advanced into the mediastinum where inspection and biopsy of the lymph nodes can then be carried out. Because these lymph nodes receive lymphatic drainage from the lungs, they are of diagnostic value for carcinoma, and granulomatous infections such as sarcoidosis. This procedure is performed in the operating theatre, and the patient usually receives a general anaesthetic.

Thoracocentesis (chest aspiration)

Thoracocentesis involves the insertion of a needle into the pleural space. Indications for a thoracocentesis include the following:
1. Removal of pleural fluid for diagnostic purposes
   a. The pleural fluid can be examined for specific gravity, white blood cell count, differential cell count, red blood cell count, protein, glucose, and amylase concentrations.
   b. The fluid can be cultured and checked for the presence of abnormal or malignant cells.

c. The gross appearance of the fluid, the quantity obtained, and the location of the site of the thoracocentesis should be recorded.
2. Biopsy of the pleura
3. Removal of pleural fluid when it is a threat to patient safety or comfort
4. Installation of medications into the pleural space.

Box 16-6 lists the nursing care for a patient having a thoracocentesis.

PREVENTION AND HEALTH EDUCATION

Disorders of the respiratory tract are probably the most common health problems for most people in the Western world.

The objectives of health education in relation to pulmonary diseases are the same as for other diseases. *Prevention, early diagnosis, prompt and often continued treatment, limitation of disability, and rehabilitation should be emphasized for all people.* Early symptoms of respiratory diseases are probably those most often ignored by the general population. Perhaps this is because, with the exception of influenza and some types of pneumonia, respiratory diseases often develop slowly and progress without the individual's awareness.

Guidelines for Care | 16-6

The patient undergoing thoracocentesis

Explain procedure. Emphasize the importance of not moving, breathing quietly, and not coughing during the procedure to avoid damage to the pleura. Although a local anaesthetic is used, discomfort may be felt when the needle enters the pleura.

Patient's respiratory status and vital signs are assessed before the procedure to collect baseline data.

If possible, the patient sits on the side of the bed with feet supported in a chair. With the use of an elevated bed table, the patient is helped to maintain a position with the head resting upon folded arms or a pillow. Patients who are unable to sit up should be turned onto the unaffected side with several pillows.

Reassure and provide physical support, such as holding patient's hand.

Monitor vital signs, general appearance, and respiratory status throughout the procedure. No more than 1500 ml of pleural fluid should be removed within a 30-minute period because of the risk of intravascular fluid shift with resultant pulmonary oedema.

After the needle is withdrawn, a sterile occlusive dressing and pressure is applied to the site.

After thoracocentesis, the patient is positioned on the unaffected side with the insertion site up.

Monitor respiratory status, vital signs, and puncture site. Observe for signs of the following complications:

Intravascular shift: hypotension, a rapid thready pulse, and increasing shortness of breath.

Lung trauma: coughing paroxysms, bloody sputum, or tracheal deviation.

Because of the deleterious effects of cigarette smoking on the cardiopulmonary systems, a concerted effort is indicated to teach people about the hazards of smoking. In recent years many organizations, most notably the Department of Health, the Health Education Authority and voluntary organizations such as the Chest, Heart and Stroke Association have launched campaigns to reduce cigarette smoking in the United Kingdom. These campaigns have been somewhat successful, and it is now estimated that only 30% of the adult population in the United Kingdom smokes. However, the number of women smokers has increased, and this is reflected in the ever-rising increase in morbidity and mortality from lung disease, especially cancer of the lung and chronic obstructive pulmonary diseases, among women. A major emphasis has been on preventing children and teenagers from beginning to smoke. Unfortunately, smoking among teenagers remains a problem. In the United Kingdom the number of manual workers who smoke (36-48% men and 32-36% women) is considerably higher than the number of non-manual workers (16-25% men and 16-27% women), and is increasing.

Primary Prevention: Prevention of Disease

Because the cause of many respiratory disorders is known, prevention is possible. The major emphasis is on avoiding respiratory infections and educating the public about the risks of cigarette smoking. Health practices helpful in preventing infection are outlined in Box 16-7.

Secondary Prevention: Early Detection

Medical attention should be sought for respiratory symptoms that do not subside within 2 weeks. Guidelines for early detection are listed in Box 16-8.

16-7

Prevention of respiratory infections

Preventing spread of infection

1. Isolate the infected person.
2. Teach the infected person to cover nose and mouth with a tissue when coughing or sneezing so that droplet nuclei are not released into the air.
3. Wash hands after coughing or sneezing.

Maintaining resistance to infection

1. Eat a balanced diet.
2. Get adequate rest and sleep.
3. Avoid crowds during periods of prevalent respiratory infections.
4. Receive annual influenza immunization and pneumonia vaccine every 3 to 5 years if over age 65 or if younger with chronic heart, lung, or renal disease.

16-8

Guidelines for early detection of major pulmonary disorders

1. Signs or symptoms requiring immediate medical follow-up
   Chronic cough
   Sputum
   Dyspnoea
2. Recommendations for screening for cancer of the lung
   Regular chest x-ray examination over age 40
   Those in high risk occupations should have yearly x-ray

MAJOR HEALTH PROBLEMS OF THE RESPIRATORY SYSTEM

There are several ways to classify disorders affecting the lung and respiration, but one of the most useful and commonly used is to divide them into restrictive and obstructive diseases.

In *restrictive lung disease, there is a restriction in lung volume and a reduction in lung compliance.* As a result there is a reduction in total lung capacity (TLC) and a decrease in vital capacity (VC) to less than the predicted norm.

In contrast, in obstructive lung disease, there is an increase in airway resistance resulting in prolonged exhalation. This results in an increase in residual volume (RV) while TLC may be normal or increased. Thus pulmonary function tests are necessary to establish the diagnosis. A comparison of the characteristic changes in pulmonary function tests for restrictive and obstructive disease is shown in Table 16-6.

There are several conditions that can cause restrictive pulmonary disease and examples of these can be found in

Table 16-7. It is impossible to discuss all of these conditions in this chapter. Atelectasis, which is the most frequent postoperative complication, is discussed in Chapter 14, Postoperative Intervention.

Conditions that result in restrictive or obstructive pulmonary disease that are discussed in this chapter are the following.

1. Restrictive pulmonary disorders
   a. Infectious diseases of the pulmonary tract
      (1) Viral: acute bronchitis
      (2) Bacterial: pneumonia, tuberculosis
   b. Occupational lung disease
   c. Adult respiratory distress syndrome (ARDS)
   d. Carcinoma of the lung
2. Obstructive pulmonary disorders
   a. Chronic bronchitis
   b. Pulmonary emphysema
   c. Asthma
   d. Cystic fibrosis

Table 16-6 Comparison of pulmonary function test results in restrictive and obstructive disease

Test	Restrictive	Obstructive
FVC	Decreased	Decreased or normal
RV	Decreased	Increased
TLC	Decreased	Normal or increased
RV/TLC	Normal or increased	Significantly increased
$FEV_{1.0}$/FVC	Normal or increased	Decreased
$FEV_{3.0}$/FVC	Normal or increased	Decreased

From Morrissey W: *Respiratory diseases.* In Kaye D, Rose LF, editors: *Fundamentals of internal medicine,* St Louis, 1983, Mosby–Year Book.

Table 16-7 Restrictive pulmonary disease

Alteration	Disease example
Parenchymal inflammation	Pneumonia, adult respiratory distress syndrome
Space-occupying lesions	Tumours, malignancies
Diffuse pulmonary disease	Silicosis, fibrosis
Pleural disease	Pleural effusion
Lung collapse	Pneumothorax, atelectasis
Resectional surgery	Pneumonectomy
Neuromuscular disorders	Poliomyelitis, Guillain-Barré syndrome, myasthenia gravis
CNS depression	Narcotics, cerebral oedema
Limitation of thoracic mobility	Abdominal tumours, ascites, paralytic ileus
Changes in bony thorax	Kyphoscoliosis

INFECTIOUS DISEASES: VIRAL DISEASES OF THE RESPIRATORY TRACT

For a viral infection of the lung to occur, pathogens must be able to enter the lower respiratory tract. This means that the defence mechanisms of the lung must be overcome in some manner. There are many lung defence mechanisms, including upper airway defences, lower respiratory tract clearance mechanisms, and intrapulmonary detoxification mechanisms.

Many respiratory diseases are probably caused by viral infections. Presently, more than 30 diseases have been found to be directly related to viral infections, and there are probably many more. Some diseases may be caused by one virus; different viruses may cause the same symptoms.

If specific signs are not evident, the clinical illness is termed a common cold, viral infection pyrexia of unknown origin (PUO), or acute respiratory illness. The most common specific respiratory diseases caused by the various viruses are epidemic pleurodynia (Bornholm's disease), acute laryngotracheobronchitis, viral pneumonia, and influenza. Most adults have developed antibodies for the more common viruses, and most viral infections are rela-

tively mild. However, they are frequently complicated by secondary bacterial infections. When new strains of the influenza virus develop, severe epidemics may ensue, and many people may die from secondary infections such as pneumonia.

ACUTE BRONCHITIS
Aetiology/Epidemiology

Bronchitis can be acute or chronic (chronic bronchitis will be discussed later in this chapter). Acute bronchitis is an inflammation of the bronchi and sometimes the trachea (tracheobronchitis). Although it occurs most often in people with chronic lung disease, it also occurs as an extension of an upper respiratory infection in people without underlying lung disease and is therefore communicable. It also may be caused by physical or chemical agents such as dust, smoke, or volatile fumes. As air pollution increases, the incidence of acute bronchitis increases. *Acute bronchitis is typically viral in origin, but bacterial pathogens such as Streptococcus pneumoniae and Haemophilus influenzae may also cause bronchitis, either as a primary or secondary infection.*

Nursing Process
Assessment

Subjective data

1. Onset and duration of symptoms (see Table 16-8)
2. Medications taken for cough and their effectiveness

Objective data

1. Vital signs—temperature may be elevated; tachypnoea frequent with severe bronchitis
2. Rasping cough with mucoid sputum
3. Chest percussion by doctor—normal
4. Auscultation by doctor—vesicular breath sounds, vocal fremitus normal, adventitious sounds—localized rales and sibilant rhonchi

Nursing Analysis

Problems are determined from analysis of patient data. Possible problems for the people with acute bronchitis may include, but are not limited to, the following:

Problems	Possible aetiologies
Airway clearance, ineffective	Tracheobronchial infection, obstruction, or secretion
Breathing pattern, ineffective	Decreased energy, fatigue
Pain	Rib or muscle trauma from coughing; inflammation of tracheobronchial tree
Knowledge deficit	Lack of exposure to information

Planning: Expected Patient Outcomes

Expected patient outcomes for the person with acute bronchitis may include, but are not limited to, the following:

1. Patient demonstrates effective cough with adequate sputum production.
   a. Both cough and sputum production decrease within 72 hours of treatment initiation.

Table 16-8 Signs and symptoms and medical therapy for acute bronchitis

Symptoms	Signs	Medical therapy
Cough	Sputum production: Viral-clear to mucopurulent: bacterial-purulent	No specific therapy for viral infection, therapy directed to relief of symptoms, i.e. cough medicine, vaporizer; fluid intake 3-4 L/day
		Bland diet
Chest pain	Tachypnoea	Antibiotics for bacterial infection (elevation in temperature and mucopurulent sputum)
	Diffuse rhonchi/wheezes	
	Chest X-ray—clear, differentiates bronchitis from pneumonia	Rest
		Avoiding exposure to further infection

b. For people with chronic lung disease, sputum becomes clear and thin (return to prebronchitis status).
2. Patient demonstrates effective breathing patterns.
3. Patient demonstrates prebronchitis vital signs.
4. Patient reports that chest pain is decreased or absent.
5. Patient describes the cause and factors contributing to the occurrence of acute bronchitis and names common symptoms of it.

Implementation
Assisting with achievement of therapeutic goals
Medications for bacterial primary or secondary infection

Therapy for bacterial primary or secondary infections may be necessary in some cases, but is controversial except in severe cases. Antibiotics that may be used include amoxycillin, co-trimoxazole (or trimethoprim) or a tetracycline such as doxycycline. The choice depends on local resistance patterns. Other antibiotics that may be used include ampicillin, a cephalosporin such as cefaclor, and erythromycin.

Interventions to achieve patient outcomes
Assisting with coughing

Assist the patient to cough effectively. Coughing is normally a mechanism that aids in the removal of inhaled foreign materials. When an infection is present the throat becomes dry and irritated and there is an increase in mucus production as part of the lung defence mechanisms.

Receptors for the cough reflex are located in the tracheal and bronchial mucosa with the largest concentration of them being found in the larynx, carina, and bifurcations of the large- and medium-sized bronchi. When these receptors are stimulated, impulses are transmitted primarily via the afferent nervous pathways (vagus, phrenic, and spinal motor nerves) to expiratory musculature (larynx, tracheobronchial tree, diaphragm, and the abdominal wall).

To produce an effective cough there must be a deep inspiration followed by maximum expiratory effort against a closed glottis. This results in a tremendous increase in intrathoracic pressure. As the glottis opens, mucus and inhaled particles are forced out of the airways at a high velocity.

Persistent coughing can be very annoying and tiring to the patient and those around him or her. Complications of persistent coughing include insomnia, exhaustion, vomiting, urinary incontinence, rib or muscle trauma, pneumo-

Table 16-9 Medications used to treat cough

Desired effect	Medications prescribed
↑ Secretions	Expectorants Ammonium chloride Ipecacuanha Squill
↓ Secretions	Anticholinergic agents Atropine
Thin secretions	Mucolytic agents Acetylcysteine Carlocysteine Methylcysteine
Depress cough reflex	Antitussives Narcotic Codeine phosphate Pholcodine Dextromethorphan hydrobramide
Soothing preparation	Simple linctus

thorax, or fainting. If cough is present, give prescribed medication. Table 16-9 lists commonly used medications and their desired effects.

Assist with coughing as necessary by supporting chest (front and back) as patient coughs. Teach patient to cough effectively to maintain a clear airway and collect required specimens. Tell patient to take a deep breath, force the air out down to residual volume, contract the diaphragm, exhale forcefully and then cough. Successful airway clearance and an effective breathing pattern should help return vital signs to prebronchitis levels.

Additional assistance in achieving therapeutic goals includes the following:
1. Provide for good drainage of tracheobronchial secretions.
2. If antibiotics are prescribed, give on time to maintain therapeutic blood levels.
3. If steam vaporization is prescribed, administer it using precautions.
4. Assist the physiotherapist and reinforce their treatment regimen.

Assisting with comfort and ADL
1. Place patient in position of comfort; an upright position should improve the patient's ability to breathe.
2. Assist with ADL as necessary during acute phase of illness.

Facilitating learning

The patient should be taught to avoid people with upper respiratory infections. If respiratory infection does occur, the patient should seek medical attention.

If the patient smokes cigarettes, he or she should be encouraged to stop smoking. Group programmes are helpful to some people and the Health Promotion unit or family doctor can supply the names of local programmes to assist people to stop smoking.

Evaluation

Evaluation is based on patient outcomes. Questions to be asked include the following:

1. Have the patient's cough and sputum production decreased?
2. Is the patient breathing effectively?
3. Have the patient's vital signs returned to prebronchitis level?
4. Has the patient's chest pain decreased?
5. Can the patient list common symptoms and describe the cause of and factors contributing to acute bronchitis?

INFECTIOUS DISEASES: BACTERIAL DISEASES OF THE RESPIRATORY TRACT

As mentioned under viral infections, the protective mechanisms of the respiratory tract must be compromised before an infection can take hold.

PNEUMONIA
Aetiology/Epidemiology

Acute pneumonias are responsible for many of the hospital admissions in the United Kingdom. Pneumonia can occur in any season but is most common during winter and early spring. People of any age are susceptible, but pneumonia is more common among infants and the elderly. Pneumonia is often caused by aspiration of infected materials into the distal bronchioles and alveoli. *Certain individuals are especially susceptible,* including *people whose normal respiratory defence mechanisms are damaged or altered (those with chronic obstructive pulmonary disease, influenza,* and *tracheostomy,* and *those who have recently had anaesthesia); people who have a disease affecting antibody response (those with multiple myeloma, hypogammaglobulinaemia, and so on);* and *alcohol misusers in whom there is increased danger of aspiration and people with delayed white blood cell response to infection.* Increasingly, nosocomial pneumonia (acquired in the hospital) is a cause of morbidity and mortality. This is the direct result of an increase in the number of patients with impaired defences resulting from certain types of therapy and of an increase in the number of patients whose lives are being prolonged with life-support therapy.

Pneumonia is a communicable disease; the mode of transmission is dependent on the infecting organism. Pneumonia is classified according to the offending organism rather than the anatomic location (lobar or bronchial)

16-9

Organisms causing infectious pneumonia in adults

Typical or classic pneumonia syndrome
Bacterial pneumonia
    Common
        Streptococcus pneumoniae empyema
    Uncommon
        Haemophilus influenzae, Staphylococcus aureus

Atypical pneumonia syndrome
Common
    Mycoplasma pneumoniae
    Viral pathogens
Uncommon
    Legionella pneumophila
    Pneumocystis carinii

Aspiration pneumonia syndrome
Hospitalized, debilitated, or antibiotic-treated patients
    Mixed anaerobic/aerobic pharyngeal flora
    Staphylococcus aureus
    Klebsiella pneumoniae
    Pseudomonas aeruginosa
    Serratia marcescens
    Acinetobacter species
    Enteric gram-negative aerobes (*Escherichia coli* and *Enterobacter* and *Proteus* organisms)
Outpatients with normal pharyngeal flora
    Mixed anaerobic/aerobic pharyngeal flora

Haematogenous pneumonia syndromes
Staphyloccous aureus
Escherichia coli
Enteric/pelvic anaerobes

Adapted from Frame PT: *Basics RD* 10:1-8, 1982.

---

as was the practice in the past. A classification of pneumonia and its causative organisms in adults is presented in Box 16-9.

Pathophysiology

Pneumonia is an inflammatory process in which there is consolidation in the lung *caused by exudate filling the alveolar spaces. Gas exchange cannot take place in consolidated areas, and blood is shunted around the nonfunctioning alveoli. Hypoxaemia* may occur depending on how much lung tissue is involved. About 60% of patients with pneumococcal pneumonia have some degree of pleural effusion. Empyema may also occur in some patients with pneumonia.[116]

Typical or Classic Pneumonia

Typical or classic pneumonia occurs in both males and females of any age. It is found both in people without underlying disease and in those with diminished defence mechanisms. *Commonly, there is a history of alcohol misuse, recent respiratory tract infection, or viral influenza* (Table 16-10).

REVIEW

Table 16-10   Signs and symptoms and drug therapy of pneumonia

Pneumonia	Risk factors	Signs and symptoms	Drug therapy
Typical syndrome S. pneumoniae, un- complicated; Streptococcus p., complicated (em- pyema, metastic infection)	Sickle cell disease Hypogammaglobulinaemia Multiple myeloma	Sudden onset with shaking, chill Fever (39° to 40°C), pleuritic chest pain, productive cough Sputum—green and purulent and may be blood tinged; "rusty" Respirations—rapid and shallow with "grunting" at end of each breath Nasal flaring, intercostal rib retrac- tion, use of accessory muscles, and cyanosis may be present	*Drugs of choice* Benzylpenicillin Amoxycillin *Other effective drugs* Erythromycin, flucloxacillin cephalosporins, aminoglyco- sides
H. influenzae, S. aureas	Advanced age COPD Alcohol misuse Recent influenza		Benzylpenicillin Ampicillin *Other effective drugs* Chloramphenicol, cefamandole, co-trimoxazole *Other effective drugs* Methicillin, oxacillin, cefazolin, cephalothin, vancomycin, clindamycin Vancomycin, IV Cefazolin, IV, plus gentamicin or tobramycin
Atypical syndrome Common causes: mycoplasma pneumoniae, viral pathogens	Childhood, young adults	Onset gradual over 3 to 5 days Malaise, headache, sore throat, dry cough May have chest wall soreness from coughing	*Drug of choice:* Erythromycin *Other effective drugs:* Tetracycline None
Uncommon causes: Legionella pneumophilia	Recent URI; influenza	Above plus abdominal pain and diarrhoea Temperature 40° C or greater Shaking chills Respiratory distress Renal failure, hyponatraemia, hypo- phosphataemia, elevated creatine phosphokinase	*Drug of choice:* Erythromycin *Other effective drugs:* Rifmapicin, gentamicin
Pneumocystic carinii	Immunological deficiency Renal transplantation Autoimmune disease Debilitation	Gradual onset with increasing dys- pnoea, dry cough, tachypnoea, hypoxaemia X-ray film—diffuse interstitial in- volvement	Co-trimoxazole Pentamidine
Aspiration Gram-negative ba- cilli; Klebsiella, Pseudomonas, Serratia, Entero- bacter, Esche- richia, Proteus, gram-positive ba- cilli	Alcohol misuse Debilitation Hospitalization (that is, nosocomial infection)	Mixed anaerobic: At first gradual onset Low-grade fever, cough Sputum—increased production, foul smelling Chest x-ray film—interstitial in- volvement in dependent portion of lung	Antibiotic therapy dependent on pathogen causing infection
S. aureus, gastric acid aspiration	Altered consciousness Aspiration of inert sub- stances: water, barium, nutritional supplements	Gram-negative or positive infec- tion: may present same clinical picture as classic pneumonia Sudden onset of respiratory dis- tress, severe dyspnoea, cyanosis, coughing, hypoxaemia, followed by signs and symptoms of sec- ondary infection	
Haematogenous Staphylococcus, E. coli, enteric anae- robes	Infected intravascular catheter Endocarditis, IV drug misuse Intraabdominal abscess Pyonephrosis Empyema of gallbladder	Pulmonary symptoms minimal compared with the symptoms of septicaemia Nonproductive cough and pleuritic pain similar to that seen in pul- monary embolism are most common complaints	*Drugs of choice* Ampicillin IV; plus gentamicin or tobramycin Clindamycin IV; plus gentami- cin or tobramycin

Atypical Pneumonia
Aetiology/epidemiology

The most common form of atypical pneumonia in adults is caused by *Mycoplasma pneumoniae*. *Legionella pneumophila* is an uncommon cause of atypical pneumonia. It occurs more commonly in older adults and in people who smoke or have abnormal pulmonary defences.[117] *Legionella pneumophila* is the agent causing Legionnaires' disease (legionellosis). It is three times more common in men than in women. *A number of conditions are believed to predispose one to legionellosis. These include chronic renal disease, chronic bronchitis or emphysema, diabetes, cancer, immunosuppressive medications, and smoking.* In the United States it is estimated that about 25,000 cases of Legionnaires' disease occur each year.

Both epidemics and sporadic cases of Legionnaires' disease occur. Epidemics have been associated with common source exposures such as air conditioning, water-cooling towers, and excavation sites. *Legionella pneumophila* has been isolated from soil and fresh water and from shower heads in hospitals.

Fine inspiratory rales may be present, but there is no evidence of consolidation. A radiograph of the chest shows patchy segmental infiltrates, which may progress from unilateral to bilateral. Pleural effusion is uncommon. Patients with legionellosis may have renal failure, hyponatraemia, hypophosphataemia, and an elevation of creatine phosphokinase.

Medical therapy

The usual treatment for both *Mycoplasma pneumoniae* and *Legionella pneumophila* pneumonia is erythromycin (see Table 16-10). If a patient is seriously ill with Legionnaires' disease, rifampicin may be added to the treatment with erythromycin. Rifampicin should never be used alone because of the great likelihood of resistant organisms developing during monotherapy. *Because relapses have occurred within 1 to 2 weeks of therapy, it is recommended that treatment for Legionnaires' disease be continued for 3 weeks.*

The overall mortality of Legionnaires' disease is 10% to 15%. Most of this is attributed to respiratory failure.

When *Mycoplasma* pneumonia is untreated, the fever and malaise generally resolve in 1 to 2 weeks. Serious systemic complications are quite rare, although haemolytic anaemia, disseminated intravascular coagulation (DIC), thrombocytopenic purpura and renal failure, myocarditis and pericarditis, meningoencephalitis and other neurological syndromes, arthritis, and hepatitis have been reported.[117] The mortality for *Mycoplasma* pneumonia is less than 1%.[117]

Pneumocystis carinii

For approximately 40 years, *Pneumocystis carinii* has been recognized as a cause of pneumonia in immunosuppressed patients. *Pneumocystis carinii* is the most common life-threatening infection to people with acquired immunodeficiency syndrome (AIDS). Malaise, fever, non-productive cough, and dyspnoea are the usual symptoms.

A radiograph of the chest shows diffuse bilateral pulmonary infiltrates, although the infiltrates may be found only in upper or lower lobes.

Medical treatment includes the intravenous administration of co-trimoxazole. Pentamidine isethionate may be used in place of co-trimoxazole in people intolerant to it. The relapse rate of *Pneumocystis carinii* in people with AIDS is estimated to be approximately 20% to 30%. Failure to respond to therapy, the necessity of mechanical ventilation, and repeated episodes of *Pneumocystis carinii* are all associated with a poor prognosis. (See Chapter 13 for further discussion of AIDS.)

Aspiration Pneumonia

The common factor in all forms of aspiration pneumonia is the aspiration of material into the airways. Aspiration pneumonia can occur while the patient is in the hospital, but diligent nursing care may prevent it. The types of aspiration pneumonia are listed in Box 16-10.

Haematogenous Pneumonia

Bacterial infections of the lung can also occur when pathogenic organisms are spread to the lungs through the bloodstream. See Table 16-10 for signs and symptoms and medical therapy of this type of pneumonia.

16-10

Types of aspiration pneumonia

Noninfectious aspiration pneumonia
1. Aspiration of gastric acid
   a. Only a small quantity of aspirated gastric acid causes severe respiratory distress within a few seconds.
   b. Bacterial superinfection, if it does occur, does not become evident for 48 to 72 hours.
2. Aspiration of large quantities of inert substances
   a. Common substances include water, barium, tube-feeding liquids, and nonacid gastric contents.
   b. Aspirated substances obstruct airways, causing respiratory distress.
   c. Secondary bacterial infection may occur in lung segments that have obstructed airways.
3. Noninfectious aspiration syndrome is witnessed or identified from suctioning of foreign material from lungs.

Bacterial aspiration pneumonia
1. High-risk people
   a. People with disorders of consciousness (for example, anaesthesia, coma, seizures, or alcohol misuse).[117]
   b. People with poor cough mechanisms (for example, laryngeal dysfunction or respiratory muscle paralysis).
2. Mixed anaerobic and aerobic flora of the upper respiratory tract is most common cause.

Nursing Process
Assessment
Subjective data

1. Onset and duration of:
   a. Cough
   b. Fever
   c. Shaking chills
   d. Chest pain
   e. Sputum production (amount, colour, and consistency; see Box 16-4, p. 298)
2. Self-care modalities used to treat symptoms
3. History of exposure to:
   a. People with infection
   b. Pulmonary irritants

Objective data

1. Observe for signs of other chronic disease and general debilitation
2. Monitor vital signs
   a. Elevated temperature (39° C to 40° C) or low-grade temperature elevation
      · Tachycardia
      Tachypnoea
3. Pulmonary examination by doctor
   a. Inspection
      (1) Accessory muscle retraction
      (2) Central cyanosis
      (3) Respiratory grunting on expiration
      (4) Guarding and restricted chest movement on affected side
   b. Palpation
      (1) Decreased expansion on affected side of chest
      (2) Increased tactile femitus
   c. Percussion
      (1) Dullness on percussion
   d. Auscultation
      (1) Bronchial breath sounds
      (2) Inspiratory crackles (rales)
      (3) Decreased vocal fremitus (pleural effusion)
      (4) Egophony (consolidation)
4. Assess investigations
   a. Chest x-ray
      Diffuse involvement—atypical pneumonia
      Lobar involvement—typical pneumonia
   b. Haematology
      (1) WBC—elevated 15 to 25×10^9/L
      (2) Cold agglutins—complement fixation/viral or *Mycoplasma pneumoniae*
   c. Arterial blood gas studies
      (1) Hypoxaemia/respiratory alkalosis
      (2) If underlying chronic pulmonary disease, respiratory acidosis

Nursing analysis

Problems are determined from analysis of patient data. Possible problems for the person with pneumonia may include but are not limited to:

Problems	Possible aetiologies
Airway clearance, ineffective	Decreased energy, fatigue, tracheobronchial inflammation
Gas exchange, impaired	Alveolar-capillary membrane changes, altered oxygen delivery
Pain	Pleural inflammation, coughing paroxysms
Infection, high risk	Compromised lung defence system
Knowledge deficit: condition and its treatment	Lack of exposure to or unfamiliarity with information
Nutrition, altered: less than body requirements	Increased metabolic needs Anorexia due to infectious process, sputum production

Planning: expected patient outcomes

Expected patient outcomes for the person with pneumonia may include, but are not limited to, the following:

1. Patient demonstrates effective cough with adequate sputum production. (Both cough and sputum production decrease within 72 hours of treatment initiation. Patient with chronic lung disease returns to prepneumonia status.)
2. Patient demonstrates improved ventilation and adequate oxygenation of tissues
   a. pH returns within normal limits.
   b. Po_2 during active disease—8 to 10.6 kPa (60 to 80 mm Hg); after resolution of disease, Pao_2 within normal limits.
3. Patient reports absence of chest pain.
4. Patient does not develop a superinfection.
5. Patient states when influenza and pneumonia vaccines should be taken.
6. Patient can state the signs and symptoms that should be reported to the doctor.
7. Patient describes the cause and factors contributing to the occurrence of pneumonia and names common symptoms indicating pneumonia.
8. Patient maintains prepneumonia body weight.
9. Patient's appetite improves and weight gain returns weight to near preillness level.

Implementation
Assisting with achievement of therapeutic goals
Medications

1. Before beginning administration of prescribed antibiotic, sputum is collected for culture. If blood culture is ordered, blood is also obtained before therapy is begun.
2. Antibiotic blood levels are monitored by giving antibiotics at scheduled times. (Table 16-10 lists the antibiotic therapy currently employed in treating pneumonia.)
3. Give medication prescribed to relieve pain. Codeine may be prescribed because it is less likely to inhibit the cough reflex than more potent narcotics.

Oxygen therapy

Oxygen by mask or cannula is usually ordered when Po_2 is less than 8 kPa (60 mm Hg).[117] When supplemental oxygen is necessary it may be administered by nasal prongs or by mask. The method used depends on the patient's condition and the concentration of oxygen required. The nurse should be familiar with the various devices used to administer oxygen, and when oxygen is in use the nurse should check the equipment frequently to be sure that it is working properly.

When the patient is having difficulty exchanging oxygen and carbon dioxide, such as occurs in pulmonary oedema, oxygen may be given under positive pressure. In some situations, such as chronic obstructive pulmonary disease, low-flow rates of oxygen are indicated. The use of low-flow oxygen is discussed on p. 362. *In all situations, the nurse should remember that a patient suffering from hypoxaemia may not be breathless or cyanotic because cyanosis does not occur until there is 5 g or more of deoxygenated haemoglobin.* In people with anaemia, all the available haeme is completely saturated with oxygen and thus they are never cyanotic even though they may be hypoxaemic. *For this reason an increase in the pulse rate may be the first indication that the patient is experiencing hypoxaemia.* Patients receiving oxygen therapy are monitored by arterial blood gas studies. These studies are explained on p. 300.

Interventions to achieve patient outcomes
Facilitating breathing

Assist the patient to breathe deeply and expand the chest to increase ventilation.

1. Place patient in position to facilitate breathing—usually upright or semi-upright position (Fig. 16-5).
2. A pillow may be placed lengthwise at patient's back to provide support and thrust thorax slightly forward, allowing freer use of the diaphragm.
3. The patient who must be upright to breathe may find it restful to rest head and arms on a pillow placed on an overbed table (Fig. 16-6).
4. For the patient with severe hypoxaemia, cotsides should be in place. Patient can use them to assist in moving about in bed.

5. Some patients may breathe best when sitting up in a large armchair while leaning on a smaller chair placed in front of them. This chair is blocked to prevent it from slipping.

Maintaining ventilation, humidity, and a comfortable temperature

1. Most patients are most comfortable if air is cool and not too humid. If available an air-conditioned room may make the patient more comfortable.
2. If patient has nose, throat, or bronchial irritation, warm moist air from a *humidifier* or *vaporizer* may be helpful.

Vaporizers. Small electric vaporizers can be purchased at most large chemist shops. However, when a patient cannot afford to purchase one, the nurse can assist in improvising equipment for inhalation and for proper humidity. An empty coffee tin or a shallow pie tin can be filled with sterile water and placed on an electric plate in the person's room to increase humidity. If the inhalation is to be directed, an ordinary steam kettle or a tea kettle with a longer improvised paper spout may be used. The paper should be changed frequently. A few drops of menthol or oil of eucalyptus can be put into the water. Benzoin causes corrosion in the kettle, which is exceedingly difficult to remove. The kettle and electric plate should be placed a safe distance from the face so that the medicated steam can be breathed freely but the person cannot be scalded or burned by accidentally tipping the kettle or by touching the hot plate. After the 25- to 30-minute treatment, equipment should be removed from the bedside.

Hydration. Dehydration results in thick, tenacious secretions. *The best liquefying agent is water, and it is preferable to adequately hydrate the patient rather than attempt to loosen secretions with mist therapy.* If the patient does not have cardiovascular disease requiring fluid restriction, a fluid intake of 3 to 4 L/day should be provided.

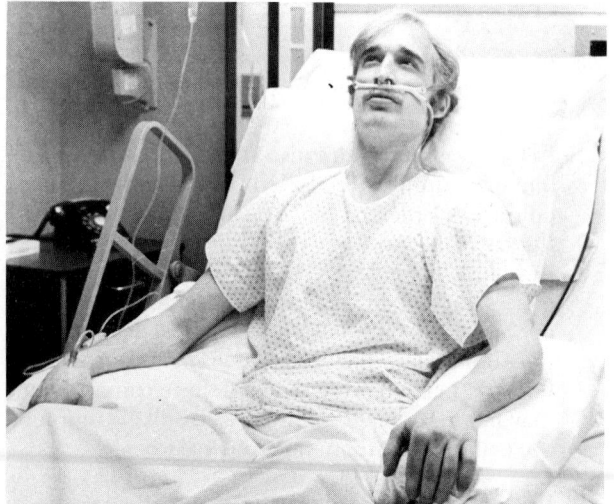

Fig. 16-5 Patient sitting upright with pillows under head and each arm to promote chest expansion and comfort.

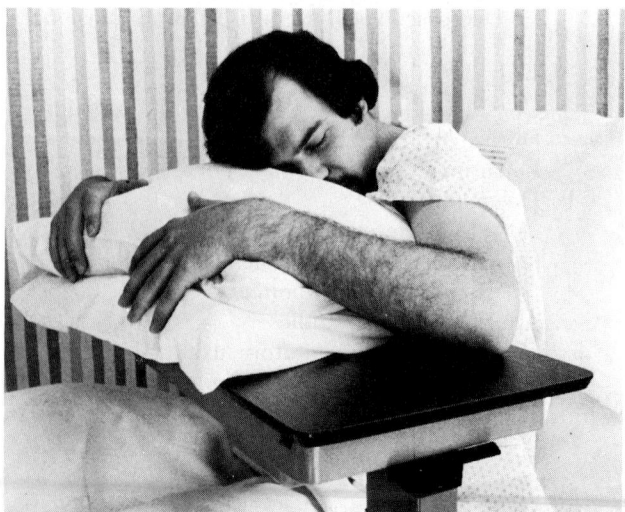

Fig. 16-6 Pillows placed on over-bed table provide comfortable support for the patient who must sleep in a sitting position.

Assisting with comfort and ADL

1. Place patient in position of comfort—patients are usually most comfortable in an upright position.
2. Support the patient's chest during coughing.

Preventing spread of infection

1. When universal precautions are used, respiratory isolation is unnecessary.
2. Hand washing is the most important way to prevent spread of pneumonia from one patient to another via the hands of hospital personnel.

Facilitating learning

The major emphasis is on prevention.

1. Two vaccines are now available to prevent respiratory infections: influenza vaccine and pneumococcal vaccine.
2. People at high risk for developing complications of influenza (pneumonia) should be immunized unless they are allergic to eggs or egg products or have had a previous reaction to vaccine.

   a. Influenza vaccine is given yearly.

   b. *Pneumonia polysaccharide* vaccine is given only every 5 years.

3. Attention needs to be paid to reducing the likelihood of gram-negative colonization patients. For this reason many hospitals have instituted tighter control policies on the use of some antibiotics except in situations where a review panel of doctors approves their use. A reduction in use of antibiotics also reduces the incidence of antibiotic-resistant hospital flora, which are the source of many nosocomial infections. (See Chapter 12.)

Complications of pneumonia

With the advent of antibiotics and better diagnostic measures such as x-ray procedures, complications during or following pneumonia are rare in otherwise healthy people. *Atelectasis, delayed resolution, lung abscess, pleural effusion, empyema, pericarditis, meningitis, and relapse are complications that were common in the past.* The fact that pneumonia and influenza remain an important cause of death in the United Kingdom is an impressive reason for strict adherence to the prescribed medical treatment. Careful and accurate observation as well as sufficient time for convalescence also helps to ensure that the average patient has a smooth recovery. Elderly people and those with a chronic illness are likely to have a relatively long course of convalescence from pneumonia, and there is a greater possibility of their developing complications. *In the United States there has been an increase in the incidence of staphylococcal pneumonia subsequent to influenza. Consolidation of lung tissue, pleural effusion, and empyema frequently occur soon after onset of this type of pneumonia and may cause death.*

Evaluation

Evaluation is based on patient outcome. Questions to be asked include the following:

1. Have the patient's cough and sputum production improved?
2. Have the patient's Pao_2 and pH returned to normal limits?
3. Does patient state that chest pain is absent?
4. Is the patient free of a superinfection?
5. Can the patient state the cause of and factors contributing to pneumonia?
6. Can the patient state the common symptoms of pneumonia?
7. Can the patient state when influenza or pneumonia vaccines should be taken?
8. Can the patient state the signs and symptoms that should be reported to the doctor?
9. Is the patient's appetite improved and weight returning to prepneumonia levels?

TUBERCULOSIS
Aetiology/Epidemiology

In 1900 tuberculosis was the leading cause of death in the developed world. It is still a major killer in other countries with 3 million deaths worldwide. It remained a major cause of death until the introduction of antituberculosis drug therapy in the late 1940s and early 1950s. The most effective of these agents is isoniazid, which first became available clinically in 1952. The use of isoniazid in combination with two agents introduced earlier, streptomycin and paraaminosalicylic acid, resulted in a striking decrease in tuberculosis mortality rates. It also made it possible for patients with tuberculosis to be treated on an outpatient basis. However, some patients still have to be hospitalized during their illness, and most nurses will care for a patient with tuberculosis at some time in their careers.

Although tuberculosis is considered a preventable and curable disease, it is a disease that demands constant public health surveillance. Pulmonary tuberculosis in the United Kingdom declined steadily from 1961, when there were 23,000 reported cases, to 1991, when there were 4,500 reported cases. From 1981 to 1991, the number of cases of respiratory tuberculosis notified in the United Kingdom remained fairly static, but recent data suggest that tuberculosis is increasing again. This increase is being seen in the elderly population and in those individuals who are HIV positive (Fig. 16-7).

Because HIV infection is an important risk factor for developing clinically apparent tuberculosis among people already infected with the tubercle bacillus, it is recommended that all HIV-infected people be screened for tuberculosis and latent tuberculous infection and, if infected, given appropriate therapy. Also, where appropriate, people with tuberculosis and known tuberculin-positive people should be evaluated for HIV infection so that appropriate counselling and treatment can be given.

Tuberculosis is caused by bacillus, *mycobacterium tuberculosis*, or tubercle bacillus, a gram-positive and acid-fast organism. If microscopic study of a slide prepared from the sputum of an individual reveals tubercle bacilli, the individual is said to have positive sputum; and this confirms the diagnosis of tuberculosis. However, most people with tuberculosis will not have positive sputum on smear, and a *positive sputum culture* will be necessary to confirm the diagnosis. Patients who have a positive culture and negative smear are less infectious than are those with both a positive smear and culture.

When a person with tuberculosis speaks, coughs, sneezes, or sings, minute droplets fall to the ground; the smaller ones evaporate, leaving *droplet nuclei* that remain suspended indefinitely in the air and are carried on air currents. Droplet nuclei are 1 to 10 μm in size and are small enough to be inhaled into the alveoli. Thus tuberculosis is transmitted by inhalation of tubercle-laden droplet nuclei.

Pathophysiology

When an individual with no previous exposure to tuberculosis (negative tuberculin reactor) inhales a sufficient number of tubercle bacilli into the alveoli, tuberculosis *infection* occurs. The body's reaction to the tubercle bacilli depends on the *susceptibility of the individual, the size of the dose, and the virulence of the organisms*. Inflammation occurs within the alveoli (parenchyma) of the lungs, and natural body defences attempt to counteract the infection.

Tuberculosis infection is unlike other infections. Usually, other infections disappear completely when overcome

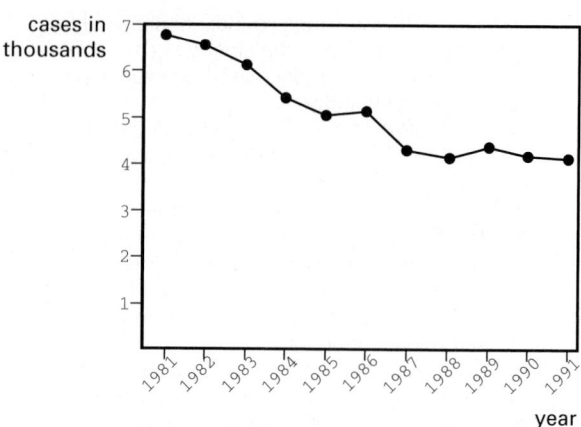

Fig. 16-7 Tuberculosis cases (numbers in thousands) 1981-1991 for the United Kingdom. (Social Trends-various dates Central Statistical Office, HMSO.)

by the body's defences and leave no living organisms and generally no signs of infection. However, a person who has been infected with tubercle bacilli harbours the organism for the remainder of his or her life unless they have received prophylactic isoniazid. Tubercle bacilli remain in the lungs in a dormant, walled-off, or so-called resting state. When a person is under physical or emotional stress, these bacilli may become active and begin to multiply. If body defences are low, active tuberculosis may develop. Most people who have active tuberculosis developed it in this manner. However, it is generally accepted that only 1 out of 10 people with a positive tuberculin test will ever develop active tuberculosis, and the incidence is expected to be much lower among those who receive preventive therapy with isoniazid.

Primary and Secondary Prevention

To eliminate tuberculosis, the organism must be prevented from being transmitted from one person to another. In the United States prevention of tuberculosis has become a major health issue with measures directed towards priority recommendations. Nurses in the United Kingdom will find parallel areas of concern. These recommendations can be found in Box 16-11.

People over 35 years of age without the risk factors listed here are not given preventive chemotherapy because of the risk of isoniazid-associated hepatitis. Although the risk is small, it is age related and increases from less than 0.2% in those under age 20 to up to 2.3% in those 50 to 64 years of age.

If isoniazid-associated hepatitis occurs, the symptoms are mild, nonspecific, and resemble those of any viral illness. (See Chapter 22 for a discussion of viral hepatitis.)

Contraindications to the use of isoniazid preventive therapy are (1) previous isoniazid-associated liver disease; (2) severe adverse reactions to isoniazid, including fever, chills, rash, and arthritis; and (3) *acute* liver disease of any cause.

People receiving isoniazid preventive chemotherapy should be seen at regular intervals by a health care provider

Priorities for preventive therapy among TB-infected people

1. People with HIV infection
2. Recent contacts of people with infectious TB
3. People with recent skin test conversions
4. People with recent TB disease who have been inadequately treated
5. People with negative sputum cultures and stable fibrotic lesions on chest radiographs consistent with inactive TB
6. People with medical conditions that increase the risk of TB
   - Leukaemia or lymphoma
   - Silicosis
   - Diabetes mellitus
   - Gastrectomy
   - End-stage renal disease
   - Antibodies to human immunodeficiency virus (HIV)

for the purpose of reinforcing the necessity of taking the chemotherapy regularly and to monitor the patient for any serious side effects. Because most cases of tuberculosis in patients with HIV infection occur in those with a history of a positive tuberculin test, people with HIV infection should be considered for preventive therapy with isoniazid. Groups that should receive particular attention are intravenous drug users, prison inmates, and the homeless, because they have an extraordinarily high incidence of HIV and tuberculosis infection.[2]

Because of the difficulty in preventing tuberculosis among homeless people special recommendations have been made for the group[12a]:

1. The highest priority should be given to (1) detection, evaluation, and reporting of homeless people who have current symptoms of active TB and (2) completion of an appropriate course of treatment by those diagnosed with active TB.
2. The second priority should be screening and preventive therapy for homeless people who have, or are suspected of having, human immunodeficiency virus (HIV) infection.
3. The third priority should be the examination and appropriate treatment of people with recent TB that has been inadequately treated.
4. The fourth priority should be screening and appropriate treatment of people exposed to an infectious (sputum-positive) case of TB. Because contacts are difficult to define in a shelter population, it is usually necessary to screen all residents of a shelter when an infectious case is identified.
5. The fifth priority should be screening and preventive therapy for homeless people with known medical conditions that increase the risk of TB, for example, diabetes mellitus and other conditions listed in Box 16-11, Number 6.

Preventive chemotherapy in the United Kingdom is isoniazid daily for 6 months. The usual adult dose is 300 mg in a single dose daily. If the person has antibodies to the human immunodeficiency virus (HIV), isoniazid is given daily for 1 year.

In 1989, the United States CDC's Advisory Committee for the Elimination of Tuberculosis (ACET) published *A Strategic Plan for Elimination of Tuberculosis in the United States*. The committee recommended that a goal be established to eliminate tuberculosis by the year 2010. To achieve the goal, a case rate of 0.1 per 100,000 people was set for the year 2010, with an interim goal of a case rate of 3.5 per 100,000 population by the year 2000. This goal may not be easy to accomplish, in view of the 1990 case rate of 10.0 per 100,000.[22]

Vaccination

Efforts continue in search of a more satisfactory tuberculosis vaccine. Presently, bacillus Calmette-Guérin (BCG) vaccine is used worldwide except in the United States and the Netherlands. The vaccine contains attenuated tubercle bacilli that have lost their ability to produce disease. It is administered only to people who have a negative reaction to the tuberculin test.

Most people who have received BCG will have a skin test reaction less than 10 mm. If a larger reaction occurs to purified protein derivative (PPD), it can be assumed that the person has a TB infection.

In the United Kingdom BCG is offered to all tuberculin negative children between the ages of 10 and 14. Additionally, it is given to health care workers, veterinary staff and those who deal with affected animal species, and tuberculosis contacts, including the newborn and immigrants from areas where tuberculosis incidence is high. The vaccine should be given only by people who have had careful instruction in the proper technique. When there is a positive reaction to skin testing with tuberculin, when acute infectious disease is present, or when there is any skin disease, BCG vaccine is not given. BCG vaccination should not be given within three weeks of a live virus, such as the rubella vaccine. Possible complications following vaccination are local ulcers, which occur in a relatively high percentage of people vaccinated, and abscesses or suppuration of lymph nodes, which occur in a small percentage.

In countries where living conditions are such that transmission of tuberculosis is to be expected, BCG vaccine may be given at birth and then repeated after 12 to 15 years. The intradermal method is used to administer the vaccine so that a uniform controlled dose can be given.

Diagnostic Tests

Each of the tests used to diagnose tuberculosis are described earlier in this chapter. The tests and the pages on which the tests are discussed are listed below.

1. Tuberculin skin testing (p. 298).
2. Chest X-ray (p. 296).
3. Sputum smear and culture (p. 298).

Establishing the diagnosis of tuberculosis

Results of chest X-rays and sputum examinations will either rule out the possibility or confirm a diagnosis of tuberculosis. Bacteriological confirmation of the presence of *M. tuberculosis* is necessary to establish the diagnosis of tuberculosis. Because it is impossible to differentiate between typical and atypical acid-fast bacilli by a sputum smear, cultures are obtained on all people. Cultures are also used for antimicrobial susceptibility (sensitivity) studies. *Despite the introduction of improved culture media, the tubercle bacillus grows slowly on artificial media, and culture reports are not available for 3 to 6 weeks.*

Blood-streaked sputum in the absence of pronounced coughing may be the first indication to the person that something is wrong. Pathological changes may have occurred in the lungs, but sputum examination may not show tubercle bacilli. However, if the nodules produced in the parenchyma of the lung become soft in the centre and then caseated and liquefied, the liquefied material may break through and empty into the bronchi and be raised as sputum. Cavities in the lung may appear on X-ray film and may be present in more than one lobe of the lung.

Medical management

Medical treatment is with antituberculosis drug therapy. The drugs used to treat tuberculosis, their classification, side effects, and tests for side effects can be found in Table 16-11. Other agents used include capreomycin and cycloserine.

The British Thoracic Society recommends an *initial phase* treatment with at least three agents for two months;

isoniazid, rifampicin and pyrazinamide are the drugs of choice. Ethambutol may be added if resistance is suspected. The *continuation phase* treatment comprises isoniazid and rifampicin for four months or longer; ethambutol or streptomycin are added if resistance is suspected.

Prevention

Preventing contamination of air with tubercle bacilli is accomplished by: (1) treating the patient with antituberculosis drugs and (2) preventing contamination of air with tubercle bacilli.

Facilitating learning

The most effective way to achieve the prevention of the transmission of tuberculosis is by patient teaching (Box 16-12).

OCCUPATIONAL LUNG DISEASES

Aetiology/Epidemiology

Many pulmonary diseases are believed to be caused by substances inhaled in the work place. They are more common (1) in manual workers than in non-manual workers, (2) in industrialized areas than in rural areas, and (3)

Table 16-11 Drugs used to treat tuberculosis

Drug	Classification	Common side effects	Tests	Remarks
Isoniazid (INH)	Bactericidal; penetrates all body tissues and fluids, including CSF	Peripheral neuritis hepatitis, rash, fever	AST, ALT (not as routine)	Daily alcohol intake interferes with metabolism of isoniazid and increases risk of hepatitis; antacids containing aluminum interfere with absorption of INH.
Rifampicin (RIF)	Bactericidal; penetrates all body tissues including CSF	Hepatitis, febrile reactions, thrombocytopenia (rare), hepatotoxicity increases when given with INH	AST, ALT platelet count (not as routine)	Urine, sweat, tears may turn orange temporarily; decrease effectiveness of oral contraceptives, anticoagulants, corticosteroids, barbiturates, hypoglycaemics, and digitalis
Ethambutol (EMB)	Bacteriostatic; does not penetrate CSF; penetrates other body fluids	Optic neuritis (reversible with discontinuation of drug; very rare at 15 mg/kg skin rash)	Visual acuity; red-green colour discrimination; GI irritation	No significant reaction with other drugs. Check vision monthly; give with food
Pyrazinamide (PZA)	Bacteriostatic or bactericidal depending on susceptibility of myocobacterium	Hyperuricaemia, hepatitis, arthralgia, GI irritation	Uric acid, AST, ALT	Obtain baseline liver function tests and repeat regularly. Give with food; Drink 2 L of fluid daily
Streptomycin (SM)	Bactericidal, aminoglycoside; disrupts protein synthesis; poor penetration into body tissues and CSF	Eighth cranial nerve damage (vestibular or cochlear; often damage is irreversible; nephrotoxicity	Vestibular function; audiograms; creatinine level determined before therapy started	Monitor kidney function monthly, monitor vestibular function with calorie stimulation test. Monitor hearing with audiograms. Meningitis treated with intrathecal or subarachnoid instillation of SM

in small and medium-sized businesses than in larger industrial plants.

In some instances it is debatable whether a person's lung disease is clearly occupation specific. This is especially so in cases of bronchitis, asthma, emphysema, or cancer because all of these conditions can be caused or aggravated by several factors found in many different occupations and by nonoccupational factors such as smoking and pollution of the atmosphere.[109]

In the United Kingdom many people are believed to be suffering from job-related diseases. Because these diseases are not always attributable to occupation, exact statistics do not exist. During 1989 there were some 2000 new cases of occupational lung disease reported for compensation purposes. Occupational asthma was the most commonly reported job-related lung disease. Any figures produced for occupational lung diseases are likely to underestimate the size of the problem as many go unreported or are misdiagnosed. Several millions of pounds a year are paid out in benefits and workers' compensation for job-related illnesses and injuries.

Prevention

Occupational lung diseases are preventable. However, there must be a concerted effort by the public, governmental agencies, and industry if these diseases are to be prevented.

Governmental action has been slow and has only occurred, in some instances, in response to environmental and health agencies, such as trade unions, that have lobbied for stricter regulation of harmful substances. What should be remembered is that whilst the health of workers is improved and health service costs are reduced there is a substantial increase in costs to industry which are eventually reflected in the prices to the consumer.

In the United Kingdom the Health and Safety Executive and Environmental Health Departments are responsible for ensuring that workplace safety legislation is enforced.

Occupational health departments in industries where workers may have exposure to harmful substances are responsible for monitoring both the workplace environment in terms of safety procedures and levels of substances, and the health and well-being of the workforce. The goal is that these job-related lung diseases become a thing of the past.

Many authorities believe that several things need to be done to reduce the incidence of occupation-related diseases: (1) education of the public about the relationship between polluted air in the work place and lung diseases; (2) general commitment to reducing, eliminating, or avoiding air pollution of the work place; and (3) elimination of the most prevalent and notorious lung hazard, cigarette smoke. (The reader is referred to reference 109 for more information.)

Education of the public includes not only employers and employees but also engineers and planners who design operations; buyers and purchasers who select ingredients, cleaning agents, and equipment; and doctors who see people with occupation-related diseases. Many times, workers who are instructed about the hazards involved in certain occupations and work places are helpful in deciding what preventive measures need to be taken to combat or minimize the effects of hazards. The commitment to reduce, eliminate, or avoid pollution of work place air requires full consideration of possible health effects whenever operations are planned, and improvement of conditions whenever possible.

It is well documented that smokers get occupation related lung diseases more often than nonsmokers and that smokers' lungs are more vulnerable to the effects of these diseases than are nonsmokers' lungs. The combined effects of cigarette smoke and industrial pollutants are very great. *The risk of developing chronic bronchitis, emphysema, lung cancer, and heart disease is much increased when a worker smokes.*[109] Some of these risks, such as lung cancer in asbestos workers who also smoke, are becoming more commonly known.

Occupation-related lung diseases can be divided into several categories. The major ones are (1) *the pneumoconioses, including silicosis and coal miner's pneumoconiosis (black lung disease);* (2) *asbestos-related lung disease;* and (3) *hypersensitivity diseases, including occupation-related asthma, allergic alveolitis (farmer's lung), and byssinosis (brown lung disease).*

The medical therapy and nursing care of these patients is dependent on the patient's signs and symptoms and complications. The reader is referred to other sections of this chapter for discussion of these topics.

The major role of nurses is to be knowledgeable about the cause and prevention of these diseases so that appropriate information and teaching can be presented to the public.

ADULT RESPIRATORY DISTRESS SYNDROME

Aetiology/Epidemiology

Adult respiratory distress syndrome (ARDS) is the name given to a syndrome of acute hypoxaemic respiratory failure without hypercapnia. The syndrome was first described by T.J. Petty in 1967. ARDS is often fatal and is characterized by severe dyspnoea, hypoxaemia, and diffuse bilateral pulmonary infiltrations after lung injury in previously healthy people. Recently, the term *hyperpermeability pulmonary oedema* (HPPE) has been used to describe the condition that affects many critical care patients yearly. Causes of ARDS are presented Box 16-13.

Prevention

Prompt treatment of the underlying cause of ARDS is the major focus of preventive care. Additionally, judicious use of the mechanical ventilator and oxygen therapy is required to avoid inducing ARDS as an untoward complication of these treatments.

Pathophysiology

The pathophysiological alterations that result in ARDS are typically initiated by a major trauma to the body, often a physical insult to a body system other than the pulmonary system.

16-13

Clinical conditions associated with ARDS/HPPE

Shock
  Septic
  Haemorrhagic
  Cardiogenic
  Anaphylactic
Trauma
  Pulmonary contusion
  Nonpulmonary, multisystem
Infection
  Pneumonia
    Viral
    Bacterial (staphylococcal or streptococcal)
      Legionellosis
  Miliary tuberculosis
Disseminated intravascular coagulation (DIC)
Fat emboli
Near-drowning
Aspiration: highly acid gastric contents (pH < 2.5)
Inhaled toxic agents
  Smoke
  Phosgene
  Oxides of nitrogen
Pancreatitis
Oxygen toxicity
Narcotic drug abuse
  Heroin
  Methadone
  Morphine
Radiation pneumonitis
Drugs
  Ethchlorvynol
  Salicylates

Adapted from Petty TL: *Adult respiratory distress syndrome.* In Kryger M: *Pathophysiology of respiration*, New York 1981, John Wiley.

Clinical Manifestations

ARDS usually occurs in a person who has had a recent physical trauma, although it can appear in people who appeared to be healthy immediately before onset (for example, someone with sudden onset of an acute infection). There is usually a latent period of 18 to 24 hours from the time of lung injury to the development of symptoms. The syndrome runs a variable course from a few days to several weeks' duration. Patients who appear to be recovering from ARDS may suddenly relapse into acute pulmonary disease from a secondary insult such as pneumothorax or an overwhelming infection. Signs and symptoms of ARDS include the following:

1. Acute respiratory distress: tachypnoea, dyspnoea, accessory muscle breathing, and central cyanosis
2. Dry cough and fever that develop over a few hours or days
3. Fine crackles throughout both lung fields
4. Altered sensorium ranging from confusion and agitation to coma

Radiological and laboratory findings include the following:

1. Chest x-rays—diffuse, bilateral, and usually symmetric interstitial and alveolar infiltrations
2. Arterial blood gases
  Hypoxaemia Po_2 less than 6.6 kPa (50 mm Hg)
  Hypocapnia
  Respiratory alkalosis
3. End-stage: hypercapnia and respiratory acidosis

Medical Management

Patients with ARDS are critically ill and are best managed in an intensive care unit. Medical management focuses on the following aspects of care:

1. Oxygenation
2. Ventilatory support
3. Fluid volume
4. Treat underlying cause of ARDS.

CANCER OF THE LUNG

Aetiology/Epidemiology

During the past 50 years there has been a startling increase in the incidence of cancer of the lung.

During 1991 there were 90 per 100,000 of the population male deaths and 42 per 100,000 female deaths from lung cancer. Lung cancer is currently the leading cause of male cancer deaths and the second highest in women. During 1986, in the United States, deaths from lung cancer overtook those from breast cancer to become the leading cause of cancer deaths in women.

The death rates for both men (decrease) and women (increase) is directly related to cigarette smoking. A history of smoking, especially for 20 years or more, is considered to be a prime risk factor. Other risk factors include exposure to certain industrial substances such as asbestos particularly in those who smoke. It is estimated that asbestos workers who smoke have six to ten times more lung cancer than the general population at large. There also is some evidence of a genetic predisposition to lung cancer.[30]

In the United Kingdom the age-adjusted death rate from cancer has been steadily increasing. Most of the increase is directly related to rise in lung cancer death rates. Age-adjusted rates for other cancer sites have been levelling off and, in some cases, declining. There has been a decline in cancer death rates for all age groups/sexes, except in people

Table 16-12 Deaths caused by lung cancer according to smoking habits*

	Deaths per 100,000 population
Nonsmoker	3.4
10-20 cigarettes per day	54.3
20-40 cigarettes per day	143.9
More than 40 cigarettes per day	217.3

* From American Cancer Society: *Cancer facts and figures.* New York, 1976. The Society.

55 years old and older, in whom the cancer death rate has been increasing.

Because of the relationship between cigarette smoking and the incidence of lung cancer, emphasis is continuing to be placed on reducing smoking. The relationship between smoking and lung cancer is shown in Table 16-12.

The mortality of people with lung cancer depends primarily on the specific type of cancer and the size of the tumour when detected. *Squamous cell carcinoma is the most common, followed by adenocarcinoma; undifferentiated small cell (oat cell) carcinoma is the least common.* Most people who develop the disease are over 50 years of age. Some of the factors believed to be involved in the increased incidence of cancer of the lung include an increase in smoking among women, more accurate diagnoses, and a tendency to name the lung as the primary site.

Less than 15% of lung cancer patients live 5 years or more after diagnosis. The survival rate is 37% for cases detected in a localized stage; only 20% of lung cancers are discovered that early. Survival rates have improved only slightly over the past 10 years.[1]

Cancer of the lung may be either metastatic or primary. *Metastatic tumours may follow malignancy anywhere in the body. Metastasis from the colon and kidney is common.* Metastasis to the lung may be discovered before the primary lesion is known, and sometimes the location of the primary lesions is not determined during the person's life.

Prevention

The cause of cancer of the lung is closely related to cigarette smoking. Table 16-12 shows the extreme increase in mortality in the United States from lung cancer in those people who smoke. Prevention is the best protection against cancer of the lung because early detection of the disease is difficult. The cancer death rates for male cigarette smokers is more than double that for nonsmokers, and the rate for female smokers is 67% higher than that for nonsmokers.[7]

Because there is no effective treatment for lung cancer, emphasis is placed on prevention. *Nearly 90% of people with lung cancer die within 5 years of diagnosis.* This figure could be lowered with early diagnosis and treatment. Unfortunately, about one third of the cases of lung cancer are inoperable when first seen by a doctor. Another one third are found to be inoperable when an exploratory thoractotomy is performed.

The goal set for year 2000 in Health of the Nation is to reduce smoking to less than 20% (baseline 1990) in an attempt to reduce lung cancer incidence and deaths.[129]

From available research data it seems evident that curtailing smoking is a primary preventive measure. The nurse should be active in teaching the dangers of smoking and should set a positive health example in this regard. It is especially important that teenagers be given specific facts about the dangers of cigarette smoking because they are not likely to be habitual smokers at that age. *Recent studies indicate that the incidence of smoking among teenagers and some groups of women is increasing.* People who are already habitual smokers should also be urged to stop smoking, although it may be difficult for them to do so. Various types of programmes are available to assist people to stop smoking. Because air pollution affects the lungs and may predispose to the development of cancer, nurses should encourage and actively support community programmes to decrease the amount of air pollution.

Pathophysiology and Clinical Manifestations

Because most new growths in the lungs arise from the bronchi, the term *bronchogenic carcinoma* is widely used. The signs and symptoms that a patient has depend on several factors including the location of the lesion.

Signs and symptoms of a *lesion in the bronchus* and lung include the following:

1. Ten percent of patients are asymptomatic and the disease is picked up on routine chest x-ray.
2. Seventy-five percent will have a cough.
3. Fifty percent will have haemoptysis.
4. Shortness of breath and a unilateral wheeze are common.

If peripheral pulmonary lesions perforate into the pleural space, there will be extrapulmonary intrathoracic signs and symptoms. These include:

1. Pain on inspiration
2. Friction rub
3. Pleural effusion
4. If the superior vena cava is involved, oedema of face and neck
5. Fatigue
6. Clubbing of fingers

Diagnostic tests include:

1. Chest x-ray (p. 296)
2. Sputum cytology test (p. 298)
3. Fibreoptic bronchoscopy (see p. 301) (sometimes biopsy taken)

In the later stage of the disease, *weight loss and debility usually indicate metastases, especially to the liver.* Cancer of the lung may metastasize to nearby structures such as the prescalene lymph nodes, the walls of the oesophagus, and the pericardium of the heart, or distant areas such as the brain, liver, or skeleton.

Medical Management

The treatment of lung cancer depends on the type and stage of the disease. *Histologically, lung cancer is divided into four major subgroups: small cell carcinoma, squamous cell carcinoma, adenocarcinoma, and large cell carcinoma.* Box 16-14 lists the types, percentage of cases in the subtypes, and recommended therapy. As with other types of cancer, lung cancer is staged (see Chapter 9 for more details about staging). The international Tumour, Node, Metastasis (TNM) Staging for Lung Cancer is presented in Box 16-15.

Because patients with early lung cancer have no symptoms, they are often inoperable by the time they are seen. Some patients with cancers of the lung are first diagnosed after chest x-ray as part of a routine physical examination. Other patients are not diagnosed until they seek medical treatment for symptoms related to metastases.

Survival rates of patients with non-small cell lung cancer (NSCLC) obviously depend on the size of the tumour, nodal status, and degree of metastases. Box 16-16 gives the 5-year survival rates for patients with non-small cell cancers.

16-14

Histological subtypes of cancer of the lung and the therapy of each type

Type	Classification and percentage of cases	Therapy
Small cell carcinoma	Small cell lung cancer (SCLC); 25% of cases	Combination chemotherapy such as (1) cyclophosphamide, doxorubicin, and vincristine, or (2) cyclophosphamide, doxorubicin, and etoposide, or (3) cisplatin plus etoposide
Squamous cell carcinoma Adenocarcinoma Large cell carcinoma	All three classified as non-small cell lung cancer (NSCLC); 75% of cases	Pulmonary resection—only one third are operable; one third inoperable because of advanced lung cancer; one third inoperable because of distant metastases

---

16-15

International TNM staging for lung cancer*

Tumour size (T)

TX = Occult carcinoma (cytologically positive; bronchoscopically and radiographically nondetectable)
T1 = Tumour 3 cm or less surrounded by lung or visceral pleura
T2 = Tumour more than 3 cm
T3 = Tumour of any size with direct extension into chest wall, or with 2 cm of the carina, or associated with atelectasis or obstructive pneumonia of the entire lung
T4 = Tumour of any size invading the mediastinal structures or vertebral body, or presence of malignant pleural effusion

Nodal status (N)

N0 = No hilar or mediastinal nodal involvement
N1 = Ipsilateral hilar anodal involvement
N2 = Ipsilateral mediastinal nodal or subcarinal nodal involvement
N3 = Contralateral hilar or mediastinal nodal involvement, supraclavicular nodal involvement (ipsilateral or contralateral)

Metastases (M)

M0 = No distant metastases
M1 = Distant visceral metastases present

Stage

Occult carcinoma	TX, N0, M0
Stage I	T1-2, N0, M0
Stage II	T1-2, N1, M0
Stage IIIA	T3, N0-1, M0
	T1-3, N2, M0
Stage IIIB	T-4, N1-3, M0
	T1-3, N3, M0
Stage IV	Any T, any N, M1

*Adapted from Mountain CF: A new international staging system for lung cancer, *Chest* 89(suppl):2255, 1986.

16-16

Five-year disease-free survival rates for surgical resection in patients with non-small cell lung cancer

	Stage	5 yr Disease-free (%)
I	T1, N0, M0	70-85
	T2, N0, M0	55-65
II	T1, N1, M0	30-50
	T1, N2, M0	25-30
IIIA	T3, N0, M0	25-35
	T3, N1, M0	15-20
	T1-2N2, M0	9-24
	T3, N2	0-5

From Bonomi P: *Primary lung cancer.* In Rakel RE, editor: *Conn's current therapy,* 1990, Philadelphia, 1990, WB Saunders.

Some patients who undergo surgical resection (pneumonectomy or lobectomy) may also receive radiation therapy or chemotherapy. These adjuvants are mainly used to treat metastases and to relieve some of the patient's symptoms. Both of these therapies are discussed in detail in Chapter 9. Because surgery is the treatment of choice, it is discussed next.

Thoracic surgery

Intelligent nursing care of patients undergoing thoracic surgery depends on knowledge of the anatomy and physiology of the chest, of the surgery performed, and of procedures and practices that assist the patient to recover from the operation. When endotracheal anaesthesia became possible, surgery of the chest was given a great impetus.

Principles of resectional surgery. Principles of resectional surgery are as follows:
 1. Endotracheal anaesthesia is used for surgery involving the lung in which the pleural space is entered.

2. With endotracheal anaesthesia it is possible to keep the uninvolved ("good") lung expanded and functioning when the chest is opened and atmospheric pressure enters the pleural space.

3. To understand resectional surgery and the purpose of chest tubes and water-seal drainage, an understanding of the following is necessary.

a. *Physiology of breathing*

(1) The pressure in the pleural space (the space between the visceral and parietal pleura) is subatmospheric (less than 101.3 kPa (760 mm Hg) and is referred to as *negative*.

(2) The pressure in the pleural space is usually 100.8 kPa (756 mm Hg) and goes down to 100.1 kPa (751 mm Hg) before inspiration. This change in pressure allows air (atmospheric pressure) to enter the lungs.

(3) When the pleura is entered surgically, atmospheric pressure enters the pleural space, and the lung collapses.

b. *Purpose of chest tubes and water-seal drainage*

(1) After resectional surgery of the lung (except pneumonectomy), one or two drainage tubes are inserted into the pleural space. Each tube is connected to a water-seal drainage bottle containing 1 to 2 cm of sterile water (see Fig. 16-8) or to another negative pressure suction system.

(2) The glass rod connected to the chest tube is under water. This "seals" the chest tube, allowing air and fluid to drain from the pleural space into the water-seal bottle, and preventing air or fluid from entering the pleural space.

(3) In all resectional surgery (except pneumonectomy), the remaining portions of the lung must overexpand and fill the space left by the resected portion.

(4) The removal of air and fluid from the pleural space accomplishes two basic purposes. These are to (1) *aid in the expansion of the remaining portion of the lung as air (positive pressure) and fluid escapes through the drainage tubes, and (2) to reestablish negative pressure in the pleural space.*

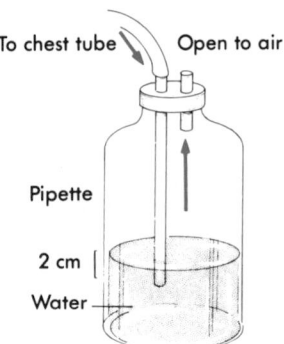

Fig. 16-8   Water-sealed closed chest drainage showing type of tube under water. (From Abels LF: *Mosby's manual of critical care*, St Louis, 1979, Mosby–Year Book.)

(5) Nursing actions necessary to maintain the integrity of the chest tubes and water-seal drainage is discussed in the section on postoperative care.

(6) Other closed chest drainage system such as Pleurevac may be used.

A closed chest drainage system is used after thoracic surgery to remove air (positive pressure) and fluid from the pleural space. Because the drainage system is closed, air is prevented from entering the chest tubes and collapsing the lung.

Today closed chest drainage system are commonly used. However, the general principles underlying this type of drainage are best understood if an older (but still used) system of water-sealed drainage bottles (under water seal) is explained first. Once the principles of water-sealed drainage are understood, this knowledge can be used to understand other types of closed drainage systems.

Type of resectional surgery. Table 16-13 presents the types of resectional surgery and the indications for the use of each type. A brief discussion of each type of resectional surgery follows.

Exploratory thoracotomy. An exploratory thoracotomy is performed to confirm a suspected diagnosis of lung or chest disease. The usual approach is by a posterolateral parascapular incision through the fourth, fifth, sixth, or seventh intercostal space. Occasionally, an anterior approach is used. The ribs are spread to give the best possible exposure of the lung and hemithorax. The pleura is entered, and the lung examined; a biopsy usually is taken; and the chest is closed. This procedure may also be used to detect bleeding in the chest or other injury after trauma to the chest. Because the pleural space was entered, a chest tube and water-seal drainage are necessary (Fig. 16-8).

Pneumonectomy. A pneumonectomy, the removal of an entire lung, is most commonly performed to treat bronchogenic carcinoma. It may also be used to treat tuberculosis. However, a pneumonectomy is only performed in those instances when a lobectomy or segmental resection will not remove all the diseased tissue. A thoracotomy is made in either the posterior or anterior chest using the method described under exploratory thoracotomy. Before the lung can be removed, the pulmonary artery and vein are ligated and then cut. The main bronchus leading to the lung is clamped, divided, and sutured, usually with black silk. To ensure an airtight closure of the bronchus, a pleural flap is placed over it and sutured into place. The phrenic nerve on the operative side is crushed, causing the diaphragm on that side to rise and reduce the size of the remaining space. Because there is no lung left to reexpand, drainage tubes are not used. Ideally the pressure in the closed chest is slightly negative. The fluid left in the space will consolidate in time, preventing the remaining lung and heart from shifting towards the operative side (mediastinal shift).

Table 16-13   Types of thoracic surgery and indications for their use

Procedure	Indications
Exploratory thoracotomy	To confirm suspected diagnosis of lung or chest disease, especially carcinoma; to obtain a biopsy
Pneumonectomy (removal of lung)	Bronchogenic carcinoma when lobectomy will not remove all of lesion; tuberculosis when other surgery will not remove all of diseased lung
Lobectomy (removal of lobe of lung)	Bronchogenic carcinoma confined to a lobe, bronchiectasis, emphysematous blebs or bullae; lung abcess, fungal infections, benign tumours; tuberculosis
Segmental resection (segmentectomy removal of one or more lung segments)	Bronchiectasis; lung abscess or cyst; metastic carcinoma
Wedge resection (removal of pie-shaped section from surface of lung)	Well-circumscribed benign tumours, metastic tumours, or localized inflammatory disease
Decortication (removal of a fibrinous peel from the visceral pleura)	Chronic empyema
Thoracoplasty (removal of ribs)	Residual air space after surgery; chronic empyema space

Lobectomy. In a lobectomy one lobe of the lung is removed. It is used to treat bronchiectasis, bronchogenic carcinoma, emphysematous blebs or bullae, lung abscess, benign tumours, fungal infections, and tuberculosis. For a lobectomy to be successful, the disease must be confined to one lobe, and the remaining lung tissue must be capable of overexpanding to fill the space of the resected lobe. One or two chest tubes are connected to water-seal bottles for postoperative drainage.

Segmental resection (segmentectomy). In a segmental resection, one or more segments of the lung are removed. This operation is used in an attempt to preserve as much functioning lung tissue as possible. It is a very taxing operation for the surgeon because the dissection between segments must be performed very carefully and slowly, and the identification of the segmental pulmonary artery and vein and bronchus is more difficult than when a lobe is involved. Because there are ten segments in the right lung and eight in the left lung, only a portion of a lobe or lobes may need to be removed. The most common indication for segmentectomy is bronchiectasis. It is also used to treat the other conditions listed in Table 16-13. Chest tube(s) and water-seal drainage are necessary postoperatively. Because of air leaks from the segmental surface, the remaining lung tissue may take longer to reexpand.

Wedge resection. In a wedge resection, a well-circumscribed diseased portion is removed without regard to the segmental planes. The area to be removed is clamped, dissected, and sutured. Chest tube(s) and water-sealed drainage are used postoperatively.

Decortication. In a decortication a fibrinous peel is removed from the visceral pleura, allowing the encased lung to reexpand and obliterate the pleural space. Chest tube(s) and chest suction are used to facilitate the reexpansion of the lung. If the lung has been encased for a long time, it may be incapable of reexpanding after decortication. In this situation thoraco-plasty may be necessary.

A newer procedure that makes it possible to preserve more lung tissue is a *bronchoplastic* or *sleeve resection.* In this procedure one lobar bronchus and part of the right or left bronchus are excised. The distal bronchus is anastomosed to the proximal bronchus or the trachea. This procedure is used to treat bronchogenic carcinoma.

Preoperative care and evaluation

Special tests are required by a patient having chest surgery, and each of these is discussed next.

Radiological procedures

The following radiological procedures are performed:
1. Posteroanterior (PA) and lateral chest films
2. Other X-ray examinations
    a. Laminograms (tomograms, planograms)
        (1) In this X-ray technique special layers of lung tissue are visualized. They are used to study neoplasms, cavities, and densities of the lung.
    b. CT scanning
        (1) CT scanning provides more accurate information than laminography in some instances. For more information see p. 296.

Bronchoscopy

Bronchoscopy is described on p. 301. It is always performed before any type of resection of the lung. Because sutures will be placed in the broncheal stump after the lung resection, it is important that the surgeon visualize the condition of the bronchi before surgery. Preparation of the patient for bronchoscopy is outlined in Box 16-17. Care of the patient following bronchoscopy is listed in Box 16-18.

Pulmonary function tests

For the patient being considered for a pneumonectomy, the preoperative evaluation is even more precise because whether the uninvolved lung will be able to sustain the

Preparation of patient for bronchoscopy

1. Doctor should explain procedure to patient and obtain patient signature on informed consent form.
2. Patients are advised not to smoke for at least 24 hours.
3. Dentures are removed. Loose teeth are noted and called to anaesthetist's attention.
4. Preanaesthetic medications are administered 30 to 60 minutes before procedure. Commonly prescribed are the following:
   a. Morphine sulphate, 5 to 15 mg IM, to suppress cough and relieve pain and anxiety. Pethidine 50 to 100 mg IM is used in people who have asthma or bronchospasm.
   b. Diazepam, 5 to 10 mg IV, for sedation and to protect against convulsive reactions to local anaesthetic agents.
   c. Atropine sulphate, 0.4 to 1 mg IM, to reduce vasovagal reflex and decrease oral secretions.

The patient following bronchoscopy under local anaesthesia

1. Patient lies flat or is placed in semi recumbent position based on doctor's preference.
2. Lying on the side facilitates removal of secretions. Usually large amounts of secretions are produced. All sputum is saved for culture and cytological examination unless otherwise ordered.
3. Patient may be hoarse and complain of sore throat. Lignocaine is often helpful in reducing discomfort.
4. Vital signs are monitored for several hours.
5. Nothing is given by mouth for at least 2 hours or until gag reflex returns.
6. Patients may receive oxygen by mask or cannula for 4 hours after bronchoscopy to improve arterial blood oxygen levels, which may become lowered during the procedure.
7. Patients are monitored for complications including the following:
   a. Massive haemoptysis (blood-tinged sputum is normal for several hours after procedure)
   b. Bronchospasm: lungs should be auscultated by doctor when vital signs are taken. If bronchospasm is present, it may be treated with aminophylline intravenously or by bronchodilator administered by aerosol.
   c. Pneumothorax: if pneumothorax is present, a chest tube is inserted and connected to water-seal drainage.
   d. Laryngeal oedema and airway obstruction: shortness of breath and laryngeal stridor are symptoms. The doctor should be notified immediately.
8. Patient should not smoke for several hours. Smoking may cause coughing and initiate bleeding.
9. Sputum may be blood streaked for a few days. Pronounced bleeding should be reported at once.

patient's respiration after surgery needs to be determined. Pulmonary function tests are usually used to determine the patient's ability to withstand pneumonectomy. In one centre, patients who are being considered for pneumonectomy are evaluated on the basis of their forced expiratory volume in the first second (FEV_1) as follows:

1. If the FEV_1 is greater than 70% of the predicted normal level (approximately 2.5 L of flow), the patient's lung function is essentially normal, and the patient should be able to tolerate a pneumonectomy as long as cardiac status and arterial blood gas levels are acceptable.
2. If the FEV_1 is less than 35% of the predicted normal level (less than 1.1 L of flow), there is severe ventilatory impairment, and *surgical resection is not feasible*.
3. If the FEV_1 is between 35% and 70% of the predicted normal level (1.2 to 2.4 L of flow) there is mild-to-moderate ventilatory impairment, and further studies will be necessary to determine the maximal tolerable resection.

The nurse should be sure that the patient understands what tests are to be performed and the preparation for them. The person's significant others are also kept informed.

Preoperative teaching

The proposed surgery is discussed with both patient and family. The goal of teaching is to prepare the patient for what he or she is expected to do postoperatively. In some hospitals nurses from the operating theatre, recovery unit, or intensive care unit do the preoperative teaching. Even when this is so, the nurse caring for the patient is responsible for determining what the patient understands about the impending surgery and to be sure that preoperative teaching is completed.

Points to be discussed in teaching include:

1. Patient's knowledge of procedure
2. Explanation of procedure as necessary, including intubation for anaesthesia, site and length of incision, and chest tube(s) and drainage system
3. Where patient will go immediately following surgery
   a. To recovery unit—for how long
   b. To intensive care unit—for how long
4. Oxygen
5. Intravenous fluid and/or blood administration
6. Pain medication
7. What patient will be asked to do
   a. Coughing and deep breathing
   b. Arm exercises
   c. Ambulation

Postoperative care

The care of the patient after thoracic surgery centres on promoting ventilation and reexpansion of the lung by maintaining a clear airway, promoting comfort by pain relief, promoting reexpansion of the lung by proper maintenance of the water-seal drainage system, promoting arm exercises to maintain full use of the patient's arm on the operated side, promoting hydration and nutrition, and monitoring the incision for bleeding and subcutaneous emphysema. These will be discussed in the implementation section.

16-19

Special care following pneumonectomy

1. Chest tubes are not necessary because there is no lung left to reexpand on the operative side.
2. Patient may lie on back or *operated side only*. Patient is not allowed to lie with operative side uppermost because of fear that the sutured bronchial stump may open, allowing fluid to drain into the unoperated side and drown the patient.
3. Pressure in the operative side will be checked in the operating theatre after the chest is closed. A pneumothorax apparatus (which can instill or remove air) will be used to check the pressure in the operative space, and air will be removed or instilled as necessary to bring the pressure to slightly negative (slightly less than 101.3 kPa, 760 mm Hg).
4. The surgeon will palpate the patient's trachea at least daily to determine if it is in midline. Deviation of the trachea towards either the operated or unoperated side is a sign of *mediastinal shift*. If pressure builds up in the operated side, the trachea will deviate towards the unoperated side. The treatment is to remove air (positive pressure) with a pneumothorax apparatus. Mediastinal shift towards the "good" lung can seriously compromise ventilation and needs to be treated promptly. Deviation of the trachea towards the operated side indicates that more pressure (air) needs to be instilled into the empty space so that the mediastinum will shift back to its normal position.
5. The patient's trachea should be palpated in the midclavicular line of the fifth intercostal space each shift and the position should be recorded. If there is a change in the position of the trachea, it should be reported immediately.
6. The patient with a mediastinal shift resembles the patient in congestive heart failure. Neck veins are distended, the trachea is displaced to one side, pulse and respirations are increased, and dyspnoea is present.

7. Serous drainage will collect in the operated space and over time will congeal to the consistency of axle grease. This is often sufficient to keep the mediastinum from shifting towards the operative side. Persistent mediastinal shift towards the operative side may have to be treated with *thoracoplasty* (removal of ribs) to reduce the size of the remaining space and assist in maintaining the mediastinum in midline. Thoracoplasty is described below.
8. It usually takes 2 to 4 days for the remaining lung to adjust to the increase in blood flow. For this reason the amount of fluids and blood given intravenously is monitored closely to prevent fluid overload. CVP monitoring is common. Rales are commonly heard over the base of the remaining lung, and vascular markings will be more prominent on x-ray films. Any increase in rales, in pulse or blood pressure, and in dyspnoea may indicate circulatory overload and should be reported immediately. Treatment may include diuretics and/or digitalization along with discontinuing intravenous fluids.
9. Deep breathing, coughing, and arm exercises are described.
10. Patients who have had a lung removed may have a lowered vital capacity, and exercise, and activity should be limited to that which can be performed without dyspnoea. Because the body must be given time to adjust to having only one lung, the patient's return to work may be delayed.
11. If the diagnosis is cancer, radiation therapy is usually given, and it may be started before the patient leaves the hospital. (See Chapter 11 for further discussion of nursing care for patients receiving radiation therapy.)
12. The patient who has had a pneumonectomy for cancer is urged to report to the doctor at once if hoarseness, dyspnoea, pain on swallowing, or localized chest pain develop because these symptoms may be signs of complications.

In most hospitals the patient will go from the recovery unit to the intensive care unit. The immediate postoperative nursing care is outlined here.

Care after pneumonectomy

The postoperative care discussed in Box 16-18 applies to all patients with resectional surgery except those having a pneumonectomy. The special care required after pneumonectomy is outlined in Box 16-19.

Complications of resectional surgery

In the immediate postoperative period (24 to 48 hours) hypotension, cardiac dysrrhythmia, pulmonary oedema, and subcutaneous emphysema may occur. Long-term complications include a residual air space, which results from failure of the remaining portions of the lung to reexpand and fill the space. If this space is small, no treatment is indicated. Two major complications of chest surgery tend to occur later in the postoperative period and require treatment: empyema and bronchopleural fistula. The patient may have empyema alone or empyema and a bronchopleural fistula.

Thoracoplasty

A thoracoplasty is an extrapleural procedure involving the removal of ribs to reduce the size of the chest cavity. Before the widespread use of resectional surgery, thoracoplasty was the basic surgical treatment for tuberculosis. Today *thoracoplasty is used infrequently and then only to prevent or treat the complications of resectional surgery.* When it is thought that a patient's lung may not be able to expand sufficiently after a resection to fill the space, a thoracoplasty is performed 2 to 3 weeks before the resection. It also may be performed before pneumonectomy. This will reduce the size of the cavity on the operative side and decrease the chance of mediastinal shift towards that side. This type of thoracoplasty is often called a *preresection* or *tailoring* thoracoplasty, that is, the chest wall is tailored to reduce its size.

If the remaining portions of the lung fail to reexpand sufficiently after resection or if another complication such as empyema occurs, a thoracoplasty is performed. *In general, it is used when there is a space in the chest that cannot be obliterated by other means.* Usually no more than three ribs are removed; therefore, paradoxical motion after thoracoplasty is seldom seen any more. Paradoxical motion is discussed under chest injuries (p. 329).

Nursing Process
Assessment
Subjective data

1. Onset and duration of signs and symptoms
2. What the patient understands about why he or she is hospitalized
   a. For diagnostic tests
   b. For chest surgery or radiation or chemotherapy
3. Whether the patient states that carcinoma of the lung is present or suspected
4. Smoking history
5. Occupational history of exposure to asbestos or other carcinogenic agents

Objective data

1. Presence of cough and whether or not productive of sputum
2. If sputum is present, whether blood-tinged
2. Haemoptysis
4. Shortness of breath when talking or on exertion
5. Unilateral wheezing on auscultation

Nursing analysis

Problems are determined from analysis of patient data. Possible problems for the person with bronchogenic carcinoma having resectioned surgery may include, but are not limited to, the following:

Problems	Possible aetiologies
Anxiety	Threat of death
	Threat/change in health status/ scocioeconomic status/role functioning environment
Gas exchange, impaired	Ventilation/perfusion impairment
Pain	Pleuritic chest pain (if pleura involved)
Knowledge deficit: about the disease and its treatment	Lack of exposure/unfamiliarity with information sources
Airway clearance, ineffective	Decreased energy/fatigue
Disuse syndrome, high risk for	Surgical incision involving trapezius muscle
Tissue integrity, impaired	Surgical incision

Planning: expected patient outcomes

Expected patient outcomes for the person undergoing resectional surgery may include, but are not limited to, the following:

1. Patient is coping effectively with anxiety.
2. Patient's gas exchange is within normal levels as evidenced by arterial blood gases.
3. Patient's postoperative pain is controlled by medication.
4. Patient is maintaining a patent airway.
5. Patient is able to put operative arm through normal range of motion.
6. Patient's incision is healing well.
7. Patient can explain regimen to follow after discharge including the following:
   a. Explain recommended changes in ADL
      (1) Which usual activities to limit and for how long
      (2) Exercise programme
   b. Explain any changes required in life-style (reason and plans for changes in occupation and habits such as smoking, activity level, and so on).
   c. State name, dose, action, and side effects of medications ordered
      (1) How and when to use PRN medications
      (2) Schedule for other medications and how to take them
   d. Describe professional and community resources necessary for structuring an environment compatible with convalescence
      (1) Plans for obtaining assistance from community nurses and or social services
      (2) Plans for necessary modifications of home
   e. Describe plans for follow-up care.
      (1) Signs or symptoms requiring immediate medical assistance
      (2) State plans for ongoing medical care

Implementation
Assisting with achievement of therapeutic goals
Maintaining chest tube(s) and drainage

All patients who have resectional surgery of the lung, except those having a pneumonectomy, will require drainage of the pleural space by one or two chest tubes connected to closed drainage. The tubes are inserted immediately after the operative incision is closed. Usually two tubes are used, although some surgeons may prefer only one tube. When two tubes are used, one catheter is inserted through a stab wound in the anterior chest wall above the resected area. This is referred to as the *anterior* or *upper tube*. It is used to remove air from the pleural space. The second tube is inserted through a stab wound in the posterior chest and is referred to as the *posterior* or *lower tube*. It is primarily for the drainage of *serosanguineous* (serum and blood) fluid that accumulates as the result of the operative procedure. The lower tube may be of a larger diameter than the upper tube to prevent it from becoming plugged with clots. Fig. 16-9 shows the placement of tubes within the pleural space. When only one chest tube is used, it is usually placed anteriorly above the resected area of the lung.

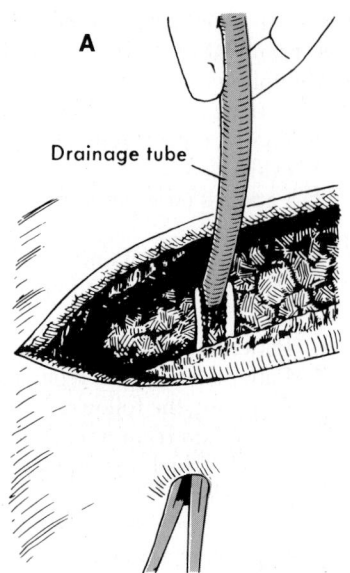

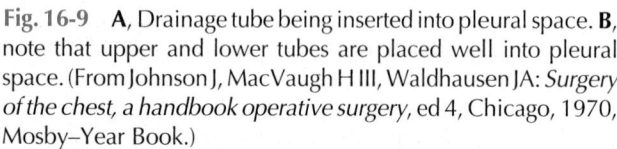

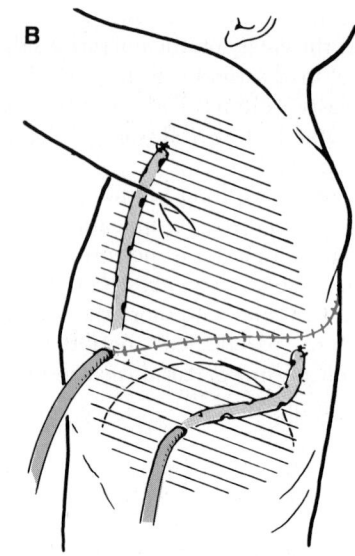

Fig. 16-9 A, Drainage tube being inserted into pleural space. **B,** note that upper and lower tubes are placed well into pleural space. (From Johnson J, MacVaugh H III, Waldhausen JA: *Surgery of the chest, a handbook operative surgery,* ed 4, Chicago, 1970, Mosby–Year Book.)

When initiating chest tube drainage, a 2 L clear glass bottle is usually used for each chest tube, although other commercial devices, such as the Pleurevac system are available. Approximately 300 ml of sterile water, or enough to fill the bottles 1 to 2 cm from the bottom, is then added. If considerable drainage accumulates in the bottle, the amount of subatmospheric (negative) pressure in the system will increase, and it will be more difficult for the patient to expel air and fluid from the pleural space. In this instance, the glass rod may be pulled up so that less of it is under water, or the surgeon may order that the drainage bottle be changed. In this case a sterile setup is prepared. When the sterile bottle with sterile water and the tubing are ready, the chest tube is clamped as close to the patient's chest as possible. The chest tube is then disconnected from the drainage tubing, the sterile setup is connected, and the chest tube is unclamped. The amount of drainage in the bottle should be measured and usually is sent to the laboratory for examination.

As the patient breathes, there will be movement of fluid in the glass tube that is under water. This is known as *fluctuation* or *oscillation,* and *the column will move up when the patient inhales or coughs, and it will fall when the patient is exhaling.*

Some thoracic surgeons wish to have the chest tubes "milked" or "stripped" to prevent formation of clots that could plug the tubes; *the practice of routinely stripping chest tube(s) is becoming less common, however, because it increases the negative pressure exerted on the pleural space.* A study by two clinical nurse specialists revealed the following: (1) The pressure generated by stripping was considerably higher than the suction pressures of −15 to −20 cm of water commonly applied to chest drainage

systems; (2) the amount of pressure was directly related to the length of the tubing stripped; and (3) even stripping only a few centimetres produced pressures near −100 cm of water, stripping the entire tube produced pressures exceeding −400 cm of water.[113] They also found that higher negative pressures resulted when a roller was used to strip the tubes rather than the hands.[113]

Undesirable side effects of increased levels of negative pressure reported in the literature include (1) lung entrapment in the thoracic tube eyelets and focal tissue infarction and (2) persistent pneumothorax.[126] The persistent pneumothorax occurs when the pleural surface of lung, which normally has air leaks at the close of the operative procedure, does not "seal off." Usually fibrin will seal the air leaks; however, the presence of an increased amount of negative pressure may prevent the air leaks from sealing off and may even increase the size of the air leaks. This is the reason why some thoracic surgeons do not attach additional suction to the water-seal drainage system for the first 24 hours or more after surgery. They believe that this amount of time is sufficient in most instances to allow the pleural surface to seal off.

In view of these findings, the nurse should consult with the thoracic surgeon about the desirability of routinely stripping chest tubes. Because the anterior (upper) tube usually evacuates mainly air, there is less reason to believe that this tube will clot up. Posterior tubes, which are commonly inserted lower in the chest, usually drain more fluid and blood and are more likely to clot up. However, gentle squeezing of the tube is usually sufficient to move the bloody drainage along in the tubing. Special caution should be used in stripping tubes of patients with a known history of fragile tissue, such as occurs in emphysema.[119] The nursing measures necessary in maintaining chest tubes and closed drainage are listed in Box 16-20.

Additional suction. Suction is usually used to speed reexpansion of the lung after surgery, using either wall suction or a suction machine. Most often -30 cm of suction

Maintaining chest tubes and closed chest drainage bottles

1. Mark water level in bottle with strip of adhesive tape so that amount of drainage can easily be determined. Write date and time on tape.
2. Fasten tubing to the bed so that there are no dependent loops between the bottles and the bed (see Fig. 20-26). Dependent loops allow fluid to collect in tubing and impede removal of air and fluid from pleural space.
3. Be sure that tip of chest tube is 1 to 2 cm under water so that if the bottle accidentally tips over, the tube will remain under water.
4. Check the glass rod in the bottle for fluctuation frequently. If the column of water is not fluctuating:
   a. Be sure patient is not lying on tubes.
   b. Check connections to be sure chest tube system is intact.
   c. Ask patient to cough or change position to see if fluctuation is restored.
   d. Fluctuation will stop when lung is reexpanded. Call the surgeon if the tubes are not patent (column of fluid not fluctuating).
5. Keep two haemostats at the bedside so that the chest tube can be clamped if a bottle is accidentally broken. When a bottle is broken, the chest catheter should be clamped and then reconnected to a sterile setup as soon as possible. Sterile water should be used in the bottle. As soon as the system is reconnected with the tip of the tube under water, the clamp should be removed. *Except in case of an emergency such as a broken bottle, most thoracic surgeons prefer that tubes not be clamped, and a specific order is written if clamping is desired.*
6. Never clamp chest tubes unless a bottle breaks (a rare occurrence) or without a written order. When chest tubes are clamped, air (positive pressure) may be trapped in the pleural space and further collapse the lung. If a patient is being transported from one place to another, such as to the x-ray department, tubes should not be clamped unless it is necessary for only a few minutes.
7. Never lift chest tube bottles above the level of the patient's chest, as this would allow fluid to be pulled into the pleural space.
8. The water-seal bottles should be placed on the floor, so that they will not be broken by a lowered cot side. When a variable height bed is being used, care is taken not to lower the bed onto the bottles.
9. If additional suction is being used, check frequently to be sure it is functioning at the prescribed level of negative pressure.

is applied, but this amount varies according to the surgeon's preference. When it is particularly important to regulate the exact amount of suction used, a "breaker" bottle may be added to the system between the suction source and the patient's drainage bottle. The use of a breaker bottle provides for control of the amount of suction that is applied

to the water-sealed bottle and thus to the patient's pleural space. The stopper in the control bottle has three openings. One is connected to the water-sealed bottle, one is connected to the suction source, and the third contains a glass rod that is under water and open to the outside (Fig. 16-10). The amount of suction produced will be determined by the distance between the surface of the water and the tip of this tube. When the suction source is turned on, the level of water in the open tube will sink in proportion to the amount of negative pressure in the system. Thus if there is 15 cm of water between the surface of the water and the tip of the tube, the amount of negative pressure in the system will be 15 cm of water pressure. Because the water will be at the bottom of the tube when this amount of pressure is reached, any increase in negative pressure will cause air to be drawn in from the outside, *breaking* the suction at this level. Therefore, it can be expected that the water in the breaker bottle will bubble almost continuously. If it fails to bubble at all, the desired level of suction is not being attained. When the water in the breaker bottle is not bubbling, the tubing should be checked for air leaks. If there are no leaks and bubbling still does not occur, the surgeon should be notified at once because the air leak in the pleura may be so great that the amount of negative pressure is not sufficient to overcome it. In this instance water may be added to the breaker bottle to increase the distance between the surface of the water and the tip of the tube, thereby increasing the amount of negative pressure being exerted on the pleural space.

The distance the tube is placed under water in the breaker bottle is determined by the surgeon. A breaker bottle and suction may be attached to one or both tubes. Most commonly it is attached to the upper tube because this is where air is most likely to be leaking from the pleural surface. A small empty trap bottle is usually attached by tubing between the breaker bottle and the suction source. The purpose of this bottle is to protect the suction motor from becoming wet should the breaker bottle overflow. See the box opposite for a summary of actions to maintain chest tubes.

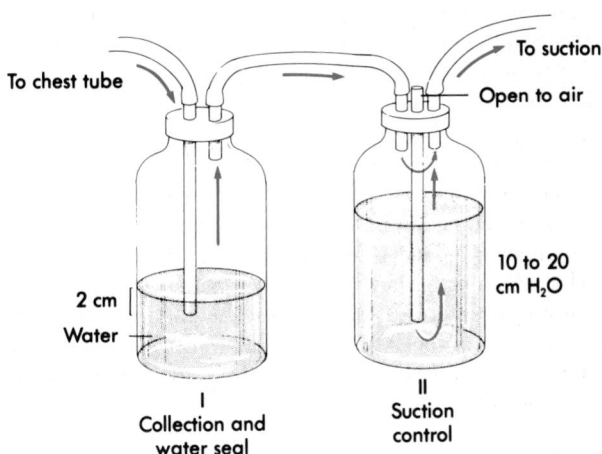

Fig.16-10   Water-sealed closed drainage system (under water seal) with suction control bottle. (From Abels LF: *Mosby's manual of critical care*, St Louis, 1979, Mosby–Year Book.)

Ambulation. There is no contraindication to ambulating with a chest tube in place. As long as the water-sealed bottle remains below the level of the chest, the patient may assume any position of comfort in bed or may be out of bed in a chair. The patient is urged to be up at least twice a day.

Removal of chest tubes. Chest tubes are removed when there is no fluctuation of fluid in the glass rod, and when x-ray films confirm the full reexpansion of the lung. Most patients have their chest tube(s) removed about 72 hours postoperatively. If there is a persistent air space in the apex of the lung, the upper tube may be left in longer. *Surgeons are concerned about leaving tubes in very long because of the risk of an ascending tube track infection.*

A well-accepted practice has been to give the patient pain medication 30 minutes before removal of chest tube(s). However, a recent study of sensations experienced by patients during chest tube removal raises questions about this practice. In this study, burning was the most frequently reported sensation, followed by pain, pulling, and pressure. The authors of the article recommend that preparing patients to experience a brief sensation of burning or pain may be the only preparation necessary. They also question the influence that the nurse's manner may have on the patient's reaction to the procedure.[48] For this reason, we recommend the nurses review this study with their surgeon colleagues to see if modification might be made in the practice in their institutions.

Surgeons vary in the exact procedure used to remove the tube, but generally a sterile scissors, 4 inch × 4 inch gauze squares, and adhesive tape are required. The suture holding the tube in place is cut, the patient is asked to exhale deeply, and the tube is removed. If a pursestring suture was used, it is retied, and a dry sterile dressing is placed over the site. Some surgeons cover the site with an occlusive dressing instead of gauze squares to ensure an airtight dressing. The dressing is covered securely by three strips of 2-inch adhesive tape.

Haemodynamic monitoring

The patient is usually attached to a cardiac monitor and a Swan-Ganz catheter and central venous pressure line may be used for haemodynamic monitoring.

Interventions to achieve patient care outcomes
Providing emotional support

All patients can be expected to be fearful and anxious, and require considerable emotional support. The nurse and surgeon should discuss the treatment plan for the patient, so that all information given to the patient and family is carefully coordinated. In addition, the patient and family should be encouraged to verbalize their fears and concerns. The nurse should be supportive without giving unrealistic reassurance.

Because of the very poor survival rate in people with lung cancer, a major role of the nurse is to teach the public how lung cancer can be prevented or at least diagnosed as early as possible. Points to be emphasized in teaching are listed in Box 16-21.

16-21

Prevention and early detection of lung cancer

1. Smoking control programmes
   a. Encourage young people not to start smoking.
   b. Educate public about hazards of smoking.
   c. Provide self-help materials to assist people to stop smoking.
   d. Refer to stop-smoking programmes sponsored by organizations such as the Health Education Authority.
   e. Stress that there is no such thing as a "safe cigarette," but that people who smoke cigarettes lower in tar and nicotine find it easier to stop smoking.[1]
   f. Support nonsmoking areas in public places such as restaurants and meeting places.
   g. Support legislation to establish nonsmoking areas in public meeting places.
2. Urge all individuals over 40 years of age to have a chest x-ray periodically in addition to regular physical examination.
3. Know the cancer detection facilities in your community or other resources to which people can be referred for evaluation.

Maintaining oxygen therapy

Oxygen is attached to the endotracheal tube. After extubation, oxygen is given by cannula, usually at 6 L/min. An oxygen mask is not used because of a need to have the patient cough and raise secretions frequently.

Promoting gas exchange by positioning of patient

The patient is kept flat in bed or with pillows to elevate slightly (20 degrees) until blood pressure is stabilized to preoperative levels. Once blood pressure is stabilized, the patient can usually breathe best in semirecumbent position with a pillow under the head and neck but not under the shoulder and back because of the subscapular incision.

Promoting abdominal breathing

Abdominal breathing exercises are a valuable adjunct to the care of the patient with chest surgery because they improve ventilation without increasing pain and assist in coughing more effectively (Fig. 16-11). The exercises should be taught *preoperatively* by the physiotherapist so that the patient has time to practise them before surgery. The patient can cough most effectively 20 to 30 minutes after receiving pain medication, and this should be capitalized on by the nursing staff.

Monitoring vital signs

Vital signs are taken every 15 minutes until the patient is well recovered from anaesthesia and then every hour until condition has stabilized. It is not unusual for blood pressure to fluctuate during the first 24 to 36 hours, and close monitoring of the patient is essential. A persistently low blood pressure is reported to the surgeon.

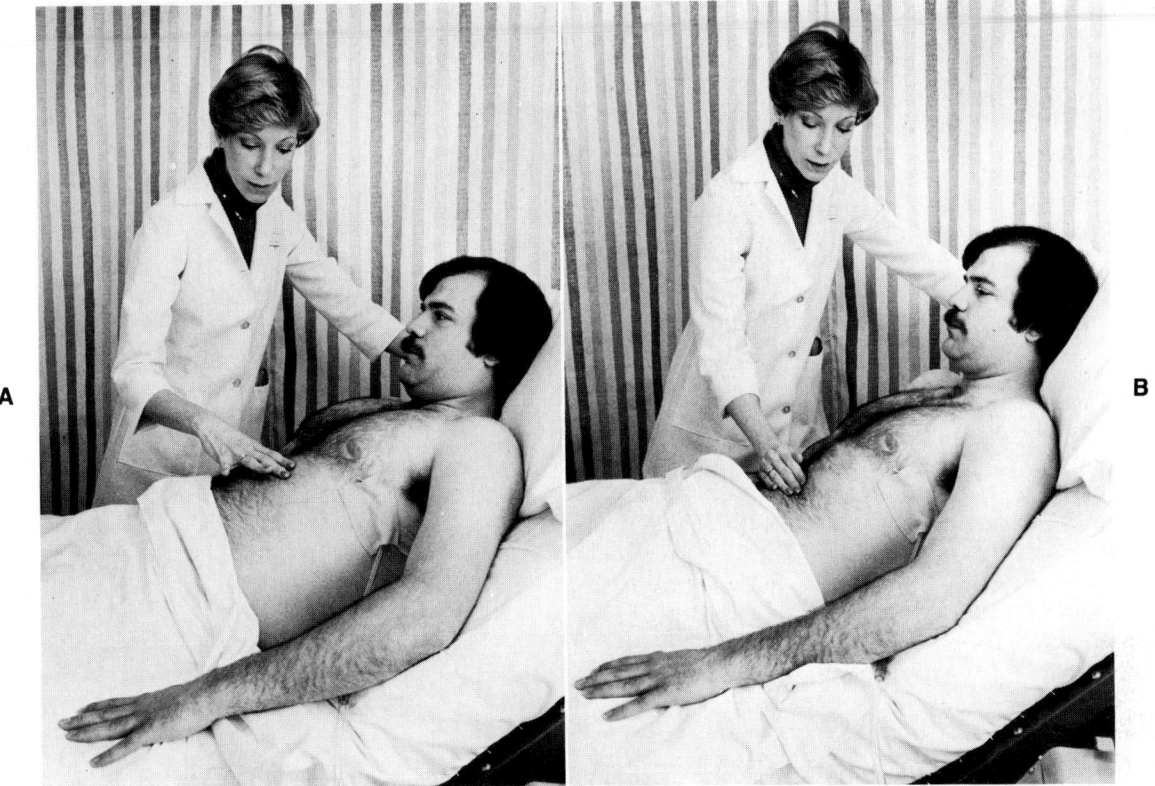

Fig. 16-11   A, Physiotherapist assists patient in learning augmented abdominal breathing. Patient is instructed to inhale through nose, using abdominal muscles and concentrate on moving lower ribs under therapist's hand. This exercise improves ventilation of bases of lungs. **B,** Physiotherapist places hand on upper abdomen in assisting patient to exhale fully.

Promoting comfort by pain relief

Morphine or pethidine hydrochloride is usually ordered for pain. Medication for pain should be given as needed and may be required as often as every 3 to 4 hours during the first 48 to 72 hours. The patient is extremely uncomfortable and will not be able to cough or turn unless there is relief from pain. In some instances the dose of the narcotic is decreased so that it may be given more frequently and yet not depress respirations. The tubes in the chest cause pain, and the patient may attempt rapid, shallow breathing to splint the lower chest and avoid motion of the catheters. This impairs ventilation, makes coughing ineffective, and causes secretions to be retained. Thus it is a nursing responsibility to make the patient comfortable, because this facilitates deep breathing and coughing. *Pain medication should never be withheld without first consulting with the surgeon because undermedication is counterproductive.* If, despite all efforts the patient's discomfort is interfering with adequate chest excursion, an intercostal nerve block may be performed.

Initiating coughing and deep breathing exercises

The patient should be assisted to cough as soon as conscious. If the blood pressure is stable, the patient is assisted to a sitting position, and the incision is supported anteriorly and posteriorly by the physiotherapist's or nurse's hands. Firm, even pressure over the incision with the open palm of the hand is a most effective method. The nurse's head should be behind the patient when the patient is coughing (Fig. 16-12). The patient is encouraged to breathe deeply, exhale, and then cough. Sips of fluids if permitted, especially of warm ones such as tea or coffee, often facilitate coughing. Mist therapy may be used to loosen secretions. Coughing *keeps the airway patent, prevents atelectasis, and facilitates reexpansion of the lung.* The patient should be assisted to cough every hour for the first 24 hours, and then every 2 to 4 hours. The patient should cough until the chest sounds clear. Otherwise, secretions will accumulate in the tracheobronchial tree.

When a patient is unable to cough effectively, tracheobronchial suctioning is performed. If suctioning fails to clear the airway, bronchoscopy may be necessary because it is crucial that the airway is kept clear. In these situations, *bronchoscopy* is performed at the bedside with a *fibreoptic bronchoscope.*

Promoting hydration and nutrition

The patient is encouraged to take fluids postoperatively and to progress to a general diet as soon as it is tolerated. Encouraging fluids helps to liquefy secretions and makes them easier to expectorate. A diet adequate in protein, zinc and vitamins (especially vitamin C) facilitates wound healing.

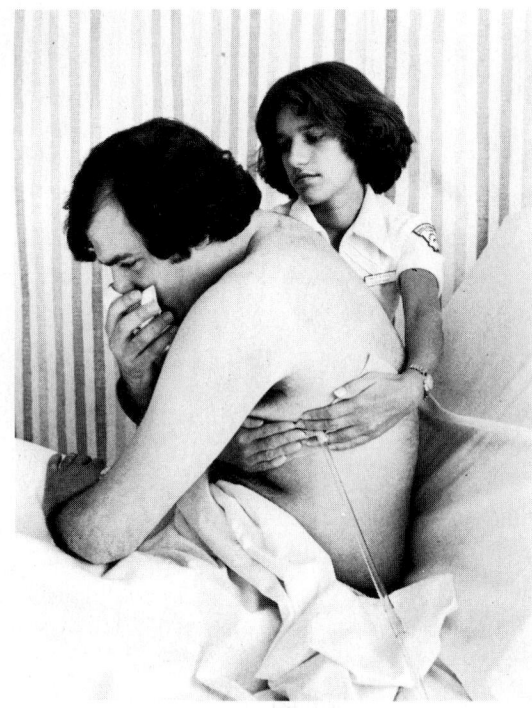

Fig. 16-12 Nurse assists patient to cough by splinting incision with firm support from hands. This lessens muscle pull and pain as patient coughs. Note that nurse keeps her head behind patient while he coughs, and patient uses tissue to cover mouth.

Promoting arm exercises

Passive arm exercises are usually started on the evening of surgery. The purpose in putting the patient's arm through range of motion is to prevent restriction of function from disuse. Most patients are reluctant to move the arm on the operative side, but with proper preoperative instruction and postoperative follow through they do so readily. *It is important for both the patient and nurse to understand that the longer the arm is unexercised, the stiffer it will become. The patient should put both arms through active range of motion two or three times a day within a few days.* The recommended exercises are similar to those done after mastectomy (see Chapter 28). The exercises are best performed when the patient is upright or lying on the abdomen. Exercises such as elevating the scapula and clavicle, "hunching the shoulders," bringing the scapulae as close together as possible, and hyperextending the arm can only be performed in these positions. Because lying on the abdomen may not be possible at first, these exercises are performed with the patient sitting on the edge of the bed or standing.

Monitoring the incision for bleeding or subcutaneous emphysema

The outer dressings are checked periodically for evidence of bleeding. *Blood on the dressings is unusual and should be reported to the surgeon at once.* The time and amount of blood is recorded in the patient's record. The surgeon may reinforce the dressing, and, in the rare instance when bleeding persists, the patient may be taken back to surgery. The chest will be reopened and the source of bleeding located and ligated.

Subcutaneous emphysema is not unusual after chest surgery. In subcutaneous emphysema, *air leaks from the pleural space through the thoracotomy incision or around the chest tubes into the soft tissues.* When palpating the chest, the presence of air under the skin is readily detected and has been described as feeling like "tissue paper" or "Rice Krispies" under the skin. Subcutaneous emphysema is most notable in the neck and chest, and, if considerable air is leaking, the patient's face and neck will become considerably enlarged. Small amounts of air will reabsorb over time and cause no problem, but if subcutaneous emphysema is worsening, the chest tube may be changed by the surgeon and a larger one inserted, because air is leaking into the tissues faster than it is being removed by the tube. Additional suction may also be applied to the chest tube(s) in an attempt to remove air more rapidly. Rarely a patient will need to return to surgery for closure of air leaks.

The patient with a pneumonectomy should have only a small amount (if any) of subcutaneous emphysema. *Progressive subcutaneous emphysema after pneumonectomy is very serious, and should be reported to the surgeon immediately because it could indicate a major leak in the bronchial stump.* This also is a rare occurrence, requiring immediate return to theatre for reclosure of the bronchial stump.

Facilitating learning

For the patient whose cancer is successfully removed at surgery and who will be discharged home, the following points need to be emphasized.

Because of early discharge, the patient will need to make

some changes in ADL. This may include taking frequent rest periods or at least a nap in the morning and afternoon for a week or two. The patient's activities are guided by fatigue. When the patient begins to get tired, he or she should stop and rest.

Exercising of the arm on the operative side should continue with the arm being put through range of motion at least twice daily. It is important that the patient understands that if the exercises are discontinued, the arm will become stiff and restricted motion will result. This is referred to by some as a *frozen shoulder*.

If the patient has not already stopped smoking, he or she will need support to do so. The patient can be referred to a support programme for those wishing to stop smoking.

The patient needs to understand the purpose, dosage, and so on of any prescribed drugs. Following successful surgery, the only medication prescribed may be an oral analgesic.

Although the patient may not appear to need the assistance of community resources at discharge, he or she should be informed of what is available. For example, a person living alone may wish to use a service such as Meals on Wheels until he or she feels more like cooking.

The patient should be able to describe plans for follow-up care including signs and symptoms such as blood in sputum, chest pain, or unexplained fever, which should be reported to the surgeon.

The patient should know the time and date of the next appointment with the surgeon. If a patient is not able to put the operative arm through full range of motion, a follow-up appointment with the physiotherapist would also be arranged.

Evaluation

Evaluation for the patient having resectional surgery is based on patient outcomes. Questions to consider may include the following:

1. Is patient's anxiety reduced?
2. Is patient maintaining adequate gas exchange?
3. Is the patient's pain under control?
4. Is the patient able to maintain a clear airway?
5. Is the patient able to move arm through full range of motion?
6. Is the patient's incision healing well?
7. Can patient explain regimen to follow at home including changes in lifestyle and plans for follow-up care with surgeon?

CHEST TRAUMA

Aetiology/Epidemiology

Trauma to the chest is a major problem most often seen first in the accident and emergency department. *Injury to the chest may affect the bony chest cage, pleurae and lungs, diaphragm, or mediastinal contents. Injuries to the chest are broadly classified into two groups—blunt and penetrating.*

Blunt, or nonpenetrating, injuries damage the structures within the chest cavity without disrupting chest wall integrity.

Penetrating injuries disrupt chest wall integrity and result in alteration in intrathoracic pressures.

A leading cause of blunt chest injuries is motor vehicle steering wheel impaction in the person not wearing a seat belt. Blows to the chest with blunt objects or as a result of a fall also cause nonpenetrating chest injury. Penetrating wounds usually result from gunshot or stabbing injuries.

Both penetrating and blunt chest injuries can be fatal. The common chest injuries and their sequelae are classified as primarily penetrating or nonpenetrating chest wounds in Table 16-14.

Prevention

Nurses can promote prevention of chest trauma through public education programmes focused on safe practices in vehicle usage and in the work place. *The major preventive measure is the use of seat belts when operating a motor vehicle.*

CHEST CAGE INJURIES: RIB FRACTURES
Pathophysiology

Rib fractures are the most common chest injury. Ribs 3 through 10 are most often fractured because they are less protected by the chest muscles. The ribs usually fracture at the point of maximal impact but may fracture at a distant site from impact. Fractures of the ribs are caused by blows, crushing injuries, or strain caused by severe coughing or sneezing spells. If the rib is splintered or the fracture displaced, sharp fragments may penetrate the pleura and the lung, resulting in a haemothorax or pneumothorax.

Common signs and symptoms of rib fracture include the following:

1. Pain at the site of injury, increasing on inspiration
2. Localized tenderness and crepitus on palpation
3. Splinting of the chest and taking shallow breaths

Medical Management

Treatment is individualized, based on the patient's age, whether there is a history of preexisting chronic pulmonary disease, and the number and location of ribs fractured. Medical treatment includes the following:

1. Stabilization of the fracture site with a rib belt or bandage
2. Analgesics as needed

Table 16-14   Types of penetrating and nonpenetrating (blunt) chest injuries

Penetrating	Blunt
Open pneumothorax (sucking chest wound)	**Closed pneumothorax**
Haemothorax	Tension pneumo-thorax
Tracheobronchial injury	Tracheobroncial injury
Pulmonary contusion	Flail chest
Diaphragm rupture	Diaphragm rupture
Mediastinal injury	Mediastinal injury
	Fractured ribs

3. For severe pain, performance of a regional nerve block

Nursing Process
Assessment
Subjective data

Subjective data include the nature of the injury and when it occurred. If patient is unable to answer questions, data are obtained from those with the patient.

Objective data

1. Pain at site of injury that increases on inspiration
2. Area tender to the touch
3. Patient splints chest and takes shallow breaths

Diagnostic tests

Fractures are confirmed by chest x-ray findings.

Nursing analysis

Problems are determined from analysis of patient data. Possible problems for the person with rib fracture may include, but are not limited to, the following:

Problems	Possible aetiologies
Pain	Trauma to the rib cage
Airway clearance, ineffective	Pain/trauma to rib cage
Anxiety	Threat to change in health status
Breathing pattern, ineffective	Pain, musculoskeletal impairment
Knowledge deficit	Lack of exposure to information or misinterpretation of information

Planning: expected patient outcomes

Expected patient outcomes for the person with fractured ribs may include, but are not limited to, the following:

1. Pain is improved.
2. Patient maintains a patent airway.
3. Patient is less anxious.
4. Patient is breathing effectively.
5. Patient understands follow-up therapy.
6. Patient understands that doctor is to be notified if shortness of breath, haemoptysis, or temperature elevation occur.

Implementation
Assisting with achievement of therapeutic goals
Initial care for fractured ribs

If ribs are fractured and the rib has not penetrated the pleura, the chest may be strapped with adhesive tape or a bandage or chest binder is applied.

1. Check strapping to be sure it is secure.
2. Give analgesics as ordered.

Interventions to achieve patient outcomes
Assisting with comfort and ADL

1. Place patient in position of comfort. May be able to breathe easier in upright or semi-recumbent position.
2. Give prescribed analgesics.

3. If pain persists despite analgesics, notify the doctor, who may infiltrate the intercostal spaces above and below the fractured rib(s) with a local anaesthetic.

Assisting with airway clearance

1. Assist patient to deep breathe and cough to clear airway.
2. If cough is ineffective, suction airway.

Providing emotional support

1. Monitor level of anxiety.
2. Check on patient frequently to reassure him or her that they are in a safe environment and their needs will be met.
3. Provide time to listen to patients' concerns and provide realistic reassurance.

Facilitating learning

1. Teach patient symptoms (increase in pain, shortness of breath) to report immediately.

Evaluation

Evaluation is based on patient outcomes. Questions to consider may include the following:

1. Is the patient's pain improved?
2. Is the patient able to breathe effectively?
3. Is the patient less anxious?
4. Can the patient state plans for follow-up care?
5. Can the patient state the signs and symptoms (shortness of breath, haemoptysis, or elevated temperature) that require immediate medical attention?

FLAIL CHEST
Pathophysiology

When multiple ribs or the sternum are fractured in more than one place, a portion of the chest wall becomes separated from the chest cage, resulting in a *flail chest*. That is, the chest wall no longer provides the rigid bony support that is necessary to maintain the bellows function required for normal ventilation. This causes *paradoxical respiratory* movement. On inspiration the dislocated segment is pulled inwards by the subatmospheric intrapleural pressure. During expiration the dislocated segment bulges outwards as intrapleural pressure becomes less negative (Fig. 16-13, C and D).

Flail chest usually causes localized atelectasis secondary to decreased ventilation, resulting in hypoxaemia. Because of the increased work of breathing, the individual may also develop hypercapnia and respiratory acidosis.

Assessment
Subjective data

Data to be collected includes the nature of the injury and when it occurred. Often the patient is too badly injured to answer questions, and data are obtained from those accompanying the patient.

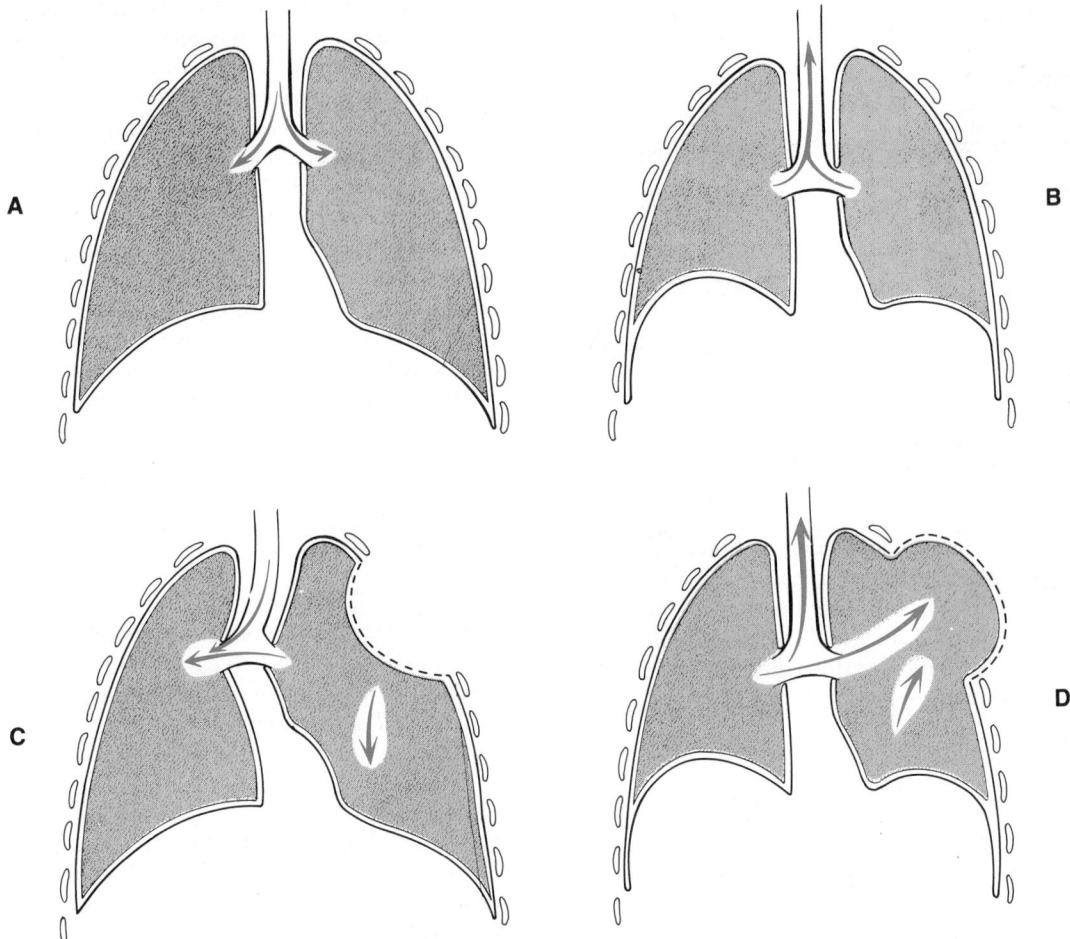

Fig. 16-13   Normal respiration. **A**, Inspiration; **B**, Expiration. *Paradoxical motion*: **C**, Inspiration, area of lung underlying unstable chest wall sucks in on inspiration. **D**, Same area balloons out on expiration. Note movement of mediastinum towards opposite lung on inspiration.

Objective data

1. Pain is severe and increases with each respiratory movement.
2. Mediastinum oscillates, or "flutters," with each respiration.
3. Breath sounds are decreased on auscultation.
4. If there is severe interference with cardiac function, neck veins will be distended.
5. Vital signs: increased pulse and respiratory rate. Blood pressure will fall if paradoxical motion is not relieved.

Diagnostic tests

1. Chest x-ray examination to determine extent of trauma.
2. Arterial blood gases to determine Pao_2 and $Paco_2$.

Medical Management

Treatment includes the following:
1. Stabilize the flail segment. After initial stabilization the individual is usually intubated and placed on a *volume-controlled ventilator*. Postive-pressure mechanical ventilation provides internal stabilization of the chest, decreases the work of breathing, and initiates the bellows function normally provided by the intact bony chest cage. If prolonged ventilatory support is required, a tracheostomy is performed.
2. Provide supplemental oxygen.
3. Correct acid-base imbalance. Mechanical ventilation is used to correct respiratory acid-base imbalance.
4. Provide analgesics for pain control.

PENETRATING CHEST WOUNDS
Pathophysiology

When a knife, bullet, or other flying missile enters the chest, a penetrating wound occurs. The major problem in penetrating injury is not injury to the chest wall but injury to the structures within the chest cavity. Penetration of the lung is associated with leakage of air from the lung into the pleural cavity (pneumothorax) (Fig. 16-14, *B*). Blood may also leak into the pleural cavity (haemothorax). As the air or

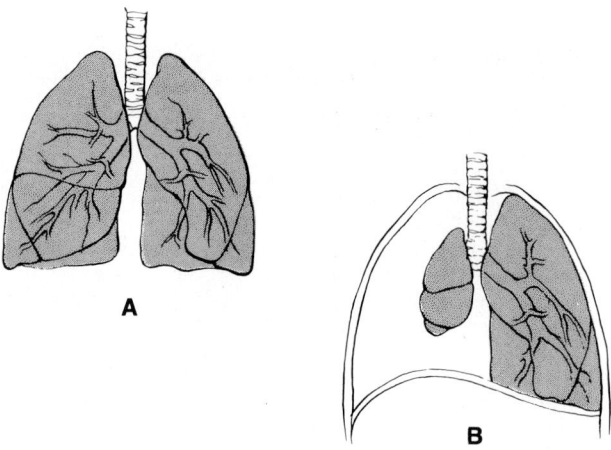

Fig. 16-14 **A**, Normal expanded lungs. **B**, Complete collapse of right lung caused by air in pleural cavity (pneumothorax).

fluid accumulates in the pleural cavity, it builds up positive pressure, which causes the lung to collapse and may cause a mediastinal shift towards the unaffected lung. This compresses the opposite lung and interferes with cardiac action. The person then has serious difficulty in breathing and may go into shock.

Assessment

Subjective data

Subjective data to collect include the nature of the injury and when it occurred. If the patient is too badly injured to answer questions, data is obtained from those accompanying the patient.

Objective data

1. Signs of shock—weak and thready pulse, falling blood pressure, and cold and clammy skin
2. Severe shortness of breath
3. Check for mediastinal shift—trachea deviated from midline

Diagnostic tests

1. Chest x-ray examination to determine extent of injury
2. Arterial blood gases to determine Pa_{O_2} and Pa_{CO_2}

Medical Management

If an open sucking wound of the chest has been sustained, it should be covered immediately to prevent air from entering the pleural cavity and causing a pneumothorax. Several thicknesses of nonporous material such as plastic food wrap may be used, and these are anchored with wide adhesive tape, or the wound edges may be taped tightly together. If an object such as a knife is still in the wound, it is *not* removed until a doctor arrives. Its presence may prevent the entry of air into the pleural cavity, and its removal may cause further damage. *The person who sustained a penetrating wound of the chest should be placed in an upright position and taken to the nearest accident and emergency department.*

Emergency treatment is directed towards *sustaining oxygen exchange and correcting circulatory failure.* Usually

the patient is intubated with an endotracheal tube and then is checked for air or blood in the pleural cavity. An emergency thoracentesis is performed, and air and fluid are removed by syringe. Usually a catheter is inserted into the pleural space and connected to water-seal drainage. If the lung fails to reexpand with this treatment or there is evidence of internal bleeding, surgical exploration may be necessary and will be performed as soon as shock and other complications are under control.

To monitor the patient for hypovolaemia, a central venous pressure (CVP) line is inserted. This line can also be used to administer intravenous fluids and blood as necessary. The CVP is a very effective way to monitor for cardiac tamponade. A pressure above 15 cm of water or a rising CVP in a patient in shock with penetrating trauma in the region of the heart often indicates cardiac tamponade.[124] If it is suspected that cardiac injury and tamponade may be present, a *pericardiocentesis* will be done.

PNEUMOTHORAX
Pathophysiology

In pneumothorax air enters the pleural space between the lung and the chest wall. It can occur spontaneously or as a result of penetrating or nonpenetrating injuries.

A *closed pneumothorax* is caused by a blunt injury resulting in fractured ribs piercing the pleural membranes or by a sudden compression of the rib cage. Air enters the pleural space, increasing intrapleural pressure, which collapses the lung (Fig. 16-14, *B*). A variant of a closed pneumothorax is a *spontaneous pneumothorax* that can result from the rupture of an emphysematous bleb on the lung surface or that may follow severe bouts of coughing in people with a chronic pulmonary disease such as asthma. Frequently, it occurs as a single or recurrent episode in an otherwise healthy young person. If large enough and left untreated, a closed pneumothorax can become a tension pneumothorax.

A *tension pneumothorax* occurs when air leaking into the intrapleural space cannot escape during expiration. *Although usually a result of a closed pneumothorax, a tension pneumothorax can be caused by a penetrating chest injury.* The accumulating air builds up positive pressure in the chest cavity, resulting in (1) lung collapse on the affected side, (2) mediastinal shift towards the unaffected side, and (3) compression of mediastinal contents (heart and great vessels), resulting in decreased cardiac output and decreased venous return.

An *open pneumothorax* occurs when a penetrating chest wound opens the intrapleural space to atmospheric pressure. Each time the patient inspires, air is sucked into the intrapleural space, increasing intrapleural pressure. An open pneumothorax is also called a sucking chest wound because the wound makes a sucking sound on inspiration and expiration. Blood also may leak into the pleural cavity creating a *haemothorax.*

The signs and symptoms and medical management of the various types of pneumothorax are presented in Table 16-15.

Table 16-15 Signs and symptoms and medical therapy for pneumothorax

Pneumothorax	Signs and symptoms	Medical management
Closed	Small or slowly developing pneumothorax may produce no symptoms Larger or rapidly developing pneumothorax results in: Sharp pain on inspiration Increasing dyspnoea Increasing restlessness Diaphoresis Hypotension Tachycardia Absence of chest movement on affected side Breath sounds absent on affected side Hyperresonance on affected side	Observation on an outpatient basis Supplemental oxygen Needle aspiration of air from pleural space Insertion of chest catheter connected to water-sealed drainage system
Spontaneous	Sudden, unexplained shortness of breath	If there are frequent recurrences, silver nitrate is instilled into the pleural space to cause adhesions between the pleurae; if this procedure fails, lung portion with defect is resected and parietal pleura is abraded
Tension	Severe dyspnoea Agitation Trachea deviated from midline towards unaffected side Jugular venous distension Absence of chest movement on affected side Hypotension, tachycardia Breath sounds absent on affected side Hyper-resonance on affected side Diminished heart sounds	Same as open pneumothorax
Open	Sucking sounds at wound site with respiration Tracheal deviation (trachea moves towards unaffected side during inspiration and returns towards midline with expiration)	Occlude open wound Same as closed pneumothorax

Nursing Process
Assessment

Subjective data

1. The nature of the injury
2. When injury occurred
3. Sudden, sharp pain in chest

Objective data

1. Dyspnoea, anxiety, diaphoresis, weak and rapid pulse
2. Cessation of normal chest movements on affected side
3. Trachea deviated towards unaffected side
4. Hyperresonance on percussion
5. Breath sounds decreased or absent
6. Vocal fremitus depressed or absent
7. No adventitious sounds

Diagnostic tests

1. Chest x-ray examination
2. Arterial blood gas determinations of Pao_2, $Paco_2$, and pH.

Nursing analysis

Problems are determined from analysis of patient data. Possible problems for the person with a pneumothorax may include, but are not limited to, those listed in Table 16-16 and the following:

Planning: expected patient outcomes

Expected patient outcomes for the person with a pneumothorax may include, but are not limited to, the following:

1. Patient is able to clear airway without difficulty.
2. Lung is reexpanded and cardiac output is normal.
3. Patient has arterial blood gases within normal limits.
4. Patient states plans for follow-up care.

Implementation
Assisting with achievement of therapeutic goals
Initial care for spontaneous pneumothorax

When a spontaneous pneumothorax is suspected, a doctor should be summoned immediately. The patient should not be left alone, should be reassured, and should be urged to remain still and not move about. Oxygen and equipment for a thoracentesis should be prepared. Air is immediately aspirated from the affected pleural space, and the intrapleural pressure is brought to normal if possible. If air continues to flow into the pleural space, a chest tube is inserted and connected to water-seal drainage. Medication is given for pain.

Table 16-16 Nursing analysis and interventions for pneumothorax

Pneumothorax type	Problems	Nursing interventions
Closed (spontaneous)	Knowledge deficit	For the outpatient or patient who has had chest tube removal, instruct patient to: 1. Report any increased dyspnoea to doctor 2. Avoid strenuous exercise or activity that increases rate and depth of breathing 3. Avoid holding breath 4. Follow doctor's instructions about resuming normal activity
	Gas exchange, impaired	1. Place in a semi-recumbent or upright position 2. Administer oxygen 3. Monitor vital signs 4. Obtain a thoracentesis tray and water-sealed drainage equipment. See p. 325 for care of the patient with chest tubes.
Tension	Knowledge deficit	Same instructions as for patient with closed pneumothorax
	Gas exchange, impaired	A tension pneumothorax is a life-threatening event. It is imperative that interventions be carried out immediately to relieve the increased intrapleural pressure. Interventions are the same as those listed for closed pneumothorax.
	Cardiac output, decreased	1. Monitor vital signs frequently. 2. Observe for cardiac dysrrhythmias. 3. Palpate for subcutaneous emphysema in upper chest and neck. 4. When pressure in the pleural space returns to normal, cardiac output will also return to normal.
Open	Knowledge deficit Gas exchange, impaired	Same instructions as for closed pneumothorax 1. Occlude wound with nonporous covering. 2. Same interventions as for closed pneumothorax. 3. Monitor arterial blood gases to determine effectiveness of treatment. Goal is to have P_{O_2} and P_{CO_2} within normal limits.

Vital signs are monitored every 15 minutes until stabilized and then every hour for the first 24 hours (see Table 16-16 for other nursing interventions).

Interventions to achieve patient outcomes

Follow-up care for spontaneous pneumothorax

When air no longer is expelled from the pleural space through the underwater drainage system and a radiograph reveals that the lung has completely reexpanded, the chest tube is removed and the person is allowed out of bed. Strenuous exertion, which increases the rate and depth of respirations, should be avoided, but relatively normal activity may be resumed rather quickly. If there are frequent recurring episodes, some doctors instil silver nitrate into the pleural space to cause adhesions to form between the visceral and parietal pleurae. If this procedure is unsuccessful, the portion of the lung containing the defect may be resected and the parietal pleura abraded so that it adheres to the visceral pleura and obliterates the pleural space.

Assisting with breathing and ADL

1. Place patient in upright position to facilitate breathing and comfort.
2. Assist patient to keep physical activity at minimum for 24 hours.

   a. Place call system and other necessary objects within easy reach of patient.
   b. Caution patient not to stretch, reach, or move suddenly.
3. Give analgesics as necessary to relieve pain.

Monitoring gas exchange and cardiac output

See Table 16-16 for interventions.

Evaluation

Evaluation is based on patient outcomes. Questions to consider may include the following:
1. Is patient able to clear airway without difficulty?
2. Has the patient's lung reexpanded?
3. Has the patient's cardiac output returned to normal?
4. Are the patient's blood gases within normal limits?
5. Can the patient state plans for follow-up care?

CHRONIC OBSTRUCTIVE PULMONARY DISEASE

Aetiology/Epidemiology

As mentioned on p. 304, *chronic obstructive pulmonary disease (COPD)* refers to diseases that produce obstruction

Table 16-17 Possible variants of COPD*

Predominant disease entity	Associated obstructive disease		
	Asthma	**Chronic bronchitis**	**Emphysema**
Chronic bronchitis	Chronic bronchitis with asthma	Pure chronic bronchitis	Chronic bronchitis with emphysema
Emphysema	Emphysema with asthma	Emphysema with chronic bronchitis	Pure emphysema
Asthma	Pure Asthma	Asthma with bronchitis	Asthma with emphysema

* In addition to the nine variants above, the individual may have a combination of asthma, bronchitis, and emphysema.

of airflow and includes *chronic bronchitis, pulmonary emphysema*, and *asthma*. The disease spectrum associated with this diagnosis ranges from pure obstructive airway disease with the presence of bronchitis but no emphysema, through various combinations, to severe emphysema without bronchitis. The pathophysiological processes that cause these changes are neither static nor are they necessarily progressive. Thus all stages are possible, from reversible abnormalities to relentlessly progressive cardiopulmonary insufficiency. There has been much confusion concerning the clinical use of the terms *chronic bronchitis, emphysema*, and *asthma*; therefore the term *chronic obstructive pulmonary disease* is now used rather than a designation of the specific disease. Frequently by the time the patient seeks medical attention, pathological changes have occurred and symptoms are often moderately severe.

During 1988 in the United Kingdom some 16% of self-reported long-standing illness was described as respiratory. It is probably safe to assume that many of these long-standing illnesses were due to COPD. These data are self-reported and were obtained via the general household survey. For employed people with these diseases frequent absences from work are likely to threaten their jobs.[30]

Both the prevalence of COPD and the death rates attributed to it have reached epidemic proportions. In 1989, COPD was the fifth cause of death in the United States, following heart disease, cancer, strokes, and accidents. Statistics for the United Kingdom show that deaths from COPD are highest in Northern Ireland and Scotland and that male deaths are twice those of females. More deaths occur during the winter months, in both manual workers and those people living in urban areas. However, the death rates from COPD in men aged 55-64 fell from 80 per 100,000 in 1977 to 60 per 100,000 in 1983.

The increase in the death rate in the United States from COPD is believed to be related to (1) the growing tendency of doctors to list it as a primary cause of death, (2) the greater use of pulmonary function testing, and (3) more emphasis in medical literature on the importance of this syndrome. Despite these facts, it is believed that the mortality is even higher than reported because many people who were reported to have died from pneumonia, asthma, or congestive heart failure probably had COPD. The major factors in this increase in mortality, in addition to improved reporting and the increased ageing of the population, is a history of cigarette smoking. These diseases are more prevalent among men than women, but death rates are

increasing in women. This is directly related to the increase in smoking among women.

Although asthma, chronic bronchitis, and emphysema are classified under the common category, it is clinically important to identify the predominant type of pulmonary disease that is the basis for the individual's COPD. Therefore, in the following presentation, COPD is divided into three major obstructive diseases: chronic bronchitis, emphysema, and asthma. Because the clinical management of chronic bronchitis and emphysema is similar, the care for patients with either of these diseases is presented together. (See nursing care plan for people with COPD on p. 354.)

CHRONIC BRONCHITIS

Chronic bronchitis is defined *clinically* by hypersecretion of mucus and recurrent or chronic productive cough for a minimum of 3 months per year for at least 2 consecutive years in patients in whom other causes have been excluded. It is characterized *physiologically* by hypertrophy and hypersecretion of the bronchial mucus glands and structural alterations of the bronchi and bronchioles.

Aetiology/Epidemiology

As indicated in Table 16-18, chronic bronchitis is caused by the inhalation of physical or chemical irritants or by viral or bacterial infections. The most common inhaled irritant is cigarette smoke, and heavy cigarette smoking is believed to be the major cause of the disease. Occupations in which dust or other irritants are inhaled may cause bronchitis, but the evidence for this is not conclusive. However, in Great Britain it has been recognized for years that the highest incidence of bronchitis occurs in large industrial cities with higher levels of air pollution.

Prevention

The overall focus for prevention of chronic bronchitis is to alleviate whatever irritant appears to be causing the associated symptoms in the individual. Of all the known risk factors, the most clearly implicated is smoking. The continued inhalation of tobacco smoke leads to worsening of bronchial inflammation and hypersecretion. Thus smoking cessation is an essential step for the prevention of chronic bronchitis. Additionally, such preventive measures as avoidance of repeated infections and prompt treatment of upper and lower respiratory infections are important steps to avoid disease progression. National standards for air quality

Table 16-18 Factors in development of COPD*

Chronic bronchitis	Emphysema	Asthma
Cigarette smoking	Cigarette smoking	Allergy
Atmospheric contaminants	Atmosphere contaminants	Hypersensitivity
Infection	Antienzyme and enzyme deficiencies (alpha, alpha$_1$, and alpha$_2$)	Infection
Chronic irritation	Advanced pulmonary fibrosis	Environment
Gastrooesophageal dysfunction	Destruction of lung parenchyma (necrosis, ischaemia)	Drugs
		Emotions
		Social conditions
		Exercise

From Tomashefski JF, editor: Chronic obstructive pulmonary disease: a perplexing and challenging spectrum: core curriculum symposium (pulmonary disease), *Postgrad Med* 62:87-151, 1977.

and governmental actions related to improving the quality of the air we breathe should be of concern to everyone.

Progress in the prevention of chronic bronchitis has been impeded by the slow and insidious onset of the disease. Recent advances in pulmonary function testing have allowed identification of abnormalities in the small airways of the lungs. It is believed that peripheral airway changes occur early in the development of obstructive lung disease. Research has indicated that some of the abnormalities associated with small airway changes may be reversible. Thus if high-risk populations could be identified and a feasible screening test developed, preventive measures could be instituted before permanent lung damage and chronic disease occur.

Pathophysiology

The two pathological changes that typify chronic bronchitis are hypertrophy of mucus-secreting glands and chronic inflammatory changes in the small airways. First, there is glandular hypertrophy. *Mucous gland hypertrophy* and *hyperplasia* from chronic irritation cause excessive mucus production. The excessive mucus and impaired ciliary movement associated with chronic bronchitis increase susceptibility to infection. Bacteria proliferate in the mucous secretions in the lumen of the bronchi. The most common infectious agents are *S. pneumoniae* and *H. influenzae*. As bacteria multiply, they exert a neutrophilic chemotaxis, and pus cells migrate from between bronchial epithelial cells to produce a mucopurulent exudate in the lumen, or the disease may progress to ulceration and destruction of the bronchial wall. The presence of granulation tissue and peribronchial fibrosis result in stenosis and airway obstruction. Small airways may be completely obliterated, and others may become dilated. This chain of events further traps secretions and promotes multiplication of bacteria. There is some evidence that the pathological changes occur initially in small airways and move to larger bronchi.[107]

Second, people with chronic bronchitis develop increased airway resistance as a result of bronchial wall tissue changes, mucosal oedema, and excessive mucus production. Excess mucus in the airways not only obstructs airflow but also often causes bronchospasm, which further increases airway resistance.

Third, there is altered oxygen-carbon dioxide exchange. Airway obstruction resulting from all the pathophysiological changes that increase airway resistance may impair the ability of the lungs to exchange oxygen and carbon dioxide. Obstructed airways cause ventilation-perfusion mismatching at the alveolar-capillary membrane by decreasing the amount of oxygenated air that reaches the alveoli. Additionally, the obstructed airways may lead to atelectasis, which further diminishes the surface area available for respiration. The result of these pathophysiological alterations is hypercapnea, hypoxaemia, and respiratory acidosis (see discussion of arterial blood gases; see p. 300).

Fourth, right ventricular decompensation (cor pulmonale) may result. The hypercapnia and hypoxaemia commonly associated with chronic bronchitis cause pulmonary vascular vasoconstriction. The increased pulmonary vascular resistance results in pulmonary vessel hypertension that in turn increases vascular pressure in the right ventricle of the heart.

Clinical Manifestations

Signs and symptoms of chronic bronchitis are manifestations of the underlying physiological abnormalities that have occurred. Table 16-19 relates normal function, primary pathophysiology, and the clinical picture observed in chronic bronchitis.

The earliest symptom of chronic bronchitis is a productive cough, especially on awakening. This symptom is often ignored by cigarette smokers who become so accustomed to an early morning cough that they take it for granted; some of them even refer to it as their "smoker's cough."

People with chronic bronchitis often unconsciously adapt their activity level to accommodate their respiratory symptoms in their daily lives. Thus they do not seek medical help until they experience a severe exacerbation of their symptoms, usually precipitated by a respiratory infection.

Pulmonary function testing reveals a limitation to airflow on expiration as evidenced by a diminished FEV$_1$. Vital capacity is also reduced, indicating diminished air movement both in and out of the lungs. Lung volumes are usually within normal limits until later in the course of the disease, when the lung volumes may be increased. There usually is no loss of diffusing capacity.

Early in the course of chronic bronchitis, the symptoms tend to be episodic in nature. As the disease progresses in severity, the patient's symptoms are constantly present to some degree. The patient appears increasingly dyspnoeic, using accessory muscles to breathe. *Chronic hypoxaemia*

Table 16-19 Normal function, primary pathophysiology, and the clinical picture in chronic bronchitis, emphysema, and asthma

Normal function/ pathophysiology	Clinical picture		
	Chronic bronchitis	Emphysema	Asthma
Bronchial mucus-secreting glands produce mucus to trap foreign particles and transport them out of lungs	Productive chronic cough, greyish-white sputum; when infected sputum is yellow, inspiratory; crackles (rales)		Inflammation, hypersecretion; eosinophils in sputum
Bronchi and bronchioles Carry oxygenated air to alveoli and carry deoxygenated air out of lungs	Inspiratory, expiratory rhonchi; dyspnoea: episodic or continual; ↓ FEV, ↓ VC with small response to bronchodilators*	Early-onset dyspnoea on exertion, which progresses to continuous dyspnoea. Rhonchi, crackles, accessory muscle breathing ↓ FEV, ↓ VC with no response to bronchodilators	Episodic dyspnoea, accessory muscle breathing; inspiratory/expiratory wheezing. ↓ FEV, ↓ VC with good response to bronchodilators. ↑ Work of breathing, pulsus paradoxus
Alveolar-capillary membrane Semipermeable membrane where oxygen diffuses from alveoli to blood and carbon dioxide diffuses from blood to alveoli	Respiratory acidosis, hypoxaemia, polycythaemia, tachycardia, cyanosis	Early stage: normal or mild hypoxaemia, respiratory alkalosis; late stage: hypoxaemia, respiratory acidosis, ↓ diffusing capacity	Respiratory alkalosis with mild hypoxaemia Status asthmaticus: respiratory acidosis with hypoxaemia
Right side of heart Carries deoxygenated blood to pulmonary vasculature for oxygen/carbon dioxide exchange	Jugular vein distention, hepatomegaly, peripheral oedema	Right ventricular decompensation	
Lung and chest wall compliance The relationship between lung and chest wall ability to expand and contract during inhalation and exhalation		↑ A-P diameter, ↓ lateral expansion, ↓ diaphragmatic excursion, ↓ breath, heart, and voice sounds, ↑ RV, ↑ FRC, ↑ TLC₃, hyperresonance, complaint of episgastric fullness	↓ Femitus, ↓ lateral expansion, hyperresonance, ↓ breath sounds, ↓ diaphragmatic excursion

* FEV, forced expiratory volume; VC, vital capacity.

resulting in polycythaemia causes the patient to appear to be cyanotic. Increased pulmonary vascular resistance caused by respiratory acidosis and hypoxaemia increases pressure on the right side of the heart, ultimately resulting in right heart failure (cor pulmonale). The person with late-stage chronic bronchitis and cor pulmonale appears stout or overweight from oedema. Because of the oedema and dusky skin colour these people are often referred to clinically as "blue bloaters." People with the preceding characteristic appearance are classified by some as having type B COPD.

Patients with chronic bronchitis complicated by cor pulmonale often have chronic respiratory failure (gradual onset of $Pao_2 < 6.6$ kPa (50) and a $Paco_2 > 6.6$ kPa (50). They are also prone to developing acute respiratory failure

(sudden onset of a $Pao_2 < 6.6$ kPa (50) and a $Paco_2 > 6.6$ kPa (50) as a complication of a respiratory infection superimposed on their already-diseased lung.

Medical Management

The process of medical diagnosis of chronic bronchitis may include any of the following:

1. Patient history
2. Physical examination
3. Diagnostic studies
   a. Chest x-ray: typical findings with chronic bronchitis increased bronchovascular markings
   b. Sputum studies for culture and sensitivity: neutrophils and bronchial epithelial cells usually present in chronic bronchitis

c. Arterial blood gas studies: see discussion under clinical manifestations
d. Haematology studies: FBC
e. Pulmonary function testing: see discussion under clinical manifestations

Effective health care management programmes for people who have chronic bronchitis or any of the variant combinations of pulmonary diseases that make up COPD requires a multidisciplinary approach. The multidisciplinary approach to the management of COPD is included in the discussion of implementation of care for patients with COPD later in this chapter.

Medical management of a person with chronic bronchitis is included in Table 16-20, which summarizes a typical multidisciplinary programme for people with COPD.

Nursing Process
Assessment
Subjective data

1. History of character of onset and duration of:
   a. Cough
   b. Sputum production (amount, colour, and consistency)
   c. Dyspnoea
   d. Pain in right upper quadrant (hepatomegaly)
2. Smoking history
3. Disease history
   a. Influenza
   b. Pneumonia
   c. Repeated respiratory tract infections
   d. Chronic sinusitis
4. Past or present exposure to environmental irritants at home or at work
5. Self-care used to treat symptoms
6. Medications taken and their effectiveness in relieving symptoms

Objective data

1. Assess general appearance
   a. Patient may appear overweight or bloated.
   b. Check for dependent oedema and jugular vein distention
   c. Abdominal assessment may indicate hepatomegaly
2. Assess vital signs
   a. Elevated temperature
   b. Tachycardia
   c. Tachypnoea
3. Pulmonary examination
   a. Inspection
      (1) Accessory muscle breathing
      (2) Forward leaning posture
      (3) Central cyanosis
      (4) Clubbing of fingers
      (5) Altered sensorium (restlessness or lethargy)
   b. Palpation by doctor
      (1) Increased tactile fremitus
   c. Percussion by doctor—normal
   d. Auscultation by doctor
      (1) Inspiratory crackles (rales)
      (2) Inspiratory and expiratory rhonchi
4. Assess laboratory findings

   a. Arterial blood gases
      (1) Respiratory acidosis
      (2) Hypoxaemia
   b. Haematology
      (1) Elevated haemoglobin and haematocrit (PCV)
      (2) Elevated WBC
   c. Pulmonary function tests
      (1) Decreased FEV_1
      (2) Normal diffusing capacity
      (3) Normal lung volumes (in end-stage chronic bronchitis lung volumes may appear similar to those found with emphysema)

Planning: expected patient outcomes

Problems and expected outcomes for patients with COPD are similar, regardless of the underlying obstructive airway disease. Thus outcomes for patients with chronic bronchitis are included later in this chapter under the outcomes for patients with COPD (p. 342).

Implementation

See Implementation section for COPD on p. 343.

Evaluation

See Evaluation section for COPD on p. 351.

EMPHYSEMA

Emphysema is defined *pathologically* by destructive changes in alveolar walls and enlargement of air spaces distal to the terminal nonrespiratory bronchioles. It is characterized *physiologically* by increased lung compliance, decreased diffusing capacity, and increased airway resistance.

Aetiology/Epidemiology

Although it is not known when emphysema actually begins, there appear to be many years between the initial pathophysiological changes and the onset of overt symptoms. Symptoms associated with emphysema usually appear in the fourth decade, and disability from disease usually occurs in the fifth or sixth decade of life. The typical individual with emphysema is a male about 55 years of age with a history of tobacco smoking.

The cause of emphysema is not known; however, recent evidence suggests that proteases released by polymorphonuclear leukocytes or alveolar macrophages are involved in the destruction of the connective tissue of the lungs. Connective tissue in the lungs is primarily composed of elastin, collagen, and proteoglycan, which can be damaged and destroyed by enzymes such as proteases and elastase. It has been demonstrated that elastase (produced by alveolar macrophages) can destroy or damage the elastin in the connective tissue of the parenchyma of the lung. Normally, inhibitors found in human serum, lung tissue, peripheral airways, and bronchial mucus protect the lung from the proteolytic enzymes. It is believed that some change in the enzyme-inhibitor balance occurs, which allows the proteolytic enzymes to attack lung tissue.

It has been known since 1965 that some people have a deficiency of alpha$_1$-antitrypsin and that these people develop severe, disabling emphysema, usually of the bullous type, early in life. Recent studies indicate that cigarette smoke increases the amount of elastase secreted by the alveolar macrophages and neutrophils and that it impairs the inhibitor functions of alpha$_1$-antitrypsin.

It is estimated that *1% of people with COPD have a congenital alpha$_1$-antitrypsin (AAT) deficiency*. The mean age for onset of dyspnoea related to COPD was 40 to 45 years in people with AAT. Their mean life expectancy was 50 to 65 years of age with smokers dying about 10 years earlier than nonsmokers.[55]

Patients with AAT can be treated with human alpha$_1$ antitrypsin, which has been approved in some countries but is very expensive. A recent study indicates that treating patients with AAT would be cost effective because it would decrease complications in those with AAT and increase their life span. Because AAT cannot be prevented, it is important that people who have it do not smoke.[55]

It is not known why some smokers develop bronchitis and others develop emphysema. Differences in susceptibility and the predominant type of disease are believed to be influenced by hereditary or environmental factors or those related to the patient's history.[106] It is established, however, that there is familial tendency to alpha$_1$-antitrypsin deficiency and that relatives of people with this type of emphysema should be screened and provided with counselling as discussed next.

Primary Prevention

The cornerstone of prevention of emphysema is education. Health education must focus on the pulmonary health risks associated with inhaled irritants, regardless of their source. Increased public awareness of the vital role clean air plays in pulmonary health is essential for the success of any legislative actions promoting air quality standards. Individuals must also be educated to understand the importance of personal responsibility to decrease their own health risk through smoking cessation.

People with a family history of emphysema should be screened for alpha$_1$-antitrypsin deficiency. It is imperative that people with this enzyme deficiency take active measures to prevent additive lung damage from smoking, air pollution, and infection. People identified as being at high risk for emphysema may require vocational counselling if their current work environment is known to have inhaled irritants. These individuals also should be counselled to receive the influenza vaccine yearly, and the pneumococcal vaccine once.

Pathophysiology

The type of emphysema can be determined only by descriptive morphology. There are two principal types of emphysema morphologically—*centrilobular* emphysema (CLE) and *panlobular* emphysema (PLE). In CLE, there is distention and damage of the respiratory bronchioles selectively. Openings develop in the walls of the bronchioles; they become enlarged and confluent and tend to form a single space as the walls enlarge. The disease tends to be unevenly distributed throughout the lung but usually is more severe in the upper portions.

In PLE, there is a more uniform enlargement and destruction of the alveoli in the pulmonary acinus. PLE

is usually more diffuse and is more severe in the lower lung. It is found in elderly people who have no evidence of chronic bronchitis or impairment of lung function.[106] It occurs just as commonly in women as in men, but PLE is less common than CLE. PLE is a characteristic finding in people with homozygous alpha$_1$-antitrypsin deficiency.[106]

The clinical diagnosis of emphysema is inferred from signs and symptoms that are manifestations of known pathophysiological changes associated with the disease. Physiological abnormalities characteristic of emphysema include the following alterations:

1. Increased lung compliance. Loss of elastic recoil resulting from destruction of elastin in lung parenchyma causes the lungs to become permanently overdistended. Thus, compared to normal lungs, emphysematous lungs have a larger increase in volume relative to the pressure change that occurs during inhalation.
2. Increased airway resistance. Destruction of elastic lung tissue causes the small airway to either collapse or narrow, particularly during expiration. Thus air becomes trapped in the distal airspaces, contributing to the lungs' overdistended state. The overdistended lungs press against the diaphragm, diminishing its ventilatory effectiveness. Accessory muscles are used to breathe as the body attempts to compensate and force the trapped air out of the lungs. This causes an increase in intrapleural pressure that increases airway collapse.
3. Altered oxygen-carbon dioxide exchange. Destruction of alveolar and respiratory bronchiole walls decreases the alveolar-capillary membrane surface area, which in turn may diminish gaseous diffusion. People with emphysema are able to compensate for these destructive changes by increasing their respiratory rate. Thus arterial blood gases remain relatively normal, although mild hypoxaemia may be present. Late in the course of the disease, extensive surface area loss coupled with ventilation-perfusion inequalities usually cause respiratory acidosis and hypoxaemia.

Normal function, pathophysiology, and clinical picture of emphysema is presented in Table 16-19.

Clinical Manifestations

Typically, the first symptoms heralding the onset of emphysema is dyspnoea on exertion, which progresses to continual dyspnoea. Sputum production tends to be scant or absent. People with emphysema usually appear thin and manifest a "barrel chest" with an increased anteroposterior (AP) diameter from hyperinflation. The characteristic breathing pattern of the emphysematous individual includes accessory muscle breathing, an increased respiratory rate, and a prolonged expiratory phase resulting from airway narrowing or collapse on expiration. These individuals will spontaneously exhibit pursed-lip breathing, which facilitates effective air exhalation. (Pursed-lip breathing elevates end-expiratory pressures, which inhibits airway collapse during expiration.)

Pulmonary function studies demonstrate an increased

residual volume, functional residual capacity, and total lung volume. Diffusing capacity is significantly reduced because of lung tissue destruction. Diminished respiratory air flow is demonstrated by a decreased forced expiratory volume (FEV) and maximal midexpiratory flow rate (MMFR). The vital capacity (VC) may be normal or only slightly reduced until late in the disease; thus the FEV_1/VC ratio is decreased. The degree of respiratory impairment may be estimated on the basis of the ratio of FEV to FVC (see Box 16-22). A significant finding that differentiates emphysema from the other obstructive airway disorders is the failure to show improvement in pulmonary function tests in response to bronchodilators.

Arterial blood gases are often near normal because of the individual's ability to compensate through increased respiratory rate and tidal volume. Indeed, many people with emphysema overcompensate and develop a mild respiratory alkalosis from hyperventilation. Because resting hypoxaemia is absent and ventilation is high, these individuals maintain a normal Pco_2 despite abnormal gas exchange and are described as "pink puffers." A person exhibiting these symptoms of pure emphysema is classified as having type A COPD. Late in the course of the disease the Pco_2 is elevated, which leads to cor pulmonale and respiratory failure.

The terms "blue bloater" and "pink puffer" represent the two extremes seen in people with chronic airway obstruction. Recently, it has been suggested that the underlying disease alone does not determine whether the person is "blue" or "pink," but rather the interaction between the lung disease and the person's drive to breathe. For example, the pink puffer may just fight harder to maintain a normal Pco_2, whereas the blue bloater settles for less work and allows the Pco_2 to rise.

Medical Management

The medical diagnosis of emphysema may include any of the following:
1. Patient history
2. Diagnostic studies
   a. Chest x-ray: positive finding = increased radiolucency of lungs with diaphragm in a low flat position
   b. Arterial blood gas studies
   c. Pulmonary function testing
   d. Haematology
      (1) alpha₁-antitrypsin assay
      (2) FBC; usually normal
   e. Sputum for culture and sensitivity

16-22

Estimate of pulmonary dysfunction based on FEV/VC ratio

Normal lung function—greater than 80% predicted values

Mild impairment—65% to 85% of predicted values

Moderate impairment—50% to 64% of predicted values

Severe impairment—49% or less of predicted values

Medical management of emphysema includes the same modalities as those used in the treatment of chronic bronchitis. Table 16-20 presents the components of medical therapy used in the treatment of both chronic bronchitis and emphysema.

Nursing Process
Assessment

Subjective data

1. History of and onset of the following:
   a. Dyspnoea—(important to investigate if patient correlates the occurrence of dyspnoea with any specific illness or other life event; establish how the patient's dyspnoea affects ADL)
   b. Cough—usually mild or may be absent
   c. Sputum production—usually scant white sputum
2. Smoking history
3. Family history of emphysema
4. Past or present exposure to environmental irritants at home or at work
5. Self-care modalities
6. Medications or other prescribed therapies and their effectiveness in relieving symptoms

Objective data

1. Assess general appearance
   a. Patient usually appears thin with a large chest. (Note: this is a normal variant in the elderly; thus it does not always signify pulmonary disease.)
2. Assess vital signs for:
   a. Tachycardia
   b. Tachypnoea
3. Pulmonary examination by doctor
   a. Inspection
      (1) Accessory muscle breathing
      (2) Forward-leaning posture
      (3) Pursed-lip breathing
      (4) Prolonged expiration
      (5) Barrel chest, increased A-P diameter
   b. Palpation by doctor
      (1) Decreased lateral expansion
      (2) Decreased fremitus
   c. Percussion by doctor
      (1) Hyperresonance
      (2) Low diaphragm
      (3) Decreased diaphragmatic excursion
   d. Auscultation by doctor
      (1) Decreased breath and heart sounds
      (2) Late inspiratory crackles
      (3) Rhonchi (Note: adventitious sounds are often not present with emphysema.)
4. Assess laboratory findings
   a. Arterial blood gases
      (1) Early stage emphysema-respiratory alkalosis with mild hypoxaemia
      (2) Late stage emphysema-respiratory acidosis with hypoxaemia
   b. Haematology

REVIEW

Table 16-20 Signs and symptoms of and medical therapy for chronic bronchitis and pulmonary emphysema

Chronic bronchitis	Pulmonary emphysema

Signs and symptoms
Early symptoms

Productive cough on awakening: often ignored by cigarette smokers who refer to it as their "smokers cough"

Dyspnoea on exertion indicating acute respiratory distress
Using accessory muscles to breathe; ruddy colour
Thin with a "barrel chest"
Usually able to maintain resting Pao$_2$
Cyanosis uncommon
Sometimes referred to as "pink puffer"

Later symptoms

Significant physical incapacity; breathlessness even when walking on a flat surface; noticeable shortness of breath (SOB) and use of accessory muscles to breathe. Cyanosis is common. Ankle oedema, bloated appearance, distended neck veins; sometimes referred to as "blue bloater"

Late in disease

Cor pulmonale (right ventricular hypertrophy), right-sided heart failure, and respiratory failure are frequent complications.

Late in disease

Paco$_2$ ↑
Cor pulmonale and respiratory failure possible complications

Pulmonary function test findings
↓ Expiratory flow rates
↓ Vital capacity
↑ Residual volume
   Total lung capacity usually within normal limits

↓ Expiratory flow rates, especially forced expiratory volume and maximal midexpiratory flow
↑ Total lung capacity
↑ Residual volume
Vital capacity may be normal or slightly reduced until late stages of disease. Change in FEV$_1$/VC ratio

Arterial blood gas findings
Low resting Pao$_2$
Elevated Paco$_2$ (if obstruction severe)
During exercise Paco$_2$ ↑ and Pao$_2$ may also ↑

Pao$_2$ normal or slightly reduced at *rest;* falls during exercise
Normal Paco$_2$
Late in disease, elevated Paco$_2$

Medical therapy
Medical therapy for chronic bronchitis and pulmonary emphysema is similar and dependent on symptoms, pulmonary function test results, and blood gas findings. Therapy may include all or some of the modalities outlined here.

Supportive measures
Education of patient and family about:
   Avoidance of cigarette smoke
   Avoidance of other inhaled irritants
   Avoidance of people with upper respiratory infections
   Control of environmental temperature and humidity
   Proper nutrition
   Adequate hydration

Specific therapy
Medications
Bronchodilators (Table 16-21)
   Antimicrobials
      Tetracycline or ampicillin usually prescribed to treat respiratory tract infections
   Corticosteroids
      May be prescribed to alleviate acute symptoms. Inhaled steroids being used more frequently. Oral prednisolone also prescribed.
   Cardiac glycosides
      May be prescribed to treat left ventricular failure.

Respiratory therapy
Aerosol therapy
Used to deliver bronchodilators through metered cartridge devices or hand-held nebulizers or by use of compressed air.
Oxygen therapy
   Required for patients who are unable to maintain a Pao$_2$ of 6.6 kPa (50 mm Hg) or more at rest or who cannot carry out ADL without becoming short of breath; 1 to 2 L of O$_2$ given by nasal cannulae

Continued.

Table 16-20 Signs and symptoms of and medical therapy for chronic bronchitis and pulmonary emphysema—cont'd

Chronic bronchitis/Pulmonary emphysema

Physical conditioning

Relaxation exercises

Progressive relaxation exercises are encouraged. Best practised before meals or 2 hours or more after eating because digestion seems to interfere with ability to relax (p. 351)

Meditation

Meditation more widely used to assist patients to relax (p. 350)

Breathing retraining by physiotherapist

Pursed-lip breathing

Leaning forward position for exhalation (Fig. 16-16)

Abdominal breathing (p. 346)

Inhalation-exhalation exercises (p. 346)

Exhalation with exertion (p. 346)

Rehabilitation

Muscle reconditioning programmes specific for the patient

---

(1) Positive alpha$_1$-antitrypsin assay

c. Pulmonary function

(1) Decreased FEV$_1$, VC, and diffusing capacity (D$_L$)

(2) Increased total lung capacity, functional residual capacity (FRC), residual volume (RV)

Nursing analysis

Problems for patients with COPD are similar regardless of the underlying obstructive airway disease.

Problems are determined from analysis of patient data. Possible problems for the person with COPD include, but are not limited to, the following:

Problems	Possible aetiologies
Gas exchange, impaired	Low ventilation/perfusion ratio
Breathing pattern, inffective	Decreased energy/fatigue, airway changes
Airway clearance, ineffective	Hypersecretion, tracheobronchial infection, decreased energy/fatigue
Nutrition altered: less than body requirements	Dyspnoea, anorexia, sputum production, medication side effects, fatigue
Infection, high risk for	Decreased lung defences
*Fluid volume excess	Pulmonary hypertension with resultant increased cardiac workload
Activity intolerance	Imbalance between oxygen demand and requirement
Sleep pattern disturbance	Dyspnoea
Fear	Long-term illness and disability, change in role functioning
Knowledge deficit: condition and its treatment	Lack of exposure/recall, cognitive limitation, unfamiliarity with information source

Planning: expected patient outcomes

The following expected patient outcomes and implementation sections apply to patients with chronic bronchitis, emphysema, or any combination of these two obstructive airway diseases.

The patient will:

1. Demonstrate improved ventilation and oxygenation
   a. Arterial blood pH and P$_{CO_2}$ that returns or stays within acceptable baseline limits
   b. Pa$_{O_2}$ at optimal level for individual
   c. Explains how and when to use oxygen therapy
2. Demonstrate an effective breathing pattern
   a. Inspiratory to expiratory ratio = 5:10 seconds
   b. Pursed-lip breathing
   c. Appropriate use of leaning forward postures
   d. Diaphragmatic breathing (abdominal muscle breathing)
   e. Exhales with activity
   f. Respiratory rate within near normal limits, moderate tidal volume
3. Demonstrate adequate airway clearance
   a. Effective methods of coughing
   b. Appropriate use of nebulizers, humidifiers, mistometers, intermittent positive pressure breathing (IPPB) machine, and medications
4. Explain dietary changes required after discharge
   a. Maintain optimal weight for height, age, and gender
   b. Explain food and fluid requirements and daily plan for achieving them
   c. List specific foods to be avoided
   d. Explain plan for frequent, small feedings that are soft and that do not require much chewing, and the need for increased time required for eating if indicated
5. Remain infection free
   a. Temperature remains normal
   b. Sputum does not change in colour, amount, or consistency
   c. If the above occur, health care provider should be informed
6. Achieve a normal fluid balance
   a. Daily weight remains stable
   b. Electrolyte levels remain within expected levels

---

* More common with bronchitis.

c. Diuretics and cardiac glycosides, if prescribed, are taken as ordered

d. If signs of oedema (weight gain, increase in dyspnoea) occur, health care provider is notified

7. Maintain or work towards an optimal activity level
   a. Pacing activities
   b. Planning for simplification of activities
   c. Participating in planned muscle conditioning programme

8. Demonstrate activities to control stress response to symptoms
   a. Muscle relaxation
   b. Meditation
   c. Participation in support group

9. Use effective measures to promote sleep
   a. Determine best position in bed (number of pillows) to minimize dyspnoea
   b. Practise methods that promote sleep (relaxation exercises, meditation, guided imagery, or soft music)

10. List common signs and symptoms that require reporting to the health care provider
    a. Change in sputum colour, amount, and consistency
    b. Increased coughing
    c. Change in behaviour
    d. Increased fatigue
    e. Increased dyspnoea
    f. Weight gain or loss
    g. Peripheral oedema
    h. Elevated temperature

11. Demonstrate how to carry out the specific exercise programme to be followed at home including:
    a. Specific exercises to be completed
    b. Frequency of each exercise
    c. Criteria for monitoring physical response to exercises such as heart rate increase or perceived fatigue

12. Demonstrate comprehension of self-care activities
    a. Explain health maintenance or therapeutic follow-up programme
    b. Describe any home medication or treatment programme
    c. Explain exercise programme to be followed at home
    d. Describe how to obtain professional and community resources necessary to structure a satisfactory environment at home
    e. State plans for ongoing follow-up care

13. Explain the following aspects of home medication or treatment regimens:
    a. State name, dose, action, and side effects of each medication to be used at home
    b. How and when to use medications ordered on an as needed basis (for example, bronchodilators, antibiotics, steroids, antacids)
    c. Techniques necessary for follow-up care (for example, segmental postural drainage, clapping and vibrating, inhalation therapy treatments)
    d. How to obtain and maintain any needed equipment or supplies such as oxygen, nebulizers, humidifiers, mistometers, IPPB machine, syringes, and medications

14. List names and telephone numbers of appropriate community services such as community nurses and a home medical equipment supplier

Implementation

COPD and all of its actual or potential impact on the individual's life are most effectively managed by a multidisciplinary team. Pulmonary health care teams consisting of doctors, nurses, respiratory workers, occupational therapists, physiotherapists, dietitians, social workers, and psychologists or psychiatrists provide a comprehensive approach to assist patients to attain or maintain their optimal level of function within the constraints of their pulmonary disability.

A typical multidisciplinary programme incorporates the areas listed in Box 16-23.

Although it is difficult to measure the physiological effects of these programmes, hospitalization of patients who have participated in them is less frequent, and most people state that they feel better.

Although the complex multidisciplinary rehabilitation team is the ideal, the nurse functioning in a small community hospital or community nursing service can provide effective rehabilitation activities for the person with COPD.

Nursing interventions for people with chronic bronchitis and pulmonary emphysema are the same and centre around the following:

Assisting with the achievement of therapeutic goals
Medications

The types of medications that may be prescribed for people with COPD include bronchodilators, expectorants, antimicrobials, corticosteroids, cardiac glycosides, diuretics, and psychopharmacological agents.

Bronchodilators. There are two basic categories of *bronchodilators*—sympathomimetic (adrenergic) agents and xanthine compounds. These bronchodilators act at different sites and appear to work synergistically when used together.[57] Table 16-21 lists the commonly used bronchodilators and their mode of action. Adrenergic agents that work at beta$_2$ sites located in smooth muscles of the airways have fewer cardiac side effects than do beta$_1$ agents whose receptor sites are in the myocardium. For this reason, salbutomol and terbutaline may be prescribed for patients with hypertension and those who have excessive palpitations or tachycardia from beta$_1$-agents.

16-23

Multidisciplinary programmes for patients with COPD[57]

Patient and family education
Pharmacotherapy
Conditioning exercises
    Cardiopulmonary conditioning
    General muscle conditioning
Pulmonary hygiene modalities
Relaxation training
Counselling
    Psychosocial counselling
    Vocational counselling

Table 16-21   Bronchodilators commonly used to treat COPD

Name	Mode of action
Methylxanthines	
Aminophylline	Block action of phosphodiesterase and interfere with degradation of cyclic AMP, resulting
Theophylline	in bronchodilation
Symphathomimetics*	
Beta$_1$-receptor sites	Activate adenylcyclase leading to increased production of cyclic AMP, resulting in relaxa-
Adrenaline	tion of smooth muscle of airway; increase in cyclic AMP also inhibits release of chemi-
Isoprenaline	cal mediators that cause bronchospasm (histamine and SRS-A)
Beta$_1$-receptor sites	
Terbutaline	
Salbutamol	
Fenoterol	

* Beta-adrenergic drugs.

Aerosol therapy. Aerosol therapy is one of the most effective ways to deliver bronchodilators and corticosteroids. The most commonly used ways to deliver an aerosol include a metered dose cartridge inhaler (MDI), hand-held nebulizer, or IPPB machine. IPPB is used less frequently and is reserved for people who cannot inhale repetitively enough to near total lung capacity (TLC) or who are unable to use a hand-held nebulizer or MDI because of lack of coordination or fatigue. Box 16-24 gives directions for using an inhaler with a spacer, and Box 16-25 gives directions for teaching patients to use a hand-held nebulizer. When administering bronchodilators, the solution should be diluted with either water or saline. Some experts recommend that the diluent be water because saline solutions already contain a solute (NaCl) in water. All bronchodilator solutions are high-molecular weight concentrated solutions and have a high solute content. When they are diluted with water, there is a maximal decrease in solute concentration; thus smaller particle size and deeper deposition of the aerosol in the smaller airways results.

Aerosol devices are excellent sites for bacterial growth, and patients using such equipment at home should be advised on how to clean them appropriately.

When a spacer (Fig. 16-15), a moulded plastic chamber, is fitted on an inhaler, medication can be delivered more safely and effectively for the following reasons. (1) Large droplets of the aerosol, which would tend to settle in the mouth and on the vocal cords, land on the walls of the spacer instead; (2) the finer droplets in the aerosol disperse more fully within the spacer and can be carried farther into the airways; (3) it is not necessary to coordinate breathing as carefully as it is with the standard inhaler and thus patients are medicated more effectively; and (4) spacers can reduce the number and volume of puffs required, thereby reducing the cost of medication because each dose is used more efficiently.[54]

After the medication is in the spacer, the patient can take several breaths, inhaling each time from the spacer, to receive the entire dose. Inhalers with spacers can be used to deliver corticosteroids, bronchodilators, and sodium cromoglycate.

Expectorants. Although expectorants are sometimes prescribed, some experts believe they do more harm than

---

Patient Teaching   16-24

Using an inhaler with a spacer

1. Exhale fully.
2. Position nebulizer in mouth without sealing lips around it.
3. Take a deep breath while releasing a puff of medication into spacer.
4. Hold breath for 3 to 4 seconds at full inspiration.
5. Exhale slowly through pursed lips.
6. Usually one or two puffs are prescribed.
7. Several breaths may be necessary to receive the entire dose from the spacer.
8. The mouth should be rinsed after completing treatment.
9. The inhaler and spacer are washed with warm soapy water, rinsed, and dried thoroughly.

Patient Teaching   16-25

Using a hand-held nebulizer

1. Exhale fully.
2. Position nebulizer in mouth *without* sealing lips around it.
3. Take a deep breath through mouth while squeezing the bulb of the nebulizer *once*.
4. Hold breath for 3 to 4 seconds at full inspiration.
5. Exhale slowly through pursed lips.
6. Usually one inhalation is sufficient. Several inhalations of a bronchodilator may cause medication overdosage and result in side effects (for instance, tachycardia, palpitation, and nervousness).

---

good.[57] Water is still considered to be the best expectorant, and adequate hydration without fluid overload should be encouraged. Usually 3 to 4 L of fluids daily are recommended unless the patient has *cor pulmonale* and is on fluid restriction.

Antimicrobials. Antimicrobials are prescribed to treat respiratory tract infections in people with COPD. The most commonly used ones are *tetracycline* and *amoxycillin*, 1 to

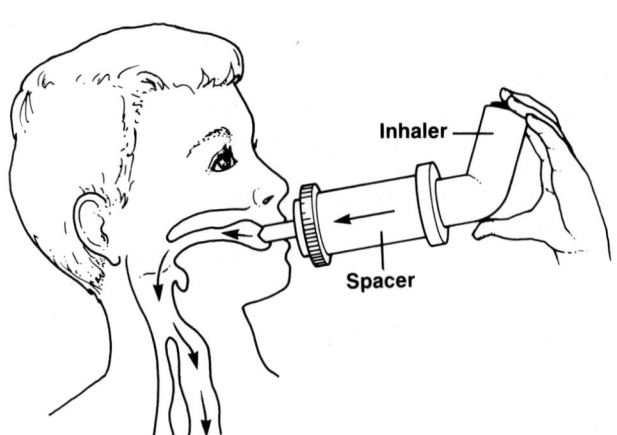

Fig. 16-15 Patient using inhaler with spacer attached to allow for better dispersal of medication.

2 g/day for 7 to 10 days. Some patients have a prescription on hand and self-administer the antimicrobial after telephone consultation with their doctor. Antimicrobials should be started within 24 hours of the first sign of a respiratory infection (increased sputum production and purulence). In patients who are febrile or have other signs and symptoms of infection that do not respond to the prescribed therapy, a sputum specimen should be sent for a Gram stain and culture and sensitivity studies. When antibiotics are used inappropriately, especially in patients who are not adequately clearing their lungs of secretions, superinfection with bacteria or fungi may occur.

Corticosteroids. Corticosteroids may be prescribed for patients with intermittent bronchial obstruction and blood or sputum eosinophilia whose condition is not controlled by bronchodilators. They can be administered orally or by inhaler with the latter becoming the most common method. Usually a short course of corticosteroids is prescribed to alleviate acute symptoms. Prednisolone is often prescribed for a total of 7 to 10 days. In some patients with asthma, a longer course of prednisolone may be prescribed and some patients are on low-maintenance doses (5 to 10 mg/day) for several months or even years. Long-term corticosteroid therapy is usually not recommended for patients with chronic bronchitis or emphysema unless their disease is rapidly progressing.[57]

People who are on long-term steroid therapy should have a tuberculin test before initiation of therapy. Those with tuberculin reaction of 10 mm induration or more are candidates for therapy. The purpose of isoniazid therapy is to prevent reactivation of tuberculosis, which is likely to occur, in people receiving prolonged steroid therapy.

Cardiac glycosides. Digoxin may be prescribed for patients with COPD and left ventricular failure. The patient receiving digoxin preparation should be carefully monitored for side effects (Chapter 17).

Patients with increased dyspnoea secondary to pulmonary oedema, or with right ventricular failure, or corticosteroid-induced fluid retention may benefit from *diuretics*. When diuretics are given, the patient should be carefully monitored for side effects. Those on thiazide diuretics need to be told to eat foods high in potassium such as bananas, oranges, prunes, and raisins.

Psychopharmacological agents. Psychopharmacological agents may need to be prescribed for some patients with severe emotional disturbances. The type of agent and size of dose are individually determined, but in general, the older the patient, the smaller the dose. When these agents are prescribed, a pharmacology book should be referred to for information about the side effects and precautions to be used in administering these agents.

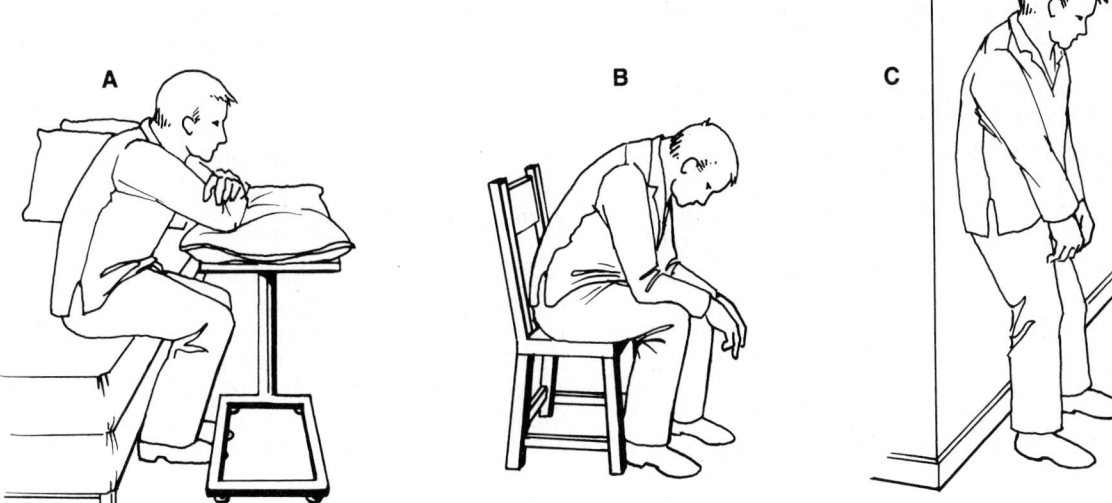

Fig. 16-16 Forward leaning position. **A,** Patient sits on edge of bed with arms folded on pillow placed on elevated bedside table. **B,** Patient in three-point position. Patient sits in chair with feet approximately 1 foot apart and leans forward with elbows on knees. **C,** Patient leans against wall with feet spread apart allowing shoulders to sag forward with arms relaxed.

Oxygen therapy

Oxygen therapy is required for patients with COPD who are unable to maintain Po_2 of greater than 7.3 kPa (55 mm Hg) or an Sao_2 of greater than 85% or more at rest and for those who cannot carry out ADL (breathing, eating, dressing, toileting) without becoming very short of breath. In these instances, 1 to 2 L of oxygen is usually given via nasal prongs to relieve hypoxaemia and decrease pulmonary hypertension, which in turn, decreases the load on the right side of the heart. It has been demonstrated that patients receive the most benefit from oxygen therapy if the oxygen is used continuously. A common misunderstanding expressed by patients requiring ongoing oxygen therapy is that they should only use their oxygen when they are symptomatic (that is, short of breath) in order to avoid becoming habituated to the oxygen and thus requiring higher levels of oxygen. It is imperative that the nurse clarify that habituation does *not* occur and that it is important to use oxygen continuously in order to receive maximal benefits of oxygen therapy.

Interventions to achieve patient outcomes
Improving gas exchange

Arterial blood gases are monitored for indications of hypoxaemia, respiratory acidosis, and respiratory alkalosis.

Hypoxaemia and hypercapnia often occur simultaneously, and the signs and symptoms of each are similar. These include headache, irritability, confusion, increasing somnolence, asterixis (flapping tremors of extremities), cardiac dysrrhythmias, and tachycardia.

If hypocapnia is developing, tachypnoea, vertigo, tingling of the extremities, muscular weakness, and spasm are commonly present. It is important to remember that the presence of signs and symptoms associated with altered levels of O_2 and CO_2 depend more on the *rate of change* than on the *degree of change. Rapidly changing signs usually indicate a rapid worsening of the patient's condition.* At the same time, patients with long-standing hypoxaemia and hypercapnia may be relatively asymptomatic because they have physiologically accommodated to increased levels of CO_2 and decreased levels of O_2.

Improving efficiency of breathing pattern
In conjunction with physiotherapist

1. Teach patient to slow respiratory frequency and to breathe slowly and rhythmically.
2. Discourage patient from taking big gulps of air.
3. Teach patient to increase inspiratory to expiratory ratio so that expiration takes twice as long as inhalation.
   a. Teach patient to count in seconds and to concentrate on increasing time taken to exhale.
   b. Count to 5 on inhalation and to 10 on exhalation.

Abdominal breathing and exercises. The physiotherapist teaches abdominal breathing, leg raising exercises, inhalation-exhalation exercises, and muscle reconditioning exercises.

Abdominal breathing improves the breathing efficiency of people with COPD because it assists the patient to elevate the diaphragm. Abdominal breathing can be taught in the sitting or lying position. In the sitting position, the patient sits on the side of the bed or in a chair and holds a cushion or a book against the abdomen. The patient then exhales slowly while leaning forward and pressing the cushion or book against the abdomen. In the lying position, a cushion or a book is placed on the abdomen and the patient is asked to "puff out" the abdomen and raise the cushion or book as high as possible. The patient then exhales slowly through pursed lips while pulling in on the abdominal muscles. Manual pressure on the upper abdomen during expiration facilitates this manoeuvre (Fig. 16-17). In addition to abdominal breathing, exercises to strengthen the abdominal muscles assist patients to use their abdominal muscles more effectively in emptying their lungs.

This same method of teaching augmented abdominal (diaphragmatic) breathing can be used to teach the patient to cough. The difference is that expiration is forced down to residual volume. This manoeuvre often stimulates the cough reflex. If it does not, the person is taught to actively cough at the end of full expiration. Physiologically, forced expiration simulates the effects of a cough and is, therefore, more effective than telling the patient to take a deep breath and then cough.

Leg-raising exercises, with each leg being raised alternately as the patient exhales, is one way to strengthen abdominal muscles. Another way is to ask the patient to raise the head and shoulders from the bed while he or she exhales. Not all patients can do all exercises, but most can do some of them on a daily or twice-daily basis. With practice and encouragement the patient can do the exercises 10 times each morning and evening after clearing the lungs as completely as possible of secretions.

Inhalation-exhalation exercises emphasize the need to prolong exhalation about four to five times longer than inhalation. Patients who walk can be taught to count in seconds and to concentrate on exhaling slowly and fully. While learning to *exhale with exertion*, the patient exhales during an activity such as bending over or sitting down.

Muscle reconditioning refers to a variety of exercises that tone muscles. For patients who are able to be out of bed, walking, using a treadmill, or riding a stationary bicycle is helpful. The exercise period is started slowly with 10 minutes twice daily three times a week, increasing to 20 minutes twice daily three times a week. The patient needs to be assessed for his or her ability to carry out such an exercise programme, and a staff member should be present during the exercise period.

Pulmonary physiotherapy. The person who has difficulty breathing may be taught how to increase the efficiency of his or her breathing pattern. Breathing exercises are usually a part of pulmonary physiotherapy, which may also include *segmental postural drainage, clapping*, and *vibrating*. Although pulmonary physiotherapy activities are performed by a physiotherapist, they may be part of a nurse's responsibility. Regardless of where the primary responsibility lies, nurses must be familiar with the techniques so that they can demonstrate and reinforce them and ensure that the individual is doing them correctly. Also, the need for pulmonary physiotherapy may occur at a time when the physiotherapist is not available to the patient.

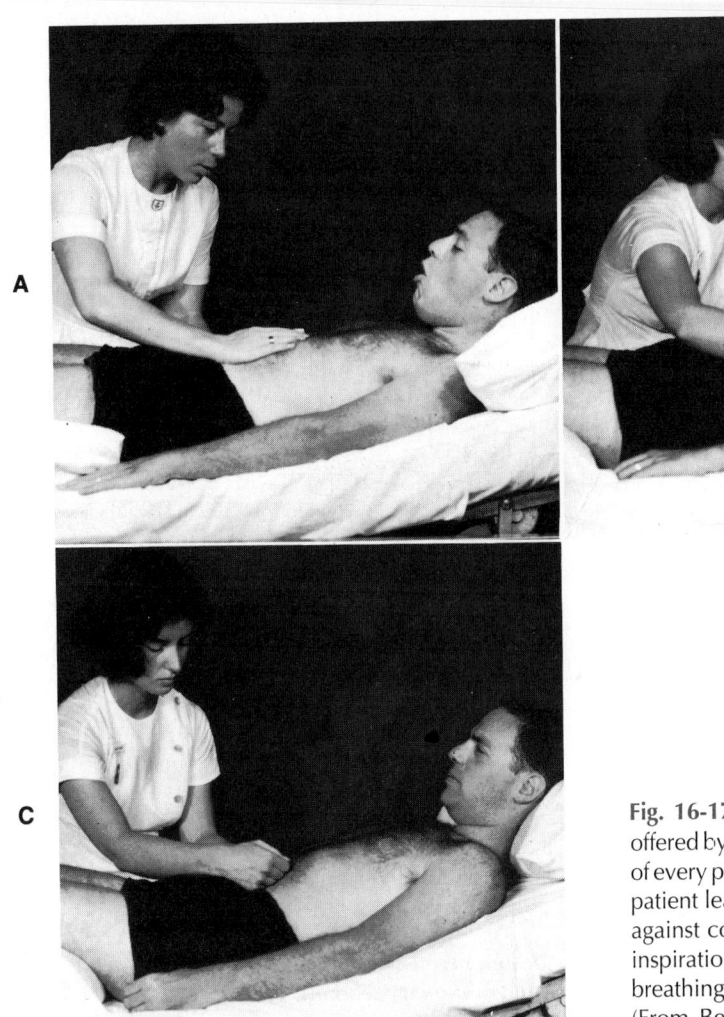

A

B

C

Fig. 16-17   A, When made to breathe against the resistance offered by the physiotherapist's hands, the patient is made aware of every phase of his respiration and use of muscle groups. **B**, The patient learns how to fully expand his lower lobes by breathing against counterpressure applied to the side of the chest during inspiration. **C**, The patient is taught diaphragmatic control by breathing against a resistance applied in the costophrenic angle. (From Bendixen HH, et al: *Respiratory care*, St Louis, 1965, Mosby–Year Book.)

Segmental postural drainage. Segmental postural drainage with clapping and vibration is a technique used to combine the force of gravity with the natural ciliary activity of the small bronchial airways to move secretions upward towards the main bronchi and the trachea. From this point the patient can cough secretions up, or they can be suctioned. In the treatment of chronic obstructive pulmonary disease, drainage of all segments is usually accomplished by placing patients in various postural drainage positions (Fig. 16-18). Treatment may also be directed at draining specific areas of the lung. While the patient is in each position, *clapping* with a cupped hand is performed over the area being drained. This manoeuvre helps to loosen secretions and stimulate coughing. After clapping the area for approximately 1 minute, the patient is instructed to breathe deeply. *Vibrating* (pressure applied with a vibrating movement of the hand on the chest) is performed during expiratory phase of the deep breath. This assists the patient to exhale more fully. The procedure is repeated as necessary. When the patient cannot tolerate a head-down position, a modified position is used.

Positions that provide gravity drainage of the lungs can be achieved in several ways, and the procedure selected usually depends on the age and general condition of the person as well as the lobe or lobes of the lungs where secretions have accumulated. A young person usually can tolerate greater lowering of the head than an elderly person whose vascular system adapts less rapidly to change of position. A severely debilitated patient may only be able to tolerate slight changes in position.

Postural drainage can be accomplished in several ways. Hospital beds can be tilted into a head-down position with little difficulty. At home blocks can be placed under the casters at the foot of the bed or a hydraulic lift can be used under the foot of the bed. If these are not available, the foot of the bed can be supported on the seat of a firm chair to provide a position in which the head is lowered.

The nurse needs to know the part of the lung that is affected and how to position the patient to drain that portion of the lung. For example, if the right middle lobe of the lung is affected, drainage will be accomplished best by way of the right middle bronchus. The patient should lie supine with the body turned at approximately a 45-degree angle. The angle can be maintained by pillow supports placed under the right side from the shoulders to the hips. The foot of the bed is raised about 30 cm (12 inches). This position can be maintained fairly comfortably by most patients for half an hour at a time. On the other hand, if the

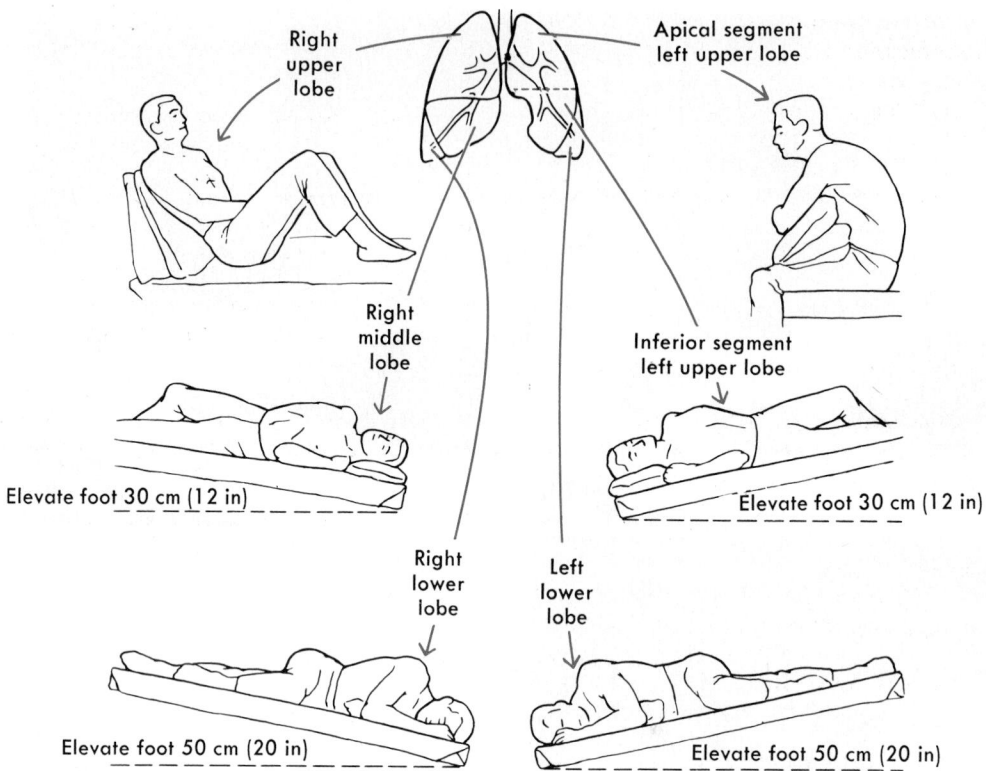

Fig. 16-18 Postural drainage requires that the patient assume various positions to facilitate the flow of secretions from various portions of the lung into the bronchi, trachea, and throat so that they can be raised and expectorated more easily. Drawing shows the correct position to drain various portions of the lung.

lower posterior area of the lung is affected, the foot of the bed can be raised 45 to 50 cm (18 to 20 inches) with the patient assuming a prone position for drainage.

Postural drainage and percussion should be planned so as to achieve maximal benefit. The best time is generally in the morning soon after arising and at night before retiring. Frequency of treatments depends on each person's needs, but care should be taken to avoid exhaustion, which results in shallow ventilation and negates the positive effects of the treatment.

Patients having postural drainage of any kind are encouraged to breathe deeply and to cough forcefully to help dislodge thick sputum and exudate that is pooled in distended bronchioles, particularly after inactivity. Humidity, bronchodilators, or liquefying agents often are given 15 to 20 minutes before postural drainage is started, because they facilitate the removal of secretions. The patient may find that sputum can best be raised on resuming an upright position even though no drainage appeared while lying down with the head and chest lowered.

Because some patients complain of dizziness when assuming positions for postural drainage, the nurse stays with the patient during the first few times and reports any persistent dizziness or unusual discomfort to the doctor. *Postural drainage may be contraindicated in some people* because of *heart disease, hypertension, increased intracranial pressure, extreme dyspnoea,* or *advanced age.* However, most people can be taught to assume the positions for postural drainage and can proceed without help after being supervised once or twice.

Chest percussion (clapping) is *contraindicated in patients* with *pulmonary emboli, haemorrhage, exacerbation of bronchospasms,* or *severe pain* and *over areas of resectable carcinoma.* Often patients with a chronic pulmonary problem need to be taught to perform postural drainage independently so that they can continue it at home. The position usually is maintained for 10 minutes at first, and the period of time is gradually lengthened to 5 to 30 minutes as the patient becomes accustomed to the position. At first, elderly people usually are able to tolerate these positions only for a few minutes. They need more assistance than other patients during the procedure and immediately thereafter. They should be assisted to a normal position in bed and asked to lie flat for a few minutes before sitting up or getting out of bed. This helps to prevent dizziness and reduces the danger of accidents from orthostatic hypotension.

The patient may feel nauseated because of the odour and taste of sputum. Therefore, the procedure should be timed so that it comes at least 1 hour before meals. A short rest period following the treatment often improves postural drainage. Teeth cleaning and mouth washes should be available for frequent use by any patient who is expectorating sputum freely.

Improving nutritional intake

People with COPD often demonstrate excessive weight loss. Some of the factors that may contribute to weight loss are:

1. A feeling of satiety with small amounts of food because of compression of abdominal contents by the flattened diaphragm
2. Dyspnoea interfering with eating
3. Increased dyspnoea when eating caused by stomach pushing up against the diaphragm
4. Decreased appetite secondary to chronic sputum production
5. Gastric irritation associated with bronchodilators and steroids
6. Increased work of breathing requiring increased caloric intake to maintain weight; makes it imperative that the patient with COPD maintain adequate nutritional levels because:
   a. A diminished total weight is correlated with a dramatic decrease in respiratory muscle (especially the diaphragm) size and strength[101]
   b. Inadequate nutritional status and in particular deficiencies in vitamins A and C decrease resistance to infection
   c. Protein insufficiency decreases colloid osmotic pressure, which increases the risk of pulmonary oedema

Nursing actions focused on assisting the patient with COPD to maintain adequate nutrition include the following:

1. Explore usual dietary habits (collect a 24-hour diet history).
2. Counsel patient to select foods that provide a high-protein, high-caloric diet (see Box 16-26).
3. Encourage vitamin supplementation. It is important to counsel the patient to select foods that provide higher calorie levels through higher fat content rather than by high carbohydrate levels. People with advanced chronic bronchitis or emphysema are unable to breathe off the excess carbon dioxide that is a natural end product of carbohydrate metabolism. Therefore, calories obtained from high carbohydrate foods may elevate arterial carbon dioxide levels in people with COPD.
4. Prepackaged food supplements such as milk shakes or snack bars taken between meals provide an excellent source of protein and calories.
5. Smaller, more frequent meals are often tolerated better than three larger meals.
6. Consider financial and ethnic background when planning for meals.

Preventing infection

The *most common complication of COPD* and cause of most hospital readmissions, is *respiratory infection*. Pulmonary system response to the infectious process includes increased respiratory rate, mucosal irritation, and increased mucus production. Because of these localized responses, patients may present with bronchospasm and a change in their pattern of sputum production (see list of signs and symptoms on p. 341). If the infection remains untreated, the end result is an overall increased work of breathing with eventual respiratory failure. Thus for the person with COPD, it is imperative that respiratory infections be avoided. The patient should be counselled to take the following steps to *decrease* the chance of contracting a pulmonary infection.

16-26

Foods to increase protein and caloric intake*

Offer frequent small feedings of foods high in protein and calories such as the following:
Milk shakes
Puddings with whipped cream
Cream soups made with single cream
Peanut butter spread on crackers, bananas, pears, or apples
Crackers and cheese, nuts, dried fruits, and ice creams readily available for snacks
High calorie protein drinks

*Excellent sources for suggestions to increase protein and calorie intake are McCauley K and Weaver R: Cardiac and pulmonary diseases-nutritional implications. *Nurs Clin North Am* 18:81-95, 1983; and Spector N: Nutritional support of the ventilator-dependent patient. *Nurs Clin North Am* 24:407-414, 1989; and Cerrato PL: The special nutritional needs of a COPD patient, *RN* 11:75-76, 1987.

---

1. Avoid large crowds, especially during known influenza seasons.
   a. Avoid contact with people who have an upper respiratory infection.
   b. Get influenza and pneumonia immunizations.
2. Contact health care provider if the following common signs and symptoms occur:
   a. Change in sputum colour, amount, and consistency
   b. Increased cough
   c. Change in behaviour (for example, more argumentative than usual) that indicates an increase in P_{CO_2}
   d. Increased fatigue
   e. Increased dyspnoea
   f. Weight gain
   g. Peripheral oedema
   h. Elevated temperature

Antimicrobial agents are prescribed to treat respiratory tract infections in people with COPD. The most commonly used antimicrobials are tetracycline or amoxycillin for 7 to 10 days. Some patients have a prescription on hand and self-administer the antimicrobial agent after telephone consultation with their doctor. Antimicrobials should be started within 24 hours of the first signs of a respiratory infection. Patients who have a fever or who have other signs and symptoms of infection that do not respond to the prescribed therapy should have a sputum specimen sent for a Gram stain and culture and sensitivity studies. When antibiotics are used inappropriately, especially in patients who are not adequately clearing their lungs of secretions, superinfection with bacteria or fungi may occur. Although these regimens of prophylactic treatment do not appear to decrease the incidence of infection, they do decrease the severity and duration of the infection.[25]

Preventing fluid volume excess

Low arterial blood oxygen is a potent pulmonary vasoconstrictor. Pulmonary vasoconstriction increases pulmonary arterial pressure. If pulmonary hypertension exists for a prolonged period of time, the increased workload on the heart's right ventricle will ultimately result in *right ventricular failure* and what is known as pulmonary heart disease or *cor pulmonale*. Depending on its severity and duration, cor pulmonale may be characterized by neck vein distention, hepatomegaly, dependent peripheral oedema, and, as oncotic pressure is exceeded, ascites and pleural effusions. Nursing interventions for fluid volume excess resulting from cor pulmonale are based on the understanding that the disease is treated by intervening with the underlying cause of the pulmonary hypertension. Therefore, nursing interventions focus on promoting adequate ventilation for optimal oxygen/carbon dioxide exchange and relieving symptoms that result from the fluid volume excess. Thus a nursing plan of care for the person with COPD that promotes optimal ventilation also intervenes with fluid volume excess resulting from cor pulmonale. Additionally, interventions focused on the symptoms of fluid volume excess include:

1. Weigh daily in the same amount of clothing and at the same time of day on the same scale.
2. Monitor intake and output accurately. (Note: Although it is unknown if fluid restriction is effective in the actual treatment of cor pulmonale, excess fluid intake may overwhelm an already compromised cardiac system.)
3. Encourage moderate exercise or change patient's position frequently to promote adequate perfusion in lung.
4. Measure abdominal girth at regular intervals to assess the possible presence or progression of ascites.
5. Administer diuretics as ordered. When diuretics are given, the patient should be carefully monitored for side effects. Those on thiazide diuretics will need to be taught about eating foods high in potassium such as bananas, oranges, prunes, and raisins.
6. Administer digoxin as ordered. (Note: Digoxin is of questionable usefulness in pure right-sided heart failure.) People receiving digoxin should be carefully monitored for side effects.

Assisting with breathing and rest

1. Place patient in position of comfort, usually upright.
2. Assist patient with progressive relaxation exercises and meditation (see Boxes 16-27 and 16-28).

Assisting with control of environment

Abrupt changes in weather or hot or cold environments can increase sputum production and bronchial obstruction.

Temperature and humidity

1. Humidity of 30% to 50% is ideal. This can be achieved by a humidifier as necessary.
2. An air conditioner may reduce dyspnoea by controlling temperature and preventing pollutants from outside air from entering.
3. Wearing a scarf over the nose and mouth in cold weather helps to warm the air and prevent bronchospasm. Masks for this purpose are also available.

16-27

Progressive relaxation exercises[84]

1. Contract each muscle to a count of 10 and then relax it.
2. Do exercises in quiet room while sitting or lying in a comfortable position.
3. Do exercise to relaxing music, if desired.
4. Have another person serve as a "coach" by giving command to contract muscle, count to 10, and relax muscle.
5. The following are examples of exercises helpful to some people with COPD.
   a. Raise shoulders, shrug them, and relax for 5 seconds; then relax them completely.
   b. Make a fist of both hands, squeeze them tightly for 5 seconds, and then relax them completely.

16-28

Meditation exercises

1. Sit or lie quietly with eyes closed and attempt to relax all muscles, beginning with feet and moving upward (see relaxation techniques above).
2. Breathe in through the nose slowly (may help to count slowly to four on inhalation), exhale slowly through pursed lips (mentally count to six) with a natural rhythm, relaxed and peaceful (this can be coached or done privately).
3. Survey the body for points of tension. Consciously relax the tense areas. The body is peaceful and relaxed.
4. Continue breathing as above, aware of the feeling of well-being throughout your body. This can be continued for 10 to 20 minutes, or after 5 minutes go to step 5.
5. Listen for (or visualize) a special relaxing sound (or image) such as relaxing sound or picture. Listen to it closely (or visualize) all the while breathing as above.
6. At this point positive suggestion can be used; for example, "I am in control of my body. When I find myself getting tense I can take a moment to stop and breathe in all the air that I need and let the tension flow away."
7. After mental suggestion continue breathing easily and slowly come back to normal alert mental state.
8. Meditation can be used at any time to induce a relaxed state of mind (for example, to promote sleep).

---

4. Moving to another climate is usually not advised unless there is some other medical indication for doing so. People living at high altitudes may be advised to move to a lower altitude or use supplemental oxygen continuously.
5. Air travel is possible. The airline needs to be informed in advance of the need for supplemental oxygen during the flight.

Avoiding inhaled irritants

Air pollution is a common problem in modern civilization and is a real threat to people with COPD who should observe the following:
1. Heed announcements on radio and television regarding air quality and avoid being outdoors when this is poor.
2. Use an air conditioner or high-efficiency particulate air filter or electrostatic filter to remove particulate matter from air.
   a. Keep filters clean.
   b. Follow manufacturer's directions for use.
3. Use an activated charcoal filter if offending odours or gas pollutants are a problem.
4. Avoid being with people who are smoking.

Improving activity tolerance

1. Allow ample time for activities; do not rush patient.
2. Provide oxygen as needed before and during activities.
3. Encourage gradual increase in activities such as walking.
4. Provide positive feedback on progress and encourage new endeavours when patient is ready.

Assisting with sleep pattern disturbance

People with COPD usually only sleep for short periods of time. Most are most comfortable sleeping in an upright position in bed or in a lounge chair with foot rest.
1. Assist with relaxation exercises at bedtime.
2. Give massage at bedtime and encourage family member to do so at home.
3. Provide relaxing music at bedtime and encourage same at home.
4. Ascertain preferred position for sleep, usually upright.
5. Establish regular bedtime to meet patient's usual routine.
6. Give bedtime snack, if desired.

Assisting with anxiety reduction

People who are short of breath are very anxious and frightened.
1. Encourage patient to talk about anxiety and fears with nurse and family members.
2. Take measures already discussed to improve airway clearance and breathing.
3. Do not leave patient alone during periods of breathlessness.
4. Explain to family reason for not leaving patient at home alone for long periods; assist them with securing community resources to assist as necessary (for instance, Home carers or the community nursing service).

Facilitating learning

People with COPD play a major role in monitoring their own condition and in maintaining their physical and psychological functioning at the maximum possible level.

For these reasons, it is imperative that the nurse thoroughly assess the patient's knowledge about COPD, including its cause and treatment. Individualized teaching plans based on the patient's knowledge level can then be developed. Areas that may be included in the teaching programme are listed in Box 16-29.

Not all people who are high risk for influenza-related complications have the annual influenza vaccination. Nurses are ideally placed to encourage uptake of this vaccine, especially in patients with COPD. The particular influenza strains included in the vaccine each year are those recommended by the World Health Organization (WHO).

Evaluation

Evaluation is based on patient outcomes. Questions to consider may include, but are not limited to, the following:
1. Are patient's arterial blood gases within acceptable baseline limits?
2. Is patient using an effective breathing pattern? Inspiratory-expiratory ratio of 5:10 seconds? Pursed-lip breathing? Using leaning forward position to empty lungs? Exhaling with activity?
3. Is patient using appropriate means to clear airway? Coughing effectively? Using MDI with spacer correctly?
4. Is patient able to explain the dietary plan to be followed after discharge?
5. Is the patient free of a superinfection?
6. Is the patient able to achieve a normal fluid balance?
7. Is patient able to maintain an optimal activity level? Pacing activities? Doing muscle conditioning exercises?
8. Is patient able to demonstrate activities to control stress response to symptoms (muscle relaxation, meditation)?
9. Is the patient successful in using measures to promote sleep?
10. Is patient able to list signs and symptoms (change in sputum, amount of coughing, fatigue, dyspnoea, elevated temperature, weight gain, peripheral oedema, or change in behaviour) that should be reported to health care provider?
11. Is patient able to demonstrate specific exercise programme to be followed at home?
12. Is the patient able to discuss how self-care activities will be accomplished after discharge?
13. Is patient able to explain home medications (name, dose, action, side effects) and how to take prescribed medications?
14. Is patient able to demonstrate how to do postural drainage and other treatments and where to obtain necessary equipment?
15. Does patient have a list of names and telephone numbers of community services?

ASTHMA

Asthma is discussed separately from bronchitis and emphysema because it results in intermittent rather than

The patient with COPD

The following areas should be addressed in a typical teaching programme for people with chronic bronchitis or emphysema:

I. Patients should be able to explain, in lay terms, the basic function and pathology of their lungs. Various leaflets exist for patient education.[130]

II. The avoidance of respiratory irritants and maintenance of a proper environment should be emphasized to people with COPD. As discussed earlier, inhaled irritants (especially cigarette smoke) pose a serious threat to these people. Steps the patient can take to reduce or avoid exposure to these irritants are listed below.

   a. Stop smoking. There are many agencies that offer programmes for people who want to stop smoking. The nurse should be familiar with community programmes and give a list of them to the patient.

   b. Ask other people not to smoke in the immediate environment. Inhalation of secondary smoke can exacerbate symptoms.

   c. Pay heed to announcements on radio and television warning of poor air quality. Do not go outside during an alert.

   d. Use an air conditioner or high-efficiency particulate air filter or electrostatic filter to remove particulate matter from air.
      1. Keep filters clean.
      2. Follow manufacturer's directions for use.

   e. Use an activated charcoal filter if offending odours or gas pollutants are a problem.

   f. Avoid abrupt environmental temperature or humidity changes because they can increase sputum production and cause bronchospasm.

      1. Use an air conditioner in hot weather.
      2. Use a face mask when going out in cold weather.
      3. Use a dehumidifier or humidifier as appropriate to maintain a humidity of 30% to 50%.

   g. If air travel is required, check with doctor about the need for supplemental oxygen.

   h. Avoid large crowds, especially during known influenza seasons.
      1. Avoid contact with people who have an upper respiratory infection.
      2. Have influenza and pneumonia immunizations.

III. The patient should be able to explain the following aspects of the home medication or treatment regimen.

   a. State name, dose, action, and side effects of each medication.

   b. Explain how and when to use medications ordered on an as needed basis (for example, bronchodilators, antibiotics, steroids, antacids).

   c. Demonstrate techniques necessary or follow-up care (for example, postural drainage, clapping and vibrating, aerosol therapy).

   d. Describe how to obtain and maintain any needed equipment or supplies such as oxygen, nebulizers, humidifiers, aerosols, IPPB machines, syringes, and medications.

IV. The patient should demonstrate how to carry out the specific home exercise programme.

   a. Specific exercises to be completed

   b. Frequency of each exercise

   c. Criteria for monitoring physical response to exercises such as heart rate increase or perceived fatigue

V. The patient should be able to list the names and telephone numbers of appropriate community support services such as the community nurse or British Red Cross.

---

continuous, irreversible airway obstruction. Its onset is sudden as opposed to the slow insidious progression of symptoms seen in bronchitis and emphysema. Asthma is characterized by increased responsiveness of the trachea and bronchi to various stimuli that cause narrowing of the airways and difficulty in breathing.

Aetiology/Epidemiology

Asthma is estimated to affect some 2 million people in the United Kingdom, of which some 750,000 are children. The prevalence of asthma in the United Kingdom, which is increasing, is about 5%, similar to that in the United States. There are around 2000 deaths from asthma each year with nearly half these deaths occurring in people under 65. Apart from being a significant cause of death, asthma leads

to serious ill-health. There is considerable time lost from school and work, with the added financial loss to individuals and employers.

The Department of Health is committed to reducing asthma deaths and the morbidity associated with the disease. It is hoped to learn more about the aetiology of the disease and standardize monitoring for deterioration and treatment regimens[131].

Table 16-22 lists the traditional classification and general causative factors associated with asthma. In any type of asthma, the airway is in a state of easy provocation, and attacks may be precipitated by a variety of factors. Although the classification listed in Table 16-22 is still the most commonly used way of differentiating types of asthma, there is a move away from using this classification system.

Table 16-22   Traditional asthma classification

Type	Immunological (allergic, extrinsic)	Nonimmunological (nonallergic, intrinsic)	Mixed (combination immunological, nonimmunological)
Onset	Usually in childhood	Usually after age 35	Any age
Causative agent/ precipitating	Any extrinsic protein (antigen)	Nonspecific stimulus	Allergen or nonspecific stimulus
Associated factors	Other allergic-based disorders (that is, eczema) Elevated IgE	Respiratory infections, influenza	Nonspecific

Table 16-23   Asthma syndromes classified by precipitating factor and response pattern

Asthma syndromes	Characteristics
Atopic asthma	Childhood onset, allergic rhinitis, allergic dermopathy, identifiable environmental precipitating events
Exercise-induced asthma	Airway contriction after exercise
Aspirin-hypersensitivity triad	Presence of nasal polyps, urticaria, and asthma after aspirin ingestion
Bronchospasm associated with nonbacterial upper respiratory tract infections	As described by patient
Industrial asthma	Bronchoconstriction associated with certain industrial precipitating factors

Clinically, most people with asthma fall into the mixed classification of asthma types; thus the traditional asthma classification is of limited usefulness in establishing individual treatment programmes. Experts in asthma treatment are recommending that asthma be grouped as *syndromes* and *classified according to precipitating factors* and *individual response patterns to precipitating factors*.[55] Table 16-23 presents some of the common syndromes of asthma using the currently recommended classification.

Prevention

Prevention of immunological (atopic) asthma is focused on identification of the allergens to which the person is sensitive. In nonimmunological or mixed asthma, factors precipitating the exacerbation of symptoms may be obscure. However, identification of causative or aggravating factors is still imperative in order to avoid or decrease the incidence of asthma attacks.

There is perhaps no disease in which knowing the patient well is more important than in asthma. Because sensitivity tests can be performed with only a very small fraction of the substances with which the patient is in contact, the doctor usually makes the diagnosis on the basis of a careful history. Knowing about the person's life-style such as the type of work, leisure-time activities, and even food preferences may give useful clues as to what precipitates the asthmatic attack. Nursing strategies for identifying causes are included in Box 16-29.

It is imperative to understand that even though psychological factors may precipitate an attack, the response to it is physiological and requires the same treatment as that prescribed for an attack precipitated by an allergen or any other factor.

Pathophysiology

An asthmatic attack results from several physiological alterations, including altered immunological response, increased airway resistance, increased lung compliance, impaired mucociliary function, and altered oxygen-carbon dioxide exchange. Each of these alterations is discussed below.

Altered immunological response

No matter what the precipitating factors are, the basis of asthma appears to be genetic or immunological factors. The basis of nonimmunological asthma is less well understood than is immunological asthma.

Immunological asthma is the result of an antigen-antibody reaction in which chemical mediators are released. The chemical mediators, which include histamine, slow-releasing substance of anaphylaxis (SRS-A), eosinophilic chemotactic factor of anaphylaxis (ECF-A), and perhaps others, cause three main reactions: (1) constriction of smooth muscles of both the large and small airways, resulting in bronchospasm; (2) increased capillary permeability that results in mucosal oedema and further narrows the airways; and (3) increased mucous gland secretion and increased mucus production. As a result, the person with an asthmatic attack struggles to breathe through a narrowed airway that is in spasm. Because breathing is laboured, the person breathes through the mouth, which dries the mucus and further occludes the airway.

Common factors triggering an asthmatic attack are presented in Box 16-30. Although allergic mechanisms are important in the pathogenesis of asthma, the many nonimmunological precipitating factors indicate that other pathophysiological processes, such as parasympathetic and sympathetic nervous system reactivity, are active in the onset of asthma. *Hypoxaemia, hypercapnia, and overuse of bronchodilators may lead to an acute asthma attack.*

Increased airway resistance

Increased airway resistance results from bronchial smooth muscle spasm, mucosal inflammation, and hypersecretion of mucus. These airway changes cause obstruction to airflow both in and out of the lungs.

Nursing Care Plan

People with COPD

DATA: Mrs D. is a 54-year-old housewife with a past medical history of severe chronic obstructive pulmonary disease with cor pulmonale. She has a 75-packet-a-year history of cigarette smoking and stopped smoking 2 years ago (husband still smokes). Patient states "I am unable to walk back from the bathroom to the living room without a 30- to 60-minute rest". Lung sounds are diminished throughout. Chest x-ray indicates overinflation of the lungs. Pulmonary function tests show severe obstructive ventilatory dysfunction with hyperinflation. Arterial blood gases are: pH = 7.34, $Paco_2$ = 6.4 kPa (48 mm Hg), Pao_2 = 9.2 kPa (69 mm Hg), oxygen saturation = 94%. Current medications include salbutamol inhaler, theophylline, terbutaline, hydrochlorothiazide, potassium and glyceryl trinitrate sublingual tablets as needed for chest pain. She is attending outpatient rehabilitation, including muscle reconditioning and education.

The nursing history identified the following:
- Mrs. D. continues to be exposed to cigarette smoke because of her husband's continued cigarette smoking. Patient stated, "He's never without a cigarette in the house."
- Mrs. D. indicated that her husband's smoking makes it hard for her not to smoke. Patient indicated that she occasionally had a cigarette.
- Mrs. D. is fearful of becoming a "bedridden invalid like my mother." Patient's mother had COPD and in her last years had a cerebrovascular accident, which left her totally dependent on her daughter for care until her death 5 years ago.

Collaborative nursing activities include those to assess (1) Mrs. D.'s current pulmonary function status, (2) establish individualized rehabilitation, and (3) evaluate current theophylline levels. Nursing actions include the following:
- Prepare patient for pulmonary function testing. Explain her role in the testing procedure and describe what she might expect to feel during testing.
- Participate in rehabilitation team meetings for planning Mrs. D.'s programme. Encourage Mrs. D. to actively participate in the planning process to establish realistic individualized programme gaols. Elicit feedback to assess her understanding of the programme activities and goals.
- Assess theophylline blood levels and presence of any medication side effects.

Nursing analysis: Activity tolerance, related to tissue hypoxia associated with impaired gas exchange/fatigue

Expected patient outcomes	Nursing interventions	Rationale
Mrs. D. demonstrates increased tolerance for activity	Provide frequent rest periods Instruct patient in energy-saving techniques Reinforce use of pursed lip breathing Gradually increase activity	Improve activity tolerance

Nursing analysis: Gas exchange, impaired, related to decrease in effective lung surface for diffusion

Expected patient outcomes	Nursing interventions	Rationale
Mrs. D.'s dyspnoea is decreased	Assess respiratory status	Obtain baseline information
	Provide low concentration oxygen as prescribed	Many people with COPD depend on hypoxaemia as stimulus to breathe
	Provide breathing training	Decreased work of breathing
	Provide rest periods	Improve tolerance

Nursing analysis: Infection, high risk for, related to increased secretions, decreased motility in lungs

Expected patient outcomes	Nursing interventions	Rationale
Mrs. D.'s infections are minimized	Restrict people with upper respiratory infections	Decrease exposure
	Teach Mrs. D. measures to prevent infections	
	Encourage Mrs. D. to have annual influenza immunization	

Nursing analysis: Self-esteem disturbance, related to changes in life-style, dependence on others

Expected patient outcomes	Nursing interventions	Rationale
Mrs. D. participates in necessary activities	Give Mrs. D. opportunities to express concerns about limitations.	Allow for communication
	Provide rationale for necessary activities	Maintain sense of control.
	Discuss with family and friends the need for patient to maintain role relationships	Increase self-esteem
	Assist patient to identify personal strengths	
	Provide information about community resources.	

Nursing analysis: Knowledge deficit, related to lack of exposure/lack of recall

Expected patient outcomes	Nursing interventions	Rationale
Mrs. D. describes therapeutic regimen and health maintenance	Teach Mrs. D.	Increase self-care abilities and self-esteem
	1. Nature of COPD and need to follow prescribed therapy and activities	
	2. Home medication and treatment plans	
	3. Home exercise plan	
	4. Avoidance of respiratory irritants and infections	
	5. Signs requiring medical attention	
	6. Professional and community resources	

Identifying factors precipitating asthma

1. Be alert for casual comments about daily activities the patient might consider insignificant.
2. Encourage patient to keep a symptom diary. Ask patient to perform the following tasks.
   a. Use a small notebook that can be carried at all times.
   b. Record everything that occurred and was present during 24 hours before and during the onset of the attack.
      When the attack began: What were you doing? Where were you? Who or what else was present? What was the weather like?
   c. Note the time and date that the attack occurred.
3. Write down what you think caused the symptoms to occur, even if it is a guess.
4. Observe patient's interaction with others and reaction to stressors that might aggravate and/or precipitate an attack.

Common factors triggering an asthmatic attack

Environmental factors
   Change in temperature, especially cold air
   Change in humidity—dry air
Atmospheric pollutants
   Cigarette and industrial smoke, ozone, sulphur dioxide, formaldehyde
Strong odours—perfume
Allergens
   Feathers, animal dander, dust mites, moulds, allergens; foods treated with sulphites (beer, wine, fruit juices, snack foods, salads, potatoes, shellfish, and fresh and dried fruits)
Exercise
Stress or emotional upset
Medications
   Aspirin and nonsteroidal antiinflammatory drugs (NSAIDs), beta-blockers (including eye drops), cholinergic drugs (to promote bladder contraction and as eyedrops for glaucoma)
   Enzymes—including those in laundry detergents
   Chemicals—toluene and others used in solvents, paints, rubber, and plastics

Increased lung compliance

The lungs become hyperinflated during an acute asthmatic attack as a result of air that becomes trapped in the distal airspaces. During the acute attack the person with asthma demonstrates the same symptoms of increased lung compliance that are observed in the patient with emphysema.

Impaired mucociliary function

Hypertrophy of mucus-secreting glands, thickened mucus, and slowed ciliary movement are common findings in people with asthma. During an asthma attack, increased mucus production combined with slowed clearance of mucus due to decreased ciliary movement results in *increased water loss from mucus*. Thus, the *mucus becomes increasingly viscous* and *can ultimately result in the development of mucous plugs, which may block airways*.

Altered oxygen-carbon dioxide exchange

Increased airway resistance and hyperinflation cause the respiratory muscles to work harder, resulting in muscle fatigue and ultimately exhaustion. In mild or short-term asthmatic attacks, the individual compensates with an increased respiratory rate, which results in respiratory alkalosis. Mild hypoxaemia from altered ventilation-perfusion ratios usually accompanies the alkalosis.

In a severe or prolonged attack, if the increased work of breathing cannot be relieved, respiratory muscle exhaustion will result in hypoventilation, which in turn causes respiratory acidosis and severe hypoxaemia. If the process cannot be reversed, the person may die.

Clinical Manifestations

The signs and symptoms associated with asthma are correlated with normal lung functions, and underlying pathophysiological origins (see Table 16-19). *The character of asthmatic attacks can vary on a continuum from chronic or acute mild intermittent attacks to life-threatening status asthmaticus.*

With chronic mild asthma, symptoms are not noticeable when the person is at rest. However, *after exertion such as laughing, singing, vigorous exercise, or emotional excitement, dyspnoea and wheezing develop rapidly*. These attacks are controlled with medications, and patients usually can continue their mode of living with a few modifications and no serious lung changes. They are not hospitalized, but they sometimes come to outpatient clinics for medical supervision.

Acute asthmatic attacks often occur at night. The person awakens with a sensation of choking caused by the mucosal inflammation and hypersecretion of mucus. Bronchospasm, with resultant increased airway resistance, causes audible *expiratory* and *inspiratory wheezing. During the acute attack patients appear to be in acute respiratory distress and typically demonstrate tachypnoea, accessory muscle breathing, and nasal flaring. They appear to be apprehensive and diaphoretic, and their attention is totally focused on their breathing.* If the treatment is successful, the attack usually ends with the coughing up of large quantities of thick, tenacious sputum. Most attacks subside in 30 minutes to 1 hour, although repeated asthmatic attacks associated with infection may continue for days or weeks. The person is usually exhausted and should rest quietly after the attack.

People who are severely affected by asthma and who have attacks that are difficult to control with the usual medications may develop *status asthmaticus*. In this case, the symptoms of an acute attack continue *despite measures to relieve them. Air trapping in the distal airspaces ultimately leads to respiratory muscle exhaustion and severe ventilation-perfusion abnormalities with resultant respiratory failure and hypoxaemia.*

Patients with *status asthmaticus* often demonstrate respiratory distress so severe that they are unable to talk. They may be moving minimal air in and out of the lungs; thus audible wheezing and adventitious lung sounds may *not* be present. *During this phase of the attack the patient will appear cyanotic and may demonstrate both pulsus paradoxis and sensorium changes.* This is a medical emergency and the patient requires immediate therapy. Most patients arrive in the accident and emergency department where treatment is begun. The patient remains in the emergency department until his or her condition is stabilized. Most patients are then admitted to the hospital for ongoing therapy and observation.

Repeated attacks of status asthmaticus may cause irreversible emphysema, resulting in a permanent decrease in total breathing capacity.

Pulmonary function studies characteristic of asthma show reduction in FEV_1 to less than 25% of predicted. The FEV is usually markedly reduced in proportion to the FVC, although the FVC may also be decreased. Improved flow rates after administration of bronchodilators indicating reversible bronchospasm is a characteristic finding with asthma.

The results of arterial blood gas studies can vary from respiratory alkalosis with mild hypoxaemia to severe respiratory acidosis with profound hypoxaemia, depending on the severity and duration of the asthmatic attack.

Medical Management

The objectives of medical management of asthma are to promote normal functioning of the individual, to prevent recurrent symptoms, prevent severe attacks, and prevent side effects from medication. The chief aim of various medications is to afford the patient immediate, progressive, ongoing bronchial relaxation. One approach is presented in Table 16-23.

Maintenance Therapy

Concern has been raised recently that many patients may be undertreated and that this may have contributed to the increase in death rates.[54]

As a result, more consideration is being given to the role of inflammation as the fundamental process in asthma. Thus, inhaled steroids along with inhaled beta$_2$-adrenergic agents are being ordered more frequently. The use of inhaled steroids ensures that the drugs reach deeper into the lung and do not cause the side effects associated with oral steroids.[54]

It is recommended that the inhaled beta$_2$-agonist must be given first to open the airway and then the inhaled steroid will be more beneficial.

In one study, patients were given peak-flow meters and taught how to use them. If their peak expiratory flow-rate (PEFR) was below 70% of normal, inhaled medication was increased; if below 50%, oral steroids were added; below 30%, emergency measures were called for and the patient called the doctor and went to the emergency department for treatment with oxygen and additional drug therapy.

In the United Kingdom the use of peak-flow meter regimen was compared with a programme based on symptoms alone. Patients were taught what to do if their breathing felt tighter, if they awoke at night with wheezing, if the inhaled bronchodilator lasted less than 2 hours or if relief lasted only 30 minutes, or if they had difficult talking. The study found that the daily use of peak-flow meters made no significant contribution. The important thing was that patients had a systematic way to evaluate their symptoms and knew what to do when they occurred. Peak flow meters are available on prescription and their use is encouraged to detect early signs of deterioration.

Table 16-23 Treatment of an acute asthmatic attack[68]

Therapy	Effects and precautions
Inhaled beta-agonist such as salbutamol or terbutaline in normal saline	Stimulates beta$_2$ receptors in bronchial smooth muscle = relaxation. Starts to act in 10 min, effects last 4-6 hours. Monitor vital signs, lung sounds, and peak expiration flow rate (PEFR) before and after each treatment
If above is not successful Methylprednisolone intravenously. Loading dose 2 mg/kg or about 125 mg every 6 hr then 60-125 mg every 6 hr for 48 hr total or until patient stable. When patient is *stabilized*, change IV to 60 mg prednisolone daily or every other day. Nebulized atropine sulphate may be tried or aminophylline may be given intravenously—a pump is used for better control of infusion. Loading dose of aminophylline 4 to 6 mg/kg over 15 to 30 min and then continuous infusion of 0.45 to 0.70 mg/kg/hr. Patients who have been on aminophylline at home will be placed on continuous IV therapy. Rate of infusion is determined by theophylline blood level. Desired level is 10 to 20 µg/ml.	Reduces inflammation and oedema of airway and decreases hyperactivity of airway. Benefit seen within 6 hours—full effect in 6-8 hours. Oral prednisolone should be tapered off by 7-10 days. Taper 60 mg × 2 days, 40 mg × 2 days, 30 mg × 2 days, and 10 mg × 2 days. Relax bronchial smooth muscle. *Too rapid an infusion may cause severe hypotension, premature ventricular contractions, and cardiac arrest.* Monitor heart rate and rhythm closely and report any changes immediately. Theophylline metabolized by the liver. For people with liver disease, smaller doses are used. Patients taking cimeidine, erythromycin, or ciprofloxacin require smaller doses. Smokers and those taking phenytoin require larger doses to maintain blood levels.

Nursing Process

Assessment

Subjective data

1. History of asthma onset and duration
2. Precipitating factors
3. Current medications
4. Medications used to relieve asthma symptoms
5. Any recent changes in medication regimen
6. Self-care methods used to relieve symptoms

Objective data

1. Assess general appearance.
   a. Does patient appear apprehensive?
   b. Is there any evidence of altered sensorium?
2. Assess vital signs.
   a. Tachycardia
   b. Pulsus paradoxus (diminished pulse with inspiration, confirmed by a 6 to 8 mm Hg drop in systolic blood pressure during inspiration)
   c. Tachypnoea
3. Pulmonary examination by doctor
   a. Inspection
      (1) Accessory muscle breathing
      (2) Forward leaning posture
      (3) Dyspnoea
      (4) Prolonged expiration
      (5) Cyanosis
   b. Palpation
      (1) Decreased lateral expansion
      (2) Decreased fremitus
   c. Percussion
      (1) Hyperresonance
      (2) Decreased diaphragmatic excursion
   d. Auscultation (Note: as *patient approaches exhaustion from increased work of breathing, breath sounds and adventitious sounds may be absent or faint*)
      (1) Inspiratory and expiratory wheezing
      (2) Rhonchi
4. Assess laboratory findings
   a. Arterial blood gases
      (1) Short-term or moderate attack—respiratory alkalosis with mild hypoxaemia
      (2) Prolonged or severe attack—respiratory acidosis with severe hypoxaemia
   b. Sputum—for eosinophilia
   c. Pulmonary function testing—decreased FEV and VC

Nursing analysis

Problems are determined from analysis of patient data. Possible problems for the person with asthma may include, but are not limited to, the following:

Problems	Possible aetiologies
Airway clearance ineffective	Ineffective technique, decreased energy/fatigue, impaired muco-ciliary clearance mechanism, inadequate fluid intake
Anxiety	Threat of unknown or death
Breathing pattern, ineffective	Bronchoconstriction, underuse of bronchodilator medications
Gas exchange, impaired	Mucus plugs, ventilation/perfusion imbalance
Knowledge deficit of predisposing factors and prevention/ treatment	Lack of exposure to information, unreceptiveness to information, unfamiliarity with information sources

Planning: expected patient outcomes

Expected outcomes for the person with asthma may include, but are not limited to, the following:
The patient will:

1. Demonstrate effective airway clearance
   a. Effective methods of coughing
   b. Appropriate use of medication and equipment
2. Demonstrate activities to control anxiety response to symptoms
   a. Muscle relaxation
   b. Meditation
   c. Appropriate use of medications
3. Demonstrate effective breathing patterns
   a. Inspiratory to expiratory ratio = 5 seconds: 10 seconds
   b. Respiratory rate within near-normal limits
4. Demonstrate improved ventilation and oxygenation
   a. Arterial blood pH and $Paco_2$ that returns or stays within acceptable limits
   b. Pao_2 at optimal level for individual
5. Patient or significant other can state the factors most likely to precipitate an asthmatic attack (for example, stress, allergens, and infections).
6. Patient or significant other can state the importance of keeping a diary of symptoms and medications (time and dose) during an asthmatic attack.
7. If the cause is allergic, state how to prepare an environmentally controlled bedroom (Chapter 33).
8. Patient or significant other can explain any home medication programme.
   a. Give name, dose, action, and side effects of each medication.
   b. State conditions under which medications might be increased (for example, infection—start or increase antibiotics; increased stress or worsening of symptoms—increase corticosteroids).
9. Patient or significant other can demonstrate how to take inhaled medications.
10. Patient or significant other can describe what to do when an acute attack occurs (for example, take medication and be quiet).
11. Patient or significant other can state signs and symptoms that indicate need for immediate medical attention (for example, asthmatic attack unrelieved by usual treatment).
12. If receiving corticosteroid therapy, patient can show card to be carried at all times giving data about the drug, dose, and name of doctor; alternative is to wear Medic-Alert bracelet.
13. Patient can state plans for ongoing follow-up care including plans for desensitization if appropriate.

Implementation

Assisting with achievement of therapeutic goals
Medications

1. Given medications as ordered. Monitor IV rates closely.
2. Monitor patient closely for side effects of medications (Table 16-24).

Interventions to achieve patient outcomes
Improving airway clearance

During an asthmatic attack secretions tend to become sticky and can plug airways, causing increased airway obstruction. By mobilizing secretions, the need for intubation and artificial ventilation can often be prevented.

1. Ensure adequate systemic fluid intake (Note: Research findings suggest that overhydration may not increase secretion clearance above levels obtained by normal hydration levels)
2. Provide adequate nutritional levels
3. Provide extra humidity
4. Medicate with bronchodilators
5. Teach effective cough manoeuvre
6. If cough ineffective to produce sputum, administer chest physiotherapy.

Providing emotional support and pre-venting anxiety

1. Do not leave patient alone during an attack
2. Encourage relaxation techniques
3. Guide/assist patient with respiratory manoeuvres
4. Assess for possible medication overuse or underuse

Improving breathing patterns

The nursing role in improving breathing patterns and gas exchange is as follows:

1. Place patient in upright position
2. Encourage slow rhythmic breathing
3. Encourage patient to breathe through nose and exhale through pursed lips
4. Administer bronchodilator and an antiinflammatory medication (corticosteroid) as ordered. Monitor patient for both therapeutic response and side effects to medications. Table 16-24 lists medications, dosage, action, and side effects of medications commonly used to treat asthma.

Improving gas exchange

Arterial blood gas results should be monitored as follows:

1. If respiratory alkalosis is present, encourage slower breathing

Table 16-24 Medications used in treatment of asthma

Medications	Dosage	Action	Side effects
Adrenaline 1 : 1000	0.3 to 0.5 ml subcutaneously, may need to repeat 2-3 times at 20-30 min intervals	Short-acting bronchodilator	Tachycardia Palpitations Elevated blood pressure
Ephedrine	25-50 mg PO q 4-6 hr	Long-acting bronchodilator	Cerebral agitation (often given with phenobarbitone)
Terbutaline	2.5 mg PO	Bronchodilator	Tachycardia Tremors Headache Spasms in extremities
Isoprenaline	1-2 inhalations, q 3 hr (max. 8 day)	Bronchodilator	Headache Tremors
Orciprenaline	20 mg PO tid or 1-2 inhalations	Bronchodilator	Tachycardia Tremors Nausea
Sodium cromoglycate	20 mg qid inhaled	Antiasthmatic mast cell stabilizer used as prophylactic against asthma attacks	Nasal congestion Nausea Bronchospasm
Corticosteroids Hydrocortisone	200-400 mg IV (up to 1 g first 24 hr) PO or IV	Antiinflammatory	Corticosteroid withdrawal syndrome, sodium retention, GI disturbance
Dexamethasone	Varies with individual response and disease severity		
Beclomethasone	Inhaled: 100 µg 3-4 times/day		
Theophylline	Dosage to maintain serum concentrations between 10-20 µg/ml	Bronchodilator	Nausea and vomiting CNS irritability Tachycardia Hypotension

2. If respiratory acidosis and hypoxaemia are present
   a. Administer O_2 as prescribed
   b. If O_2 does not relieve the attack, intubation and ventilatory assistance may be required

Facilitating learning

After the patient has recovered from an acute attack, the patient's knowledge about asthma is assessed, and the following points are stressed.

1. Keep a symptom diary to help identify:
   a. Possible precipitating factors
   b. Symptom patterns
   c. Efficacy of self-treatment modalities (include time and dose of any medications self-administered)
2. Signs and symptoms
   a. Tightness in chest
   b. Restlessness or vague feeling of uneasiness
   c. Dyspnoea
   d. Increased wheezing
   e. Productive cough
3. Self-treatment of signs and symptoms
   a. Take bronchodilator as ordered.
   b. Take adrenaline if prescribed by doctor.
   c. State conditions under which medication might be increased (infection—start or increase antibiotics; increased stress or worsening of symptoms—increase inhaled corticosteroid)
   d. If another person is not present, call someone so patient will not be alone.
   e. Try to remain calm and breathe slowly; use relaxation techniques at first sign of attack
   f. If symptoms are not relieved, call doctor or go to nearest accident and emergency facility.
4. Know how to use special equipment (metered dose inhaler [Box 16-31], inhaler with spacer [Box 16-24], nebulizer [Box 16-25], and peak flow meter if one is prescribed).

Evaluation

Evaluation is based on patient outcomes. Questions to consider may include the following:

1. Can the patient demonstrate ways to maintain a clear airway?

16-31

Correct way to use a metered-dose inhaler

1. Inhale through nose, then slowly breathe out completely.
2. Place mouthpiece in mouth.
3. Press down on inhaler, while simultaneously inhaling one puff deeply. Breathe in air from around the mouthpiece while inhaling.
4. Hold breath for a few seconds, then exhale.
5. Repeat second puff if one is ordered.

Caution: Some people with asthma may experience bronchoconstriction after using a metered-dose inhaler. Patients who complain of chest tightness after using a metered-dose inhaler may be reacting to the propellant.

---

2. Can the patient demonstrate muscle relaxation and meditation exercises used to control anxiety?
3. Does the patient demonstrate a respiratory rate that is within near-normal limits?
4. Are the patient's arterial blood gas findings at acceptable levels?
5. Can the patient state factors that need to be avoided to prevent an asthmatic attack?
6. Does the patient have a symptom diary so that he or she can record time of regular medications and the onset of symptoms?
7. Can the patient discuss what he or she has done to prepare an environmentally controlled bedroom?
8. Can the patient state the purpose, dosage, and side effects of each prescribed medication?
9. Can the patient state conditions under which medication might be increased or changed? Infection—start or increase antibiotics; increased stress—increase dose of inhaled corticosteroid.
10. Can the patient state what to do if usual therapy does not improve symptoms (call doctor or go to an accident and emergency facility, preferably one where the patient and his or history and treatment are known).
11. Does the patient carry a card stating drugs, doses, and name of doctor or does the patient wear a Medic-Alert bracelet?
12. Can the patient state time of next medical appointment?

CYSTIC FIBROSIS

Aetiology/Epidemiology

Cystic fibrosis (CF) continues to be the most common lethal genetic disease among whites but is rare in Asian and black people. It is an autosomal recessive disease, and one in 20 to 25 individuals carries the CF gene. When both parents are carriers (heterozygotes), there is a one in four chance with each pregnancy that their child will have CF (Fig. 16-19).

In the United Kingdom CF occurs in about 1 in 2000 live births. Over recent years the number of adults with CF has increased steadily because of increased life expectancy and diagnostic advances.

Reaching adulthood is now a realistic expectation for infants and children with CF. The average life expectancy is 24 years with a maximum survival of 30 to 40 years. The major contributing factors to this increased life expectancy include diagnostic advances and therapeutic interventions.

Prevention

Because CF is a genetically inherited disease, identification of carriers who may pass on the defect and disease to offspring remains the most important preventive strategy. Early identification of carriers combined with genetic counselling minimizes the chance of offspring inheriting this lethal genetic disease. Family histories of possible incidences of CF should be followed up by genetic testing.

Inheritance possibilities

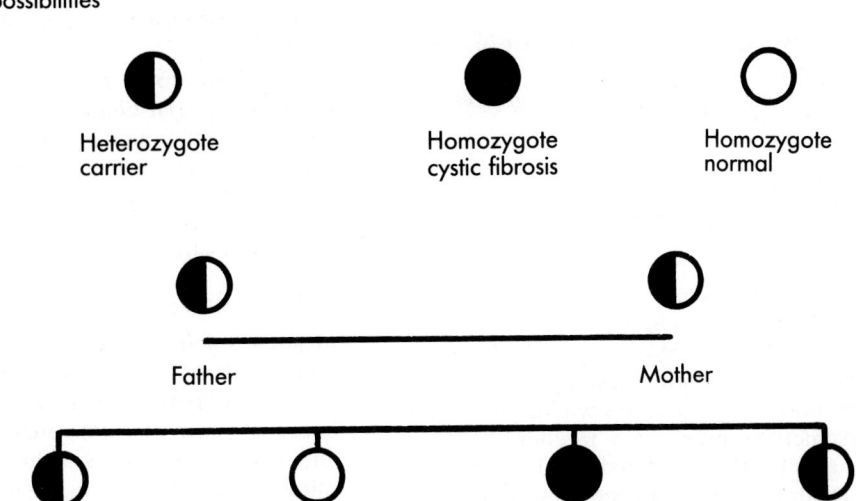

Fig. 16-19   Inheritance of cystic fibrosis when both mother and father are carriers of cystic fibrosis gene (Modified from CF Foundation Fact Sheet, 1980, Bethesda, Maryland).

Pathophysiology

Cystic fibrosis is an exocrine gland disease involving various systems (pulmonary, pancreatic/hepatic, gastrointestinal, and reproductive). Obstruction of the exocrine gland ducts or passageways occurs in nearly all adult patients with CF.[128] Exocrine gland secretions are known to have a decreased water content, altered electrolyte concentration, and abnormal organic constituents (especially mucus glycoproteins); yet the specific biochemical or physiological defect that leads to obstruction is not known.

The following physiological alterations are found in adults with CF.

1. Pulmonary damage. Mucus obstruction, inflammation, oedema, and smooth muscle restriction of airways are found in this chronic obstructive pulmonary disease. Changes in the airways predispose the person to respiratory infection, which can be life-threatening. Frequent, recurrent pulmonary infections erode blood vessels. Brachial arteries branching from the aorta and the lung at high pressures are most at risk for bleeding (haemoptysis).

   Other complications of damage to the airways include *pneumothorax, respiratory insufficiency,* and *cor pulmonale.* These complications account for 95% of the deaths in adults with CF.

2. Gastrointestinal and pancreatic involvement. Intestinal obstruction occurs in 20% of adult patients with CF. Generally, pancreatic insufficiency predisposes to intestinal obstruction. Cramps and abdominal pain in adults with CF should arouse suspicion of intestinal obstruction. Pancreatic insufficiency is reported in 80% to 90% of adults with CF. The pathological lesions in the pancreas decrease pancreatic enzyme production and lead to malabsorption of fat.

3. Glucose intolerance. About 40% of adults with CF have glucose intolerance caused by obstruction of islets of Langerhans by pancreatic fibrosis.[128]

Clinical Manifestations

Three major clinical symptoms are associated with CF: *recurrent respiratory infections, malnutrition,* and *excessive salt losses.* Early identification of CF often rests on the presence of several otherwise unexplained clinical symptoms. In infants, clinical symptoms of CF may include meconium ileus and failure to thrive. Excessive salt losses in infants may first be detected by the infant's mother who reports that the child tastes salty when kissed. Older children should be suspected of having CF when *recurrent respiratory infections* and *failure to thrive despite large appetites cannot otherwise be explained. Excessive salt losses* in older children and young adults with CF may be manifested by *heat exhaustion after exercise or exposure to hot weather,* or *dehydration after fevers.* In young adults, the *only* clinical manifestation of CF may be *infertility.*

Specific clinical manifestations by system are listed below. *Pulmonary signs and symptoms of CF include:*

1. Chronic productive cough and/or recurrent bronchitis or pneumonia
2. Rales and rhonchi, decreased pulmonary compliance, digital clubbing
3. Shortness of breath and dyspnoea on exertion, wheezing, and weight loss occur with respiratory complications and usually indicate need for vigorous therapy

Gastrointestinal signs and symptoms include:

1. Frequent, bulky, greasy stools
2. Weight loss
3. Cramps and abdominal pain—should make one suspect an obstruction is present

Glucose intolerance signs and symptoms include:
1. Polyuria, polydipsia, and polyphagia
2. Absence of ketoacidosis even with above signs

Diagnostic Tests

The diagnosis of CF is confirmed by the presence of *at least two* of the *following:*
1. A positive sweat test with a chloride level greater than 60 mmol/L (60 mEq/L)
2. COPD
3. Exocrine pancreatic insufficiency
4. A positive family history of CF

Medical Management

The goals of medical management of CF are to *minimize bronchial plugging and to inhibit bacterial colonization.*[111]
Measures to minimize bronchial plugging include:
1. Chest physiotherapy with chest percussion and postural drainage for 20 minutes two to three times daily and sometimes much more frequently.
2. Mucolytic agents may be ordered to thin secretions, although ensuring that the patient is well hydrated may be sufficient to thin secretions.
3. Humidification of air is controversial because it has been associated with bronchospasm and bacterial colonization. It may be helpful for some patients, however, and some doctors may prescribe it.

To minimize bacterial colonization during acute phases of the disease, sputum should be cultured and tested for sensitivity. Antibiotics are prescribed based on the results of these tests. Combination therapy with two or three antibiotics is recommended to prevent bacterial resistance and is usually prescribed for 14 days. *Shorter courses of antibiotic therapy are associated with reexacerbation of symptoms.* Oral antibiotics may be prescribed for long-term therapy to inhibit bacterial colonization, although there is little scientific basis for this practice. *Inhaled antibiotics are given in very high doses because only about 10% of the inhaled drug is absorbed.*

Respiratory Failure

Patients with CF eventually succumb to progressive respiratory and cardiac failure. Because these patients have a fatal disease they usually have "do not resuscitate" orders and are not intubated or placed on mechanical ventilation. The patient and family have to be involved in this decision, and nurses play an important role in supporting the patient and family in their decision. The median age of death of adults with CF is 22 for women and 28 for men.

Research

There is considerable ongoing research on CF. The indentification of the CF gene, in 1989, was a major breakthrough and has raised hopes for future progress in preventing and treating CF.

RESPIRATORY INSUFFICIENCY AND RESPIRATORY FAILURE

Aetiology/Epidemiology

The term *respiratory insufficiency* is usually used to indicate that the exchange of oxygen and carbon dioxide is not adequate to meet the needs of the body during normal activities. *Respiratory failure* is said to occur when ventilation is not sufficient to achieve adequate gas exchange even at rest. Many disorders can lead to or are associated with both respiratory insufficiency and failure; these are listed in Table 16-25.

The diagnosis of respiratory insufficiency or failure is based on arterial blood gas studies, pulmonary function testing, and the clinical status of the patient. The criteria listed in Box 16-30 are generally used in defining a state of failure. However, it cannot be overemphasized that these parameters are only *guidelines* and must be applied in light of the individual's history, age, and overall condition.

Pathophysiology and Clinical Picture

Regardless of the underlying condition, the resultant events or processes that occur in respiratory failure are the same. With inadequate ventilation, the arterial Po_2 falls and tissue cells become hypoxic. The Pco_2 increases, leading to a fall in pH, and the patient becomes acidotic. The nurse must keep in mind while working with the patient with COPD who has developed respiratory failure that this patient normally exists in a compensated state with decreased Pao_2 levels and elevated $Paco_2$ levels. Thus the parameters in Box 16-30 are not applicable; the pH level, however, is a useful guide in assessing the degree of insufficiency. When the pH begins to fall below 7.3, it is an indication that the patient is no longer able to compensate for the elevated $Paco_2$ level.

Respiratory insufficiency and failure can result from a worsening in the condition of the patient with any of the disorders already mentioned.

Interventions

Intervention for the patient who has respiratory insufficiency or failure always begins with a recognition of the underlying disease state or cause of the disturbance in ventilation. Therapy is first directed at improving the underlying condition, such as sepsis, or by removing the cause, such as fluid overload.

The goals of intervention are to improve oxygenation and ventilation to restore the person's Pao_2 and $Paco_2$ to their previous levels. The initial medical management can often be conservative if the diagnosis is made early enough.

Oxygen

Particular care is needed in working with the patient who has chronic lung disease. As mentioned earlier, *individuals with COPD normally are CO_2 retainers and exist with elevated $Paco_2$ levels and have lost the usual respiratory drive, carbon dioxide stimulation.* They no longer respond to increased carbon dioxide levels by increasing their rate and depth of respiration; rather, the elevated $Paco_2$ depresses the respiratory centre. Their respiratory drive is now derived from their low Pao_2 levels; therefore, even though these people lack oxygen, it is extremely dangerous to raise their Pao_2 to normal levels. If the arterial Po_2 is normal and there is retention of carbon dioxide (*hypercapnia*), the person will have no respiratory drive. Hypoventilation becomes more severe and $Paco_2$ continues to rise. This situation results in *carbon dioxide narcosis*, a markedly elevated carbon dioxide level that causes coma or semicoma. People with COPD are, therefore, treated with low-flow

Table 16-25 Dissorders associated with respiratory insufficiency and failure

Pulmonary disorders	Nonpulmonary disorders
Severe infection	CNS disturbance secondary to drug overdose, anaesthesia, head injury
Pulmonary oedema	Neuromuscular disorders (for example, Guillain-Barré syndrome, myasthenia
Pulmonary embolus	gravis, multiple sclerosis, poliomyelitis, muscular dystrophy, spinal cord
COPD	injury)
Adult respiratory distress syndrome (ARDS)	Postoperative reduction in ventilation following thoracic or abdominal surgery
Cancer	Prolonged mechanical ventilation
Chest trauma	
Severe atelectasis	
Airway compromise secondary to trauma, infection, or surgery	

16-30

Criteria for diagnosis of respiratory failure

Pa_{O_2}	<8 kPa (60 mm Hg) when breathing room air
Pa_{CO_2}	>6.6 kPa (50 mm Hg)
Vital capacity	<15 ml/kg
Respiratory rate	>30/min or below 8/min

or controlled-flow oxygen; that is, inspired oxygen concentrations of 24% to 30%. These concentrations can easily be obtained by using a Ventimask (Fig. 16-20) or a two-pronged nasal cannula with a 1 to 2 L oxygen flow. This amount of oxygen can significantly increase the amount of oxygen carried by haemoglobin without a significant increase in arterial Po_2; therefore, the patient's blood carries much more oxygen even though hypoxaemia is still present. The person continues to have respiratory drive, and the Pa_{CO_2} does not rise.

By the use of low-flow concentration oxygen, the amount of oxygen carried in the patient's blood can often be increased enough to maintain basic body functions without further reduction of ventilation. People who do not have COPD, who have a normal Pa_{CO_2}, but who are hypoxic are usually able to tolerate high flow rates of oxygen (5 to 10 L/min). Oxygen is an integral part of the therapy of patients with respiratory insufficiency and failure; however, some hazards are associated with prolonged use.

Oxygen toxicity is the term used to describe the damage to lung tissue that results from prolonged exposure to high concentrations of oxygen. Although the exact effects of oxygen in any one individual may depend on the person's underlying pathological condition, it is believed that exposure to greater than 60% oxygen for a period of more than 36 hours, or exposure to 100% oxygen for a period of more than 6 hours, results in atelectasis and alveolar collapse. Breathing very high concentrations of oxygen (80% to 100%) for prolonged periods (24 hours or more) is often associated with the development of ARDS (p. 315). Thus it is a firm general principle that the lowest amount of oxygen that will achieve an acceptable Po_2 is the amount that should be given.

Airway management

In addition to providing supplemental oxygen, care of the people with respiratory insufficiency usually includes aggressive airway management and attempts to improve ventilation. Suctioning, IPPB, ultrasonic mist therapy, and postural drainage with clapping and vibrating are all employed in an attempt to halt the progression of insufficiency. When the patient develops respiratory failure and can no longer maintain his or her own respirations, an artificial airway is necessary.

Types of artificial airways

An endotracheal tube is usually chosen initially as a means of providing an airway; tracheostomy is only performed if airway maintenance is necessary for a prolonged period of time or if trauma to the airway prevents the use of an endotracheal tube. Although a tracheostomy has the *disadvantage* of a higher risk of infection, it is often elected for long-term airway management because it is *much more comfortable than an endotracheal tube and allows the person to eat.*

In endotracheal intubation a tube is passed through either the nose or mouth into the trachea; in a tracheostomy an artificial opening is made in the trachea into which a tube is inserted (Fig. 16-21). These procedures are used (1) to establish and maintain a patent airway, (2) to prevent aspiration by sealing off the trachea from the digestive tract in the unconscious or paralyzed person, (3) to permit removal of tracheobronchial secretions in the person who cannot cough adequately, and (4) to treat the patient who requires positive pressure ventilation that cannot be given effectively by mask. Whether an intubation or a tracheostomy is performed initially depends on the facilities available and the preference of the doctor. Most doctors now consider it safer to do an emergency endotracheal intubation and then perform a tracheostomy as a nonemergency procedure in the operating theatre if prolonged support of the airway is needed. In this instance the endotracheal tube is not removed until after the tracheostomy opening is made.

A tracheostomy is necessary when an endotracheal tube cannot be inserted or when it is contraindicated, as in severe burns or laryngeal obstruction caused by tumour, infection, or vocal cord paralysis. Tracheostomy may also be required when a patient is conscious and cannot tolerate an endotracheal tube. Once the airway is secured either by intubation or by tracheostomy, secretions are aspirated and well-humidified oxygen is usually given. If the patient is unable to sustain respiration, a mechanical ventilator is attached to the endotracheal tube or the tracheostomy tube. When mechanical ventilation is required, a cuffed

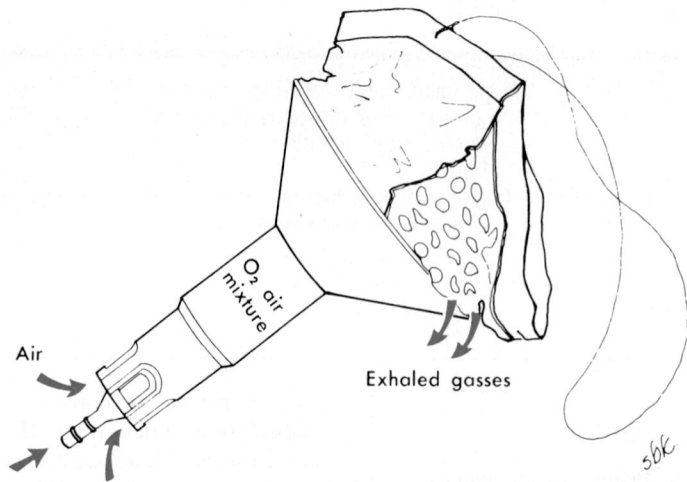

Fig. 16-20 Ventimask allows air to be mixed with oxygen to provide diluted oxygen to patient. (From Wade JF: *Comprehensive respiratory care*, ed 3, St Louis, 1982, Mosby–Year Book.)

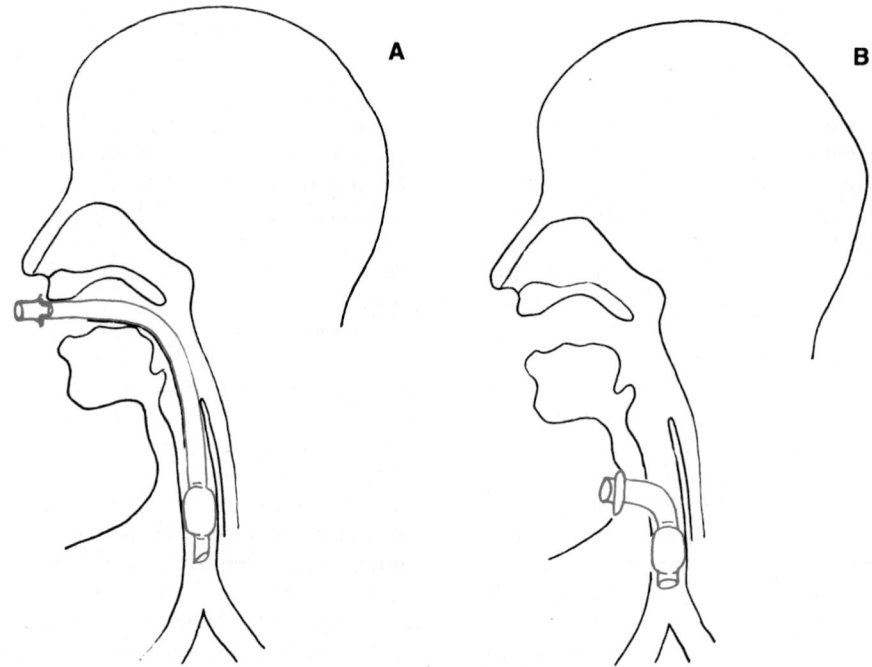

Fig. 16-21 **A,** Position of endotracheal tube. **B,** Position of tracheostomy tube.

tube is used. Usually an endotracheal tube is not left in place longer than 10 to 14 days. If the patient is unable to maintain an open airway after this period of time, a tracheostomy is performed.

The endotracheal tube is made of plastic, with an inflatable cuff so that a closed system with the ventilator may be maintained (Fig. 16-22). The tube is inserted via the mouth or nose through the larynx into the trachea. If an oral endotracheal tube is used, a rubber airway or bite block is often necessary to prevent the patient from biting down on the tube and obstructing the airway.

The tracheostomy tube is usually made of plastic or metal. It may be either a single-lumen or double-lumen (Jackson) type (Fig. 16-23). Both types of tubes may be

cuffed, and the newer plastic tubes come with high-volume, low-pressure cuffs that are less likely to cause damage to the trachea. Single-lumen tubes must be changed about every 72 hours, because they are more difficult to clean and more likely to become plugged than are double-lumen tubes.

Metal tubes are commonly available in sizes 00 to 8 (No. 00 is used for the premature or newborn infant; a No. 6 or 7 is used for most adults). The metal tracheostomy tube consists of two parts, an inner and an outer cannula. The outer cannula is removed only by the doctor, whereas the inner cannula is removed regularly by the nurse for cleaning. The metal tracheostomy tube has a lock that must be turned to remove the inner cannula. The lock should be secured when the inner cannula is reinserted after clean-

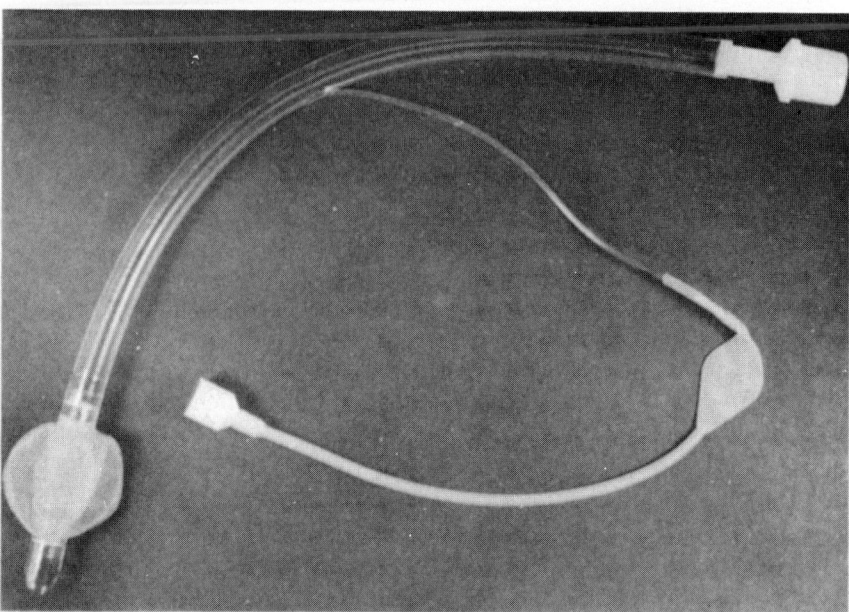

Fig. 16-22 Forregar high-volume, low-pressure cuffed endotracheal tube. Cuff shown here is not inflated. Low-pressure cuff is preferred because it is less likely to cause tracheal damage.

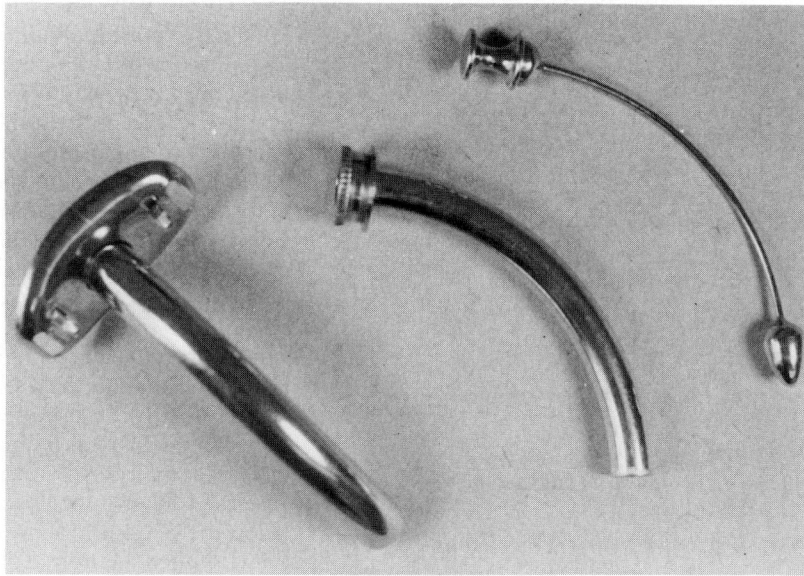

Fig. 16-23 Metal tracheostomy tube showing, from left to right, outer cannula, inner cannula, and obturator.

ing. Twill tapes attached to either side of the tube are tied securely behind the neck to prevent the tube from becoming dislodged when the patient coughs or moves about.

Should the tube be coughed out, the opening may close, and the patient will be unable to breathe. Therefore, a tracheal dilator or curved haemostat is always kept at the bedside so that the opening can be held open if the tube is dislodged. Some surgeons prefer to place a retention suture on each side of the tracheostomy opening and tape the end of the suture to the skin. If the opening shows signs of closing, tension can be placed on the sutures to widen the opening.

The operative wound may be sealed with a plastic spray, or a small dressing may be placed around the tracheostomy tube. Although drainage should be minimal, the wound is inspected frequently for bleeding during the immediate postoperative period. The dressings are changed as they become soiled with mucus drainage.

Depending on the patient's condition, a tracheostomy can be either temporary or permanent; the person who has a laryngectomy will have a permanent tracheostomy. Any patient who has had a tracheostomy is apprehensive and is often fearful of choking. Thus when feasible, the procedure is thoroughly explained to the patient before surgery. Both patient and family need to understand that the *patient will be unable to speak* and that *constant attendance will be provided until the patient can give self-care safely.*

A fenestrated tracheostomy tube has an opening on the upper surface of the outer cannula that allows air inspired through the nose and mouth to pass through the tube. When the external opening is plugged, air can pass over the vocal cords, allowing the individual to talk. If ventilatory assistance is required, the inner cannula can be inserted so that the patient can be connected to a ventilator.

General care of the patient with an endotracheal or tracheostomy tube

An endotracheal or tracheostomy tube provides a direct route for introduction of pathogens into the lower airway, increasing the risk of infection. It is essential that the following preventive nursing interventions be consistently implemented.

1. Minimize infection risk
   a. Endotracheal tubes irritate the trachea, resulting in increased mucus production. Assess the patient regularly for excess secretions, and suction as often as necessary to maintain a patent airway. See Box 16-34 for sterile suctioning procedure.
   b. Provide constant airway humidification. Endotracheal airways bypass the upper airway that normally humidifies and warms inspired air. An external source of warmed, humidified air must be provided to avoid thickening and crusting of bronchial secretions.
   c. All respiratory therapy equipment should be changed every 24 hours. In addition:
      (1) Replace any equipment that touches the floor.
      (2) Remove water that condenses in equipment tubing. Do not pour condensed water back into humidifier reservoir.
   d. Provide frequent mouth care. Secretions tend to pool in the mouth and in the pharynx, particularly if the cuff of the tube is inflated. There is an increased risk of ulceration or abrasion of the lips and oropharynx when an endotracheal tube or oral airway is present.
      (1) Gently suction oropharynx as needed.
      (2) Inspect the lips, tongue, and oral cavity regularly.
      (3) Clean the oral cavity with swabs soaked in saline.
      (4) Apply moisturizing agent to cracked lips.

   e. Maintain adequate nutritional levels.
      (1) The patient with an endotracheal tube is allowed nothing by mouth. Nourishment will be given parenterally or by gastrointestinal feedings. Gastrointestinal supplemental feedings pose less infection risk and are more economical. See Box 16-31 for guidelines for administering gastrointestinal feedings to the intubated patient.
      (2) The patient with a tracheostomy tube is usually able to swallow and have a normal oral intake. Some experts prefer that the cuff on the tracheostomy tube be inflated while the patient is eating to prevent aspiration. Others believe that the inflated cuff bulges into the oesophagus and makes swallowing more difficult, and they therefore prefer that the cuff be deflated. Nursing assessment will determine which technique to use. Methylene blue dye can be swallowed before each feeding or mixed with the tube feeding. If the dye does not appear in tracheal secretions, it is safe to proceed with the meal.

2. Ensure adequate ventilation and oxygenation.
   a. The doctor will assess lung sounds regularly. Unless the individual's underlying lung pathology alters lung ventilation, breath sounds should be heard bilaterally, and chest expansion should be symmetric. If a cuffed tube is inserted too far, it will slip into one of the main-stem bronchi (usually the right) and occlude the opposite bronchus and lung, resulting in atelectasis on the obstructed side. Even if the tube is still in the trachea, airway obstruction will result if the end of the tube is located on the carina (area at lower end of trachea at point of bifurcation of main-stem bronchi). This will result in dry secretions that obstruct both bronchi. Although these complications are more common with the use of an endotracheal tube, they can occur with a tracheostomy tube, especially in a small person with a short neck. In either case the tube is pulled back until it is positioned below the larynx and above the carina. The tube is then fastened securely in place with adhesive tape or twill ties.
   b. Turn and reposition the patient every 2 hours for maximum ventilation and lung perfusion.
   c. Assess respiratory frequency, tidal volume, and vital capacity.
   d. Perform postural drainage, cupping (clapping), and vibrating as appropriate (p. 347).

3. Provide safety and comfort.
   a. Most endotracheal and tracheostomy tubes have cuffs for the following reasons:
      (1) To provide a sealed airway for positive-pressure ventilation
      (2) To prevent aspiration in the unconscious person, during meals or during tube feedings
      (3) To exert pressure on bleeding sites following throat or neck surgery
   b. Assess tube placement at regular intervals.

16-31

Care of the intubated patient receiving gastrointestinal feedings (not continuous)

1. Assess for the presence of bowel sounds.
2. Elevate the head of the bed at least 30 degrees.
3. Inflate the tube cuff.
4. Administer the gastrointestinal feeding to which methylene blue dye has been added.
5. Assess at regular intervals for aspiration. The presence of methylene blue in secretions indicates aspiration.
6. Regularly assess for tube placement and residual stomach contents.

(1) The tube is secured around neck with tape or specially designed ties.

(2) The endotracheal tube is marked to establish a landmark for position comparison and to measure and document the length of tube that extends beyond the patient's lips

c. Change tapes or ties whenever soiled to decrease skin irritation.

d. Always keep a spare tube and tracheal dilators at the bedside.

e. Minimize sensory deprivation.

(1) Patients with endotracheal tubes or tracheostomy tubes with the cuff inflated cannot talk. Therefore an acceptable communication mode must be established.

(a) Organize questions so that the patient can use a simple "yes" or "no" response, nodding head or using hand signals.

(b) The patient may be able to use an erasable board (Magic Slate) or note pad to communicate.

(c) Always talk to the patient and explain all procedures.

(d) Reorient the patient frequently.

(e) Encourage family and friends to talk to the patient.

(f) Keep call light (or bell) within patient's reach.

(g) Reinforce that the ability to speak will return when the tube is removed.

4. Observe special considerations during immediate extubation period.

a. Monitor for signs such as increased respiratory distress, increased hoarseness, and laryngeal stridor, indicating upper airway obstruction secondary to laryngeal oedema.

b. Assess for adequacy of cough and gag reflex.

c. After removal of a tracheostomy tube there is a temporary air leak at the incision site.

d. The stoma can be suctioned. However, frequent use of the stoma for suctioning can delay closure and healing of the tracheostomy incision.

Although the low-pressure cuffs used today reduce the risk of tracheal wall damage, it is important to inflate the cuff with the correct amount of air (Box 16-32).

Care of the patient with a tracheostomy

Although nursing care of patients with endotracheal and tracheostomy tubes is similar, patients with tracheostomies have additional nursing care needs. Analgesics and sedatives are given judiciously so as not to depress the respiratory centre. The patient is suctioned as often as necessary, possibly every 5 minutes during the first few postoperative hours. The need for suctioning can be determined by the sound of the air coming from the tracheostomy tube, especially after the patient takes a deep breath. *When respirations are noisy and pulse and respiratory rates are increased, the patient needs to be suctioned.* Patients who are conscious can usually indicate when they need to be suctioned. With any sign of respiratory distress, the tube should be suctioned. If mucus is blocking the inner cannula

---

16-32

Inflating an endotracheal or tracheostomy cuff

The cuffs should be inflated to a volume that provides adequate occlusion around the tube without increasing the risk of tracheomalacia, tracheal stenosis, tracheooesophageal fistula, or erosion through a major blood vessel. Many experts recommend the "minimal leak technique," which is described below.

1. Using a 10- or 20-ml syringe, slowly inject air into cuff.

2. As air is introduced, assess for air leak around tube. This is determined (1) by ability of patient to talk or make sounds, and (2) being able to feel air coming from patient's nose or mouth.

3. When the airway is sealed and no passage of air around the tube can be detected, remove 0.5 ml of air. This creates a "minimal leak" and ensures that the lowest possible pressure is being exerted on the tracheal wall.

4. The doctor may auscultate over the trachea while ventilating the patient with either an Ambu bag or mechanical ventilator. A small amount of air should be heard gurgling past the cuff.

5. If an adequate seal cannot be obtained with 25 ml of air, notify the doctor.

---

of a metal tube and cannot be removed by suction, the inner cannula is removed to open the airway. When the mucus is thick, the inner cannula should be cleaned and replaced at once because the outer tube may also become blocked. If, despite these measures, the patient becomes cyanotic, the doctor should be summoned at once. A patient who is able to cough up secretions probably will require suctioning less frequently. The amount of mucus subsides gradually, and the patient eventually may go for several hours without being suctioned. However, even when secretions are minimal, the patient is apprehensive and needs constant attendance. Box 16-33 describes routine tracheostomy care.

See p. 369, Box 16-34, for the details of suctioning an endotracheal or tracheostomy tube.

Care of the patient discharged with a tracheostomy

Patients to be discharged with a tube in place are taught to care for and change the tube while in the hospital. A mirror will be necessary to perform this procedure, which may be begun a few days after surgery.

Patients who go home with the tracheostomy tube in place must be provided with necessary supplies or with instructions as to where to secure them and with knowledge of how to care for themselves. They should have suction equipment, which is provided for home use. Suction can be provided by attaching a suction base to a tap. Many hardware stores carry the necessary equipment. The amount of suction is controlled by the stream of water.

Maintaining air humidification

Because the insertion of the endotracheal or tracheostomy tube bypasses the upper airway, the patient's ability to

16-33

Routine tracheostomy care

Materials: Suction catheter, cleansing solutions (usually sodium bicarbonate, hydrogen peroxide and saline), tracheostomy care pack or two sterile bowls, sterile applicators, sterile gloves, tracheostomy dressing (must be a nonshredding material), twill tape, disposable bag, and antibiotic ointment.

1. Wash hands and apply nonsterile gloves.
2. Explain procedure.
3. Suction mouth or oropharynx if needed.
4. Prepare sterile work field.
5. Remove soiled tracheostomy dressing and discard in disposable bag.
6. Put on *sterile gloves*. If tracheostomy has an inner cannula, remove and clean it in hydrogen peroxide solution or sodium bicarbonate. Rinse with saline solution.
7. Inspect inner cannula lumen for patency before reinserting it.
8. Replace tracheostomy ties if soiled. Always hold tracheostomy in place with one hand while ties are being changed. If possible, a second nurse can assist to ensure that tube is not accidentally dislodged.
9. Tie end of twill tapes in a square knot on one side of neck.
10. Using sterile technique, clean tracheostomy incision. Apply antibiotic ointment.
11. Apply sterile tracheostomy dressing.

humidify and warm inspired air is lost. Therefore, whether the patient is on or off the respirator, the inspired air should be heated and humidified to prevent mucosal irritation and drying of secretions. *Large-bore* tubing is needed to provide this mist because water particles condense in *small-bore* tubing. A noticeable difference in the viscosity of secretions is evident in patients who do not receive mist for even as short a period as 30 minutes. Other important nursing care measures and observations vary with the route of intubation—via the larynx or from below the larynx. The patient who has an endotracheal tube in place usually has an increased volume of oropharyngeal secretions because of irritation from the tube. The patient also has great difficulty in swallowing (especially if an oral tube is used), necessitating frequent oropharyngeal suctioning.

Providing nourishment

The patient with an endotracheal tube is allowed nothing by mouth. Nourishment is given intravenously or by nasogastric tube feedings. The patient with a tracheostomy tube in place is usually able to swallow and have a normal oral intake. As mentioned earlier, some experts prefer that the cuff on the tracheostomy tube be inflated while the patient is eating to prevent aspiration. Others believe that the inflated cuff bulges into the oesophagus and makes swallowing more difficult, and therefore, they prefer the cuff to be deflated. Nursing assessment determines which technique to use. In determining if the patient aspirates food, it is often helpful to feed the patient red gelatin. The consistency of gelatin makes it easier to swallow than water, and the red colour makes it easy to detect if aspirated into the lower airway.

Maintaining precautions to protect airway

People who have a permanent tracheostomy must take some special precautions. They must not go swimming and must be careful while bathing or taking a shower that water is not aspirated through the opening into the lungs. They are advised to wear a scarf or a shirt with a closed collar that covers the opening, yet is of porous material. This material performs some of the functions normally assumed by the nasal passages, such as the warming of air and the screening out of dust and other irritating substances.

Providing adequate rest

The patient who is subjected to many treatments can become excessively fatigued, further compromising ventilatory capacity. Frequent rest periods must be interspersed with treatments, and it is the nurse's responsibility to see that the patient has a quiet environment and is not disturbed by unnecessary interruptions at rest times. Unfortunately, people who have severe respiratory insufficiency must have frequent treatments and interventions; it is *not appropriate, although the person may be quite tired, to allow the patient to sleep through the night and to omit treatments*. This inevitably leads to a worsened status.

Although people with respiratory insufficiency are often anxious and frightened, sedation is contraindicated because it depresses respirations. Therefore, it is especially important that the nurse be supportive of the patient and be skilful in assisting the patient to breathe effectively. The patient can be extremely demanding, and the nurse must understand the fear and anxiety that is often the basis for the patient's behaviour.

Monitoring ventilation

Aggressive, constant nursing care is essential for these patients. The nurse must be continually alert to clinical changes that represent changes in the patient's ventilation. Increasing confusion and behavioural changes often indicate an elevated $Paco_2$. The behavioural changes may range from pugnacious, combative behaviour to lethargy. Other clinical signs of *hypercapnia* are flushed skin caused by reflex vasodilation, muscle twitching, and headache. Signs commonly seen in hypoxaemia include tachycardia, increased pulse rate, cyanosis, changes in blood pressure, and changes in behaviour. In *early* stages of hypoxaemia the blood pressure is elevated as a result of vasoconstriction and increased peripheral resistance. In *later* stages, the blood pressure falls to hypotensive levels and circulatory arrest can occur. It is important to point out that cyanosis is not an early sign of hypoxia because it does not occur until arterial oxygen saturation is less than 85%; thus the nurse needs to be alert to the earlier signs of hypoxaemia mentioned earlier.

Mechanical Ventilation

If the patient is unable to maintain ventilation (as indicated by a rising arterial Pco_2), mechanical ventilation is neces-

---

16-34

Suctioning a patient with an endotracheal or tracheostomy tube

1. All patients with tubes require suctioning and should be suctioned as often as necessary. The frequency of suctioning is determined by listening/auscultation. Much of the ability to produce an effective cough is lost because it is impossible for the person who is intubated to build up the pressure needed to create an expulsive cough.

2. The mouth and oropharynx above the cuff are suctioned first. This catheter is discarded, and a *sterile catheter* and sterile technique are used to suction the trachea.

   It is not necessary to deflate the cuff each time the patient is suctioned. The nurse may wish to deflate the cuff once per shift to remove secretions pooled on top of the cuff and to ensure that it is properly sealed. Deflation should be performed when the nurse is ready to suction the trachea.

3. Suction as deeply as possible. In an adult, a catheter can be introduced through an endotracheal tube approximately 45 to 55 cm (18 to 22 inches). The recommended depth through the tracheostomy tube is 20 to 30 cm (8 to 12 inches). The catheter should be approximately one-half the diameter of the tube.

4. A fenestrated catheter with a whistle tip is attached to the suction outlet. The catheter is always inserted without suction being applied. Once the catheter is in place, suction is applied by placing the thumb over the fenestration in the catheter.

5. Before suctioning, the patient is hyperoxygenated with 100% oxygen. An Ambu, anaesthesia, or Laerdal bag is used to deliver 6 to 10 breaths of 100% oxygen. Preoxygenation with 100% oxygen is necessary because oxygen will be removed during suctioning.

6. The suction catheter is lubricated with sterile water or a water-soluble lubricant. In the person with a tracheostomy, suctioning usually stimulates coughing. If the patient coughs, the catheter is removed because its presence obstructs the trachea and the patient must exert extra pressure to cough around it. As coughing occurs, the nurse or the patient should have tissues ready to receive mucus, which may be ejected with force.

7. If mucus is thick, sticky, and difficult to remove, sterile saline solution may be instilled into the tube just before suctioning. From 5 to 15 ml is commonly used.

8. Although some clinicians recommend that the patient's head and shoulders be turned to the right when suctioning the left bronchus and vice versa, there is no objective evidence that this technique improves suctioning of the desired bronchus. In most people the right main-stem bronchus is easier to enter anatomically and thus is suctioned more often than the left bronchus. The catheter is rotated as it is withdrawn with the suction on.

9. To prevent hypoxia, the patient must **not** be suctioned longer than 10 to 15 seconds at a time and should rest 1 to 3 minutes between aspirations, and 100% oxygen should be administered between suctioning. If secretions are interfering with breathing, suctioning may have to be more frequent.

10. The patient is monitored for signs of hypoxia such as tachycardia, bradycardia, or ectopic beats.

---

sary. The ventilator will be attached either to an endotracheal or to a tracheostomy tube (p. 363).

The goal of mechanical ventilation is to deliver a minute ventilation (respiratory rate × tidal volume) with an enriched concentration of oxygen sufficient for adequate tissue oxygenation.[96] The usual tidal volume delivered by a ventilator is in the range of 10 to 15 ml/kg, compared with a spontaneous tidal volume of 5 ml/kg.

Because of the complexity of mechanical ventilation, the ideal place for these patients is in the intensive care unit where experienced nursing staff can care for them. Additionally, ventilators are constantly being improved and new models are introduced periodically. For this reason, an ongoing staff development programme is mandatory. However, it must be stressed that a nurse can only become proficient in working with the patient after repeated experience under the preceptorship of more experienced nurses.

Many different kinds of ventilators are available. *Volume-cycled ventilators* are currently the most commonly used positive pressure ventilators. They provide a wide range of flexibility to meet individual requirements for adequate oxygen and carbon dioxide exchange. The functions that can be adjusted on the volume-cycled ventilator are listed in Box 16-35.

With a *volume-cycled* machine a *constant volume* of air is delivered with each breath. The volume is preset and is delivered to the patient at whatever pressure is necessary to attain that volume. A volume-cycled machine should have a pressure cutoff valve. Such a mechanism allows a pressure limit to be set. If the pressure required to deliver the set volume exceeds the pressure limit, the machine will turn off before the entire volume is delivered. *The pressure limit on a volume-cycled machine usually has an audible alarm. The nurse can set the limit slightly above (approximately 5 cm of water) the pressure required to ventilate the patient. The alarm will then go off if the patient coughs, accumulates secretion, or starts to resist the machine.*

Regardless of which type of ventilator is used, mechanisms for various regulations are necessary if the machine is to be adjusted to each patient. It is preferable to have a respirator that can be used to assist or control the patient's breathing. *"Assist" means that the patient's own inspiratory effort triggers (turns on) the machine.* Most respirators have

---

16-35

Functions that can be adjusted with volume-cycled ventilators

Tidal volume—volume of air in a normal breath

Sigh—periodic deep breath; used to prevent microatelectasis and decreased lung compliance; decreased need for sigh function because ventilating with large tidal volumes

FiO_2—oxygenation concentration delivered through the ventilator

Alarm systems—vary from machine to machine; basic alarms usually present are:
1. High-pressure alarm—increased resistance somewhere in system from lungs to machine
2. Low-pressure alarm—system not reaching minimal pressure required for ventilation
3. Low-volume alarm—when volume of ventilation does not equal the amount set

Control modes—Degree of ventilation that is controlled by the ventilator; can vary from complete ventilator control to almost total patient control

---

a *sensitivity control knob* that can be adjusted to respond to weak inspiratory efforts. *"Control" implies the use of automatic cycling.* The patient may be apnoeic and the machine set at the desired rate; the patient's own respiratory rate may be too slow, and the automatic cycling can be used to force an increase in the rate; or the patient's own respiratory efforts can be ignored and an automatic rate used to ventilate the patient. (Some machines with automatic cycling do not allow for the latter adjustment). It is also helpful to be able to regulate the flow rates at which the gas is delivered to the patient. For example, patients breathing at rapid rates and high volumes need faster flow rates than those breathing slowly and at moderate volumes. A final necessity is the ability to regulate the inspired concentration of oxygen from 20% (room air) to 100%.

All mechanical ventilators must do the following:
1. Provide for the heating and humidification of inspired air
2. Provide a means for measurement of expired volumes
3. Be dependable for long periods of use
4. Be easily cleaned

Any patient on continuous mechanical ventilation should be "sighed" (given a deep breath) several times an hour. Some ventilators automatically "sigh" the patient, while with others the patient is "sighed" manually using a self-inflating (Ambu) or anaesthesia bag. This periodic deep breathing is necessary to prevent alveolar collapse and resultant atelectasis.

Positive End-Expiratory Pressure

Positive end-expiratory pressure (PEEP) is a ventilator mode that has been shown to increase the effectiveness of mechanical ventilation in certain patients. PEEP involves the maintenance of positive pressure, at the end of expiration, rather than allowing airway pressure to return to normal (atmospheric) as usually occurs. By maintaining positive pressure, alveoli that would otherwise collapse on expiration are held open, thus increasing the opportunity for gas exchange across the alveolar-capillary membrane. This is accomplished by the increase in functional residual capacity. The result is a decrease in physiological shunting and the ability to achieve a higher level of PaO_2 with lower concentrations of delivered oxygen (FiO_2). PEEP has its greatest use in the treatment of adult respiratory distress syndrome (ARDS), but is also used in treating any patient who would otherwise require unacceptably high concentrations of oxygen.

The hazards of PEEP are related to the increase in intrathoracic pressure. Most serious of the dangers related to this technique is the increased incidence of pneumothorax, particularly in those with friable lung tissue, as seen in people with emphysema or lung cancer. *The sudden disappearance of breath sounds on one side, in conjunction with signs of respiratory distress, in the patient being ventilated with PEEP must be taken as an indication of a pneumothorax.* This can develop into a life-threatening episode if the pneumothorax is large, and the doctor must be called immediately. Another *less serious consequence* of PEEP may be a *reduction in venous return, which is impeded by the increased intrathoracic pressure, and a subsequent fall in cardiac output.* This effect seems to be particularly common in patients who are relatively dehydrated and can sometimes be avoided by careful fluid administration.

Continuous Positive Airway Pressure

Continuous positive airway pressure (CPAP) is a technique that maintains positive pressure in the lung during spontaneous ventilation.[36]

CPAP is used most often with spontaneously breathing patients, although it also can be delivered through the tubing circuits of a volume-controlled ventilator. CPAP maintains positive pressure at the end of expiration. In this way it is similar to PEEP, which is used only for patients being mechanically ventilated. With CPAP, expiration is controlled by a valve in the expiratory circuit that measures airway pressure and stops expiration before airway pressure returns to zero.

One disadvantage of CPAP is that the work of breathing may be increased because of resistance in initiating gas flow.[96] The level of CPAP chosen should be as low as possible to obtain a PO_2 greater than 8 kPa (60 mm Hg) with a relatively safe FiO_2 of less than 0.6. With CPAP there is lack of backup mandatory ventilation and careful monitoring of O_2 saturation with oximeters is very important. Respiratory rates, level of agitation, and blood gases must be monitored to prevent unrecognized hypercapnia.[96]

Pressure Support Ventilation

Pressure support ventilation (PSV) is another mode of ventilation. It relies on patient effort to determine tidal volume and frequency. This mode differs from CPAP in that the patient's inspiratory efforts trigger ventilator air flow until a preset airway pressure is reached. Air flow continues as long as the patient is making sufficient inspiratory effort to keep airway pressure below the preset limit. The advantages of pressure support ventilation may include overcoming the circuit-resistance breathing associated with spontaneous breathing through a ventilator. By decreasing the level of "pressure support" over time, this mode of ventilation can be an effective weaning technique.[96]

Biphasic Airway Pressure

A recent addition to the ventilator mode is biphasic airway pressure (BiPAP), which delivers pressure support ventilation (PSV) for inspiration and CPAP on expiration. It is used primarily to assist breathing during sleep for patients with neuromuscular disorders such as muscular dystrophy and central sleep apnoea. To deliver BiPAP, a small mask is fitted over the nose. The use of BiPAP during sleep allows the patient to obtain a restful night's sleep and to awake feeling more refreshed.

Suctioning the Patient

When the patient on a ventilator needs suctioning, a closed system is preferred. In closed system endotracheal suctioning, an adaptor is inserted at the endotracheal tube-ventilatory circuitry interface. This allows patients to be suctioned without disconnecting them from the ventilator. The potential benefits of this form of suctioning are (1) the maintenance of positive-pressure ventilation, (2) the continuation of oxygen supply, and (3) the stability of PEEP.

General Care of the Patient on a Ventilator

In planning care for the patient on a mechanical ventilator, it is imperative to know the patient's ability to breathe spontaneously in the event of accidental disconnection from the ventilator. In most facilities, respiratory technicians regularly monitor ventilator function and settings, but the nurse is also responsible for ensuring that the ventilator settings are maintained. Usually a checklist is used to verify the ventilator settings on an hourly basis.

The patient should be assessed on a regular basis and any time a ventilator alarm sounds. The cause of an alarm sounding can be a dysfunction anywhere from the person's lungs to the machine. Trouble-shooting should be carried out in a systematic fashion, starting with the patient and moving towards the machine. Assessment should include the following:

1. Patient assessment
   a. Inspection
      (1) Does the person appear to be in respiratory distress?
      (2) Is the person's chest moving with machine-cycled inspiration?
      (3) Is the chest moving bilaterally?
   b. Auscultation (usually by doctor)
      (1) Are breath sounds present?
      (2) Are adventitious sounds present?
      (3) Are breath sounds coordinated with ventilator inspiration?
2. Tubing to machine assessment
   a. Inspection

(1) Is there an air leak around the endotracheal cuff?
(2) Is there excess condensation in the tubing? (Always remove water from tubing system. Do not empty back into humidifier reservoir.) Note: Not all ventilators have humidifiers.
(3) Check all ventilator settings and readouts.

If the alarm continues to sound and the cause cannot be determined or the patient is in respiratory distress, the patient is disconnected from the machine and manually ventilated with an Ambu bag with oxygenated air until the problem can be resolved.

Weaning From the Ventilator

The decision to wean a person from the ventilator is based on clinical evidence of improved physical status. Weaning is most successful when performed by a nurse who has developed a trusting relationship with the patient. The underlying condition that compromised the patient's respiratory status must be stabilized. Weaning is initiated when the patient meets certain physiological criteria, such as:

1. Acceptable arterial blood gases
2. Tidal volume greater than 10 ml/kg
3. Vital capacity greater than 15 ml/kg
4. Fio_2 less than 0.5
5. Maximal inspiratory pressure greater than 20 cm of water

The patient should be able to breathe on his or her own through the endotracheal tube for at least 30 minutes.

Nursing interventions during the weaning process include the following:

1. Before initiating weaning, prepare the patient. Teach effective breathing techniques. Inform the patient that weaning may take several attempts.
2. Obtain baseline vital signs, tidal volume, and vital capacity.
3. Stay with the patient during the initial weaning process.
4. Coach the patient as needed to breathe slower and deeper.
5. Suction as needed.
6. Monitor for the clinical signs of hypoxaemia and hypercapnia (tachycardia, dysrrhythmias, increased blood pressure, agitation, diaphoresis, or increased somnolence).
7. If patient is unable to breathe on own, reconnect to ventilator.
8. Weaning may require several attempts for increasingly longer periods of time before the ventilator can be disconnected.

Care of the Patient Discharged on a Ventilator

It is becoming more common for patients who cannot be weaned from the ventilator to be sent home on the ventilator. Before discharge, careful planning is required to assure that the home can accommodate the patient and the necessary equipment.

SUMMARY

1. In restrictive lung disease, there is a restriction in lung volume and a reduction in lung compliance. In obstructive lung disease, there is an increase in airway resistance resulting in prolonged exhalation.
2. Acute bronchitis, pneumonia, tuberculosis, fungal infections, occupational-related lung diseases, adult respiratory distress syndrome, and cancer of the lung are examples of restrictive lung diseases.
3. Chronic obstructive lung disease refers to diseases that produce obstruction of airflow and includes asthma, chronic bronchitis, pulmonary emphysema, and cystic fibrosis.
4. Primary prevention of respiratory infections includes prevention of the spread of infection by teaching the infected person to cover nose and mouth with a tissue when coughing or sneezing so that *droplet nuclei* are not released into the air.
5. Adult respiratory distress syndrome is often fatal and is characterized by severe dyspnoea, hypoxaemia, and diffuse bilateral pulmonary infiltrations following lung injury in previously healthy people.
6. The cause of cancer of the lung is closely related to cigarette smoking. From available research data, it seems evident that curtailing smoking is a primary preventive measure.
7. Efforts to detect malignant lesions of the lungs early, while curative treatment may be possible, are critical. The nurse should encourage all people over the age of 40 to have an x-ray examination of the chest periodically in addition to a regular physical examination.
8. Postoperative care of the patient after thoracic surgery centres on promoting ventilation and reexpansion of the lung by maintaining a clear airway; promoting comfort by pain relief; promoting reexpansion of the lung by proper maintenance of the water-seal drainage system; promoting arm exercises to maintain range of motion; and monitoring the incision for bleeding and subcutaneous emphysema.
9. If an open sucking wound of the chest has been sustained, the wound should be covered immediately to prevent air from entering the pleural cavity and causing a pneumothorax.
10. Cystic fibrosis is an inherited disease that causes airway obstruction. It usually develops in childhood.
11. Because of better treatment, more patients with CF are living into their twenties.
12. Asthma results in intermittent rather than continuous airway obstruction.
13. Respiratory failure is said to occur when ventilation is not sufficient to achieve gas exchange even at rest.
14. Patients in respiratory failure require intubation and mechanical ventilation.

STUDY QUESTIONS

- What is the quality of air in the community in which you reside? If air pollution is a problem, what are the major contributing factors (industries, motor vehicle exhaust, and so on)? Are the community groups working to improve the problem? If so, what activities are they involved in and how might a nurse be helpful to their efforts?
- Where is the branch of the National Asthma Campaign and the Chest, Heart and Stroke Asociation nearest your community? What services do they provide for health professionals and for patients?
- What is the tuberculosis case rate in the area in which you live? Is this higher or lower than the national rate? List the factors that contribute to a higher or lower case rate in your community.
- List the services available in your community to assist people who wish to stop smoking and to which you could refer patients or friends.
- Design a teaching plan or project that you believe would help convince teenagers they should not smoke. Would you use a different approach for females than for males?
- Plan a 3000-kilocalorie, high-protein diet for a 60-year-old man with pulmonary emphysema who is very short of breath and finds eating to be a chore.

REFERENCES AND SELECTED READINGS

1. American Cancer Society: *Cancer facts and figures* 1991, Atlanta, Ga, 1992, The Society.
2. Barnes P et al: Tuberculosis in patients with human immunodeficiency virus infection, *New Engl J Med*, 324(23):1644-1649, 1991.
3.* Barry MA et al: Tuberculosis infection in urban adolescents: results of a school-based testing program, *Am J Pub Health* 80:439-441, 1990.
4. Bates D: *Respiratory function in disease*, ed 3, Philadelphia,1989, WB Saunders.
5. Bonomi P: *Primary lung cancer*. In Rakel RE, editor: *Conn's current therapy 1990*, Philadelphia, 1990, WB Saunders.
6. Bradley RB: Adult respiratory distress syndrome, *Focus on Critical Care* 14:48-59, 1987.
7. Brisette S, Zinman R, Reidy M: Nursing care plans for lessons in young adults with advanced cystic fibrosis, Issues in contemporary pediatric nursing 10(2):87-97, 1987.
8. Callahan M: A prudent pulmonary rehabilitation program, *Am J Nurs* 85:1368-1369, 1985.
8a.* Carroll PL: What's new in chest-tube management, *RN* 54(5):34-40, 1991.
8b. Carroll P: Nursing the thoractomy patient, *RN* 55(6): 34-42, 1992.
9.* Carroll PL: Cyanosis: the sign you can count on, *Nurs 88* 18(3):50, 1088.
10.* Carroll PL: Lowering the risks of endotracheal suctioning, *Nurs 88* 18(5):46-50, 1988.
11.* Caruthers DD: Infectious pneumonia in the elderly, *Am J Nurs* 90(2):56-60, 1990.
12. Centers for Disease Control: CDC Surveillance Summaries, Dec 1991, Tuberculosis morbidity in the United States: final data, 1990, *MMWR* 40 (no. SS3):23-28, 1992.
12a.* Centers for Disease Control: Prevention and control of tuberculosis among homeless persons. Recommendations of the Advisory Council for the Elimination of Tuberculosis, *MMWR* 41(no. RR5):1-23, 1992.
13. Centers for Disease Control: Nosocomial transmission of multi-drug resistant tuberculosis among HIV-infected persons—Florida and New York, 1988-1991, *MMWR* 40(34) 585-591, Aug 20, 1991.

14. Centers for Disease Control: State tobacco prevention and control activities: results of 1989-1990 association of state and territorial health officials (ASTHO) survey—final report, *MMWR* 40(RR-11):1-41, Aug 16, 1991.

15. Centers for Disease Control: Purified protein derivative (PPD)—tuberculin anergy and HIV infection, *MMWR* 40 (no. RR-5); 27-33, April 28, 1991.

16. Centers for Disease Control: Influenza activity-world-wide, 1990-1991, *MMWR* 40(41):709-712, 1991.

17. Centers for Disease Control: Prevention and control of influenza, *MMWR* 40 (no. RR-6):1-15, May 24, 1991.

18. Centers for Disease Control: Summary of notifiable diseases, United States, 1990, *MMWR* 39 (53):1-62, Oct 4, 1991.

19. Centers for Disease Control: Tuberculosis among foreign-born people entering the United States, *MMWR* 39 (RR-18), Dec 28, 1990.

20. Centers for Disease Control: The surgeon general's 1990 report on the health benefits of smoking cessation—ecutive summary, *MMWR* 39 (no RR-12):1-12, Oct 5, 1990.

21. Centers for Disease Control: Screening for tuberculosis and tuberculosis infection in high-risk populations and the use of preventive therapy for tuberculosis infection in the United States, *MMWR*, 29 (no RR-8):1-12, May 18, 1990.

22. Centers for Disease Control, Morbidity and Mortality Weekly Report: update: tuberculosis elimination—United States, *MMWR* 39 (10):153-156, 1990.

23. Centers for Disease Control, Morbidity and Mortality Report: Cigarette smoking—behavioural risk factor urveillance system, *MMWR* 38(49):845-848, 1989.

24. Centers for Disease Control, Morbidity and Mortality Weekly Report—Summary of notifiable disease United States 1988, *MMWR* 37(54):41-43, 1988.

25. Cherniack RM: Current therapy of respiratory disease—two, Toronto, 1986, BC Dekker.

26.* Chulay M, Graeber GM: Efficacy of a hyperinflation and hyperoxygenation suctioning intervention, *Heart Lung* 17:1:15-22, 1988.

27. Cobb N, Etzel RA: Unintentional carbon monoxide related deaths in the United States, 1979 through 1988, *JAMA* 266(5):659-663, 1991.

28.* Cornell C: Tuberculosis in hospital employees, *Am J Nurs* 88(4):484-48, 1988.

29. Davis PB: Pathophysiology of pulmonary disease in cystic fibrosis, *Semin Resp Med* 6(4):261-269, 1985.

30. Dept of Health and Human Services: *Healthy people 2000: national health promotion and disease prevention objectives*, Washington, DC, 1990, US Govt Printing Office.

31. DeVito AJ: Rehabilitation of patients with chronic obstructive pulmonary disease, *Rehab Nurs* 10:12-15, 1985.

32.* Dooley SW et al: Guidelines for preventing the transmission of tuberculosis in health care settings, with special focus on HIV-related issues, *MMWR* 39 (no. RR-17):1-26, 1990.

33.* Dougherty S: The malnourished respiratory patient. *CritCare Nurs* 8:13-15, 18-22, 1988.

34.* Douglas RG: Prophylaxis and treatment of influenza, *N Engl J Med* 322(7):443-449, 1990.

35. Dowling PT: Return of tuberculosis: screening and preventive therapy, *AFP* 43(2):457-467, 1991.

36. Dupuis YG: Ventilators theory and clinical application, ed 2, St Louis, 1991, Mosby–Year Book.

37.* Durham E, Frost-Hartzer P: Relaxation therapy works, *RN* 54(8):40-42, Aug 1991.

38.* Engelking C: CE lung cancer therapy, *Am J Nurs* 87: 1438-1439, 1987.

39.* Engelking C: Teaching, counseling, and caring, *Am J Nurs* 87:1439-1440, 1987.

40.* Engelking C: CE lung cancer: the language of staging, *Am J Nurs* 87:1434-1437, 1987.

41. Ferland PA: Are you ready for ventilator patients? *Nurs 91*, 21(1):42-47, Jan 1991.

42.* Finesilver C: Perfecting the art of respiratory assessment, *RN* 55(2):22-30, Feb 1992.

43. Forouzesh M, Price JH, Taylor C: Pulmonary disease, *Nurs Care* 15:19-22, 1992.

44. Fraser RG et al: *Diagnosis of disease of the chest*, vol 3, ed 3, Philadelphia, 1990, WB Saunders.

45.* Freedberg PD et al: Effect of progressive muscle relax-ation on the objective symptoms and subjective responses associated with asthma, *Heart Lung* 16:24-30, 1987.

46.* Fuchs Carroll P: Caring for ventilator patients, *Nursing 86* 16(6):34-39, 1986.

47.* George MR: CF not just a pediatric problem anymore, *RN* 53(9):60-65, Sept 1990.

48. Gift AG, Bolgiano CS, Cunningham J: Sensations during chest tube removal, *Heart Lung* 20(2):131-137, 1991.

49. Hahn DL, Dodge RW, Golubjatnikov R: Association of *Chlamydia pneumoniae* (strain TWAR) infection with wheezing, asthmatic bronchitis, and adult-onset asthma, *JAMA* 266 (2):225-230, 1991.

50. Handwerger S et al: Tuberculosis and the acquired immunodeficiency syndrome at a New York city hospital, *Chest* 91(2):176-180, 1987.

51. Hanley MV, Tyler ML: Ineffective airway clearance related to airway infection, *Nurs Clin North Am* 22(1):135-149,1987.

52. Hartman B et al: Pneumocystis carinii pneumonia in the acquired immunodeficiency syndrome (AIDS)—diagnosis with bronchial brushings, biopsy, and bronchoalveolar lavage, *Chest* 87:603-607, 1985.

53. Harvard Medical Health Letter: *Asthma*, part 1, Harvard Medical School, 16(7):5-7, May 1991.

54. Harvard Medical Health Letter: *Asthma*, part 2, Harvard Medical School, 16(8):1-4, June 1991.

55. Hay JW, Robin ED: Cost-effectiveness of alpha1 anti-trypsin replacement therapy in treatment of congenital chronic obstructive pulmonary disease, *Am J Pub Health* 81(4): 427-433, 1991.

56.* Hefts D: Chest trauma, *RN* 54(5):28-32, 1991.

57. Hodgkin JE, Petty RL: *Chronic obstructive pulm-onary disease: current concepts*, Philadelphia, 1987, WB Saunders.

58.* Hoffman LA: Airway management for the critically ill patient, *Am J Nurs* 87(1):39-43, 1987.

59.* Hoffman LA, Maskiewicz RC: The specifics of suctioning, *Am J Nurs* 87(1):44-53, 1987.

60.* Irwin M, Openbrier D: A delicate balance—strategies for feeding ventilated COPD patients, *Am J Nurs* 3:274-280, 1985.

61. Janson-Bjerklie S, Shnell S: Effect of peak flow information on patterns of self-care in adult asthma, *Heart Lung* 17: 543-549, 1988.

62. Johnson A: The elderly and COPD, *J Gerontol Nurs* 14: 20-24, 1988.

63.* Jordan K: Chest trauma, *Nursing* 90(9):34-42, 1990.

64.* Kersten LD: *Comprehensive respiratory therapy*,Philadelphia, 1989, WB Saunders.

65. Klinger JR, Nichols NS: Right ventricular dysfunction in chronic obstructive pulmonary disease, *Chest* 90(3): 715-723, 1991.

66.* Knebel AR: Complications in critical care weaning from mechanical ventilation: current controversies, *Heart Lung*, 20(4):321-331, 1991.

67.* Krokosky NJ: Black lung and silicosis, *Am J Nurs* 85: 883-886, 1985.

68. Larson EB, Ramsey PG, editors: *Medical therapeutics*,Philadelphia, 1989, WB Saunders.

69. Lewis MI, Belman MJ: Nutrition and respiratory muscles, *Clin Chest Med* 9:337-348, 1988.

70. Lordi GM, Reichman LB: Tuberculosis and other myco-bacterial disease. In Rakel RE, editor: *Conn's current therapy 1990*, Philadelphia, 1990, WB Saunders.

71.* Madsen LA: Tuberculosis today, *RN* 53 (3):44-50, 1990.

72. Mapp CS: Trach care—are you aware of the danger? *Nurs 88* 18(7):34-42, 1988.

73. Marx JL: The cystic fibrosis gene is found, *Science* 245: 923-925, 1989.

74.* Mathews PJ, Mathews LM, Mitchell RR: Artificial airways resuscitation guidelines you can follow, *Nurs 92*, 22(1): 53-59, Jan 1992.

75.* McNaull FH: CE lung cancer: tobacconism in America, *Am J Nurs* 87:1430-1432, 1987.

76.* McNaull FW: CE lung cancer: What are the odds? *Am J Nurs* 87:1428-1429, 1987.

77. Norton LC et al: Common problems and state of the art in nursing care of the mechanically ventilated patient, *Crit Care Nurs* 6:23-37, 1986.

78.* Openbrier DR, Hoffman LA, Weismiller SA: Home oxygen evaluation, *Am J Nurs* 88(2):192-197, 1988.

79.* Openbrier DR, Fuoss C, Mall CC: What patients on home oxygen therapy want to know, *Am J Nurs* 88(2):198-202, 1988.

80. Orsi AJ: Asthma—the danger is real, *RN* 54(4):58-62, April 1991.

81.* Preucser BA et al: Effects of two methods of preoxy-genations on mean arterial pressure, cardiac peak airway pressure, and past suctioning hypoxemia, *Heart Lung* 17(3):290-298, 1988.

82. Ramsdell JW: *Bronchodilator drugs*. In Bordow RA, Moser KM: *Manual of clinical problems in pulmonary medicine*, Boston, 1988, Little Brown.

83. Ray JW, Robin ED: Cost-effectiveness of alpha$_1$-antitrypsin replacement therapy in treatment of congenital chronic obstructive pulmonary disease, *Am J Pub Health*, 81(4): 427-433, 1991.

84.* Renfroe KL: Effect of progressive relaxation on dyspnea and state anxiety in patients with chronic obstructive pulmonary disease, *Heart Lung* 17:408-413, 1988.

85. Roberts SL: High-permeability pulmonary edema: nursing assessme diagnosis and interventions, *Heart Lung* 19(3):287-299, 1990.

86. Rogge JA et al: Effectiveness of oxygen concentrations of less than 100% before and after endotracheal suction in patients with chronic obstructive pulmonary disease, *Heart Lung* 18:64-71, 1989.

87. Schmidt GA, Hall JB: Acute and chronic respiratory failure assessment and management of patients with COPD in the emergent setting, *Concepts Emerg Crit Care* 261: 3444-3453, 1989.

88. Schumann L, Parsons GH: Tracheal suctioning and ventilator tubing changes in adult respiratory distress syndrome: use of a positive end-expiratory pressure valve, *Heart Lung* 14, 362-367, 1985.

89. Shapiro BA, Harrison RA, Trout CA: *Clinical application of respiratory care*, ed 3, Bowie, Md, 1985, The Charles Press.

90. Shekelton ME: Coping with chronic respiratory difficulty, *Nurs Clin North Am* 22(3):569-581, 1987.

91.* Slonim NB, Hamilton LH: *Respiratory physiology*, ed 5, St Louis, 1987, Mosby–Year Book.

92.* Sonnesso G: Are you ready to use pulse oximetry? *Nurs 91* 21(8):60-64, August 1991.

93. Spector N: Nutritional support of the ventilator-dependent patient, *Nurs Clin North Am* 24:407-414, 1989.

94.* Stevens SA, Becher KL: Respiratory assessment, *Nurs 88* 18(1):57-63, 1988.

95.* Stiesmeyer JK: What triggers a ventilator alarm? *Am J Nurs* 91(10):61-64, 1991.

96. Struve SW, Dean NC: *Acute respiratory failure*. In Rakel RE, editor: *Conn's current therapy*, Philadelphia, 1991, WB Saunders.

97. Taggart JA, Dorinsky NL, Sheahan JS: Airway pressure during closed suctioning, *Heart Lung* 17(5):536-542, 1988.

98. Tiep BL et al: Pursed-lip breathing training using ear oximetry, *Chest* 90:218-221, 1986.

99. Traver G, Mitchell JT, Flodquist Prestley G: *Respiratory care: a clinical approach*, Gaithersburg, Md, 1991, Aspen.

100.* Walsh LM, Johnson CC: Update on microbial agents, *Nurs Clin North Am* 26(2):341-360, June 1991.

101. West JB: *Pulmonary pathophysiology—the essentials*, ed 3, Baltimore, 1987, Williams & Wilkins.

102. Whitney E: Chronic bronchitis and emphysema, *Nurs 92*,22(3):34-42, 1992.

103. Yeaw EMJ: Good lung down? *Am J Nurs* 92(3):27-32, 1992.

104. Youmans GP, Patterson PY, Sommers HM: *The biologic and clinical basis of infectious diseases*, ed 3, Philadelphia, 1986, WB Saunders.

105. Alford RH: Histoplasmosis. In Conn HF: *Current therapy 1982*, Philadelphia, 1982, WB Saunders.

106.* American Lung Association: *Chronic obstructive pulmonary disease*, New York, 1981, The Association.

107. American Lung Association: *Diagnostic standards and classification of tuberculosis*, New York, 1981, The Asso-ciation.

108. American Lung Association: *The asthma handbook*, New York, 1984, The Association.

109. American Lung Association: *Occupational lung disease: an introduction*, New York, 1979, The Association.

110. Centers for Disease Control: *Humidifiers: tips given on trimming hazards*, Atlanta, 1979, The Centers for Disease Control.

111. Davis PB, diSant' AP: Diagnosis and treatment of cystic fibrosis—an update, *Chest* 85(6):802-808, 1984.

112. DeTrayer A, Estenne M: Coordination between rib cage muscles and diaphragm during quiet breathing in humans, *J Appl Physiol* 57:899, 1984.

113.* Duncan C, Erickson R: Pressures associated with chest tube stripping, *Heart Lung* 11:166-171, 1982.

114.* Erickson R: Solving chest tube problems, *Nursing 81* 11(6):62-68, 1981.

115.* Erickson R: Chest tubes: they're really not that complicated, *Nursing 81* 11(5):34-43, 1981.

116. Fletcher CM, Pride NB: Definition of emphysema, chronic bronchitis, asthma, and airflow obstruction: 25 years from the CIBA symposium, *Thorax* 39:81-85, 1984 (editorial).

117.* Frame PT: Acute infectious pneumonia in the adult, *Basics RD* 10:3, 1982.

118. Godfrey S: *Exercise-induced asthma*. In Clark TJH, Godfrey S, editors: *Asthma*, ed 2, London, 1983, Chapman and Hall.

119.* Gold W: Restrictive lung disease, *Phys Ther* 48(5): 455-466, 1982.

120. Hagarty E: Weaning your COPD patient from the ventilator *RN* 47(7):36-40, 1984.

121. Harris B, Hyman RB: Clean vs sterile tracheostomy care and level of pulmonary infection, *Nurs Res* 33:80-85, 1984.

122. Kryger M, editor: *Pathophysiology and respiration*, New York, 1981, John Wiley.

123. Langston HT, Barker WS: *The adult thoracic surgical patient*. In Neville WE, editor: *Intensive care of the cardiopulmonary patient*, ed 2, Chicago, 1983, Yearbook.

124. Leininger BJ: *Thoracic trauma*. In Neville WE: *Intensive care of the surgical cardiopulmonary patient*, Chicago, 1983, Yearbook

125.* Matthews LW, Drotar DD: Cystic fibrosis—a challenging long-term chronic disease, *Pediatr Clin North Am* 31(1):133-152, 1984.

126. Stahley TL, and Trench WD: Lung entrapment and infarction by chest tube suction, *Radiology* 122:307, 1977.

127. Treoloar D, Stechmiller J: Pulmonary aspiration in tube-fed patients with artificial airways, *Heart Lung* 13:667-671, 1984.

128. Wood RF, Boot TF, Doershuk CF: Cystic fibrosis: state of the art, *Am Rev Resp Dis* 113:833-877, 1976.

129. Department of Health: *The health of the Nation. A strategy for health in England*. Presented to Parliament by the Secretary of State for Health,London, 1992, HMSO.

130. Bagnall P, Sigsworth J: Living with lung problems, *Professional Nurse* 3(12): 514-517, 1988.

131. Department of Health: *The health of the Nation. A consultative document for Health in England*. Presented to Parliament by the Secretary of State for Health, London, 1991, HMSO.

FURTHER READING

Greener M: Gene therapy: the dawn of a revolution, *Professional Nurse* 8(12): 784-787, 1993.

Howard P: *Respiratory medicine in clinical practice*, London, 1991, Edward Arnold.

Kendrick AH, Smith EC: Simple measurements of lung function. *Professional Nurse* 7(6): 395-404, 1992.

Kendrick AH, Smith EC: Respiratory measurements 2: interpreting simple measurements of lung function, *Professional Nurse* 7(11): 748-754.

Kendrick R: Night School, *Nursing Times* 89(30): 44-45, 1993.

Macleod Clark J, Haverty S, Kendall S: Helping people to stop smoking: a study of the nurse's role, *Journal of Advanced Nursing* 15(3): 357-363, 1990.

Osman LM, Russell IT, Friend JAR, Legge JS, Douglas JG: Predicting patient attitudes to asthma medication, *Thorax* 48(8): 827-830, 1993.

Rees J, Price J: *ABC of Asthma*, ed 2 (third impression), London, 1992, British Medical Association.

Wrightson N, Thompson A, Blake A: Breathing new life: Lung transplantation in cystic fibrosis, *Nursing Times* 89(23): 38-41, 1993.

17

The Patient with Cardiovascular Problems

Terri Abraham
Mary A. (Sandy) Wyper

After studying this chapter, the learner should be able to:

- Identify life-threatening dysrhythmias.
- Describe treatment modalities for cardiac dysrhythmias.
- Identify risk factors for coronary artery disease.
- Explain the pathophysiological basis, therapeutic modalities, and nursing interventions for angina pectoris, myocardial infarction, and congestive heart failure.
- Plan teaching needs of patients with angina, myocardial infarction, and congestive heart failure, and patients undergoing cardiac surgery.
- Describe the pathophysiological bases for pulmonary oedema and cardiogenic shock and the relation of the therapeutic modalities for these conditions to those for congestive heart failure.
- Explain the pathophysiological bases for disorders of the various layers of cardiac tissue (pericardium, myocardium, endocardium), the cardiac valves, and the aorta.
- Describe surgical intervention for repair of cardiac valves and aortic aneurysms and the pre-/postoperative nursing care required.

Cardiovascular disorders are a major health problem in Britain, although deaths from myocardial ischaemia and its complications have decreased significantly since the 1970s. Key factors contributing to this decline include (1) advances in medical and surgical treatment of coronary disease, (2) reduction in cigarette smoking, (3) improved screening and treatment of hypertension, and (4) an overall increase in health awareness, notably increased interest in exercise or fitness and improved nutritional habits.

Every year in the U.K., coronary artery disease causes more than 50,000 premature deaths in people under age 70. More than 20% of these people die before they reach hospital.[57] These statistics strongly support the need for public education about the early recognition of cardiac emergencies and basic cardiac life support measures. It is hoped that effective application of the increased knowledge of cardiovascular disease and its risk factors will enable healthcare professionals to assist people more effectively in achieving and maintaining optimal health.

ANATOMY AND PHYSIOLOGY
Basic Structure of the Heart

The heart is a small organ (about the size of a fist) located in the middle and slightly to the left of the mediastinum, where it is partially overlapped by the lungs. The heart is wider at the top (base) than at the bottom (apex) and is positioned in the chest so that the blunt tip of the apex projects forward and to the left. The lower border of the heart rests on the diaphragm.

The heart is enclosed by the *pericardium*, which consists of two layers: the inner layer (visceral pericardium) and the outer layer (parietal pericardium). The two pericardial surfaces are separated by a pericardial space that normally contains approximately 10 to 20ml of thin, clear pericardial fluid. This lubricating fluid moistens the contacting surfaces of the pericardial layers and reduces the friction produced by the pumping action of the heart. If too much fluid collects in the pericardial space (pericardial effusion), pressure is exerted on the heart muscle, leading to decreased pumping efficiency.

There are three layers of cardiac tissue:

Epicardium: Outer layer of the heart
   Same structure as the visceral pericardium
Myocardium: Middle layer of the heart
   Composed of striated muscle fibres
   Responsible for the heart's contractile force
Endocardium: Inner layer of the heart
   Consists of endothelial tissue
   Lines the inside of the chambers and covers the heart valves

Chambers

The heart is divided into two halves by a muscular wall (septum) (Fig. 17-1). Each half has an upper collecting chamber (atrium) and a lower pumping chamber (ventricle), for a total of four chambers. Oxygen-poor venous blood enters the right atrium, flows from the right atrium to the right ventricle (mainly by gravity) when the tricuspid valve is opened, and is pumped to the lungs through the pulmonary artery. Oxygen-rich blood returns from the lungs to the left atrium, enters the left ventricle when the mitral valve is opened, and is ejected into the aorta for distribution to the peripheral tissues.

The *right atrium* is a thin-walled structure that serves as a reservoir for venous blood returning to the heart via the superior and inferior vena cava and the coronary sinus. The right atrium stores this blood during right ventricular systole (contraction). The *right ventricle* receives venous blood from the right atrium during ventricular diastole (relaxation) and then propels this blood through the pulmonary valve into the pulmonary artery and then to the lungs. The overall workload of the right ventricle is less than that of the left ventricle because the pulmonary system is a low-pressure system.

The thin-walled *left atrium* receives oxygenated blood from the four pulmonary veins and serves as a reservoir during left ventricular systole. Blood flows by gravity from the left atrium into the *left ventricle* through the opened mitral valve during ventricular diastole. Blood is then ejected from the left ventricle through the opened aortic valve into the systemic arterial circulation during ventricular systole. The left ventricle has thick walls because it must contract against a high-pressure systemic circulation to deliver blood to the peripheral tissue.

Valves

The four cardiac valves are flap-like structures that function to maintain unidirectional (forward) blood flow through the heart chambers. These valves open and close in response to pressure and volume changes within the cardiac chambers. The cardiac valves can be classified into two types: the atrioventricular (AV) valves, which separate the atria from the ventricles, and the semilunar valves, which separate the pulmonary artery and the aorta from their respective ventricles.

Atrioventricular valves

The AV valves are the *tricuspid* valve, located between the right atrium and the right ventricle, and the *mitral* (bicuspid) valve, located between the left atrium and left ventricle. The tricuspid valve contains three leaflets held in place by fibrous cords called the *chordae tendinae*, which in turn are anchored to the ventricular wall by the papillary muscles. The mitral valve on the left side of the heart has two valve cusps or leaflets. It is attached in the same manner as the tricuspid valve. The chordae tendineae are important because they support the AV valves during ventricular systole to prevent valvular prolapse into the atrium. A degree of leaflet overlapping during closure of the AV valves helps prevent the backward flow of blood. Damage to the chordae tendineae or to the papillary muscles would permit blood to regurgitate (flow backward) into the atrium during ventricular systole. The AV valves are *closed during ventricular systole (contraction) and open during diastole (relaxation)*.

Semilunar valves

The semilunar valves include the *aortic* and *pulmonary* valves. The structural design of the semilunar valves is quite different from that of the AV valves; each consists of three

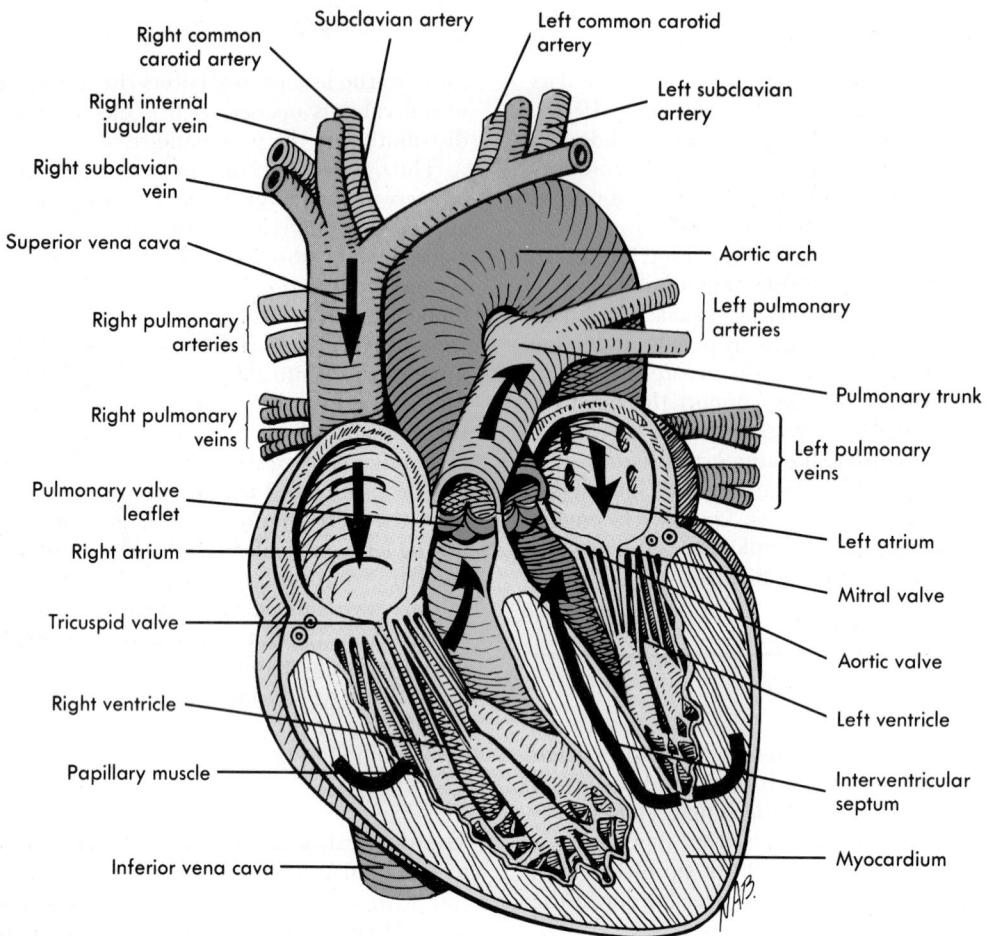

Fig. 17-1   Heart in frontal section: course of blood through the chambers.

cup-like cusps. They lie between each ventricle and the great vessel into which it empties. These valves are *open during ventricular systole* to permit blood flow into the aorta and pulmonary arteries and *closed during diastole* to prevent retrograde flow from the aorta and pulmonary artery back into the ventricle when it is relaxed.

Coronary arteries

The coronary arteries arise at the beginning of the aorta right behind the aortic valve (Fig. 17-2). The function of the coronary artery system is to provide an adequate blood supply to the myocardium.

There are two main coronary arteries—the left and the right. The left coronary artery, which supplies the left side of the heart, divides into two main branches, the *left anterior descending* (LAD) and the *circumflex coronary arteries* (CCA). The right coronary artery (RCA) supplies the right side of the heart. There are few connections (anastomoses) between the main coronary arteries; therefore, blockage of a coronary artery or one of its branches will cause diminished blood flow (ischaemia) to the portion of cardiac muscle supplied by that vessel and may result in angina pectoris or a myocardial infarction. Such blockages may be caused by coronary artery spasm, clots or, more commonly, by fatty deposits in the walls of the arteries

(coronary atherosclerosis).

The venous system of the heart has three subdivisions: the thebesian veins drain a portion of the right atria and right ventricular myocardium; the anterior cardiac veins drain a large portion of the right ventricle; and the coronary sinus and its branches drain the left ventricle (the greatest portion of the myocardial venous return).

Conduction system

The mechanical contraction of the heart is the product of a stimulus response process. Properties that are integral components of the electromechanical events in the heart are automaticity, excitability, conductivity, and contractility (Box 17-1). These properties allow the heart to initiate impulses (either spontaneously or from a stimulus), to transmit impulses, and to respond by muscle contraction.

Action potential

The resting myocardial cell has a membrane potential (that is, an electrical charge) as a result of the relative distribution of extracellular and intracellular sodium and potassium ions. Whenever the cell is stimulated, the membrane potential changes. A graphic record of this change forms the basis for an electrocardiogram (ECG). The

CORONARY ARTERIES

CORONARY VEINS

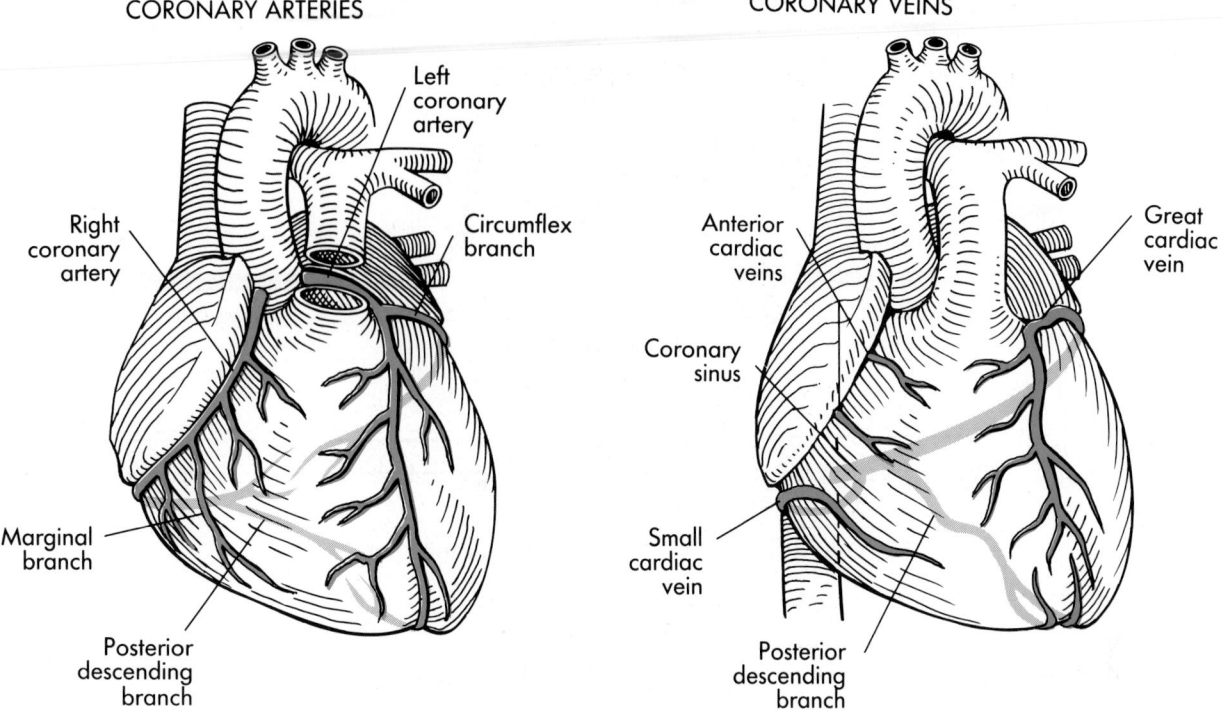

Fig. 17-2   Coronary blood vessels.

change in electrical potential in response to a stimulus is known as the action potential. The two components of the action potential are *depolarization* (generation of the impulse) and *repolarization* (return of cell to resting state). The electrical current stimulates the release of calcium ions, which catalyse the reaction of myocardial contraction.

Resting membrane potential

In the resting state, the inside of the cell is negative with respect to the outside (Fig. 17-3). Initiation and conduction

of cardiac impulses depend on the cell's ability to maintain an electrical potential gradient when the cell is at rest. The main factor that contributes to the −90mV resting membrane potential (see Fig. 17-3) is the cell's permeability to potassium and nonpermeability to sodium. Because more sodium is pumped out of the cell via the sodium–potassium exchange pump so potassium is moved in; a net outward current of positive ions further enhances the cell's negativity during the resting phase.

Depolarization

The initiation of a cardiac impulse begins with the process of depolarization, which indicates the rapid reversal of the resting membrane potential. Depolarization results from increased cell membrane permeability to sodium and subsequent rapid intracellular sodium influx as well as potassium movement out of the cell. This movement of ions across the membrane creates an electrical current. When the amount of sodium entering the cell reaches a critical level, an electrical impulse is generated. The impulse may spread as a wave of depolarization to adjacent cells.

Repolarization

Repolarization is the process by which the cell returns to the resting state. The following sequence occurs: (1) cell membrane permeability to sodium decreases, and (2) sodium leaves the cell while potassium returns through an active ion transport system.

Sequence of cardiac activation

The primary structures of the conduction system are listed in Box 17-2 and illustrated in Fig. 17-4. The sequence of cardiac activation is as follows:

17-1

Properties of cardiac cells

Automaticity
The ability of the heart to initiate impulses regularly and spontaneously. (Although most cardiac cells have this ability, it is the primary function of the sinoatrial node, designating it the dominant pacemaker in the normal heart.)

Excitability
The ability of cardiac cells to respond to a stimulus by initiating a cardiac impulse.

Conductivity
The ability of cardiac cells to respond to a cardiac impulse by transmitting the impulse along cell membranes.

Contractility
The ability of cardiac cells to respond to an impulse by contracting. (Contractile cells comprise the largest mass of the myocardium.)

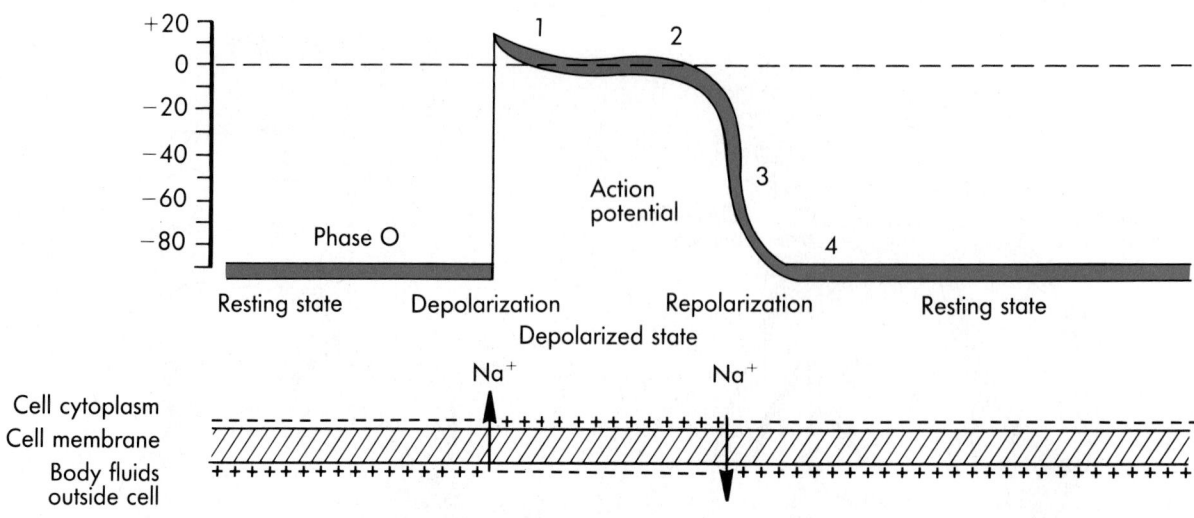

Fig. 17-3   Phases of the action potential of cardiac muscle.

1. Depolarization is initiated by an impulse from the sinoatrial (SA) node.
2. The impulse spreads through both atria.
3. The impulse reaches the AV node, which delays the impulse about 0.1 second.
4. The impulse is transmitted along the branches of the bundle of His to the Purkinje fibres, activating both ventricles almost simultaneously.
5. Activation of ventricular muscle proceeds from apex towards base of heart.

17-2

Structure of the conduction system of the heart

Sinoatrial (SA) node
Pacemaker node located in right atrium near opening of superior vena cava

Bachmann's bundle
Facilitates spread of impulse to left atrium

Internodal tracts
Connect SA and AV nodes

Atrioventricular node (AV)
Located on right side of interatrial septum

Bundle of His
Thick cable of fibres starting at the AV node, bifurcating into left and right bundle branches (LBB and RBB) down the two sides of the interventricular septum; the LBB bifurcates into anterior and posterior divisions

Purkinje fibres
Network of fibres at end of bundle of His that transmits impulse to both ventricular walls

---

Cardiac Cycle

The cardiac cycle has two phases—diastole and systole. Relaxation and filling of the chambers take place during diastole. Contraction and emptying occur during systole.

Diastole

It is useful to envisage the cardiac cycle starting at a point immediately after ventricular systole. At this time the AV valves are closed, and the atria are rapidly filling with blood (atrial diastole). Ventricular diastole is conceptualized in the following phases:

1. *Isovolumetric ventricular relaxation*: ventricular muscle relaxed but not yet filling
2. *Rapid ventricular filling*: passive gravity flow of blood from atria to ventricles; starts when atrial pressure exceeds ventricular pressure and AV valves open
3. *Slow ventricular filling*: occurs as increasing blood volume causes ventricular pressure to rise, which slows further filling
4. *Atrial systole*: atrial musculature contracts, propelling an additional 20 to 30% of blood into the ventricle before ventricular contraction. Atrial contraction occurs following electrical depolarization of the atria.

Systole

Electrical activation (depolarization) precedes mechanical contraction of both atria and ventricles. The ventricular systolic phase is comprised of the following:

1. *Isovolumetric ventricular contraction*: increase in myocardial tension and intraventricular pressure without change in blood volume; AV valves closed
2. *Maximal ventricular ejection*: greater pressure in ventricles than in aorta or pulmonary artery forces open semilunar valves, and blood is pumped into pulmonary and systemic circulation
3. *Reduced ventricular ejection*: ventricles remain contracted and a small quantity of blood is ejected from momentum built up by contraction; higher pressure

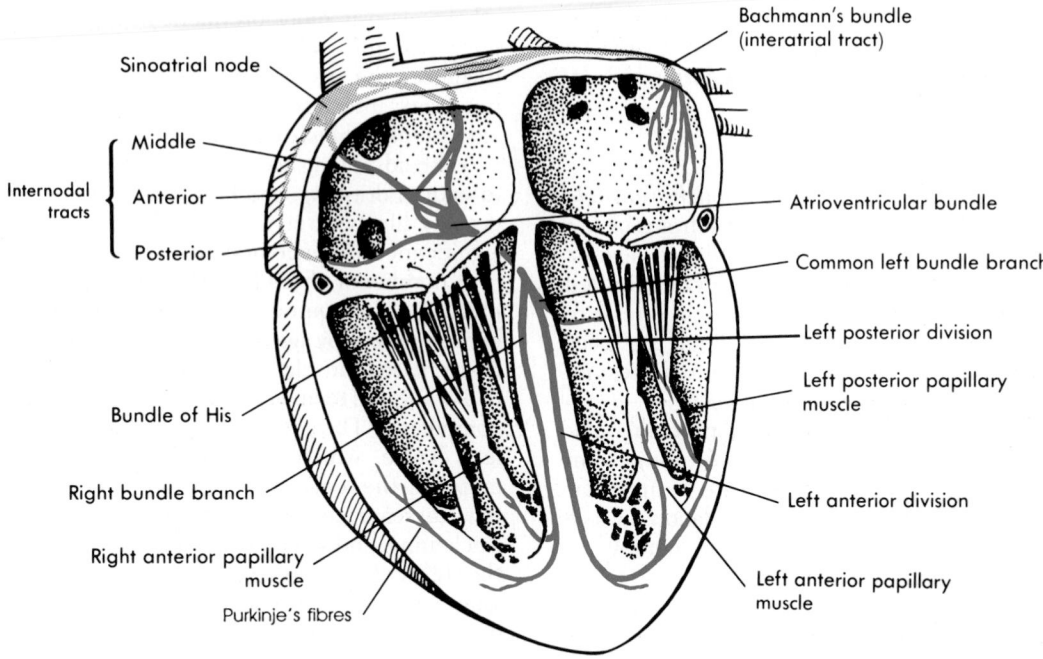

Fig. 17-4   Schematic diagram of heart illustrating the conduction system.

in the aorta and pulmonary artery than in ventricles causes closure of semilunar valves—the end of ventricular systole

The familiar "lub-dub" heard when listening to the heart corresponds with the closure of the valves. The first sound results from closure of the atrioventricular valves at the beginning of ventricular systole. The second sound results from closing of the semilunar valves at the end of ventricular systole.

Cardiac Output

The amount of blood ejected from the left ventricle into the aorta per minute is called *cardiac output* (CO). Cardiac output is equivalent to *stroke volume* (SV) (volume of blood ejected from the left ventricle with each contraction) multiplied by *heart rate* (HR) (number of heart beats per minute):

$$CO = SV \times HR$$

The average adult CO is 5.6 L/min. However, during periods of strenuous exercise the CO may reach 20 to 25 L/min.

Cardiac output therefore depends on the relationship between stroke volume and heart rate. Despite fluctuations in one of these two variables, CO can be maintained at relatively constant levels by compensatory adjustments made in the other variable. For example, if the heart rate slows, the time for ventricular filling (diastole) is lengthened. This allows for an increase in preload and a subsequent increase in stroke volume. Conversely, if the stroke volume falls, the heart rate can increase to compensate temporarily and to maintain cardiac output. There-

fore, the actual determinants of cardiac output are the mechanisms regulating stroke volume and heart rate.

Control of stroke volume

Three significant factors affecting stroke volume and thus cardiac output are preload, contractility, and afterload.

Preload

Starling's law of the heart states that myocardial fibre responds with a more forceful contraction when it is stretched. An example of this phenomenon is that of increasing the stretch of a rubber band to obtain a more forceful recoil when the rubber band is released. Myocardial fibres can be stretched by increasing the volume of blood delivered to the ventricles during diastole. The degree of myocardial stretch before contraction is expressed in terms of preload. *Preload is related to the volume of blood distending the ventricles at the end of diastole.* It is determined by the amount of venous return and the ejection fraction. The ejection fraction is the portion of the end-diastolic volume that is actually ejected (normally about two-thirds). A decrease in the ejection fraction results in a greater amount of blood left in the ventricle at the end of systole.

Since Starling's length–tension relationship is functional only within certain physiological limits, it is important to note that prolonged, excessive stretching of the myocardial fibres will eventually lead to a *decrease* in cardiac output by reducing the stroke volume.

Contractility

Contractility refers to a change in the inotropic state (force of contraction) of the muscle without a change in myocardial fibre length or preload. Contractility can be increased by sympathetic stimulation or by the administration of substances such as calcium or adrenaline. Increased contractility improves ventricular emptying during systole, thereby increasing the stroke volume.

Afterload

Afterload is defined as *the amount of tension the ventricle must develop during contraction* to eject blood from the left ventricle into the aorta. The major impedance against which the left ventricle must pump is primarily determined by *peripheral vascular resistance*. Increase in pressure resulting from hypertension or vasoconstriction produces an increased resistance to pumping and requires an increase in ventricular tension to eject blood.

Ventricular tension is also directly proportional to ventricular size. Dilation of the ventricles resulting from increased ventricular volume will elevate ventricular tension and thus afterload. Excessive elevation of the afterload may impair ventricular emptying, thereby reducing stroke volume and cardiac output.

Control of heart rate

Under normal circumstances, heart rate is regulated by the activity of the sinoatrial SA node. The number of electrical impulses initiated per minute by this pacemaker is primarily the result of its innervation by fibres from both the sympathetic and the parasympathetic branches of the autonomic nervous system (ANS). Impulses from the sympathetic branch have a positive chronotropic effect (increase heart rate), and those from the parasympathetic branch have a negative chronotropic effect. Parasympathetic innervation occurs by way of the vagus nerve and is commonly thought to act as a "brake" that maintains resting heart rate at 65 to 75 beats per min. Some of the common conditions associated with increased or decreased impulse initiation by the SA node are listed in Box 17-3. In addition to factors that influence the SA node, disturbances in the heart's conduction system and excitation of other pacemaker cells can affect heart rate. These will be discussed in more detail in the next section on cardiac dysrhythmias (p. 383).

In summary, ventricular function and therefore CO are influenced by heart rate and stroke volume. Heart rate is primarily controlled by the ANS, and stroke volume depends on the three distinct variables of preload, contractility, and afterload.

Physiological Changes with Ageing

Age-related changes take place in the chemical composition, cells, and tissues of the heart and blood vessels and influence many aspects of cardiovascular functioning.[21, 33] However, despite the physiological changes of ageing, the heart is able to meet the average day-to-day demands and function adequately. It is only under unusual circumstances or increased stress (such as sudden demands for more oxygen or the presence of cardiac pathological conditions) that the deteriorating function of the heart is most apparent. For instance, *asymptomatic ischaemia* may cause

significant functional impairment. Not only is coronary atherosclerosis more prevalent in the elderly, but it frequently manifests as an occult (hidden) disease. It is crucial to detect the occult form of this disease to determine necessary interventions, such as pharmacotherapy and alterations in lifestyle.

With advancing age, lifestyles often change with regard to eating, drinking, smoking, and physical activity. A sedentary lifestyle versus habitual exercise can produce a significant difference in cardiac output.

A number of physiological factors reduce the efficiency of the heart as a pump as evidenced by a 30% reduction in cardiac output by age 65. Atrophy of muscle cells may lead to decreased muscle mass. Increased amounts of connective tissue add to myocardial stiffness and decrease cardiac compliance. The aorta and the major arteries also become less elastic, which compounds problems in filling and emptying the ventricles. The amount of subendocardial fat may increase, and the endocardium undergoes fibrosis, thickening, and sclerosis. In addition, delays may occur in the ability of myocardial cells to recover following electrical stimulation. The efficiency of the cardiac pump is also diminished because of decreased production of enzymes that influence the force and speed of ventricular contractions.

The aorta and its branches and the major pulmonary arteries and their branches undergo progressive dilation and elongation with age. Because the enlargement is transverse and longitudinal, the aorta tends to become tortuous. These alterations are caused by fragmentation, degeneration, and reduction in the amount of elastic tissue, as well as by increased collagen deposits and structural changes. Because of decreased vascular distensibility, arterial pulse pressure increases secondarily to increased systolic pressure (with less change in diastolic pressure).

Increased amounts of connective tissue in the SA node, internodal tracts, AV node, and bundle branches may cause conduction defects and a less effective heart rate response to exercise. The heart rate tends to return to normal more slowly following any type of exertion. In addition, the elderly may be more prone to dysrhythmias because of increased sensitivity to stimulation of the carotid sinus and an overall reduction in coronary blood flow.

The cardiac valves are also affected by the ageing process. The mitral and aortic valves seem particularly vulnerable to fibrosis and calcification and can become somewhat rigid. Distortion of the aortic valve cusps can occur and may actually interfere with blood flow to the coronary arteries. These rigid valves can lead to audible systolic murmurs, usually of an ejection nature.

Confusion or decreased mental alertness may be early signs of a significant decrease in cardiac output in the elderly. These findings may mask other pertinent symptoms of decreased cardiac functioning, such as pain, fatigue, or dyspnoea. Therefore, thorough evaluation of cardiovascular functioning should always be included in the assessment of changes in mental status.

Age-related changes in the cardiovascular system are significantly more pronounced in response to *exercise*. The overall increase in heart rate during vigorous exercise is less in elderly people. Older people without significant coro-

17-3

Factors affecting sinus node
Increase heart rate
Emotions (fear, anger)
Pain
Decreased blood pressure
Increased body temperature
Exercise
Adrenaline
Decrease heart rate
Stimulation of baroreceptors in carotid sinus or aortic arch
Decreased body temperature
Increased intracranial pressure
Digitalis excess
Beta-blockers

nary artery disease (AD) may demonstrate increases in stroke volume greater than those in younger individuals. These increases compensate for the lesser increases in heart rate. Left ventricular ejection fraction has been shown to decrease, or fail to increase, with more exercise in people with coronary artery disease.

CARDIAC DYSRHYTHMIA

People with heart disease or with conditions that can affect heart function may experience cardiac dysrhythmias, which in certain situations may lead to cardiac arrest. Although the term dysrhythmia is preferred to denote a disturbance or variation from normal heart rhythm, the term *arrhythmia* can be used interchangeably with dysrhythmia.

The discussion of dysrhythmias is intended as a brief introduction to the more common dysrhythmias.

The haemodynamic consequences of dysrhythmias are extremely variable. Some cause no significant alteration in cardiac output (CO), although they may produce annoying symptoms such as a "fluttering" feeling in the chest or the sensation that the heart has "flipped over." Other dysrhythmias cause reductions in CO that result in symptoms of decreased perfusion. This is particularly likely if the dysrhythmia is associated with a very fast or very slow heart rate. Two dysrhythmias, ventricular fibrillation and ventricular stand-still, cause death if not promptly treated, because they result in *no* CO. There are many causes of dysrhythmias, some of which are not primarily related to a cardiovascular disease.

Accurate assessment of heart rate and rhythm and comparison of findings with baseline data will allow the nurse to detect some changes in the heart's electrical activity, but not all dysrhythmias are easily noted by physical assessment. A visual display of cardiac electrical activity on the oscilloscope of a cardiac monitor or a graphical record such as an ECG is always required for definitive identification of cardiac dysrhythmias.

Detection of Cardiac Rhythms
Electrocardiogram (ECG)

An ECG is a graphical record of the electrical activity of the heart muscle. The recording is made at a standard speed on a grid that allows measurement of both the intensity of electrical events (voltage) and their duration. Intensity is measured on the vertical axis in millivolts (mV), and time is measured on the horizontal axis in seconds. Each small square on the grid is equivalent to a known unit of time (0.04 second) and voltage (0.1mV), which allows rapid calculation of both these parameters.

The ECG may be recorded by a special technician or by healthcare professionals who have been trained in the procedure. It is essential that the patient be relaxed and cooperative, so the nurse must be able to explain both the purpose of this test and the procedure itself. It is important to emphasize that the ECG machine is merely *recording* electrical energy produced by the body and is not delivering any electrical current to the body. The patient's comfort and safety are maintained by preventing unnecessary exposure and by ensuring adequate grounding of the ECG machine.

In brief, recording electrodes are placed on the patient's four extremities and on the anterior thorax. A conductive substance (jelly, paste, or a specially prepared disposable pad) is placed between the skin and the electrodes to facilitate high-quality recording. The patient must lie still during the procedure, which is not painful and takes less than five minutes. The operator controls the ECG machine, which is designed to record electrical activity in several planes.

Typically, 12 different views are recorded, hence the term *12-lead ECG*, When cardiac electrical activity occurs in a normal manner, a *cardiac complex* such as the one schematically depicted in Fig. 17-52 is produced.

The nature of cardiac dysrhythmias can be inferred by observing the presence, rate, and regularity of the various components of the cardiac complex and the relationship between the component parts. Ischaemia, injury, or infarction of the myocardium, as well as an assortment of other conditions (some of which do *not* represent cardiac pathology), may alter the size, shape, or configuration of various components of the cardiac complex.

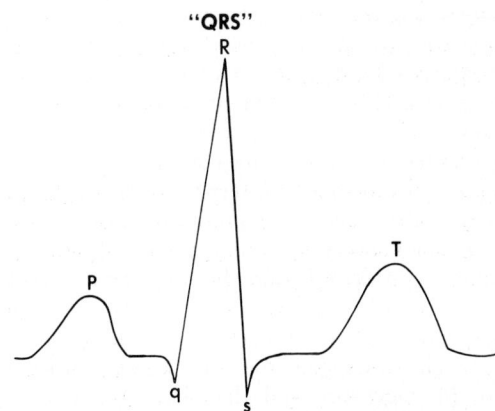

Fig. 17-5   Normal cardiac complex as seen in lead II.

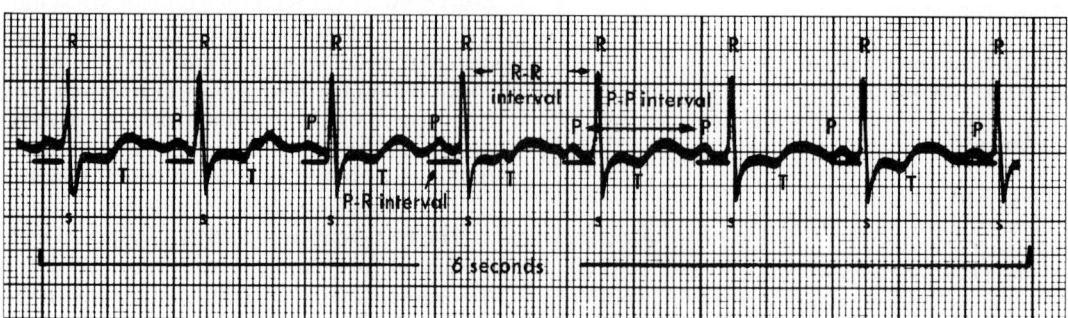

Fig. 17-6   Normal sinus rhythm showing R-R, P-P, and P-R intervals

In summary, the ECG shows only the electrical activity of the heart, which may or may not be disturbed by a pathological process. It does not show the actual physical state of the heart or indicate its ability to function as a pump. Its most important diagnostic uses are the interpretation of abnormal cardiac rhythms and the identification of ischaemia or pathology resulting from coronary atherosclerotic heart disease (AHD).

Cardiac monitors

It is common practice to assess on a continuing basis the cardiac electrical activity of people who are known or suspected to have dysrhythmias or who are prone to develop dysrhythmias. This assessment is performed with a cardiac monitor that displays information from *one* electrocardiographical lead on an oscilloscope. The lead chosen for display varies with the condition of the patient, but standard lead II or MCL$_1$ (a close facsimile of V$_1$) is frequently used.

Most monitors provide a visual display of cardiac electrical activity and the current heart rate. Preset alarms warn of heart rates that exceed or drop below limits considered acceptable for each patient. More sophisticated monitors are designed to detect and tentatively interpret dysrhythmias and their frequency with a computer.

Acutely ill people are monitored in intensive-care settings, but the increased use of battery-powered ECG transmitters that do not require direct connection of the patient to the oscilloscope (*telemetry monitoring equipment*) has expanded the use of such equipment to other patients as well. This development has resulted in the need for nurses working on general medical–surgical units to become familiar with monitoring equipment and to acquire some basic skills in rhythm interpretation.

Attachment to a cardiac monitor does not significantly alter a person's need for nursing care. Placement of the monitoring electrodes on the anterior thorax rather than the extremities leaves the patient relatively free to carry on usual activities. Special attention should be paid to the electrode sites to ensure a constant tight seal between the electrode and the skin and to note the development of any skin irritation. If a rash appears, the electrodes must be switched to alternate sites. Instruc-

tions supplied by individual electrode manufacturers guide the nurse in the application procedure and in necessary routine maintenance. Periodic checking of the monitoring system to ensure proper grounding and secure connection of all component parts is another general nursing responsibility.

Normal Sinus Rhythm

The term *normal sinus rhythm* (NSR) implies that cardiac electrical activity is within normal limits as indicated by the following criteria (Fig. 17-6).

1. P waves present and regular. If the SA node is initiating electrical activity in a rhythmical manner, atrial depolarization should occur in a rhythmical manner.
2. Atrial rate (P waves) between 60 and 100 beats per minute. This represents the range of normal rates for SA node.
3. Each P wave is followed by a QRS complex. This verifies conduction of the impulse initiated by the SA node into the ventricles and implies that the heart rhythm is regular and the heart rate is also between 60 and 100 beats per minute.
4. In addition, normal P-R interval and QRS duration indicate normal functioning of all components of the conduction system.

Types of Dysrhythmias

The many types of dysrhythmias are grouped in the following discussion according to anatomical origins.

Dysrhythmias originating in the sinus node
Sinus dysrhythmia

Sinus dysrhythmia is the most frequently noted dysrhythmia. It is typically found in young adults and the elderly. The P waves are of sinus origin and have a constant morphology. There are two forms of sinus dysrhythmia—respiratory and nonphasic. In the respiratory form, the cyclic pattern of changing P-P or R-R intervals correlates with the patterns of inspiration and expiration. During inspiration, the intervals shorten as the heart rate increases. Conversely, the intervals lengthen during expiration. These phenomena result from a reflex inhibition of vagal tone, an enhancement of sympathetic tone, or both. The nonphasic form has no correlation to respiration. It may be caused by vagal stimulation from other vagally innervated organs.

Sinus dysrhythmia is a benign rhythm that usually requires no treatment. With slow heart rates, some people may experience palpitations or dizziness. In such cases, exercises or medications that increase the heart rate will abolish the dysrhythmia.

Sinus tachycardia

Sinus tachycardia is the result of the SA node firing at a faster than normal rate (that is, greater than 100 beats per minute). Any condition that increases the body's demand for oxygen may cause this dysrhythmia, which is a normal response to exercise, excitement, and fever. Sinus tachycardia may also be a compensatory response to anaemia, heart failure, and haemorrhage. The ECG appearance (Fig. 17-7) is the same as with normal sinus rhythm except for the faster atrial and ventricular rates (usually 100 to 150 beats per minute). The general result of sinus tachycardia is an increased CO, although a prolonged episode may precipitate ventricular failure caused by decreased ventricular filling time and therefore decreased cardiac output. When the underlying cause has been treated, the SA node returns to a normal rate.

Sinus bradycardia

Sinus bradycardia is the result of the SA node firing at a slower than normal rate (that is, less than 60 beats per minute). This dysrhythmia may be a normal finding in athletes or others whose heart muscles contract at peak efficiency. It may also be the result of stimulation of the parasympathetic nervous system, increased intracranial pressure, myocardial infarction, or lack of blood and oxygen in the SA node. The ECG appearance (Fig. 17-8) is the same as for normal sinus rhythm except for the slower

atrial and ventricular rates (usually 40 to 60 beats per minute).

Generally, sinus bradycardia is a benign rhythm. Often in association with myocardial infarction, it is a compensatory rhythm because it reduces myocardial oxygen demand. If the heart rate is too slow to maintain adequate CO, the person may be predisposed to syncope and congestive heart failure. Administration of atropine or isoprenaline is usually effective in increasing the heart rate. The person with refractory bradycardia who is symptomatic may require a permanent implantable pacemaker.

Sick sinus syndrome

Sick sinus syndrome (SSS) is a term describing several clinical disorders of SA node function. The tachycardia–bradycardia syndrome is the most common type of SSS. It is characterized by the presence of a sinus bradycardia with intermittent episodes of atrial tachy-dysrhythmias. Complications of this inefficient rhythm include congestive heart failure and cerebrovascular accidents resulting from thromboembolisms. Some individuals may remain asymptomatic or complain only of palpitations. For the severely symptomatic person, the heart rhythm should be stabilized by a permanent implantable pacemaker.

Dysrhythmias originating in the atria
Premature atrial beat

The premature atrial beat (PAB) is initiated by an ectopic focus (outside the SA node) in the atria (Fig. 17-9). It is characterized by a premature P wave with a contour different from that of a sinus P wave. The QRS complex may or may not be normal, and the PAB is followed by a pause approximately equal to the sinus cycle (measured R to R). The atrial impulse may be nonconducted (blocked) because of refractoriness of the ventricles at the time the impulse arrives. The nonconducted atrial beat (blocked

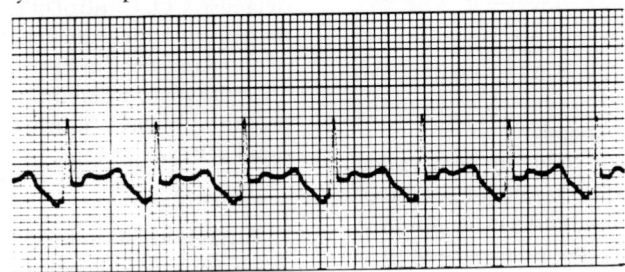

Fig. 17-7 Sinus tachycardia. Lead II showing heart rate of 115 beats per minute, regular rhythm, normal PR interval, and normal QRS duration.

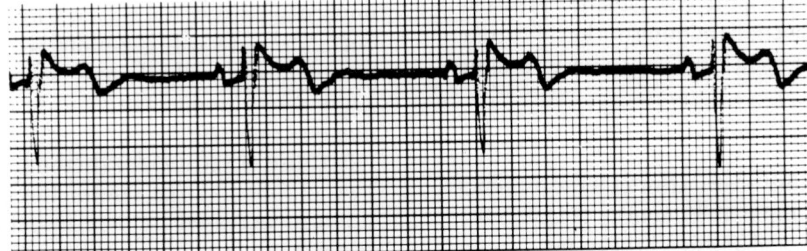

Fig. 17-8 Sinus bradycardia (lead V_1). P waves are present and regular. Atrial and ventricular rates are 44 beats per minute. Each P is followed by a QRS.

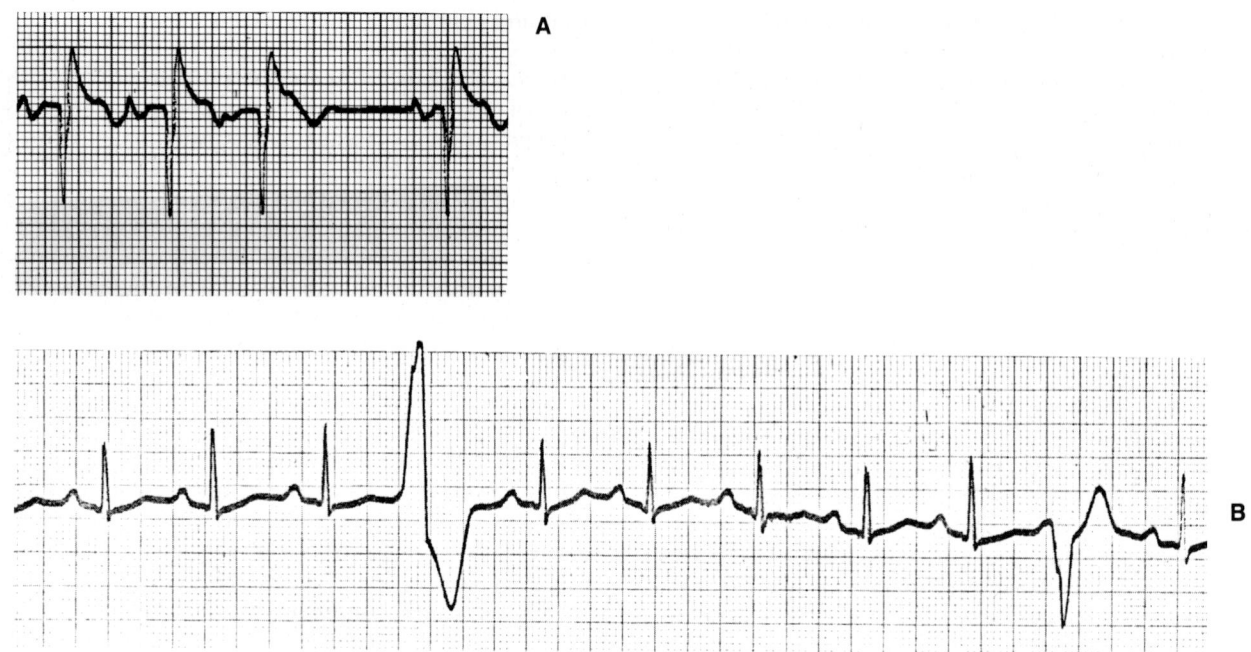

Fig. 17-9   A, Premature atrial beat (lead V₁). Third beat is premature atrial beat with abnormal early P wave followed by normal QRS complex. **B,** Premature ventricular beats (lead II). Fourth and tenth beats are premature with no P wave and wide, bizarre QRS. Different shapes of premature ventricular beats indicate two different ectopic sites in ventricles.

PAB) is the most common cause of irregularities in the heart rhythm.

In the absence of organic disease, such as ischaemia, no treatment is required. Often the omission of caffeine and tobacco will suppress the atrial focus. If symptoms are present or organic disease is known, PABs may be suppressed by digitalis, quinidine, or procainamide.

Atrial tachycardia

In atrial tachycardia, the atrial rate is approximately 150 to 250 beats per minute. The QRS complex is generally normal, and the ventricular rate is regular.

When atrial tachycardia occurs suddenly, it is called paroxysmal atrial tachycardia (PAT). Transient episodes of PAT may occur in children and young adults in the absence of heart disease. When underlying disease is present, it is usually rheumatic heart disease. The person may complain of palpitations and experience anxiety during a tachycardic episode. Short, infrequent episodes require no treatment. Lengthy occurrences may require carotid sinus pressure, vagal stimulation, or intravenous administration of cardiac glycosides, verapamil, or beta-blockers to restore sinus rhythm.

Atrial flutter

The characteristic feature of atrial flutter is the presence of a sawtooth pattern of rapid atrial activity (Fig. 17-10). The atria depolarize at a rate of 250 to 350 beats per minute. These atrial depolarizations produce flutter (F) waves that give the baseline a sawtooth appearance. The QRS con-

figurations are normal. Physiologically, the AV node usually prevents conduction of each atrial impulse to the ventricles. Despite this protective mechanism, ventricular rates of greater than 150 beats per minute can occur. There is no true PR interval, and it is impossible to discern which atrial impulse is actually conducted to the ventricles.

The potentially rapid ventricular rate of atrial flutter may decrease CO. Control of the ventricular rate or conversion to sinus rhythm is the major treatment goal. Direct-current cardioversion is the treatment of choice in the patient with an acute myocardial infarction to protect an already compromised myocardium from the metabolic demands of a rapid ventricular rate.

Atrial fibrillation

Atrial fibrillation (Fig. 17-11) is the most rapid of atrial dysrhythmias. The atria beat chaotically at rates of 350 to 600 beats per minute. The baseline is characteristically composed of irregular undulations without definable P waves. The QRS complex is usually normal, but the ventricular rhythm is irregularly irregular. If untreated, the ventricular rate will generally be 100 to 180 beats per minute. Atrial fibrillation may be paroxysmal and transient, or it may be chronic. The latter generally indicates underlying heart disease.

Because of ventricular rhythm irregularity and the loss of synchronous atrial contractions (atrial kick), cardiac output is decreased and a pulse deficit often exists. In the presence of mitral stenosis, thrombi may form in the atria and cause embolisms affecting the lungs or periphery. The goal of therapy is to prevent these complications by control-

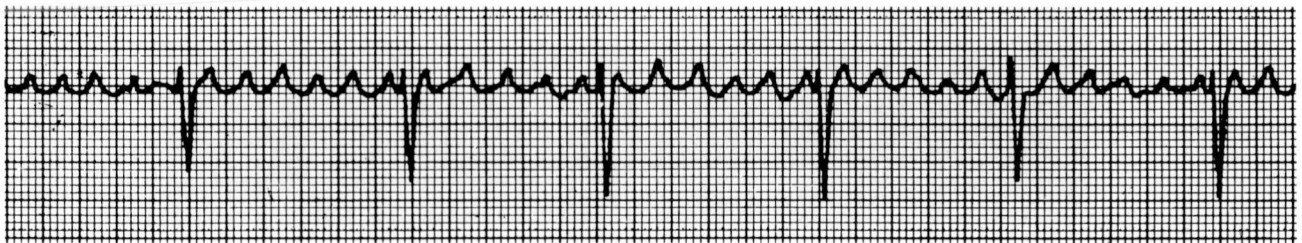

Fig. 17-10   Atrial flutter (V₁). Rate of atrial flutter waves is 300 per minute. Ventricular rate is 50 to 75 beats per minute.

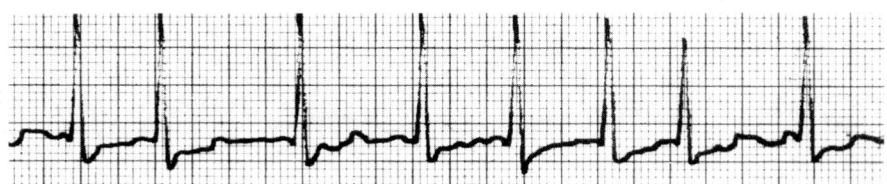

Fig. 17-11   Atrial fibrillation (lead II). Atrial rate is rapid with varying conduction to ventricles, rhythm is irregular, QRS complex is normal, and no definite P waves are visible.

ling the ventricular rate and giving anticoagulants to certain patients.

Dysrhythmias originating in atrioventricular junction

Premature junctional beats

The premature junctional beat (PJB) arises from an ectopic focus near the junction of the AV node and the bundle of His. These PJBs may occur in the normal heart; they are also associated with digitalis toxicity, congestive heart failure, ischaemia, and hypokalaemia. The P waves may occur before, during, or after the QRS. The QRS is normal, and the ventricular rhythm is regular.

When the automaticity of a junctional pacemaker increases to a rate greater than 60 per minute, it may override the SA node as the pacemaker of the heart. This rhythm is called *accelerated junctional rhythm* if it occurs at 60 to 100 beats per minute. A *junctional tachycardia* exists when the rate exceeds 100 beats per minute.

Treatment should correct the underlying cause. Quinidine, propranolol, and procainamide may suppress PJBs. Phenytoin is particularly effective in suppressing PJBs secondary to cardiac glycoside toxicity.

Dysrhythmias originating in the ventricles

Premature ventricular beats

The premature ventricular beat (PVB) arises from an ectopic focus in the ventricles. The characteristic wide, bizarre QRS complex (usually greater than 0.12 second) makes the PVB readily recognizable on the ECG tracing (Fig. 17-12). No associated P wave precedes the QRS complex, and the T wave is in the opposite direction from the main QRS deflection. Frequently PVBs are followed by a compensatory pause so that the interval from the beat preceding to the beat following the PVB is equal to two sinus cycles.

Even in the absence of heart disease, PVBs occur often and increase in number with a person's age. The incidence and frequency of occurrence are higher, however, for the population with heart disease. Clinically, PVBs are associated with myocardial infarction, congestive heart failure, digitalis toxicity, drug therapy, and electrolyte imbalances. Pharmacological suppression of PVBs is most often accomplished with lignocaine, procainamide, and quinidine.

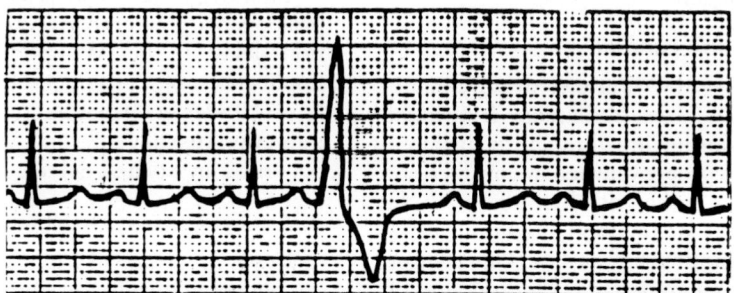

Fig. 17-12   Premature ventricular beat (PVB). Lead II showing fourth beat is a PVB with wide early QRS complex; no P wave associated with beat.

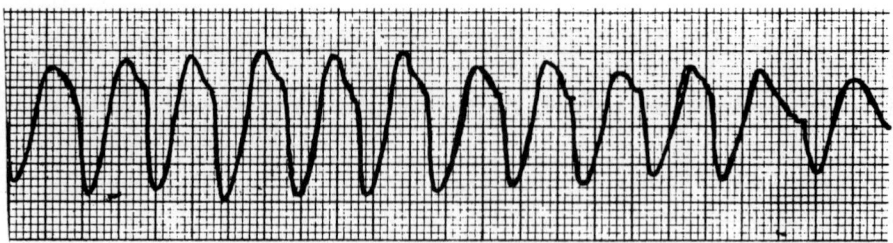

Fig. 17-13   Ventricular tachycardia at a rate of approximately 150 beats per minute; rhythm is slightly irregular.

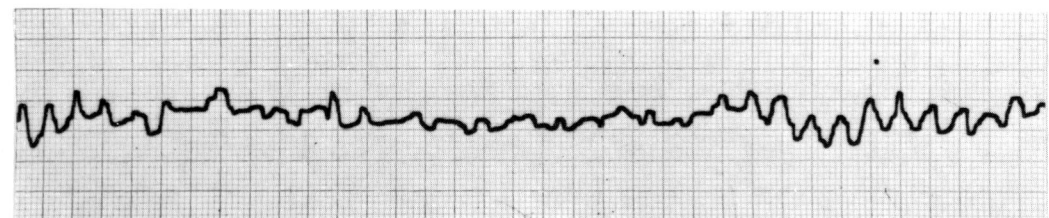

Fig. 17-14   Ventricular fibrillation (lead II). Tracing shows electrical chaos in myocardium. There are no QRS complexes and no definite P waves visible.

Ventricular rhythms and tachycardia

If the SA node and AV junction fail to initiate impulses, a ventricular pacemaking cell will automatically begin to initiate impulses at an inherent rate of 20 to 40 beats per minute. This is known as *idioventricular rhythm*. If the ventricle-initiated rhythm increases to 40 to 100 beats per minute, it is known as *accelerated idioventricular rhythm*. It may be seen in digitalis toxicity or as a complication of an acute myocardial infarction. Generally, neither of these rhythms is treated except to correct underlying abnormalities.

By definition, three or more successive PVBs constitute *ventricular tachycardia* (Fig. 17-13). The ventricular rate is usually 150 to 250 beats per minute. Although P waves may be present, they are not associated with the QRS complexes. Ventricular tachycardia may complicate any form of heart disease. If the patient remains stable, treatment may include intravenous lignocaine, procainamide, or bretylium. If pharmacological measures are unsuccessful, the alternative is cardioversion.

Ventricular fibrillation and standstill

In *ventricular fibrillation*, the ventricles twitch chaotically, much as they do in atrial fibrillation. Individual muscle fibres are depolarizing but in a disorganized fashion. Thus, they fail to produce a proper ventricular contraction. Common causes for this lethal dysrhythmia include ischaemia in the ventricles, electrocution, drowning, electrolyte imbalances, and toxic doses of cardiac glycosides or quinidine. The ECG tracing consists of a bumpy line of unidentifiable waves (Fig. 17-14).

In *ventricular standstill* (asystole), the ECG tracing is a flat line. No electrical activity is noted; all pacemaking cells have failed. Clinically, ventricular fibrillation and standstill cannot be differentiated without an ECG. Both are fatal dysrhythmias requiring immediate measures. The patient has no blood pressure, pulse or audible heartbeat, or respirations and quickly loses consciousness. CPR must be instituted immediately and defibrillation performed within one minute to prevent biochemical derangements that further compromise the patient.

Conduction abnormalities
Atrioventricular block

A block to impulse conduction may occur anywhere along the conduction pathways. One common area of block is the atrioventricular (AV) junction. The severity of the block is identified by degrees: first-, second-, or third-degree AV block.

First-degree atrioventricular block

First-degree AV block is present when the PR interval is prolonged to greater than 0.20 second, indicating a conduction delay in the AV node (Fig. 17-15). The clinical implications of a prolonged PR interval depend upon the level of the lesion. It may be associated with acute myocardial infarction (usually inferior). When a first-degree AV block occurs as an isolated defect, no treatment is necessary.

Second-degree atrioventricular block

In second-degree AV block, some of the atrial impulses are not conducted to the ventricles. There are two types of second-degree AV block: type I (Wenckebach or Mobitz I), when pathology is in the AV node, or type II (Mobitz II),

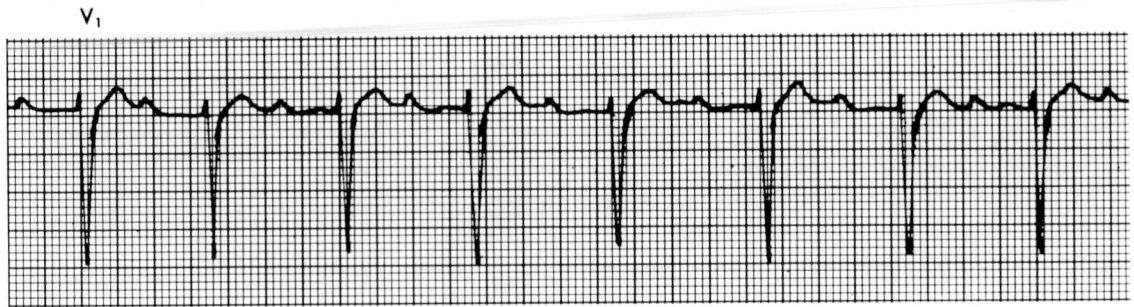

Fig. 17-15   First-degree atrioventricular block; the PR interval is 0.33 second (too long). (From Conover MB: *Cardiac arrhythmias*, ed 2, St Louis, 1978, Mosby–Year Book.)

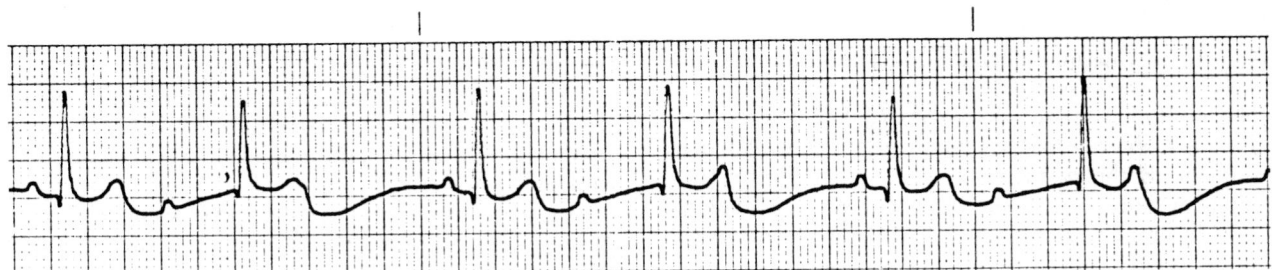

Fig. 17-16   Second-degree atrioventricular block, type I (Wenckebach). Every third P wave is hidden in preceding T wave; conduction is 3 : 2. Note progressive lengthening of PR interval before dropped QRS.

when the lesion is within or below the bundle of His. Each type has different clinical implications, treatment, and prognosis.

Type I second-degree AV block is characterized by a PR interval that progressively lengthens until a P wave is not followed by a QRS complex (Fig. 17-16). The nonconducted beat is the result of the arrival of the impulse during the refractory period of the AV node. The ratio of P waves to QRS complexes may vary. Any drug that slows AV conduction may cause a type I block. It often occurs in patients with acute inferior wall myocardial infarction. Type I blocks are often transient and reversible and generally require no treatment unless the patient becomes symptomatic.

Type II second-degree AV block is less common but more serious than type I. A type II block is characterized by nonconducted sinus impulses despite constant PR intervals. Usually the QRS complexes are widened because of a bundle branch block (BBB). The dropped beat represents a form of intermittent blockage of both bundle branches. Type II blocks are most often seen with acute anterior wall myocardial infarction and may progress to third-degree or complete heart block. A temporary pacemaker is often used prophylactically until the condition stabilizes.

Third-degree atrioventricular block

In third-degree AV block (complete heart block), all the sinus or atrial impulses are blocked, and the atria and ventricles are forced to beat independently. The ventricles are driven by a junctional or ventricular pacemaker cell. The rate and dependability of the ventricular rhythm are related to the level of the lesion. If a junctional pacemaker drives the ventricles, ventricular rate will be at least 40 to 60 beats per minute (Fig. 17-17). Atropine may be useful in restoring conduction.

If a ventricular pacemaker controls the ventricles, the rate will be 20 to 40 beats per minute, and the patient may experience syncope, congestive heart failure, altered mentation, or angina. Generally the patient will require a permanent artificial pacemaker. Intravenous adrenaline or isoprenaline may increase the ventricular rate temporarily until artificial pacing can be instituted.

Bundle branch block

A bundle branch block (BBB) occurs as a transient block or permanent defect secondary to tachydysrhythmias, congestive heart failure, acute myocardial infarction, pulmonary embolus, hypoxia, or metabolic derangement. The electrical impulse spreads from one ventricle to the other by abnormal pathways producing distinct ECG tracings and widened QRS complexes.

A BBB may occur in the right bundle branch, the more delicate structure of the two bundles. In the younger person, right bundle branch block (RBBB) often results from right ventricular hypertrophy, whereas coronary artery heart disease is usually the cause in the older

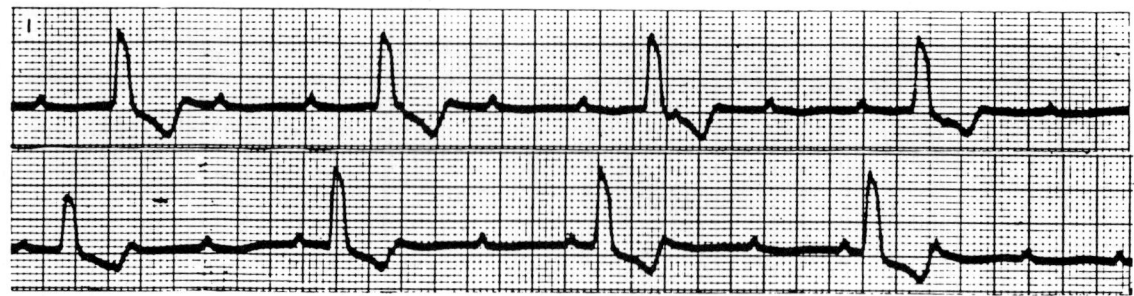

Fig. 17-17   Complete (third-degree) atrioventricular block. The strips are continuous. In the presence of sinus tachycardia (rate 108 per minute), an independent idioventricular rhythm occurs (rate 36 per minute). Note that the ventricular rhythm is absolutely regular, whereas the PR relationship is constantly changing, (From Marriott HJL, Conover MB: *Advanced concepts in arrhythmias,* ed 2, St Louis, 1989, Mosby–Year Book.)

person. In the absence of other conduction defects, no intervention is necessary.

The left bundle branch has a main trunk that bifurcates into the left anterior and left posterior divisions. A block may occur in the main trunk or in either of the two divisions. A block in the main trunk produces a complete left bundle branch block (LBBB). LBBB is associated with severe coronary atherosclerotic heart disease, valvular disease, hypertensive disease, cardiomegaly, and acute anterior wall myocardial infarction. For in-depth discussion on this topic, see specific cardiology textbooks.

Treatment Modalities

Three major treatment modalities are employed for cardiac dysrhythmias:

1. Therapy aimed at relieving the underlying cause of the dysrhythmia (Box 17-4)
2. Drug therapy aimed at suppressing impulse formation by ectopic sites or enhancing impulse formation by the SA node
3. The use of electrical stimuli to suppress ectopic impulse formation or to initiate impulse formation in a regulated manner

Antiarrhythmic agents

The list of *antiarrhythmic drugs* in current use appears to grow almost daily. The development of drugs that are effective and free of dangerous or annoying side effects has been a challenge to the pharmaceutical industry. See pharmacology texts for specific information regarding antiarrhythmic agents.

17-4

Therapies to relieve underlying cause of dysrhythmias

Oxygen to relieve hypoxia
Provision of depleted serum electrolytes (especially potassium)
Treatment of heart failure
Relief of anxiety
Removal of noxious stimuli (for example, caffeine)

Pacemakers

The use of various forms of electrical stimuli in the treatment of cardiac dysrhythmias has a number of nursing implications; therefore, these modalities will be discussed in detail.

An artificial pacemaker is a mechanical device that electronically stimulates impulse initiation within the heart. The pacemaker system is composed of a battery-powered energy source (technically called a *pulse generator* but more commonly called a *pacemaker*) and a wire or catheter that delivers the electronic stimulus to a point of contact in the atrial or ventricular myocardium or both. The purpose of artificial pacing is control of heart rate.

Pacemakers are primarily used to treat conduction defects, in which case the catheter is placed in the atria, ventricle, or both to ensure adequate depolarization beyond the site of impulse blockage (Fig. 17-18, A). These devices are also employed to remedy inadequate impulse initiation by the SA node and to suppress myocardial irritability that does not respond to antiarrhythmic therapy. In these instances the catheter may be placed in the atrium, since the underlying problem does not involve failure of the conduction system (Fig. 17-18, B). Ventricular pacing is "nonphysiological," since it does not result in coordination between atrial and ventricular mechanical activity. The CO thus achieved, however, is adequate for most people requiring pacemakers.

Pulse generators

The pulse generator has a number of controls that can be easily manipulated in a temporary system. These are more easily manipulated than those in permanent systems because of improvements in technology. These controls include energy output, heart rate, and pacing mode (asynchronous or demand).

Temporary pacemakers

Temporary pacemakers are used in the following situations:

1. Emergency treatment of ventricular standstill
2. Short-term treatment of conduction defects causing decreased CO

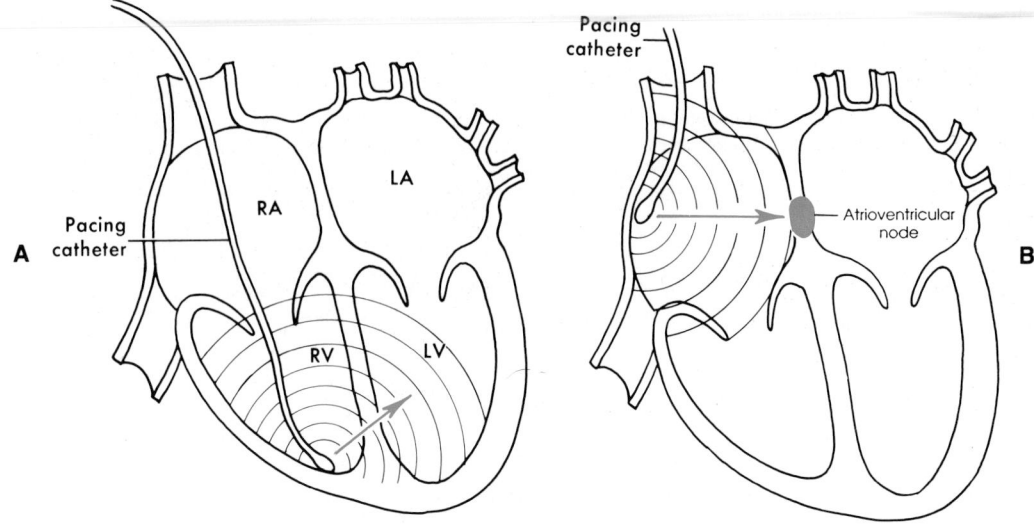

Fig. 17-18 **A,** Ventricular pacing: impulses are initiated in ventricle. **B,** Atrial pacing: impulses are initiated in atrium and travel to ventricles by normal conduction system.

3. Prophylactic management of people who are prone to the sudden development of complete heart block

A temporary pacing system is characterized by an *external* pulse generator attached to the distal end of the pacing catheter. The catheter may be advanced through the venous system to make contact with the endocardial surface of the heart, or it may be sutured directly to the epicardial surface. The transvenous approach can be employed at the bedside under ECG guidance or in a special procedure room under fluoroscopy. Direct suturing of the catheter to the epicardium is performed during cardiac or thoracic surgery.

If the patient is connected to a cardiac monitor, the presence of the pacing stimulus (a small vertical spike that indicates that the pulse generator has sent a stimulus to the heart) and evidence that the stimulus actually causes depolarization (either a P wave or a QRS complex immediately following the stimulus, depending on where the catheter has been placed) will be noted.

The pulse generator may be secured to an arm if the antecubital fossa is the insertion site of the pacing catheter. If a subclavian site is used (an approach that has become more common because it leads to greater catheter stability), the pulse generator may be taped to the chest or placed in a chest pocket on specially prepared hospital gowns. Nursing care of patients with temporary pacemakers is summarized in Box 17-5.

Permanent pacemakers

Permanent pacemakers are used in the long-term treatment of persistent dysrhythmias that are amenable to this type of therapy. The pacing system is totally implanted, with the pulse generator generally placed in a subcutaneous "pocket" beneath the clavicle (Fig. 17-19). As with temporary pacing systems, the catheter may be placed in contact with the heart by the transvenous or epicardial approach.

Permanent pacemakers are inserted in the operating room or in a special procedure room. The transvenous approach to insertion does not require general anaesthesia, a fact that decreases the risk of this procedure. The generator is powered by a battery that has an expected life of 4 to 10 years.

Manipulation of heart rate and energy output has been difficult at best once the permanent unit was implanted; however, recent technological advances have resulted in programmable pulse generators that allow variation in both the present heart rate and the energy output. The latter manipulation has proved useful in reducing battery drain.

After several years of research and development, Mirowski

Guidelines for Care 17-5

The patient with a temporary pacemaker

Assessment of pacemaker function
- Assess heart rate to verify that it has not fallen below the present level; if it has, notify doctor
- If patient is connected to cardiac monitor, monitor presence of pacing stimulus and that a P wave or a QRS complex immediately follows the stimulus

Maintenance of system integrity
- Ensure that catheter terminals are securely connected to pulse generator
- Ensure that pulse generator is attached to person in such a way that accidental dislodgement of the system does not occur

Maintenance of patient safety and comfort
- Assess for signs of infection at catheter insertion site
- Encourage range of motion in extremity to which pulse generator is attached, as permitted
- Ensure that patient avoids contact with any electrical machinery that is not properly earthed
- Explain the purpose of the pacing system and any prescribed restrictions on physical activities to prevent anxiety

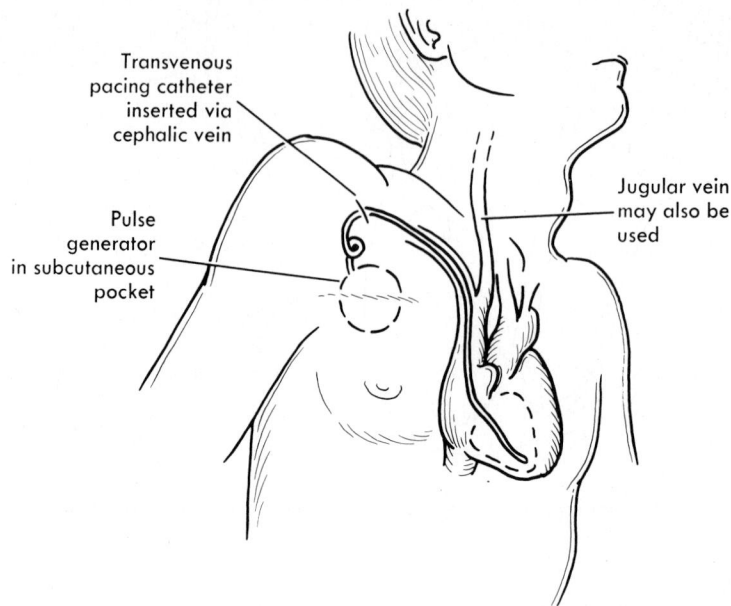

Transvenous
pacing catheter
inserted via
cephalic vein

Pulse
generator
in subcutaneous
pocket

Jugular vein
may also be
used

Fig. 17-19 Thoracic placement of a permanent pulse generator (pacemaker) and transvenous pacing catheter.

and others implanted the first permanent *automatic* defibrillator in 1980.[59] This device automatically senses ventricular fibrillation and, within approximately 15 to 20 seconds, delivers an electrical countershock. It is also capable of identifying and correcting ventricular tachycardia with cardioversion. Defibrillatory energy requirements are considerably less because the shock is being applied directly within the heart.

The automatic implantable cardioverter defibrillator (AICD) consists of a pulse generator and two lead or sensing systems. The device is implanted surgically through a median sternotomy or lateral thoracotomy approach. This device has been approved by the Department of Health, and the Home Office[58] for two categories of patients: (1) those who have experienced recurrent life-threatening ventricular dysrhythmias, inducible into sustained hypotensive ventricular tachycardia or ventricular fibrillation despite conventional antiarrhythmic drug therapy, and (2) those who have survived one or more episodes of sudden cardiac death resulting from ventricular tachycardia or ventricular fibrillation not associated with acute myocardial infarction.

Immediate postinsertion care of a person with a permanent pacemaker includes relief of incisional discomfort, monitoring for infection, and assessment of the system's functioning. Attaching the person to a cardiac monitor for 24 to 48 hours following insertion is the usual practice. Long-term follow-up of these people is essential and is especially important within the last year of anticipated battery life. Pacemaker clinics have been established to facilitate follow-up, and in some instances, telecommunications systems allow telephone assessment of functioning.

Patient Teaching | 17-6

The patient with a permanent pacemaker

Count pulse daily for 1 full minute; report rate significantly above or below programmed rate to the doctor

Report signs of infection (pain, redness, drainage over incision site) to the doctor.

Report signs of decreased cardiac output (dizziness, fatigue, "palpatations," dyspnoea) to the doctor.

Avoid handling electrical equipment (such as blow dryers, battery-operated toothbrushes) next to pacemaker (may cause interference, place the pacemaker in a fixed mode or shut it off[65]).

Carry an identification card that states:
  Pacemaker's manufacturer, model, and serial number
  Implant date
  Programmed rates
  Doctor's name and phone number.

Show pacemaker identification card to security guards before passing through metal detectors (detector will not affect pacemaker but will trigger the alarm).

Report regularly for pacemaker evaluation, as instructed.

Literature published by pacemaker manufacturers and by the The British Heart Foundation* can be incorporated into teaching plans (Box 17-6) for people with per-manent pacemakers.

MAJOR HEALTH PROBLEMS OF THE HEART

Alterations in cardiovascular structure or function affect circulation and may therefore be life threatening. Disease of the heart and major blood vessels may be classified in a variety of ways such as congenital versus acquired, identification of the structure involved (valvular heart disease, myocarditis, endocarditis), aetiology of the disease (inadequate coronary artery blood flow, hypertensive cardiovascular disease, rheumatic heart disease), disruption of cardiac physiology (dysrhythmias), and disruption of cardiac function (heart failure, cardiogenic shock). The following common cardiac and aortic disorders are discussed in this chapter.

1. Interference with coronary blood flow: coronary artery disease (angina pectoris, myocardial infarction)
2. Failure of the heart as a pump: congestive heart failure, cardiogenic shock
3. Diseases of specific portions of the cardiac tissue: pericarditis, myocarditis, endocarditis
4. Diseases that are secondary to other diseases or conditions: cardiovascular syphilis, alcoholic cardiomyopathy, rheumatic heart disease, cocaine abuse
5. Inadequate valvular functioning: stenosis or insufficiency
6. Weakening of aortic wall: aortic aneurysms.

CORONARY ARTERY DISEASE

Pathophysiology

Coronary artery disease (CAD) refers to a variety of pathological conditions that obstruct blood flow through the arteries that supply the heart (Box 17-7). Atherosclerosis is the most common aetiological factor leading to coronary atherosclerotic heart disease (CAHD).

Atherosclerosis, the predominant type of arteriosclerosis in humans, is characterized by the accumulation of fatty materials (lipids) and fibrous tissue within the arterial walls. As these atherosclerotic changes progress, the lumen of the vessel becomes narrowed, and blood flow is obstructed to those areas of the myocardium supplied by the artery. Since this is a form of arteriosclerosis, the arterial wall also loses its elasticity and becomes less responsive to changes in blood volume and pressure.

Although several theories have been postulated to explain the pathogenesis of atherosclerosis, the aetiology of this condition remains unclear. Atherosclerotic lesions usually develop near the origin and bifurcation of the main coronary arteries. The left coronary artery is more often affected than the right coronary artery. The disease process is initially localized but then becomes diffuse with advancing coronary atherosclerosis.

The first lesion to form within the coronary arterial wall is called a fatty streak (Fig. 17-20). This lesion begins to appear in coronary vessels as early as 15 years of age. Lipid-filled cells, or "foam cells," invade the intimal wall

17-7	**Conditions that obstruct coronary blood supply**
	Atherosclerosis
	Arteriosclerosis
	Arteritis
	Coronary artery spasms
	Coronary thrombosis
	Embolism

and produce a fatty streak. As the disease progresses, raised thick fibrous plaques form and with increasing size limit the luminal capacity of the vessel. These lesions are typically characteristic of advancing atherosclerosis.

An even more advanced stage of atherosclerosis is represented by a calcified fibrous plaque or complicated lesion. This calcified deposit can rupture and hence greatly increase the risk of spasm, thrombus formation, and embolization. It is this final type of atherosclerotic lesion that gives rise to the symptoms of CAHD. The arterial lumen becomes so narrowed that a great imbalance exists between myocardial oxygen supply and myocardial oxygen demand. Manifestations of myocardial ischaemia do not usually occur until the artery is about 75% occluded. They include the following:

1. Angina pectoris
2. Myocardial infarction
3. Sudden death

Risk Factors

Extensive clinical research has identified several contributing factors that place an individual at risk for the development of coronary artery disease. The cumulative effect of these risk factors accelerates the atherosclerotic process. Risk factors are grouped into two basic categories: those that cannot be altered by the individual (nonmodifiable) and those that the individual has the capacity to change (modifiable) (Box 17-8).

17-8	**Risk factors for coronary artery disease**
	Nonmodifiable risk factors
	Age
	Sex
	Race
	Family history
	Modifiable risk factors
	Cigarette smoking
	Hyperlipidaemia
	Diabetes mellitus
	Hypertension
	Obesity
	Lack of exercise
	Stress
	Oral contraceptives

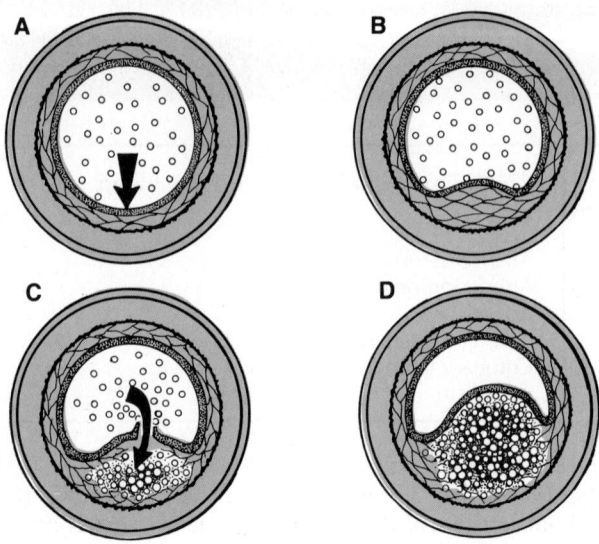

Fig. 17-20 Progressive development of coronary atherosclerosis. **A,** Injury to intimal wall. **B,** Lipoprotein invasion of smooth muscle cells. **C,** Development of fatty streak and fibrous plaque. **D,** Development of complicated lesion.

Nonmodifiable risk factors

Age

Both morbidity and mortality of coronary artery disease increase with age. Clinical symptomatology may be seen as early as the second decade of life, but the incidence of CAHD steadily rises in the 30- to 50-year age group. As reported by the Framingham Heart Study, 5% of all heart attacks occur in people under age 40, and 45% occur in people under age 65.[3] In essence, 50% of heart attacks occur in individuals over the age of 65. Although improvements in diet and reduction of other risk factors may alter this trend in the aged of the future, most people in this risk category today are a reflection of yesterday's poor health practices.[21]

Sex

Men are at a greater risk for the development of CAHD. Women are usually not affected by this disease until after menopause. The postmenopausal increase has been attributed to decreased levels of oestrogens and rising blood lipids. The incidence of CAHD in women has been rising, and it is now a leading cause of death in women as well as men.

Race

Black Americans have a higher risk for CAHD than do whites. One possible explanation for this finding is their increased incidence of hypertension (33% higher than in the white population).[3]

Family history

A familial tendency towards the development of CAHD has been demonstrated. The presence of coronary atherosclerosis in a parent or sibling under 50 years old is associated with the same finding in another family member. The extent to which genetic and environmental factors contribute to this disorder, however, is still not known.

Modifiable risk factors

Cigarette smoking

Cigarette smoking is a major contributing factor of CAHD. Cigarette smokers have a two to three times greater risk of death from CAHD than nonsmokers. This risk is related to the number of cigarettes smoked per day; the more cigarettes smoked, the greater the risk. Individuals who give up smoking are at less risk than smokers.

Although the exact relationship between cigarette smoking and coronary atherosclerosis is unclear, it is thought to be associated with the effects of nicotine and the higher content of carbon monoxide produced by the smoker. Nicotine increases myocardial workload and subsequent oxygen demand. Carbon monoxide interferes with oxygen transport. The combination of these two factors may place an inordinate demand on a diseased heart.

Hyperlipidaemia

Hyperlipidaemia refers to the elevation of cholesterol and triglyceride levels within the blood. Cholesterol can be obtained directly from animal dietary sources (see Chapter 4) or manufactured by the liver and intestine. Triglycerides are derived from fatty acids found in adipose tissue or the diet. Cholesterol and triglycerides are involved in the transportation, digestion, and absorption of fats.

Individuals with cholesterol levels in excess of 300mg/dl have four times the risk of CAHD of those with levels less than 200mg/dl. There is also clinical evidence that high levels of a specific type of lipid–protein complex, the *low-density lipoproteins*, are indicative of CAHD. These lipoproteins transport plasma lipids and contain approximately 50% cholesterol. In contrast, the high-density lipoproteins are thought to have an antiatherogenic effect.

A diet high in saturated fat, cholesterol, and calories is thought to be a major factor in the development of hyperlipidaemia. Dietary management, therefore, is an essential component in the prevention of this risk factor. Changes in long-established dietary patterns do not come easily, however. Awareness of the link between diet and the development of CAHD is frequently not sufficient motivation for modifications in diet that require a great deal of determination and creativity.

Diabetes mellitus

Individuals with diabetes mellitus are at much greater risk for CAHD. Coronary atherosclerosis has been found to be two to three times more prevalent in people with diabetes, regardless of blood lipid levels. The mechanisms by which impaired glucose tolerance increases the risk for CAHD is unclear. A predisposition to vascular degeneration has been noted in diabetics, and abnormal lipid metabolism may also play a role in the development of atheromas.[45] Adherence to a prescribed medical regimen for glucose regulation may diminish the effect of this risk factor and is within the realm of individual responsibility.

Hypertension

The relationship between high blood pressure and CAHD has been attributed to acceleration of the process that results in coronary atherosclerosis. In addition, increased peripheral vascular resistance associated with hypertension increases afterload and the demand on the left ventricle. The result is an increased demand for myocardial oxygen in the face of a diminished supply. The effects of hypertension are potentially modifiable through adherence to a medical regimen for control of systolic and diastolic blood pressure.

Obesity

Obesity or excess body weight in relation to height increases the workload and hence the oxygen demand of the heart. Its effect as a risk factor is questionable, although obesity highly correlates with hypertension, hyperlipidaemia, and diabetes. Specifically, obesity tends to be associated with increased caloric intake and elevated levels of low-density lipoproteins.

Lack of exercise

The lack of exercise has not been clearly linked to CAHD. It has been demonstrated, however, that exercise can improve the efficiency of the heart by the reduction of heart rate and blood pressure. Other physiological effects of regular exercise, such as decreased levels of low-density lipoproteins, lowered blood glucose levels, and improved cardiac output, have been associated with a lesser chance of CAHD. The psychological benefits of exercise, reduced anxiety and depression, may also be of significance.

Stress

The effect of stress on the pathogenesis of CAHD is controversial. Stress stimulates the cardiovascular system by the release of catecholamines, which in turn increase the heart rate and produce vasoconstriction. Stress also plays a major role in those individuals with type A behaviour. Behaviours including ambitiousness, aggressiveness, competitiveness, impatience, muscle tenseness, vigorous speech, and rapid pace in all activities are indicative of the type A behaviour pattern.[61] In early studies, people with type A personality characteristics were found to have twice the risk of developing CAHD compared with the type B personality, which has totally opposite characteristics. However, several recent prospective studies fail to confirm these earlier findings. In fact, it now appears that not only is the global type A behaviour pattern not a reliable indicator of subsequent development of CAHD, but some aspects of this behaviour pattern may even represent a positive and healthy coping pattern.[26]

Oral contraceptives

The use of oral contraceptives (birth control pills) has been associated with an increased risk of CAHD. The nature of the association is not clearly understood. It is possible that this risk factor acts synergistically with others.

ANGINA PECTORIS
Aetiology

Although angina pectoris is usually caused by atherosclerosis of the coronary vessels, the incidence is high in people with hypertension, diabetes mellitus, thromboangiitis obliterans, aortic regurgitation caused by rheumatic heart disease or syphilis, periarteritis nodosa, and polycythaemia vera. Other causes of anginal pain include aortic insufficiency, severe anaemia, and coronary arterial spasm. Typically, angina is triggered by cold, exercise, or anything that increases cardiac workload and myocardial oxygen consumption.

Pathophysiology

Angina pectoris or chest pain is a clinical syndrome produced by insufficient coronary blood flow. An imbalance exists between myocardial oxygen supply and myocardial oxygen demand, which creates transient myocardial ischaemia. The underlying mechanism to account for the experience of pain is probably related to the change from aerobic to anaerobic metabolism. By-products from anaerobic metabolism, specifically lactic acid, may initiate sensory receptors and cause pain. The release of other substances from the ischemic cells may also produce pain in this manner. Since the basic problem in angina is an imbalance between oxygen supply and demand, the primary goals of therapy are directed to the restoration of this balance (Table 17-1).

Two subcategories of angina should be distinguished from the classic condition. These are unstable angina and variant angina. A brief description of these forms of angina is presented here. For further information, consult a cardiology textbook.

Unstable angina

Unstable angina is also referred to as preinfarction angina, crescendo angina, or intermittent coronary syndrome. This type of angina is characterized by an increase in the severity, frequency, or duration of symptoms without infarction.

Variant angina

Variant angina, or Prinzmetal's angina, is thought to develop from intermittent coronary artery spasm with or without atherosclerotic heart disease. This type of anginal pain can occur during normal activities and is not necessarily precipitated by exercise or stress. Anginal pain in this condition often develops at the same time of day or night, demonstrating a cyclic pattern. Some people with variant angina may also have typical exertional angina.

Nursing Process
Assessment
Subjective data

Collect data concerning the person's knowledge about the disorder, presence of risk factors, and perception of the anginal pain. Specific data related to pain include the following:

1. Location and radiation to other sites: the pain is most often substernal or retrosternal. Pain may radiate to other sites (Fig. 17-21) or may occur *only* in one of those sites.
2. Quality of the pain: the pain is frequently described as a tightness or heaviness in the chest. Pressure, or a squeezing sensation, may also be part of the

Table 17-1   Coronary artery disorders

Disorder	Signs and symptoms	Medical therapy
Angina pectoris	Chest pain (substernal, retrosternal), may radiate to neck, jaw, arm, back; usually brought on by exertion, emotional upsets; relieved by rest, nitroglycerin	Avoidance of precipitating factors Reduction of modifiable risk factors Medications: nitrates, beta-adrenergic blocking agents, calcium channel blockers Oxygen therapy Electrocardiogram monitoring
Myocardial infarction	Severe, crushing chest pain; may radiate as with angina; not relieved with rest, nitroglycerin May be associated with dyspnoea, diaphoresis, apprehension, nausea	Relief of pain (O$_2$, morphine, other analgesics) Electrocardiogram monitoring Reduction of O$_2$ demand (rest) Prevention of complications (stool softeners, anticoagulants) Treatment of complications (dysrhythmias, congestive heart failure)

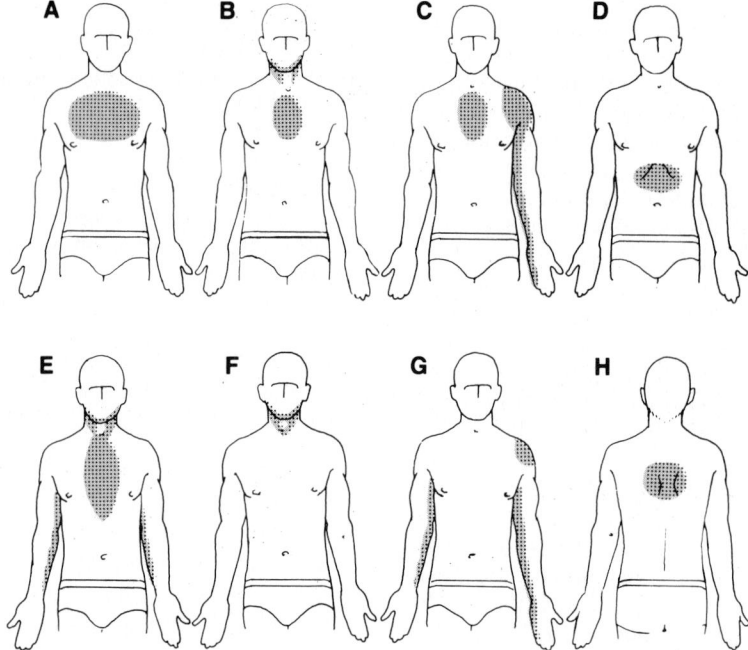

Fig.17-21   Sites where ischaemic myocardial pain may be referred. **A,** Upper chest. **B,** Beneath sternum radiating to neck and jaw. **C,** Beneath sternum radiating down left arm. **D,** Epigastric. **E,** Epigastric radiating to neck, jaw, and arms. **F,** Neck and jaw. **G,** Left shoulder, inner aspect of both arms. **H,** Intrascapular.

description. The person may complain only of a vague discomfort that is sometimes misinterpreted as indigestion. Angina is *not* usually described as a "sharp" pain.

3. Onset and duration of the pain: usually of brief duration.
4. Precipitating factors: often identified as exertion, exposure to extreme hot or cold, stress or emotional upset, or a heavy meal. *No* precipitating factor may be identified with variant angina.
5. Associated symptoms: apprehension, nausea, diaphoresis may be noted but are not common.
6. Relieving factors: angina is usually relieved by rest and/or nitroglycerin.

The nurse should be especially alert to reports of *change* in the frequency, severity, precipitating factors, or duration of anginal attacks, as these may be warnings of worsening ischaemia.

Objective data

1. Patient behaviour: note presence of diaphoresis, apprehension. People with angina are sometimes seen pressing a fist against the sternum during an attack.
2. Changes in vital signs: increases in pulse rate, blood pressure, and respiratory rate may be noted.
3. Changes in cardiac rhythm.
4. Pattern of anginal attacks with particular attention to changes.

Diagnostic tests

The diagnosis of ischaemic heart disease is frequently made on the basis of the patient's history. Diagnosis of angina may also be facilitated by carrying out an electrocardiograph (ECG) (p. 383), Holter monitor, coronary angiography, and stress testing.

Electrocardiogram

Characteristic findings of ischaemia, ST segment depression, and T wave inversion may be seen during chest pain. The absence of ECG changes does not exclude the diagnosis of ischaemia.

Holter monitor

A Holter monitor is a small portable ECG monitor about the size of a large transistor radio. In nonacute situations, a patient can be connected to this monitor to evaluate chest pain during performance of daily activities. Two wires are attached to the patient's chest and connected to the monitor. The patient wears the monitor for 24 hours, during which time the ECG tracing is recorded on tape and the patient maintains a log of daily activities, medications, and unusual sensations. Compare the log with the corresponding segment of the ECG tracing.

Coronary angiography

Selective coronary angiography may be carried out as part of a catheterization of the left side of the heart. Injection of contrast medium into the coronary arteries is followed by cineangiographical films to monitor the progression of the "dye." The contrast medium outlines the entire coronary circulation and enables the examiner to evaluate the anatomy of the coronary arteries, as well as note the location and nature of any lesions (that is, areas in which the arteries are narrowed or obstructed) and the presence of collateral circulation.

Stress testing

Stress testing or exercise electrocardiography is a noninvasive test used to evaluate cardiovascular response to controlled physical work loads. The indications for performing a stress test are identified in Box 17-9.

During stress testing, the patient pedals a stationary bicycle or walks on a treadmill. Throughout the testing, the patient's blood pressure and ECG are recorded. Conditions that require termination of the testing are listed in Box 17-10. The risk of developing a myocardial infarction is less than 1 in 500; the risk of death is less than 1 in 10,000.[8]

Adequate patient preparation is extremely important. The patient should do the following:

1. Get adequate rest the night before the test
2. Avoid coffee, tea, and alcohol on the day of the test
3. Avoid smoking and taking nitroglycerin during the two-hour period immediately before the test
4. Eat a light breakfast or lunch at least two hours before the test
5. Wear comfortable, loose-fitting clothes; women need to wear a bra for support
6. Wear sturdy, comfortable walking shoes

17-9

Indications for stress testing

Evaluate symptoms of coronary atherosclerotic heart disease (CAHD).
Determine physical work capacity and aerobic capacity.
Determine functional capacity following a myocardial infarction.
Determine limitations for exercise programming.
Evaluate dysrhythmias that develop during exercise.
Screen patients over age 40 and at risk for CAHD.
Evaluate effect of pharmacological agents on dysrhythmias and angina.

17-10

Conditions requiring termination of stress testing

Ventricular tachycardia
Marked decrease in peak systolic blood pressure
Marked decrease in heart rate
Vertigo
Frequent premature ventricular beats
Anginal pain
Severe dyspnoea
Severe anxiety
Diagnostic ST segment depression on electrocardiogram

---

7. Consult with the doctor regarding the taking of medications before the test (digoxin, propranolol, and vasodilators may affect the results of the stress test)
8. Inform the doctor if any unusual sensations develop during the test (for example, chest pain, dizziness)
9. Rest after the test; do *not* take a hot shower; a warm bath one or two hours after the test is permitted

Nursing analysis

Determine nursing analyses from assessment of patient data. Possible nursing analyses for the person with angina may include, but are not limited to, the following:

Problem	Possible aetiologies
Pain	Myocardial ischaemia, coronary artery occlusion, vasospasm, hypoxia, overactivity
Tissue perfusion, altered: cardiovascular	Hypertension, angina, coronary artery occlusion
Activity intolerance	Imbalance between oxygen supply and demand, sedentary lifestyle, immobility, pain, fatigue, generalized weakness
Anxiety	Threat or actual change in health status, diagnosis of pathology involving a major organ, threat to self-concept, threat of death
Knowledge deficit	Lack of exposure/recall, information misinterpretation, unfamiliarity with information resources, cognitive limitation, lack of interest

Planning: expected patient outcomes

Expected patient outcomes for the person with angina may include, but are not limited to, the following:

1. States feeling more comfortable.
2. Demonstrates cardiac tolerance to increased activity (stable pulse and blood pressure).
3. Identifies factors that reduce activity tolerance and progresses to highest level of mobility possible.
4. Uses effective coping mechanisms in managing anxiety.
5. Identifies factors that increase cardiac workload.
6. Describes the following:
   a. Disease process, causes, variables contributing to symptoms, and interventions for disease or symptom control
   b. Events that may precipitate anginal attacks
   c. Medical regimen
   d. Plans to participate in a regular exercise programme
   e. Rationale for and type of surgery to be performed, if surgery is indicated
   f. Plans for medical follow-up

Implementation

Assisting with achievement of therapeutic goals

The major medical therapy is pharmacological. Medications are prescribed to dilate coronary arteries and decrease the workload on the heart. The drugs include the following:

1. Nitrates (glyceryl trinitrate, and isosorbide dinitrate): given to dilate coronary arteries and collateral vessels of the heart and to dilate peripheral vessels, especially the veins.
2. Beta-adrenergic blocking agents (propranolol, nadolol, metoprolol, and atenolol): lower oxygen demands during exercise, improve the oxygen supply/demand balance, and lower heart rate and blood pressure. Beta-blockers should be withdrawn gradually.
3. Calcium channel blockers (nifedipine, diltiazem, verapamil): decrease heart rate and improve oxygen supply by dilating coronary arteries.

If angina is present, give glyceryl trinitrate sublingually. Repeat dosage in five minutes if pain does not subside. Repeat two or three times at five-minute intervals.

Other activities include the following:

1. Monitor for dysrhythmias.
2. Administer oxygen per nasal cannula as prescribed.
3. Monitor effects of daily activities on cardiac status, occurrence of dysrhythmias, and need for oxygen.

Interventions to achieve patient outcomes

Promoting comfort

Reduce or remove any known factors (physiological or psychological) that are contributing to increased pain. Assess for causes of decreased pain tolerance, such as anxiety, fatigue, or lack of knowledge. Fatigue from increased oxygen demands with a decreased oxygen supply increases pain perception. Therefore take measures to reduce fatigue, such as providing rest periods if fatigue is present during physical activities. Provide a calm environment to decrease stress and anxiety that can increase the pain experience. Give nitroglycerin if angina is present.

Promoting tissue perfusion

Instruct patient to avoid becoming overly fatigued and to stop activity immediately in the presence of chest pain, dyspnoea, faintness, or light-headedness, which indicate low tissue perfusion. Decreased tissue perfusion causes cellular hypoxia with subsequent ischaemia, cellular swelling, and cellular death.

Promoting activity and rest

Enhance the patient's activity tolerance by encouraging slower activity or shorter periods of activity with more rest periods. Pulse increases of 50 per minute occur with strenuous activity; this rate is safe provided it returns to the resting pulse within three minutes. Most people with angina pectoris can tolerate mild exercise such as walking and playing golf, but exertion such as running or climbing stairs rapidly causes pain. Anginal pain occurs more easily in cold weather. Some people may have to take nitroglycerin prophylactically before they engage in exercise or sexual activity, but the key to healthful activity is to avoid overexertion.

Promoting relief of anxiety and feeling of wellbeing

Help the patient reduce the level of anxiety. Because excessive emotional strain also causes vasoconstriction by releasing adrenaline into circulation, the patient should minimize emotional outbursts, worry, and tension. People with angina may need continuing help in accepting situations as they find them. See Chapter 5 for approaches to assist people to cope with stress and anxiety.

Teaching patient/family

Delay teaching until the individual is ready. The patient needs to be relatively free of pain and excessive anxiety in order to learn. Promote a positive attitude and active participation of patient and family to encourage compliance. The teaching plan includes information about medications, approaches to minimize precipitating events, effects of exercise on reduction of myocardial oxygen needs, and the need for regular medical follow-up (Box 17-11).

Evaluation

Evaluation will be based on expected patient outcomes. Questions to ask may include the following:

1. Is patient able to control pain by use of prescribed medication?
2. Can patient describe ways to minimize events that may precipitate anginal pain?
3. Is patient engaged or planning to engage in a regular exercise programme?
4. Does the patient use effective coping mechanisms to manage anxiety?
5. Does the patient know action, usage, and side effects of prescribed medications?
6. Does the patient know CAHD risk factors that can be modified?

MYOCARDIAL INFARCTION
Aetiology

Acute myocardial infarction (AMI) is caused by sudden blockage of one of the branches of a coronary artery. It

Patient Teaching   17-11

The patient with angina pectoris

Use of nitrate medications
  Use glyceryl trinitrate prophylactically to avoid pain known to occur with certain acivities
  Burning sensation on tongue indicates nitroglycerin is activated
  Throbbing sensation in head and flushing may occur
  Sit and stand slowly after taking nitroglycerin
  Place glyceryl trinitrate tablets under the tongue at the onset of anginal pain; second tablet can be taken after 5 minutes and third tablet after another 5 minutes if pain is unrelieved
  Call doctor if pain does not subside after third tablet; go to nearest casualty department; do not drive yourself
  Always carry glyceryl trinitrate
  Store glyceryl trinitrate in dark bottle and keep in dry place
  Replenish glyceryl trinitrate supply every 6 months or before expiration date
  Remove all old nitrate ointment just before application of new cream
Ways to minimize percipitating events
  Avoid overexertion
  Try to reduce stress and anxiety, which cause blood vessels to constrict
  Avoid overeating, as it places an increased work load on the heart
  Avoid cold weather (constricts coronary vessels to conserve body heat, hence anginal pain can develop more easily)
  Dress warmly in cold weather
  Avoid hot, humid conditions (increases work load of heart)
  Walk downhill with wind since walking uphill and against wind increase work load of heart
Effects of exercise programme in reduction of myocardial oxygen needs
  Engage in regular exercise programme
  Exercise conditions heart muscle and can decrease oxygen demand during exercise
  Space exercise period with rest periods
  Take glyceryl trinitrate before exertion
Need for regular medical follow-up

may be extensive enough to interfere with cardiac function and cause immediate death, or it may cause necrosis of a portion of the myocardium with subsequent healing by scar formation or fibrosis. Coronary occlusion is a general term for blockage of a coronary artery. The blockage may be caused by formation of a thrombus in the coronary artery (coronary thrombosis), sudden progression of atherosclerotic changes, or prolonged constriction of the arteries.

Pathophysiology

Prolonged ischaemia lasting more than 35 to 45 minutes produces irreversible cellular damage and necrosis. The contractile properties of cardiac muscle within the necrotic areas become permanently impaired (Fig. 17-22). The final extent of the infarct depends on the ability of the sur-

rounding ischaemic tissues to recruit collateral circulation. Collateral circulation is the development of new vessels within the heart to compensate for the damaged artery.

The clinical features of a myocardial infarct are determined by the site and extent of the disease process. An occlusion in the *left anterior descending* coronary artery (LAD) typically results in an *anterior wall infarction*. Depending on the exact site of the occlusion, the area involved may be limited or massive. Substantial loss of left ventricular muscle mass is associated with severe haemodynamic consequences.

An occlusion in the *right* coronary artery (RCA) may result in an *inferior* or *posterior* wall infarction. Although the loss of muscle mass may not be as extensive as in anterior infarctions, the person with an inferior infarction may be predisposed to dysrhythmias and conduction defects because of the proximity of the RCA to the conduction system. A lateral wall infarction is usually caused by an occlusion of the *left circumflex* coronary artery. The signs and symptoms and medical therapies to curtail the complications of myocardial infarction are outlined in Table 17-1 (p. 396).

Nursing Process
Assessment
Subjective data

Myocardial infarction (MI) can be equated with irreversible myocardial ischaemia; hence many of the associated signs and symptoms are similar to those found with angina. Typically the symptoms are more severe and of longer duration than the person's usual angina attacks, although they may occur in a person who has never previously complained of angina. Symptoms are absent or unreported in about 15% of all myocardial infarctions. Data to be collected include the following:

1. Patient's perception of the pain
   a. Location and radiation to other sites (see Fig. 17-21)
   b. Quality of the pain: often described as crushing or vice-like; often more severe than angina
   c. Onset and duration of pain: may be of sudden onset or may build up over a period of a few minutes; duration is longer than angina—may be several minutes to several hours
   d. Precipitating factors: often occurs with intense emotion or exertion but may also occur at rest
   e. Relieving factors: not relieved by rest, nitroglycerin, changes in body position.
2. Associated symptoms: may include nausea, dyspnoea, dizziness, weakness, and a sense of impending doom.

Ojective data

1. Behaviour: often very apprehensive
2. Changes in vital signs: pulse rate may increase in response to pain or diminished cardiac output; may decrease if conduction defects develop; blood pressure may decrease if the extent of myocardial damage is significant; vital sign changes in elderly people are noted in the box entitled "The elderly with cardiovascular problems."

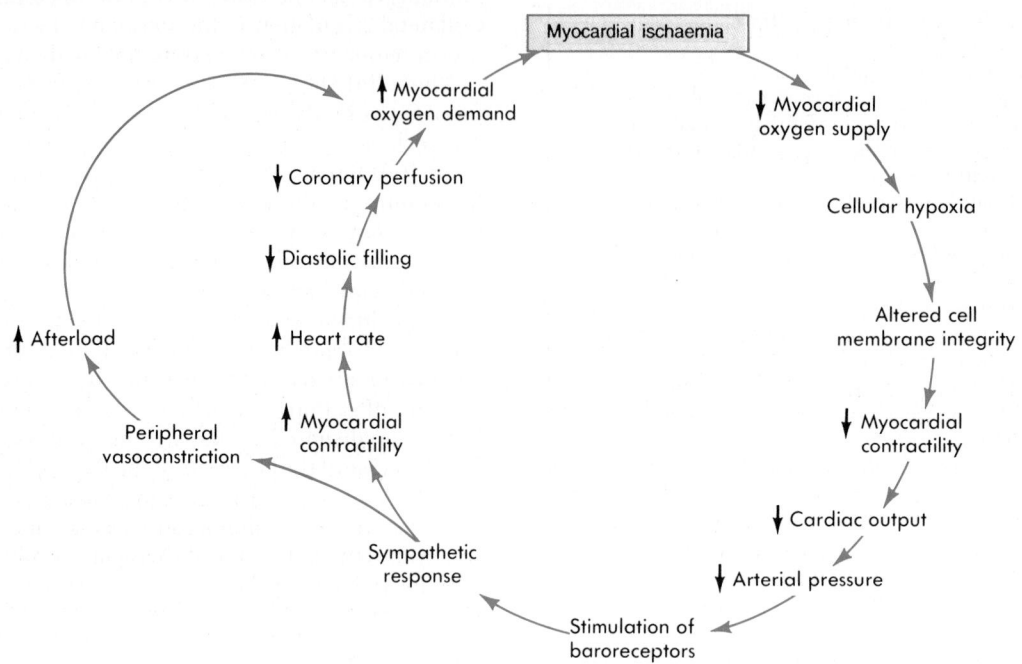

Fig. 17-22   Effects of prolonged myocardial ischaemia.

3. Associated signs: may include diaphoresis, vomiting, pallor, cold clammy skin, cardiac dysrhythmias, laboured respirations
4. Breath sounds: no change may be noted, but if pulmonary oedema develops, rales will be present
5. Presence of risk factors

Diagnostic tests

Although the clinical picture of severe crushing chest pain, pallor, diaphoresis, and apprehension or a sense of impending doom is the classic description of a person having a myocardial infarction, it by no means describes *all* infarction patients. About 15% of myocardial infarctions occur without the characteristic signs and symptoms (called "silent infarctions"), and individual variation in the symptoms is to be expected. A variety of diagnostic tests are used, therefore, to verify the diagnosis. These tests include blood tests that detect both nonspecific and specific changes caused by the infarction, an ECG, radiological tests, and scintigraphical studies.

Blood tests

A nonspecific reaction to myocardial injury is an elevation in white blood cell count (12,000 to 15,000/mm³). This increase begins a few hours after the onset of pain and lasts for three to seven days. In general, high white blood cell counts are associated with larger infarcts. Also, the erythrocyte sedimentation rate (ESR) rises during the first week after the infarction and remains elevated for several weeks.

Serum enzymes. As infarcted cardiac muscle cells die, cellular components are released into the vascular system. Some of these components are enzymes that can be

evaluated by blood levels. Creatine phosphokinase (CPK), serum glutamic-oxaloacetic transaminase (SGOT) (also termed serum aspartate amino-transferase [AST]) and lactic dehydrogenase (LDH) are found to be elevated at varying times following a myocardial infarction (Fig. 17-23).

Since these enzymes are not exclusively found in the heart, measurements of enzyme fractions or *isoenzymes* are more diagnostic of myocardial insult. Isoenzymes levels of CPK are the most reliable indicators of cardiac damage. The CPK isoenzyme that contains the mycardial band (MB) subunits, CPK (MB)₁, is elevated for 48 hours after a transmural infarction. Lactic dehydrogenases can be fractionated into five distinct isoenzymes. Of these, LDH₁ and LDH₂ are most important: LDH₂ is found more abundantly in serum, whereas heart muscle is rich in LDH₁. An elevation in serum LDH₁, therefore, is confirmation of a myocardial infarction.

Electrocardiogram

Characteristic findings of infarction include ST segment elevation in leads overlying the infarcted area (an early finding) and the development of pathological Q waves (a later finding). As the infarction "evolves," the ST segments return to baseline and the T waves become inverted. The electrocardiogram is considered to be one of the most reliable tools for diagnosing a myocardial infarction, but occasionally the "typical" changes do not develop, and serum enzymes must be relied upon to a greater extent.

Radiological tests

An X-ray film of the chest may be taken to determine overall size and configuration of the heart as well as individual cardiac chamber size. Most abnormalities of

Enzyme	Onset (h)	Peak (h)	Duration (d)
Creatine phosphokinase (CPK)	3–6	12–18	3–4
Serum glutamic-oxaloacetic transaminase (SGOT).	4–6	24–36	4–7
Lactic dehydrogenase (LDH)	12	48	10–14

Fig. 17-23 Patterns of serum enzyme levels following myocardial infarction.

heart size can be detected with a standard posteroanterior and lateral view of the chest. Calcifications in the large blood vessels, heart muscle, valves, and pericardium can also be visualized.

Cardiac fluoroscopy facilitates observation of the heart from varying views while the heart is in motion. Fluoroscopy can be used to detect ventricular aneurysms, which appear as a paradoxical bulging during systole.

Scintigraphical studies

Myocardial imaging. Myocardial imaging is a noninvasive procedure that aids in evaluating the myocardium and coronary arteries. The two most commonly used techniques are pyrophosphate scanning and thallium scanning. Even though these scans involve radioactive materials, they are safe for patients and hospital personnel.

Echocardiograph. Echocardiography is an examination of the structures and movements of the heart by means of reflected pulsed ultrasound. As a noninvasive investigation employing nonionizing energy, echocardiography has become established as a useful additional method of evaluating almost all forms of heart disease. It is of particular value in pericardial effusion, in mitral valve lesions, and in hypertrophic obstructive cardiomyopathy.

Thallium scanning. Thallium 201 is an intracellular ion that is actively transported into normal cells. If the cell is ischaemic or infarcted, the thallium will not be picked up, and a "cold spot" image is produced. This radioisotope is injected intravenously with the patient at rest or during stress testing.

Multiple-gated acquisition scanning. Another way of imaging myocardial function is with a *dynamic* scan to assess cardiac wall motion and global left and right ventricular function. Multiple-gated acquisition cardiac blood pool imaging (MUGA scanning) can demonstrate cardiac wall motion, which permits assessment of injury as well as capacity of cardiac function.

A small amount of technetium 99m (attached to human serum albumin or to autologous red blood cells) is injected intravenously. MUGA scanning reflects mild injury of the cardiac wall as hypokinesia versus a more severe disturbance producing akinesia or dyskinesia. It also reveals other important events, such as right ventricular infarction and aneurysm formation. In addition, it permits evaluation of

---

The Elderly with Cardiovascular Problems

Assessment

Count the pulse for a full minute at rest and after exertion. The pulse is often slower and may be irregular because elderly are more prone to decreased cardiac output and dysrhythmias.

Monitor changes in blood pressure:

Systolic blood pressure in elderly may normally be as high as 160mm Hg (as compared with 140mm Hg in younger adults). A widened pulse pressure may also be observed.

Check blood pressure in a lying, sitting, and standing position to detect postural hypotension because vasomotor control is decreased in the elderly.

When assessing the heart, the apical impulse may be harder to locate. Murmurs are common from thickening and calcification of the valves.

Monitor for signs of mental confusion, lethargy, indigestion, and weakness in the elderly person; these may be early signs of cardiac disease. Angina is commonly noted with ischaemic heart disease.

Assess elderly patient with myocardial infarction for signs of congestive heart failure, a common complication.

Intervention

Prevent falls in elderly that may be associated with bradycardia, postural hypotension, or myocardial infarction.

Teach the elderly to move and stand slowly to prevent falling because of hypotension (drop attacks).

Teach the patient who is taking diuretics or antihypertensives to move slowly and cautiously.

Teach the elderly to avoid standing for long periods (blood pooling), especially over a hot stove or in the shower (heat causes vasodilation thus lowering blood pressure).

Teach the foot-pumping exercises, which are performed before rising from bed or chair, to increase venous return.

Teach patient and significant others to seek early medical attention for unexplained illness, unrelieved indigestion, or sudden changes in behaviour.

Common disorders in elderly

Congestive heart failure
Angina pectoris
Myocardial infarction
Dysrhythmias

---

the effects of pharmacotherapeutics (for example, nitroglycerin, vasodilators) on ventricular function.

Positron emission tomography. Positron emission tomography is a radionuclide-based imaging technique that uses short-lived radionuclides as tracers to report perfusion and metabolic events. These tracers are generally given by intravenous injection or inhalation and only occasionally by intraarterial injection. The trace elements readily pass through the tissues. Under normal circumstances, the well-perfused, aerobically metabolizing myocardium prefers free fatty acids for energy production from oxidative metabolism. When ischaemia is present, more glucose and less fatty acid tends to be utilized.

Nursing analysis

Nursing analyses are determined from the assessment of patient data. Possible nursing analyses for the people with myocardial infarction may include, but are not limited to, the following:

Problem	Possible aetiologies
Pain: chest	Persistent myocardial ischaemia, hypoxia, immobility, overactivity, diagnostic tests, improper positioning
Tissue perfusion, altered: cardiovascular	Decreased cardiac output, pulmonary oedema, congestive heart failure, angina, vasospasm or vasoconstriction
Cardiac output, decreased	Reduced stroke volume, cardiogenic shock, bradycardia, tachycardia
Constipation	Immobility in postinfarction period, opiate pain medication

Problem	Possible aetiologies
Activity intolerance	Imbalance between oxygen supply and demand, immobility, angina, sedentary lifestyle
Anxiety	Change in health status, threat of death, threat to self-concept, situational crisis
Knowledge deficit	Lack of exposure/recall, information misinterpretation, ineffective coping patterns

Planning: expected patient outcomes

Expected outcomes for the people with myocardial infarction may include, but are not limited to, the following:
1. States feeling more comfortable
2. Demonstrates cardiac tolerance to activity (stable pulse and blood pressure)
3. Identifies factors that increase cardiac workload
4. States breathing is easier and fatigue is decreased
5. Stools are soft and formed
6. Identifies factors that reduce activity tolerance in a programme of progressive activity
7. Participates in a programme of progressive activity
8. Uses effective coping mechanisms in managing anxiety
9. Describes the following:
    a. Nature of myocardial infarction and how the healing process relates to the treatment regimen
    b. Variables contributing to symptoms and interventions for disease or symptom control
    c. Risk factors that can be modified and plans to alter lifestyle
    d. Plans to participate in a regular exercise programme
    e. Rationale for and type of surgery, if indicated
    f. Any dietary restrictions
    g. Plans for ongoing medical care

Implementation
Assisting with achievement of therapeutic goals

Medical interventions include promoting oxygenation of the tissues, relieving pain, preventing further tissue damage, promoting improved coronary circulation, and preventing complications. Analgesic drugs, such as morphine sulphate, can be administered for the relief of pain. Myocardial tissue oxygenation can be improved with supplemental oxygen. When relaxation occurs with pain relief and with improved tissue oxygenation, cardiac workload is reduced. Cardiac monitoring is used to detect the occurrence of dysrhythmias.

When complications are inevitable, the therapeutic aims are early detection and control. Healing of the myocardium is a natural process that is promoted by rest and reduction of myocardial oxygen demands. The trend towards early ambulation under carefully monitored conditions has reduced the incidence of complications, such as thromboembolic phenomena and psychological manifestations of depression and hopelessness, which were largely related to a prolonged period of immobility.

In recent years, considerable attention has been directed toward therapies that limit the size of the infarcted area and prevent further tissue injury. One approach to this goal is reperfusion of the occluded coronary artery. To be effective, reperfusion must be attained within three to five hours following the onset of symptoms. Administration of fibrinolytic agents either systemically or directly into the coronary arteries activates mechanisms that lyse existing blood clots. Streptokinase, urokinase, alteplase, and anistreplase are currently used in reperfusion therapy. The use of laser angioplasty may also promote reperfusion and has the advantage of acting locally rather than initiating a more widespread fibrinolytic response.[45,49,52] Beta-adrenergic blocking agents reestablish the balance between myocardial oxygen supply and demand.

Nursing interventions include the following:
1. Administer medications as prescribed:
    a. Intravenous lignocaine is usually given prophylactically to prevent ventricular fibrillation
    b. Anticoagulants (heparin or warfarin) may be prescribed to decrease incidence of thrombophlebitis and pulmonary embolism
    c. *Avoid giving intramuscular injections* because these alter serum enzyme levels
2. Monitor for signs of complications of myocardial infarction (See relevant sections in this chapter for an expanded discussion of these conditions.):
    a. Congestive heart failure (crackles, tachycardia and tachypnoea, dyspnoea and increased respiratory effort, S_3 heart sound, weight gain, oliguria)
    b. Thromboembolic phenomena (pain in chest or legs)
    c. Pericarditis
    d. Mitral insufficiency
    e. Cardiogenic shock (decreased blood pressure, tachycardia, cold clammy skin, mental confusion, severe oliguria)
3. Maintain patient on prescribed low-cholesterol, low-salt diet without caffeine-containing beverages

Interventions to achieve patient outcomes
Promoting comfort

Perception of pain and discomfort by an individual is highly variable. After vascular access is established, morphine sulphate may be administered for relief of pain and apprehension and to produce vasodilation. Continued episodes of chest pain may be related to infarct size, insufficient collateral circulation, and increased myocardial consumption. Provisions for comfort and rest are essential to reduce sympathetic stimulation and subsequent myocardial oxygen demand.

Promoting tissue perfusion

Decreased tissue perfusion causes cellular hypoxia with subsequent ischaemia, cellular swelling, and cellular death. Instruct the patient to avoid excessive fatigue and to stop activity immediately in the presence of chest pain, dyspnoea, light-headedness, or faintness. Administer oxygen for 24 to 48 hours and longer if persistent pain, hypotension, dyspnoea, or dysrhythmias occur.

Promoting adequate cardiac output

1. Monitor the patient for the following parameters:
   a. Dysrhythmias on ECG tracings
   b. Vital signs
   c. Effects of daily activities on cardiac status, as evidenced by occurrence of dysrhythmias and need for oxygen
   d. Signs of fluid overload and electrolyte imbalance
2. Document rate and rhythm of pulse.
3. Administer pharmacotherapy, as prescribed.
4. Plan nursing strategies to promote rest and minimize unnecessary disturbances.

Promoting elimination

Constipation is common from the effects of narcotics and decreased activity; a stool softener is usually prescribed. Avoid using bedpans and straining at stool because Valsalva's manoeuvre causes changes in blood pressure and heart rate, which may trigger ischaemia, dysrhythmias, pulmonary embolus, or cardiac arrest.

Providing rest

The patient is usually placed on bedrest and ask to use a commode for 24 to 48 hours. Assist with activities of daily living during this period. Sedation with diazepam or an equivalent may be prescribed to relieve anxiety and restlessness and to promote sleep.

Promoting activity

After the first 24 to 48 hours, patients are usually encouraged to increase their activity gradually, depending on the extent of the infarction. During this period, the person is continually monitored for signs of dysrhythmias, presence of cardiac pain, and changes in vital signs.

Promoting relief of anxiety and feeling of wellbeing

During hospitalization, many patients experience denial, depression, and anxiety. Depression may occur several days later and may continue after the patient is discharged. Generally, patients tend to become more anxious on the second day of hospitalization after the immediate threat of death from infarction has passed. Anxiety varies in intensity contingent on the severity of the threat as perceived by the individual, as well as the person's success in coping. Most people who have a myocardial infarction, however, adjust extremely well. Over 85% of all patients with uncomplicated myocardial infarctions are able to return to work. This, along with resuming normal sexual functioning, aids tremendously in the adjustment process. Provide the patient and family with opportunities to explore their concerns and to explore alternative methods of coping, if appropriate.

Promoting patient/family learning

Education of the patient and family enables them to assume a more active role in the patient's healthcare. A great deal of anxiety and apprehension can be allayed by providing information about the cardiac condition and its management. Major points for teaching are outlined in Box 17-12.

The patients and their partners may need teaching and reassurance regarding resuming *sexual activities*. Many feel that their sex life is over after a myocardial infarction. Education should aim at supplying information and dispelling misinformation. Once patients with an uncomplicated myocardial infarction are capable of walking two flights of stairs without difficulty, they are generally able to perform sexual intercourse safely. Approximately 80% of all postcoronary patients will be able to resume sexual activity without serious risk. The other 20% need not totally abstain, but their sexual activity should be limited according to their cardiac capacity.

Evaluation

Evaluation will be based on the expected patient outcomes. Questions to consider include the following:
1. Was chest pain decreased?
2. Was need for additional oxygen decreased?
3. Are stools soft and formed?
4. Is activity tolerance increasing as evidenced by absence of fatigue, dyspnoea, or discomfort with increasing activity?
5. Does the patient use effective coping mechanisms to manage anxiety?
6. Does the patient know the nature of the disorder, ways to decrease possibility of further ischaemic attacks, activity prescription?
7. Has the patient made plans for follow-up medical care?

CARDIAC SURGERY FOR MYOCARDIAL ISCHAEMIA

Surgical intervention is often necessary for patients with severe myocardial ischaemia that is uncontrolled by medical therapy. Recommendation for surgery is based on the assessment of the expected benefits of the procedure and the inherent surgical risks. Patients with cardiomegaly, severe congestive heart failure, recent myocardial infarction, high left ventricular end-diastolic pressure, and an inadequate ejection fraction are at higher risk.

The patient with myocardial infarction

Effect of myocardial infarction, the healing process, and treatment regimen

Effect of medications in the treatment of myocardial infarction

Association between risk factors and coronary artery disease

Indentify nonmodifiable risk factors

Identify modifiable risk factors (especially cigarette smoking)

Effect of dietary restrictions on coronary atherosclerosis heart disease: low salt, low cholesterol, no caffeine, fluid restrictions

Effect of activity on heart and need to participate in a progressive activity plan

Resumption of sexual activity (if appropriate)

Abstention of sexual intercourse as directed, usually for 4–6 weeks (sexual closeness, for example, cuddling may be started earlier as desired)

Reporting to doctor the following symptoms occuring during or following intercourse

Dyspnoea or increased heart rate continuing for more than 15 minutes after intercourse

Extreme fatigue

Chest pain during intercourse

Palpitations for more than 15 minutes after intercourse

Insomnia after intercourse

Coronary Artery Bypass Graft

Surgical correction of myocardial ischaemia is usually done through a bypass procedure in which a graft is sutured above and below the area of blockage in the coronary artery. Any number of bypasses can be performed, depending on the location and extent of the blockages. Blood flow to the ischaemic areas of the heart is then conducted through the new grafts, thus "bypassing" the obstruction.

Bypass grafts are obtained from sections of the saphenous vein or the internal mammary artery. The saphenous vein is harvested from the inner thigh and sectioned. Removal of this vein does not compromise circulation in the leg, since there are numerous other vessels to assist in this function.

The heart is exposed through a median sternotomy or anterolateral thoracotomy; retractors are used to spread the chest wall. Saphenous vein sections are grafted from the aorta to the point beyond the blockage. The internal mammary artery remains attached proximally to the subclavian artery. The distal portion is grafted to the coronary artery beyond the occlusion. Cardiopulmonary bypass is often used during cardiac surgery to allow the surgeon easier access to the operative site while maintaining perfusion of vital organs.

Cardiopulmonary bypass

Most heart surgeries require partial or total cardiopulmonary bypass. In *partial* bypass, pulmonary circulation is not interrupted. Oxygenated blood is drained from the left side of the heart, passed through a pulsatile pump, and returned through the descending aorta or common femoral artery. *Total* cardiopulmonary bypass involves both circulation and oxygenation of the extracted blood. Cannulas are placed in the right atrium to drain venous blood. The machine oxygenates this blood and pumps it back into the ascending aorta or femoral artery.

Besides the capability of the heart–lung machine to provide extracorporeal circulation, it also serves as a direct route for medication administration and systemic hypothermia. Cooling of the machine solutions and subsequent body cooling lowers oxygen consumption by decreasing cellular metabolism.

Types of equipment

Many types of equipment are used during cardiac surgery. Some of these and their uses are described in the following list:

1. Endotracheal tube, ventilator: to maintain open airway, ventilation, and access to secretions
2. Cardiac monitor: to identify dysrhythmias
3. Intravenous line: to replace fluids, monitor central venous pressure, administer medications
4. Arterial line: to monitor blood pressure, obtain arterial blood samples
5. Pulmonary artery catheter (Swan Ganz): to monitor pulmonary artery pressure, capillary wedge pressure, and cardiac output
6. Chest tube: to drain blood and air from chest
7. Epicardial pacing wires: to facilitate temporary cardiac pacing, if necessary
8. Urinary catheter: to monitor fluid status

Preoperative care

Preoperative care consists of (1) altering medications, (2) preparing the operative site, and (3) providing patient teaching. Digitalis preparations are discontinued on the day of surgery. Diuretics are also withheld so that the patient is adequately hydrated. Anticoagulants (warfarin, heparin) and other medications with anticoagulant effects (aspirin) are discontinued 48 hours before surgery.

In preparing the operative site, the patient showers with a special antimicrobial soap on the night before surgery. The chest and abdomen are shaved from neck to groin and from the left to the right midaxillary lines. If saphenous veins are needed for grafting, the inner aspects of the legs are also shaved.

Preoperative teaching is essential for a patient undergoing cardiac surgery. Involvement of the patient's family or significant others is also of importance in preparing the patient for surgery. The initial preoperative teaching is frequently done by nurses from the surgical intensive care unit. All nurses caring for the patient should be familiar with the content, however, so they may reinforce major points, be alert to areas of special concern, and answer questions posed by patients and family members. An outline of content specific to coronary bypass surgery is summarized in Box 17-13.

Postoperative care

Postoperative care includes the following goals: promotion of oxygenation and comfort, maintenance of fluid and elec-

Patient Teaching 17-13

The patient undergoing coronary artery bypass surgery

Simple explanation of anatomy of heart, function of coronary arteries, and effect of coronary atherosclerosis heart disease (use of heart drawings and models is helpful)

Explanation of surgery
  Removal of saphenous vein or use of internal mammary artery
  Effect on cardiac function

Definition of terms: *bypass, graft*

Explanation of events on day of surgery
  Preoperative medications
  Length of time in surgery (depends on number of arteries to be bypassed)
  Length of time until able to see family (usually 1.5–2 hours after surgery)

Explanation of the intensive-care unit
  Description of physical facilities and layout
  Nurse will be available at all times
  Visiting hours for family
  Length of stay in unit (2–3 days)

Explanation of monitors
  Round patches on chest connected to cardiac monitor
  Beeping sounds from monitors may be heard

Explanation of lines
  Intravenous routes for fluid and medications
  Central venous line in chest or groin to monitor fluid status
  Pulmonary artery line in chest or neck to measure pulmonary pressure
  Plastic connector line to obtain blood samples without a needle prick

Explanation of drainage tubes
  Catheter draining urine from bladder
  Chest tube draining bloody fluid from incision (usually removed day after surgery)

Explanation of breathing tube
  Tube in windpipe connected to machine called ventilator
  Tube prevents speech (can mouth words or write notes to communicate)
  Tube removed when patient is fully awake and stable
  Secretions in lungs or tube removed by nurse using a suction catheter

Explanation and demonstration of activity and exercises
  Purpose of activity and exercises is to promote circulation, keep lungs clear, and prevent infection
  Activity will include:
    Turning from side to side in bed
    Sitting on edge of bed on night of surgery
    Sitting in chair night or morning after surgery
  Range of motion exercises to arms and legs
  Effective deep breathing (use of sustained maximal inspiration, holding breath for 3–5 seconds at end of deep inspiration)
  Use of incentive spirometer (similar technique used to take deep breath)

Relief of pain
  Pain will be present at chest incision and leg incision
  Frequent pain medication will be given, but patient should always tell nurse when pain is present

Explanation of diet
  Will receive iced water to sip after removal of breathing tube
  Clear liquids with gradual progression to regular diet

---

trolyte balance, and prevention or early detection of complications (thrombophlebitis, pulmonary embolus, cardiac tamponade, cardiac dysrhythmias, and cardiac failure).

Promoting oxygenation

1. Ventilate with supplemental oxygen
2. Turn from side to side
3. Keep head of bed elevated at least 10 to 20 degrees
4. Assess quality of breath sounds
5. Monitor arterial blood gases
6. Encourage performance of range of motion exercises
7. Encourage progressive activity level
8. Daily chest X-ray films will be obtained
9. Monitor patency and drainage from chest tube
10. Assist with deep breathing, coughing, and use of incentive spirometer

Maintaining fluid and electrolyte balance

Give crystalloid fluids intravenously to maintain adequate circulating blood volume. Administration of colloids (whole blood, packed cells, plasma, or plasma expanders) depends on the haemoglobin and total protein concentrations. Potassium is frequently required after heart surgery, and the patient is monitored for signs of hypokalaemia. Nursing activities include the following:

1. Maintain prescribed flow rate of parenteral fluids
2. Maintain patency of chest tube and urinary catheter
3. Record amount of drainage accurately
4. Assess for signs of fluid loss (dry skin, dry mucous membranes, decreased skin turgor) and fluid overload (peripheral oedema, neck vein distention, moist respirations)
5. Monitor central venous pressure (CVP) readings
6. Monitor daily weight
7. Assess serum electrolytes (especially potassium) and haematocrit
8. Monitor pulmonary artery parameters: pulmonary artery pressure, pulmonary capillary wedge pressure

Promoting comfort

1. Administer narcotic analgesics (morphine sulphate or pethidine) every three hours during first 24 hours, then as needed
2. Provide frequent mouth care until patient is taking fluids regularly

3. Eliminate unnecessary environmental stimuli (noise, lights) that impair ability to rest/sleep
4. Provide backrub for backache
5. Change linens if profuse nights sweats occur; assure patient that this commonly occurs
6. Group daily activities to allow for periods of uninterrupted rest/sleep
7. Encourage use of splinting devices (pillow, blanket) during coughing
8. Provide explanations for activities, as necessary
9. Monitor patient for changes in behaviour and encourage patient to express concerns

Preventing/detecting complications

1. Thrombophlebitis/pulmonary embolism
   a. Encourage leg exercises until patient is ambulatory
   b. Encourage use of elastic stockings
   c. Encourage ambulation when permitted
2. Tamponade (compression of heart from accumulation of blood or fluid under pericardium)
   a. Monitor colour and amount of chest tube drainage (change in colour to bright red, sustained bleeding, or sudden cessation of drainage)
   b. Assess for increase in bleeding from midsternal incision
   c. Assess for other signs (restlessness, diaphoresis, hypotension, increased CVP, decreased urinary output)
3. Cardiac dysrhythmias
   a. Maintain continuous ECG monitoring
   b. Assess cardiac rhythm
   c. Monitor daily electrolyte values (especially potassium)
   d. Medicate with antiarrhythmic drugs as prescribed
   e. Assist in treatment of other underlying causes of dysrhythmias (decreased oxygenation)
4. Cardiac failure
   a. Monitor for signs of low cardiac output (hypotension, increased heart rate, restlessness, lethargy)
   b. Monitor CVP readings
   c. Monitor hourly urine output during initial period
   d. Monitor pulmonary artery
   e. Administer blood products and volume expanders as prescribed

Discharge planning

The usual hospital stay is 7 to 10 days after surgery, barring any complications. Before discharge, the patient and family need specific guidelines for physical activity level. Encourage activities at a slow progressive pace unless overexertion occurs. Daily walking and gradually increasing weekly distance are highly recommended. Caution patients to avoid heavy lifting (greater than 14 kilograms) and activities that require repetitive arm movements, such as vacuuming and playing golf. Instruct patients not to drive a car or perform heavy labour until permitted by the doctor.

Sexual intercourse can be resumed within the third or fourth postoperative week. Caution couples to avoid sexual positions in which the patient would be supporting weight.

Patients should avoid large meals or the consumption of alcohol before sexual activity.

In summary, the following patient outcomes are expected:

1. Describe extent of permissible activity
   a. Describe plans for progressive return to physical activity as recommended by the doctor
   b. State awareness of when sexual activity may be resumed
   c. Describe criteria to use as a guide in determining if overexertion occurs (fatigue, dyspnoea, pain)
   d. Describe plans to return to work if employed
2. Plan meals incorporating a balanced diet with any prescribed modifications
3. Describe any medication regimen
4. Describe plans to return to work if employed
   a. Explain basis of any symptoms that may persist (dyspnoea, pain, night sweats)
   b. Describe signs or symptoms requiring immediate medical attention (fever, increasing dyspnoea, chest pain with minimal exertion)
   c. State plans for ongoing medical care

Percutaneous Transluminal Coronary Angioplasty

An alternative approach to coronary bypass surgery for selected patients with myocardial ischaemia is percutaneous transluminal coronary angioplasty (PTCA). This procedure consists of dilating the coronary vessel wall by mechanical compression of the atheromatous plaque. The method is attractive because of a short recovery period, discharge within three days barring complications, and a shorter return-to-work time than with bypass surgery.[33]

Selection criteria for PTCA include persistent angina despite medical treatment and a lesion that is single, non-calcific, and located in a portion of a proximal vessel that does not involve a point of bifurcation; PTCA is not usually considered for lesions in the left main coronary artery. The procedure may also be used following thrombolytic therapy for myocardial infarction and to dilate areas of stenosis in bypass grafts.

During PTCA, a pacemaker catheter is inserted as a precautionary measure through the femoral vein, and a specially designed catheter in the femoral artery. The catheter is advanced under fluoroscopy (similar to cardiac catheterization) to the site of the coronary obstruction. Once the catheter is in position, a balloon on the catheter is inflated to provide compression and rupture the atheromatous plaque. Heparin is infused during the procedure. Anticoagulation may be continued for several months after the procedure.

Following PTCA the patient may return to the general medical unit or may be admitted to an intensive-care unit. In either case, nursing care includes immobilizing the legs for 6 to 12 hours, monitoring for bleeding at the catheter insertion sites, monitoring pedal pulses for indications of femoral artery thrombosis, and monitoring for chest pain that could be caused by an abrupt occlusion of the coronary vessel, restenosis of a dilated artery, coronary artery spasm, or pulmonary embolism. In the case of pulmonary embolus, the site of thrombus formation is usually the femoral vein puncture site. Chest pain requires an immediate ECG and the use of nitrates or calcium channel blockers as prescribed. The ECG results may indicate the need for repeat PTCA or emergency coronary bypass surgery.

About 5 to 10% of patients who undergo PTCA have a major complication such as a myocardial infarction, the need for emergency coronary bypass surgery, or in-hospital death.[33] Minor complications include prolonged angina, bradycardia or transient ventricular dysrhythmias, and excessive blood loss. Over the long term, restenosis of the vessel is a significant complication and occurs in about 25 to 30% of patients, usually within the first eight months following the procedure.

Intravascular Stenting

Restenosis persists as the single greatest limitation of PTCA. Stenosis recurs in 30 to 60% of patients, depending on the dilatation location within the graft. A recent approach to solving the problem of restenosis has been to seek ways of "stenting," or maintaining the cylindrical lumen produced by the balloon. Two techniques are being investigated. The first is to produce a "biological stent" during balloon dilatation through coagulation of collagen, elastin, and other tissues in the vessel wall by laser photocoagulation or radiofrequency-induced heat. The second method consists of prosthetic intravascular cylindrical stents capable of maintaining a cylindrical lumen after balloon deflation and withdrawal.

Laser Therapy for Cardiovascular Disease

Light is a form of electromagnetic energy that lasers use under controlled conditions. As laser light interacts with tissues, it is transmitted, scattered, reflected, or absorbed. A thermal reaction occurs when target tissue absorbs the laser light. This thermal reaction produces necrosis, haemostasis, coagulation, evaporation of tissue, cutting, or vaporization, depending on the time of application, power density, and focusing of spot size.

Nursing care after laser angioplasty is similar to postcatheterization care. Cardiac rehabilitation after laser therapy is important to heighten patients' awareness of the value of risk-factor reduction to prevent the advance of coronary artery disease.

CONGESTIVE HEART FAILURE

Heart failure (also known as cardiac insufficiency) is a state in which the heart is no longer able to pump an adequate supply of blood to meet the demands of the body. *Congestive heart failure* refers to a state of circulatory congestion resulting from heart failure and its compensatory mechanisms.[45] Heart failure may develop rapidly after a specific insult to the myocardium (such as an acute myocardial infarction) or may develop more gradually in response to a prolonged stress (such as hypertension). In the latter case, the person may initially seek medical attention with milder symptoms because the circulatory system has had more time to adjust to the heart's decreased performance and the resultant compensatory responses.

Aetiology

The causes of heart failure can be categorized to correspond to the three determinants of stroke volume: myocardial contractility, preload, and afterload (see p. 381). Heart failure can also be the result of conditions that reduce ventricular filling. Examples of specific aetiologies of heart failure are summarized in Box 17-14.

Pathophysiology

Compensatory responses to inadequate cardiac output

Inadequate cardiac output triggers a number of compensatory responses that are geared towards maintaining adequate perfusion to vital body organs (Box 17-15). The initial response is stimulation of the sympathetic nervous system, which has two main effects: (1) increased rate and force of myocardial contraction and (2) peripheral vasoconstriction. Peripheral vasoconstriction shunts arterial blood away from less vital organs such as the skin and kidneys and towards more vital organs such as the brain. Constriction of the veins increases venous return to the heart, which increases cardiac volume and dilates the ventricles. The increased stretch of myocardial muscle fibres enhances contractility.

Initially these responses may result in improvements in cardiac output, but, in the long term, afterload and myocardial oxygen demands are also increased, and stretch of myocardial fibres moves beyond a point where contraction is enhanced. Unless the person was in a state of fluid depletion to start with, the increased ventricular volume aggravates preload and compounds the failure.

A second type of compensatory response involves activation of the renin–angiotensin system (Chapter 25). A decrease in renal blood flow and, subsequently, of glomerular filtration rate, triggers the release of renin, which interacts with angiotensinogen to form angiotensin I. Conversion of angiotensin I to angiotensin II results in further peripheral vasoconstriction and increased reabsorption of sodium and water by the kidneys. These events increase fluid volume and maintain blood pressure in the short term but increase both preload and afterload in the long term.

17-14

Causes of heart failure

Direct damage to the heart (reduction in contractile ability)
  Myocardial infarction, myocarditis, myocardial fibrosis, ventricular aneurysm
Ventricular overload
  Volume overload (increased preload): aortic regurgitation, ventricular septal defect
  Pressure overload (increased afterload): aortic or pulmonary stenosis, systemic hypertension, pulmonary hypertension
Restriction to ventricular diastolic filling
  Constrictive pericarditis or cardiomyopathy, rapid rate dysrhythmias, cardiac tamponade, mitral stenosis

From Spann JF, Hurst JW: *The recognition and management of heart failure.* In Hurst JW: *The heart, arteries and veins,* ed 6, New York, 1986, McGraw-Hill.

<table>
<tr><td>17-15</td><td colspan="2">Compensatory responses to inadequate cardiac output</td></tr>
</table>

Response	Initial effect
Stimulation of sympathetic nervous system	Increased rate and force of myocardial contraction
	Peripheral vasoconstriction—shunting of blood to vital organs, increased venous return, increased blood pressure
Activation of renin–angiotensin system	Increased reabsorption of sodium and water—increased blood volume; peripheral vasoconstriction
Ventricular hypertrophy	Increased myocardial contractility

A third type of compensatory mechanism involves changes in the structure of the myocardium itself. Over time, the ventricular myocardium thickens or hypertrophies to improve contraction, but this too results in increased myocardial oxygen demands.

Initially, one side of the heart fails. Since the left ventricle is most often affected by coronary atherosclerosis and hypertension, heart failure usually begins there. However, since both ventricles are part of the same system, the right ventricle often becomes impaired as well. The symptoms of heart failure are the result of decreased cardiac output and congestion that involves the venous system or the pulmonary system or both. The symptoms are summarized in Box 17-16. In general, the symptoms of heart failure are considered relative to the amount of associated physical exertion. A classification scheme developed by the New York Heart Association ranges from "asymptomatic with ordinary physical exertion" (Class I) to "symptomatic at rest" (Class IV).[45]

Left ventricular failure

Failure of the left ventricle to pump adequate amounts of oxygenated blood to meet the demands of the body results in two major consequences: (1) signs and symptoms of decreased cardiac output (see general symptoms of heart failure) and (2) pulmonary congestion (sometimes called backward failure). The reduced ejection fraction leads to increased end-diastolic volume (preload) and increased left ventricular end-diastolic pressure (LVEDP). This increased pressure is reflected backward into the pulmonary circulation, which is normally a low pressure, high capacitance circuit. Ultimately, increased pressure in the pulmonary circulation causes fluid to be forced into the alveoli and interstitial tissue. In severe cases, fluid may reach the bronchioles or the pleural space. The symptoms may range from mild dyspnoea to those of frank pulmonary oedema (p. 414) or pleural effusion.

Dyspnoea

Dyspnoea, or laboured breathing, is an early symptom of left ventricular failure. It is caused by interference with gas exchange as a result of the fluid in the alveoli. It may occur or become worse only on physical exertion, such as climbing stairs, walking up an incline, or walking against the wind, since these activities require increased amounts of oxygen.

<table>
<tr><td>17-16</td><td>Signs and symptoms of congestive heart failure</td></tr>
</table>

Signs and symptoms caused by decreased cardiac output to systemic tissues

Fatigue	Oliguria
Angina	Decreased
Anxiety	gastrointestinal
S_3 heart sound	motility
	Skin cool, pale

Signs and symptoms caused by congestion backward from left ventricle

Dyspnoea	Pulmonary rales (crackles)
Cough	
Orthopnoea	X-ray evidence of pulmonary congestion

Signs and symptoms caused by congestion backward from right ventricle

Peripheral oedema	Liver engorgement
Distended neck veins	Elevated central venous pressure

Orthopnoea

Difficulty in breathing when lying flat may be present, and people often must sleep propped up in bed or in a chair. When the person is lying flat, ventilation is decreased and the blood volume in the pulmonary vessels is increased. Orthopnoea is often described by the number of pillows required for the patient to rest comfortably when in bed, for example, "three-pillow orthopnoea."

Although orthopnoea may occur immediately after lying down, it often does not occur for several hours. At that time, it causes the person to wake with severe dyspnoea and coughing. This condition is known as *paroxysmal nocturnal dyspnoea* and results from the accumulation of fluid in the lungs as the person is lying in bed. The patient usually has a feeling of suffocation and often awakens in panic.

Apnoea and hyperpnoea (Cheyne-Stokes)

The patient with heart failure may have alternating periods of apnoea and hyperpnoea called Cheyne-Stokes respirations. Pulmonary congestion results in decreased oxygenation of the blood, and altered cardiac function may cause an abnormally long circulation time between the lungs and respiratory control centres in the brain. Periods of hyperpnoea cause carbon dioxide levels to fall to such an extent that the respiratory centre is not stimulated. A period of apnoea results that may last as long as 30 seconds. During this time the carbon dioxide levels build up again until respirations resume and another period of hyperpnoea begins. This phenomenon often begins as the patient goes to sleep and decreases as sleep deepens and ventilation decreases.

Cough

A persistent hacking cough is often a symptom of left-sided heart failure. It results from congestion of trapped fluid, which is irritating to the mucosal lining of the lungs and bronchi. The cough is usually productive of large quantities of frothy sputum, which is occasionally blood tinged. On auscultation *rales* (crackles) may be heard. Rales are the moist popping and crackling sounds heard most often at the end of inspiration.

Right ventricular failure

Right ventricular failure occurs when this chamber is unable to pump effectively against increased pressure in the pulmonary circulation. Most often the increased pressure is the result of blood backing up from a failing left ventricle, but right ventricular failure can also be a consequence of chronic pulmonary disease and pulmonary hypertension.

Inability of the right ventricle to pump blood forward into the lungs results in congestion that is reflected backward into the systemic circulation. Increased venous volume and pressure force fluid out of the vasculature into interstitial tissue (*peripheral oedema*). This oedema is first likely to appear in dependent areas of the body such as the feet, ankles, and sacrum. It is usually nontender and may become pitting (easily depressed by the pressure of an examiner's thumb). As right ventricular failure worsens, oedema progresses up the legs into the thighs, external genitalia, and lower trunk. Extremely engorged tissue causes the skin to crack, and fluid may "weep" from the tissues.

The *liver* may also become engorged with intravascular fluid, resulting in enlargement and tenderness in the right upper abdominal quadrant. As venous stasis increases, pressure within the portal system becomes so great that fluid is forced through the blood vessels into the abdominal cavity (ascites). The ascitic fluid can reach volumes of more than 10L, displacing the diaphragm and resulting in severe respiratory distress. A paracentesis (see Chapter 22) may be required to relieve the pressure on the diaphragm. *Distended neck veins* are a result of the increased systemic venous pressure and are usually observed when the patient is in a sitting position (see Fig. 7-3).

General symptoms of heart failure

Fatigue

People with heart failure commonly note fatigue following activities that ordinarily are not tiring. The fatigue results from impaired blood circulation to tissues as a result of the decreased CO. The reduction in tissue oxygen decreases the production of adenosine triphosphate (ATP), the immediate energy source for muscle contractions. In addition, the impaired circulation causes a decrease in the removal of metabolic waste products; the result of this is further decreased muscle function.

Anginal pain

Cardiac pain is *not* a typical symptom of heart failure; however, angina pectoris can occur from the decrease in CO. It is most likely to occur in patients with CAHD, which increases the patient's sensitivity to a deficiency in the oxygen content in the circulating blood. As heart failure develops, the blood is less effectively oxygenated and angina occurs. As the fluid overload state is corrected, the chest pain resolves.

Anxiety

Most people are aware of the importance of an effectively functioning heart. Awareness that one has signs and symptoms of heart failure may therefore be anxiety producing, especially if the symptoms have occurred suddenly or are clearly getting worse. The frequent association of dyspnoea with heart failure is another reason why anxiety is a common finding. Perceived difficulty with breathing can be a stressful experience, and anxiety may make the dyspnoea worse. In extreme cases, anxiety may also increase oxygen demands on an already compromised heart.

Nursing Process
Assessment
Subjective data

Collect data concerning the occurrence of signs and symptoms that may indicate the presence of heart failure, the person's ability to cope with the physical limitations, knowledge of the condition and treatment regimen, and ability to adhere to the treatment regimen. Also elicit patient concerns and anxieties. Specific areas for assessment include the following:

1. Respiratory status-dyspnoea, orthopnoea (precipitating factors, severity, relieving factors).
2. Signs of fluid retention—recent weight gain, pedal oedema (shoes too tight), skin feels tight.
3. Ability to perform daily activities—fatigue, lack of endurance (precipitating factors, extent).
4. Comfort—anginal or abdominal pain.
5. Knowledge of condition and treatment regimen.
6. Ability to adhere to any prescribed treatment regimen; factors that make adherence difficult.
7. Measures taken to compensate for physical limitations.
8. Usual coping skills.
9. Specific concerns related to condition.

Objective data

1. Neck vein distention: presence, degree.
2. Oedema: site, degree of pitting.
3. Abdominal distention.
4. Daily weights: weigh on litter scale if severe heart failure present; weigh at same time of day (usually in morning after emptying bladder, before breakfast) and with same amount of clothing.
5. Adventitious breath sounds.
6. Gallop rhythm of heart on auscultation.

7. Level of consciousness.
8. Pulse changes and respiratory effort with activity.

Diagnostic tests

Heart failure is typically diagnosed based on the clinical signs and symptoms and the presence of a precipitating cause. An electrocardiogram is usually done to determine the presence or absence of an acute myocardial infarction, to assess for dysrhythmias, and to identify compensatory responses such as ventricular hypertrophy. Chest X-ray films are done to assess pulmonary congestion and cardiac enlargement. Actual cardiac output may be determined by a variety of techniques, but this assessment is usually reserved for the more critically ill patient. A number of other tests have been devised to provide data about cardiac functioning and are discussed briefly below. They include echocardiograms, gated pool imaging, and pulmonary artery catheterization.

Echocardiogram

Information about the shape, size, and movement of the cardiac muscle and valves can be obtained through the use of ultrasonic sound waves directed to the heart. These waves are reflected by cardiac structures and can be visualized as an electronic waveform on an oscilloscope. The use of this noninvasive test to detect valvular abnormalities is discussed more fully on p. 424.

Gated pool imaging

Gated pool imaging involves the intravenous injection of technetium 99m. Three and five minutes after injecting the technetium, the patient is placed in a supine position, and computer outlines of the left side of the heart during all cardiac cycles are obtained. This procedure is used to evaluate left ventricular function and specifically to calculate the ejection fraction.

Pulmonary artery catheterization

The development of a balloon-tipped, flow-directed pulmonary artery catheter (commonly called a Swan-Ganz catheter in recognition of the doctors who developed it) has made possible significant advances in the diagnosis and treatment of cardiac failure. Specifically, its uses include the assessment of right and left ventricular function and evaluation of the effect of various cardiovascular drugs and other treatment modalities such as increasing or restricting intravenous fluids.

A flexible multilumen catheter is inserted into a major vein by means of a cutdown. The catheter is threaded through the superior vena cava, the right atrium, right ventricle, and pulmonary artery, and into a small branch of this artery (pulmonary wedge position).

Representative waveforms are viewed on an oscilloscope and pressure readings can be obtained from various cardiac chambers (see normal pressures on p. 425). Pulmonary wedge pressure reflects left ventricular pressure and allows monitoring of preload. In addition, the thermistor port allows determinations of CO.

Nursing analysis

Nursing analyses are determined from the assessment of patient data. Possible nursing analyses for the people with heart failure may include, but are not limited to, the following:

Problem	Possible aetiologies
Cardiac output, decreased	Reduced stroke volume, cardiogenic shock, tachycardia, hypertension, valvular insufficiency
Fatigue	Decreased oxygenation, muscle weakness, inadequate rest, inadequate nutrition
Gas exchange, impaired	Ventilation/perfusion imbalance
Nutrition, altered: less than body requirments	Oedema, dyspnoea, fatigue, drug therapy

Problem	Possible aetiologies
Self-care deficit	Activity intolerance/fatigue, pain/discomfort, anxiety
Skin integrity, impaired, high risk for	Immobility, decreased tissue perfusion to skin, oedema
Anxiety	Threat of death; threat/change in health status, socioeconomic status, role; threat to self-concept
Knowledge deficit	Lack of exposure/recall, information misinterpretation, cognitive limitation

Planning: expected patient outcomes

Expected outcomes for the patient with heart failure may include, but are not limited to, the following:
1. Identifies factors that increase cardiac workload.
2. Performs ADL without undue fatigue.
3. Achieves normal respiratory rate without use of supplemental oxygen; states breathing is easier; confusion is decreased.
4. Demonstrates cardiac tolerance to increased activity (pulse and blood pressure are stable).
5. Eats prescribed diet.
6. Performs ADL within symptom limitations.
7. Skin remains intact.
8. Uses effective coping mechanisms in managing anxiety.
9. Describes the following:
   a. A modified plan for activity that avoids fatigue or dyspnoea
   b. Plans for a diet in accordance with prescribed sodium or fluid restrictions
   c. Medication therapy, including adverse side effects
   d. Usage and precaution of supplemental oxygen therapy, if prescribed for home use
   e. Plans for follow-up healthcare

Implementation
Assisting with achievement of therapeutic goals

Treatment of congestive heart failure has the overall aim of restoring a supply of blood and oxygen that is equal to the demands of bodily tissues. Approaches to treatment therefore may focus on increasing oxygen supply, decreasing oxygen demand, or both (Box 17-17). A second aim of treatment is reducing pulmonary and/or systemic congestion and the associated symptoms. Identification and treatment of the underlying aetiology and factors that may have precipitated a particular episode of heart failure (that is, caused excessive demands on the heart) are important therapeutic goals.

At many acute-care hospitals, patients with acute congestive heart failure are admitted to medical or cardiac intensive-care units. Occasionally, the doctor may elect to place the patient in the usual room accommodations, where the environment is less stressful and where family members can visit more routinely.

Medications

Cardiac glycoside therapy. Digitalis and its derivatives (cardiac glycosides) usually are effective in improving myocardial function in people with congestive heart failure. The positive inotropic action of digitalis preparations enhances mechanical performance by strengthening the force of myocardial contractions. This leads to increased cardiac output and increased blood flow to the kidneys. Digitalis preparations also decrease heart rate (automaticity) and cardiac conduction velocity, which permits the ventricles to relax more and allow for better filling of the ventricles with blood.

When acute congestive heart failure occurs, the doctor usually orders an *optimal therapeutic dose* of a digitalis preparation to slow the ventricular rate and decrease symptoms. This larger dose given over a short period of time, usually 24 to 48 hours, is called a *loading* or *digitalizing* dose. In some instances the dose may approach the toxic level, and the patient then requires careful observation for signs and symptoms of toxicity (Box 17-18). After the optimal therapeutic dose has been determined, give the patient a daily maintenance dose of digitalis.

Two types of digitalis preparations (cardiac glycosides) may be used. Digoxin or digitoxin is most commonly used for maintenance drug therapy. Digoxin has a more rapid effect than digitoxin yet has sufficient duration for adequate maintenance therapy. If digoxin is given intramuscularly, inject it deeply and massage the area after injection because the drug is a tissue irritant.

Before giving a cardiac glycoside, take the apical pulse rate. If this rate is below 60, withhold the medication until the doctor has been consulted. Also evaluate the pulse for changes in rhythm. Always take the pulse rate of people with irregular rhythm for a full minute for accuracy. Evaluate the response to digitalis on the basis of relief of symptoms, that is, decreased oedema, loss of weight, fluid output greater than fluid intake, and no dyspnoea or cyanosis.

Diuretic therapy. Diuretic therapy is the most effective approach for symptomatic relief to patients with moderate to-severe congestive heart failure.[55] The purpose of diuretic therapy is to decrease cardiac workload by reducing circulating volume and thus reduce preload.

Essential to proper initiation of diuretic therapy is

17-17

Medical therapy for congestive heart failure

Reduction of oxygen requirements
    Treatment of precipitating causes
    Rest
Improvement of oxygen supply/reduction of
    congestion
    Oxygen therapy
    Positioning of patient to facilitate breathing
    Increase myocardial contractility (positive
        inotropic drugs)
    Reduce preload (sodium restriction, diuretics,
        venous-dilating drugs)
    Reduce afterload (arterial dilating drugs, mixed
        arterial/venous-dilating drugs, angiotensin-
        converting enzyme inhibitors)

17-18

Signs and symptoms of cardiac glycoside toxicity

Cardiovascular effects

Bradycardia
Tachycardia
Bigeminy (double beats)
Ectopic beats
Pulse deficit (difference between apical and radial
    pulse)

Gastrointestinal effects

Anorexia
Nausea and vomiting
Abdominal pain
Diarrhoea

Neurological effects

Headache
Double, blurred, or coloured vision
Drowsiness, confusion
Restlessness, irritability
Muscle weakness

---

determining how much fluid should be removed from the patient by establishing a "dry weight." This can be accomplished by gradually removing fluid with diuretics and assessing the patient's blood pressure. When the patient becomes hypotensive, particularly orthostatic, this signals the doctor that too much fluid has been removed. The patient is then permitted to reaccumulate a small amount of fluid until hypotension no longer occurs. The weight at which this occurs is then considered the patient's dry weight.

Currently, thiazides (Table 17-2) are the diuretics of choice in the treatment of heart failure. The major complication is hypokalaemia, which can be prevented by the intake of foods high in potassium or by potassium supplements. The most potent diuretics available are the loop diuretics (frusemide, bumetanide). These medications are reserved for severe congestive heart failure or when other

Table 17-2   Diuretics used in treatment of heart failure

Type	Example	Side effects
Thiazide	Hydrochlorothiazide Chlorothiazide	Gastrointestinal upsets (can be minimized by taking medication with meals); hypokalaemia; hyperglycaemia
Loop	Frusemide Bumetanide	Similar to thiazide diuretics; also ototoxicity and blood dyscrasias
Potassium-sparing	Spironolactone Triamterene	Gastrointestinal irritation; hyperkalaemia

forms of treatment are ineffective in relieving symptoms. These agents also increase renal blood flow and therefore may prove effective in treating heart failure when renal function is also impaired.

Other drugs. Vasodilators may be used to decrease afterload by decreasing resistance to ventricular emptying. Commonly used agents include sodium nitroprusside, hydralazine, and prazosin. Nifedipine, a calcium channel blocker, also has vasodilator effects. Captopril, an angiotensin-converting enzyme inhibitor with hypotensive properties, is also a vasodilator and blocks sodium retention by suppressing aldosterone. Vasodilators are more effective in the treatment of acute rather than chronic heart failure.

Sodium-restricted diet

Oedema is often effectively controlled in patients with heart failure by restricting sodium intake. The degree of restriction depends on the severity of the failure and the extent of diuretic therapy. The severely restricted sodium diet is rarely prescribed because this diet is unpalatable and expensive, which results in poor patient compliance.

The amount of sodium in the normal diet is 3 to 10g/d. Sodium restriction in people receiving diuretics may not be dropped below 3 to 5g/d because of the dangers of hyponatraemia. In mild cardiac failure, sodium may be restricted to 1 to 2g/d; this is known as a no-added-salt (NAS) diet. It is essentially a normal diet, except that no extra salt is added to prepared foods and, obviously, salted foods such as crisps are omitted. For moderate or severe heart failure, the amount of sodium permitted is specifically prescribed.

Low-sodium diets can be made more appealing by adding salt substitutes to food in place of table salt. Since many salt substitutes contain potassium, the patient's need for potassium must be assessed. Often the increased potassium is beneficial when the patient is on diuretic therapy. The use of herbs often makes the food more appetizing.

Fluid restriction is less commonly instituted than in the past as long as the person is on a sodium-controlled diet and is receiving diuretics or digitalis. If fluids are restricted, the amount of fluid permitted is prescribed by the doctor and a plan is made, in conjunction with the patient if possible, to space the fluids over the day.

Interventions to achieve patient outcomes

Guidelines for nursing interventions for a person with congestive heart failure are summarized in Box 17-19.

Promoting rest and activity

Reducing the requirement for oxygen can best be effected by providing the patient with the degree of activity that does not compromise myocardial function, as demonstrated by the presence of symptoms. For mild heart failure, the patient may be treated on an ambulatory basis with only a regimen of less strenuous activity and more rest than usual.

For severe heart failure, a programme of bed rest or limited activity may be necessary until symptoms abate. Permissible activity will be based on symptoms such as dyspnoea and fatigue. A careful assessment must be made each day to determine the amount of rest required. If the patient has difficulty relaxing because of apprehension or anxiety, a tranquillizer may be prescribed.

Ambulation is started slowly to avoid overloading the heart. The regimen varies with individual patient response. When a patient has been on restricted bedrest, activities progress slowly from dangling, to sitting, to walking increased distances under close supervision. If signs of dyspnoea, fatigue, or increased pulse rate that does not stabilize readily occur, the patient returns to bed. Oxygen is given for dyspnoea, and the doctor is notified.

The plan for increased activity is explained to the patient and family. They should understand that if activity tires the person excessively, it may be curtailed. Overactivity can produce physical and mental setbacks that delay ultimate recovery.

Rest to the heart is also promoted by preventing constipation, since straining at defecation places an extra burden on the heart. During straining against a closed glottis (Valsalva manoeuvre), venous return to the heart is decreased as a result of increased intrathoracic pressure. When this pressure is released after straining, a large amount of venous return creates an increased work load on the heart. The faeces can be kept soft by stool softeners or bulk-forming laxatives. If an enema is necessary, it should be of low volume.

Providing oxygenation

In heart failure, the oxygen content of the bloodstream may be markedly reduced because of the less effective oxygenation of the blood as it passes through the congested lungs. The patient may be more comfortable and better able to rest when receiving oxygen, since it helps in reducing dyspnoea and fatigue. Oxygen is usually administered by nasal cannula at 2 to 6L/min. Obtain baseline arterial blood gases when oxygen therapy begins and intermittently during therapy to assess effectiveness of the treatment.

Breathing is often made easier by maintaining the patient in a supported sitting position. These positions maximize oxygenation by permitting greater lung expansion. The patient is often orthopnoeic and tends to breathe more easily sitting than lying in bed. If the patient is sitting in a chair, elevate the feet to reduce pooling of fluid in the dependent limbs. When the patient is in a sitting position in bed, place a pillow lengthwise behind the shoulders and back so that full expansion of the rib cage is possible. The arms may be supported on pillows to reduce the pull on the shoulder muscles. An over-the-bed table may be placed close to the patient to allow resting of the head and arms.

Promoting nutrition

During the acute stage of congestive heart failure, the diet should be bland, low-calorie, low-residue with vitamin supplement (in addition to any sodium restrictions (see p. 412). Anorexia is often present because of oedema in the gastrointestinal tract, dyspnoea, fatigue, and the effect of medications. Frequent small feedings minimize exertion and reduce gastrointestinal blood requirements, which can tax the failing heart. Care must be taken to provide a diet that meets the metabolic demands of the body so that body wasting does not occur.

Although careful records of intake and output are kept on most patients with cardiac failure, the best method to estimate progress and response to prescribed diet, medications, and other forms of treatment is *daily monitoring of the patient's weight*. Weight gain indicates fluid retention. Carefully record the weight on admission and then daily while the patient is hospitalized. Weight loss in the patient stabilized at dry weight indicates inadequate nutrient intake.

Facilitating self-care and skin integrity

Careful daily assessments determine the extent to which the person can perform ADL such as eating and bathing. Most patients prefer to maximize their independence, and this is encouraged within the limitations of their symptoms.

Oedematous skin is poorly nourished and very susceptible to breakdown. Oedema of the sacrum is prevalent in patients with heart failure who are restricted to bed rest, and decubiti can develop quickly. Institute measures to prevent skin breakdown early.

Facilitating coping with anxiety

Because anxiety increases the symptoms of heart failure, take measures to help the person decrease anxiety. These measures include the following:

1. Identifying the feelings and the content related to these feelings
2. Identifying strengths that can be used for coping
3. Learning what can be done to decrease the anxiety, (for example, learning about measures to control heart failure and measures to reduce stress; see Chapter 6)

Guidelines for Care   17-19

The patient with congestive heart failure

Provide oxygenation
  Administer oxygen by nasal cannula at 2–6 L/min as prescribed
  Give oxygen as needed for dyspnoea
  Patient should be well supported in a sitting position
Provide rest and activity
  Reinforce importance of conservation of energy and planning for activities that avoid fatigue
  Encourage activity within prescribed restrictions; monitor for intolerance to activity (dyspnoea, fatigue, increased pulse rate that does not stabilize)
  Assist with ADL as necessary; encourage independence within patient's limitations
  Provide diversional activity that will assist in conservation of energy
Monitor for signs of fluid and potassium imbalance; record daily weights
Provide skin care, particularly over oedematous areas; use prophylactic measures to prevent skin breakdown
Assist in maintaining an adequate nutritional intake while observing prescribed dietary modifications (sodium restrictions)
Monitor for constipation; give prescribed stool softeners
Give prescribed medications
  Digitalis (take apical pulse before administration)
  Diuretics (assess for hypokalaemia)
  Vasodilators
  Drugs to reduce anxiety and promote sleep
Provide patient/family opportunities to discuss their concerns
Teach patient about the disorder and self-care (Box 17-20)

Working with family members in the same manner is also helpful to decrease their anxiety so they can be of greater support to the patient.

Facilitating patient/family learning

Patients who will be receiving oxygen therapy at home need to know how to manage the therapy. Instructions include the following:

1. Indication for initiating oxygen therapy
2. Method of initiating oxygen therapy
3. Precautions necessary when oxygen therapy is being used

Start teaching patients their dietary restrictions early during hospitalization to permit time for learning and asking questions. The patient may need frequent interactions with the dietitian and nurse before being able to follow a prescribed diet. Additional teaching includes the signs and symptoms that indicate recurring congestion, avoidance of fatigue and need for rest periods at home, and the medication regimen (Box 17-20).

Evaluation

Evaluation will be based on the expected patient outcomes. Questions to ask may include the following:

1. Is the patient breathing more easily?
2. Is the patient more comfortable?
3. Is the patient less fatigued?
4. Does the patient know how to plan activities to prevent fatigue and dyspnoea?
5. Is peripheral oedema decreased?
6. Is the patient using effective coping mechanisms to manage anxiety?
7. Can the patient describe components of the treatment regimen?
8. Can the patient explain the rationale for the treatment regimen?
9. Can the patient state plans for follow-up care?

Pulmonary Oedema

Acute pulmonary oedema is the rapid effusion of serous fluid from plasma into the pulmonary interstitial tissue and alveoli. It is a medical emergency that requires immediate care. The causes of pulmonary oedema include the following:

1. Severe left ventricular failure
2. Inhalation of irritating gases
3. Rapid administration of intravenous fluids (whole blood, plasma, crystalloid fluids)
4. Barbiturate or opiate overdose

Pathophysiology

In pulmonary oedema caused by heart failure, cardiac output decreases, resulting in increased left atrial pressure. This increases pulmonary vein and capillary pressure. As the pulmonary capillary pressure exceeds the intravascular osmotic pressure, serous fluid is rapidly forced into the alveoli. Fluid rapidly reaches the bronchioles and bronchi, and patients literally begin to drown in their own secretions. As oxygenation decreases, the person shows signs of respiratory distress (Box 17-21). The sputum is frothy from air mixing with the fluid in the alveoli and blood-tinged from blood cells that have exuded into the alveoli.[44]

Medical therapy

Treatment for acute pulmonary oedema involves a number of simultaneous interventions to promote oxygenation, improve CO, and reduce pulmonary congestion.[56] Whenever possible, identify the underlying cause. The components of treatment are similar to those discussed for congestive heart failure but are applied more vigorously. Common interventions include patient positioning, intravenous morphine sulphate, oxygen, rapid digitalization, and intravenous aminophylline (Box 17-22). Other measures to reduce circulating blood volume may include administering diuretics such as frusemide and ethacrynic acid, rotating tourniquets on three extremities, and performing a phlebotomy.

Cardiogenic Shock

Cardiogenic shock is a shock state of primary cardiac origin. It is most frequently caused by myocardial infarction but

---

Patient Teaching 17-20

The patient with congestive heart failure

Monitor for signs and symptoms of recurring congestive heart failure and report these signs and symptoms to the doctor or clinic:
  Weight gain of 1–1.5kg (2–3lb) over a short period of time (about 2 days)
  Loss of appetite
  Shortness of breath
  Orthopnoea
  Swelling of ankles, feet, or abdomen
  Persistent cough
  Frequent nighttime urination
Avoid fatigue and plan activity to allow for rest periods
Plan and eat meals within prescribed sodium restrictions
  Avoid salty foods
  Avoid drugs with high sodium content (for example, some laxatives and antacids)—read the labels
  Eat several small meals rather than three large meals per day
Take prescribed medications
  If several medications are prescribed, develop a method to facilitate accurate administration
  Digitalis: check own pulse rate daily: report a rate of less than 60 per minute to the doctor
  Diuretics
    Weigh self daily at same time of day
    Report weight gain to the doctor
    Eat foods high in potassium and low in sodium (such as oranges, bananas)
  Vasodilators
    Report signs of hypotension (light-headedness, rapid pulse, syncope) to the doctor
    Avoid alcohol when taking vasodilators
Report to the doctor for follow-up as directed

17-21

Signs and symptoms of pulmonary oedema

Restlesness
Vague uneasiness
Dyspnoea
Tachycardia
Pallor or cyanosis
Cough productive of large quantities of blood-tinged frothy sputum
Audible wheezing

---

also may result from other cardiac disorders that lead to low cardiac output (Box 17-23).

Pathophysiology

Cardiogenic shock occurs when cardiac function is severely impaired and cardiac output is low. As the shock progresses, coronary artery perfusion decreases, leading to cardiac muscle ischaemia that leads to further decreased function (Fig. 17-24). The mortality rate is high. (See Chapter 7 for further discussion on shock.)

Nursing Care Plan	**Person with congestive heart failure**

DATA: Mr G is a 59-year-old factory worker with a long history of hypertension. He has taken his antihypertensive medications only sporadically and frequently fails to keep follow-up appointments at the hypertension clinic. His blood pressure has never been under good control, and readings have typically been 160–190/96–100mm Hg. Mr G has felt fatigued for several weeks and has noticed increasing difficulty with breathing, particularly when moving heavy equipment at work. At times he awakens during the night and feels like he is suffocating. He came to the clinic to get something to help him sleep better and was admitted to the hospital for evaluation. Tests revealed that he has hypertensive cardiovascular disease and congestive heart failure. Following loading doses of digoxin, he is being maintained on 0.25mg orally, twice a day. He is also on a low-sodium diet and hydrochlorothiazide 50mg orally, four times daily. His activity has been restricted to "up in room as tolerated."

The nursing history identified the following:
1. He and his wife have little understanding of the low-sodium diet that was prescribed years ago. He remembers the diet instructions as "not adding too much salt at the table." He frequently eats sandwiches of luncheon meat and cheese at work or has canned soup from the vending machine.
2. The episodes of nocturnal dyspnoea have been very frightening to both Mr G and his wife. They have tried various preventive measures such as more fresh air, but nothiing seems to work. Mrs G states that she is almost afraid to go to bed anymore.
3. He sees little need to take "medicine" if he doesn't feel sick. Now the doctor has prescribed more medicine for his heart when the trouble is his breathing.
4. He is reluctant to tell his boss about the dyspnoea he encounters at work because he doesn't want to be labelled a "cry baby"—"It's better to just tough things out."

Collaborative nursing activities include those to assess (1) Mr G's response to the therapeutic regimen and (2) the presence of any complications associated with the regimen. Nursing actions include monitoring the following:
1. Response to exertion—especially heart rate and respiratory effort
2. Breath sounds—location and extent of adventitious sounds such as rales (crackles)
3. Daily weights and intake/output
4. Blood pressure
5. Heart rate and rhythm; abnormal cardiac sounds such as an S_3 gallop
6. Serum electrolytes—especially potassium.

Nursing analysis: Cardiac output, decreased, related to reduced stroke volume, resulting in a compromised state.

Expected patient outcomes	Nursing interventions	Rationale
Mr G's pulse and respirations are within normal limits.	Organize care to provide scheduled periods for rest and to minimize unnecessary disturbances.	Exercise and physical activity increase cardiac output, heart rate, and blood pressure
Mr G identifies factors that increase cardiac workload.	Explain and encourage increases in activity and ambulation to prevent a sudden increase in cardiac workload.	Regular exercise makes the heart more efficient, so stroke volume increases and is not appreciably altered.
	Monitor respirations every four hours for increased effort, pulse for tachycardia.	
	Monitor heart sounds every four hours for presence of gallop rhythm	Surge of blood to heart after intrathoracic pressure decreases causes increase in cardiac workload.
	Teach Mr G to avoid Valsalva's manoeuvre.	

Nursing Care Plan

Person with congestive heart failure—cont'd

Nursing analysis: Tissue perfusion, altered, related to decreased blood flow to tissues and oedema

Expected patient outcomes	Nursing interventions	Rationale
Mr G demonstrates improved circulation (decreased neck vein distention, decreased peripheral oedema, decreased weight).	Assess neck vein distention, oedema of extremities, and coolness of skin every four hours; weigh daily.	Provides information on fluid retention from decreased circulation.
	Encourage movement and activity as tolerated.	Movement promotes circulation to tissues.
Skin breakdown does not occur.	Eliminate or reduce pressure points by changing position frequently, use of pressure mattress, etc. Give diuretics and sodium-restricted diet as prescribed.	Oedema interferes with diffusion of O_2 to cells. Cellular nutrition depends on adequate blood flow.

Nursing analysis: Activity intolerance related to imbalance between oxygen supply and demand

Expected patient outcomes	Nursing interventions	Rationale
Mr G complains of less dyspnoea on exertion.	Plan activities to conserve energy; allow for rest periods; provide assistance with aspects of physical care that are tiring; discuss ways to conserve energy at home and at work.	Pacing of activities will lessen myocardial oxygen demand. Any factor that compromises cardiovascular function reduces tolerance to activity

Nursing analysis: Anxiety (Mr G and his wife) related to perceived change in health status (onset of frightening symptoms) and uncertainty regarding cause or measures to control

Expected patient outcomes	Nursing interventions	Rationale
Mr G and wife express less anxiety about paroxysmal nocturnal dyspnoea (PND) episodes.	Explain basis for symptoms and expectations of therapeutic regimen; suggest sleeping with head of bed slightly elevated.	Providing structure in a situation of uncertainty allows people to gain control and feel less anxious.

Nursing analysis: Knowledge deficit (low-sodium diet, pathophysiology of heart failure, rationale for therapeutic regimen) related to lack of recall and lack of exposure

Expected patient outcomes	Nursing interventions	Rationale
Mr G and wife can describe congestive heart failure and explain the basis for symptoms.	Teach about the heart as a pump and effect of hypertension; select an appropriate analogy from Mr G's home or work life regarding pumps and pressure.	Learning is easier when content can be related to something familiar.
Mr G can explain rationale for low-sodium diet, diuretic, digoxin.	Teach relationship between sodium, fluid retention, and hypertension; explain effect of digoxin on heart.	Understanding of the rationale for therapeutic regimen may improve compliance.
Mr G and/or wife can describe basic elements of a low-sodium diet.	Provide and discuss information on foods to avoid and foods that may be eaten liberally on this diet.	Providing information on activities that are allowed, as well as those that must be avoided, gives people resources for coping with restrictions.

Nursing analysis: Noncompliance (previously) with therapeutic regimen possibly related to absence of physical symptoms or inability to cope with taking on any aspect of the "sick role"

Expected patient outcomes	Nursing interventions	Rationale
Mr G adheres to therapeutic regimen.	Explore previous noncompliance to determine reasons from Mr G's perspective; identify difficulties foreseen with new regimen; help Mr G explore acceptable alternatives.	Data are insufficient to guide specific plan; Mr G's perceptions of difficulties with therapeutic regimen provide avenues for intervention by nurse.

17-22 Medical therapy for acute pulmonary oedema	
Intervention	**Rationale**
Patient in high supported sitting position or over side of bed with arms supported on bedside table	Promotes expansion of lungs; legs in dependent position causes venous pooling and reduction in venous return (preload)
Morphine sulphate, 4–8mg, intravenously	Decreases anxiety; slows respirations; reduces venous return
Oxygen at 40–70% by face mask; intubation as needed	Promotes oxygenation; increased tidal volume also promotes removal of secretions from alveoli
Rapid digitalization if patient not previously taking digitalis	Improves contractility; increases cardiac output and reduces heart rate; converts rapid rate dysrhythmias such as atrial fibrillation
Aminophylline 250mg, given intravenously over approximately 30 minutes	Relieves bronchospasm and wheezing; acts as diuretic

17-23 Causes of cardiogenic shock
Myocardial infarction Critical aortic stenosis Intractable dysrhythmias Ruptured aortic aneurysm Severe congestive heart failure Massive pulmonary embolism Cardiac tamponade

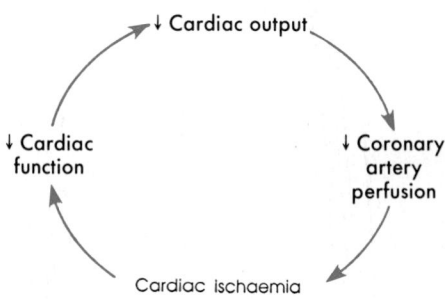

Fig. 17-24   Sequence of events in cardiogenic shock.

Medical therapy

Cardiogenic shock is a medical emergency that requires immediate intervention and constant attention to prevent irreversible cell damage and death. Therapy is aimed at correcting factors that contribute to decreased tissue perfusion, such as cardiac dysrhythmias, hypoxaemia, and pain.

Invasive monitoring lines that are usually placed include catheters in the pulmonary artery, systemic artery, and urinary bladder. The left ventricular end-diastolic pressure (LVEDP) is reflected in the pulmonary capillary wedge pressure, which is used as a guide to fluid therapy.

The following therapy may be initiated:

1. Vasopressors and cardiotonic agents (for example, dopamine, noradrenaline) to raise systemic arterial pressure without increasing cardiac work load; vasopressors are titrated to maintain systolic pressure, preferably above 90mm Hg
2. Hyperventilation and buffering agents (for example, sodium bicarbonate) to counteract lactic acidosis
3. Intravenous fluids if hypovolaemia is present: care must be taken to prevent fluid overload with resulting pulmonary oedema
4. Use of intraaortic balloon counterpulsation, if necessary (see discussion below)

General care of the patient in shock is described in Chapter 7.

Intraaortic balloon counterpulsation

A counterpulsation device facilitates blood circulation by decreasing aortic pressure during systole and increasing it during diastole. The overall effects include the following:

1. Increase in coronary artery perfusion
2. Decrease in preload (degree to which the myocardium is stretched before contracting)
3. Decrease in afterload (resistance against which blood is expelled).

In addition to being used in the situations producing cardiogenic shock, the intraaortic balloon pump may be used in unstable patients with cardiac disease before and during open heart surgery and in assistance when removing these patients from cardiopulmonary bypass following surgery.

Technique

The intraaortic balloon is inserted percutaneously or by cutdown into the right or left femoral artery. It is advanced into the thoracic aorta and sutured into place at the insertion site after the balloon tip has been correctly positioned just distal to the left subclavian artery (Fig. 17-25). The end of the balloon catheter is attached to a pump console, which alternately inflates and deflates the balloon using helium or carbon dioxide gas.

The timing of the inflation–deflation sequence is of the utmost importance in obtaining maximal counterpulsation effect. Using the ECG to trigger the pumping mechanism and the arterial waveform to determine the effectiveness of the counterpulsation, the balloon is timed to inflate just at the beginning of ventricular diastole, immediately after closure of the aortic valve and thus enhances coronary

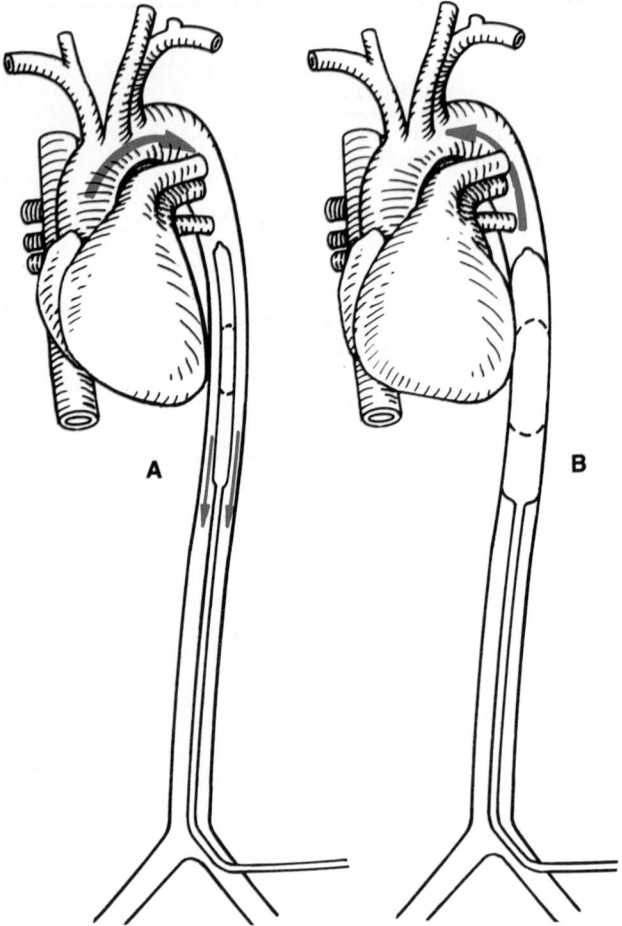

Fig. 17-25 Representation of intraaortic balloon positioned just distal to left subclavian artery. **A,** Balloon is deflated allowing forward blood flow during systole. **B,** Balloon is inflated to increase coronary perfusion during diastole.

artery filling. The balloon remains inflated during diastole and is then timed to deflate immediately before the next ventricular systolic ejection or just before the aortic valve reopens, thereby reducing afterload and secondarily decreasing preload. Improper timing of the balloon not only defeats the purpose of counterpulsation, but also could directly damage the myocardium. This is particularly true in early inflation or late deflation, in which the heart would be ejecting blood against a partially inflated balloon.

Nursing management

1. Monitor vital signs and indices of cardiac function at frequent intervals as specified
2. Position patient:
   a. Head of bed elevated no more than 30° to prevent balloon migration upward in aorta
   b. Reposition patient every two hours on alternate sides to prevent skin breakdown and other consequences of immobility
   c. Avoid hip flexion on catheterized side; restrain leg if necessary.
3. Monitor circulation of both legs before catheter insertion and hourly thereafter until balloon is removed

4. Keep dressing on balloon insertion site clean and dry; change every 24 to 48 hours using sterile technique
5. Administer prescribed heparin or low-molecular-weight dextran to prevent blood clotting or emboli

Considerable psychological support is necessary for the patient and family during such critical therapy. Not only are the physical size and noise of the pump console very intimidating, but its presence only reinforces everyone's awareness of the frailty of the patient's heart and uncertainty about the future. Careful but simple explanations of the pump's action are necessary for patients who are alert enough to understand; it is important that they not get the mistaken idea that the pump is working instead of their heart. Some patients with this type of misunderstanding fear that they will die if the pump stops even momentarily. Such fear makes them anxious and restless and further increases the body's demand for oxygen. Continuous reassurance and repeated simple explanations are essential. Some patients may benefit from mild sedation.

INFLAMMATORY HEART DISORDERS

This section will discuss a group of cardiac conditions that are generally the result of inflammation. All cardiac tissues are susceptible to inflammation, and heart failure can be a serious and rapid result of the inflammatory process. The specific pathological mechanisms for each disorder are discussed below, and in Table 17-3, signs and symptoms and medical therapy are summarized.

PERICARDITIS

Pericarditis may result from bacterial, viral, or fungal infection. In addition, it may occur as a complication of a systemic disease, such as rheumatoid arthritis, systemic lupus erythematosus, scleroderma, uraemia, or myocardial infarction, or may result from trauma or neoplasm.

Pericarditis is an inflammatory process of the visceral or parietal pericardium or both. It may be acute or chronic, and infection may spread from or to the myocardium. *Acute pericarditis* is further classified as fibrinous or exudative. The exudate may be serous, purulent, or haemorrhagic. When fluid accumulates in the pericardial sac, *cardiac tamponade* (compression of heart from blood or fluid) causes decreased venous return to the heart and decreased ventricular emptying. Symptoms result from interference with ventricular functioning (Box 17-24).

A known aetiological disease process is treated specifically, such as with antibiotic therapy, if indicated. Salicylates or indomethacin may be used to decrease inflammation. If the accumulation of pericardial fluid or effusion is large, the doctor may remove the fluid by *pericardiocentesis*. A *pericardial fenestration* (pericardial window) may be performed to provide continuous drainage of pericardial fluid.

Chronic pericarditis is referred to as chronic constrictive or adhesive pericarditis. It is three times more prevalent in

REVIEW

Table 17-3 Inflammatory heart disorders

Disorder	Signs and symptoms	Medical therapy
Pericarditis	*Acute*: Severe precordial chest pain referred to neck, shoulder, left arm; intensified when lying supine, coughing or breathing deeply or swallowing Pericardial friction rub Fever, leukocytosis, electrocardiogram changes Cardiac tamponade *Chronic*: Dyspnoea, fatigue, congestive heart failure	*Acute*: Treatment of underlying condition Supportive care: salicylates, indometha-cin, corticosteroids Pericardiocentesis for injection of anti-biotic or sclerosing agent Pericardial fenestration *Chronic*: Digitalization, diuretics Low-sodium diet Pericardiectomy for severe cases
Myocarditis	May be asymptomatic Nonspecific complaints of dyspnoea on exertion, palpitations, precordial chest pain, fever, tachy-cardia	Antibiotics Corticosteroids for severe cases Antiarrhythmic drugs for disrhythmias
Endocarditis	Gradual onset: malaise, achiness, fever Splenomegaly, clubbing of fingers, Osler's nodes on fingers, petechiae in conjunctiva and mouth, cardiac murmur, anaemia	Bedrest Antibiotics (intravenous) Prolonged antibiotic therapy Incision and drainage of abscesses Valve replacement
Rheumatic fever/rheumatic heart disease	Symptoms follow pharyngeal infection in 1–4 weeks Joint pain—recurrent Heart murmur, friction rub, cardiac arrhythmias, congestive heart failure	Antibiotics Anti-inflammatory drugs (salicylates, corticosteroids) Early ambulation
Cardiovascular syphilis	Signs of aortic aneurysms, aortitis, aortic valve in-sufficiency, congestive heart failure	Penicillin Surgery for aneurysm or aortic valve insufficiency, if feasible Treatment of congestive heart failure, if it develops

men than women. It may result from fibrosing of the pericardial sac secondary to trauma or neoplastic disease. In the majority of cases, no specific pathogen can be identified as the causative agent. Chronic pericarditis is often associated with other disease processes (Box 17-25). If the pericardium becomes a constrictive band surrounding the heart, it will prevent adequate filling and emptying of the ventricles, thus decreasing CO and ultimately producing cardiac failure.

Removal of the pericardium (*pericardiectomy*) may be necessary to restore cardiac function. Postoperative care is similar to that of other surgery. Other measures to restore more efficient pumping include digitalization, diuretic therapy, and a low-sodium diet.

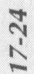

17-24

Symptoms of cardiac tamponade

Diminished or absent point of maximal impulse (PMI)
Diminished peripheral pulses
Distended neck veins (secondary to increased central venous pressure)
Decreased blood pressure (secondary to ineffective pumping action)
Narrowing pulse pressure (difference between systolic and diastolic blood pressure)
Paradoxical pulse (decrease in pulse strength during inspiration)
Diminished heart sounds

MYOCARDITIS

Myocarditis is an inflammatory disease of the myocardium that causes an infiltrate in the myocardial interstitium and injury to adjacent myocardial cells that is atypical of infarction. Myocarditis may be primary, with an unknown aetiology, or secondary, from an identifiable cause such as drug hypersensitivity or toxicity and infection. In Britain, infection is most often caused by a virus, including coxsackievirus, echovirus, viral encephalitis, influenza virus, and herpes simplex.[57]

Myocarditis is difficult to study in human beings, because it frequently remains undiagnosed until chronic cardiac dysfunction and congestive heart failure become

clinically obvious. Very often this inflammatory process develops secondary to acute endocarditis or pericarditis. Myocarditis may be classified as acute (benign or fulminant) or chronic.

Patients with myocarditis are often treated with bedrest and digitalis to prevent heart failure and cardiogenic shock. Immunosuppression may be beneficial in reducing myocardial inflammation.

ENDOCARDITIS

Endocarditis is an infection of the endocardium and most often of the heart valves. The more recent method of

17-25

Disorders associated with chronic pericarditis

Rheumatic heart disease
Congenital heart disease
Hypertensive heart disease
Systemic lupus erythematosus
Rheumatoid arthritis
Sclerodema
Myxoedema
Renal failure

classification of infective endocarditis is on the basis of the causative organism, for example, enterococcal endocarditis or streptococcal endocarditis. It may occur in acute or subacute forms. Acute endocarditis occurs rapidly, often on normal heart valves, and if untreated may cause death within days or weeks. The subacute form develops more gradually, usually on previously damaged heart valves, and responds well to treatment.

Major causes of underlying cardiac pathological conditions include rheumatic valvular disease, congenital heart disease, and degenerative heart disease. Endocarditis may also be preceded by intrusive procedures, such as gynaecological examinations or minor surgery. Other people at high risk are intravenous drug abusers because of the possibility of bacteraemia from contaminated needles and syringes.

The infecting organisms are carried by a turbulent blood flow and deposited on the heart valves or elsewhere on the endocardium. The turbulent blood flow occurs in areas of myocardial anomalies, such as prolapsed mitral valves or ventricular septal defects. The organisms bombard the heart valves, become embedded in the valve matrix, and result in vegetative growths that may scar and perforate the leaflets. Further risk results if the vegetative growths break free of the valves, enter the bloodstream, and cause emboli. If the vegetative emboli enter organs such as the spleen or kidney, abscesses may form.

Prevention of infective endocarditis includes correction of any underlying cardiac defect, as well as measures to prevent bacteraemia. For people with underlying cardiac disease, early and vigorous treatment of infections, good oral hygiene, and prophylactic antibiotic therapy when undergoing dental care or a surgical procedure are important. When infective endocarditis occurs, prolonged antibiotic therapy may be required after the organism is identified. Abscesses may require surgical drainage.

RHEUMATIC HEART DISEASE

Rheumatic fever is an acute inflammatory reaction. It is important in the discussion of inflammatory heart disease, as it has tremendous potential for causing chronic heart problems. Over the last 50 years, rheumatic fever has become less frequent and less severe in the U.K.[31a] Symptoms of cardiac involvement usually follow a group A beta-haemolytic streptococcus pharyngeal infection. Ninety percent of the victims are between the age of 5 and 15.

Rheumatic fever may progress with mild symptoms and go undiagnosed, or the disease may be subclinical with no symptoms. The patient develops cardiac manifestations years later. On careful history taking, a recollection of a childhood illness confirming the likelihood of rheumatic fever is usually found.

The pathophysiology of rheumatic heart disease remains unclear. The pericardium, myocardium, or endocardium can be involved. The affected tissue develops small areas of necrosis (*Aschoff bodies*), which heal, leaving scar tissue. Myocardial changes are usually reversible. In the pericardium and endocardium, however, the disease process is usually not reversible and produces the disabling effects of rheumatic heart disease. The valves are typically most affected and become fibrous and incompetent. The leaflets of a valve may fuse during the healing phase (p. 422).

VALVULAR HEART DISEASE

Pathophysiology

Valvular heart disease is a general term that refers to any one of a variety of conditions that affect the valves within the heart. Normal valves function to maintain a unidirectional flow of blood through the cardiac chambers by passively opening and closing in response to variant pressure gradients. The mitral and tricuspid valves (atrioventricular valves) prevent the backflow of blood from the ventricles into the atria during systole. Movement of the atrioventricular valves is facilitated by the chordae tendinae and papillary muscles (see Fig. 17-1). Similarly, the aortic and pulmonary valves (semilunar valves) prevent the backflow of blood from the aorta and pulmonary artery into their respective ventricles during diastole.

The two basic problems that compromise the normal function of the valves are stenosis and insufficiency. *Stenosis* is a thickening of the valvular tissue, which causes a narrowing of the valvular orifice. *Insufficiency* refers to the inability of the valve to close completely. An insufficient or incompetent valve allows blood to flow in a retrograde or regurgitant manner.

The predominant aetiological factor in the development of a stenosed or insufficient valve is rheumatic fever. Throughout the course of this disease, large haemorrhagic and fibrinous lesions vegetate along the inflamed edges of the valves.[29] These lesions frequently develop on adjacent valve leaflets so that the edges adhere together. As the disease process progresses, the leaflets become so scarred there is permanent leaflet fusion and limited valvular movement of the normally free-flapping edges.

Since these underlying pathological changes occur over a period of time, the clinical signs and symptoms of a stenosed or insufficient valve do not usually show up until 10 to 40 years after the onset of rheumatic fever. Furthermore, the extent of valvular damage is largely dependent on its normal degree of motion. Since the pressures and consequent valvular movement on the left side of the heart are greater than those on the right, the mitral and aortic valves are more susceptible. The tricuspid and pulmonary valves are much less frequently affected by rheumatic fever.

The signs and symptoms and medical therapy of valvular heart disorders are outlined in Table 17-4 for each type of disorder. Additional information about specific valvular disorders is provided in the sections that follow.

REVIEW
Table 17-4 Valvular heart disorders

	Signs and symptoms	Medical therapy
Mitral insufficiency	Excessive fatigue, weakness, exhaustion Weight loss Exertional dyspnoea, orthopnoea, paroxysmal nocturnal dyspnoea, rales Late stages: pulmonary oedema, right-sided heart failure *Auscultation:* Palpable thrill at apex S_1 absent, soft, or buried in murmur Murmur: high pitched blowing, swishing, throughout systole (at apex) S_3 low pitched	Activity limitations Sodium-restricted diet Diuretics Digoxin Treatment of atrial dysrhythmias Surgery: valvuloplasty, valvular replacement, annuloplasty
Mitral stenosis	Excessive fatigue, weakness Dyspnoea, exertional dyspnoea, orthopnoea, paroxysmal nocturnal dyspnoea Dry cough, bronchitis, rales Pulmonary oedema Recurrent pulmonary emboli Haemoptysis Right-sided heart failure *Auscultation:* Palpable thrill at apex S_1 snapping, increased, loud Murmur: soft, low pitched, rumbling, diastolic (at apex)	Sodium-restricted diet Diuretics Activity limitations Oxygen therapy Anticoagulant therapy Surgery: valvulotomy, valve replacement
Aortic insufficiency	Palpitations, sinus tachycardia Exertional dyspnoea, orthopnoea, paroxysmal nocturnal dyspnoea Excessive diaphoresis Angina Late stages: left- and right-sided heart failure *Auscultation:* Murmur: high pitched, blowing, diastolic (third intercostal space) Systolic ejection murmur at base	Digoxin Sodium-restricted diet Diuretics Nitroglycerin (angina) Penicillin therapy (if syphilis a cause) Surgery: valve replacement, valvuloplasty
Aortic stenosis	Angina Syncope Fatigue, weakness Exertional dyspnoea, orthopnoea, paroxysmal nocturnal dyspnoea Pulmonary oedema, rales Late stages: right-sided heart failure *Auscultation:* Murmur: low pitched, rough, rasping, systolic (at base or carotids) Systolic thrill at base of heart	Activity limitations Sodium-restricted diet Diuretics Digoxin Nitroglycerin (angina) Surgery: valve replacement
Tricuspid stenosis	Pulmonary congestion, dyspnoea Right-sided heart failure Decreased cardiac output: weakness, fatigue, weight loss, hypotension Late stages: cirrhosis, jaundice, malnutrition	Sodium-restricted diet Digoxin Diuretics Surgery: valvuloplasty, valve replacement
Tricuspid insufficiency	Right-sided heart failure Decreased cardiac output: weakness, fatigue, weight loss, hypotension *Auscultation:* Murmur: blowing, throughout systole (left sternal border, increases with inspiration)	Sodium-restricted diet Digoxin Diuretics Surgery: narrowing of annulus, valve replacement

Mitral stenosis

Mitral stenosis is more often found in women than men. As rheumatic fever is the primary factor in its development, the progressive destruction of the valve occurs over a 20-year period. Mitral commissures (junctions between adjacent cusps) fuse, and the valvular leaflets or cusps thicken and calcify. The chordae tendinae also become short and thick. These underlying changes result in a narrow mitral valve that impedes the normal blood flow. Nonrheumatic causes include atrial myxomas, bacterial vegetation, thrombus formation, or calcification of the mitral annulus.

To accommodate the increased work load required to move blood through this narrowed orifice, the left atrium hypertrophies. The resultant left atrial pressure exerts further pressure onto the pulmonary vasculature, causing pulmonary hypertension and pulmonary congestion. Eventually these conditions result in right ventricular failure and right-sided heart failure.

Another common complication of mitral stenosis is atrial fibrillation. Structural changes in the atrial wall from the increased pressure predispose to this dysrhythmia. The coupling of atrial fibrillation and pooling of blood in the atria increases the likelihood of thrombus formation and arterial embolization.

Mitral insufficiency

In contrast to mitral stenosis, mitral insufficiency is more commonly seen in men than women. Although the same pathological processes occur as a result of rheumatic fever, several other acquired and congenital conditions, such as papillary muscle dysfunction, ruptured chordae tendinae, prolapsed mitral valve, bacterial endocarditis, and congenital abnormalities, can contribute to its development. The result is that the mitral valve leaflets fail to close fully. Consequently, a variable amount of blood leaks back through the valve from the left ventricle into the atrium.

The left atrium dilates and hypertrophies to compensate for the increased volume and pressure. The left ventricle also hypertrophies in response to the increased preload (blood that was regurgitated into the atrium during systole is returned to the ventricle during diastole). In other words, the ejection fraction is reduced and the end-diastolic volume is increased.

Aortic stenosis

Aortic stenosis constitutes 25% of all valvular heart diseases. Diseases of the aortic valve do not usually occur as a single entity; most often there is also involvement of the mitral valve. Aortic stenosis develops as a congenital or acquired condition (rheumatic fever, arteriosclerosis). Clinical symptoms of aortic stenosis are not manifested until the size of the opening in the valve has been reduced to approximately one-third of normal. This situation may not occur until many years after the inception of the disease process. The asymptomatic nature of this disease is largely caused by the tremendous compensatory abilities of the left ventricle.

The left ventricle must generate an abnormally high pressure to eject blood through the narrowed aortic orifice. This added pressure requirement results in ventricular hypertrophy with a concomitant increase in myocardial oxygen demand. The oxygen demand may exceed the supply because of reduced cardiac output and inadequate coronary artery perfuson. Classic symptoms of angina may result.

The progressive stenosis accompanied by ventricular hypertrophy in the presence of mitral valve disease causes a decrease in CO. Symptoms of pulmonary congestion and eventually right-sided heart failure ensue.

Aortic insufficiency

Rheumatic fever accounts for approximately 80% of all cases of aortic insufficiency. In this instance the valve fails to close completely, and this results in a retrograde blood flow from the aorta into the left ventricle during diastole. The ventricle hypertrophies to hold all the regurgitant blood. Over time, the left ventricle cannot withstand the added work load, leading to the development of decreased CO, left ventricular failure, and right-sided heart failure. Other causes of aortic insufficiency include Marfan's syndrome, congenital anomalies, syphilis, severe hypertension, bacterial endocarditis, traumatic valve rupture, and dissecting aortic aneurysm.

Tricuspid stenosis

Tricuspid stenosis is a relatively uncommon valvular lesion that usually coexists with stenosis of the mitral or aortic valves. The major cause of this disease is rheumatic fever. The leaflets become thick and fuse together, and the chordae tendinae also become short and thick. Hence during diastole blood flow is reduced through the compromised valve. This blockage further causes a backflow of blood in the systemic circulation. Engorgement of the superior and inferior vena cava precede the development of right-sided heart failure.

Tricuspid insufficiency

Tricuspid insufficiency is a rare disorder that is more prevalent in children than adults. The disease usually develops secondary to marked dilation of the right ventricle and tricuspid valve ring.[8] The valve itself widens and the leaflets are unable to close properly. Therefore, there is regurgitant blood flow to the right atrium during systole. The right atrium hypertrophies to accommodate the increased volume, but invariably the CO decreases with the concomitant decreased blood flow to the left side of the heart. Eventually the excess volume in the atrium causes right-sided heart failure.

Pulmonary valve disease

Lesions of the pulmonary valve are extremely rare in adults. This valve is less likely to be affected by rheumatic fever and bacterial endocarditis. For a more detailed discussion of congenital pulmonary stenosis, refer to a standard paediatric text.

Nursing Process
Assessment

Assessment data that the nurse obtains are essentially the same for any patient with valvular heart disease. Many of the symptoms are related to decreased CO.

Subjective data

1. Ability to carry out ADL and other desired activities: changes in endurance, fatigue, weakness
   These symptoms result from inadequate CO with subsequent impairment in cellular oxygenation
2. Shortness of breath: occurrence, type
   The patient may have dyspnoea on exertion (DOE), orthopnoea, or paroxysmal nocturnal dyspnoea (PND) (p. 408), depending on the degree of heart failure
3. Pain in chest (angina): occurrence, measures used to relieve pain
4. Palpitations: occurrence

Palpitations are a sensation in the chest described as a bounding or pounding of the heart

5. Syncope: occurrence
   A patient may verbalize feelings of light-headedness, dizzy spells, or fainting; these symptoms can be associated with a decrease in CO
6. Peripheral oedema: site, extent, time of day
   Swelling of legs during the day with decreased swelling at night when legs are elevated is usually reported
7. Body weight: perceived pattern of weight gain
8. Diet and medications: ability to carry out therapeutic regimen

Table 17-5 Findings in valvular heart disorders

Disorder	Chest radiograph	Electrocardiogram	Echocardiogram	Cardiac catheterization
Mitral stenosis	Left atrial enlargement Mitral valve classification Right ventricular enlargement Prominence of pulmonary artery	Left atrial hypertrophy Right ventricular hypertrophy Atrial fibrillation	Thickened mitral valve Left atrial enlargement	Increased pressure gradient across valve Increased left atrial pressure Increased PCWP Increased right heart pressures Decreased cardiac output
Mitral insufficiency	Left atrial enlargment Left ventricular enlargement	Left atrial hypertrophy Left ventricular hypertrophy Atrial fibrillation Sinus tachycardia	Abnormal mitral valve movement Left atrial enlargement	Mitral regurgitation Increased atrial pressure Increased LVEDP Increased PCWP Decreased cardiac output
Aortic stenosis	Left ventricular enlargement Aortic valve calcification May have enlargement of left atrium, pulmonary artery, right ventricle, right atrium	Left ventricular hypertrophy	Thickened aortic valve Thickened ventricular wall Abnormal movement of aortic leaflets	Increased pressure gradient across valve Increased LVEDP
Aortic insufficiency	Left ventricular enlargement	Left ventricular hypertrophy Tall R waves Sinus tachycardia	Left ventricular enlargement Abnormal mitral valve movement Increased movement of ventricular wall	Aortic regurgitation Increased LVEDP Decreased arterial diastolic pressure
Tricuspid stenosis	Right atrial enlargement Prominence of superior vena cava	Right atrial hypertrophy Tall peaked P waves Atrial fibrillation	Abnormal valvular leaflets Right atrial enlargement	Increased pressure gradient across valve Increased right atrial pressure Decreased cardiac output
Tricuspid insufficiency	Right atrial enlargement Right ventricular enlargement	Right ventricular hypertrophy Atrial fibrillation	Prolapse of tricuspid valve Right atrial enlargement	Increased atrial pressure Tricuspid regurgitation Decreased cardiac output

LVEDP, Left ventricular end-diastolic pressure; *PCWP,* pulmonary capillary wedge pressure.

Objective data

1. History of rheumatic fever
2. Observation/inspection
   a. Position and comfort level of patient
   b. Character and rate of breathing
   c. Use of supplemental oxygen
   d. Skin colour and temperature
   e. Nailbed colour and blanching (capillary filling)
   f. Diaphoresis
3. Auscultation
   a. Cardiac rate and rhythm
   b. Presence or change in heart sounds (murmurs, S_3, S_4, friction rub)
   c. Character of heart sounds at all auscultatory sites (aortic, pulmonary, tricuspid, mitral)
   d. Character and distribution of breath sounds
   e. Presence of adventitious breath sounds (rales, rhonchi)
4. Palpation
   a. Warmth of extremities
   b. Equality of symmetry of pulses
   c. Presence of oedema, pitting or nonpitting
   d. Signs of phlebitis (increased calf diameter, positive Homans' sign)
   e. Pulse rate and rhythm
5. Change in body weight

Diagnostic tests

Four major diagnostic tests are used to determine the presence of valvular heart disease: chest radiograph, ECG, echocardiogram, and cardiac catheterization. Table 17-5 summarizes the findings that are indicative of each specific type of valvular disease.

Chest radiograph

A chest radiograph demonstrates the overall size and configuration of the heart and its chambers. Calcification in the pericardium, myocardium, valves, or large blood vessels is also evident on the film. Most cardiac abnormalities that are discernable on a chest X-ray can be detected with standard anterioposterior and lateral views of the chest.

Electrocardiogram

An ECG (p. 410) is helpful in the diagnosis of valvular heart disease. Hypertrophy of either chamber, as well as specific dysrhythmias, can be detected.

Echocardiography

Echocardiography is most useful in the detection of abnormalities in the mitral and aortic valves. It is some benefit in the diagnosis of tricuspid valve disease.

Echocardiography is a noninvasive technique that uses ultrasound to assess the structures and motions within the heart. A small transducer is placed on the patient's anterior left chest and moved in various directions to visualize specific cardiac areas. This small transducer functions as a transmitter and receiver. It transmits high-frequency sound waves to the heart and then receives the reflected or echoed ultrasonic beams from the patient's heart. The ultrasonic beam is converted into electrical energy so that lines and spaces are displayed on the oscilloscope. These lines and spaces represent bone, cardiac chambers, valves, the septum, and muscle. A representative copy of the echocardiogram is obtained on paper to become a permanent record of the findings.

Since echocardiography is a noninvasive procedure, it is safer than cardiac catheterization. Hence, whenever possible, it precedes the cardiac catheterization. No special preparation is required for the test. The patient can eat and take medications as usual. Most importantly, the patient should be told about the purpose and procedure of this test. The patient must be aware of the importance of lying still for approximately 30 to 60 minutes. After the test the patient may resume normal activities, since there are no adverse effects from this test.

Cardiac catheterization

Cardiac catheterization is an extremely valuable diagnostic procedure that provides information about the structure and the function of the cardiac chambers, valves, and vessels. Since this is an invasive procedure, it is usually performed after several other diagnostic tests. A catheterization is performed on either the right or left side of the heart depending on the suspected valvular dysfunction. The purpose and procedure of each type are outlined in Box 17-26.

17-26

Cardiac catheterization

Right side	**Left side**
Purpose	Evaluate pressures on left side of heart
Confirm suspected valvular heart disease—congenital or acquired	Assess competency of valves
	Assess left ventricular function
Procedure	Cutdown made in large artery in patient's arm or groin
Cutdown made in large vein in patient's arm	Catheter threaded via flouroscopy through descending aorta, aortic arch, ascending aorta, aortic valve, and left ventricle
Catheter threaded via fluoroscopy through superior vena cava, right atrium, right ventricle, pulmonary artery and pulmonary capillaries	Blood sample obtained to determine oxygen content and saturation
Blood sample obtained to determine oxygen content and saturation	Pressure recorded for each chamber/vessel
Pressures recorded for each chamber/vessel	Pressure gradient measurement across valves obtained

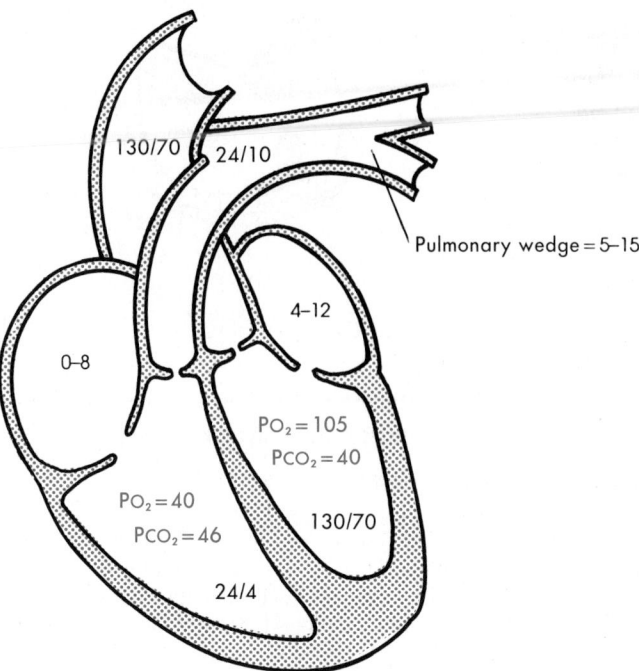

130/70   24/10

Pulmonary wedge = 5–15

4–12

0–8

$PO_2 = 105$
$PCO_2 = 40$

$PO_2 = 40$
$PCO_2 = 46$

130/70

24/4

Fig. 17-26   Pressure readings and blood gases in millimetres of mercury (mmHg) in chambers of heart and major blood vessels.

Normal pressure readings and oxygen concentrations for the chambers and great vessels are listed in Fig. 17-26. The right side of the heart is a low-pressure system with less oxygen saturation, since the blood there is going to the lungs. In contrast, the left side of the heart is a relatively high-pressure system with full oxygen saturation, as the blood there is returning from the lungs. Any changes in normal pressures and oxygen saturation are significant. Abnormalities in pressure gradients across valves are also indicative of valvular heart disease.

Nursing analysis

Nursing analyses are determined from assessment of patient data. Possible nursing analyses for the people with valvular disease may include, but are not limited to, the following:

Problem	Possible aetiologies
Activity intolerance	Imbalance between oxygen supply and demand, weakness
Breathing pattern, ineffective	Decreased cardiac output, fatigue
Pain	Angina, organ congestion
Fluid volume, excess	Decreased cardiac output
Knowledge deficit	Lack of exposure/recall

Planning: expected patient outcomes

Expected therapeutic outcomes for the patient with valvular heart disease centre around relief of symptoms and adequate cardiac functioning. Signs of pulmonary congestion and systemic venous congestion should be decreased, and improvement in cardiac output should be noted. The extent to which these outcomes are realized depends on the severity of the underlying problem, the presence or absence of other medical conditions, and the response of the patient to the treatment regimen. Outcomes related to the possible nursing analyses may include, but are not limited to, the following:

1. Rests between activities.
2. States that breathing is easier and fatigue occurs less frequently with activity.
3. States feeling more comfortable.
4. Coughs less frequently; pitting oedema decreases.
5. Describes the following:
   a. Nature of valvular disease
   b. Medication regimen
   c. Prescribed dietary sodium modifications
   d. Work, rest, and activity programme to conserve energy and decrease exertional dyspnoea
   e. Rationale for and type of surgery to be performed, if indicated
   f. Plans for continued medical therapy.

Implementation
Assisting with achievement of therapeutic goals

1. Administration of medications, as prescribed (diuretics, digoxin, antiarrhythmics)
2. Continued monitoring for signs of decreased CO
   a. Daily intake and output
   b. Daily weights
   c. Respiratory rate and rhythm
   d. Auscultation of breath sounds and heart sounds
   e. Condition of skin and mucous membranes
   f. Capillary perfusion
   g. Equality and strength of peripheral pulses
   h. Presence and extent of oedema
   i. Blood pressure
3. Sodium restricted diet for fluid control of pulmonary or systemic venous congestion

Interventions to achieve patient outcomes
Assisting with comfort and ADL

1. Identify those activities of daily living which are fatiguing and for which patient may need some assistance
2. Design with patient a plan that will allow for completion of daily activities
3. Incorporate rest periods between activities
4. Maintain use of supportive oxygen therapy during activities, as necessary

Facilitating patient/family teaching

1. Effect of a sodium-restricted or fluid-restricted diet on cardiac function, as appropriate
2. Effects of medications: diuretics, cardiac glycosides, anticoagulants
3. Prophylactic use of antibiotics before and after dental work
4. How to check for build-up of fluid in legs
5. Purpose of procedure for diagnostic tests (echocardiogram, cardiac catheterization)
6. Purpose and nature of surgical intervention, if appropriate.

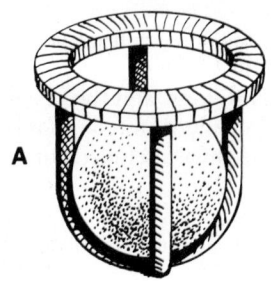
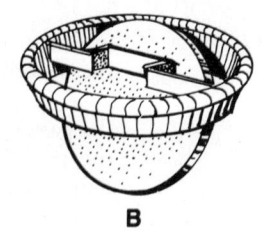
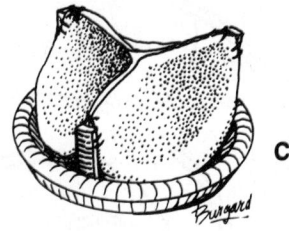

Fig. 17-27 Heart valve replacements. **A,** Caged-ball valve. **B,** Tilting-disk valve. **C,** Biological valve.

17-27

Types of valve repair

Valvuloplasty
Repair of valve, suturing of torn leaflets

Annuloplasty
Repair of ring or annulus of incompetent valve, tightening and suturing of annulus

Valvulotomy/commissurotomy
Repair of a leaflet or commissure, fibrous band or ring

Evaluation

Evaluation will be based on expected patient outcomes. Questions to consider to include the following:
1. Is patient able to describe a work, rest, and activity programme to conserve energy?
2. Can patient describe the nature of the valvular disorder?
3. Is patient able to explain any required dietary changes?
4. Can patient explain medication regimen?
5. Does the patient understand the plans for continued medical follow-up?

Surgical Intervention

Surgical intervention is indicated for a patient whose lifestyle is severely compromised by valvular heart disease. If a patient has haemodynamically debilitating symptoms that are unsuccessfully managed by conventional medical therapies, surgery is then the recommended treatment modality. There are two basic surgical procedures: repair of the valve problem or replacement of the valve.

Repair of valve

Several terms are used to describe the specific anatomical structure undergoing repair (Box 17-27). Valvulotomy or commissurotomy can be done as a closed or open procedure. A closed approach involves removing a rib with a small incision into the left atrium. A dilator is then used to widen the narrowed valve and free the stenosed leaflet. The atrium is also palpated for thrombi. In the open technique, used also for valvuloplasty and annuloplasty, the thorax is incised and the heart completely exposed.

17-28

Guidelines for Care

The patient undergoing valvular surgery

Preoperative care
Give medications as ordered
  Digitalis preparations and diuretics are often discontinued before surgery to avoid dysrhythmias associated with digitalis toxicity that may be precipitated by cardiopulmonary bypass
  If the patient has been receiving anticoagulants, vitamin K may be administered before surgery to return prothrombin time to normal
  Antibiotics may be given to decrease incidence of postoperative endocarditis
Prepare patient for surgery by providing explanation of procedure and usual postoperative routines, addressing specific concerns of patient and family

Postoperative care
Administer anticoagulant therapy as prescribed
Assess apical heartbeat: a "click" sound is usually heard; reassure patient that this sound is normal; assess for development of murmur
Explain medication regimen to patient
  Need for antibiotics for approximately 1 month following valve replacement
  Need for cardiac glycosides to improve cardiac function and control dysrhythmias for prescribed time (usually 3–6 months after surgery)

Replacement of valve

Many types of valves can be used for replacement. A valve is selected on the basis of location of the incompetent valve, the underlying pathological changes, and the age of the patient. The size of the prosthetic valve is of major importance. Valves are grouped according to their design and function: caged-ball, caged-disk, titling-disk, and biological valves (Fig. 17-27).

Caged-ball valves are the most durable. Their use, however, is restricted to patients with a large enough annulus and chamber to accommodate the cage itself. It is never used for tricuspid valve replacement because of the limited capacity of the right ventricle.

Caged-disk valves occupy less space in the ventricles than other valves and require less force to move the occluding disk. This type of valve creates more obstruction to blood flow than other type of valves. If the disk "sticks" in the cage, causing total obstruction of blood flow, haemodynamics are seriously compromised.

Tilting-disk valves have occluders that tilt or pivot within a ring rather than balls or disks that pop back and forth in a cage (Fig. 17-27, B). This type of valve produces nearly central blood flow through its orifice, providing more normal blood flow. However, the valve may develop areas under the pivoting points, where thrombi can form as a result of the blood stasis.

Biological valves are derived from animal cardiac tissue or human cadaver donors. Animal valves carry less risk for thromboembolism; however, they tend to degenerate over time. Improvements in organ procurement and storage may make more human valves available in the future. These valves are less prone to infection and rejection than other replacements.

Preoperative and postoperative nursing care

Nursing care for the patient undergoing valvular heart surgery is essentially the same as that for patients undergoing coronary bypass surgery (p. 598). Specific nursing care related to valvular surgery is listed in Box 17-28.

ANEURYSMS

Pathophysiology

An aneurysm is a local or diffuse dilation of an artery. It occurs secondary to a variety of disease processes such as infections, hypertension, or syphilis, although arteriosclerosis is the predominant aetiological factor. Regardless of the pathogenesis, the musculoelastic middle (media) layer of the artery becomes weakened, and it produces stretching of the inner (intima) and outer (adventitia) layers. Blood pressure within the vessel continues to weaken its walls and to enlarge the aneurysm.

The extent of arterial damage and clinical symptomatology vary greatly according to the type, size, and location of the aneurysm. An aneurysm is classified on the basis of its shape and subsequent damage to the affected artery (Fig. 17-28). The *fusiform aneurysm*, the most common type, assumes a spindle shape around the entire circumference of the vessel. In contrast, a *saccular aneurysm* affects only a part of the arterial circumference. This type of aneurysm appears as a unilateral sac or outpouching on the side of the artery. Also, a saccular aneurysm is more likely to rupture. A *dissecting aneurysm* develops from a split or tear in the intimal wall overlying a diseased media. This relatively uncommon occurrence leads to the accumulation of blood in a newly formed cavity between the vessel layers.

Although these types of aneurysms can develop in any artery, the major site for aneurysm formation is the aorta. Since the aorta has such a large diameter and is subject to great pressures, it is often the location for underlying disease processes. Aortic aneurysms are found in the thoracic segment and, more commonly, in the abdominal portions. Since there is some difference between aneurysms in these locations, they are discussed as separate entities.

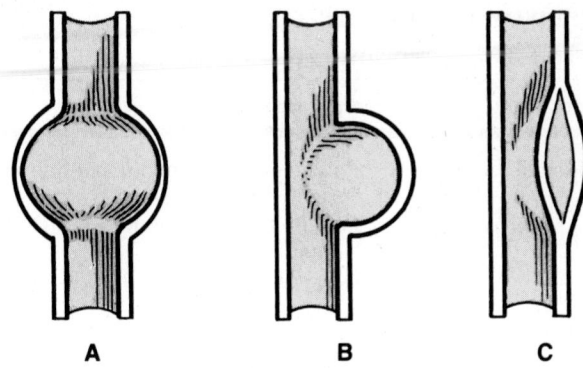

Fig. 17-28   Types of aneurysms. **A,** Fusiform. **B,** Saccular. **C,** Dissecting.

Thoracic aortic aneurysms

Aneurysms within the thoracic area can develop in the descending, ascending, or transverse section of the aorta. Hypertensive men between 50 and 70 years of age are typically subject to this disease.

Aneurysms in the *descending aorta* are usually fusiform and originate just distal to the left subclavian artery. A patient with this form of aneurysm is asymptomatic. Symptoms of chest pain are associated with aneurysms of the *ascending aorta* (Table 17-6). Less frequent are aneurysms of the *transverse aorta* or aortic arch. Symptoms of this type directly relate to the aneurysm's compression on surrounding structures, such as the lungs, trachea, and larynx. Operative mortality is highest in people who have an acute onset of symptoms and in whom a dissecting aneurysm begins in the ascending aortic arch and causes insufficiency of the aortic valve.

Abdominal aortic aneurysms

Aneurysms of the abdominal aorta are more prevalent in hypertensive men over 60 years of age. The vast majority of these aneurysms develop just below the renal arteries but above the iliac bifurcation. An abdominal aneurysm grows slowly, hence the patient is usually asymptomatic. At other times the person may have pain or tenderness in the mid or upper abdomen. The aneurysm can leak into the retroperitoneal or pelvic cavity, or dissect into the duodenum. As the aorta exceeds its normal 3 to 4 cm diameter at this point, there is an increased probability of rupture.

The prognosis for a patient with an abdominal aortic aneurysm depends not only on the size of the defect but, more importantly, on the extent of arteriosclerotic heart disease. The aneurysm may extend to impinge on the renal, iliac, or mesenteric arteries. The stasis of blood favours thrombus formation along the wall of the vessel, and if the aneurysm is large, the most feared complication is aneurysmal rupture. More than half of those with untreated abdominal aneurysm die within two years of diagnosis; over 85% die within five years.

Diagnostic Tests
Radiography

An aneurysm is most often detected accidentally by routine chest or abdominal X-ray, since symptoms are rarely mani-

REVIEW

Table 17-6 Aneurysms

Type	Signs and symptoms	Medical therapy
Abdominal aortic	Pulsating mass in mid-upper abdomen Systolic bruit over aorta Pain in mid-upper abdomen or in lower back or groin Long-standing cramps in buttocks, thighs, calves	Antihypertensive medications Pain medications Inotropic agents (for example, propranolol) Surgery: resection of aneurysm with graft replacement
Thoracic aortic	*Ascending aorta:* Chest pain: deep, diffuse, aching *Transverse aorta:* Dyspnoea, cough, hoarseness *Dissecting aneurysm:* Tearing sensation in chest, pain radiating to neck, shoulders, lower back, abdomen	Antihypertensive medications Negative inotropic agents (for example, propranolol) Surgery: Resection of aneurysm with graft replacement Aortic valve replacement (if aortic insufficiency)

fested. Radiological findings show widening of the aorta with a ring of calcification outlining the aneurysm and displacement of surrounding structures.

Angiography

An aortogram reveals the size and location of an aneurysm. This test determines whether an aneurysm is leaking, expanding, or dissecting. An aortogram is performed by insertion of a catheter into the femoral, bronchial, or axillary artery. The patient may feel a burning sensation when the contrast dye is injected. Following injection of the contrast material, a series of radiograms is taken at intervals to determine an accurate flow study.

After the procedure, the patient must remain resting in bed for 6 to 12 hours with only minimal flexion of the cannulated joint. Monitor vital signs every 15 minutes for two hours. Assessment of pulses, skin colour, temperature, movement, and numbness distal to the site is also important. Inspect the injection site whenever vital signs are taken for the presence of bleeding, swelling, or haematoma.

Sonography

Ultrasound is also helpful in determining the shape and location of the aneurysm. Special conducting gell is applied to the skin, and the Doppler probe head is placed over the gel to intensify sounds of pulse vibration. This procedure detects blood flow and presence of bruit. Since this a noninvasive procedure, there are no special precautions or posttest care.

Surgery

Surgery is the treatment of choice for patients with large or dissecting aneurysms or with those aneurysms that produce symptoms with a significant risk of rupture. Elective resection at the time of the first symptoms is often advised, since emergency surgery increases surgical risks. Complications of surgery include massive haemorrhage, injury to adjacent structures (duodenum, ureters, kidneys), myocardial infarction, renal failure, stroke, or graft infection.

Procedures
Thoracic aorta

Surgical intervention for the patient with an aneurysm of the thoracic aorta is comparable to open heart surgery. A midline thoracic incision is made, and the aneurysm is exposed. Cardiopulmonary bypass (p. 404) maintains tissue oxygenation during clamping of the aorta. Hypothermia may also be indicated to decrease the metabolic requirements of the tissues. While the aneurysm itself is being rejected, cross-clamps are placed above and below the aorta to prevent blood flow into the operative area. An artificial patch or tube (Teflon or Dacron) is grafted on the area.

Abdominal aorta

Surgical intervention for the removal of an abdominal aortic aneurysm is performed without use of heart and lung bypass, since arterial blood flow to lower extremities can be interrupted safely during the operative procedure. An abdominal incision is made, the aneurysm is opened, and any clots and debris are removed. A synthetic graft in the form of a patch or tube is sutured onto the tissues. Once the graft is replaced, the remaining arterial wall is sutured over the graft.

Preoperative preparation

The doctor explains the surgical risks when obtaining informed consent for the surgery. The nurse provides support for the patient during the decision-making process, since the surgery is associated with some mortality and morbidity.

The preparation and postoperative care for resection of a thoracic aortic aneurysm are similar to that for cardiac surgery (p. 404). Resection of an abdominal aortic aneurysm is similar to other abdominal surgery. Some surgeons additionally require a bowel preparation for optimal preparation, should bowel surgery be necessary. Heparin is usually given during surgery, before clamping the artery.

Postoperative care (abdominal aortic aneurysm)

1. Monitor the following parameters:
   a. Vital signs until stable
   b. Central venous pressure, pulmonary artery pressure, pulmonary capillary wedge pressure; observe for decrease indicating hypovolaemia
   c. Dysrhythmias
   d. Hourly circulation checks with assessment of all pulses distal to graft site
      (1) Absent pulses more than 6 to 12 hours indicate arterial occlusion
      (2) Poor peripheral perfusion: marked decrease in blood pressure, weak thready pulses, cool skin temperature, diaphoresis
      (3) Advanced occlusion: pain, cramping, numbness in extremities; legs may be white or blue and cool to cold
   e. Neurological check level of consciousness and ability to move lower extremities every one to two hours
   f. Blood loss: monitor chest tube output every hour; report drainage of > 100 ml/h × 3 hours
   g. Electrolytes: hypokalaemia, hypocalcaemia; supplement when necessary
   h. Postoperative ileus or distention: nasogastric output, bowel sounds, abdominal pain or discomfort
   i. Renal function (since aorta was clamped during surgery, preventing blood flow to kidneys)
      (1) Hourly urine flow greater than 25 to 30ml through indwelling catheter
      (2) Urine colour (haematuria may occur with renal damage)
      (3) Daily blood urea nitrogen (BUN)
2. Keep patient flat in bed without sharp flexion of hip and of knee to avoid pressure on femoral and popliteal arteries; turn patient gently side to side
3. Give medication for pain
4. Institute pulmonary ventilatory measures (deep breathing and coughing, and so on); use firm abdominal support to incision during coughing
5. Prevent postoperative thrombophlebitis
   a. Check for pain or cramps in calf, tenderness in specific areas of leg, redness along course of vein
   b. Encourage dorsiflexion and plantar flexion of feet
   c. Use elastic stockings
6. Encourage ambulation, when permitted

SUMMARY

1. Cardiac output is a function of heart rate and stroke volume.
2. Heart rate is generally under the control of the autonomic nervous system.
3. Stroke volume is determined by preload, contractility, and afterload.

4. A normal cardiac complex consists of a P wave, a QRS complex, and a T wave. The exact configuration of each component will vary according to the view or lead that is being recorded.
5. Normal sinus rhythm is characterized by a rhythm that is regular, a rate between 60 and 100 beats per minute, and a cardiac complex that is within established criteria for configuration and duration of the components and intervals.
6. Dysrhythmias may originate in the sinus node, atria, atrioventricular junction, or ventricles. Conduction abnormalities include atrioventricular blocks and bundle branch block.
7. Two life-threatening dysrythmias are ventricular fibrillation and ventricular standstill. CPR must be initiated and maintained until definitive treatment is effective.
8. Components of a teaching plan for patients with permanent pacemakers include the rationale for insertion, activities to avoid, the method for monitoring the function of their particular pacemaker, and symptoms to report to their doctor.
9. Nonmodifiable risk factors for CAHD include advancing age, being of the male sex or black race, and a positive family history of CAHD.
10. Major modifiable risk factors for CAHD include cigarette smoking, hyperlipidaemia, diabetes mellitus and hypertension. A diet high in cholesterol and saturated fats contributes to the risk factors.
11. Angina pectoris is chest pain caused by reversible myocardial ischaemia. Treatment involves increasing myocardial blood and oxygen supply (either with medication or surgical intervention) and reducing myocardial oxygen demands.
12. Teaching plans for patients with angina should include CAHD risk factor identification and reduction, interventions to use when chest pain occurs, methods of reducing myocardial oxygen demands, and symptoms to report to the doctor.
13. A myocardial infarction is the result of prolonged myocardial ischaemia that causes irreversible cellular damage and necrosis.
14. The clinical consequences of a myocardial infarction depend on the location of the coronary artery occlusion and the extent of necrosis.
15. Medical therapy for myocardial infarction includes measures to reduce the size of the infarcted area, to reduce myocardial oxygen demands, and to prevent or treat complications.
16. Possible nursing analyses for the patient with myocardial infarction include activity intolerance, decreased cardiac output, chest pain, anxiety, knowledge deficit, and diagnoses related to psychosocial adjustment of the patient and the family.
17. The two most common complications of myocardial infarction are cardiac dysrhythmias and left ventricular failure.
18. Teaching plans for patients with myocardial infarction should include content on the pathophysiology of myocardial infarction, the healing process, the treatment regimen, risk factors for coronary artery disease, the relationship between the treatment regimen and risk factor reduction, and resumption of activities (including sexual activity) following the acute phase of illness.
19. Heart failure is a state in which the heart is no longer able to pump an adequate supply of blood to meet the demands of the body.

20. Congestive heart failure refers to a state of circulatory congestion resulting from heart failure and its compensatory mechanisms. Symptoms of congestion may involve the pulmonary circulation, the systemic venous circulation, or both.

21. Signs and symptoms associated with congestive heart failure include those resulting from decreased cardiac output (forward failure) and those resulting from the subsequent congestion (backward failure).

22. Treatment for congestive heart failure involves improving oxygen supply to the tissues, decreasing oxygen demands on the myocardium, and relieving the symptoms of congestion. Common elements of treatment include oxygen, rest, positioning to facilitate optimal respiration, positive inotropic drugs, diuretics, sodium-restricted diet, and arterial/venous-dilating drugs.

23. Teaching plans for patients with congestive heart failure include content on the pathophysiology of the condition, approaches to regulating and monitoring the effect of activity, avoidance of precipitating factors, rationale for the treatment regimen, approaches to implementing the treatment regimen, and signs and symptoms to report to the doctor.

24. Pulmonary oedema represents the most severe form of congestion resulting from left ventricular failure, and cardiogenic shock represents the most severe form of decreased cardiac output. Both conditions are medical emergencies and require immediate, intensive medical and nursing intervention.

25. Inflammation of the pericardium, myocardium, or endocardium may be a consequence of infectious diseases, neoplasms, and other metabolic disorders. Patients with these conditions have the usual signs and symptoms associated with the inflammatory process and may also develop heart failure. Measures to prevent further episodes are important aspects of the treatment regimen.

26. Cardiac murmurs are a common physical finding in patients with valvular heart disease. Depending on the severity of the disease, the patient may or may not develop clinical symptoms such as those associated with heart failure.

27. Treatment for cardiac valvular disease involves management of the clinical symptoms. Surgical repair of the valve or replacement of the valve with an artificial prosthesis may be necessary.

28. An aneurysm is a local or diffuse dilation of an artery. Atherosclerosis is a common cause of this problem. Aneurysms may be fusiform, saccular, or dissecting and may form in the thoracic or abdominal aorta.

29. Depending on the location and size of the aneurysm, surgical resection may be necessary. An artificial tube is grafted onto the resected area.

STUDY QUESTIONS

- Using box 21-5 (Rhythm strip analysis) as your guide, analyse Fig. 21-18 (Sinus tachycardia). How do your findings compare with those in the legend?

- Review the process of wound healing in Chapter 18. How can this process be applied to a myocardial infarction?
- What is being done in your community to increase the public's awareness of risk factors for CAHD? How would you go about teaching the lay public about this heath problem?
- Examine the chart of a patient who has had a myocardial infarction. What ECG changes did you note? What changes occurred in the serum enzymes? How do the changes you noted compare to the usual pattern for myocardial infarction? What significance do these changes have for nursing interventions?
- Mr N is scheduled for CABG surgery. He has never had surgery before and is very apprehensive. He lives out of town; his wife is staying at a nearby hotel. What should be included in a preoperative teaching plan for Mr N?
- Examine the chart of a patient who has congestive failure. How do the patient's symptoms compare with the usual symptoms for congestive heart failure? Did the patient have left- or right-sided failure or both? What was the aetiology of congestive heart failure in this patient? What data would indicate an improvement in the pumping capabilities of this patien's heart? What nursing analyses did you identify for the patient? Could other analyses have been appropriate?

REFERENCES AND SELECTED READINGS

1. ABC of Resuscitation Edited by TR Evans (on behalf of the Resuscitation Council), *BMJ*, 1986.
1a.* Alpert JS: The pharmacologic management of coronary artery disease, *Heart Lung* 15:558-561, 1986.
2. Alpert JS, Rippe JM: *Manual of cardiovascular diagnosis and therapy*, ed 3, Boston, 1988, Little, Brown.
3. American Heart Association: *Heart facts*, Dallas, 1991, The Association.
4. Ayres SM: The prevention and treatment of shock in acute myocardial infarction, *Chest* 93:17S-21S, 1988.
5.* Baggs JG, Karch AM: Sexual counseling of women with coronary heart disease, *Heart Lung* 16:154-159, 1987.
5a.* Bavin TK, Self MA: Weaning from intra-aortic balloon pump support, *Am J Nurs* 91(10):54-59, 1991.
6. Berne RM, Levy MN: Cardiovascular physiology, ed 6, St Louis, 1991, Mosby-Year Book.
6a. Bernstein AD, Camm AJ, Fletcher RD, et al: The NASPE/BPEG Generic code for antibradyarrythmia and adaptive rate pacing and antitachyarrythmia devices, *PACE* 10:794, 1987.
7.* Borders CR: When the bypass patient returns home: problems your bypass patients face after discharge, *Patient Care* 19(13):65-76, 1985.
8. Braunwald E, et al: *Harrison's Principles of internal medicine*, ed 12, New York, 1991, McGraw-Hill.
9. Breithardt G, Borggrefe M: Recent advances in the identification of patients at risk of ventricular tachyarrhythmias: role of ventricular late potentials, *Circulation* 75:1091-1096, 1987.
10.* Burgess AW, Hartman CR: Patients' perceptions of the cardiac crisis, *Am J Nurs* 86:568-571, 1986.
11.* Carpenito LJ: Nursing diagnosis: application to clinical practice, ed 4, Philadelphia, 1991, JB Lippincott.
12. Cohn LH: Surgical treatment of acute myocardial infarction, *Chest* 93:13S-16S, 1988.
12a. Colling A, et al: Tee side coronary survey: An epidemiological study of acute attacks of MI, *BMJ* 2:1169-1173, 1976.
13. Conner WE, Bristow JD: Coronary heart disease: prevention, complications, and treatment, Philadelphia, 1985, JB Lippincott.

*Recommended for student reading.

14.* Conover MB: *Understanding electrocardiography,* ed 6, St Louis, 1991, Mosby–Year Book.

15.* Conti CR: Advances and controversies: laser therapy for cardiovascular disease, *Heart Lung* 16:465-473, 1987.

16. Cosgrove D, et al: Results of mitral valve reconstruction, *Circulation* 74 (suppl 1):182-187, 1986.

17.* Darovic GO: *Hemodynamic monitoring: invasive and noninvasive clinical application,* Phiadelphia, 1987, WB Saunders.

18.* Deans K, Hartshorn J: Use of antithrombotic agents in valvular heart disease, *J Cardiovasc Nurs* 1(3):65-69, 1987.

19. Duncan C, et al: Effect of chest tube management on drainage after cardiac surgery, *Heart Lung* 16:1-9, 1987.

20. Dunn DL, Gregory JJ: Noninvasive temporary pacing: ex-perience in a community hospital, *Heart Lung* 18:23-28, 1989.

21. Ebersole P, Hess P: Toward healthy aging: human needs and nursing response, ed 3, St Louis, 1990, Mosby–Year Book.

22.* Finesilver C, Metzle DJ: Right ventricular infarction: the critically different MI, *Am J Nurs* 91(4):32-36, 1991.

23. Gardin JM, et al: Effects of aging on peak systolic left ventricular wall stress in normal subjects, *Am J Cardiol* 63:998-999, 1989.

23a.* Gawlinski A, Jensen G: The complications of cardiovascular aging, *Am J Nurs* 91(11):26-30, 1991.

24. Gold HK: Thrombolysis in acute myocardial infarction, *Chest* 93:10S-12S, 1988.

25. Gottleib SV: Ischemia as an indicator of future adverse events in patients with coronary artery disease, *J Myocard Ischemia* 1:20-28, 1989.

26. Groer MW, Shekleton ME: Basic pathophysiology: a holistic approach, ed 3, St Louis, 1989, Mosby–Year Book.

27. Guyton AC, et al: *Textbook of medical physiology,* ed 8, Philadelphia, 1991, WB Saunders.

28.* Hall LT: Cardiovascular lasers: a look into the future, *Am J Nurs* 90(7):27-30, 1990.

29. Hurst JW: *The heart, arteries, and veins,* ed 6, New York, 1986, McGraw-Hill.

30. Izor-Povenmire K, House AA: Acute crack cocaine intoxication: a case study, *Focus Crit Care,* 16:112-119, 1989.

31.* Joseph DL, Bates S: Intraaortic balloon pumping: how to stay on course, *Am J Nurs* 90(9):42-47, 1990.

31a. Jullian DG: *Cardiology,* ed 5, London, 1988, Ballière Tindall.

32. Kerber RE, et al: Energy, current, and success in defi- brillation and cardioversion, *Circulation* 77:1038-1046, 1988.

33. Kinney MR, et al: *Comprehensive cardiac care,* ed 7, St Louis, 1991, Mosby–Year Book.

34.* Kleinhenz TJ: The inside story on preload and afterload, *Nurs* 15(5):50-55, 1985.

35. Krone R: Valvular heart disease. In Ahumadr G: *Cardiovas-cular pathophysiology,* New York, 1988, Oxford University Press.

36. Lakatta EG, et al: Human aging: changes in structure and function. *J Am Coll Cardiol* 10(2):42A-47A, 1987.

37.* Loan T: Nursing interaction with patients undergoing coronary angioplasty, *Heart Lung* 15:368-375, 1986.

37a.* Lothian CL: Laser angioplasty: vaporizing coronary artery plaque, *Nurs 92* 22(1):63-64, 1992.

38. Loveys VJ: Physiologic effects of cocaine with particular reference to the cardiovascular system, *Heart Lung* 16: 175-182, 1987.

39.* Marrie TJ: Infective endocarditis: a serious and changing disease, *Crit Care Nurs* 7(2):31-46, 1987.

40. McGill HC Jr: The cardiovascular pathology of smoking, *Am Heart J* 115:250-257, 1988.

41.* Mickus D, Monahan KJ, Brown C: Exciting external pacemakers, *Am J Nurs* 86:403-405, 1986.

42.* Misenski M: Pathophysiology of acute myocardial infarction: a rationale for thrombolytic therapy, *Heart Lung* 17:743-750, 1988.

43.* Norsen LH, Fox GB: Understanding cardiac output and the drugs that affect it, *Nurs 86* 16(5):43-45, 1986.

44. Porth CM: *Pathophysiology: concepts of altered health status,* ed 3, Philadelphia, 1990, JB Lippincott.

45. Price SA, Wilson LM: Pathophysiology: clinical concepts of disease processes, ed 3, New York, 1986, McGraw-Hill.

46.* Purcell JA, Burrows SG: A pacemaker primer, *Am J Nurs* 85:553-568, 1985.

47. Purdy RE, Boucek RJ: *Handbook of cardiac drugs,* Boston, 1988, Little, Brown.

48. Roberts WC: The aging heart, *Mayo Clin Proc* 63:205-206, 1988.

49.* Rodriguez SW, Reed RL: Thrombolytic therapy for MI, *Am J Nurs* 87:632-640, 1987.

50. Roubin GS: Intracoronary stenting, percutaneous place-ment of intracoronary prosthesis: new solutions and new problems, *J Invasive Cardiol* 1(1):1-6. 1988.

51.* Runions J: A program for psychological and social enhancement during rehabilitation after myocardial infarction, *Heart Lung* 14:117-125, 1985.

52.* Sakallaris BR: Advances and controversies: laser therapy for cardiovascular disease, *Heart Lung* 16:464-473, 1987.

53. Saul L: Arrhythmia mimics. I. *Am J Nurs* 91(3):41-43, 1991.

54. Saul L: Arrhythmia mimics. II. *Am J Nurs* 91(5):41-45, 1991.

55. Schroeder SA, et al: *Current medical diagnosis and treatment,* ed 30, Norwalk, Conn, 1991, Appleton & Lange.

56. Spann JF, Hurst JW: The recognition and management of heart failure. In Hurst JW: *The heart, arteries, and veins,* ed 6, New York, 1986, McGraw-Hill.

57. Timms AD, Nathan W: *Essentials of cardiology,* London, 1992, Blackwell Scientific Publications.

58. Walton J: *Oxford companion to medicine,* Oxford, 1986, Oxford University Press.

59. Wetherall DJ *et al; Oxford textbook of medicine* Oxford, oxford University Press.

60.* Witherell CL: Questions nurses ask about pacemakers, *Am J Nurs* 90(12):20-26, 1990.

61.* Chesney MA, Rosenman RH: Type A behavior: obser-vations on the past decade, *Heart Lung* 11:12-18, 1982.

62. Mirowski M, et al: Termination of malignant ventricular arrhythmias with an implanted automatic defibrillator in human beings, *N Engl J Med* 303:322-324, 1980.

FURTHER READING

Hickey M: Controlling cor pulmonale, *Nursing* 20(5):32E, 32H, May 1990.

McRae ME: Care plan for the patient undergoing intra-cardiac myxoma excision, *Critical Care Nurse* 10(9):58-60, 62-63, October 1990.

Wingate S: Rehabilitation of the patient with valvular heart disease, *J Cardiovascular Nursing* 1(3):52-64, May 1987.

The Patient with Peripheral Vascular Problems

Eileen Walsh

After studying this chapter, the learner should be able to:

- Identify risk factors associated with the development of peripheral vascular disorders.
- Compare pathophysiology, problems, expected outcomes, and interventions for patients with arterial and venous disorders.
- Describe nursing interventions for patients having surgery for arterial and venous disorders.
- Describe the pathophysiology and nursing interventions for patients with leg ulcers and lymph disorders.
- Identify problems and nursing interventions to prevent and control hypertension.

Problems of the peripheral vascular system refer to a number of disorders that disrupt blood flow through the blood vessels. This classification generally excludes those conditions that affect the aorta and coronary arteries, which have a more direct relationship to the heart (see Chapter 17) and the cerebral vessels (see Chapter 29). Specific alterations in arterial and venous blood flow in the lower and upper extremities are discussed in this chapter. Lymphoedema is included because the lymphatic system complements the function of the vascular system. In addition, a section on hypertension is included because it is a major contributing factor to peripheral vascular problems.

ANATOMY AND PHYSIOLOGY

All the cells of the body depend on an intact and functioning vascular system. This vascular system is a closed circuit consisting of the systemic and pulmonary circulations. Blood circulates from the left side of the heart to the tissues and back to the right side of the heart. It then flows through the lungs and back to the left side of the heart. The main components of the vascular system are the arteries, capillaries, and veins. The vascular system is aided by the lymphatic system, which contains lymph vessels and nodes.

Arteries

Arteries are thick-walled vessels that transport oxygenated blood via the aorta away from the heart and to the tissues. As the arteries approach the tissues, they branch into smaller vessels called arterioles (Fig. 18-1). All arteries are composed of the following three basic tissue layers:

1. Inner layer of endothelium (intima).
2. Middle layer of connective tissue, smooth muscle, or elastic fibres (media).
3. Outer layer of connective tissue (adventitia).

The media comprises the major part of the vessel wall. In the large arteries the media is primarily composed of elastic and connective tissue, which enables the artery to respond to alterations of blood volume while maintaining a constant flow. Arterial constrictions (decreased arterial diameter) increases resistance to blood flow. There is much less elastic fibre in the smaller arteries and arterioles; these vessels have smooth muscle that contracts and relaxes through nervous, chemical, and hormonal factors.

Capillaries

The capillaries are minute, thin-walled vessels located in the tissues and are composed of a single layer of cells. The capillaries connect the arterioles to the smallest veins and venules, allowing for the exchange of essential cellular products. Nutrients, oxygen, and regulatory substances move into the cells, whereas waste products, carbon dioxide, and cellular secretions move from the cells into the blood.

Veins

Veins are thin-walled vessels that transport deoxygenated blood from the capillaries back to the right side of the heart. They are composed of three layers: intima, media, and adventitia. Unlike the arterial walls, there is little

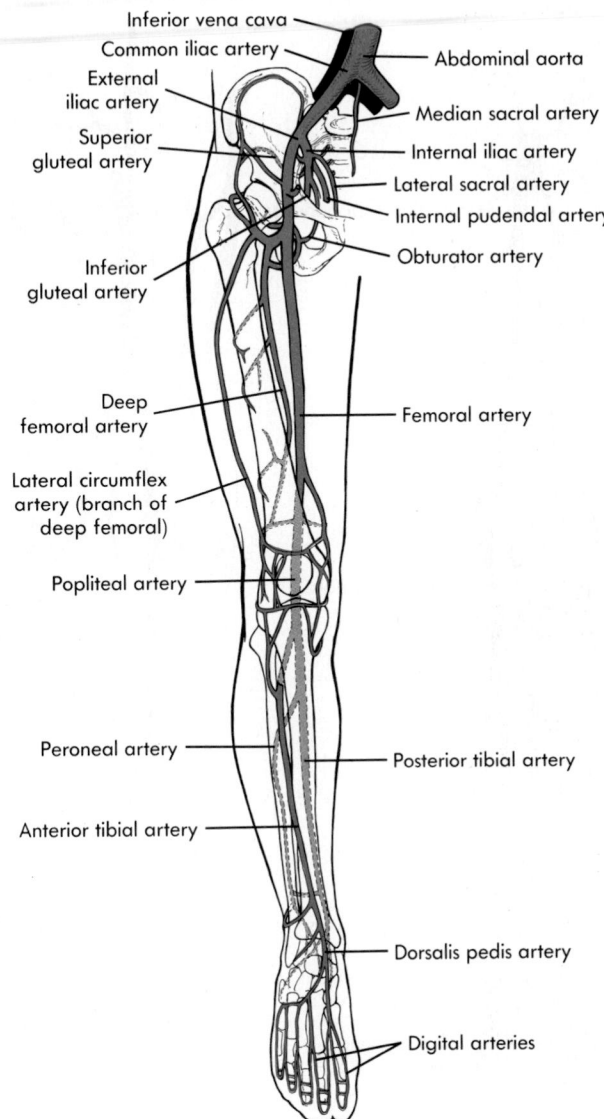

Fig. 18-1   Major arteries of lower limb. (From Seeley RR, Stephens TD, and Tate P: *Anatomy & physiology*, ed 2, St. Louis, 1992, Mosby–Year Book.)

smooth muscle and connective tissue. This makes the veins distensible, enabling larger volumes of blood to accumulate. The sympathetic nervous system innervates the veins, causing vasoconstriction, decreased venous volume, and increased circulating blood volume. Major veins, particularly those in the lower extremities (Fig. 18-2) have oneway valves that allow blood to flow against gravity.

Lymphatics

The lymphatic vessels carry lymph from the tissues back into the venous circulation. This system is made up of small thin vessels located throughout the body in close proximity to the veins (Fig. 18-3). The lymphatics begin as capillaries that drain the tissues of lymph (a fluid similar to plasma) and tissue fluid containing cells, cellular debris,

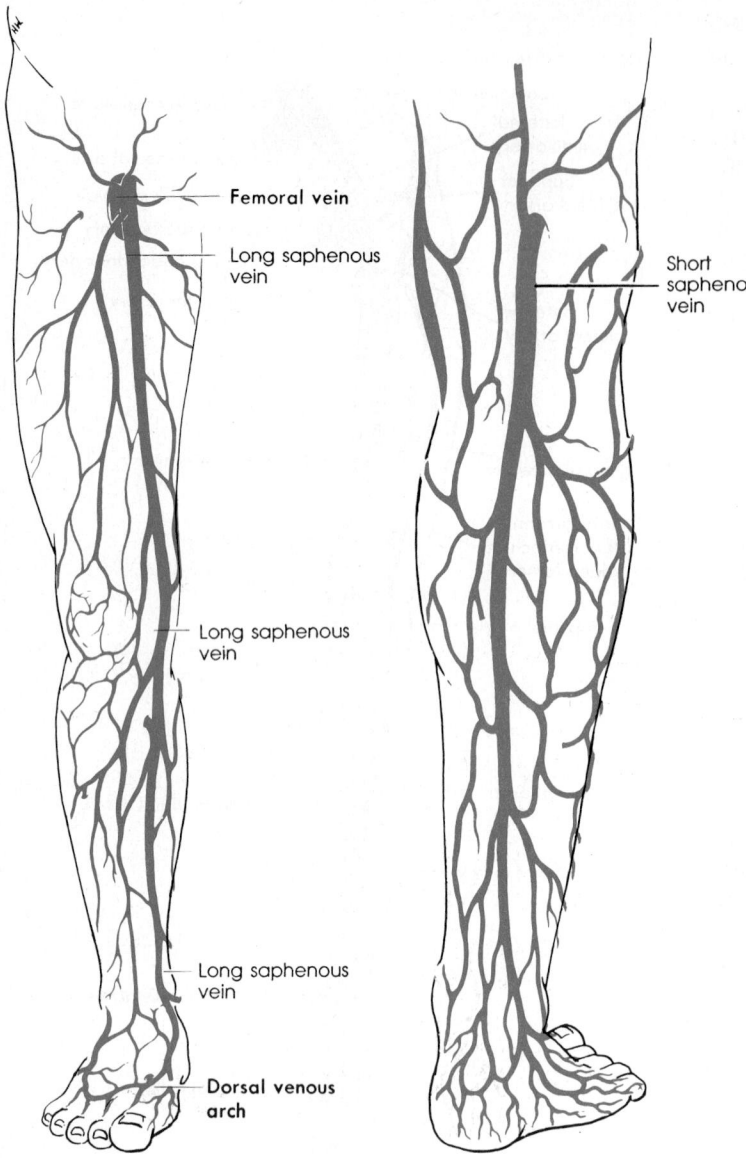

Femoral vein

Long saphenous vein

Long saphenous vein

Long saphenous vein

Dorsal venous arch

Short saphenous vein

Fig. 18-2 Superficial veins of the leg and foot. (From Anthony CJ, Thibodeau GA: *Textbook of anatomy and physiology,* ed 12, St. Louis, 1987, Mosby–Year Book.)

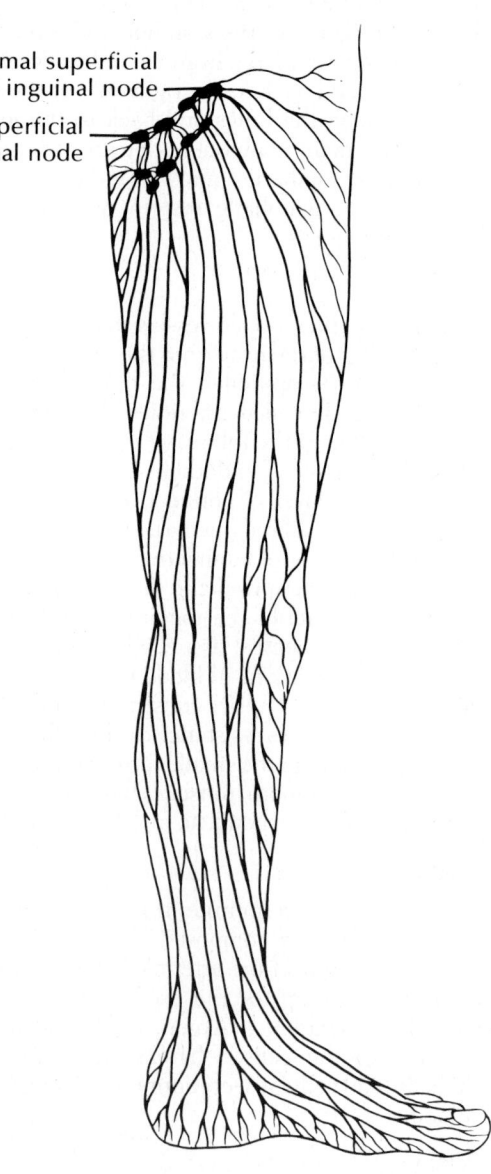

Proximal superficial inguinal node

Distal superficial inguinal node

Fig. 18-3 Superficial lymphatics of medial aspect of lower extremity (after Sappey). (From Francis CC, Martin AH: *Introduction to human anatomy,* ed 7, St. Louis, 1975, Mosby–Year Book.)

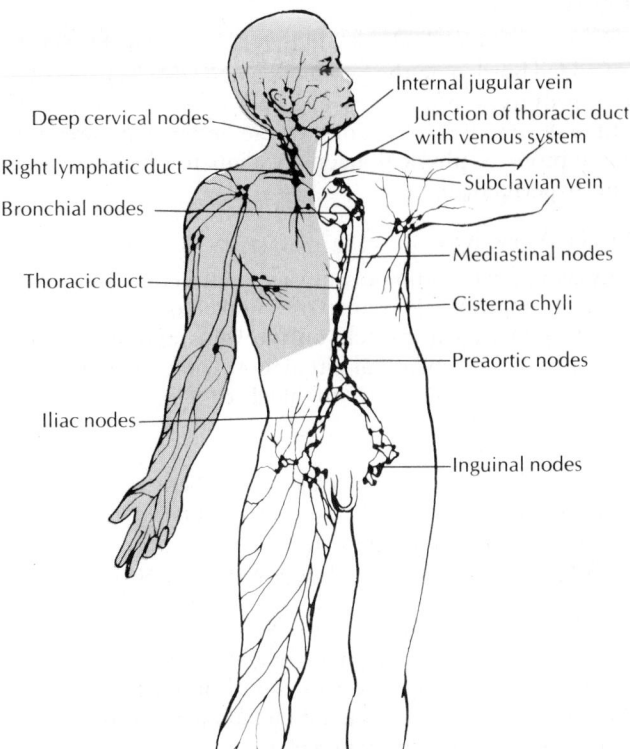

Fig. 18-4 Lymphatic drainage pathways. Shaded area of the body is drained through the right lymphatic duct, which is formed by the union of three vessels: the right jugular trunk, the right subclavian trunk, and the right bronchomediastinal trunk. Lymph from the remainder of the body enters the venous system by way of the thoracic duct. (From Malasanos L, Barkauskas V, and Stoltenberg-Allen K: *Health assessment*, ed. 4, St Louis, 1990, Mosby–Year Book.)

and proteins. The lymph flows through oval bodies called *lymph nodes*, which remove noxious agents such as bacteria and toxins. The lymph then drains into the thoracic duct and the right lymphatic duct, which empty into the junction of the internal jugular vein and subclavian vein (Fig. 18-4).

Physiological Changes with Ageing

Degenerative changes occur in the vascular system as part of the normal ageing process. These changes affect the walls of the blood vessels and predispose people to problems in the transport of blood and nutrients to the tissues. There is an increased thickness in the intima wall resulting from fibrosis. Further wall stiffness is caused by an accumulation of collagen and calcium in the intima and media. The elastic fibres of the media become thin and calcified. These changes markedly decrease the elasticity and flexibility of the vessels and hence increase peripheral vascular resistance, causing a rise in blood pressure. There is less blood flow through the vessels, leading to a decreased supply of oxygen and nutrients coupled with the accumulation of cellular secretions, waste products, and carbon dioxide. Gerontological considerations for care are described in the box entitled "The elderly with peripheral vascular problems."

The Elderly with Peripheral Vascular Problems

Assessment

Assess peripheral pulses and skin of lower extremities of all elderly people because of decreased vasomotor response and changes in arterial walls that decrease peripheral circulation and tissue oxygenation.

Assess extent of activities that produce intermittent claudication and occurrence at night; symptoms are more pronounced with age.

Assess ability to ambulate and carry out ADL when peripheral vascular problems are present.

Assess blood pressure. Normal systolic blood pressure in elderly may be 160mm Hg (as compared with 140mm Hg in younger adults). A widened pulse pressure may be present.

Assess ability to comply with pharmacological therapy if patient has hypertension.

Intervention

Carry out measures to decrease infection potential; the decreased immune response of elderly places a higher risk of infection when circulation is compromised.

Use measures to increase circulation to compromised area: lower the legs for arterial problems and elevate legs for venous problems.

Teach patient and significant other:
　Foot care to decrease infection potential; if necessary place lamb's wool between toes to prevent rubbing.
　Location and palpation of peripheral pulses to monitor arterial circulation.
　Need to examine skin of legs closely and report signs of decreased skin temperature, changes in skin appearance, and cuts or scratches that do not heal.

Facilitate patient compliance with pharmacological therapy of hypertension. Decreased vision and remembering when to take medications are common factors that affect compliance of the elderly.

Common disorders in elderly

Arteriosclerosis obliterans
Leg ulcers from chronic deep vein insufficiency
Hypertension

18-1

Risk factors for peripheral vascular disorders

Cigarette smoking
Hypertension
Hyperlipidaemia
Obesity
Physical inactivity
Emotional stress
Diabetes mellitus
Family history of atherosclerosis

PREVENTION AND HEALTH EDUCATION

Primary Prevention

Primary prevention is the most important means for reducing the incidence of peripheral vascular disorders. Nurses in all clinical settings can provide health education about the risk factors that affect development of peripheral vascular disorders. Because these disorders normally develop with advancing age, all individuals can benefit from this information, particularly those in the elderly age groups.

The risk factors associated with the development of peripheral vascular disorders are listed in p. 435. These factors are similar to those of other forms of cardiovascular diseases (Chapter 17). Specific health teaching is discussed on p. 439.

Cigarette smoking

Smoking is one of the major contributory factors in the development of peripheral vascular problems. Nicotine causes vasoconstriction and spasms of the arteries, thus reducing circulation to the extremities. The carbon monoxide inhaled in cigarette smoke reduces oxygen transport to the tissues.

Hypertension

Hypertension causes the elastic tissue in the arteries to be replaced by fibrous collagen tissue. This makes the arterial wall less distensible and increases the resistance to blood flow (p. 454).

Hyperlipidaemia

Hyperlipidaemia refers to the elevation of lipids, such as cholesterol and triglycerides, within the blood. Cholesterol and triglycerides contribute to the development of atherosclerotic plaques in the vessels (see Chapter 17).

Obesity

Obesity, or excess body weight in relation to height, places an added burden on the heart and blood vessels. Excess fat compromises blood vessels and contributes to increased venous congestion. Obese individuals are also more prone to physical inactivity, diabetes, hypertension, and hyperlipidaemia.

Physical inactivity

Physical activity promotes muscle contraction and relaxation. It improves the return of venous blood to the heart by the pumping of muscle on the veins and aids in the development of collateral circulation, which is useful for venous return when veins are blocked.

Emotional stress

Emotional stress stimulates the sympathetic nervous system and causes peripheral vasoconstriction. Stress can also cause increased cholesterol and platelet levels, decreased clotting time, and sustained high blood pressure.

Diabetes mellitus

The exact mechanism by which diabetes contributes to the development of peripheral vascular disorders is unknown. The changes in glucose and fat metabolism are thought to affect the atherosclerotic processes.

Secondary Prevention

Secondary prevention is important because peripheral vascular disorders can become chronic and potentially disabling diseases. People with peripheral vascular disorders are subject to periods of exacerbation and complications such as infection, injury, thrombosis, and amputation. People with early symptoms are encouraged to seek medical care. Increasing the person's knowledge of the specific disorder and prevention of future occurrences is essential.

MAJOR HEALTH PROBLEMS OF THE PERIPHERAL VASCULAR SYSTEM

Changes in the peripheral vascular system may cause local arterial or venous disorders or may result in a systemic effect (for example, hypertension). Major peripheral vascular disorders that are discussed in this chapter include the following:
1. Arterial disorders
   a. Atherosclerosis
   b. Arteriosclerosis obliterans
   c. Thromboangiitis obliterans (Buerger's disease)
   d. Arterial embolism
   e. Aneurysm of lower extremity
   f. Raynaud's disease.
2. Arteriovenous fistula.
3. Venous disorders
   a. Thrombophlebitis
   b. Varicose veins.
4. Leg ulcers.
5. Lymphoedema.
6. Hypertension.

ARTERIAL DISORDERS

Any disturbance in the structure of the arteries interferes with transport of blood from the heart to the tissues. The result is diminished blood and decreased oxygen and nutrients to the tissues. The symptoms of arterial disease are not caused by the degree of obstruction or narrowing but by the degree to which the involved body part is deprived of circulation. This in turn is affected by such factors as blood pressure and presence or absence of collateral circulation.

Signs and symptoms, and medical therapy for the various types of arterial disorders, are listed in Table 18-1.

<u>REVIEW</u>

Table 18-1 Arterial disorders

Disease	Signs and symptoms	Medical therapy
Arteriosclerosis obliterans	Early: intermittent claudication, low skin temperature, diminished or absent arterial pulses distal to the obstruction, audible bruits Late: burning pain at rest, pallor or cyanosis, persistent reddish-blue discolouration, dry shiny skin, loss of hair on legs, deformed toenails, numbness and tingling, ulceration and gangrene of toes and foot	Cessation of cigarette smoking Regular exercise programme Drug therapy with vasodilators (controversial) Weight reduction Low-fat and low-cholesterol diets, antilipaemic medications Control of hypertension and diabetes Surgery: removal of occlusion, bypass of occlusion Percutaneous transluminal angioplasty
Thromboangiitis obliterans	Pain in digits at rest, sensitivity to cold, intermittent claudication in arm or hand, reduced or absent distal pulses, digits pale or persistently red, numbness and tingling, ulceration and gangrene of digits	Cessation of smoking Keep body warm Prevent injury to feet and hands Drug therapy with vasodilators (controversial) Surgery: sympathectomy to decrease arterial spasms, amputation of areas of ulceration and gangrene
Arterial embolism	Sudden onset of pain, coldness, and numbness Burning or aching pain distal to occlusion Muscular weakness Diminished or absent pulses distal to occlusion Skin pallor or cyanosis Signs and symptoms of shock	Bed rest Drug therapy: anticoagulants, fibrinolytics (streptokinase) Treatment of shock Surgery: embolectomy
Aneurysm of the extremity	May be asymptomatic Large pulsatile mass in area of artery Audible bruit Pain, coldness, and numbness distal to aneurysm	Drug therapy to control hypertension Surgery: removal of aneurysm
Raynaud's disease	Chronically cold hands and feet Vasospastic attack in digits: pallor, cyanosis, coldness, numbness, occasional pain After attack: intense redness, tingling, or throbbing Symptoms intensify with cold and emotional stress Ulcerations of fingertips in advanced cases	Protection against exposure to cold Cessation of cigarette smoking Drug therapy: calcium channel blockers, vascular smooth muscle relaxants, vasodilators Biofeedback Surgery: sympathectomy, amputation of areas of ulceration and gangrene

OBSTRUCTIVE ARTERIAL DISORDERS

Arterial disorders that may lead to arterial obstruction include arteriosclerosis obliterans, thromboangiitis obliterans, arterial embolism, and aneurysm of lower extremity.

Aetiology/Epidemiology
Arteriosclerosis obliterans

Arteriosclerosis obliterans is a disorder in which there is segmented arteriosclerotic narrowing or obstruction of the intima and media of vessel walls. It results from advanced atherosclerotic plaque formation, and the risk factors are similar to those for atherosclerosis. Arteriosclerosis obliterans is the most common cause of arterial obstructive disease in the extremities of people over age 30. It affects men more than women, with clinical symptoms evident in people between ages 50 and 70. In the people with diabetes, the disease becomes more progressive, affecting the smaller arteries, primarily below the knee.

Thromboangiitis obliterans

This disorder, also called Buerger's disease, is an episodic and segmental obstructive and inflammatory disorder of the arteries and veins. It typically occurs in men between ages 20 and 40 and has been reported in all races. Although the cause is unknown, it almost always occurs in men who smoke.

Arterial embolism

Arterial emboli are blood clots floating in arterial blood. These clots most commonly originate in the heart as a result of atrial fibrillation, myocardial infarction, or congestive heart failure. The clots may also be associated with immobility, anaemia, and dehydration.

Aneurysms of lower extremity

An aneurysm is an enlarged, dilated portion of an artery. Although it may follow trauma, such as a motor vehicle accident, it is most commonly associated with atherosclerosis. Aneurysms of the lower extremity, particularly in the popliteal area (Fig. 18-5), arc more common in people over age 60 who have pronounced arteriosclerosis.

Pathophysiology
Atherosclerosis

Atherosclerosis is generally viewed as a type of arterio-sclerosis or as a part of the ageing process. This disease involves the development of lesions in the intimal wall.

Three types of lesions have been identified: (1) fatty streaks, which consist of smooth-muscle cells and lipid deposits that are present in all individuals, although they do not necessarily progress to produce disease; (2) fibrous plaques, which involve a thickening of the intima and are surrounded by lipids, collagen, smooth-muscle cells, and plasma components; and (3) the complicated lesion that is a large mass consisting of calcified fibrous plaques.

The result of atherosclerosis is narrowing of the artery, which progresses to obstruction, thrombosis, aneurysm development, and rupture. In addition, nutrients and oxygen to the tissues can be reduced, resulting in ischaemic necrosis of the tissue cells. (For further information on atherosclerosis, see Chapter 17.)

Arteriosclerosis obliterans

The primary lesion of arteriosclerosis obliterans is plaque formation on the intimal wall that causes partial or com-plete occlusion. In addition, there is calcification of the media and the gradual loss of elasticity that further weakens the arterial wall and predisposes the patient to aneurysmal dilation or thrombus formation. As a result, the artery is unable to transport an adequate blood volume to the tissues during exercise or at rest. Symptoms appear when the blood vessels can no longer supply the tissue with required nutrients and remove wastes.

The most common symptom of arterial insufficiency, *intermittent claudication*, occurs with exercise and consists of pain that develops during exercise in a muscle that has an inadequate blood supply. It is described as a cramp that disappears within one to two minutes of cessation of exercise. The pain is usually bilateral but may be unilateral. The muscles of the calf are more frequently affected because the femoral artery is often involved.

A gnawing or burning pain occurring at rest, especially at night, is indicative of severe disease. Feelings of coldness, numbness, and tingling may also occur concurrently with pain. In advanced disease, the ischaemia may lead to necrosis, ulceration, and gangrene (particularly of the toes and distal foot) because of the decreased circulation.

Thromboangiitis obliterans (Buerger's disease)

In contrast to arteriosclerosis obliterans, this disorder develops in the small arteries and veins, primarily in the feet and hands, although the wrists and lower leg may also be involved. Symptoms are most always a result of occlusion of the arteries, leading to ischaemia, complicated in later stages by infection. The main characteristic is inflamma-tory infiltration of vessel walls. Different segments of arteries may be involved. The process is intermittent, and arteries may recannulize during quiescent periods.

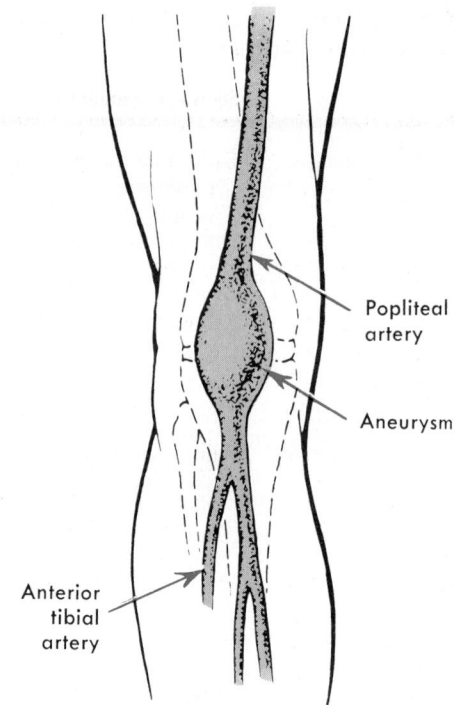

Fig. 18-5   Posterior view of the knee with an aneurysm of the popliteal artery. (From Anderson HC: *Newton's geriatric nursing,* ed 5, St Louis, 1971, Mosby–Year Book.)

The most common symptom is pain with exercise in the arch of the foot or instep claudication. With involvement of the hands, the pain is usually bilaterally symmetrical. Pain at rest is frequent and persistent, particularly in the people with atherosclerosis. Changes in skin colour or temperature, sensitivity to cold, and ulcers or gangrene of the digits may be present. Superficial thrombophlebitis is a common early sign.

Arterial embolism

A blood clot may become detached from the site of origin and travel through the arterial circulation. The embolus is frequently a fragment of arteriosclerotic plaque loosened from the aorta. Emboli tend to lodge in the bifurcation of arteries, especially in the femoral or popliteal arteries causing obstruction. Blood flow to sites distal to the lodged embolus is impaired, and ischaemia occurs. Signs and symptoms depend on the size of the embolus, the presence of collateral circulation, and the proximity to a major organ. Abrupt cessation of blood flow causes severe pain. Distal pulses are absent, and the extremity becomes cold, numb, and pale. Shock may develop if an embolus blocks a large artery.

Aneurysm of lower extremity

Destruction of the medial layer of an artery leads to weakening of the arterial wall and to the eventual formation of an aneurysm. Thrombi form at the site of the aneurysm and break off, forming emboli that may travel and obstruct more distal portions of the artery. Symptoms of an aneurysm may be absent. A large pulsating mass may be palpated at the site of the aneurysm.

Nursing Process
Assessment

Data collection for the people with arterial insufficiency focuses on noted changes in the circulation of the extremities and possible causative factors.

Subjective data

1. Onset of symptoms: slow and progressive or sudden.
2. Changes noted in skin colour and temperature of extremities.
3. Discomfort or pain in extremities: onset, location, quality, and occurrence with exercise or at rest.
4. Effect on extremities of cold temperatures, cigarette smoking, or emotional stress.
5. Effectiveness of measures used to relieve discomfort or pain.
6. Presence of risk factors: cigarette smoking; physical inactivity; obesity; emotional stress; history of hypertension, hyperlipidaemia, or diabetes; family history of atherosclerosis.

Objective data

1. Skin changes indicating tissue anoxia:
   a. Appearance: shiny, taut, absence of hair on extremities (indicates lack of tissue oxygen)
   b. Colour: pallor, redness, cyanosis
   c. Temperature: coldness
   d. Presence of ulcerations or gangrene.
2. Condition of nailbeds: opaque, thickened, capillary refill greater than three seconds.
3. Peripheral pulses: presence and quality (*Note*: compare bilaterally).
4. Presence of audible bruit or palpable thrill over artery indicating turbulent flow through a narrowed vessel.
5. Symmetry of extremities.
6. Sensation in extremities: numbness, tingling.
7. Muscle tone: weakness, loss of tone.
8. Effectiveness of prescribed medications.

Diagnostic tests

Several tests may be used in the diagnosis of arterial disorders. Noninvasive diagnostic tests such as segmental limb pressure and pulse volume recordings are often used. These diagnostic tests are outlined in Table 18-2.

Nursing analysis

Problems are determined from analysis of patient data. Possible problems for the people with an obstructive arterial disorder may include, but are not limited to, the following:

Problem	Possible aetiologies
Activity intolerance	Imbalance between oxygen supply and demand; immobility
Infection, high risk for	Lack of knowledge
Injury, high risk for	Sensorimotor deficits
Knowledge deficit	Lack of exposure, recall
Skin integrity, impaired, high risk for	Immobility, tissue anoxia

Problem	Possible aetiologies
Tissue perfusion, altered peripheral	Decreased arterial blood flow

Planning : expected patient outcomes

Expected patient outcomes for the people with an obstructive arterial disorder may include, but are not limited to, the following:

1. Performs measures to increase peripheral perfusion.
2. Participates in activity, with a balance between activity and rest.
3. Describes ways to prevent skin lesions, infection, and injury.
4. Describes risk factors that may compromise arterial circulation and plans to avoid these factors, follows prescribed medication regimen, and plans for ongoing care.

Implementation
Assisting with achievement of therapeutic goals
Medications

The most frequently used medications to treat obstructive arterial disorders include anticoagulants, fibrinolytics, and vasodilators. *Anticoagulants* are used to prolong clotting time, thus preventing extension of a clot and inhibiting further clot formation. Heparin and warfarin sodium (Table 18-3) are the most commonly administered anticoagulants. *Fibrinolytics*, or thrombolytics, are useful in dissolving existing thrombi when rapid dissolution of the clot is required to preserve organ and limb function. Streptokinase and urokinase (Table 18-4) impair haemostasis by increasing fibrinolytic activity. After infusion of fibrinolytics, the patient is started on heparin or oral anticoagulants to prevent clot extension or formation. Guidelines for the care of the patient receiving anticoagulant or fibrinolytic therapy is described in Box 18-2. The use of *vasodilators* is controversial; most studies indicate that these drugs are not effective.

Interventions to achieve patient outcomes
Promoting tissue perfusion

Nursing interventions are directed towards activities that promote tissue oxygenation and include the following:

1. Maintain a warm environmental temperature of about 21°C. (70°F.).
2. Place legs in *slight dependency* (uses gravity to enhance tissue perfusion) and avoid elevating legs (impedes arterial flow).
3. Avoid pressure on affected extremity; use padding for severe ischaemia.
4. Avoid vigorous massage of extremities (may promote embolus formation).
5. Teach patients to carry out above activities in addition to the following:
   a. Avoid chilling (causes vasoconstriction) and exposure to cold; layer clothing in cold weather.
   b. Avoid constrictive clothing that impedes circulation: rolled stockings, socks with tight banding, girdles, tight waistbands, and tight shoelaces.
   c. Avoid crossing legs at knees (places pressure on arteries of legs).
   d. Stop smoking (nicotine causes vasoconstriction

Table 18-2 Diagnostic tests for arterial disorders

Test	Purpose	Procedure	Comments
Doppler ultrasonography	Evaluate vascular network (arteries, veins) Measure blood flow through vessels Monitor status of bypass grafts	High-frequency sound waves directed to artery or veins through hand-held transducer moved evenly across skin surface; audible tone produced proportional to blood velocity	No discomfort experienced Noninvasive Explain to patient that noise will be heard
Segmental limb pressure	Evaluate arterial occlusion	Systolic pressure readings from each limb segment obtained by pneumatic pressure cuffs and Doppler probe; readings compared	Noninvasive
Pulse volume recordings	Substantiate diagnosis of arterial stenosis and occlusion	Pneumatic pressure cuffs attached to extremities; pressure changes recorded by pressure transducer as waveforms during cuff inflation and deflation	Useful to assess areas such as foot and toes, not easily evaluated by segmental limb pressure
Exercise testing	Determine amount of exercise that precipitates ischaemia and claudication	Ankle pressure, pulse volume, and blood pressure measured while person walks on treadmill at specific speed for about 5 minutes or until onset of leg pain	Exercise should be stopped at onset of pain
Radionuclide scan	Visualize vascular system and detect changes in blood vessels Assess arterial blood flow; determine perfusion pressure Identify arterial obstruction or vascular abnormality Determine patency of bypass graft	Injection of radionuclide followed by scanning of area at predetermined intervals to determine accumulation of radionuclide	Explain to patient that radiation dose is usually less than that received from diagnostic X-rays Check for allergy to iodine, shellfish
Arteriography (angiography)	Visualize arterial system and detect vascular changes Assess arterial blood flow Indentify arterial obstruction, vascular abnormality, or aneurysm	Dye injection through catheter inserted into femoral or brachial artery followed by X-ray films	Transient flushing and burning sensation felt when dye is injected Post-test assessment includes the following: 1. Injection site for bleeding, haematoma, and swelling, especially thigh 2. Peripheral pulses distal to site hourly for 4–8 hours 3. Allergic reaction to dye (dyspnoea, flushing, urticaria, nausea, vomiting) 4. Sensation distal to site Encourage patient to drink fluids to facilitate excretion of dye
Digital subtraction angiography	Visualize vascular system Determine presence and extent of occlusion	Dye injected through catheter inserted into blood vessel; X-ray signals are digitized	Same as for arteriography
Transcutaneous oxymetry	Evaluate severity of limb ischaemia Assess healing of ulcers Determine level of amputation	Sensors placed on skin to measure oxygen diffusion gradient between electrode and capillaries	Explain to patient that measurements may be taken in several positions
Magnetic resonance imaging (MRI)	Evaluate vascular network (arteries, veins) Measure blood flow velocities Assess stages of vascular disease	Radiofrequency pulses excite protons, which give a signal creating an image	Explain to patient that the space is very tight Noise level may be high; ear plugs provided

Table 18-3   Anticoagulants used in treatment of vascular disorders

Drug	Action	Dosage	Side effects
Heparin	Forms complex with antithrombin III which inhibits thrombin action Intravenous route produces immediate action; duration is 2 hours Subcutaneous route used for maintenance and prophylaxis	Intravenous: Loading dose 5,000u Continuous drip: 1,000–2,000u/h at 14–28u/kg/h in 5% dextrose or NS Intermittent: initial loading dose, then 5,000–10,000u every four hours Subcutaneous: 5,000u 2 hours before surgery and every 8–12 hours thereafter Other: 10,000–12,000u every 12 hours NOTE: dosage adjusted to maintain activated partial thromboplastin time (APTT) at 2–2.5 times laboratory control Normal APTT = 33–45 seconds Prolonged APTT = 60–100 seconds	Haemorrhage, spontaneous bleeding, epistaxis, bleeding gums, haematoma, gastrointestinal bleeding with black tarry stools
Warfarin sodium	Inhibits vitamin K-dependent clotting factor synthesis (factors II, VII, IX and X) Depressess prothrombin activity Peaks in 36–72 hours Duration is 2–5 days	Oral 10–15mg/d until prothrombin time within therapeutic range Then 3–9mg/d NOTE: dosage adjusted to maintain prothrombin time reported as the international normalised ratio	Same as for heparin

Table 18-4   Fibrinolytics used in treatment of vascular disorders

Drug	Action	Dosage	Side effects
Streptokinase	Synthetic protein derived from streptococcal bacteria Activates plasminogen by forming streptokinase–plasminogen complex	Intravenous: Loading dose 250,000iu over 30 minutes Then 100,000iu/h for 24–72 hours (arterial thrombosis) or 72 hours (deep vein thrombosis)	Bleeding, bronchospasm, rash, urticaria
Urokinase	Human proteolytic enzyme derived from cultured kidney cells and urine Directly converts circulating plasminogen to plasmin	Intravenous: Loading dose 4,100iu/kg over 10 minutes Then 4,400iu/kg/h for 12–24 hours	Same as for streptokinase

The patient on anticoagulant or fibrinolytic therapy

Monitor the infusion accurately; maintain desired therapeutic rate of units per minute or hour.

Assess skin for signs of bleeding: bleeding gums, nosebleeds, petachiae (pinpoint red areas on skin), ecchymosis (bruising), haematoma formation, and venepuncture sites.

Monitor urine, stool, vomit, and gastric secretions for blood.

Avoid administration of medications by intramuscular route to prevent bleeding.

Avoid unnecessary bleeding.

Use a soft toothbrush and brush teeth gently.

Use an electric razor rather than razor blade for shaving.

Avoid use of rectal thermometers (may cause mucosal bleeding).

Special care with *anticoagulant therapy*

Give heparin by deep subcutaneous injection; use a fine gauge needle at a 90° angle; do not aspirate nor massage site after injection (can result in bleeding); rotate sites on a regular basis.

Administer protamine sulphate if necessary, as a heparin antagonist to reverse anticoagulant effects.

Hold pressure for 3–5 minutes on venepuncture sites.

Monitor results of blood tests: a partial thromboplastin time should be 2 times normal level (normal activated partial thromboplastin time is 33–45 seconds); a prothrombin time (PT) should be 1.2–1.5 times normal level (normal PT is 11–12 seconds).

Avoid use of aspirin; aspirin inhibits platelet adhesion, thus having an anticoagulant effect; also interacts with anticoagulants.

Special care with *fibrinolytic therapy*

Assess patient for signs of intracranial bleeding: headache, vomiting, disorientation, mental confusion.

Assess patient for signs of retroperitoneal bleeding: low back pain, muscle weakness, or numbness in lower extremity.

Avoid insertion of unnecessary venous and arterial lines; insert before initiation of therapy if necessary.

Hold pressure on all venepuncture or other bleeding sites for 20–30 minutes to promote blood clotting.

Give antiulcer medication, if prescribed, as a prophylactic measure.

General exercises

1. Engage in a regular aerobic exercise programme that includes activities such as walking, swimming, jogging, or cycling (see Chapter 4).
2. Do 30 to 45 minutes of activity with warm-up and cool-down activities on three alternate days.
3. Walk at a slow pace on a daily basis.

Special exercises

1. Perform the following Buerger-Allen exercises on a daily basis
   a. Lie flat with legs elevated above heart level for two to three minutes
   b. Sit for 2 to 3 minutes with legs relaxed and slightly dependent
   c. Flex, extend, invert, and evert feet for 30 seconds in each position
   d. End by lying flat with legs at heart level and cover with warm blanket for five minutes
2. Perform other exercises such as ankle rotations, ankle pumps, and knee extension on a daily basis.

Maintaining skin integrity and preventing infection

Because of decreased tissue oxygenation from decreased circulation, the skin is at high risk for breaking down and becoming infected. Nursing activities include examining the skin on a daily basis when the patient is hospitalized and encouraging the patient to be as mobile as possible. If redness or other signs of infection are noted, notify the doctor. Teach the patient to monitor and protect the skin:

1. Assess skin on a daily basis for intactness, dryness, redness, and lesions; use mirror to inspect areas that are difficult to see, such as heels and plantar surface of toes.
2. Take a daily bath in tepid water (three times per week if skin is very dry)
   a. Use a neutral pH soap to prevent skin irritation
   b. Wash gently; avoid scratching and vigorous rubbing
   c. Dry skin gently
   d. Lubricate skin with moisturizing agent; avoid using alcohol (dries skin).
3. Take meticulous care of feet
   a. Bathe each toe and dry well
   b. Use only prescribed foot powders
   c. Wear clean cotton socks and change daily (synthetic fibres can cause irritation and do not absorb moisture).
4. Avoid wearing shoes that do not "breathe", such as those made of synthetic materials (prevents evaporation and contributes to fungal infections).
5. Avoid application of direct heat such as hot water.
6. Contact healthcare professional at onset of skin breakdown such as abrasions, lesions, or ulcerations.
7. See chiropodist at regular intervals.

Preventing injury

With decreased circulation to the extremities, sensation may decrease. Injuries may include cuts or abrasions, burns, and excessive pressure (leading to further ischaemia). Teach the patient to carry out the following activities:

---

and vasospasms; inhaled carbon dioxide reduces oxygen-carrying capacity of blood).

Promoting activity

Activity improves circulation through muscle contraction and relaxation. Exercise also stimulates collateral circulation that increases blood flow to the ischaemic area. Teach the patient to carry out general and specific exercises and to allow adequate time for rest between vigorous activities. Exercises include the following:

1. Wear comfortable protective shoes at all times (do not go barefoot); alternate shoes on a daily basis to allow for airing.
2. Trim nails carefully: Cut at regular intervals, soak in warm water to soften nails, use straight nail clippers, and avoid using scissors to prevent cutting skin.
3. Avoid scratching and rubbing feet to prevent abrasions.
4. Check water temperature carefully (ability to sense temperature may be decreased).
5. Seek advice from a chiropodist for thickened or deformed nails, blisters, corns, calluses, and ulcerations (self-treatment may cause infection).

Facilitating patient learning

The patient is taught how to promote tissue perfusion, maintain skin integrity, and prevent infection and injury as described previously. In addition, teach the patient the medication regimen and importance of taking the prescribed medications. Special instructions for the patient receiving oral anticoagulant therapy at home are listed in Box 18-3. The patient also needs to know that arterial disorders are usually chronic disorders and that medical follow-up is important to help prevent advanced disease with necrosis and ulcerations.

Evaluation

Questions to consider may include the following:
1. Does the patient perform measures to increase peripheral perfusion?
2. Is the patient able to tolerate activity and balance activity with rest?
3. Is the skin intact?
4. Have infection and injury been prevented?
5. Can the patient describe:
   a. Daily physical activity to be carried out?
   b. Risk factors to be avoided?
   c. Medication regimen?
   d. Plans for continued medical follow-up?

Surgery

Surgery is indicated for patients who have advanced arterial disease in which ischaemic changes are present or for patients with severe pain that impairs their activities. These surgical procedures include arterial bypass surgery, embolectomy, percutaneous transluminal angioplasty (PTA), removal of aneurysm and closure of a fistula, sympathectomy, and amputation.

Arterial bypass surgery and reconstruction

If *arteriosclerosis obliterans* is rapidly progressing and intermittent claudication has become gravely disabling, surgery to correct the obstruction is indicated. The most common procedure is a bypass of the obstructed arterial segment, using prosthetic material such as Teflon or Dacron or autogenous (the patient's own) artery or vein, such as the saphenous vein (Fig. 18-6). The bypass may involve the aorta itself, as with an aortofemoral bypass, or more distal vessels, such as the femoral–popliteal bypass. Procedures that are performed either in conjunction with a bypass or by themselves include *patch grafting* (replacing

---

Patient Teaching   18-3

The patient receiving oral anticoagulant therapy

Know general action and side effects of prescribed drug; avoid taking medications containing aspirin, which also has an anticoagulant effect.

Take the anticoagulant at the same time every day; do not stop taking it until advised by the doctor.

Check for signs of bleeding (gum bleeding, nose bleeds, bruising, cuts that do not stop bleeding with direct pressure, blood in urine or stool); report these signs promptly to healthcare professional.

Wear a Medic-Alert bracelet or carry an identification card containing the drug name, drug dosage, and doctor's name in case of emergency.

Report for prescribed blood tests (activated partial thromboplastin time, prothrombin time) used to adjust drug dosage.

Do not add dark green and yellow vegetables to diet (contain vitamin K, which counteracts the anticoagulant drug effect).

Restrict alcohol intake (increases anticoagulant effect).

Guidelines for Care   18-4

The patient following arterial surgery of limbs

Monitor skin colour and temperature distal to the graft site every hour.

Assess sensation and movement in the distal limb.

Assess peripheral pulses in the involved limb.
   Sudden absence of pulse may indicate thrombosis.
   Mark location of peripheral pulse with a pen to facilitate frequent assessment.
   Use a Doppler if pulses are difficult to palpate.
   Compare pulses of involved limb with pulses of noninvolved limb.

Monitor extremity for oedema.

Check incision for redness, swelling, and drainage.

Monitor and immediately report signs of complication, such as increasing pain, fever, changes in drainage, absent or weakening pulse, change in skin colour, limitation of movement, or paraesthesia.

Promote circulation.
   Reposition patient every 2 hours.
   Ask patient not to cross legs.
   Use a footboard and or bed cradle to keep bed clothes off extremity.
   Encourage progressive activity when permitted.

Avoid sharp flexion in the area of the graft.

Monitor for signs of bleeding secondary to anticoagulation therapy.

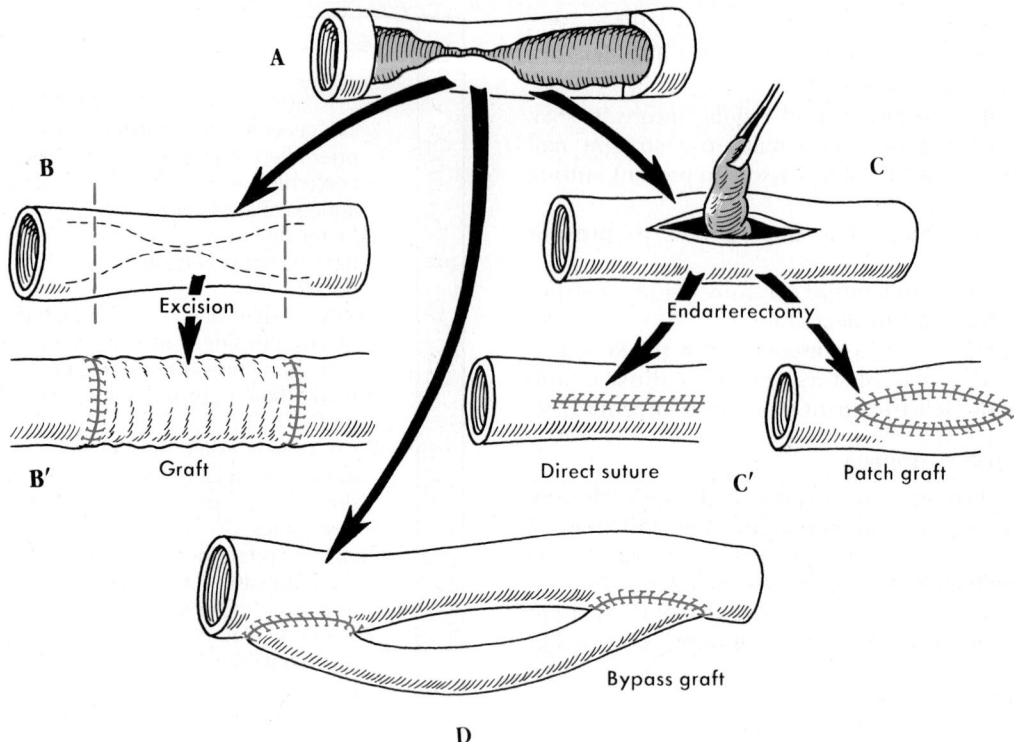

Fig. 18-6   **A,** Obstructed artery. Methods of restoring arterial blood flow include: **B** and **B'**, excision followed by grafting; **C** and **C'**, endarterectomy followed by either direct suture or patch graft; and **D,** bypass graft. (Redrawn from Juergens JL, et al: *Peripheral vascular disease,* Philadelphia, 1980, WB Saunders. By permission of Mayo Foundation.)

a damaged segment of the arterial wall with a vein patch) and *endarterectomy* (stripping arteriosclerotic plaques from the intima and inner media using balloon catheters or other instruments). Care of the people with an aortic bypass graft is discussed under abdominal aneurysms in Chapter 17. Care following femoral–popliteal bypass is the same as for other arterial surgery (Box 18-4).

Embolectomy

An embolectomy is the surgical removal of a blood clot and is most often used when large arteries are obstructed. Success of the surgery depends on the length of time the extremity was ischaemic; surgery must be performed within 6 to 10 hours to prevent muscle necrosis and loss of the extremity. Nursing care after embolectomy is described in Box 18-4. An endarterectomy, to remove the blood clot and strip the atherosclerotic plaque from the inner arterial wall, may also be performed.

Percutaneous transluminal angioplasty

Percutaneous transluminal angioplasty may be used as surgical treatment for atherosclerotic obliterans or in the removal of a stenotic arterial graft. A specially designed catheter is inserted under fluoroscopy and advanced to the site of the obstruction. The balloon tip of the catheter is inflated to provide compression and rupture the atherosclerotic plaque. Thrombosis may occur after treatment; therefore, anticoagulants are usually prescribed. Care following percutaneous transluminal angioplasty is similar to that following arterial surgery (Box 18-4).

Removal of aneurysm and closure of fistula

The blood vessel may be ligated unless the procedure is incompatible with the life of tissues distal to the lesion. Homografts or Teflon or Dacron grafts may be used in larger blood vessels of the extremities, either to replace the portion of the artery that contains the aneurysm or to bypass the abnormality. Popliteal function is better at the flexion crease when the patient's own vein is used. Perioperative care is similar to that for the patient undergoing an embolectomy.

Amputation

Although a partial or complete amputation of an extremity may be necessary as a result of sarcoma or trauma, most amputations are indicated for patients with advanced atherosclerosis and gangrene of the extremities. The majority of amputations are of the lower extremity; the toes are the most amputated part of the body. An amputation may also be offered as an option to improve functional ability with a prosthesis.

The surgical goal is to remove the least amount of tissue possible and to create a stump adequate for the fitting of a prosthesis. The specific level of amputation is determined by the extent of the disease process. Below-knee (BK) amputations maintain knee function and allow for greater stability with a prosthesis. A BK amputation is usually done in the lower third of the leg, leaving a 12 to 18cm stump. An above-knee (AK) amputation may be made at any level although it is frequently below the middle of the thigh to preserve an adequate stump for satisfactory use of a prosthesis. Above-knee amputations are often performed after unsuccessful BK amputations.

Amputation involves loss of a body part; therefore, feelings of grief related to loss are usually experienced. (For further discussion on loss and grief see Chapter 11). Before and after surgery the patient should exercise to strengthen arm and leg muscles to promote movement and ambulation and to prevent knee and hip contractures.

After surgery, most people experience phantom sensations, or feelings related to the removed limb. About 10% of patients experience uncomfortable sensations (*phantom limb pain*) similar to the pain experienced before amputation or the sensation of a cramped or uncomfortable position. In most instances, this discomfort disappears with time, but the pain may become chronic for some people. Even though the limb is removed, the pain is a real sensation and should not be dismissed as illusionary.

A *prosthesis* may be used immediately after or within five weeks of surgery. A plaster may also be applied over the dressing to allow for attachment of a metal pylon prosthesis. A permanent prosthesis is made six months after surgery to allow for stump shrinkage and moulding.

Preoperative care includes the following:

1. Assist patient to express feelings, concerns, and fears; accept patient reaction of anger, discouragement, and grief.
2. Discuss postoperative regimen with patient and family.
   a. Frequent positioning to promote circulation
   b. Exercises to strengthen arm muscles for the use of crutches: push-ups and weightlifting
   c. Exercises to strengthen leg muscles to prevent knee and hip contractures and to promote ambulation: ankle rotations, ankle pumps, and quadriceps sets
3. Teach crutch walking if appropriate (usually done by physiotherapist).
4. Ensure adequate pain relief to lessen incidence of phantom limb pain.

Postoperative care is described in Box 18-5.

VASOMOTOR ARTERIAL DISEASE— RAYNAUD'S PHENOMENON/DISEASE
Aetiology/Epidemiology

Raynaud's *phenomenon* is characterized by episodic arterial spasms of the extremities, predominantly of the hands. It occurs secondary to other disorders, such as occlusive arterial diseases, connective tissue diseases, or neurogenic lesions. Raynaud's phenomenon develops more frequently in women between ages 20 and 40, and is more common during winter months. Raynaud's *disease* has no known cause, although immunological factors, alterations in sympathetic innervation, emotional stress, and a hypersensitivity to cold have been suggested.

Pathophysiology

Symptoms of Raynaud's phenomenon or disease result from the episodic arterial spasms, usually in the fingers. Few pathological changes occur in the early stages; with

---

Guidelines for Care   18-5

The patient after an amputation

Assess stump and monitor wound drainage for colour and amount; report signs of increased drainage.

Position patient with no flexion at hip or knee to avoid contractures; encourage prone position.

Maintain patient in semi-recumbent or flat position after above-knee amputation.

Support stump with pillow for first 24 hours (according to doctor preference and avoiding flexion); place rolled blanket along outer aspect to prevent outward rotation.

Encourage exercises to prevent thromboembolism.
   Active range of movements of unaffected leg, ankle rotations and pumps
   Use of overhead trapeze when moving in bed
   Push-ups from sitting position and bed
   Quadriceps sets (see Chapter 32)
   Lifting stump and buttocks off bed while lying flat on back to strengthen abdominal muscles

Teach care of stump.
   Inspect for redness, blister, and abrasions
   Wash stump with mild soap, rinse with water, and pat dry
   Avoid use of oils and creams
   Remove stump bandage or stump sock and reapply as needed; use firm smooth figure-eight wrapping (Fig. 18-7) to reduce swelling and shape stump (if rigid dressing not used)

Encourage patient to ambulate using correct crutch-walking technique.
   Keep elbows extended; limit elbow flexion to 30° or less
   Avoid pressure on axilla
   Bear weight on palms of hands, not on axilla.
   Maintain upright posture (head up, chest up, abdomen in, pelvis in, foot straight).

Monitor patient's abillity to use a prosthesis

---

advancing stages, the intimal wall thickens and there is hypertrophy of the medial wall. The person typically complains of chronically cold hands and feet. During arterial spasms, sluggish blood flow causes pallor, coldness, numbness, cutaneous cyanosis, and pain. After the spasms, the involved area becomes reddened with tingling and throbbing sensations. With advanced disease, ulcerations can develop on the fingertips and toes.

Assessment

Subjective data include the following information:

1. Feelings in hands and feet: coldness, numbness, tingling.
2. Measures used to relieve symptoms: effect of warmth.
3. Presence of associated factors: emotional stress, cigarette smoking, exposure to cold.

Objective data include observations of the hands and feet: temperature, skin colour changes (white, blue, red), and presence of ulcerations on fingertips and toes.

A *diagnostic test* used for Raynaud's disease is the cold stimulation test. Skin temperature changes are recorded by a thermistor attached to each finger. The patient's hand is submerged in an ice-water bath for 20 seconds and ongoing temperatures are recorded. A comparison is made for baseline data.

Interventions

Medical therapy for the people with Raynaud's disease is primarily preventive. Drug therapy with calcium channel blockers, vascular smooth muscle relaxants, and vasodilators may be prescribed to promote circulation and reduce pain. Biofeedback techniques to increase skin temperature and thereby prevent spasms have been beneficial in some cases. A *sympathectomy* may be indicated to relieve symptoms in the early stage of advanced ischaemia. Sympathectomy involves removal of the sympathetic ganglia or a division of their branches. If the disease is advanced with ulcerations and gangrene, the involved area may have to be amputated.

Nursing interventions are similar to those for other arterial disorders in terms of preventing injury and promoting tissue perfusion (p. 439). Teaching the patient includes the following:

1. Effects of smoking on arterial flow (nicotine causes vasoconstriction); recommend techniques to stop smoking, such as behaviour modification, stimulus control, biofeedback, nicotine gum or patches, and hypnosis.
2. Ways of avoiding exposure to cold:
   a. Wear adequate clothing to promote warmth
   b. Layer clothes as needed (several layers provide more warmth than one heavy layer)
   c. Wear gloves and warm socks during winter months
   d. Use caution when cleaning refrigerator and freezer
   e. Wear gloves when handling frozen foods
   f. Avoid occupations that require constant exposure to cold.
3. Avoidance of drugs that can cause vasoconstriction, such as oral contraceptives, beta-adrenergic blockers, and ergotamine.
4. Use of anti-inflammatory analgesics to promote comfort.

ARTERIOVENOUS FISTULA

An arteriovenous fistula involves both arteries and veins and consists of an abnormal direct communication between an artery and vein.

Aetiology

Arteriovenous fistulas may be congenital or acquired. Most acquired arteriovenous fistulas develop secondary to penetrating injuries from trauma; a single fistula is rare. More often, multiple fistulas affect circulation to an entire region or area such as an arm or leg.

Pathophysiology

In an arteriovenous fistula, the high arterial blood flow bypasses the capillary network and goes into the veins. This causes an increase in venous pressure that predisposes to venous engorgement, dilatation, and aneurysm develop-

ment. The veins become thickened as the artery thins and loses its elastic and muscular properties.

Symptoms resulting from the increased venous pressure may include pain at the site of a fistula; oedema, varicosities, and asymmetry of an extremity; tortuous, dilated superficial veins; and venous pulsations. Venous bruit and thrill may be heard from the turbulent blood flow. Testing includes arteriography and Doppler ultrasonography.

Interventions

Small peripheral arteriovenous fistulas may not require intervention. *Surgical* intervention may be indicated when ulceration, bleeding, or severe arterial or venous insufficiency occur. The most common procedure is embolization consisting of closing the fistula with embolic material such as Gelfoam, glass beads, or muscle. Large fistulas may be repaired or resected, or the involved artery may be ligated.

Nursing management is primarily support and teaching. Elastic stockings can help prevent discomfort and oedema. Postoperative care includes assessing skin colour and temperature and peripheral pulses distal to the surgery. Teaching includes information about the underlying disease and measures to prevent symptoms of venous insufficiency and to promote venous return (p. 449).

VENOUS DISORDERS

Venous disorders arise when there is alteration in transport of blood from capillary beds back to the heart. Changes in smooth muscle and connective tissue make the veins less distensible with limited recoil capacity. Valves in the veins may malfunction, causing backflow of blood. The major venous disorders are thrombophlebitis and varicose veins (Table 18-5).

THROMBOPHLEBITIS

Aetiology/Epidemiology

The primary factors associated with development of thrombophlebitis include venous stasis, damage to the vessel wall, and blood hypercoagulability. This disorder is common in hospitalized patients, particularly those who have undergone major surgery (especially pelvic surgery and total hip replacement) or who have sustained a myocardial infarction. Hypercoagulability may also occur with the use of oral contraceptive drugs (especially in women over age 35) and with adenocarcinoma. Thrombophlebitis occurs most frequently in women and affects people of all races. The incidence increases with advancing age.

Pathophysiology

Thrombophlebitis of the legs develops in deep veins (femoral, popliteal, small calf veins) and in superficial veins (usually the saphenous vein, Fig. 18-2). Thrombi form in the veins from accumulation of platelets, fibrin, white blood cells and red blood cells. Deep vein thrombophlebitis (DVT) tends to occur at bifurcations of the deep veins,

REVIEW
Table 18-5   Venous disorders

Disease	Signs and symptoms	Therapy
Thrombophlebitis	Entire limb may be pale and cold Area along vein may be reddened and feel warm to touch Homan's sign: pain in calf on dorsiflexion Superficial veins feel hard and thready and are sensitive to pressure Difference in circumference of extremities	Bedrest during acute phase Warm moist heat to reduce discomfort and pain Elevation of extremity Elastic bandage Heparin and warfarin Vasodilator to combat arterial spasms and improve circulation Fibrinolytics to dissolve and break up the thrombus Exercise programme after acute phase

Varicose veins	Veins appear as darkened, tortuous, raised blood vessels; more pronounced on prolonged standing
	Feeling of heaviness in legs
	Fatigue
	Pain and muscle cramps
	Oedema
		Conservative treatment:
		  Elevate legs at least every 2–3 hours
		  Wear elastic stocking
		  Avoid standing for long periods of time
		  Weight reduction if obese
		Surgery: venous ligation and stripping

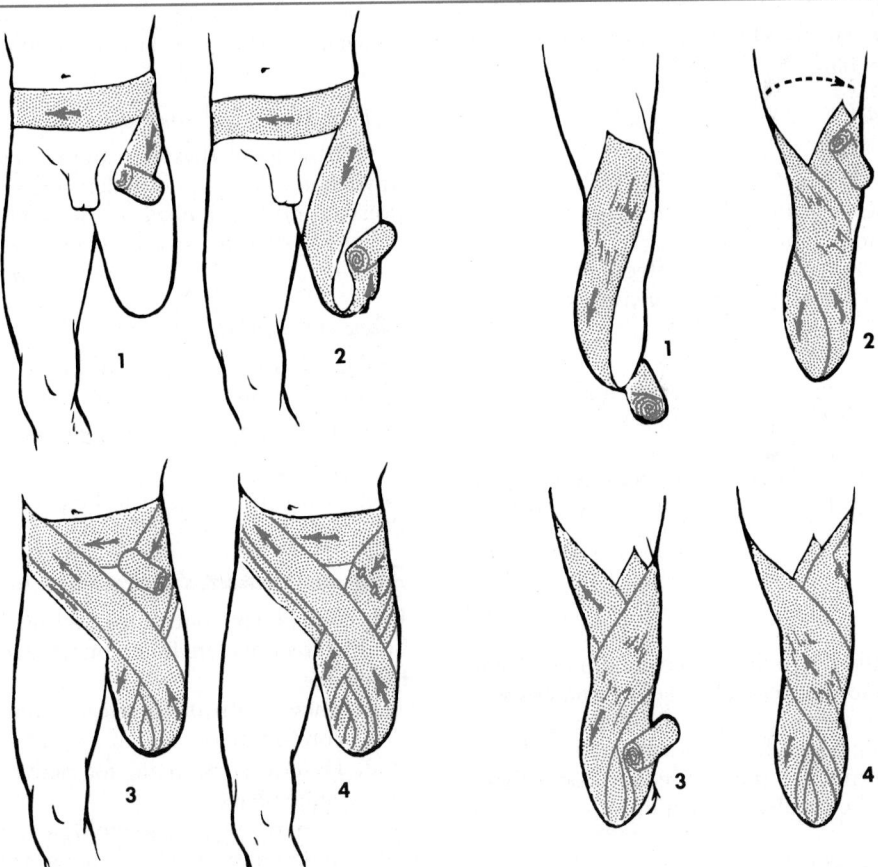

Fig. 18-7   *Left,* correct method of badaging midthigh amputation stump. Note that the bandage must be anchored around patient's waist. *Right,* correct method for bandaging midcalf amputation stump. Note that bandage need not be anchored about waist.

which are sites of turbulent blood flow. A major risk during the acute phase of DVT is dislodgement of the thrombus, which can migrate to the lungs, causing a pulmonary embolus (Fig. 18-8).

Pain and oedema result from the vein obstruction. An increase may be noted in circumference of the calf or thigh at the site of the thrombus. Active dorsiflexion may produce calf pain (Homan's sign); however, this action should be avoided because of increased risk of embolization. Because superficial veins are closer to the surface, signs of inflammation (redness, warmth, tenderness along the course of the vein) may be noted with superficial thrombophlebitis.

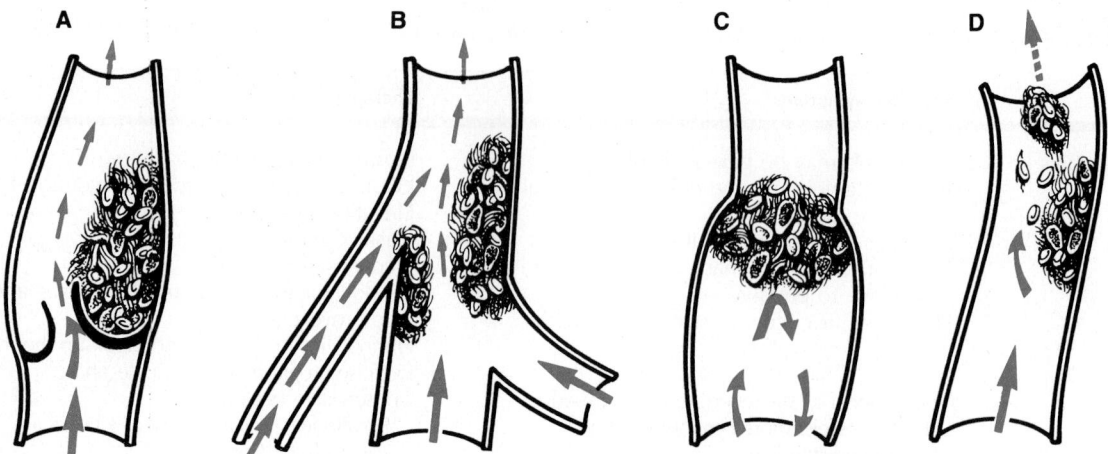

Fig. 18-8 Development of thromboemboli with arrows indicating direction of blood flow. **A,** Thrombus in a valve pocket of a deep vein with blood flowing beside thrombus. **B,** Thrombi tend to form at bifurcations of deep veins with some slowing of blood flow. **C,** Complete occlusion of vein by thrombus, forcing back flow of blood. **D,** Embolus, which has broken off from thrombus and is floating in bloodstream, could migrate to lungs and cause pulmonary embolus.

Nursing Process
Assessment
Subjective data

1. Characteristics of pain in the extremity.
2. Onset and duration of symptoms.
3. History of venous disorders, effects of previous therapies, and use of preventive measures.

Objective data

1. Colour and temperature of extremity (pale and cold if vein is occluded; red and warm if superficial vein is inflamed).
2. Oedema of calf or thigh: Use tape measure and mark site of measurement for future measurements; measure both legs for comparison.

Diagnostic tests
Venography

Venography is used to assess the condition of the deep leg veins and to diagnose deep vein thrombosis. A radiopaque contrast dye is injected through a catheter placed in a foot vein. Serial films are obtained to detect filling defects. Injection of the dye can cause a brief inflammatory response or allergic reaction.

Doppler ultrasonography

Doppler ultrasonography is used to measure flow through vessels. A probe or electronic stethoscope is placed over the patient's femoral and popliteal veins. The flow probe directs an ultrasound beam at the involved areas; the beam is reflected off the red cells that circulate through the blood vessels. The reflection varies according to the rate of flow in the vessel. This change in the frequency of reflected sound according to velocity of the flow is referred to as a Doppler effect (Fig. 18-9). Both extremities are compared for diminished or absent readings over the veins.

Impedance plethysmography

Impedance plethysmography is used to measure changes in venous volumes and to detect deep vein thrombosis. A pressure cuff is applied to the thigh and electrodes are attached to the patient's leg. Venous volume tracings during inflation and deflation of the cuff are compared.

Nursing analysis

Problems are determined from analysis of patient data. Possible problems for the people with thrombophlebitis may include, but are not limited to, the following:

Problem	Possible aetiologies
Knowledge deficit	Lack of exposure/recall
Pain, leg	Inflammation, oedema, venous stasis

Planning: expected patient outcomes

Expected patient outcomes for the person with thrombophlebitis may include, but are not limited to, the following:

1. Shows signs of decreased pain; states feeling more comfortable.
2. Describes rationale for activity limitation during acute phase.
3. Describes pharmacological therapy, signs of pulmonary embolus, and preventive measures.

Implementation
Assisting with achievement of therapeutic goals
Acute care for thrombophlebitis

Bedrest is prescribed during the acute phase for *deep vein thrombosis* to prevent embolus. The affected extremity is elevated periodically above heart level to prevent venous stasis and to reduce oedema. Specific activity orders depend on doctor preferences. When the patient begins to ambulate, elastic stockings or an elastic bandage is used to compress the superficial veins, increase blood flow through

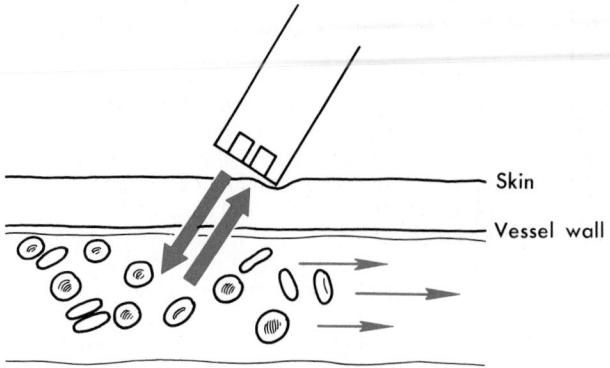

Fig. 18-9   Doppler effect showing red blood cells reflecting sound.

the deep veins, and prevent venous stasis. Anticoagulants are routinely given (p. 441), and vasodilators or fibrinolytics may also be prescribed.

Superficial thrombophlebitis is usually treated by rest; however, doctors differ in regard to the amount. Some doctors believe that complete immobilization is necessary to prevent emboli formation; others believe that clots are sufficiently adherent to vein walls and that mobility improves general circulation and prevents further venous stasis. Anti-inflammatory drugs may be prescribed.

Surgery

Surgical intervention for venous thrombosis is indicated only when other conservative measures are unsuccessful. If the thrombosis is recurrent and extensive, or if the patient is at high risk for pulmonary embolism, surgery may be necessary. A thrombectomy or a vena caval interruption may be performed. Vena caval interruption consists of transvenous placement of a grid or umbrella in the vena cava to block the passage of emboli.

Preoperative care includes monitoring peripheral pulses and signs of bleeding from anticoagulant therapy and pulmonary emboli (for instance, sudden chest pain and cough). Postoperative nursing care is described in Box 18-6.

Interventions to achieve patient outcomes
Promoting comfort

Analgesics reduce pain and discomfort in the people with acute thrombophlebitis. Anti-inflammatory medication decreases the inflammation, thereby contributing to increased comfort. Warm moist heat, heating pads, or ice packs may be prescribed to enhance resolution of the inflammation.

Teaching the patient

The major emphasis of nursing interventions for the person with a chronic venous disorder is patient teaching. Important topics for teaching are measures to increase tissue perfusion by preventing venous stasis (and thereby preventing pain) and measures to prevent recurrences.

1. Prevention of venous stasis
   a. Avoid prolonged sitting or standing
   b. Elevate legs when sitting
   c. Avoid crossing the legs at the knee
   d. Wear elastic stockings (Box 18-7)
   e. Avoid constriction on leg veins by tight bands (socks and garters)
   f. Carry out daily exercises and physical activity (promotion of blood flow by contraction of leg muscles)
      (1) Practise dorsiflexion of both feet while sitting or lying down
      (2) Walk daily; increase distance as tolerated
      (3) Swim several times weekly if possible
      (4) Use stationary bicycle.
2. Prevent recurrence
   a. Maintain desired weight for height.
   b. Modify lifestyle (both at work and at home) as necessary to prevent long periods of standing or sitting.
   c. Follow activity programme as described above.
   d. Take special precautions if pregnant (because of increased pressure on veins) or for any surgical procedure (especially pelvic surgery).

Evaluation

Evaluation is based on expected patient outcomes. Questions to consider may include:
1. Does patient state that leg pain is decreased?
2. Did patient remain inactive during acute phase?
3. Can patient describe the medication regimen, preventive measures, and signs to report to doctor?

VARICOSE VEINS
Aetiology/Epidemiology

Varicose veins can develop from the congenital absence of a valve or acquired valve incompetence. They often occur as a result of external pressure on the veins from pregnancy, ascites, or abdominal tumours. Other associated factors are prolonged standing, constricting clothing, and marked obesity. They may also occur from sustained elevations in venous pressure from heart disease or cirrhosis. From 10% to 20% of the world's population is affected. The highest incidence is in women aged 40 to 60.

Prevention

People with varicosities, especially if there is a family history of varicosities, should wear elastic stockings during activities that require prolonged standing or when pregnant. Moderate exercise and elevation of the legs when sitting help to prevent venous congestion. No continual pressure should be applied to the legs.

Pathophysiology

Varicose veins are abnormally dilated veins with incompetent valves occurring most often in the legs and lower trunk. The long and short saphenous veins are most often involved (Fig. 18-10). The precipitating factor is weakness of the vessel wall. The weakened area dilates, stretching the valves, which then become incompetent. This results in inability to support a column of blood, and venous pooling.

Varicose veins may be primary or secondary. *Primary* varicosities have a gradual onset and affect superficial veins. Often there are no symptoms except the appearance of darkened tortuous veins. Symptoms include dull aches, muscle cramps, heaviness, or fatigue arising from

18-6

Guidelines for Care

18-6

The patient after venous surgery

Monitor for signs of bleeding, especially on first postoperative day; if incisional bleeding occurs, elevate the leg, apply pressure over the wound, and notify the surgeon.

Assist patient to ambulate as soon as permitted; instruct patient to avoid sitting or bending at hip (restricts venous return).

Check elastic bandage several times a day to maintain even pressure on leg veins.

Give analgesics as necessary for pain and discomfort.

Patient Teaching

18-7

The use of elastic stockings

Use correct size (see instructions on box or consult medical supply person) and length (to knee or groin) as prescribed.[48]

Apply stocking before getting out of bed.

For ease of application, turn foot of stocking inside out, slide foot into stocking, and pull stocking over leg.

Remove stocking at bedtime if desired; if leg aches at night, stocking may be of benefit if worn in bed.

Keep a second stocking to hand for use when the other is being washed.

decreased blood flow to the tissues. *Secondary* varicosities affect the deep veins and result from chronic venous insufficiency or venous thrombosis. Symptoms of oedema, pain, changes in skin colour, and ulceration may occur from venous stasis.

Diagnostic Tests

Trendelenburg's test is a simple noninvasive diagnostic tool to assess the competency of the venous valves through measurement of venous filling time. The patient lies down with the affected leg raised to allow for venous emptying. A tourniquet is then applied above the knee, and the patient stands. The direction and filling time of the veins are recorded both before and after the tourniquet is removed. Incompetent valves are evident when the veins fill rapidly from backward blood flow.

Interventions

Sclerotherapy consists of injection of a sclerosing solution at the sites of the varicosities. It produces permanent obliteration of the collapsed veins. Elastic bandages are applied for continuous pressure for one to two weeks. The procedure is performed as ambulatory surgery and offers good cosmetic results.

Surgical intervention is indicated for oedema, recurrent leg ulcers, pain, or cosmetic reasons. Surgery consists of vein ligation and stripping. The long saphenous vein is ligated (tied) close to the femoral junction, if possible. The long and short saphenous veins are then stripped out through small incisions at the groin, above and below the knee, and at the ankle (Fig 18-11). An elastic bandage is applied firmly.

Postoperative nursing care includes the following:

1. Monitor for signs of bleeding: if bleeding occurs, elevate leg, apply pressure on wound, and notify surgeon.
2. Keep patient flat in bed for first four hours; elevate leg to promote venous return when lying or sitting.
3. Medicate 30 minutes before ambulation.
4. Keep elastic bandage snug and wrinkle free; do not remove bandage for daily care.

Because varicosities are chronic conditions, the person must know how to prevent venous stasis and encourage venous return. Preventive measures are listed on p. 449.

LEG ULCERS

Aetiology

Most leg ulcers occur from chronic deep vein insufficiency or severe varicose veins, and less frequently from arterial obstruction. Other causes include burns, leg trauma, and neurogenic disorders. People with diabetes mellitus are at high risk for development of leg ulcers because of vascular insufficiency.

Pathophysiology

A leg ulcer is an open necrotic lesion that results from inadequate exchange of oxygen and other nutrients to the tissues because of decreased circulation. The same underlying pathophysiological changes that contribute to chronic venous or arterial insufficiency are involved. Secondary bacterial infection occurs because of the decreased circulation that limits the body's response to infection. The infection, in turn, delays healing.

Clinical signs vary, depending on the underlying problem. A *venous ulcer* (stasis ulcer) is usually moderately painful and located on the medial aspect of the ankle. Oedema and pigmentation are common around the ulcer because of venous stasis. Most venous ulcers heal with therapy. An *arterial ulcer* (ischaemic ulcer) causes more pain and has a more necrotic, pale grey base because of lack of oxygen to the tissues. Pale or mottled skin is common around the ulcer base. Oedema is infrequent. Peripheral pulses are diminished or absent. Arterial ulcers frequently develop on the heel, lateral malleolus, toes, and dorsum of the foot.

Nursing Process
Assessment

Subjective data

1. Onset and duration of symptoms.
2. Extent and characteristics of pain.
3. Limitations in mobility and activity.
4. History of deep vein thrombosis, varicose veins, arterial insufficiency, or diabetes.

Objective data

1. Appearance and temperature of the skin.
2. Location and appearance of the ulcer.
3. Presence and quality of all peripheral pulses.
4. Presence of oedema, eczema and "ankle flare".

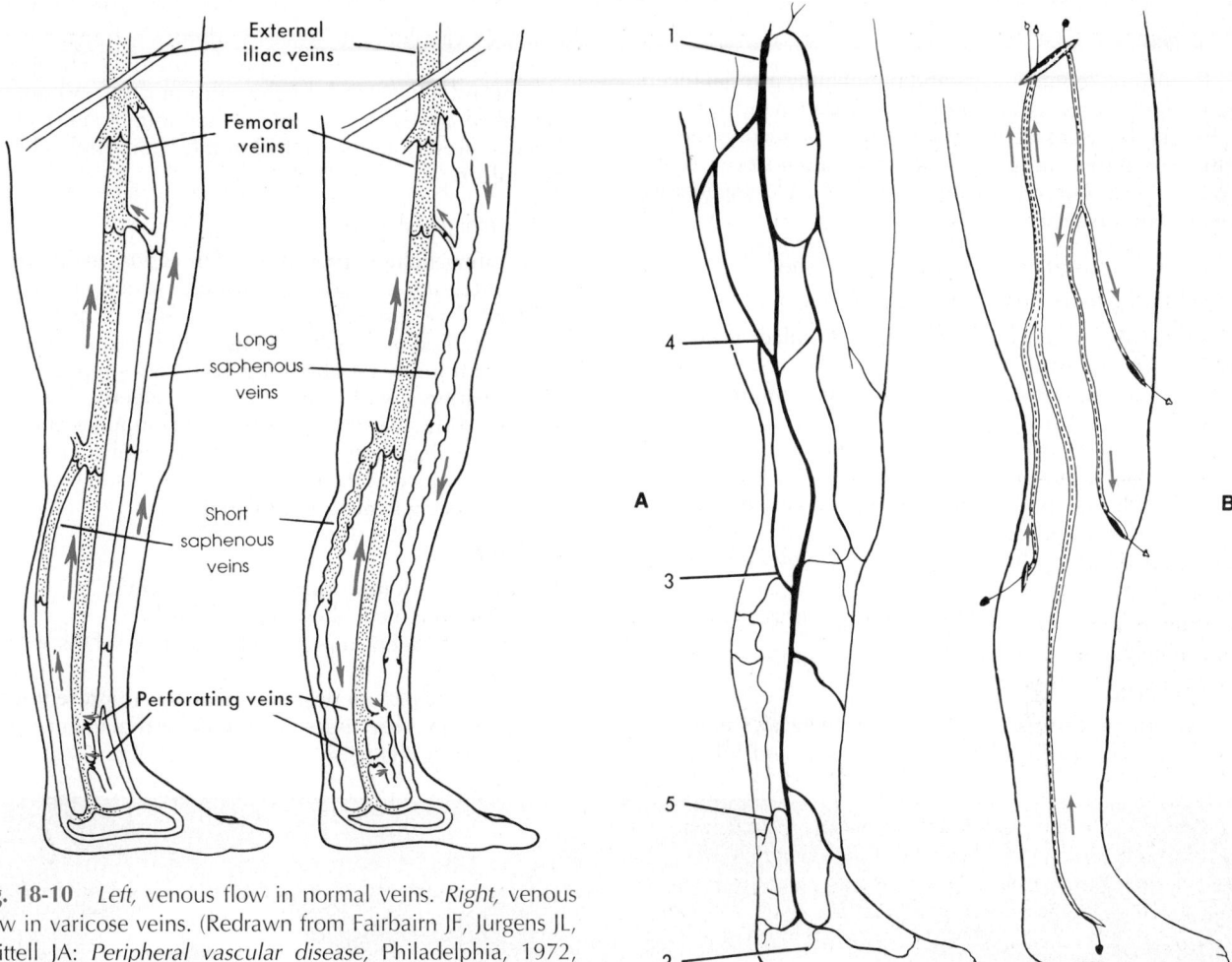

Fig. 18-10   *Left,* venous flow in normal veins. *Right,* venous flow in varicose veins. (Redrawn from Fairbairn JF, Jurgens JL, Spittell JA: *Peripheral vascular disease,* Philadelphia, 1972, WB Saunders.)

Fig. 18-11   **A,** Outline of incompetent long saphenous system with numerals indicating main tributaries. **B,** Passing of strippers in preparation of removal of incompetent veins.

Nursing analysis

Problems are determined from analysis of patient data. Possible problems for the people with leg ulcers may include, but are not limited to, the following:

Problem	Possible aetiologies
Tissue perfusion, altered peripheral	Decreased blood flow (arterial or venous)
Pain, ulcer	Inflammation, necrosis
Knowledge deficit	Lack of exposure/recall

Planning: expected patient outcomes

Expected patient outcomes for the person with leg ulcers may include, but are not limited to, the following:

1. Ulcer shows signs of healing and absence of further breakdown.
2. Patient participates in activities of daily living (ADLs) without discomfort or pain.
3. Patient describes measures to prevent infection and increase tissue perfusion, and care of the ulcer.

Implementation
Assisting with achievement of therapeutic goals

The primary goal in treating leg ulcers is to promote wound healing and prevent infection. Necrotic tissue is debrided by chemical, or surgical means. The choice of dressing is of vital importance, and a leg ulcer assessment chart such as that in *Leg Ulcer Management*[10a] should be used. *Chemical* beads, such as dextranomer paste pad, and hydrocolloid dressings, may be placed over the ulcer (avoiding healthy tissue) to break down the debris. Occasionally necrotic tissue can also be cut away with the aid of *surgical* instruments, usually a scalpel.

Topical and systemic *antibiotics* may be prescribed to prevent infection. Systemic antibiotic therapy is the most effective route in the treatment of leg ulcers. Periodic culture of wound drainage may be ordered to monitor the effectiveness of the antibiotics.

A *boot* may be applied to cover small, newly formed ulcers in ambulatory people (Fig. 18-12). This boot protects the ulcer and provides constant and even support to the area. The boot is made from a special type of impregnated gauze that hardens after it is wrapped around the patient's leg. The boot is generally left on for one to two weeks, although it may be changed more often if there is copious drainage. Elastic bandages are applied to the leg after the ulcer has healed.

Surgery

Recurrent venous ulcers and nonhealing arterial ulcers may require surgical intervention. Ligation of incompetent veins may be necessary. Arterial bypass and reconstruction can be used to revascularize the artery and restore circulation (p. 443). Amputation may be required if less aggressive means are unsuccessful.

Interventions to achieve patient outcomes

Promoting tissue perfusion

Circulation of tissue surrounding the ulcer is encouraged by the following actions:

1. Maintain proper body positioning to improve circulation by gravity:
   a. Elevate head of bed on three- to six-inch blocks for an *arterial* ulcer
   b. Elevate lower extremities to decrease oedema for a *venous* ulcer.
2. Use a bed cradle to protect leg from pressure of bedclothes.
3. Use cotton between toes to prevent pressure on a toe ulcer.

Promoting comfort

Encourage the use of prescribed analgesics and anti-inflammatory medication to reduce pain and inflammation. Medicate for pain 30 to 45 minutes before a dressing change. Use aseptic technique in dressing changes to prevent infection and further discomfort. Administer prescribed antibiotics on time to maintain blood levels for effective prevention or control of infection, thus relieving discomfort.

Teaching the patient

Teaching includes prevention of infection, maintenance of skin integrity, and measures to increase peripheral tissue perfusion (see pp. 439 and 449). Teach the patient the correct method of dressing changes and discuss resources in the community for obtaining necessary supplies. Many of the patients with leg ulcers are elderly; therefore, ascertain if the patient is able to obtain supplies and carry out the dressing changes. If not, other people in the home must be included in the teaching. If the person lives alone, other approaches must be explored.

Evaluation

Questions to ask may include the following:

1. Does the ulcer show signs of healing?
2. Is the patient able to participate in ADLs without pain?
3. Can the patient describe measures to prevent infection, increase tissue perfusion, and make necessary dressing changes?

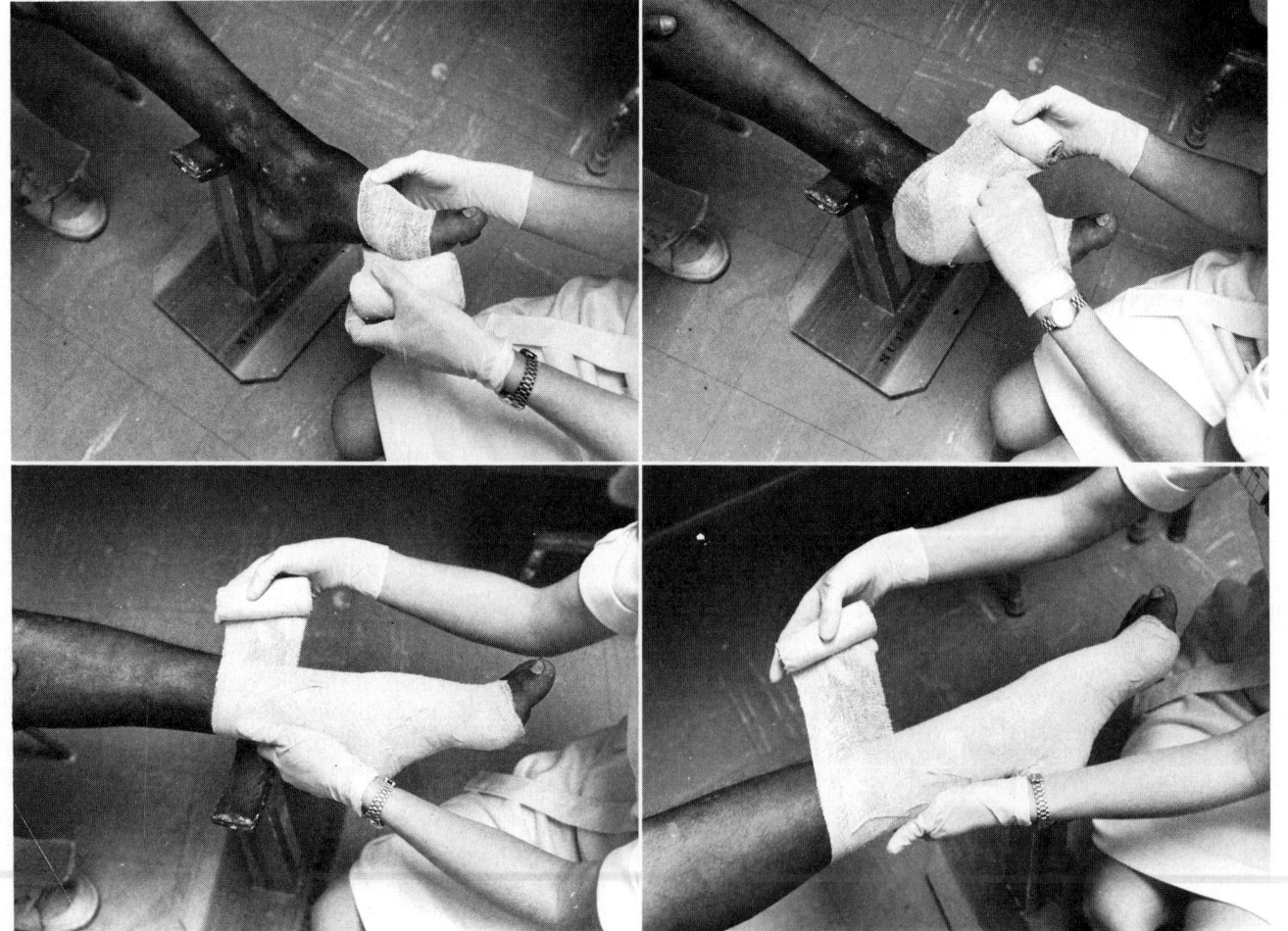

Fig. 18-12   Nurse applying Unna paste boot using specially impregnated gauze. Note ulcers on inferior aspect of patient's foot.

18-8

Causes of secondary lymphoedema

Obstruction
    Malignant tumours
    Postsurgical removal of lymph nodes
    Mechanical trauma
    Postirradiation
Inflammation
Infection (parasitic)

LYMPHOEDEMA

AETIOLOGY

Lymphoedema is an abnormal collection of lymph in tissues. It may be *primary*, congenital or developing at puberty as a result of hypoplastic development of lymph vessels; or *secondary*, developing from obstruction, inflammation, or parasitic infection (Box 18-8). The most common causes are neoplastic obstruction and surgical removal of lymph nodes, such as with radical mastectomy.

Pathophysiology

Lymphoedema results when lymphatic vessels or lymph nodes become obstructed and cannot return tissue lymph to the circulation. Obstruction may result from inflammation or mechanical blocking of lymph flow. The obstruction may lead to incompetence of valves in the lymph vessels with resulting stasis of lymph flow and eventual fibrosis. The limb becomes enlarged. *Oedema* is initially pitting; but over time, it becomes brawny (nonpitting) as the tissue hypertrophies. Inflammation (cellulitis or lymphangitis) may occur with minor limb injuries. Lymphoedema of the lower extremities begins with mild swelling on the dorsum of the foot, usually at the end of the day, and gradually extends to involve the entire limb. The condition is aggravated by prolonged standing, pregnancy, obesity, warm weather, or menstruation.

Nursing Process
Assessment
Subjective data

1. Onset of swelling in affected extremity.
2. History of secondary cause of lymphoedema (Box 18-8).
3. Effectiveness of current therapy to reduce oedema.

Objective data

1. Observation of extremities for oedema: unilateral, pitting or nonpitting.
2. Comparison in size of extremities.
3. Quality of peripheral pulses.

Diagnostic tests

Lymphangiography consists of injection of a radiopaque dye directly into the lymphatic vessels. An X-ray examination is made after injection and 24 hours later. The lymph nodes can also be visualized. Periodic X-ray examinations can be made for up to six months because the dye remains in the lymph system.

Nursing analysis

Problems are determined from analysis of patient data. Possible problems for the person with lymphoedema may include, but are not limited to, the following:

Problem	Possible aetiologies
Body image disturbance	Change in body appearance
Knowledge deficit	Lack of exposure/recall

Planning: expected patient outcomes

Expected patient outcomes for the person with lymphoedema may include, but are not limited to, the following:

1. Expresses confidence in self, despite change in appearance of extremity.
2. Describes measures to decrease infection, maintain intact skin, and improve lymph drainage.

Implementation
Assisting with achievement of therapeutic goals

Therapy for lymphoedema is conservative. The goal is to reduce oedema and to maintain skin integrity. Therapy includes the following:

1. Passive and active exercises.
2. Elevation of affected extremity.
3. Elastic stocking to reduce oedema of leg.
4. Restriction of dietary sodium to reduce fluid retention and thereby decrease oedema.
5. Diuretic therapy to decrease limb size temporarily by decreasing total body fluid.
6. Long-term antibiotic therapy to control recurrent cellulitis and infection.

Most patients respond to conservative medical therapy and do not require surgical intervention. If indicated, surgery consists of removal of the oedematous lymph tissues or reconstruction of the lymphatic drainage channels.

Interventions to achieve patient outcomes
Promoting positive body image

Lymphoedema may cause a limb to become excessively large, which greatly alters the patient's appearance. Although the limb can be covered by clothing, the size cannot be hidden (except with a long skirt for women). The change in appearance can lead to a poor self-concept. The patient should be given opportunities to express feelings and encouragement to follow through on measures to decrease some of the oedema. Positive attributes are emphasized.

Teaching the patient

Patient teaching includes measures to prevent infection and improve lymph drainage:

1. Take antibiotics for as long as prescribed to prevent infection.
2. Take measures to promote skin integrity and thus prevent infection:
    a. Monitor skin for intactness, swelling, redness, and lesions

    b. Seek medical assistance if skin changes occur

    c. Carry out special foot care (for leg oedema) to prevent minor infection.

3. Take measures to improve lymph drainage and decrease oedema:

    a. Elevate affected extremity above heart level at frequent intervals

    b. Avoid prolonged standing

    c. Sleep with foot of bed elevated four to eight inches

    d. Wear elastic stockings from arising until retiring at night

    e. Avoid constrictive clothing

    f. Exercise on a regular basis

    g. Take diuretics as prescribed

    h. Follow prescribed sodium-restricted diet.

4. Carry out instructions for continued medical follow-up

Evaluation

Questions to ask may include the following:

1. Is patient able to discuss feelings about altered appearance of the extremity?

2. Is patient taking measures to facilitate control of oedema and thereby promote a more positive body image?

3. Can the patient describe ways to prevent infection and to improve lymph drainage?

4. Is the patient making plans for follow-up care?

HYPERTENSION

Hypertension can be considered with peripheral vascular disorders because they both involve problems of peripheral circulation and are affected by similar factors. Hypertension itself is a risk factor in atherosclerosis, the major cause of peripheral vascular disease.

Aetiology/Epidemiology

Hypertension is defined as a consistent systolic blood pressure greater than 140mmHg and/or a consistent diastolic blood pressure greater than 90mmHg. (Traditionally blood pressure is measured in millimetres of mercury (mmHg) although the correct SI unit is pascals (Pa)). A more complete classification of blood pressure which was developed in the United States to assist in establishing a more universal diagnosis of hypertension, is listed in Table 18-6. It must be emphasized that the categorical classification is based on the average of two or more blood pressure readings, not a single elevated reading.

Many millions of Britains have been diagnosed with elevated blood pressure or are taking antihypertensive medications. It is estimated that some 15% of the population of the United Kingdom has an elevated blood pressure, with many individuals being undiagnosed. The exact number is unknown because most individuals are symptom-free and others avoid pursuing treatment .

The incidence of hypertension increases with age and varies considerably among different groups. Hypertension occurs more often in men than in women and is nearly twice as prevalent among Afro-Caribbean individuals than in Caucasians. Hypertension in Afro-Caribbean individuals is usually more severe than it is in similar hypertensive Caucasians. There is an increased incidence and severity of hypertension in black Americans in the southeastern United States, compared with those residing in other areas.

There are two types of hypertension, essential (primary, idiopathic) and secondary. *Essential* hypertension accounts for 85 to 90% of all types of hypertension. Although there is no generally accepted cause of essential hypertension, several theories have been suggested, including arteriolar changes, alterations in sympathetic tone, hormonal influence, and genetic factors. *Secondary* hypertension develops as a consequence of an underlying disease or condition (Table 18-7). In most instances, the hypertension will subside when the disease is treated or corrected.

Prevention
Primary prevention

Primary prevention is aimed at reducing risk factors associated with hypertension (Box 18-9). Health education programmes include teaching about moderate sodium intake, a decreased saturated-fat diet, maintenance of optimal body weight for height, cessation of cigarette smoking, moderate consumption of alcohol, and the use of effective coping strategies to minimize stress.

Secondary prevention

Secondary prevention consists of identification and control of hypertension in high-risk groups, such as blacks (especially males), obese people, and blood relatives of known hypertensives. A major effort should be made to contact people who have limited access to healthcare because of geographical or other constraints. Follow-ups should be made after initial blood pressure measurements depending on the range of initial findings (Table 18-8). Mass blood pressure screenings are currently not recommended. Most often these screenings occur at large-scale gatherings where environmental conditions may cause inaccurate blood pressure readings. In addition, these sites tend to be frequented by the same people.

Pathophysiology

Blood pressure is the pressure exerted by the blood on the vessels through which it flows. Systolic pressure is the pressure exerted during ventricular contraction; diastolic pressure is pressure during ventricular relaxation. Blood pressure is regulated by two factors: blood flow and peripheral vascular resistance. Factors that determine *blood flow* are the volume of blood ejected from the left ventricle with each contraction (stroke volume) and the heart rate (see Chapter 17). *Peripheral vascular resistance* is affected primarily by the diameter of the blood vessel and, to a lesser degree, by the viscosity of the blood. Increased peripheral vascular resistance as a result of narrowing of the arterioles is the most common characteristic in hypertension.

Dilation and constriction of the peripheral arterioles are controlled by several mechanisms, primarily the sympathetic nervous system and the renin–angiotensin system. The vasomotor centre in the medulla can be stimulated by the baroreceptors or by psychogenic stress. Impulses are

Table 18-6   Classification of blood pressure* (age 18 and older)

Range (mmHg)	Classification
Diastolic	
less than 85	Normal blood pressure
85–89	High–normal blood pressure †
90–104	Mild hypertension
105–114	Moderate hypertension
greater than or equal to 115	Severe hypertension
Systolic	
less than 140	Normal blood pressure
140–159	Borderline isolated systolic hypertension ‡
greater than 160	Isolated systolic hypertension ‡

* Based on average of two or more readings on two or more occasions.
† High–normal blood pressure takes precedence over normal (systolic) blood pressure when both occur in same person.
‡ Borderline isolated systolic hypertension or isolated systolic hypertension take precedence over high–normal blood pressure when both occur in same person.

Table 18-7   Causes of secondary hypertension

Disorder/condition	Mechanism
Kidney	
Renal parenchymal disease (glomerulonephritis, renal failure)	Most often cause a renin or sodium dependent hypertension; physiological changes relate to type of disease and severity of renal insufficiency
Renovascular disease	Decrease in renal perfusion from atherosclerotic or fibrotic narrowing of renal arteries; causes marked increase in peripheral vascular resistance and cardiac output
Adrenal cortex	
Cushing's syndrome	Increase in blood volume
Primary aldosteronism	Increase in aldosterone, causing sodium and water retention that increase blood volume
Phaeochromocytoma	Excess secretion of catecholamines (noradrenaline increases peripheral vascular resistance)
Coarctation of aorta	Causes marked elevated blood pressure in upper extremities with decreased perfusion in lower extremities
Head trauma or cranial tumour	Increased intracranial pressure reduces cerebral blood flow; resultant ischaemia stimulates medullary vasomotor centre to raise blood pressure
Pregnancy-induced hypertension	Cause unknown; generalized vasospasm may be a contributing factor

then carried through the sympathetic nervous system, causing the release of catecholamines. Noradrenaline is released from the postganglionic fibres, causing blood vessel constriction and increased peripheral resistance. Adrenaline is secreted by the adrenal medulla and causes vasoconstriction. Adrenaline also increases ventricular contraction force and cardiac output.

Renal regulation is an essential component of blood pressure control. Activation of the renin–angiotensin system occurs when there is reduced bloodflow to the kidneys. Renin leads to the formation of angiotensin, a potent vasoconstrictor. Angiotensin stimulates the secretion of aldosterone, which promotes retention of sodium and and water.

Hypertension is essentially a disease without symptoms. When symptoms do occur, they are usually indicative of advanced hypertension. Signs and symptoms may include early morning headache, blurred vision, and spontaneous nosebleeds. Evidence of the effects of advanced hypertension may include nausea, vomiting, and confusion (hypertensive encephalopathy), and exertional dyspnoea and dysrhythmias (left ventricular hypertrophy).

Complications

With prolonged hypertension, the elastic tissue in the arterioles is replaced by fibrous collagen tissue. The thickened arteriole wall becomes less distensible, creating even greater resistance to blood flow. This process leads to decreased tissue perfusion, especially in the target organs, the heart, kidneys, and brain.

In the cardiovascular system, decreased coronary perfusion may lead to *angina pectoris* or *myocardial infarction*. As the heart is forced to work against consistently elevated aortic pressure, left ventricular hypertrophy and *congestive heart failure* may result.

As the renal vessels thicken and perfusion diminishes, the glomerulus is deprived of its blood supply. Permanent kidney damage and *renal failure* may result. Cerebral ischaemia and arteriosclerosis can result from the progressive effects of hypertension; *stroke* or *cerebral haemorrhage* may occur.

Malignant hypertension is a severe, rapidly progressive elevation in blood pressure that causes damage to the small arterioles in major organ systems (heart, kidneys, brain, eyes). A primary distinguishing finding is inflammation of the arterioles (arteriolitis) in the eyes. Retinitis and papilloedema occur in later stages. This type of hypertension is most common in Afro-Caribbean males under age 40. Unless medical treatment is successful, the course is rapidly fatal. The most common causes of death are myocardial infarction, congestive heart failure, stroke, or renal failure.

18-9

Risk factors in essential hypertension

Age: advancing
Sex: male
Race: Afro-Caribbean
Family history: hypertension
Obesity: associated with increased intravascular
volume
Atherosclerosis: narrowing of arteries increases
blood pressure
Smoking: nicotine constricts blood vessels
High-salt diet: sodium causes water retention,
increasing blood volume
Alcohol: increases plasma catecholamines
Emotional stress: stimulates sympathetic nervous
system

Table 18-8   Recommendations for follow-up of initial blood pressure measurements in adults (over age 18)

Range (mmHg)	Recommended follow-up*
Diastolic	
less than 85	Recheck within 2 years
85–89	Recheck within 1 year
90–104	Confirm within 2 months
105–114	Evaluate or refer to source of care within 2 weeks
greater than or equal to 115	Evaluate or refer immediately to source of care
Systolic	
less than 140	Recheck within 2 years
140–199	Confirm within 2 months
greater than or equal to 200	Evaluate or refer to source of care within 2 weeks

* If recommendations for follow-up of diastolic and systolic blood pressure are different, the shorter recommended time for recheck should take precedence.

Nursing Process
Assessment
Subjective data

Subjective data are collected about the presence of any symptoms, history of hypertension, and patient knowledge of hypertension. These data may include the following:

1. Presence of early morning headache, blurred vision, confusion, exertional dyspnoea.
2. Presence of risk factors (Box 18-9) including stress in occupation or daily life.
3. Course and compliance with therapy for previously diagnosed hypertension.
4. Current knowledge of hypertension: definition, meaning of systolic and diastolic readings, and effects of high blood pressure on heart, kidneys, and brain.

Objective data

Two or more blood measurements are taken in both arms with the patient in both supine and sitting positions. Additional data include:

1. Height and weight (identification of obesity).
2. Examination of neck by doctor for carotid bruits and abdomen for abdominal bruits (sound of blood flow through narrowed passageways).
3. Auscultation of heart by doctor for abnormal heart sounds: S_3 and S_4, murmurs (evidence of left ventricular hypertrophy).
4. Palpation of peripheral pulse by doctor: rate, amplitude, bilateral symmetry (signs of peripheral vascular narrowing).
5. Funduscopic eye examination by doctor (presence of arteriolar narrowing or haemorrhage).

Diagnostic tests

Diagnostic tests used to determine the possible cause of hypertension, to assess the effect of the disease on other organ systems, or to provide baseline information may include the following:

1. Serum levels of sodium, potassium, calcium, and creatinine as well as haemoglobin and haematocrit (severity and possible causes).
2. Urinalysis, urea, and renal function tests (effect on kidneys and baseline for drug therapy).
3. An electrocardiogram, chest X-ray, and possibly echocardiography (extent of left ventricular hypertrophy or aortic calcification).

Nursing analysis

Problems are determined from analysis of patient data. Possible problems for the people with hypertension may include, but are not limited to, the following:

Problem	Possible aetiologies
Knowledge deficit: nature of hypertension, risk factors, drug therapy	Lack of exposure/recall, unfamiliarity with information resources
Noncompliance: drug regimen, ongoing care	Patient value system, treatment side effects
Sexual dysfunction	Lack of information of effects of medications

Planning: expected patient outcomes

Expected patient outcomes for the people with hypertension may include, but are not limited to, the following:

1. Explains nature of hypertension and effects of hypertension on heart, kidney, brain.
2. Demonstrates correct procedure for self-management and recording of blood pressure.
3. Maintains blood pressure within desirable range.
4. Describes therapeutic regimen.
5. Describes plan to participate in other measures to promote normal blood pressure (dietary changes, exercise, stress reduction).
6. Explains effects of prescribed antihypertensive

medication on sexual function (as appropriate).

7. Takes antihypertensive medications as prescribed.

Implementation

Assisting with achievement of therapeutic goals

Medical therapy is directed at the control of hypertension and the prevention of associated diseases. The primary goal is to maintain a systolic blood pressure of less than 140mmHg and a diastolic pressure of less than 90mmHg. The decision to treat hypertension is based on degree of the blood pressure elevation, presence of risk factors, and extent of damage to associated organ systems. *Nonpharmacological* means, such as dietary programmes of weight control and reduction of sodium and saturated fats, as well as exercise programmes, are prescribed. Most people with hypertension have difficulty maintaining the desired blood pressure with these measures alone; therefore drug therapy is usually prescribed.

Pharmacological therapy

Antihypertensive medications have a protective effect against damage to the heart, kidneys, and brain in patients with mild hypertension. Drug treatment has been shown to successfully lower a consistent diastolic blood pressure from higher than 94mmHg to less than 90mmHg. When a diastolic blood pressure is between 90 and 94mmHg, an individualized approach to drug therapy is used.

Commonly used hypertensive drugs are listed in Table 18-9. Drug selection is determined by use of a step-care approach. Therapy is started with a small dose of a less potent drug. Additions and substitutions of drugs, and dosage adjustments are based on the patient's response. The step-care approach is as follows:

Step 1: Use a diuretic, beta-blocker, alpha-blocker, calcium antagonist, or angiotensin-converting enzyme (ACE) inhibitor.

Step 2: If ineffective after one to three months, increase dosage of drug, add a second drug of a different class, or substitute another drug.

Step 3: Add a third drug of a different class or substitute a second drug.

Step 4: Add a fourth drug of a different class or substitute a third drug: evaluate further and refer to a specialist if ineffective.

After one year of satisfactory blood pressure control, a stepdown approach may be effective in patients also adhering to nonpharmacological measures.

Hypertensive crisis

Hypertensive emergency or crisis refers to a situation that requires immediate blood pressure lowering. Although such cases are relatively uncommon, prompt recognition and management are essential to prevent organ dysfunction. Clinical conditions that may precipitate a hypertensive crisis include hypertensive encephalopathy, intracranial haemorrhage, left ventricular heart failure, dissecting aortic aneurysm, severe hypertension of pregnancy, head injury, extensive burns, unstable angina, or acute myocardial infarction. It may also occur in patients with poor hypertensive control and in those who abruptly discontinue their medications. Parenteral drug administration through intravenous and intramuscular routes is used to quickly lower markedly elevated blood pressure. Intravenous medications are administered by drip and titrated according to the patient's response. Common drugs used in the treatment of hypertensive emergencies are listed in Table 18-10.

Interventions to achieve patient outcomes

The major nursing strategies in the care of the people with hypertension are patient teaching and counselling. Teaching is directed towards increasing knowledge about hypertension, risk factors, associated diseases, and the treatment regimen. Counselling includes assisting the

---

Table 18-9 Oral medications for treatment of hypertension

Drug	Action*	Side-effects*
Thiazide/thiazide-like diuretics		
Bendrofluazide	Block sodium reabsorption in cortical portion of ascending tubule; water excreted with sodium, producing decreased blood volume. NOTE: thiazides ineffective in renal failure	Increased urea, uric acid, blood glucose, calcium, cholesterol, and triglycerides
Benzthiazide		Decreased potassium
Chlorothiazide		Possible postural hypotension in summer from sodium loss
Chlorthalidone		
Clopamide		Gastrointestinal upset, dry mouth, thirst, weakness, muscle aches, fatigue, tachycardia
Hydrochlorothiazide		
Hydroflumethiazide		Sexual dysfunction (impotence)
Indapamide		
Mefruside		
Methyclothiazide		
Metolazone		
Polythiazide		
Xipamide		
Loop diuretics		
Bumetanide	Block sodium and water reabsorption in medullary portion of ascending tubule; causes rapid volume depletion	Decreased potassium
Ethacrynic acid		Thirst, skin rash, postural hypotension, nausea, vomiting
Frusemide		

Table 18-9 Oral medications for treatment of hypertension—cont'd

Drug	Action*	Side-effects*
Potassium-sparing diuretics Amiloride Spironolactone Triamterene	Inhibit aldosterone; sodium excreted in exchange for potassium	Dry mouth, confusion Increased potassium levels Diarrhoea Gynaecomastia with spironolactone
Adrenergic inhibitors **Beta-adrenergic blockers** Acebutolol Atenolol Metoprolol Nadolol Pindolol Propranolol Timolol	Block beta-adrenergic receptors of sympathetic nervous system, decreasing heart rate and blood pressure NOTE: beta-blockers should not be used in patients with asthma, chronic obstructive pulmonary disease, congestive heart failure, and heart block; use with caution in diabetes and peripheral vascular disease	Bronchospasms Bradycardia, fatigue, insomnia Sexual dysfunction Peripheral vascular insufficiency Increased triglycerides
Centrally acting alpha-blockers Clonidine Methyldopa	Activate central receptors that suppress vasomotor and cardiac centres, causing a decrease in peripheral resistance. NOTE: rebound hypertension may occur with abrupt discontinuation of drug (except with methyldopa)	Drowsiness, sedation Dry mouth Fatigue Sexual dysfunction Orthostatic hypotension Positive Coomb's test with methyldopa
Peripheral-acting adrenergic antagonists Bethanidine Detrisoquine Guanethidine	Deplete noradrenaline in peripheral sympathetic postganglionic fibres Block noradrenaline release from adrenergic nerve endings	Orthostatic hypotension Lethargy, depression Sexual dysfunction
Alpha-1-adrenergic blockers Doxazosin Prazosin Terazosin	Block synaptic receptors that regulate vasomotor tone; reduce peripheral resistance by dilating arterioles and venules	"First dose" syncope, orthostatic hypotension, weakness, palpatations, decreased low-density lipoproteins
Combined alpha- and beta-adrenergic blockers Labetalol	Same as for beta-blockers	Bronchospasm, orthostatic hypotension, peripheral vascular insufficiency
Vasodilators Hydralazine Minoxidil	Dilate perpheral blood vessels by directly relaxing vascular smooth muscle NOTE: usually used in combination with beta-blocker and diuretic as they increase sodium and fluid retention and can cause reflex cardiac stimulation	Headache, dizziness Tachycardia, palpitations, fatigue, oedema
Angiotensin-converting enzyme inhibitors Captopril Enalapril Lisinopril	Inhibit conversion of angiotensin to angiotensin II thus blocking the release of aldosterone, thereby reducing sodium and water retention	"First dose" hypotension, headache, dizziness, fatigue Increased potassium Cough, skin reactions
Calcium antagonists Dilitiazem Felodipine Isradipine Nicardipine Nifedipine Verapamil	Inhibit influx of calcium into muscle cells; act on vascular smooth muscles (primary arteries) to reduce spasms and promote vasodilation	Dizziness, fatigue, nausea, headache, oedema

Table 18-10 Medication for treatment of hypertensive emergencies

Drug	Action*	Side-effects*
Vasodilators		
Sodium nitroprusside	Dilate peripheral blood vessels by	Headache, dizziness
Glyceryl trinitrate	relaxing vascular smooth muscle	Tachycardia, palpitations, fatigue, nausea,
Diazoxide		oedema
Hydralazine		NOTE: thiocyanate toxicity may occur with
		sodium nitroprusside
Adrenergic inhibitors		
Phentolamine	Block adrenergic receptors of sympathetic	Tachycardia, orthostatic hypotension
Trimethaphan camsylate	nervous system, thereby dilating	
Labetalol	peripheral blood vessels and reducing	
Methyldopa	peripheral vascular resistance	

* Primary action and common side effects are included and are related to entire drug category; consult drug reference or drug package insert for more specific information.

people in making behavioural changes to further reduce, control, or maintain blood pressure at acceptable levels, and in coping with sexual dysfunction.

Increasing knowledge of hypertension

The individual needs to understand the concepts of blood pressure and hypertension. Use simple words to define systolic and diastolic blood pressure. Explain the effects of hypertension on the heart, kidneys, and brain. Teach the people self-monitoring of blood pressure, as appropriate, and advise the people to purchase a reliable instrument. Ask the people to keep a written record of blood pressures, including date and any pertinent information if elevated or lowered.

Teaching about risk factors

Dietary modifications. Explain that excess salt intake will contribute to fluid retention; more fluid in the circulating blood will increase the blood pressure. Teaching should include the following:

1. Avoid adding salt to foods during preparation and at the table; substitute herbs for flavour.
2. Avoid highly salted foods, such as crisps, crackers, nuts, canned soups, and packaged luncheon meats.
3. Minimize eating in fast food restaurants (most of these foods have increased salt and fat content).
4. Reduce intake of saturated fats to maintain body weight and control atherosclerotic changes (see Chapter 4).
5. Use moderation in alcohol consumption: alcohol may potentiate certain antihypertensive medications in addition to raising blood pressure.

Other risk factors. Other behavioural changes to discuss include cessation of cigarette smoking, participating in exercise programmes, and reducing stress.

1. Explain the effects of *nicotine* on blood vessels (p. 44\5); suggest use of behaviour modification (Chapter 4), group therapy, or hypnosis as means of stopping smoking.
2. Discuss need to participate in a regular *aerobic* exercise programme three times a week (see Chapter 5), consisting of 20 to 45 minutes of activity with warm-up and cool-down periods.

3. Help patient identify sources of *stress*; demonstrate relaxation techniques such as deep breathing, progressive muscle relaxation, and imagery that can help lower blood pressure; suggest use of biofeedback techniques (see Chapter 5).

Teaching about medications

Patients who are prescribed medications to control their blood pressure should know the name and type of drug, general action, dosage, and administration timing. Common side effects include potassium depletion, orthostatic hypotension, and sexual dysfunction. *Potassium depletion*, seen mostly with use of diuretics, can be avoided by eating foods high in potassium (see Chapter 6) or by taking a potassium supplement as prescribed. *Orthostatic hypotension* is often worse in the mornings (when blood pressure is normally lower), after alcohol ingestion (vasodilator), and during immobility that follows exercise (pooling of blood in muscles). Orthostatic hypotension may be avoided by the following:

1. Rise slowly from a lying or sitting position to standing.
2. Sit down immediately if feeling faint; lower head.
3. Avoid long periods of standing (blood pools in legs, thereby temporarily causing hypovolaemia).
4. Avoid very hot showers or baths (cause vasodilation, temporarily decreasing blood pressure).
5. Take medication at bedtime if drug can cause "first dose" hypotension or syncope.

Maintaining sexual function

Sexual dysfunction is a potential side effect of adrenergic inhibitors. In general, beta-adrenergic blockers and alpha-blockers decrease ejaculation ability. Beta-blockers also depress libido. Specific drugs, such as clonidine, interfere with erection. The patient needs to know about these effects. Do not make assumptions that the patient is not sexually active, despite marital status or age. Define terms of sexual dysfunction, such as libido, erection, and ejaculation, in simple language. Encourage the patient to report promptly any problems to a healthcare professional, and include the sexual partner in the teaching process, if possible (see Chapter 26). Suggest patient consult the doctor concerning substituting an alternate medication.

Preventing noncompliance

Noncompliance with the therapeutic regimen is a major reason for inadequate hypertension control. One reason is that symptoms are usually absent until advanced stages; hence the individual may not perceive a need to adhere to therapy. A second factor is the experience of unpleasant medication side effects and hesitancy to seek professional follow-up. If several medications are prescribed, it is sometimes difficult to remember to take the medications correctly. Well-controlled hypertensives have been found to have fewer hypertension-related problems and lower blood pressures.

Measures to help increase compliance with therapy include the following:

1. Be sure that patient understands that absence of symptoms does not indicate control of blood pressure; remind patient that symptoms do not occur until advanced stages of the disease.
2. Advise patient against abrupt withdrawal of medication; rebound hypertension can occur.
3. Encourage patient to discuss unpleasant side effects of medication and other nonpharmacological therapies with a healthcare professional.
4. If remembering to take medications is a problem, discuss alternate ways to remember, such as taking them with certain meals or placing medication in separate containers labelled with times of day.
5. Suggest patient participate in an exercise programme with a friend (see Chapter 4) or pay for the programme (more likely to participate "to get money's worth").
6. Include family and significant others in the teaching process to provide support and promote adherence to regimen.
7. Explain reason for regular healthcare follow-up (high blood pressure is a chronic disorder).
8. Contact patients who consistently cancel follow-up appointments .

Evaluation

Questions to ask may include the following:

1. Can patient explain the nature of hypertension and effects on heart, kidney, and brain?
2. Can patient or significant other demonstrate correct procedure for self-measurement and recording of blood pressure?
3. Is blood pressure maintained within desirable range?
4. Can patient describe the drug regimen?
5. Is patient participating in dietary regimen, aerobic exercise programme, and stress reduction activities?
6. Can patient explain effects of adrenergic inhibitors on sexual function, if indicated?
7. Is patient taking antihypertensive medication as prescribed?

SUMMARY

1. Risk factors associated with the development of peripheral vascular disorders include cigarette smoking, hyperlipidaemia, hypertension, obesity, physical inactivity, emotional stress, diabetes mellitus, and a family history of atherosclerosis.
2. Primary prevention through health education about risk factors is the most important means to reduce the incidence of peripheral vascular disorders.
3. Arterial disorders occur when any disturbance in the structure of the arteries causes diminished blood flow and decreased oxygen and nutrients to the tissues.
4. The symptoms of arterial disorders are not caused by the degree of obstruction but by the extent to which the involved body part is deprived of circulation.
5. Medical therapy for patients with atherosclerosis include smoking cessation; low-fat, low-cholesterol diet; weight reduction; regular exercise; control of associated diseases (for example, diabetes and hypertension); and management.
6. Intermittent claudication is a symptom of arterial disorders. This term is used to describe a cramp-like muscle pain that develops during exercise and is relieved after one to two minutes after stopping the exercise. It is usually unilateral and primarily affects the calf muscles.
7. Peripheral pulses may be absent or diminished in patients with arterial disorders.
8. Important nursing interventions for the patient undergoing arterial bypass surgery include frequent assessment of peripheral pulses and the graft site, avoiding flexion in the area of the graft, and position changes to promote circulation.
9. Positioning a patient with an arterial disorder may include placement of the extremity flat in bed or in a slightly dependent (that is, 15°) position to promote circulation. Elevation is contraindicated in arterial disorders.
10. An important nursing intervention for the patient undergoing amputation surgery is to avoid flexion at the hip or knee to prevent contractures.
11. A teaching plan for a patient with arterial problems includes measures to prevent infection and injury, interventions to maintain skin integrity and to increase peripheral tissue perfusion, and methods to alter risk factors.
12. Thrombophlebitis can affect the superficial or deep veins. Thrombophlebitis in a deep vein can lead to a pulmonary embolus.
13. Deep vein thrombosis is treated by bedrest with periodic elevation of the affected extremity above heart level to prevent venous stasis and reduce oedema.
14. Patients with chronic venous disorders such as varicose veins should be taught measures to increase perfusion. Measures to avoid include wearing restrictive clothing, crossing legs at the knee, and sitting or standing for long periods; measures to practise include elevating legs when sitting, wearing elastic stockings, and using good posture.
15. Leg ulcers can develop secondary to arterial or venous disorders. The primary goal in treating these ulcers is to promote wound healing and to prevent infection.
16. Debriding chemicals remove necrotic tissue from leg ulcers. A special protective boot may be applied over ulcers for ambulatory patients. Arterial bypass surgery

or amputation may be necessary for nonhealing chronic ulcers.

17. Lymphoedema results from interference with the drainage of interstitial fluid from the tissues; the affected part becomes greatly oedematous.

18. Counselling and teaching the patient with lymphoedema includes elevation of the affected extremity, wearing elastic stockings, taking diuretics as ordered, and avoiding an excess intake of foods high in sodium.

19. Hypertension is generally considered to be present when blood pressure levels persistently exceed 140/90mmHg. Most hypertension is idiopathic. It is a major cause of coronary artery disease, cardiac failure, strokes, and renal failure.

20. Drugs to control hypertension include diuretics (especially thiazides), peripheral- and central-acting adrenergic blockers, beta-blockers, and vasodilators. Medications are added in steps, as necessary, to control the blood pressure within normal limits.

21. People with hypertension should monitor their own blood pressure, continue prescribed medications, exercise, avoid salty foods, stop smoking, and continue with follow-up healthcare.

STUDY QUESTIONS

- What is the physiological basis for the difference in leg positioning for arterial and venous disorders?
- What are the similarities and differences in patient teaching with arterial and venous disorders?
- Examine the notes of a patient with an arterial disorder. What diagnostic tests were done, and how would you explain these tests to a patient? What specific patient teaching is indicated? Is there notation of patient teaching on the notes?
- If you were directed to plan for hypertension screening in the community, which of the following sites would be most effective for identifying silent hypertension: shopping centre, senior citizen centres, churches in black communities, blue collar workers in industrial centres? Give a rationale for your selection(s).
- Your 45-year-old neighbour tells you that she had her blood pressure taken by a friend and that it was 140/96mmHg. She says she's not worried because many of her family members also have high blood pressure. What actions would you take and why?

REFERENCES AND SELECTED READINGS

1.* Adelman EM: When the patient's blood pressure falls: what does it mean, what should you do? *Nurs 87* 17(10) 66-73, 1987.

2.* Bartucci MR, et al: Factors associated with adherence in hypertensive patients, *ANNA J* 14:245-248, 1987.

3.* Beaver BM: Health education and the patient with peripheral vascular disease, *Nurs Clin North Am* 21: 265-272, 1986.

4. Bergan JJ, Yao JT: *Venous disorders*, Philadelphia, 1991, WB Saunders .

5. Bernstein EF: *Noninvasive diagnostic techniques in vascular disease*, St Louis, 1990, Mosby–Year Book.

5a. Cornwall JV, Dore CJ, Lewis D: Graduated compression and its relation to venous filling times, *Br Med J* 295:1087-1090, 1987.

6. Cotran RS, et al: *Robbin's pathologic basis of disease*, Philadelphia, 1989, WB Saunders.

7. Craeger MA: Preventing and treating deep vein thromb-ophlebitis, *Drug Ther* 15:16-25, 1985.

8. Crockett F: Varicose veins as a cause of venous ulceration, *Pract Cardiol* 11:191-199, 1985.

9.* Cunningham SG: Nonpharmacologic management of blood pressure, *J Cardiovasc Nurs* 23(4):18-22, 1987.

10.* Daeschner SA: Pulmonary embolism, *Nurs 88* 18(9):33, 1988.

10a. Dale JJ, Gibson B: Leg ulcer management, *Professional Nurse* 8(5):3-15 (supplement), 1993.

11.* David JA: Wound management update, *Nurs 88* 18(6):33–37, 1988.

12.* Dixon MB, et al: Arterial reconstruction for atherosclerotic occlusive disease, *J Cardiovasc Nurs* 1(2):36-49, 1987.

13. Douglas MK, Shinn JA: *Advances in cardiovascular nursing*, Rockville, 1985, Aspen Systems.

14.* Doyle JE: Treatment modalities in peripheral vascular disease, *Nurs Clin North Am* 21:241-253, 1986.

15.* Ekers MA: Psychosocial considerations in peripheral vascular disease: cause or effect? *Nurs Clin North Am* 21:255-263, 1986.

16. Foreman MD: Arterial prosthetic graft injections: the pathophysiologic basis of nursing care, *Focus Crit Care* 12:23-28, 1985.

17. Ganong WF: *Review of medical physiology*, ed 15, Norwalk, Conn, 1991, Appleton & Lange.

18.* Gerdes L: Recognizing the multisystemic effects of embolism, *Nurs 87* 17(12):34-41, 1987.

19. Goldberg K, editor: *Vascular problems*, Springhouse, Penn, 1986, Springhouse.

20. Haimovici H, et al: *Vascular surgery: principles and techniques*, ed 3, Norwalk, Conn, 1989, Appleton & Lange.

21.* Henneman EA, Henneman PL: Intricacies of blood pressure measurement: reexamining the rituals, *Heart Lung* 18(3): 263-271, 1989.

22.* Herman JA: Nursing assessment and nursing diagnosis in patients with peripheral vascular disease, *Nurs Clin North Am* 21:219-231, 1986.

23.* Hill MN, Cunningham SL: The latest words for high BP, *Am J Nurs* 89:504-509, 1989.

24.* Keller KB, Lemberg L: Vignettes in coronary care: hypertensive crisis, *Heart Lung* 20(4):421-424, 1991.

25.* Kleven MR: Comparison of thrombolytic agents: mechanisms of action, efficacy, and safety, *Heart Lung* 17(6):750-755, 1988.

26. Krakosky JN, Vanscoy GJ: Running an anticoagulation clinic, *Am J Nurs* 89: 304-306, 1989.

27.* Massey JA: Diagnostic testing for peripheral vascular disease, *Nurs Clin North Am* 21:207-218, 1986.

28. McCarthy WJ, Williams LR: Femoral artery reconstruction, *Crit Care Q* 8:39-48, 1986.

29.* McMahan BE: Why deep vein thrombosis is so dangerous, *RN* 51:20-23, 1987.

30.* Miller RA, Evans WE: Immediate postop prosthesis, *Am J Nurs* 87:310-311, 1987.

31.* Moore LD, Pulliam CB: An on-the-spot guide to antihypertensive drugs, *Nurs 86* 16(1):54-57, 1986.

32. Moore WS: *Vascular surgery: a comprehensive review*, Philadelphia, 1991, WB Saunders.

33. Pender NJ: *Health promotion in nursing practice*, ed 2, Norwalk, Conn, 1987, Appleton & Lange.

34.* Ramsey R: Adjusting drug dosages for critically ill elderly patients, *Nurs 88* 18:47-49, 1988.

35. Report of the Joint National Committee on Detection, Evaluation, and Treatment of High Blood Pressure, US Department of Health and Human Services, Public Health Services, Bethesda, Md, 1988, National Institutes of Health.

36. Schmieder RE, Rockstroh JK, Messerli FH: Antihypertensive therapy: to stop or not to stop? *JAMA* 265(12):15661571, 1991.

37. Schroeder SA, et al: Current medical diagnosis and treatment, Norwalk, Conn, 1991, Appleton & Lange.

38. Schwartz SL, et al: *Principles of surgery*, ed 5, New York, 1989, McGraw-Hill.

39. Sobel BE: Fibrinolysis and activators of plasminogen, *Heart Lung* 17(6):775-779, 1987.

40.* Swithers CM: Tools for teaching about anticoagulants, *RN* 51(1):57-58, 1988.

41.* Turner JA: Nursing interventions in patients with peripheral vascular disease, *Nurs Clin North Am* 21: 233-240, 1986.

*Recommended for student reading.

42.* Vitello-Ciccio K: Thrombolytic therapy: urokinase, *J Cardiovasc Nurs* 1(2):59-62, 1987.

43.* Wagner MM: Pathophysiology related to peripheral vascular disease, *Nurs Clin North Am* 21:195-205, 1986.

44. Way LW: *Current surgical diagnosis and treatment*, ed 9, Norwalk, Conn, 1991, Appleton & Lange.

45. Wyngaarden JB, Smith LJ: *Cecil textbook of medicine*, ed 18, Philadelphia, 1988, WB Saunders.

46. Yec BH, Zorb SL.: *Critical care nursing*, Boston, 1986, Little, Brown.

47. Young JR, et al: *Peripheral vascular disease*, St Louis, 1991, Mosby–Year Book.

FURTHER READING

Caroll D, Rose K: Treatment leads to significant improvement. Effect of conservative treatment on pain in lymphoedema, *Professional Nurse* 8(1):32-36, 1992.

Galvin KT, Gorst KL, Kester RC: Overcoming the threat of cardiovascular disease. Health education programme among people with intermittent claudication, *Professional Nurse* 6(9):493-497, 1991.

Sneddon M: Creating educational opportunities to improve care. Management of the oedematous limb, *Professional Nurse* 7(12):818-822, 1992.

19

The Patient with Haematological Problems

Kathryn Sabo Thompson
Rosemarie M. Hogan

After studying this chapter, the learner should be able to:

- Differentiate among the functions of red blood cells, white blood cells, platelets, and the lymphatic system.
- Compare and contrast different types of anaemia in terms of pathophysiology, assessment, and interventions.
- Contrast bone marrow aspiration and biopsy and the related care.
- Explain the genetic factors of sickle cell disease and describe sickle cell crisis.
- Compare and contrast disorders of coagulation (thrombocytopenia, haemophilia, DIC).
- Describe the four types of leukaemia and their therapeutic modalities and nursing interventions.
- Differentiate between Hodgkin's disease and non-Hodgkin's lymphomas and related treatment modalities and nursing interventions.

Table 19-1 Normal adult values of cellular blood components

Type	Normal values
Red blood cells	Male: $4.6\text{-}6.2 \times 10^{12}/L$
	Female: $4.2\text{-}5.4 \times 10^{12}/L$
White blood cells	$4\text{-}10 \times 10^9/L$
Neutrophils	38%-70%
Eosinophils	1%-5%
Basophils	0%-2%
Monocytes	1%-8%
Lymphocytes	15%-45%
Platelets	$150\text{-}400 \times 10^9/L$
Haematocrit/Packed cell volume (PCV)	Male: 42%-53%
	Female: 38%-46%
Haemoglobin	Male: 13.4-17.6 g/dL
	Female: 12-15.4 g/dL
Mean corpuscular volume (MCV)	81-96 fL
Mean corpuscular haemoglobin concentration (MCHC)	30-36 g/dL (30%-36%)

Neutrophils through Lymphocytes bracketed: Differential blood count—totals 100%

Disorders related to the haematological system are usually the result of problems in the normal production, development, and function of the components of blood or alterations in the rate of blood cell destruction. The illness can be chronic, acute, or a combination of both.

ANATOMY AND PHYSIOLOGY

The haematopoietic system includes blood and its components as well as the mononuclear phagocytic system (reticuloendothelial system), which is located throughout the body. The mononuclear phagocytic system function is phagocytizing foreign materials and lysing (breaking down) red blood cells.

Components of the Haematopoietic System
Blood

Blood is a suspension of particulate materials in an aqueous colloid solution. The aqueous component of blood (plasma) is 91% to 92% water and 7% to 9% solids such as proteins, inorganic substances such as sodium, potassium, and calcium, and organic constituents such as urea, uric acid, and glucose.[26]

The cell components of blood include erythrocytes (or red blood cells [RBC]), leukocytes (or white blood cells [WBC]), and thrombocytes, or platelets (Table 19-1). All normal cells are derived from a single stem cell located throughout the bone marrow. The stem cell can divide into lymphoid and blood stem cells, which in turn become progenitor cells that divide along a specific single pathway (Fig. 19-1). This process is known as *haematopoiesis* and takes place in the bone marrow of the skull, vertebrae, pelvis, sternum, ribs, and proximal epiphysis of long bones. Production may take place in all the long bones during periods of increased demand, such as with haemorrhage or during blood cell destruction (haemolysis).

Red blood cells

A RBC is a nonnucleated biconcave disc that is soft and pliable. This property enables the RBC to change its shape during passage through the microcirculation. The RBC's major component is haemoglobin (Hb), a protein that transports oxygen and approximately 20% of carbon dioxide and maintains normal pH through a series of intracellular buffers (see Chapter 7). The Hb molecule contains globin (two pairs of polypeptide chains) and four haem groups. Each haem group contains an atom of ferrous iron. Oxygen is loosely and reversibly combined with haemoglobin to form oxyhaemoglobin. Each molecule of haemoglobin can carry four bound molecules of oxygen, one oxygen molecule to each of the four haem groups. At the tissue site, the oxygen is released into the plasma and diffuses into the tissue cells to supply their needs.

Maturation of RBCs requires adequate amounts and use of vitamin B_{12}, folic acid, proteins, enzymes, and minerals such as iron or copper. *Erythropoietin*, a glycoprotein hormone believed to originate in the kidney, appears to stimulate RBC production (*erythropoiesis*). Tissue hypoxia resulting from changes in oxygen stimulates erythropoietin production. The stem cells involved in RBC production then initiate formation and maturation of the erythrocytes.

RBCs circulate for 120 days. Their cell membranes become fragile and rupture during passage through tight spots in the circulation. Many RBC fragments in the spleen are phagocytized and digested by mononuclear phagocytic cells. *Energy* in the form of ATP is required to maintain cell membrane integrity and the relatively low sodium and high potassium content of the red cell and for defence against oxidation and other environmental stressors.

White blood cells

WBCs may be classified into two groups: *granular leukocytes* (also called *polymorphonuclear* [PMN] *leukocytes*), consisting of neutrophils, eosinophils, and basophils; and *nongranular leukocytes*, consisting of monocytes and lymphocytes. The granulocytes contain enzymes that kill and digest bacteria upon degranulation of the cells.

Eosinophils have a weak phagocytic action and function in antigen-antibody reactions. Levels are elevated in

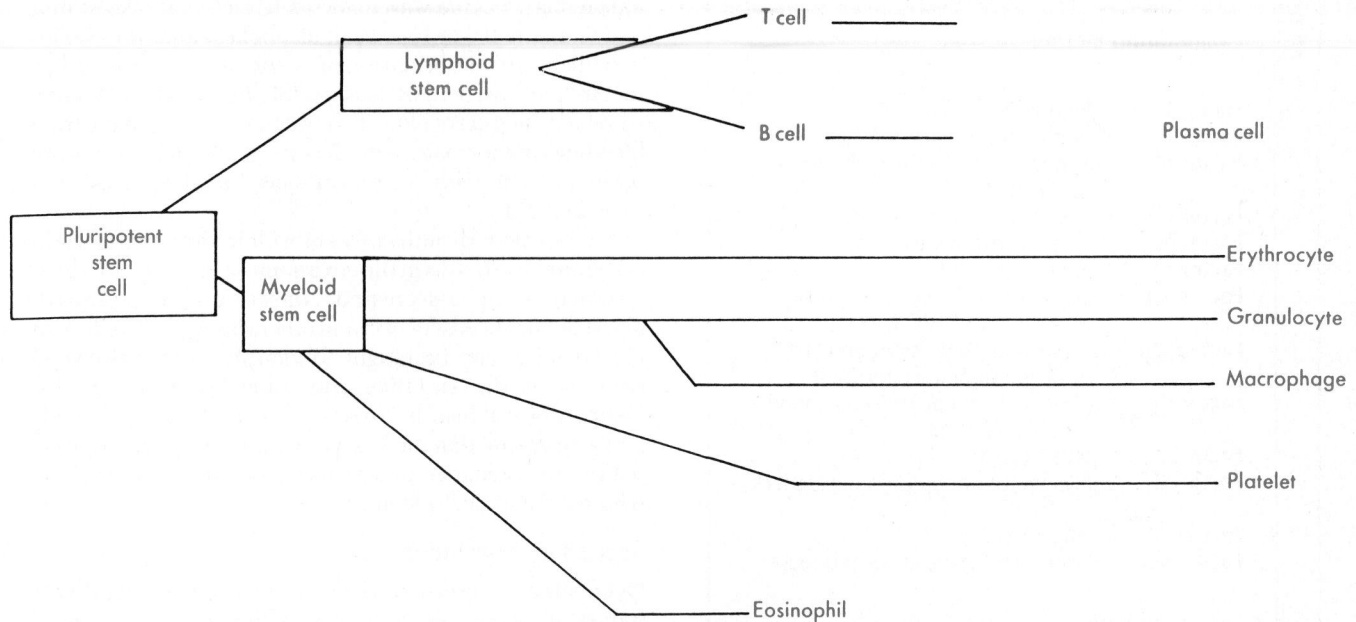

Fig. 19-1   Diagram of stem cell differentiation showing common progenitor cell for lymphoid cells, erythrocytes, granulocytes, and platelets. (Modified from Clinc M, Golde D: Blood 53:157-164, 1979.)

asthmatic attacks, drug reactions, and certain parasitic infections. *Basophils* contain histamine and heparin; they release histamine in allergic responses. Elevated basophil levels may be found in immunological reactions and proliferative disorders of blood-forming cells.[26]

Neutrophils are present in the circulation or along the capillary walls (the margination pool). They move into the tissues and mucous membranes and serve as the body's primary defence against bacterial infection through the process of phagocytosis.

Monocytes are larger than neutrophils and have one large folded or indented nucleus. They leave the circulation and become tissue *macrophages*, which also have phagocytic action, removing dead and injured cells, cell fragments, and microorganisms.

Lymphocytes are mononuclear with a round or oval nucleus. They originate primarily in lymphoid tissue (lymph nodes) but also in the bone marrow. There are two types of lymphocytes—T lymphocytes and B lymphocytes. T lymphocytes initiate the cellular immune response, while B lymphocytes (immunoglobulins) initiate the humoral immune response.

Laboratory tests have been developed to measure the amounts and functioning of all cellular components of the blood.

Platelets

Platelets (thrombocytes) are not cells but are granular disc-shaped, nonnucleated cell fragments. One third of the platelets are in the spleen as a reserve pool and the remainder in circulation. Platelets are derived from the stem cells that differentiate into the megakaryoblast, which in turn maturates into megakaryocytes. These cells eventually break up into individual platelets that are essential to haemostasis and coagulation.

Haemostasis results from the adhesion and aggregation (clumping) capabilities of platelets to plug small breaks in blood vessels. Platelets also release *thromboplastin* (factor III), which, in the presence of calcium ions, converts prothrombin into thrombin in the first step of the coagulation mechanism. In the second step of the coagulation mechanism, thrombin promotes the conversion of fibrinogen (a soluble plasma protein) into fibrin (an insoluble strand). Step one requires coagulation factors IV, V, VIII, IX, X, XI, and XII; whereas step two requires factors IV and XIII (Box 19-1).

Clot destruction occurs when fibrin is split by the enzyme *plasmin* (fibrinolysin) into fibrin degradation products (FDP). Plasmin is formed from plasminogen (a plasma protein) by the action of plasminogen activators (such as streptokinase, urokinase, tissue kinase, and factor XIIa). FDP interferes with thrombin activity, platelet functioning, and fibrin formation, thus dissolving the clot.

Mononuclear phagocytic system

The mononuclear phagocytic system, also called the monocyte-phagocyte system or reticuloendothelial system, includes circulating monocytes and their precursor cells in the bone marrow. It also includes more or less fixed mononuclear phagocytic cells found in blood channels in the spleen and liver (Kupffer cells) and in the lymphatic system, serosal cavities of the body, lungs, general connective tissue, and bone marrow.

The important function of the mononuclear phagocytic system is *phagocytosis*, that is, cleaning the blood, lymph, and intestinal spaces of foreign material, especially bacteria, that are removed in a few hours by macrophages (phagocytic cells) located throughout the body. This removal of foreign materials is the first step—essential in the chain of events leading to the immune response .

<table>
<tr><td colspan="2">**19-1** Coagulation factors</td></tr>
<tr><td>Factor I</td><td>Fibrinogen</td></tr>
<tr><td>Factor II</td><td>Prothrombin</td></tr>
<tr><td>Factor III</td><td>Thromboplastin, tissue thrombo-plastin</td></tr>
<tr><td>Factor IV</td><td>Calcium</td></tr>
<tr><td>Factor V</td><td>Proaccelerin, labile factor</td></tr>
<tr><td>Factor VI</td><td>No longer used</td></tr>
<tr><td>Factor VII</td><td>Serum prothrombin conversion accelerator (SPCA)</td></tr>
<tr><td>Factor VIII</td><td>Antihaemophilic globulin (AHG) Antihaemophilic factor (AHF)</td></tr>
<tr><td>Factor IX</td><td>Plasma thromboplastin component (PTC); Christmas factor</td></tr>
<tr><td>Factor X</td><td>Stuart factor</td></tr>
<tr><td>Factor XI</td><td>Plasma thromboplastin antecedent (PTA)</td></tr>
<tr><td>Factor XII</td><td>Hageman factor</td></tr>
<tr><td>Factor XIII</td><td>Fibrin-stabilizing factor, fibrinase</td></tr>
</table>

In addition to phagocytosis, the mononuclear phagocytic system removes the Hb of RBCs that have reached the end of their life span, splitting Hb into an iron-containing substance and bilirubin (see Chapter 22).

Physiological Changes with Ageing

The total number of leukocytes and differential counts show no variation through middle age and no gross changes in old age. In general the leukocyte count does not rise as high in response to infection, and studies suggest that the elderly have a diminished marrow granulocyte reserve.

The Hb level decreases after middle age, although the decrease in women seems to be relatively less than that in men. Unexplained anaemia in the elderly has been noted, but iron absorption is not impaired. However, use of orally administered iron is reduced. This anaemia does not appear to be related solely to age.[47] Serum iron and iron-binding capacity decrease in the elderly, and low serum vitamin B_{12} and folic acid levels occur in a significant proportion of elderly people but without anaemia.

No age-related changes in platelets have been reported. RBC sedimentation rate increases significantly, but this rate is of limited value in detecting disease in the elderly. Some of the plasma coagulation factors have been reported to increase with age (factors I, V, VII, and IX). Partial thromboplastin time may be shortened.[18] Changes in lymphocyte (T cells and B cells) function are described in Chapter 33.

PREVENTION AND HEALTH EDUCATION
Primary Prevention

Health promotion for haematological disorders includes health teaching to prevent the disorders, when possible. Exposure to certain chemicals and drugs places individuals at high risk, especially for aplastic anaemia and the leukaemias. People with inadequate dietary intake of iron and vitamins B_{12} or folic acid, alcoholics, and others with poor dietary habits because of inadequate knowledge or low income, are particularly susceptible to anaemia. Women who have long-term blood loss because of heavy menstrual bleeding (menorrhagia) are also at risk for anaemia, as are other persons with long-term slow blood loss, as with haemorrhoids.

Occupational health nurses provide information to workers about health risks in the environment and ways in which risk factors can be decreased. Nurses in all settings teach about dietary needs for iron and other vitamins. People with low incomes can be taught to identify inexpensive food sources of the vitamins and minerals necessary for haematological health. Nurses can also become politically active to ensure that there is adequate government funding for the maintenance of adequate benefit levels for those who have marginal incomes.

Secondary Prevention

Occupational health nurses are involved in identifying industrial chemicals or processes that place workers in danger and in screening employees as pertinent. Screening for anaemias in any setting occurs during routine physical examinations with blood tests.

Diseases such as sickle cell anaemia, the thalassaemias, and haemophilia are hereditary; therefore, marriage between carriers of defective genes may result in children with the disease. One of the most difficult and sensitive roles for nurses is that of genetic counsellor, communicating to individuals with hereditary problems the risk factors involved and possibility of having children with severe haematopoietic disease. Couples will make their own decisions after information has been shared with them. The decision to conceive a child, given the hereditary risk, is extremely difficult and can prove to be devastating to a couple.

MAJOR HEALTH PROBLEMS RELATED TO BLOOD AND LYMPH SYSTEMS

Disorders associated with the haematopoietic system are diverse in their underlying pathological manifestations, disease course, and response to treatment. Most often, the symptoms are the result of interference with the normal development and function of the blood components and with altered haematopoiesis (blood cell production). Normally homeostasis is maintained through a balance between the rate of production of normal blood cells and the rate of destruction. Disorders of the blood are manifested when this haemostatic balance is lost. Disturbances in the coagulation mechanism also result in blood disorders.

In addition to primary haematological disorders, secondary effects from disease of another body system may also manifest themselves in abnormal haematological findings. For example, the anaemia that is associated with azotaemia is the consequence of disease existing outside of the haematopoietic system. Major health problems include the following:

1. RBC disorders
   a. Anaemias
   b. Erythrocytosis: polycythaemia
2. Coagulation disorders
   a. Platelet disorders: thrombocytopenia
   b. Haemophilia
   c. Disseminated intravascular coagulation (DIC)
3. WBC disorders: agranulocytosis, leukaemia
4. Lymph system disorders: lymphadenopathy, lymphomas (Hodgkin's and non-Hodgkin's)
5. Plasma cell dyscrasias: multiple myeloma

DISORDERS ASSOCIATED WITH ERYTHROCYTES

Anaemia (decreased RBCs) and erythrocytosis (increased RBCs) are the general categories of red cell disorders. Sickle cell anaemia, a form of anaemia, is discussed separately from the other types of anaemia because of differences in nursing care.

ANAEMIA

Anaemia refers to a deficiency of RBCs as reflected in a decreased haemoglobin level, packed cell volume (haematocrit), and red cell count.

Aetiology

Anaemias may be divided into those that are the result of blood loss, impaired production of RBCs, increased destruction of RBCs, or nutritional deficiencies (Table 19-2).

Blood loss is a major cause of anaemia. The anaemia may be due to acute blood loss by haemorrhage or to blood loss over a period of time, as from slow bleeding from a peptic ulcer, GI tumour, bleeding haemorrhoids, or menorrhagia.

Impaired production of RBCs leads to *aplastic anaemia*. Causes of aplastic anaemia may be antineoplastic or cytotoxic agents, certain drugs, and viral infections. At times no causative agent can be found (idiopathic aplastic anaemia).

Anaemias that result from destruction of RBCs are termed *haemolytic anaemias*. Many are of *genetic* origin, including hereditary spherocytosis, and the haemoglobinopathies, including sickle cell disease, thalassaemia, and enzyme-deficiency anaemia. *Acquired* haemolytic anaemia may be caused by a drug (methyldopa, penicillin) or an autoimmune response or may be idiopathic or secondary to lymphocytic lymphoma or chronic lymphocytic leukaemias.

The final group of anaemias are due to *nutritional deficiencies*. A major example of this type of anaemia is *iron deficiency anaemia*, which may result from chronic blood loss or from inadequate dietary intake. *Vitamin B_{12} deficiency* anaemia usually occurs from decreased absorption rather than decreased intake. *Folic acid deficiency anaemia* results from inadequate dietary intake (often associated with alcoholism), malabsorption syndromes, and certain medications.

Pathophysiology

Anaemia secondary to blood loss

Anaemia associated with blood loss may be acute or chronic. *Acute anaemia* is the direct result of the decrease

in a large amount of circulating RBCs. An adult of average build can lose 500 ml of blood (out of a total of 6000 ml) without serious or lasting effects. Losses of 1000 ml or more can cause acute consequences. The severity of symptoms depends on the severity of blood loss and the resulting degree of hypoxia (inadequate tissue oxygenation); as the number of RBCs decreases, less oxygen is delivered to tissues. Sudden acute haemorrhage with loss of 30% or more of blood volume causes symptoms of diaphoresis, restlessness, tachycardia, tachypnoea, shortness of breath and, without intervention, shock. The body's compensatory responses to hypoxia include the following[37]:

1. Increased cardiac output and respirations increasing oxygen delivery to the tissues
2. Increased release of oxygen by haemoglobin
3. Expanded plasma volume by pulling fluid from tissue spaces
4. Redistribution of blood to vital organs.

Compensatory vasoconstriction to shunt blood to vital organs is responsible for some of the signs and symptoms of anaemia, such as pallor or cold or clammy extremities. Cerebral hypoxia causes symptoms of mental confusion, bizarre behaviour and drowsiness, headache, dizziness and tinnitus (ringing of the ears).

Chronic anaemia secondary to blood loss is the most common cause of iron-deficiency anaemia (p. 469). The body has remarkable adaptive powers and may adjust fairly well to a marked reduction in RBCs and Hb, provided the condition develops gradually. An individual may remain asymptomatic even though the total RBC count may drop to almost half of its normal level or the Hb level to below 7 g/dL. When blood loss is continuous and moderate in amount, the bone marrow may be able to keep up with the losses by increasing RBC production. If the cause of chronic blood loss is not found and corrected, eventually the bone marrow will not be able to keep pace with the loss, and symptoms of anaemia will appear: fatigue and weakness, tachycardia, and exertional dyspnoea. In addition, gastrointestinal symptoms (anorexia, nausea, constipation or diarrhoea, stomatitis) may also occur as a result of chronic hypoxia.

Aplastic anaemia

The word aplastic means no tendency to develop into new tissue. The defect leading to aplastic anaemia is most likely injury or destruction of a common stem cell (see Fig. 19-1) that affects all subsequent cell populations. This produces a deficiency in blood cell production in bone marrow. Aplastic anaemia is characterized not only by impaired RBC production but also by impairment of all blood-producing elements. A decrease in WBCs (leukopenia) and in platelets (thrombocytopenia) occurs. Loss of RBCs leads to symptoms of chronic anaemia. Fewer WBCs increase the risk of infection, and decreased platelets may lead to bleeding in the tissue (ecchymoses), as well as GI, GU, and CNS bleeding.

Haemolytic anaemias

Haemolytic anaemia results when the RBCs are destroyed at such a rapid rate that the bone marrow is unable to compensate for the loss. The severity of the anaemia is determined by the degree of lag between the rate of RBC

Table 19-2 Disorders of red blood cells

Disorder	Signs and symptoms	Medical therapy
Anaemias		
Secondary to blood loss Acute	Hypovolaemic and hypoxaemic symptoms (weakness, stupor, irritability, cool moist skin, hypotension, tachycardia, ↓ Hb and PCV, pallor)	Treat for shock: IV fluids, whole blood or packed cells; identify source of loss; administer iron
Chronic	Depends on degree of ↓ in Hb; if less than 8.0 g/dl: weakness, fatigue, ↑ pulse, pallor, exertional dyspnoea	Packed cells, iron; identify source of loss
Aplastic anaemia	As in chronic anaemia plus those related to ↓ WBC and platelets (ecchymoses), petechaie, GI, GU, CNS bleeding, increased risk of infection	Remove causative agent; supportive care until bone marrow is regenerated: transfusions; bone marrow transplantation, antithymocyte therapy
Haemolytic anaemia Congenital Sickle cell anaemia	↓ Hb; ↓ PCV; pain (bones, joints, back): generalized, localized or migratory; vomiting; fever; infections; chronic leg ulcers; cardiomegaly; murmurs; CHF; delay in growth and sexual maturation; swollen hands and feet (dactylitis); jaundice	No specific therapy; analgesics, oxygen, adequate hydration, treatment of infection, polyvalent pneumococcal vaccine to prevent pneumococcal infections, antisickling agents (experimental), therapeutic apheresis
	Thrombotic crisis: severe pain in abdomen and musculoskeletal system	Adequate hydration, exchange transfusions (replacing person's blood with packed red cells, unit for unit)
	Aplastic crisis: rapid ↑ in anaemia	
Thalassaemia	Thalassaemia minor: mild anaemia Thalassaemia major: severe anaemia	No therapy required; transfusions with severe symptoms or to maintain Hb near normal
Enzyme deficiency	Anaemia when person exposed to oxidant drugs (aspirin, sulphonamides, antimalarial)	Remove causative drug
Acquired haemolytic anaemia	Same as with other anaemia	Corticosteroids, splenectomy in those who do not respond to drug therapy
Nutritional anaemia Iron deficiency anaemia	Gradual development; may have few signs; fatigue, exertional dyspnoea, severe anaemia, brittle spoon-shaped (concave) nails with longitudinal ridges, atrophy of tongue papillae, smooth shiny tongue, cheilosis (cracks in corner of mouth); low serum iron, pallor, weakness	Determine and correct cause Oral iron administration (ferrous sulphate); parenteral iron if oral not tolerated or not absorbed via GI tract; adequate balanced diet
Megaloblastic anaemia	Low serum B_{12} and folate levels, neurological abnormalities (peripheral neuropathies, loss of balance), symptoms associated with underlying disease and anaemia	Parenteral administration of vitamin B_{12}, usually once a month
Erythrocytosis		
Polycythaemia vera (primary)	Absent in early stages; headache, tinnitus, blurred vision, reddened skin, nosebleeds, ecchymoses, GI bleeding caused by platelet dysfunction, thrombosis, hepatomegaly, splenomegaly, ↑ total RBC volume, ↑ or normal plasma volume	Periodic phlebotomy (removal of blood), radioactive phosphorus, chemotherapeutic agents such as busulphan
Secondary polycythaemia	↑ RBC, ↑ PCV; symptoms may be similar to but less severe than those in polycythaemia vera	Correct underlying condition
Pseudopolycythaemia	As above; is self-limiting; symptoms are mild	Stress reduction

destruction (haemolysis) and the rate of bone marrow production of red cells (erythropoiesis). *Hereditary spherocytosis*, an inherited autosomal dominant trait, is characterized by a membrane abnormality leading to osmotic swelling of the red cell and susceptibility to destruction by the spleen. It is most commonly detected in childhood but may be noted initially in adulthood. Severe anaemia (aplastic crisis, p. 473) may occur if bone marrow production is impaired, as by infection. Jaundice may result from the chronic RBC haemolysis in the spleen.

Haemoglobinopathies

Haemoglobinopathies are a group of haemolytic diseases in which one or more amino acids are substituted in the globin chain of the Hb molecule, leading to the formation of abnormal Hb (for example, haemoglobins S and C). The most common haemoglobinopathy is sickle cell anaemia (p. 472).

Thalassaemia, which is a haemoglobinopathy, is an inherited disorder characterized by a decreased synthesis of one of the globin chains of haemoglobin. The beta (β) chain is most often affected (β-thalassaemia). As a result, haemoglobin synthesis decreases, although haemoglobin accumulates in the erythrocyte of the unaffected globin chain. These alterations result in decreased red cell production and a chronic haemolytic anaemia. The red cells are characteristically hypochromic and microcytic. Hb electrophoresis is diagnostic.

There are two types of thalassaemia: thalassaemia minor, which is usually asymptomatic, and thalassaemia major, which is characterized by severe anaemia. Lifespan is significantly shorter, and frequent transfusion therapies may produce iron overload, a problem that can be ameliorated by an iron-chelating drug such as desferrioxamine.

Another type of haemoglobinopathy is *enzyme deficiency*. Deficiency of enzymes in the pathways that metabolize glucose and generate ATP frequently leads to premature red cell destruction. The most common clinically significant enzyme abnormality is that of *glucose-6-phosphate dehydrogenase*. This disorder is of two types—mild African type and the more severe Mediterranean type, both of which may cause chronic haemolytic anaemia. When an oxidant drug puts the cells under stress, acute haemolysis results.

Acquired haemolytic anaemia

Haemolytic anaemia may be drug induced or may be caused by an autoimmune disorder. In the latter case an antibody develops that is directed against an antigen on the individual's own RBCs. The antibody-coated red cells are destroyed prematurely by the cells of the mononuclear phagocytic system, particularly in the spleen. Diagnosis is confirmed by demonstrating the presence of the antibody on the red cells (antiglobin or Coombs' test).

Drugs produce haemolysis in a variety of ways. Methyldopa is associated with production of an autoantibody and a positive Coombs' test in approximately 20% of patients. More rarely, high-dose penicillin causes haemolysis by producing an antibody that requires the presence of penicillin on the red cell membrane for its effects to occur. This disorder is often fatal, in part because transfusion is often made difficult and dangerous by the fact that the autoantibody reacts not only with the patient's red cells but also with all donor cells.

Anaemia secondary to nutritional deficiency

The nutritional anaemias include iron-deficiency anaemia and the megaloblastic anaemias.

Iron deficiency anaemia

Iron is a fundamental part of the Hb molecule, and its deficiency leads to production of red cells with a decreased amount of Hb and ultimately to a decreased number of red cells. The average adult body contains approximately 4 g of iron, 3 g of which are in Hb. Average daily loss of iron by the body is approximately 1.5 mg, which is compensated for by absorption from the diet of approximately that amount of iron daily. This tenuous balance may be compromised by chronic blood loss, which may be physiological, as in menstruation, or pathological, as in GI or other bleeding.

It is also common in menstruating women, pregnant women, and growing children. Aged individuals may eat an imbalanced diet because of limited income, mobility, and isolation from those people who might help with preparation or purchase of food.

The anaemia is characteristically hypochromic and microcytic.

Megaloblastic anaemia

Megaloblastic anaemia is characterized by the presence of megaloblasts (immature progenitors of abnormal RBCs) in the bone marrow. The red cells are macrocytic. There is a deficit in the nucleus of the maturing red cell as a result of interference with DNA synthesis from a nutritional deficiency, primarily vitamin B_{12} or folic acid.

Vitamin B_{12} requires the presence of an intrinsic factor from gastric secretion for absorption in the ileum. Two interferences with absorption are lack of intrinsic factor or direct interference with the transport of vitamin B_{12} across the membrane in the ileum. Intrinsic factor may be absent as a result of genetic factors (*pernicious anaemia*) or from surgical resection of the stomach. Malabsorption in the ileum may result from malabsorption syndromes, small bowel diverticuli, intestinal inflammations, or intestinal resection.

Because vitamin B_{12} can be stored in the body, deficiencies may not produce symptoms for many years. Diagnosis of pernicious anaemia is confirmed by an abnormal Schilling test, which demonstrates the inability to absorb vitamin B_{12} unless intrinsic factor is administered.

Folic acid is a vitamin of the B complex that is involved in the synthesis of amino acids and DNA and therefore in the maturation of RBCs. Certain medications inhibit the enzyme that is involved in normal absorption of folate through the intestinal wall. Vitamin B_{12} deficiency and folic acid deficiency often occur together.

Nursing Process
Assessment

Subjective data

Collect the following subjective data from patients with anaemia:

1. Knowledge of cause of the anaemia
2. Feelings of weakness or fatigue and ability to carry out ADL
3. Feelings of dyspnoea and precipitating activities
4. Factors that appear to exacerbate symptoms
5. History of exposure to chemicals (insecticides, benzene products) or drugs that may cause aplastic anaemia
6. Family history of anaemia

Objective data

Physical examination of the person with anaemia usually shows normal findings. The skin and mucous membranes may appear pale and cool. If haemolytic anaemia is present, the skin and eyeballs may appear yellowish from bile deposits. Laboured breathing may be observed, especially with exertion. The pulse may be rapid. With severe anaemia, monitor the patient's ability to respond to questions and for signs of confusion.

If blood loss has occurred or if the person has severe aplastic anaemia, monitor and report signs of bleeding, external or internal (bleeding gums, melaena). For aplastic anaemia, monitor for signs of infection (from the leukopenia).

Diagnostic tests
Laboratory tests

Clinical significance of abnormal blood counts are noted in Table 19-3. RBCs are usually decreased but are not good indicators of anaemia: haematocrit and haemoglobin (Hb) tests are better indicators. Normal values are listed in Table 19-1. The *haematocrit* (packed RBC volume) is the ratio of RBC volume to the whole blood volume. The haematocrit rarely falls below 25% in chronic anaemia.[30] An Hb test measures the amount of Hb in circulation.

RBC indices provide a differential diagnosis of the type of anaemia. The RBC indices include *the mean corpuscular volume* (MCV) and *mean corpuscular Hb concentration* (MCHC). The MCV estimates the average size of the RBC. The MCHC measures the content of Hb in RBCs. (The significance of changes in these indices are listed in Table 19-3.)

Peripheral blood smears provide information on the aetiology of the anaemia. Observe the size and shape of the RBC, as well as extent of cell maturity and ratio of the various cell types to each other. WBCs can also be examined to provide information about adequate bone marrow production.

Bone marrow aspiration

Bone marrow aspiration is appropriate when the diagnosis is not clearly established by peripheral blood smears or when further information is needed. Aspiration is the most common procedure for obtaining a bone marrow sample. The procedure is possible because normal bone marrow is soft and semifluid and can therefore be removed by aspiration through a needle. Bone marrow aspiration is also used in the diagnosis of acute leukaemia and thrombocytopenia.

The skin surrounding the puncture site is shaved, if necessary, and cleansed with an antiseptic such as povidine-iodine. Sterile towels are placed around the site. The skin and periosteum are anaesthetized to avoid pain. First, the most superficial layer of the skin is infiltrated with lignocaine. After a few seconds the needle is further advanced until bone is touched. Procaine is then injected to anaesthetize the periosteum.

The marrow aspiration needle is inserted, and when the marrow cavity is entered, the marrow stylet is removed from the needle and a sterile syringe is attached. The syringe plunger is drawn back until marrow appears in the syringe. As the plunger is drawn back the person will experience a brief, sharp pain, sometimes described as a burning sensation. The pain is caused by the suction exerted as the plunger is pulled back. Some persons may complain of tenderness at the aspiration site for a few days. Most often no pain or discomfort is experienced following the procedure.

Nursing care with bone marrow aspiration includes the following:

1. Explain procedure to patient, stating that there may be brief discomfort when the marrow is aspirated.
2. To prevent movement, place hands on patient's shoulders and instruct patient to remain still at the time of aspiration.
3. Apply pressure over aspiration site after needle is removed to prevent bleeding; apply pressure for 3 to 5 minutes if patient is thrombocytopenic.
4. Assess for bleeding from aspiration site.
5. Provide comfort measures to help patient relax.

Bone marrow biopsy

When a large sample of bone marrow is needed, a bone marrow biopsy may be performed. Persons most likely to undergo a bone marrow biopsy are those with pancytopenia (more than one altered cell type), metastatic tumour, lymphoma, and multiple myeloma.

The most common site for bone marrow biopsy is the posterosuperior iliac spine, although the sternum may also be used. The initial steps in the biopsy procedure are similar to those outlined for bone marrow aspiration. The use of a Jamshidi needle allows for a core of marrow to be collected. Nursing care following a bone marrow biopsy is similar to that of bone marrow aspiration.

From microscopic examination of the bone marrow, iron stores can be determined, as can the morphology of the progenitor cell. Megaloblastic (RBC precursor) changes and the absence of cells may be observed. Infiltration with leukaemic cells may also be determined.

Nursing analysis

Problems are determined from analysis of patient data. Possible problems for the person with anaemia may include, but are not limited to, the following:

Problem	Possible aetiologies
Fatigue	Decreased tissue oxygenation, inadequate rest
Injury, high risk for falls, bleeding	Decreased cerebral oxygenation, decreased coagulation
Infection, high risk for	Decreased WBC, decreased immune response
Decisional conflict	Threat to health of future children
Knowledge deficit	Lack of exposure or recall

Table 19-3   Clinical significance of abnormal blood counts

	Increased values	Decreased values
RBC	Polycythaemia (erythrocytosis)	Leukopenia
WBC	Neutrophilia	Leukopenia
	Leukaemias	Aplastic anaemia
		Neutropenias
Platelets	Polycythaemia	Aplastic anaemia
		Thrombocytopenia
		Disseminated intravascular coagulation (DIC)
Haematocrit/packed cell volume (PCV)	Polycythaemia	Anaemias
		Haemorrhage
Haemoglobin	Polycythaemia	Anaemias
		Haemorrhage
Mean corpuscular volume (MCV)	Pernicious anaemia	Iron deficiency anaemia
	Folic acid deficiency	Chronic blood loss
Mean corpuscular haemoglobin concentration (MCHC)		Iron deficiency anaemia
		Chronic blood loss

Planning: expected patient outcomes

Expected patient outcomes for the patient with anaemia may include, but are not limited to, the following:

1. States feeling more rested and less fatigued.
2. No injuries have occurred from falls.
3. Bleeding is controlled.
4. No infection is present.
5. Makes decisions with spouse concerning conception based on knowledge of illness (haemolytic anaemia).
6. Explains nature of anaemia, measures to prevent injury and bleeding, replacement therapy, and follow-up care.

Implementation

Assisting with achievement of therapeutic goals

Transfusion therapy may be given for anaemias from acute blood loss. With chronic blood loss, packed cells (plasma reduced blood) are more appropriate, if indicated, because the patient has had time to replace the plasma. Monitor the patient for signs of transfusion reactions (see Chapter 33).

Bone marrow transplantation is the treatment of choice for people with severe aplastic anaemia (aplastic crisis) who are under age 30 and who have HLA-matched siblings[30] (p. 485). Those over age 30 or without HLA-matched siblings are treated with immunosuppressive therapy such as antithymocyte globulin (see Chapter 33).

The medical treatment for nutritional anaemias is primarily drug replacement (Table 19-2). Oral ferrous sulphate is the drug of choice for iron deficiency anaemia or anaemia from chronic blood loss. Parenteral iron may be given if GI disease is present or if blood loss continues. Iron therapy should be taken for 3 to 6 months after normal haematological levels are restored to replenish iron stores.[30] Vitamin B_{12} replacement therapy must be given parenterally because of the decreased oral absorptive capabilities. Life-long therapy is necessary for persons with pernicious anaemia. Folic acid replacement therapy is given orally.

Interventions to achieve patient outcomes
Promoting rest

Fatigue is a major problem for people with anaemia because of the decreased oxygenation to tissues from the decreased Hb. For the hospitalized patient, plan care so that there is a balance between activities and rest to prevent increased oxygen expenditure and hypoxemia. Those at home need to plan ADL to allow rest periods.

Preventing injury

When muscle weakness or confusion is present with severe anaemia (because of the decreased oxygenation to muscles and brain), supervise patient ambulation to prevent falls. Keep the room uncluttered. Encourage the patient to use handrails if present.

Remember that the patient with aplastic anaemia is susceptible to bleeding because of decreased platelets. Apply direct pressure for 5 minutes after injection or if any external bleeding occurs. Encourage patient to use a soft toothbrush to prevent bleeding of the gums. Suggest that patient use an electric shaver to prevent skin breaks. Encourage fluids and dietary fibre to promote a soft stool, thus decreasing irritation of the rectum or haemorrhoids, which cause bleeding. Avoid drugs such as aspirin that have anticoagulant properties.

Preventing infection

Patients with severe aplastic or haemolytic anaemia may be susceptible to infection because of decreased WBCs or decreased immune response. Persons with colds or other infections should avoid contact with the patient. Provide and teach good hygiene care. Avoid injections and other intrusive procedures, if possible.

Counselling patients

People who have a hereditary haemolytic anaemia (hereditary spherocytosis, haemoglobinopathies, or enzyme deficiency) have the potential to transmit the trait to their children. It is therefore important for these people to seek genetic counselling to assist them and their spouses in making decisions about bearing children. As cited in the discussion on prevention of haemotological disorders (p. 466), this is not an easy decision to make. The nurse can provide opportunities for the couple to explore their feelings and to help them use problem-solving techniques in coming to a conclusion. The decision is ultimately up to the couple.

Facilitating patient learning

Because anaemia is often a chronic condition, patient teaching is an important part of nursing care and includes the following:

1. Knowledge about the cause of the anaemia, preventive measures (if any), and therapeutic modalities.
2. Measures to prevent infection and bleeding (see above).
3. Replacement therapy when indicated for anaemia from chronic blood loss or nutritional anaemia.
   a. Iron
      (1) Take ferrous sulphate after meals to prevent GI irritation.
      (2) Stools will be black from digested iron.
      (3) Report signs of nausea or diarrhoea to doctor.
      (4) Eat iron-rich foods: organ meats (especially liver), seafood, whole or enriched grains, legumes, green leafy vegetables, and nuts.[36]
      (5) Take iron for 3 to 6 months after blood levels are restored, to build up iron stores.
   b. Vitamin B_{12}
      (1) Must be given parenterally because of decreased absorption.
      (2) Life-long therapy is necessary.
   c. Folic acid
      (1) Take prescribed oral folic acid.
      (2) Eat foods rich in folic acid: green leafy vegetables, liver, kidney, asparagus.[36]
4. Follow-up care
   a. Report for blood tests as directed to determine progress.
   b. Report signs of increasing weakness or fatigue, increased dyspnoea, or signs of infection or bleeding.

Special considerations for care of elderly people with haematological problems are described in the box entitled, "The Elderly with Haematological Problems."

The Elderly with Haematological Problems

Assessment
Assess adequacy of iron and folic acid intake.
Assess presence and extent of fatigue and ability to carry out ADL.

Intervention
Assist patient with nutritional deficiency anaemia to plan diet that includes food rich in iron and folic acid, as appropriate.
Assist patient to plan for rest periods when fatigue is present.
Teach patient and significant others:
   Importance of prescribed replacement therapy and ways to facilitate compliance.
   Need to report signs of increasing fatigue to doctor.
   Measures to prevent infection with leukaemia. Elderly people have the added risk factor of decreased immune response and are highly susceptible to pneumonia.

Common disorders in elderly
Nutritional deficiency anaemia
Leukaemia (ANLL, CLL)
Lymphoma

Evaluation

Questions to consider include the following:

1. Does patient state feeling more rested and less fatigued?
2. Has the patient been free from falls?
3. Is bleeding absent or controlled?
4. Is the patient free of infection?
5. Can the patient explain the nature of the anaemia and the correct method for taking medications?
6. Is the patient eating foods rich in the deficient nutrient (if appropriate)?
7. Are haemoglobin and haematocrit levels increasing towards normal?

SICKLE CELL ANAEMIA
Aetiology/Epidemiology

Sickle cell anaemia is a haemolytic anaemia (see p. 468) with a genetic origin. It is a common genetic disorder in the United Kingdom. It occurs predominantly in Afro-Caribbean individuals and in some of Mediter-

---

Table 19-4 Types of sickle cell disorders

Term	Characteristics	Hb Molecule
Sickle cell trait	Carrier of Hb S People are asymptomatic	Hb SA
Sickle cell disease	Presence of sickling with associated symptoms	Hb SS
Sickle cell syndromes	Diseases associated with presence of Hb S	Hb SC (sickle cell Hb C) Hb SD (sickle cell Hb D) Hb Sβ (sickle cell thalassaemia)

ranean origin. Sickle cell disease affects around 4000–5000 people in the United Kingdom and some 150 affected babies are born each year.[48] An unknown number of people have sickle cell trait caused by the presence of one abnormal gene.

Pathophysiology

The basic abnormality lies within the globin (protein) fraction of the Hb, where a single amino acid is substituted for another in one of the polypeptide chains. This single amino acid substitution profoundly alters the properties of the Hb molecule. Hb S is formed instead of the normal Hb A. The tendency towards sickling depends on both the relative quantity of Hb S in the RBCs and the levels of oxygen tension within the tissues of the body.

Different terminologies are used with sickle cell anaemia: sickle cell trait, sickle cell disease, and sickle cell syndromes (Table 19-4). A person with sickle cell trait (Hb SA) has received an Hb S gene from one parent and an Hb A gene (normal) from the other.

The clinical manifestations of the disease result from the sickling phenomenon. Sickling occurs when red cells containing Hb S are deoxygenated; this is the result of the poor solubility of the Hb S, which crystallizes in the RBCs. The RBCs elongate and become rigid and crescent- or sickle-shaped (tactoid formation). Sickling is always present to some extent in the person with sickle cell anaemia. Because of increased RBC destruction, patients are often jaundiced and may develop gallstones (cholelithiasis secondary to increased bilirubin).

Sickle cell crises

Basically, any event that increases the body's need for oxygen or that alters the transport of oxygen may lead to the exacerbation of symptoms called *crisis*. Symptoms may be exacerbated by pregnancy, infection, surgery, trauma, and dehydration. Sickle cell crises are primarily thrombotic or aplastic.

Thrombotic crisis is the most common sickle cell crisis. Signs and symptoms occur as a result of occlusions in the microvasculature by sickled cells causing deoxygenation of tissues with pain and infarctions in organs such as the kidney, lung, bones, and central nervous system (Fig. 19-2). The sites most frequently affected in crises are the abdomen, back, chest, and joints.

Aplastic crisis, usually secondary to infection, involves cessation of bone marrow function and decrease in erythropoiesis and reticulocyte count. Signs of severe anaemia are often present.

Megaloblastic crisis, the result of depletion of bone marrow stores of folic acid, is prevented or treated by folic acid administration. *Splenic sequestration* crisis, pooling of blood in the spleen, causes splenic enlargement and hypovolaemia with signs of shock.

Nursing Process
Assessment

Subjective data

Data to be obtained from the patient with sickle cell disease include the following:

1. Knowledge of the disease and family history
2. Factors that precipitate crises or exacerbate symptoms
3. Presence of fatigue.
4. Presence of pain and measures taken for pain relief
5. Feelings of dyspnoea and precipitating activities
6. Ability to carry out ADL

Objective data

Objective data collected by physical assessment and patient observation may include the following:

1. Skin: pale (anaemia) or jaundiced (RBC destruction)
2. Legs: presence of infected ulcers on lower leg
3. Overt signs of pain
4. Temperature: elevation from infection (low-grade fever)
5. Pulse rapid (from decreased oxygenation)
6. Laboured breathing, especially with activity

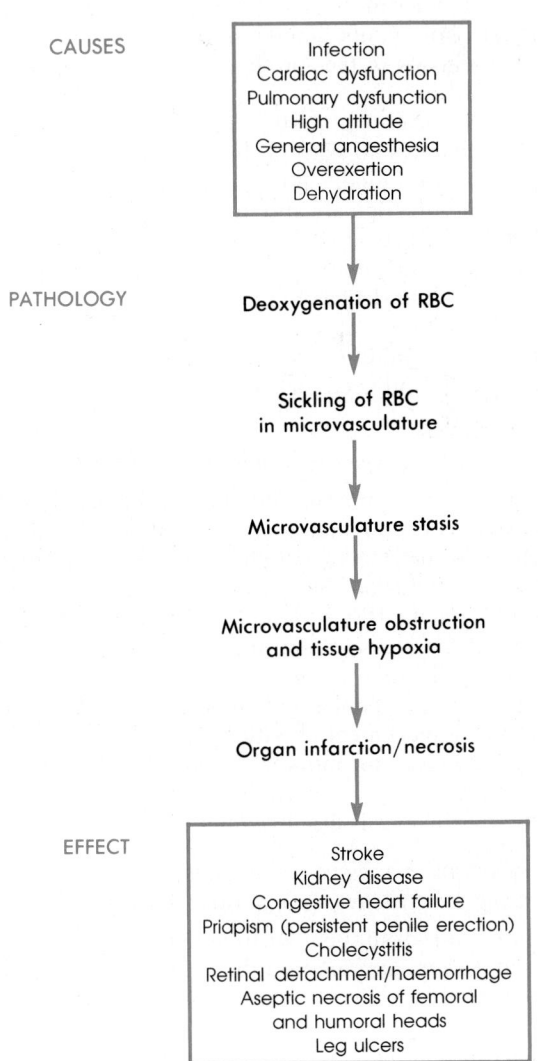

Fig. 19-2 Pathophysiology of sickle cell crisis.

Nursing analysis

Problems are determined from analysis of patient data. Possible problems for the patient with sickle cell disease may include, but are not limited to, the following:

Problem	Possible aetiologies
Activity intolerance	Decreased oxygen transport
Tissue perfusion (peripheral, renal, pulmonary), altered	Dehydration, interrruption of blood flow
Pain: joints, chest	Decreased tissue oxygenation, inadequate pain management techniques
Infection, high risk for	Anaemia tissue destruction, knowledge deficit
Anxiety	Threat to self-concept or life, situational crisis
Decisional conflict	Decision making regarding childbearing
Knowledge deficit	Lack of information or recall, poor motivation, anxiety

Planning: expected patient outcomes

Expected outcomes for the patient with sickle cell disease may include, but are not limited to, the following:
1. States feeling rested and that exertional dyspnoea is lessened.
2. Drinks at least 4 L of fluid daily.
3. Demonstrates no signs of thrombosis.
4. States pain is modified or absent.
5. Signs of infection are absent.
6. Signs of anxiety are decreased.
7. Makes decisions with spouse concerning conception based on knowledge of illness.
8. Explains nature of sickle cell disease, factors that precipitate painful crises, fluid needs, counselling resources, and need for follow-up care.

Implementation

Assisting with achievement of therapeutic goals

Because there is no specific therapy for sickle cell disease, treatment is symptomatic. Transfusions may be given; the blood products generally used are packed RBCs. The goal of transfusion therapy depends on the specific condition: replacing RBCs for anaemia; lowering the percentage of Hb S in an infarction; and increasing the amount of circulating Hb and thus oxygen in overwhelming infections, leg ulcers, pregnancy, and preoperatively. Exchange transfusions (replacement of patient's blood with normal blood) may be given for intractable crises, stroke, or as a preventive measure preoperatively.[30] Care of the patient receiving transfusions is discussed in Chapter 33.

Interventions to achieve patient outcomes
Promoting activity tolerance and tissue perfusion

Fatigue and dyspnoea with activity result from decreased tissue oxygenation because of decreased oxygen-carrying capabilities of the haemoglobin. Assist and teach patient to maintain a balance between rest and exercise to prevent increased oxygen expenditure. Oxygen may be given during crises to increase oxygen blood saturation.

The vas-occlusive nature of painful episodes requires adequate *hydration* to decrease blood viscosity. During a crisis, the patient requires 6 to 8 L of fluids daily and at least 4 to 6 L at all other times. If IV fluids are necessary, use of small-bore (No. 23) needle avoids multiple punctures and infiltration.[46]

Promoting comfort

Pain of sickle cell crisis is excruciating and involves all the principles of pain management (see Chapter 8). Pain medications (narcotics and nonnarcotics) must be given continuously—orally, intramuscularly, or intravenously. Evaluation of pain therapies is very important.

Preventing infection

The person with sickle cell disease is especially prone to respiratory infections and ulcers of the lower leg. Good hygiene is essential. The patient should avoid those with upper respiratory infections; pneumococcal vaccine may be prescribed. The patient should examine the legs daily for signs of skin breakdown.

Counselling patients

Many people with sickle cell disease display anxiety about recurring crises and the nature of their chronic illness. Provide counselling and suggest ongoing counselling (if needed) and the use of support groups. Information about local services can be obtained from the Sickle Cell Society. Assist the patient to be as independent and productive as possible in a difficult situation when sickle cell crises are frequent. *Genetic* counselling (p. 472) is also important to assist the couple in making informed decisions about procreation.

Facilitating patient learning

The family as well as the patient needs to know about the disease to dispel myths and misconceptions, to decrease anxiety, and to provide optimal care. Teaching includes the following:
1. Nature of sickle cell disease
2. Avoidance of situations that cause crisis (infection, overexertion, emotional stress, alcohol, cigarette smoking)[28]
3. Importance of adequate fluid intake (at least 4 to 6 L/day)
4. Availability of counselling and support services
5. Need for medical follow-up

Nursing care of the patient with sickle cell crisis is summarized in Box 19-2. A sample nursing care plan is described opposite.

Evaluation

1. Does patient state feeling more rested and comfortable?
2. Is patient drinking at least 4 to 6 L/day?
3. Is patient free of thrombosis and infection?
4. Are signs of anxiety decreased and does patient state plans for counselling and support services as needed?
5. Have patient and spouse begun to deal with the problem of childbearing?

Nursing Care Plan	**People with sickle cell crisis**

DATA: Mr. S. is a 24-year-old Afro-Caribbean individual, married, works as a postman, who is father of one child. He was diagnosed at age 10 as having sickle cell disease but has been largely asymptomatic until 2 years before this admission. When he was first admitted with symptoms of sickle cell crisis, he had severe joint pain in upper and lower extremities, moderate fever (38.1°C), shortness of breath.

PHYSICAL EXAMINATION: Coarse rales in both lower lobes, cyanosis of lips and nailbeds, dry scaly skin on both legs, 2 + pitting oedema with a small (2 cm) reddened area over each medial malleolus. No hair was visible on toes. His Hb was 9 g/dl.

MEDICAL ORDERS: Oxygen by nasal cannula, 4L/min, bed rest but allowed up to toilet, morphine sulphate 15 mg IM 3-4 hourly prn. Mr. S. was given two units of packed cells to be followed by IV fluids. Sickle cell crisis with congestive heart failure was diagnosed.

The nursing history identified the following:
1. Mr. S. is very "worried" about the outcome of the hospitalization and his ability to "catch his breath."
2. He expresses his concern about his liability to support his family and be a "father" to his son and especially to take part in athletic events: "I'm hardly a man." His wife has assumed responsibility for the garden, formerly his responsibility.
3. He continues to exercise and jogs several times a week. He smokes 20 cigarettes per day and states he has never been "a big fluid drinker," although he does have a pint of beer a day. He states that he does not know what brings on the crisis.
4. He is concerned about his sexual relationship with his wife because of his general fatigue. They had one child before he was aware of the genetic nature of the disease and expresses concern about having other children who might inherit the disease.

Collaborative nursing action includes those to maintain fluid and electrolyte balance and peripheral and pulmonary oxygen/carbon dioxide balance as well as to prevent further vascular occlusion.

Nursing actions include monitoring for the following:
1. Signs of infection: pyrexia, abnormal fluid, positive blood and sputum cultures, tachy-cardia, tachypnoea.
2. Signs of increased fluid/electrolyte imbalance, CHF and renal failure; haematocrit, electrolyte levels, intake and output, skin turgor; respiratory status (rate, depth of respiration, presence of crackles, skin colour, level of consciousness), renal function: creatinine, blood urea.

Nursing Analysis: Anxiety: related to threat to self-concept, health status and role functioning

Expected patient outcomes	Nursing interventions	Rationale
Signs of anxiety are decreased	Give Mr. S. opportunities to explore concerns about the effects of the disorder.	Making the unknown known may decrease anxiety.
	Assess his knowledge of sickle cell anaemia and correct misunder-standings.	
	Teach relaxation measures.	Relaxation decreases the psycho-motor responses to anxiety.

Nursing Analysis: Potential for infection: related to spleen dysfunction, inadequate primary defence (broken skin) and inadequate secondary defences (decreased haemoglobin)

Expected patient outcomes	Nursing interventions	Rationale
Infection does not occur.	Use good medical asepsis.	Aseptic technique decreases pa-tient's contact with pathogenic or-ganisms; infection is predicted on type and number of organisms to which individuals are exposed and patient resistance to infection.
	Restrict people (staff/visitors) with any type of infection.	Restricting people with infection decreases patient's contact with infectious agents. *continued.*

Nursing Care Plan | **People with sickle cell crisis—cont'd**

Nursing analysis: Pain in joints and chest related to poor pain management techniques, lack of knowledge

Expected patient outcomes	Nursing interventions	Rationale
Mr. S. states feeling comfortable.	Give prescribed analgesics on a regular basis and evaluate effectiveness of medication: obtain prescriptions for increased doses if necessary.	Pain of sickle cell crisis is excruciating: large doses of medication may be required.
	Identify measures Mr. S. has found helpful and include these measures in the care.	Patients often have the most accurate information for their pain control.
	Support joints gently when assisting patient to do range of movement exercises.	Improper support increases stress on joints and increases pain.
	Use moist heat or massage, if helpful.	Heat dilates blood vessels and increases circulation to the area. Massage may increase circulation, relax tense muscles.
	Use other pain-relieving measures; person with frequent crises may benefit from learning special techniques such as biofeedback or self-hypnosis.	Biofeedback, self-hypnosis decrease the physiological responses to pain (muscle spasm, increased pulse).

Nursing analysis: Activity intolerance related to decreased oxygen transport

Expected patient outcomes	Nursing interventions	Rationale
No dyspnoea occurs with activity. Mr. S. states feeling rested.	Provide prescribed oxygen as needed.	High concentration of O_2 in alveoli increases diffusion across membranes.
	Limit activities and provide periods of rest.	Decreased activity decreases O_2 needs of body.
	Administer prescribed transfusion (packed red cells).	Packed cells increase the number of RBCs available to carry O_2 to tissue cells in the anaemic person.

Nursing analysis: Potential sexual dysfunction: related to fatigue, pain, fear of pregnancy

Expected patient outcomes	Nursing interventions	Rationale
Mr. S. and wife state the sexual relationship is satisfying.	Discuss coital positions that require less energy for the person who becomes tired easily.	Coitus requires energy and involves neuromuscular activity; on side or male-inferior position is less demanding for male patient.
	Suggest coitus at times of day when Mr. S. is less fatigued (morning, afternoon).	Fatigue increases with continued daily activities and demand on cardiovascular system.
	Discuss genetic counselling and contraceptive methods	Knowledge of and use of reliable methods to prevent pregnancy reduce fear that may cause sexual dysfunction.

Nursing analysis: Self-esteem disturbance: related to loss of body function, change in life-style and masculine role

Expected patient outcomes	Nursing interventions	Rationale
Mr. S. states satisfaction with life and self.	Provide opportunities for Mr. S. to discuss feelings about inability to fulfil expected roles.	Verbalization of concerns decreases their impact and assists in problem solving.
	Assist Mr. S. to identify personal strengths.	Focusing on strengths and positive factors provides the baseline for personal growth.
	Assist Mr. S. to explore alternative ways to meet role expectations.	Concern over losses may immobilize patient; assistance in exploring alternatives is a therapeutic role of the nurse.
	Suggest joining a support group or obtaining counselling to minimize dependency behaviours.	Research shows that increased social support from family and groups increases recovery from disease and disability and facilitates rehabilitation.

Nursing analysis: Knowledge deficit: related to lack of exposure/recall and unfamiliarity with information sources

Expected patient outcomes	Nursing interventions	Rationale
Patient/family describe the nature of the disorder and care requirements.	Review with Mr. S. the basis of sickle cell disease and genetic effects.	Knowledge of causes of disease is *one* factor in ensuring patient compliance with medical regimen and adherence to preventative measures.
	Provide resources for family planning and genetic counselling.	Individuals and groups with in-depth knowledge of family planning methods help patients identify a family planning method that conforms to the patient's cultural and religious values.
	Encourage Mr. S. to avoid situations that cause crises (see text).	(See first rationale and text.)
	Encourage Mr. S. to drink 4 to 6 L fluid daily; explain rationale.	Dehydration is a primary cause of RBC sickling.

Care of the patient with sickle cell anaemia during crisis

Promoting adequate hydration
  Maintain intake of at least 4000 ml, unless contraindicated
  Maintain IV fluids as ordered
Maintaining tissue oxygenation
  Avoid overexertion by patient
  Maintain oxygen by mask or cannula as ordered
Preventing infection (same as for leukaemia, p. 485)
Providing comfort
  Give pain medication continuously during crisis
  Evaluate response to medication to determine if increased dosage is needed
  Do not discount severity of pain
Promoting psychological comfort
  Encourage independence and productive life
  Be a good listener and give information to decrease anxiety

6. Can patient and family describe the nature of sickle cell disease, precipitating factors, and need for follow-up care?

ERYTHROCYTOSIS (POLYCYTHAEMIA)
Aetiology and Pathophysiology

Polycythaemia, an abnormal increase in RBCs, may be primary or secondary. *Primary polycythaemia* (*polycythaemia vera*) is a proliferation disorder of unknown aetiology. It is characterized by hyperplasia of the bone marrow; there is usually a simultaneous increase in WBCs and platelets.

Secondary polycythaemia may result from cardiac, pulmonary, or renal disorders, or it may be stress related. Chronic hypoxia is a major cause of secondary polycythaemia; it stimulates the production of the enzyme erythropoietin, which then stimulates the bone marrow to increase RBC production. More red cells are then available to carry oxygen.

The signs and symptoms of polycythaemia (headache, dizziness, blurred vision, fatigue) are secondary to increased blood viscosity and total blood volume. Pruritus results from the increased number of basophils. Vasodilation occurs as a result of increased RBCs. There is also marked leukocytosis and thrombocytosis/thrombocythaemia, which, along with the increased RBC count, predispose the person to thrombosis, tissue hypoxia, and bleeding (Table 19-2).

Nursing Process
Assessment
Subjective data and objective data

Subjective data include reports of headache, blurred vision, fatigue, and pruritus. Assess the person's knowledge about the nature of polycythaemia. *Objective data* include observations for signs of bleeding, such as nosebleeds or areas of ecchymosis. Principal laboratory tests to determine the nature of the erythrocytosis consist of determination of the arterial oxygen concentration, red cell volume, and plasma volume.

Nursing analysis

Problems are determined from analysis of patient data. Possible problems for the person with polycythaemia include, but are not limited to, the following:

Problem	Possible aetiologies
Knowledge deficit	Lack of exposure to pertinent information

Planning: expected patient outcomes

Expected patient outcomes for the person with polycythaemia may include, but are not limited to, the following:

1. Explains the nature of the disorder, importance of continued medical care, and reason for therapy.
2. Describes foods to avoid.
3. Describes signs of thrombosis.

Implementation

Patient teaching is the primary care for persons with polycythaemia and includes the following:
1. Nature of the disorder
2. Importance of continued blood tests and medical care
3. Phlebotomy therapy
   a. Removal of 500 ml blood per week until haematocrit level reaches 45%
   b. Repeat phlebotomy when haematocrit level rises over 50% (usually every 2 to 3 months)
4. Avoidance of foods high in iron content (liver, oysters, legumes) because patient already has increased iron from increased RBCs
5. Signs of extremity thromboses (swelling, redness, pain) requiring medical attention

Evaluation

1. Can the person explain the nature of the disorder and rationale for therapy?
2. Does the person describe plans to avoid iron-rich foods?
3. Does the person know signs of thrombosis requiring medical intervention?

COAGULATION DISORDERS

PATHOPHYSIOLOGY

Platelets are formed in the bone marrow. In the normal adult approximately 80% of the platelets are in free circulation and 20% are stored in the spleen. It is estimated that the normal life span of platelets is approximately 10 days. Laboratory values for a normal adult platelet count range from $150-400 \times 10^9$/L.

Refer to p. 465, if necessary, for a discussion of the coagulation process. Remember that platelets release thromboplastin (factor III); therefore, changes in platelet *function* will interfere with coagulation. Platelets also plug

Table 19-5   Disorders of coagulation (platelets)

Disorder	Signs and symptoms	Medical therapy
Idiopathic thrombocytopenia purpura (ITP)	Petechiae, ecchymoses, easy bruising; platelet count below 10×10^9/L, prolonged bleeding time	Corticosteroids, splenectomy, therapeutic plasmapheresis
Secondary thrombocytopenia	Same as above	Correct underlying cause
Thrombocytosis/thrombocythaemia	Bleeding (mucosal areas, especially GI tract); thrombosis (primarily venous, but may be arterial)	Cytotoxic drugs to decrease bone marrow activity; platelet pheresis, aspirin
Haemophilia	Life-long bleeding into any part of body, spontaneously or after trauma; may be into joints or retroperitoneal, intracranial areas; signs of blood loss	Replacement of deficient coagulation factor VIII or IX; topical coagulants (fibrin foam or thrombin); concentrated preparations of fibrinogen; plasmapheresis to remove antibody inhibitors against factor VIII
Disseminated intravascular coagulation (DIC)	Diffuse bleeding into mucous membranes and tissues, wound sites; renal failure; prolonged prothrombin time	Correct underlying problem, cardiovascular support, platelet packs, cryoprecipitate, fresh whole blood; haemodialysis for renal failure

small breaks in blood vessels by adhesion and clumping. Aspirin inhibits the release of intrinsic platelet ADP and produces a defect in platelet aggregation. The defect remains for the life of the platelet, and clot formation is inhibited.

Changes in circulating platelet *numbers* can also affect coagulation. *Thrombocytosis* or *thrombocythaemia* (increase in number of circulating platelets) is usually seen in association with other diseases. The danger of thrombocytosis is that it may lead to thrombosis of abnormal bleeding (Table 19-5). Care of the patient is similar to that for those receiving anticoagulation therapy. *Thrombocytopenia* (decrease in number of circulating platelets) leads to bleeding.

Coagulation disorders may be congenital or acquired. The most common *congenital* coagulation disorders are the haemophilias. *Liver disease* is the most common *acquired* coagulation disorder. The liver produces most of the clotting factors: II, V, VII, IX, X, and fibrinogen. Liver disease may produce impaired production of these clotting factors and an elevated prothrombin time. A deficiency in vitamin K can also affect clotting since vitamin K is a cofactor in the synthesis of clotting factors II, VII, IX, and X. Approximately 50% of required vitamin K is obtained from a normal diet, and the remainder is produced by intestinal bacteria. *Inactivation of intestinal bacteria* by intestinal antibiotics can lead to vitamin K deficiency. Disseminated intravascular coagulation (DIC) is also an acquired disorder of coagulation.

THROMBOCYTOPENIA
Aetiology

Thrombocytopenia, a decrease in number of circulating platelets, can result from decreased platelet production or increased platelet destruction. Decreased production is usually caused by drugs (Box 19-3) or bone marrow suppression from chemotherapy or radiotherapy.

Pathophysiology

The most common thrombocytopenia from increased platelet destruction is *idiopathic thrombocytopenia purpura* (ITP). It occurs most commonly in the second and third decades of life and is caused by production of an autoantibody (IgG), which is directed against a platelet antigen. It is manifested by excessive bleeding, which may be reflected in purpuric lesions on the skin or by visceral bleeding (Table 19-5).

Assessment
Subjective data and objective data

Subjective data include eliciting a history of recent viral infection, as this may produce transient thrombocytopenia. Also obtain a detailed history of drug and alcohol use.

Objective data include observing the patient for the presence of ecchymoses (bruises or black and blue marks caused by bleeding into the subcutaneous tissues and skin) and petechiae (1- to 4-mm flat, round, purple-red haemorrhagic bruises in the skin), bleeding gums, vaginal bleeding, GI bleeding, or haematuria.

Diagnostic tests

Diagnostic tests include laboratory studies and bone marrow examination (p. 470). Commonly used tests for assessment of platelets include platelet count, peripheral blood smear, and bleeding time, which is usually prolonged. The bone marrow is examined for the presence of *megakaryocytes* (precursors of platelets in the bone marrow). Their presence suggests that the thrombocytopenia is caused by peripheral platelet destruction, and their absence or decrease suggests a failure of thrombopoiesis.

Implementation

The medical management of idiopathic thrombocytopenic purpura includes corticosteroid therapy, plasmapheresis, and splenectomy. Steroids appear to decrease the autoantibody that is directed against the platelet antigen. Splenectomy removes the organ primarily responsible for destruction of the antibody-coated platelets. Danazol, immunoglobulin, or immunosuppressive drugs also may be administered.

Nursing management is primarily teaching the patient with thrombocytopenia. Of primary concern is the bleeding tendency and measures taken to prevent haemorrhage and injury (see Box 19-4). Bleeding associated with trauma is likely with a platelet count less than 60×10^9/L. The need for avoidance of trauma is obvious. Spontaneous haemorrhage looms as a life-threatening possibility in individuals with a platelet count of less than 20×10^9/L. Teaching also includes signs of decreased platelets (petechiae, ecchymosis, haematuria, menorrhagia) and the need for continuous follow-up medical care.

HAEMOPHILIA

Aetiology and Pathophysiology

Haemophilia is a hereditary coagulation disorder. Both haemophilia A (factor VIII deficiency) and haemophilia B, also called Christmas disease (factor IX deficiency), are inherited as sex-linked recessive disorders and are therefore almost exclusively limited to males. An example of the inheritance pattern of haemophilia is shown in Fig. 19.3.

The degree of bleeding is related to the amount of factor activity and the severity of injury. Spontaneous bleeding, joint bleeding (haemarthrosis), and deep tissue haemorrhage occur with factor levels less than 1%. Retroperitoneal and intracranial bleeding may also occur and may be life-threatening. Patients may experience bleeding after tooth extraction, minor trauma, or during surgical procedures. Any body system may be affected.

Assessment

Subjective data and objective data

Subjective data include the patient's and family's knowledge of the disorder, measures taken to prevent injury, and coping mechanisms. If pain or bleeding is present, explore possible causes to ascertain if these could have been prevented (data useful for teaching future prevention). *Objective data* include presence of bleeding or swelling of joints (indicating joint bleeding).

Diagnostic tests

A diagnosis of haemophilia is made by specific assays for factors VIII and IX. The partial thromboplastin time (PTT) is prolonged in both types of haemophilia. The platelet count and prothrombin time are normal.

Implementation

Assisting with achievement of therapeutic goals

Bleeding disorders may require local treatment such as ice bags, manual pressure or dressings, immobilization, and elevation of a body part. Joint aspiration may be necessary. Muscle stretching exercises are begun after pain and bleeding have subsided (usually within 3 to 5 days). Active range of motion exercises are encouraged when swelling has subsided.

With major haemorrhages, careful monitoring is necessary to avoid fluid overload if large plasma volumes are given. Concentrates (Table 19-6) provide the deficient factors and prevent fluid overload and fewer side effects (such as urticarial or febrile reactions) in some patients. High cost and contamination with the virus of serum hepatitis are drawbacks, however, to the use of some of the concentrates. The heat treatment of factor VIII now reduces the likelihood of AIDS transmission.

Factor replacement therapy may be given on an outpatient basis, either in a clinic or in the home. Home infusion programmes have gained interest and are seen as a way of controlling bleeding episodes more quickly, thereby decreasing the need for hospitalization and a long absence from school or work.

A synthetic drug that is effective against mild haemophilia and von Willebrand's disease (deficiencies in factor VIII and in platelet adhesion) is desmopressin. It is administered intravenously and can cause a threefold to sixfold increase in factor VIII activity.

The outlook for the person with haemophilia has been greatly improved by the availability of transfusion therapy.

Table 19-6 Blood factor replacement therapy for haemophilia

Type	Clotting factors	Comments
Fresh frozen plasma	All	Thawed to 37° C before infusion; allergic reactions are common; fluid overload possible, especially in older people
Cryoprecipitate	VIII, fibrinogen	Thawed at 37° C before infusion; occasional allergic reactions; low risk of hepatitis transmission, administer at 12-hour intervals
Lyophilized factor VIII concentrate	VIII	Stable at room temperature; possible haemolytic reactions for people with blood types A, B, AB when given over prolonged period; allergic reactions rare
Vitamin K dependent complex	VII, IX, X, prothrombin	Keep refrigerated; higher risk of hepatitis transmission and thrombus formation (heparin usually given concurrently)

In the past many people with factor VIII deficiency died in the first 5 years of life. Today people with moderate or mild haemophilia may live normal, productive lives.

Counselling and teaching

Threat of spontaneous bleeding episodes and pain control are ongoing stressors the individual must confront. Important points for teaching are listed in Box 19-5. Those individuals who are able to meet the demands of their illness and adapt their life-styles accordingly are able to live productive lives as individuals, spouses, parents, and employees.

Genetic counselling, aimed at explaining the pattern of inheritance of haemophilia, may be of great value to adults contemplating parenthood. Such counselling can assist potential parents in evaluating realistically their ability to raise a child afflicted with haemophilia and to anticipate ways to meet the demands placed on both of them and the child.[18]

The Haemophilia Society is an organization established for people with haemophilia and their families. The basic function of the Haemophilia Society is to support people with haemophilia, carriers of the abnormal gene and affected families. It is also concerned with ensuring that high quality treatment and local facilities are available. Another important role is that of public education, especially since the contamination of Factor VIII with the AIDS virus in the early 1980s. Unfortunately, this led to various fears and prejudices in the general public against individuals with haemophilia.

DISSEMINATED INTRAVASCULAR COAGULATION

Aetiology

Disseminated intravascular coagulation (DIC) is a pathophysiological response of the body's haemostatic mechanisms to disease or injury. DIC is a complicated and potentially fatal syndrome that is characterized initially by clotting and secondarily by haemorrhage.

It occurs in any condition where tissue thromboplastin is liberated subsequent to tissue destruction. One of the most common causes is abruptio placentae, or premature separation of the placenta. Tumour products, crushing trauma, burns, leukaemia, vasculitis, sepsis and shock, as well as surgery (especially prostatic, orthopaedic or open heart) may also initiate DIC.[26]

Defective gene is found on X chromosome.
When faulty X chromosome is present in a male,
the male will be a haemophiliac.

When faulty X chromosome is present in a female,
she will be a carrier of haemophilia.

In conception between a normal male and a carrier female, four possibilities arise:

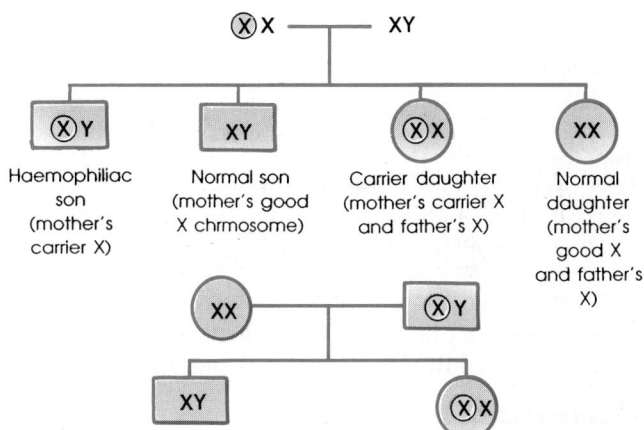

In conception between a haemophiliac male and a normal female, son will be normal but daughter will be carrier.

Fig. 19-3   Pattern of inheritance of haemophilia.

Pathophysiology

DIC is essentially an imbalance between the processes of coagulation and anticoagulation. The normal balance of clotting factors and fibrinolytic factors, which under normal conditions prevent bleeding while maintaining the fluidity of the blood, are altered.

The primary disease or injury initiates the clotting process. This response is generalized and occurs throughout the vascular system, creating a state of *hypercoagulability*. The fibrinolytic processes, which normally operate to limit clot extension and dissolve clots, are then stimulated. As clotting factors are depleted and fibrinolysis continues, a state of *hypocoagulability* develops.

19-5

Patient Teaching

The patient with haemophilia

Nature of disease: genetic basis
Prevention of haemorrhage
Possibility of bleeding after dental extraction
Avoidance of contact sports
Importance of carrying a card or wearing a
    Medic-Alert tag with name, blood type,
    doctor's name and phone number, and
    diagnosis
Community resources (Haemophilia Society)
Family planning techniques if desired
Need for medical follow-up

Guideline for Care

19-6

The patient with DIC

Monitor continually for bleeding sites or changes
    in amount of bleeding (especially if heparin
    therapy is given)
Assess and record amount of drainage from chest
    and nasogastric tubes and oozing from incisions
Monitor fluid rates; be alert for signs of fluid over-
    load (increased pulse rate, distended jugular
    veins, and increased CVP)
Provide care for the critically ill patient
Explain to family what is occurring and provide
    opportunities for expressions of feelings

The most common sequela of DIC is haemorrhage. This paradox is caused by decreased platelets and the depletion of clotting factors, II, V, VIII, and fibrinogen and the production of fibrin degradation products (FDP) through fibrinolysis. FDP act as anticoagulants, which increase the haemorrhagic tendency (p. 465).

Assessment

The first signs and symptoms may be those of haemorrhage (oral, vaginal, rectal, after injection and venepuncture, petechiae, and ecchymosis). Pain may be present from joint bleeding.

Diagnostic tests

Laboratory findings, which may be the only indications of the syndrome in the early stages, may include the following:

1. Decreased circulating platelet count
2. Prolonged prothrombin time
3. Prolonged partial thromboplastin time
4. Decreased factors V and VIII
5. Decreased fibrinogen levels
6. Increased fibrin split products (fibrinolysis)
7. Abnormal RBCs on peripheral blood smear

Implementation

Medical management is aimed at correcting the underlying problem. Antibiotics, chemotherapeutic agents, and cardiovascular support may be used. Fresh-frozen plasma and packed RBCs may be administered to restore clotting factors and blood volume.

Nursing intervention in the care of the patient with DIC is extremely challenging (Box 19-6). The person is critically ill and frequently has numerous sites of bleeding before DIC becomes evident. Frequently the patient is comatose, and the presence of purpura, numerous intravenous lines, and drainage tubes makes the patient's appearance especially upsetting to the family. Most of the primary conditions associated with DIC are of a sudden nature, and the family requires help in understanding this catastrophic occurrence and support during the long period of treatment.

Interventions for thrombocytopenia (p. 479) are applicable to the patient with DIC. The patient requires careful monitoring of fluid replacement therapy, renal function and fluid output, and signs and symptoms of further bleeding.

DISORDERS ASSOCIATED WITH WHITE BLOOD CELLS

NEUTROPENIA (LEUKOPENIA)

Neutropenia is defined as a neutrophil count of less than 2×10^9/L. It may occur as a primary haematological disorder but is seen more often in association with other disorders, including malignant disease of the bone marrow, aplastic anaemia, megaloblastic anaemia, use of chemotherapeutic agents, starvation, and viral infections. Severe neutropenia can also occur as a reaction to drugs, particularly in the patient with aplastic anaemia secondary to cytotoxic drugs. The degree of susceptibility to infection is in direct proportion to the degree of neutropenia. Individuals with marked neutropenia are at risk for contracting a life-threatening infection.

Agranulocytosis is an acute disease in which the number of WBCs suddenly decreases, usually as the result of chemicals or drugs (sulphonamides, propylthiouracil, chloramphenicol, and bone marrow depressant drugs such as chemotherapeutic agents). Clinical signs include infection, malaise (discomfort, headache, lassitude, muscle aches), ulceration of mucous membranes, chills, and fever. A sepsis may develop, which may lead to death. Care is directed towards removing the causative agents and resolving infection. If bone marrow is not destroyed, the prognosis for recovery is good.

Granulocyte transfusions may be used for the patient with severe neutropenia. Nursing interventions focus on preventing infections (see Box 19-7) and careful monitoring for early signs of infection so that therapy can begin promptly. Because neutrophil count is low, some of the classic signs of infection and the inflammatory response (purulent drainage, abscess formation, sequestration of a local infection) may be absent (Chapter 33). Fever may also be absent because of a lack of the endogenous pyrogens that are produced by neutrophils in response to infection.

NEUTROPHILIA

Neutrophilia is defined as a neutrophil count greater than 10×10^9/L. Such an increase is a normal response to infections, primarily bacterial. It may also increase with strenuous exercise. Prolonged elevation of the neutrophil count, especially in the absence of an apparent cause, is a reason for a diligent search for the underlying cause. Persistent elevated neutrophil counts are associated with leukaemia, polycythaemia vera, myeloid metaplasia, and a variety of systemic and inflammatory disorders. Treatment consists of therapy for the primary condition.

LEUKAEMIA

Aetiology

The cause of leukaemia is unknown. An increased incidence of leukaemia in siblings has led to hypotheses of genetic predispositions or viral origins. Radiation and chemicals (including benzene, arsenic, chloramphenicol, and antineoplastic drugs) have also been implicated.

Pathophysiology

Leukaemias are malignant disorders of the haematopoietic system involving the bone marrow and lymph nodes; they are characterized by uncontrolled proliferation of leukocytes and their precursors. The large number of cells accumulate first at the site of origin (granulocytes in the bone marrow, lymphocytes in the lymph nodes), then spread to haematopoietic organs, leading to organ enlargement (splenomegaly, hepatomegaly). The proliferation of one type of cell often interferes with the normal production of other hematopoietic cells, leading to the development of immature cells and to cytopenias (decreased numbers). The immaturity of the white cells leads to decreased immunocompetence with increased susceptibility to infections.

Classification

The leukaemias are classified as acute or chronic and further subdivided according to cell type or maturity of the cell.

Acute leukaemias

Acute leukaemias involve immature cells and are classified according to the predominant cell in the bone marrow, either lymphoblasts (acute lymphoblastic leukaemia) or myeloblasts (acute myeloblastic leukaemia). Acute leukaemias have a rapid onset and a short course, ending in death if untreated. The immaturity of the white cells leads to numerous infections, such as ulcerations of the mucous membranes, pneumonias, and septicaemias. Early symptoms include fever, lymphadenopathy, pallor, and fatigue from anaemia, and ecchymoses (Table 19-7). The WBC count may be normal or decreased.

Acute lymphoblastic leukaemia (ALL)

ALL arises from a single lymphoid stem cell (see Fig. 19-1) with impaired maturation and accumulation of the malignant cells in the bone marrow. It is common to find different stages of lymphoid development in the bone marrow from very immature to almost normal cells. The degree of immaturity is a guide to prognosis; the more immature the cells, the poorer the prognosis. Leukocytes in the bloodstream are predominantly in the blast form. The WBC count is often decreased, but a blood smear will show immature lymphoblasts. It is primarily a disease of children, but adults may develop it. Complete remissions are achieved in 70% to 90% of all newly diagnosed patients.

Acute myeloblastic leukaemia (AML)

AML arises from a single myeloid stem cell (see Fig. 19-1) and is characterized by the development of immature myeloblasts in the bone marrow. The WBC count is usually in the low ranges of normal, and bone marrow aspiration reveals an increased number of myeloblasts. In the untreated patient or the person who is nonresponsive to therapy, the median survival time is approximately 2 to 3 months. Complete remission occurs in 50% to 75% of treated patients, and the median survival time is approximately 2 to 3 years. Approximately 20% of patients are in complete remission at 5 years and are capable of prolonged disease-free periods (remissions).

Chronic leukaemias

Chronic leukaemias are classified according to the predominant mature white cell, either lymphocytes (chronic lymphocytic leukaemia) or granulocytes (chronic myelogenous leukaemia). Chronic leukaemias have a more insidious onset and a median survival time of 4½ to 5½ years. Initially there are fewer infections than in acute leukaemias because of the maturity of the white cells in the chronic disorder, but eventually infections of the skin and pneumonias result from decreased immunocompetence. Early signs of chronic leukaemias include fatigue, weakness, anorexia, and weight loss characteristic of a hypermetabolic state. An enlarged spleen and liver can usually be palpated. The WBC count is usually elevated.

Chronic lymphocytic leukaemia (CLL)

CLL is characterized by a proliferation of small, abnormal, mature B lymphocytes, leading to decreased synthesis of immunoglobulins and depressed antibody response. The accumulation of abnormal lymphocytes begins in the lymph nodes, then spreads to other lymphatic tissues. There is a marked increase in the number of leukocytes and mature

Table 19-7   Leukaemias

Type	Signs and symptoms	Medical therapy
Acute lymphoblastic leukaemia (ALL)	Respiratory infections, anaemia, bleeding of mucous membranes; proliferation of lymphoblasts in bone marrow, lymph nodes, spleen; hepatomegaly; splenomegaly; bone pain; CNS symptoms (headache, vomiting, seizures)	Combined chemotherapy, radiotherapy and immunotherapy; drugs: vincristine, prednisolone, crisantaspase
Acute myeloblastic leukaemia (AML)	Same as above	Chemotherapy with cytarabine, doxorubicin, thioguanine
Chronic lymphocytic leaukaemia (CLL)	Painless and massive lymphadenopathy and splenomegaly; hepatomegaly with disease progression; anaemia; thrombocytopenia; fatigue; weakness, pruritic vesicular lesions	Chemotherapy with alkylating agents (chlorambucil) and glucocorticoids (only when symptoms appear)
Chronic myelogenous leukaemia (CML)	Fatigue, weakness, anorexia, weight loss; blastic (accelerated) phase: anaemia, thrombocytopenia, fever, adenopathy, splenomegaly with sensation of abdominal fullness	Chemotherapy with agents used in AML; also vincristine, busulphan

lymphocytes. At the time of diagnosis the bone marrow is often filled by lymphatic infiltrations. The WBC count rises to a level between $20\text{-}100 \times 10^9/L$. Bone marrow biopsy shows infiltration of lymphocytes.

Chronic myelogenous leukaemia (CML)

The primary defect in CML is an abnormal stem cell leading to an uncontrolled proliferation of the granulocytic cells. As a result of this proliferation, the number of circulating granulocytes increases markedly. In most cases, a characteristic chromosomal abnormality, the *Philadelphia chromosome*, is present. Diagnosis of CML is made on the basis of an elevated WBC count of $15\text{-}500 \times 10^9/L$, granulocytes on the peripheral blood smear that range in maturity from blast cells to mature neutrophils, granulocytic hyperplasia in the bone marrow, and the presence of the Philadelphia chromosome.

Nursing Process
Assessment
Subjective data and objective data

Subjective data include eliciting feelings of weakness and fatigue and a history of predisposition to infection. The person's knowledge of the nature of leukaemia and concerns related to the disease are also obtained. The type of *objective data* depends on the type of leukaemia and may include monitoring for lymphadenopathy, splenomegaly, fever, pallor, and bleeding. The mouth is examined for breaks in the mucous membranes. The person is also observed for behavioural signs of anxiety.

Diagnostic tests

Laboratory tests include bone marrow biopsy or aspiration, and WBC counts for differentiation of the type of leukaemia.

Nursing analysis

Problems are determined from analysis of patient data. Possible problems for the person with leukaemia may include, but are not limited to, the following:

Problem	Possible aetiologies
Infection, high risk for	Decreased WBCs, chemotherapy, radiation
Injury, high risk for: haemorrhage	Disease process, trauma, chemotherapy
Anxiety	Threat of death, change in health status
Coping, ineffectual, individual/family	Situational crisis, prolonged disability, ineffective problem solving
Knowledge deficit	Lack of exposure or recall

Planning: expected patient outcomes

Expected patient outcomes for the person with leukaemia may include, but are not limited to, the following:

1. Shows no signs of infection or excessive bleeding.
2. Shows evidence of problem solving and finding satisfying solutions.
3. Assumes activities of daily living.
4. Describes the nature of the disease, the therapeutic progamme, symptoms requiring follow-up, and available community resources.

Implementation

Many of the interventions for the listed problems are discussed in the chapter on cancer (see Chapter 9).

Assisting with achievement of therapeutic goals

Leukaemia, by its nature, is a diverse illness. The varied courses and response or lack of response to treatment also add to the diversity. Complete and prolonged remission of the disease is the goal of medical therapy. Complete remission exists when all tests are normal, and all symptoms have disappeared. Partial remission occurs when symptoms have disappeared, but the disease remains in the bone marrow.

Chemotherapy

Chemotherapy is the primary treatment modality. The first phase of chemotherapy is termed *induction chemo-*

<table>
<tr><td>19-8</td><td>Chemotherapeutic agents commonly used in leukaemia therapy</td></tr>
</table>

Crisantaspase	Melphalan
Busulphan	Azathioprine
Chlorambucil	Methotrexate
Cyclophosphamide	Prednisolone
Cytarabine	Thioguanine
Doxorubicin	Vincristine

therapy and consists of combination chemotherapy (use of more than one chemotherapeutic agent, see Chapter 9). Commonly used agents in the treatment of leukaemias are listed in Box 19-8. Bone marrow studies are conducted 2 and 3 weeks following initiation of therapy. A different drug regimen will be given if evidence of disease in the marrow is still present after 3 weeks.

During induction therapy, the patient is at high risk for haemorrhage or infection. Nursing care of the patient during this phase includes the following:

1. Monitor vital signs every 4 hours
2. Use bleeding precautions
   a. Use soft toothbrush or swabs for mouth
   b. No rectal temperatures, medications, or enemas
   c. Use electric razor
   d. Avoid aspirin
3. Monitor for signs of bleeding (observation of skin, testing urine with haemastix and stool for guaiac)
4. Give antibiotics on time to maintain blood levels if fever occurs
5. Monitor administration of whole blood or blood component therapy, if given
6. Assess intravenous site of chemotherapy for redness, swelling, tenderness, extravasation of drugs (Chapter 9)
7. Provide immediate care of extravasation of chemotherapeutic drugs (discontinue infusion, apply ice to area, infiltrate subcutaneous area with sodium bicarbonate or steroids)[39]

Maintenance therapy, the second phase of therapy, is usually required to maintain a complete remission. This therapy is often given on an outpatient basis. Appropriate duration of therapy in patients who continue free of disease varies, depending on the type of the disease and the patient's response to therapy. Chemotherapy is discussed in more detail in Chapter 9.

Bone marrow transplantation

Bone marrow transplantation, using HLA-identical bone marrow, has been used with increasing frequency and promises to have an increasing impact on the progress of AML. In addition to leukaemia, bone marrow transplantation is being used for patients with lymphoma, aplastic anaemia, thalassaemia, and immunodeficiency disorders.

Pretransplant preparation is necessary for bone marrow transplantation. It has two goals: *immunosuppression* to allow acceptance of an immunologically nonidentical graft and *cytoreduction* to kill all tumour cells. This is accomplished by chemotherapy followed by total body irradiation.[15]

The procedure consists of taking 600 to 1000 to 2500 ml[30] of marrow cells by multiple needle aspiration from the posterior iliac crest of the donor under general or spinal anaesthesia. After processing, the marrow is placed in a blood transfusion bag and administered intravenously through a Hickman catheter (see Chapter 9) at the same rate as RBC administration (about 4 hours).

Patients over 30 may develop severe acute graft-versus-host reaction (Chapter 33), which may be fatal. One approach being used to prevent graft-versus-host reaction is to treat the donor marrow with monoclonal antibodies before transplantation. This removes mature T cells, which cause the reaction, but leaves immature T cells to prevent infection (Chapter 9).

Another method to prevent graft-versus-host reaction is *autologous* bone marrow transplantation. Some of the *patient's* bone marrow is removed during a period of remission and is frozen. It is stored for transplantation when needed by the patient. Recombinant human granulocyte-macrophage stimulating factor (GM-CSF), produced by recombinant DNA technology, is being given to patients after undergoing autologous bone marrow transplantation to accelerate myeloid engraftment, decrease infectious episodes, and shorten hospital stay.

Nursing care is focused on preventing infection, providing emotional support and skin care, and maintaining fluid, electrolyte, and nutritional balance. Protective isolation (Chapter 9) may be used.

Interventions to achieve patient outcomes
Preventing infection

Patients with leukaemia are at high risk of infection as a consequence of leukopenia. They may suffer from recurrent perirectal abscesses, pneumonia, and septicemias. Measures to prevent infection include the following:

1. Place patient in a side room; avoid contact with visitors and staff who have infection.
2. Place patient in protective isolation (see Chapter 9).
3. Provide meticulous hygiene, including daily bath, careful oral hygiene, and perineal care; use antiseptic creams.
4. Avoid catheterizations.
5. Use povidone iodine skin cleansing for 1 minute before parenteral injections (or other preparations as prescribed).
6. Maintain a clean environment.
7. Provide emotional support for anxiety when infection occurs.

Preventing excessive bleeding

Patients with leukaemia have fewer platelets, which causes bleeding, as evidenced by petechiae, ecchymosis (bleeding into the skin), epistaxis (nosebleeds), and GI and urinary tract haemorrhage. Measures to prevent excessive bleeding include the following:

1. Assess all sites for bleeding.
2. Test urine (Haemastix) and stool (guaiac) for blood.
3. Keep venepuncture and intramuscular injections to a minimum.
4. Apply pressure to venepuncture sites for 5 minutes, arterial sites for 10 minutes.

5. Use soft toothbrush or swab for mouth care.
6. Keep mouth clean and free of debris with normal saline rinse if bleeding occurs.
7. Avoid taking rectal temperatures, administering rectal medications, or giving enemas.
8. Avoid invasive procedures.

Counselling patient and family

Each person with leukaemia responds in a different way. It cannot be predicted for certain whether an individual will respond to a prescribed treatment or how long a remission will last. Leukaemia is a threat to life, a situational crisis. Both patient and family, therefore, can experience anxiety, especially when the diagnosis is first made and during acute phases. Even the patient in remission may experience periods of anxiety when other illnesses occur and be concerned that the acute phase has returned. Anxiety is also high during chemotherapy and bone marrow transplantation. Give patients and family members opportunities to talk, to share fear and concerns, to ask questions. Help them explore alternative methods of coping, if appropriate. Carefully explain therapies and planned activities. Include the family in all aspects of patient care.

Facilitating patient learning

How the individual incorporates the illness into life is also unique to each person. Nursing has the key role in patient education (Box 19-9). Of utmost importance in learning is the ability of the person to identify the body's signals that blood abnormalities exist. Bone pain, often severe, may signal blast crisis (acute proliferation of immature cells).

Individuals whose illness runs the course of several months to years often become very knowledgeable about their disease, blood components, related symptoms, and specific chemotherapeutic drugs. These patients sometimes discuss their progress in terms of changes in their blood counts. Over time many individuals become attuned to how such changes affect them. For example, they often can predict their count by how they feel. Many such people respond well to being included in their plan of care during hospitalization and in preparation for discharge.

Evaluation

Questions to consider include the following:
1. Is the patient free of infection?

2. Is the patient assuming activities of daily living?
3. Is the patient free from anxiety?
4. Do the patient and family say they are coping with the illness?
5. Is the patient knowledgeable about the disease, its effects, and the treatment regimen?
6. Can the patient describe symptoms that require medical intervention?
7. Can the patient state importance of and schedule for chemotherapy and periodic blood tests?

DISORDERS ASSOCIATED WITH THE LYMPHATIC SYSTEM

LYMPHADENOPATHY

Lymph node enlargement (lymphadenopathy) may be caused by infection in the area drained by the lymph vessel containing the node or by systemic infection. Enlargement of the node, which in this situation is usually painful, is a positive sign indicating immune responsiveness to the invading microorganisms. Lymphadenopathy may also occur when the node is invaded by cells normally not present (leukaemic cells, cancer cells) and is a pathophysiological sign of lymphomas such as Hodgkin's disease. Some body areas where lymph nodes may be palpated are illustrated in Fig. 19-4.

Lymphangiography is a radiological technique used for evaluation of lymph nodes to detect the presence of disease. This procedure is especially valuable in assessing those nodes that are anatomically too deep to allow for evaluation by palpation. For this procedure a small incision is made on the dorsal surface of each foot so that the small lymph glands are made accessible. A dye is slowly instilled over several hours, filling all lymph chains and nodes. Radiographs are usually done immediately after the dye is absorbed and again at intervals of 24 and 48 hours after the procedure. In addition, because the dye remains in the lymph nodes for as long as 6 months after the initial study, disease status and response to therapy can be periodically evaluated with routine abdominal x-ray films.

LYMPHOMAS

Lymphomas are malignant disorders of the lymph system. Hodgkin's disease is considered separate from other lymphomas (Table 19-8).

Aetiology and Pathophysiology
Hodgkin's disease

Hodgkin's disease, which was considered fatal until fairly recently, is now potentially curable. Although the cause is unknown, it is thought that viruses may be implicated. The person has *defective cellular immunity* (*T cell disease*) and is therefore at high risk for infections. Four pathological variants of Hodgkin's have been recognized: *lymphocyte predominant, nodular sclerosis, mixed cellularity,* and

---

Box 19-9   Patient Teaching

The patient with leukaemia

Nature of the disease process and its effects
Prevention of infection
Drug regimen: name, side effects, (see Chapter 9)
Method of arranging for chemotherapy administration and periodic blood counts
Symptoms requiring immediate medical attention (fever, bleeding)
Available community resources (Leukaemia Care Society, Leukaemia Research Fund)
Need for continual medical follow-up

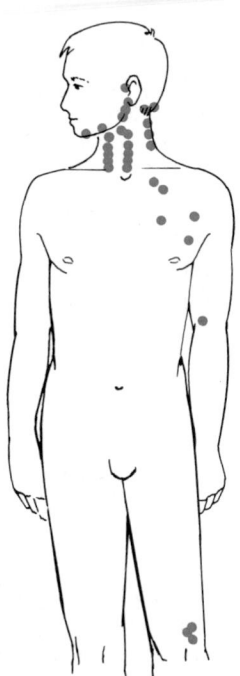

Fig. 19-4   Diagram of body areas where enlarged lymph nodes may be palpated.

lymphocyte depletion. The lymphocyte predominant and nodular sclerosis types have the best prognosis, and lymphocyte depletion, the worst. Hodgkin's disease is usually characterized by the presence of the Reed-Sternberg cell, a large macrophage-derived cell.

The most important prognostic indicator is the stage of disease at the time of diagnosis. Accurate staging (see Box 19-10) is crucial to the subsequent treatment regimen. All stages are subclassified further, as follows:

A: No symptoms
B: Presence of weight loss, fever, profuse night sweats

Non-Hodgkin's lymphomas

Non-Hodgkin's lymphomas (NHL) include a broad spectrum of lymphoid malignancies with different histopathologies, disease courses, and responses to therapy. Accurate identification of the histopathology is crucial to the determination of the treatment plan. NHL can be categorized as *lymphocytic, histiocytic,* or *mixed cell types.* A lymphocytic cytology has the most favourable prognosis, and the histiocytic has the least favourable. Immature lymphocytes are produced, leading to impaired B-cell (humoral) immune response. These patients are therefore also at high risk for infections.

Nursing Process
Assessment

Subjective data and objective data

Subjective data include the following:
1. Knowledge of the disorder
2. Effect of fatigue on the ability to carry out ADL

Staging of Hodgkin's disease	
Stage	**Definition**
I	Single abnormal lymph node
II	Two or more abnormal lymph nodes on the same side of the diaphragm
III	Abnormal lymph node regions on both sides of the diaphragm, which may also be accompanied by involvement of the spleen
IV	Diffuse or disseminated involvement of one or more extralymphatic organs or tissues with or without lymph node involvement

19-10

3. Discomfort from night sweats or pruritus
4. Appetite and present nutritional status

Objective data include weight and condition of skin from scratching (for example, excoriations).

Diagnostic tests

Diagnostic tests for lymphomas may include a chest x-ray film to identify a mediastinal mass and lymphangiography to evaluate the retroperitoneal nodes. The liver and spleen are evaluated by radionuclide scanning or by computed tomography (CT scan). A staging laparotomy may be performed to obtain a biopsy specimen of retroperitoneal lymph nodes and of both lobes of the liver and to remove the spleen. The diagnosis is often arduous and difficult, and explanation of the diagnostic procedures helps provide the patient with the emotional support so often needed during this time.

Slides may be sent to major cancer centres for consultation regarding the classification of the disease. Once the diagnosis is made, the extent of the disease (staging) must be determined for planning the treatment regimen.

Nursing analysis

Problems are determined from analysis of patient data. Possible problems for the person with lymphomas may include, but are not limited to, the following:

Problem	Possible aetiologies
Comfort, altered: night sweats, pruritus	Hypermetabolism
Infection, high risk for	Defective immune response
Coping, ineffective individual	Situational crisis
Knowledge deficit	Lack of exposure or recall

Planning: expected patient outcomes

Expected patient outcomes for the person with lymphomas may include, but are not limited to, the following:
1. States feeling more comfortable without itching.
2. Is free from infection.
3. Discusses effects of illness on life's activities and methods of coping.
4. Describes the nature of the disorder, the therapeutic regimen, and community resources.

Table 19-8 Disorders of the lymphatic system

Disorder	Signs and symptoms	Medical therapy
Hodgkin's disease	Lymph node enlargement (firm, nontender, painless), fever, weight loss, night sweats, pruritus, fatigue	Radiation therapy for stages IA and IIA, radiation and chemotherapy for stage IIIA, combination chemotherapy for stage IIIB and IVB
Non-Hodgkin's lymphoma	Nontender "bulky" lymphadenopathy, moderate hepatomegaly and splenomegaly, fever, night sweats, weight loss	Initial localized radiotherapy; total nodal radiation and chemotherapy for multifocal lesions
Multiple myeloma	Severe disabling bone pain (especially in weight-bearing areas), hypercalcaemia, renal failure, anorexia, CHF, bleeding tendency, coma	Radiation for bone pain, chemotherapy, hydration, ambulation, blood transfusions for anaemia, analgesics

Implementation

Assisting with achievement of therapeutic goals

Chemotherapy and radiation therapy are the primary treatment modalities for the lymphomas (Table 19-8). For Hodgkin's disease, treatment yields a cure rate of approximately 90% for stage I and 80% for stage II. Combination chemotherapy is the treatment of choice for stages IIIb and IV. The most commonly used combination is the MOPP regimen (see Chapter 9). It is administered in a 2-week course each month with prednisolone added during the first and fourth course. The drugs are administered for at least 6 months or for two or three courses following the attainment of complete remission. Complete remissions are achieved in approximately 80% of these patients, and long-term, disease-free remissions and probable cures occur in half of this group.

When nodal radiation is used, only those areas of the body to be irradiated are exposed; the other areas are protected by a mantle.

Varying approaches are used for non-Hodgkin's lymphomas. Single alkylating agents, such as chlorambucil, or combination chemotherapy may be used. Local or total nodal radiation therapy may be given. Explanation of the treatment regimen is important to ensure patient understanding and compliance to achieve therapeutic goals.

Interventions to achieve patient outcomes
Promoting comfort

Fever, pruritus, and profuse night sweats may lead to general discomfort. Comfort measures for pruritus, such as baths and antipruritic medication (see Chapter 34), may be instituted. Frequent changes of night clothing or bed clothes may be necessary, and high fluid intake is encouraged to replace fluid lost with sweating.

Preventing infection

Because of decreased immunity, the person with a lymphoma needs to avoid sources of infection, such as persons with upper respiratory infections. Thoroughly wash any breaks in the skin with soap and water, apply a topical antibiotic such as polymyxin B, and keep the area clean until healed. Report signs of infection to the doctor.

Counselling patients

Hodgkin's disease most often affects young adults. Therefore special attention needs to be given to minimize the impact of the illness and its treatment on their lives, not only during the treatment period but beyond. Before treatment begins, discuss therapy-induced sterility. For young women receiving radiation therapy alone, ovaries may be surgically relocated outside the field of radiation. Sterility frequently occurs in association with chemotherapy. For women this is often temporary, and the ability to conceive and bear normal children often returns after therapy is completed. For men, sterility is more frequently permanent. For this reason the option of sperm banking should be discussed before beginning either radiation or chemotherapy.

To allow for work and career development, every effort should be made to schedule treatment at those times and days of the week that least interfere with work and other important events in the person's life. The nurse has a crucial role in assisting individuals to develop a realistic approach to the illness and in successfully meeting the demands and limitations imposed by the illness and its treatment.

Individuals with lymphomas may have periods of remission and recurrence. Such peaks and valleys are stressful and disruptive. Many patients describe subsequent courses of treatment following a recurrence as more stressful than the initial treatment. Comments include, "Is it worth it? I don't have the same faith." Other patients, realistically encouraged by the initial response to treatment, are able to express an optimistic outlook, "It worked the first time. It will work again." Recognition of the stress involved in therapy requires that support systems be available to the individual. The health care team can provide some of the needed support and guidance as the individual learns to incorporate the illness into daily life.

Facilitating patient learning

Teaching the patient includes the following:
1. Nature of the disorder
2. Importance of the extensive diagnostic testing in identifying the treatment plan
3. Effects of therapy on sterility
4. Need for periodic blood counts
5. Side effects of radiation and chemotherapy and how to cope with them (see Chapter 9)
6. Need for continued medical follow-up
7. Community resources

Evaluation

Questions to consider include the following:

1. Is the patient comfortable?
2. Is the patient infection free, with normal temperature and no abnormal discharges?
3. Is the patient making plans to resume activities?
4. Can the patient describe the disease process, therapeutic regimen, and identify community resources?

MULTIPLE MYELOMA

Aetiology and Pathophysiology

Multiple myeloma is a lymphoproliferative disorder associated with plasma cells, the most mature form of activated B lymphocytes that are responsible for immunoglobulin synthesis (see Chapter 33). This is a malignant neoplastic disease that arises in the bone marrow and involves bones primarily.

Plasma cell proliferation suppresses normal marrow elements resulting in "punched out" bone lesions that are visible on x-ray examination. Functionally abnormal immunoglobulin production suppresses formation of normal immunoglobulins needed to prevent infections.[26]

Because of changes in the bone, patients develop severe disabling bone pain (especially in weight-bearing bones), pathological fractures, neurological symptoms from cord compression, hypercalcaemia (because of bone destruction), with symptoms of renal failure, anorexia, confusion, and coma. Renal tubules may be damaged by myeloma proteins (Bence-Jones proteins).

Pneumonia, urinary tract infections, and bacteraemia occur because of the decrease in normal immunoglobulins. Expanded plasma volume may lead to congestive heart failure. Increased plasma viscosity leads to visual problems, headache, immobility, and confusion. Haemorrhage may occur because the myeloma proteins interact with plasma coagulation factors and also coat platelets, decreasing their function.

Assessment

Subjective data and objective data

Subjective data include the presence of bone pain, anorexia, and neurological symptoms such as numbness, tingling, and weakness. *Objective data* include skin colour, urinary output, signs and symptoms of infection, level of consciousness, and signs of bleeding.

Diagnostic tests

Diagnostic tests include x-ray evaluation of bones, haematological studies (serum protein electrophoresis and immunoelectrophoresis), Bence-Jones proteins, and calcium levels.

Implementation

There is no cure for multiple myeloma, and treatment is primarily palliative. The median survival is 5 to 6 years.[30] Combination chemotherapy is given for bone pain or other symptoms. Localized radiotherapy may also be used. During therapy, monitor renal and cardiac function.

Pain control includes analgesic administration and careful handling of extremities when mobilizing or turning the patient. Because immobility increases bone demineralization and osteoporosis, it is essential that the patient maintain mobility to prevent fractures. Use of splints, braces, and walking aids may facilitate activity.

If the patient is prone to infection or bleeding, initiate interventions that prevent their occurrence (see p. 488). Counselling and teaching about these side-effects are essential, as well as providing psychological support for an individual with a chronic debilitating disease.

SUMMARY

1. Major health problems of the hematopoietic system include RBC disorders (anaemias, polycythaemia), WBC disorders (leukaemias), coagulation disorders (platelet disorders, haemophilia, DIC), lymphatic system disorders (Hodgkin's disease, non-Hodgkin's lymphoma), and plasma cell disorders (multiple myeloma).
2. Anaemia may be caused by blood loss, impaired RBC production, increased RBC destruction, or nutritional deficiency.
3. Weakness and fatigue are major signs of anaemia. They result from decreased oxygenation from lack of haemoglobin and increased energy needs required by increased RBC production.
4. Bone marrow samples may be obtained by aspiration or biopsy from the sternum, iliac crest, or tibia.
5. Sickle cell anaemia is a haemolytic anaemia with a genetic basis; a sickle cell crisis occurs when the RBCs become deoxygenated and sickle-shaped, thus causing stasis and obstruction of the microvasculature, leading to organ infarction and necrosis.
6. Ingestion of iron compounds is part of the therapy for iron-deficiency anaemia or anaemia from chronic blood loss only; it will not help the other types of anaemias.
7. Thrombocytopenia is a decrease in the number of circulating platelets and leads to bleeding; persons with thrombocytopenia need to learn how to prevent injury and haemorrhage.
8. Haemophilia is a hereditary coagulation disorder; haemophilia A is a lack of coagulation factor VIII, and haemophilia B is a lack of factor IX; maintenance therapy consists of blood factor replacement therapy and prevention of injury.
9. Disseminated intravascular coagulation (DIC) is a coagulation disorder characterized initially by clotting and secondarily by haemorrhage. It results from an alteration in the balance between clotting factors and fibrinolytic factors; the person is usually critically ill.
10. Persons with alterations of WBCs are at high risk of infection, because leukocytes are a major factor in the body's defence against invading microorganisms.
11. The leukaemias are malignant disorders characterized by uncontrolled proliferation of WBCs and their precursors; the cause is unknown.
12. Leukaemias may be lymphocytic or myelogenous, and acute or chronic. Acute leukaemias have a rapid onset

and a short course, if untreated; chronic leukaemias have a more insidious onset and longer course. The major therapies for leukaemias are chemotherapy and bone marrow transplantation.

13. Lymphomas are malignant disorders of the lymphatic system. Persons with Hodgkin's disease have defective cellular immunity and are therefore at high risk for infection. Non-Hodgkin's lymphoma is a group of lymphoid malignancies. Chemotherapy and radiation are the primary treatment modalities for lymphomas.

14. Multiple myeloma is a lymphoproliferative disorder associated with plasma cells (B lymphocytes); it is a malignant disorder arising in the bone marrow and affects primarily bones. The person is at high risk for pathological fractures.

STUDY QUESTIONS

- From your knowledge of physiology, explain why the patient who is anaemic may have dyspnoea, tachycardia, and fatigue.
- What is the difference between sickle cell anaemia and nutritional deficiency anaemia? How does treatment differ?
- Why does WBC count increase during infection? Why is a person with leukopenia more susceptible to infection?
- What are the differences in the four major forms of leukaemia in terms of course and treatment?
- Why are patients with leukaemia and multiple myeloma at high risk for infection, even though WBC counts may be elevated?

REFERENCES AND SELECTED READINGS

1.* Baker LS: You and leukemia: a day at a time, Philadelphia, 1988, WB Saunders.
2. Baum K, et al: The painful crisis of homozygous sickle cell disease, Arch Intern Med 147:1231-1234, 1987.
3.* Borley D: Oncology nursing: leukemia and bone marrow transplant. 3. Nurs Mirror 160(6):30-34, 1985.
4. Brain MC, Carbone PP: Current therapy in hematology-oncology, ed 4, St Louis, 1991, Mosby–Year Book.
5. Brannan D, Guthrie T: Idiopathic thrombocytopenia purpura in adults, South Med J 81(1):43-44, 1989.
6.* Cerrato PS: Could you spot the other anaemia? RN 49(10):63-64, 1986.
7.* Coyle MK: Organic illness mimicking psychiatric episodes, J Gerontol Nurs 13(1):31-35, 1987.
8. Dalton W, Miller T: Multidrug resistance, principles and practice of oncology, Updates 5(7):1-13, 1991.
9. DeVita V, Hellman S, Rosenberg S: Cancer: principles and practice of oncology, ed 3, Philadelphia, 1989, JB Lippincott.
10.* France-Dawson M: Sickle cell disease: implications for nursing care, J Adv Nurs 11(6):729-737, 1986.
11.* Fraser M, Tucker M: Second malignancies following cancer therapy, Semin Oncol Nurs 5(1):43-45, 1989.
12.* Freedman SL: An overview of bone marrow transplantation, Sem Oncol Nurs 4(1):3-8, 1988.
13.* Froberg J: The anemias: causes and courses of action, RN 52(1):24-29, 1989.
14.* Gallagher MT, Wyland N: Leukemia: when white cells run wild, RN 49(10):33-37, 1986.

15.* Gibson L: Bone marrow transplant: the process, Nurs Times 83(3):36-38, 1986.
16.* Goodman M: Managing the side effects of chemotherapy, Semin Oncol Nurs 5(2):29-52, 1989.
17. Haskell C: Cancer treatment, ed 3, Philadelphia, 1990, WB Saunders.
18.* Huckstadt A: Haemophilia: the person, family and nurse, Rehab Nurs 11(3):25-28, 1986.
19.* Lakhani AK: Current management of acute leukemias, Nursing 88 (London) 3:755-758, 1987.
20. Lamb C: Managing sickle cell emergencies, Patient Care 19(1):92-95, 1985.
20a. Leach M: Anaemia—nursing care and intervention, Professional Nurse 6(8):454-456, 1991.
21. Mauer AM: Acute lymphoblastic leukemia in a young adult, Hosp Pract 22(9):145-156, 1987.
22.* McConnell EA: Leukocyte studies: what the counts can tell you, Nursing 86 16(3):42-43, 1986.
23.* Moeller KI: Suppressing the risks of bone marrow suppression, Nursing 87 17(3):52-54, 1987.
23a. Morgan G: Nursing the patient with leukaemia, Nursing 3(40):19-22, 1989.
23b. Pallister CJ, A 'crisis' that can be overcome. Management of sickle cell disease, Professional Nurse 7(8):509-513, 1992.
23c. Pallister CJ, Thalassaemia: a preventable disease? Professional Nurse 7(10):666-669, 1992.
24. Pittiglio D, Sacher R: Clinical hematology and fundamentals of hemostasis, Philadelphia, 1987, FA Davis.
25. Post-White J: Glucocorticoid-induced suppression in the patient with leukemia or lymphoma, CA Nurs 9(1):15-22, 1986.
26. Price SA, Wilson LM: Pathophysiology, ed 3, New York, 1986, McGraw-Hill.
27. Ratnoff OD, Forbes CD: Disorders of hemostasis, ed 2, Philadelphia, 1991, WB Saunders.
28. Rifkind R, et al: Fundamentals of hematology, ed 3, Chicago, 1986, Year Book.
29.* Rooney A, Haviley C: Nursing management of disseminated intravascular coagulation, Oncol Nurs Forum 12(1):15-22, 1985.
30. Schroeder SA et al: Current medical diagnosis and treatment, Norwalk, Conn., 1991, Appleton & Lange.
31.* Simonson GM: Caring for patients with acute myelocytic leukemia, Am J Nurs 88:304-309, 1988.
32.* Smith D: Sexual rehabilitation of the cancer patient, Cancer Nurs 12(1):10-15, 1988.
33.* Terry BA: Hodgkin's disease and non-Hodgkin's lymphomas, Nurs Clin North Am 20(1):207-217, 1985.
34. Thomas ED: Bone marrow transplantation: present states and future expectations. In Isselbacker KJ et al: Harrison's Principles of internal medicine, ed 11, New York, 1987, McGraw-Hill.
35.* Trotta P: Nursing assessment of symptoms associated with hyperviscosity syndrome, Oncol Nurs Forum 14(1):21-27, 1987.
36. Williams SR: Essentials of nutrition and diet therapy, ed 5, St Louis, 1990, Mosby–Year Book.
37. Wyngaarden JB, Smith LH: Cecil's Textbook of medicine, ed 18, Philadelphia, 1988, WB Saunders.
38. Alcorn R, et al: Fluid therapy and exercise in the management of sickle cell anemia, Phys Ther 64:1520-1522, 1984.
39.* Campbell VB, Preston R, Smith KY: The leukemias: definition, treatment, and nursing care, Nurs Clin North Am 18(3):523-542, 1983.
40.* Gibbons PT: Transfusion therapy in sickle cell disease, Nurs Clin North Am 18(3):563-568, 1983.
41.* Hutchinson MM: Aplastic anemia: care of the bone marrow failure patient, Nurs Clin North Am 18(3):543-552, 1983.
42.* Hutchinson MM, King AH: A nursing perspective on bone marrow transplantation, Nurs Clin North Am 18(3):511-522, 1983.
43.* Lopez JA, Hausz M: Therapeutic apheresis, Am J Nurs 82:1572-1578, 1982.
44. Miller VG: The sickle cell anemia patient in surgery, AORN J 31:1080-1090, 1979.
45. Nausef WM, et al: A study of the value of simple protective isolation in patients with granulocytopenia, N Engl J Med 304:448-452, 1981.
46.* Rozell MS, Hijazi M, Pack B: The painful episode, Nurs Clin North Am 18(1):185-199, 1983.
47.* Williams I, Earles AN, Pack B: Psychological consider-ations in sickle cell disease, Nurs Clin North Am 18(1): 216-230, 1983.
48. Midence K, Davies S, Foggie F: Courage in the face of crisis (Sickle cell disease). NT 88(22): 46-48, 1992.

---

*Recommended for student reading.

Metabolic and
Endocrine Problems

Unit Seven

The Patient with Diabetes Mellitus

Dorothy Blevins
Virginia L. Cassmeyer

After studying this chapter, the learner should be able to:

- Differentiate between the two major types of diabetes mellitus (DM).
- Describe prevention and health education for DM.
- Explain the pathophysiological bases for hyperglycaemia, nonketotic coma, diabetic ketoacidosis, macrovascular and microvascular changes, neuropathy, and lower extremity changes.
- Identify assessment parameters of DM.
- Describe dietary recommendations and systems for learning dietary requirements.
- Explain the role of exercise in DM.
- Describe medication regimens for DM.
- Describe therapy for correcting acute metabolic crises.
- Explain the effect of surgery on the person with DM.

Diabetes mellitus (DM) is a complex chronic disease involving (1) disorders in carbohydrate, protein, and fat metabolism and (2) the development of macrovascular, microvascular, and neurological complications. It is classified as an endocrine or hormonal disease because of its central feature of hyperglycaemia, which results from a deficit in production or utilization of insulin.

ANATOMY AND PHYSIOLOGY

Insulin deficiency hampers the metabolism of carbohydrates, proteins, and fats. The deficit may occur because the pancreatic beta cells do not secrete insulin properly or because hepatic or peripheral cell receptors are resistant to the binding of insulin or transfer of insulin across the cell membrane. Diabetes mellitus has been described as "cellular starvation in the midst of plenty"; cells are deprived of glucose while hyperglycaemia exists. When glucose is not available for cellular function, cells use other fuels; these are derived from glycogen, amino acids, lactate, glycerol, and ketones. These energy substrates are stored chiefly in muscle, hepatic, and adipose cells.

Hormonal Regulation of Blood Glucose

The pancreatic hormone, *insulin*, has a major metabolic role during fed states; it promotes the use of available glucose and promotes the storage of fuels for later use. See Box 20-1 for the actions of insulin that are *hypoglycaemic, antilipolytic, and anabolic*. Of the several hormones involved in the regulation of blood glucose levels, insulin is the only one that lowers blood glucose. In diabetes, an insulin deficit raises blood glucose above normal levels.

Glucagon, another hormone produced in the pancreas, maintains normal blood glucose levels during fasting states. Glucagon is called a counterregulatory hormone which acts "counter to insulin"; that is, it raises blood glucose. The major role for glucagon is during fasting states when it promotes the use of stored fuels by these processes: *glycogenolysis, gluconeogenesis, ketogenesis, and lipolysis*. The liver is a chief site for producing new glucose from glycogen and amino acids and releasing this into the blood.

Free fatty acids are released from triglyceride stores and can be used as energy sources. In diabetes, excessive amounts of glucagon contribute to the hyperglycaemia and other metabolic alterations of the disease.

People with normal metabolism are able to maintain blood glucose levels of 3.6–5.3 mmol/L (euglycaemia) under markedly different conditions of food intake. In nondiabetic people, blood glucose levels may rise to 7–8 mmol/L after eating (postprandial), but these then rapidly return to normal, as excess glucose is extracted from the blood and stored as glycogen in liver and muscle cells (glycogenesis).

Other counterregulatory hormones affect metabolism much as glucagon does. These include *growth hormone*, produced in the anterior pituitary gland, *adrenaline*, produced in the adrenal medulla, the *glucocorticoids*, produced in the adrenal cortex, and *thyroid hormone*. They also raise blood glucose and promote the use of stored fuels by one or more of the same processes listed above. The secretion of the counterregulatory hormones often increases during the stress response, thus providing glucose for increased energy needs. If there is sufficient insulin in stress states, blood glucose levels will stay within normal limits or be only slightly elevated for a short time. In diabetes, the insulin deficit is made worse by the effects of the counterregulatory hormone, and blood glucose levels can rise greatly during the stress response.

Anatomy

Insulin and glucagon are produced by the islet cells in the pancreas, which is both an exocrine and an endocrine gland. It lies retroperitoneally behind the stomach, with its head and neck in the curve of the duodenum, its body extending horizontally across the posterior abdominal wall, and its tail touching the spleen. More than 1 million islet cells are located throughout the organ. Three types of endocrine cells are alpha (α), which secrete glucagon, beta (β), which secrete insulin, and delta (Δ), which secrete gastrin and pancreatic somatostatin.

Physiology

Insulin is necessary for the transport of glucose, amino acids, potassium, and phosphate across cell membranes, especially those of adipose and resting muscle cells. Insulin is also needed to activate enzymes that promote intracellular metabolism.

It should be apparent that when there is a deficit of insulin, as in diabetes mellitus, *hyperglycaemia, increased fat metabolism*, and *decreased protein synthesis* occur.

A small amount of insulin is secreted continually (basal secretion), and a bolus (surge) amount is secreted in response to intake of glucose and amino acids. Insulin is also secreted in response to a rise in hepatic glucose output (HGO), which is stimulated by glucagon and/or other counterregulatory hormones. This surge in HGO normally occurs at approximately 4 AM; it is reflected in rising blood glucose levels (*dawn phenomenon*).

Physiological Changes with Ageing

Diabetes mellitus affects about 15% to 20% of persons over the age of 65. The disease of diabetes in the elderly must be

20-1	Actions of insulin	
Hypoglycaemic	Decreases blood glucose level
	Increases uptake and utilization of glucose by adipose and muscle cell
	Increases phosphorylation of glucose by liver
	Increases glycogenesis
Suppresses fat metabolism	Increases lipogenesis (antilipolytic)
Promotes protein synthesis	Increases amino acid incorporation into protein (anabolic)

differentiated from the normal changes of ageing that affect glucose tolerance.[42]

Carbohydrate tolerance gradually declines as people age. Glucose ingestion results in higher levels of blood glucose and longer durations of hyperglycaemia in the elderly. After a loading dose of glucose, the 2-hour glucose blood level can be expected to increase approximately 0.6–0.8 mmol/L for each decade of life. The change in fasting blood glucose levels related to age is less marked—only 0.1 mmol/L per decade.

This age-related carbohydrate intolerance has been variously attributed to reduced insulin release from beta cells, a delay in insulin release, and/or a decrease in peripheral sensitivity to insulin.

A second physiological change associated with ageing that is important in diabetes management is a rise in the renal threshold for glucose above the average of 8.9–10 mmol/L blood glucose.

CLASSIFICATION OF DIABETES MELLITUS

This chapter focuses on insulin-dependent diabetes mellitus (IDDM, type 1) and non-insulin-dependent diabetes mellitus (NIDDM, type 2). These are two of eight diagnoses of glucose intolerance. Table 20-1 describes five of these, including IDDM and NIDDM and the criteria for their diagnoses. These are part of a classification system developed in 1979 by an international work group and adopted for use in United States and by the World Health Organization. This classification made labels previously used to categorize persons with diabetes (borderline, latent, juvenile, and adult onset) obsolete. The older terms were discontinued because they were not associated with clear diagnostic criteria. This classification specifies two other diagnoses of glucose intolerance:

1. Potential abnormality of glucose tolerance (in people with known risk factors)
2. Previous abnormality of glucose tolerance (in people who have had transient hyperglycaemia)

In IDDM, little or no insulin is secreted by the beta cells, whereas in NIDDM, the beta cell defect and the amounts of insulin secreted are variable, depending on the course of the disease.

A major characteristic of IDDM is the therapeutic need for insulin for survival. This insulin deficiency is often termed absolute, in comparison with a relative deficit of insulin in NIDDM. Because of the complete dependency on exogenous insulin, persons with IDDM disease tend to have more severe and unstable glucose intolerance. In addition, they are prone to acute metabolic complications of ketosis and ketoacidosis (p. 499).

In NIDDM, hyperinsulinaemia may be present, or normal or low amounts of insulin may occur in the blood. Although much is still unknown about NIDDM, it is understood that *insulin resistance plays a major role in NIDDM*. In this condition there are deficient numbers of

Table 20-1   Diagnoses of diabetes mellitus and other categories of glucose intolerance

Disorder	Description	Criteria for diagnosis
Diabetes mellitus Insulin dependent (IDDM), type 1	Insulin deficiency caused by islet cell loss; often associated with specific HLA types, predisposition to viral insulitis or autoimmune phenomena; *ketosis prone*; occurs at any age, common in youth	Unequivocal elevation of plasma glucose (≥11.1 mmol/L and classic symptoms of diabetes (polydipsia, polyuria, polyphagia, weight loss), or Fasting plasma glucose (FPG) ≥7.8 mmol/L on two occasions, or FPG <7.8 mmol/L and 2 hr plasma glucose ≥11.1 mmol/L with one intervening value ≥11.1 mmol/L after a 75 g glucose load (OGTT)
Non-insulin-dependent (NIDDM), type 2	*Ketosis resistant;* more frequent in adults, but occurs at any age; majority of patients overweight; familial tendency; may require insulin for hyperglycaemia during stress	Same as above
Diabetes associated with certain conditions or syndromes	Hyperglycaemia occurring in relation to other disease states: pancreatic disease, drugs or chemicals, endocrinopathies, insulin receptor disorders, certain genetic syndromes	Same as above
Impaired glucose tolerance (IGT)	Abnormality in glucose levels intermediate between normal and overt diabetes; may progress to diabetes (25%), improve to normal, or remain unchanged	FPG <7.8 mmol/L and 2 hr plasma glucose ≥140 mg/dl and <11.1 mmol/L with one intervening value ≥11.1 mmol/L after a 75 g glucose load
Gestational diabetes (GDM)	Glucose intolerance with recognition of onset during pregnancy related to placental hormones antagonistic to insulin; 35% to 50% develop NIDDM within 8 years	Two or more of following plasma glucose concentrations met or exceeded using a 100 g glucose load: FPG 5.8 mmol/L; 1 hr, 10.6 mmol/L; 2hr, 9.2 mmol/L; 3 hr, 8 mmol/L

Adapted from Shuman, CR, and Spratt, IL: Office guide to diagnosis and classification of diabetes mellitus and other categories of glucose intolerance, Diabetes Care 4(2):335, 1981. With permission from the American Diabetes Association, Inc.

> **Recommended health behaviours for people at risk for or with diabetes mellitus**
>
> Use dietary patterns to avoid hyperlipoprotein-aemia, obesity
> Develop pattern of consistent exercise
> Seek detection and control of glucose intolerance, and hypertension
> Avoid cigarette smoking

effective insulin receptors, postreceptor defects or both. Early in NIDDM, insulin levels may be high as the pancreas responds to the failure of insulin and glucose to cross the cell membrane. Insulin secretion may be delayed in response to a glucose load; thus postprandially, blood glucose rises higher and stays higher than normal. The beta cell defect may worsen as the course of NIDDM progresses and result in low levels of insulin.[39]

Note that both forms of the disease may occur at any age; however, IDDM is more commonly associated with onset in childhood, adolescence, or young adulthood, whereas NIDDM is more commonly associated with onset after 40 years of age. Both forms of the disease are associated with vascular and neurological complications; however, they differ in the organs most frequently affected.

Gestational diabetes mellitus (GDM) has its onset during pregnancy. If glucose tolerance remains impaired after the pregnancy, the disease is reclassified as IDDM or NIDDM. Pregnancy stresses glucose tolerance in all women, particularly in the latter half of pregnancy when placental hormones are secreted in increasing amounts. These hormones increase the supply of amino acids and glucose.

Pancreatectomy and chronic pancreatitis are obvious reasons why people might develop hyperglycaemia. So, too, are diseases or treatments that induce an excessive secretion of one or more counterregulatory hormones. Commonly used drugs that can induce hyperglycaemia include frusemide and thiazide diuretics, glucocorticoids, adrenaline, phenytoin, and nicotinic acid.

PREVENTION AND HEALTH EDUCATION
Primary Prevention

It has been long known that three factors increase the risk of diabetes: a *family history* of the disease, *obesity*, and, for women, the *birth of a large-weight baby* (over 9 lb). Avoiding obesity and, if necessary, reducing weight under medical supervision are the major focuses in primary prevention of NIDDM (type 2).

Health behaviours recommended to modify the risk of diabetes mellitus or its complications are similar to those that modify the risk of cardiovascular disease (see Box 20-2).

Cardiovascular disease is the leading cause of death among people with diabetes. It is estimated that the cardiovascular disease risk in diabetics could be decreased by more than one third if the following goal was achieved.

Genetic counselling is hindered by the current state of knowledge about modes of transmission. People with diabetes may be told that the rates of transmission from parent to child are low (2% to 5% for IDDM and 10% to 15% for NIDDM).[5] Current research is directed towards investigation of whether the expression of IDDM can be prevented in first-degree relatives of people with diabetes. Previous research has demonstrated that insulin requirements can be minimized or delayed in those with recent onset of IDDM by the use of immunosuppressants.[54] However, some subjects experienced nephrotoxicity. Long-term side effects may pose constraints on the widespread use of immunosuppressants.

Secondary Prevention: Detection of Diabetes Mellitus

The prevalence of clinically diagnosed diabetes is estimated to be around 1% of the total population at any one time. Approximately one-half million people in England have been clinically diagnosed as having diabetes. The prevalence is considerably higher for certain groups of the population, particularly people from Asian and Afro-Caribbean origin. In those of Asian origin, the prevalence of NIDDM is nearly five times that of a comparable European population.[42a, 58a]

The majority (90%) of people with diabetes mellitus have NIDDM (type 2). Forty percent to 50% of these individuals have mild hyperglycaemia and glucose intolerance and are relatively asymptomatic, and *the disease is undiagnosed*. However well they feel, they are at risk for developing more severe glucose intolerance and vascular and neurological complications. NIDDM is a risk factor for heart disease, peripheral vascular disease, stroke, and hypertension. Although in some patients diabetes is diagnosed only when vascular or neurological complications ensue, increasing evidence points to a relationship between the duration of the disease and metabolic control of blood glucose and the development of long-term complications of diabetes.

Screening programmes

Screening programmes are directed chiefly towards detection of NIDDM (type 2) for two reasons: (1) the incidence of NIDDM is greater, and (2) screening programmes currently available are not effective in identifying IDDM before the actual onset, which is very sudden and severe. Many authorities believe screening of high-risk populations (elderly, poor, nonwhite, pregnant women) to be a better use of resources than screening entire populations.

Tertiary Prevention

Measures to prevent, detect early, and to treat acute and chronic complications of diabetes mellitus form a major portion of diabetes education for individuals and groups of patients and for health professionals. Table 20-2 shows a brief listing of measures used to detect early and to treat some of the long-term complications. These complications are more completely described later in the chapter. Basic to the prevention of all complications is the control of

Table 20-2 Prevention of long-term complications of diabetes mellitus[60]

Complication	Early detection	Early intervention
Eye problems	Ophthalmoscopic examination	Care by an ophthalmologist Control of hyperglycaemia Control of hypertension Laser photocoagulation Referral for low vision evaluation, optical aids, and rehabilitation
Kidney problems	Examination of urine for albumin and/or protein excretion Measurement of serum creatinine and creatinine clearance	Control of hyperglycaemia Control of hypertension and other cardiovascular risk factors Consultation with a nephrologist Limiting protein intake Avoiding nephrotoxic agents Early treatment of urinary tract infections
Atherosclerosis	History for risk factors and symptoms Examination: ECG and serum lipids measurements, peripheral pulses	Control of hyperglycaemia Control of hypertension Weight control Exercise Consultation with specialist: cardiologist, neurologist, vascular surgeon
Neuropathy	History of symptoms of pain, numbness and so forth Examination: orthostatic blood pressures, muscle strength, reflexes, and sensory function	Control of hyperglycaemia Avoidance of neurotoxic agents Education about the importance of routine evaluation, foot care, and specific treatments of neuropathy
Foot problems	History of symptoms of numbness, infection and peripheral vascular insufficiency Complete foot examination	Control hyperglycaemia Control of atherogenic risk Education about the importance and methods of foot care Referral to a chiropodist and vascular surgeon Referral for special shoes, shoe inlays, assistive mobility devices and rehabilitation services

hyperglycaemia. Because long-term complications involve vascular and neurological changes, it is not surprising to see that measures to decrease risk factors for cardiovascular and neurological disease are given high priority.

AETIOLOGY/EPIDEMIOLOGY

Diabetes mellitus is not a single entity but a heterogenous group of diseases with diverse causes that are incompletely understood.[51] Both genetic and environmental factors have been implicated and are under study. A combination of factors is most likely responsible for both IDDM and NIDDM. Although the same aetiological factors relate to both NIDDM and IDDM, the relative importance of individual factors differ. A *family history of diabetes* is a risk factor for developing the disease; however, the relationship of genetic transmission to diabetes mellitus is not yet well understood.

IDDM is considered an *autoimmune disorder that destroys the beta cell*. Evidence for an autoimmune basis of the disease includes the immunogenetic association of IDDM with HLA haplotypes, lymphocytic infiltration of beta cells in persons with IDDM, the experimental reversal of IDDM by immunosuppressant therapy, and increased rate of other autoimmune diseases in patients with IDDM.[54] Three *immunological markers* are *islet cell antibodies* (ICAs), *insulin autoantibodies* (IAAs), and *autoantibodies* to a 64,000M, islet protein.[47] These markers are present several years before the onset of hyperglycaemia, when most of the B cell functional reserve is lost.[47]

Multiple environmental agents have been proposed as important in the development of IDDM: viruses, diet, and toxins.[54]

An association between acute viral infections and the occurrence of IDDM in some communities has been noted. Certain viruses (coxsackie virus B, rubella, and mumps) have been implicated in particular cases.

The aetiology of NIDDM is not well understood. Overweight adults, especially those with a family history of diabetes, are at high risk for NIDDM. About 25% of persons with impaired glucose tolerance (IGT) and 30% to 35% of women with gestational diabetes develop NIDDM. Controversy persists about whether a pancreatic islet cell disorder or insulin resistance at peripheral and hepatic cell membranes is the primary disorder.

Epidemiological studies have *identified populations* of the *poor, the elderly*, and *the nonwhite* to be at *high risk for NIDDM*. The nonwhite populations also have higher incidence of diabetic complications and diabetes mortality rates that are double those of the white population.

PATHOPHYSIOLOGY

To understand the complex changes that diabetes causes throughout the body, it is helpful to consider those that occur when insulin deficit induces hyperglycaemia, those that occur when there is an acute metabolic crisis, and those that occur as a result of vascular and neurological defects. Each is discussed below.

Hyperglycaemia

Normally, when insulin is present, glucose intake (or glucose production) in excess of caloric needs is stored as glycogen in the cells of the liver and muscle or as fat. These processes of glycogenesis and lipogenesis prevent *hyperglycaemia* (blood glucose concentration > 6.1 mmol/L). When *insulin deficit* is present, four metabolic derangements lead to hyperglycaemia:

1. Transport of glucose across cell membranes diminishes.
2. Glycogenesis diminishes, and excess glucose remains in the blood.
3. Glycolysis increases; thus glycogen stores are reduced and "liver" glucose is added to the blood continually rather than when needed.
4. Gluconeogenesis increases, and more "liver" glucose is added to the blood from the breakdown (catabolism) of amino acids and glycerol from triglycerides.

The five classic signs of hyperglycaemia are:

1. Polydipsia
2. Polyuria
3. Polyphagia
4. Weight loss
5. Fatigue

Associated with the hyperglycaemia from the insulin deficit are abnormal levels of free fatty acids, cholesterol, and triglycerides in the blood.

Cellular Starvation

Blood glucose concentration is high in uncontrolled diabetes mellitus, yet cells are subjected to starvation conditions. Insulin deficiency impairs the uptake of glucose in insulin-dependent peripheral tissues (skeletal muscle and adipose tissue). If glucose is not available, muscle cells metabolize their own glycogen supply, and in prolonged fasting, they may use free fatty acids and ketones. Brain cells are not insulin-dependent and must have a constant supply of glucose; they can utilize ketones for part of their energy requirement.

Similarly, the uptake of amino acids is impaired. Instead of protein synthesis, *proteins are catabolized* and the amino acids are used to provide the substrate necessary for gluconeogenesis in the liver. Because of impaired metabolism, fatigue, loss of weight, and loss of strength may occur, with stunting of growth in children. Insulin deficiency can lead to the increased mobilization and metabolism of fats. Instead of lipogenesis, lipolysis occurs when insulin deficiency is severe, as in IDDM. Increased fatty acids, triglycerides, and glycerol circulate and provide the liver with substrates for ketogenesis and gluconeogenesis. There is a resultant production of ketones (highly acidic, intermediate metabolites of fat). *Ketosis* is the condition of ketone excess in the blood. If severe enough, ketosis can lead to a form of metabolic acidosis and coma, *diabetic ketoacidosis*.

In NIDDM ketosis is usually absent. There seems to be enough effective insulin to suppress the breakdown of fats, but not enough or not enough effective insulin to control blood glucose at normal levels.

Insulin Resistance

Insulin can be present in the blood in normal and even in abnormally high amounts, yet be unable to effect cellular processes. In this condition, called *insulin resistance*, peripheral and hepatic cells are insensitive to insulin. Insulin resistance may be caused by any of several factors: decreased number of insulin receptors, decreased insulin binding, and/or postreceptor defects and hyperglycaemia. *Insulin resistance is a major component of obesity and NIDDM.*

An exogenous source of animal insulin, particularly beef insulin, leads to the development of insulin antibodies. A rare *syndrome* of insulin resistance occurs in which insulin requirement exceeds 200 u/24 hr.

Hyperosmolality

A major pathophysiological alteration associated with hyperglycaemia is hyperosmolality. Blood glucose concentrations of 3.3–5.6 mmol/L correlate with normal blood osmolality values of 280 to 290 mosmol/kg. Hyperglycaemia increases blood osmolality. Increases in blood glucose content and blood osmolality lead to *dehydration* by two mechanisms.

1. Glycosuria and osmotic diuresis ensue when blood glucose concentrations exceed the renal threshold. Large amounts of water and electrolytes may be lost, along with loss of calories.
2. Fluid shifts from the intracellular compartment to the more highly concentrated extracellular compartment, resulting in intracellular fluid deficit.

Osmotic diuresis increases urine volume (*polyuria*). Thirst is stimulated, and the patient drinks large amounts of fluid (*polydipsia*). Because of the calorie loss and cellular starvation, the appetite increases, and the person eats more (*polyphagia*). When combined with *loss of body weight* and *fatigue*, the "three p's" (polyuria, polydipsia, and polyphagia) are the classic signs of hyperglycaemia. These symptoms are usually less severe in NIDDM, but the risks of dehydration are still present.

Polydipsia is important in preventing hypovolaemia because the resultant increase in fluid intake compensates for excess fluid losses caused by polyuria. As long as intravascular fluid volume is sufficient to maintain renal perfusion and glomerular filtration, the osmotic diuresis continues. When the fluid deficit is great enough to contract the intravascular fluid space and thus impair kidney function, *oliguria may signal a very severe fluid deficit.*

Hyperglycaemic, Hyperosmolar, Nonketotic Coma (HHNC)

Blood glucose levels may exceed 55.6 mmol/L, urinary glucose may be 5% to 10%, and serum osmolality may exceed 370 to 380 mosmol/kg in the absence of blood ketones. Coma in these circumstances is termed hyperglycaemic, hyperosmolar, nonketotic coma (HHNC) and occurs in NIDDM. Most frequently, HHNC occurs in the elderly, debilitated, and those who have impairments of mobility or cognition. So long as persons with hyperglycaemia and glycosuria can respond to thirst and replace fluids lost by glycosuria and osmotic diuresis, the risk of HHNC is diminished.

If fluid intake is diminished and dehydration ensues, the risk becomes greater. Frequently an associated illness increases fluid losses (fever, diarrhoea, vomiting) and insulin-antagonist hormones. Often, HHNC develops slowly over a period of days, and patients or carers may not identify the need for increased fluid intake. The elderly have less accurate thirst sensations, and they and people who are acutely ill may not have access to fluids.

HHNC may also develop in nondiabetic people receiving enteral or parenteral nutrition if hyperglycaemia is induced. Adequate fluid intake and prompt recognition and treatment of hyperglycaemia reduce the risk of HHNC in these people. In some studies,[51] the mortality rate from HHNC is reported to be as high as 40% to 60%.

Blood hyperosmolality, marked dehydration, and resultant fluid shifts decrease intracellular fluid volume. Cerebral dysfunction reflects cell dehydration and is manifested by changes in neurological parameters. Laboratory findings reflect the fluid deficit and hyperosmolar state: normal to high serum sodium and chloride concentrations, elevated glucose concentration, elevated haematocrit, and elevated blood urea level.

Diabetic Ketoacidosis (DKA)

Diabetic ketoacidosis (DKA), a severe metabolic disorder, is characterized by hyperglycaemia, hyperosmolality, and *metabolic acidosis*. The acidosis differentiates DKA from HHNC, as can be seen in Table 20-2. Six clinical signs are characteristic of DKA: dehydration, lethargy, Kussmaul's breathing, flushed face, fruity breath odour, and nausea and vomiting.

DKA is preventable and treatable. The mortality rate of 100% in the preinsulin era has steadily decreased. It is most frequently seen in people with IDDM but can occur in NIDDM. It is usually precipitated in the known diabetic by stressors that increase insulin needs, although it may occur when diabetes is out of control because of noncompliance with prescribed therapy.

A frequent precipitating factor is an *infection*, such as those of the urinary or respiratory tracts. Other major stressors that can precipitate diabetic ketoacidosis are surgery, trauma, major illnesses, therapy with steroids, and emotional upset. Occasionally diabetic ketoacidosis is the initial symptom in adults with undiagnosed diabetes, and it is often the initial problem in children with diabetes.

Increased lipolysis, oxidation of fats, and ketogenesis result in increased levels of organic acid (ketones) in body fluids. As ketones "use up" the body's alkali reserve for buffering, the pH of the blood decreases. Kussmaul breathing is stimulated to compensate for the metabolic acidosis. The *osmotic diuresis* is *made worse* by the *ketonaemia* and from *protein catabolism*, which increases the nitrogen load to the kidney. *Ketones give the breath a fruity odour.* When the *extracellular fluid deficit is severe*, polyuria may decrease, and *anuria may be seen*. The detection of signs and symptoms of hyperglycaemia, urinary ketones, sleepiness, "air hunger," nausea, and vomiting can alert diagnosed patients to seek medical help early so that prompt treatment can be given.

Macrovascular Changes

Atherosclerosis is a macrovascular disease. The vascular changes occur in the large arteries and are the same as those seen in nondiabetics. It is well known, however, that diabetics are prone to develop atherosclerosis at an earlier age, that the disease progresses faster, and that it is more severe and extensive in diabetics than in nondiabetics. In addition, the complications of athersclerosis occur more frequently in diabetics than in nondiabetics. Coronary artery disease and cerebrovascular disease are three times more common, and peripheral disease is five times more common. People with NIDDM develop macrovascular changes more frequently than do people with IDDM. Diabetes is associated with various atherogenic factors: abnormal lipid metabolism, changes in platelet adhesion, and hormonal changes (Chapter 17).

Insulin plays a major role in the metabolism of fats. *Lipid disorders* are frequently found in people with diabetes mellitus. *Hyperinsulinism* also may be an atherosclerogenic factor.[34] In IDDM, peripheral hyperinsulinism may occur as a result of sufficient exogenous insulin given to suppress hepatic glucose output. In NIDDM, insulin resistance is often accompanied by excessive pancreatic secretion of insulin. Persistently elevated insulin levels have been associated with hypertension, elevated very low density lipid (VLDL) and decreased high density lipid (HDL) cholesterol concentrations, as well as with atherosclerosis.[34] *Hypertension* has long been known to accelerate atherosclerosis; in diabetes, the combination of uncontrolled hyperglycaemia and uncontrolled hypertension is particularly damaging to the vasculature.

Decreased lumens of large blood vessels compromise the delivery of oxygen to tissues and can cause tissue ischaemia, resulting in *cerebrovascular disease, coronary artery disease, renal artery stenosis*, and *peripheral vascular disease*. Approximately three fourths of all cerebrovascular accidents are related to diabetes; and cardiovascular disease is the most common cause of death among older diabetics.

Microvascular Changes

Microvascular changes occur in both IDDM and NIDDM and are unique to diabetes; that is, the microvascular lesions do not occur in nondiabetics. These changes occur most frequently in people with IDDM. Tissue damage in organs is caused by a combination of atherosclerotic changes in large vessels and the defects in the microcirculation. *Changes in the microvasculature are particularly damaging to the retina, kidney, and nerves.* Two structural changes in the capillary are *thickening of the basement membrane* and *increased glycosylation of the collagenous* and *reticular fibres of the blood vessels.*[28] Increased rigidity of the vessel wall, decreased permeability of the vessel wall, capillary hypertension, and changes in blood flow through the capillary are some of the changes that interact to affect organ perfusion. Organ perfusion is increased early in the disease process, and the resultant haemodynamic changes may play a role in further structural damage. Later in the disease process, blood flow is impeded, and decreased organ perfusion results. *A history of hyperglycaemia is thought to play a major role in the development of microvascular lesions.*

Nephropathy

One of the major results of microvascular changes is alterations in renal structure and function. Four types of lesions can occur: pyelonephritis, glomerular lesions, arteriosclerosis of the renal arteries and the afferent and efferent arterioles, and tubular lesions. *Diabetic nephropathy* is characterized by *albuminuria, hypertension,* and *progressive renal insufficiency.*[28]

The progression of nephropathy has been well documented in people with IDDM. The usual pattern begins with a silent period, with no clinically observable signs of nephropathy, that exists for about 15 years. However, researchers have demonstrated that microvascular changes occur soon after diagnosis. *Glomerular hypertrophy* related to mesangial capillary enlargement is often associated with increased kidney size.[41] An *increase in glomerular filtration rate* is typically found after the onset of hyperglycaemia. There is early onset of *microalbuminaemia,* defined as albuminuria of 30 to 300 mg/24 hr, that precedes by many years clinically detectable proteinuria (over 300 mg/24 hr).

Clinical period

Tests to detect *microalbuminaemia* are not yet widely available,[45] whereas tests to measure larger amounts of albumin or protein are commonly used. The clinical onset of detectable *proteinuria* can thus be quite late in the course of nephropathy. As renal insufficiency develops, the *serum creatinine concentration* and *the blood urea increase,* and other signs and symptoms of renal insufficiency and failure appear (Chapter 25).

Diabetes is present in approximately 17% of patients treated for end-stage renal disease in Britain. The incidence is much higher in patients who develop diabetes before age 20 years. After a duration of 20 years, the chance of a diabetic person developing renal disease is estimated at 40% for those whose diabetes was diagnosed before age 20 years, and 2% to 4% in those diagnosed after age 20.[60] About equal numbers of people with each type of diabetes develop ESRD each year. This occurs because of the greater number of people with NIDDM (90%) than with IDDM (10%). Attention is directed towards control or prevention of factors known to increase the progression of renal disease in diabetics.

The *normalization of blood glucose levels* and the *control of hypertension* are high priorities. Recently, the use of a *lowered protein intake* (40 g/24 hr) and decreased use of animal protein are being evaluated in research studies for their effectiveness in slowing the progression of microalbuminaemia, hyperfiltration, and further renal damage.[28] *All nonpregnant adults with diabetes currently are encouraged to limit their daily protein intake to 0.8 g/kg of body weight.* This early intervention is an attempt to modify the haemodynamic changes occurring in the glomeruli by reducing the nitrogen load of the glomerular filtrate. ACE inhibitors have been shown to reduce microalbuminaemia and are being evaluated for their effectiveness in decreasing the rate of development of nephropathy.[45] The value of controlling hyperglycaemia in reversing some of the haemodynamic changes that occur within the glomerulus has been shown in animal and human volunteer studies;

reversal of hyperfiltration and renal hypertrophy that were induced by amino acids in diabetic subjects occurred when hyperglycaemia was corrected.[20]

The treatment and nursing care of renal insufficiency in people with diabetes are similar to that in nondiabetics. It is important to remember that as renal insufficiency develops, the patient receiving insulin may require *less* insulin because it will be excreted more slowly. Renal transplantation is the treatment of choice, because diabetic complications progress rapidly in many patients who receive dialysis. If transplantation is not possible, dialysis is necessary to maintain life. Dialysis is often instituted earlier for those with diabetes and renal failure than for nondiabetics because renal failure causes progression of other complications such as neuropathy and retinopathy in the diabetic. There have been improved survival rates with dialysis for diabetic patients over the last decade. The improved rates may be due to beginning dialysis earlier, to improved control of hypertension, and to improved technical management of dialysis. Short-term survival rates at 5 years or less are now equivalent to those attained by transplantation.[41] Islet cell transplantation or pancreatic transplantation are being performed at the time of kidney transplantation in some medical centres.

Diabetic Retinopathy

Two percent of diabetic people are likely to develop difficulty in seeing as a result of diabetic retinopathy and diabetic macular oedema,[8a] the latter seen most frequently in those with NIDDM.[17] After 10 years, half of all patients with IDDM have diabetic retinopathy, whereas after 15 to 20 years, 1 in 10 patients with NIDDM will have retinopathy.[28]

Macular oedema is characterized by retinal thickening, hard exudates, and/or areas of nonperfusion in the macular area. Destruction of the macular retina results in loss of central vision. Diabetes is the leading cause of blindness in people between the ages of 20 and 65 years. In addition to retinopathy, the diabetic person is also subject to increased *cataract* formation. *Cataracts may be caused by prolonged hyperglycaemia that results in swelling of the lens and opacity formation.*

There are no symptoms of early retinal changes, and there may be no symptoms even when retinopathy is advanced. Early detection requires a complete ophthalmological examination. All patients with NIDDM should be referred at diagnosis to an ophthalmologist, and then seen yearly. (The disease of NIDDM usually has been present long before diagnosis.) All patients with IDDM should be referred to an ophthalmologist for follow-up 5 years after diagnosis and yearly thereafter.

Vitrectomy, the removal of vitreous humour that has been infiltrated by haemorrhage, is another treatment for retinopathy. The removed vitreous humor is replaced by saline solution; unfortunately improved vision does not always result. Refer to Chapter 30 for a discussion of care, assistive devices, and referral sources for rehabilitative services for the blind and for those with low vision. See page 509 for modifications useful in helping the visually impaired individual manage the diabetes regimen.

Neuropathy

Diabetes may affect peripheral sensory and motor nerves, the autonomic nervous system, or the central nervous system. Multiple and varied symptoms may result, depending on the neurons involved. The most common type of diabetic neuropathy is *symmetric peripheral polyneuropathy*.

Approximately 12% of patients display neuropathy on diagnosis of diabetes, and over 60% will have neuropathy after 25 years.[60] It is seen in both IDDM and NIDDM. As with all neuropathological syndromes, the pathology includes altered nerve conduction that is related to ischaemia and/or impaired neural metabolism. Usually the first symptom is *bilateral sensory loss in the distal lower extremities;* later, the upper extremities may be affected in a "stocking and glove" distribution. This sensory loss impairs the ability of the patient to detect pressure or pain. It is a major risk factor for amputation of the lower extremities. *The inability to detect pressure or pain in the feet often leads to neuropathological ulcers, infections, gangrene, and trauma. It is essential that patients with sensory loss be vigilant in performing foot care* and in protecting the feet from injury (for example, not walking barefoot).

Treatment includes *control of hyperglycaemia.* When neuropathy is painful, treatment includes one or more psychotherapeutic agents such as amitriptyline, or drugs usually used for anticonvulsant therapy (such as carbamazepine).

All neuropathological syndromes cause considerable distress to patients; on the whole, treatment is palliative. Safety issues become a major concern when patients develop orthostatic hypotension, hypoglycaemic unawareness, or both.

Two *autonomic neuropathies* are of special concern in the management of hyperglycaemia. *Delayed gastric emptying* slows the delivery of glucose to the blood from food intake. Insulin timing in relation to meals may need to be altered to prevent the occurrence of hypoglycaemia. In addition, measures may include small, liquid, low-fibre, low-fat meals, and metoclopramide. *Hypoglycaemic unawareness* impairs the person's ability to detect and treat early hypoglycaemia. It may necessitate maintaining an increased level of blood glucose as a therapeutic goal. It is essential that patients with these disorders, and their families, be well educated about the prevention and treatment of hypoglycaemia.

Lower Extremity Changes

Macrovascular changes, microvascular changes, and neuropathies cause changes in the lower extremities. The interrelationships of vascular and nerve changes in diabetic foot lesions, which often result in amputation because of gangrene.

Amputation occurs 15 times more frequently in diabetic persons than in nondiabetic persons; 16% of diabetic patients require a lower-leg amputation at some time.[46, 60a] Survival rates after amputation are very low (50% for the first 3 years; 40% after the first 5 years).[36]

The *three most common causes of amputation in diabetes* are *gangrene* (90%), *infection* (71%), and *nonhealing ulcer* (65%).[36] *Dry gangrene* occurs when tissue death is not associated with inflammatory changes; *autoamputation* (spontaneous detachment) is often the treatment of choice for toes affected by dry gangrene. The area is kept dry during the process with close monitoring of the integrity of proximal tissues. In contrast, *wet gangrene* is tissue death coupled with inflammation. Septicaemia and septic shock may occur. Antibiotic therapy, debridement, and, often, amputation are treatment measures. Infections and nonhealing ulcers often lead to gangrene.

Infections of the lower extremity start in cracks in hypertrophied and dry skin, from ingrown toenails, under corns and calluses, and in traumatized tissues. A *neurotropic ulcer* is one that develops under corns or calluses and is insensitive to pain. Fifteen percent of people with diabetes have skin ulcers.[36] Infections in ulcers can appear superficial but be quite invasive. A recent clinical study found "clinically silent" osteomyelitis in 68% of ulcers; 64% of the ulcers had no associated signs of inflammation.[46]

Accurate diagnosis of osteomyelitis has been reported with the use of 24-hour leukocyte scanning. This new noninvasive test has more sensitivity in identifying osteomyelitis than roentgenograms, bone scans, or 4-hour leukocytic scanning tests.[46]

In addition to antibiotics, *ulcer debridement* and *vascular reconstruction are commonly used to facilitate wound repair in diabetic foot ulcers.*

Absence of weight-bearing is often necessary for healing of diabetic foot ulcers. Extra-depth shoes with custom-designed plastic insoles may help prevent recurrent ulcers.

Foot care

Prevention of ulcers, trauma, and infections of the lower extremities is the key to prevention of amputation. The need for daily foot care, including inspection, cannot be overemphasized. The patient can use a mirror to examine soles of the feet. The nurse's effectiveness in teaching about foot care will be greater if the patient has previously included foot care as a part of daily care. Box 20-3 contains guidelines for instruction. Also teach patients to take shoes and stockings off at each medical visit and ask the doctor to examine the feet. Foot evaluation is recommended for all diabetic patients; chiropodist services are essential when there are vascular changes, neuropathy, or foot lesions such as calluses, corns, or bunions.

Nursing Process

Assessment

Subjective data

If the patient is acutely ill, the priority assessment is focused on the extent of metabolic imbalance and its effects on the patient's well-being. Does the patient complain of lethargy, air hunger, or the classic signs of hyperglycaemia? Collect specific data about nausea, vomiting, abdominal pain, last food intake, and time and dosage of oral hypoglycaemic agents, insulin, or both.

Take a thorough history to determine whether any conditions are present that affect blood glucose concentrations:

1. Food intake in excess of energy requirements
2. Infection or other acute illness
3. Stress related to psychological or social factors
4. Drugs or other treatments that affect blood glucose
5. Omission of required insulin or oral hypoglycaemic agent

Guidelines for Care 20-3

Diabetic foot care

Wear well-fitting shoes and clean stockings at all times when walking, and *never walk bare-footed.*

Bathe feet daily and dry them well, paying particular attention to area between the toes.

Do not self-treat calluses, corns, or ingrown toe-nails; a chiropodist should be consulted if these are present.

Bath water should be 29.5° to 32° C (85° to 90° F) and should be tested with a bath thermometer or the elbow before immersing the feet.

Avoid heating pads, hot water bottles, and warming feet against radiator or close to fireplace.

Institute measures that help increase circulation to the lower extremities:

Avoid smoking.

Avoid crossing legs when sitting.

Protect extremities when exposed to cold.

Avoid immersing feet in cold water.

Use socks or stockings that do not apply pressure to the legs at specific sites.

Institute a regimen of exercises (Chapter 4).

Inspect feet daily and report any cuts, cracks, redness, blisters, or other signs of trauma to health care provider so that early treatment can be instituted.

If feet are dry, use a lubricating lotion or cream; if moist, use powder.

Do not limit nursing assessment to the determination of metabolic status. It is also important to assess, soon after admission, the patient's knowledge and coping ability in diabetes management. Unless the patient is acutely ill, it is usually wise to complete a general nursing assessment before focusing on diabetes and its related care. There are two reasons for this. First, the nurse can learn a great deal about the patient's perspective of diabetes self-care during the general interview. Does the patient specify the disease, the regimen of therapy, and state special needs relating to diabetes? Is the patient concerned about how the plans for diet, activity, monitoring, medications, and foot care will differ from home schedules? A person well educated in diabetes management will be assertive in planning with the nurse how to minimize disruption of care while in the hospital.

The second reason to do a general assessment before focusing on diabetes is related to the reason for which the patient was admitted. Most newly diagnosed adults are not hospitalized; instead, they are treated in ambulatory settings. The primary concern at the time of hospitalization may be related to fears of blindness, amputation, heart attack or stroke, or a non-diabetes-related medical problem. These concerns and expectations about treatment need to be explored before those of diabetes for the patient who believes diabetes problems to be secondary in importance.

Begin to explore how well the patient copes with this chronic illness with questions such as: How easy or difficult is it to stay on the diet? What is difficult or easy about diabetes or its treatment for you? Asking the patient to describe a typical day (meal intake and times, sleep and work schedules, social activities, exercise and monitoring schedules) will help the nurse understand how the therapeutic regimen is incorporated into the patient's life-style and help identify areas of conflict and strengths of the patient.

Assess for the presence of vascular and neuropathological complications: How is your vision? Do you have any problems with blood pressure, eyes, kidney, circulation, sensation? Ask these questions during the general nursing history. Most importantly, if the patient answers yes to any of these questions, what special care is needed?

In assessing learning needs, whenever possible observe actual self-care practices: insulin injection, urine or SBM testing, foot care, and so on.

Because education is an integral part of the treatment, assess the *learning needs* related to self-care of *all* patients who are diabetic. Do this assessment early in the hospitalization in order to increase the time available for teaching. Unfortunately, many patients who have had diabetes for a long time may have inadequate knowledge, skills, or attitudes to manage their diabetes at optimal levels. The development of vascular or neurological complications may require learning modifications of self-care measures.

Objective data

Objective data to be collected include the following:
1. Level of consciousness
2. Blood and urinary glucose concentrations
3. Blood and urinary ketone concentrations
4. Blood urea nitrogen
5. Blood pressure, pulse, and respiratory pattern
6. Body temperature
7. Body weight
8. Urinary volume (per timed period)
9. Appearance of mucous membranes and skin
10. Presence of skin lesions
11. Skin turgor
12. Breath odour

When an acute metabolic crisis is suggested by the patient's clinical findings, further assessment is related to *metabolic acidosis* and *fluid imbalance* (p. 499).

Assessment of any adult patient with diabetes mellitus also includes data for identifying *abnormalities related to vascular or neurological changes.* Measures directed towards prevention or treatment of these complications may be required. In addition, the patient often needs assistance with activities of daily living and modification of diabetes self-care activities. Assessment should always include attention to the *lower extremities, vision, cardiovascular-renal status,* and *neurological status.*

Diagnostic tests

Fasting blood glucose and *glucose tolerance* tests are most commonly used in diagnosis. Directions about timing and fasting requirements for a particular test must be explained to the patient. For the glucose tolerance test, give the patient specific, written directions because many variables interfere with the accuracy of this test.

The table lists other tests that are used less commonly. Cortisone- and ACTH-stimulating tests are provocative tests that challenge the capacity to maintain normal blood glucose levels when a counterregulatory hormone is administered. The C-peptide test can be used to differentiate whether the source of circulating insulin is endogenous or exogenous, as well as to evaluate pancreatic secretion. C-peptide tests and serum insulin measurements are used more frequently in research than in clinical practice.

Monitoring glucose control

In the past, good to excellent control was defined by higher levels of blood glucose than is now thought to be ideal. Previously 5% to 10% of daily calorie loss through glycosuria was considered acceptable. Patients who received their diabetes education before 1980 may need reeducation about desired levels of control.

Once the diagnosis of diabetes mellitus is made, measurements of blood glucose are essential in evaluating the effectiveness of treatment measures. Tests that measure blood glucose levels may be ordered to be *fasting; postprandial* (1 hour, 2 hours or 3 hours after eating); and *preprandial* (½ to 1 hour before meals). All give useful information about control of blood glucose in relation to food, fasting, exercise, and the particular insulin or oral hypoglycaemic agent being used.

Laboratory tests

For the hospitalized patient, a fasting blood glucose test often is ordered daily. Tests by the laboratory may be ordered at other times. In addition, capillary blood glucose obtained by fingerstick is often ordered before meals and at bedtime—more frequently for the person in acute metabolic crisis or if on sliding scale insulin.

When trying to correlate test results of laboratory and bedside meters, it is helpful to consider that normal values for glucose differ according to whether measurement is made using whole blood or plasma/serum, to the source of the whole blood, and to whether the patient was fasting or not. Laboratory tests of blood glucose are often performed on samples of plasma or serum, whereas capillary whole blood is tested in bedside meters. Plasma/serum glucose levels are usually 10% to 15% higher than simultaneously measured whole blood glucose levels. In addition, capillary whole blood in the fasting patient is normally 0.3 to 0.6 mmol/L higher than venous whole blood; capillary whole blood postprandially is normally 1.1-3.9 mmol/L higher than venous whole blood.[33]

Self-monitoring of blood glucose (SBM)

The technology now available for self blood glucose monitoring (SBM) has made it possible for people with diabetes to manage their blood glucose at near physiological levels.

Increasingly, those with diabetes mellitus are using SBM to determine their metabolic status rather than testing urine for glucose. Various types of tests for home blood glucose monitoring correlate well with laboratory measurement of blood glucose level. A reflectance meter adds to the cost and inconvenience of monitoring but gives a precise numerical value. Some test strips (Chemstrip bG, Visiden) do not require a meter and indicate only the *range* of blood glucose. For many patients, knowing the range is sufficient.

Self-monitoring has been found to facilitate glycaemic control in all people with diabetes. It is essential for patients who are pregnant, for those who use multi-injection insulin regimens or pump therapy, and for all those who want ideal glycaemic control.

SBM is very helpful to the patient in making decisions about exercise and food and in preventing hypoglycaemia or severe hyperglycaemia and metabolic crisis. Analysis of the patient's log of blood glucose levels, food intake, medication usage, and so on can uncover specific problems in blood glucose control. Patients can modify insulin timing or dosage, food intake, and/or exercise. Some patients, after learning the use of insulin dosage algorithms, adjust insulin dosages according to a given protocol.

Certain factors should be considered before recommending blood glucose monitoring to a particular patient. Those with neuropathy or vascular or inflammatory conditions of the fingers may be at risk for tissue injury from repeated pricking of the finger. Patients may not perceive the expense, discomfort, and inconvenience as barriers. Visual acuity must be adequate to "read" the colour changes of the test strips or to read the digital display of the meter or a "talking" meter must be used. Those who believe that they have managed their diabetes well in the past with urine testing may have little incentive to do blood glucose monitoring. The most important factor, perhaps, is that the patient and the health care provider intend to use the information gained to achieve better blood glucose control than can be obtained with urine testing.

Doctors' recommendations for frequency of testing vary greatly. Some patients are advised to test before and after meals and at bedtime. For others who have established stable control, doctors may recommend testing frequently during one day of the week and whenever they feel ill.

To do the testing, the person sticks a finger and applies a drop of blood to a commercially prepared glucose oxidase stick. The timing for the reading and the preparation of the specimen are very important in obtaining accurate results.

Monitoring of glycosylated proteins

Glycosylation results in the binding of glucose to proteins, and the amount of glycosylation of a particular protein correlates with blood glucose levels. Tests most frequently measure glycosylated haemoglobin A or Al_c to monitor past blood glucose control.

Glycosylated haemoglobin accumulates during the lifespan of red blood cells and reflects the *average* glucose level over several weeks. In normal people the level of Hb Al_c is 3% to 6%. The goal of therapy is for the person with diabetes mellitus to be able to maintain Hb Al_c within normal or at least no greater than one and one half times normal.

This test is the first measurement of how well patients have controlled blood glucose over a period of time. It is also used in research studies of blood glucose control and to differentiate noncompliance from an acute illness that results in an elevated level of blood glucose. Findings can be summarized as follows:

1. Any level of blood glucose with a high Hb Al$_c$ value suggests poor compliance over the previous 6 to 12 weeks
2. A high blood glucose level with a low Hb Al$_c$ value indicates recent onset of a hyperglycaemic process, such as an infection or frequent episodes of hypoglycaemia

The glycosylation of other proteins can also be measured. One test, fructosamine assay, indicates blood glucose control over the past 2 or 3 weeks. This assay is useful in pregnant women with IDDM or gestational diabetes and in puberty, when body changes are frequent and rapid.

Urine testing

Some patients monitor glucose levels by urine testing, even though the information obtained is imprecise and difficult to use in daily decision making about ways to achieve "strict" control. Nurses can help patients to understand that negative results of urine tests (in a patient with a renal threshold of ≥ 10 mmol/L) may mask significant hyperglycaemia. In contrast, some patients, often children, have low renal thresholds and can control blood glucoses at optimal levels with urine tests alone. Some patients combine urine testing with blood glucose testing to monitor blood glucose in time periods between blood tests.

Urine testing for the presence of ketone bodies should be encouraged for the following people:
1. All patients with IDDM (type I) with blood glucose over 13.9 mmol/L
2. All diabetics who feel ill

Often, a "double-voided" specimen is ordered as the sample to be obtained for urine testing of glycosuria. The patient is directed to empty the bladder one-half hour before the desired time of the specimen, drink water, and then void and test the freshly formed urine.

Patients should record and report the extent of glycosuria by *percentage* rather than by plus signs (+, ++, +++, ++++); plus marks do not correlate with the same percentage of glycosuria on all urine tests. This can lead to errors in interpretation of the test results.

The age of the individual, stability of disease, and renal threshold affect the doctor's decision in advising the patient to use urine testing. The nurse can assist the person in interpreting the urine test results and in understanding the rationale for the specific regimen.

Nursing analysis

Nursing analyses are determined from assessment of patient data. Possible nursing analyses for the person with diabetes mellitus may include, but are not limited to, the following:

Problems	Possible aetiologies
Altered nutrition: more than body requirements	Excessive intake in relation to metabolic needs, established eating patterns, knowledge deficit, noncompliance
Self-care deficit in one or more activities	Perceptual impairment (visual, sensory), motor impairment
Impaired skin integrity or high risk for impaired skin integrity	Pressure from ill-fitting shoes, lack of chiropody services, knowledge deficit about foot care, visual or mobility impairment hampering inspection
Fluid volume deficit: actual or high risk for	Polyuria, other fluid losses, decreased fluid intake, insulin deficit
Knowledge deficit (diabetes management)	Lack of exposure, poor recall, new diagnosis or new treatment, cognitive limitation
Noncompliance (with one or more aspects of diabetes regimen)	Cultural influences, established daily patterns of eating, activity, lack of resources

Planning: expected patient outcomes

Expected patient outcomes for the person with diabetes mellitus may include, but are not limited to, the following:
1. Blood glucose is at optimal level.
2. Ideal weight is maintained or achieved.
3. Is able to perform health care skills accurately, including insulin administration, test monitoring and interpretation of results, foot care, diet manipulation, and so forth.
4. Skin integrity is maintained; proper foot care is implemented.
5. Hydration is adequate.
6. Repeats accurate information about diabetes mellitus and measures for its control.
7. Can explain signs and symptoms of hypoglycaemia and hyperglycaemia and what to do when they occur.
8. Knows when to seek medical assistance.
9. Identifies one goal of improved health maintenance and states behaviour necessary to achieve goal.

Implementation

Assisting with achievement of therapeutic goals
Promoting nutrition

Diet is considered to be the keystone of therapy in both IDDM and NIDDM with three nutritional goals[1]:
1. Control of blood glucose and blood lipid levels
2. Achievement and maintenance of desirable body weight
3. Provision of adequate nutrition and balanced diet

Dietary recommendations
1. Calories should be sufficient to promote normal growth and activity in the child and to maintain *ideal* weight and activity in the adult.
2. Calorie intake should be as follows:
   a. Protein, 12% to 20% (0.8 g/kg body weight)
   b. Carbohydrate, 55% to 60%
   c. Fat less than 30%
3. The amount of carbohydrate is individualized and depends on the impact of carbohydrate on blood glucose and lipid levels and individual eating patterns.

4. No more than 10% of calories from fat should be from saturated fats and the remainder from unsaturated fats. Cholesterol should be restricted to less than 300 mg daily.
5. Foods with unrefined carbohydrates and foods with fibre should be incorporated into the diet. The amount of highly refined carbohydrates low in fibre should be reduced; the diet should include 25 to 30 g of plant fibre/1000 kcal.
6. Consistency in timing and the distribution of calories, carbohydrates, protein, and fat for each meal are most important in IDDM and in patients with NIDDM on insulin.
7. Weight control is more important in obese persons with NIDDM; balanced meals at consistent times aid in achieving this goal.
8. Sodium intake should be limited to 1000 mg/1000 kcal of total intake, not to exceed 3000 mg/day.
9. A variety of nutritive and nonnutritive sweeteners should be encouraged.
10. Alcohol should be used in moderation, if at all. Alcohol has 7 kcal/g when metabolized and must be included in calorie calculations. Patient should be aware of potential severe hypoglycaemia from alcohol.

Some evidence indicates that *water-soluble fibre* helps to reduce blood glucose levels and blood lipids and to enhance bowel function. Fibre content should be increased gradually to prevent abdominal discomfort. Additional fluids should be recommended when fibre intake is increased. Foods containing water-soluble fibre include the following:

1. Legumes
2. Oats
3. Barley
4. Fruit

Individualization of dietary recommendations for a particular patient has always been a principle of dietary therapy. This principle has been reinforced by recent knowledge about the many factors that influence the effect of specific starches on blood glucose levels. Beginning research indicates that some starches (complex carbohydrates) may raise blood glucose more than previously thought.

The term *glycaemic index* is used to describe the change in blood glucose levels from ingestion of specific foods compared with that induced by a standard glucose load.

Many factors, including the preparation of foods and the combination of foods, influence the glycaemic index. Too little is known at this time to make generalized recommendations using the glycaemic index. However, individual patients may use blood glucose monitoring to assess the effect of particular food intake. A second benefit of the knowledge gained by research on the glycaemic index is less reliance on *total* restriction of simple CHO. Small portions of foods containing sucrose can be eaten with meals, provided blood glucose levels are controlled.[19]

Patients may choose to include four "sweeteners" in their food. Aspartame and saccharin are nonnutritive sweeteners; fructose and sorbital are nutritive sweeteners, with a caloric value of 4 cal/g.

Principles of dietary planning. Should a nutritional history reveal that the patient's food intake and patterns of eating incorporate the above recommendations, few changes would be recommended. It is often said that the diet needed by a diabetic person is that needed by all persons. However, most people find it necessary to change dietary habits to reduce hyperglycaemia and maintain ideal weight. Recommendations need to be made with awareness of the difficulty with which people change established eating habits. It is best to start with the patient's current diet and make as few modifications as necessary to achieve therapeutic goals.

Dietary planning should include considerations of the following factors:

1. The patient's personal, cultural, or religious food preferences
2. Life-style: working hours, family composition, financial resources
3. Activity: activity patterns; timing and level of exercise; periods of exercise, work, and sleep
4. Hypoglycaemic drugs; onset, duration, and peak activity of insulin or oral hypoglycaemic agents
5. Other modifications needed in consistency or nutrient content
6. Personal perceptions of ideal body weight

Promoting exercise

Exercise is the second treatment modality of diabetes mellitus. Glucose can enter *active* muscle cells without the action of insulin and can then be oxidized to carbon dioxide and water in most patients; thus *exercise has a hypoglycaemic action*. Exercise also decreases insulin resistance by increasing the number or activity of insulin receptors and promoting weight loss in the obese diabetic.

People with type 2 diabetes (NIDDM) benefit from regular exercise for 30 minutes three or four times a week. Results of exercise are improved glucose tolerance, insulin sensitivity, and weight loss. In addition, aerobic exercise improves cardiovascular function and lipid profiles.[22]

There are some cautions about exercise that patients must know. Exercise in the presence of hyperglycaemia above 250 mg/100 ml can increase the hyperglycaemia and even promote ketosis. Very intense exercise, even in people with well-controlled blood glucose, can increase blood glucose levels.

Before an exercise programme begins, the patient should have a complete cardiovascular examination, including a stress ECG if over age 35. Working capacity can be evaluated to determine the level of exercise that can be instituted safely. The person with diabetes mellitus should be evaluated for retinopathy, neuropathy, and hypertension because particular types of exercises should be avoided in these conditions.[22]

Those people receiving insulin or oral hypoglycaemic agents should understand that diet and medications are planned around the usual activity level and pattern of exercise. Decisions about timing and duration of exercise are safer if the patient uses SBM. Optimal timing of exercise would be during periods of hyperglycaemia (but with blood glucose levels below 14.8 mmol/L) and *not* during the peak action of insulin. Hypoglycaemia is more likely to occur when exercise and peak action of insulin coincide. Encourage patients to use SBM one-half hour before beginning vigorous exercise and, if blood glucose is low (below 3.8 mmol/L), to eat a snack of complex carbohydrates and protein. Also encourage them to eat at 30-minute intervals during prolonged exercise. The increased sensitivity to insulin induced by exercise can last several hours and up to 3 days; inadequate food during this time can precipitate an episode of hypoglycaemia. Changes in activity level require changes in diet or medication.

Activity. In addition to stressing the importance of exercise, the nurse can assist the patient in planning how to incorporate regular exercise into the life-style after discharge. Previously sedentary adults should be encouraged to *gradually* increase activity and work up to 30 minutes of brisk walking, swimming, or low-impact aerobic exercises. Plans need to be reasonable and take into account previous activity level, cardiopulmonary status, mobility, and interests. For example, an elderly hemiplegic patient could be encouraged to do range-of-motion and leg-raising exercises, and a younger person with no disabilities could be encouraged to develop interest in a specific exercise or sports programme. Sports that are contraindicated for patients receiving insulin include those in which the dangers of hypoglycaemia increase the hazard of the sport (for example, scuba diving or sky diving).

Medications

Insulin. Insulin is necessary for the survival of patients with IDDM. It is also used to treat NIDDM in some patients in whom other measures have not achieved a desired level of blood glucose control.

The current trend in treatment is to achieve the best control of blood glucose possible for each individual, that is, to achieve blood glucose levels near normal limits if this can be done without significant hypoglycaemia.

Properties of insulin. Insulin preparations have four major properties that are incorporated into the prescription: (1) type of action, (2) strength, (3) species source, and (4) purity.

TYPE OF ACTION. All insulins are hypoglycaemic, but they differ in the speed with which they begin to act (*onset*), the period of time they have the strongest action (*peak*), and how long they act (*duration*). Insulins are classified as short,

intermediate, and long acting. Table 20-3 gives the characteristics of seven standard insulin preparations. Nurses need to know the characteristics of each in order to coordinate food and activity with insulin action. This coordination is necessary so that (1) insulin is available for optimal metabolism when food is taken, and (2) food is available while insulin is acting to prevent hypoglycaemic reactions.

Three principles are useful in coordinating food and hypoglycaemic medications:
1. Food must be taken after insulin (or oral agent) within the time of onset; for example, with regular insulin, food must be taken within 1 hour after injection.
2. Intermediate- or long-acting insulins require that a supplemental feeding be given, timed to match the peak action of the insulin, for example, an afternoon feeding if NPH insulin given at 7 AM.
3. With intermediate- or long-acting insulin a bedtime feeding is required so that glucose is available through the night.

STRENGTH. Insulin preparations are available in the concentration of insulin units in 1 ml volume, U-100 insulin, or 100 units/ml.

It is very important that the insulin concentration and the insulin syringe calibration match in units per millilitre to prevent errors in dosing.

SPECIES. In the past, most insulin was prepared from a combination of beef and pork pancreas. Single-species insulin (usually pork) could be obtained for patients with beef-insulin allergy or antibodies. (Pork insulin most closely resembles human insulin and is considered the least antigenic animal insulin.) Insulins available are highly purified to reduce hypersensitivity reactions.

"Human" insulin is either porcine (pork insulin modified enzymatically to structurally resemble human insulin) or bacterially produced by recombinant DNA techniques. It is increasingly prescribed in place of animal insulin, because it has less antigenicity than animal insulin, and it greatly expands the insulin resources of the world. The insulins available in Britain today appear in Table 20-4.

Insulin administration. Increasingly, doctors are attempting to simulate the normal bodily secretion of insulin that occurs in nondiabetics, that is, a continuous basal level of insulin that rapidly increases with food intake. In addition, they try to mimic the tendency for glucose to reach its lowest peak between 3 AM and 4 AM and a tendency for blood

Table 20-3 Action of insulin preparations

Type of insulin	Time of onset (hr)	Peak of action (hr)	Duration of action (hr)	Insulin appearance
Short acting				
soluble insulin	0.5-1	2-5	6-8	Clear
Intermediate acting				
Biphasic insulin	<2	4-12	Up to 24	Cloudy
Insulin suspension,				
isophane	<2	4-12	Up to 24	Cloudy
Long acting				
Insulin zinc suspension	2-3	6-15	Up to 30	Cloudy

glucose and basal insulin secretion to rise between 5 AM and 8 AM before breakfast (dawn phenomenon). A description of various regiments is presented in Box 20-4; regimens 3 to 6 are designed to mimic the normal endogenous secretion pattern. These regimens are termed *intensive therapy* and are aimed at "tight control" of blood glucose. Obviously the risk of hypoglycaemia is increased with intensive therapy.

The insulin type and dosage are ordered in anticipation of food, activity, and other factors that balance or affect the insulin requirements. Regardless of the particular regimen, consider the following information before administering insulin:

1. Time of onset, peak, and duration of the insulin
2. Availability of food or adequate glucose at these times of action
3. Plans for treating hypoglycaemia should it occur

Thus if a patient were ordered nothing by mouth for several hours, insulin should not be given until provision is made for an intravenous infusion of a dextrose solution.

ROTATION OF NEEDLE INSERTION SITES. The subcutaneous tissue of the upper arms, the anterior and lateral aspects of the thigh, most of the abdomen, and the buttocks may be used for insulin injections.[1a] It is very important that the site of injection of insulin be rotated to assure proper absorption of insulin and to prevent lipodystrophy.[1a] No injection site should be used more than once a month.

The older practice of randomly rotating sites between *anatomical areas such as the arms, thighs, buttocks, and abdomen* with each injection is no longer recommended. If possible *only one anatomical area is used throughout the patient's life* because the absorption rate of insulin varies among these sites.[1a] The rate of absorption of insulin from fastest to slowest is abdomen, arms, and legs. Some specialists are recommending that only the abdomen be used.[6,63] However, in a majority of instances it is not possible to use only one anatomical area.[13a] The abdomen or any other anatomical area might not provide a large enough surface area for multiple injections in a small person. Remember no one site should be used more than once a month and some persons will be on three to four injections a day, thus requiring 90 to 120 sites per month in one anatomical area. Some people have an aversion to injecting themselves in the abdomen, and others find it difficult to use arms or legs.

The most commonly used recommendation is rotation of sites within one *anatomical area until no more sites are available*, and then movement to another anatomical area.[13a,23a,23c] For most people, if this recommendation is followed a patient will use one anatomical area for 3 to 4 days up to several weeks. In some instances the person may use only two of the anatomical areas.[13a] That is, all sites in the arms will be used, then all sites in the abdomen will be used, and then the person will switch back to the arms.

Table 20-4 Examples of insulins available in the United Kingdom

Duration/source	Product	Manufacturer	Strength
Short acting			
Human	Humulin Actrapid	Novo Nordisk	U-100
	Humulin Velosulin	Novo Nordisk Wellcome	U-100
	Human Actrapid Penfill	Novo Nordisk	U-100
	Humulin S	Lilly	U-100
Pork	Velosulin	Novo Nordisk Wellcome	U-100
Beef	Hypurin Neutral	CP	U-100
Beef/Pork	Rapitard MC	Novo Nordisk	U-100
Intermediate-acting/Long-acting			
Human	Humulin Lente	Novo Nordisk	U-100
	Human Monotard	Lilly	U-100
	Human Ultratard	Novo Nordisk	U-100
	Humulin Zn	Lilly	U-100
	Human Insulatard	Novo Nordisk	U-100
	Human Protaphane	Novo Nordisk	U-100
	Humulin I	Lilly	U-100
	Pur-in Isophane	CP	U-100
Pork	Semitard MC	Novo Nordisk	U-100
	Insulatard	Novo Nordisk	U-100
Beef	Hypurin Lente	CP	U-100
	Hypurin Isophane	Novo Nordisk	U-100
	Hypurin Protamine Zinc	CP	U-100
Beef/Pork	Lentard MC	Novo Nordisk	U-100
Biphasic (all are U-100, Isophane/soluble)			
Human	Human Actraphane	Novo Nordisk	70/30
	Humulin M1	Lilly	90/10
	PenMix 10/90	Novo Nordisk	90/10
Pork	Initard 50/50	Novo Nordisk	50/50

Insulin therapy regimens

1. One injection of intermediate-acting insulin per day
   Most frequently used in people with NIDDM who are not controlled with diet and/or oral hypoglycaemic agents
   Does not mimic the normal endogenous pattern
   May be used with oral hypoglycaemic agents
2. Two injections of intermediate-acting insulin per day
   Used mostly in people with NIDDM
   Does not mimic the normal endogenous pattern
3. Split and mixed insulin regimen: injection of rapid-acting insulin and intermediate-acting insulin at breakfast and supper
   Used in many people with IDDM
   Theoretically, the morning rapid-acting insulin covers breakfast and early morning, the morning intermediate-acting insulin covers lunch and afternoon, the evening rapid-acting insulin covers the evening meal, and the evening intermediate-acting insulin covers the bedtime snack and the *basal level needed* during the night
4. Split and mixed insulin regimens (similar to No. 3 above), except that the evening intermediate-acting insulin is given at bedtime instead of at supper time
   Used in people with IDDM
   Theoretically provides better basal nighttime coverage and provides coverage for the natural prebreakfast elevation in glucose
5. Multidosage regimen: three injections of rapid-acting insulin, one before each meal; and one injection of intermediate insulin given at bedtime
   The rapid-acting insulin provides coverage for each meal
   The bedtime intermediate-acting insulin provides the nighttime basal level and coverage for the natural prebreakfast glucose elevation
6. Multidosage regimen: three injections of rapid-acting insulin, one before each meal; and an injection of long-acting insulin given at breakfast or at supper or split between breakfast and supper (provides the same coverage as No. 5 above)

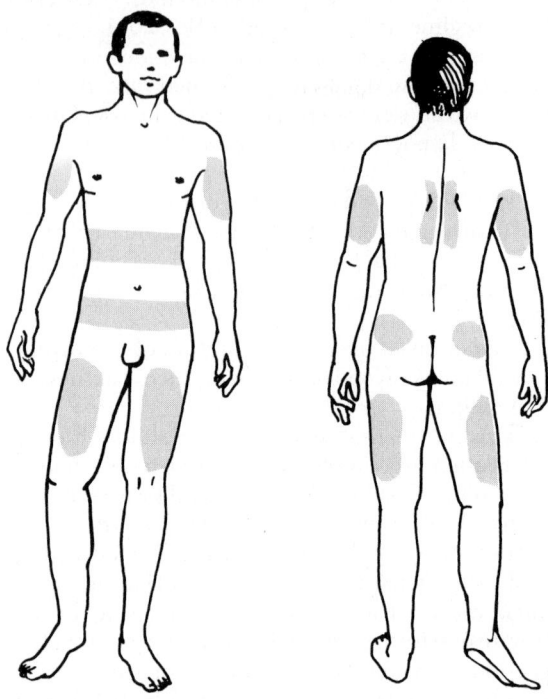

Fig. 20-1   Rotation of sites for insulin injection.

Important to remember is that the best, most effective plan for rotation of sites should be individualized for each person. The major areas for injection and the multiple sites within these areas are depicted in Fig. 20-1.

Two forms of *lipodystrophy* can occur: hypertrophy and atrophy. *Hypertrophy* is thickening of an injection site because fibrous scar tissue develops from repeated injections in the same site. A hypertrophic area is usually devoid of nerve endings, and the patient likes to reuse it because injections are painless. Absorption from this area is slow and erratic.

Atrophy is loss of subcutaneous fat. The cause is unknown. It is thought to result from repeated injections in the same site, faulty injection technique, or

impurities in the insulin. Some researchers have successfully treated atrophy by injecting purified insulin into atrophic areas.

SELF-INJECTION OF INSULIN. Most people are fearful of self-injection and would prefer to postpone learning this task; yet repeated practice is necessary if they are to safely administer an accurate dose using sterile technique. The nurse must teach this skill early and with attention to the patient's fear, whether that fear is or is not expressed.

One study supports the belief that adults can learn this skill most readily and cope best if the first self-injection is not delayed for practice with syringe, vials of medicine, or any other equipment.[64] Traditionally, the patient has been given an orange to inject as practice before self-injection. Instead, the researcher suggests that the patient perform self-injection first.

The nurse should firmly encourage the patient to hold the syringe, cleanse and pierce the skin, and inject the ordered insulin (or an equivalent dosage of sterile saline) from the syringe previously prepared by the nurse. Verbal encouragement and a guiding hand may be necessary for the patient to self-inject successfully. After adults experience self-injection, they are better able to focus on preparation of the insulin syringe (see Box 20-5 for guidelines in insulin administration).

Help patients to determine the quantity of disposable syringes and needles and other supplies needed for at least a month. Cotton wool balls purchased in bulk and a bottle of 70% ethyl alcohol, as compared with individually wrapped alcohol pledgets, can reduce costs.

Set up typical trays for injection at home to use in demonstrations and for patient practice. Discuss boxes or

---

20-5	### Guidelines for insulin administration

1. Always use an insulin syringe calibrated in the same units as the insulin.
2. Select insulin according to type, strength, species, purity, and brand name as specified by the prescription.
3. Rotate or gently roll or shake the bottle if it is other than soluble insulin.
4. Do not inject cold insulin; allow it to come to room temperature if it is stored in the refrigerator before using.
5. Examine intermediate- and long-acting insulin vials for suspension of insulin (cloudy, appearance); do not use if it is *not* cloudy. Examine human insulin for a frosty or clumping of precipitate—do not use if present.
6. Check for and remove any air bubbles after insulin is drawn into the syringe (do not use an air bubble to clear the needle after the injection).
7. When mixing insulins, do not vary the sequence in which two insulins are drawn into the same syringe; inject air into both bottles—first into intermediate and then into soluble; withdraw the insulin first from the soluble vial and then from the longer-acting insulin vial. Commercially premixed isophane and soluble insulin may be prescribed.
8. Insert the needle into fatty tissue closer to muscle than to skin; if there is little subcutaneous tissue, "pinch" up the skin and use a 45-degree angle and a ³/₈ or ¹/₂ inch needle. Use a 90-degree angle when the fat pad is large.

---

trays that can be used at home to keep all equipment together. The equipment should be stored on a shelf or closet, out of reach of children and out of sight.

INSULIN PUMPS. Very close control of blood glucose can be achieved for some patients with IDDM with an insulin infusion pump. External insulin pumps, which are battery operated and portable, deliver regular insulin at a basal rate (continuously) and a bolus dose at meal times. The insulin is delivered from a reservoir through tubing to a needle placed in subcutaneous tissue. The external pump is only disconnected to change the needle (every 2 to 3 days).

About the same size as a small calculator, the external pump can be worn on a belt at the waist or in a pocket. The patient requires considerable education to ensure safe and effective insulin delivery. Complications include hypoglycaemia, infection at the site of needle insertion, and rapid onset of ketoacidosis if the pump becomes disconnected. Pumps do not decrease the amount of attention the patient must give to diabetes management; pumps require the use of frequent SBM and decisions about food, exercise and insulin dosage. Insulin pumps are expensive; however blood glucose levels must be carefully monitored, and the insulin delivery rate set manually by the nurse or doctor.

Insulin pumps now in use are open-loop systems. These pumps enable patients to avoid multiple insulin injections; however, blood glucose levels must be monitored and the insulin delivery rate manually set.

EXPERIMENTAL THERAPIES. Internal (implantable) pumps are now being used for some patients who are participating in clinical research trials. These devices are computerized and have a reservoir of insulin from which the programmed dose is injected into the peritoneal cavity. The patient transmits directions to the pump by radiotelemetry. Advantages of internal pumps are avoidance of peripheral hyperinsulinaemia and suppression of hepatic glucose output. The reservoir is refilled every 40 to 60 days by transcutaneous injection.[55]

ALTERNATIVE DELIVERY SYSTEMS OF INSULIN. Over the years, there has been interest in developing systems to deliver insulin: by nasal spray, by skin patches, and by specially protected encapsulated forms for oral use.[7] To date, none of these have been satisfactorily developed for widespread clinical use.

Storage of insulin. Patients should be taught to give insulin at room temperature to decrease the risk of lipodystrophy and to decrease the antigenicity of the insulin. The current practice is to keep the currently used vial at room temperature if it can be used within 1 month, even though insulin vial labels direct the refrigeration of all insulin. It is known that regular insulin will remain stable for 12 months at 37° C (modified insulins for 24 months). Teach travellers to carry insulin with them rather than to pack it in baggage that might be subjected to extreme temperatures in car boots or cargo compartments of planes or trains.

Refrigeration is recommended for additional vials and when prefilled syringes are used, to decrease the potential bacterial growth from contamination.

Measures to assist the visually impaired diabetic. Blind patients or those with hand disability may be able to self-inject if the syringes are prepared for them. Often a family member or neighbour who has been taught by a community nurse prefills a 1-week supply of syringes. It is important that the patient gently rotate the prefilled syringe before administering the insulin and allow it to come to room temperature.

In addition to prefilled syringes, the visually impaired patient may be able to see the darker and larger markings on the 0.5 ml syringe. This syringe can only be used for doses of <50 units of U-100 insulin. Similarly, a magnifier that clamps on the insulin syringe may aid the patient in withdrawing an accurate dosage.

Many other aids for the visually impaired diabetic are advertised in publications for diabetics. Special syringes with plunger locks or attachable devices for locking the plunger and devices for measuring predetermined dosage can be supplied.[27]

People with poor vision risk drawing air instead of insulin into the syringe. Caution them to invert the bottle completely and to insert the needle only a short distance. Often they are advised to use only about two thirds of the bottle of insulin and to have on hand another full bottle. Some persons have a community nurse or a friend withdraw the last doses in a bottle of insulin for them or go to a clinic for the last few injections.

Table 20-5 Oral hypoglycaemic agents

Agent	Range of daily dose
Sulphonylureas	
Chlorpropramide	100 to 500 mg
Tolazamide	100 mg to 1 g
Tolbutamide	500 mg to 2 g
Glibenclamide	2.5 to 15 mg
Gliclazide	40 to 320 mg
Glipizide	2.5 to 15 mg
Biguanides	
Metformin	500 mg to 3 g

Oral hypoglycaemic agents. Orally administered agents are available for controlling blood sugar levels in people with diabetes mellitus; they are sulphonylurea and biguanides compounds (Table 20-5). Glipizide and glibenclamide, are more potent than the first-generation compounds; thus doses are smaller. These drugs have fewer drug–drug interactions, because they are not so easily displaced (unbound) from albumin by other drugs.

The sulphonylurea compounds increase the ability of the islet cells of the pancreas to secrete insulin, although other methods of action are being studied. With long-term use, they may increase the number of insulin receptors and correct defects in postreceptor insulin action.

Complications of oral hypoglycaemic agents are infrequent (see Box 20-6). Oral hypoglycaemic agents differ in routes of excretion; the presence of liver or kidney dysfunction may increase the risk of complications. Chlorpropramide may prolong hypoglycaemia because of its long half-life (36 hours) and duration of action (24 to 60 hours). See Table 20-5 for information about the hypoglycaemic agents.

Chlorpropramide is usually given in one dose per day; Tolbutamide has the shortest duration of action (6 to 12 hr) and is ordered two to three times a day.

The drugs are not hormones, and it is inaccurate to refer to them as oral insulin.

Doctors vary in their use of these agents because of the controversial study conducted in the 1970s by the University Group Diabetes Programme (UGDP) in the U.S. It is recommended that orally administered hypoglycaemic agents be limited to people with symptomatic adult-onset nonketotic diabetes mellitus that cannot be adequately controlled by diet or weight loss alone.

These medications are not used to treat IDDM or in pregnant women. They are useless in the treatment of diabetic ketoacidosis. A few patients may be treated with a combination of insulin and oral agents.[8]

People taking oral hypoglycaemia medications need to be as careful about taking the prescribed dosage, following the prescribed diet, maintaining the usual amount of exercise, testing by SBM, and taking general health precautions as do those taking insulin.

Preventing, detecting, and treating hypoglycaemia

Hypoglycaemia (plasma glucose level <3.3 mmol/L) occurs in at least two circumstances in diabetes mellitus. It

---

20-6

Complications of oral hypoglycaemic agents

Hypoglycaemia
Allergic skin reactions
Gastrointestinal complaints
Haematological disorders
Water detention and dilutional hyponatraemia (with chlorpropramide)

20-7

Signs and symptoms of hypoglycaemia

Sympathetic nervous system activity

Pallor	*Perspiration
Piloerection	Hunger
Tachycardia	Palpitation
*Nervousness	Irritability
*Weakness	Trembling

Central nervous system activity

Headache	Blurred vision
Diplopia	Incoherent speech
Emotional changes	Fatigue
*Mental confusion	Numbness of lips,
Convulsions	tongue
	Coma

* Four signs most commonly reported by patients.

---

occurs by far more frequently in the patient receiving insulin or an oral hypoglycaemic agent in whom there is an insulin excess relative to food intake or energy expenditure. Hypoglycaemia in this situation occurs for the following reasons:

1. Too large a dosage taken in relation to the need for insulin
2. Too little food taken (meals delayed or omitted) or delayed gastric emptying
3. Exercise excessive in relation to food intake and hypoglycaemic agent or insulin
4. Emotional stress
5. Vomiting, diarrhoea, or decreased food absorption

A less common instance is hypoglycaemia occurring in the early phase of NIDDM, when a sluggish release of insulin allows peak insulin activity to occur hours after food has been ingested.

The symptoms of *hypoglycaemia* can occur when blood glucose level falls rapidly: that is, the blood glucose level may be >3.3 mmol/L, but the patient has the symptoms of hypoglycaemia. Symptoms of hypoglycaemic reaction can vary among patients and from time to time in one patient.

Symptoms of sympathetic nervous system (SNS) activity usually precede those of the CNS and are related to adrenaline action. Signs of cerebral dysfunction reflect hypoglycaemia that interferes with the glucose supply of nerve cells (see Box 20-7). Prolonged attacks of severe hypoglycaemia can cause brain damage.

20-8

Nursing Research

Paulk LH. Hypoglycaemic reactions: from the diabetic's perspective, unpublished master's thesis, Kent, Ohio, 1983, Kent State University.

A description of the responses to hypoglycaemic episodes and self-care measures used to prevent and treat hypoglycaemic episodes was gained by the interview of 30 insulin-requiring adult patients with diabetes.

Their ages ranged from 19 to 76 years and the duration of treatment with insulin ranged from 1 to 47 years.

Sixty percent of the sample reported the three most frequent symptoms of hypoglycaemia to be: nervousness, weakness, and sweating (all early symptoms related to epinephrine activity).

Mental confusion was the most frequently reported symptom related to change in central nervous system activity. Sixty-two percent of the sample reported nocturnal reactions and severe reactions involving memory loss.

Thirty-six percent of the subjects reported that they did nothing to prevent attacks and used the same substance (juice, sweets) to treat all attacks. The recommendations of the researcher were that (1) the most frequently reported symptoms be used in initial teaching, (2) patients be taught to treat at the earliest symptom, (3) measures to prevent hypoglycaemia be reinforced in patient teaching, and (4) patients learn to use more than one treatment substance. For the subset of patients with fear, hypoglycaemic unawareness or severe reactions, an alternative plan for treatment must be developed with patient's significant others. Family members should be taught not to put food in mouth of the unconscious patient. A trained layperson can be taught to administer 1 mg glucagon (adult dose) into muscle or subcutaneous tissue.

20-9

Carbohydrates (10 to 15 g) for relief of hypoglycaemia

½ Cup fruit juice
½ Cup cola drink (not diet)
½ Cup jelly dessert (not diet)
4 Cubes sugar
1 Digestive biscuit

hypoglycaemia, give an intravenous bolus of 50% dextrose.

After recovery the patient should eat a snack consisting of complex carbohydrates and proteins (for example, milk and digestive biscuit) or eat the next meal if it is due. Ascertain the reason for hypoglycaemia if possible, and monitor the patient more frequently, until duration of the action of the hypoglycaemic agent is completed.

The nurse should not hesitate to treat the patient if symptoms of hypoglycaemia occur. Hospital protocols should clearly describe prompt treatment of hypoglycaemia in patients who cannot take anything by mouth.

To facilitate prompt treatment for unconsciousness, diabetic persons should carry identification cards with the insulin or hypoglycaemic agent and dosage listed. Medic-Alert bracelets or necklaces can also alert others to the diabetic status.

Patients who are receiving insulin or orally administered hypoglycaemic agents must know how to prevent, detect, and treat hypoglycaemic reactions before discharge. The nurse provides and explains the following:

1. Written material describing symptoms and treatment
2. Written material describing exercise related to hypoglycaemia
3. Diabetic identification card
4. Sample of quickly absorbed glucose to carry

Somogyi phenomenon. Some patients have great difficulty in stabilizing blood glucose levels. One cause of instability is the Somogyi phenomenon, a sequence of increasing peaks and valleys in blood glucose levels. It is often triggered by an insulin dosage in excess of true insulin requirements.

Very frequently the signs and symptoms of hypoglycaemia are not obvious enough to be detected. In many instances the hypoglycaemia occurs at night and is undetected. The hyperglycaemia is not recognized until early morning, and it is assumed that the patient needs higher doses of insulin, but this treatment just makes the problem worse.

The signs and symptoms of the Somogyi phenomenon can be those normally seen with hypoglycaemia, but frequently they consist only of nighttime sweats, nightmares, and a headache on arising. There may be weight gain in the presence of glycosuria, no glucose but ketone bodies in the urine (counterinsulin hormones stimulate lipolysis and beta-oxidation of fats), and wide fluctuations in blood and urine glucose levels unrelated to meals.

Monitoring the blood glucose once or twice during the night can help identify undetected hypoglycaemia and help

For some patients, a disturbing development is a diminished ability to perceive hypoglycaemic symptoms, particularly the early SNS symptoms. This dysfunction is associated with duration of disease, development of neuropathy, and use of certain drugs that affect the SNS (for example, beta blockers). Patients find this loss frightening because they no longer are able to intervene early in the reaction, but only when signs of cerebral dysfunction alert others or themselves to a more severe hypoglycaemic reaction. If a hypoglycaemic reaction is suspected, obtain a blood glucose level if it can be done quickly. Encourage patients to use SBM and not to rely on subjective feelings alone. At the same time, encourage them to take action—to use SBM and ingest glucose when subjective feelings first occur. See Box 20-8 for a description of a research study of hypoglycaemic reactions from the patient's perspective.

Hypoglycaemia in a *conscious patient* is treated by administering a quickly absorbed sugar; 10 to 15 g carbohydrate should be given promptly (see Box 20-9). With this amount of food, the patient usually feels better within 5 to 15 minutes. Should symptoms not decrease, give another feeding after this time. With unconsciousness or severe differentiate early morning hyperglycaemia from the *dawn phenomenon* from elevated hyperglycaemia from insulin-induced hypoglycaemia (*Somogyi phenomenon*).

Treatment of Somogyi phenomenon consists of decreasing the insulin dosage. A primary nursing role is to document complaints of hypoglycaemia, glucose intake, and laboratory results, and in particular to look for complaints of night sweats, nightmares, and early morning headaches. Correlating these complaints and laboratory results with the time of meals and insulin type and dosage will also help to identify the phenomenon.

Correcting acute metabolic crises

Diabetic ketoacidosis (DKA) and hyperosmolar nonketotic coma (HHNC) are medical emergencies that require intensive nursing care. Therapy is directed towards correction of hyperglycaemia, dehydration, electrolyte imbalances, acidosis, and precipitating factors. All of these interventions should occur simultaneously. Intense monitoring is necessary to evaluate treatment effects.

Insulin. Insulin replacement is based on one or a combination of several indices of insulin deficit (see Box 20-10).

A low-dose insulin system of treatment is usually used for DKA. It includes the use of intravenous push and continuous intravenous infusion of regular insulin. *Regular insulin is the only insulin that may be given intravenously.* The low-dose regimen includes a bolus of 10 to 20 units of regular insulin given by intravenous push and then regular insulin infused continuously at a rate of 10 to 12 units/hour. Most patients respond well to this regimen. Blood glucose levels should decrease by 2.8-5.6 mmol/L/hour. In a few patients, insulin resistance may be present, and the hyperglycaemia and blood glucose levels do not decrease. This insulin resistance is treated with another bolus of regular insulin or by an increase in the infusion rate. If blood glucose decreases more rapidly than 5.6 mmol/L, the infused rate will be decreased or even stopped temporarily and then restored at a lesser dosage. In the past, *high-dose* therapy consisting of an intravenous bolus of 50 to 150 units of regular insulin followed by repeated doses given either intravenously or subcutaneously was used. This form of therapy is not used frequently.

Patients with HHNC will usually be treated with the same low-dose insulin regimen. However, smaller doses of insulin are required.

As blood glucose level decreases and nears 11.1-16.7 mmol/L, close attention must be given to preventing and detecting the onset of hypoglycaemic reactions. As hyperglycaemia subsides, insulin resistance decreases and insulin sensitivity increases. For this reason the nurse should be more alert at this time for the symptoms of hypoglycaemia and expect changes in insulin dosage that reflect the decreasing blood glucose levels.

Fluid and electrolyte replacement. The patient with HHNC may have a fluid deficit of 8 to 12 L, and the patient with DKA a deficit of 3 to 5 L. To correct the *dehydration and sodium deficit*, normal saline solution or 0.45% saline (half-strength normal saline) solution is given intravenously. Initially, the solution is infused rapidly and at a rate of 1 to 3 L/hr or more in adults without cardiac or renal failure. When the urine output is 1 to 2 ml/min and the blood pressure is stable, the rate is reduced to 1 L in 2 to 4 hours. When the blood glucose level falls to 16.7 mmol/L, 5% glucose solutions are used. Monitor the patient very carefully for signs of fluid overload.

Potassium is not initially added to the intravenous fluids because the serum potassium level is usually *elevated* at the beginning of therapy in the patient with DKA, even though total body stores of potassium are depleted. With correction of the dehydration, acidosis, and insulin deficit, potassium moves back into cells and urinary excretion of potassium increases. *Hypokalaemia* can develop rapidly. Serum potassium levels and ECG tracings are monitored to determine when potassium should be added.

The administration of fluids and insulin usually corrects the acidosis in DKA so that bicarbonate administration is seldom needed. Bicarbonate is not usually given unless serum bicarbonate is 5 mmol/L and blood pH is <7.

An additional electrolyte imbalance that may develop during ketoacidosis is *hypophosphataemia*. Without adequate phosphorus, decreased peripheral oxygen delivery and additional tissue anoxia may result. Phosphorus in the form of potassium phosphate may be given.

Nursing interventions planned for the patient depend on the severity of the clinical findings and the prescribed therapy. In all patients, careful and frequent monitoring of the following is necessary:

1. Vital signs
2. Level of consciousness
3. Intake and output
4. Resolution of other signs of dehydration and acidosis
5. Serum potassium levels and ECG changes
6. Signs and symptoms of fluid overload
7. Blood glucose and ketone bodies

The nurse must make sure that the specimens are collected as ordered and that the appropriate tests are done. It is important to document test results. The assessments made by the nurse and the results of laboratory tests will be used to make appropriate adjustments in therapy. A flow sheet with all pertinent laboratory and assessment data is instituted so that all changes in the patient's status are displayed in a readily comprehensible manner.

Treatment of precipitating condition. As therapy for acute metabolic imbalance begins (insulin, fluid and electrolyte replacement), attention is given to detecting and treating concurrent illness. Sometimes the precipitating factor is not determined until treatment is well under way and the patient is recovered from coma sufficiently to give

---

20-10

Indices of insulin deficit

pH value <7.35
Blood glucose level
Degree of ketonaemia
Clinical findings, including degree of coma

a history of preceding events. Sometimes family members can give insight into possible aetiology. A common cause of DKA and HHNC is infection. Antibiotic therapy should begin after specimens for culture and sensitivity of urine, sputum, wound drainage, or blood are obtained.

Should lack of knowledge or of compliance be implicated in DKA or HHNC, begin patient education or counselling as soon as the patient has recovered enough to be comfortable and is feeling well enough to learn or to explore causes of noncompliance.

Promoting safety and well-being. The patient with severe insulin deficit is critically ill and requires excellent nursing. Skilled care involves attending to the following:

1. Required monitoring (as discussed previously)
2. Prescribed therapeutic measures
3. Maintenance of airway in an unconscious patient
4. Frequent turning, mouth care, and skin care
5. Side rails and hand restraints, if necessary, to maintain intravenous lines and ensure patient safety
6. Attention to discomforts of abdominal pain, nausea, and vomiting usually present in the conscious patient
7. Maintenance of nutrition
   a. Fluids first when able to take something by mouth
   b. Solid foods as soon as possible to improve gastric tone
8. Maintenance of the flow sheet
9. Reassurance about care
10. Meeting psychological needs of patient and family

Minimizing disruption of diabetes treatment

Disruption of blood glucose control often occurs when patients with diabetes are scheduled for surgery or diagnostic tests or when there is an intercurrent illness. This is particularly so when insulin or oral hypoglycaemics are a part of the daily regimen. Medication, glucose intake, and frequency of monitoring are three measures that may need to be modified so that optimal metabolic balance can be achieved.

Effects of surgery on the person with diabetes. Surgery is a physical and psychological stressor for anyone. For the person with diabetes mellitus there are additional risks. The stress of surgery can disrupt metabolic control. People with diabetes are at increased risk for the following:

1. Infection
2. Impaired wound healing
3. Age-related complications (many people with NIDDM are elderly)
4. Postsurgical complications from macrovascular and microvascular changes

The person with diabetes mellitus is at risk for developing *hypoglycaemia or hyperglycaemia* during the perioperative period. During this period, patients usually are not given anything by mouth and are given fluid intravenously. This decreases total calorie intake and may also decrease insulin needs. However, the effects of surgery on counterregulatory hormones may increase the need for additional insulin. The stressors of surgery cause the release of ACTH, glucocorticoids, and catecholamines, all of which can elevate serum glucose levels.

Guidelines for Care 20-11	**The person with diabetes during the perioperative period**
	
	Diabetics who receive insulin
	  Preoperative
	    Intravenous infusion of glucose on morning of surgery
	    One-half usual insulin dose subcutaneously
	  Intraoperative
	    Monitoring of blood glucose levels if surgery is lengthy
	    Additional insulin or glucose as needed
	  Postoperative
	    Intravenous infusion of glucose until food can be taken orally
	    Insulin given subcutaneously in equally divided doses over 24 hours or added to intravenous fluids
	    Blood glucose and urine ketones monitored every 4 to 6 hours
	    Additional insulin given if indicated from monitoring
	Diabetics not normally given insulin
	  Preoperative
	    Intravenous infusion of glucose on morning of surgery
	  Postoperative
	    Blood glucose and urine ketone levels monitored every 4 to 6 hours
	    Insulin given if indicated from monitoring
	All diabetics
	  125 to 250 g CHO/day until normal diet resumed
	  Normal regimen reinsituted as soon as possible
	  Continued monitoring of blood glucose and urine ketone levels even after usual diet resumed (increased insulin may be needed because of catabolism from surgery)

Management of the diabetic person undergoing surgery. See Box 20-11 for modifications of therapy during the perioperative period. To minimize the disruption in metabolic control, the patient's metabolism should be thoroughly regulated before surgery. Maintain the normal food, fluid, and medication routine until the night before surgery. After surgery, perform blood glucose checks on an every 4 to 6 hour schedule; the results are used to determine the amount of insulin needed. Urine checks for ketones may also be done. To prevent starvation ketosis, all diabetic patients should receive 125 to 250 g carbohydrate/day until they resume a normal diet.

Care during surgery and diagnostic tests. When fasting is necessary, take care to avert hypoglycaemia in the person who takes insulin or an oral hypoglycaemic agent. Clarify orders as necessary to ensure that glucose is available while insulin is acting. Sometimes insulin administration is delayed until the patient finishes a specific test and can resume eating. When fasting must be prolonged for a diagnostic test or for surgery, provide caloric intake by intravenous infusion. The minimum intake recommended to prevent hypoglycaemia and starvation ketosis and to provide basic energy requirements is 250 g/24 hr. An intravenous flow rate of a 5% glucose solution at a rate of 5 to 10 g of glucose per hour is commonly used. Frequent monitoring of blood glucose levels is very helpful in determining proper rates and concentrations of intravenous fluids containing glucose and the required dosages of insulin to maintain metabolic control.

It is routine to schedule diagnostic tests or surgery for diabetic patients early in the morning to minimize the amount of disruption in their regimen.

Disruption of metabolic control places diabetic patients at higher risk for infection and for problems in wound healing. Compromised wound healing may occur because of impairments in cellular repair, phagocytosis, and fibroplastic proliferation.[58]

There are several protocols for perioperative management of insulin, fluids and electrolytes, and caloric intake in the patient with diabetes. Differences in management may occur because of the nature of the surgery (inpatient/outpatient, short/long, minor/major); the nature of anaesthesia (type, length), and whether patients have used insulin or hypoglycaemic agents before surgery. For example, the patient with well-controlled NIDDM, scheduled early in the day for outpatient tooth extraction, may not require any special modification of the diabetic regimen except fasting after midnight, delay of insulin or oral hypoglycaemic agent, and no food intake until after the surgery. (Intermediate-acting insulins are not acting during early morning; thus, the patient might be instructed to take the usual dose of NPH insulin and omit regular insulin before coming to the surgical centre.)

In contrast, a patient with IDDM scheduled for cardiac bypass surgery requires significant modification of insulin and caloric intake throughout the perioperative period. Not only can extended length of surgery, anaesthesia, and recovery be expected; but this type of surgery markedly increases requirements for insulin.[29]

Controversy exists about the best way to manage insulin regimens for patients undergoing major surgery. Still common is the practice of giving about 50% of the intermediate insulin dosage by subcutaneous injection before surgery and supplementing it with regular insulin during and after surgery as indicated by glucose monitoring. Increasingly recommended is intravenous administration of regular insulin only. The absorption of insulin from subcutaneous tissue becomes even more erratic when fluid shifts and haemodynamic changes occur as a result of anaesthesia and surgery.[29]

Controversy also exists about the best way to administer insulin intravenously during the operative period and postoperatively. Surgeons may order regular insulin to be given by bolus or by fixed-rate or variable-rate infusions. Better metabolic control has been reported with variable-rate infusions of glucose containing insulin and potassium.[29]

Three factors that affect the postoperative recommendations for management of insulin dosage are (1) postoperative dietary intake, (2) postoperative nausea and vomiting, and (3) the ability to use the results of capillary blood glucose monitoring. Although sliding scale insulin protocols are still in common use, the use of insulin logarithms, which better predict the doses of insulin required,[29] is increasing.

Care during concurrent illness. Concurrent illness may also disrupt diabetes control. All illnesses influence the status of diabetes control. In most instances the person with diabetes needs increased insulin in the presence of a concurrent illness, especially infection. Yet many mistakenly believe that if they cannot eat they do not need to take the prescribed insulin or oral hypoglycaemic agent. *Failure of patients with IDDM to take insulin when ill is a frequent cause of ketoacidosis.* These patients should take their insulin and *carbohydrate* in some form.

"Sick days" is the name given to times when the person with diabetes feels ill and may have anorexia, nausea, and malaise and yet have no defined illness. For one or two sick days, teach the patient to maintain metabolic balance by the following guidelines:

1. Take prescribed dose of insulin.
2. Spread 50% of the daily CHO allowance over 24 hours.
3. Increase fluid intake.
4. Include food items with more simple sugars than regularly allowed, such as custard, nondiet soft drinks, nondiet gelatin.
5. Advance diet towards the normally prescribed diet as soon as possible.
6. Institute blood glucose and urine ketone monitoring on a more frequent basis.

The person must know when to call the primary health care provider. Each person will receive individual instructions, but in general the primary health care provider should be called if any of the following occur:

1. A full day's urine glucose test results are at maximum readings or blood glucose levels are consistently elevated beyond a specified level, often 11.1 mmol/L
2. Ketone bodies persist in the urine for 6 hours or more
3. The person is not able to take *any* food or fluids for longer than 4 hours
4. The person is febrile

Interventions to achieve patient outcomes
Preventing fluid deficit

Dehydration is a potentially dangerous sequella of hyperglycaemia, and it is a corollary to the metabolic crises of diabetes: DKA and HHNC. An insulin deficit is the basic feature of both of these life-threatening states. The usual monitoring of fluid balance for any patient includes measuring weight, intake and output, and excessive losses from polyuria, vomitus, diarrhoea, drainage, and so on. These measurements are as important in the diabetic patient as they are in any patient; however, in the diabetic patient, the monitoring of blood glucose and urinary ketones also is essential in order to detect, prevent and correct an insulin deficit. Report evidence of dehydration or hyperglycaemia above 11.1 mmol/L to the doctor and obtain directions for fluid replacement and insulin coverage.

Oral or intravenous fluids are necessary to compensate for excess losses that occur in the osmotic diuresis of glycosuria. When fluid intake is adequate, and when the renal threshold for glucose is normal, the patient can maintain a normal glomerular filtration rate (GFR) and is able to clear excess glucose and, to some extent, ketoacids from the extracellular fluids.[37] Decreases in GFR caused by volume depletion lead quickly to metabolic decompensation.

Patients who have age-related high renal thresholds for glucose or who have renal disease lack this "safety valve" of glycosuria and are at higher risk for developing hyperosmolar imbalance. Teach patients experiencing sick days to attempt to drink at least 8 ounces of fluids every hour they are awake.[37] Because they need to replenish electrolytes as well, these fluids should include soups, broths, colas, and so on, and not just water. It is essential to provide frail elderly or disabled people with access to an adequate fluid intake, because they are at particular risk for HHNC.

Facilitating learning

An integral part of the treatment of diabetes mellitus is education of patients so they can assume responsibility for required self-care, including seeking medical advice or treatment when needed. Teaching should begin at the time of diagnosis and continue until the patient is competent in maintaining an optimal level of wellness. Educational programmes for diabetic people can be planned in the following three phases:

1. *Initial management*, in which the knowledge and skills needed to survive are emphasized
2. *Home management*, in which patients learn to be self-sufficient in the daily management of the disease
3. *Improvement of life-style*, in which patients learn how to enrich their lives by gaining flexibility in management, insight, and self-determination

Each phase is specified by objectives and the requisite knowledges, skills, and attitudes. The nurse should begin teaching about initial management before introducing more complex home management content. Evaluation of learning and reinforcement should be part of the plan.

It is important to set priorities in teaching and begin with the most basic information.

For example, when insulin is newly prescribed, teaching the patient how to administer insulin safely and accurately takes precedence over the other components, and related survival skills must be taught before more advanced content.

The nurse would focus first on teaching the patient to:

1. Identify the prescribed insulin
2. Check the expiration date
3. Prepare and administer an accurate dose using sterile technique
4. Never change the insulin dosage, strength, type, species without the doctor's direction
5. Plan the purchase, storage, and disposal of insulin and syringes and needles
6. Prevent, recognize, and treat hypoglycaemia

It would be inappropriate when first introducing insulin therapy to teach about the various kinds of insulin or the different insulin regimes that are used.

It is also important to individualize the teaching plan according to the assessed needs for learning. All patients with diabetes need to be assessed for learning needs. It is important to understand that many patients who have had diabetes for years may not have adequate education or have not updated their knowledge and skills for some time. It is only through an individual assessment that the nurse can identify the specific knowledge, skills, and attitudes that require intervention.

There are usually assessment guides and teaching tools within a nursing department or agency that can facilitate teaching. Often, diabetes educators who can provide access to teaching materials and serve as consultants are available. If there is a centralized diabetes education programme, promptly refer the patient and plan for collaborative efforts between staff nurses and the teaching team.

With short hospital stays, begin teaching as soon as the patient is judged ready to learn. Some interventions must be planned early by making appointments for specific times. These include:

1. Dietary consultation
2. Attendance at groups classes, if available
3. Involvement of family members in particular sessions

The teaching plan should clearly delineate when initial instruction and reinforcement is to take place for each of the components selected for teaching. If specific outcomes

Table 20-6   **Phases of diabetes education**

Initial management	Home management	Improvement of life-style
Survival knowledge and skills	Self-sufficiency in daily management of diabetes	Enrichment of life by flexibility in management, insight, and self-determination
Objectives for the component—definition of diabetes		
States need for insulin in body	Lists symptoms of diabetes	Identifies significance of hyperglycaemia in relation to other metabolic problems and long-term complications
Describes what happens in body when insulin is deficient	Explains relationship of symptoms to insulin deficiency	States significance of hyperglycaemia and glycosuria, or vice versa, relative to changes in renal threshold
States simple working definition of diabetes	States how diagnosis of diabetes is made	Lists main differences between insulin-dependent and non–insulin-dependent diabetes
States role of food, activity, and medication in treatment of diabetes	IDDM: States relationship of under-nutrition to insulin deficiency	States current knowledge of hereditary aspects of diabetes
	NIDDM: States relationship between state of overnutrition, inactivity, and relative insulin deficiency	Verbalizes concerns about diabetes in other family members

From A Joint Task Force for the American Diabetes Association and the American Association of Diabetes Educators, Spring 1979, American Diabetes Association.

The Elderly with Diabetes Mellitus

Assessment

Assess for signs of diabetes mellitus; the elderly may have a history of recent weight loss, decreased vision, urinary tract infection, or mental changes rather than classic symptoms of diabetes mellitus.

Assess vision and ability to ambulate.

Monitor weight of elderly people; Type 2 diabetes mellitus (NIDDM) is associated with obesity.

Monitor glucose levels; glucose levels may be tolerated at higher levels than in younger adults.

Intervention

Encourage regular exercise, such as paced walking, to decrease hyperglycaemia and increase calorie expenditure.

Encourage a diet that promotes weight reduction if obesity is present.

Be aware that the elderly person with diabetes mellitus may have vision changes and plan care accordingly.

Teach patient to maintain hydration and eat prescribed diet (even when not hungry) to prevent hypoglycaemic episodes (anorexia is common in the elderly).

Teach patient or significant other management of oral hypoglycaemics (or insulin if used), diet, and blood sugar testing.

Teach importance of foot care to decrease potential of gangrene; the elderly person may have concurrent peripheral vascular problems.

Common complications in elderly

Vascular degeneration in kidneys, eyes, heart, and legs from lipidaemia (causing atherosclerosis) and hyperglycaemia

Infections and ulcers of the lower extremeties

Cerebal vascular accidents

---

are clearly identified for the individual patient, evaluation can be facilitated and needed modifications put in place as necessary.

Initial instruction for a hospitalized patient with newly diagnosed diabetes should encompass three factors:

1. Expected length of stay
2. Specific referrals for further teaching
3. Other concerns and teaching needs not related to diabetes self-care

Teaching sessions should include mutual planning and goal setting. Patients with diabetes often report that their education was "too much and too fast." Teaching approaches and methods need to be modified according to the learning style, motivation, and comfort level of the patient. Eliciting feedback from the patient during the instruction will help identify correct pace and depth and allow modifications to be made as needed.

Some teaching can focus on ongoing care activities: for example, plans should specify that foot care instruction be given along with foot care and that instruction related to blood glucose monitoring and medications be gradually introduced as these tasks are performed. Flow sheet information relating to status of diabetes and its treatment can

be shared to illustrate the interactions of food, medication, illness, and so on. The patient can be helped to keep his or her own flow sheet at the bedside. This can serve as an introduction to the type of records to be kept after discharge.

Written materials should be selected carefully for accuracy and relevance to the individual's learning needs and reading level. For example, the patient with NIDDM need not be given materials that discuss the management of IDDM. Written materials should always be introduced to reinforce or amplify previous instruction. After the patient has read the materials, provide an opportunity to answer questions and clarify any misconceptions.

Follow-up. The many teaching needs of the person with diabetes mellitus have been discussed. Education is an integral part of therapy and must be planned over a period of time if the patient is to be capable of diabetes management. The knowledge and skills necessary for self-care are summarized in Box 20-12. Teaching usually begins at the time of diagnosis, but the nurse must be aware that everything cannot be learned during the first contact. Priorities need to be set: teach the person the skills necessary to meet immediate needs, and then refer to an ambulatory setting or home health care agency. Follow-up might take place in a G.P. clinic or hospital.

In addition to securing follow-up education appointments, the nurse can do the following:

1. Reinforce the value and need of continued learning
2. Encourage family members to participate
3. Give the patient written instructions and educational literature
4. Ensure that the patient has a resource person to call if assistance is needed before the next appointment

Give the patient local sources of information, such as the public library and the local diabetes association, as well as specific appointment information.

Promoting adherence to diabetic regimen

The ability of the patient with diabetes mellitus to manage self-care at an optimal level on a daily basis is not only based on knowledge and skills, but on motivation, willingness, and ability to make behavioural changes. Many of these changes include those that are recommended for all people and are related to food intake, regular exercise, and participation in regular screening examinations. For the person with diabetes, however, failure to integrate the diabetes regimen into daily life leads to more frequent and more severe complications.

Inability to make these changes independently and to maintain the changed behaviour may be related to emotional responses, family conflicts, economic barriers, and perceived problems in communication with health care providers.

The emotional impact of the disease on the patient and the family can lead to nonadherence. Emotional responses to diabetes affect the patient's motivation and capacity to make changes. One researcher has described three phases of health and functioning in NIDDM[30]:

1. Up to 1 year post diagnosis. This phase involves a sense of helplessness, anxiety, and/or anger. During

20-12

Summary of knowledge and skills for adequate self-care of diabetes mellitus (survival level)

Basic understanding of diabetes mellitus and how metabolism is changed by it

Therapeutic regimen prescribed and how it works to keep the blood sugar level normal

Diet ordered (calories, CHO, and such), how to to calculate diet requirements for each meal, ability to incorporate personal preferences

Exercise and its effect on calorie and insulin needs, and how to manage if exercise level is increased above usual

If receiving insulin:
  Type, amount, timing, method of administration
  Ability to give the insulin accurately
  Ability to care for equipment properly

If receiving oral hypoglycaemic agents:
  Type, dosage, time schedule
  Potential side effects
  What to do if new or unexpected symptoms occur

Self-monitoring routine for glucose status (urine ketone and serum glucose monitoring):
  How to do the tests accurately
  What to do if the results show hyperglycaemia, ketonuria, or hypoglycaemia
  How to care for equipment and supplies

Signs and symptoms of hypoglycaemia, how to treat them, and what to do if they occur frequently

Signs and symptoms of hyperglycaemia and what to do when they occur

How to manage diabetes mellitus on days when usual diet cannot be eaten because of illness

Measures to prevent lower extremity trauma or injury

Type of follow-up care necessary and whom to contact with questions

---

knowing that most people experience emotional distress on learning that they are diabetic, and that they may expect to feel more comfortable as they experience living with this chronic disease and becoming proficient in its management. Referral to a specialized counsellor is helpful when severe or prolonged emotional responses interfere with quality of life or with carrying out the prescribed treatment measures.

Adherence is best promoted when the family and the patient work collaboratively on the tasks involved in managing this chronic illness. Integration of a diabetes regimen into one's life-style involves not only the people with diabetes, but also the family members. Sometimes compliance with the diabetic regime serves as a focal point for interpersonal conflicts. This is typically illustrated by the teenage patient's noncompliance being the focus for parent-teen conflicts about independence. Conflicts may be just as overt in the adult people and family; food often serves as an available forum for focusing interpersonal conflicts. Family members can be helped to assume supportive roles by involvement in educational programmes and support groups. Specialized counselling can also be useful to patients and family members if dysfunctional behaviour persists.

Adherence to diabetic regimens may be made more difficult when there are economic barriers. Restriction of access to health care and employment are problems for many patients with diabetes. Sometimes the problem can be ameliorated when the doctor can document that the diabetes is under excellent control and that measures to prevent complication are being used. Encourage patients to consult the diabetic association to obtain information about these issues and to seek guidance from their specific carers.

Effective interpersonal communication is necessary between the patient and the health care provider in any chronic illness. A barrier to adherence exists if the patient perceives goals or recommendations as not achieveable yet is unable to share this perception with the health care provider. Help the patient to be assertive in asking questions, describing barriers, and seeking resources to improve their ability to maintain health.

There has been an increasing trend in diabetes treatment and education to use behavioural modification techniques and contracting, particularly in approaches to diet and exercise. Steps include selecting an achievable goal, selecting one or two behavioural changes, and using monitoring and positive reinforcement of the behaviour.[32,49]

People can be referred to groups focused on weight loss, or support groups sponsored by local diabetes associations, where the focus arises out of the expressed needs of the group participants. These groups often include topics such as psychological responses, socioeconomic strategies and handling of interpersonal conflicts, and information about current therapy. Formal programmes in diabetes education may include follow-up group sessions for reinforcement of learning. At some agencies, recheck clinics are held at intervals and include laboratory testing, consultation, and planned instruction.

In addition to attending community-run diabetic clinics, patients can obtain up-to-date information from the Irish and British Diabetic Associations.*

---

this time, increased feelings of vulnerability to illness, loss of function, amputation, and disabilities occur along with decreases in self-esteem. Depression may occur. Anxieties about work and marital roles and social functioning may persist. Patients who are over 40 may for the first time be confronted with a sense of their own mortality.

2. Middle phase of management. Characterized by relative well-being and functioning.

3. Final phase, for some. Adjustment to one or more permanent physical complications and physical impairments. Feelings of depression, anxiety, and helplessness coincide with the stressors associated with learning to adapt to the complication(s).

Patients and family members may receive some comfort by learning how adherence to blood glucose control can lead to benefits such as increased vigour and sense of well-being and a decrease in acute illness episodes. In addition, blood glucose control is the best means for preventing vascular and neurological damage. Patients may be reassured by

Nursing Care Plan

People with diabetes mellitus

DATA: Mrs. T. is an obese, 52-year-old married woman with NIDDM diagnosed 3 years ago. She was referred to a short-term ambulatory diabetes education programme by her G.P. for instruction on insulin administration, since she had not achieved blood glucose control with dietary measures and oral agents.

The nursing history identified the following:

1. Mrs. T. saw referral as necessary but perceived it and the inability to control weight and blood glucose as a personal failure.

2. She maintained inconsistent sleep/activity schedule. (Worked as an LPN 8 PM to 8 AM Saturday and Sunday with 2 to 4 hours sleep during day; arose at 8 AM and retired at 11 PM on other days.)

3. She had accurate knowledge about dietary modifications and had participated successfully in several weight reduction programmes with 20- to 40-pound weight loss each time.

4. She does not exercise consistently.

5. She has performed blood glucose monitoring on others and once or twice on self.

6. She state that work is important to her; she derives satisfactions from work group socialization and says it "keeps me busy."

7. She fears that her husband will die suddenly at home. Two years ago she performed CPR when he had a cardiac arrest at home. Realizes that she maintains work schedule "to keep me from worrying about my husband."

Objective data included blood glucose, 12.2 mmol/L; weight, 91 kg; height, 5'4"; BP 134/84; urine glucose 2% with no ketones present.

Collaborative nursing actions include teaching Mrs. T. those measures that would help her achieve control of blood glucose (insulin, diet, and exercise) and to detect, prevent, and treat hypoglycaemic reactions. The nurse reported Mrs. T.'s work schedule to the doctor and asked for insulin dosage alterations on weekends. The doctor was unaware of her work schedule and stated that blood glucose control could not be optimum with this schedule.

Nursing analysis: Knowledge deficit: self-injections, self-blood glucose monitoring related to lack of exposure

Expected patient outcomes	Nursing interventions	Rationale
Mrs. T will independently administer to self	Support Mrs. T. as necessary to self-inject insulin	Adults who perform this task have minimal discomfort and realize they are capable of giving own insulin
Mrs. T. will perform blood glucose monitoring (BGM) accurately	Observe patient's skill in BGM; correct as necessary	Evaluation of patient technique is necessary to ensure accuracy
Mrs. T. will use measurements obtained by BGM to achieve fasting blood glucose below 7.8 mmol/L	Review with Mrs. T. the effect of activity, dietary intake, and insulin on blood glucose. Instruct patient on frequency and timing of BGM	BGM gives immediate feedback about previous behaviours and reinforces value of therapeutic measures
Mrs. T. can detect and treat hypoglycaemia	Review with Mrs. T. signs and symptoms and treatment measures	This knowledge assures that patient can safely give own insulin and decreases fear of a reaction
	Refer to dietitian for modification of diet necessary with insulin, and for verification of diet knowledge	The dietitian is the appropriate person to teach about diet

Nursing analysis: Altered health maintenance: related to ineffective coping skill

Expected patient outcomes	Nursing interventions	Rationale
Mrs. T. will state at least one change that will improve blood glucose control	Teach Mrs. T. effects of stress, lack of exercise, and activity pattern on blood glucose	If Mrs. T. understands how stress impairs health, likelihood of change is more likely
	Explore with Mrs. T. willingness and ability to change behaviours: sleep/activity, coping, and exercise	Goals are more likely to be achieved if Mrs. T. makes realistic choices after considering cost and benefits
	Engage Mrs. T. in mutual problem solving; refrain from prescribing	Increasing Mrs. T.'s sense of control can help with self-esteem and enhance attitudes towards change
	Explore sources for long-term support in learning more effective coping skills. Suggest support groups: 1. For spouses of patients with myocardial infarction 2. For weight loss *and maintenance* of weight loss 3. Available at work in health service programme	Changing life-style, eating behaviours, and coping skills are very difficult; support over long periods of time is usually required
	Suggest to Mrs. T. that she seek a trial period on day shift on weekends	Trial period can help Mrs. T. make informed choices about work schedule in attaining goals

Evaluation

Questions that guide the nurse's evaluation derive from an understanding of potential effects of diabetes mellitus on physical well-being, the importance of education for self-management of blood glucose control, and the psychological impact of this chronic disease and its treatment.

Specific goals or objectives for each patient identify the intended outcomes of health care.

1. What level of blood glucose control has been achieved?
2. Has ideal weight been achieved or maintained?
3. Has the patient developed sufficient skill to be independent and safely carry out self-management of the disease in terms of administration of insulin injections or oral hypoglycaemic agents, treatment of hypoglycaemic reactions, and foot care?
4. Is proper foot care practised? Is skin integrity present?
5. Has the patient maintained fluid balance?
6. Is the patient equipped with knowledge and skills to make decisions about food, exercise, medications, and when to seek medical advice?
7. Is the patient committed to prevention of short- and long-term complications (follow-up, self-management)?
8. Is the patient coping with diabetes self-care measures, fears and concerns, and life-style changes?

SUMMARY

1. Diabetes mellitus is a complex metabolic disorder and may be clinically expressed as non-insulin dependent diabetes mellitus (NIDDM) and as insulin-dependent diabetes mellitus (IDDM) in persons with onset generally before age 40.
2. Insulin deficit is a central feature of the disease; insulin deficit may be *absolute* when beta cells do not secrete insulin; or *relative*, when beta cell defect and peripheral resistance to insulin is present.
3. Glucagon excess and increase in other antagonists to insulin contribute to the hyperglycaemia; these are increased during the stress response.
4. Measures to prevent and treat obesity are the focus of primary prevention of NIDDM; screening to detect people who are undiagnosed (50%) is the focus of secondary prevention.
5. Insulin deficit and hyperglycaemia lead to many immediate alterations in metabolism: hyperosmolarity and osmotic diuresis, glycosuria, cellular starvation, calorie loss, and increased fat metabolism and catabolism.
6. Diabetic ketoacidosis (*DKA*) and hyperglycaemic, hyperosmolar, nonketotic coma (*HHNC*) are two life-threatening situations that occur in diabetes mellitus.
7. The duration of hyperglycaemia seems a major predictor of the development of microvascular lesions (nephropathy, retinopathy), macrovascular lesions (atherosclerotic disease), and neuropathy.
8. Amputation in diabetes mellitus can result as a consequence of alterations in blood vessels and nerves,

tissue trauma, and infection occurring in people with inadequate skin integrity and insensitivity to pain or pressure. Proper foot care can reduce the risk of amputation.

9. Because patients must be capable in diabetes management, nursing assessment must address the knowledge and coping skills of a patient early in hospitalization so that appropriate education and counselling can proceed.
10. A well-educated person with diabetes will be assertive in describing special needs relating to patterns of food intake, exercise, monitoring, medications, and foot care.
11. Assessment of the person with diabetes includes collecting objective data about metabolic status, cardiovascular-renal status, vision, and nerve function. The lower extremities should be carefully examined.
12. Dietary recommendations in diabetes mellitus include the following: calorie distribution of CHO (55% to 60%), fat (20% to 30%) with restriction in saturated fat to 10%, and protein (20%); limitation of cholesterol, sodium, and refined simple CHO; and increased use of complex, unrefined CHO.
13. The three primary modalities of treatment of diabetes mellitus are diet, exercise, and hypoglycaemic agents; education for self-management of these modalities is an integral part of treatment.
14. Exercise has a hypoglycaemic action in most instances; but, it can increase hyperglycaemia if blood glucose levels are very high or if exercise is intense. Exercise also aids in cardiovascular fitness and weight reduction and weight maintenance programmes, and it decreases peripheral resistance.
15. Nurses and patients must be careful to use prescribed insulin: strength, species, length of action, purity.
16. The oral hypoglycaemic agents used in NIDDM stimulate pancreatic beta cell secretion and decrease peripheral resistance. They may induce hypoglycaemia.
17. Patients using insulin pump therapy or multiple injections always self-monitor blood glucose. These technologies make it possible to achieve normoglycaemia in well-educated patients.
18. Haemoglobin Al_c measures the amount of glycosylation of normal haemoglobin A; it correlates with average blood glucose levels over the past 2 to 3 months.
19. The treatment of hypoglycaemia must be prompt; give 10 to 15 g of simple CHO as soon as symptoms are detected. The first signs present are those of adrenaline excess; later signs are those of cerebral dysfunction.
20. Insulin or oral hypoglycaemic agents should not be omitted when short illness occurs; about 50% of daily CHO intake should be distributed over 24 hours.
21. The impact of the diagnosis of diabetes mellitus and living with this chronic illness may be expressed by patients emotionally, in concerns about the future, in patient-family conflicts, and in noncompliance.
22. The treatment of DKA and HHNC requires replacement of insulin, fluids, and electrolytes; treatment of precipitating conditions; and monitoring and supportive nursing care of these acutely ill patients.

---

* British Diabetic Association, 10 Queen Ann St, London, WIM 0BD. Irish Diabetic Association, 82-83, Lower Gardiner St, Dublin 1. Republic of Ireland.

23. Patients fasting or undergoing surgery require modifications of insulin and food intake and increased monitoring of metabolic status.
24. Foot care includes daily inspection, measures to maintain integrity of skin, and prevention of injury. Referral to chiropody services is highly recommended.
25. Diabetes education must be individualized and planned over time. Initial instruction should be restricted to "survival skills" and beginning home management skills with referral for continued education.
26. Evaluation of nursing interventions includes assessment of whether the metabolic balance is improved, whether the patient has the requisite knowledge and coping skills for self-management, and whether appropriate referrals were made.

STUDY QUESTIONS

• What are the major differences between insulin-dependent (IDDM) and non-insulin-dependent (NIDDM) diabetes mellitus?
• What information needs to be included on an assessment guide to elicit information about risks for metabolic crises, vascular and neurological complications of diabetes mellitus, and nonadherence to prescribed regimen?
• What would be included in a teaching plan for a 22-year-old newly diagnosed person with IDDM and how would this differ for a 68-year-old person with NIDDM?
• What are the patient problems posed by "strict" versus "loose" control of blood glucose?

REFERENCES AND SELECTED READINGS

1. American Diabetes Association: Principles of nutrition and dietary recommendations for individuals with diabetes mellitus, *Diab Care* 10(1):126-132, 1987.
2. American Diabetes Association and American Dietetic Association: *Exchange lists for meal planning*, Alexandria, Va, 1986, The Association.
3. American Diabetes Association: A Position Statement: standards of medical care for patients with diabetes mellitus, *Diab Care* 12:365-368, 1989.
4. Andreoli FE, et al: *Cecil's essentials of medicine*, Philadelphia, 1986, WB Saunders.
5. Benson JW: In Metz R, Larson E (editors): *Blue book of endocrinology*, Philadelphia, 1986, WB Saunders.
6. Bantle JP: Injection site rotation: the downside, *Practical Diabetol* 9(5):1-3, 1990.
7. Beaser RS, Weir GC, Hill J: Diabetes research update, *Diabetes in the News*10(1):7-1, 1991.
8. Bingham PR, Riddle MC: Combined insulin-sulfonylurea treatment of type II diabetes, *Diab Educator* 15:450-455, 1989.
8a. British Diabetic Association, Diabetes in the UK. London: BDA, 1988.
9.* Brown S: Effects of educational interventions in diabetes care: a meta-analysis of findings, *Nurs Res* 37:223-230, 1988.
10.* Byrnes CA: What's new in the diabetic diet, *Nurs* 87 17(8):58-59, 1987.
11.* Callahan M, Bradley DJ: Why you should teach your diabetic patients to chart, *Nurs* 88 18(3):48-49, 1988.
11a. Christensen MH et al: How to care for the diabetic foot, *Am J Nog* 91(3):50-58, 1991.
12. Davidson MB: Aging: relation to diabetes and carbohydrate metabolism: conclusions, *Diab Spectrum* 2:190-192, 1989.
13. Davidson MB: How to get the most out of insulin therapy, *Clin Diab* 8:565-73, 1990.
14. DeAtkine D, Surwit R, Feinglos M: Stress and diabetes, *Practical Diabetol* 10(5):1-8, 1991.
15. DeFronzo RA: From research to practice: conclusions, *Diab Spectrum* 3:325-328, 1990.
16. Engerman RL, Kern TS: Progression of incipient diabetic retinopathy during good glycemic control, *Diabetes* 36: 808-812, 1987.
17. Ferris FL, Early Treatment Diabetic Retinopathy Study Research Group: Photocoagulation for diabetic retinopathy, *JAMA* 266:1263-1265, 1991.
18.* Fondiller S: Meeting the growing challenge of diabetes, *Am J Nurs* 91(11):57-66, 1991.
19. Franz MJ: Evaluating the glycemic response to carbo-hydrates, *Clin Diab* 11:129-130, 1986.
20.* Gluck SL, Klahr S: Enlarging our view of the diabetic kidney, *N Engl J Med* 324:1662-1664, 1991.
21. Goetz FC, Moudry-Munns K, Sutherland DER: Whole-organ pancreas transplantation in the 1990's, *Clin Diab* 9:33-41, 1991.
22.* Graham C: Exercise in the elderly patient with diabetes, *Practical Diabetol* 10(5):8-11, 1991.
23.* Graham C, Lasko-McCarthey P: Exercise options for persons with diabetic complications, *Diab Educator* 16: 212-219, 1990.
23a. Guthrie DW, Guthrie RA: *Nursing management of diabetes mellitus*, ed 3, New York, 1991, Springer.
23b. Guthrie RA: New approaches to improve diabetes control, *Am Family Physician* 43:570-578, 1991.
24. Hanefeld M et al: Therapeutic potentials of acarbose as first-line drug in NIDDM insufficiently treated with diet alone, *Diab Care* 14:732-737, 1991.
25. *Healthy People 2000: National Health Promotion and Disease Prevention Objectives*, US Dept of Health and Human Services, Public Health Service, Washington, DC, 1991.
26. Heins JM, Rosett JW, Davis SG: The new look in diabetic diets, *Am J Nurs* 87:196-199, 1987.
27.* Herget M, Williams A: New aids for low-vision diabetics, *Am J Nurs* 89:1319-1322, 1989.
28. Hernandes CG: The pathophysiology of diabetes mellitus; an update, *Diab Educator* 15:162-168, 1989.
29. Hirsch B, McGill B: Role of insulin in management of surgical patient with diabetes mellitus, *Diab Care* 11: 980-991, 1990.
29a. Holmes CS, editor: *Neuropsychological and behavioural aspects of diabetes*, New York, 1990, Springer-Verlag.
30. Holmes DM: The person and diabetes in psychosocial context, *Diab Care* 9:194-206, 1986.
31. Jeweler D, Steinburg C: Finding more clues, *Diab Forecast* 43(9):31-38, 1990.
32. Horton ES: Exercise and decreased risk of NIDDM, *N Engl J Med* 325:196-198, 1991.
33.* Johnson CKH: Measuring blood glucose: does your meter agree with the lab, *Diab Forecast* 44(10):71-72, 1991.
34. Kaplan N: Hyperinsulinemia in diabetes and hypertension, *Clin Diab* 9(1):1-8, 1991.
35. Keegan DJ et al: Fighting diabetes: a global effort, *Diab Forecast* 44(9):35-40, 1991.
35a. King Edwards Hospital Fund for London: The Nation's Health: A strategy for the 1990's, The King's Fund Centre, London, 1991.
36.* Knighton DR et al: Treating diabetic foot ulcers, *Diab Spectrum* 3:51-56, 1990.
37.* Ley B, Goldman D: Sick-day management: preparing for the expected, *Diab Spectrum* 4:173-176, 1991.
38. Levin ME, O'Neal LW, editors: *The diabetic foot*, ed 4, St Louis, 1988, Mosby—Year Book.
39. Lorber DL: Commentary: what is type II diabetes . . . and what else is it, *Practical Diabetol* 9(5):9, 1990.
40. Lorber DL: Nonketotic osmolarity in diabetes, *Practical Diabetol* 10(1):5-9, 1991.
41. Matson MD, Kjellstrand CM: Long-term follow-up of 369 diabetic patients undergoing dialysis, *Arch Intern Med* 148:600-604, 1988.
42. Messana I, Beizer JL: Diabetes in the elderly, *Practical Diabetol* 10(1):1-4, 1991.
42a. Nabarro JDN: Diabetes in the UK: Some facts and figures, *Diabetic Med* 5:816-822, 1987.
43. National Institutes of Health: *The national long-range plan to combat diabetes*, DHHS Pub. No. PHS 87-1587, Bethesda, Md, US Dept of Health and Human Services, 1987.
44. Nelson RL: The OBTT: its practical use, *Diab Spectrum* 2:219-223, 1989.
45. Neuman RG, Cohen MP: Testing for microalbuminuria, *Diab Professional*, 90:1-4, 1989.
46.* Newman LG et al: Unsuspected osteomyelitis in diabetic foot ulcers, *JAMA* 266:1246-1251, 1991.

47. Palmer JP: From research to practice: commentary, *Diab Spectrum* 4:211-213, 1991.

47a. Peterson A, Drass J: Managing acute complications of diabetes, *Nursing 91* 21(2):34-40, 1991.

48.* Pfeifer M: Cardiovascular autonomic neuropathy, *Diab Spectrum* 3:18-19, 45-48, 1990.

49. Powers MA: Facilitating nutritional changes in difficult patients, *Diab Spectrum* 4(4):186-192, 1991.

50. Rickabaugh TE: Plan of attack is needed to scale exercise walls, *Diab in News* 10(4):50-51, 1991.

51. Rifkin H, Porte D, editors: *Ellenberg and Rifkin's diabetes mellitus, theory and practice*, ed 4, New York, 1990, Elsevier.

52. Rimoin DL, Rotter JI: Genetics and genetic counseling, *Diab Spectrum* 4:194, 1991.

53. Rost K: Research needs and strategies for the meantime. *Diab Dateline: Bull National Diab Information Clearing House* 9(2):1-2, 1988, US Depart of Health and Human Services, Public Health Service, NIH, Bethesda, Md, 1988.

54. Rossini AA, Mordes JP, Handler EW: A tumbler hypothesis: the autoimmunity of insulin-dependent diabetes mellitus, *Diab Spectrum* 2:195-200, 1989.

55. Saudek MD, Zacur HAA, Pitt HA: Implanted insulin pumps: a status report, *Practical Diabetol* 9(2):18-20, 1990.

56. Scharp DW, Lacy PE: The clinical feasibility of human islet transplantation, *Clin Diab* 9(4):42-45, 1991.

57.* Schwarts MJ et al: Unsuspected osteomyelitis in diabetic foot ulcers, *JAMA* 266:1246-1251, 1991.

58. Shuman CR: Controlling diabetes during surgery, *Diab Spectrum* 2:263-269, 1989.

58a. Simmons D, Williams DRR, Powel MJ: Prevalence of Diabetes in a predominant Asian Community: Preliminary findings of the Coventry Diabetes Study, *BR Med J* 298: 18-21.

59. Sorbinil Retinopathy Trial Research Group: A randomized trial of Sorbinil, an aldose reductase inhibitor, in diabetic retinopathy, *Diab Spectrum* 4:131-141, 1991.

59a. Tandan R et al: Topical capsaicin in painful diabetic neuropathy, *Diabetes Care* 15:8-14, 1992.

60. *The prevention and treatment of complications of diabetes: a guide for primary care practitioners*, Atlanta, 1990, 6-1 to 6-4, US Department of Health and Human Services, Centers for Disease Control.

60a. Walkirn PJ: Diagnoses and Management of Diabetic nephropathy, *Medicine International* 65:2,705, 1986.

61. Warshaw H: Sweet nothings; update on sugar substitutes, *Diab Self-Management* 8(2):34-37, 1991.

61a. Wetherall DJ, Lidingham JPG, Warrel DA: Oxford Text Book of Medicine, Oxford University Press, 1984.

62.* Winter W: Atypical diabetes in blacks, *Clin Diab* 9(4): 49-56, 1991.

63.* Zehrer MS, Hansen R, Bantle J: Reducing blood glucose variability by use of abdominal insulin injection sites, *Diab Educator* 16:474-477, 1990.

64. Carlyon PE: Diabetic self-injections: analysis or two teaching/learning approaches, unpublished masters thesis, Kent, Ohio, 1980, Kent State University.

*Recommended for student reading.

FURTHER READING

Bateman J: An extra source of conflict? Diabetes in adolescence, *Professional Nurse* 5(6):290-292, 294, 296, March 1990.

Cradock S: Nurse... I'm going on holiday: considerations for people with diabetes, *Professional Nurse* 5(11):600-602, Aug 1990.

McEvilly A: Diabetic home care, *Nursing Standard* 6(6):20-21, Oct 30-Nov 5 1991.

Samanta A, Denham J, Jowett NI, Burden AC: Management of the acutely ill diabetic patient, *Intensive Care Nursing* 1(4): 194-203, 1986.

Siddons H, McAughey D: Professional development brings specialist knowledge: the role of the diabetes specialist nurse... The Manchester model, *Professional Nurse* 7(5):321-324, Feb 1992.

Walker R: Dire care for diabetes, *Nursing Standard* 6(43):53, July15-21 1992.

21

The Patient with Endocrine Problems

Virginia L. Cassmeyer
Dorothy Blevins

After studying this chapter, the learner should be able to:

- Describe the anatomy and physiology of the endocrine system.
- Describe the nature of hormonal imbalances in terms of hyposecretion and hypersecretion.
- Describe the pathophysiological bases, signs, and symptoms of dysfunction of the endocrine glands.
- Develop a plan of care, including identification of appropriate problems, patient outcomes, and interventions for patients with selected endocrine problems.
- Specify learning needs of patients receiving long-term hormonal replacement therapy.

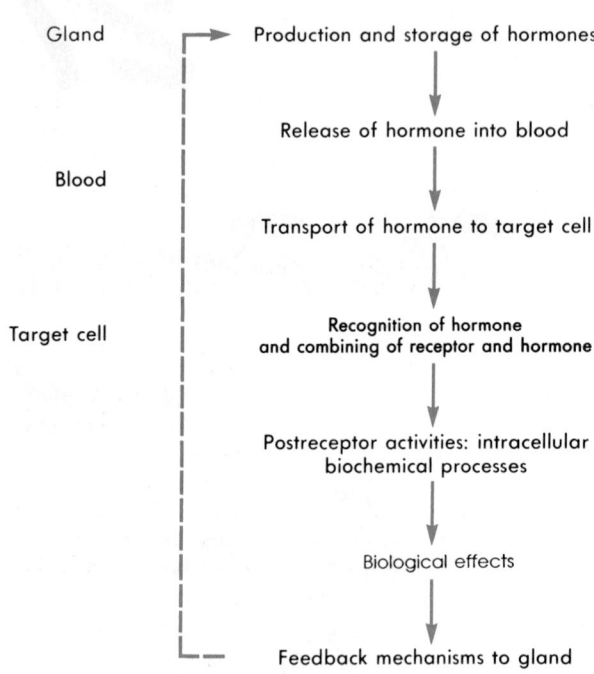

Fig. 21-1   Processes of endocrine system.

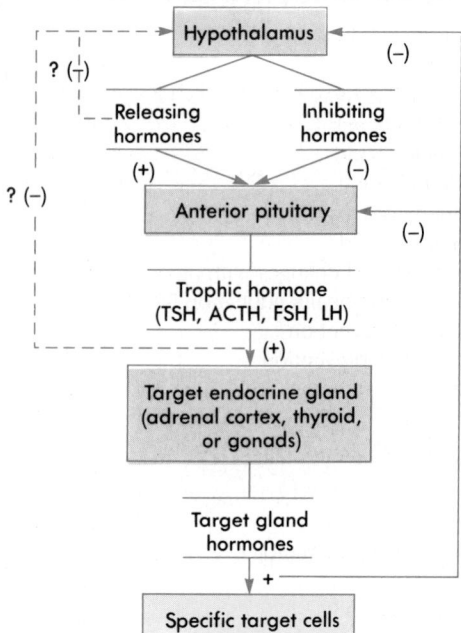

Fig. 21-2   Deficit amount of a target gland hormone allows development of more trophic hormone. This system controls the levels of some hormones secreted by the adrenal cortex (glucocoticoids), thyroid (T₃ and T₄), and the gonads. (Redrawn from Harvey, AM, et al: *The principles and practice of medicine,* ed 20, New York, 1980, Appleton-Century-Crofts.)

The endocrine system functions as the regulator of multiple body processes, primarily through the actions of hormones. Hormones are chemical compounds that are synthesized in glands under genetic control and then secreted into the blood. They affect specific target cells in the body and control diverse physiological functions. Alterations in the function of the endocrine glands, hormones, or target cellular activities usually result in a wide variety of effects. Many endocrine diseases have a slow and subtle onset of signs and symptoms; yet, because many of the functions controlled by the endocrine system are vital, dysfunction can be serious and even fatal.

Research is advancing the knowledge of complex cellular activities that result from the presence of hormones. Fig. 21-1 illustrates a simple schema of the components of the endocrine system, that is, the series of processes that are now considered integral to the endocrine system. This chapter discusses the health problems related to the hormones of the anterior and posterior pituitary, adrenal cortex and medulla, thyroid, and parathyroid. The endocrine functions of the pineal and thymus glands are poorly understood. The gonads are discussed in Unit IX, the endocrine secretions of the gastrointestinal tract are discussed in Chapters 23 and 24, and pancreatic endocrine dysfunction is discussed in Chapter 20.

ANATOMY AND PHYSIOLOGY

Hormone levels are finely regulated in healthy people. For hormones to initiate changes in cellular function the hormone must combine with a specific receptor located on the cell membrane or within the cell. Before the discussion of the anatomy and physiology of the specific endocrine glands, some information on hormonal regulation and receptor activity will be reviewed.

Hormonal Regulation

The amount of hormone available to receptors is critical for health. The amount is kept within definite limits by a number of factors. One factor, the closed-loop negative-feedback system, is shown in Fig. 21-2. It is an important regulating mechanism for hormones secreted by the hypothalamus, anterior pituitary, thyroid, adrenal cortex, and gonads. In this regulatory system, the hypothalamus stimulates gland A to produce trophic hormone X, which stimulates gland B to produce hormone Y; hormone Y then inhibits the secretion of hormone X by gland A and the hypothalamic hormone that started the stimulation. This regulating mechanism for cortisol secretion is called the hypothalamic-pituitary-adrenal cortex (HPA) axis.

A simpler and more direct feedback control is exhibited by other glands. For these glands feedback is exerted by the level of a particular substance in the blood on a particular hormone's production or secretion. For example, a lowered serum calcium concentration stimulates the secretion of parathyroid hormone (PTH) and a higher serum calcium level inhibits the secretion of PTH.

Other factors influencing secretion patterns of hormones include sleep-wake patterns, age, and growth and development. Hormones are not secreted at a uniform rate or steady flow but are released in bursts. Some hormones have cyclic rhythmic patterns of secretions, and thus rhythmic patterns of serum hormone levels can be noted; for example, cortisol has a diurnal pattern and oestrogen has a monthly pattern.

The rate of excretion or metabolic inactivation also affects the levels of circulating hormones. Usually hormones have a very short activity period before they are degraded and excreted by the liver or kidneys. Diseases of these two organs can change hormone levels and activity.

Receptor Activity

It is hypothesized that hormones initiate cellular activity in one of two ways. In the *mobile receptor* model the hormones are thought to cross the plasma cell membrane and combine with receptors in the cytoplasm of the cell. The hormone-receptor complex then crosses the nuclear membrane and reacts with particular proteins in the chromatin of the nucleus or binds with deoxyribonucleic acid (DNA). In general, steroid hormones, such as adrenal cortical steroids, and androgen(s), oestrogen, and progesterone act in this manner. Thyroid hormone may also act in the same way.

In the second model or the *fixed receptor* model, the hormone combines with a receptor on the plasma membrane of a cell and initiates a sequence of events coordinated by a second messenger causing the cell to initiate whatever activity it is equipped to do. Adrenocorticotrophin hormone (ACTH), thyroid stimulating hormone (TSH), glucagon, insulin, PTH, and the catecholamines may initiate cellular activity in this manner.

Hypothalamus

The hypothalamus is a very small area of the brain consisting of numerous poorly defined nuclei. It lies above the anterior and posterior pituitary. The hypothalamus receives input directly or indirectly from almost every part of the brain and is a major controller of both the anterior and posterior pituitary.

Pituitary Gland

The pituitary gland (hypophysis) is approximately 1 cm in size and weighs 500 mg. The pituitary gland is actually two glands, the larger anterior pituitary or adenohypophysis and the posterior pituitary or neurohypophysis. The small size of the pituitary gland should not be misleading. The pituitary is often called the *master gland* because of its major influence on other glands and thus on the entire body. This influence is exerted by six hormones that are produced by different cells of the anterior pituitary gland and by two hormones released by the posterior pituitary gland. See Table 21-1 for the specific name and functions of each hormone.

Thyroid-stimulating hormone (TSH), adrenocorticotrophic hormone (ACTH), and the gonadotrophic hormones are called trophic hormones because the target cells

Table 21-1 Pituitary hormones

Hormone	Function
Anterior pituitary	
Growth hormone (GH)	Target organ: whole body, possibly works on most tissue through action of somatomedin
	Concerned with growth of cells, bones, and soft tissue
	Increases mitosis
	Affects carbohydrate, protein, and fat metabolism
	Increases blood glucose by decreasing glucose utilization; insulin antagonist
	Increases protein synthesis
	Increases free fatty acid levels, lipolysis, and ketone formation
	Increases electrolyte retention and extracellular fluid volume
Prolactin (PRL)	Target organ: breast and gonads
	Necessary for breast development and lactation
	Regulator of reproductive function in males and females
Thyroid-stimulating hormone (TSH)	Target organ: thyroid
	Necessary for growth and functions of thyroid; controls all functions of thyroid
Adrenocorticophic hormone (ACTH; corticotrophin)	Target organ: adrenal cortex
	Necessary for growth and maintenance of size of adrenal cortex
	Controls release of glucocorticoids (cortisol) and adrenal androgens
	Minor role in release of mineralocorticoids (aldosterone)
Ganodotrophins	
Follicle-stimulating hormone (FSH)	Target organs: gonads
	Stimulates gametogenesis and sex steroid production in males and females
Luteinizing hormone (LH)	
Posterior pituitary	
Antidiuretic hormone (ADH)	Target organ: kidney tubular cells
	Effects changes in kidney tubular membrane to increase water absorption; stimulates smooth muscle of intestines and blood vessels
Oxytocin	Target organs: breast, uterus
	Stimulates uterine contractions and breast milk ejection

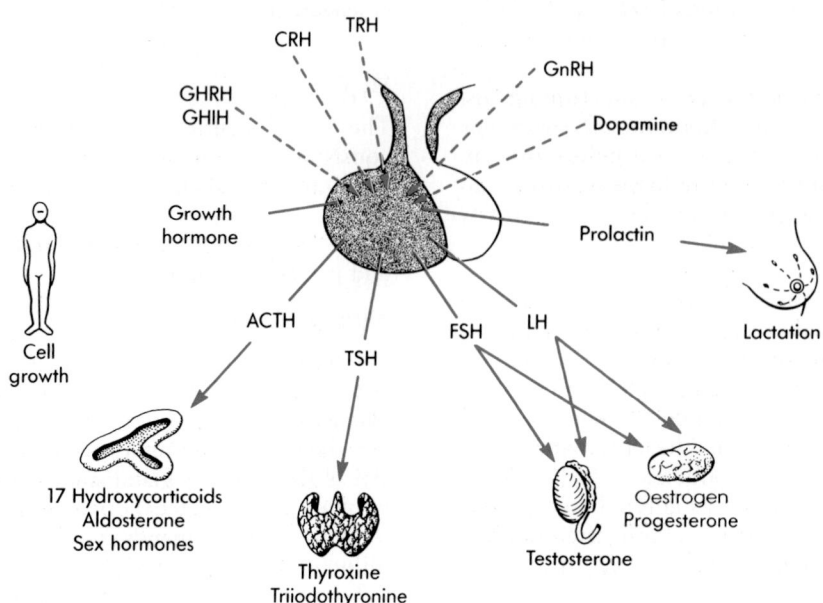

Fig. 21-3   Relationships between hormones of the hypothalamus, anterior pituitary gland, and target tissues are depicted. Six releasing or inhibiting hormones have been chemically identified: growth hormone–releasing hormone *(GHRH)*; growth hormone–inhibiting hormone *(GHIH,* somatostatin); thyrotrophin-releasing hormone *(TRH)*; corticotrophin–releasing hormone *(CRH)*; gonadotrophin-releasing hormone *(GnRH)*; and dopamine, which acts as a prolactin inhibiting hormone *(PIH)*. Each anterior pituitary hormone is shown with its respective target tissues: body cells *(GH)*; adrenal cortex *(ACTH)*; thyroid stimulating hormone *(TSH)*; testes and ovaries *(FSH and LH)*; and breasts *(prolactin)*.

for these hormones are other endocrine glands. As trophic hormones these hormones are necessary for the growth and maintenance of the size of the targeted endocrine glands, as well as functioning as major regulators of the synthesis and secretion of hormones from these targeted endocrine glands. The other pituitary hormones exert their influence directly on body cells.

Relationship between hypothalamus and pituitary gland

The hypothalamus serves as a vital link between the neurological and hormonal regulatory mechanisms. The hypothalamus and the anterior pituitary are connected by the hypothalamic-hypophyseal portal blood system, by which neurosecretory-releasing hormones and neurosecretory-inhibiting hormones are carried from the hypothalamus to the anterior pituitary. The exact number of releasing and inhibiting hormones is not known. At present, six of these hypothalamic hormones have been identified. These hormones are depicted in Fig. 21-3. The interactions between the hypothalamus, anterior pituitary, and other endocrine glands or target organs are also summarized in the legend in Fig. 21-3. The hypothalamus also exerts control over the posterior pituitary gland to which it is structurally connected. ADH and oxytocin are produced in the hypothalamus in the paraventricular and supraoptic nuclei and are carried down neurones by axonal transport to the terminal branches that are located in the posterior pituitary lobe. There they are stored and then released.

Adrenal Gland

The two adrenal organs lie in the retroperitoneal area, each capping the upper pole of a kidney. There are two glands in each adrenal organ: the adrenal cortex, or outer layer, and the adrenal medulla, or central portion. The *adrenal cortex* secretes two groups of hormones that are necessary for life: the *glucocorticoids* of which cortisol is the principal hormone, and the *mineralocorticoids* of which aldosterone is the principal hormone. The third group of hormones secreted by the cortex in both men and women is the androgens. Although these androgens do not have much intrinsic biological activity, they can be converted to testosterone or oestrogen in the periphery. This source of androgens is an important consideration in certain pathological conditions or when treatments require the absence of a particular sex hormone.

Table 21-2 lists the specific effects of each adrenal hormone. Although the glucocorticoids have other important functions, they have a major role in *nutrition* (cortisol has hyperglycaemic, catabolic, and lipolytic effects) and in *biological defences* (cortisol has antiinflammatory and immunosuppressive effects).

The secretion of cortisol is regulated by ACTH (a pituitary hormone) under the influence of corticotrophin-releasing hormone (CRH). Cortisol has a circadian diurnal pattern of release with peak levels occurring in the early morning following release of ACTH. This pattern of release follows sleep-wake cycles. Through a negative feedback system, serum levels of cortisol also are primary regulators for inhibition or stimulation of ACTH release. Low serum levels of cortisol stimulate the release of ACTH and then, as a result, the release of cortisol. High serum levels of cortisol inhibit the release of ACTH and thus its own release. However, during the stress response, hypothalamic stimulation (by CRH) of the pituitary results in increased ACTH secretion and stimulation of the adrenal glands that release cortisol. This stress response overrides the usual negative feedback system.

Mineralocorticoid secretion is increased during the stress response; however, the primary regulator at all times is the renin-angiotensin system (see Chapters 6 and 25). An increased serum potassium level also stimulates the adrenal cortex to increase its release of aldosterone. Mineralocorticoids are necessary for the maintenance of sodium, potassium, and water balance; they act on the kidneys to increase the retention of sodium and water and the excretion of potassium.

The *adrenal medulla* secretes adrenaline and noradrenaline, which augment the catecholamines produced by the sympathetic nervous system. These *catecholamines* secreted by the adrenal medulla are not necessary for life but, in excess, can be responsible for serious hypertension.

A small amount of the catecholamines is released at all times, but during the stress response, increased amounts are released as part of the *physiological stress response*. Table 21-3 lists the multiple effects of increased adrenal-medullary stimulation. Different effects in the body are seen as a result of stimulation of different receptors located on target organs. Receptors are classified as:

alpha (α)-adrenergic:

α_1-adrenergic receptors are on various target organs throughout the body and are excitatory.

α_2-adrenergic receptors are at presynaptic sites on nervous tissue and are inhibitory.

Beta (β)-adrenergic:

β_1-adrenergic receptors are located primarily in the heart.

β_2-adrenergic receptors are located elsewhere in the body.

Noradrenaline stimulates only alpha (α) receptors; adrenaline stimulates both beta (β) and α receptors.

Parathyroid Gland

The *parathyroid gland* consists of four minute glands that are variously located on the posterior aspect of each thyroid lobe. Occasionally extra glands are located on the thyroid, in the mediastinum, or behind the oesophagus. Parathyroid hormone (PTH) regulates calcium and phosphorus metabolism by its effect on gastrointestinal absorption, kidney excretion, or bone resorption. A low serum calcium level stimulates the release of PTH. The specific functions of PTH are listed in Table 21-4.

Thyroid Gland

The thyroid gland is located in the anterior aspect of the neck and weighs about 20 g. It consists of two lobes connected by an isthmus and lies just below the larynx. The thyroid gland stores iodine and secretes the thyroid hor-

Table 21-2 Functions of the adrenal hormones

Gland	Hormones	Functions
Adrenal cortex	Glucocorticoids (cortisol)	Overall effect is to maintain blood glucose level by increasing gluconeogenesis and decreasing rate of glucose use by cells
		Increases level of protein catabolism
		Promotes lipolysis
		Promotes sodium and water retention
		Antiinflammatory
		Degrades collagen
		Decreases T lymphocyte participation in cellular-mediated immunity by decreasing circulating level of T lymphocytes
		Increases serum level of neutrophils by increasing release and decreasing destruction but neutrophils are prevented from migrating to sites of injury
		Decrease new antibody release
		Decreases eosinophils, basophils, and monocytes
		Decreases scar tissue formation
		Increases RBC formation and possibly increases platelet formation
		Stimulates appetite
		Increases gastric acid and pepsin production
		Maintains emotional stability
	Mineralcorticoids (aldosterone)	Primary stimulus is the renin-angiotensin system
		Primarily responsible for maintenance of normovolaemic state by increasing sodium and water retention in distal kidney tubules
		Causes potassium excretion
		Causes increased excretion of ammonium and magnesium ions
	Androgens	Same functions as gonadal sex hormones
Adrenal medulla	Adrenaline and noradrenaline	Necessary for maintenance of neuroendocrine integrating functions of body
		See Table 21-3 for a summary of the effects of these two catecholamines

Table 21-3 Effects of adrenal-medullary-sympathetic stimulation on body organs*

Organ	Effect	Organ	Effect
Heart	Increased conduction velocity, automaticity, contractility, rate, and stroke volume caused by β_1-stimulation	Gallbladder	Relaxation
		Kidney	Increased renin secretion caused by β_2-stimulation
Blood vessels		Urinary bladder	Relaxation of detrusor muscle and contraction of internal spincter
Coronary vessels, brain, lungs	Dilation caused by β_2-stimulation and autoregulatory phenomena	Skin	Pilomotor muscle contraction and localized sweating
Skin, mucosa, abdominal viscera, renal and salivary gland vessels	Constriction caused by α-stimulation; renal vessels also have dopaminergic receptors	Liver	Glycogenolysis and gluconeogenesis caused by β_2-stimulation
Veins	Constriction caused by α-stimulation	Pancreas	Decreased secretion of acini cells; β_2-stimulation causes increased secretion of islet β-cells but α-stimulation causes decreased secretion of islet cells; α-effect predominates so insulin secretion decreased
Bronchial muscles	Relaxation caused by β_2-stimulation		
Gastrointestinal tract	Inhibition of production of gastrointestinal secretions; decreased motility and contraction of sphincters caused by β_2-stimulation	Fat cells	Lipolysis
		Brain	Increased alertness, restlessness
		Eyes	Dilation of pupils and relaxation of ciliary bodies

* These total effects would be seen in the physiological response to stressors.

Table 21-4 Functions of parathyroid hormone (PTH)

Organ	Effects of PTH
Kidney tubule	Decreases urinary excretion of calcium
	Increases urinary excretion of phosphorus
	Inhibits H^+ ion secretion
	Decreases reabsorption of sodium bicarbonate
	Increases renal threshhold for glucose
Gut	Increases calcium and phosphorus absorption from intestinal tract (requires vitamin D)
Bone	Converts osteogenic osteocytes to osteolytic osteocytes
	Decreases the number of osteoblasts
	Decreases bone formation and increases bone breakdown

Table 21-5 Functions of thyroid hormone

Hormones	Functions
Thyroxine (T_4) Triiodothyronine (T_3)	Regulates protein, fat, and carbohydrate catabolism in all cells
	Regulates metabolic rate of all cells
	Regulates body heat production
	Insulin antagonist
	Maintains growth hormone secretion, skeletal maturation
	Affects CNS development and function
	Necessary for muscle tone and vigor
	Maintains cardiac rate, force, and output
	Maintains secretions of gastrointestinal tract
	Affects respiratory rate and oxygen utilization
	Maintains calcium mobilization
	Affects RBC production
	Stimulates lipid turnover, free fatty acid release, and cholesterol synthesis
Calcitonin	Lowers serum calcium and phosphorus levels
	Decreases calcium and phosphorus absorption in gastrointestinal tract
	Inhibits bone resorption

mones and calcitonin. The two thyroid hormones are thyroxine (tetraiodothyronine, T_4) and triiodothyronine (T_3).

The production of the thyroid hormones is under the control of thyroid-releasing hormone (TRH) from the hypothalamus and thyroid-stimulating hormone (TSH) from the anterior pituitary. A primary regulator of T_4 and T_3 is the negative-feedback system depicted in Fig. 21-2. Calcitonin is primarily regulated by serum levels of calcium; elevated serum levels of calcium promote the release of calcitonin, and lowered serum levels of calcium inhibit calcitonin release.

The functions of the thyroid hormones and calcitonin are presented in Table 21-5. Overall, T_3 and T_4 regulate metabolic rate, growth and tissue differentiation. Calcitonin helps maintain serum calcium levels.

Physiological Changes with Ageing

Changes in the endocrine system are associated with normal ageing. Endocrine dysfunction may result from cellular damage resulting from ageing, wear and tear on the endocrine tissue from long-term use, or genetically programmed cellular changes. Endocrine changes may result in altered synthesis and secretion of hormones, altered metabolism of hormones, altered circulatory levels of hormones, altered biological activity, altered target cell and target tissue responsiveness, or altered intrinsic rhythms.

Although findings are not consistent, the following is a summary of the major alterations in endocrine function that are most frequently reported.*

1. The most commonly seen change is decreased ovarian functioning in females, resulting in increased gonadotrophins and changes in reproductive and sexual functioning. No similar change in males has been reported.

2. Impaired secretion of hypothalamic hormones or impaired response to feedback may influence endocrine system responsiveness to alterations in the internal environment, and thus to stressors.

3. The anterior pituitary gland shows morphological changes with increased fibrosis and microadenoma formation, a decrease in basal levels of prolactin in females and a decrease in growth hormone and somatomedins.

4. Antidiuretic hormone secretion in response to changes in serum osmolality is increased, resulting in increased levels of ADH. However, elderly people also have alterations in renal function that decrease the ability to concentrate urine and can result in hyponatraemia. Nocturia is commonly present.

5. Various changes in thyroid gland structure, including glandular atrophy, fibrosis, nodularity, and infiltrates have been found. The following changes in thyroid hormone levels have been reported:
   a. Decreased T_4 secretion and metabolism.
   b. Decreased plasma T_3 levels.
   c. Increased basal plasma TSH levels.
   d. Decreased responsiveness in TSH secretion to TRH

   Hypothyroidism is very common in the elderly. Whether all these changes in thyroid structure, function, or disease can be attributed to the ageing process is unclear. Some of the early clinical manifestations of hypothyroidism, such as skin and hair changes, neurological changes, or gastrointestinal change can be seen in elderly people for other reasons, leading health care professionals to ignore or potentially misdiagnose the changes.

6. Calcium homeostasis is altered in the older adult. Changes found include decreased intake of calcium, negative calcium balance, bone loss, decreased intestinal adaptation to varied calcium intake, hypercalciuria, and decreased vitamin D levels. Age-related alterations in PTH may explain some of the changes in calcium homeostasis, but more research is needed.

7. The adrenal cortex, which is small and contains fibrous tissue, responds to feedback mechanisms and maintains circadian patterns of cortisol secretion in response to circadian patterns of ACTH. However, the amount of cortisol secreted is decreased because of decreased metabolic clearance and decreased usage. Thus increased blood cortisol levels result in decreased secretion. The amount of androgens secreted by the adrenal cortex is decreased, and the renin-aldosterone response to postural changes and volume depletion is depressed.

---

*References 3, 4, 6, 8, 10, 34.

If the endocrine changes described in the preceding section are ignored, the elderly may be misdiagnosed. That is, endocrine disease may not be diagnosed. Changes in serum sodium and potassium such as hyponatraemia and hypokalaemia must be carefully evaluated to differentiate changes related to endocrine changes with ageing from those that might be due to drugs such as diuretics, other diseases such as congestive heart failure, or diet. The potential role of changes in PTH in development of metabolic bone disease contributing to osteoporosis needs more exploration. It is important to remember that the hypothalamic-pituitary-adrenal axis and the hypothalamic-pituitary-thyroid axis, which are important in daily living and response to stressors, are intact but may be slower to respond thus explaining in part the decreased ability to respond to physiological and psychological stressors.

Besides the changes listed above, changes in response to actual endocrine pathology have been reported. Some elderly people with hyperthyroidism have subtle signs and symptoms that make diagnosis difficult. Elderly people tolerate hypothyroidism better, and there may be a greater insufficiency of thyroid hormones when they are first diagnosed. Also, early signs and symptoms of hypothyroidism such as skin changes, change in hair, increased diastolic pressure, decreased memory and so forth may be overlooked because they are seen in many elderly people even in the absence of thyroid pathology.

PREVENTION AND HEALTH EDUCATION
Primary Prevention

Few primary endocrine diseases can be prevented at this time. *Simple goitre*, a disease characterized by an enlargement of the thyroid gland, is an exception. This condition may occur because of a lack of ingested iodine. The nurse can participate in primary prevention by teaching the importance of eating foods that contain iodine, such as seafoods and leafy vegetables.

Diseases similar to endocrine hypersecretory states may be caused by inappropriate use of hormones for nonmedical purposes. This abuse of hormones is termed *factitious* and is often concealed from health care providers. Primary prevention education programmes should focus on the use of gonadal steroids and growth hormones by athletes, glucocorticoids for mood elevating effects, and thyroid drugs by dieters.

Secondary Prevention

Malignant tumours of the endocrine gland are less prevalent than other forms of cancer. The thyroid gland can be easily palpated, and people should be encouraged to have regular physical examinations to help in early detection of thyroid carcinoma. This cancer appears in all age-groups and especially in those with a history of irradiation to the neck structures. In recent years, there has been a concerted search in many countries for adults who received irradiation of the upper thorax, head, or neck for conditions such as thymus conditions, enlarged tonsils and adenoids, acne, dysfunction of the eustachian tube and so forth during early childhood years. These individuals are urged to seek medical attention for detection of thyroid cancer.

Heart disease can be induced or aggravated by certain hormonal alterations. Thyroid and adrenocortical dysfunction are two disorders in which early detection and treatment can minimize cardiovascular disease. The nurse can assist in the early detection of these disorders by encouraging people to seek medical attention for persistent vague complaints of decreased well-being that may include the following:

1. Fatigue
2. Altered nutritional intake
3. Changes in skin and hair appearance and condition
4. Changes in excretory patterns

Although endocrine diseases are not the only cause of these signs and symptoms, it is true that these are early signs and symptoms of many endocrinopathies.

Tertiary Prevention

A major contribution of the nurse to patients with diagnosed endocrinopathies is that of assisting them to learn self-management of their chronic diseases. The progression of many hormonal deficiency diseases can be halted or slowed by patients who are educated and motivated to follow prescribed regimens. Hormonal replacement, when necessary, is an important method of treatment that must be handled by the patient over a long period of time. It should be stressed that failure to maintain adequate hormonal replacement and other parts of the regimen can result in illness and death.

MAJOR HEALTH PROBLEMS OF THE ENDOCRINE SYSTEM

The classifications of hypersecretion and hyposecretion of hormones help organize the information in this chapter. Only those endocrine problems encountered most frequently are discussed; these are listed in Table 21-6. The most frequent endocrine disorder in the United Kingdom is diabetes mellitus, which is discussed in Chapter 20. The next most frequent disorder is thyroid dysfunction. All endocrine disorders can lead to significant health problems in individuals.

Regardless of the pathological process involved, endocrine disorders are characterized by an alteration in *amount* of effective hormone, either an excess or a deficiency. Hormonal alterations *may result from* the following:

1. Change in the integrity of glandular tissue
2. Dysfunction of regulating mechanisms
3. Decrease in excretion or inactivation of hormones
4. Peripheral resistance to the action of the hormones

Aetiological factors of endocrine glandular disorders are classified as primary, secondary, or iatrogenic:

Primary: disorder of the gland
Secondary: disorder of a target gland because of disorder in the pituitary gland or the hypothalamus
Iatrogenic: hormonal disorders that occur because of treatment

Hyposecretory states may occur when there is absence of glandular tissue or when there is *hypoplasia* (decrease in number of functioning cells). *Atrophy* (decrease in gland size) and hypoplasia often occur together. Hypersecretory states may occur when there is *hyperplasia* (increase in number of active secreting cells) or a tumour. For example, pituitary hyperplasia might be a response to hypothalamic stimulation. *Hypertrophy* (increase in gland size) is not always accompanied by an increased secretion of hormone. One pathological cause of hypersecretory states is the secretion of hormones by tissues in quantities not related to body needs. These tissues are not responsive to the regulating mechanisms, for example, to the negative feedback loops or to the trophic hormone stimulation or lack of stimulation. Affected endocrine glands are said to be autonomous when this escape from regulation occurs.

ANTERIOR PITUITARY DYSFUNCTION

Dysfunction of the anterior pituitary may involve increased or decreased secretion of one or more than one hormone. Important information related to hypersecretory and hyposecretory states is presented first followed by a discussion of the nursing process as it pertains to the most common situations affecting the anterior pituitary gland.

Table 21-6   Health problems caused by imbalances in the endocrine system

Gland	Hyposecretion	Hypersecretion
Pituitary	Panhypopituitarism, hypopituitarism, dwarfism, pituitary adrenal insufficiency, thyroid deficiency secondary to pituitary deficiency, hypoprolactinaemia, diabetes insipidus	Hyperpituitarism, acromegaly, gigantism, pituitary Cushing's syndrome, thyroid excess secondary to pituitary excess, hyperprolactinaemia, syndrome of inappropriate ADH secretion (SIADH)
Thyroid	Hypothyroidism, cretinism, myxoedema	Hyperthyroidism
Parathyroid	Hypoparathyroidism	Hyperparathyroidism
Adrenal cortex	Addison's disease	Adrenal Crushing's syndrome, hyperaldosteronism
Adrenal medulla		Phaeochromocytoma
Pancreas (endocrine)	Diabetes mellitus (see Chapter 20)	Hypoglycaemia (see Chapter 20)

HYPERSECRETION

Hypersecretion of the anterior pituitary may involve one or more hormones.

Aetiology/Epidemiology

The causes of hypersecretion of anterior pituitary hormones are multiple. Hypersecretion may be:

1. A primary problem (tumour or hyperplasia) in the anterior pituitary gland.
2. Secondary to hypothalamic dysfunction (increased secretion of releasing hormones or decreased secretion of inhibiting hormones).
3. Secondary to target gland dysfunction (lack of negative feedback).
4. Mimicked by excessive secretion of hormone by ectopic nonendocrine tissue.
5. Iatrogenic from drug therapy.

Pituitary adenomas are the most common cause of hyperpituitarism. Pituitary adenomas of the anterior pituitary gland account for 6% to 18% of all intracranial tumours.[42] In most patients the cause of the adenoma is unknown and no family history exists. Pituitary adenomas are almost always *secreting* or *functioning* tumours. These tumours are usually benign, but some can grow very aggressively.

Prolactin-secreting tumours[42] (prolactinomas) account for 60% to 80% of all pituitary tumours. The next most frequently occurring tumour secretes growth hormone (GH) (somatotroph tumour). Tumours that secrete adrenocorticotrophic hormone (ACTH) (corticotroph tumours) are the third most frequently occurring tumours.

Pathophysiology

Secreting pituitary tumours cause two clinical problems depending on the size, location, and *secreting capacity* of the tumour. These are (1) neurological alterations resulting from pressure on surrounding nervous system structures and (2) hypersecretion of one or more anterior pituitary hormones (see Table 21-1, for a review of functions of anterior pituitary hormones).

The major effects of hypersecretion of anterior pituitary hormones are presented in Table 21-7. The effects of growth hormone (GH) and prolactin excess are presented in more detail because these are the most common hypersecretory conditions seen in adults.

Growth hormone excess

An excess of GH is almost always caused by a secreting pituitary tumour, although occasionally there is no distinct tumour. Hypersecretion of GH that occurs in children before fusion of the epiphysis results in *gigantism*. Such children reach enormous proportions because of massive growth in both the length and width of bones. Soft tissue enlarges along with the skeleton.

Table 21-7 Anterior pituitary dysfunction

Alterations in secretion	Signs and symptoms	Medical therapy
GH excess	Gigantism in children; acromegaly in adults: growth of soft tissues, cartilages, bones; enlargement and coarsening of facial features; enlarged tongue; visceral enlargement (liver, spleen, heart, kidneys); warm, moist, coarse skin,husky voice; prominent muscle development;insulin resistance	Removal of tumor: adenectomy, hypophysectomy; irradiation; medications that suppress GH: bromocriptine mesylate or long-acting somatostatin analog, octreotide.
GH deficiency	Dwarfism in children; sensitivity to insulin; fasting hypoglycaemia	Growth hormone replacement in children
ACTH excess	Similar to Adrenal Cushing syndrome (adrenocortical excess) Table 21-9)	Pituitary ablation: adenectomy, hypophysectomy; radiation; surgical removal of ectopic sourse of ACTH
ACTH deficiency	Similar to Addison's disease (primary adreno-cortical deficit) (Table 21-9); asthenia (weakness); nausea, vomiting; hypotension; hypoglycaemia; hyperkalaemia	Glucocorticoid replacement
TSH exess	Same as primary hyperthyroidism (thyroid hormone exess) (Table 21-12)	Removal of tumor: adenectomy, hypophysectomy
TSH deficit	Same as primary hypothyroidism (thyroid hormone deficit) (Table 21-12)	Thyroid hormone replacement
Prolactin exess	Amenorrhoea; galactorrhoea; depressed libido; osteopenia, hirsutism and acne in women; importence and oligospermia in men	Removal of tumor: adenectomy, hypophysectomy; irradiation; drugs to suppress prolactin; bromocriptine mesylate
Prolactin deficit	Failure of postpartum lactation	
Gonadotrophic hormone exess	Precocious sexual development in children; changes in secondary sex characteristics: hirsutism in women; gynaecomastia in men	Removal of tumor: adenectomy, hypophysectomy
Gonadotrophic hormone deficit	Delayed sexual development in children; in adults: female—amenorrhoea, infertility; male—importence; in both—changes in secondary sex characteristics	Replacement of gonadotrophins in cyclic pattern

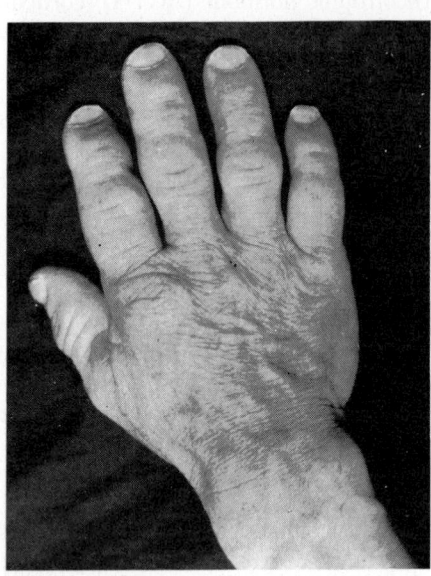

Fig. 21-4 Hand showing characteristics of acromegalic condition. (From Schottelius BA, Schottelius DD: *Texbook of physiology*, ed 18, St Louis, 1978, Mosby–Year Book.)

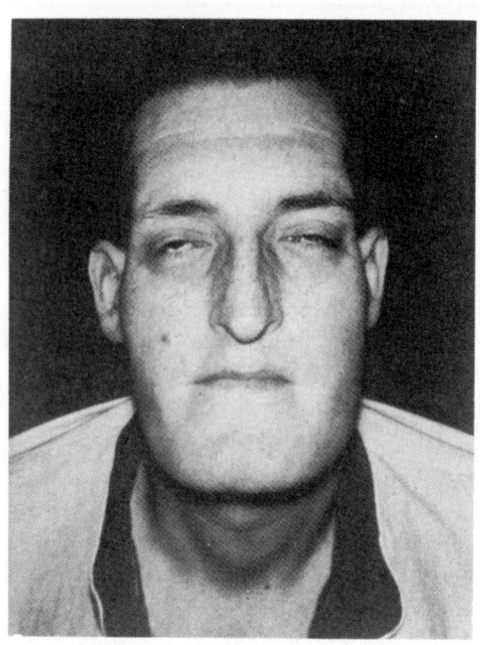

Fig. 21-5 Acromegaly. Note large head, exaggerated forward projection of jaw, and protrusion of frontal bone.

Hypersecretion of GH that occurs after the fusion of the epiphysis results in *acromegaly*. This disorder affects men and women equally and most frequently begins between the second and fourth decades of life. The changes are slow and progressive and frequently go unrecognized for some time. The adult with acromegaly may note an increase in ring, shoe, glove, and hat size. The hands become spadelike in appearance (Fig. 21-4). The enlargement of the mandible causes an under bite and increased spacing of the lower teeth. The forehead and orbital ridges become prominent (Fig. 21-5). Widening of spaces between joints occurs with increased cartilage growth. This leads to osteoarthritis with pain and limitation of joint motion. Changes in the spine may cause nerve root and cord compression.

The following systemic changes can result from excess in growth hormone:

1. Increased metabolic rate
2. Increased sweating and sebaceous gland activity
3. Glucose intolerance (50% of patients) and insulin resistance that can lead to diabetes mellitus
4. Hypertension (25% of patients) and cardiomegaly can lead to congestive heart failure (CHF)

Many patients with GH excess eventually develop neurological alterations resulting from an expanding lesion. Frequently they do not seek help until neurological signs and symptoms occur. Common neurological alterations are described below.

Prolactin excess

Prolactin excess is usually caused by pituitary adenomas, usually microadenomas (tumours less than 1 cm in diameter), or hypothalamic dysfunction. Dopamine is the primary hypothalamic inhibitor of prolactin release; interruption of dopamine transmission to the pituitary can result in prolactin excess. Other causes are hypothyroidism, renal failure, and side effects of drugs. Levels of serum prolactin over 300 μg/ml suggest a prolactinoma.[20] Prolactin excess interferes with normal gonadal function by disturbing the hypothalamic-pituitary-gonadal axis. People usually seek help for gonadal dysfunction or changes in breast tissue before neurological signs and symptoms from an intrapituitary mass are present. Women may complain of amenorrhoea or galactorrhoea. They often complain of depressed libido. Men may give a history of depressed libido, infertility, or impotence. Other signs and symptoms of hypogonadism, such as changes in secondary sex characteristics, may be present.

Neurological alterations

Tumours larger than 1 cm in diameter (macroadenomas) cause compression of the pituitary and enlargement of the sella turcica; as they expand, they can invade or compress nearby tissue. Patients experience progressive loss of vision, and if untreated, permanent blindness results. Other symptoms include headaches that are characteristically bitemporal or bifrontal and result from pressure on the sella turcica. Confusion and impaired memory may occur but are rare. Symptoms of increased intracranial pressure may develop as lesions expand in size.

HYPOSECRETION

Hyposecretion of the anterior pituitary gland may involve one or more of the anterior pituitary hormones and is referred to as *hypopituitarism*. If all anterior pituitary hormones are deficit, as well as antidiuretic hormone from the posterior pituitary, the condition is called *panhypopituitarism*.

Aetiology/Epidemiology

The cause of hypopituitarism or panhypopituitarism is most frequently the presence of a nonsecreting tumour of the pituitary that is compressing normal secretory tissue. Other causes of hyposecretion of anterior pituitary hormones include ischemia and necrosis after haemorrhage or trauma, infection, autoimmune problems, radiation, and developmental problems. Gonadotropin hormone deficits can result from severely malnourished states such as anorexia nervosa. In hypopituitarism or panhypopituitarism, unless due to removal of the pituitary or massive destruction of the pituitary, the hormone deficits of the anterior pituitary do not usually appear simultaneously. Deficits of GH and gonadotrophins occur first, followed by deficits of TSH, and then ACTH.

Pathophysiology

The signs and symptoms associated with anterior pituitary deficiency vary widely depending on the hormones that are deficient and the cause of the deficiencies (see Table 21-1, p. 525 for a review of functions of anterior pituitary hormones). If a tumour is the cause of the problem, neurological alterations as described on page 532 can be present. Signs and symptoms associated with specific hormone deficiencies are summarized in Table 21-7.

Although growth hormone deficiency occurs first in hypopituitarism in the adult, it causes no striking effects except that it may aggravate hypoglycaemia related to other problems. However, congenital deficiency of growth hormone in the child results in short stature (dwarfism). Pituitary dwarfism is a rare disorder and is characterized by short stature that is apparent at about 4 years of age (Fig. 21-6). The child typically appears immature and has increased truncal fat. Bone age and height age are usually approximate, and as the child matures, the body proportions approach those of an adult.

Deficiency of gonadotrophins will result in various alterations in sexual and reproductive functioning. In adult women, amenorrhoea and infertility occur. In adult males infertility and impotency occur. Changes in secondary sexual characteristics will also be present. Lack of TSH and ACTH results in signs and symptoms of primary hypothyroidism and primary adrenocortical insufficiency, which are discussed later in this chapter.

Nursing Process
Assessment

The application of the nursing process to patients with either *hypersecretion* or *hyposecretion* of the *anterior pituitary* focuses on patients with secreting pituitary tumours, pituitary surgery, and potential hormonal imbalances related to the surgery. Many of the descriptions of assessment, data analysis, and planning discussed in this section can be applied to later sections in the chapter. The following are some common clinical problems seen in the various endocrine disorders discussed in this chapter:

1. Fatigue
2. Nutritional alterations
3. Fluid and electrolyte imbalances
4. Cardiovascular changes
5. Changed body characteristics

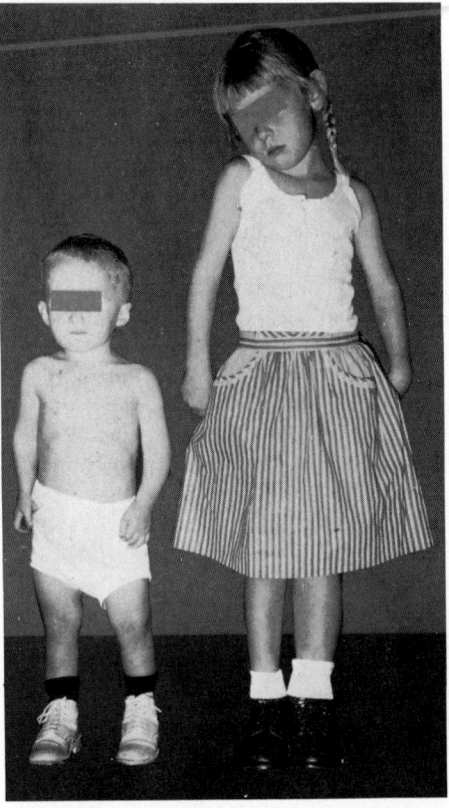

Fig. 21-6 Hypopituitary dwarfism in a 4-year-old boy whose height is 25 inches. Girl is also 4 years old and has a normal height of 39 inches. Dwarf has normal face, as well as head, trunk, and limbs of approximately normal proportions. (From Brashear HR, Raney RB: *Handbook of orthopaedic surgery,* ed 10, St Louis, 1986, Mosby–Year Book.)

6. Intolerance to stressors
7. Emotional instability
8. Reproductive alterations

Nursing assessment should include the following:

1. Assessing for clinical signs and symptoms that indicate the extent of hormonal imbalances
2. Assessing for manifestations of potential complications of the endocrine disorder or its treatment
3. Eliciting the patient's and family's perceptions of health problems, their management, and the assistance needed
4. Determining the resources needed by the patient and family to cope with the disorder and to manage it in the hospital and after discharge

Assessment of psychological and social factors is important for several reasons. The endocrine diagnostic process can be lengthy and frightening. Stressors in the patient with pituitary hormonal imbalances should be avoided as much as possible, because the stress response places an additional burden on the impaired endocrine function. Body image changes and physical problems may influence the person's goals, activities of daily living, and relationships with others. The person's coping abilities may also be diminished because of energy depletion or physiological crisis. Learning to incorporate a treatment regimen into daily life is often necessary for optimal treatment and sometimes necessary to maintain life.

Subjective data

Because anterior pituitary dysfunction can potentially affect almost every other endocrine gland, the assessment focuses on a variety of areas. The collecting of information regarding changes in body characteristics is important not only in defining the physiological problem, but also in identifying potential or present emotional or psychological problems. Some of the changes that occur with pituitary endocrine disorders are irreversible even when the physiological problem is controlled. Body characteristics are part of the identity of the person, and the patient may have problems dealing with the changes.

The patient's or other's description of the following factors helps define the needs for assistance:

1. Fatigue, rest, and sleep patterns
2. Eating patterns (frequency of food intake)
3. Fluid intake and output patterns
4. Cardiovascular history
5. Special hygiene or grooming needs (hirsutism, perspiration, obesity)
6. Discomforts
7. Emotional response
8. Reproductive history
9. Medication usage
10. The endocrine disorder and its treatment

Objective data

Initially, inspection is used to assess the patient's body growth and developmental status and should include the following:

1. Height and weight
2. Body proportions
3. Amount and distribution of muscle mass
4. Fat distribution
5. Skin pigmentation
6. Hair distribution

A great variation exists in these characteristics in the general population, and often changes are not obvious. Inspection of family members for like characteristics provides information as to whether the characteristics seen in the patient are caused by heredity or pathophysiological alterations. The patient's alertness and speech patterns can be assessed when the history is being collected. Physical assessment should be thorough in these patients because of the wide spectrum of bodily effects that occur with pituitary dysfunction.

The minimum baseline data should include the following:

Nutritional status: presence or absence of fat pads, truncal obesity, abnormal fat depositions; muscle mass, strength; serum levels of lymphocytes, albumin, glucose

Fluid and electrolyte status: vital signs, urine output, fluid intake; signs of fluid excess (oedema, jugular vein distension [JVD], adventitious lung sounds) or deficit (orthostatic blood pressure, poor skin turgor, sunken eyeballs, dry mucous membranes); serum levels of electrolytes, urea, creatinine

Cardiovascular status: blood pressure level including postural BP; pulses, skin colour; signs of hypotension or cardiac failure; serum levels of electrolytes, triglycerides, cholesterol; ECG.

Diagnostic tests

Usually target organ function is first studied to confirm the presence of a hormonal deficit or excess suggested by the patient's history and clinical findings. Thus measurement of cortisol, T_3 and T_4, and oestrogen or testosterone are usually the first tests performed when pituitary disorders are suspected. These are followed by measurements of ACTH, TSH, and FSH and LH. The nontrophic hormones (GH and prolactin) will also be measured.

Further studies may be needed for exact diagnosisl. Provocative tests involve the use of a stimulant or suppressant of the hormone and measurements of the effects on hormonal serum levels. Provocative tests are not used in prolacting exess or deficit because serum levels give confirming data about pituary function.

Skeletal and skull X-ray examinations are used to assess changes in bone structure and the size of the pituitary gland and sella turcica. Computed tomography (CT) scanning may be used to demonstrate the presence of intrasellar masses and to differentiate a pituitary tumour from an "empty" sella turcica. An enlarged sella turcica may be described as "empty," a condition resulting from herniation of the arachnoid and subarachnoid cistern into the pituitary fossa. The displacement of the pituitary gland is not always clinically significant.

Nursing analysis

Problems are determined from the analysis of patient data. Possible problems for the person with anterior pituitary dysfunction (secreting pituitary tumours and/or postoperative pituitary surgery) may include, but are not limited to, the following:

Problem	Possible aetiologies
Infection, high risk for	Leakage of spinal fluid throgh incisional site in dura
Fluid volume deficit	Compromised regulatory mechanism; inadequate conservation of sodium and/or water
Knowlege deficit: disorder, diagnostic or treatment measures, self-care measures	Lack of exposure, cognitive limitation
Impaired physical mobility	Intolerance to activity: decreased strength, pain
Body image disturbances	Change in body appearance or function
Sensory/perceptual alterations: visual	Altered sensory transmition

Planning: expected patient outcomes

Expected patient outcomes for the person with anterior pituitary imbalance may include, but are not limited to, the following:

1. Restoration of physiological well-being, as evidenced by:
   a. Normal body temperature
   b. No evidence of CSF leakage
   c. Desired weight
   d. Balance of intake and output
   e. Stable blood pressure and pulse within optimal limits
   f. Prompt recovery from crisis

2. Explains planned diagnostic and therapeutic measures.
3. Explains rationale for medications and prescribed modification of food and fluid intake.
4. Demonstrates requisite knowledge, skill, and resources for self-management of treatment measures:
   a. Describes the hormonal imbalance and relates to signs and symptoms.
   b. Explains the planned treatment measures and effects of treatment.
   c. Explains the prescribed medication programme.
      (1) Awareness of the need for lifelong replacement therapy
      (2) Drugs, dosage, and frequency of therapy
      (3) Desired effects and side effects of therapy
      (4) What to do when signs and symptoms of undertreatment or overtreatment occur
   d. Describes the times when extra hormonal therapy is necessary.
   e. Describes need to obtain MedicAlert symbol to wear.
   f. States plans for regular follow-up care.
5. Physical mobility increases. Receives needed assistance for activities unable to do because of decreased mobility.
6. Speaks of self in positive terms, listing strengths and ways to deal with deficits.
7. Explains to others the assistance needed because of visual defect or weakness.

Implementation

Assisting with achievement of therapeutic goals

Untreated GH-secreting tumours can result in major neurological alterations as well as continual systemic changes if the hormone level is not returned to normal and if tumour growth is not inhibited. Treatment consists of surgery, radiation, or pharmacological agents. The primary treatment is neurosurgery using a transsphenoidal approach. Radiation therapy may be used as an adjunct to surgery or as an alternative. Radiation lowers hormone levels much more slowly and is associated with a high incidence of hypopituitarism. Bromocriptine, a dopamine agonist, is effective in lowering GH levels but not always to the level needed, and therefore it is used mainly if surgery and radiation have not been effective.

Interventions to assist with patient outcomes

Preventing infection

The transsphenoidal approach is most frequently used to resect an adenoma. The sella turcica is entered through the sphenoid sinus, and the tumour is removed with the aid of a surgical microscope. The incision is made between the gums and upper lip. This approach may also be used to implant ^{39}Y. The opening made in the dura mater on entering the sella turcica is frequently patched with a piece of fascia taken from the leg; thus the patient must be prepared for the leg incision. The patch is to prevent a cerebrospinal fluid (CSF) leak. Leaking of CSF may occur for a few days postoperatively but should then stop. The nose may be packed and a gauze sling placed under it to absorb drainage.

Monitoring for the presence of CSF leak is important. The following data should be noted:
1. Complaint of postnasal drip
2. Constant swallowing
3. Evidence on the nasal sling or gauze pads of a "halo ring" (clear CSF fluid marking around a darker centre of serous fluid)
4. Presence of glucose in the nasal drainage CSF fluid contains glucose, whereas nasal drainage does not. If the glucose test is positive, a specimen should be sent to the laboratory for confirmation.

If a persistent leak occurs, bed rest with the patient's head elevated to decrease CSF pressure and place pressure against the patch is prescribed. Most often CSF leaks heal spontaneously, but occasionally surgical repair is necessary. Activities that increase intracranial pressure should be avoided.

Headache may be present and is treated with non-narcotic analgesics or codeine. Persistent headache or nuchal rigidity (neck stiffness) may indicate the presence of meningitis and should be reported immediately. Because of the risk of infection, prophylactic antibiotics may be ordered preoperative or postoperatively.

Other nursing interventions for the patient with transsphenoidal surgery include the following:
1. Encourage oral fluids and a clear liquid diet as soon as the patient is alert and no longer nauseated from the anaesthesia.
2. Increase the diet as tolerated (anorexia may result from a decreased sense of smell).
3. Reassure the patient that the loss of smell is temporary and should improve as soon as the nasal packing and sling is removed.
4. Provide oxygen and humidity as ordered to keep the nasal and oral mucous membranes moist.
5. Provide mouth care:
   a. Avoid toothbrushing to prevent disruption of the suture line.
   b. Use soft cotton swabs to cleanse the teeth.
   c. Offer mouth rinses frequently.

Monitoring of fluid, electrolyte, and hormonal status

The patient with panhypopituitarism after surgery or other intracerebral problems requires lifelong replacement of cortisol, thyroid, and in most instances, gonadotrophins or sex hormones. The exception to replacement of gonadotrophins or sex hormones is the patient with cancer whose pituitary was removed to eliminate gonadotrophic stimulation of tumour growth, which is not being done very frequently.

ACTH deficiency and thus glucocorticoid deficiency occurs immediately if the total pituitary has been removed. Although it occurs rarely after transsphenoidal adenectomy, a temporary ACTH deficiency can result in adrenocortical insufficiency and even *adrenal crisis*. The patient is treated with replacement therapy as long as necessary. Plasma levels of cortisol will be assessed before discharge to make sure that the deficit has been corrected.

To detect adrenocortical deficiency and to determine adequacy of cortisol replacement, frequent monitoring of any patient with potential for adrenocortical insufficiency is necessary. Actions include the following:

1. Taking vital signs every hour and PRN after surgery until stable, then every 4 hours
2. Tabulating intake and output every 8 hours
3. Weighing patient daily

Electrolyte levels are ordered at least daily to monitor sodium and potassium levels. Signs of insufficient cortisol replacement are usually vague and nonspecific. Maintaining the patient's blood pressure at optimal levels is a major clinical guideline that determines the amount of cortisol replacement.

Progression of symptoms can be rapid, and profound shock can develop. The treatment of adrenal crisis is discussed on p. 542. The critical treatment measure is the replacement of cortisol and administration of volume expanders.

The removal of the pituitary gland or oedema of surrounding tissue can precipitate the sudden onset of *diabetes insipidus* from the lack of ADH. Disruption of the hypothalamic secretion of ADH can also result in ADH alterations. Diabetes insipidus is usually not permanent, even if all of the pituitary gland has been removed—ADH is produced in the hypothalamus and adequate amounts can be released from there.

Monitoring for patients who may develop diabetes insipidus includes the following:

1. Intake and output tabulated every 4 hours
2. Specific gravity determined on each urine specimen (continuously dilute urine with specific gravity of 1.000 to 1.005 is a sign of diabetes insipidus)

Polyuria makes it imperative that fluid intake be maintained to balance the urinary output. When diabetes insipidus occurs, thirst is a frequent complaint. It can usually be managed by providing ice chips and adequate water intake. If fluid deficit is severe, vasopressin is administered.

Deficiency of TSH and of thyroid hormones usually does not occur on a temporary basis, and it is not seen immediately even after the total pituitary has been removed, because the thyroid stores enough hormone to last for several weeks. If the total pituitary has been removed, the patient will eventually require thyroid replacement.

Gonadotrophin deficiency requires lifetime therapy to maintain normal sexual characteristics and reproductive ability. To maintain libido, secondary sexual characteristics, and well-being, men are given testosterone and women receive oestrogen-progesterone preparations. If childbearing is desired, the gonadotrophins (LH and FSH) must be replaced.

Facilitating learning

Nurses will be instituting various types of patient education interventions. First, patients will need to be prepared for laboratory tests (hormonal, chemical, and electrolyte studies) and X-ray procedures. Once the diagnosis is made, patients will need to be prepared for surgery or other therapy.

Nurses make an important contribution to patients with hypopituitarism resulting from the tumour or the surgery when they help them and their families understand the prescribed regimen for hormonal replacement. The serious nature of adrenocortical insufficiency should be stressed.

ADH deficiency following surgery is usually temporary. The patient does need to understand the replacement therapy and why signs and symptoms occur (thirst, polyuria). If other deficiencies (TSH or gonadotrophins) occur, the patient will need to know how to manage replacement therapy.

Patients treated with bromocriptine alone or as adjunctive therapy must know how to self-administer the drug. For prolactin-secreting tumours, 2.5 to 15 mg of bromocriptine daily usually is effective. Higher doses may be necessary for growth-hormone-secreting tumours. The primary side effects are mild nausea, vomiting, and postural hypotension. Repeated hormonal analysis is carried out to monitor the effectiveness of therapy.

Assisting with adaptation to changes in body image and bodily functions

The changes in appearance that result from GH excess and sometimes the changes associated with other hormonal excesses or deficits are not always reversible with treatment. Additionally some of the losses in body function are not reversible. When dealing with changes in body image, nurses must help patients develop realistic images and maximize their ability to attain the desired images by strengthening the remaining functional abilities. Patients need to be shown that not all changes are negative and must be helped to see themselves in positive terms. Sometimes consultation with people who specialize in make-up, clothing, and colours can be used to help accentuate the patient's best physical attributes.

Developing progressive activity plans with patients will assist them to regain some of the lost physical mobility and also will help to increase self-esteem. Increasing physical activity should be started as soon as possible. Referral to physiotherapy may be helpful for some patients. Visual alterations, although usually not severe, require that first and foremost the patient is assessed to determine any special needs to maintain the patient's safety. Depending on the amount of loss, the patient may need care as described in Chapter 30 for the visually impaired.

Evaluation

Evaluation is based on the expected patient outcomes. Key questions to consider include the following:

1. Are a stable weight, blood pressure, intake and output, and temperature achieved?
2. Can the patient describe self-care needs?
3. Does the patient speak of self in positive terms?
4. Is the patient able to get around safely?

POSTERIOR PITUITARY DYSFUNCTION

The two hormones of the posterior pituitary are oxytocin and antidiuretic hormone (ADH). (See Table 21-1, p. 525 for a review of the functions of oxytocin and ADH). Refer to midwifery texts for further information about oxytocin. The two alterations of ADH secretion, ADH excess and deficit, are described in Table 21-8.

Table 21-8   Alterations in ADH (posterior pituitary) secretion

Alteration	Signs and symptoms	Medical therapy
ADH deficit: Diabetes insipidus	Polyuria, polydipsia, dilute urine (specific gravity 1.000 to 1.005); if fluid intake is insufficient; dehydration, vascular collapse; weakness, anorexia	Fluid intake to balance fluid output; vasopressin, lypressin, desmopressin; surgical removal of tumor; drug therapy: thiazide diuretics, chlorpropamide
ADH excess: SIADH	*Dilutional hyponatraemia:* Serum Na below 130 mmol/L; weakness; lethargy; confusion; convultions; weight gain; oedema	Surgical removal of ADH secreting tissue (pituitary or nonpituitary); water restriction of 800 to 1000 ml/day; hypertonic saline with diuretics (for critical levels of sodium); demeclocycline

HYPOSECRETION OF ANTIDIURETIC HORMONE

Aetiology

Pituitary diabetes insipidus (DI) results from a lack of sufficient ADH. The cause may be a brain or pituitary tumour, head trauma, encephalitis, meningitis, adenectomy or hypophysectomy, or other cranial surgery. The cause is often idiopathic, although a rare hereditary form of the disease occurs. Nephrogenic DI is a second form of the disorder and results from failure of the renal tubules to respond to ADH.

Pathophysiology

The secretion of ADH is an important and normal response to stressors or plasma hyperosmolality. ADH effects changes in the kidney tubular membrane to increase water absorption to dilute the hyperosmolality and to provide an adequate blood volume during the stress response. In the presence of ADH, the urine is concentrated. When ADH is absent, water is not reabsorbed in the tubules and a large amount (7 to 11 L/day) of dilute urine is produced.

When the posterior pituitary does not release ADH or the hypothalamus does not secrete ADH in response to a hyperosmolar state, diabetes insipidus results. The potential is great for severe dehydration and vascular collapse if the patient does not replenish fluids lost by the excessive urination. The three classic symptoms that should alert the nurse to diabetes insipidus are *polyuria, dilute urine*, and *polydipsia.*

Often the patient complains of insatiable thirst. Ice water is preferred, although the reason for this is unknown. Voiding may occur so often that there is interference with sleep and the patient complains of tiredness.

HYPERSECRETION OF ANTIDIURETIC HORMONE

Aetiology

The causes of syndrome of inappropriate antidiuretic hormone (SIADH) are many (see Box 21-1). This disorder is associated with various pathological processes as well as with drug therapy.

Pathophysiology

In the syndrome of inappropriate antidiuretic hormone (SIADH), the patient is unable to excrete dilute urine and therefore retains water. Normally, ADH secretion is self-limiting; in SIADH, there is a continual release of ADH unrelated to plasma osmolality. Haemodilution results in depressed levels of solutes and electrolytes. CNS dysfunction occurs as a result of the hyposmolar state in which fluid shifts between intracerebral fluid compartments.

Medical Management

See Table 21-8 for a summary of the medical therapy for SIADH.

21-1

Aetiological factors associated with SIADH

Pulmonary disorders: malignant neoplasms such as oat cell adrenocarcinoma of the lung, tuberculosis, ventilator patients receiving positive pressure

Other malignancies: duodenum, pancreas, prostate lymhoma, sarcoma, leukaemia

CNS disorders: tumors, infection, trauma
  Endocrine disorders that result in hypovolaemia and impaired free water excretion, particulary if associated with fluid replacement (adrenal insufficiency, anterior pituitary insufficiency)

Drugs such as colfibrate, cyclophosphamide, morphine

Sressors: fear, acute infections, pain, anxiety, trauma surgery

---

ADRENAL GLAND DYSFUNCTION

Dysfunction of the adrenal gland can be manifested as an increased or decreased function of the cortex or an increased function of the medulla (Fig. 21-7). The three major hormones of the adrenal cortex are cortisol, aldosterone, and androgens. The adrenal medulla produces

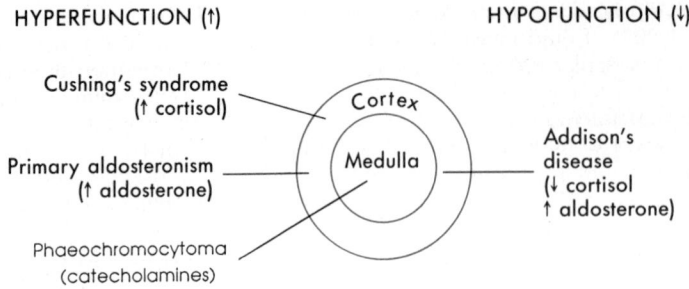

HYPERFUNCTION (↑)   **HYPOFUNCTION (↓)**

Cushing's syndrome
(↑ cortisol)   Cortex

Primary aldosteronism
(↑ aldosterone)   Medulla   Addison's
disease
(↓ cortisol
↑ aldosterone)

Phaeochromocytoma
(catecholamines)

Fig. 21-7 Dysfunction of the adrenal cortex and adrenal medulla.

Table 21-9   Adrenal gland dysfunction

Alteration in secretion	Signs and symptoms	Medical therapy
Adrenocortical excess	**Cortisol excess** Body appearance change Hyperglycaemia, hypernatraemia, hypokalaemia Increased susceptibility to infections Emotional changes Hypertension, oedema Weakness, fatigue	Surgery: adrenalectomy (unilateral, bilateral), excision of adrenal or pituitary tumour Irradiation of pituitary Drugs to suppress cortisol synthesis: metyrapone, aminoglutethimide
	Aldosterone excess Hypertension Hypokalaemia Hypernatraemia Metabolic alkalosis Headache, oedema Severe muscle weakness	Surgery: adrenalectomy, excision of tumour Spironolactone and antihypertensive agent
	Androgen excess Hirsutism, virilization, amenorrhoea in females, precocious sexual development in young boys	Surgery: adrenalectomy, excision of tumour
Adrenocortical deficiency	**Cortisol lack** Weight loss, asthenia Hypoglycaemia, hyponatraemia, hyperkalaemia Intolerance to stressors Hyperpigmentation GI complaints: nausea, vomiting, abdominal pain, diarrhoea Addisonian crisis: hypotension, vasomotor collapse, coma, hyperpyrexia	Replacement therapy: glucocorticoids (cortisone, hydrocortisone); mineralocorticoids, (fludrocortisone) For Addisonian crisis: hydrocortisone phosphate (IV), normal saline solution IV, rest
	Aldosterone lack Hypotension, hyponatraemia, hyperkalaemia	Replacement therapy: mineralocorticoids (fludrocortisone)
Adrenal medulla excess	Hypertension, episodic or sustained (usual) Occasional hypotension and tachycardia Headache, episodic Diaphoresis (sweating), pallor Palpitations Hyperglycaemia during attacks Constipation or diarrhoea	Surgery: excision of tumour Drugs to suppress catecholamine actions: Phenoxybenzamine, metyrosine, nitroprusside, propranolol or metoprolol

adrenaline and noradrenaline. The nursing process that starts on p. 541 applies to the various types of adrenal gland dysfunction that are discussed in this section.

HYPERSECRETION

Hypersecretion of the adrenal cortex can be of one hormone or all three. See Table 21-2, p. 527 for a review of functions of the hormones of the adrenal cortex. See Figure 21-2, p. 526 for a review of control mechanisms for glucocorticoids. Hypersection of adrenal medullary secretions can be adrenaline alone, noradrenaline alone, or both.

Cortisol Excess

Aetiology

Excessive production of cortisol, regardless of the cause, results in a group of signs and symptoms classified as *Cushing's syndrome*. The causes of Cushing's syndrome may be classified into four categories.

1. *Primary or adrenal Cushing's syndrome*: adrenal adenomas, adrenal hyperplasia, or adrenal carcinomas that produce excessive cortisol.
2. *Secondary or pituitary Cushing's syndrome* (also called Cushing's disease): excessive pituitary ACTH secretion resulting in excessive cortisol.
3. *Ectopic Cushing's syndrome* (also called secondary Cushing's syndrome): excessive secretion ACTH from nonpituitary sites, such as bronchogenic carcinoma, pancreatic carcinoma, bronchial adenoma, and so forth, resulting in excessive secretion of cortisol.
4. *Iatrogenic Cushing's syndrome*: excessive cortisol resulting from chronic therapeutic use of exogenous glucocorticoids.

Excessive pituitary secretion of ACTH is the most frequent pathological cause of Cushing's syndrome. Iatrogenic Cushing's syndrome is the most frequently seen syndrome in clinical practice. Therapeutic doses of glucocorticoids are prescribed for a variety of conditions including:

1. Treatment of autoimmune diseases such as rheumatoid arthritis and lupus
2. Prevention of rejection in organ transplantation
3. Prevention of excessive fibrosis (scarring) after certain surgeries or diseases particularly of the eye
4. Reduction of acute increased intracranial pressure or immediately after spinal cord injury
5. Treatment of inflammatory process associated with COPD, regional ileitis enteritis, and ulcerative colitis.

Pathophysiology

Whether the cause is pathological or iatrogenic, cortisol excess has widespread effects (Table 21-9). The changes in body appearance may be quite striking:

1. The *adipose deposition* is classic in its distribution to trunk, facies (moon face), and intrascapular areas ("buffalo hump").
2. *Muscle wasting* is most obvious in the legs, thighs, and buttocks.
3. Pale, purplish *striae* result from thinning of skin and weakening of collagenous fibres that expose subcutaneous tissue.
4. Tissue *bruises* easily with ecchymosis formation from lack of collagen support of the blood vessels.

21-2	Conditions for which people with cortisol excess are at high risk
	Hypertension
	Diabetes mellitus
	Osteoporosis
	Peptic ulcer
	Psychose
	Infection

The effects of excessive cortisol place the patient at higher risk for many chronic illnesses (see Box 21-2). Increased gastric secretion and altered mucosal defence mechanisms increase the risk of peptic ulcers. In addition, the effects of cortisol excess on emotional stability are marked. Patients may report insomnia, nightmares, and mood swings. Frank psychoses can develop.

Many of the signs and symptoms of cortisol excess are related to its diabetogenic, catabolic, and ketogenic effects:

1. Loss of bone matrix and calcium from bones
2. Decreased glucose intolerance, decreased glucose use, and increased gluconeogenesis
3. Increased ketogenesis and fatty acid mobilization

Because cortisol has some mineralocorticoid-like activity, excessive sodium and water retention can occur.

Cortisol is immunosuppressive as a result of decreased lymphocyte production and cell-mediated immunity (Chapter 33). Although the number of neutrophils may be increased, the migration and thus activity of these cells are decreased and there are decreased fibrin deposits that limit localization of infections and allow systemic spread.

The potency of anti-inflammatory action and mineralocorticoid activity vary among the many preparations. The side effects of glucocorticoids place a limit on the dosage employed over time.

Beside the problems caused by corticosteroid therapy (cortisol excess), the patient is also at risk for an episode of *adrenocortical insufficiency* (cortisol deficit) should the medication be stopped suddenly or a severe stressor be encountered shortly after the medication is stopped (see section on adrenal corticoid insufficiency).

Aldosterone Excess

Aetiology/epidemiology

The cause of excessive aldosterone secretion can be primary, resulting from an aldosterone secreting adrenal adenoma, or secondary. Secondary increases in aldosterone can follow increased renin production by the kidney and are associated with renal and hepatic disease and congestive heart failure. Primary aldosteronism is rare.

Pathophysiology

Three major effects of aldosterone excess are *hypertension*, *hypokalaemia*, and *hypernatraemia*. Hypertension results from the increased blood volume as a result of sodium reabsorption. As the sodium is retained, potassium is excreted and results in hypokalaemia. Hypokalaemia can result in the following:

1. Changes in excitability of muscle membrane, causing weakness, paraesthesia, hypoactive bowel sounds, and hypoactive deep tendon reflexes
2. Cardiac arrhythmias, changes in ECG patterns (depressed or inverted T-wave is a major change), and increased sensitivity to cardiac glycosides
3. Loss of the kidneys' concentrating ability: dilute urine, polyuria, and nocturia
4. Metabolic alkalosis

See Table 21-9 for a summary of signs and symptoms and medical therapy for aldosterone excess.

Androgen Excess

Aetiology/epidemiology

Androgen excess can result from adrenal adenomas or carcinomas or adrenal hyperplasia. Androgen excess may occur in ovarian disease or as a side effect of some medications. Androgen excess often occurs in combination with cortisol excess in adrenal hyperplasia and with cortisol and aldosterone excess in adrenal carcinoma.

Pathophysiology

Androgen excess does not produce clinically significant signs in adult men. Two signs of androgen excess in women are *hirsutism* and *virilization*.

1. *Hirsutism*: an increase in coarse, dark hair on the face, abdomen, axillae, and pubes; increased sebceous gland activity leading to oily skin and acne
2. *Virilization*: symptoms of amenorrhoea or oligomenorrhoea, clitoromegaly, frontal balding, deepening voice, and muscle hypertrophy

Catecholamine Excess

Aetiology/epidemiology

Although rare, the most common cause of excess catecholamines in adults is *phaeochromocytoma*, a catecholamine-producing tumour of the adrenal medulla. Approximately 10% of tumours of the medulla will be bilateral.[9a] These tumours arise from chromaffin cells which are derived from neural crest cells and thus similiar tumours can be found in the head, neck area, mediastinum, abdomen, bladder, testes, or anywhere along the sympathetic nervous system trunk. Ten per cent or greater number of tumours are extra-adrenal.[9a] Phaeochromocytomas can be benign or malignant. Approximately 10% are malignant and the malignancy rate increases in extra adrenal tumours and in children.[9a]

Pathophysiology

Although hypotension and tachycardia can be the major signs of an adrenaline secreting tumour, the *prominent sign of catecholamine excess is hypertension*, which may be labile, depending on blood levels of the catecholamines, or the blood pressure may stay persistently elevated. Most patients have an elevated blood pressure reading at least 50% of the time.[42] Headache is abrupt, severe, throbbing, and generalized; it usually is of short duration. The headache is often associated with sweating and palpitations. If hypertension is longstanding, the patient may develop hypertensive retinopathy. Other signs and symptoms along with the medical therapy are summarized in Table 21-9. An impor-

tant point to remember is that a large percentage of patients remain hypertensive even after surgery.[9a]

Frequently the patient has a history of paroxysmal attacks that are precipitated by multiple factors. Postural changes (especially flexion or bending of the body), sneezing, abdominal pressure, sexual activity, eating, urination, Valsalva manoeuvre, exercise, pain, and changes in environmental or body temperature are some of the major precipitating factors. In phaeochromocytoma, the serum levels of catecholamines and their metabolites (metadrenalines, vanillylmandelic acid [VMA]) in the urine are increased. The localization of the tumour is done with use of I-metaiodobenzylguanidine (^{131}I-MIBG) scintigraphy. CT scanning and MRI, which were once the major tools to localize tumours, are used to further delineate tumours.

HYPOSECRETION

The adrenal cortex is essential to life. Without its hormones, cortisol and aldosterone, the body's metabolic processes would respond inadequately to even minimal physical and emotional stressors, such as changes in temperature, exercise, or excitement. The normal functions of the adrenal cortex hormones are presented in Table 21-2, p. 527.

Adrenocortical Insufficiency

Aetiology/epidemiology

The causes of adrenocortical insufficiency include the following:

1. Primary causes: adrenocortical destruction from infection, haemorrhage, or autoimmune processes; idiopathic atrophy; or congenital hypoplasia. Also called Addison's disease.
2. Secondary causes: adrenal hypoplasia resulting from lack of pituitary ACTH.
3. Iatrogenic: bilateral adrenalectomy, metyrapone therapy, or sudden withdrawal of long-term glucocorticoid therapy.

Pathophysiology

Hypotension, hyponatraemia, and hyperkalaemia are characteristically seen in patients with primary adrenocortical insufficiency because of a lack of mineralocorticoids. These patients are subject to changes in cardiovascular status because of fluid and electrolyte alterations. A low circulating vascular volume and a decreased heart size develop. ECG changes (peaked T-wave is a major change) may occur with hyperkalaemia.

Conversely, when there is hypoplasia secondary to decreased ACTH secretion, aldosterone secretion is not impaired. This occurs because ACTH has minimal influence on aldosterone secretion, which is under control of the renin-angiotensin system. However, there may be evidence of hyposecretion of other pituitary hormones.

Table 21-9 explains many of the signs and symptoms that occur with the lack of cortisol in primary, secondary, and iatrogenic insufficiency because of diminished protein, carbohydrate, and fat metabolism. These pathophysiological changes may lead to:

1. Hypoglycaemia
2. Weight loss
3. Weakness, fatigue

Gastrointestinal symptoms (for example, anorexia, nausea and vomiting, or diarrhoea) are often the reason that the person initially seeks help. Symptoms of adrenocortical insufficiency most often have a gradual onset and are vague. Asthenia (weakness) is a cardinal complaint, the intensity of which is out of proportion to other overt symptoms. It is usually more severe when stressors are present and eventually may force the patient to stay in bed.

The decreased cortisol level is often associated with mental and emotional changes: loss of vigour, depression, irritability, and loss of ability to concentrate. Apathy and generalized weakness contribute to decreased activity.

Hyperpigmentation with a bronzelike discoloration of skin and mucous membranes is a common sign in primary adrenal insufficiency. This is caused by increased levels of melanocyte-stimulating hormone (MSH) from the anterior pituitary. In normal people, cortisol causes negative feedback inhibition of MSH, one of the precursors of ACTH. This lack of cortisol in adrenal insufficiency allows the MSH level to increase along with the ACTH. People with secondary insufficiency do not usually have hyperpigmentation because their levels of MSH and ACTH are low (see Figure 21-2, p. 527 for a review of the negative feedback control of cortisol).

Iatrogenic adrenocortical insufficiency results from hypothalamic-pituitary-adrenal changes that are induced by corticosteroid therapy. An elevation of serum cortisol levels inhibits the secretion of ACTH and CRH; thus the responsiveness of the hypothalamic-pituitary-adrenal (HPA) axis and the stimulation of the cells of the adrenal cortex are decreased. This form of insufficiency shows up when the corticosteroid therapy is withdrawn. This suppression of the responsiveness of the HPA axis may persist for up to 1 year, if corticosteroid therapy is used in large doses or if therapy is prolonged. During the period of HPA axis suppression, stressors may precipitate acute adrenocortical insufficiency (adrenal crisis). Measures to reduce the suppression of the HPA axis include administering cortisol on alternate days in the morning or in a larger dose in the morning and a smaller dose in the early afternoon. Topical administration of corticosteroids causes less suppression than does systemic administration. Tapering with withdrawal is used to prevent reactivation or flare-up of the underlying disease and to determine the lowest adequate dosage.

Addisonian Crisis (Adrenal Crisis)

Adrenal crisis is a *severe* and *sudden* exacerbation of adrenal insufficiency. It can quickly lead to death unless it is treated promptly. It is usually precipitated by stressors. Adrenal crisis (*Addisonian* crisis) can occur in any person with adrenal insufficiency and is manifested by acute exaggeration of signs and symptoms and vascular collapse. (See Box 21-3.)

Nursing Process
Assessment

Subjective data

Common considerations in assessing patients with pituitary dysfunction (p. 533) are also pertinent for adrenal

---

21-3	**Signs and symptoms of adrenal crisis**

Hypotension
Shock
Fever
Nausea and vomiting
Confusion
Electrolyte imbalances ($\downarrow$ sodium, $\uparrow$ potassium)
Hypoglycaemia

---

dysfunction because of the effect of the anterior pituitary on the adrenal glands.

Diagnostic tests

Diagnosis in adrenocortical dysfunction relies heavily on measurements of serum and urinary levels of hormones and metabolites.

Nursing analysis

Problems are determined from the analysis of patient data. Possible problems for the person with adrenal dysfunction may include those identified on p. 533 (with the exception of sensory/perceptual alterations) because anterior pituitary dysfunction may result in adrenal cortex dysfunction.

Planning: expected patient outcomes

Expected outcomes for the person with adrenal hormonal imbalances include those listed on p. 534. In addition, expected outcomes include, but are not limited to, the following:

1. Patient with Cushing's syndrome:
   a. Explains ways to avoid infections and describes what to do if infections occur.
   b. Describes dietary restrictions.
   c. Intake equals output, oedema decreases, body weight decreases.
   d. Fatigue is decreased as rated by patient.
   e. States needs (if unable to meet by self because of fatigue) are met.
   f. Describes self in positive terms.
   g. Describes any therapeutic regimens prescribed for hypertension or diabetes mellitus, if appropriate.
2. Patient with aldosterone excess:
   a. Sodium and water balance return to normal.
   b. Blood pressure is within normal limits.
   c. Describes any therapeutic regimens prescribed for hypertension and hypokalaemia.
3. Patient with androgen excess:
   a. Describes self in positive terms.
4. Patient with phaeochromocytoma:
   a. Mental status and sensory and motor function remain normal.
   b. Describes what can and should do if attack occurs.
   c. Describes any diagnostic tests, planned therapy.
5. Patient with *adrenocortical insufficiency*:
   a. Blood pressure and pulse are returned to normal and are maintained; urine output is normal; skin warm and dry; mental status normal.

Table 21-10 Comparison of clinical problems of Cushing's disease and Addison's disease

Cushing's syndrome	Addison's disease
Hypertension	Hypotension
Hyperglycaemia	Hypoglycaemia
Hypervolaemia	Hypovolaemia
Hypokalaemia	Hyperkalaemia
Immunosuppression	Intolerance to stressors
Osteoporosis	

b. Intake equals output and is within normal limits; body weight is returned to normal and maintained.

c. Stressors are decreased until patient stable.

d. Explains the effects of stressors on the need for medication.

e. Identifies stressors in own life and ways to control them.

f. States awareness of the need for additional medication in times of severe stress response.

g. Describes any therapeutic plans and self-care needs.

Implementation

The interventions designed to assist in achievement of therapeutic goals and to achieve patient outcomes are presented together for each type of patient.

Certain nursing measures are appropriate regardless of the type of adrenal dysfunction. The *maintenance* of medication regimens is a high priority. Other measures include those that achieve the following:

1. Provision of adequate rest
2. Regulation of blood pressure levels within desired limits
3. Maintenance of fluid and electrolyte balance
4. Maintenance of adequate nutrition to maintain or achieve desired weight and to keep blood glucose levels within normal limits
5. Provision of an environment that is as restful and as free of stressors as possible

The reasons for the above nursing measures are shown in Table 21-10.

The patient with Cushing's syndrome

Nurses can assist patients with specific therapy directed towards correcting the hormonal imbalance caused by disease. Measures may include one or more of the following:

1. Pituitary surgery or radiation
2. Unilateral or bilateral adrenalectomy
3. Drug therapy to suppress or block synthesis of cortisol (see Table 21-9)
4. Surgery to remove an ectopic source of ACTH

In iatrogenic Cushing's syndrome or when corrective treatment is not feasible, measures include those that control the side effects of the glucocorticoid therapy, that

is, hypertension, hypokalaemia, hyperglycaemia, hypercalciuria, hypervolaemia, infections, and osteoporosis.

Nurses can assist patients with the following:

1. Nutrition: calorie and sodium restrictions and potassium supplements to deal with the fluid volume excess, fatigue, and altered nutrition
2. Fluid and electrolyte balance: diuretics and potassium supplements; restriction of fluids to deal with fluid volume excess and fatigue
3. Blood glucose control: calorie restriction and insulin replacement to deal with the altered nutrition and help with body image changes
4. Blood pressure control: antihypertensive agents and sodium restrictions to deal with the fluid volume excess
5. Ambulation to prevent osteoporosis and safety measures to prevent pathological fractures when osteoporosis is present

People with Cushing's syndrome are at particular risk for *nosocomial infections* because of their immunosuppressed states. Immunosuppression combined with metabolic imbalance and obesity impairs wound healing. Careful handwashing and aseptic technique are essential. Patients must not be exposed to infection, and they should be separated from other patients with infections. Staff members who have *any* signs or symptoms of infection should not care for these patients.

Body image changes are numerous. They are reversible once the hypersecretion of glucocorticoids is controlled. However, for the patient with iatrogenic Cushing's syndrome counselling and care as described on page 536 is necessary.

The patient with pituitary, adrenal or ectopic Cushing's syndrome will need explanations about the disease, treatment, and expected outcomes. These patients are usually very ill and tire easily so teaching needs to be spaced at intervals. Adrenal surgery causes many problems the patient must be prepared for. Considerable haemodynamic and metabolic changes occur rapidly. A temporary cortisol deficit may occur after unilateral adrenalectomy or resection of an adenoma. The cortisol deficit results from the depressed responsiveness of the HPA axis and the atrophy of the normal adrenal gland, which is caused by HPA axis suppression by the previously high blood-cortisol levels. Bilateral adrenalectomy results in permanent cortisol deficit because surgery changes the hormonal imbalance from cortisol excess to cortisol deficit. After adrenal surgery the patient has iatrogenic adrenal insufficiency and is at risk for adrenal crisis. Hormonal replacement is essential for maintenance of life. After bilateral adrenalectomy, ACTH levels rise in the absence of the negative feedback control of cortisol-blood levels.

For the patient with iatrogenic Cushing's syndrome, the major focus of nursing care is patient teaching. The patient must be prepared for all potential side effects. They will need teaching about diet, fluid and electrolytes, blood glucose control, blood pressure control, ambulation, and avoidance of infection. Because the information and self care is so tremendous, several teaching sessions should be planned and written, verbal and audio-visual materials should be used.

The patient with primary aldosteronism

The fluid and sodium excess and hypertension associated with primary aldosteronism are usually treated with surgical resection of the adrenal adenoma or unilateral adrenalectomy. Bilateral hyperplasia is usually treated with sodium restriction, potassium replacement, and the aldosterone antagonist, spironolactone. These same measures may be used preoperatively.

After surgery a temporary suppression of renin-induced aldosterone production may be present and fluid deficit can occur. If the aldosterone deficit is severe, fludrocortisone may be necessary. If the deficit is mild, treatment of acidosis and hyperkalaemia may be achieved with sodium carbonate and sodium polystyrene sulphonate after surgery. Usually aldosterone production returns to normal within 6 months. Surgery reverses hypertension in a majority of patients.

Patients will require teaching for the diagnostic test and for the adrenal surgery (see opposite) or for life-long medications and dietary treatment. Written materials should be used to supplement verbal information.

The patient with androgen excess

Body image change is the major problem for the person with androgen excess. Nursing care will focus on helping patients manage and cope with these changes (see p. 536).

The patient with phaeochromocytoma

The primary treatment of phaeochromocytoma is surgical removal of the tumour. The priority of preoperative care is control of hypertension. Medication to control hypertension includes alpha and beta adrenergic blocking agents (see Table 21-9). During a hypertensive crisis, the patient should be admitted to an intensive care unit. Cardiac monitoring and frequent monitoring of vital signs are necessary. When the patient's blood pressure reaches the desired level, medication can be gradually decreased.

Maintaining blood pressure at a desired level is a major concern during anaesthesia, surgery, and the postoperative period. The antihypertensive medication used preoperatively may influence the choice of anaesthetic agent; manipulation of the tumour during surgery may release large bursts of hormones causing elevation of the blood pressure. When the tumour is removed sudden hypotension may occur. Hypotension is usually treated with plasma or a plasma substitute. Appropriately administered volume expanders (normal saline) usually control the hypotension, making vasopressors unnecessary.

On the first postoperative day, hypertensive episodes are common and caused by the response to pain and to hypervolaemia caused by the treatment of hypotension after surgery. Currently, the most effective therapy for this hypertension is a rapidly acting diuretic such as frusemide.

The patient will need careful preparation for diagnostic tests so that the tumour can be identified as quickly as possible. Preoperatively the blood pressure must be controlled for at least 1 week before surgery so patients will need to know self-care measures. Postoperatively, many patients remain hypertensive so the patient will need to know how to take any prescribed medications and the side effects to monitor for. The patient will be followed and reassessed for reoccurrence. The patient must understand the importance of this follow-up.

The patient with adrenal insufficiency

The primary nursing activities for a patient with severe adrenocortical insufficiency are directed towards improving and maintaining cardiac output and fluid volume and decreasing the number of stressors. Actions required include:

1. Hormonal replacement of glucocorticoids and mineralocorticoids
2. Administering sodium and fluids as ordered
3. Monitoring fluid status including intake and output, daily weights, urine specific gravity, blood pressure and pulse, mental status, and skin temperature and moisture
4. The number of stressors are decreased by using a side room, limiting disturbances, keeping temperature controlled, decreasing noise, and promoting physical and mental rest.

Fatigue will be partially relieved as cardiac output and fluid status are improved. The patient does need an adequate intake of carbohydrates and protein to meet glucose and protein needs.

The patient's adrenal insufficiency may be partial or complete, thus the doses of hormonal replacement will vary. In mild adrenocortical insufficiency, cortisol may be needed only during periods of stress, and mineralocorticoid insufficiency can be managed with high sodium intake. When cortisol and aldosterone deficit is absolute, as after bilateral adrenalectomy, the usual hormonal replacement is as follows:

1. Cortisone: 37.5 mg daily (25 mg in the early morning and 12.5 mg in the early evening)
2. Fludrocortisone: 0.1 to 0.2 mg daily

Synthetic preparations of cortisol may be used instead of cortisone.

Adrenal insufficiency after surgery of the pituitary gland or associated with other disease of the anterior pituitary gland was discussed on p. 536.

Once the patient is stable, patient education to promote self-care will be necessary. Additionally the patient will have to institute monitoring to detect signs and symptoms of excess of glucocorticoids and mineralocorticoids because the needs vary from day to day (see page 538). Last the patient must be able to identify stressors, ways to minimize stressors, and how to change the medication at times of increased stressors.

Surgery

The patient undergoing adrenal surgery usually has a preoperative state of hormonal excess (cortisol, aldosterone, or catecholamines) that is suddenly reversed by surgery. This rapid change is associated with instability in haemodynamic and metabolic functions and varies according to the hormones involved and the amount of functional adrenal tissue that remains. The patient must be given constant nursing attention until hormonal stability is regained or a maintenance regimen established.

When cortisol deficit is expected after surgery, glucocorticoid replacement is first given by intravenous infusion throughout the perioperative period and then changed to oral doses. The dosage is adjusted by evaluating measurements of blood pressure, blood glucose, electrolyte, and serum cortisol levels. Monitoring for signs of adrenal insufficiency and adrenal crisis should be frequent. An increase in glucocorticoid medication is often required when blood pressure levels are less than adequate.

Along with hormonal, fluid, and electrolyte replacement, vasopressors may be necessary to maintain adequate blood pressure in the immediate postoperative period. Orthostatic hypotension is not unusual as the patient begins ambulation.

The patient is also observed carefully for signs of hypoglycaemia (weakness, sweaty, nervous, tachycardia, skin moist, sluggish, increased appetite). This condition is most likely to occur if the patient had diabetes mellitus as a symptom, but it can occur in any patient who has adrenal gland surgery. Intravenous solutions containing glucose are usually ordered. If the patient is able to eat, the nurse should check to see that all food on the tray is consumed. A balanced diet of carbohydrates, proteins and fat is encouraged.

Teaching the patient about adrenocortical insufficiency and the importance of hormonal replacement was discussed previously for the patient having surgery on the pituitary. It is not unheard of for patients to be admitted to the hospital in adrenal crisis because they did not understand the need to take their medication as ordered.

Evaluation

Evaluation is based on the expected patient outcomes. Questions to consider may include the following:
1. For the patient with Cushing's syndrome:
   a. Were infections avoided?
   b. Were dietary restrictions maintained?
   c. Did intake and output stay in balance? And was an appropriate weight attained?
   d. Was fatigue controlled?
   e. Could patient accurately describe self-care?
2. For the patient with aldosterone excess:
   a. Was sodium and water balance restored and maintained?
   b. Was blood pressure kept within normal limits?
   c. Could the patient describe the self-care needs for elevated blood pressure and low potassium?
3. For the patient with androgen excess:
   a. Did patient describe self in positive terms?
4. For the patient with phaeochromocytoma:
   a. Did mental status and sensory and motor function remain normal?
   b. If changes occurred, were they detected and reported immediately?
   c. Did the patient know what to do for paroxysmal attacks?
   d. Could the patient describe:
      (1) Purpose of diagnostic test?
      (2) Planned surgery and care associated with surgery?
      (3) Self care needs after discharge?
5. For the patient with adrenocorticoid insufficiency:
   a. Was blood pressure, pulse, urine output, intake and body weight returned to normal and maintained?
   b. Was fatigue decreased?
   c. Could the patient identify stressors and describe what to do when stressors increased?
   d. Could patient describe self care needs?

PARATHYROID DYSFUNCTION

Parathyroid hormone (PTH) is involved with maintenance of calcium and phosphorus levels (Table 21-4, p. 528 presents an overview of functions of the PTH). PTH and vitamin D are two major regulators of calcium metabolism. PTH excess results in increased blood calcium levels, whereas PTH deficit leads to hypocalcaemic states. PTH excess leads to hypophosphataemia, whereas PTH deficit is associated with elevated serum levels of phosphorus.

PTH and vitamin D work together to promote absorption of calcium from the intestine. They both promote bone resorption of calcium. In hypoparathyroidism, PTH deficiency impairs the synthesis of vitamin D to its active form $(1,25[OH]_2D)$, and thus vitamin D deficiencies accompany PTH deficits. Calcitonin, a third regulator of calcium metabolism, has actions antagonistic to PTH and vitamin D. It is not involved in parathyroid disorders; however, it may be used for treatment of severe hypercalcaemia. Calcitonin inhibits bone resorption. The signs, symptoms, and medical therapy for people with various types of dysfunctions are summarized in Table 21-11. The nursing process for parathyroid dysfunction starts on p. 546.

PARATHYROID HORMONE (PTH) EXCESS

Aetiology

Parathyroid hormone excess results from primary causes such as parathyroid gland adenomas and carcinomas and parathyroid hyperplasia. Secondary causes of parathyroid hormone excess include renal failure, rickets, PTH-resistant nephropathy, vitamin D intoxication, and ectopic secretion by parathyroid-like tumours. Parathyroid abnormalities in people with renal failure are a common clinically seen cause of excess.

Pathophysiology

Normally, a low serum calcium level stimulates secretion of PTH, whereas a high serum level inhibits its secretion. In primary hyperparathyroidism, PTH does not become suppressed with the elevated serum calcium level (dysfunctional negative-feedback system), thus hypercalcaemia results. In many instances elevated serum calcium is the only sign of parathyroid dysfunction and is detected on routine examination. Mild symptoms of weakness and easy fatigability may be present. In some patients severe effects of hypercalcaemia (renal or bone disease) may be evident.

Most of the symptoms seen in PTH excess are a result of the hypercalcaemia. The effect of increased calcium on the muscles leads to hypotonicity of gastrointestinal muscles, skeletal muscles, and tendon reflexes. Thus decreased bowel mobility, abdominal pain, nausea, vomiting, and anorexia are common and lead to weight loss and fatigue. Some patients have histories of peptic ulcer disease and GI bleeding. The fatigue associated with the weight loss is worsened by skeletal muscle weakness. Mental changes may vary from confusion to depression or psychosis. Relatively small elevations of calcium may cause major mental changes, especially in elderly people.

Table 21-11   Parathyroid dysfunction

Signs and symptoms	Medical therapy
PTH hormone excess Hypercalcaemia and hypophosphataemia: Anorexia, nausea, vomiting, fatigue, depression, polyuria, polydipsia, dehydration; bone pain, muscle hypotonia and hypore flexia; constipation	Hydration, normal saline infusion Frusemide Phosphate infusion or oral salts Calcitonin Plicamycin Dialysis Surgical excision of tumor or parathyroidectomy Antacids (phosphate-binders) for patients with renal failure

PTH hormone deficiency
Hypocalcaemia:
  Paraesthesia, Chvostek's sign, Trousseau's sign, carpopedal spasm, marked anxiety, seizures, laryngeal stridor, dyspnoea, cyanosis, arrhythmias
Hyperphosphataemia:
  Soft tissue calcifications; nausea, vomiting, abdominal pain; dry scaling skin, brittle nails; patchy, thin hair
	Calcium salts: give with food but not dairy products; calcium gluconate, calcium chloride
	Vitamin D supplements
	Dietary calcium and vitamin D

The continued removal of calcium phosphate from the bones results in a variety of bone lesions. Bone pain may be severe, and bone fragility can predispose the patient to fractures. In primary hyperparathyroidism, hypophosphataemia occurs.

Secondary hyperparathyroidism develops from chronic hypocalcaemic states, such as renal failure. Hyperplasia of the parathyroid glands develops with an increase in PTH. The hyperplasia and excessive production of PTH may be enough to keep the serum calcium normal, but this is at the expense of bone integrity. In some patients, the parathyroid glands become autonomous and lose their responsiveness to serum calcium levels (tertiary hyperparathyroidism). In renal failure the chronic hypocalcaemia results from ↑ phosphorus, inability to activate vitamin D, and poor calcium intake and absorption.

Primary and most causes of secondary hyperparathyroidism result in *hypercalcaemia* and *hypophosphataemia*. The patient has increased urinary excretion of both calcium and phosphorus with the following effects:
1. Inability of the kidney to concentrate urine
2. Polyuria
3. Increased risk of renal calculi with subsequent urinary obstruction or infection
4. Calcification of renal tubules

In hyperparathyroidism secondary to renal failure, the changes in urinary and kidney function as described in the preceding paragraph are not seen and hyperphosphataemia occurs.

When the serum calcium level rises above 4.0–4.5 mmol/L, acute hypercalcaemic crisis occurs. Severe intractable vomiting leads to dehydration and electrolyte imbalances. Fever, severe mental changes, coma, and cardiac arrhythmias may result, ending in death if untreated.

PARATHYROID HORMONE (PTH) DEFICIENCY
Aetiology
Parathyroid hormone deficiency results from autoimmune destruction of the gland, from idiopathic changes, or secondary to excision of the glands. Temporary hypoparathyroidism is a risk for every person undergoing thyroidectomy or surgical exploration of the neck.

Pathophysiology
With a diminished level of parathyroid hormone, there is decreased bone resorption, and the serum calcium level falls. Because parathyroid hormone is involved in the renal clearance of phosphate, serum phosphate levels increase. The decreased level of serum calcium results in neuromuscular irritability.

Nerves show decreased thresholds of excitation, repeated responses to a single stimuli, and in severe cases, continuous activity. The neuromuscular irritability is manifested in both peripheral sensory and motor nerves and is responsible for the signs of latent tetany (see Box 21-4). Convulsions, laryngeal stridor and bronchospasm, and cardiac arrhythmias are possible if treatment is not instituted for the latent tetany.

Acute hypocalcaemia (tetany) is life threatening, and the signs of latent tetany should always be promptly reported to the doctor (see Box 21-4 and Table 21-11). Changes in electroencephalographic (EEG) patterns may be present, and a prolonged Q-T interval is frequently seen on the cardiac monitor.

It is important for the nurse to recognize that the clinical findings of hypocalcaemia are more reliable than the total serum calcium level, which measures (1) the ionized (unbound) blood calcium, which is the active metabolic calcium, and (2) the nonionized (bound) calcium, which

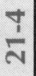

21-4

Signs of latent tetany

Paraesthesia in fingertips and around the mouth
Chvostek's sign (facial contraction on tapping facial nerve near jaw angle)
Trousseau's sign (carpal spasm after compression of upper arm with a cuff)
Carpopedal spasm (spasm of wrist and fingers and/or feet and toes)

does not affect neuroactivity. A low serum albumin results in a decrease in nonionized (bound) calcium and total serum calcium. But because ionized calcium levels are normal, signs and symptoms of hypocalcaemia do not occur.

The principal problem in acute hypoparathyroidism is hypocalcaemia. In prolonged hypoparathyroidism, there may be other problems of calcium imbalance, such as cataracts, malabsorption, and decreased growth of skin and nails. Hyperphosphataemia is indicated by calcifications in blood vessels, nerves, and soft tissues.

Nursing Process
Assessment

The signs and symptoms of calcium excess and deficit are priority observations when patients are assessed for parathyroid dysfunction.

Subjective data

The following subjective data are obtained from the patient:
1. Presence of discomfort (bone pain), fatigue, or paraesthesia
2. Elimination patterns (constipation, polyuria)
3. Gastrointestinal symptoms (anorexia, nausea, vomiting,↑ abdominal pain, or history of constipation or ulcers)
4. Emotional changes (anxiety)
5. Medication usage
6. Dietary history
7. Knowledge of condition

Objective data

Objective data include the following:
1. Mental status (signs of behaviour changes)
2. Intake and output every 8 hours
3. Daily weight
4. Changes in reflexes (hypo- or hyper-reflexia)
5. Respiratory status
6. Muscle weakness or twitching
7. Electrolyte levels (calcium, phosphorus)
8. Condition of skin, hair, and nails

Diagnostic tests

Because the maintenance of normal calcium and phosphorus metabolism involves multiple systems besides the parathyroid (skeletal, gastrointestinal, and urinary), when parathyroid function is being assessed, the patient also undergoes diagnostic tests of these other systems. This is necessary to determine whether the problem with calcium and phosphorus metabolism is caused by parathyroid metabolism or other disease states. In addition, ECG, EEG, and sometimes nerve conduction studies may be performed in an effort to detect hypotonicity or neuromuscular irritability.

Planning: expected patient outcomes

Expected patient outcomes for the person with parathyroid disorders may include, but are not limited to the following:
The patient with *hyperparathyroidism* and *hypercalcaemia* should be able to:
1. Maintain optimal mobility by pacing activities and scheduling analgesics.
2. Maintain adequate nutritional intake.
3. Maintain adequate bowel elimination.
4. Be up without falls or other injuries.
5. List signs and symptoms of calcium imbalance.
6. Describe symptoms requiring medical follow-up.
7. Explain planned medication regimen, if appropriate.
8. Describe plans for follow-up care.

The patient with *hypoparathyroidism* and *hypocalcaemia* should be able to:
1. Maintain adequate air exchange, shown by adequate blood gases and absence of stridor and dyspnoea.
2. Maintain adequate cardiac output as shown by blood pressure and perfusion to CNS, kidney, and periphery; experience no undetected cardiac arrhythmias.
3. Not experience any undetected increase in neuromuscular irritability and, if convulsions occur, not experience injury.
4. State plans for self-care:
   a. Explain the prescribed drug therapy (calcium, vitamin D)
   b. State reasons for lifelong calcium and vitamin D therapy, if total parathyroid function is lost.
   c. Plan a diet high in vitamin D.
   d. Describe symptoms for tetany or hypercalcaemia that require immediate attention.
   e. State plans for ongoing follow-up care.

Implementation

The interventions to assist with achievement of therapeutic goals and achieve patient outcomes are discussed together for each specific pathological state.

Hyperparathyroidism

Correction of hypercalcaemia and treatment of hyperparathyroidism

Definitive treatment of hyperparathyroidism requires surgical removal of the adenoma or of all but a part of one gland, if hyperplasia is the cause. Treatment varies depending on whether symptoms are present. In mild asymptomatic hypercalacemia when renal function, urinary calcium excretion, and skeletal system X-ray films are normal, surgery may be withheld until abnormalities occur. This type of patient should be evaluated every 6 to 12 months.

Medical treatment of hypercalcaemia may be performed preoperatively and in some patients who are not suitable candidates for surgery. Normalization of electrolyte levels reduces the risk of surgery.

Hypercalcaemia greater than 3.5 mmol/L requires immediate therapy if cardiac arrhythmias and coma are to be avoided.[20] Several measures can be used. The first step is diuresis; this involves hydration followed by a potent diuretic, such as frusemide, for the excretion of several grams of calcium per day. This therapy can be used only in patients with adequate renal function. Intake and output must be monitored closely in all patients receiving this treatment. Replacement of electrolytes other than calcium may be necessary. This may include potassium, phosphorus (phosphate), and magnesium. Drugs that inhibit bone resorption include salmon calcitonin, plicamycin, and phosphates.

Calcimar may be given in acute hypercalcaemia. It acts rapidly and causes an abrupt inhibition of bone resorption. Sensitivity skin testing may be performed with 1 MRC unit applied to the forearm. A rapid fall in the serum calcium level may occur after injection. Plicamycin is a cytotoxic antibiotic that has a potent effect on serum calcium levels; often only one dose is ordered. See Table 21-11 for other agents that are used as adjunctive therapy in selected instances of hypercalcaemia.

Improving mobility and preventing injury

Activities that provide stress to long bones are known to increase bone formation, whereas immobilization fosters demineralization; thus ambulation should be promoted in these patients. A programme of progressive activities should be planned with the patient, with attention to his or her level of weakness and pain. Activities should be spaced to lessen fatigue, and pain medication should be given before ambulation. Safety measures to prevent injury from falling are a high priority in these patients, who are weak, may have impaired cognitive function, and often have increased bone fragility.

Maintaining adequate nutritional intake and managing constipation

The hypercalcaemia results in several problems that disrupt normal GI function, fluid and nutritional intake, and elimination. Nursing care to manage these needs includes:

1. Promoting urinary elimination by ensuring a fluid intake of 3 L/day unless contraindicated
2. Providing appetizing, small meals and liquids that the patient enjoys
3. Providing symptomatic relief and administering prescribed agents for bone pain or gastrointestinal distress
4. Preventing faecal impaction by careful attention to elimination patterns and use of dietary fibre, fluids, activity, and stool softeners, laxatives, or enemas
5. Monitoring for signs of renal calculi (Chapter 29)

Facilitating learning

This patient will first need explanations of the therapeutic interventions (fluids, medications) to elicit the patient's cooperation. The patient will then need information about the various diagnostic tests (blood, urine) that will be carried out. Lastly the patient will need information related to the surgery and the self-care after surgery. The information related to surgery is explained in the next section.

Parathyroid surgery

Partial parathyroidectomy is usually the treatment of choice in primary hyperparathyroidism. The usual surgery involves removing three glands totally and part of the fourth gland. An alternative approach involves removing all four glands and implanting some of the removed tissue into the muscle of the forearm. Implantation avoids vascular failure and death of residual parathyroid tissue left in the neck. If no glandular abnormality is found at the time of surgery, extensive exploration of the neck and surrounding areas for additional glands that could be the cause of the symptoms is necessary.

Postsurgical hypocalcaemia. The serum calcium level decreases within 24 hours after successful surgery. The patient must be monitored carefully for signs of tetany. Parathyroid function usually returns to normal in 5 to 7 days after subtotal resection. By this time the remaining parathyroid tissue resumes normal secretion. If mild hypocalcaemia occurs, oral calcium is given. If hypocalcaemia is severe, calcium gluconate or calcium chloride is given intravenously. Calcium replacement is continued until the serum calcium level returns to normal, usually within a few days. If signs and symptoms of hypocalcaemia continue to be present, calcium and/or vitamin D replacement therapy in the same amount as that used to treat hypoparathyroidism will be necessary. While patients are receiving replacement therapy, they must be monitored carefully for signs and symptoms of hypercalcaemia.

If total parathyroidectomy is performed, hypoparathyroidism will develop, and the patient will need the same treatment as any other patient with hypoparathyroidism.

Hypoparathyroidism

Decreasing neuromuscular excitability and the resultant respiratory and cardiac problems and tetany that results in injury

When the patient has a known risk of tetany, nursing interventions include the following:
1. Prompt reporting to doctor of any signs of hypocalcaemia
2. Maintenance of emergency equipment (tracheostomy set and intravenous calcium) at bedside
3. Frequent assessment of signs of latent tetany (opposite site)
4. Administering prescribed calcium and vitamin D replacement, and aluminium-based antacids to patient with hyperphosphataemia
5. Maintaining a quiet, nonstressful environment

The symptoms of hypocalcaemia are more severe in patients with alkalosis because alkalosis causes more of the dissolved calcium to bind to serum albumin. If more calcium is bound, less is ionized, and hypocalcaemic symptoms occur more readily. Attention to acid-base balance includes the prevention and treatment of causes of alkalosis: hypokalaemia and respiratory alkalosis (hyperventilation). Caution should be used with agents that promote alkalosis, such as certain drugs and gastrointestinal intubation.

Providing a nonstressful environment for the patient with hypoparathyroidism is a major nursing responsibility because stressors can promote hyperventilation, which can precipitate alkalosis and tetany and ineffective breathing. Actions might include the following:

1. Frequent contacts by nursing staff
2. Explanations of treatments geared to patient's level of understanding and concern
3. Plan visitations that are most calming for patient
4. Discussion with family members about avoiding disturbing discussions

If tetany develops, the nurse assists as needed in emergency treatment of airway obstruction, cardiac arrhythmia, and seizures.

After the patient has been stabilized and the risk of tetany is past, the patient will be started on long-term maintenance therapy to maintain serum calcium levels. Long-term maintenance of normal serum calcium levels can usually be achieved by daily calcium and vitamin D supplements. Replacement of PTH is not possible.

Large doses of vitamin D_2 or D_3 are required to overcome the effect of the lack of PTH on the synthesis of vitamin D. Use of one of the more potent vitamin D preparations such as calcifediol or calatriol necessitates frequent measurements of serum and urinary calcium.

Dietary intake of calcium may be limited by the necessity for restricting phosphorus intake. When a low phosphorus intake is required, dairy products and egg yolks (good sources of phosphorus and vitamin D) are avoided. Phosphate-binders (such as aluminium-based antacids) may be prescribed to increase excretion of phosphorus. The amounts of elemental calcium contained in calcium preparations varies, depending on the salt. Calcium salts may be given as lactate, gluconate, or carbonate; calcium phosphate is contraindicated.

Dosages of vitamin D and calcium are adjusted to maintain a normal serum calcium and to minimize urinary calcium excretion, to avoid the risk of renal calculi. The lack of PTH results in excessive urinary calcium levels. Thiazide diuretics and a restricted sodium intake are helpful in decreasing hypercalcinuria.

Medical follow-up with monitoring of laboratory tests of serum and urinary calcium levels is necessary to prevent hypercalcaemia, renal colic, and metastatic calcifications. The patient must be well educated for self-management of the illness.

Table 21-12 Thyroid gland dysfunction

Signs and symptoms	Medical therapy
Thyroid hormone deficit	

Hypothyroidism (early signs):
  Weight gain; weakness, fatigue, lethargy; sluggishness; sleepiness; slowed mental process; slurred speech; intolerance to cold; constipation; dry skin; dry sparse hair; infertility; decreased libido; decreased body temperature; menorrhagia in young women
(late):
  Lethargy; periorbital puffiness; nonpitting oedema of feet and hands; large tongue; dull facies; pale, cool, rough, "doughy" skin; coma
  Decreased urine flow and urine concentration; proteinuria (see text for cardiac, musculoskeletal, and gastrointestinal symptoms)
	Replaces therapy of thyroid hormones
	  Thyroxine sodium
	  Liothyronine sodium

Thyroid hormone excess	

Hyperthyroidism
Loss of weight, fatigue, hyperthermia, change in fat metabolism
Mental status: anxiety, poor concentration, restlessness, emotional lability, irritability, restlessness
Nervous system: fine tremors, rapid tendon reflexes, decreased fine coordination
Cardiovascular system: tachycardia, increased blood pressure, angina, arrhythmias, cardiac hypertrophy
Respiratory system: decreased vital capacity and dyspnoea
Gastrointestinal system: increased frequency of stools, increased appetite, hepatic dysfuction
Muscle and bone changes: muscle weakness, atrophy, osteoporosis
Skin changes: warm, moist skin, intolerance to heat, fine hair
Dermopathy: pretibial myxoedema, vitiligo, hyperpigmentation
Sexual changes: amenorrhoea, decreased libido
Enlarged thyroid
	Reduction of thyroid hormone
	  Antithyroid drugs; aqueous iodine oral solution propylthiouracil, carbimazole
	Radioactive iodine
	Surgery: subtotal or total thyroidectomy
	
	Thyroid crisis:
	  Antithyroid drugs; oxygen, hypothermia to reduce fever, IV fluids, hydrocotisone, propranolol

Facilitating learning

Vitamin D appears to be the principal regulator of the level of calcium ions in the body and therefore increases the absorption of calcium. The person with hypoparathyroidism needs a diet high in vitamin D. The amount of calcium and vitamin D is gradually adjusted until the serum calcium level is normal. Recognition of symptoms of hypocalcaemia and hypercalcaemia is important so that adjustment in dosage can be instituted.

Evaluation

Questions that the nurse can use to evaluate the nursing care of the patient with parathyroid dysfunction may include the following for the patient with hypercalcaemia and hyperparathyroidism:

1. Was mobility maintained?
2. Was nutritional status maintained?
3. Was normal bowel elimination maintained?
4. Is patient prepared to manage treatment measures at home?
5. Is patient aware of need for lifelong replacement therapy, if indicated?

For the patient with hypocalcaemia and hypoparathyroidism, evaluate on the following:

1. Were complications (tetany, impaired air exchange, decreased cardiac output) prevented by early detection and reporting of signs and symptoms?
2. Was the patient free of injuries?
3. Could the patient explain medications, diet, follow-up care, and signs and symptoms to report immediately?

THYROID DYSFUNCTION

Alterations in the thyroid gland may be associated with hyperthyroid, hypothyroid, or euthyroid metabolic states (Table 21-12). A review of the normal functions of the thyroid are presented in Table 21-5, p. 528.

A brief discussion of goitre and thyroiditis will be presented before an examination of the major problems of hypothyroidism and hyperthyroidism. This section concludes with the nursing process for patients with either hypersecretion or hyposecretion of the thyroid hormone or surgery of the thyroid gland.

GOITRE

Any enlargement of the thyroid gland is called a goitre. A goitre may be caused by various disorders that prevent the synthesis of normal quantities of thyroid hormones or when there is increased stimulation of the thyroid gland by thyroid stimulating hormone (TSH) or TSH-like substances. These disorders include the following:

1. Iodide deficiency
2. Congenital metabolic defects preventing synthesis of thyroid hormones
3. Blocking of hormone synthesis by chemical agents (e.g., substances in cabbage, turnips, soybeans)
4. Blocking of hormone synthesis by drugs (for example, thiocarbamides, sulphonylureas, and lithium)
5. Selected types of hyperthyroidism

Goitre occurs in the first four categories because of an impairment in hormonal synthesis associated with a reduction of the thyroid hormones T_3 and T_4. It is believed that this reduction prevents the normal feedback inhibition of TSH. The TSH level is increased, which in turn causes an increase in thyroid mass. This thyroid enlargement (Fig. 21-8) may be sufficient to allow for adequate hormonal synthesis. In the last category there is an increase in TSH or TSH-like substance from the disease with resultant thyroid enlargement and excessive production of T_3 and T_4.

Not all patients with goitre demonstrate an elevated level of TSH. Another hypothesis is that goitre results from the stimulation of the thyroid gland by thyroid growth immunoglobulins. Goitre may be diffuse or nodular; nodules are caused by an adenoma, a carcinoma, inflammatory processes, or a haemorrhage.

Simple goitre is the term used for thyroid enlargement that is not associated with hyperthyroidism, hypothyroidism, malignancy, or inflammation. It is frequently seen in females, appearing at puberty or during pregnancy.

THYROIDITIS

Inflammation of the thyroid gland may be acute, subacute, or chronic and is characterized by painful swelling of the thyroid gland. Acute thyroiditis following infections by a pyogenic organism and subacute thyroiditis that follows a viral infection are rare.

The most common form of thyroiditis is Hashimoto's thyroiditis, in which the thyroid is infiltrated with lymphocytes and plasma cells. Autoimmunity is considered to be the pathological basis of this chronic thyroiditis. Early in the disease when functioning thyroid tissue is still present, excessive stored thyroid hormone may be released, resulting in signs and symptoms of transient

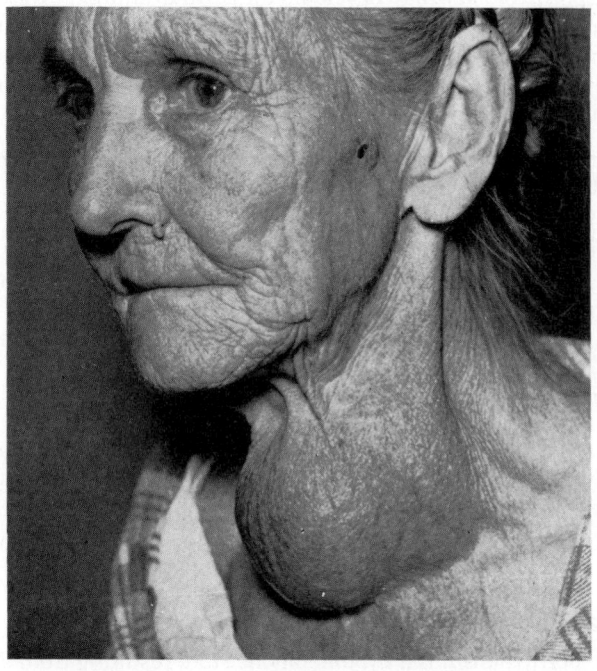

Fig. 21-8 Simple goitre. (From Prior JA, Silberstein JS, Stang JM, *Physical diagnosis: the history and examination of the patient,* ed 6, St Louis, 1981, Mosby–Year Book.)

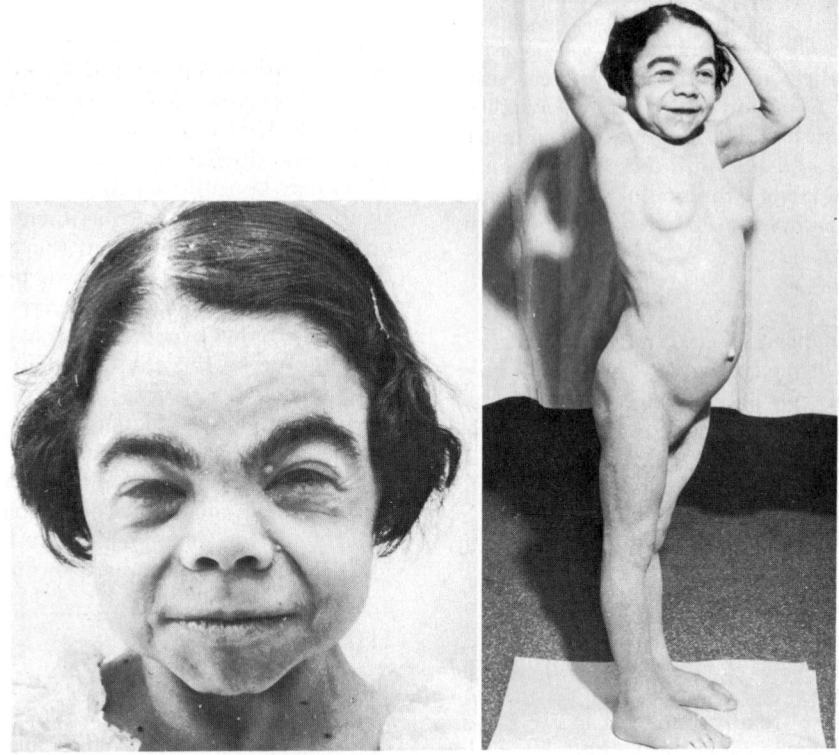

Fig. 21-9 Adult cretin (33 years old, untreated). Note characteristic cretinoid features, dwarfism (height of 44 inches), absent axillary and scant pubic hair, poorly developed breasts, potbelly, and small umbilical hernia. (From Schneeburg NG: *Essentials of clinical endocrinology*, St Louis, 1979, Mosby–Year Book.)

hyperthyroidism. As the disease progresses, the thyroid gland may be destroyed, and signs and symptoms of hypothyroidism may develop. Antithyroid antibodies are present in the serum. Although TSH levels may be elevated in the early stages of the disease, serum T_4 and T_3 levels gradually decrease. There is diffuse enlargement of both lobes of the thyroid gland.

HYPOTHYROIDISM
Aetiology

The causes of hypothyroidism may be primary, secondary, tertiary, or iatrogenic. Primary hypothyroidism can result from:
1. Congenital atrophy or congenital defect in enzyme production.
2. Idiopathic causes.
3. Iodine deficiency.
4. Chronic thyroiditis.

Secondary and tertiary causes of hypothyroidism include hypothalamic-pituitary dysfunction. Treatment with radioactive iodine, antithyroid drugs or surgery of the thyroid are iatrogenic causes of hypothyroidism.

Pathophysiology

Hypothyroidism is a hypometabolic state resulting from a deficiency of thyroid hormone that may occur at any age. Signs of infantile (congenital) hypothyroidism, or *cretin-*

ism, are not usually seen until several months after birth; by then, mental and physical retardation are usually irreversible. Figure 21-9 shows an adult who had untreated infantile hypothyroidism.

In adults the most frequent causes of hypothyroidism are autoimmune thyroiditis, ablative therapy, and idiopathy. It may be secondary to pituitary failure and TSH lack or may result from hypothalamic disease that causes a deficiency of thyroid-releasing hormone. In hypothyroidism resulting from pituitary or hypothalamic problems, TSH is depressed and no hyperplasia occurs. In primary hypothyroidism, hyperplasia is present because a lack of T_4 and T_3 result in an increase in TSH.

The signs and symptoms of hypothyroidism result from a deficiency of T_3 and T_4, leading to a decrease in the normal metabolic functions that are under the control of these hormones. Usually the pathophysiological changes develop slowly and early symptoms are vague (fatigue, weakness, lethargy, and intolerance to cold). Table 21-12 lists some other early signs and symptoms of hypothyroidism.

The characteristics of hypothyroidism vary with the age of onset and the severity of the deficiency. There is an accumulation of hyaluronic acids and alteration of ground substances that result in mucinous oedema. This development is responsible for the thickened tissues of hands, feet, and tongue and around the eyes and for effusions in the pleura, pericardium, and joints.

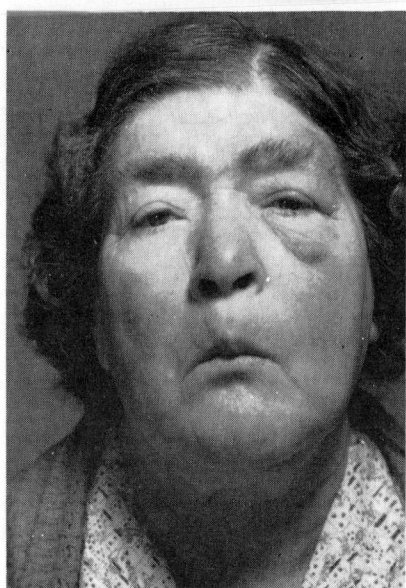

Fig. 21-10   Person with myxoedema. (From Schottelius BA, Schotteliusm DA: *Textbook of physiology*, ed 18, St Louis, 1978, Mosby–Year Book.)

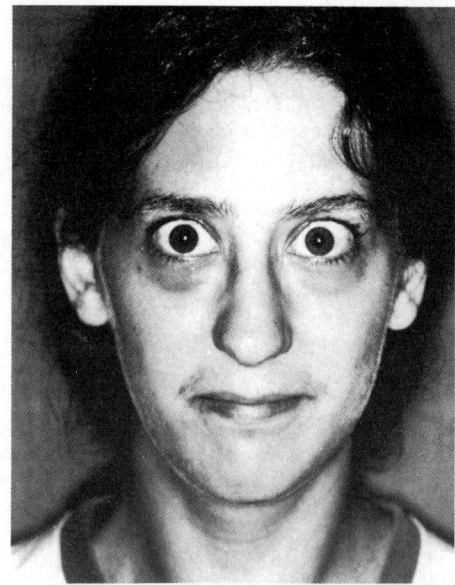

Fig. 21-11 Ophthalmopathy of Graves' disease. (From Kaye D, Rose LF: *Fundaments of internal mediocine*, St Louis, 1993 Mosby–Year Book.)

See Fig. 21-10 for an example of the facies characteristic of hypothyroidism. These patients often have coarse skin that bruises easily (because of increased capillary fragility) and is pale and yellow (because of anaemia and hypercarotenaemia). Hair becomes sparse, dry, and brittle. Mental processes slow, with loss of initiative, memory deficit, and slurred speech; somnolence, confusion, and even dementia may occur. Muscular and joint stiffness are common. Appetite decreases and decreased peristaltic activity lead to constipation. Despite these marked changes, some individuals do not seem to be aware of the changes in their physical functioning, appearance, or behaviour.

Cardiovascular dysfunction is a serious outcome of untreated hypothyroidism. Besides bradycardia, there may be elevation of diastolic blood pressure, cardiomegaly, and changes in cardiac output. Hypercholesteraemia is often present. Angina or cardiac failure may occur. Diminished heart sounds may represent pericardial effusion. *Pleural effusion* and ascites can develop.

Myxoedema coma occurs as the hypothyroidism worsens. The patient becomes less responsive and goes into a coma. An infection such as pneumonia, cellulitis, or pyelonephritis may precipitate the coma in a poorly treated patient.

HYPERTHYROIDISM

Aetiology

The causes of hyperthyroidism include primary, secondary, tertiary, and iatrogenic causes. The primary causes include:
  1. Toxic diffuse goitre (Graves' disease)
  2. Toxic multinodular goitre
  3. Toxic adenoma
  4. T_3 thyrotoxicosis

  5. Secreting thyroid cancer
  6. Early stage of thyroiditis (temporary)
Secondary and tertiary causes of hyperthyroidism include hypothalamic-pituitary hyperfunction and some ovarian tumours. Factitious use of thyroid medication is an iatrogenic cause of hyperthyroidism.

Pathophysiology

Hyperthyroidism, a hypermetabolic state, is also called thyrotoxicosis. Hyperthyroidism results from excessive secretion of thyroxine (T_4) or triiodothyronine (T_3). The most common causes are toxic diffuse goitre (Graves' disease) and toxic nodular goitre. In both of these conditions, secretion of T_4 and T_3 becomes autonomous, and the thyroid gland is no longer regulated by TSH.

Hyperthyroidism is more common in women than in men, and there is a higher incidence between 20 and 40 years of age. It often appears after episodes of emotional trauma, infection, or increased stressors and occurs frequently in people who have had other endocrine disturbances.

The cardiovascular system is seriously affected by hyperthyroidism because of the increased metabolic rate and the direct effects of thyroid hormones on the heart.

Sympathetic nervous stimulation is responsible for many of the symptoms of hyperthyroidism listed in Table 21-12. Atrial fibrillation and congestive heart failure may evolve in hyperthyroidism if not treated. Other symptoms are related to a chronic catabolic state or interactions with other hormones.

Because the pathophysiology of the two major causes of hyperthyroidism differ somewhat, each will be discussed individually.

The Elderly with Endocrine Problems

Assessment

Assess for signs and symptoms of decreased alertness, decreased mobility, or increased susceptibility to cold, which may be signs and symptoms more typicaly noted with hypothyroidism in elderly.

Assess signs of myxoedema, seen with untreated hypothyroidism.

Assess for signs of drug toxicity because of decreased metabolic activity from diminished endocrine function.

Assess for signs of infection because thymic activity is decreased.

Intervention

Assist elderly patient to plan a way to remember taking replacement therapy; without a plan, the apathetic patient may forget to take the thyroid hormone replacement.

Teach patient and significant others the following:
Monitor for drug side effects,
Report signs of angina or congestive heart failure that may result from initial doses of thyroid hormone replacement.
Take precautions to avoid infections.
Take measures to prevent constipation, which often occurs with hypothyroidism, especially in the elderly.

Common disorders in the elderly

Hypothyroidisum
Infections

Graves' disease (toxic diffuse goitre)

Graves' disease, which is characterized by a triad of symptoms—*goitre, hyperthyroidism,* and *exophthalmos* (abnormal protrusion of the eyes, Fig.21-11)—is thought to be an autoimmune disease and is the result of thyroid-stimulating immunoglobulins (TSI), also called long-acting thyroid stimulator (LATS). The cause of the abnormal development of the immunoglobulins is unknown. People with specific haplotypes and monozygotic twins have a higher frequency of Graves' disease.

Retro-orbitally, there is oedema with infiltration (fat, mucopolysaccharides, and lymphocytes) that results in proptosis. This process *is not closely correlated* with the severity of hormonal excess. The forward protrusion intensifies other signs related to the eye that result from increased sympathetic nervous sytem (for example, stare and lid lag). In severe *exophthalmos*, there may be an inability to close the eye and extraocular muscle weakness.

The amount of thyroid enlargement varies in Graves' disease, but it is diffuse and usually symmetrical. An important sign of Graves' disease is a *bruit* heard over the thyroid; this sign reflects increased vascularity.

Toxic multinodular goitre

Milder hyperthyroidism and nodular disease are typical of toxic multinodular goitre. This condition usually occurs after age 50 and is most commonly seen in the elderly. Usually nontoxic nodular disease has been present for many years before health care is sought. In the elderly, signs of increased sympathetic activity (for example, tremors, hyperactivity, and heat intolerance) may not be as marked and can make diagnosis more difficult. Unexplained tachycardia or a decrease in mental status may lead to the diagnosis.

Thyroid crisis

Thyroid storm crisis may occur in people with uncontrolled hyperthyroidism. It is believed that in thyroid crisis, increased amounts of hormones are released into the bloodstream and metabolism is markedly increased. It may be precipitated by infection, stressors, or thyroid surgery undertaken on a patient who was not adequately prepared with antithyroid drugs. The onset often occurs spontaneously. The patient's temperature may rise to 41°C (106°F) as the body becomes unable to release the heat formed with increased metabolism. The pulse will be rapid, and there is marked respiratory distress, apprehension, restlessness, irritability, and prostration. The patient may become delirious and finally comatose, with death resulting from heart failure.

Nursing Process
Assessment
Subjective data

Hypersecretion or hyposecretion of the thyroid gland has marked effects on the patient's ability to function, as well as on physiological processes. The nurse collects data from the patient or a family member about the factors listed below. It is important to ask if there has been a change in any of these factors and when the change was first noted.

Energy level
Mood and mental ability
Ability to carry out activities of daily living
Ability to manage stressors
Intolerance to heat or cold
Food intake
Elimination patterns
Weight changes
Skin and hair changes
Changes in reproduction function

The interview should help the nurse determine the patient or family's understanding of the disease and its treatment and learn about the care needs of the patient.

Objective data

Initial physical examination by the doctor and observation by the nurse should provide the following baseline information about the patient:

Mental status (ability to follow directions)
Nervous system status
Nutritional status

Cardiovascular status
Body characteristics
Skin appearance and texture
Hair quality and amount
Eye appearance and extraocular motion
Presence and location of oedema
Neck appearance and range of motion
Abdominal girth
Muscle mass/strength

Diagnostic tests

Testing for thyroid function can be made at the hypothalamic, pituitary, thyroid, serum, or peripheral tissue levels. Table 21-13 presents the major test procedures and preparations and their interpretation. The most commonly used tests are serum T_4 and T_3 concentrations, and TSH levels. T_3 resin uptake is also frequently used. The T_3 resin uptake test evaluates changes in serum protein concentrations that can alter the binding of T_3 and T_4. Changes in thyroxine-binding globulins (TBG) and prealbumin may alter free T_4 concentrations and, to a lesser extent, T_3. The T_3 resin uptake along with the serum T_4 can be used to determine free T_4 levels.

An elevated T_4 level often confirms clinical findings of overt hyperthyroidism, whereas T_3 testing is more sensitive in discerning mild hyperthyroidism. TSH radioimmunoassay and stimulation testing can help differentiate primary and secondary hypothyroidism, hyperthyroidism, and the effectiveness of treatment. Investigation of thyroid nodules may require needle biopsy or surgical exploration.

Nursing analysis

Problems are determined from the analysis of patient data. Possible problems for the person with thyroid hormone imbalance may include, but are not limited to the following:

Planning: expected patient outcomes

Expected patient outcomes for the person with thyroid disorders may include, but are not limited to the following. Specifically, the patient with *hypothyroidism* should be able to perform the following:
1. Gradually increase independence in self-care abilities.
2. Employ measures to prevent constipation.
3. Blood pressure and cardiac output will be returned to normal and maintained within normal limits.
4. State plans for follow-up care:
   a. State symptoms of hypothyroidism requiring immediate follow-up.
   b. State plans for regular medical appointments.
   c. State need for daily replacement therapy.

The patient with *hyperthyroidism* should be able to perform the following:
1. Employ coping measures to decrease anxiety and interpersonal friction.
2. Describe ways to increase caloric and protein intake.
3. State ways to help improve sleep.
4. Cardiac output will be maintained.

5. State plans for follow-up care:
   a. State symptoms requiring immediate follow-up (signs of remission, thyroid crisis, hypothyroidism).
   b. State plans for regular medical appointments.
6. Describe eye care if exophthalmos is present.

Implementation

Assisting with achievement of therapeutic goals
Medications

Medications may be used to treat goitre, hyperthyroidism, or hypothyroidism.

The drugs used most commonly to treat *hypothyroidism* are listed in Box 21-5. It is important that dosages be increased gradually because a sudden increase in metabolic rate can cause cardiac failure.

Thyroid hormone replacement. Thyroxine sodium is initiated at a dose of 100 to 200 µg daily as a single dose before breakfast; in the elderly and patients with heart disease, the initial dose is 25 to 50 µg daily. The dose is increased by 25 to 50 µg daily every four weeks, and the usual maintenance dose is 100 to 200 µg daily. The daily maintenance dose of thyroid hormones varies widely. The correct dose is determined by clinical status and assay of TSH levels. Diuresis with weight loss and regression of puffiness is an early response. Increased pulse rate, improvement of appetite, and relief of constipation are usually seen next. Most signs of hypothyroidism are eventually reversed.

Adults with hypothyroidism respond quickly to the administration of thyroid hormones. Changes in appearance and physical symptoms occur within 2 to 3 days. Treatment must be continued throughout life. Medication dosage may need periodic adjustment to avoid symptoms of hyperthyroidism or recurrence of hypothyroidism.

Antithyroid drugs. Propylthiouracil or carbimazole block thyroid hormone synthesis, thus they reduce the output of thyroid hormone in hyperthyroidism (see Table 21-13). Usually antithyroid drugs are used before ablation of thyroid tissue by radioactive iodine or surgery.

The patient usually is started on a relatively large dose of an antithyroid drug, then the dosage is gradually reduced to a level sufficient to maintain the euthyroid state. When antithyroid drugs are used as the primary therapy, they commonly are continued for 6 to 18 months or longer. Some patients stay in remission without further therapy. Others require longer drug therapy, additional therapy, or lifelong therapy.

The patient should see the doctor at regular intervals after drugs are discontinued so that early signs of recurrence are noticed. It is important to give the drugs at regularly spaced intervals, because the blood levels are reduced in about 8 hours. Some people may not tolerate continued use of antithyroid drugs. Toxic side effects include agranulocytosis and cholestasis. Skin rashes, joint pains, and diarrhoea may also occur.

Iodides. Aqueous oral iodine solution can rapidly reduce the patient's metabolic rate. It is given for short

<table>
<tr><td>21-5</td><td>

Replacement therapy for hypothyroidism
Thyroxine sodium (synthetic T_4)
Liothyronine sodium (synthetic T_3)

</td></tr>
</table>

<table>
<tr><td>21-6</td><td>

Possible complications after thyroid surgery

Haemorrhage
Oedema about vocal cords and larynx
Laryngeal nerve injury
Tetany

</td></tr>
</table>

periods only. Its principal use is to decrease thyroid vascularity before surgery. Iodide administration saturates the thyroid gland with iodine and interferes with ablation of the thyroid by ^{131}I; therefore the administration of iodides is contraindicated before ^{131}I therapy. See Table 21-13 for important activities relevant to iodide administration.

Iodide may be used in concert with antithyroid therapy preoperatively; it is given *after* propylthiouracil has reduced the hyperthyroidism.

Radioactive iodine

Ablation of the thyroid gland may be achieved by radiation. The most commonly used isotope is ^{131}I. It is the treatment of choice for most people with hyperthyroidism. A radioactive isotope of iodine, ^{131}I is given by mouth, is absorbed rapidly in the stomach, and becomes concentrated in the thyroid. Usually, a single dose is given in a radioactive "cocktail." It takes about 3 weeks for the symptoms of hyperthyroidism to subside, and more than 2 months for thyroid function to become normal. Occasionally, remission is not achieved with one dose, and the treatment is repeated after an interval of several months.

<table>
<tr><td rowspan="2">21-7</td><td rowspan="2" style="writing-mode:vertical">Guidelines for care</td><td>

The patient after thyroid surgery

Monitor for postoperative complications.
  Larygeal damage: hoarseness, weak voice, stridor
  Haemorrhage or tissue swelling:
    Bleeding: check dressing and back by slipping hand gently behind neck and shoulders
    Choking sensation
    Difficulty in swallowing or coughing
    Sensation of dressing being too tight even after it is loosened
  Hypocalcaemia (tetany):
    Paraesthesias
    Trousseau's and Chvostek's signs
    Carpopedal spasm
    Seizure activity
  Respiratory distress:
Maintain equipment at bedside for treatment of laryngeal obstruction (tracheostomy set) and tetany (calcium gluconate).
For acute respiratory distress:
  Call for imediate medical asstance.
  If a doctor is not readily available, remove clips and sutures as previously instructed.
Encourage high-carbohydrate fluids by mouth and a soft diet as tolerated.
Provide comfort.
  Use·prescribed analgesics.
  Local agents (analgesic throat lozenges or gels) ease swallowing; give 30 minutes before meals.
  Avoid placing tention on suture line.
  After 5 to 7 days, gradual range of motion may be promoted.
Teach patient about required drugs (dosage, side effects) and importance of medical follow-up.

</td></tr>
</table>

Table 21-13 Antithyroid drugs

Drug	Actions	Interventions

Iodide solutions
  Aqueous iodine oral
  solution (Lugol's Solution)
	Rapid action, block synthesis and release of thyroid hormone; less sustained action; reduce vascularity of the thyroid gland, thus often used in preparation for surgery; saturate(s) thyroid with iodide, thus radioactive iodine studies or treatment of thyroid cannot be carried out	Explain to patient that compliancewith prescribed dosage is necessary; give through a straw to avoid staining of teeth; give in milk or fruit juice; teach patient to report toxic symptoms: brassy taste, sore teeth and gums

Propylthiouracil	Blocks synthesis of thyroid hormone and the release of stored hormone	Explain to patient that 2–4 weeks are necessary before improvement is noticed; teach patient to report toxic symptoms: fever, sore throat, skin eruptions; leukopenia or pancytopenia may occur
Carbimazole	Blocks synthesis of thyroid hormone, not the release of stored hormone	

Nursing Care Plan

Person with hyperthyroidism

DATA: Mrs. T., a 28-year-old housewife, is admitted for diagnostic evaluation before a thyroidectomy, which is planned for 2 weeks. Graves' disease was diagnosed 2
days ago; hospitalization was delayed until child-care arrangements were made for her 6-
year-old step-son. (The marriage occurred 3 months ago.) Initial therapy, started 2 days
ago, is carbimazole and aqueous oral iodine solution. The ECG report is sinus tachycardia
(rate 132).

The nursing history identified the following about the patient:
1. Mrs. T. feels overwhelmed, cries frequently, and fears losing control of temper.
2. She has lost a stone in 2 months and is always hungry, although she is eating large
amounts of food.
3. She is bothered by heat, others' noisiness, and her own clumsiness.
4. She expects medicine to keep her feeling better and dreads surgery.

The physical examination revealed the following: BP: 140/90; T: 38.0°C pulse: 136, R:24.
Staring gaze of eyes with proptosis (equal bilaterally); right eye slightly reddened. Skin
warm and perspiration present. Increased muscle tone; quick muscle response to sudden
noise; fine tremor of both hands. Diffuse enlargement of thyroid visible. *Bruit* present
over thyroid.

Collaborative nursing actions include those to prevent further environmental stressors that
could make the patient more uncomfortable and increase her signs and symptoms.

Nursing actions include monitoring for the following: temperature, pulse, respiration, blood
pressure, weight, excessive hunger, and tremulousness.

Problem: Decreased cardiac output: related to environmental stimulation

Expected patient outcomes	Nursing interventions	Rationale
Pulse rate is less than 10 above baseline during first 72 h Pulse rate decreases gradually after 72 h Undetected cardiac arrhythmias do not occur	Assess vital signs, especially heart rate and rhythm at least 4 hourly Instruct Mrs. T. to report palpitations, chest pain, and dizziness Assess daily weight, daily intake and output; assess for signs of oedema Decrease known stressors; explain all interventions, and listen to Mrs. T. Balance periods of activity with rest Administer prescribed drugs and monitor therapeutic response	The early detection of cardiac changes such as atrial fibrillation or thyroid crisis allows prompt treatment and prevents cardiovascular crisis

Problem: Coping ineffective individual: related to personal vulnerability to environmental stimuli

Expected patient outcomes	Nursing interventions	Rationale
Explains reason for change in behaviour Emotional lability is minimized Identifies at least one coping mechanism that will help during periods of nervousness	Discuss reasons for emotional lability Maintain calm, relaxed environment Encourage visitors who are calm and will not upset her Provide privacy (such as a single room) Suggest that others avoid sharing distressing news with her Explain all interventions Avoid stimulants such as coffee, tea, caffeine, and alcohol Help her identify previous coping mechanisms or explore new ones	A supportive environment can reduce environmental stimuli and stressors and assist patient in coping

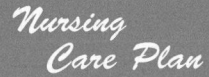

Person with hyperthyroidism—cont'd

Problem: Altered nutrition: less than body requirements related to increased metabolic needs

Expected patient outcomes	Nursing interventions	Rationale
Normal weight is maintained Mrs. T. gains at least 0.5 kg/wk, if weight is below normal	Monitor weight weekly Monitor serum albumin, haemoglobin, and lymphocyte levels Help her plan for high-calorie, high-protein, high-carbohydrate diet with selection from all food groups Suggest six meals per day or between-meal snacks	Increase nutrient intake to meet increased metabolic demand

Problem: Sensory/perceptual alterations: high risk for visual related to environmental agents

Expected patient outcomes	Nursing interventions	Rationale
Vision does not worsen Explains measures to protect eyes	Assess visual acuity, ability to close eyes, and photophobia Protect eyes from irritants: Use patches or glasses when in high wind Use artificial tears, if prescribed Elevate head of bed at night	These measures can prevent corneal injury and minimize risk of loss of vision

Problem: Hyperthermia: related to increased metabolic rate

Expected patient outcomes	Nursing interventions	Rationale
States that she feels more comfortable	Control environmental temperature for comfort (fans may be helpful) Suggest that she take frequent showers Encourage adequate fluid intake and monitor fluid losses	These measures keep her comfortable by increasing heat loss and preventing problems of increased fluid loss

Problem: Activity intolerance: related to generalized weakness and decreased cardiac reserve

Expected patient outcomes	Nursing interventions	Rationale
States fatigue is decreased	Assess activity programme Suggest ways to modify fatiguing activities Identify activities that can be done by others until condition is controlled Plan for rest periods Encourage activities that promote sleep at night	Reduction of energy expenditure is necessary to reduce fatigue; in people with increased metabolism

Problem: Impaired home maintenance management: related to activity intolerance, fatigue, and emotional lability

Expected patient outcomes	Nursing interventions	Rationale
States plan for home maintenance management	Assist her to identify home maintenance difficulties Assist her to identify people who can provide temporary help Make referrals as needed, such as to social services Identify people who can help monitor her compliance with medical regimen	These measures increase resources available to patient and reduce stress from inability to meet expectations of role

Problem: Knowledge deficit: therapeutic regimen related to lack of exposure to information

Expected patient outcomes	Nursing interventions	Rationale
Explains medical regimen and care needs	Explain how and when to take prescribed medications Describe symptoms of infection to be reported to doctor, such as sore throat or fever Describe ways to plan prescribed dietary intake Provide required teaching about care needs (comfort, sleep, and rest)	These measures increase likelihood of compliance with therapy used to achieve euthyroid state and optimal physical status before surgery

Hypothyroidism frequently develops after ^{131}I therapy, and the onset can occur years after treatment.

Radioactive iodine is not used in pregnant women because iodine readily crosses the placenta and may affect the foetus. Some doctors do not prescribe ^{131}I for people in the childbearing years because of the belief that there is a potential for damage to the gonads, although this belief is not supported by research.

Patients who receive radioactive iodine for hyperthyroidism need to have the treatment explained to them with special care, and they usually need repeated reassurance that the radioactive properties are quickly dissipated. Because people with hyperthyroidism may be more emotional than other people, they sometimes think they are experiencing reactions to the drug long after this is possible.

Surgery

Surgery of the thyroid is the procedure of choice for removal of goitre-causing pressure, and for cancer of the thyroid. Part or all of the thyroid gland may be removed surgically. Total thyroidectomy (complete removal of the thyroid) may be performed for cancer of the thyroid, and the patient must then take thyroid hormone regularly for the remainder of his or her life. Hyperthyroidism may be treated surgically by removing approximately five sixths of the gland (subtotal thyroidectomy). In most cases this operation permanently alleviates symptoms, while the remaining thyroid tissue provides enough hormones for normal function. Hypothyroidism, if present, is treated with replacement doses of thyroid hormone. The remaining tissue can hypertrophy, however, and hyperthyroidism can recur.

Before thyroid surgery is undertaken, a normal (euthyroid) state must be produced by drug therapy. An ECG is made before surgery to detect evidence of heart damage.

Postoperative complications. The complications after thyroid surgery are extremely serious. Monitoring for these complications has the highest priority in postoperative care (see Box 21-6).

Haemorrhage can result in incisional bleeding or in compression of the trachea and surrounding tissue. Haemorrhage is most common in the first 12 to 24 hours after surgery.

Although slight hoarseness is normal, the patient is observed for any increase in hoarseness and accompanying respiratory difficulty. To reveal early symptoms of laryngeal nerve injury, patients are asked to speak as soon as they have emerged from anaesthesia and at intervals of 30 to 60 minutes.

Respiratory obstruction can occur for many reasons. These include laryngeal nerve injury, compression of the trachea by haemorrhage, vocal cord oedema or spasm, and tetany. Emergency measures for these complications are outlined in Box 25-17. Injury to the parathyroids is uncommon but may occur. Surgery or inflammation may block the normal release of parathyroid hormone, and symptoms of tetany caused by calcium deficiency may appear from 1 to

7 days after surgery. Serum calcium levels are usually monitored, and hypocalcaemia is treated by replacement of calcium intravenously. Daily oral doses of calcium are then given until normal function returns.

Postoperative nursing interventions are summarized in Box 21-7.

Interventions to achieve patient outcomes

Interventions to assist in meeting the various outcomes are presented for each pathological state separately.

Hyperthyroidism. Since the advent of antithyroid drugs and ^{131}I therapy, most people with hyperthyroidism can be cared for at home. Although these people usually are not particularly hyperactive, they are likely to be nervous and irritable. It is important that family and friends understand that extreme sensitivity and irritability are part of the disease; otherwise, they may become upset with the individual and aggravate the situation. It may be necessary to assist these persons with activities requiring fine motor coordination and concentration, although they may appear physically able to perform the activities themselves. They will need an explanation about why they require such assistance.

The patient's cardiac status needs to be monitored closely. Rest periods need to be provided and encouraged. As activity is changed the patient's cardiac status needs to be reassessed.

Other interventions by nurses or caregivers at home indicated for the person with hyperthyroidism include:
1. Maintain a cool, quiet environment.
2. Assist person to obtain sufficient rest.
3. Encourage quiet activities that require gross motor movements (for example, weaving and reading), which the person can do without assistance.
4. Assist person with tasks requiring fine motor coordination (for example sewing and washing dishes).
5. Provide a high-calorie, high-protein diet; snacks between meals may be necessary to maintain weight and meet energy requirements.
6. Discourage the use of caffeinated drinks.
7. If exophthalmos is present:
   a. Encourage use of dark glasses, which afford some protection from wind, sun, and dust.
   b. Administer soothing eye drops, such as hypromellose, which may prevent drying of the eye and provide comfort.

The patient with hyperthyroidism requires education about the disease, diagnostic tests, treatment, and self-care needs (medications, eye care, diet). Educational sessions should be spaced, and written material should supplement verbal information.

Hypothyroidism. The patient's slowed mental and physical functioning requires understanding and patience on the part of caregivers. A thorough explanation of the cause of the changes in the patient's physical and mental responses also should be given to family or friends. As thyroid hormone levels return to normal, the patient's physical and mental state will return to normal and the patient will be able to take over own self-care.

Other nursing care includes the following:

1. Minimize environmental stressors, because the patient is less able to respond to them.
2. Administer replacement therapy and monitor patient for effectiveness of therapy and side effects.
3. Provide complete care at first and gradually increase patient's self-care.
4. Prevent constipation and faecal impaction by administering fluids, fibre, and stool softeners and by encouraging activity.
5. Monitor cardiac response to therapy and any increase in activity.

Patient education is an important part of the patient care. Because the patient has impaired cognitive functioning at the beginning of therapy, instructions need to be simple, concise, and repeated frequently. The patient needs to be taught about the need for life-long therapy and given suggestions on how to manage constipation. Other information on self-care must be discussed. The planned follow-up needs to be explained.

Evaluation

Evaluation is based on expected patient outcomes. Questions useful in evaluating nursing care of patients with thyroid dysfunction may include the following:

For the patient with hypothyroidism:

1. Were self-care needs met?
2. Was the patient able to maintain normal bowel elimination?
3. Was cardiac output returned to normal and maintained?
4. Is the patient prepared to manage self-care at home (diet, medications)?
5. Does the patient know plans for follow-up?

For the patient with hyperthyroidism:

1. Was the patient able to identify several coping measures to decrease anxiety?
2. Did the patient maintain adequate nutritional intake?
3. Did the patient attain adequate sleep/rest patterns?
4. Was cardiac output returned to normal and maintained?
5. Can the patient describe ways to meet self-care needs (handling medicines, eye care, rest/activity needs, diet)?
6. Does the patient know plans for follow-up care?

SUMMARY

1. Normal physiology depends on the proper amounts of hormones being available to act on cell receptors of target tissues.
2. Many factors influence secretory patterns and rates of secretion of hormones. Atrophy and hypoplasia of a gland result in hyposecretion, whereas hypertrophy and hyperplasia result in hypersecretion.
3. The hypothalamic-pituitary-target gland axis is a principal regulator of hormonal secretion of the adrenal, thyroid, and gonad glands.
4. Parathyroid hormone, vitamin D, and calcitonin are three regulators of calcium and phosphorus balance. The serum level of calcium is the principal regulator of parathyroid hormone secretion.
5. *Giantism* in children and *acromegaly* in adults are conditions resulting from growth hormone excess. Tumours or pituitary hyperplasia may be treated with surgery, irradiation, or growth hormone suppressants.
6. The most common pituitary tumour is a prolactinoma that may present with symptoms of galactorrhoea or reproductive dysfunction.
7. Pituitary tumours may cause compression of normal tissue, resulting in hyposecretion of anterior pituitary hormones. They may also compress the optic chiasma and cause visual field defects.
8. Life-long replacement of cortisol is necessary to maintain life after a bilateral adrenalectomy or pituitary ablation or when disease or injury has destroyed the pituitary or adrenal cortex (for instance, in Addison's disease).
9. Administration of *therapeutic* doses of glucocorticoid medications produce iatrogenic Cushing's syndrome and place the patient at risk for adrenocortical insufficiency or crisis if abruptly stopped.
10. Diabetes insipidus results from ADH deficit and is characterized by polyuria and low specific gravity of urine. Overdosage of ADH replacement can induce weight gain and reduce urinary volume.
11. Cardiac problems may develop from several hormonal alterations: growth hormone, cortisol, thyroid hormone, and catecholamines. Cardiac arrhythmias may occur in hypoparathyroidism and hyperthyroidism.
12. Fluid and electrolyte imbalances are predominate features of disorders of the posterior pituitary and adrenal cortex.
13. Hypertension may result from adrenal medullary or adrenal cortical hypersecretion.
14. Nutritional problems are common with hormonal disorders. Excesses of growth hormone and cortisol can induce states of catabolism, ketogenesis, and hyperglycaemia. Hyperthyroidism increases the amounts of nutrients required. Hypothyroidism decrease the calories required.
15. Disorders of growth may be a reflection of hormonal alterations, for instance, in *pituitary dwarfism* and *congenital cretinism* (hypothyroidism). Skin, hair, and nails may be changed in appearance in several of the hormonal disturbances.
16. Skeletal abnormalities and loss of bone integrity is a hallmark of parathyroid dysfunction. *Osteoporosis* from excessive bone resorption of calcium may limit the amount of corticosteroid medications given in chronic inflammatory diseases. *Acromegaly* (growth hormone excess) induces bony growth, which alters the patient's appearance and may cause joint problems and compression syndrome.
17. Hypotension is of particular concern in deficits of ADH, glucocorticoids, and mineralocorticosteroids. Volume expanders may be required immediately after

adrenal surgery or to treat Addison's crisis. Large doses of cortisol have mineralocorticoid effects.

18. Both vitamin D and calcium supplements are necessary to maintain serum calcium levels in *hypoparathyroidism* and to prevent *tetany*.

19. Neuromuscular irritability in hypocalcaemia gives rise to the symptoms of latent tetany and to cardiac arrhythmias, laryngeal obstruction, and convulsions. *Trousseau's sign, Chvostek's sign, carpopedal spasm,* and *paraesthesia* should be reported promptly.

20. The first priority in treatment of hyperparathyroidism is reducing severe hypercalcaemia (that is, levels greater than 3.5 mmol); cardiac arrythmias and coma can result if treatment is delayed.

21. Thyroid enlargement (goitre) may be detected by inspection and palpation and described as diffuse or nodular, and the qualities of symmetry and presence of pain or tenderness noted. *Simple goitre* is the term used to describe enlargement without thyroid hormone alteration.

22. *Hyperthyroidism* has many causes; excesses of T_3 and T_4 induce a hypermetabolic state and excessive sympathetic nervous system stimulation.

23. *Graves' disease* is characterized by hyperthyroidism, goitre, and exophthalmos. The presence of thyroid-stimulating antibodies confirms the diagnosis.

24. *Hypothyroidism* often has an insidious onset. A decrease in the metabolic functions under the control of T_4 and T_3 gives rise to multiple symptoms. Fluid retention results in weight gain, changes in appearance of skin, and effusions.

25. Hypothyroidism in the elderly may not be detected until severe changes in cardiac or mental status occur.

26. Thyroid hormone replacement reverses most signs of hypothyroidism in the adult; thyroxine is a common drug used for maintenance therapy.

27. Treatment of Graves' disease, the most common disease associated with hyperthyroidism, may include medications, ^{131}I, or surgery.

28. Complications of thyroid surgery include haemorrhage, tetany, laryngeal nerve injury, and respiratory obstruction.

STUDY QUESTIONS

- What is the role of the adrenal gland in response to stressors?
- Giving a large amount of hormone such as cortisone to a person who is producing that hormone affects endogenous production in what way? Why does this change occur?
- How would you explain to a patient with hyperthyroidism that increased amounts of food are needed?
- Are there other patient situations where increased foods are needed for the same reason as occurs in hyperthyroidism?
- What potassium problems are caused by disorders of the adrenal cortex and anterior pituitary? Why do these problems occur?
- What nutritional guidelines should be taught to people with hypersecretion and hyposecretion of the adrenal cortex or of the thyroid gland?

REFERENCES AND SELECTED READINGS

1. Bagdale JD: Endocrine emergencies, *Med Clin North Am* 70(5):1111–1128, 1986.
2. Barkan A: Acromegaly and gigantism. In The Endocrine Society: *41st post graduate annual assembly syllabus*, Bethesda, Md, 1989, The society.
3. Blackman M: Pituitary hormones and aging, *Endocrinol Metab Clin North Am* 16(4):981–994, 1987.
3a. Blondell R: Hypopituitarism, *AFP* 43:2029–2036, 1991.
3b. Brunader RE, Moore DC: Education of the child with growth retardation, *AFP* 35:165–176, 1987.
4. Davis PJ, Davis FB: Endocrinology and aging. In Reichel W, editor: *Clinical aspects of aging*, Baltimore, 1985, Williams and Wilkins.
5. DeGrootl et al: *Endocrinology*, ed 2, New York, 1989, Grune and Stratton.
6.* Ebersole P, Hess D: *Toward healthy aging*, ed 3, St Louis, 1990, Mosby-Year Book.
7. Endocrine Society: *43rd post graduate assembly syllabus*, Bethesda, Md, 1991, The society.
8.* Feit H: Thyroid function in the elderly, *Clin Geriatr Med* 4:151–161, 1988.
9. Guyton AC: *Human physiology and mechanisms of disease*, ed 4, Philadelphia, 1987, WB Saunders.
9a. Hart JJ: Pheochromocytoma, *AFP* 42:163–169, 1990.
10. Ingbar SH: The effects of aging on the thyroid hormone economy in man, *Prog Clin Biol Res* 74:135–145, 1985.
11.* Lancaster LE: Renal and endocrine regulation of water and electrolyte balance, *Nurs Clin North Am* 22:761–772, 1987.
12. Lennquist S: The thyroid nodule: diagnoses and surgical treatment, *Surg Clin North Am* 67:213–232, 1987.
13.* Lockhart J: Actionstat, *Nurs 88* 18:33, 1988.
14. Loriauy DL: Cushing's syndrome. In the Endocrine Society: *41st Post graduate annual assembly syllabus*, Bethesda, Md, 1989, The society.
15. Marx SH: Familial multiple endocrine neoplasia type 1. In The Endocrine Society: *41st post graduate annual assembly syllabus*, Bethesda, Md, 1989, The society.
16.* Mathewson MK: Thyroid disorder, *Crit Care Nurse* 7(1):74–85, 1985.
17. Mazzaferri E et al: Solitary thyroid nodule: diagnoses and management, *Med Clin North Am* 72:1177–1211, 1988.
18. McCance K, Huether SE: *Pathophysiology: the biologic basis for disease in adults and children*, St Louis, 1990, Mosby-Year Book.
19. Melmed S, Fagin JA: Acromegaly update—etiology, diagnoses, and management, *West J Med* 146:328–336, 1987.
20. Metz R, Larson EB: *Blue book of endocrinology*, Philadelphia, 1985, WB Saunders.
21. Molitch M: Lactation and prolactinomas. In The Endocrine Society: *41st post graduate annual assembly syllabus*, Bethesda, Md, 1989, The society.
22. Nabarro JD: Acromegaly, *Clin Endocrinol* 26:481–512, 1987.
23.* O'Neil I: Thyroid crisis, *Nurs 87* 17(1):335–338, 1987.
24. Robinson AG, Amico JA: Non-sweet diabetes of pregnancy, *N Engl J Med* 324:556–558, 1991.
25. Sakiyama R: Common thyroid disorders, *AFP* 38(1):227–238, 1988.
25a. Salman K, Miller JL, Rose LI: Selection of thyroid preparations, *AFP* 40:215–219, 1989.
26.* Sarsany S: Thyroid storm, *RN* 51(7):46–48, 1988.
27. Sawin CT: Hypothyroidism, *Med Clin North Am* 69:989–1003, 1988.
28.* Schira M: Steroid dependent states and adrenal insufficiency, *Nurs Clin North Am* 22:837–841, 1987.
28a. Shulman L, Miller JL, Rose LI: Growth hormone therapy, *AFP* 41:1541–1546, 1990.
29. Singer FR: Calcitonin: actions and therapeutic uses. In The Endocrine Society: *41st post graduate annual assembly syllabus*, Bethesda, Md, 1989, The society.
30. Sitges-Serra A, Caralps-Riera D: Hyperparathyroidism associated with renal disease, *Surg Clin North Am* 67:359–377, 1987.
31. Sivula A, Ronni-Sivula H: Natural history of treated primary hyperparathyroidism, *Surg Clin North Am* 67:329–341, 1987.
32. Snyder PJ: Gonadotroph cell adenomas of the pituitary, *Endocr Rev* 6:552–630, 1985.
33. Snyder PJ: The myth of the nonsecreting pituitary adenoma. In The Endocrine Society: *41st post graduate annual assembly syllabus*, Bethesda, Md, 1989, The society.
34. Spaulding S: Age and the thyroid, *Endocrinol Metab Clin North Am* 16(4):1013–1025, 1987.
35. Svee F: Steroid usage: too much of a good thing. In The Endocrine Society:

*Suggested for student reading.

41st post graduate annual assembly syllabus, Bethesda, Md, 1989, The society.

36. Thomas C, Groom RD: Current management of the patient with autonomously functioning nodular goitre, *Surg Clin North Am* 67:315–328, 1987.

37. Thompson N, Cheung P: Diagnoses and treatment of functioning and non-functioning adrenocortical neoplasms including incidentalomas, *Surg Clin North Am* 67:423–436, 1987.

38. Vance ML, Thorner MO: Prolactinomas, *Endocrinol Metab Clin* 16:731–753, 1987.

39. Verbalis JG: SIAD and other hyponatremic states. In The Endocrine Society: *41st post graduate annual assembly syllabus*, Bethesda, Md, 1989, The society.

40. Wilson JD, Foster DW, editors: *Williams' textbook of endocrinology*, ed 7, Philadelphia, 1985, WB Saunders.

41. Wolf PG, Meek JC: Practical approach to the treatment of hypothyroidism, *AFP* 45:722–731, 1992.

42. Wyngaarden JB, Smith LH, editors: *Cecil textbook of medicine*, ed 18, Philadelphia, 1988, WB Saunders.

43.* Camunas C: Pheochromocytoma, *Am J Nurs* 83:887–891, 1983.

44.* Evangelisti JT et al: Thyroid storm: a nursing crisis, *Heart Lung* 12:183–194, 1983.

45.* Gotch PM: Teaching patients about adrenal corticosteroids, *Am J Nurs* 81:78–85, 1981.

46.* Hoffman JT: Syndromes of ectopic hormone production in cancer, *Nurs Clin North Am* 15:499–509, 1980.

47. Hoffman JT, Newby TB: Hypercalcemia in primary hyperparathyroidism, *Nurs Clin North Am* 15:469–480, 1980.

48. Honigman RE: Deciphering diagnostic studies: thyroid function tests, *Nurs 82* 12(4):68–71, 1982.

49. Hurley JR: Thyroid disease in the elderly, *Med Clin North Am* 67(2):497–516, 1983.

50. Jones SG: Adrenal patient: proceed with caution, *RN* 45(2):69–72, 1982.

51.* Jones SG: Bilateral adrenalectomy: postop dangers to watch for, *RN* 34(2):66–69, 1982.

52.* Larson CA: The critical path of adrenocortical insufficiency, *Nurs 84* 14(10):66–69, 1984.

22

The Patient with Hepatic Problems

Virginia L. Cassmeyer
Dorothy Blevins

After studying this chapter, the learner should be able to:

- Describe the physiological functions of the hepatic system.
- Differentiate between diffuse and focal hepatocellular disorders.
- Differentiate between acute and chronic hepatitis.
- Explain the pathophysiological basis for common manifestations of diffuse liver disorders and the signs and symptoms of cirrhosis.
- Discuss the care of the patient with diffuse liver disorders such as cirrhosis or hepatitis or their sequelae.
- Describe the care of patients with liver abscesses, tumours, or trauma.

The hepatic system is affected by a variety of pathological processes that may severely affect normal metabolic processes. Many of the disorders of the hepatic system are chronic and require patients to make changes in their lifestyles, if optimal health is going to be maintained. These patients need nursing support to deal with their chronic health problems in the most effective ways.

ANATOMY AND PHYSIOLOGY

The hepatic system is a major system involved in regulation of body functions. The liver, which consists of two lobes, is one of the largest organs of the body and is located in the right upper quadrant of the abdomen under the diaphragm. It extends up under the ribs and is 4 to 8 cm in height in the midsternal line and 6 to 12 cm in height in the midclavicular line. It normally extends from the fifth intercostal space to just below the costal margin. The gallbladder lies under the inferior surface of the liver.

The liver is made up of small liver lobules composed of hepatic cellular plates. Each hepatic cellular plate is usually two cells thick, and between these cells run biliary canaliculi. Venous sinusoids (also called hepatic sinusoids), which are capillaries of the liver that receive blood from both the portal vein and the hepatic artery, lie on the opposite sides of the hepatic cells. After flowing through the venous sinusoids, blood is emptied into the central vein and from there flows into the hepatic vein. The venous sinusoids are lined with Kupffer's cells, which are reticuloendothelial cells that phagocytize bacteria and other foreign products.

The liver is ideally structured to receive large supplies of blood to carry out its multiple functions, which are summarized in Box 22-1. Although only 25% of its blood supply is oxygenated, oxygen extraction by the liver is so efficient that there is little variation in oxygen consumption regardless of the rate of oxygen flow. The liver contains about 15% of the total blood volume and can quickly expel about half of this blood in situations of haemorrhage. The liver can also increase the percentage of blood volume it stores in the presence of vascular excess. Thus, the liver serves as a blood reservoir.

It is helpful to think of the liver as a metabolic factory and a waste disposal facility. The portal vein brings to the liver raw materials absorbed from the gastrointestinal tract, finished products are manufactured by the liver, and then the hepatic venules and biliary canaliculi act as the distributors of these products through blood and bile flow. Waste products that are produced through these metabolic processes are eliminated through bile flow or carried by blood to other parts of the body for elimination.

Carbohydrate, Protein, and Fat Metabolism

The liver has a major role in the metabolism of the major food nutrients. Through various enzymatic activities, the liver can oxidize carbohydrates, proteins, and fats for energy or use these nutrients to produce needed compounds, or to produce storage forms of these compounds for future use.

The liver helps maintain a normal blood glucose level. Immediately after meals, the liver cells extract glucose and other sugars from the sinusoidal blood and use them to

---

22-1

Summary of functions

Carbohydrate, protein, and fat metabolism
  Carbohydrate metabolism
    Glycogen formation and storage
    Glucose formation from glycogen (glycogenolysis) and from amino acids, lactic acids, and glycerol (gluconeogenesis)
  Protein metabolism
    Protein catabolism
    Protein synthesis
      Albumin
      Globulin
      Clotting factors C-reactive protein
      Transferrin
      Enzymes
      Ceruloplasmin, etc.
    Formation of needed amino acids
  Fat metabolism
    Oxidation of fatty acids for energy
    Ketone formation
    Synthesis of cholesterol and phospholipids
    Formation of triglycerides from dietary fats and excessive dietary carbohydrates and proteins
    Formation of lipoproteins
Production of bile salts
Bilirubin metabolism
Detoxification of endogenous and exogenous substances
  Ammonium
  Steroid hormones (aldosterone, oestrogen, testosterone, etc.)
  Drugs
Storage of minerals and vitamins
Protection (Kupffer cells)

---

form glycogen (glycogenesis). Between meals, or in longer fasting states, the liver provides glucose to the blood by breaking down glycogen (glycogenolysis) or by forming new glucose from amino acids, glycerol, and lactic acids (gluconeogenesis).

The liver provides needed amino acids through the process of transamination. In addition, it is the only source of albumin, which is necessary for the maintenance of osmotic pressure. The liver is the source of several clotting factors (I–XIII). Although some of these may be produced elsewhere in the body, the levels decrease significantly with liver disease. The production of factors II, VII, IX, and X requires vitamin K. Because vitamin K is a fat-soluble vitamin, it requires adequate production and excretion of bile for its absorption. In addition to protein synthesis, the liver catabolizes proteins as necessary for energy.

The liver is involved in multiple aspects of fat metabolism. Fatty acids that are metabolized by the liver are released from adipose tissue or derived from food. Triglycerides in the diet are absorbed in chylomicrons and metabolized to fatty acids. Fatty acids may be (1) oxidized, (2) metabolized to ketones, (3) converted to phospholipids, (4) used to form cholesterol esters, or (5) reesterified to triglycerides and combined with protein, cholesterol, and phospholipids to form lipoproteins.

Production of Bile Salts

Bile production is one of the major functions of the liver. Bile is a complex compound composed of cholesterol, phospholipids, bile salts, bile pigments (bilirubin), and a very small amount of proteins and electrolytes. Ninety-seven percent of bile is water. Metabolites of drugs and other substances that need to be excreted are also found in bile. Bile salts are necessary for the absorption of fats, cholesterol, and fat-soluble vitamins. Bile is released from the liver and concentrated and stored in the gallbladder. The liver secretes approximately 700 ml of bile daily. The bile salts released during each meal are reabsorbed into the enterohepatic circulation and recycled two or three times during a meal.

Bilirubin Metabolism

Bilirubin is a by-product of the haem portion of red blood cells and is released when red blood cells are destroyed. The bilirubin at this point is not water soluble (*unconjugated/indirect*) and is carried in the blood attached to protein. The liver is responsible for picking up this unconjugated bilirubin, for converting it into a water-soluble form (*conjugated/direct*) and for secreting conjugated bilirubin into the bile. The bilirubin in bile is emptied into the duodenum and is broken down by bacteria into *urobilinogen*. Some of the urobilinogen is excreted with the faeces, giving stool its brown colour; some is eliminated in the urine; and the majority returns to the liver and is recycled.

Detoxification

The liver has a prime role in detoxification of both exogenous and endogenous substances. Ammonia, from protein metabolism or from intestinal production, is one of the major toxic products handled by the liver. Because the liver extracts almost all the ammonia produced in the gut via the enterohepatic circulation and detoxifies this ammonia and the ammonia liberated in the liver itself, peripheral blood levels are kept very low. The ammonia is detoxified by conversion into urea, which is then excreted by the kidneys. The liver also has a major role in the detoxification of many drugs. All barbiturates (except phenobarbitone and barbitone) and many other sedatives are inactivated by the liver. The status of the liver plays an important role in the effectiveness of toxicity of these and other drugs. The liver also serves a function in metabolizing aldosterone, corticosterone, oestrogen, and testosterone steroid hormones.

Storage of Minerals and Vitamins

The liver stores reserves of various minerals and vitamins. This storage prevents abnormal internal levels from occurring, although the intake may be very irregular. Vitamins A, D, and B_{12} are stored in sufficient quantities to prevent deficiencies for months. Vitamins E and K are also stored. Iron in the form of *ferritin* is stored and can be used to resupply iron for haemoglobin formation as needed; copper is stored as well.

Blood Reservoir

The liver, because of its tremendous vascular supply and sinusoidal system, can act as a reservoir for blood. When the venous vascular volume becomes greater than the right side of the heart can handle, blood will accumulate in the liver.

Protection

The Kupffer cells, which line the sinusoids of the liver, are phagocytic cells. These cells are very efficient in removing infective organisms and other foreign substances from the blood as blood flows through the liver. The phagocytic activity of the liver is very important in protecting the body from infections.

Physiological Changes with Ageing

Most of the functions of the liver do not seem to be affected by ageing, even though the weight of the liver lessens and there are identifiable microscopic changes in liver cells. However, enzymes involved in the metabolism of drugs such as anticonvulsants, psychotropics, and oral anticoagulants are decreased.[44] Nurses need to be alert to signs and symptoms of excesses of these and other drugs metabolized by the liver.

PREVENTION AND HEALTH EDUCATION

Primary Prevention

Both hepatitis and cirrhosis, the two major diffuse hepatocellular problems, are preventable. Every nurse has a responsibility to be involved in preventive care in whatever ways possible to promote appropriate health care that reduces the incidence of these diseases as well as others.

Cirrhosis

The term *cirrhosis* refers to several diseases that are characterized by diffuse inflammation and fibrosis resulting in major structural changes and functional loss. Although the incidence of deaths from cirrhosis has decreased for all people, cirrhosis was still the ninth leading cause of death in 1985.[14] Table 22-1 presents the number of deaths attributed to cirrhosis and liver diseases over a 5 year period in Great Britain.

The major cause of cirrhosis is excessive alcohol consumption.[14] Thus, interventions designed to prevent the incidence of cirrhosis must focus primarily on controlling the ingestion of alcohol. Nurses need to work to identify preventive strategies and early interventions for excessive alcohol consumption.

Hepatitis

Hepatitis refers to acute or chronic inflammation of the liver. It may be induced by toxins, including alcohol, viruses, or bacteria. Both toxic and viral hepatitis are preventable.

Toxic hepatitis

Toxic hepatitis may be induced by industrial toxins, household agents, alcohol, and prescription and nonprescription drugs. Toxic hepatitis due to alcohol is called *alcoholic hepatitis*. Nurses can assist in the prevention of toxic hepatitis by teaching the dangers of the injudicious use of materials that are known to be injurious to the liver and by emphasizing the need for a well-balanced

Table 22-1 Deaths caused by chronic liver disease and cirrhosis

	1987	1988	1989	1990	1991
England and Wales	2709	2801	3023	3063	3012
Scotland	401	429	427	490	476
Northern Ireland	58	59	70	70	60
Total	3168	3289	3520	3623	3632

From *International statistical classification of diseases, injuries and causes of death,* Office of Population Censuses and surveys, 1993.

diet with recommended dietary requirements of nutrients and minimal or *no alcohol.* Interventions designed to control ingestion of alcohol should be emphasized.

Some drugs that are known to cause mild liver damage must be used therapeutically. However, the nurse should warn the public about the use of preparations that are available without prescription that may be injurious

Viral hepatitis

The term *viral hepatitis* refers to five distinguishable forms of hepatitis: hepatitis A, B, C[7,9] (previously called *non*-A, *non*-B [parenteral form]), D, and E (previously called *non*-A, *non*-B [nonparenteral form]). Viral hepatitis is the most serious infection of the liver. It is

a notifiable disease in the United Kindom. In 1990, 9005 cases were reported, from Emgland and Wales, to the office of Population Censuses and Surveys. This was an increase of more than 25% compared with 1989.[9a] It is well accepted that the figures for any given year may be grossly underestimated, because people with subclinical manifestations are often not reported as having active disease.

The three major forms of hepatitis are hepatitis A, B, and C. These three forms of hepatitis are the focus of current health initiatives. Information about the viral agents and routes of transmission, along with information about measures to prevent hepatitis, is presented in detail in conjunction with other information about viral hepatitis (see pages 570 to 571).

Secondary Prevention: Detection of Disease

Most of the diseases of the hepatic system result in early signs and symptoms that are vague and nonspecific. Early detection of these signs and symptoms can result in more rapid initiation of effective nursing and medical interventions. Because of their holistic assessment nurses can identify people with life-style patterns that would put them at high risk for hepatic dysfunction, and can encourage and refer people who have vague signs and symptoms to seek additional evaluation as appropriate.

MAJOR HEALTH PROBLEMS OF THE HEPATIC SYSTEM

Disorders of the hepatic system that are encountered in clinical practice include not only those caused by infectious organisms and toxins, but also abnormalities from changes in structure and function. The more common disorders are discussed in this chapter and outlined below.

1. Diffuse hepatocellular disorders
   a. Cirrhosis of the liver
   b. Hepatitis
2. Focal hepatocellular disorders
   a. Liver abscess
   b. Trauma to the liver
   c. Tumours of the liver

The nursing process discussion that concludes this chapter applies to all the above disorders.

DIFFUSE HEPATOCELLULAR DISORDERS

Regardless of the specific pathological condition, disorders secondary to diffuse parenchymal damage result in problems that are common to all these conditions. These problems will be discussed before the specific disorders of cirrhosis and hepatitis are discussed.

Common Manifestations of Diffuse Hepatocellular Disorders

Jaundice

Jaundice is a symptom complex caused by a disturbance of physiology of bilirubin metabolism and the excretion of bile and is present in many hepatic problems as well as in disorders of the pancreatic and biliary systems. Regardless of the course of jaundice, there is an *excess of bilirubin* in the blood that eventually is distributed to the skin, mucous membranes, and other body fluids and tissues, giving them a yellow discoloration. If bilirubin has been processed by the liver (extracted, conjugated, and secreted), it is water soluble and can be excreted in urine, which will be darker than usual. The presence of bilirubin in the skin causes *pruritus (itching)* in about 20% to 25% of the patients who have jaundice. Regardless of the type of jaundice, there will be an *increase in the total serum bilirubin* (normal: 0.1 to 1 mg/dl). Jaundice can usually be detected when bilirubin concentrations exceed 2.5 mg/dl. The changes in concentration of bilirubin and bilirubin metabolites in the serum, urine, or stool help in determining the type of jaundice. Serum bilirubin levels must be combined with other laboratory and diagnostic tests and interpreted in view of the history and clinical findings.

Jaundice can result from haemolysis and obstruction of extrahepatic and intrahepatic biliary ducts. Table 22-2

Table 22-2   Types of jaundice

Category	Pathology	Possible findings
Obstructive		
Intrahepatic	Suppression of bile flow in canaliculi or small biliary ductiles (cholestasis)	Direct* bilirubin elevated; alkaline phosphatase elevated; no enlargement of bile ducts seen on scan or ultrasound
Extrahepatic (biliary tract obstruction)	Obstruction of bile flow in large bile ducts	Direct* bilirubin elevated; alkaline phosphatase elevated; enlargement of bile ducts documented by scan, ultrasound; absence of urobilinogen in urine
Hepatocellular	Hepatocyte injury from toxins (toxic/alcoholic hepatitis), viruses (viral hepatitis) or as part of syndrome of cirrhosis	Transaminases (ALT, AST) elevated 10- to 15-fold; both direct* and indirect† bilirubin may be elevated (direct more than indirect); prolonged prothrombin time
Haemolytic	Excessive amounts of bilirubin are released from RBCs as would be seen in sickle-cell anaemia; liver is unable to excrete bilirubin as rapidly as it forms	Usually mild elevation of total bilirubin (indirect more than direct)

*"Direct" measures conjugated bilirubin.
†"Indirect" measures unconjugated bilirubin.

compares the different causes of jaundice. A common cause of *intrahepatic cholestasis* (stasis of bile within the small biliary canniculi of the liver) is drug reactions such as from phenothiazines. Clay-coloured (greyish-white) stools indicate that bile is not reaching the intestine and suggest *extrahepatic obstruction* (obstruction of hepatic, gallbladder, or common bile duct). An absence of urobilinogen in the urine supports this inference because bile and bilirubin must reach the intestines for the normal formation of urobilinogen, some of which is usually excreted in the urine. Frequent causes of extrahepatic obstruction are gallstones lodged in the common bile duct, pancreatitis, and carcinoma of the head of the pancreas, all of which are discussed in Chapter 24.

In hepatocellular damage, there is interference with uptake, conjugation, and excretion of bilirubin into bile. Excretion is the most profoundly affected process and a predominantly *conjugated hyperbilirubinaemia* is seen. *The level of jaundice does not correlate with the severity of hepatitis; however, in cirrhosis, jaundice suggests a poorer prognosis.*

Bleeding tendencies and anaemia

Bleeding tendencies and anaemia are common complications of hepatic disease. They may occur in people with advanced cirrhosis or hepatitis. These tendencies are a result of deficiencies in the formation of clotting factors, thrombocytopenia, and a deficiency of erythrocytes. In patients with obstructive jaundice and hepatic disease, the synthesis of various clotting factors is impaired. If the patient's bile duct is obstructed, absorption of fat and vitamin K (fat soluble) is reduced. Even if vitamin K is absorbed, severely damaged liver cells may not synthesize adequate amounts of clotting factors, especially prothrombin. Other vitamin deficiencies (A, B complex, D) may also result from decreased absorption of fat-soluble vitamins or the inability to store the vitamins.

The patient with hepatic disease may also develop an enlarged spleen as a result of portal hypertension. This is believed to be a primary factor in thrombocytopenia and increased red blood cell destruction. In addition, alcohol has a direct toxic effect on bone marrow, which can cause thrombocytopenia and anaemia.

Various other factors contribute to the anaemia, including blood loss from gastrointestinal bleeding and decreased red blood cell production secondary to folic acid deficiency and poor protein intake.

Infection

The patient with diffuse hepatocellular disease is at risk for infection. Depressed protein synthesis, lymphatic obstruction of the splanchnic organs, impaired Kupffer cells, and depressed bone marrow all contribute to the increased risk. Leukopenia may be present.

Fluid and electrolyte alterations

Fluid volume deficit results when body losses exceed body gains and should be considered when the following symptoms are seen:

1. Vomiting
2. Anorexia with decreased intake
3. Haemorrhage
4. Diarrhoea

It is important that nurses understand that patients with *hypoalbuminaemia* (serum level below 4 g/dl) may have a contracted intravascular volume, *even in the presence of oedema and ascites.* This phenomenon is seen most often in cirrhosis and results from the decreased production of albumin and the continued loss of this protein into the peritoneal cavity. As a result, the colloidal osmotic pressure of the blood is decreased (leading to increased fluid filtration through the capillary wall) while the return of fluid to the capillary is impaired. The patient is less able to maintain adequate perfusion of tissues should blood volume decrease further.

The sequence of these mechanisms and how they interact to intensify ascites is not well established. A vicious cycle is established as the albumin lost into the peritoneal cavity further decreases the patient's serum albumin levels, resulting in an increase in interstitial fluid. As a result, hydrothorax, and ankle and presacral oedema may accompany the ascites. The patient with cirrhosis frequently is unable to excrete normal amounts of urinary sodium. *Hyponatraemia* is frequent and reflects the disproportional retention of water in comparison to sodium.

Alterations in renal function may occur because of decreased blood volume, portal hypertension, and increased circulating hormones. Decreased excretion of water, sodium, and metabolic wastes is common. Oliguria, azotaemia (nitrogen wastes in the blood), and low urinary sodium (less than 10 mEq/L) may occur abruptly and signal hepatorenal syndrome. Although renal medullary blood flow is maintained in this condition, there is a marked decrease in renal cortical blood flow. Precipitants of hepatorenal syndrome, which has a mortality rate of nearly 90%, are the following:

1. Diuretic therapy
2. Paracentesis
3. Gastrointestinal haemorrhage

CIRRHOSIS OF THE LIVER

Cirrhosis of the liver is the term applied to chronic disease of the liver characterized by diffuse inflammation and fibrosis of the liver that result in drastic structural changes and significant loss of hepatic function. The basic processes leading to cirrhosis are liver cell death with scar tissue formation and regeneration of cell mass that causes distortion of the structure with a resultant change in circulation. Primary prevention of cirrhosis is discussed on p. 564.

Aetiology/Epidemiology

Laënnec's cirrhosis is most frequently caused by chronic alcoholism. Malnutrition associated with other diseases such as pancreatitis and ulcerative colitis may also cause Laënnec's cirrhosis. The major hepatotoxin leading to postnecrotic cirrhosis is viral hepatitis.

Postnecrotic cirrhosis, usually caused by viral hepatitis, is the most common type of cirrhosis on a worldwide basis. More rare nonspecific types of cirrhosis account for about 10% of the deaths resulting from cirrhosis. In England and Wales it is the 14th and 17th leading cause of death for men and women, respectively.

Pathophysiology

Cirrhosis secondary to excessive alcohol consumption and other causes is usually preceded by fatty infiltration of the liver, which is reversible if the causative factor is removed. The fatty infiltration is followed by acute inflammation (alcoholic hepatitis if due to alcohol) and finally cirrhosis, if the degenerative process continues. Fatty liver and alcoholic hepatitis are described on p. 569.

The end result of cirrhosis is loss of normal physiological functions of the liver and obstruction of hepatic portal blood flow. Alterations in physiological functioning are seen late in the disease because the liver has a large reserve capacity and remarkable powers of regeneration.

The fibrosis in the liver resulting from the continual destruction distorts the hepatic structures and obstructs splanchnic veins and portal blood flow. This vascular obstruction can worsen the fluid and electrolyte problems, bleeding, anaemia, and other problems resulting from loss of normal physiological function of the liver. Additionally, this vascular obstruction can cause new problems. The portal hypertension associated with the obstruction of blood flow will cause vascular haemostasis, varicose veins, hemorrhoids, and oesophageal varices.

A variety of signs and symptoms can be seen in people with cirrhosis, regardless of the cause of cirrhosis. Frequently, the patient will have a long history of vague, nonspecific early symptoms such as failing health, nausea, vomiting, anorexia, indigestion, flatulence, and constipation. Malnutrition and the resultant weight loss may not be obvious because of abnormal water retention or because of the calories obtained from alcohol. Abdominal pain may be present and is variable in character. It may be dull, mild, sharp, steady, or wavelike. It may be confined to the right upper quadrant by the liver or referred to the lower abdomen. Late signs and symptoms such as jaundice, ascites, and oedema usually occur together.

Once cirrhosis is established it usually advances slowly to death. However, its progression can often be halted if prescribed therapeutic interventions are followed. Unfortunately, at times rapid deterioration occurs. Continued progression of the cirrhotic process will result in total liver failure, bleeding oesophageal varices, portal-systemic encephalopathy, or renal failure.

Because of the severity of portal hypertension, oesophageal varices, portal-systemic encephalopathy, and hepatorenal syndrome, these four problems will be discussed in more detail.

Portal hypertension

As structural damage occurs and portal circulation is obstructed, portal hypertension occurs. This hypertension results in a back flow of blood into the veins emptying into the portal veins. These veins in turn develop collateral channels of circulation. Collateral channels are most likely to occur in the paraumbilicus veins, the haemorrhoidal veins, and the veins at the cardia of the stomach that extend into the oesophagus. These veins become distended and tortuous because they are not anatomically equipped to handle large volumes of blood. This results in haemorrhoids, oesophageal varices, and a ring of varicosities surrounding the umbilicus (caput medusae). In addition, the spleen enlarges (splenomegaly) and sodium and water retention worsen, causing more oedema. The increased pressure in the portal system results in transudation of albumin and fluid from the vascular compartment of the liver and other organs into the peritoneal cavity, worsening ascites. Lymphatic flow also is obstructed by the increased pressure, and this adds to the ascites.

Bleeding oesophageal varices

Bleeding oesophageal varices (Fig. 22-1) occur frequently in patients with cirrhosis of the liver and portal hypertension. The small vessels of the oesophagus become tortuous and fragile and may be affected by mechanical trauma from ingestion of coarse foods and acid pepsin erosion, which may result in bleeding. Bleeding may also occur as a result

<u>REVIEW</u>
Table 22-3 Diffuse disorders of the liver

Disorder	Signs and symptoms	Medical therapy
Cirrhosis of the liver	Malaise	Rest
	Gastrointestinal symptoms: anorexia, indigestion, nausea, vomiting, flatulence, altered bowel function	Diet: high calorie, normal to high protein (unless ammonia toxicity is present), low fat, vitamin supplement (A, B, C, D)
	Malnutrition: muscle wasting, muscle weakness, possible loss of weight depending on fluid status	Bile salts
Abstinence from alcohol
	Fluid retention: oedema, ascites, abdominal distention, hydrothorax (often on right), weight gain	Sodium and water restriction
Furosemide, spironolactone
Albumin infusion (salt-poor)
Peritoneal-jugular shunt (PJS)
	Jaundice: pruritus, hypoprothrombinaemia, steatorrhoea, light-coloured stools, dark urine	Paracentesis
Antihistamines
	Hepatomegaly, splenomegaly	
	Increased oestrogen: palmar erythema, gynaecomastia, spider angiomas, sparse body hair, testicular atrophy	
	Portal hypertension: caput medusae, haemorrhoids, oesophageal varices, oedema of lower extremities	Surgical procedures that shunt blood away from liver
	Gastrointestinal bleeding	Fresh blood transfusion, plasma expanders, normal saline (IV)
	Oesophageal varices	Saline lavage
Vasopressin or other pharmacological therapy
Injection of sclerosing agents
Oesophageal tamponade
Other therapy as described in text
	Bleeding tendencies, purpura, haematuria, gingival bleeding, epistaxis, melaena, haematemesis	Vitamin K
Transfusions of whole blood, plasma, platelets
	Anaemia: pallor, fatigue, and decreased RBC, haematocrit and haemoglobin	High protein diet with supplements of vitamins and folic acid
Splenectomy
	Portal-systemic encephalopathy: impaired attention span, impaired concentration, apathy, insomnia, slurred speech, yawning, asterixis, fetor hepaticus, coma, muscular rigidity, hyperreflexia, myoclonus seizures	Protein-free diet
Enemas, cathartics
Lactulose, neomycin
Dialysis, exchange transfusion
Corticosteroids
Amino acid (arginine) or levodopa replacement
	Hepatorenal syndrome: oliguria, azotaemia, blood pressure, oedema, hyponatraemia, neurological changes, anorexia, fatigue, and weakness	Improve hepatic function
Stop nephrotoxic drugs
Maintain haemodynamic status
Dialysis/ultrafiltration
Liver transplantation
Viral hepatitis	**Preicteric stage**
Anorexia, nausea and vomiting, chills and fever, arthralgia, right upper quadrant tenderness, fatigue	Rest
Diet: high calorie, high protein, low fat
Avoidance of toxins
	Icteric stage
Jaundice (yellow sclera and skin), dark urine, light-coloured stools	Vitamin K
Diet as above
Rest
Avoidance of toxins
	Posticteric stage
Fatigue	Rest
Diet as above
Avoidance of toxins

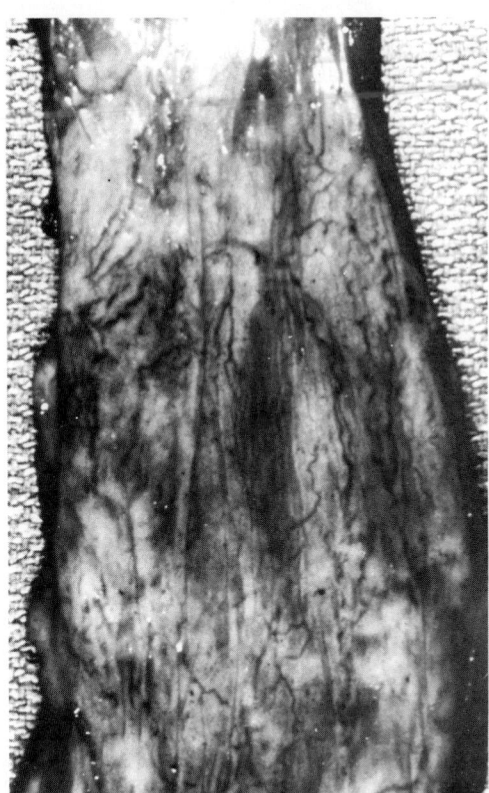

Fig. 22-1   Oesophageal varices. Swollen varices and extensive collateral circulation are evident in segment of oesophagus from patient whith Laënnec's cirrhosis. (From Groer ME, Shekleton ME: *Basic pathophysiology: a conceptual approach,* ed 2, St Louis, 1983, Mosby–Year Book. Courtesy department of pathology, University of Tennessee, Knoxville.)

of coughing, vomiting, sneezing, straining at stool (Valsalva's manoeuvre), or any physical exertion that increases abdominal venous pressure. Bleeding is frequently abrupt and without pain. Severe haematemesis and resultant shock may follow, requiring immediate emergency treatment. Treatment for this complication is summarized in Table 22-4.

Portal systemic encephalopathy

Portal systemic encephalopathy (PSE), formerly called *hepatic coma* or *ammonia toxicity*, is a metabolic encephalopathy associated with liver failure. This dysfunction of the central nervous system is thought to be related to several factors. Many patients with PSE have an increase in blood ammonia concentration. Normally, ammonia, which is formed in the intestines from the breakdown of protein by intestinal bacteria, is converted to urea in the liver. When liver failure occurs the detoxification ability of the liver may be decreased and thus ammonia is not converted into urea and ammonia concentration in the circulating blood is increased. Additionally, in liver failure, ammonia levels may be increased because blood is shunted past the liver. There are many factors that can increase blood ammonia levels.

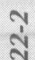

22-2

Common hepatotoxins

Drugs: chlorpromazine, isoniazid, tetracycline, thiazides, paracetamol
Organic solvents: carbon tetrachloride, methylenedianiline (MDA)
Phosphorus, heavy metals
Plant poisons
Alcohol

Hypokalaemia, alkalosis, sedation, and *gastrointestinal bleeding,* as well as other factors, are common precipitants of PSE. Treatment for PSE is started when the earliest signs are detected. The interventions for portal systemic encephalopathy are summarized in Table 22-4.

Hepatorenal syndrome

Hepatorenal syndrome is the sudden onset of renal failure from unknown causes in people with progressive hepatic failure. A major factor is thought to be vasoconstriction of the renal vessels from an increase in renin, decrease in prostaglandins, release of endotoxins, or increase in sympathetic activity. The decreased renal blood flow can result in ischaemic damage and cell death. Oliguria, increased nitrogen waste products, and fluid and electrolyte imbalances occur. The patient will have the fatigue, anorexia, neurological changes, and weakness commonly seen in other causes of renal failure (see Chapter 25). The treatment for this problem is summarized in Table 22-3.

HEPATITIS

Hepatitis may be defined as an acute or chronic inflammatory disease of the liver. Although the term *hepatitis* is most commonly used in conjunction with viral hepatitis, the disease can be caused by toxic injury to the liver, including by alcohol, viruses, or bacteria.

Toxic hepatitis

The primary prevention of toxic hepatitis is discussed on p. 564. Box 22-2 lists some common hepatotoxins. Two types of chemical hepatotoxicity occur: direct toxic and idiosyncratic. In direct toxic hepatitis, the agent causes toxicity with predictable regularity and is dose dependent, such as with paracetamol, tetracycline, alcohol, and carbon tetrachloride. The reactions in idiosyncratic toxic hepatitis are sporadic and not dose dependent, such as with isoniazid and chlorpromazine, which suggests idiosyncrasy in the host.

The pathological changes in the liver will depend on the toxic agent. For example, necrosis and fatty infiltrates are present when the causative agent is carbon tetrachloride, whereas cholestasis with portal inflammation is seen when the toxic agent is chlorpromazine.

Fatty liver and alcoholic hepatitis

The leading cause of hepatic disease in Britain is alcohol.[48] There are two reversible conditions for alcoholic liver damage: *fatty liver* and *alcoholic hepatitis*. In fatty liver, fatty deposits are seen within hepatocytes and the patient may complain of right quadrant tenderness. Hepatomegaly and elevated levels of transaminases are often present.

In alcoholic hepatitis, histological examination reveals deposits of hyalin within hepatocytes, leukocytic infiltration and development of connective tissue surrounding hepatocytes and the central vein. The clinical presentation is varied; it can be asymptomatic or reflect liver failure. Anorexia, nausea, vomiting, weight loss, and abdominal pain are common.

Alcohol has at least two toxic effects on fat metabolism that lead to fatty liver:
1. Increased NADPH generation, which promotes fatty acid synthesis and triglyceride formation
2. Inhibition of the release of triglycerides

In addition, acetaldehyde may be directly toxic to the hepatocytes. Factors that may enhance hepatotoxicity of alcohol include malnutrition, genetic susceptibility, and immune processes.

Viral Hepatitis

Viral hepatitis refers to several clinically similar but aetiologically and epidemiologically distinct infections.

Aetiology/epidemiology

There are currently five types of hepatitis: hepatitis A; hepatitis B; hepatitis C[7,9] (formerly called non-A, non-B hepatitis [parenterally transmitted form]); hepatitis D and hepatitis E[7]. The vast majority of cases of hepatitis that are seen clinically are caused by hepatitis A or hepatitis B viruses. Most cases of all types of hepatitis occur in young adults. Factors such as viral agent, transmission, and high-risk groups vary for the types of hepatitis.

Prevention of incidence or transmission of hepatitis
General preventive measures

The major activity that can assist in the general prevention of viral hepatitis is thorough handwashing by all people. All faeces, urine, blood and other body fluids should be considered potentially infectious for a wide variety of organisms and disposed of properly. Nurses should be involved in the promotion of the development of adequate sewage disposal systems to prevent contamination of food and water supplies that may result in endemic forms of hepatitis A.

Because hepatitis B, hepatitis C, and possibly hepatitis A, as well as carrier states of some types of hepatitis can be spread by contaminated needles and other equipment that comes in contact with infected blood and other body fluids, disposable and nondisposable needles, syringes, and other equipment used in patient care must be handled with great care. *All equipment should be treated as if it had been used on an infected person and handled using universal precautions or body substance precautions (an extension of universal precautions because it focuses on all body substances) no matter who the patient.*

Needles should *not* be recapped. They should be discarded in puncture resistant containers designed for this purpose. Other disposable equipment should also be discarded in appropriate containers; the containers are marked "Contaminated" to alert people handling the rubbish.

Nondisposable equipment should be rinsed, packaged so sharp objects do not accidentally puncture someone, and sterilized by dry heat and steam under pressure (autoclaving), or by gas sterilization. If invasive reusable equipment is used in an environment in which autoclave sterilization is not available and boiling is the only available way to sterilize, the nurse should see that everything placed in the water sterilizer is covered completely and boiled for at least 30 minutes. The nurse should realize that the boiling time needed to destroy hepatitis virus is unknown and that water sterilization of invasive equipment, such as catheters, to be used for another patient is *not* an acceptable method for preventing the transmission of hepatitis.

Preventive measures used with people with known hepatitis

Patients with known hepatitis A should be placed on *enteric precaution* (which is really an extension of universal precautions because it focuses on appropriate handling of contaminated gastrointestinal secretions). Children should be in private rooms, but responsible adults do not require one. Good handwashing after faecal and urine elimination is the major isolation measure. Anyone who must handle faeces or potentially contamined articles (bedpan, nappies, rectal thermometer) should wear gloves and gowns and wash hands thoroughly after completing care. Separate toilet facilities are sometimes used, but this is not necessary if faecal contamination, which might occur in a person who is confused, is not a problem. The toilet should be cleansed thoroughly daily. All disposable and nondisposable equipment and linens should be bagged properly and labelled correctly before being removed from the patient's room.

For patients with hepatitis B, and C, good hand washing and body substance precautions (an extension of universal precautions because it focuses on appropriate handling of *all* body substances) are used any time blood or other body fluids are handled. Gowns and gloves should be worn when the amount of potential contamination with blood or other body fluids is great (such as in the theatre or in intensive care). If splattering of contaminated blood and other body fluids is likely, goggles and a mask are worn. Care must be taken to avoid contact between the blood and other body fluids of an infected person and open cuts, the mucous membranes, or eyes of another person. All invasive equipment such as needles, lancets, and dental drills should be disposed of properly or sterilized properly. All contaminated linens and other items should be bagged and labelled correctly. People who have had viral hepatitis should not be blood donors. The patient with acute hepatitis B and hepatitis C, should not have intimate sexual contact during the period of infection. Protection of household and sexual contacts of people who become hepatitis B carriers is discussed later in this chapter.

Prophylaxis

Prophylaxis can be instituted either before exposure for people at high risk and/or after exposure. The recommendations for prophylaxis vary for the different types of hepatitis and are reevaluated on a continual basis.

Pathophysiology

Viral hepatitis causes diffuse inflammatory infiltration of hepatic tissue. With typical acute viral hepatitis, there is no collapse of lobules, no loss of lobular architecture, and minimal or no fibrosis. Inflammation, degeneration, and regeneration may occur simultaneously, distorting the normal lobular pattern and possibly creating pressure about the portal vein. Laboratory findings include elevations in serum levels of transaminases (ALT and AST), prothrombin time, alkaline phosphatase, and bilirubin. Symptoms may vary in severity; many patients have very mild symptoms and do not have jaundice. Because the pathological process is usually distributed evenly throughout the liver, biopsy in most cases is diagnostic for viral hepatitis.

In most instances of nonfatal viral hepatitis, regeneration begins almost with the onset of the disease. The damaged cells are removed by phagocytosis and enzymatic reaction, and the liver returns to normal.

The outcome of viral hepatitis may be affected by such factors as the following:

1. Virulence of the virus
2. Amount of hepatic damage sustained before exposure to the virus
3. Natural barriers to damage and disease of the liver
4. Supportive care the patient receives when symptoms appear

The majority of patients recover normal liver function, but the disease may take several courses; different terms describe each of these courses (Box 22-3).

Signs and symptoms of the various types of viral hepatitis are not clinically distinctive from each other except that acute symptoms may be more severe in hepatitis A. Serological tests are used to validate the type of viral hepatitis. Symptoms appear before jaundice is apparent. Anorexia is one of the most frequent symptoms. This preicteric stage lasts for approximately 1 week and then subsides as hepatocellular jaundice occurs.

The icteric stage usually reaches its intensity in 2 weeks and may last from 4 to 6 weeks. The *posticteric* or convalescent stage begins with the disappearance of jaundice and may last from a few weeks to several months. Complete recovery is usually expected in 6 months. The disease may relapse during the posticteric stage, with recurrence of previous symptoms but to a milder degree. See Table 22-3 for a summary of the signs and symptoms of viral hepatitis and an overview of the medical therapy.

Chronic Hepatitis

If hepatitis lasts 6 months, it is classified as chronic hepatitis. Viral hepatitis is only one cause, but it is the most common aetiology of chronic hepatitis (drugs, toxins, metabolic liver disease, and autoimmune processes are other causes).

Chronic viral hepatitis

Chronic viral hepatitis is not seen with hepatitis A. *Chronic active hepatitis* is the most serious form of chronic hepatitis. Twenty percent of cases follow HBV infection. There is extension of the necrosis with loss of normal

22-3	**Atypical courses of hepatitis**	
	Submassive hepatic necrosis	Destruction of substantial group of adjacent cells but without destruction of the greater part of a lobule; most patients recover
	Massive hepatic necrosis	Destruction of whole lobule; most patients recover
	Fulminant viral hepatitis	Sudden and severe degeneration of the liver resulting in hepatic failure
	Subacute fatal viral hepatitis	Severe but slower degeneration of the liver

structure and function. Very frequently the disease progresses to cirrhosis. If left untreated, most patients will die within 4 to 5 years; about 75% respond well to corticosteroid treatment.

Chronic persistent hepatitis and *chronic lobular hepatitis* are characterized by abnormal liver function tests, fatigue, and hepatomegaly for greater than 6 months, but there is no necrosis and no increase in mortality.

FOCAL HEPATOCELLULAR DISORDERS

The three most common focal disorders of the liver, their aetiologies, signs and symptoms, and medical therapies are listed in Table 22-4. Each disorder will be discussed briefly.

LIVER ABSCESS

Aetiology/Epidemiology

Liver abscesses may result from a variety of organisms, including *Escherichia coli*, *Staphylococcus*, *Streptococcus*, *Pseudomonas*, *Proteus*, and *Klebsiella*. In patients with depressed immune functioning, such as those with neutropenia or leukaemia, systemic candidiases with multiple hepatic abscesses have been found. Many people with abscesses have multiple bacteria involved.[44] *Entamoeba histolytica* is an important worldwide cause of amoebic liver abscess and dysentery. It most frequently is found in tropical and subtropical regions.

Pathophysiology

Pyogenic abscesses can occur as either a singular large abscess or multiple small and/or microscopic abscesses. Amoebic liver abscesses are typically large and singular.

Liver abscesses are usually a secondary site of infection. Pyogenic organisms originating in various areas of the body reach the liver through the biliary, vascular, or lymphatic systems. In addition, pyogenic organisms may be introduced by penetrating injuries to the liver or by direct contiguous extension. In amoebic abscesses, the vegetative form of the organism moves from the gut to the small portal vessels and into the hepatic tissue, where it becomes activated and causes tissue destruction and abscess formation.

Table 22-4 Focal disorders of the liver

Disorder	Signs and symptoms	Therapy
Liver abscess	Fever, chills Vague abdominal discomfort, tenderness over liver, palpable liver Jaundice, leucocytosis ↑ Serum alkaline phosphatase ↑ ALT, AST	Surgical incision and drainage and broad spectrum antimicrobial therapy for pyogenic abscess Amoebic abscess: chloroquine, metronidazole
Trauma to liver	Variable signs: pain, shock, abdominal rigidity Blood and bile with peritoneal tap	Drainage Suture and drainage Resection Blood volume management Antimicrobial therapy
Carcinoma of liver	Weight loss, weakness Jaundice, anaemia Ascites, oedema Upper right quadrant pain, hepatomegaly Unexplained fever Elevated liver enzymes (ALT, AST) Elevated sedimentation rate Elevated AFP	Surgical excision Chemotherapy: methotrexate, fluorouracil, doxorubicin, mitomycin C; often administered by hepatic artery perfusion Homotransplantation Decompression of biliary tract Palliative radiation

The abscess formation may disrupt hepatic function, but most of the altered physiological functioning is caused by the presence of an acute infective process. If liver abscesses are not identified, they continue to increase in size and can perforate into the pleural cavity, the peritoneal cavity, or the pericardial cavity. The clinical manifestations of liver abscess are often nonspecific and are related to the infectious process. Patients present with tenderness of the right upper quadrant, hepatomegaly, and persistent fever; 20% to 40% show pleural involvement (effusion, pain on breathing, cough, crackles). The mortality rate for untreated liver abscess is 100%. Complications include sepsis, peritonitis from rupture of abscess, and respiratory complications (emboli, infection). See Table 22-4 for a summary of signs and symptoms of liver abscesses and the proposed medical therapy.

TRAUMA TO THE LIVER

Aetiology/Epidemiology

Because of its location and size, the liver is frequently subjected to trauma, which may be either penetrating (gunshot wounds, stab wounds) or blunt (collision with steering wheel during road traffic accidents, falls). If the injury is severe, rupture of the liver may occur with severe internal haemorrhage.

Pathophysiology

The pathophysiology seen varies with the types of injury. Liver injuries are graded on a scale of one to five.[37] In grade one there is laceration and capsular tear with minimal damage to the parenchyma. In grades two through five

there is increasing parenchymal damage with fracture of the liver. In grade five, the damage extends into the retrohepatic vasculature. The liver is a highly vascular organ, and severe haemorrhage that results in hypovolaemic shock may occur. Stab wounds often make a relatively superficial incision and may do no more damage than a needle biopsy of the liver. Gunshot wounds and blunt trauma often result in significant haemorrhage that results in hypotension or shock and leakage of bile from the biliary canaliculi. Hypovolaemic shock may occur. If the peritoneal cavity has been contaminated by blood or bile, *peritonitis* (abdominal tenderness, rebound tenderness, muscle rigidity or spasm, decreased bowel sounds, increased white blood cell level, and fever) occurs. Less severe blunt trauma may result in subcapsular haematoma only.

Late complications of liver trauma may include the following:

1. Severe haemorrhage, resulting from disseminated intravascular coagulation that often accompanies shock during the total course of treatment
2. Degeneration and sloughing of segments of the liver that have had disruption in circulation with resultant haemorrhage
3. Intrahepatic abscess formation
4. Traumatic hepatic cyst formation
5. Infections of other areas of the body following hepatic trauma
6. Subphrenic abscess formation
7. Biliary fistulas

The mortality rate for liver trauma has decreased over the years. The mortality rate depends on type of injury (highest for blunt trauma because of the larger portion of liver damaged and because of other associated injuries), severity of the injury (highest for those requiring resection of a large amount of liver), and the presence of associated injuries (increasing mortality with each additional injury to another organ). See Table 22-4 for an overview of signs and symptoms of and medical therapy for trauma of the liver.

TUMOURS OF THE LIVER

Aetiology/Epidemiology

Tumours of the liver may be either malignant or benign. Benign lesions include haemangiomas, cysts, and, rarely, adenomas. These benign tumours occasionally enlarge enough to become symptomatic and present problems in differentiation from a malignant tumour. Malignant tumours may be metastatic or primary. *Metastatic tumours* are common; they occur 20 times more frequently than primary tumours and rank second to cirrhosis as a cause of fatal liver disease.

Primary hepatic carcinomas may arise within the liver (hepatocellular) or the bile duct cell (cholangiocellular) or may be of mixed origin. Hepatocellular tumours are the most common, but primary liver cancer accounts for only 1% to 2% of malignant tumours found at death in Britain. They are more common in men and usually occur in the fifth and sixth decades of life.[50]

Pathophysiology

The liver most commonly receives metastatic cells from tumours in the gastrointestinal tract, the lungs, the breast, the kidney, and melanomas of the skin. See Table 22-4 for common signs and symptoms of metastatic lesions of the liver. Metastatic carcinoma of the liver varies from a few small nodules to large nodes. Adjacent nodes may eventually grow together and compress the surrounding liver tissue. Usually different parts of the liver are uniformly involved so that liver biopsy may be a useful diagnostic aid.

Primary lesions may be multiple or singular, diffuse or nodular, and may spread to only a lobe or to the entire liver. The cancerous cells appear to compress the surrounding normal liver cells and to spread quickly by invading the portal vein branches. Spread may be by direct extension to surrounding tissue. Primary cancers also tend to cause haemorrhage and necrosis. The most common site for metastasis of the primary liver lesion is the lung, but it may metastasize elsewhere. Primary lesions tend to grow rapidly, sometimes without signs or symptoms, and the patient may live only a short time after onset.

Jaundice and ascites are signs that the metastatic or primary process is quite far advanced. Extreme weakness is also usually an outstanding symptom. Ascites occurs secondary to compression of the portal vein. Gastrointestinal bleeding may also be present and may confuse the diagnosis. A special blood test that may be used to help diagnose primary liver carcinoma is a high serum concentration of alpha-fetoprotein (AFP). AFP in concentrations of 500 mg/ml is found in 70% of patients with hepatocellular cancer. (Lower levels may be found in patients with metastatic carcinoma or viral hepatitis.)

Nursing Process

Assessment

Subjective data

The patient's description of complaints or symptoms and course of illness yields useful data for the nurse who is planning care for the patient with hepatic disease. Among the potential symptoms, the following are explored:

1. Level of fatigue and amount of rest needed
2. Extent of pruritus and measures used to relieve it
3. Severity of anorexia; food intake patterns and likes and dislikes
4. Nausea or vomiting
5. History of oedema or ascites
6. Changes noted in mood, alertness, and mental ability
7. Pain: onset, location, measures used to relieve it
8. Episodes of bleeding, lightheadedness, or syncope
9. Known allergies or toxic agents

When viral hepatitis is a potential medical diagnosis, the past history often contributes clues as to the time and type of contact (blood or sera, polluted water, food, shellfish, and so on). The past history is also vital in determining the injurious agent in toxic hepatitis. The patient's description of the course of illness in chronic hepatitis or cirrhosis can be helpful in giving the nurse insight into the patient's understanding of the disease, its prognosis, and whether the patient believes there is control over its progress.

When alcohol ingestion is a factor, data from the patient should include the patient's knowledge of the effect of the alcohol and the person's desire to abstain from drinking.

Objective data

A thorough physical assessment is required on admission to obtain data for baseline comparisons. There is a possibility that any of the manifestations listed in Box 22-4 will be present in a patient with a hepatic disease; in the patient with cirrhosis, these manifestations will be chronic

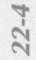

22-4	Common manifestations of liver disease
	Ascites and oedema
	Bleeding tendencies
	Oesophageal varices with gastrointestinal bleeding
	Malnutrition
	Jaundice
	Portal-systemic encephalopathy (hepatic coma)

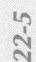

22-5	Parameters of mental functioning
	Attention span
	Ability to concentrate
	Presence of irritability, apathy, or restlessness
	Writing patterns
	Speech patterns
	Level of consciousness

in nature and subject to progressive worsening.

The patient with hepatic dysfunction can deteriorate rapidly, and many factors can depress hepatic function. It is helpful to have the same nurse responsible for the care of the patient and for documenting changes in mental functioning that can occur as hepatic dysfunction worsens (see Box 22-5).

Asterixis (liver flap) is a characteristic sign elicited by asking the patient to dorsiflex the wrist while the arm is extended. The patient's hand has a peculiar flapping tremor. *Fetor hepaticus* is a sweet but fetid breath odour. Asterixis, fetor hepaticus, and decreasing consciousness indicate progressing portal-systemic encephalopathy.

Ascites and peripheral oedema are monitored by daily measurements of the abdomen and extremities. All patients with abdominal wounds or bleeding tendencies are monitored for signs of internal haemorrhage (shock). The liver may be examined while the abdomen is examined. The abdomen is first observed for the following signs:

1. Striae caused by stretching of skin with ascites
2. Engorged veins caused by obstruction of portal flow
3. Abdominal distention caused by ascites

Auscultation of the abdomen for bowel sounds is done before percussion or palpation. Percussion is used to assess the size of the liver as well as for ascites.

Percussion is used to check for the presence of *shifting dullness*. Ascites causes dullness and bulging of flanks when the patient is supine (Fig. 22-2); tympany may be found centrally. If the patient is turned to the side, the bulging and dullness is shifted to the dependent side.

While the patient is lying supine, the abdomen can be examined for presence of a *fluid wave*.

The liver may also be palpated by deep palpation. The liver edge, if palpable, presents a firm, sharp, regular ridge with a smooth surface. It is considered abnormal when felt more than 1 cm below the costal margin.

When caring for the patient with hepatic disease, the nurse should make ongoing observations about each of the following:

1. Body weight
2. Vital signs
3. Intake and output
4. General appearance: muscle mass, nutritional status, colour of skin and sclera
5. Mental status
6. Breath sounds and respiratory effort
7. Abdomen, including abdominal girth
8. Skin: colour, presence of spider angiomas, bleeding sites, excoriations, palmar erythema
9. Extremities: oedema
10. Colour of urine and stools

Diagnostic tests

Multiple tests may be necessary to determine the extent and seriousness of hepatic disease. Additional studies may include abdominal films, barium swallow and enema, and endoscopic examinations. The diagnostic workup will frequently include one or several tests for examination of the biliary tract (see Chapter 24).

Liver biopsy

Biopsy of the liver presents the risk of haemorrhage because of the vascularity of the liver and the bleeding tendencies that often occur with liver disease. The procedure may be open or closed. The open procedure is done in the theatre, and the usual preoperative procedure is required.

The closed procedure is often done at the patient's bedside. This procedure is contraindicated if the patient has an infection of the right lower lobe of the lung, ascites, or a blood dyscrasia, or is unable to cooperate by holding a breath. The procedure consists of inserting a specially designed needle through the chest or abdominal wall into the liver and removing a small piece of tissue for study. Movement by the patient may tear the liver covering. Although no physical preparation is necessary for a closed procedure, written consent is usually required, a current haematological and coagulation profile should be available, and food and fluids may be withheld after midnight the night before. Importantly, the patient needs teaching, time to have questions answered, and support.

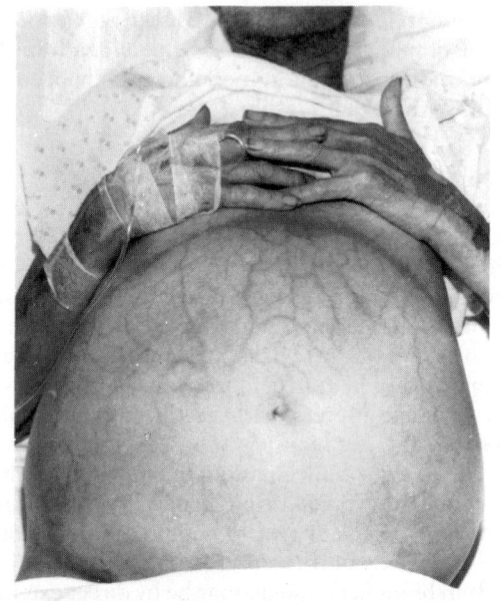

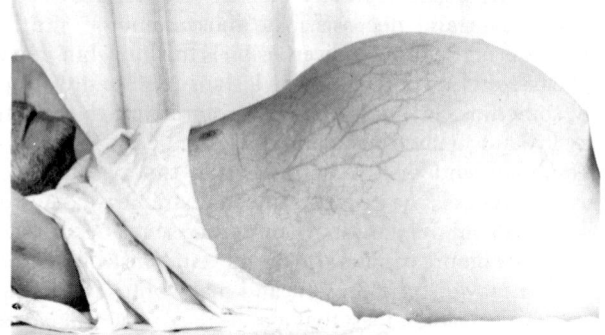

Fig. 22-2   Massive ascites. Note bulging flanks, dilated upper abdominal veins, and everted umbilicus. (From Prior JA, Silberstein JS, Stang JM: *Physical diagnosis: the history and examination of the patient,* ed 6, St Louis, 1981, Mosby–Year Book.)

Nursing analysis

Nursing analyses are determined from assessment of patient data. Possible nursing problems for the person with diseases of the liver may include, but are not limited to, the following:

Problem	Possible aetiologies
Fatigue	Generalized weakness, imbalance between supply and demand of energy
Fluid volume excess or deficit	Compromised regulatory mechanisms, inappropriate fluid and sodium intake
Infection, high risk for	Decreased immune response, pruritus, skin lacerations, intrusive procedures, inadequate measures to prevent transmission of infection
Injury: high risk for: falls	Sensory/perceptual deficits, tremors, weakness, impaired cognition
Cardiac output, decreased (potential)	Potential for haemorrhage, potential for fluid deficit in response to diuretic therapy
Nutrition, altered: less than body requirements	Anorexia, inadequate intake, increased metabolic needs
Pain	Jaundice and pruritus, ascites
Breathing pattern, ineffective	Ascites, coma
Knowledge deficit: diagnostic tests, treatment, home care, follow-up care	Lack of exposure, potential cognitive limitations
Health maintenance, altered	Inability to make appropriate judgements because of excessive alcohol consumption

Planning: expected patient outcomes

Expected patient outcomes for the person with hepatic dysfunction may include, but are not limited to, the following:

1. Demonstrates an increase in self-care ability each day.
2. Develops no undetected oliguria; does not exceed 1 kg loss of body weight per day.
3. Develops no new infections; temperature remains at a normal level.
4. Does not fall or suffer any injury.
5. Does not develop undetected bleeding and/or hypotension.
6. Eats diet high in calories and carbohydrates, with adequate vitamins, minerals, and protein as appropriate for pathophysiological state.
7. States that itching is reduced and has no skin lacerations.
8. Normal breath sounds and a normal chest X-ray examination are present.
9. Explains the disorder and relationships to relevant symptoms and treatment.
10. Describes plans for self-care (activity, rest, sleep)
11. Gives detailed description about ways to manage diuretic therapy, water restriction, diet prescription, and avoidance of alcohol.
12. Describes signs and symptoms to report to doctor.
13. If alcohol abuse is a problem, is able to make conscious decision about the use of services such as Alcoholics Anonymous.

Implementation

The patient with hepatic disease should be considered to have multisystem disorders and to be at risk for fluid and electrolyte imbalances, infection, alteration in mental status, and haemorrhage. Thus, regardless of the specific medical or nursing analysis or severity of distress, the nurse should institute a monitoring schedule that ensures early detection of these clinical findings.

The frequency of monitoring depends on the current status of the patient, the medical and nursing analysis, and the estimation of risk. For example, the patient who is actively bleeding from liver trauma or oesophageal varices requires continuous monitoring in an intensive care unit. In contrast, the patient who has bleeding tendencies because of a mild increase in prothrombin time may be monitored by routine vital signs, daily guaiac tests for occult blood in the stool, and daily prothrombin time, partial thromboplastin time, and haematocrit. Institution of new therapeutic agents, a change in therapy (dosage of medication, amount of food, or fluid intake), or the onset of complications necessitates review of the monitoring plan to assess its adequacy.

Assisting with achievement of therapeutic goals

Rest, nutrition, and absence of toxin use are principal treatments for patients with hepatic disorders. Before the nurse's role in implementing these treatments is discussed, this section will discuss other treatments for specific hepatic lesions or dysfunctions.

Medications

The drugs to be described are antimicrobial and chemotherapeutic agents. Diuretics and drugs used to treat bleeding will be discussed later.

Antibiotics. The nurse will be involved in the administration of antibiotics to patients with bacterial infections of the liver (liver abscess, wound infections). The specific antibiotic therapy is based on culture and sensitivity studies of material obtained by percutaneous or surgical aspirations of the abscess or on studies of wound drainage. Blood cultures are usually done to determine if septicaemia is present. Anaerobic organisms alone or in combination with aerobic organisms account for 50% of liver abscesses; common organisms are *Escherichia coli*, *Klebsiella*, and *Staphylococcus aureus*. Appropriate broad-spectrum antibiotics may be administered for 4 to 6 weeks to a patient with pyogenic liver abscess. Surgical drainage of the abscess is also frequently necessary. See Chapter 12 for details about administration of antibiotics.

Because patients with liver dysfunction may be immunosuppressed, they are subject to a variety of infections including superinfections and nosocomial infections. Therefore, the nurse may be involved in the administration of antibiotics to patients with liver disease who have infections of the urinary tract, pneumonia, peritonitis, or other infections. There is no antibiotic therapy for hepatitis. The patient with amoebic abscess is treated with amoebicidal agents. Usually surgery is not done.

Chemotherapy. Chemotherapy is used to induce regression of primary and metastatic lesions of the liver; it also may be part of other therapy such as radiation or surgery.

Fluorouracil (FU) and doxorubicin (Adriamycin) have been used as single-drug therapy. Combination chemotherapy with FU and carmustine, lomustine, or streptozotocin have also been tried. Chemotherapeutic agents have been given intravenously or by infusion into the hepatic artery.

Hepatic arterial infusion can be accomplished by one of two methods. In the first method, a percutaneous catheter is inserted into the hepatic artery using fluoroscopy. The catheter is attached to an external infusion pump that is filled with the appropriate chemotherapeutic agent and programmed to deliver the agent over a desired period of time. The catheter is removed after each drug treatment cycle. In the second method, a catheter is surgically inserted into the hepatic artery and connected to an implanted infusion pump.

The implanted pump can be filled with the correct amount of drug and programmed to deliver the chemotherapeutic agent over a desired time interval and at a desired dosage. In chemotherapy-free intervals the pump is filled with a heparin solution, so that patency of the hepatic artery catheter is maintained. Depending on flow rates and drug schedule, the chamber is refilled at various intervals that are scheduled so that the chamber never empties completely.

The implanted infusion pump allows the patient to be treated at home. The patient comes into an outpatient site at prescribed times for addition of drugs or heparin solution and a recheck of pump flow rate. The patient will need physical care before and after surgery similar to that of any patient having surgery (Chapter 14). Instructions regarding self-care and needs related to the chemotherapeutic agent being used (see Chapter 9 and a pharmacology text) are also needed. The nurse will also be involved in refilling the pump at the prescribed intervals.

Reduction of oedema and ascites

Oedema and ascites are typically found in patients with cirrhosis; however, they may occur in any patient whose hepatic dysfunction results in (1) hypoalbuminaemia; (2) dilutional hyponatraemia; and (3) portal hypertension. Under these circumstances, diuresis occurs slowly and is more difficult to accomplish than it would be in a patient with a normal serum colloidal osmotic pressure, a normal serum sodium-to-water ratio, and relatively similar hydrostatic pressures in portal and systemic venous circulations.

Sodium restriction and bed rest are usually the first approach to reducing oedema. These measures and an adequate diet often result in a spontaneous diuresis that reflects improved hepatic function. The amount of sodium restriction may be based on 24-hour urinary excretion of sodium but is generally not less than 1 g daily. The lack of salt in food makes it less palatable, and the patient may not consume adequate protein and calories. Inadequate intake is reported to the doctor and dietition because adjustments

may need to be made in sodium restriction. Salt substitutes may be permitted.

A second intervention that may be used, if hyponatraemia is present, is fluid restriction. Fluids may be restricted to as little as 500 ml/day and will usually not exceed 1500 ml/day. The fluid restriction may affect the patient's food intake. The patient is encouraged to assist in planning the distribution of fluid intake. It is not unusual for fluid and sodium to be restricted and bed rest continued when diuretic therapy is ordered.

Nursing assessments to monitor fluid and electrolyte balance in patients with oedema or ascites are listed in Box 22-6. These assessment measures enable the nurse to detect the onset of hypokalaemia, oliguria, azotaemia, and PSE (all of which are complications of diuresis in patients with hepatic dysfunction and are related to excessive fluid and potassium losses).

Ascites cannot be mobilized at rates greater than 900 ml/day (approximately 900g/day of weight loss).[36] Hypovolaemia can occur if amounts greater than this are diuresed (unless peripheral oedema is contributing the additional fluid). Azotaemia and oliguria result from decreased renal perfusion in hypovolaemic states. PSE may be precipitated by azotaemia, hypovolaemia, and hypokalaemia.

Diuretic therapy. Frusemide alone or with spironolactone is commonly used to promote diuresis in people with hepatic dysfunction who do not respond to sodium restriction and bedrest. Spironolactone provides the benefit of retention of potassium along with the excretion of sodium.

Potassium supplements are often prescribed along with the frusemide and, at times, may be necessary for the patient treated with spironolactone. The nurse should monitor the patient's potassium level and be alert for signs of potassium imbalance (see Chapter 6). Magnesium levels also need to be monitored carefully. Magnesium may be low because of a poor nutritional history, and diuretics will worsen the loss of magnesium. However, if hepatorenal failure is present, both potassium and magnesium may be high.

Infusions of salt-poor albumin in 25-g units may be given to increase the effectiveness of diuretic measures. These infusions expand the blood volume, thus increasing renal blood flow and serum osmotic pressure. They may also decrease the risk of oliguria, azotaemia, and encephalopathy. The effects are short term and protein loss into the ascitic fluid continues. Albumin is very viscous and must be infused with a large-bore needle, such as a No. 18. It is often used to improve the patient status during acute crises or to prepare the patient for surgery. The administration of

22-6	**Assessment for patients with oedema or ascites**
	Daily weights Intake and output Measurement of abdominal girth Blood pressure Mental status Serum electrolytes

salt-poor albumin may expand the blood volume rapidly. During and following administration, the patient is monitored carefully for signs of pulmonary oedema.

Paracentesis. A peritoneal tap may be done to obtain fluid for laboratory study but paracentesis places the patient at risk for complications such as shock, hypovolaemia, azotaemia, encephalopathy, and infection. Although once a standard mode of therapy, paracentesis is now used with caution and usually only as a last resort in patients with severe and chronic liver disease.

If the abdomen is taut with fluid and is producing dyspnoea and anorexia, paracentesis may be necessary. In general, only enough fluid to relieve symptoms is removed; this decreases the risk of rapid fluid shifts and additional protein loss. One litre of ascitic fluid contains as much protein as 200 ml of whole blood. Salt-poor human albumin may be administered following this procedure to counteract the shift of fluid and protein into the peritoneal cavity. When paracentesis is done, the patient must be monitored for signs and symptoms of all complications. Monitoring would include blood pressure, pulse, temperature, skin colour and temperature, urine output, mental status, and abdomen (for signs of peritonitis).

Peritoneal venous shunt. In chronic and resistant ascites caused by cirrhosis, a LeVeen peritoneal venous shunt may be used. The shunt allows for the continuous reinfusion of ascitic fluid back into the venous system through a silicone catheter with a one-way pressure sensitive valve. One end of the catheter is implanted in the peritoneal cavity, and the tube is channelled through subcutaneous tissue to the superior vena cava where the other end is implanted. The valve opens when there is a pressure differential greater than 3 mm of water between the abdominal cavity and the thoracic vein, allowing fluid to move from the peritoneal cavity into the superior vena cava.

People treated with a shunt may also receive frusemide therapy, and the two together have been successful in relieving ascites in some patients. People who have a shunt may still have severe problems, including disseminated intravascular coagulation, bleeding varices, and congestive failure.[5]

When shunts are first implanted and functioning, there can be dramatic changes such as haemodilution of intravascular fluid, decreased abdominal girth, and increased renal output. The rapid addition of ascitic fluid back to the vascular compartment can result in fluid overload with signs and symptoms of pulmonary oedema. As peritoneal fluid is removed, less of a pressure gradient exists between the peritoneal fluid and the jugular vein. To force the valve open, deep breathing is encouraged at regular intervals with the patient in the supine position.

Control of bleeding

Bleeding tendencies or actual haemorrhage is common in patients with hepatic disorders. See p. 566 for the specific factors that may decrease coagulation ability in hepatocellular or biliary tract disease. Also, see p. 567 for the reason that dilated haemorrhoidal, gastric, and oesophageal veins are frequent sites of bleeding when portal hypertension is present.

Gastrointestinal bleeding is not uncommon in patients with jaundice and/or portal hypertension. Patients with cirrhosis or recent alcohol intake may have bleeding from gastritis or peptic ulcers, as well as from haemorrhoidal or oesophageal venous rupture.

Bleeding may also be prolonged in tissue injury and in surgical wounds. Assessment measures for bleeding and measures to minimize bleeding are presented in Boxes 22-7 and 22-8.

The nurse assists with specific medical therapies to improve the status of coagulation. A trial of vitamin K (usually daily for 3 days) may be ordered to determine whether the liver is able to manufacture prothrombin and other clotting factors when an adequate supply of vitamin

---

22-7

Assessment for bleeding

Check the following for blood:
  Urine, stool, vomitus, or gastrointestinal drainage
Assess the following for bleeding:
  Mouth
  Wounds
  Skin (for purpura, haematoma, or petechiae)
Monitor vital signs for the following:
  Hypotension
  Postural hypotension
  Tachycardia
Monitor results of the following:
  Prothrombin or partial thromboplastin times
  Platelet count
  Haematocrit level in concert with assessment of sodium and fluid status

---

22-8

Measures to minimize bleeding

1. Arrange with the laboratory to minimize number of venepunctures.
2. Start IV infusions when blood samples are drawn.
3. Apply pressure for 5 minutes to sites of veniepunctures or injections, for 10 minutes to sites of arterial puncture.
4. Suggest patient use a soft toothbrush or cotton swab for brushing of teeth to prevent bleeding gums.
5. Serve the patient with oesophageal varices only soft foods (for example, bread rather than toast).
6. Avoid taking temperatures rectally, and use gentle pressure and well-lubricated enema tips if haemorrhoids are present.
7. If injection must be given, use the smallest-gauge needle possible.
8. Instruct patient not to strain at stool and to avoid vigorous coughing or blowing of the nose.
9. Avoid clutter in patient's room and give adequate assistance in ambulating to prevent falls.

K is given. Recall that shunting of blood around the liver or the absence of bile or bacteria in the intestine reduces the supply of vitamin K available to the liver. Vitamin K will not help if hepatic cell damage is the cause of reduced prothrombin formation. If this is the case, whole blood or plasma may be given to replace clotting factors at least temporarily. If the patient has a reduced platelet level, platelet transfusions may be given.

Table 22-3 lists some of the treatment measures used with bleeding oesophageal varices. This haemorrhage is often massive and life-threatening; mortality rates are 30% to 60%.

Shunts and nonshunting operations

The first priority in the management of bleeding is to establish the source of bleeding. After diagnosis the goal is to control bleeding and to replace the blood volume. Bleeding may be controlled with:
1. Gastric lavage (see Chapter 23 for discussion of this procedure)
2. Pharmacological therapy
3. Injection sclerotherapy
4. Balloon tamponade of varices
5. Endoscopic oesophageal varix ligation (banding)
6. Surgery: shunts and nonshunting operations

Pharmacological therapy. Vasopressin is usually given intravenously (may be given into the mesenteric artery) at a dose of 0.2 µ to 0.8 µ/minute on an intermittent basis or as a continuous infusion. It lowers portal pressure by causing splanchnic vasoconstriction and thus can stop or control oesophageal bleeding. Side effects, which the nurse will monitor for and report immediately, include hypertension, bradycardia, abdominal cramping and pallor. Coronary artery vasoconstriction as well as mesenteric artery vasoconstriction can occur; thus vasopressin must be used with caution in people with coronary artery disease and in the elderly.[5,18] Glyceryl trinitrate (transdermal, sublingual, or intravenous) has been combined with vasopressin to decrease the systemic vasoconstriction, including coronary vasoconstriction, while maintaining the decrease in portal pressure. The combination therapy has been effective in controlling bleeding while decreasing side-effects. With vasopressin water retention can also occur. Careful monitoring of blood pressure, pulse, fluid status, and for recurrence of bleeding must be carried out while the therapy is withdrawn. Argipressin, an analogue of vasopressin, given intravenously has been shown to be effective with fewer cardiac effects in preliminary studies.

Injection sclerotherapy. For emergency treatment of varices and longer-term control or for control and prevention of rebleeding in patients who may not be candidates for surgery, injection sclerotherapy may be used. In this procedure a fibreoptic endoscope is introduced into the oesophagus by the doctor; and, once the bleeding site is identified, a sclerosing agent is injected into the varices. This agent causes thromboses and sclerosis of the vessel and should result in haemostasis in 3 to 5 minutes. If haemostasis does not occur, a second injection may be given. The procedure may be repeated as necessary and can be initiated while the patient is bleeding or as an elective procedure. Before the procedure the patient and significant others need an explanation of the procedure, and the patient should receive nothing by mouth for at least 6 hours. A mild sedative and a local anaesthetic will be given. After the procedure the nurse will monitor the patient for complications (perforated oesophagus, aspiration pneumonia, pleural effusion, and worsening of ascites). Respiratory support to ensure adequate air exchange must be provided. *Retrosternal pain* is often present and is treated with analgesics; fever is common for several days. The procedure has shown very favourable results in some patients.

Oesophageal tamponade. The original Sengstaken-Blakemore tube is a three-lumen tube with two balloon attachments. One lumen serves as a nasogastric suction tube, the second is used to inflate the gastric balloon, and the third is used to inflate the oesophageal balloon (Fig. 22-3). The addition of a fourth lumen to aspirate hypopharyngeal secretions resulted in a 4-lumen Sengstaken-Blakemore tube.[6a] These two tubes are most frequently used and are the focus of this discussion. Another tube, the Linton tube, has no oesophageal balloon and has a lumen for the aspiration of stomach and lower oesophageal contents; it is less frequently used.[6a] The tube is passed through the nose or mouth into the stomach with the balloons deflated. When the tube is in the stomach, the gastric balloon is inflated with 150 to 250 ml of air or 25% gastrograffin[6a] and the lumen is clamped; the tube is then pulled out slowly until resistance is met. A cube of foam rubber (nasal cuff) is placed between the tube and the nares and secured to the face with pressure-sensitive tape. The nasal cuff absorbs excess nasal secretions and reduces trauma to the nostril, or the tube is taped directly to the side of the mouth. Although only rarely used, a device shaped like a motorbike helmet may be used to provide traction on the tube to keep it in the proper position.

If bleeding continues after the gastric balloon is inflated, the oesophageal balloon, which is connected by a Y tube to a manometer, is inflated to a pressure of 30 to 40 mm Hg and then clamped. To stop the bleeding, the pressure must be greater than the patient's portal venous pressure. If bleeding is from oesophageal varices, blood will no longer be aspirated from the stomach. If there is still blood present, the stomach may be lavaged with room temperature or cold saline.

The nasogastric lumen and the oesophageal lumen are usually connected to suction, which permits easy appraisal of cessation of bleeding and also keeps the stomach and oesophagus empty. It is important to remove all blood from the stomach because the presence of blood may precipitate PSE from ammonia produced from the digested blood. Cathartics, antacids, and neomycin or lactulose may be given through the gastric lumen with suction temporarily discontinued (20 minutes). It is important to remove secretions from the hypopharyngeal space to prevent aspiration.

The oesophageal balloon can be left inflated up to 48 hours without tissue damage or severe discomfort. However, the oesophageal balloon is usually deflated in approximately 12 hours to assess if bleeding has stopped. The fully inflated gastric balloon with or without traction exerted on it can compress the stomach wall between the balloon and

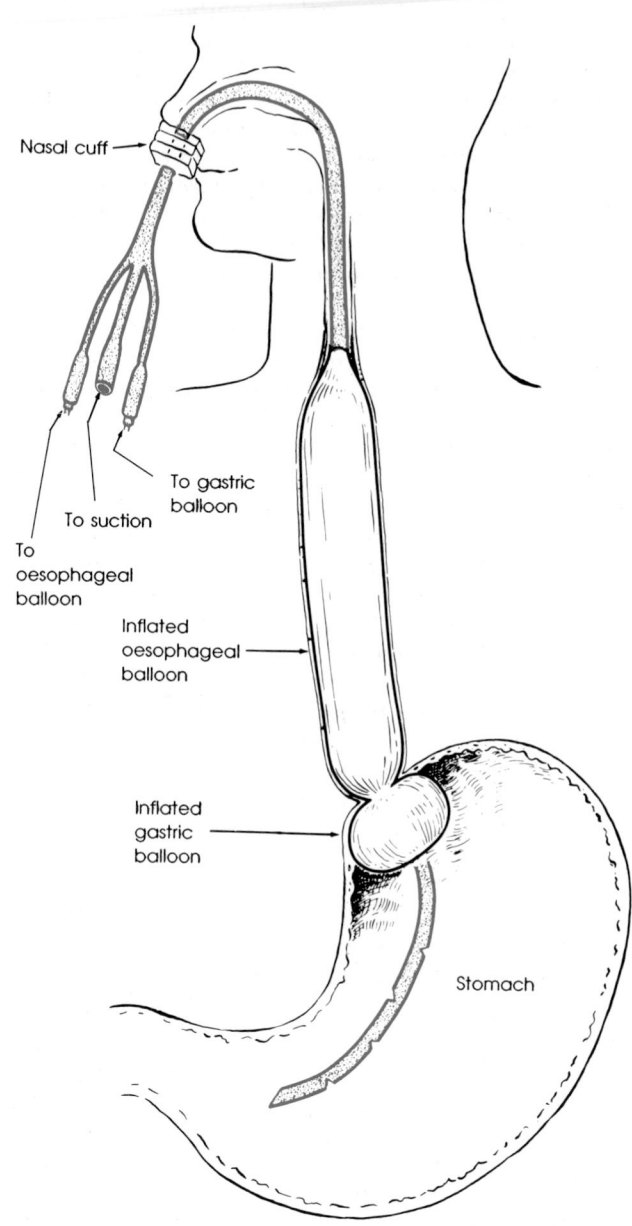

Nasal cuff

To gastric
balloon

To suction

To
oesophageal
balloon

Inflated
oesophageal
balloon

Inflated
gastric
balloon

Stomach

Fig. 22-3   Sengstaken-Blakemore tube with oesophageal and gastric balloons inflated. (Redrawn from *Rubber appliances in surgery and therapeutics*, Providence RI, Davol, Inc.)

the diaphragm causing ulceration of the gastric mucosa and severe discomfort. To offset the possibility of necrosis, the doctor may release the traction and balloon pressures periodically.

The nurse must stay with the patient while balloons are deflated to secure the tube's position and to detect recurrence of bleeding. Intensive monitoring of the patency of the airway also is necessary when the balloons are inflated. *Asphyxiation* is a hazard if the inflated oesophageal balloon moves into the upper airway. This can happen if the gastric balloon deflates or ruptures and the inflated oesophageal balloon moves upward. If this happens, the oesophageal

balloon is deflated at once and the entire tube is removed. A scissors, which can be used to cut the tube and deflate balloons rapidly, must be at the bedside.

The nurse will be assisting with therapeutic measures aimed at restoration of blood volume and coagulation factors and the prevention and treatment of PSE.

Surgery

Focal liver disease. Treatment of liver abscess consists of incision and drainage of the abscess or abscesses and treatment with broad-spectrum antibiotics for pyogenic abscesses. Portal hypertension occurs in rare instances from scarring of the liver as part of the healing process. These patients require close follow-up after discharge from the hospital.

If trauma to the liver has occurred, blood volume replacement is usually required. Emergency surgery may be needed to repair the ruptured liver and local pressure may need to be applied to stop the bleeding. Removal of necrotic tissue may also be indicated, as well as drainage of any bile that may be leaking from the liver surface. The patient may require long-term follow-up to check for signs and symptoms of residual liver damage.

In most instances there is no corrective medical surgical treatment for metastatic or primary carcinoma of the liver because the disease is too far advanced when first diagnosed. Patients are usually alert at this time and will know the prognosis. The patient and family are assisted to live with the prognosis and to do the things they wish to do in the time remaining for the patient (see Chapter 9).

In a few patients with primary tumours, surgery may be possible. If the tumour is limited to a single lobe and there is no evidence of metastases elsewhere, a hepatic lobectomy may be done to remove metastatic as well as primary carcinoma. The remarkable regenerative capacity of the liver permits resection of 70% to 80% of the organ.

Homotransplantation of the liver has been performed in a few medical centres. Rapid advances in technology and pharmacological agents are occurring; however, availability of donor organs and high costs are major limitations.

Hepatic transplantation is done in selected cases of biliary atresia in children and chronic aggressive hepatitis, cirrhosis, and malignancy in adults.

Portalcaval shunts. The only way to achieve permanent lowering of portal pressure is by surgical treatment to reduce blood flow through the portal system. Fig. 22-4, *A* and *B*, shows two different techniques to decompress the portal vein and one technique, *C*, to decompress the oesophageal veins. It must be remembered that the patient with hepatic damage severe enough to cause bleeding oesophageal varices is not a good operative risk.

The mortality rate when surgical shunts are used as immediate intervention for bleeding oesophageal varices is 50%; it is 10% when performed in well-selected patients with portal hypertension who are not actively bleeding. It is generally believed that a prophylactic shunt is not justified. Shunts are recommended only when there has been at least one haemorrhage from oesophageal varices and the patient does not respond to other therapy.

The shunts shown in Fig. 22-4, *A* and *B* create a connection between the high-pressure portal system and the low-pressure vena caval system, thereby decompressing the portal system. A major complication is PSE resulting from less venous blood passing through the liver. Nursing care of the patient having liver surgery is discussed in Box 22-4.

Interventions to achieve patient outcomes

The nursing care directed towards many of the nursing analyses such as fluid volume changes, high risk for infection, high risk for injury, decreased cardiac output, and ineffective breathing pattern are collaborative in nature and were discussed in the preceding section. This section focuses on the other nursing analyses that are more independently cared for.

Promoting optimal balance between rest and activity and assisting with comfort

Hepatic repair and regeneration can be promoted by rest, nutrition, and avoidance of toxins and infection. The liver can best be allowed time for repair and regeneration by decreasing the metabolic demands of activity, of infection, of catabolism, and of the stress response.

The doctor usually prescribes the desired amounts of rest and activity. In hepatitis, serum enzyme levels may indicate necrosis and may serve as a guide (the higher levels indicate a need for more rest and restricted activity). It is believed that activity and maintaining an upright position decrease hepatic blood flow, thus preventing optimal circulation to the already compromised liver. Relapses are frequently attributed to premature increases in activity.

Although the doctor's prescriptions define whether complete bedrest or some ambulation is allowed, the nurse must use judgment in determining activity levels within these limits. The patient with hepatic dysfunction has overwhelming fatigue and benefits from a paced schedule, alternating self-care activities with rest. The schedule should include rest before meals and before family visits. The nurse can use the patient's rating of fatigue and the serum transaminase levels as guide to increases in activity. As patients recover and acute discomfort recedes, patients may need assistance in finding diversional activities that will dispel boredom, yet not be tiring. Boredom and social isolation are particularly difficult for patients who are placed in isolation. Recurrence of anorexia, enlargement or tenderness of the liver, or lack of progress as indicated by laboratory studies indicate a need to return to bed rest.

There are many sources of discomfort for patients with hepatic disorders. The nurse can promote rest by assisting patients to reduce discomfort by direct physical care measures:

1. Assist patients with ascites to shift position frequently. They often require a high supported sitting position for ease in breathing.
2. Provide assistance for acute symptoms of chills, fever, diaphoresis, nausea, vomiting, and diarrhoea.
   a. Apply blankets to provide comfort during chills, yet not so many that temperature is increased.
   b. Use tepid sponge baths to lower temperature and apply cool cloths to the forehead.
   c. Change linens or dressings as frequently as necessary.
   d. Provide clean receptacles for emesis and diarrhoea and remove them promptly.
   e. Provide quiet, cool, and pleasant environment.
3. Provide measures to decrease pruritus:
   a. Use cool, light, and nonrestrictive clothing and dry, soft bed linens.
   b. Avoid extremes of temperature in baths or compresses.
   c. Avoid stimulating perspiration.
   d. Maintain a cool environment.
   e. Administer prescribed antihistamines or cholestyramine.
   f. Use distraction to decrease patient's perception of pruritus.

Assisting with nutrition

Good nutritional intake is necessary for repair and regeneration of the liver. Rest and nutrition are key treatments for hepatitis, alcoholic lesions of the liver, cirrhosis, and during recovery from infections, surgery, or trauma of the liver. The patient with a malignant tumour of the liver also needs a focus on nutrition and rest. The liver's ability to excrete toxins and to carry on its many other functions may be seriously hampered by inadequate intake of protein and vitamin B complex. If hepatic damage has occurred, the organ's ability to store glycogen and vitamins A, B complex, C and D may also be decreased.

Although fat is a concentrated source of calories, most patients with diffuse hepatic disorders but not focal hepatic disorders have some fat intolerance. Oral bile salts may improve the digestion and absorption of fats and fat-soluble vitamins.

A diet high in calories, protein, and vitamins; fairly high in carbohydrates (unless weight reduction is desired); and with moderate amounts of fat is often ordered for patients with diffuse or focal hepatic disease.

However, a high-protein diet may not be possible if there is potential or actual PSE. In this case, protein restriction becomes necessary. If protein needs to be restricted for some time, the doctor may prescribe an enteral or parenteral supplement that has selected BCAAs and a low content of SCAAs.

Because alcohol is thought to interfere with hepatic conversion of folic acid to its active metabolites, many people with cirrhosis have a folic acid deficiency anaemia that usually responds well to treatment with oral doses of folic acid. Other nutritional anaemias requiring nutritional supplements include vitamin B_{12} and iron deficiency anaemias (see Chapter 19).

Anorexia and fatigue interfere with adequate food intake. Although large amounts of food may be prescribed, it is exceedingly difficult for patients to eat these amounts. The person with diffuse or focal liver disease is often anorexic, and it can become a challenge for the nurse to identify ways to encourage the person to eat the prescribed

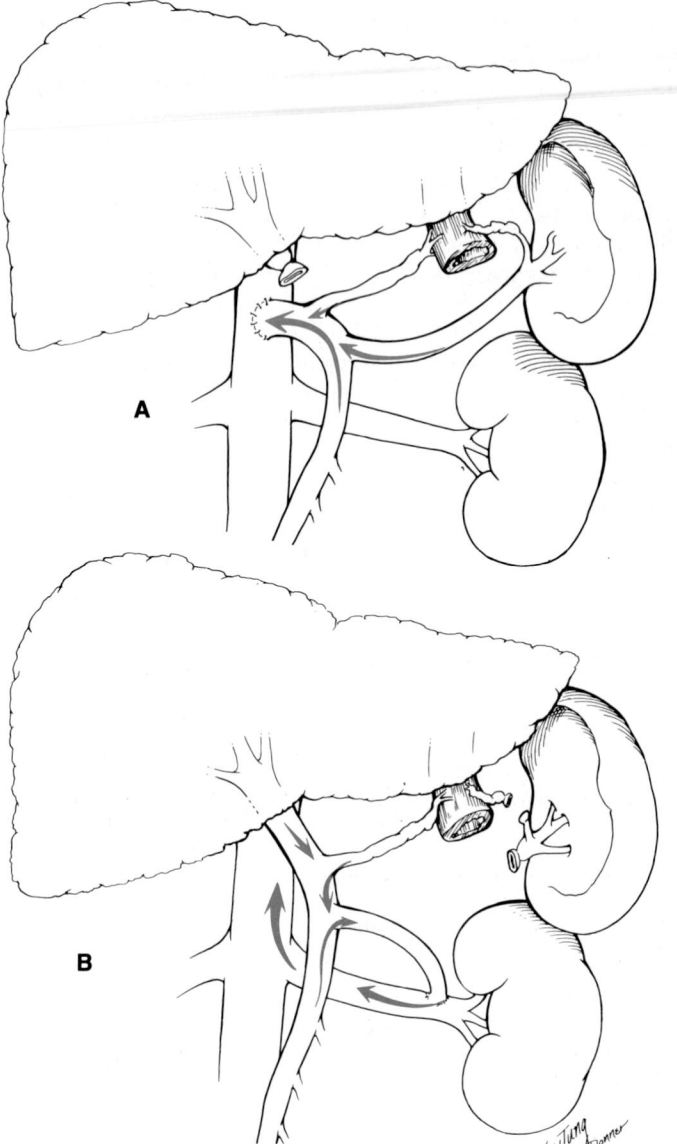

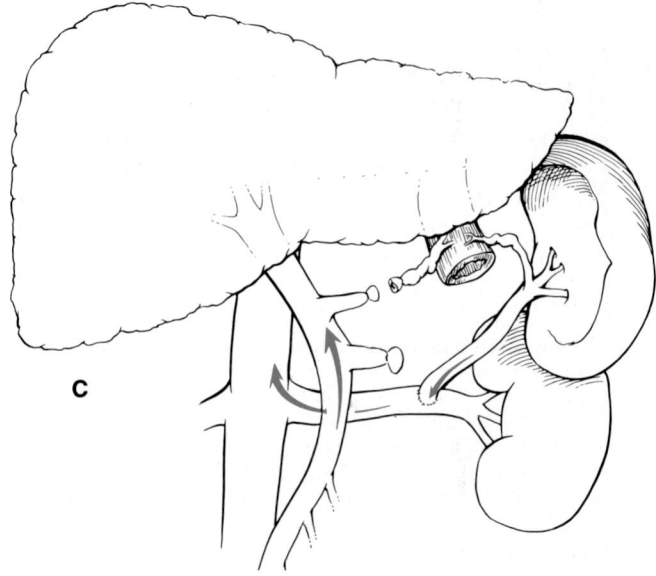

Fig. 22-4 Decompression operations for portal hypertension. **A,** End-to-side portacaval shunt. **B,** Splenorenal shunt. **C,** Distal splenorenal shunt.

diet. It is important to remember that the nurse is the health team member who provides this direct assistance to the patient. The following are specific measures to promote nutritional intake:

1. Provide frequent oral hygiene.
2. Provide a pleasant atmosphere.
3. Incorporate patient's food preferences.
4. Serve small, frequent feedings.
5. Increase caloric content by adding calories to prepared foods (for example, powdered milk, sauces, butter).
6. Use calorie-rich juices and drinks as fluid allowance, particularly if fluids are restricted.
7. Request use of salt substitutes, herbs, and spices if sodium is restricted.

Facilitating learning and promoting health maintenance

All patients need to be prepared for diagnostic tests, to understand their treatments, and to learn how to implement their therapeutic regimens at home. Patients with chronic hepatic dysfunction need to under-stand long-term care needs for changes in life-style, diet, fluid intake, and avoidance of toxins, including alcohol. All patients should be taught how to prevent further hepatic damage from insults of inadequate food, toxins, including alcohol, and infections.

The patient with malignant tumours, whether primary or metastatic, needs help to deal with self-care needs and to deal with cancer (see Chapter 9). A major focus for many patients with cirrhosis is helping them to confront the effect of alcohol on their well-being. It requires willing-ness to engage in discussion about alcohol. Denial is a major part of excessive alcohol consumption and "breaking through" denial is a part of treatment that occurs over time. Discussion of past alcohol intake and its effects on physical health, and social functioning (family, job, in-volvement with police, and accidents) is a necessary early part of improving health maintenance. Confrontation by family members, employers, and friends may be part of intervention.

The nurse can assist patients with alcoholism and cirrhosis due to alcoholism or other causes by giving

Nursing Care Plan	**Person with cirrhosis**

DATA: Mr. S. is a 55-year-old salesman with portal hypertension who is admitted to the hospital with upper gastrointestinal bleeding. Endoscopy revealed enlarged oesophageal and upper gastric veins and a bleeding ulcer. Gastric lavage with iced saline controlled bleeding; 1 U of packed red blood cells was given. Treatment orders included protein (20 g day) and sodium (1000 mg day) restrictions, fluid (1000 ml day) restriction, neomycin 1 g orally every 4 hours, thiamine 1 ml intramuscularly once a day for 3 days, vitamin K subcutaneously once a day for 3 days, and spironalactone 25 mg twice a day. A physical exam revealed slight jaundice of sclera and skin; ascites and peripheral oedema; thin legs and arms with poor musculature; signs of increased oestrogen; orientation to person, place, and time; and coherence; blood pressure of 116/60 mm Hg; pulse of 90 beats min; and respiratory rate of 32.

The nursing history identified the following:

- Mr. S. has participated in Alcoholics Anonymous (AA) for 1 year; he has not been drinking since then.
- Mr. S. has had influenza-like symptoms the past 2 weeks but continued with his busy schedule. He complains of fatigue, anorexia, and itching.

Collaborative nursing actions include interventions to prevent further impairment of physical status from haemorrhage and ammonia toxicity and to assist in treatment of the gastric ulcer and fluid excess. Nursing actions include monitoring for the following:

- Signs of haemorrhage: haematemesis, decreased blood pressure, tachycardia, restlessness, stools testing positive for guaiac, and cool, moist skin
- Signs of portal systemic encephalopathy: change in mental status, asterixis, and change in handwriting or tremors

Nursing analysis: Fatigue related to muscle wasting, blood loss, and potential anaemia

Expected patient outcomes	Nursing interventions	Rationale
Mrs S. will indicate on a weekly basis that he is less fatigued He will show improved rating of fatigue on a scale of one (no fatigue) to 10 (severe fatigue) Mr. S. will show a gradual increase in activities on a weekly basis	Ensure or maintain bed rest as prescribed during the acute phase After acute phase, encourage increasing activity interspersed with rest periods as tolerated; coordinate with patient Intervene if patient shows fatigue after or during visits by family or friends Make sure diet is well balanced nutritionally and that patient takes calories, protein, and sodium within proper restrictions	Graduated increase of activity is important so as not to overtax patient who has poor nutritional status and activity tolerance

Nursing analysis: Nutrition, altered: less than body requirements related to anorexia and flu-like symptoms

Expected patient outcomes	Nursing interventions	Rationale
Mr. S. ingests required nutrients and adequate calories on a daily basis; signs of muscle wasting lessen	Assess knowledge of nutrient needs On a daily basis, plan and implement well-balanced, high-carbohydrate, low-protein diet with adequate vitamins Decrease roughage in diet Encourage use of salt substitute or alternative seasonings such as Mrs. Dash Give antiemetics as prescribed and extra mouth care if nausea is present Suggest small, frequent meals, 6 meals day Use measures that encourage eating such as a clean environment and making sure patient is rested and comfortable Support continuation of AA activities while patient is hospitalized	Food intake within prescribed limitation can influence liver regeneration; nursing measures can influence amount of intake in anorectic patient. Low-fibre diet is necessary because of oesophageal varices It is important that patient continue AA participation as he has for the past year. AA representatives should be allowed to see patient as condition permits and patient desires.

Nursing analysis: Fliud volume excess related to impaired metabolism of aldosterone and hypoalbuminaemia

Expected patient outcomes	Nursing interventions	Rationale
Mr. S.'s weight and abdominal girth decrease daily Oedema resolves Serum sodium and potassium levels remain within normal limits	Monitor weight daily, blood pressure every 4 hours, assess oedema every shift, and measure abdominal girth daily Monitor intake and output on every shift until excess fluid is excreted Teach patient the rationale for sodium restriction as the patient shows interest Provide best rest for ascites Give the patient prescribed diuretics Restrict fluids; provide those that are best tolerated, and space the fluids throughout 24 hours with greatest volume in daytime and least at night	Diuresis in cirrhosis is undertaken slowly using very conservative measures because of the contracted intravascular fluid volume. Diuresis in excess can jeopardize renal perfusion and precipitate portal-systemic encephalopathy, so careful monitoring is necessary

Nursing analysis: Breathing pattern, ineffective related to ascites and immobility and potential stasis of secretions

Expected patient outcomes	Nursing interventions	Rationale
Mr. S.'s dyspnoea is decreased or does not worsen as indicated on a scale of 1 (no dyspnoea) to 5 (severe dyspnoea) Breath sounds are clear	Monitor respirations and breath sounds every 4 hours Place in supported sitting position Encourage patient on bed rest to turn frequently, every 2 hours Encourage deep breathing every 2 hours	Nursing measures to encourage deep chest excursions are important when ascites and immobility are present . A sitting position can relieve pressure on diaphragm, which can decrease chance of stasis of secretions

Nursing analysis: Skin integrity, impaired, high risk for, related to immobility, poor nutrition, oedema, and jaundice

Expected patient outcomes	Nursing interventions	Rationale
Mr. S.'s skin remains intact	Assess patient's skin daily for signs of possible breakdown Use measures such as egg crate mattress and routine turning schedule to prevent skin breakdown Keep skin clean and moisturized Clean and apply lotion every shift Keep nails short and clean Provide soft cloth to rub skin	Patient has poor nutrition, oedema, immobility; all of these are risk factors for decubitus ulcers requiring preventive care. Jaundice could lead to scratching and requires preventive care

Nursing analysis: Itching related to jaundice and environmental stimuli

Expected patient outcomes	Nursing interventions	Rationale
Mr. S. states that he feels more comfortable and that itching is decreased. Mr. S. is not observed scratching	Avoid heat and heavy clothing; provide a cool environment Apply antipruritic lotion as prescribed to skin as needed at least every shift Give prescribed antihitamines Use diversional activities such as music Keep patient's fingernails cut short and clean If patient must scratch, provide soft cloth to prevent excoriations Use tepid water for bathing	Nursing measures relieve or lessen the effects of environmental stimuli, reduce itching, and promote comfort

*Nursing
Care Plan*   **Person with cirrhosis—cont'd**

Nursing analysis: Infection, high risk for, related to immunosuppression

Expected patient outcomes	Nursing interventions	Rationale
Mr. S. develops no infections; temperature remains normal	Monitor patient for signs of infection every shift Use sterile technique for all invasive procedures Encourage pulmonary hygiene such as turning and deep breathing every 1 to 2 hr Restrict exposure to people with infections	Infections in patient with cirrhosis can be life threatening because they can cause sepsis and can precipitate failure, which may result in portal systemic encephalopathy Measures to prevent infection are essential in people whose immune systems are suppressed Early detection is important for early treatment

Nursing analysis: Coping, ineffective individual, related to health crisis

Expected patient outcomes	Nursing interventions	Rationale
Mr. S. will describe at least one coping mechanism to deal with health crisis	Assess patient's perception of health and present illness Identify and support patient's coping strategies such as prayer, music, conversation, etc Listen actively if patient expresses feeling of powerlessness, fears, or spiritual distress. Plan time daily for listening Assess and facilitate family support. Meet with family or significant other on a scheduled basis	Support of patient undergoing a health crisis can facilitate use of intrapersonal family resources. One can expect this patient to be discouraged and fearful. Ineffective coping may precipitate return to alcohol.

Nursing analysis: Injury, high risk for bleeding and falls related to decreased metabolic function of liver

Expected patient outcomes	Nursing interventions	Rationale
No undetected bleeding occurs Vital signs return to normal	Monitor the following for blood: urine, stool, skin, and mucous membranes Check patient's vital signs q4h and prothrombin and PTT levels and thrombocytes daily Avoid injections if possible; apply pressure at all puncture sites for 5 min Give prescribed vitamin K Teach patient to use soft toothbrush and to avoid straining or coughing	Patient's oesophageal varices and cirrhosis make him a candidate for bleeding and falls; surveillance is the major nursing focus, as well as decreasing precipitating factors
No falls occur	Provide support when patient is ambulating to prevent falls Maintain safe environment	

Nursing Care Plan — Person with cirrhosis—cont'd

Nursing analysis: Self-esteem disturbance related to inability to accept physical changes of increased abdominal girth, jaundice, and change in secondary sexual characteristics and potential changes in role

Expected patient outcomes	Nursing interventions	Rationale
Mr. S. describes self in realistic terms, which include positive characteristics	Encourage patient participate in goal setting and decision making Help patient identify personal strengths and give positive feedback Assist family to understand patient's need for a positive self-concept and how they can help Assist patient to explore ways to diminish overt signs of jaundice and ascites and thus help body image	Poor self-esteem can lead to poor coping, causing the patient to resume alcohol consumption

Nursing analysis: Knowledge deficit: follow-up care and home care related to change in health status and previous inability to cope with information

Expected patient outcomes	Nursing interventions	Rationale
Mr. S. describes nature of cirrhosis and therapeutic regimen	Assess patient's knowledge and clarify the following, as necessary: basis of signs and symptoms and therapeutic regimen, dietary and fluid restrictions, medication therapy, avoidance of infection and bleeding, and signs (increased temperature, bleeding worsening jaundice, change in mental status, etc) requiring immediate medical follow-up	Patient has had the medical problem for some time, so first assess his knowledge; he may not need teaching. The assessment will help identify other reasons for the delay in seeking help

them as much control as possible. This could include the following:

1. Involve the patient in goal setting and decision making.
2. Give positive feedback for accomplishments.
3. Support the patient in times of failure.
4. Help the patient recall past accomplishments.
5. Help significant others provide positive feedback.
6. Help the patient find ways to disguise jaundice or ascites.

A different set of issues is the focus of teaching and promotion of health maintenance in the patient with toxic or viral hepatitis. Often, patients with hepatitis are young adults who find that fatigue and slow recovery interfere with personal and career goals. The nurse can assist the patient and family to cope with these concerns by listening actively and supporting their coping mechanisms. Accurate information about rest requirements and infectiousness of viral hepatitis, as well as about measures that must be used at home to prevent transmission of viral hepatitis and further recovery should be provided. The patient and family need an opportunity to express their fears and concerns about care requirements, prognosis, and infectiousness.

Evaluation

Evaluation will be based on the identified patient outcomes. For the person with acute hepatic dysfunction, questions to consider may include the following:

1. Are signs and symptoms of fluid changes, infection, bleeding, or jaundice decreasing?
2. Have complications (infection, bleeding, respiratory dysfunction, skin breakdown) been avoided?
3. Have falls or other injuries been avoided?
4. Is the patient getting sufficient rest?

For people with chronic hepatic dysfunction, do the patient and family know the following:

1. The nature of the disorder and need for continued medical follow-up?
2. Measures to prevent exacerbations and complications?
3. Signs and symptoms to be reported to the doctor?
4. All information related to diet and medications?

SUMMARY

1. The anatomic structure of the liver has several specialized characteristics: the organization of cellular plates;

the portal vein and hepatic arterial blood supply into the sinusoids; the biliary canaliculi emptying into the larger biliary ductules, ducts and common bile duct; and Kupffer's cells lining the blood vessels.

2. The liver is important for proper metabolism of fat, protein, and carbohydrate, for production of plasma proteins, for bilirubin metabolism and bile production, and for detoxification.

3. Physiological changes that occur in ageing may change the metabolism of drugs.

4. All types of jaundice are associated with increased serum levels of bilirubin; haemolytic jaundice is a problem of excessive red blood cell breakdown; obstructive jaundice is associated with an elevation of conjugated bilirubin (direct) and an absence of urinary urobilinogen, and hepatocellular jaundice is often associated with elevated serum transaminases.

5. An increased prothrombin time may be associated with a decrease in vitamin K or hepatocellular inability to form prothrombin even if vitamin K is adequate.

6. Increasingly severe histological changes in liver cells are seen in alcoholic fatty liver, alcoholic hepatitis, and Laënnec's cirrhosis; the latter condition is not reversible.

7. In Britain, cirrhosis is most commonly a result of chronic alcoholism and is characterized by multiple changes in hepatic function. Portal hypertension, bleeding oesophageal varices, and hepatorenal syndrome are three problems that threaten life.

8. The incidence of toxic hepatitis could be reduced by decreased use or proper use of toxins such as petroleum distillates; alcoholic hepatitis is the major type of toxic hepatitis in Britain.

9. There are five known types of viral hepatitis. Measures to control hepatitis A and hepatitis E are directed towards hand washing and interrupting the faecal-oral route of transmission. The other three types are spread through infected blood and other body fluids.

10. Anorexia and influenza-like symptoms are often more acute in hepatitis A but these symptoms occur in all types of hepatitis. They occur before icterus (jaundice) appears.

11. Most people with viral hepatitis recover within 6 months and have no residual hepatic damage. Hepatitis B and C may lead to a carrier state, atypical course of illness, chronic hepatitis, or cirrhosis.

12. Preexposure and postexposure prophylaxis for hepatitis include immune globulin and HBIG (passive immunity) and hepatitis B vaccine (active immunity).

13. The CDC in the United States is the national authority for information about the prevention of infectious diseases.

14. There are many tests that use serological markers (antigens, antibodies) for differentiating the type of hepatitis: HBsAg is one test for hepatitis B. Hepatitis A is detected by the presence of IgM-class anti-HAV, and hepatitis C is detected by anti-HCV.

15. The CDC considers hepatitis B to be the greatest occupational hazard for health workers. Measures to decrease risk include hepatitis B vaccination, hand washing, and universal or body substance precautions used with all patients.

16. Common problems of diffuse hepatocellular disease are jaundice, bleeding tendencies, anaemia, infection, and fluid and electrolyte imbalances.

17. Diuresis of ascitic fluid is slow and can induce complications: hypokalaemia, magnesium deficit, oliguria, azotaemia, and portal systemic encephalopathy. One kg of loss of body weight per day is the maximum safe amount of ascitic fluid loss.

18. Portal systemic encephalopathy (PSE) is associated with elevations of serum ammonia or other metabolic abnormalities. Central nervous system dysfunction is manifested in a sequential pattern leading to coma. Asterixis is an early sign.

19. Common precipitants of PSE are hypokalaemia, alkalosis, sedation, and gastrointestinal bleeding.

20. Measures to control bleeding in oesophageal varices include use of the Sengstaken-Blakemore tube, pitressin infusion and other drugs, injection sclerosis, oesophageal variceal ligation, or surgery. Measures to prevent PSE are also started when there is gastrointestinal bleeding.

21. After oesophageal haemorrhage unresponsive to other measures, elective surgical decompression of the portal vein may be done by creating a connection between portal and systemic venous circulation (liver bypass or shunting procedures); elective nonshunting procedures may also be done.

22. Portal-systemic encephalopathy may be treated by neomycin, lactulose, and no- or low-protein diet. These measures may be used as prophylaxis when there is gastrointestinal bleeding.

23. Liver abscesses may be pyogenic and treated with broad-spectrum antibiotics and surgery, or they may be amoebic and treated with amoebicidal drugs.

24. Metastatic tumours of the liver are 20 times more prevalent than primary tumours of the liver. Symptoms occur late; jaundice, ascites, and weakness are common.

25. Malignant lesions of the liver are treated by resection, palliative use of radiation, and chemotherapy by systemic routes or portal arterial infusion.

26. Assessment techniques of value in people with hepatic diseases include percussion and palpation of the liver, and inspection, auscultation, and percussion of the abdomen. Palpating for fluid wave is helpful when ascites is present.

27. In liver biopsy, aseptic technique and assisting the patient to hold his or her breath during the procedure reduce risks of infection and haemorrhage.

28. Rest, nutrition, and abstinence from toxins are three major treatments of focal or diffuse hepatic disorders.

29. Patients with chronic diffuse hepatic disease will require extensive teaching to assist them to master self-care skills.

30. The patient with hepatic disease may need to make major changes in life-style (avoidance of alcohol or changes in sexual practices).

STUDY QUESTIONS

- Why does gastrointestinal bleeding, low serum potassium, or alkalosis increase the risk of portal-systemic encephalopathy?
- Why are people with diffuse hepatic disease at greater risk for infection?
- What measures are needed to decrease incidence and transmission of hepatitis B?
- Why do people in high-risk groups for hepatitis B not receive the correct primary preventive care?

REFERENCES

1.* Advisory Committee Immunization Practices (ACIP): Recommendation for protection against viral hepatitis, *MMWR* 39(S-2):1–26, 1990.
2.* Adinaro D: Liver failure and pancreatitis: fluid and electrolyte concerns, *Nurs Clin North Am* 22:843–852, 1987.
3. Alter MJ et al: The changing epidemiology of hepatitis B in the United States, *JAMA* 263:1218–1222, 1989.
4.* Anderson FP: Portal-systemic encephalopathy in the chronic alcoholic, *Crit Care Q,* 8(4):40–52, 1989.
5. Arora S, Kaplan MM: Cirrhosis. In Rakel RE, editor: *Conn's current therapy,* ed 28, Philadelphia, 1989, WB Saunders.
6. Berne R, Levy M, editors: *Physiology,* ed 2, St Louis, 1988, Mosby-Year Book.
6a. Blumgart LH, editor: *Surgery of the liver and biliary tract,* New York, 1988, Churchill Livingstone.
7. Bradley DW: Hepatitis non-A, non-B viruses become identified as hepatitis C and E viruses, *Prog Med Virol* 37:101–135, 1990.
8.* Brown M: Gastroesophageal varices, *Prim Care* 15:175-186, 1988.
9. Deinstag JL: Hepatitis non-A, non-B: C at last, *Gastroenterology* 99(4):1177–1180, 1990.
9a. Department of Health: *On the State of the public health for the year 1990,* London, 1990, HMSO.
10.* Dobberstein K: The liver: to know it is to love it, *Am J Nurs* 87:74, 1987.
11. Franks AL et al: Hepatitis B virus infection among children born in the U.S. to Southeast Asian refugees, *New Engl J Med* 321:1301–1305, 1989.
12. Frey CF et al: Liver abscesses, *Surg Clin North Am* 69:259–271, 1989.
13.* Gillham MB, Southworth K, Dollahite J: Nutritional treatment for the alcoholic patient, *Crit Care Q* 8(4):20–28, 1986.
14.* Healthy People 2000: National Health Promotion and Disease Prevention Objectives, US Dept of Health and Human Services, Public Health Service, Washington, DC, 1990, US Government Printing Office.
14a. Heeg JM, Coleman DA: Hepatitis kills, *RN* 55(4):60–68, 1992.
15. Hoofnagle JH: Toward universal vaccination against hepatitis B virus, *New Engl J Med* 321:1333–1334, 1989.
16. Hoofnagle JH: Type D (Delta) hepatitis, *JAMA* 261:1321–1325, 1989.
17. Jensen DM: Portal-systemic encephalopathy and hepatic coma, *Med Clin North Am* 70:1081–1092, 1986.
18.* Keith JS: Hepatic failure: etiologies, manifestation, and management, *Crit Care Nurse* 5(1):60–86, 1985.
19. Korniewicz DM, Kirwin M, Larson E: Do your gloves fit the task? *Am J Nurs* 91(6):38–40, 1991.
20.* Korniewicz DM et al: Integrity of vinyl and latex procedure gloves, *Nurs Res* 38:144–146, 1989.
20a. Levine BA, Sirinek KR: The portacaval shunt-is it still indicated? *Surg Clin North Am* 70:361–377, 1990.
20b. Lillemoe KD, Cameron JL: The interposition mesocaval shunt, *Surg Clin North Am* 70:379–393, 1990.
21. Ludwig J: Etiology of biliary cirrhosis: diagnositic features and a new classification, *Zentralbl Allg Pathol* 134:132–141, 1988.
22. Maddrey WC, Thiel DHV: Liver transplantation: an overview, *Hepatology* 8:948–959, 1988.

23.* Maloney JP: Surgical intervention in the alcoholic patient with portal hypertension, *Crit Care Q* 8(4):63–73, 1986.
24. Mattsson L, Weiland O, Glaumann H: Long-term follow-up of chronic posttransfusion non-A, non-B hepatitis: clinical and histological outcome, *Liver* 8:184–188, 1988.
25. Maxwell AJ, Mamtora H: Fungal liver abscesses in acute leukemia—a report of two cases, *Clin Radiol* 39:197–201, 1988.
26. Metzger U: Intraportal chemotherapy for colorectal hepatic metastases, *Antibiot Chemother* 40:51–60, 1988.
27. MMWR: Changing patterns of groups at high risk for hepatitis B in the United States, *MMWR* 37:429–437,1988.
28.* MMWR: Hepatitis A among drug abusers, *MMWR* 37:297–305, 1988.
29.* MMWR: Hepatitis B among parenteral drug abusers North Carolina, *MMWR* 35:481–483, 1986.
30. MMWR: Inadequate immune response among public safety workers receiving intradermal vaccination against hepatitis B-United States, 1990-1991 *MMWR* 40:569–571, 1991.
31. MMWR: Public Health Service inter-agency guidelines for screening donors of blood, plasma, organs, tissues, and semen for evidence of hepatitis B and hepatitis C, *MMWR* 40(RR-4):1–17, 1991.
32. MMWR: Recommendations for preventing transmission of human immunodeficiency virus and hepatitis B virus to patients during exposure-prone invasive procedures, *MMWR* 40(RR-8):1–9, 1991.
33. MMWR: Update on hepatitis B prevention, *MMWR* 36:353–366, 1987.
34. Price SA, Wilson LM: Pathophysiology: clinical concepts of disease processes, ed 4, St Louis, 1992, Mosby-Year Book.
34a. Rector WG, Jr: *Complications of chronic liver disease,* St Louis, 1992, Mosby-Year Book.
34b. Russell B: Score: hepatitis viruses 5, vaccines 1, *Amer Nurse* 24(8):2, 11, 1992.
35. Schreeder M: Viral hepatitis, *Prim Care* 15:157–173, 1988.
36. Schroeder SA, et al, editors: *Current medical diagnosis and treatment: 1990,* Norwalk, Conn, 1990, Appleton & Lange.
37.* Semonin-Holleran R: Critical nursing care for abdominal trauma, *Crit Care Nurse* 8(3):48–58, 1988.
38. Solomon J, Harrington D, Gogel HF: When the patient suffers from esophageal bleeding, *RN* 50(2):24–27, 1987.
39. Starzel TE, Iwatsuki S: Transplantation of the liver. In Schiff L, Schiff ER, editors: *Diseases of the liver,* ed 6, Philadelphia, 1987, JB Lippincott Co.
40. Steven CE et al: Epidemiology of hepatitis C Virus, *JAMA* 263:49–53, 1990.
40a. Stiegmann GV, Goff JS: Endoscopic esophageal varix ligation: preliminary clinical experience, *Gastrointestinal Endoscopy* 34:113–117, 1988.
41. Stone MD, Benotti PN: Liver resection: preoperative and postoperative care, *Surg Clin North Am* 69:383–391, 1989.
42. Vitale G, Heusen LS, Polk H: Malignant tumours of the liver, *Surg Clin North Am* 66:723–741, 1986.
42a. Wexler MJ, Stein BL: Nonshunting operations for hemorrhage, *Surg Clin North Am* 70:425–448, 1990.
43. Widmann F: *Goodall's Clinical interpretation of laboratory tests,* ed 10, Philadelphia, 1987, FA Davis.
44. Wyngaarden JB, Smith LH, Bennett JC, editors: *Cecil Textbook of medicine,* ed 19, Philadelphia, 1992, WB Saunders.
45. Zimmerman HJ, Maddrey WC: Toxic and drug-induced hepatitis. In Schiff L, Schiff ER, editors: *Diseases of the liver,* ed 6, Philadelphia, 1987, JB Lippincott.
46.* Freditti SL: When the liver fails, *Am J Nurs* 84:64-67, 1984.
47.* Gullate MM, Foltz AT: Hepatic chemotherapy via implantable pump, *Am J Nurs* 83:1674–1678, 1983.
48. Klopp A: Shunting malignant ascites, *Am J Nurs* 84:212–213, 1984.

---

* Recommended for student reading.

FURTHER READING

49. King Edwards Hospital Fund for London: *The nation's health: A strategy for the 1990s,* London, 1991, King's Fund Centre.
50. Kew M.: Hepatic Tumours: *Medicine International* 29: 1201–1205, 1986.
51. Alleyne GAO, Hay RW, Picou DI, Whitehead RG: *Protein energy and malnutrition,* Edward Arnold, 1977: London.
52. Office of Population Censuses and Surveys: Population and vital statistics. Deaths per 100,000, 1990.
53. Maxwell M: The liver, *Nurs Mirror* 157(11): 18–20, 1983.
54. Marta MT: Endoscopic retrograde cholangiopancreatography-its role in diagnosis and treatment, *Focus on Critical Care* 14(5): 62–63, 1987.

Problems with Digestion or Elimination

Unit Eight

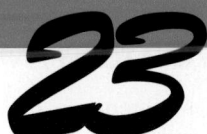

The Patient

with

Gastrointestinal

Problems

Barbara C. Long
Rebecca Roberts

After studying this chapter, the learner should be able to:

- Compare and contrast obesity and protein-energy malnutrition and their nursing interventions.
- Compare and contrast the nature of common inflammatory disorders of the mouth, stomach, intestines, and appendix and nursing interventions for them.
- Describe the cause of dysphagia and heartburn and related therapeutic interventions.
- Differentiate gastric and duodenal ulcers and required medical and nursing care.
- Explain malabsorption syndrome and nursing interventions.
- Differentiate ulcerative colitis, Crohn's disease, and diverticular disease and the care required for each.
- Describe the nature and care of the patient with intestinal obstruction and with hernias.
- Differentiate preventive and therapeutic modalities for patients with cancer of the mouth, stomach, and bowel.
- Describe the care of people with a stoma for faecal diversion.
- Differentiate types of surgery and nursing care for people with anorectal lesions.

ANATOMY AND PHYSIOLOGY

Maintenance of adequate nutrition and elimination requires an intact and functioning gastrointestinal tract. Normally, food and fluids are placed in the mouth, chewed (if solid), pushed to the pharynx by the tongue, and swallowed by automatic reflex activity down the oesophagus into the stomach. Digestion starts in the mouth and ends in the small intestine, although fluids continue to be reabsorbed in the colon. Fig. 23-1 shows the anatomic structures of the gastrointestinal tract. The gallbladder and pancreas, which are also involved with digestion, are discussed in Chapter 24.

Mouth and Oesophagus

Salivation

The cortical thought of food initiates saliva production from the salivary glands. The salivary secretions consist of *serous secretion*, containing salivary amylase for starch digestion, and *mucous* secretion for lubrication. These two secretions account for one half of the upper gastrointestinal tract secretions.

Mastication

The teeth initiate food breakdown; no other part of the gastrointestinal tract can perform this function if the teeth are missing. Enzymes can act only on the exposed surfaces of the food particles. Very fine particulation prevents excoriation of the lining of the tract, and the rate of digestion depends on the total surface area of food particle exposed. General health teaching for children and adults should stress the reason behind thorough mastication of all food substances that are ingested.

Swallowing

Swallowing must be accomplished without compromising respiration. The tongue forces the bolus of food into the pharynx, from which point the food moves to the upper oesophagus and then down into the stomach. Food is prevented from passing into the trachea by the closing of the epiglottis over the trachea and the opening of the oesophagus.

The oesophagus is a hollow tube. The upper one third is composed of skeletal muscle and the remainder of smooth muscle. It is lined with mucous membrane, which secretes a mucoid substance for protection. The bolus of food arrives at the cardiac sphincter of the stomach usually within 5 to 10 seconds of ingestion.

The *cardiac sphincter* (at the junction of the oesophagus with the stomach) prevents reflux of stomach contents into the lower oesophagus. This area is heavily layered with mucoid glands. The secretions adhere to the food particles and prevent actual contact with the wall mucosa. The coated particles adhere to each other, forming a bolus for digestion. These secretions act as a protective mechanism for the sphincter zone, since they themselves are strongly resistant to digestion.

Stomach

The food bolus enters the stomach, the largest dilated portion of the tract. The stomach has relatively little muscular tone, which permits increased distention. *Peristalsis*, the alternate contraction and relaxation of the muscle fibres, propels the substance in a wavelike motion through the stomach and intestines.

The mucous membrane lining the stomach is arranged in thick folds known as *rugae* that provide an increased surface area for exposure and contain the openings of the gastric glands. The gastric secretions are clear and colourless and contain water, salts, enzymes, and hydrochloric acid. The amount of enzymes produced is in direct proportion to the amount needed, and the actual food substance stimulates the release of a particular enzyme. The gastric mucosa releases gastrin, which stimulates the production of *pepsinogen* (the precursor of pepsin), and *lipase*. Pepsin digests protein, and lipase splits fats. The production of hydrochloric acid (HCl) does not appear to depend on the presence of any particular food.

As the food moves towards the *pyloric sphincter* at the distal end of the stomach, peristaltic waves increase in force and intensity. The fluid bolus now becomes a substance known as *chyme*. Chyme is pumped through the pyloric sphincter into the duodenum. Two factors regulate emptying of stomach contents: consistency of the fluid chyme and receptiveness of the duodenum. The average length of time food remains in the stomach after a meal is 2 to 6 hours.

Intestines

The small intestine has three parts: the *duodenum*, which connects to the stomach, the *jejunum* or middle portion, and the *ileum*. The large intestine also has three parts: the *caecum*, which connects to the small intestine, the *colon*, and the *rectum*. The primary function of the intestines is to receive the chyme from the stomach and move the chyme forward to facilitate proper absorption of water, nutrients, electrolytes, and bile salts (Fig. 23-2). Secondary functions include secreting mucus and serving as a storage area before waste discharge.

Movement

Peristaltic movements that mix the intestinal contents propel the contents of the small intestine towards the anus. Chyme moves slowly and normally takes 3 to 10 hours to move from the stomach to the ileocaecal valve (see Fig. 23-1). In the colon, the faecal contents are pushed forward by *mass movements* that occur only a few times each day. These mass movements are stimulated by gastrocolic reflexes initiated when food enters the duodenum from the stomach, especially after the first meal of the day. This is therefore the most frequent time of the day for defaecation to occur.

The defaecation reflex occurs when faeces enter the rectum. Afferent impulses are transmitted to the sacral segments of the spinal cord, from which reflex impulses are transmitted back to the colon and rectum, initiating relaxation of the internal anal sphincter.

Secretion

Secretions of the small intestine, biliary, and pancreatic systems provide for the final digestion of food. As chyme enters the small intestine, gastric secretion of hydrochloric acid is slowed. Mucous secretion throughout the tract

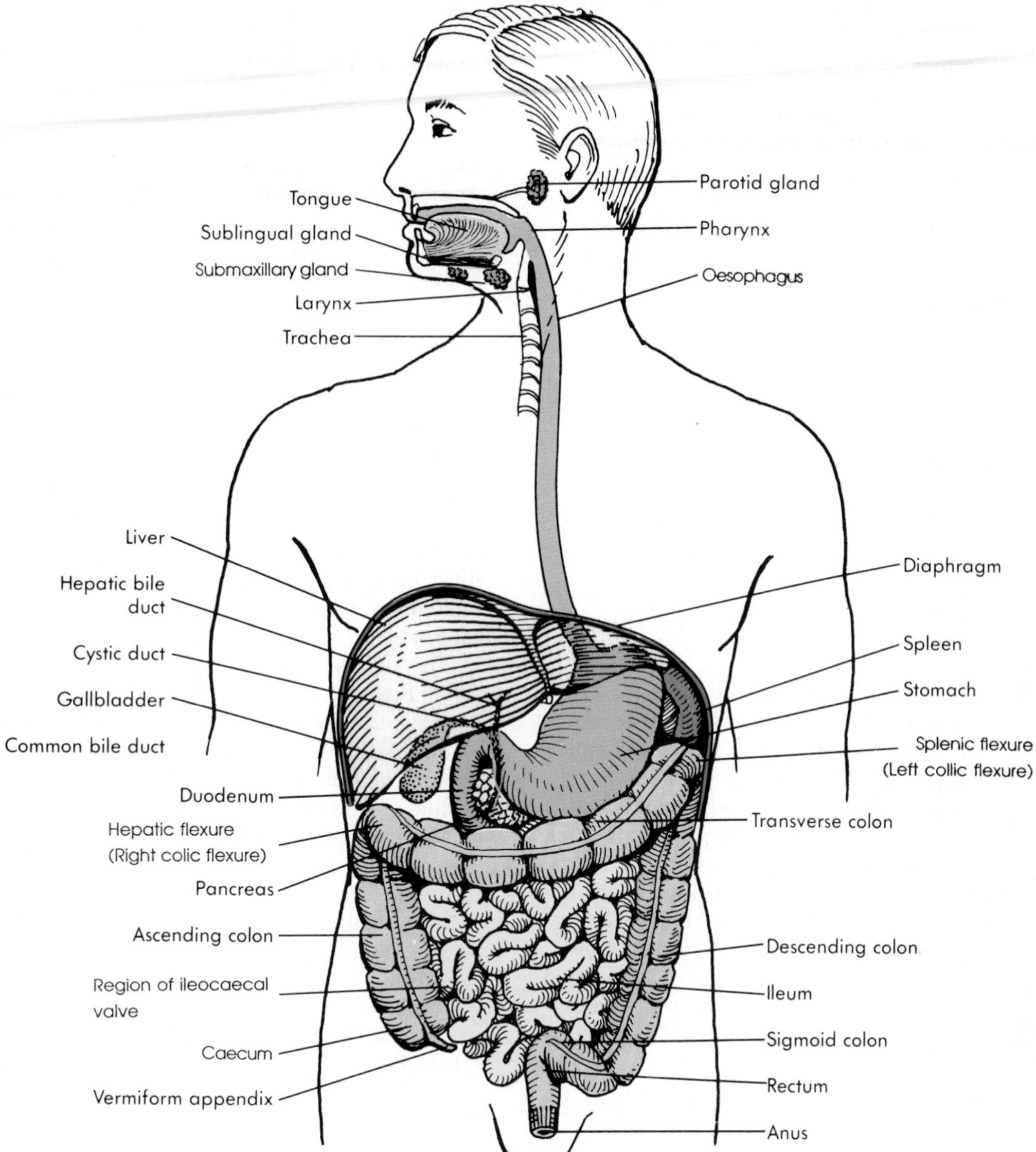

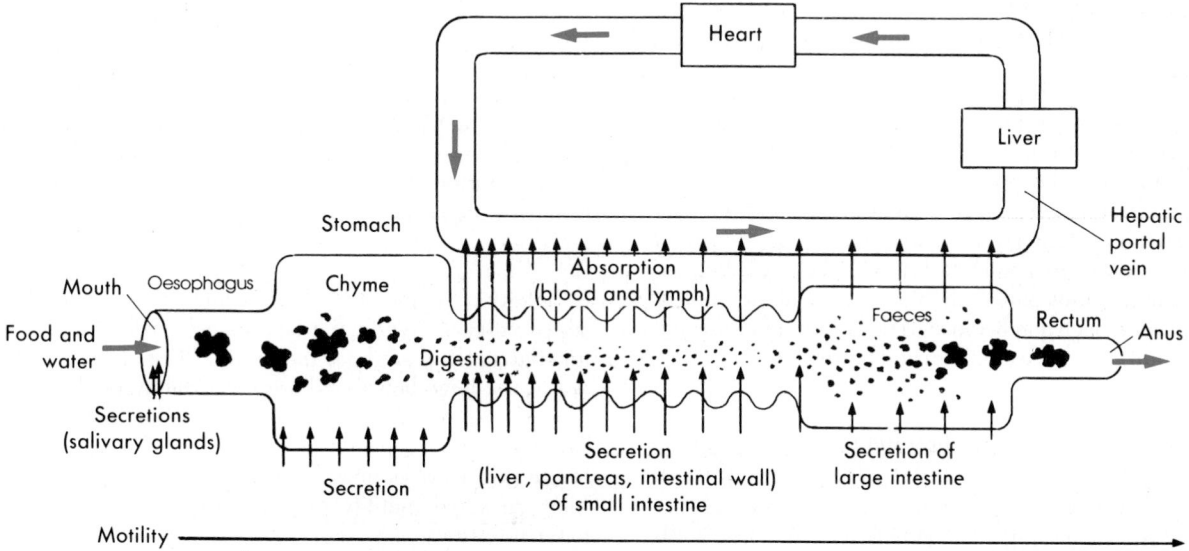

Fig. 23-1   Organs of digestive system and associated structures.

Fig. 23-2   Summary of gastrointestinal activity involving motility, secretion, digestion, and absorption. (From Vander AJ, et al: *Human physiology*, ed 3, New York, 1980, McGraw-Hill. Used with the permission of McGraw-Hill.)

Table 23-1 Digestive enzymes

Enzyme	Location	Conversions
Salivary amylase	Saliva	Starch → disaccharides
Pepsin	Gastric juice	Protein → polypeptides
Lipase	Pancreatic juice (small amount in gastric juice)	Fats → glycerol and fatty acids
Trypsin	Pancreatic juice	Polypeptides → peptides and amino acids
Amylase	Pancreatic juice	Disaccharides → monosaccharides
Sucrase	Intestinal juice	Sucrose → glucose and fructose
Lactase	Intestinal juice	Lactose → glucose and galactose
Maltase	Intestinal juice	Maltose → glucose

Table 23-2 Fluid composition of gastrointestinal secretions

Site	Secretion	Approximate amount (ml/day)
Mouth	Saliva	1500
Stomach	Gastric juice	2500
Intestines	Bile	500
	Pancreatic juice	1500
	Intestinal juice	1000
	TOTAL	7000

increases food adhesion, prevents contact of the food with the wall of the mucosa, enhances free passage of the food, neutralizes the small amounts of acid or alkali, and makes some particles more resistant to digestion.

Emptying into the duodenum are the common bile duct (from the liver and gallbladder) and the pancreatic duct. *Bile*, which is produced in the liver and stored in the gallbladder, drains into the duodenum to assist in absorption of fats by emulsifying the fat and breaking down large fat droplets into small droplets. *Pancreatic juice* contains three digestive enzymes, trypsinogen (which is converted into trypsin by the enzyme enterokinase in the small intestines), amylase, and lipase. The actions of the various digestive enzymes are described in Table 23-1.

Digestion

The digestion of *carbohydrate* begins in the mouth, where the breakdown of polysaccharides (starches) to disaccharides (sucrose, lactose, maltose) occurs by the action of amylase. The disaccharides are then broken down into monosaccharides (glucose, galactose, and fructose) by the action of the enzymes within the intestinal mucosa and by pancreatic amylase.

Protein digestion begins in the stomach, when pepsin breaks down proteins into polypeptides (an intermediate step). In the small intestine, trypsin further breaks down the polypeptides into peptides and amino acids.

Fat requires emulsification into small droplets before it can be broken down into glycerol and fatty acids. Most fat digestion occurs in the small intestine with the emulsification by bile and action of pancreatic lipase. A small amount of lipase in the stomach may begin digestion of some fats that are already emulsified, such as cream and butter.

Absorption

Ninety per cent of nutrient absorption occurs within the small intestine, either by active transport or diffusion. Many nutrients, such as amino acids, monosaccharides, sodium, and calcium, are transported by active transport, requiring metabolic energy expenditure. Other nutrients, such as fatty acids and water, diffuse passively across the cell membrane. Pancreatic lipase and conjugated bile salts must be present in the intestinal lumen for hydrolysis of fats into fatty acids to permit diffusion across the cell membrane.

The GI tract secretes approximately 7000 ml of fluids daily (Table 23-2); about 2000 ml are usually ingested daily. Therefore, the GI tract processes approximately 9000 ml of fluid daily. The jejunum and ileum absorb the largest amount of fluid (7500 ml); thus, approximately 1500 ml of fluid reaches the caecum daily.

The transit time in the large bowel is slow, taking about 12 hours for material to reach the rectum. Reabsorption of water, electrolytes, and bile salts occurs predominantly in the ascending colon. The colon has the capacity to absorb six to eight times more fluid than is delivered to it daily. Approximately 200 ml of fluid contents remains to be mixed with the residue of faeces. Normally, this residue (faeces) is evacuated on a fairly regular basis. The evacuation schedule differs for each individual and may vary from one to three times per day to once every 3 to 4 days.

Fluid and electrolyte balance

Pathological changes occur with the loss of particular segments of small or large bowel or when reabsorption is impaired. The loss of small bowel contents precipitates metabolic acidosis and hypokalaemia from the loss of bicarbonate and potassium. This problem may occur with drainage of small bowel contents through a suction tube or fistula or with persistent vomiting of intestinal contents. Losses from the large intestine comprise mainly loss of water, sodium, and to a lesser extent chloride, resulting in dehydration and hyponatraemia. This occurs in conditions in which the rate of peristalsis is increased.

Bacteria

In addition to its role in nutrition, the intestinal tract supports bacterial growth that enhances digestive processes and has a role in antibody formation. Most of the organisms are in the large bowel and are responsible for the production of vitamin K, which is necessary for blood clotting. Antibiotic enemas decrease the number of organisms, thus interfering with vitamin K synthesis. Conditions that inhibit intestinal motility may lead to bacterial overgrowth in the intestines.

The Elderly with GI problems

Assessment

Assess for dry mouth (from decreased salivation), missing teeth, or poorly fitting dentures that may interfere with eating.

Assess mouth for early signs of periodontal disease (bleeding or receding gums, loose teeth) or oral cancer (white patches or red granular patches, especially on anterior side of tongue or floor of mouth).

Assess dietary intake for adequate fluid intake (at least 1500 ml daily), for adequate food intake, and for fibre-containing foods. Elderly people, especially those living alone, often drink and eat less than adequate amounts; their diet may also be deficient in fibre, which is needed to maintain normal bowel elimination and help prevent colon cancer. Convenience foods are usually low-fibre.

Assess usual activity level; activity in the form of some type of exercise (based on the person's capabilities) facilitates normal bowel elimination.

Assess laxative use; if needed, bulk laxatives or stool softeners provide for normal stools without affecting bowel function.

Test stool for guaiac (occult blood), which may result from diverticular disease, GI cancer, or haemorrhoids, all commonly seen in elderly people.

Intervention

Use measures that encourage eating when patient is anorexic (commonly seen in elderly people).
    People are more likely to eat types of food they usually eat (especially ethnic foods). Suggest family provide favourite foods.
    If patient lives alone and is eligible, Meals on Wheels is available in the community to provide a daily nourishing meal.
    More spices, sugar, and salt (or substitute) may be needed in foods because elderly tend to lose their sense of smell and taste.

Assist elderly to complete hospital menu, if necessary, because of poor vision or loss of fine motor control.
    Suggest hospitalized patient sit in chair when possible to eat meals (usual pattern for eating).
    Offer food supplements between the usual three times daily meal pattern; smaller more frequent meals are better tolerated. Offer substitutes for missed meals.

Following GI diagnostic procedures, provide oral fluids (if permitted) and opportunity to rest (these procedures are often lengthy and tiring). Monitor stools for barium excretion and constipation.

Promote normal bowel function with adequate fluid intake, dietary fibre, ambulation, and bulk laxatives or stool softeners.

If diarrhoea is present, which may result in dehydration and hypokalaemia in elderly people, do the following:
    Monitor fluid balance and serum potassium levels.
    Report oliguria (less than 50 ml/hr for 2 to 3 hours) and abnormal serum potassium level to doctor.
    Encourage fluid intake.
    Monitor perianal skin for excoriations; keep the skin clean and apply a soothing ointment such as white soft paraffin (elderly skin is more fragile and susceptible to breakdown).

Teach patient:
    Adequate fluid intake (use juices when possible for additional nutrient intake) and regular exercise to prevent constipation.
    High-fibre diet to help prevent constipation, diverticulitis, and colon cancer. Omit fibres if symptomatic diverticulitis is present.
    Avoid overuse of laxatives.

Common disorders in elderly

Hiatus hernia
Cancer of mouth, stomach, and colon
Constipation
Diverticulosis
Faecal incontinence

Physiological Changes With Ageing

Changes in the gastrointestinal tract structure and function may occur with ageing but vary among individuals and may or may not cause altered functioning.

In the mouth, ageing teeth become darker and may loosen from loss of supporting bone and gums. Teeth may become uneven or develop fractures, and circulation of the gums is reduced. Gum changes affect denture fit. Salivary gland output decreases, leading to increased dryness of mucous membranes and making them more susceptible to breakdown. Dryness of the mouth may also interfere with chewing.

Changes in the ability to digest and absorb foods are related to decreased secretion of most digestive enzymes and bile production. Absorption of fats and fat-soluble vitamins becomes impaired. The increased residue resulting from decreased digestion and absorption may lead to increased flatulence. Gas-forming foods may be less well tolerated than when the person was younger.

Decreased intestinal motility may result from decreased peristalsis, decreased muscular tone of the intestinal wall, and decreased abdominal muscle strength. Decreased anal sphincter tone may also be present. These changes contribute to the increased occurrence of constipation or loss of sphincter control in the older person. Considerations for the care of elderly people with GI problems are listed in the special box.

PREVENTION AND HEALTH EDUCATION

Disorders of the digestive system are among the most commonly encountered health problems. Symptoms produced by digestive disorders are numerous and often lead to decreased employment productivity. Gastrointestinal symptoms, such as nausea and vomiting or diarrhoea, often result from disorders of other body systems. Interference with functioning of the gastrointestinal system leads to temporary or long-term nutritional imbalances.

Primary Prevention: Prevention of Disease

Because the cause of many gastrointestinal disorders is unknown, prevention may not be possible. Some health practices that are either known to be or are thought to be helpful in preventing disorders include good oral hygiene and nutrition and avoidance of tobacco use and stress.

Secondary Prevention: Early Detection

Early detection of major gastrointestinal health problems can prevent serious complications such as a ruptured appendix with peritonitis. People at high risk for cancer of the colon (p. 894) need careful screening to detect early signs of cancer because the cancer may be in an advanced stage before any symptoms occur. Guidelines for early detection are listed in Box 23-1.

MAJOR HEALTH PROBLEMS OF THE GASTROINTESTINAL SYSTEM

Nutritional excess (obesity) and deficit (protein-energy malnutrition) are disorders that relate to ingestion of food. Gastrointestinal disorders may be classified according to their overall effect on gastrointestinal function or according to the function of specific areas.

CLASSIFICATION BY GENERAL FUNCTION

Disorders of the gastrointestinal (GI) tract may interfere with function in one of three ways: interference with motility and control, with digestion and absorption, and with mechanical passage of food, chyme, and faeces.

Disorders of Motility

Interference with GI motility may ocur in any part of the GI tract. Oesophageal disorders interfere with swallowing and movement of food to the stomach. Vomiting is reverse peristalsis and may result from delayed gastric emptying. Surgical removal of part of the stomach leads to rapid emptying (dumping syndrome). Intestinal hypermotility produces diarrhoea. Faecal incontinence results from loss of control. Decreased intestinal motility may lead to flatulence and constipation. Paralytic ileus is failure of intestinal peristalsis.

Disorders of Digestion and Absorption

Disorders that interfere with the digestion and absorption of food include inflammatory disorders, ulcerations, or malabsorptions. *Inflammatory* disorders may occur in any part of the GI tract (Fig. 23-3) and may be acute or chronic. Acute inflammations are painful and produce swelling of the mucosa that may interfere with absorption. Chronic inflammations create changes in the muscular walls, as well as in the mucosa. *Ulcerations* may also extend through the mucosa into the muscular wall and cause pain. *Malabsorption* disorders may alter digestion when nutrients are not broken down into a form that can be transported across cell membranes, or they may alter absorption of the nutrients across the cell membranes and into the lymphatic or circulatory system.

Obstructive Disorders

The GI tract may become obstructed at any point from the portal of entry (mouth) to the exit (rectum). Obstruction may occur from mechanical causes that physically impede passage of intestinal contents or from paralytic causes, in which the passageway is open but peristalsis ceases. Mechanical obstructive disorders include tumours, hernias, adhesions, twisting or telescoping of the intestines, and interferences with the vascular supply.

CLASSIFICATION BY SPECIFIC FUNCTION

GI disorders can also be grouped by functions of specific areas: ingestion via the mouth and oesophagus, digestion in

---

23-1

Early detection of major gastrointestinal disorders

Signs requiring immediate medical follow-up

Mouth
A sore that bleeds easily and does not heal
A lump or thickening
A persistent red or whitish patch
Difficulty chewing, swallowing, or moving tongue or jaws

Abdomen
Persistent heartburn, indigestion
Abdominal pain, especially if accompanied by nausea and vomiting

Elimination
Change in bowel habits
Blood in the stool

In the United States the American Cancer Society recommendations for screening for cancer of colon and rectum
Digital rectal examination by doctor every year after age 40
Stool guaiac test done by patient at home every year after age 50
Sigmoidoscopic examination every 3 to 5 years after age 50; following two initial negative tests, 1 year apart.
Some of these tests, e.g. digital examination form part of a routine health screening in the United Kingdom and trials are currently underway regarding the efficacy of other measures.

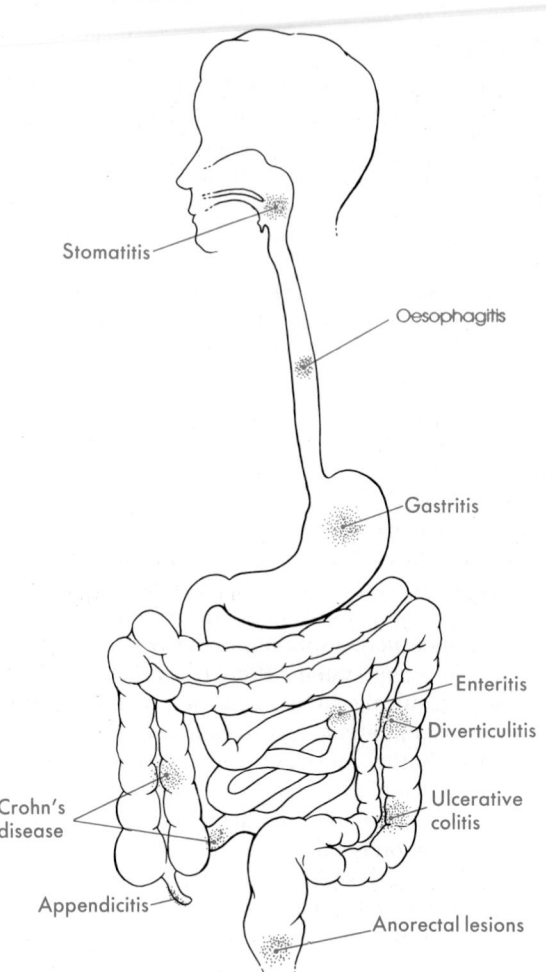

Stomatitis

Oesophagitis

Gastritis

Enteritis

Diverticulitis

Ulcerative colitis

Crohn's disease

Appendicitis

Anorectal lesions

Fig. 23-3   Inflammatory disorders of gastrointestinal system.

the stomach and duodenum, and elimination via the intestines. Common GI disorder classifications (as discussed in this chapter) are:

1. Ingestive disorders
   a. Inflammations of the mouth
   b. Oesophageal disorders
   c. Cancer of the mouth and oesophagus
2. Digestive disorders
   a. Gastritis
   b. Ulcerations of stomach and duodenum
   c. Cancer of the stomach
   d. Malabsorption syndromes
3. Elimination disorders
   a. Acute inflammatory intestinal disorders
   b. Chronic inflammatory intestinal disorders
   c. Ileus: paralytic, intestinal obstruction
   d. Hernias
   e. Anorectal lesions
   f. Colorectal cancer

NUTRITIONAL EXCESS AND DEFICIT

Ingesting more calories than are burned off by metabolism or activity leads to weight gain. Overweight (up to 20% above standard weight tables) does not in itself usually cause health problems, although the person is not at an optimal level of health (see Chapter 4). Obesity, however, does cause physiological problems. Nutritional deficiencies also cause problems, the most common deficiency being protein-energy malnutrition. Both obesity and protein-energy malnutrition may require therapy.

OBESITY

Obesity is generally defined as weight greater than 20% of standard weight tables. In the United Kingdom some 37% of men and 24% of women were overweight in 1986/87 and a further 12% of women and 8% of men were classified as being obese.[20b] Gross obesity is extremely hazardous to health.

Aetiology

Obesity results from a complex interrelationship of genetic, psychological, social, and environmental factors. Although "fatness" seems to occur in some families, much of this may be a result of learned eating behaviours of high caloric foods rather than genetic influence. Old age is not a factor; few elderly persons are obese. Mild overweight can be beneficial to elderly people, as it provides nutrient stores during periods of stress and illness.

Pathophysiology

Obesity results from the intake of foods in amounts exceeding body needs; the excess is stored as fat. In people

Table 23-3   Physiological effects of obesity

Parameter	Metabolic effect	Associated disorder
Increased fatty acid utilization	Hypertriglyceridaemia	Atherosclerosis, hypertension, emboli
	Increased cholesterol synthesis	Gallstones
Increased glucose	Hyperinsulinism leading to pancreatic β-cell failure	Diabetes mellitus
Increased body mass	Cumulative trauma to weight-bearing joints	Osteoarthritis
	Increased workload for heart	Angina, sudden death
	Decreased thorax expansion with decreased tidal volume	Respiratory insufficiency

of normal weight who gain weight, fat is deposited by *hypertrophy* of existing fat cells in adipose tissue. These people respond well to weight reduction regimens. Fat cells can also increase in number (*hyperplasia*). Excess food intake has been shown to stimulate hyperplasia. Hyperplasia is irreversible and conditions people to be overweight throughout their lives.[31] Weight reduction in people with hyperplastic obesity is difficult to achieve and to maintain.

Table 23-3 lists the physiological effects of obesity. Increased fatty acid utilization, glucose, and body mass may contribute to the development of atherosclerosis, hypertension, emboli, gallstones, diabetes mellitus, osteoarthritis, angina and sudden death, and respiratory insufficiency.

Interventions

Nursing diagnoses, expected outcomes, and implementation of nursing actions to help the overweight person are described in Chapter 4. People with severe or massive obesity often have difficulty losing weight or maintaining weight loss by the usual dietary, behaviour modification, and exercise approaches. These people may require more drastic therapy.

Very low calorie diets

A variety of very low calorie diets (VLCD) have been used to treat obesity. VLCD consists of powdered formulas of egg and milk proteins that provide 400 to 800 kcal/day. People taking VLCD lose 2 to 4 lb/week over a 4- to 6-month programme. Achievement of long-term weight loss requires a significant change in eating and exercise behaviours; therefore, the patient must follow behaviour modification and exercise programmes concurrently. Positive results of VLCD are rapid improvement in obesity-related diseases, but these benefits are offset by the potential for serious complications. Medical supervision is therefore essential. Side effects include hair loss, fatigue, cold intolerance, orthostatic hypotension, fluid and electrolyte disturbances, and other signs of protein-energy malnutrition. Long-term results are generally disappointing; the majority of these people regain considerable weight.[16,60]

Surgery

When the person is grossly obese and when other methods have been diligently tried and have failed, the doctor may consider surgery. Criteria for surgery include morbid obesity for at least 5 years, no major illness, evidence of serious dietary efforts, and high motivation. Obese people are a high surgical risk, however, and the surgery itself adds more risks.

The more common surgical approaches are *gastroplasty*, which reduces food intake (horizontal gastroplasty or vertical banding gastroplasty), and *gastric bypass*.

PROTEIN-ENERGY MALNUTRITION

Aetiology

Protein-energy malnutrition is a common form of nutritional deficiency in the United Kingdom. Causes include decreased nutrient intake, increased nutrient loss, and increased nutrient requirements (see Box 23-2). Approximately 50% of hospitalized adult patients have protein-energy malnutrition.[75] In developing countries, this disorder is a major health problem. It may occur in two forms, *Kwashiorkor* (protein deficiency when calorie intake is inadequate) and *marasmus* (deficiency

of both proteins and calories). The typical child with kwashiorkor has thin extremities and ascites of the abdomen.

Pathophysiology

If diets contain sufficient carbohydrates and fats, the body will use these nutrients for energy needs. When the caloric intake is reduced, however, increased amounts of body proteins will be used for energy. The body will meet energy requirements at the expense of protein needs.

A deficiency of both calories and protein is characteristic of protein-energy malnutrition in adults. Proteins are constantly being synthesized and broken down into amino acids in the body to be reformed into other proteins. Amino acids that are not used are excreted. The body can synthesize certain amino acids (nonessential) but depends on ingested proteins to supply the eight essential amino acids. When more nitrogen (the end product of amino acid breakdown) is excreted than is ingested in proteins, the body is said to be in *negative nitrogen balance*, and weight loss, decreased muscle mass, and weakness result from tissue catabolism.

With weight loss of more than 10% of body weight, loss of physiological function usually begins to develop, and loss of 35% to 40% usually results in death.[60] Protein loss leads to *decreased muscle mass*, especially in the liver, heart, lungs, GI tract, and immune system. Protein synthesis in the liver decreases, resulting in a decrease in serum proteins (hypoproteinaemia) that cause oedema. Cardiac output decreases. Respiratory muscles atrophy, leading to *decreased vital capacity*. Atrophy of GI mucosa and loss of intestinal villi cause *malabsorption*. Because lymphocytes are protein, a major complication is a decrease in lymphocyte production, especially T cells; this places the individual at high *risk for infection*. Haemoglobin levels may also decrease, because both haemoglobin and transferrin (which binds iron in haemoglobin) are proteins.

Nursing Process
Assessment

Subjective data

Obtain the following information from the patient:
1. Patient's perceptions about the weight loss
2. Dietary history
3. Foods that can be tolerated; likes and dislikes
4. Ability and desire to eat
5. Facilities and ability for purchasing, storing, and preparing food
6. Financial resources, if appropriate

Objective data

Objective data include the following:
1. Weight and height
   Underweight is considered to be less than 90% of desirable weight (Chapter 4); severe weight loss is less than 75% of desirable weight
2. Signs of infection or skin breakdown

Diagnostic tests

1. Low haemoglobin levels in absence of blood loss
2. Plasma albumin level of less than 30 g/L on two or more determinations, indicating decreased protein synthesis

Causes of protein-energy malnutrition

Decreased nutrient intake

Anorexia	Financial distress
Nausea	Inability to shop or
Dysphagia	cook
Mouth disorders	Decreased desire to
Pain	cook
	Depression
	Substance abuse

Increased nutrient losses

Vomiting	Diarrhoea
Malabsorption	Immobility

Increased nutrient requirements

Surgery	Infection
Fever	Cancer

3. Urinary creatinine of less than 20 mg/kg in 24 hours for males or less than 16 mg/kg in females, with a normal plasma creatinine level, indicating decreased muscle mass. N.B. Normally the urinary excretion of creatinine in 24 hours is 20 mmol (2g) in men and 10 mmol (1g) in women.

Nursing analysis

Problems are determined from analysis of patient data. Possible problems for the person with protein-energy malnutrition may include, but are not limited to, the following:

Problem	Possible aetiologies
Fatigue	Muscle weakness, inadequate nutrition
Infection, high risk for	Decreased nutrition, decreased immune response
Nutrition, altered: less than body requirements	Inadequate nutrient intake, increased nutrient losses, increased nutrient requirements

Planning: expected patient outcomes

If oral intake is permitted, the patient's fullest cooperation will be needed to increase the possibility of adequate nutritional intake. Patient participation in the planning is therefore a vital part of the care.

Expected patient outcomes for the person with protein-energy malnutrition may include, but are not limited to, the following:

1. The patient includes rest periods in the day's activities.
2. Infection does not occur.
3. If eating is permitted, the patient:
   a. Participates in menu selection.
   b. Eats all food on tray, if hospitalized.
   c. Eats six small meals per day plus supplementary foods and vitamins, as planned, at home.
4. If tube feedings are given:
   a. Feedings are given at a slow, constant rate.
   b. Patient is hydrated.
   c. Patient states feeling comfortable.
   d. Complications do not occur or are quickly corrected.

5. If total parenteral nutrition (TPN) is given:
   a. Fluid and electrolyte balance is maintained.
   b. Hypoglycaemia or hyperglycaemia do not occur.
   c. Infection and air embolism do not occur.
   d. Patient states feeling comfortable.

Implementation

Assisting with achievement of therapeutic goals

Gastrostomy

Method. Gastrostomy is an alternative approach to nasogastric tube feedings when the person is unable to swallow for a long period. The procedure takes place under local or general anaesthesia and involves the creation of an opening into the abdomen and insertion of the catheter through the stomach wall.

The *percutaneous endoscopic gastrostomy* (PEG) does not require incision into the abdominal cavity and is a safer and more rapid method. It is performed under local anaesthesia; the patient is mildly sedated. A small incision is made in the skin of the abdomen, and a cannula is pushed through the adjacent abdominal and gastric walls while the site is observed through a gastroscope. A long silk suture is threaded through the cannula, grasped through the endoscope, and pulled up through the endoscope, which is then removed. The exit end of a specially prepared mushroom catheter is attached to the thread, and the catheter is then pulled in retrograde fashion through the oesophagus and stomach and out the abdominal wall. Internal and external dams hold the catheter in place. A jejunostomy tube may be inserted by the same method.

Food and fluids. After gastrostomy tube insertion, the doctor may order the tube to be attached to low intermittent suction for 24 hours, or fluids may begin the first day. The following method may be used for giving the initial feedings, as tolerated:[16]

Day 1: One half concentration of feeding solution at 25 ml/h by continuous drip

Day 2: Full-strength feeding solution at 50 ml/h by continuous drip

Day 3: Full-strength solution at 75 ml/h by continuous drip

After day 3, as tolerated: change to bolus feeding of 500 ml every 4 to 6 hours for gastrostomies; jejunostomies require continuous infusions

Principles of administration are the same as for tube feedings. A dressing is not generally used to prevent the possibility of skin maceration, breakdown, or infection. Clean the skin with a suitable solution to remove crusts and rinse with normal saline or water.

The psychological trauma of not being able to eat normally is usually severe. The patient may become depressed and needs a great deal of encouragement. However, as most patients become proficient in feeding themselves, they gradually accept this method of obtaining nourishment as inevitable and adjust remarkably well.

Interventions to achieve patient outcomes

Preventing fatigue

The loss of muscle mass and the decreased utilization of nutrients lead to decreased energy production and fatigue.

Table 23-4   Tube feedings

	Elemental	Supplemental	Liquid whole foods
Content	Simple carbohydrates, amino acids	Complex carbohydrates, peptides	Complex carbohydrates, proteins
Advantages	Given through small-bore tube Well tolerated for prolonged use	Can be given through small-bore tube More effective protein content than elemental	Lower osmolality Moderate price Acceptable flavour More nutritionally complete
Disadvantages	Unpalatable High osmolality Not well tolerated by bolus feeding Excellent culture media for bacteria Expensive Require monitoring of blood glucose and electrolytes	More expensive than liquid whole foods Tend to coagulate in tube Require monitoring of blood glucose and electrolytes	High fat content Tend to coagulate in tube May require a large-bore tube

Rest periods are therefore essential to decrease energy expenditure. Dyspnoea with exertion and pulse rates that take longer than 5 minutes to stabilize are signs that activities need to be modified.

Preventing infection

Maintenance of medical and surgical asepsis is particularly important for the person with protein-energy malnutrition. These individuals should avoid any person with upper respiratory infections. If the patient is relatively immobile in chair or bed, good skin care is essential to prevent skin breakdown and subsequent infection. Surgical wounds may heal more slowly, and they require strict surgical asepsis.

Encouraging oral intake

Adequate nutrients to meet nutritional requirements can be taken orally, enteraly (tube feedings, gastrostomy), or as TPN. The best way to receive nutrients is the oral route. People with inadequate nutrition stores need encouragement to eat, although forced feeding may lead to frustration or nausea and vomiting. Motivating a person with anorexia to eat can be a challenge. Interventions that can correct the cause will lead to improved appetite. Providing an environment conducive to eating and providing several small meals rather than three large meals per day may facilitate an adequate nutritional intake.

A high-calorie, high-protein diet is indicated if the patient can eat. The diet is essentially a normal one with added protein and supplementary high-calorie feedings. High-protein diets are contraindicated if there is liver disease.

Facilitating tube feedings

Nasoenteral tubes are used to provide nutrients when a person with normal intestinal function is unable to ingest sufficient nutrients by oral ingestion, has difficulty swallowing, or has mild to moderate malabsorption (short bowel syndrome). The tube is inserted through the nose and terminates in the stomach, duodenum, or jejunum.

Feeding tubes are soft polyurethane or silicone tubes with a narrow lumen (usually No. 5F to No. 8F), although in some instances a larger bore tube (No. 12F or No. 14F) may be necessary. Some tubes have a monofilament or stainless steel stylet for easy passage. A tube with a weighted end may be used to help pass the tube through the pylorus into the intestine, if desired.

Technique. Administration of tube feedings may be by bolus, gravity drip, or infusion pump. *Bolus* delivery consists of infusing 300 to 400 ml of feed over several minutes four to six times daily.[28] It is appropriate only for people who can eat and are receiving supplemental tube feedings. The sudden influx of the feeding may cause nausea, cramping, diarrhoea, or aspiration. The *gravity* method consists of placing the feeding in a feeding bag attached to the nasoenteral tube and allowing the fluid to run in by gravity. Disadvantages of this method include erratic fluid flow and greater potential of tube blockage. The gravity method may be used for intermittent or continuous administration. Most people can tolerate 250 to 400 ml per feeding given over 20 to 30 minutes. The *infusion pump* is the preferred method for more constant administration rate and less probability of tube blockage or of diarrhoea; however, it is more expensive. Pump accuracy must be checked routinely by comparing the actual drop count with the preestablished rate.

Solutions. Different types of fluids may be given by tube feedings (Table 23-4). Liçvidized whole foods may be used; these are nutritious and less expensive, but they require large-bore tubes and are good culture media for bacteria. Elemental and semielemental feedings are more easily digested and can be given through small-bore tubes, but they are more expensive and less nutritionally complete than liquid whole foods.

Complications. Methods of preventing complications include the following:
1. Regurgitation with aspiration
   a. Keep head elevated to at least 30 degrees at all times.
   b. Monitor tube position every 4 hours.
2. Tube dislodgement: tape tube to nose.

3. Tube clogging
   a. Give fluid at a constant rate (by pump, if possible).
   b. Give water before and after intermittent feedings and medications, and 4 hourly during continuous feedings.
   c. Give medications by *liquid* form; crushed tablets may clog tube.
4. Bacterial contamination
   a. Do not let feeding of freshly liquidized feeds (perish-able) hang for more than 6 hours, ready-to-use feeds more than 24 hours, and all other feeds more than 12 hours.
   b. Use prefilled delivery sets if possible; if unavailable, use ready-to-use feeds that do not have to be diluted or reconstituted (the less the handling, the less the potential for contamination).
   c. Rinse delivery set before adding new feed.
5. Dehydration
   a. Give water as necessary; total fluid intake should equal urinary output.
   b. Iso-osmolality is 300 mOsm; the greater the osmolality of the feeding, the more water is needed.
   c. Give extra water if the need is increased, as with fever.
   d. Monitor for signs of dehydration: thirst, oliguria, decreased skin turgor, dry mucous membranes.
6. Diarrhoea
   a. When starting tube feedings, initiate feedings slowly at half-strength, then increase concentration and rate gradually (at different times).
   b. Dilute elixirs and hypertonic oral suspensions before inserting through feeding tube.
   c. If diarrhoea occurs:
      1. Check concurrent medications for those that may be causing the diarrhoea; consult with doctor.
      2. If medication is not a cause, decrease rate of fluid flow.
      3. Administer prescribed antidiarrhoeal medication through tube.
7. Hyperglycaemia
   a. Monitor urine for glucose and acetone every 4 to 6 hours until stable.
   b. If urine tests positively, decrease rate of feeding flow and notify doctor.

Home tube feedings. Patients can maintain home tube feedings after receiving instruction in insertion and care of the tube, in feed care and insertion, and in monitoring for complications. An enteral feeding pump may be borrowed or purchased. The person needs to know where in the community to obtain materials (tubes, administration sets, and feed bags).

Facilitating total parenteral nutrition

Total parenteral nutrition (TPN) is a method of giving concentrated solutions intravenously to maintain protein synthesis. Indications for this therapy are (1) major gastrointestinal diseases, fistulas, or inflammatory diseases; (2) extensive negative nitrogen balance, such as occurs with major body burns, extensive wounds, or cachexia; and (3) gastrointestinal side effects from radiation therapy.

Technique. Under strict aseptic conditions, a central venous catheter is inserted into the subclavian vein through the chest wall or into the basilic vein in the antecubital fossa and then threaded through to the superior vena cava. The large amount of blood in the superior vena cava helps to dilute the highly concentrated solution rapidly and thus prevent phlebitis or vein occlusion.

A Hickman catheter is commonly used in place of a standard intracatheter. This catheter is designed so that the end of the catheter can be capped between infusions. When infusion is complete, fill the catheter with heparinized saline solution to prevent clotting and cap it until the next infusion.

The catheter is secured with one suture and covered by an air-occlusive dressing. The dressing may be transparent or a gauze dressing covered entirely with adhesive tape. Start the infusion with a standard intravenous fluid (5% dextrose) until a radiograph confirms the location of the catheter tip in the superior vena cava.

Solutions. Solutions for TPN are good culture media and are prepared under strict aseptic conditions in the pharmacy under a laminar airflow hood. The doctor orders the solution contents based on the person's nutritional needs. Keep the solutions refrigerated until ready for use and then warm them to room temperature before infusion. Use prepared solutions within 48 hours to prevent contamination.

TPN solutions usually consist of 25% to 35% dextrose, 3% to 5% amino acids, electrolytes, minerals, and vitamins. Fat emulsions (10% to 20%) may also be added through a separate peripheral IV over 4 to 12 hours or through a Y connector in the main line.[71] Dextrose and fat are given for caloric value to spare the proteins for anabolism. Fat provides twice the caloric value of glucose, exerts minimal osmotic pressure, and prevents fatty acid deficiency. Regular insulin may be added to the TPN solution or may be given by injection for glucose utilization.

Complications. Complications of TPN may be mechanical, infectious, or metabolic. *Mechanical* problems may include pneumothorax, haemothorax, air embolism, catheter misplacement, brachial plexus injury, and thromboembolism. These complications are rare with correct catheter insertion and maintenance. *Infection* is a serious complication but can be prevented by using conscientious aseptic technique during catheter insertion and subsequent care.

The major *metabolic* alterations are hyperglycaemia or, more rarely, hypoglycaemia. Other possible alterations include fluid imbalances; electrolyte imbalances in sodium, potassium, calcium, magnesium, and phosphates; and acid-base imbalances (primarily acidosis). Vitamin D deficiency and vitamin A excess may also occur. Monitor serum levels several times a week, and test blood sugar and urine for sugar and acetone. Weigh the patient daily for the first 2 weeks and three times a week thereafter. Early satiety may occur for several days after TPN is discontinued.

Patient care. Care of the patient receiving TPN consists of preventing infection and air embolism, maintaining fluid and electrolyte balance, encouraging ambulation and activities of daily living, and promoting comfort (see Box 23-3).

Patients may have many fears and concerns about being fed

The patient receiving total parenteral nutrition

Prevent infection
  Maintain strict aseptic technique
  Keep solutions cold until ready for use; use within 24 to 36 hours
  Change dressings according to established protocols
Prevent air embolism
  Position patient as flat as possible during dressing and tubing changes
  Tape all connections of the system
  Clamp catheter when opening system
  Cover insertion site with an air-occlusive dressing (covered with adhesive tape) or transparent dressing
Maintain fluid and electrolyte balance
  Maintain a continuous uniform infusion rate
  If rate is too *slow*:
    Return rate to prescribed rate
    If prescribed rate does not resume, ask person to change position
    Monitor and report to doctor signs of *hypoglycaemia* (pallor, diaphoresis, tachycardia, hunger, trembling, behavioural changes)
  If rate is too *fast*:
    Slow infusion to prescribed rate
    Monitor for signs of *overhydration* (neck vein distension, cough, weight gain)
    Monitor for signs of *hyperglycaemia* (blood sugar in urine, nausea, weakness, thirst, headache)
  Monitor daily weights and intake and output
  Monitor serum electrolyte, glucose, and blood urea levels
Encourage ambulation, activities of daily living
Promote comfort
  Provide for good oral hygiene
  Provide emotional support to enhance coping

---

by intravenous fluids over a long period of time. They should understand what is occurring and the reason for the frequent dressing changes. Encourage them to sit at the dinner table to participate in the social interaction. If food is not permitted orally, people may need aid in coping with stress incurred by the smell of food or watching others eat. If receiving TPN over a long period of time, they may be concerned about regaining taste or normal eating patterns. Being fed only by tube, even though temporary, may create stress from a change in body image. Encourage patients to express their feelings and support them in developing coping patterns to deal with these stresses (see Chapter 5).

Home total parenteral nutrition. Since the advent of home total parenteral nutrition (HTPN) many people have been able to lead more nearly normal lives—going to work or school and participating in selected activities, including sexual. These people infuse the solutions over a 12-hour period overnight and then participate in normal daily activities. Their lives are somewhat limited by being connected to the infusing equipment for the 12 hours, although there are vest systems that support the HTPN solution, tubing, and pump to provide increased mobility. There are also 24-hour battery packs to provide more freedom for the person who is connected to a pump that requires an electrical outlet.

Learning to mix, infuse, and disconnect the infusion and care for the equipment may be overwhelming at first for both patient and family. The hospital nurse begins teaching in the hospital well before the patient is discharged; the community nurse continues the process at home. Teaching includes the following:

1. Principles of aseptic technique
2. Opening and setting up bags
3. Starting pump, stopping infusion, flushing tubing, clamping tube
4. Maintaining and troubleshooting equipment
5. Catheter care
6. Monitoring for signs of complications
7. Where to obtain supplies and need for storage space for supplies in the home

Companies that supply HTPN equipment and supplies often have a nutrition support nurse who can provide information as necessary and may have an instruction manual for patient use.[18]

Nutrition teams are available to assist the person or family member to carry out TPN care at home. Before the patient is discharged, the community nurse meets the other team members and the patient to facilitate the move home. The community nurse then assists the person with HTPN at home until the person becomes self-sufficient and can manage independently. The patient maintains contact with the health team for assistance with changes that are needed and with problems that may arise. The person often requires changes in solution content depending on response to therapy.

Complications of HTPN are similar to those of TPN. However, risk of infection increases, mostly from *Staphylococcus aureus*. Catheter damage may occur from repeated cross-clamping; however, the catheter may be repaired with a catheter repair kit. An occluded catheter may be opened by instillation of urokinase or streptokinase into the catheter. Unusual metabolic deficiencies may occur with long-term therapy, such as deficiencies in chromium, selenium, molybdenum, and vitamins A and E.

HTPN is expensive, but the cost is considerably less than the similar care provided in a hospital. In addition, the person can remain at home and have continuity in activities of daily living.

Evaluation

Evaluation is based on expected patient outcomes. Questions to consider include the following:

1. Does the patient include rest periods in the day's activities?
2. Has infection been avoided?
3. If eating is permitted, does the patient participate in menu selection?
4. If tube feedings are given, is patient hydrated?
5. If TPN is given, have infection, air embolism, and other complications been avoided?

INGESTIVE DISORDERS

VOMITING

Although vomiting is a symptom rather than a disorder per se, it is a common disruption of motility of the upper GI tract and therefore is discussed here.

Pathophysiology

Vomiting is often preceded by nausea but may occur alone. It may be a symptom of a disease process (such as infection or uraemia) or a response to drugs, visceral injury, pain, psychic trauma, radiation, or motion. Vomiting is initiated by the vomiting centre in the brain. It is reverse peristalsis. Vomiting can be defined as forceful ejection of stomach contents. If the pyloric end of the stomach is obstructed, the vomitus will project away from the person (projectile vomiting).

Prolonged and severe vomiting will interfere with nutrition and cause fluid and electrolyte imbalance, specifically dehydration and metabolic alkalosis with loss of potassium, chloride, and hydrogen ions. The act of vomiting produces a strain on the abdominal muscles, and in some postoperative patients it may cause wound dehiscence or bleeding. Vomiting is especially dangerous for anaesthetized patients, comatose people, and infants because they are likely to aspirate the vomitus into the lungs. Aspiration may block oxygen intake (asphyxia) or lead to inflammation of the lung (atelectasis, pneumonitis), especially in an elderly person whose nasopharyngeal reflexes are less acute than those of a younger person.

Assessment

Subjective data: onset of vomiting, patient's perception of cause

Objective data: examination of vomitus
1. Greenish yellow: bile
2. Bright red: overt bleeding of recent origin
3. Brownish "coffee-ground": blood has been in the stomach for a period of time and is partly digested
4. Faecal odour: intestinal contents from an intestinal obstruction

Vomiting of blood is termed *haematemesis*. It is important to ascertain whether the content expelled from the mouth has been vomited from the stomach or coughed up from the lungs. Bloody sputum usually has a more frothy appearance than haematemesis. "Dry" emesis or retching may occur when the stomach is empty.

Implementation

1. Assisting with achievement of therapeutic goals
   a. If vomiting is anticipated (such as with radiation or motion), give prescribed antiemetic 30 minutes before the event.
   b. If vomiting is present, give prescribed antiemetic by suppository or intramuscular injection.
2. Assisting with comfort
   a. Provide a calm environment to decrease anxiety.
   b. Suggest deep breaths through the mouth if nausea or gagging occurs.

   c. Remove vomitus as soon as possible and provide oral hygiene.
   d. Provide fluids in small amounts after vomiting subsides; effervescent drinks are usually well tolerated.
   e. Provide solid foods (after vomiting subsides) that are well tolerated, such as plain biscuits, baked potato, or apple.

INFLAMMATORY DISORDERS OF THE MOUTH

Aetiology

The mouth is an excellent barometer of general health, reflecting general disease and debility as well as good health. Specific diseases of the mouth most often occur when general nutrition and oral hygiene are poor, when people neglect their teeth, and when smoking is excessive.

In the mouth, inflammation may occur on the mucous membranes, gum, or tongue from viruses, bacteria, fungi, or irritants.

Pathophysiology

Several factors contribute to the development of oral inflammatory disorders: (1) poor oral hygiene, (2) stress, (3) nutritional deficiencies, (4) debilitating diseases, (5) heavy smoking, and (6) chemotherapy. Poor oral hygiene leads to mouth debris that can irritate the mucous membranes. Other irritants include smoke, broken teeth, and irritating foods. Stress, malnutrition, and chemotherapy interfere with the body's immune response, leading to breakdown of body defences.

Inflammation of the mucous membranes (*stomatitis*) often results in small, painful ulcerations. Scarring rarely occurs, as only the mucous membrane is usually involved. Inflammation of the gums may cause teeth to loosen. Causative organisms include bacteria, viruses, or fungi.

Aphthous stomatitis (Table 23-5) occurs frequently, especially among young adults. The lesions are painful but usually heal in about 1 to 3 weeks. *Herpetic* stomatitis may occur only once or be recurrent. People receiving immunosuppressive drugs have increased susceptibility.

Thrush frequently occurs when antibiotics are given over a period of time to control other infections. It is thought that the elimination of bacteria permits growth of the existing fungus, causing thrush. People at higher risk include denture wearers, people with debilitating or acute illnesses, or those with impaired immune response.[60]

The parotid gland that drains into the mouth may also become inflamed (parotitis). Acute communicable parotitis (mumps) is caused by a virus that is transmitted by direct contact with the saliva. Noncommunicable parotitis occurs in debilitated people whose oral hygiene is poor, whose mouths have been permitted to become dry, and who have not chewed solid foods regularly. Elderly people are more susceptible than younger ones. Usually the *staphylococcus* organism is not present.

Nursing Process
Assessment

In patients at high risk of developing infections, assess the mouth daily for developing or healing inflammations.

REVIEW

Table 23-5 Inflammatory disorders of the mouth

Disease	Signs and symptoms	Medical therapy
Aphthous stomatitis (canker sores)	Ulcer on mucous membranes becomes covered with opaque material; pain	Hydrocortisone pellets
Herpetic stomatitis (cold sore, fever blister)	Painful vesicle formation on junction of lips to mucosa, lymphadenopathy, crusting, malaise	Symptomatic treatment: analgesics, bland mouth rinses; rest; avoidance of stress; acyclovir
Vincent's gingivitis (ulceromembranous stomatitis)	Malaise, acute painful bleeding gums, fetid breath, ulceration on margins of gums, dysphagia	Gentle debridement by dentist; mouthwashes with warm normal saline or 3% hydrogen peroxide; rest; antibiotics if severe
Candidiasis (thrush)	White patches (like mike curds) over inflamed membranes	Nystatin, miconazole, amphotericin
Gingivitis (gums)	Red inflamed gums, bleeding with minimum injury, swelling of interdental spaces	Good oral hygiene and dental care
Periodontitis (loss of bone supporting teeth	Same as for gingivitis, loose teeth, recession of gums, possible abscess formation	Dental care, dental surgery

Subjective data

Question the patient about the presence and extent of the following symptoms: (1) pain in the mouth, (2) loss of appetite, (3) nausea, (4) foul taste in the mouth, and (5) increase or decrease of salivation. The inflammatory response causes the pain, which restricts ability or desire to keep the teeth and mouth clean. This leads to the foul taste and loss of appetite. Swallowing of inflammatory debris may produce nausea.

Objective data

1. Mouth inspection
   a. Cleanliness
   b. Condition of teeth (caries, loose teeth, debris)
   c. Signs of inflammation (redness, oedema, ulceration, or white curdlike patches of thrush)
   d. Bleeding of mucous membranes or gums
2. Ability of patient to carry out oral hygiene
   a. Mental status (decreased consciousness or confusion)
   b. Ability to open mouth (pain may limit mouth movement)
   c. Cleanliness of mouth after oral hygiene
3. Ability to ingest and swallow food

Nursing analysis

Problems are determined from analysis of patient data. Possible problems for the person with a mouth infection may include, but are not limited to, the following:

Problem	Possible aetiologies
Oral mucous membrane, altered	Poor oral hygiene, inflammation
Pain, mouth	Inflammation of mouth
Fluid volume deficit, high risk for	Foul taste, mouth discomfort
Nutrition, altered: less than body requirements	Difficulty chewing, foul taste, mouth discomfort
Knowledge deficit	Lack of exposure/recall

Planning: expected patient outcomes

Expected patient outcomes for the person with a mouth infection may include, but are not limited to, the following:

1. Mouth is clean; mucosa is pink and moist.
2. Says mouth feels comfortable.
3. Has a fluid intake greater than 1500 ml/day; skin turgor is good.
4. Eats a balanced diet; weight remains stable.
5. Describes risk factors to be avoided to prevent recurrence of oral inflammations.

Implementation

Assisting with achievement of therapeutic goals

If antibiotics are ordered, give them on time on a regular basis to maintain blood levels. If the patient has difficulty swallowing tablets, crush the tablets, if possible, or give the antibiotics intramuscularly or intravenously. If nystatin is prescribed for oral thrush, the patient should hold the suspension and swish it through the mouth for as long as possible before swallowing it.

Interventions to achieve patient outcomes

Providing mouth care

Thorough and frequent mouth care is a must to remove the debris and to permit healing of the oral mucosa.

1. Frequency
   a. Mild stomatitis: at least every 4 hours
   b. Severe stomatitis: at least every 2 hours
2. Types of solutions
   a. Alkaline mouthwashes, such as sodium bicarbonate or sodium perborate
   b. Hydrogen peroxide diluted 1:4 with normal saline (mix just before use to prevent decomposition)
   c. Lignocaine gel rinses may be prescribed for stomatitis resulting from chemotherapeutic drugs

3. Removal of dentures if causing pain
4. Use foam-sponge toothbrushes
5. If the toothbrush causes pain, gently wipe gum and teeth with moistened gauze wrapped around a tongue depresser; rinse with solution followed by water

Promoting pain relief

Pain may be partially relieved by good oral hygiene. Smoking is contraindicated. Cold drinks or sucking on an ice lolly may be soothing. Analgesic drugs may be necessary, and lignocaine may be applied to provide topical anaesthesia.

Facilitating eating and drinking

If the mouth is very sore and painful, eating may be difficult, and the patient may need considerable encouragement. Patients can best tolerate soft foods, including strained meats and fish, pureed vegetables and fruits (except citrus), cooked cereals, soups, fruit jelly, and ice cream. Hot spicy foods are to be avoided; cold drinks may be soothing. High-protein, high-calorie drinks such as eggnog serve both nutritional and fluid needs.

Patient teaching

People at high risk for developing recurrent oral infections need to know about contributing factors that may be controlled, such as poor oral hygiene, poor nutrition, irritating foods, heavy smoking, and stress (see preventive measures, p. 596).

Evaluation

Evaluation is based on the expected patient outcomes. Interventions may have to be modified based on the severity of the oral infection. Assess mouth daily for cleanliness and extent of healing and comfort. Questions to consider include

1. Are mucous membranes clear and pink?
2. Does the patient state mouth feels comfortable?
3. Is the patient hydrated?
4. Has the patient's weight remained stable?
5. Can the patient describe ways to avoid recurrent infection?

CANCER OF THE MOUTH

Epidemiology

Cancer of the mouth (Table 23-6) accounts for about 2% of all cancers.[66a] Men are affected more often than women, and occurrences are more frequent after age 45; the average patient age is about 55. In the United States an increasing number of teenagers are developing oral cancer from chewing tobacco or betel leaf. Although any part of the mouth may be affected, the lips and the anterior tongue and floor of the mouth are the most common sites.

Pathophysiology

Most oral cancers are squamous cell carcinomas; occasionally the tumour may be a basal cell carcinoma that starts on the skin and spreads to the lips. Risk factors include heavy tobacco and alcohol use; the combination causes an apparent breakdown in the immune system. Ultraviolet rays from the sun are a risk factor for cancer of the lips.

Oral cancers can be classified according to four stages. In stages I and II, there is no lymph node spread or metastasis; tumour size varies from less than 2 cm (I) up to 4 cm (II). In stage III, the tumour size is greater than 4 cm, and there may be a palpable node on one side. In stage IV, the tumour is invasive, and there may be metastasis to the liver or lungs. Surgery or radiation may be used to treat stage I cancers, and both therapies are used for stages II and III. Stage IV therapy is usually palliative.

Premalignant lesions (that may or may not become malignant) include *leukoplakia* (white patches), *erythroplasia* (red granular patches), and *erythroplakia* (white plaques within red patches). The red patches have a higher potential for malignancy than leukoplakia.[60]

The cure rate for cancer of the *lips* is high because the lesion is easily apparent to the patient and to others. Metastasis to regional lymph nodes has occurred in many people when the case is diagnosed. In some instances a lesion may spread rapidly and involve the mandible and the floor of the mouth by direct extension.

Table 23-6   Cancer of mouth and oesophagus

Place	Contributing factors	Signs and symptoms	Medical therapy
Mouth			
Lips	Smoking, alcohol, sunlight	Fissure or painless indurated ulcer	Excision, jaw reconstruction if extensive
Anterior tongue and floor of mouth	Smoking, alcohol, chewing tobacco	Ulcer or growth	Local tissue perfusion with antimetabolites; Partial or total excision of tongue; Radical neck dissection (if extensive); Radiation therapy instead of or following surgery
Oesophagus	Alcohol, heavy smoking	Dysphagia, regurgitation, aspiration of fluids, foul breath odour	Upper and middle one third: oesophagogastrostomy; Lower one third: oesophagogastrectomy

Cancer of the *anterior tongue* and *floor of the mouth* may seem to occur together because their spread to adjacent tissues is so rapid. Metastasis to the neck has already occurred in more than 50% of people when the diagnosis is made because of the tongue's abundant vascular and lymphatic drainage. The mortality rate is high in stages III and IV. Lesions about the base of the tongue may go unnoticed by the patient and may be far advanced when treatment begins.

Prevention and Health Education

Primary prevention includes the following:
1. Avoid excess exposure to sun and wind on lips; use lip balm with sunscreen.
2. Eliminate smoking or chewing tobacco or betel leaf.
3. Maintain good oral hygiene and dental care.

Secondary prevention includes frequent dental examinations (the dentist may identify early lesions) and consulting the doctor for a mouth lesion that does not heal within 2 to 3 weeks.

Nursing Process

Assessment

Subjective data

1. Eating patterns: changes may occur in the ability to eat certain foods, especially solids.
2. Discomfort in mouth (only seen with extensive lesions).
3. Concerns: the person's facial appearance will usually change, depending on the amount of tissue to be removed during surgery. Even with reconstructive surgery, noticeable changes will be present.

Objective data

Condition of mouth: people with oral cancer frequently have poor dental hygiene; chemotherapy or radiation threatens intactness of mucous membranes; breath may be foul.

Nursing analysis

Determine problems from analysis of patient data. Possible problems for the person receiving therapy for cancer of the mouth may include, but are not limited to, the following:

Problem	Possible aetiologies
Oral mucous membranes, altered	Oral cavity radiation, decreased salivation
Nutrition, altered: less than body requirements	Chewing or swallowing difficulties, anorexia
Verbal communication, impaired	Resection of oral tissue
Body image disturbance	Actual/threat of facial/head disfigurement with therapy, foul breath

Planning: expected patient outcomes

Expected patient outcomes for the person receiving therapy for cancer of the mouth may include, but are not limited to, the following:
1. Incisions heal without infection.
2. Patient feeds self through appropriate means and consumes a nutritionally balanced fluid or soft diet.

3. Patient has a means of communication and is working to improve speech.
4. Patient interacts with others and states plans for gradual resumption of activities involving others.

Implementation

Assisting with achievement of therapeutic goals
Surgery

The tongue may be partially excised (hemiglossectomy) or totally excised (glossectomy). If the lymph nodes are involved, a radical neck dissection (Chapter 15) may be performed.

Antibiotics may be given *preoperatively* to decrease the number of bacteria present in the mouth. Prostheses of the palate and jaw may be designed to replace portions of tissue that have been resected. If a prosthesis is to be made, impressions will be taken during the preoperative period; the prosthesis will be fitted when healing has occurred postoperatively. If a composite resection including a radical neck dissection is to be performed, reconstructive surgery will be done, if possible, during the initial procedure; it may also be performed at a later date. *Postoperative* care of the patient is focused on promoting an adequate airway, mouth drainage, oral hygiene, comfort, nutrition, and speech (see Box 23-4).

Facilitating oral hygiene. Good mouth care is essential for comfort, prevention of infection, and promotion of healing. Teeth brushing is usually contraindicated because of discomfort and potential trauma. Use sterile equipment to prevent introduction of exogenous organisms, and encourage patients to assist in their oral hygiene as soon as possible.

Facilitating nutrition. Most patients can suction and feed themselves a few days after mouth surgery and are happier doing so. Chewing is difficult without the tongue, and the person has a problem getting the food to the posterior pharynx. Sensation in the mouth is decreased, and the patient has difficulty locating the position of the food in the oral cavity. One method of eating is for the person to use the forefinger to push the food to the posterior pharynx.

Facilitating communication. The patient commonly loses the ability to speak for short or long periods after surgery, but if the vocal chords are intact, speech will eventually return. A magic slate, letter board or flash cards may be used for communication; however, some patients have difficulty using these methods because of visual impairments. Conversation can be carried out so that the patient's responses can be limited to affirmative or negative gestures. Loud noises are disturbing to the patient because the oral tissue loss may create a channel that amplifies sound; therefore address the patient in a soft, clear voice. Speech retraining may be necessary, and a tape recorder may be useful for the patient to hear his or her own voice to work on improvements.

Radiation

Tumours of the mouth may be treated by radiation in various forms. Needles containing radium, radioactive cobalt, or other radioactive substances may be inserted and left in place for a prescribed time. Seeds containing emanations from

The patient undergoing mouth surgery for cancer

Preoperative care

Clarify patient's knowledge of expected changes after surgery.

Explain expected postoperative measures (including suctioning, nasogastric tube).

Provide opportunities for patient and family to begin to express feelings about changes in body image.

Postoperative care

Monitoring

Assess facial movement for facial nerve damage (if parotid gland excised): ask patient to raise eyebrows, frown, smile, show teeth, pucker lips.

Assess degree and character of drainage.

Amount of drainage and presence of blood should be minimal.

Haemorrhage may occur with wide resection of tongue.

Maintaining adequate airway/promoting drainage

Have patient lying on side initially.

Have patient in upright position when fully alert.

Suction mouth (except for lip surgery).

Gauze wick may be used to direct saliva into a vomit bowl.

Maintain patency of drainage tubes, if used.

Promoting oral hygiene and comfort

Clean involved areas of mouth with cotton applicator moistened with hydrogen peroxide and saline.

Mouth irrigations

Use sterile equipment.

Use solution of sterile water, diluted hydrogen peroxide, normal saline, or sodium bicarbonate (avoid commercial mouthwashes).

Protect any dressings from getting wet.

A catheter may be inserted along the side of cheek and the solution injected with gentle pressure; a spray may also be used.

Give analgesics as indicated (pain is usually mild).

Promoting nutrition

Tube feedings will be used initially with hemiglossectomy.

Oral fluids: place in back of throat with suitably modified syringe or feeding cup with attached tubing.

Eating soft foods

Encourage patient to feed self when possible.

Teach patient to follow all meals with clear water to cleanse mouth.

Avoid using fork, which may traumatize new tissue.

Foods

Avoid long-term use of commercial preparations such as instant breakfast drinks (may cause diarrhoea or constipation).

Fruit-flavoured yogurt preparations are less irritating than fruit jelly and easier to swallow.

Avoid very hot or cold foods (hot foods irritate new tissue; cold foods may cause facial pain or paralyze oral functions).

Promoting speech

Limit patient responses initially to yes–no questions that can be answered by gestures.

Encourage patient when speech returns to speak slowly.

Listen carefully and validate communication before initiating action on requests.

Speak in a soft clear voice.

Refer patient to speech therapist if necessary.

Encourage socialization with others.

---

radium or radioactive cobalt may be used and left in place indefinitely or else removed. External radiation treatment using X-rays or other radioactive substances may be prescribed.

Radiation therapy produces secondary effects in the mouth that include mucositis, dryness, dental decay, and tightening of the jaw muscle. Some of the changes may be permanent. The initial reaction is an inflammation of the mucous membrane. Sloughing of the tissues may occur and cause a fetid odour. Dentures are not tolerated for some time thereafter because of the sensitivity of the tissues. Dryness of the mouth begins 1 to 2 weeks after radiation therapy begins and may persist throughout life. The dryness makes the mouth feel uncomfortable and gives an unpleasant taste.

Decreased salivary secretion and altered pH of the saliva contribute to rapid dental decay, especially at the gingival margins. The patient should begin an active dental control programme before radiation therapy starts. Fluoride treatments to the teeth may be given and a conscientious toothbrushing regimen is instituted.

The general care of the patient receiving radiation therapy is discussed in Chapter 9. Specific considerations for the patient receiving radiation of the mouth include the following:

1. Provide good oral hygiene.
2. Remove dentures at night; check dentures for fit.
3. Encourage fluid intake of at least 2500 ml/day unless contraindicated.
4. Encourage chewing sugar-free gum or lozenges to stimulate salivation.
5. Provide humidity in air for added moisture and comfort.
6. Avoid very hot or cold food, dry bulky foods, or smoking to decrease irritation of sensitive mucous membranes.

Palliative care

Tissue necrosis and severe pain occur in advanced cancer of the mouth, either from failure of treatment or from death of tissue as a result of radiation. The patient usually experiences difficulty in swallowing, fear of choking, and the constant accumulation of foul-smelling secretions. Good mouth care is extremely important. The danger of severe and even fatal haemorrhage must always be considered. It is very difficult to induce these patients to take sufficient nourishing fluids. A gastrostomy (p. 599) may be done to permit direct introduction of food into the stomach. Family members caring for the person at home need considerable support from hospice or other community nurses.

Table 23-7   Oesophageal disorders

Disease	Signs and symptoms	Medical therapy
Achalasia (aperistalsis of oesophagus)	Dysphagia for liquids and solids, weight loss, substernal chest pain	Forceful dilatation of lower oesophageal sphincter with pneumostatic or mechanical dilators
	Later: regurgitation	Cardiomyotomy
Oesophageal strictures	Dysphagia	Oesophageal dilatation, resection of stricture
Oesophageal diverticulum (pouch in mucosa)	Dysphagia, fetid breath	Surgery for severe symptoms (excision of herniated sac)
Gastro-oesophageal reflux	Heartburn	Antacids; histamine-2 blockers (cimetidine), ranitidine;
Hiatal hernia (sliding, paraoesophageal)	50% asymptomatic, heartburn, dysphagia	No treatment if asymptomatic
		Heartburn: high-protein, low-fat diet; antacids
		Surgery for incarcerated hernias through thorax or abdomen

Interventions to achieve patient outcomes

Counselling

The person with cancer of the mouth faces two threats: threat to life and possible disfigurement. Because the face and neck are readily visible to others, one of the major problems that the person will have to cope with and adapt to is the change in body image. The impact of the loss may be slightly minimized when the grieving process begins early. The full emotional impact of the loss, however, occurs after therapy.

Withdrawal because of not wanting to be viewed by others or because of foul breath odour is often observed in these patients. The patient needs to experience acceptance by health professionals. The family members may need help in understanding patient behaviour and in coping with their own feelings concerning the patient's appearance. Patients are encouraged to identify their feelings and are provided with support and explanations as appropriate. Patients are encouraged to mingle with others as soon as clues indicating readiness are observed.

Evaluation

Evaluation is based on expected patient outcomes. Questions to consider include:

1. Have incisions healed without infection?
2. Can patient feed self, and is patient consuming a nutritionally balanced diet?
3. Does patient have a means of communication, and is patient working to improve speech?
4. Does patient interact with others and state plans for resumption of activities involving others?

COMMON OESOPHAGEAL DISORDERS

A number of oesophageal disorders delay motility in the oesophagus. Table 23-7 describes some of these disorders.

Aetiology and Pathophysiology

Oesophageal motility may be impaired by physiological dysfunction or lack of peristalsis (achalasia), by a narrowed tract (stricture), by lack of structural integrity (diverticulum), or by irritation of the oesophageal lining, particularly at the gastro-oesophageal junction (gastro-oesophageal reflux, hiatus hernia).

Various degrees of *achalasia* can exist; the cause is unknown. In addition to the absent peristalsis, the lower oesophageal sphincter does not relax with swallowing. In severe conditions the portion of the oesophagus above the achalasia dilates, and the person may have difficulty swallowing food and fluids past that point. Chest pain results from oesophageal spasms. Increased hydrostatic pressure (as with the Valsalva manoeuvre) helps to overcome the increased lower oesophageal pressure.

Strictures may be corrosive or benign. Corrosive strictures occur from ingestion of a strong alkali (such as caustic soda) or strong acid (such as toilet bowl cleaner) that causes severe oesophageal burns. Benign strictures develop following inflammatory lesions (such as those occurring with gastro-oesophageal reflux), acute viral or bacterial diseases, or mucosal injury from prolonged presence of indwelling nasogastric tubes.[60] Narrowing of the oesophagus makes swallowing difficult.

An *oesophageal diverticulum* is a bulging of the oesophageal mucosa and submucosa through a weakened portion of the oesophageal muscle. As food is ingested, some of it may collect in the pouch formed by the weakened area. After a sufficient amount of food has collected in the pouch, it overflows into the oesophagus and is regurgitated. There is always danger that some of the regurgitated food may be aspirated in the trachea during sleep.

Gastro-oesophageal reflux occurs when the lower oesophageal sphincter (LES), at the junction of the oesophagus and stomach, becomes incompetent and permits reflux of gastric material into the oesophagus. The acidity of the gastric juice irritates the oesophageal mucosa, creating a muscle spasm. Chronic reflux may lead to stricture of the LES (as a result of fibrosis from the inflammatory process), delaying passage of food into the stomach. An incompetent LES may be idiopathic (no known cause) or may be exacerbated by anticholinergic drugs, caffeine, theobromine (chocolate), alcohol, or smoking. Gastro-oesophageal reflux may also occur with *hiatus*

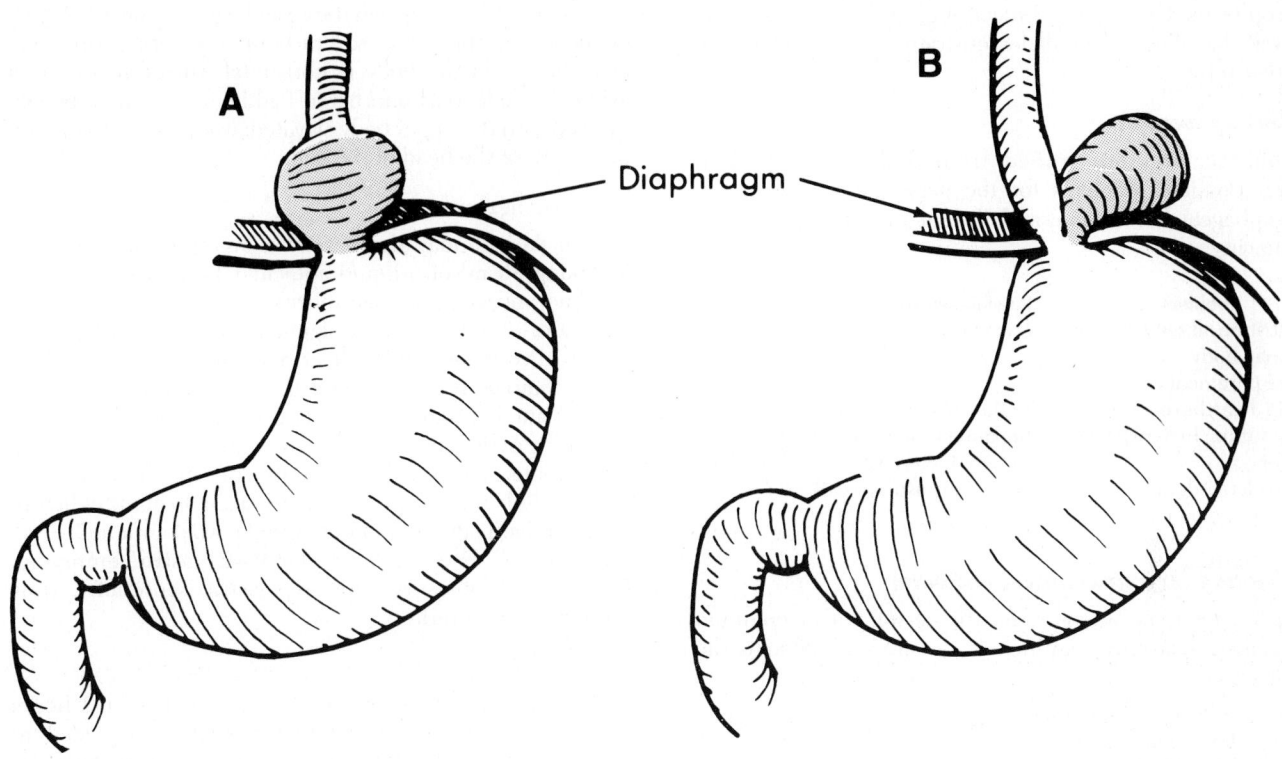

Fig. 23-4 Hiatus Hernia. **A,** Sliding hernia. **B,** Paraoesophageal hernia.

hernia, a protrusion of part of the stomach through the diaphragm into the thoracic cavity (Fig. 23-4). Obesity and ageing are contributing factors to the development of hiatal hernias.

Nursing Process
Assessment

Subjective data

Dysphagia is a primary symptom of oesophageal disorders. Oesophageal dysphagia of motor origin characteristically produces dysphagia for both solids and liquids. This differs from dysphagia that results from paralysis of neurological origin (difficulty swallowing liquids) or dysphagia caused by obstruction of the oesophageal lumen (difficulty swallowing solids). If the patient has had dysphagia for a period of time, it is helpful to know what approaches to eating the person has found most useful.

Ask the patient who experiences *regurgitation* if it occurs at night (staining of the pillow may have been observed), and if there is a foul odour of the regurgitated material (seen with oesophageal diverticulum).

Heartburn is a substernal "burning" sensation resulting from gastro-oesophageal reflux. The pain may be referred to the neck or back if severe. It is frequently accompanied by a sour regurgitation of gastric contents but is not accompanied by nausea.

Objective data

Assess the ability to swallow by placing three fingers over the thyroid cartilage of the larynx (Adams apple) and ask the person to swallow or by observing the movement of the larynx. Elicit the gag reflex by touching the posterior tongue or pharynx lightly with a tongue depresser. Do *not* check the gag reflex if there is no laryngeal movement. People who have diffiulty swallowing may still have a gag reflex.[21] Make a further assessment, if necessary, by placing 4 to 5 ml of water in the oropharynx and asking the patient to swallow.

Diagnostic tests

The diagnosis of oesophageal disorders is facilitated by X-ray films of the oesophagus taken after barium swallow. The patient may be placed in Trendelenburg's position during the X-ray examination or fluoroscopy to identify gastro-oesophageal reflux.

A water siphon test is a fluoroscopic examination in which barium is swallowed followed by plain water. If the LES is incompetent, the barium will be seen to reflux into the oesophagus. Overnight pH recordings measured from swallowed glass electrodes will demonstrate periods of increased gastric reflux.

Nursing analysis

Problems are determined from analysis of patient data. Possible problems for the person with a common oesophageal disorder may include, but are not limited to, the following:

Problem	Possible aetiologies
Nutrition, altered: less than body requirements	Dysphagia
Pain: heartburn	Reflux of acid gastric contents
Aspiration, high risk for	Impaired swallowing, incompetent LES
Knowledge deficit	Lack of exposure/recall

Planning: expected patient outcomes

Expected patient outcomes for the person with a common oesophageal disorder may include, but are not limited to, the following:

1. Eats a nutritionally balanced diet.
2. Describes any recommended dietary changes.
3. States feeling comfortable.
4. Does not aspirate.
5. Describes body-position and activity requirements.

Implementation

Assisting with achievement of therapeutic goals

The doctor may dilatate the oesophagus with dilators (bougies) or inflatable bags for *achalasia* or *oesophageal strictures*. The procedures may be performed under fluoroscopy to prevent damage to the mucosa. Postoperatively, monitor the patient for *chest pain*, indicating oesophageal perforation. Fluids and soft foods are indicated when swallowing produces pain. Most patients will require pain medication in the early postoperative period.

People with symptomatic *hiatal hernias* usually have gastro-oesophageal reflux with resultant heartburn. Measures to reduce heartburn are described below. H_2 receptor blockers (p. 615) may be prescribed for hiatal hernias. If these measures are ineffective, surgery may be necessary. The fundus of the stomach is wrapped around the lower oesophagus (Nissen fundoplication). Increases in intragastric pressure are thereby transmitted to the lower oesophagus, facilitating closure of the oesophageal sphincter.[68] Oesophageal surgery is discussed on p. 611.

Interventions to achieve patient outcomes

Facilitating nutrition

People with oesophageal disorders who experience *dysphagia* have difficulty swallowing both solids and liquids. Frequent small feedings may alleviate this difficulty. Some patients drink large amounts of fluid while swallowing solids to increase oesophageal pressure, thus pushing the food into the stomach. The Valsalva manoeuvre can also be used to help push the food past the sphincter. Eating with the head elevated encourages movement of food through the oesophagus by gravity. Regurgitation of food may occur several hours after eating, especially at night, when the body is horizontal (therefore eating is avoided for at least 2 hours before bedtime). Encourage people to sleep with the upper body elevated; wooden blocks may be used to raise the head of the bed.

Promoting comfort

The patient may decrease discomfort from heartburn by taking 30 ml of a liquid antacid 1 hour after meals, at bedtime, and whenever heartburn occurs. Gaviscon, which is a mixture of antacids with alginic acid, has been found to be effective in alleviating heartburn. Two to four tablets, when *chewed* thoroughly and then swallowed, produce a viscous antacid foam that coats the oesophagus and floats on the gastric contents. If antacids are not effective, medications that increase LES contraction may be prescribed; these include metoclopramide to be taken 30 minutes before meals and at bedtime. Patients should avoid anticholinergic medications, because they decrease gastric emptying. Histamine-2 blockers suppress gastric secretions, thus preventing night reflux.

Preventing aspiration

Tell the patient to remain upright for at least 2 hours after eating to prevent regurgitation that may lead to aspiration. Also suggest that the patient sleep with the head elevated. The head of the bed can be raised on 15 cm blocks.

Facilitating patient learning

Prevention is the best approach to treatment of heartburn. Encourage a high-protein, low-fat diet. Protein stimulates gastrin release that increases LES pressure. Fats, however, stimulate release of the hormone cholecystokinin that decreases LES pressure. Other foods that decrease LES pressure include caffeine products, chocolate, peppermint and spearmint oils, and alcohol; therefore, these foods should be avoided.

Evaluation

Evaluation is based on expected patient outcomes. Questions to consider include:

1. Does the patient eat a nutritionally balanced diet?
2. Can the patient describe recommended dietary changes?
3. Does the patient state that he/she feels comfortable?
4. Has aspiration been avoided?
5. Can the patient state (1) body-position and activity requirements, (2) how to achieve comfort and an adequate diet when at home, (3) medication, dosage schedule and side effects, and (4) signs and symptoms that must be reported to the doctor?

CANCER OF THE OESOPHAGUS

Epidemiology

Carcinoma is the most common condition causing obstruction of the oesophagus and accounts for about 2% of all cancers in the United Kingdom.[66a] In the United Kingdom most cases occur in men. Smokers, alcoholics, and people with achalasia are at high risk.

The only possible hope for successful treatment lies in very early diagnosis and treatment. Any person who has difficulty in swallowing, no matter how trivial it may seem, should be urged to seek medical advice at once. This applies particularly to people over 40 years of age because cancer of the oesophagus occurs more often in middle and later life than at younger ages.

Pathophysiology

Cancer may develop in any portion of the oesophagus but is most common in the middle and lower thirds. The tumour may be a squamous cell carcinoma originating in the oesophagus or an adenocarcinoma that spreads upward from the stomach. The cancer may spread to adjoining areas by local invasion or by lymphatic spread. Symptoms depend on the area and extent of metastasis.

Implementation

The treatment for cancer of the oesophagus is usually surgery, although radiation may be used. An *oesophagogastrostomy* is a resection of a portion of the oesophagus with anastomosis to the stomach. An *oesophagogastrectomy* is resection of a lower oesophageal section together with a proximal portion of the stomach, followed by anastomosis of the remaining portions of oesophagus and stomach. Adjuvant chemotherapy enhances the prognosis.

Considerable psychological support is usually required as the patient and family begin to cope with the diagnosis, prognosis, and physical debility of the patient. Encourage the patient to stop smoking, to avoid others with upper respiratory infections, and to seek medical help for even minor illnesses. Provide palliative and supportive care, as described in Chapter 9, as indicated.

OESOPHAGEAL SURGERY

Preoperative Care

The care of the person undergoing surgery of the oesophagus is described in Box 23-5. Improving the nutritional status is particularly important before surgery because the person is usually malnourished because of dysphagia and anorexia from the foul taste. Total parenteral nutrition is often prescribed, although a temporary gastrostomy may be performed to supply food in the preoperative or early postoperative period.

Good mouth care is essential, especially when the patient is spitting up decomposed food, blood, or pus. Mouthwashes are useful in making the mouth feel fresher; offer them to the patient before meals. Vary the mouthwashes from time to time unless the patient has a preference, because sometimes the flavour of the solution may be identified with the unpleasant throat secretions and becomes almost as distasteful as the secretions.

Preoperative patient teaching includes the care of the patient experiencing chest surgery (Chapter 16) if this is appropriate. A nasogastric tube will be in place after surgery.

23-5

Guidelines for Care

The patient undergoing oesophageal surgery

Preoperative care

Encourage improved nutritional status.
    Encourage high-protein, high-calorie diet if oral diet is possible.
    Total parenteral nutrition (TPN) may be necessary for severe dysphagia or obstruction.
Provide mouth care; vary the solution used.
Give preoperative preparation appropriate for thoracic surgery (Chapter 16).
Give prescribed antibiotics before oesophageal resection or bypass.

Postoperative care

Promote good pulmonary ventilation.
Maintain chest drainage system as prescribed.
Maintain gastric drainage system.
Maintain nutrition.
    Start clear fluids at frequent intervals when oral intake is permitted.
    Introduce soft foods gradually with several small meals of bland foods.
    Have patient keep head elevated for 2 hours after eating and while sleeping if heartburn occurs.

Postoperative Care

The immediate postoperative care centres on prevention of respiratory complications and maintenance of chest and gastric drainage systems. Postoperatively the nasogastric tube is usually left in place until complete healing of the oesophageal anastomosis has occurred because oesophageal tissue is very friable and because the anastomosis may be under tension. The nasogastric tube is not disturbed to prevent traction on the suture line. Small amounts of bright red blood may drain from the nasogastric tube for 6 to 12 hours after surgery. The colour of the drainage then changes to greenish yellow.

When oral intake is permitted, give clear fluids first until well tolerated; then the diet progresses to soft foods. If part of the stomach has been pulled up into the thoracic cavity, the patient may complain of a feeling of fullness in the chest or difficulty in breathing after eating. Smaller, more frequent meals may alleviate this problem. Heartburn (p. 609) may result from gastric reflux if the oesophageal sphincter has been removed or made incompetent.

DIGESTIVE DISORDERS

Most digestion takes place in the stomach, duodenum, and jejunum. Gastritis, peptic ulcer, cancer of the stomach, and malabsorption syndrome are the major digestive disorders (Table 23-8).

REVIEW
Table 23-8   Digestive disorders

Disorder	Signs and symptoms	Medical therapy
Gastritis	Anorexia, epigastric fullness, nausea/vomiting, epigastric discomfort, haematemesis, or melaena Shock and oesophageal strictures	Mild: antacid, rest Severe: correction of fluid/electrolyte imbalances, sedatives, antacids, H_2 blockers
Peptic ulcer	Epigastric pain relieved by food or antacids	Antacids, H_2 blockers, sucralfate, surgery for intractable ulcers or complications
Gastric cancer	Few early symptoms: anorexia, weight loss, anaemia Late symptom: palpable abdominal mass	Subtotal gastrectomy, chemotherapy, radiation therapy
Malabsorption syndrome	Steatorrhoea, flatulence, abdominal distension, anorexia, weight loss, signs of vitamin and protein deficiencies	Elimination of foods that cannot be tolerated; TPN when necessary; packed RBC for severe anaemia

Table 23-9   Types of peptic ulcers

Type of Ulcer	Location	Comment
Oesophageal	Lower third of oesophagus	Usually result from gastro-oesophageal reflux
Gastric	Usually on antrum or lesser curvature of stomach	Larger and deeper than duodenal ulcers; gastric malignancy must be ruled out
Duodenal	Usually in first part of duodenum	More common than gastric ulcers; not as well defined
Marginal	Jejunum near site of gastrojejunal anastomosis	Difficult to heal

GASTRITIS

Aetiology

Gastritis (inflammation of the stomach) is a common disorder characterized by anorexia, epigastric fullness and discomfort, and nausea and vomiting. The cause is often undetermined, but gastritis commonly results from stress, alcohol, or drugs (especially salicylates, antibiotics, indomethacin, sulphonamides, steroids). The disorder may also occur with bacterial or viral infections, from irritation by backflow of bile or pancreatic secretions, with radiation, or from corrosive substances.

Pathophysiology

Drugs, alcohol, bile salts, or pancreatic enzymes may damage the gastric mucosa (erosive gastritis), disrupting the gastric mucosal barrier and allowing a back-diffusion of acid and pepsin into the gastric tissue, causing inflammation. The gastric mucosa responds to most irritating agents by regeneration of the mucosa; therefore the disorders are often self-limiting. With continued irritation, the tissue becomes inflamed and bleeding may occur.

Ingestion of corrosive acids or alkalies can result in inflammation and necrosis of the stomach wall (corrosive gastritis). The necrosis may lead to perforation of the stomach wall with subsequent haemorrhage and peritonitis.

Chronic gastritis may be associated with atrophy of gastric glands and the appearance of patches of thin, grey, or greenish grey mucosa (atrophic gastritis). The loss of gastric mucosa will eventually reduce gastric secretion and lead to pernicious anaemia. Atrophic gastritis may be a precursor to gastric carcinoma. Chronic gastritis may also be associated with peptic ulcer disease or may occur following gastrojejunostomy.[40]

Nursing Process
Assessment

Subjective data include presence of anorexia and nausea and the extent of abdominal discomfort. *Objective data* include (1) vomit (frequency, amount, presence of blood) and (2) signs of fluid and electrolyte imbalance (thirst, decreased skin turgor, dry mucous membranes, oliguria, muscle weakness).

Nursing analysis

Problems are determined from analysis of patient data. Possible problems for the person with gastritis may include, but are not limited to, the following:

Problem	Possible aetiologies
Pain: epigastric	Gastric irritation
Fluid volume deficit	Vomiting

Planning: expected patient outcomes

Expected patient outcomes for the person with gastritis may include, but are not limited to, the following:

1. States epigastric pain is minimized or relieved.

Implementation

Assisting with achievement of therapeutic goals

Mild gastritis is treated with antacids and rest. With severe gastritis, intravenous fluids and electrolytes are prescribed to maintain fluid balance until symptoms subside. Then give tea, clear soup, and ginger ale orally at frequent intervals. The patient can usually tolerate bland feedings of custard, jelly, and cream soups after 12 to 24 hours, and then can tolerate other foods that are added gradually. People with chronic superficial gastritis will usually respond to a diet that avoids highly seasoned or greasy foods. Carbonated liquids are well tolerated.

Histamine H_2 blockers (p. 615) may be prescribed to inhibit gastric acid formation and thus decrease gastric irritation. Sucralfate (p. 615) may also be prescribed to protect the gastric mucosa by coating it to prevent back diffusion of acid and pepsin that causes irritation.

Interventions to achieve patient outcomes

Assisting with comfort

Antacids usually help to decrease epigastric discomfort. Good mouth care is indicated if vomiting is present. Rest and a calm environment help to decrease the effects of stress.

23-6

Factors contributing to development of peptic ulcers

Smoking

Cigarette smokers have increased incidence of peptic ulcers and delayed healing of gastric ulcers.

Drugs

Prolonged aspirin intake may lead to peptic disease. Corticosteroids, salicylates, indomethacin, and phenylbutazone in high doses may cause acute ulcers or exacerbate an already existing chronic peptic ulcer.

Emotional tension

No direct relationship has been demonstrated between personality and peptic ulcer, but emotional tension can alter gastric functioning. Stress may lead to a stress ulcer.

Genetic factors

A tendency for gastric or duodenal ulcers may be inherited.

Blood group

Duodenal ulcers occur more frequently in people with type O blood.

Micro-organism

Presence of the bacteria *Helicobacter pylori*.

Evaluation

Evaluation is based on expected patient outcomes. Questions to consider include:

1. Does patient state that epigastric pain is minimized or relieved?
2. Is patient hydrated?

STRESS EROSIONS/STRESS ULCERS

Stress erosions or ulcers are a form of gastritis that may occur with stressful disorders such as shock, severe trauma, major surgery, sepsis, or severe burns. The lesions are usually superficial. The gastric mucosa becomes eroded or superficially ulcerated in multiple sites. Possible causative factors have been identified as mucosal ischaemia or mucus deficiency. Stress erosions associated with the central nervous system, such as with brain tumours or injury or with cerebrovascular accidents, are termed *Cushing's ulcers* and are characterized by gastric hyperactivity. However, stress erosions from other causes do not demonstrate hyperacidity, and they may result from increased acid back-diffusion (similar to gastric ulcers).

Stress erosions can be prevented in high-risk people, such as those in intensive care units, by administration of antacids and H_2 blockers or sucralfate. Stress erosions develop within 24 to 48 hours of the stressful episode. Note signs of upper GI bleeding (haematemesis, melaena). Pain is not a prominent symptom. If bleeding is severe, the patient receives blood transfusions. Therapy consists of administration of antacids and H_2 blockers or sucralfate.

PEPTIC ULCER

Aetiology/Epidemiology

A peptic ulcer is an acute or chronic ulcer that occurs in the area accessible to gastric secretions (lower oesophagus, stomach, duodenum, jejunum) (Table 23-9). Peptic ulcers occur in the presence of gastric acid, but the cause of most peptic ulcers is unclear.

A number of environmental, psychological, and genetic factors may contribute to the development or delay of healing of peptic ulcers (see Box 23-6). A common belief is that people exhibiting certain traits such as tenseness or a striving for perfection or success are more likely to develop peptic ulcers. Conclusive evidence to support this belief is lacking. Diet does not appear to be a predisposing factor, although caffeine-containing foods may exacerbate an ulcer. Cigarette smoking and regular use of aspirin are strongly associated with chronic peptic ulcers.

Ulcers in the duodenum occur more frequently than gastric ulcers and have a greater incidence in people 20 to 45 years of age. Gastric ulcers occur more frequently in people over age 40.

Pathophysiology

An *acute peptic ulcer* is usually superficial, involving only the mucosal layer. In most cases it heals within a relatively short time, but it may bleed, perforate, or become chronic. A *chronic peptic ulcer* is a deep crater with sharp edges and a "clean" base. It involves both the mucosa and the submucosa. If the

Table 23-10   Comparison of duodenal and gastric ulcers

	Duodenal ulcer	Gastric ulcer
Pathophysiology	Normal back diffusion of gastric acid; increased gastric secretion and emptying rate	Increased back diffusion of gastric acid; normal gastric secretion and emptying rate
Epidemiology	2 to 5 times more common than gastric ulcers; most common in men 20 to 45 years of age	Less common than duodenal ulcers; most common in people 40 to 60 years of age
Pain	Epigastric pain 45 to 60 minutes after eating and	Epigastric pain about 30 minutes after eating and on an empty stomach
Diagnostic studies	Upper GI series	Upper GI series; gastroscopy with biopsy to determine if ulcer is benign or malignant
Course	Can usually be controlled by medical therapy	More difficulty to control medically; and recurs more frequently than duodenal ulcer

ulcer penetrates the stomach wall and becomes adherent to an adjacent organ such as the pancreas, the organ may become the base of the ulcer.

Ulceration of the stomach and duodenum occur through different mechanisms. People with *gastric* ulcers have a normal gastric secretion and a normal emptying rate of the stomach but an increased diffusion of gastric acid *back* into the tissue. Free acid that has been secreted into the stomach normally diffuses back slowly into the tissue. Rapid diffusion causes an inflammatory reaction in the tissue leading to tissue breakdown and bleeding. Gastric mucosa is normally protected from autodigestion by a thick layer of gastric mucus and by a gastric mucosal barrier.[55] Bile acids, alcohol, and salicylates can break down the natural barrier that slows the back diffusion. Cigarette smoking has been shown t increase bile reflux from the duodenum into the stomach.[72]

People with *duodenal* ulcers have a normal back diffusion of gastric acid but an increased gastric acid secretory rate and a markedly increased rate of gastric emptying. Thus there is an increase in the amount of gastric acid in the gastric lumen, and if not buffered with a food such as protein or an antacid, the acid is propelled rapidly into the duodenum. The increased amount of acid in the duodenum irritates the duodenal mucosa, leading to tissue breakdown. Table 23-10 lists differences between duodenal and gastric ulcers.

Zollinger-Ellison syndrome refers to peptic ulceration associated with a non-insulin-producing islet cell tumour of the pancreas. The syndrome is characterized by one or more peptic ulcerations in the lower end of the oesophagus, stomach, duodenum, and jejunum and by enormous gastric hypersecretion and acidity.

Nursing Process
Assessment

Subjective data

Pain, which is the major symptom of peptic ulcer, has the following characteristics:
1. Usually described as gnawing, aching, or burning
2. Usually confined to a small area of the upper abdomen near the midline
3. May radiate around the costal area to the back
4. Starts 1 to 2 hours after eating when the stomach begins to empty
5. May disappear with ingestion of food or an antacid

6. Frequently occurs at night when the stomach is empty

Assess the patient with a peptic ulcer for the presence, location, and character of pain as well as time of occurrence in relation to food and effectiveness of antacids. Some people never experience pain, and the peptic ulcer may be discovered accidentally by X-ray or postmortem examination.

Objective data

Monitor the patient for signs of haemorrhage (haematemesis, tarry stools), perforation (severe abdominal pain, abdominal rigidity), or pyloric obstruction (weight loss, projectile vomiting).

Diagnostic tests

The diagnosis of peptic ulcer is made from the patient's history, a gastrointestinal series, gastric juice analysis, and stool examinations for occult (hidden) blood (p. 630). Direct visualization of the ulcer by gastroscopy differentiates gastric ulcer from gastric carcinoma.

Selective *angiography* is becoming useful in the diagnosis and evaluation of treatment of gastric haemorrhage when angiography is combined with endoscopy. With angiography a contrast medium is injected through an arterial catheter for better visualization of bleeding areas and for differentiation between normal and tumour vessels. Following the procedure, observe the femoral insertion site for signs of bleeding, and take vital signs at frequent intervals.

Nursing analysis

Problems are determined from analysis of patient data. Possible problems for the person with a peptic ulcer may include, but are not limited to, the following:

Problem	Possible aetiologies
Pain: epigastric	Ulceration of mucosa
Coping, ineffective individual	Situational stressors
Knowledge deficit	Lack of exposure/recall

Planning: expected patient outcomes

Expected patient outcomes for the person with a peptic ulcer may include, but are not limited to, the following:
1. States pain is decreased, minimal, or absent.
2. Identifies life stressors and describes useful stress management techniques.
3. States plans to modify health-risking behaviours (smok-

Table 23-11   Drug therapy for peptic ulcer

Drug	Action	Comments
Antacids	Neutralize gastric acid	Generally heal ulcers in 4 to 6 weeks Side effects limited to diarrhoea or constipation Lack of adherence to regimen by many patients
Histamine H2 receptor antagonists (cimetidine, ranitidine, famotidine, nizatidine)	Inhibit acid secretion	Generally heal ulcers in 4 to 6 weeks Side effects may interfere with administration
Sucralfate	Coats ulcer, prevents action of acid and pepsin on ulcer	Generally heal ulcers in 4 to 6 weeks Longer time span before recurrence Large capsule; may be difficult to swallow
Anticholinergics	Decrease gastric secretions, delay gastric emptying	Less effective than other drugs; now rarely used Side effects usually occur with therapeutic doses.

ing, alcohol ingestion) if pertinent.

4. Describes factors that contribute to healing, medication plan to be followed, and plans for follow-up care.

Implementation

Assisting with achievement of therapeutic goals

The pain of peptic ulcer is directly related to periods of the day when gastric acidity is high, particularly several hours after meals and at bedtime, when acid secretion is high and the stomach is empty. Measures to decrease ulcer pain and promote healing include drug therapy (antacids, histamine H_2 blockers, sucralfate) (Table 23-11) and food to buffer the gastric acidity.

Antacids

Antacids are the most effective therapy for relieving peptic ulcer pain; they act by decreasing gastric acidity. Antacids of choice are the nonsystemic antacids, which are poorly absorbed from the stomach and therefore do not alter the pH of the blood or interfere with normal acid-base balance. Sodium bicarbonate is readily absorbed and therefore should be avoided as an antacid for relief of ulcer pain. Also, the reaction of sodium bicarbonate and hydrochloric acid forms carbon dioxide, which may cause distension.

Antacids may be administered frequently, and if symptoms are severe, it may be necessary to give them as often as every 30 to 60 minutes. When antacids are given to a person in a fasting state, the buffering power is usually transitory. For maximal effectiveness, antacids should be given 1 and 3 hours *after* meals; this produces a buffering effect that lasts approximately 3 to 4 hours. Aluminium hydroxide becomes less reactive over time and should not be given with anticholinergic drugs or with tetracycline because it interferes with absorption of these drugs. Liquids are more effective than tablets; if tablets are used, they are chewed slowly to permit complete pulverization.

Histamine H_2 receptor antagonists

One of the major stimulants of hydrochloric acid secretion in the stomach is histamine (in addition to gastrin and acetylcholine). In the body, histamine has two types of receptors, H_1 receptors, which mediate histamine action in the smooth muscle (and are blocked by antihistamines), and H_2 receptors, which mediate secretion of hydrochloric acid in the stomach. Histamine H_2 receptor antagonists, therefore, are drugs that block histamine's stimulation of gastric acid, either in the fasting state or the stimulated state.

Histamine H_2 receptor antagonists that are available for peptic ulcer therapy include cimetidine, ranitidine, famotidine, and nizatidine. The overall side effects are low but may include confusion, dizziness, and weakness (most common in elderly people); diarrhoea and abdominal cramps; bradycardia or tachycardia; impotence and gynaecomastia; itching and rash; and thrombocytopenia. The patient needs to know about the possibility of a decreased libido and to monitor for signs of bleeding (from the thrombocytopenia). Cimetidine has increased toxicity when given concurrently with benzodiazepines, metoprolol, propanolol, phenytoin, theophylline, and tricyclic antidepressants.

Sucralfate

Sucralfate helps to heal ulcers and decrease pain by coating the ulcer, thus preventing irritation by gastric acid and pepsin (Table 23-11). Sucralfate decreases the absorption of tetracycline and phenytoin; therefore, administer these drugs at least 2 hours apart from sucralfate administration. Give antacids at least 30 minutes before or after sucralfate.

Interventions to achieve patient outcomes
Promoting comfort

Although modifying the diet has not been shown to accelerate healing of an uncomplicated ulcer, regulation of food may promote comfort. Food in the stomach, especially protein, buffers gastric acid; however, food also stimulates gastric acid secretion, which may irritate the ulcer and cause pain. Controversy exists concerning whether ulcer pain is better relieved by three regular meals or six small meals a day. The person with the pain can best judge which approach provides the maximum comfort. Suggest the following eating guidelines:

Table 23-12   Comparison of different types of vagotomy procedures for peptic ulcer

Type of surgery	Advantages	Disadvantages
Truncal vagotomy with pyloroplasty	Low operative mortality and morbidity	High recurrence rate
Selective vagotomy with pyloroplasty	Preservation of vagal innervation of viscus; fewer side effects than truncal vagotomy	More difficult to perform than truncal vagotomy
Proximal vagotomy	Preserves gastric emptying; low recurrence rate; fewer side effects; no intrusion of GI tract	Requires greater expertise
Vagotomy with antrectomy	Lower recurrence rate than for vagotomy with pyloroplasty	Higher operative mortality Greater side effects

---

Guidelines for Care 23-7

The patient with a peptic ulcer

Medications
Know dosage, administration, action, and side effects.
Continue drug for prescribed time, even when symptoms abate.
Keep antacids available at all times.
Anticipate increased need for antacid during periods of stress.
Avoid self-medication with systemic antacids (bicarbonate of soda) that alter acid-base balance.
Avoid ulcerogenic drugs such as salicylates, ibuprofen, corticosteroids.
Use paracetamol or buffered aspirin (if tolerated) for relief of pain.

Smoking
Stop smoking if possible.
If stopping smoking increases discomfort from stress, try to decrease amount smoked.

Eating
Eat three balanced meals a day.
Eat between-meal snacks if this helps to relieve pain.
Avoid any foods that increase discomfort.
If alcohol is taken, drink in moderation and not on an empty stomach.
Avoid stress at mealtimes and plan for a quiet time after eating.

Relaxation and reduction of stress
Participate in recreation and hobbies that promote relaxation.
Provide for a good night's sleep on a regular basis.
Use relaxation techniques to decrease effects of stress.
Participate in a reasonable exercise programme to promote well-being.
Structure home and work environment to keep stressors at a reasonable level.
Avoid factors found to increase symptoms, if possible.

1. Eat meals slowly to prevent overdistension and gastric acid reflux.
2. Eat snacks if pain occurs between meals.
3. Restrict foods that stimulate gastric acid secretion (coffee, tea, cola).
4. If alcohol is consumed (stimulating gastric acid secretion), it should be taken in moderate amounts or less and not on an empty stomach.
5. Restrict bedtime snacks that may increase nocturnal pain.
6. Avoid any foods that increase discomfort.

Counselling and teaching

Ulcer pain typically appears in a cyclic manner, with periods of days to weeks of pain interspersed with periods of little or no pain. Patients therefore need to know what to do at home to prevent or modify the pain. A summary of patient teaching is given in Box 23-7.

In addition to knowing measures for relief of pain, the person with a peptic ulcer needs to understand about factors that contribute to healing and to preventing ulcer recurrence. These factors include preventing stress, avoiding irritating substances that are poorly tolerated, avoiding ulcerogenic drugs, avoiding smoking, and maintaining the medical regimen.

Stress plays a role in the pathogenesis of peptic ulcers, probably by increasing acid secretion from vagal stimulation.[55] Thus actions that avoid stressful situations or minimize the effect of stress can promote healing or prevent recurrence. If removal from stressful environmental influences is impossible, the person must learn to cope with the stressful situations without reactivating the ulcer. (Measures to decrease stress are described in Chapter 5.) Occasionally the person requires psychological counselling to better understand the problems and develop more effective coping behaviours.

Since there seems to be a relationship between *smoking* and irritation of a peptic ulcer, most doctors believe that the person who has a peptic ulcer should give up smoking permanently. To do so is sometimes very difficult, since often the person's life and work situations as well as personality are such that a change of this sort is a major one. Encourage those few people whose ulcers are reactivated when they attempt to give up smoking to at least moderate the habit.

If every consideration is given to adjusting the prescribed regimen to fit the appropriate physical, economic, and social pattern, the person with an ulcer will be better able to follow the medical treatment.

Evaluation

Questions to consider for the person with a peptic ulcer include the following:

1. Has epigastric pain been relieved or minimized?
2. Does the person know measures to minimize the effects of stress in daily living?
3. Has the person made plans to avoid or modify activities that delay healing?
4. Can the person describe
   a. Correct administration of prescribed medications?
   b. Specific actions to take to promote healing of the ulcer and decrease recurrence?
   c. Plans for follow-up care?

Surgery for Peptic Ulcer

Emergency surgery is necessary when a peptic ulcer perforates and causes peritonitis or erodes a blood vessel, causing severe haemorrhage. Elective surgery may be performed if the ulcer does not respond to the medical regimen and continues to produce symptoms, if it causes pyloric obstruction, or if a chronic recurring gastric ulcer is thought to be premalignant. The basic surgical procedures for treatment of peptic ulcers are subtotal gastrectomy, vagotomy, and pyloroplasty. Subtotal gastrectomy is now rarely performed alone but is usually combined with a form of vagotomy. Pyloroplasty is also combined with a vagotomy. The several common surgical combinations are listed in Table 23-12.

Table 23-13 describes *subtotal gastrectomies*. The Billroth II is usually preferred for duodenal ulcers because of decreased duodenal recurrence. The duodenal stump is preserved to permit bile flow into the jejunum to mix with the food but may develop infection from stasis.

Part of the vagus nerve innervating the stomach is severed in a *vagotomy* for the purpose of decreasing gastric acidity. There are three types of vagotomies currently in use: truncal, selective, and proximal. With both *truncal* and *selective* vagotomies, gastric emptying is inhibited; thus a pyloroplasty or antrectomy (removal of antrum or lower portion of stomach) must be performed to prevent gastric stasis by enlarging the pyloric opening. The *proximal* vagotomy severs only the branches of the gastric portion of the vagal nerve that innervate the upper two thirds of the stomach, thus maintaining effective gastric emptying. Because a pyloroplasty or antrectomy is unnecessary with a proximal vagotomy, there is no intrusion into the gastric lumen and side effects, especially diarrhoea, are reduced.

A *pyloroplasty* or drainage procedure widens the pyloric outlet. It is performed with a truncal or selective vagotomy to prevent gastric stasis. One type of pyloroplasty is the Heineke-Mikulicz procedure.

Care of the patient experiencing gastric surgery is described on p. 622.

Complications of Peptic Ulcer

A peptic ulcer may perforate a major blood vessel and cause haemorrhage, perforate the stomach or duodenal wall, or cause an obstruction at the pyloric end of the stomach.

Haemorrhage

Peptic ulcer is the most common cause of massive upper gastrointestinal bleeding. Duodenal ulcers have a higher incidence of bleeding than gastric ulcers. In some cases bleeding is slight, and the only symptoms are tarry stools and a developing iron deficiency. When a major blood vessel erodes, bleeding is massive.

The medical management of haemorrhage is summarized in Table 23-14. If endoscopy shows a bleeding ulcer, endoscopic haemostatic therapy (heater probe, electrocautery, or Nd:YAG laser) may be used.[68] Surgery is indicated for uncontrolled bleeding or for recurrence of haemorrhage. Vagotomy with pyloroplasty is preferred to gastrectomy. The drainage from the nasogastric tube is usually dark red for 6 to 12 hours after surgery but should turn greenish yellow within 24 hours. The patient may continue to pass tarry stools for several days postoperatively, but this is usually because the blood from the haemorrhage before surgery has not yet completely passed through the gastrointestinal tract. Stools may be guaiac positive for several days after bleeding stops.

If gastric lavage is indicated, saline is usually used to minimize loss of electrolytes. No evidence supports the use of iced solutions.[56]

Nursing interventions during the phase of *severe gastric bleeding* include the following actions:

1. Assisting with achievement of therapeutic goals
   a. Monitor vital signs and urinary output for response

Table 23-13   Comparison of subtotal gastrectomy procedures

	Gastroduodenostomy	Gastrojejunostomy
Common term	Billroth I	Billroth II
Procedure	Removal of lower part of stomach (antrectomy) with anastomosis to remaining segment of duodenum	Removal of lower part of stomach (antrectomy) with anastomosis to side of the proximal jejunum
Common use	Gastric ulcer	Duodenal ulcer
Side effects	Decreased gastric capacity, rapid emptying with decreased effect of pancreatic enzymes (malabsorption)	Same as Billroth I; stasis with subsequent infection in the blind duodenal loop

Table 23-14 Complications of peptic ulcer

	Haemorrhage	Perforation	Pyloric obstruction
Clinical picture	Haematemesis, tarry stools, shock	Sudden severe abdominal pain, usually several hours after eating; abdominal rigidity; decreased abdominal sounds; increased pulse and respiratory rate	Partial obstruction; epigastric fullness, anorexia, weight loss; complete obstruction: projectile vomiting of undigested food, dehydration
Diagnostic findings	Blood in vomitus and stool	Leukocytosis X-ray film; air under diaphragm	Anaemia, hypochloraemia, hypokalaemia, hyponatraemia X-ray film: large gastric fluid level
Medical treatment	Bed rest, sedation, blood transfusions, gastric lavage treatment for shock, cimetidine After bleeding stops: antacids hourly or by continuous drip	Gastric decompression, parenteral fluids, antibiotics, surgery	Gastric decompression, correction of metabolic alkalosis and dehydration Antacids and liquids after 72 hours if obstruction decreased Surgery if obstruction persists

to therapy for shock.

   b. Monitor nasogastric drainage, emesis, and stools for amount of blood loss (stools may be red or tarry depending on the length of time required for passage).

   c. Test stools daily for occult blood (guaiac) until bleeding has completely stopped.

   d. Assist with medical treatments (blood transfusions, saline gastric lavage) and monitor patient's response.

   e. Prepare patient for surgery if indicated.

2. Assisting with patient comfort

   a. Provide special mouth care after vomiting (a weak solution of hydrogen peroxide will help remove blood from the oral mucosa).

   b. Administer prescribed sedative/narcotic regularly to decrease apprehension.

   c. Remove all evidence of bleeding as quickly as possible.

   d. Tell patient rationale for blood transfusion.

   e. Tell patient that rest and quiet will help stop the bleeding.

   f. Maintain a calm approach.

   g. Restrict activities only to those deemed necessary until massive bleeding has slowed down or stopped.

Perforation

Perforation is an erosion of a peptic ulcer through the muscular wall, providing an opening from the gastrointestinal tract into the peritoneal cavity. Most perforated ulcers are located on the anterior duodenal wall. Immediately on perforation a chemical peritonitis results from contact with the gastrointestinal contents, and bacterial peritonitis results within 12 hours. Symptoms and medical management are listed in Table 23-14. People taking corticosteroids may develop a peptic ulcer and perforation without exhibiting any of the usual symptoms.

Some perforations are minor and close within a short time or wall themselves off. However, most perforations require surgery and should be closed surgically as soon as possible. Surgery may consist of simple laparotomy with closure (oversewing) of the perforation and aspiration from the peritoneum of all escaped GI fluid. Most people who have had a perforated ulcer, however, continue to have recurrences of ulcer symptoms. Therefore, most surgeons now perform definitive ulcer surgery, such as vagotomy with gastric resection or pyloroplasty, if the patient's condition permits. A pelvic abscess may require incision and drainage.

Nursing interventions for the person with a *perforated ulcer* include the following activities:

1. Assisting with achievement of therapeutic goals

   a. Connect the nasogastric tube initially to continuous suction until stomach is empty, then maintain at intermittent suction.

   b. Place patient in appropriate position for condition, e.g. degree of pain present.

   c. Prepare patient for surgery, if indicated.

   d. Monitor postoperatively for continuing peritonitis and abscess formation (fever, respiratory distress, increased abdominal pain, distension, hyperactive or absent bowel sounds, inability to pass flatus or stool).

2. Assisting with patient comfort

   a. Give analgesic medications at regular intervals for pain control during acute phase.

   b. To decrease apprehension, explain what is being done.

Pyloric obstruction

Pyloric obstruction may be caused by oedema of tissues around an ulcer or by scar tissue from a healed ulcer located near the pylorus. It may be only a partial obstruction and cause dilation of the stomach, or it may be complete. Obstruction caused by oedema and spasm generally responds to medical management (Table 23-14).

At the end of a 72-hour period of gastric decompression, a *saline load test* is performed to assess the degree of gastric emptying: 700 ml of normal saline at room temperature is introduced through the nasogastric tube over a 3- to 5-minute period, and the tube is then clamped. After 30 minutes the stomach is aspirated. A residual volume of more than 350 ml indicates continued pyloric obstruction, and surgery consisting of either a vagotomy with pyloroplasty or gastrectomy is considered. If the saline load test demonstrates improved gastric emptying, oral liquids and antacids are introduced with continued assessment of gastric emptying for several days.

Nursing interventions for the person with a *pyloric obstruction* include the following activities:

1. Monitor for signs of increased severe abdominal pain and decreased abdominal sounds.
2. Assist with achievement of therapeutic goals.
   a. Assist with gastric lavage and maintain gastric decompression.
   b. Explain saline load test, when pertinent.
   c. Prepare patient for surgery as necessary.

CANCER OF THE STOMACH

Aetiology/Epidemiology

Almost all gastric tumours are malignant. The incidence of cancer of the stomach has decreased in recent years; nevertheless, gastric cancer still had a mortality rate of 20 per 100,000 in men and 10 per 100,000 in women in 1991.[18a] It occurs more frequently in men than women. It rarely occurs in people under the age of 40 and is most frequent between the ages of 60 and 70. The cause is unknown, although the incidence is higher when gastric acid is low. Contributing factors, symptoms, and usual medical therapy are summarized in Table 23-8 (p. 612).

Pathophysiology

Cancer may develop in any part of the stomach but is found most often in the distal third. Most gastric cancers are adenocarcinomas and occur in polypoid, ulcerative, or infiltrative forms. The ulcerative form is the most common and may produce peptic ulcer-type symptoms that, unfortunately, tend to delay diagnosis and encourage self-treatment. Growths located at the entrance or exit of the stomach may lead to signs of oesophageal or pyloric obstruction (heartburn or early satiety). In general, however, early signs of gastric cancer are absent.

Gastric cancer may spread directly through the stomach wall into adjacent tissues, to the lymphatics, to the regional lymph nodes of the stomach, to other abdominal organs, or through the bloodstream to the lungs or bones. Involvement of the regional lymph nodes occurs early, followed by involvement of the more distal nodes. There is a tendency towards intraperitoneal seeding, particularly to the peritoneal cul-de-sac. Prognosis depends on the depth of invasion and extent of metastasis.

Medical Therapy

Surgery is the primary therapy for gastric cancer. If the tumour has not spread beyond the stomach, a subtotal gastrectomy (gastroduodenostomy or gastrojejunostomy) is usually performed. Tumours high in the cardia of the stomach may require a total gastrectomy (oesophagojejunostomy).[68] Palliative subtotal gastrectomy may be performed when haemorrhage or obstruction occurs.

Chemotherapy and radiotherapy may be given for metastatic disease to decrease symptoms and prolong survival. Only about 12% of people with gastric cancer survive for 5 years.[68]

GASTROINTESTINAL INTUBATION

GI intubation consists of inserting a tube through the nose into the stomach (nasogastric) or beyond the stomach into the intestine (intestinal). Common uses of GI intubation include the following:

1. Nasogastric (N/G)
   a. Decompression of stomach
   b. Tube feedings, including medication administration (p. 600)
   c. Removal of gastric contents (gastric haemorrhage or perforation)
   d. After oesophageal or gastric surgery to permit healing of suture line
   e. Gastric analysis (test meal)
2. Intestinal: intestinal decompression

The following section discusses the use of GI intubation for decompression and drainage and the care of people with a GI tube.

Types of Tubes

Different types of tubes are used depending on the purpose and site (Table 23-15). A *Ryle's tube* is used for gastric intubation; however, because it is a single-lumen tube, damage to the mucosa may result even with intermittent suction. A less traumatic approach is the double-lumen Salem *sump tube*. The larger lumen of the sump tube drains the area, while the smaller lumen provides a continuous flow of air at atmospheric pressure, thus maintaining the suction at a lower level and preventing adherence of the tube against the tissue wall. The air vent should never be clamped off or connected to suction.

Two tubes that may be used for intestinal decompression are the Miller-Abbott tube and the Cantor tube. The length of these tubes permits their passage through the entire intestinal tract. A small balloon on the tip of each tube acts like a bolus of food when inflated with air or injected with water or mercury. This balloon stimulates peristalsis, which advances the tube along the intestinal tract. If peristalsis is absent, the weight of the mercury in the balloon will usually carry it forward. When a Miller-Abbott tube is used, the mercury is inserted into the balloon of the tube after the tube is passed.

Insertion of Tubes

Nasogastric tubes may be inserted by the nurse or the doctor. *Intestinal* tubes are more difficult to insert because of the addition of the balloon. The intestinal tube can be mechanically inserted only into the stomach. Its passage along the remainder of the GI tract depends on gravity and peristalsis.

Nursing Care Plan | **Person with peptic ulcer**

DATA: Mr. J. is a 42-year-old single computer operator with a history of duodenal ulcer (diagnosed 4 years ago). He has had periods of epigastric distress for the past month with partial relief from an antacid. He was admitted 2 days ago with haematemesis, tarry stools, faintness, and a blood pressure of 96/54 mm Hg (usual 124/84). Intravenous fluids were initiated. Endoscopy revealed a bleeding duodenal ulcer. A nasogastric tube was inserted and antacids prescribed hourly per tube. Cimetidine was started by intravenous push. His blood pressure is now stable and the nasogastric tube was removed early today. He is taking oral fluids and has been started on a soft diet. Current prescriptions include cimetidine 300 mg with meals and at bedtime and antacid 30 ml 1 and 3 hours after meals.

The nursing history identified the following:
1. He is vague about the nature of peptic ulcer or possible complications.
2. He takes aspirin for headaches "from computer eyestrain."
3. He smokes 30 cigarettes per day; he has tried several times, unsuccessfully, to stop.
4. He spends two to three evenings a week at a local pub and "has a few pints."

Collaborative nursing actions include those to prevent further injury from haemorrhage or perforation. Immediate reporting of and treatment of early signs may prevent serious effects (loss of blood, peritonitis, or death).

Nursing actions include *monitoring* for the following:
1. Signs of haemorrhage: haematemesis, decreased blood pressure, restlessness, cool moist skin, stools that test positive for guaiac
2. Signs of perforation: severe, sudden, sharp abdominal pain

Nursing analysis: Pain: epigastric related to irritation of gastric acid on duodenal ulcer

Expected patient outcomes	Nursing interventions	Rationale
Mr. J. states epigastric pain is decreased	Give prescribed cimetidine with meals and at bedtime (8 AM, 12 noon, 5 PM, and 9 PM)	Cimetidine encourages healing by decreasing gastric acid secretion; give with meals to inhibit food-stimulated HCl secretion
	Give prescribed antacid 1 and 3 hours after meals (9 AM, 11 AM, PM, 3 PM, 6 PM, and 8 PM)	Antacids neutralize HCl; they interfere with absorption of cimetidine if given concurrently
	Teach relaxation measures as appropriate,	Relaxation facilities rest to promote healing

The weight of the mercury in the balloon helps propel the tube through the intestines.

The intestinal tube is passed in the same manner as the nasogastric tube. After the intestinal tube reaches the stomach its passage through the pylorus into the duodenum is facilitated by positioning and activity.

1. Encourage the following patient positions;
   a. Right side for 2 hours, then
   b. Lying on back with head elevated for 2 hours, then
   c. Left side for 2 hours
2. Encourage patient ambulation following passage of tube into the pylorus (often assessed by X-ray film)
3. Advance the tube 2 to 10 cm (1 to 4 inches) at specified intervals to provide slack for peristaltic action

4. Secure tube to face *only* when desired point has been reached; coil extra tubing on bed or pin to clothing

The intestinal tube is usually monitored daily by X-ray film for signs of coiling or telescoping of the tube. Telescoping is movement of bowel along with the tube resulting in intussusception (p. 634), a serious complication.

Facilitating Drainage

Because the gastric or intestinal fluid must move against gravity to be removed, suction is required. *Intermittent low-pressure suction* is used for single-lumen tubes; constant suction could damage the mucosal wall if a section of the wall were to be pulled continually against the drainage holes of the tube. Intermittent suction permits the wall to drop away from the tube when suction is not occurring. Constant low-pressure suction is used for a sump tube.

Nursing analysis: Altered health maintenance: related to lack of knowledge

Expected patient outcomes	Nursing interventions	Rationale
Mr. J. states plans to decrease smoking and drinking and to avoid aspirin	Teach effects of aspirin, smoking and alcohol on ulcer formation	Aspirin is ulcerogenic; smoking delays healing; alcohol stimulates HCl and may further irritate ulcer
	Discuss previous efforts at discontinuing smoking: explore additional ways, especially group programmes such as those provided by local health groups	Programmes that include group support are often more successful than trying to stop smoking by oneself
	Explore with Mr. J. reasons for frequent visits to the pub, then explore other ways of meeting his needs (such as nonalcoholic drinks or substituting other social activities)	Assisting Mr. J. to think about reasons and alternate approaches will increase the potential for a behavioural change
	Suggest Mr. J. get his eyes tested (if appropriate); describe analgesics that do not contain aspirin (such as paracetamol	Headaches may be caused by strain from decreased vision; fewer headaches will decrease need for analgesics

Nursing analysis: Knowledge deficit: related to lack of recall or exposure

Expected patient outcomes	Nursing interventions	Rationale
Mr. J. describes nature of and therapy for peptic ulcer	Review nature of peptic ulcer and possible recurrence; review factors that contribute to healing (see Box 27-8); review methods of pain relief, including administration and side effects of cimetidine and antacids; review need to report symptoms of bleeding, perforation, or pyloric obstruction to doctor immediately	Reinforcement of earlier teaching will help promote retention

Use normal saline to irrigate the tube because a hypotonic solution such as water would increase electrolyte loss. It is difficult to aspirate irrigating solution from *intestinal* tubes because of the tube's length. If no return flow can be obtained, use only a small amount of fluid and record the amount instilled.

PREVENTING INJURY

Pressure of the tube against the nares may lead to irritation and tissue breakdown. The oropharyngeal mucosa or the parotid glands may become inflamed as a result of dry mucous membranes from oral breathing (nares plugged) or from GI bacteria that travel up the tube by capillary action. Discomfort at the jaw angle may indicate a parotitis. Methods to prevent injury from gastric intubation include the following:

1. Tape tube securely to nostril so that it does not press against nostril
2. Pin tube loosely to clothing to support weight of tube and permit free head movement
3. Prevent oral inflammations
   a. Keep oral mucous membranes moist
   b. Give frequent mouth care
   c. Use ice chips sparingly (ingestion of large amounts of hypotonic water from the melted ice may produce electrolyte loss through suction)
   d. Provide boiled sweets (e.g. fruit drops) for sucking to stimulate flow of saliva

Table 23-15   Nasogastric and intestinal tubes

Tube	Purpose	Characteristic	Use
Nasogastric			
Ryle's	Removes fluid and gas from stomach (decompression); may also be used to give tube feedings	Single lumen; easy to maintain; may cause trauma to stomach wall	Use intermittent suction at low pressure setting or open drainage into bag
Salem sump	Same purpose as Ryle's tube	Double lumen, one for drainage and one to provide an air vent to prevent tube adherence to stomach wall	Use low (30 mm Hg) *constant* suction; attach the larger lumen of tube only to suction
Entron	Tube feedings for gastric feedings only	No. 6 Fr (small bore); has a stylet for easier insertion but no weighted end	Clamp off when not in use; do not attach to suction (collapses)
Dobbhoff enteric	Tube feedings for gastric or intestinal feedings	No. 8 Fr (small bore); has a stylet for easier insertion and a weighted end to pass into intestines	Same as for the Entron tube
Intestinal			
Miller-Abbott	Removes fluid and gas from intestines (decompression)	Double lumen, one for balloon inflation and one for drainage	Use low pressure intermittent suction; clamp off balloon tube and attach drainage tube only to suction
Cantor	Same purposes as Miller-Abbott tube; (used less frequently)	Single lumen; mercury is injected into balloon with needle and syringe prior to suction	Use low pressure intermittent suction

N.B. Other examples of tubes are in use and nurses should be familiar with those used in their location.

Promoting Comfort

The presence of the tube in the nasopharynx causes local discomfort, and the person may complain of a lump in the throat, difficulty in swallowing, sore throat, hoarseness, earache, or irritation of the nostril. Methods to promote comfort include the following:

1. Remove excess secretions around nares.
2. Apply *water-soluble* lubricant (K-Y jelly) to tube at nostril to prevent secretion buildup.
3. Provide for relief of sore throat with:
   a. Warm saline gargles
   b. Ice bag to neck
   c. Prescribed throat lozenges
   d. Frequent position changes to relieve pressure of tube on throat
4. Use semi-recumbent or upright position (unless contraindicated) to prevent oesophageal reflux (heartburn).

Monitoring for Complications

In addition to inflammations of the mouth and parotid glands, the person with GI intubation may experience fluid and electrolyte and pulmonary complications. *Fluid and electrolyte imbalances* result from loss of GI secretions and include dehydration, hyponatraemia, and hypokalaemia. Loss of acid *gastric* contents may lead to metabolic *alkalosis*, whereas loss of alkaline *intestinal* contents may produce metabolic *acidosis* (Chapter 7). Monitor the person for signs and symptoms of these imbalances, and record the amount and character of drainage from the tubes accurately.

Aspiration pneumonia may result from regurgitation of the stomach contents or placement of fluids in an incorrectly positioned tube. Observe for respiratory infection—increased respiratory rate and temperature. Ascertain positioning of nasogastric tubes in the stomach before introducing fluids.

SURGERY OF THE STOMACH

A number of different surgical procedures may be performed on the stomach (Table 23-16). The suffix *-ostomy* means "an opening into," thus *gastrostomy* refers to an opening into the stomach. If only one prefix precedes the term *-ostomy*, then the surgical opening is made from the exterior, such as gastrostomy. When two prefixes precede *-ostomy*, the surgery consists of an opening made between two organs (*anastomosis*); for example, a gastroenterostomy is an anastomosis of a portion of the stomach (*gastro-*) with a portion of the small intestine (*entero*). The surgical procedures are more commonly used for cancer of the stomach are gastroduodenostomy (Billroth I) and gastrojejunostomy (Billroth II).

Preoperative Care

If the nutritional status of the patient is poor, an attempt is made to improve nutrition preoperatively. Total parenteral nutrition (p. 601) or a temporary gastrostomy (p. 599) may be necessary. If the patient is to have surgery for an ulcer, any

Table 23-16　Surgeries of the stomach

Name	Description	Comments
Oesophagogastrostomy	Anastomosis of oesophagus and stomach	Usually involves the removal of lower one third of oesophagus; tissue graft may be used
Oesophagojejunostomy	Removal of stomach (total gastrectomy) and anastomosis of oesophagus to jejunum	Two portions of jejunum meeting oesophagus are sometimes joined to form a reservoir for food
Gastrectomy	Removal of part (subtotal) or all (total) stomach	Remaining portions are anastomosed to small intestine of stomach
Gastrostomy	Insertion of the tube through abdominal wall into stomach	Permits oesophageal bypass allowing for nutritional feedings into GI tract
Gastroduodenostomy	Formation of new opening between stomach and duodenum	In Billroth I surgery part of stomach is removed and remaining portion is anastomosed to duodenum
Gastrojejunostomy	Anastomosis of stomach with jejunum	In Billroth II surgery duodenal stump is closed after excision of lower part of stomach
Antrectomy	Removal of entire antrum (lower portion) of stomach	Usually followed by gastroduodenostomy
Pyloroplasty	Repair of pyloric opening of stomach	To enlarge opening and facilitate stomach emptying
Gastric partitioning	Stapling of stomach to reduce size	Staples applied in two rows partially across stomach for control of massive obesity

Table 23-17　Postgastrectomy complications

Complications	Symtoms	Therapy
Bleeding in anastomotic suture line	Large quantity of blood in nasogastric tube drainage during day 1; may also occur on days 4 to 7	Treatment for upper GI haemorrhage (p. 617)
Duodenal stump leakage	Severe upper abdominal pain that may radiate to shoulder, fever, leukocytosis; usually occurs on days 3 to 6	Surgery
Gastric retention	Abdominal fullness, nausea, and vomiting after nasogastric tube is removed	Nasogastric suction for 48 hours then feedings resumed slowly; surgery if no improvement
Dumping syndrome	Weakness, faintness, tachycardia, diaphoresis during eating or from 5 to 30 minutes later	Small frequent feedings (low carbohydrate, high fat and protein); fluids only between meals
Blind loop syndrome (stasis in blind loop with bacterial proliferation	Abdominal pain 15 to 30 minutes after eating; steatorrhoea, diarrhoea, weight loss	Antibiotics; surgery to change a Billroth II to a Billroth I may be necessary

special dietary prescriptions are continued through the preoperative period.

The major focus of preoperative nursing care is teaching the patient. Since the incision for gastric surgery is high in the abdomen, emphasize breathing exercises preoperatively (see Chapter 14). The patient should know that a nasogastric tube may be in place for several days postoperatively because of decreased peristalsis from manipulation of the gastrointestinal tract organs during surgery and to prevent trauma or pressure on suture lines.

Postoperative Care

The care of the patient after gastric surgery centres on promoting pulmonary ventilation, nutrition, and comfort and teaching the patient. Specific nursing care is listed in Box 23-8.

Promoting pulmonary ventilation

Patients with high abdominal incisions are at high risk of developing postoperative pulmonary complications because they are inclined to lie still and breathe shallowly to limit incisional pain. Measures to encourage movement and deep breathing take high priority.

Facilitating gastric drainage

Drainage from the nasogastric tube after surgery usually contains some blood for the first 6 to 12 hours, but bright red blood, large amounts of blood, or excessive bloody drainage

The patient undergoing gastric surgery

Preoperative care

Teach breathing exercises and leg exercises.
Explain special postoperative measures: nasogastric tube and parenteral fluids until peristalsis returns.

Postoperative care

Promoting pulmonary ventilation
   Encourage patient to turn and deep breathe at least every 2 hours or less until patient is ambulating well.
   Give pain medication before activities to encourage active patient participation (thus increasing ventilation).
   Position patient to promote chest expansion (upright).
Promoting nutrition
   Measure nasogastric tube drainage accurately for determination of fluid and electrolyte replacement.
   Monitor patient for signs of leakage of the anastomosis (pain, fever) when oral fluids are initiated.
   Add small amounts of bland food at frequent intervals until foods are well-tolerated.
   Monitor patient for early satiety and regurgitation.
   If regurgitation occurs:
      Tell patient to eat less food at a slower pace.
      Report persistent regurgitation to surgeon.
   Report signs of dumping syndrome (weakness, faintness, palpitations of heart, diaphoresis, feeling of fullness, nausea, diarrhoea) to surgeon.
   Monitor weight.
Providing comfort
   Provide special mouth care until oral fluids are resumed (p. 604).
   Provide analgesic medications on a regular basis during first few days to prevent pain.
   Splint incision before patient coughs.
   Encourage ambulation.
Patient teaching
   Gradually increase amount of food until able to eat three meals a day, if possible.
   If discomfort occurs after eating, decrease size of meals and amount of fluids with meals and eat more slowly.
   Avoid stress, if possible, during and immediately after meals; plan a rest period after eating.
   Elevate head when lying down (if cardia of stomach removed) to prevent gastro-oesophageal reflux (heartburn).
   Use measures to modify effects of stress (see Chapter 5).
   Monitor weight regularly; report weight loss to surgeon.
   Report signs of complications to surgeon (vomiting after meals, increasing feeling of abdominal fullness, increasing weakness, haematemesis, tarry stools, pain, persistent diarrhoea).

is reported to the surgeon immediately (Table 23-16). *If the nasogastric tube stops draining, notify the surgeon*, since a buildup of gas or fluid can cause pressure on the suture line resulting in rupture or dislodgement of the sutures. Do not irrigate the N/G tube without surgeon approval. It is the *responsibility of the surgeon to adjust the placement of the nasogastric tube* so that inadvertent dislodgement of the sutures is prevented. Report signs of return of GI functioning (bowel sounds heard, passage of flatus) to the surgeon.

Promoting nutrition

Until the nasogastric tube is removed and the patient is able to drink enough nutritious fluids, fluids are given parenterally. The average patient requires about 3000-3500 ml of fluids intravenously each day (2500 ml for normal body needs plus enough to replace fluids lost through the gastric drainage and vomitus).

Fluids by mouth are restricted for about 12 to 24 hours or according to the wishes of the surgeon. Fluids are then introduced slowly until well tolerated. Small amounts of bland food may be added until the patient is able to eat six small meals a day and to drink 120 ml of fluid every hour between meals. The dietary regimen must be adapted to the individual, since some people tolerate increasing amounts of food and fluids better than others. Vitamins may be prescribed until the patient is eating a full, well-balanced diet.

Early satiety and regurgitation after meals are common problems after gastric surgery. Eating less food more slowly and chewing thoroughly is usually effective. Persistent early satiety or regurgitation may be caused by oedema of the suture line. A nasogastric tube may need to be reinserted until the oedema subsides.

Dumping syndrome

After a gastric resection, the dumping syndrome occurs to some extent in most patients.[68] It may also occur in patients who had a vagotomy, antrectomy, or gastroenterostomy. The onset may occur during the meal or from 5 to 30 minutes after the meal. The attack may last 20 to 60 minutes. The patient complains of weakness, faintness, tachycardia, and diaphoresis. Other symptoms include a feeling of fullness, discomfort, nausea, and diarrhoea.

The symptoms are thought to be caused by the entrance of hypertonic food directly into the jejunum without undergoing usual changes and dilution in the stomach. The food mixture, more hyperosmolar than the jejunal secretions, causes fluid to be drawn from the bloodstream to the jejunum. The reaction appears to be greater after the ingestion of sugar, since sugar is the most osmotically active food. The symptoms are also attributed to the sudden rise in blood sugar (hyperglycaemia), with the entrance of glucose into the bloodstream, and the subsequent fall in the blood sugar level. The rapid gastric emptying and the propulsion of chyme into the small intestine are felt to initiate an intensive gastrocolic reflex and cause diarrhoea and a feeling of fullness and discomfort.

Reactive hypoglycaemia, sometimes called "dumping," has some of the same symptoms. It occurs 3 to 4 hours after eating.[68] Symptoms are relieved by ingestion of sugar.

Table 23-18　Causes of intestinal malabsorption

Factors affecting absorption	Mechanism	Examples
Altered digestion (intraluminal phase)	Decreased gastric function	Subtotal gastrectomy
	Decreased pancreatic lipase	Pancreatic insufficiency: pancreatitis, cancer of pancreas, cystic fibrosis, Zollinger-Ellison syndrome
	Decreased conjugated bile salts	Liver disease, biliary tract obstruction, enteric fistulas
		Drugs that precipitate bile salts (neomycin, cholestyramine)
Altered mucosal cell transport (mucosal phase)	Genetic abnormalities	Lactase deficiency
	Small bowel disease	Crohn's disease, glutensensitive enteropathy (coeliac disease), tropical sprue, Whipple's disease, infectious or allergic enteritis, parasitic infections, small bowel ischaemia
	Inadequate surface	Intestinal resection or bypass
	Drugs	Para-aminosalicylic acid, colchicine, irritant laxatives, neomycin
	Radiation	Radiation enteritis
Altered lymph/blood transport (transit phase)	Lymphatic obstruction	Lymphoma
	Altered blood supply	Superior mesenteric thrombosis

Teaching for the patient who experiences dumping syndrome includes the following:
1. Eat a low-carbohydrate, moderate-fat, high-protein diet
2. Drink fluids only between meals
3. Avoid eating large amounts of food at one time
4. Rest after meals (recumbent position for 30 minutes)
5. Take anticholinergic drugs before meals as prescribed

Total Gastrectomy

Total gastrectomies are now rarely performed. The nursing care of the patient who has had a total gastrectomy (oesophagojejunostomy) differs in some ways from that of patients undergoing other types of gastric surgery. A thoracic approach is used, and the nursing care will be the same as that for the patient who has had chest surgery. Drains are usually inserted from the site of the anastomosis, and there may be serosanguineous drainage. There is little or no drainage from the nasogastric tube because there is no longer any reservoir in which secretions may collect, and there is no stomach mucosa left to secrete.

Following a total gastrectomy the maintenance of good nutrition is difficult because the patient can no longer eat regular meals and because the food that is taken is poorly digested and therefore poorly absorbed from the intestines. Since the patient also becomes anaemic, ferrous sulphate, folate, and vitamin B_{12} (injections) are often prescribed. These patients rarely regain normal strength.

MALABSORPTION SYNDROME

Aetiology

Malabsorption syndrome is a group of signs and symptoms resulting from inadequate absorption of fat in the small intestine. Because fat-soluble vitamins (A, D, E, and K) require fat for absorption, decreasing absorption of these vitamins usually accompanies fat malabsorption. In addition, fat malabsorption often is accompanied by decreased absorption of protein, carbohydrate, and minerals. Different signs and symptoms specific to various nutrients result from malabsorption of nutrients other than fat.

Adult lactase deficiency is a common disorder found among most populations of the world with the exception of northern European Caucasians and their descendants. In the United Kingdom it is seen in individuals of Asian or Afro-Caribbean descent. In North America, Blacks, Jews, Orientals, American Indians, Eskimos, and Mexicans are frequently affected. Lactase deficiency is usually a congenital disorder, although symptoms may not occur immediately. It also occurs occasionally after a subtotal gastrectomy.

Some adults have an intolerance to gluten found in grains (wheat, rye, barley, oats). The disorder may be termed *gluten sensitive enteropathy*. These people often have a history of childhood coeliac disease or evidence of disease in relatives. Tropical sprue is different than coeliac disease and is endemic to the Caribbean, Southeast Asia, and India.

Pathophysiology

Malabsorption results when there are (1) alterations of digestion so that nutrients are not broken down into a form that can be transported across the cell membranes of the villi; (2) alterations in the transportation of nutrients across the cell membranes of the villi so that nutrients cannot be absorbed; and (3) alterations in the transport of nutrients, particularly fat, from the villi through the lymphatic or circulatory systems (Table 23-18).

Lactase deficiency results from a lack of the enzyme lactase, which hydrolyzes lactose (a disaccharide found in milk) into glucose and galactose for absorption. The undigested lactose acts as an osmotic agent drawing water into the intestinal lumen and a substrate for bacterial fermentation, producing abdominal distension and pain.

Intolerance to gluten found in grains leads to atrophy of the intestinal villi and microvilli. The proximal jejunum is the area most affected. This disorder is thought to be a hypersensitivity response. Tropical sprue has both a nutritional and infectious basis and responds to treatment with antibiotics, as well as to diet therapy.

Nursing Process

Assessment

The stool is assessed for presence of light, greasy, bulky, mushy appearance and a foul odour. This is a sign of *steatorrhoea* (excess fat in the stool). The stools float because of their low specific gravity and because of gas produced by action of intestinal bacteria on the undigested fat. Bowel movements may be limited to one bulky stool a day or may be frequent. If the malabsorption is caused by a lactase deficiency, the patient will have a watery, foul-smelling diarrhoea. Malabsorption causes *flatulence* and abdominal distension. Decreased fat absorption leads to weight loss, weakness, fatigue, and anorexia.

If malabsorption is severe, the person will have signs of *vitamin deficiency* (bleeding, bone pain and fractures, hypocalcaemia, anaemia, inflammation of the tongue, muscle tenderness, peripheral neuritis, and dermatitis). *Protein deficiency* will be evidenced by oedema, hypoalbuminaemia and loss of muscle mass. The skin will be dry and scaly and may be hyperpigmented.

If acute generalized malabsorption is present, the patient is monitored for signs of *bleeding* (ecchymosis, haematuria), tetany, and skin breakdown.

Nursing analysis

Determine problems from analysis of patient data. Possible problems for the person with a malabsorption syndrome may include, but are not limited to:

Problem	Possible aetiologies
Nutrition, altered: less than body requirements	Malabsorption
Pain: abdominal, bone, muscle, dry mucous membranes	Malabsorption
Knowledge deficit	Lack of exposure/recall

Planning: expected patient outcomes

Expected patient outcomes for the person with a malabsorption syndrome may include, but are not limited to, the following:
1. Consumes nutrients that can be tolerated
2. States feeling comfortable
3. Describes diet to be followed and signs indicating need for dietary reevaluation

Implementation

Promoting nutrition

If intolerance to a specific substance is present, omit that substance from the diet. Thus, in adult *lactase deficiency*, all foods containing milk products or added lactose are avoided. Milk substitutes are available, and vegetable oils are used instead of butter. Some people can tolerate some cheeses and yogurt. Calcium substitutes are required.

If *gluten intolerance* is present, exclude all cereal grains and their products (except for rice). This is a difficult diet to follow because many commercial foods, including some instant coffees, contain some wheat filler. Corn, soybean, and gluten-free flour are available for cooking.

If *generalized acute malabsorption* is present, the patient may require total parenteral nutrition or intravenous albumin, calcium, magnesium, and potassium. Packed red blood cells may be necessary if anaemia is severe.

Providing comfort

Mouth care

Dry mucous membranes and enlarged tongue lead to oral discomfort. Good mouth care every 4 hours to maintain hydration will ease discomfort.

Bone and muscle pain

Analgesics may relieve bone or muscle pain. Aspirin may be contraindicated because of the bleeding tendency from vitamin deficiencies. Gentle handling of the extremities is indicated.

Anal care

The anorectal area may become irritated with diarrhoea. Provide for gentle personal hygiene after *each* loose stool.

Counselling and teaching

Because there is no "cure" for malabsorption syndrome, people with these problems must learn to adjust their diets for life. Teaching the person includes the following:
1. Avoid all foods containing that which is not tolerated.
2. Read carefully the labels of prepared foods.
3. Follow the appropriate diet (lactose-free or gluten-free) for life.
4. Re-evaluate diet if symptoms reoccur.

Evaluation

Evaluation of the care of the person with malabsorption syndrome is based on the expected patient outcomes. Questions to consider are:
1. Is the patient consuming nutrients that can be tolerated?
2. Is the patient comfortable?
3. Does the patient know the types of food to be avoided?

FLATULENCE

Pathophysiology

Gas collects in the GI tract as a result of swallowed air, as gas formed by the action of intestinal bacteria, and as carbon dioxide formed by the action of hydrogen carbonate with hydrochloric acid or fatty acids. Normally the gas is either reabsorbed or is expelled. When gastrointestinal motility is decreased, the gas collects in the stomach or intestines, causing abdominal distension and pain.

Assessment

"Wind pains" can cause severe abdominal discomfort. The abdomen is distended over the entire area (as differentiated from lower abdominal distension occurring from a full bladder). The abdomen has a drumlike sound if percussed.

Implementation

Some of the following interventions may help decrease the intestinal gas volume when a pathological condition is not present:
1. Avoid activities that increase repetitive swallowing of air such as gum chewing.
2. Maintain an erect position after meals to facilitate gas rising to the fundus of the stomach and being expelled.

3. Eat a low-fat diet to decrease carbon dioxide production.
4. Take antacids containing aluminium hydroxide and simethicone 1 hour after meals to neutralize acid and reduce flatus.
5. Avoid gas-forming carbohydrates that produce more discomfort (for example, selected vegetables, fruit, or bran).
6. Ambulate to increase peristalsis to move the gas through the intestinal tract, if discomfort is present.

ELIMINATION DISORDERS

The major disorders of the intestines are inflammatory disorders (acute and chronic) that may interfere with absorption and disorders that interfere with passage of the chyme and faecal matter (paralytic ileus, intestinal obstruction, hernias, and tumours). Anorectal lesions, which may be inflammatory or vascular (haemorrhoids), may interfere with passage of faeces because of the discomfort produced.

ACUTE INFLAMMATORY INTESTINAL DISORDERS

Aetiology

Inflammation of the intestines (enteritis) is a common occurrence and may occur alone or in combination with gastritis (p. 612). Gastroenteritis is often of viral origin. Some foods may irritate the intestinal mucosa, which leads to mild symptoms of belching, abdominal discomfort, and diarrhoea.

Food poisoning occurs after the ingestion of food that is contaminated by bacteria containing toxins. Some examples of

bacteria that cause food poisoning, along with the foods in which they are found or food preparation methods that produce the bacteria, are: (1) *Staphylococcus aureus*: enterotoxin in fish, meats, unrefrigerated mayonnaise or cream-filled foods; skin and respiratory tract of food handlers; (2) *Salmonella*: inadequately cooked pork, poultry, eggs; (3) *Campylobacter jejuni*: poultry, unpasteurized milk and water, and (4) *Clostridium botulinum*: improperly canned or smoked foods. Bacteria and parasites may also cause intestinal inflammations (Table 23-19). The appendix may become inflamed (appendicitis); appendicitis is most common in males aged 10 to 30.

Pathophysiology

Enteritis

Acute enteritis can be caused by direct bacterial or viral infection or by the effect of neurotoxins produced by bacteria. This produces either an increased secretion of water and salt into the gut lumen or an increase in motility, causing large amounts of undigested food and fluid to be excreted. In the latter case, large amounts of gas and foul-smelling stool result. With profuse diarrhoea, large amounts of fluid and electrolytes may be lost, leading to dehydration, hyponatraemia, and hypokalaemia (see Chapter 6).

Parasitic infections

The most common parasitic infections are amoebiasis and trichinosis (Table 23-19). *Amoebiasis* is caused by the protozoan parasite that primarily invades the large intestine and secondarily the liver. The active motile form of the protozoan, the trophozoite, is not infectious and, if ingested, is easily destroyed by digestive enzymes. However, the inactive form (cyst) is highly resistant to extremes in temperature, most chemicals, and the digestive juices. When the cyst is swallowed in *faecally contaminated food or water*, it easily passes into the

REVIEW

Table 23-19

Disease	Signs and symptoms	Medical therapy
Gastroenteritis	Abdominal cramps, nausea and vomiting, diarrhoea, headache vomiting subside, then fluids and	Nothing by mouth until nausea and bland diet; rest
Food poisoning	*Staphylococcus aureas:* Nausea and vomiting, abdominal pain, decreased temperature; diarrhoea is variable	Bed rest, fluids
	Salmonella: Nausea and vomiting, abdominal pain, chills, fever, weakness	Bed rest, fluids
	Campylobacter jejuni: Abdominal pain, blood in faeces, nausea and vomiting, abdominal pain, diarrhoea	Bed rest, fluids, erythromycin
	Clostridium botulinum: Nausea and vomiting, double vision, flaccid paralysis of face and throat, dryness of skin and mucous membranes	Botulinum antitoxin, maintenance of ventilation and oxygen, parenteral fluids
Amoebiasis	Early: abdominal cramps, intermittent diarrhoea/constipation, flatulence	Amoebicidal drugs
	Late: frequent liquid stools containing blood, mucus; fever, colicky abdominal pain	
Trichinosis	Oedema of eyelids, muscle stiffness, weakness, fever, pain on eye motion, dyspnoea	Symptomatic: bed rest, analgesics, steroids, thiabendazole
Appendicitis	Sudden onset, pain in umbilical region becomes localized in right iliac fossa, nausea and vomiting, low grade fever, leukocytosis	Appendicectomy when diagnosis confirmed

intestines, where the active trophozoite is released and enters the intestinal wall. Here it feeds on the mucosal cells, causing ulceration of the intestinal mucosa. Although the disease exists chiefly in tropical countries, it also prevails wherever sanitation is poor. The cyst can survive for long periods outside the body.

Trichinosis is caused by the larvae of a species of roundworm, which become encysted in the striated muscles of humans, pigs, and other animals (rodents) that eat infected pork in garbage. Trichinosis has a worldwide distribution with the highest incidence occurring in Europe and the United States. It occurs more often in pigs that have been fed garbage than in those fed on grain. The larvae do not form cysts in pork; therefore, they are not visible to the naked eye and cannot be seen by food inspectors.

Trichinosis is transmitted through inadequately cooked food. *Pork* is the most common source of infection. When infected food is eaten, live encysted larvae develop within the intestine of the host; they mate and produce eggs that hatch in the uterus of the female worm. The larvae are discharged in huge numbers into the lymphatics and lacteals of the host's small intestine at the rate of about two every hour for about 6 weeks. They pass to the muscles of the host, where they become encysted by the reaction of the host's body and may remain for many years.

The trichinosis parasite can be killed by cooking at the recommended temperature of 77°C (170°F) or by freezing at a temperature of -15°C (5°F) for 20 days.[60] They are not killed by smoking, pickling, or other methods of processing. Sausage and other infected pork products carelessly prepared are a source of infection in humans.

Appendicitis

Appendicitis is an inflammation of the vermiform appendix, located near the ileocaecal valve. The inflammation may be initiated by obstruction from a faecalith (a stonelike mass formed from faeces), infection from colon bacilli or streptococcus, or appendiceal kinking or occlusion. A small part of the appendix may be oedematous or necrotic, or the entire appendix may be involved. Pressure within the appendix builds up rapidly, leading to early necrosis of the appendiceal walls with subsequent perforation. Heat and external pressure (such as that resulting from enemas) increase the appendiceal pressure, facilitating rupture of the appendix.

Although the typical symptoms of acute appendicitis (anorexia, nausea, and vomiting combined with abdominal pain that becomes located at McBurney's point halfway between the umbilicus and right ileal crest) are common findings, many variations of these symptoms may occur. The pain may be located in other parts of the abdomen as a result of the stretching of the appendix or the location retrocaecally or adjacent to the ureter. Low-grade fever and leukocytosis result from the inflammation.

Peritonitis

If peritonitis (inflammation of the peritoneum) results from a perforated appendix, adhesions form quickly in an attempt to wall off the infection, and the omentum helps to enclose areas of inflammation, forming an abscess. As healing occurs, fibrous adhesions may form, leading to intestinal obstruction

at a later date. At other times the fibrous adhesions may disappear completely. Local inflammatory reactions of the peritoneum include redness, oedema, and the production of large amounts of fluid containing electrolytes and proteins. Hypovolaemia, electrolyte imbalance, dehydration, and finally shock develop from loss of circulating fluid if the infection is not contained. Intestinal peristalsis is halted by a severe peritoneal infection.

Nursing Process
Assessment

Subjective data to be collected from the person with an acute inflammatory disorder of the intestines include anorexia, nausea, and presence and extent of abdominal discomfort. If food poisoning is suspected, question the person about possible sources of food contamination. Abdominal pain is usually diffuse except if acute appendicitis is present. With appendicitis, there is often rebound tenderness over McBurney's point if pressure is applied lightly, then released suddenly.

Objective data to be collected include the following:
1. Vomit: frequency, amount, presence of blood
2. Stools: frequency, character, amount if liquid, presence of foul odour
3. Flatulence
4. Signs of fluid and electrolyte imbalance (thirst, dry mucous membranes, haemoconcentration, oliguria, muscle weakness)

Nursing analysis

Problems are determined from analysis of patient data. Possible problems for the person with an acute inflammatory disorder of the intestines may include, but are not limited to, the following:

Problem	Possible aetiologies
Fluid volume deficit	Diarrhoea
Pain: abdominal	Intestinal inflammation
Infection: high risk for spread	Lack of knowledge

Planning: expected patient outcomes

Expected patient outcomes for the person with an acute inflammatory disorder of the intestines may include, but are not limited to, the following:
1. Patient is hydrated (moist skin and mucous membranes, good skin turgor).
2. Patient states feeling more comfortable.
3. Infection is not spread.

Implementation
Assisting with achievement of therapeutic goals

When *appendicitis* is suspected, the patient usually is hospitalized at once and placed on bed rest for observation and the necessary diagnostic procedures (serum WBC, urinalysis, flatplate abdominal X-ray film) that must be performed. Because an operation may be performed shortly after admission, do not give the patient anything by mouth until blood count reports are available. Parenteral fluids may be given during this time. Do not give narcotics until the cause of the pain has been determined because they would mask signs or

REVIEW

Table 23-20   Chronic inflammatory bowel disorders

Disease	Signs and symptoms	Medical therapy
Crohn's disease	Periods of exacerbation and remission Acute: colicky or steady right lower quadrant pain, malaise, moderate fever, mild diarrhoea, mucus or pus in stool Chronic: weight loss, anaemia, fistula formation, intestinal obstruction	Diet: high-calorie, high-protein, high-vitamin Sulphonamides, azathioprine Surgery for fistulas or intestinal obstruction (colectomy or colostomy)
Ulcerative colitis	Periods of exacerbation and remission Severe diarrhoea (15 to 20 stools/day containing blood, mucus, pus); anorexia; weight loss; anaemia; low grade fever Severe: weakness, debility, cachexia, dehydration, hypokalaemia, hypoproteinaemia	Diet: high-calorie, high-protein, high-vitamin (avoid milk) Sulphonamides, corticosteroids Surgery for refractory disease or complications (total colectomy with permanent ileostomy)
Diverticulitis of colon (inflamed mucosal pouches)	May be asymptomatic Intermittent lower left quadrant pain aggravated by emotional tension or eating Constipation alternating with diarrhoea	Diet: high in vegetable fibre, wholegrain cereals Bulk stool additives; opioid analgesics, anticholinergics (dicyclomine, propantheline) Bed rest, sedation, and parenteral or oral fluids for severe episode Surgery for complications of perforation or obstruction (colectomy, temporary colostomy)

symptoms. Sometimes an ice bag to the abdomen is ordered to help relieve pain. *Heat and enemas are contraindicated*, as they may cause the appendix to rupture. Explain to the patient that a rectal examination (done by the doctor) is necessary to help establish the diagnoses. Surgery consists of an appendicectomy (removal of the appendix).

Interventions to achieve patient outcomes

Promoting hydration

When nausea and vomiting are present, give the person nothing by mouth until symptoms subside. With severe vomiting, replace fluids and electrolytes intravenously. A sedative such as diazepam or an antiemetic such as prochlorperazine may be prescribed parenterally or by suppository. When vomiting subsides, give tea, clear soup, and ginger ale orally every hour. Bland feedings of custard, jelly, and cream soups are usually tolerated after 2 to 24 hours. Carefully measure and record intake and output.

Assisting with comfort

Abdominal cramping from diarrhoea may be relieved by constipating agents containing an opiate, which is chemically related to pethidine, or loperamide. Belching and defaecation also often relieve the discomfort. If appendicitis is ruled out, heat to the abdomen may offer some relief.

Preventing spread of infection

Universal precautions help to control spread of infection in the hospital. Stress cleanliness, and advise patients that it is important to wash their hands well after bowel movements and before meals to prevent spread of infection.

Evaluation

Evaluation is based on expected patient outcomes. Questions to consider include:

1. Is patient hydrated, with moist skin and mucous membranes and good skin turgor?
2. Is the patient more comfortable?
3. Has the spread of infection been avoided?

CHRONIC INFLAMMATORY BOWEL DISEASE

Chronic inflammations of the bowel include two disorders, Crohn's disease and ulcerative colitis, that are fairly similar and are referred to as chronic inflammatory bowel disease. Another chronic inflammatory disorder is diverticulitis (inflammation of colon diverticula), but because it is a different entity, it is discussed separately. Table 23-20 lists signs and symptoms and usual medical therapies of these disorders.

Aetiology/Epidemiology

Chronic inflammatory bowel disease occurs primarily in young adults aged 15 to 30 but may occur up to age 70. The cause is unknown, although both genetic and environmental factors have been implicated. There is a higher incidence of inflammatory bowel disease in Western Europe and the United States. Ulcerative colitis occurs twice as often as Crohn's disease, but incidence of the latter is increasing.

Pathophysiology

Ulcerative colitis and *Crohn's disease* differ in terms of location and type of lesions. Ulcerative colitis starts in the rectosigmoid colon and spreads upward. Crohn's disease can affect both the small and large intestines, and the areas of inflamed tissue are often separated by normal tissue. The lesions of ulcerative colitis are mucosal ulcerations that bleed easily. As the lesions advance, the bowel mucosa becomes oedematous and thickened with scar formation. The colon may lose its elasticity and absorptive capability. The lesions of Crohn's disease are granulomatous ulcers that may involve deeper structures. The ulcers may perforate and form fistulas. Scar tissue may lead to intestinal obstruction.

The loss of absorptive capability in both ulcerative colitis and Crohn's disease leads to anorexia, weight loss, malaise, and diarrhoea. Severe diarrhoea leads to dehydration from fluid loss, hypokalaemia from loss of potassium-rich intestinal secretions, and hypoproteinaemia from loss of protein through the damaged intestinal epithelium.[72]

Nursing Process
Assessment

Collect subjective and objective data about the patient's knowledge of the disorder, nutritional status, pattern of elimination, comfort, and ability to cope with stress.

Subjective data

1. Patient's understanding of the disorder
2. Patterns of bowel elimination: frequency, character, amount; presence of blood, fat, mucus, or pus
3. Pain: location, character, frequency, relief with passage of stools, relief measures taken
4. Nutritional status
   a. Intolerance to certain foods
   b. Intake of caffeinated drinks, alcohol
   c. Appetite, presence of nausea
   d. Usual weight, recent weight loss
   e. Weakness, fatigue
5. Sleep: interference because of diarrhoea or pain
6. Stress
   a. Perceived sources of stress in daily life
   b. Occupation: nature, hours of work, job satisfaction
   c. Usual coping methods and present effectiveness
7. Social relationships
   a. Extent of social activities and interferences as a result of illness
   b. Availability and perceived support of significant others
8. Sexual: effect of illness on sexual relationships
9. Medications taken at home: type, dosage, effect

Objective data

1. Weight
2. Temperature
3. Observable eating patterns
4. Signs of dehydration with severe ulcerative colitis (decreased skin turgor, dry mucous membranes)
5. Stool: number, character, amount, presence of blood (overt, positive guaiac test), pus, mucus
6. Condition of perianal skin with severe diarrhoea
7. Behaviour: signs indicating stress or anxiety (for example, restlessness, pacing, twisting hands, verbal comments indicating concerns)

Information about the patient's understanding of the nature and precipitating factors is helpful in planning necessary teaching. Analyze the diet of the person with ulcerative colitis or Crohn's disease for nutritional adequacy. Compare the person's usual daily intake to the basic four food groups to determine quality of nutrient intake. Anorexia and intolerance to milk products are characteristic of ulcerative colitis. With severe ulcerative colitis or Crohn's disease, there is weakness from loss of weight because of the decreased nutrient intake and decreased absorption. Cachexia may result.

The pattern of bowel elimination for the person with chronic bowel inflammation may vary as follows:

Ulcerative colitis	Severe diarrhoea (15 to 20 stools/day) stool may contain blood, pus, mucus
Crohn's disease	Mild diarrhoea; stool may contain mucus, fat or pus; no blood
Diverticulitis	Constipation or constipation alternating with diarrhoea; stool may contain blood

With ulcerative colitis, abdominal cramps may occur with or without bowel movements. The colicky right lower quadrant abdominal pain of Crohn's disease is often relieved by a bowel movement. The pain of diverticulitis may be aggravated by eating.

Symptoms of chronic inflammatory bowel disorders may be exacerbated by stress or tension. Knowledge of the patient's perception of the effect of stress on the onset of symptoms and of the patient's usual coping patterns is useful for planning measures to relieve or reduce effects of stress.

Diagnostic tests

Laboratory tests are conducted for the presence of anaemia and for blood in the stools. Inflammatory bowel disease is diagnosed by means of radiographs, sigmoidoscopy, or colonoscopy. A biopsy of tissue may be taken during sigmoidoscopy or colonoscopy.

Stool examination for occult blood

Occult blood may be identified by one of three tests: guaiac, benzidine, or orthotoluidine. The *guaiac* test is the least sensitive but does not require special preparation. With the *benzidine* or *orthotoluidine* tests, false readings may be obtained if the patient ingests meat (false-positive) or vitamin C in quantities greater than 500 mg/day (false-negative). Ask patients about whether they have taken these substances before performing the benzidine or orthotoluidine tests.

Radiographs

The barium enema, also called lower GI series, helps identify the lesions of inflammatory bowel disease, as well as complications such as fistulas, strictures, polyps, and megacolon of perforation.

Endoscopy

Sigmoidoscopy is a common procedure for visualizing the rectum and sigmoid colon just past the sigmoid flexure. Colonoscopy is a more exacting procedure and is usually performed only when clinically necessary.[72] Neither sigmoidoscopy nor colonoscopy is performed during acute episodes of inflammatory bowel disease.

Nursing analysis

Problems are determined from analysis of patient data. Possible problems for the person with chronic inflammatory bowel disease may include, but are not limited to, the following:

Problem	Possible aetiologies
Nutrition, altered: less than body requirements	Loss of nutrients in diarrhoea, anorexia
Fluid volume deficit, high risk for	Diarrhoea
Pain: abdominal, anus	Diarrhoea, anal skin irritation
Skin integrity, impaired, high risk for	Malnutrition
Coping, ineffective individual, family	Chronicity of disorder, situational crises
Fatigue	Anaemia, malnutrition, inflammatory response, stress
Sexual dysfunction	Malnutrition, diarrhoea
Knowledge deficit	Lack of information or recall

Planning: expected patient outcomes

Expected patient outcomes for the person with a chronic inflammatory bowel disorder may include, but are not limited to, the following:

1. Eats a high-protein, high-calorie, high-vitamin, well-balanced diet.
2. Drinks 2500 ml/day; skin and mucous membranes are moist.
3. States feeling more comfortable.
4. Skin of elbows, sacrum, and anorectal area is intact.
5. Describes alternative coping measures, if appropriate.
6. Plans activities to permit rest periods when fatigued.
7. Expresses concerns regarding sexuality and explores alternative ways of meeting sexuality needs, if appropriate.
8. Describes nature of illness and prescribed therapy, measures to promote relaxation and rest, symptoms requiring medical attention, and plans for regular follow-up care.
9. Family/friends describe:
    a. Approaches to promote patient independence and control of own daily activities.
    b. Approaches to cope with own feelings regarding patient's illness.

Implementation

Assisting with achievement of therapeutic goals

Therapy for inflammatory bowel disease during exacerbations is primarily supportive and includes nutritional therapy and rest. Medications include the following:

1. Sulphasalazine: the most commonly prescribed drug. Patient instructions include drinking 2000 to 2500 ml/day to prevent crystallization in kidneys and avoiding sunlight or using sunscreen because of photosensitivity. Infertility may occur.
2. Mesalazine (5-ASA, the active ingredient of sulphasalazine): given rectally for ulcerative colitis; oral forms are available; has fewer side effects than sulphasalazine.
3. Corticosteroids: given in high dosages over a limited time for severe disease to suppress inflammation; dosages are decreased gradually before drug is discontinued.
4. Antibiotics: given to acutely ill patients with signs of peritoneal irritation or with a fistula.
5. Bulk forming agents in preference to the antimotility drugs for diarrhoea.
6. Vitamin supplements, particularly when anorexia and nausea are present; replacement of vitamin B_{12} when there is a marked loss of ileum.
7. Iron dextran: given by Z-track for anaemia (oral iron intake is ineffective because of intestinal ulceration).

Interventions to achieve patient outcomes

Promoting nutrition

A low fibre diet to promote bowel rest and to avoid irritation of the mucosal lining is recommended during exacerbations. The diet should be high in proteins and calories to replace lost nutrients. With inflammatory bowel disease, large amounts of proteins are lost through the intestinal wall by exudation or bleeding. Calories are needed for energy to spare the protein for healing. Fats are sometimes not well tolerated because of malabsorption. Some people with ulcerative colitis have an intolerance to lactose, and these people should avoid milk products. In acute stages, give an elemental diet that is almost residue free (products that are generally used for tube feedings but are here given orally). Palatability may be a problem; serving fluids chilled and offering a variety of flavours increases patient acceptance. For severe exacerbations, total parenteral nutrition (TPN) is commonly used.

Promoting fluid balance

Profuse diarrhoea leads to loss of fluids and electrolytes. Encourage fluids to 2500 ml/day for people on oral diets. Keep the mouth moistened and apply lotion to the skin. Monitor weight for marked changes resulting from fluid losses or gains. Monitor fluid intake and output daily in the hospitalized patient.

Promoting comfort and skin integrity

Encourage patients to use the toilet or commode whenever possible, but a weak, acutely ill person usually wants the bedpan accessible at all times. Dispose of bedpans as often as they are used, which may be frequently for patients with ulcerative colitis. Room deodorizers may be necessary. Patients who brace themselves on the bedpan by leaning on their elbows may develop pressure areas; these areas will need to be protected and examined frequently.

The anal region often becomes excoriated from the frequent stools. Painful anal fissures and fistulas may also develop. Keep the anal area clean and dry. Medicated wipes can provide greater comfort than toilet tissue. Frequent baths or use of bidet also promote comfort and cleanliness. Ointments may be used to protect the perianal skin.

Facilitating coping

Ulcerative colitis and Crohn's disease are lifelong illnesses with periods of exacerbation and remission that can disrupt the person's life. Emotions and stress have been noted to play a role in exacerbations. If the disease is of long duration, the patient is usually thin, nervous, and apprehensive and is inclined to be preoccupied with physical symptoms. Insecurity, dependency, and depressed or hostile behaviour may be present. Family and friends may take over control of the person's life, adding to the person's feelings of loss of self-control.

The caregiver may also experience feelings of frustration and dissatisfaction. Empathetic communication over time is usually needed to establish a helping relationship. It may be necessary to plan to spend time with the person and with the family on a regular basis.

Help the person with chronic inflammatory bowel disease to identify possible sources of life stressors and to examine ways to possibly reduce or modify the stress. Assess the person's usual coping mechanisms for effectiveness, and discuss alternate coping strategies as appropriate (see Chapter 5). Knowledge about the illness, diagnostic tests, and therapy may help to decrease anxiety. Patients need to be included in planning of activities to gain some control over their lives. During periods of remission, the person may need to be encouraged to participate in social activities.

Promoting rest

Fatigue is common because of increased energy demands from the inflammatory process and decreased energy supply from malnutrition and anaemia. Include planned rest periods in the daily activities. When fatigue subsides, encourage progressive activity. During periods of remission, encourage the person to participate in social activities but not overextend to the point of fatigue.

Promoting sexuality

Sexual response may be decreased by chronic inflammatory bowel disease and may interfere with sexual relationships. Malnutrition and frequent diarrhoea lead to decreased libido. Give the person an opportunity to discuss any sexual concerns, and assist the person to communicate these concerns with the involved party. Alternate ways of meeting sexuality needs can be explored (see Chapter 26).

Facilitating patient learning

Patient teaching is important on an ongoing basis to help the person learn effective self-care. Main points to be included in teaching are listed in Box 23-9. Pamphlets about inflammatory bowel disease to be used in patient teaching can be obtained from the Crohn's in Childhood Research Association and Ileostomy Association.

Evaluation

Evaluation is based on expected patient outcomes. Questions to ask may include the following:

1. Is the patient eating a well-balanced, high-protein, high-calorie diet and drinking 2000 to 2500 ml/day?
2. Does the patient feel comfortable and rested?
3. Is skin intact on elbows, sacrum, and anorectal area?

Patient Teaching **23-9**

The patient with a chronic inflammatory bowel disease

Diet
> Eat high-protein, high-calorie, high-vitamin diet (avoid milk products with ulcerative colitis).

Elimination
> Take medications as prescribed.
> Drink at least 8 glasses fluid daily.
> Keep rectal area clean; use analgesic rectal ointment or take bath or use bidet for anal discomfort.

Promotion of rest
> Use relaxation measures (such as breathing exercises) when emotional tension is present.
> Identify sources for an ongoing supportive relationship.
> Maintain a regular sleep schedule.
> Plan daily activities to avoid fatigue; rest as necessary.

Health maintenance programme
> List signs indicating possible exacerbation or complications (abdominal pain, increasing diarrhoea or constipation, presence of blood or pus in the stool, fever, progressive weight loss).
> Plan for regular follow-up.

---

4. Are patient and family coping with the changes caused by inflammatory bowel disease?
5. Does the patient plan activities to permit for rest periods?
6. Has the patient expressed concerns regarding sexuality and explored alternative ways of meeting sexual needs?
7. Can the patient describe the nature and therapy for inflammatory bowel disease and need for medical follow-up?
8. Can family and friends describe their approaches to promote patient's independence?

Surgery

Ulcerative colitis can be treated by surgery. The trend is towards earlier surgical intervention for the acutely ill person and for people experiencing frequent exacerbations. Surgery is clearly indicated when complications are present, including massive haemorrhage, perforation of the colon, strictures, and medically unresponsive toxic megacolon (dilation and hypertrophy of the colon).

Different types of surgery may be performed. A common procedure is removal of the diseased colon and rectum, with the end of the ileum being brought out through the abdominal wall (*ileostomy*). If the rectum is only mildly diseased, an ileorectal anastomosis may be performed with preservation of rectal function.

A different type of surgical approach is the *continent ileostomy* or Kock's pouch. An intraabdominal reservoir with a nipple valve is formed from the distal ileum to provide continence. The capacity of the pouch increases slowly over months until it can hold approximately 500 ml. Contents of the pouch are removed several times a day by catheterization.

Difficulties have occurred with valve failure and in keeping the ileal contents from becoming too thick and plugging up the stoma.

Total colectomy and mucosal proctectomy with *ileoanal anastomosis* (with or without a valveless pouch) consists of resection of the colon, removal of rectal mucosa leaving rectal muscle intact, and anastomosis of ileum with the anal sphincter. A J-pouch, an S-pouch, and a W-pouch are approaches that can be used. These methods are now used more frequently than the continent ileostomies. A 2-month temporary ileostomy is performed to permit healing of the anastomosis. Bowel incontinence may be a sequela.

Crohn's disease does not respond well to surgery and has a high recurrence rate. Surgery is indicated when complications occur (bowel obstruction, fistulas, abscesses). Types of surgery include (1) segmental *resection* of the diseased bowel with anastomosis (preferred method) or (2) bowel *bypass* by anastomosing the ileum to the disease-free colon, leaving the diseased bowel intact. A newer procedure is *strictureplasty*, in which blocked or narrowed bowel segments are widened, leaving the bowel intact.

Ileostomy care

The general care of the patient with an ileostomy is similar to that of the patient with a colostomy (p. 643).

Faecal drainage from the ileostomy stoma begins within 72 hours. It is liquid and may be constant. Within 10 to 15 days, the ileostomy output will be a soft, slightly formed stool. The terminal ileum adapts to the loss of the colon and begins to reabsorb water. Patients with ileostomies have "toothpaste" consistency stools within 3 to 6 months after the adaptation of the ileum. Drainage usually occurs 2 to 4 hours after a meal, although there may be a small amount of output intermittently throughout the day.

Exceptions to this pattern of ileostomy elimination are seen in patients who have had previous bowel resections or resections of the ileum for Crohn's disease. The more small intestine that is lost, the greater the chance of a high volume of very liquid output with resultant dehydration.

Maintaining fluid and electrolyte balance

An excessive loss of fluid through the ileostomy, usually from 1000 ml to 2000 ml daily, may occur during the initial postoperative period. The amount of fluid output then diminishes to 500 to 800 ml/day.[68] Sodium and potassium losses are greater with an ileostomy than the amounts normally lost in faeces. The person with an ileostomy is therefore at greater risk for dehydration, hyponatraemia, and hypokalaemia during periods of decreased fluid intake or of increased fluid output. Potassium supplements may be necessary. After the initial period, a large amount of output — requiring the pouch to be emptied hourly or more frequently — is considered to be diarrhoea. During these periods, monitor the person for signs of fluid and electrolyte imbalance. Teach the patient how to promote fluid and electrolyte balance (see Box 23-10).

Promoting nutrition

The patient may be kept on a low-fibre diet for 6 weeks to decrease the amount of bulky and undigested foods as the intestinal tract recovers from the surgical intervention. As the person begins to add foods, it is recommended that only one high-fibre food be added at a time and that the person chew the food well. Foods should not be eliminated from the diet unless the person is unable to tolerate them after two or three trials.

Food blockage (a large mass of undigested food, especially high-fibre foods) may occur with an ileostomy. The food becomes lodged at a kink, or narrowing, in the bowel and blocks the lumen. The result is a mechanical bowel obstruction. Blockage most commonly occurs when a person eats several high-fibre foods in one meal or does not chew the foods properly.

If the ileostomy becomes blocked, the person should get into a knee-chest position and gently massage the area below the stoma. Stomal oedema will develop with a food blockage, and the pouch should be changed to accommodate the swelling. Diarrhoea usually follows the removal of the obstruction, and the patient will need fluid replacement. Abdominal pain in the peristomal area is generally present for 3 to 5 days after obstruction. If the obstruction is not passed following the use of the knee-chest position, the patient should notify the doctor.

DIVERTICULAR DISEASE OF THE COLON

Diverticula, or pouches, form when increased pressure within the colon pushes weakened areas of the colon outward. The cause is thought to be a low intake of dietary fibre, which is often typical of diets in industrialized societies. Diverticula usually occur after age 40, and the incidence increases with age. The nonsymptomatic condition is called diverticulosis.

Patient Teaching   23-10

The patient with an ileostomy

Promoting fluid and electrolyte balance
 Look for signs of dehydration (dry skin and mucous membranes, thirst).
 Increase fluid intake if stool output markedly increases or signs of dehydration occur. Drink fluids containing electrolytes or clear soup.
 Avoid routine laxatives.
 Monitor closely for increased faecal output when taking antibiotics.
 In areas where "traveller's" diarrhoea is a high risk, drink bottled water and avoid uncooked fruits and vegetables.
Promoting nutrition and absorption
 Start with bland low-residue foods.
 Introduce new foods (especially high-fibre foods) one at a time.
 Avoid several high-fibre foods at one meal to prevent blockage.
 Chew foods thoroughly.
 Avoid foods that cause problems such as wind or obstruction (these may include coconut, corn, celery, Chinese foods).
 Avoid foods that cause odours (these may include onions, cabbage, fish, spicy foods).
 Use liquid or chewable medications rather than enteric-coated, time-released, or hard tablets, if possible.

Diverticulitis

Symptoms appear when the diverticula become inflamed (diverticulitis), creating painful spasms, or when complications such as perforation, obstruction, or haemorrhage occur. Bowel motility may be slow because of insufficient fibre, leading to constipation, or fast because of the inflammation, leading to diarrhoea.

With acute diverticulitis, intravenous fluids or a clear liquid diet may be prescribed to allow the bowel to rest. Antibiotics are also prescribed. Recurrent attacks of diverticulitis or occurrence of complications usually require surgical resection of the involved colon with an end-to-end anastomosis. Bowel surgery is described on p. 639. A temporary colostomy may be necessary for 6 to 8 weeks.

Diverticulosis

When the person is asymptomatic, encourage a diet high in vegetable fibre (fruits and vegetables, whole grain cereals). Patients should avoid foods with seeds and nuts, as these irritate the diverticula. Individuals may add unprocessed wheat bran to foods, but initially only in small amounts that increase slowly to a quarter cupful daily in fruit juices or soups. Bran initially causes abdominal distension and excess flatus. N.B. Bran added to food may cause malabsorption of minerals such as iron, calcium and zinc. The purpose of the high-fibre diet is to increase stool bulk and bowel transit time, thus increasing the diameter of the colon and decreasing intraluminal pressure.

Bulk forming agents and stool softeners such as docusate sodium may be prescribed for people with diverticular disease. Anticholinergic drugs may be given to slow peristalsis and to decrease spasms in the sigmoid colon.[60]

Because emotional tension often precipitates diverticulitis, the person may need assistance in learning how to reduce emotional tension. Relaxation techniques, planned rest periods, and regular sleeping hours may prove helpful.

INTESTINAL OBSTRUCTION

Aetiology

Intestinal obstruction (ileus) occurs when there is impedance to the normal flow of intestinal contents, either because of disturbance to neural stimulation of bowel for peristalsis (paralytic ileus) or because of something interfering with normal flow of bowel contents (mechanical/organic ileus). *Paralytic ileus* results mainly from handling of the bowel during abdominal surgery, from peritonitis, or from pain of thoracolumbar origin (see Box 23-11). *Mechanical obstructions* of the small intestines are primarily adhesions, whereas in the large bowel, neoplasms are the major cause. A *volvulus* is a twisting of the bowel. *Intussusception* is a telescoping of a segment of the bowel within itself. *Hernias* may cause bowel obstruction when a loop of bowel becomes strangulated in the weakened ring or incision (p. 636). In *cancer of the bowel*, the growth narrows the lumen of the bowel. The clinical manifestations and medical therapy of intestinal obstruction are outlined in Table 23-21.

Pathophysiology

When peristalsis ceases, the involved intestinal area becomes distended by gas and fluid. Approximately 7 L of fluid are secreted into the stomach and small intestines per day; most of this fluid is normally reabsorbed in the colon. When peristalsis ceases, however, much of the fluid remains in the stomach and small intestine. The retained fluid increases pressure on the mucosal wall and, if not removed, results in ischaemia, necrosis, bacterial invasion, and eventually peritonitis. Loss of the fluids leads to hypovolaemia (shock) and dehydration. Loss of sodium and chloride ions causes a shift of potassium from the cells, leading to hypokalaemic alkalosis.

When mechanical obstruction occurs, peristaltic waves proximal to the affected area increase in an effort to move the intestinal contents past the obstruction. These peristaltic movements create a high-pitched abdominal sound.

As the abdomen distends from the distended gut, pulmonary ventilation may become impaired from pressure on the diaphragm. Pressure on the bladder may cause urinary retention. Constipation occurs with mechanical obstruction because some faeces usually pass around the obstruction. When peristalsis ceases completely, as with paralytic ileus or complete organic obstruction, no bowel movement occurs (absolute constipation).

23-11

Causes of intestinal obstruction

Paralytic ileus

Manipulation of abdominal viscera during abdominal surgery
Peritoneal irritation (peritonitis)
Pain of thoracolumbar origin
    Rib or spinal fractures
    Myocardial infarction
    Pneumonia
    Pyelonephritis
    Ureteral or biliary calculi
    Retroperitoneal haemorrhage
Sepsis
Hypokalaemia causing decreased muscle tone of bowel
Intestinal ischaemia

Mechanical intestinal obstruction

Adhesions
Hernias
Neoplasms
Inflammatory bowel disease
Foreign bodies, gallstones
Faecal impaction
Strictures: congenital, radiation
Intussusception
Volvulus

REVIEW

Table 23-21   Obstructive disorders of the intestinal tract

Disorder	Signs and symptoms	Medical therapy
Paralytic ileus	Continuous abdominal pain, distension, vomiting, absolute constipation, decreased or absent bowel sounds	Restricted oral intake, IV fluids, GI suction
Mechanical intestinal obstruction	Colicky abdominal pain, vomiting, constipation, high-pitched bowel sounds	Same as above; surgery
Hernia	Lump in weakened area, especially with straining; pain with incarceration	Herniorrhaphy
Cancer of the bowel	Blood in stool, changes in bowel habit	Resection of bowel, with or without stoma

Nursing Process
Assessment

The following parameters need to be monitored in the patient who is thought to be developing an intestinal obstruction:
1. Bowel sounds: presence and character
    a. Loud, frequent, high-pitched sounds are heard as obstruction is developing.
    b. Bowel sounds are not heard when peristalsis ceases.
    c. Weak bowel sounds and passage of flatus occur as peristalsis returns (flatus is a more significant sign).
2. Vomiting: assess type and frequency
    a. Profuse, nonfaecal vomiting is seen with obstruction of the proximal small bowel.
    b. Occasional faecal-type vomitus is seen with obstruction of the distal bowel.
3. Abdominal pain: location and character
    a. Cramping pain occurs as obstruction develops.
    b. Pain becomes more constant and diffuse with distension.
4. Abdominal distension: use a tape measure to determine change in size; always measure at the same site (usually across the umbilicus).
5. Urinary output: amount
    a. Monitor total output (decrease seen with dehydration).
    b. Monitor amount of urine at each voiding for signs of urinary retention.
6. Vital signs
    a. Fever, tachycardia, and hypotension with dehydration.
    b. Fever may also indicate more obstruction or peritonitis.

Diagnostic tests

X-ray films of the abdomen (flat plate and upright) identify air- and fluid-filled areas of obstruction. Serum blood tests indicate alterations from normal (haemoconcentration) when dehydration occurs. There will be a decrease in sodium and potassium and an increase in haematocrit, plasma bicarbonate, serum pH, and blood urea.

Nursing analysis

Problems are determined from analysis of patient data. Possible problems for the person with an intestinal obstruction may include, but are not limited to, the following:

Problem	Possible aetiologies
Fluid volume deficit	Abnormal loss of GI fluids
Ineffective breathing pattern	Abdominal distension
Pain: abdominal	Abdominal distension

Planning: expected patient outcomes

Expected patient outcomes for the person with an intestinal obstruction may include, but are not limited to, the following:
1. Patient is hydrated (moist skin and mucous membranes, good skin turgor).
2. Breath sounds are clear; respirations are easy and regular.
3. Patient states feeling more comfortable.

Implementation
Assisting with achievement of therapeutic goals

Conservative medical therapy consists of oral intake restrictions, parenteral fluids and electrolytes, and gastric or intestinal suctioning until bowel function returns.

Interventions to achieve patient outcomes
Promoting hydration

Give fluids containing electrolytes parenterally in large quantities (3000 to 4000 ml/day) to prevent dehydration. The doctor determines the amount to be given based on the amount of gastric drainage from nasogastric or intestinal intubation; thus it is important to measure gastric drainage accurately. Flow sheets are helpful for careful monitoring of intake and output. Monitor the patient for signs of fluid overload (bounding pulse, neck vein distension, cough). Central venous pressure (Chapter 9) may be monitored in high-risk patients (elderly, cardiac disease).

Promoting pulmonary ventilation

Abdominal distension creates pressure on the diaphragm, inhibiting chest expansion. Nursing measures to promote aeration of the alveoli include the following:

1. Upright position to release pressure on diaphragm
2. Deep breathing exercises
3. Encouraging patient to breathe through the nose and not swallow air to prevent further distension

Promoting comfort

Pain and vomiting often leave the patient physically and emotionally exhausted. Assistance in simple activities such as turning in bed may be necessary. Comfort measures associated with nasogastric intubation (p. 622) are helpful. The patient may need reassurance that the decompression will ease the discomfort from the distension.

Because oral fluids are usually restricted, mouth care is important for preventing infection and increasing comfort. If the patient is poorly nourished, measures to keep the skin soft and intact and free from pressure are indicated.

Surgery

Surgery is usually performed to relieve mechanical and vascular obstruction. The operative procedure varies with the cause and the location of the obstruction and the general condition of the patient. If constricting bands or adhesions are found, they are cut, and it may be necessary to resect the occluded bowel and anastomose the remaining segments. Care of the patient undergoing intestinal surgery is described on p. 639.

Evaluation

Evaluation is based on expected patient outcomes. Questions to consider are:
1. Is the patient hydrated?
2. Have pulmonary complications been avoided?
3. Is the patient relatively comfortable?

HERNIAS

Hernias account for a large number of intestinal obstructions. A hernia is a protrusion of an organ or structure from its normal cavity through a congenital or acquired defect. In addition to a loop of bowel, a hernia, depending on its location, may contain peritoneal fat, a section of bladder, or a portion of the stomach.

If the protruding structure of the organ can be returned by manipulation to its own cavity, it is called a *reducible* hernia. If it cannot, it is called an *irreducible* or *incarcerated* hernia. When the blood supply to the structure within the hernia becomes occluded, the hernia is said to be *strangulated*. Some types of hernias are described below.

Types of hernias

Inguinal
  Indirect Loop of intestine passes through abdominal ring and follows course of spermatic cord into inguinal canal
  Direct   Loop of intestine passes through posterior inguinal wall
Femoral   Loop of intestine passes through femoral ring down into femoral canal
Umbilical   Loop of intestine passes through umbilical ring
Incisional Loop of intestine or other organ protrudes through weakened scar

A hernia that is not incarcerated can very often be reduced by the person lying down with the feet elevated or by lying in a bath of warm water and pushing the mass gently back towards the abdominal cavity.

Surgery is frequently performed for large hernias or when there is a high risk of incarceration. A *herniorrhaphy* consists of suturing the defect in the fascia. In the postoperative period following repair of an *umbilical* or large *incisional* hernia, a nasogastric tube may be used to prevent postoperative vomiting and distension with subsequent strain on the suture line.

Because of postoperative inflammation, oedema, and haemorrhage, *swelling of the scrotum* often occurs after repair of an indirect inguinal hernia. This complication is extremely painful, and any movement of the patient causes discomfort. Ice bags help relieve pain. The scrotum is usually supported with a suspensory or is elevated on a rolled towel. Urinary retention may occur because of the discomfort in movement, which produces hesitancy in urination. Ecchymosis of the lower abdominal wall or upper thigh may occur after extensive manipulation during surgery. The ecchymosis fades in a few days. Sexual functioning is not affected.

The patient who has had elective surgery for a hernia should not drive for at least 2 weeks. Physical activities should not include any heavy lifting, pulling, or pushing for at least 6 weeks.

CANCER OF THE BOWEL
Epidemiology

Malignant tumours of the colon and rectum are among the most commonly occurring malignancies in the United Kingdom, third following cancer of the lung and skin in men and second following cancer of the breast in women.[20b] The incidence of bowel cancer is significantly higher in developed countries whose inhabitants are of Northern European descent, and it is lower in Japan, India, Africa, and some Latin American countries. The incidence of bowel cancer also increases with age and reaches a peak in people in their late 70s. Clinical manifestations and types of surgery are outlined in Table 23-22.

Aetiology

Although the cause of cancer of the bowel remains unknown, environmental and genetic factors and preexisting disease appear to be influential (see Box 23-12). The high incidence of

---

23-12	**Risk factors for colorectal cancer**
	Age: over 40
	Past history
	Colon polyps (adenomas)
	Cancer: colorectal, breast, genital
	Ulcerative colitis
	Polyposis syndromes
	Immunodeficiency disease
	Family history: colorectal cancer, polyposis syndromes

Table 23-22 Cancer of the colon

Location	Signs and symptoms	Surgery
Ascending colon	Occult blood in stool, anaemia, nausea/vomiting, right upper quadrant pain, palpable mass	Right colectomy with anastomosis
Descending colon	Gross blood in stool, progressive constipation with increased frequency, pencil-shaped stools	Left colectomy with anastomosis
Sigmoid colon and rectum	Rectal bleeding, constipation and increased frequency, sensation of incomplete bowel evacuation	Sigmoid: left colectomy with anastomosis Upper rectum: resection with anastomosis Lower rectum: abdominoperineal resection with colostomy

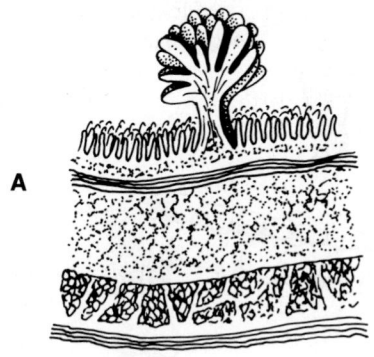

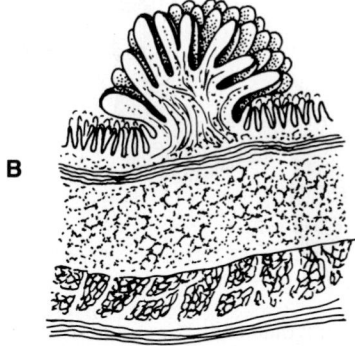

Fig. 23-5 Colon polyps. **A,** Tubular adenoma (note peduncle). **B,** Villous adenoma.

colorectal cancer in industrial countries relates to a diet high in animal fat, protein, and refined carbohydrates that are low in dietary fibre. Although a direct causative relationship has not been established, high fat and low-fibre diets may be significant causative factors. Low-fibre diets decrease colonic transit time and potentially increase contact of endogenous or exogenous carcinogens with the bowel mucosa. Popular literature often suggests that certain foods are carcinogenic; however, research has not yet identified specific foods as carcinogenic for bowel cancer. Genetically, some "cancer families" have been identified in which cancers of certain body areas, including the bowel, are transmitted as dominant traits.

Prevention and Health Education

Primary prevention for colon cancer includes reducing fat intake to 35% or less of calories and increasing fibre intake to 12 to 24 g/day with an upper limit of 32 g.[20a] These

guidelines for fat intake established by the Department of Health,[20a] correlates with the national risk factor targets set out in Health of the Nation 1992.[20c]. Studies show that diets high in vegetable fibre offer the most protection. Little is yet known about the mechanisms for cancer protection by fibre; therefore, a fibre intake from a variety of foods (whole grains, vegetables, fruits) rather than fibre supplements is recommended.

Secondary prevention involves early detection. Because colorectal cancer develops over time, detection is possible before symptoms appear. In the United States, many lives could be saved if everyone followed the following guidelines recommended by the American Cancer Society.

1. Digital rectal examination yearly after age 40
2. Occult blood stool test yearly after age 50
3. Sigmoidoscopy every 3 to 5 years after age 50, following two negative yearly examinations

Some of these tests, e.g. digital examination, form part of a routine health screening in the United Kingdom and trials are currently underway regarding the efficacy of other measures. Anyone who develops a change in bowel habits, a change in the shape of the stool, or the passing of blood should consult their doctor.

Pathophysiology

Polyps are *benign* growths (adenomas) on the colonic mucosa; they are considered to be premalignant. The two major types of polyps are the more common *tubular adenoma*, a globelike structure attached to the bowel wall by a "stem" (peduncle), and the *villous adenoma*, a large soft polyp that has several fingerlike projections but no peduncle (Fig. 23-5). Villous adenomas are more likely to become malignant.

Cancer of the colon may develop in one of two ways. In the caecum and *ascending* colon, the lesions tend to develop as polyps that grow as cauliflowerlike masses protruding into the lumen of the colon. These lesions may ulcerate, but obstruction of the colon is uncommon. Eventually, the lesions penetrate the colon wall and extend into surrounding tissue.

In the *descending* colon, especially the rectosigmoid portion, an annular lesion is more common. The early lesion is a small polypoid mass that becomes plaquelike. The plaque grows circumferentially, encircling the colon wall, and then contracts, causing narrowing of the lumen. Obstruction may result from formed stool on the left side that is unable to pass through the narrowed lumen. These lesions also eventually penetrate the colon wall and extend into adjacent tissue.

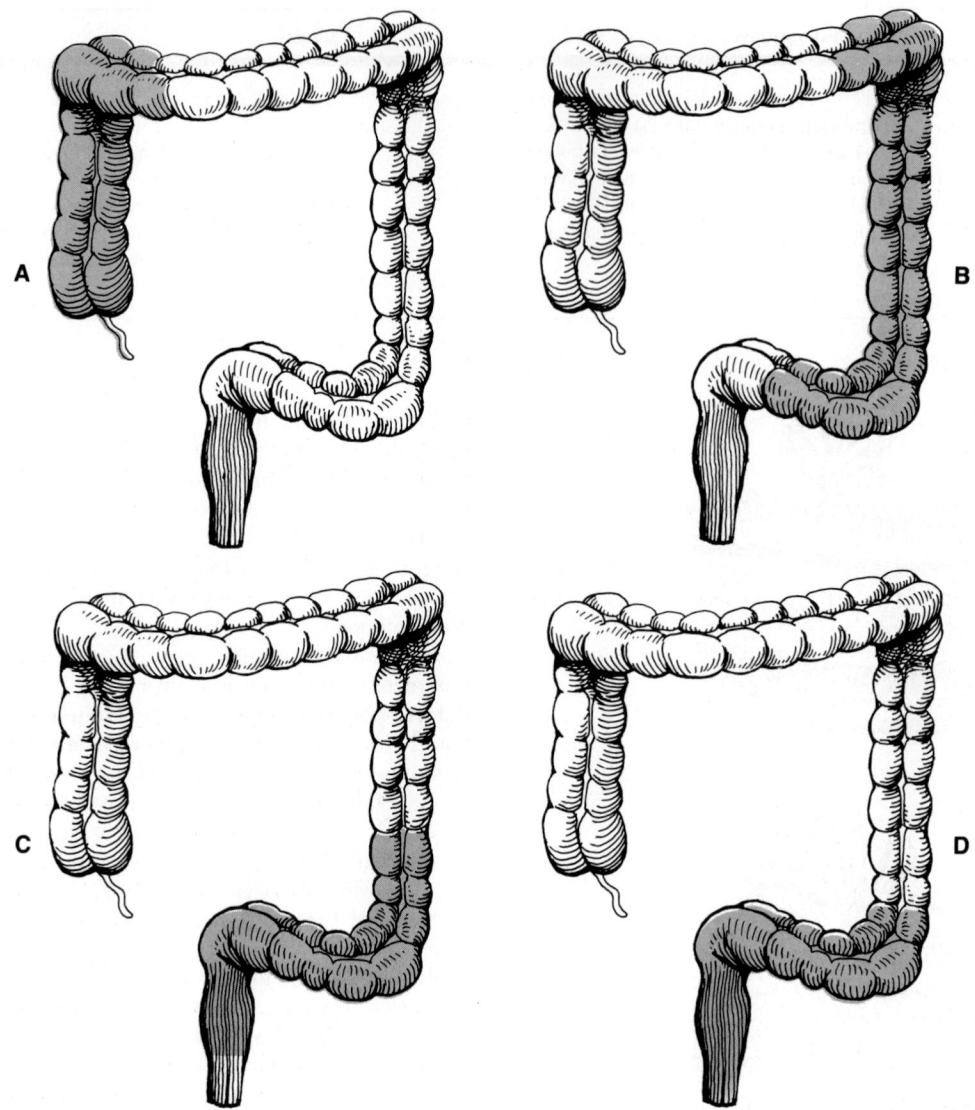

Fig. 23-6 Bowel resection. **A,** Right hemicolectomy. **B,** Left hemicolectomy. **C,** Anterior rectosigmoid resection. **D,** Abdominoperineal resection.

Cancer of the colon may spread by direct extension or through the lymphatic or circulatory systems, seeding at distant points in the peritoneum or at distant points in the colon. The liver is the major organ of metastasis because the colonic blood vessels empty into the hepatic portal vein leading to the liver.

Diagnostic Tests

Diagnosis of cancer of the colon is made by physical examination, sigmoidoscopy, colonoscopy, and barium enema examination. Cancer of the rectum can be accurately diagnosed by pathological examination of a biopsy specimen taken during a proctoscopic examination. Stools are examined for occult blood (p. 630).

Carcinoembryonic antigen monitoring

Carcinoembryonic antigen (CEA) is an antigen seen in foetal life. It was originally isolated from patients with colonic cancer, but it is also seen in people with ulcerative colitis, cirrhosis, and other forms of cancer and in chronic cigarette smokers.

The CEA test is not useful as a screening test for colonic cancer; however, it is useful as an indicator of the effects of therapy. For example, a drop in CEA level suggests the effectiveness of the therapy. A continued high level or rise in level suggests recurrence or spread of the tumour.

Medical Therapy

Surgery

Treatment of cancer of the colon is always surgical, and the tumour, surrounding colon, and lymph nodes are resected. The amount of bowel resected is based on removal of all tissue supplied by the blood vessel of the diseased tissue. Sugery is performed in one of the following ways: (1) the diseased portion of the bowel is removed (resected), and the remaining ends are joined together in an end-to-end anastomosis (EEA), or (2) the diseased portion of the bowel is removed, and the functioning end is brought out onto the abdominal surface forming a stoma (p. 641). Only 10% of people with rectal cancer require a stoma.

Resection with anastomosis can be performed for cancer of the ascending, descending, or sigmoid colon and upper rectum (Fig. 27-24 *A, B,* and *C*). These surgeries are performed through abdominal incisions, and natural defaecation is maintained. The anastomosis may be done by suturing or stapling techniques. A greater amount of rectal tissue can be removed with the stapling technique for anastomosis.

Growths in the lower rectum require removal of the entire rectum and sigmoid colon by an abdominoperineal resection (p. 640); this surgery requires formation of a stoma. Care of the person experiencing bowel surgery is described below.

Obstruction or perforation of the colon usually requires a temporary colostomy, followed later by closure of the colostomy. Prognosis after surgery depends on the stage and location of growth. Patients with low-lying colorectal stage C cancers have a lower survival rate than those with high-lying colonic cancers.[72] Duke's stages of colorectal cancer are listed below:

Stage A: Confined to bowel mucosa
Stage B: Invading muscle wall
Stage C: Lymph node involvement
Stage D: Metastases or locally unresectable tumour

Other therapies

Radiation therapy is generally ineffective in treating colon cancer but may be used to treat some rectal cancers. It may be used preoperatively in large, locally extensive growths to retard growth; this prevents cells that may accidentally be dislodged during surgery from seeding themselves at other locations. Radiation may be given postoperatively to decrease recurrence.

Chemotherapy is used for metastatic disease and for people with a high risk of recurrence.[72] It is most effective in preventing liver metastasis. The chemotherapeutic agent of choice is fluorouracil, alone or in combination with other agents.

BOWEL SURGERY

Surgery of the bowel may be performed for different reasons, including bowel obstruction, ulcerative colitis, and bowel cancer. The major concern with any type of bowel surgery is contamination by faecal contents. Preoperative preparations are directed towards minimizing this problem. Many of the people experiencing bowel surgery are elderly, because the largest number of bowel surgeries are performed for bowel cancer. Elderly people have a higher risk for postoperative pulmonary embolism and fluid imbalances. If the procedure is performed by laparoscopic surgery, the risks and length of recovery are decreased.

Preoperative Care

Preoperative care consists primarily of preparing the bowel to decrease intestinal bacteria and to remove faeces. This

---

Guidelines for Care   23-13

The patient undergoing bowel surgery

Preoperative care

Preventing infection
  Give low-residue diet several days before surgery.
  Give clear liquids day before surgery.
  Give prescribed antibiotic.
  Give prescribed enemas, washouts and laxatives.
Teaching
  Explain special postoperative procedures (for example, nasogastric intubation, parenteral fluids for several days).
  Teach deep breathing exercises and leg exercises.
  Teach how to facilitate turning in bed without exerting pull on abdomen.

Postoperative care

Promoting oxygenation
  Encourage turning and deep breathing exercises.
  Encourage patient to be active.
Maintaining fluid and electrolyte balance
  Maintain patency of GI tube.
  Record amount of drainage accurately.
  Maintain prescribed flow of parenteral fluids.
  Monitor for signs of fluid loss (dry skin and mucous membranes, decreased skin turgor) or overhydration, especially in the elderly.
Promoting elimination
  Monitor for signs of returning peristalsis (passage of flatus, return of bowel sounds).
  Encourage increasing ambulation.
  Monitor character of initial stools.
Promoting comfort
  Give good oral hygiene until oral fluids are taken freely.
  Lubricate nares with water-soluble lubricant.
  Use measures to maintain moisture of oral mucous membranes (rinse mouth, chew gum, suck hard sweets).
  Give analgesics on a regular basis during the first 48 hours to minimize severe pain.
Teaching
  Drink at least 2000 ml of fluid daily to avoid constipation.
  Avoid use of laxatives without medical approval; stool softeners or bulk forming agents may be used.
  Avoid heavy lifting for at least 6 weeks after surgery.

---

is accomplished by (1) a low-residue diet for several days followed by clear liquids the day before surgery, (2) bowel cleansing with enemas, washouts and laxatives for several days before surgery, and (3) oral antibiotic therapy. Neomycin is usually the chosen antibiotic because it is not absorbed through the intestinal tract, has low toxicity, and has broad-spectrum activity against colonic bacteria. Vigorous mechanical cleansing or purging may be poorly tolerated by some people, such as the acutely ill or elderly; therefore, these approaches may be modified.

Patient teaching includes preparing the patient for postoperative procedures, such as nasogastric intubation and the need for parenteral fluids for several days until peristalsis returns. Ventilatory measures, as well as leg exercises (Chapter 14), will also be important postoperatively, especially for the elderly patient.

Postoperative Care

Extensive handling of the GI organs during surgery markedly inhibits peristalsis. Care during the early postoperative period emphasizes (1) preventing a buildup of fluid and gas by the use of nasogastric intubation, (2) preventing pulmonary complications, (3) maintaining fluid and electrolyte balance, (4) promoting elimination, and (5) promoting comfort.

Atelectasis, pulmonary embolism, and deep vein thrombosis may result from decreased respiration and circulation. Incisional pain may limit chest expansion and the patient may require much encouragement to move, ambulate, and breathe deeply. There is a high risk of pulmonary embolism after perineal resection. Venous congestion in the pelvic veins leads to stasis of circulation; platelets adhere to the vessel walls, especially at the bifurcation of pelvic blood vessels, leading to formation of blood clots with possible embolism.

The length of time required for peristalsis to return depends on the extent of bowel manipulation. Presence of bowel sounds and passage of wind signal the return of function. It is not unusual after a resection of the bowel for diarrhoea to occur after peristalsis returns. Usually it is temporary and soon disappears. When stool consistency becomes normal, advise the patient to avoid becoming constipated, because a hard stool and straining to expel it could possibly injure the anastomosis, depending on its location.

The care of the patient experiencing bowel surgery is summarized in Box 23-13.

Abdominoperineal Resection

Malignant growths in the lower two thirds of the rectum are removed by abdominoperineal resection (Fig. 23-6, D). The operation is performed through two incisions: a low midline incision of the abdomen and a wide elliptic incision about the anus. Through the abdominal incision, the sigmoid colon is divided and the lower portion is freed from its attachments and temporarily left beneath the peritoneum of the pelvic floor. The proximal end of the sigmoid is then brought out through a small stab wound on the abdominal wall and becomes the permanent colostomy. Through the perineal incision, the anus, rectum and distal portion of sigmoid are removed. The perineal wound may be closed around Penrose drains, or it may be left wide open to heal slowly from the inside outward. The open perineal wound will take longer to heal than a usual incision. Care of the patient with an abdominoperineal resection is summarized in Box 23-14.

Many patients complain of *phantom rectal sensations* and of feeling the necessity to defaecate. An explanation of cortical perception and transmission of nerve impulses often helps the patient cope with these sensations.

Guidelines for Care   23-14

The patient with an abdominoperineal resection

Preoperative care

Prepare patient as for other bowel surgery.
Prepare patient for a stoma (p. 641).
Prepare patient for a perineal incision: wound may be open and, if so, will take longer to heal.

Postoperative care

Provide care as for other bowel surgery.
Preventing complications
 Shock: monitor for early signs and institute shock measures.
 Haemorrhage
  Check perineal dressing frequently: initial drainage is profuse and serosanguineous.
  Reinforce initial dressings as necessary.
  Report excessive bleeding to surgeon.
Thrombophlebitis/pulmonary embolism
 Encourage leg exercises (Chapter 14) until patient is ambulatory.
 Encourage use of elastic stockings with elderly patients or those with poor leg circulation.
 Encourage ambulation when permitted.
Promoting healing
 Maintain low continuous suction of sump catheters, if present.
 Change perineal dressing as frequently as needed after first 24 hours.
  Record precise directions for dressing change on nursing care plan.
  Irrigate wound with normal saline solution by use of catheter.
  Cover with dry dressings and hold in place with a T-binder (the T "top" is wrapped around the waist and the T strap is brought up between the legs).
 Substitute baths for irrigation when patient is ambulatory; maintain free flow of water on perineal wound in bath (rubber ring may be helpful).
 Provide stoma care (p. 643).
Promoting urinary elimination
 Maintain patency of indwelling catheter.
 Monitor for residual urine when catheter is removed.
  Keep accurate intake and output records.
  Monitor for lower abdominal distention, patient discomfort, restlessness.
 Use measures to encourage voiding if patient has inability to initiate stream.
Promoting comfort
 Assist patient to find a comfortable position in bed: lying on side is usually preferred.
 Assist patient to turn frequently.
 Try a foam pad under buttocks for supine position.
 Give narcotics at regular intervals until severe pain decreases (about 3 days postoperatively).
 Give patient/family opportunities to express

Urinary retention is a common occurrence following rectal excision. Factors that influence urinary retention include loss of pelvic support, chronic urinary tract infection, enlarged prostate, or nerve injury. Loss of pelvic support increases problems with micturition when the patient is supine; thus micturition may improve with ambulation. If nerve injury is present, problems with urinary retention and urinary tract infections may persist for several months with partial resolution of retention but with urinary incontinence experienced at night.

Sexual difficulties may occur in about 40% of males following abdominoperineal resection. Difficulty with ejaculation is more commonly seen than impotence (difficulty with erection), but they may occur together. Convalescence after an abdominoperineal resection is prolonged and may require many months. Support is usually needed during this time.

FAECAL DIVERSION: STOMAS

Diversion of the faecal stream may be performed for GI diseases or for trauma. Common reasons for ostomy surgery include the following:

Type	Reason
Ileostomy	Ulcerative colitis, familial polyposis
Temporary colostomy	Trauma: gunshot wounds, stab wounds, road traffic accident
	Complications of diverticulitis, volvulus, bowel ischaemia, perforation
Permanent colostomy	Cancer of colon and rectum

Diversion of the faecal stream may be temporary or permanent. In a *temporary diversion* the faecal stream is rerouted to allow the GI tract an opportunity to heal or to provide an outlet for the stool when an obstruction is present. A *permanent diversion* implies that the intestine cannot or will not be reconnected; thus, a return to a normal elimination mode will not occur.

Surgical Sites

When the small bowel (ileum) is the site of diversion, the ostomy is called an *ileostomy*. The surgical diversion of the large colon will result in a *colostomy*. The anatomical location of the colostomy will determine the name, that is, *ascending colostomy*, *transverse colostomy*, or *sigmoid colostomy*. The effects are different for each type of ostomy (Table 23-23).

The two main types of functioning stomas are the end stoma and the loop stoma. A nonfunctional end stoma is referred to as a *mucous fistula*.

When an *end stoma* is created surgically, the proximal bowel is brought out through an incision in the abdominal wall, folded over on itself (forming a cuff), and sutured. The stomal surface is the mucosal lining or inner layer of the intestinal wall. The remaining *distal* bowel may be surgically removed, oversewn to form a Hartmann's pouch, or brought to the skin surface to form another stoma, the mucous fistula (Fig. 23-7). If the proximal and distal stomas are adjacent (Fig.23-8), they are referred to as a *double-barrelled ostomy*.

The *loop stoma* is created by bringing the bowel through an abdominal incision, sliding a support under the bowel, and opening the upper wall of the bowel (Fig. 23-9). The posterior wall remains intact. There is one stoma, but there are two openings: proximal and distal. The loop ostomy is generally a temporary procedure.

Patients who do not receive adequate bowel preparation before a loop or double-barrelled procedure may have a bowel evacuation through the rectum. Patients should be told this may occur. Mucus may continue to be passed through the rectum.

Psychological Response to Ostomy Surgery

When the surgeon tells the person of the probable need for an ostomy, the immediate reaction is likely to be shock and disbelief. Whether the ostomy is to be temporary or permanent, it is difficult for most people to accept. It is not unusual for the person to be sad, withdrawn, and depressed after learning of the need for ostomy surgery.

Removal of any part of the body involves a sense of loss. Thus, the person facing ostomy surgery may experience grief

Table 23-23 Comparison of ileostomy and colostomies

	Ileostomy	Ascending colostomy	Transverse colostomy	Sigmoid colostomy
Location	Ileum	Ascending colon	Transverse colon	Sigmoid colon
Type of drainage	Liquid-to-paste consistency	Liquid-to-soft	Soft	Soft-to-formed
Bowel regulation	No	No	No	Only with irrigations (if desirable)
Fluid imbalance	Monitor for dehydration if high-output diarrhoea	Same	May occur with bouts of diarrhoea	Usually not a problem unless there were previous resections
Skin irritation	Occurs easily because of digestive enzymes	Same	Can occur from exposure to stool	Same as transverse colostomy
Other complications	Food blockage Prolapse of stoma Stricture	Prolapse Stricture	Prolapse Stricture	Prolapse Stricture Constipation

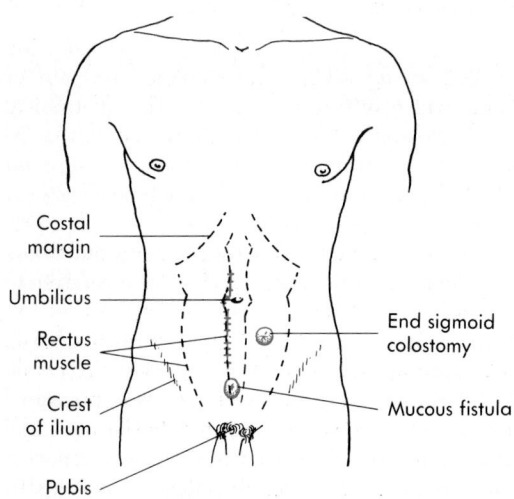

Fig. 23-7   End sigmoid colostomy and mucous fistula.

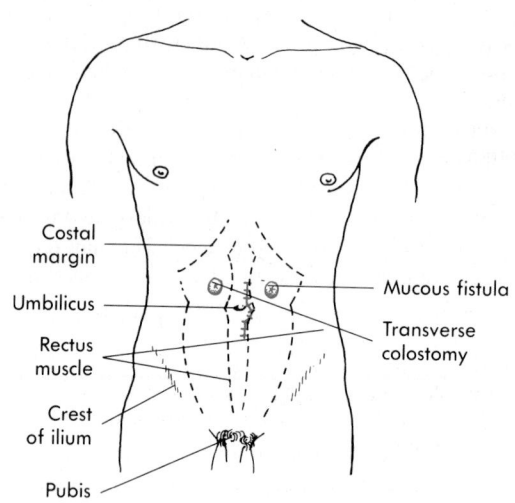

Fig. 23-8   Transverse colostomy; adjacent mucous fistula.

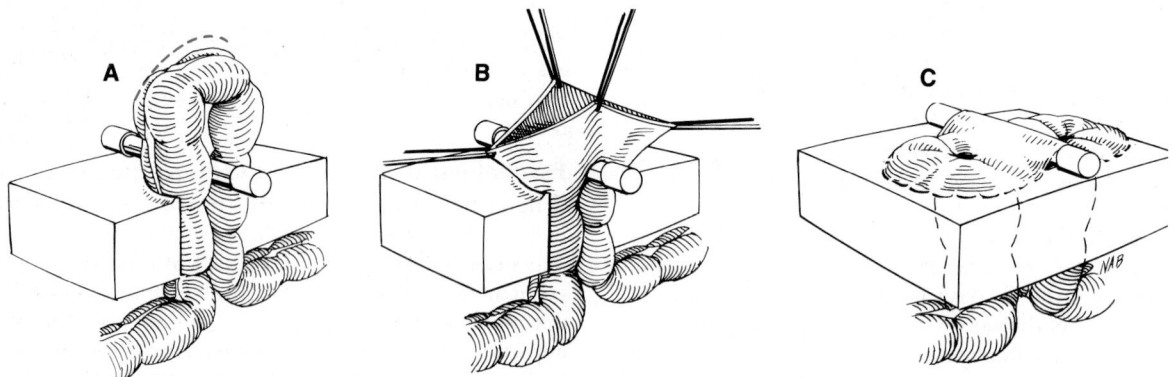

Fig. 23-9   Loop colostomy. **A,** Bowel brought through incision and supported with rod.
B, Incision in anterior wall. **C,** Edges are folded over to make two openings in one stoma.

and mourning over the lost part, which includes shock, denial, anger, and depression. (See Chapter 11 for a discussion of these reactions.) The change in body image may result in feelings of guilt, shame, or disgust. Usually the formation of the stoma is viewed as mutilating surgery, but for some individuals the surgery may be a relief or release from coping with chronic pain, diarrhoea, or debility. No matter what reaction is expressed, patients need time and the support of others to work through their feelings.

Preoperative Care

The general preoperative and postoperative care for bowel surgery is followed for the person scheduled for ostomy surgery. Guidelines for ostomy care are summarized in Box 23-15.

Counselling and teaching are important aspects of preoperative care. Assist the patient and family and friends to identify their feelings and reactions to the proposed surgery. Assess the patient's knowledge of the surgery, as

The patient with a colostomy or ileostomy

Prepare the person for surgery by describing the ostomy, answering questions, and dispelling misconceptions.

Monitor the stoma postoperatively for swelling, colour, function, and intactness of mucocutaneous suture line.

Assess the readiness of the person to view the stoma and to begin learning about care of the ostomy.

Promote acceptance of the change in the body through own facial expressions and empathetic interactions.

Instruct the person in the care of the ostomy through use of a detailed and individualized care plan.

Provide the person with written instructions and supplies.

Provide necessary follow-up care.

Provide information concerning support services such as the Ileostomy Association and the British Colostomy Association.

Suggested preoperative teaching for the patient requiring a stoma

Simple explanation with drawings of anatomy of the GI tract

Explanation of surgery
  Areas to be removed
  Effect on bowel function

Definition of terms: colostomy (or ileostomy), stoma, bag

Explanation of appearance/sensation of stoma and basic management

Availability of nurse/stoma therapist after surgery to teach patient the care of the stoma both in hospital and in the community

well as responsiveness to information. Some people are very upset by the impending surgery and want little information. However, it is important for each person to know at least what is meant by ostomy surgery and the type of management it will require. Many people have misconceptions about the ostomy that add to the preoperative anxiety. Dispelling these myths and giving correct information can lessen the fears of an ostomy. Some suggested information is listed in Box 23-16.

Postoperative Care

Stoma drainage

Assess the stoma regularly for colour and to ensure intactness of the stoma-skin suture line. A red colour denotes viability. A stoma that has impaired circulation will appear dark, dusky, or black.

The stoma secretes mucus immediately following surgery and will continue to do so. During the first 24 to 48 hours, the stomal drainage is mucoid and serosanguineous. As intestinal function returns, flatus will be produced. Faecal drainage is initially liquid for all ostomies. Drainage from a colostomy may then change quickly, depending on its location (Table 23-23).

Protecting the skin

Faecal drainage from the stoma can be very irritating to the skin surrounding the stoma; therefore, the skin needs protection. *Skin barriers* are substances that are applied to protect the skin. The most commonly used barriers are 4 × 4 inch squares or pectin-based *wafers* that are cut to fit snugly around the stoma. *Pastes* are useful to fill in creases or folds in poor locations and to supplement wafers for a longer seal. Powders must be covered with a *sealant* (spay, liquid, gel, wipe) before a pouch can be applied.

Peristomal skin infections may be bacterial or fungal. The most common is a yeast infection from *Candida albicans*. The skin becomes bright red with papular lesions in an irregular area; secondary skin changes occur as the process continues, and dry, scaling areas develop. Treatment involves the use of nystatin powder sealed with a skin sealant.

Changing the bag/pouch

Products for ostomy care are available in a variety of styles, shapes, and sizes. Bags are available in clear and opaque plastics, and covers are designed to make the wearing of a pouch more comfortable.

An effective bag system protects the skin, contains the stool, moulds to the body contour, allows comfortable bending and movement, and is inconspicuous and odourproof. Selection of an effective bag system is crucial to the rehabilitation process.

Preparing the patient to care for the stoma facilitates incorporation of the body changes into the new body image. Most people do not wish to look at the stoma immediately. Do not push them to look at the stoma, but gently encourage them to look at it as they show interest in doing so.

A patient may be unable (or may refuse) to participate in self-care, which creates a management problem. The patient, family member or friend, nurse, and surgeon need to discuss the problem openly. Someone must be prepared to care for the stoma after the patient is discharged from the hospital. If the patient is unwilling to assume an active role, an early psychiatric referral may be helpful.

Teach the patient the steps of changing the bag (Box 23-17) and give written instructions before discharge. A minimum of three lessons is generally needed. Lessons should begin when the patient is receptive to instruction.

During the first lesson, the patient observes the steps of the procedure. The nurse informs the patient that the stoma has no touch sensation, and the red colour means the stoma has healthy blood supply. Address questions and concerns. During the second lesson, the patient assists with preparing the bag, cleansing the skin and stoma, and centring the bag around the stoma. The patient changes the bag with supervision as needed for the third lesson. Some people need more practice, and additional

23-17

Changing the bag/pouch

Pattern

1. The pattern should be 1/8 inch larger than the stoma.
2. Always label the pattern for "top" or "skin" side. •

Skin barrier

1. Use either a quarter, a half, or a full wafer, depending on the size of the stoma and the abdomen.
2. Round the corners to conform to the shape of the adhesive on the pouch bag.
3. Trace the pattern on the paper side.
4. Cut hole on pattern line (line will not be visible when it is cut).
5. Smooth sides of the opening with your finger.

Bag

1. Bag opening should be slightly larger than the opening of the skin barrier (paper can cut the stoma).
2. Trace pattern on the paper side of the bag (use the opening from the skin barrier that has already been cut).
3. Cut the hole larger than the line of the pattern (cut outside the line).
4. Smooth edges around the opening.
5. Remove paper backing from the bag, centre the openings, and apply the shiny side of the skin barrier to the bag.

Applying the system

1. Remove the old bag and skin barrier carefully.
2. Cleanse the skin with warm water.
3. Pat the skin dry.
4. Warm the skin barrier (the bag is already attached).
5. Remove the backing; save this paper (it can be used as a pattern in the future).
6. Centre opening with stoma; press and seal to the skin; hold hand against the bag to help seal the skin barrier to the skin.
7. Close the bottom of the bag.

From Broadhurst BB, Broadwell DC: Ostomy care for children. Unpublished material, 1981.

A patient who is free of stool between irrigations can wear a closed-end bag with a gas-relief valve or stoma "cap," a small square bag with an absorbent dressing. The stoma will continue to secrete mucus and expel flatus between irrigations, so an ostomy covering with a gas filter is desirable. Some people are unable to regulate the colostomy with irrigations and decide to wear drainable bags instead of irrigating.

People who have irrigated their colostomies successfully for years may develop irregular results with irrigation secondary to ageing. As one ages, there is a decrease in mucus production and peristalsis. This is often frustrating for patients who may feel they have failed because the elimination pattern is unpredictable.

Various types of commercial irrigation sets are available, and they all require similar supplies: an irrigation sleeve that fits over the stoma and is long enough to drain into the toilet, a cone tip for the insertion of water into the stoma, an enema bag to contain the solution, and clips to close the top and bottom of the sleeve.

When prescribed, irrigations are begun after the bowel has begun to function and the stool is beginning to become soft, usually about the seventh postoperative day. The procedure for irrigation is outlied in Box 23-18.

The irrigation procedure is usually performed in the toilet. The patient may wish to sit on a chair on a pillow and face the commode until the perineal wound heals. Subsequently the patient sits on the toilet. Cramping during an irrigation may be caused by inserting the water too rapidly or from water that is too cold. Rate of flow varies with the pressure (height of the bag) and calibre of the tube.

Promoting nutrition

Anyone with an ostomy should eat balanced meals at regular intervals, and chew foods slowly and thoroughly. Patients need to be informed that certain foods such as seeds, kernels, and other undigested residue will be visible in the stool.

People with a *colostomy* do not need a restricted diet, although many people develop their own food preferences. They should be informed which foods tend to cause wind in order to avoid these foods as desired. Most bags are odour-proof, and some are available with gas-relief valves that make wind less of a problem.

People with an *ileostomy* need to avoid high-fibre or high-residue foods for 4 to 6 weeks after surgery. High-fibre foods can then be added one at a time in small amounts. If the person is unable to tolerate the food after two or three trials, the food can be eliminated from the diet.

Promoting return to normal activity

Most people achieve optimal recovery within 3 months, and they can return to their normal activities, including work. Discuss questions about activities before the patient goes home. Travelling is possible for the ostomate. Preparations to be considered are listed in Box 23-19. With careful planning the person with an ostomy can participate in activities enjoyed before the surgery.

Promoting sexuality

The opportunity for the patient and significant other to ask questions regarding the return to normal sexual functioning

sessions are planned. A community nurse referral may be needed for assessment of the patient's ability to adapt to the ostomy in the home environment.

Before discharge, the patient needs a supply of bags and skin barriers, a list of what supplies to order, and the names of local suppliers. A prescription for ostomy supplies is needed for their local chemist shop.

Promoting regular elimination: colostomy irrigation

People with descending or sigmoid colostomies may decide to manage the colostomy with regular irrigations. The purpose of regular colostomy irrigations is to stimulate emptying of the colon at a convenient and regular time.

23-18	Colostomy irrigation

1. Remove old bag.
2. Clean skin and stoma with water.
3. Apply irrigating sleeve and belt.
4. Fill bag with desired amount of tepid water (250 to 1000 ml).
5. Hang bag so bottom of bag is at shoulder height.
6. Remove air from tubing.
7. Gently insert irrigating cone snugly into stoma, holding it parallel to floor.
8. Let water run in slowly until patient identifies need to expel stool.
9. Remove cone and allow solution to drain into container.
10. When most of stool is expelled (about 15 minutes) rinse sleeve with water and close up bottom end.
11. Encourage activity to complete bowel emptying (about 30 to 45 minutes).
12. Remove sleeve and apply clean bag.

Patient Teaching 23-19	The patient with a stoma

Promoting nutrition and elimination

Eat a balanced diet. Avoid foods that cause diarrhoea or constipation.
Drink at least 2500 ml of fluids daily (6 glasses).
Avoid foods that cause flatus, as desired.

Promoting return to normal activities

Participate in activities enjoyed before surgery.
Avoid direct contact sports such as rugby. Activities such as swimming, tennis, and planned exercise programmes are all possible.
When travelling:
  Wear seat belt above or below stoma.
  Hand-carry regular ostomy supplies to facilitate care if baggage is misplaced.
  Use disposable bags.
  Carry plastic bags for disposal of used supplies.
  Take extra supplies for unexpected events requiring extra days.
  Eat moderately. Use restraint when eating new foods.
  Use caution about water intake in areas where "traveller's diarrhoea" is a high risk.

Promoting sexuality

Allow time to ease into sexual relations.
Resume sleeping in bed with partner if this was habit before surgery.
Talk with partner about the stoma.
Empty the bag before intercourse.
Use an attractive cover over the bag.
Tape bag to abdomen or groin.
Experiment with different positions.

Preventing complications

Report the following symptoms to surgeon or nurse stoma therapist:
  Changes in configuration, colour, consistency, or odour of stool
  Bleeding through stoma or rectum
  Persistent diarrhoea or lack of stool evacuation despite medications, treatment, fluids, diet, and exercise programme
  Persistent skin irritation despite treatment
  Changes in contour of stoma (prolapse, inversion)
  Persistent leakage around appliance
  Signs of dehydration and electrolyte imbalance

needs to be provided. It is most often the nurse who hears cues such as, "I guess I'll never be able . . . ," or, "I wonder what my spouse . . . ." The nurse takes this opportunity to clarify this concern with the person. Arrangements can be made, if desired by the patient, for the significant other to be present when the nurse or surgeon frankly discusses sexual functioning. Many people will not verbalize their concerns about sexuality so that a deliberate meeting must be planned to facilitate expression of these concerns. The patient and sexual partner can be assisted to consider sexual positions that may be more facilitating and less problematic if a bag is worn.

About 15% of men with ostomies have decreased sexual activity that may be related either to nerve injury or to psychological reasons. The successful return to sexual activity depends on psychosexual functioning before surgery and adaptation and coping following surgery. Other ways of expressing affection may be considered. Counselling may be helpful if nerve injury is not present and sexual difficulties are being experienced. Women have a decreased incidence of nerve injury because of the larger pelvis. Ostomy surgery does not interfere with contraception, pregnancy, or delivery.

Community resources

During and after hospitalization, the patient and significant others have additional resources available to assist in adapting and coping with the ostomy. A representative from the local branch of the appropriate Ostomy Association can be requested to visit the patient either preoperatively or postoperatively. This visitor can share how he or she has learned to live well with the ostomy. The patient may wish to become a member of the Association and through meetings learn how others in the community are effectively dealing with the ostomy.

The stoma therapist, a nurse with additional education in providing ostomy care, should be consulted (if available) to assist or coordinate instruction. Consult the social worker, clinical nurse specialist, dietitian, and clergy as needed.

It is essential that the patient and significant other know that they must obtain a prescription, from their family doctor, to obtain further stoma care products. The local pharmacist should be informed of the patient's likely needs to arrange to carry stock and avoid situations where items run out.

Closure of Colostomy

If the colostomy was created to relieve obstruction or to divert the faecal stream to permit healing of a portion of the bowel, the person will be readmitted to the hospital at a later date for a further examination and for possible resection of any diseased portion of the bowel. The ostomy subsequently may be closed.

In preparing to resect the bowel and close the colostomy, the surgeon may order irrigation of the colostomy and probably both openings of a loop colostomy. The irrigation fluid, usually normal saline solution, is instilled into each opening as ordered. For irrigation of the distal stoma, the patient should sit on the bedpan or the toilet. Unless the distal bowel is obstructed, the solution instilled into the distal loop will be expelled through the rectum. The returns are inspected before being discarded.

Requirements Before Discharge

Give the following instructions to the patient before discharge from the hospital:
1. Written information about the ostomy
2. Written instructions for application of the bag
3. A list of supplies to order
4. A temporary supply of items needed for bag changes
5. A measuring guide and instructions for determining the size of bags to order
6. List of chemists in the area
7. Information about the appropriate Ostomy Associations and the local branch
8. Phone numbers of the primary nurse, the stoma therapist, the surgeon, and the community nurse service

---

ANORECTAL DISORDERS

Pathophysiology

The anorectal area may develop fissures, abscesses, or fistulas (Table 23-24). A *fissure* is usually the result of trauma caused by passage of hard-formed stool that overstretches the anal lining. It does not heal readily. An *anal abscess* may develop in an anal fissure, and if the sinus tract draining the abscess does not close, a chronic draining *fistula* may develop.

Haemorrhoids occur frequently as a result of congestion in the veins of the haemorrhoidal plexus. Heredity, occupations requiring long periods of standing or sitting, the erect posture assumed by human beings, structural absence of valves in the haemorrhoidal veins, increase of intraabdominal pressure caused by constipation, straining at defaecation, and pregnancy are factors that predispose to development of haemorrhoids. Haemorrhoids may be internal (above the internal sphincter) or external (outside the anal sphincter). Many people have both internal and external haemorrhoids.

Nursing Process
Assessment

Pain, bleeding, and itching are the major symptoms of haemorrhoids. Data to be collected include the following:
1. Pain
   a. Onset: with defaecation, sitting, or walking
   b. Character: constant or episodic; sharp or throbbing
2. Bleeding: presence, amount, colour (bright or dull red)
3. Stool: consistency (hardness), streaked with blood or pus
4. Itching: frequency, onset

Bleeding is usually bright red because of proximity of the bleeding site. Internal haemorrhoids often bleed with defaecation, whereas external haemorrhoids rarely bleed. Rectal bleeding must not be confused with menstrual bleeding in women.

Nursing analysis

Problems are determined from analysis of patient data. Possible problems for the person with an anorectal lesion may include, but are not limited to, the following:

Problem	Possible aetiologies
Constipation	Anal discomfort
Pain: rectal	Anal surgery

Table 23-24 Common anal lesions

Lesion	Description	Symptoms	Treatment
Anal fissure	Slitlike ulceration in epithelium of anal canal	Pain with defaecation; bleeding; constipation	Stool softeners; analgesic ointments; baths, bidet; surgical removal of fissure if medical therapy ineffective
Anal abscess	Abscess in tissue around anus	Persistent throbbing anal pain with walking, sitting, defaecation; systemic signs of infection	Incision and drainage of abscess
Anal fistula	Hollow track leading through anal tissue from anorectal canal through skin near anus	Purulent discharge near anus	Fistulectomy or fistulotomy
Haemorrhoids	Varicosities of lower rectum and anus	Bleeding with defaecation; pain if thrombosed	Analgesic ointments for mild discomfort; injection, ligation, or haemorrhoidectomy for severe discomfort

Planning: expected patient outcomes

Expected patient outcomes for the person with an anorectal lesion may include, but are not limited to, the following:
1. Stool is soft and formed.
2. States feeling more comfortable after surgery.

Implementation

Assisting with achievement of therapeutic goals
Anorectal surgery

Preoperative care. Give the patient a laxative if needed and encourage a full, normal diet until a few hours before administration of local anaesthetic. Stool softeners are often given to facilitate passage of the stool through the rectum postoperatively, and a bulk laxative may be given to increase the bulk of the stool. An enema may be prescribed 1 to 2 hours before surgery.

Postoperative care. Because the operations are often considered minor, there may be a tendency to minimize anorectal surgery. In reality, the surgery may cause as much discomfort as many major surgeries. The pain, which results from rectal spasms, may inhibit urination and defaecation. Patients worry considerably about passing the first stool, which can be uncomfortable. Pain can be minimized by the use of analgesics, baths, bidets and stool softeners.

During the first 12 hours after surgery, haemorrhage is a possibility and again after 7-10 days (secondary haemorrhage). Blood may collect in the anal canal and not be expelled; therefore, monitor other signs of haemorrhage (vital signs, restlessness, thirst). Avoid moist heat (baths) during this period, as moist heat will encourage further bleeding by dilating the blood vessels. The postoperative care of the patient experiencing anorectal surgery is summarized in Box 23-20.

Interventions to achieve patient outcomes
Promoting normal stools

Chronic constipation may precipitate anal lesions. Once the lesion is present, defaecation may initiate rectal spasms, causing the person to delay defaecation. This leads to formation of a hard stool as water is reabsorbed in the colon, causing further discomfort. Therefore, institute measures to promote passage of a soft stool, including activity, adequate fluids (at least 2000 ml/day), and dietary fibre. A stool softener may be prescribed.

Promoting healing

Abscesses are incised and drained. Dressing containing purulent drainage must be changed frequently to protect the skin. Haemorrhoids may be injected, ligated, coagulated, or excised (see Table 23-25).

Evaluation

Evaluation is based on the expected patient outcomes. Questions to consider include:
1. Is stool soft and formed?
2. Is the patient comfortable?

Guidelines for Care   23-20

The patient following anorectal surgery

Assessment
Monitor vital signs every 4 hours for 24 hours.
Monitor for signs of restlessness, thirst.
Inspect rectal area or dressing every 2 to 3 hours for 24 hours.
Monitor urinary output.

Promotion of comfort
Assist patient to a position of comfort; lying on side is often preferred.
Use floatation pad under buttocks for sitting.
Give analgesic medications as needed during first 24 hours
Use moist heat after 12 hours: rectal compresses, bidets or baths 3 to 4 times/day.

Promotion of elimination
Give stool softener as prescribed.
Give an analgesic shortly before first bowel movement, if possible.
If an enema is prescribed, use a well-lubricated catheter or small rectal tube.

Patient teaching
Take a bath or use bidet after each bowel movement for at least 1 to 2 weeks after surgery.
Eat adequate dietary fibre; drink at least 2000 ml of fluids/day, and exercise moderately.
A stool softener may be desired every day or every other day until healing is completed.
Report the following symptoms to doctor: rectal bleeding, continued pain on defaecation, suppurative drainage.

FAECAL INCONTINENCE

Pathophysiology

Voluntary emptying of the rectum occurs when the external anal sphincter (under cortical control) relaxes and the abdominal and pelvic muscles contract. Conditions that interrupt transmission of messages to and from the brain (cortical lesions, spinal cord lesions) cause injury to the sphincter (trauma, fistulas, abscess) or cause perineal muscle relaxation (childbirth, perineal surgery, ageing) and may lead to faecal incontinence.

Assessment

Faecal incontinence is characterized by involuntary passage of stool. Data to be collected include the following:
1. Frequency of defaecations
2. Nature of the stool
3. Awareness of need to defaecate
4. Ability to contract abdominal and perineal muscles
5. Willingness of person to participate in exercise or bowel control programme.

Implementation

1. Assisting with bowel control
   a. Provide a high-fibre diet to facilitate a formed stool.

Table 23-25 Treatment of haemorrhoids

Procedure	Description	Comments
Injection	Sclerosing solution injected into submucosal area	Bleeding stops in 24 to 48 hours
Ligation	Constriction of haemorrhoids by rubber bands	Destroyed tissue sloughs off within 1 week
Infrared photocoagulation	Radiation for 1.5 sec by an infrared photo-coagulator probe	Tissue becomes necrotic and sloughs off
Haemorrhoidectomy	Excision of haemorrhoids	Preoperative: stool softener Postoperative: dressings may be omitted; stool softeners; first defaecation is painful; monitor for excessive bleeding

b. Provide a fluid intake of about 3000 ml/day to promote a soft stool.

c. Administer a stool softener daily, if necessary.

d. Plan a bowel training programme to prevent incontinence if control is not feasible. Within a few days the patient will probably defaecate only once a day when stimulated. If the stool remains soft, the programme may be changed to every other day. Consistency in carrying out the plan is important for success (see Box 23-21).

e. If faecal incontinence is uncontrollable, identify the defaecation pattern. Place the patient on the toilet or commode at the time that defaecation is anticipated. Protective disposable pants are available to provide the person with a sense of security and dignity. A rectal pouch may be used to collect liquid stools.[29]

2. Assisting with comfort. Assist the person to cleanse the anal and perineal areas as soon as possible after faecal incontinence to eliminate odour and prevent skin breakdown.

3. Counselling and teaching

a. Provide empathetic communication. The person may have feelings of regression, inadequacy, or uncleanliness as a result of the loss of control. The person needs to feel accepted as an adult and accept the condition as a situational physical condition and not personal inadequacy.

b. Encourage patients to participate in all or some of their own management to the extent that is possible, thus providing them with a sense of control.

c. Teach perineal exercises for weak perineal muscles (Chapter 25).

SUMMARY

1. GI signs requiring immediate medical follow-up include (1) a sore that bleeds easily and does not heal, (2) a lump or thickening or a persistent red or whitish patch in the mouth, (3) persistent heartburn or indigestion, (4) abdominal pain accompanied by nausea and vomiting, and (5) a change in bowel habits or the presence of blood in the stool.

2. Protein-energy malnutrition leads to decreased muscle mass, decreased vital capacity, oedema, malabsorption,

---

23-21

Bowel training programme

1. Include patient and family/friend in the planning.
2. Determine when bowel evacuation usually occurs (most frequent times are after breakfast or dinner).
3. Determine whether a morning or evening programme is more suitable for patient.
4. Insert glycerine or bisacodyl *suppository* 30 minutes before expected time of defaecation; give suppository at *same time every day*.
5. Ask patient to sit on toilet if possible for defaecation.
6. If necessary, massage abdomen towards the sigmoid area (left lower quadrant) to encourage defaecation; digital rectal stimulation may also stimulate defaecation.

---

and risk for infection. Special therapies include tube feedings, total parenteral nutrition, or gastrostomy feedings.

3. Common inflammatory disorders of the mouth include aphthous or herpetic stomatitis, Vincent's angina, thrush, gingivitis, and periodontitis.

4. Contributing factors to cancer of the mouth and oesophagus include alcohol and heavy smoking or chewing tobacco.

5. A hiatus hernia consists of herniation of the upper part of the stomach through the diaphragm, causing heartburn.

6. Heartburn is relieved by taking antacids; eating a high-protein, low-fat diet in small frequent feedings; avoiding smoking; avoiding lifting, bending, or lying down immediately after eating; and sleeping with upper body elevated.

7. Acute gastritis is a common occurrence; stress erosions (or ulcers) are a form of gastritis resulting from stress; chronic gastritis may lead to pernicious anaemia or gastric cancer.

8. Gastric ulcers result from increased back diffusion of gastric acid into the tissues; gastric acid and emptying rate are normal. Duodenal ulcers result from increased gastric acid emptied more rapidly into the duodenum.

9. Dumping syndrome occurs from entrance of a hyperosmolar mixture directly into the jejunum after gastric surgery.

10. Malabsorption syndrome is a group of disorders resulting from inadequate absorption of fat in the small intestine; common malabsorption syndromes include lactase deficiency and gluten sensitive enteropathy.

11. Inflammation of the intestines (enteritis) may result from viruses, bacteria, or parasites. Common parasitic infections include amoebiasis (from faecally contaminated food or water) or trichinosis (from improperly cooked pork).

12. Although symptoms of appendicitis may be atypical, a common site of abdominal pain is McBurney's point (halfway between the umbilicus and right iliac crest).

13. Ulcerative colitis affects primarily the left colon with a continuous area of mucosal involvement; the liquid stools contain blood, but not fat. Crohn's disease affects segmental areas of the ileum, caecum, and right colon, involving submucosal layers; the frequent semisoft stools contain fat but not blood. Surgery may be useful for ulcerative colitis and sometimes for Crohn's disease.

14. Care of the person with ulcerative colitis or Crohn's disease includes a low-residue, high-protein, high-calorie diet, medications (corticosteroids, sulphasalazine), comfort measures following diarrhoea and to protect skin, and promotion of sexuality.

15. Diverticular disease involves outpouching of the colon wall; diverticulitis is the inflammatory condition, diverticulosis the quiescent phase. Encourage a high-fibre diet to increase bowel transit time and stool bulk.

16. Intestinal obstruction may result from inhibition of peristalsis (paralytic ileus) or from mechanical obstruction, such as by adhesions, volvulus, intussusception, hernias, or cancer. Therapy consists of inserting a nasogastric tube, restricting oral intake, and removing the source of obstruction, if possible.

17. Hernias may occur in the inguinal, femoral, or umbilical areas from mural defects or in weakened scars from previous abdominal surgeries. Of concern is the possible entrapment (incarceration) of a loop of bowel. The treatment is surgical.

18. Colon polyps (adenomas) are benign growths that are premalignant; the villous adenomas are more likely to become malignant than the pedunculated tubular adenomas.

19. Cancers of the ascending colon are of the cauliflowerlike mass type, and because the chyme is liquid, there is less probability of obstruction. Cancer of the descending colon is usually an annular lesion that may narrow the lumen and obstruct the more solid faeces.

20. Surgery for cancer of the colon and upper rectum usually consists of resection with anastomosis; surgery for the lower rectum consists of an abdominoperineal resection with a colostomy.

21. Stoma care includes cleaning the skin to prevent skin breakdown, early treatment of excoriated skin, and application of bags to prevent leakage.

22. Teaching the person with a colostomy includes promoting nutrition and elimination, promoting return to normal activities and sexuality, and preventing complications.

STUDY QUESTIONS

Gastrointestinal disorders alter function of the GI tract. What changes can occur in functioning? What general effects can result from the altered functioning?

What are the differences in electrolyte and acid-base imbalances resulting from loss of gastric secretion versus loss of intestinal secretions? Explain the rationale.

What are the differences and similarities among the infections of the mouth, stomach, and intestines?

What types of obstructions can occur in the GI tract? What are the effects?

Compare and contrast cancer of the mouth, oesophagus, stomach, and bowel in terms of occurrence, incidence in males and females, methods of prevention (if any), and types of surgery performed.

REFERENCES AND SELECTED READINGS

1.* Alterescu V: Colostomy, *Nurs Clin North Am* 22:281–290, 1987.

2.* Alterescu V: The ostomy: What do you teach the patient? *Am J Nurs* 85:1250–1253, 1985.

3. Altman DF: Gastrointestinal diseases in the elderly, *Med Clin North Am* 67(2):1250–1253, 1985.

4. American Cancer Society: *Cancer facts and figures 1991*, New York, 1991, The Society.

5.* Atkins JM, Oakley CW: A nurse's guide to TPN, *RN* 49(6):20–24, 1986.

6. Atkinson RL: Low and very low calorie diets, *Med Clin North Am* 73(1):203–214, 1989.

7.* Backer CL, LoCicero J: Surgical management of esophageal disorders, *CCQ* 9(3):12–19, 1986.

8. Bates B: *A guide to physical examination*, ed 5, Philadelphia, 1991, JB Lippincott.

9.* Beck ML: Nutritional support: percutaneous endoscopic gastrostomy, *Nursing 89* 19(4):76–77, 1989.

10.* Becker KL, Stevens SA: Performing in-depth abdominal assessment, *Nursing 88* 18(6):59–63, 1988.

11.* Benedict P, Haddad A: Postop teaching for the colostomy patient, *RN* 52(3):85–90, 1989.

12. Binder V, Riis P: Lifelong control with inflammatory bowel disease patients, *Med Clin North Am* 74(1):219–227, 1990.

13.* Bockus S: Troubleshooting your tube feedings, *Am J Nurs* 91(5):24–28, 1991.

14. Bongiovanni GL: *Essentials of clinical gastroenterology*, ed 2, New York, 1988, McGraw-Hill.

15.* Broadwell D: Peristomal skin integrity, *Nurs Clin North Am* 22:321–322, 1987.

16.* Bruckstein DC: Percutaneous endoscopic gastrostomy, *Geriatr Nurs* 9(2):32–33, 1988.

16a.* Bryant GA: When the bowel is blocked, *RN* 55(1):58–67, 1992.

17. Butrum RR, Clifford DK, Lanza E: NCI dietary guidelines: rationale, *Am J Clin Nutr* 48:888–895, 1988.

18.* Carr P: When the patient needs TPN at home, *RN* 49(6):25–30, 1986.

18a. Central Statistical Office: *Social trends* 23, London, 1993, HMSO.

19.* Cerrato PL: How safe are modified fasts, *RN* 52(11):79–81, 1989.

20.* Dalton-Loehman D, Connor PA: Beyond ileostomy: surgery for a normal life, *RN* 52(7):29–34, 1989.

20a. Department of Health: *Dietary reference values for food energy and nutrients for the United Kingdom*. Report on Health and Social Subjects, no. 41. Report of the Panel on Dietary Reference Values of the Committee on Medical Aspects of Food Policy. London, 1991, HMSO.

20b. Department of Health, *The Health of the Nation. A consultative document for health in England. Presented to parliament by the Secretary of State for Health*, London, 1991, HMSO.

20c. Department of Health, *The Health of the Nation: A strategy for health in England. Presented to parliament by the Secretary of State for Health*, London, 1992, HMSO.

*Recommended for student reading.

21.* DiIorio C, Price ME: Swallowing: an assessment guide, *Am J Nurs* 90 (7):38–41, 1990.

22.* Dobkin KA, Broadwell DC: Nursing considerations for the patient undergoing colostomy surgery, *Sem Oncol Nurs* 2:249–255, 1986.

23.* Doughty DB: Colorectal cancer: aetiology and pathophysiology, *Sem Oncol Nurs* 2:235–241, 1986.

24. Eisenberg P: Enteral nutrition: indications, formulas, and delivery techniques, *Nurs Clin North Am* 24(2):275–337, 1989.

25.* Erickson P: Ostomies: the art of pouching, *Nurs Clin North Am* 22:271–320, 1987.

26.* Feickert DM: Gastric surgery: your crucial pre- and postop role, *RN* 50(1):24–35, 1987.

27.* Feickert DM, Jillson E, Palazzo T: Gastrectomy for stomach carcinoma, *AORN J* 47:1396–1406, 1988.

28.* Foltz AT: Nutritional factors in the prevention of gastrointestinal cancer, *Sem Oncol Nurs* 4:239–245, 1988.

29. Freedman P: The rectal pouch: a safer alternative to rectal tubes, *Am J Nurs* 91(5):105–106, 1991.

29a.* Fritsch DE, Klein DG: Ludwig's angina, *Heart Lung* 21:39–47, 1992.

29b. Goodinson SM: Assessment of Nutritional Status, *Professional Nurse* 2(11):367–369, 1987.

30.* Greitzu S: Closeup on cancer care: colorectal cancer, when a polyp is more than a polyp, *RN* 49(9):22–30, 1986.

31. Groer MW, Shekleton ME: *Basic pathophysiology: a conceptual approach*, ed 3, St Louis, 1989, Mosby-Year Book.

32.* Hennessy K: Now TPN therapy begins at home, *RN* 51(6):81–84, 1988.

33. Hennessy K: Nutritional support and gastrointestinal disease, *Nurs Clin North Am* 24(2):373–380, 1989.

34.* Irwin M: Managing leaking gastrostomy sites, *Am J Nurs* 88:359–360, 1988.

35.* Joachim G et al: Inflammatory bowel disease: effects on life-style, *J Adv Nurs* 12:483–487, 1987.

36.* Johndrow PD: Making your patient and family feel at home with TPN, *Nursing 88* 18(10):65–69, 1988.

36a.* Johns JL: When the patient has an ulcer, *RN* 54(11):44–50, 1991.

37.* Johnson S: A safer gastrostomy for the high-risk patient: percutaneous endoscopic gastrostomy, *RN* 49(3):29–32, 1986.

38. Kennedy-Caldwell C: The morbidly obese surgical patient, *Crit Care Nurs* 7(5):87–89, 1987.

39. Kohn CL, Keithley JK: Enteral nutrition: potential complications and patient monitoring, *Nurs Clin North Am* 24(2):339–351, 1989.

40.* Konopad E, Noseworthy T: Stress ulceration: a serious complication in critically ill patients, *Heart Lung* 17(4):339–348, 1988.

41. McConnell EA: Auscultating bowel sounds, *Nursing 90* 20(5):106, 1990.

42. McCrae AD, Hall NH: Current practices for home enteral nutrition, *J Am Dietetic Assoc* 89:233–239, 1989.

43.* Medvec BR: Esophageal cancer: treatment and nursing intervention, *Sem Oncol Nurs* 4:246–256, 1988.

44.* Meize-Grochowski AR: When the diagnosis is Crohn's disease, *RN* 54(2):52–55, 1991.

45. Mendeloff AI: Diet and colorectal cancer, *Am J Clin Nutr* 48:780–781, 1988.

46. Metheny NM: *Fluid and electrolyte balance: nursing considerations*, Philadelphia, 1987, JB Lippincott.

47.* Moore MC: Do you still believe these myths about tube feedings? *RN* 50(5):51–55, 1987.

48.* Neufeldt J: Helping the inflammatory bowel disease patient cope with the unpredictable, *Nursing 87* 17(8):47–49, 1987.

49.* Olender L: Why tube feedings may be the wrong answer, *RN* 52(6):43–45, 1989.

50. O'Toole MT: Advanced assessment of the abdomen and gastrointestinal problems, *Nurs Clin North Am* 25(4):771–776, 1990.

51. Pagana KD, Pagana TJ: Diagnostic testing and nursing implications: a case study approach, ed 3, St Louis, 1989, Mosby-Year Book.

52. Petrosino BM et al: Implications of selected problems with nasoenteral feedings, *Crit Care Nurs Q* 12(3):1–18, 1989.

53. Podiasky P, Budzinski HM: Percutaneous endoscopic gastrostomy, *AORN J* 45:1403–1411, 1987.

54.* Price ME, DiIorio C: Swallowing: a practice guide, *Am J Nurs* 90(7):42–46, 1990.

55. Price SA, Wilson LM: *Pathophysiology: clinical concepts of disease processes*, ed 3, New York, 1986, McGraw-Hill.

56. Rakel RE: *Conn's current therapy 1989*, Philadelphia, 1989, WB Saunders.

57.* Rideout BW: The patient with an ileostomy: nursing management and patient education, *Nurs Clin North Am* 22(2):253–262, 1987.

58. Ruderman WB: Newer pharmacologic agents for inflammatory bowel disease, *Med Clin North Am* 74(1):139–154, 1990.

59. Schreiber H, Guyton DP: Gastric bubble: therapy for obesity, *Ohio State Med J* 82:476–479, 1986.

60. Schroeder SA et al: *Current medical diagnosis and treatment 1991*, ed 30, Norwalk Conn, 1991, Appleton & Lange.

61.* Schulmeister L: Join the fight against oral cancer, *Nursing 87* 17(5):66–67, 1987.

62.* Shipes E: Psychosocial issues: the person with an ostomy, *Nurs Clin North Am* 22:291–302, 1987.

63. Sleisinger M, Fordtran JS: *Gastrointestinal disease: pathophysiology, diagnosis, and management*, ed 4, Philadelphia, 1989, WB Saunders.

64.* Smith CE: Assessing bowel sounds, *Nursing 88* 18(2):42–44, 1988.

65. Smith DB: Continent diversions: an overview, *Dimens Oncol Nurs* 3(4):18–23, 1990.

66.* Starkey JF, Jefferson PA, Kirby DF: Taking care of a percutaneous endoscopic gastrostomy, *Am J Nurs* 88:42–45, 1988.

66a. Thomson AD, Cotton RE: *Lecture notes on pathology*, ed 3, Oxford, 1983, Blackwell Scientific Publications.

67. Turnball GB: Dealing with sexuality after ostomy surgery, *Progressions* 1(1):15–18, 1989.

68. Way LW: *Current surgical diagnosis and treatment*, ed 9, Norwalk, Conn, 1991, Appleton & Lange.

69. Wang JF: Stomach cancer, *Sem Oncol Nurs* 4:257–264, 1988.

70. Williams SR: *Essentials of nutrition and diet therapy*, ed 5, St Louis, 1990, Mosby–Year Book.

71. Worthington PH, Wagner BA: Total parenteral nutrition, *Nurs Clin North Am* 24(2):355–369, 1989.

72. Wyngaarden JB, Smith LH: *Cecil's textbook of medicine*, ed 18, Philadelphia, 1988, WB Saunders.

73.* Young CK, White S: Preparing patients for tube feedings at home, *Am J Nurs* 92(4):46–53, 1992.

FURTHER READING

Dyer S: Stoma Care: Choosing the Right Appliance, *Professional Nurse* 3(8):278–283, 1988.

Fawcett HV: A superior method of tube placement. Percutaneous endoscopic gastrostomy, *Professional Nurse* 6(2):92–96, 1990.

Finnegan S, Oldfield K: When eating is impossible: TPN in maintaining nutritional status, *Professional Nurse* 4(6):271–275, 1989.

Finnegan S: Mechanical Complications of Parenteral Nutrition, *Professional Nurse* 4(7):325–327, 1989.

Goodwin K: An insight into patient satisfaction. Evaluation of a stoma care service, *Professional Nurse* 8(3):153–156, 1992.

Kelly M: Loss and grief reactions as a response to surgery, *Journal of Advanced Nursing* 10:517–525, 1985.

Taylor SJ: A Guide to Enteral Feeding, *Professional Nurse* 4(4):195–200, 1989.

Taylor SJ: Preventing Complications in Enteral Feeding, *Professional Nurse* 4(5):247–249, 1989.

Truswell AS: *ABC of nutrition*, London, 1986, British Medical Association.

24

The Patient with Biliary and Pancreatic Problems

Virginia L. Cassmeyer
Dorothy Blevins

After studying this chapter, the learner should be able to:

- Describe the anatomy and physiology of the biliary system and pancreas.
- Discuss the treatment approaches for cholecystitis, cholelithiasis, and cancer of the biliary system.
- Describe the treatment for acute and chronic pancreatitis and pancreatic tumours.
- Contrast the nursing care of the patient experiencing acute and chronic problems of the pancreas.

The biliary system and pancreas are affected by various pathological processes that alter normal metabolism. Some of the disorders are chronic and require that the patient make changes in life-style to keep the disorder under control. Patients with biliary system or pancreatic problems need nursing support to deal with acute problems as well as chronic health problems.

ANATOMY AND PHYSIOLOGY

Biliary System

The gallbladder, a pear-shaped organ, lies on the inferior surface of the liver. The biliary system consists of the gallbladder and its associated ductal system (Fig. 24-1). The ductal system provides a pathway for the bile that is formed in the liver to be transported to the gallbladder or to the intestine and also functions to regulate bile flow. The liver produces up to 1 L of bile per day. As it is formed, bile is excreted into the hepatic ducts, where it passes into the cystic duct to be stored in the gallbladder.

The capacity of the gallbladder is usually 50 ml but can increase under normal conditions. In the gallbladder, bile is concentrated to a solution that is 5 to 10 times as concentrated as that produced in the liver.

Bile contains cholesterol, phospholipids, bile salts, bilirubin, and a very small amount of protein and electrolytes; 97% of bile is water. Some toxins, drug metabolites, and hormones are excreted in bile. Because bile can be released directly into the duodenum through the common bile duct, the removal of the gallbladder has no long-term consequences.

Neural and hormonal mechanisms control the secretion of bile from the gallbladder. Food, particularly lipids in the duodenum, causes the release of *cholecystokinin* (CCK), also sometimes still called cholecystokinin-pancreozymin, from the mucosa of the duodenum. CCK is released into the blood and travels to the gallbladder. One of its activities is to stimulate the gallbladder musculature to contract. At the same time it causes the muscle of the sphincter of Oddi (at the end of the common bile duct) to relax and permit entry of bile into the duodenum. Gastrin, another gastrointestinal hormone, and vagal stimulation can also cause the gallbladder to contract.

Bile acids are predominantly composed of a cholesterol derivative, and they function in intestinal metabolism of fats and other substances as follows:

1. Facilitate fat digestion by emulsifying fats for action by intestinal lipases
2. Facilitate absorption of fats, fat-soluble vitamins, iron, and calcium
3. Activate the release of pancreatic and intestinal enzymes

Most of the bile salts secreted into the duodenum are reabsorbed into the enterohepatic circulation from the terminal ileum or other parts of the intestines. These bile salts are recirculated two to three times per meal. The reabsorption from the intestinal tract is so efficient that only 15% to 25% of the bile salts need to be replaced per day.

Pancreatic Exocrine System

The pancreas, an elongated flattened organ, is located in the posterior abdomen with its head lying in the curvature of the duodenum and its tail resting against the spleen. The pancreatic exocrine system includes the exocrine glands of the pancreas (acinar cells) and a ductal system (Fig. 24-1). (The endocrine functions of the pancreas are described in Chapter 20.) Acinar cells release their secretions into ducts that converge to form the main pancreatic duct (duct of Wirsung). Lining the ducts are cells (ductal cells) that secrete a bicarbonate-rich fluid. In most people, the pancreatic duct merges with the common bile duct at the entry into the duodenum, but in some persons the common bile duct and pancreatic duct do not merge.

The acinar cells of the pancreas secrete multiple digestive enzymes.

1. Proteolytic enzymes: trypsinogen, chymotrypsinogen, and procarboxypeptidase
2. Amylolytic enzyme: amylase
3. Lipolytic enzymes: lipases
4. Nucleolytic enzymes: ribonuclease and deoxyribonuclease

The pancreatic exocrine secretions are released under the influence of the *vagus nerve, secretin, cholecystokinin* (CCK), and *gastrin* during digestion. Gastrin is released during the gastric phase and stimulates the release of bicarbonate-rich solution. The entry of chyme and acids into the small intestines stimulates the release of secretin and cholecystokinin. *Secretin* then *stimulates* further secretion of the pancreatic *bicarbonate-rich solution,* and *cholecystokinin stimulates* the release of the *pancreatic enzyme-rich* solution.

Physiological Changes with Ageing

The gallbladder and ductal system do not show changes with ageing. The composition of bile is increasingly lithogenic, which may be related to an increase in biliary cholesterol.[24] Cholelithiasis and cholecystitis increase in the aged. The pancreas shows anatomic and physiological changes with ageing. Ductal hyperplasia and fibrosis occur. These anatomical changes are not always associated with altered physiological function, although the volume of stimulated pancreatic secretion decreases after age 40 and the enzyme output and the activity of lipase decrease.[24] One last change in pancreatic function noted in the elderly is an increase in pancreatitis after surgery.[34]

PREVENTION AND HEALTH EDUCATION

Primary Prevention
Gallstones

Preventing gallstones, the most prevalent disorder of the biliary tract, is not currently possible. Populations at higher risk are those who are obese and those with certain metabolic and haemolytic disorders. Patients who tend to form stones in the ducts are usually advised to be careful of their fat intake and to drink generous amounts of fluids unless contraindicated for some reason.

Pancreatic disease

A major cause of chronic pancreatitis is excessive alcohol consumption. Thus a major focus of primary prevention for pancreatic disease is preventing or controlling excessive alcohol consumption. This is a very difficult undertaking. Interventions appropriate for the prevention and control of excessive alcohol consumption are essential. The second major cause of pancreatitis is gallbladder disease. Thus measures helpful in decreasing gallstone formation would also help to prevent pancreatitis.

Secondary Prevention

Early detection of disease allows for the most beneficial treatment. Many disorders of the biliary system and pancreas are associated with vague, persistent, nonspecific gastrointestinal symptoms long before more specific or severe symptoms occur. Nurses can encourage people who complain of vague but persistent symptoms to seek medical evaluation and can discourage the use of home remedies and over-the-counter preparations that delay the seeking of professional help.

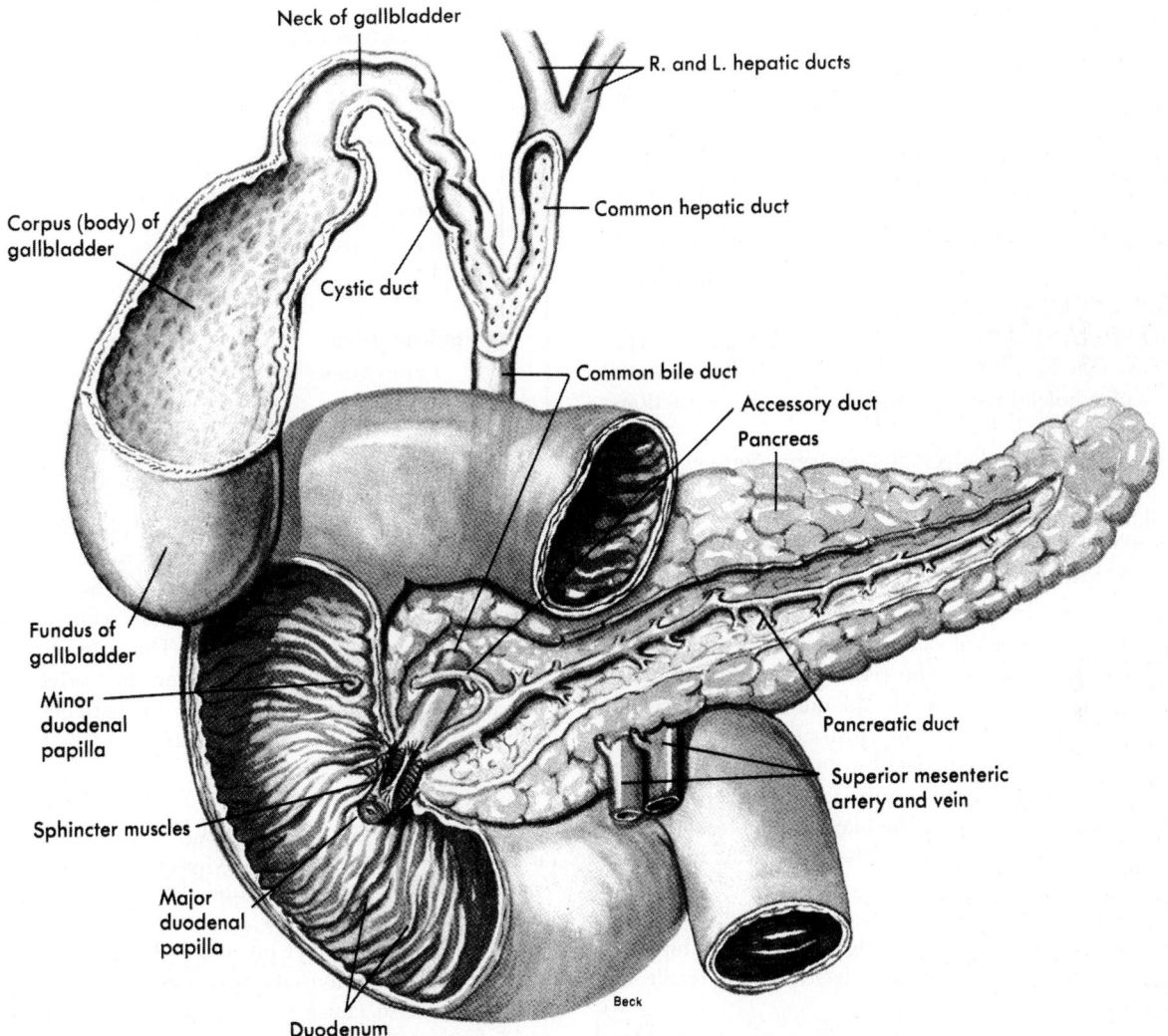

Fig. 24-1   Anatomical schemata of biliary and pancreatic ductal systems. Note head of pancreas surrounds common bile duct. (From Thibodeau GA: *Anthony's textbook of anatomy and physiology*, ed 13, St. Louis, 1990, Mosby–Year Book.)

MAJOR HEALTH PROBLEMS OF THE BILIARY SYSTEM AND PANCREAS

Disorders encountered in the biliary system and pancreas include obstruction and inflammatory problems as well as tumours. The disorders to be discussed include:

The biliary system
1. Cholecystitis
2. Cholelithiasis
3. Carcinoma

The pancreas
1. Pancreatitis
2. Tumours of the pancreas

The nursing process that relates to the above disorders concludes the discussion of biliary system and pancreatic disorders respectively.

DISORDERS OF THE BILIARY SYSTEM

Stone formation, inflammation, and carcinoma are the major disorders of the biliary system. The signs, symptoms and medical therapy are summarized in Table 24-1.

CHOLELITHIASIS/CHOLECYSTITIS

Aetiology/Epidemiology

Cholelithiasis is gallstone formation in the gallbladder. Gallstones are composed primarily of *cholesterol, bile salts,* calcium, *bilirubin,* and proteins. The specific factors contributing to the formation of gallstones can be categorized into *metabolic factors* and factors that cause stasis or inflammation. See Box 24-1 for a list of factors increasing the risk of cholelithiasis. About 75% of gallstones in Western cultures are cholesterol stones. The remaining 25% consist of bilirubin pigment stones.

Cholecystitis is inflammation of the gallbladder. The symptoms may be acute or chronic and usually are associated with cholelithiasis or other causes of obstructions of the bile passages.

Cholelithiasis and cholecystitis are very common health problems. Both occur more frequently in women who are in the middle and older age groups.

Pathophysiology

Why gallstones form is not completely understood. Although many pathological states associated with increased serum cholesterol increase the risk of developing cholelithiasis, serum cholesterol levels do not always correlate with the presence of cholesterol gallstones. It appears that a proper relationship among lecithin (a phospholipid), bile salts, and cholesterol is necessary for cholesterol to be soluble in bile. A reduction in the bile salt pool (reabsorbed in the terminal ileum) decreases the amount of bile salts and thereby the solubility of cholesterol.

Increased serum bilirubin associated with various pathophysiological states can change the relationship between bile salts, cholesterol, and lecithin and result in stone formation.

Biliary stasis leads to stagnation of bile in the gallbladder and to excessive absorption of water, allowing the salts to precipitate easily. Fasting states reduce the normal stimulation of bile flow. *Inflammation* of the biliary system results in the absorption of more of bile salts with a reduction in the solubility of cholesterol.

Gallstones may be present for years without signs and symptoms, which may only occur when a stone becomes lodged in a biliary duct. However, a history of *postprandial indigestion* is common. The indigestion is due to impaired metabolism of fatty foods and may be associated with *flatus, diarrhoea, abdominal distension,* and *nausea* and *vomiting.* Eructations occur immediately after a meal, in contrast to several hours later with gastric ulcers. If fat absorption is impaired for some time, fat-soluble vitamins, including

	Factors increasing the risk of cholelithiasis

24-1	**Metabolic**
	Biliary cholesterol saturation
	  Oestrogens
	  Oral contraceptives
	  Obesity
	  Terminal ileal disease or resection
	Increased levels of serum bilirubin
	  Haemolytic anaemias
	  Cirrhosis
	Increased serum cholesterol
	  Obesity
	  Pregnancy
	  Diabetes mellitus
	  Hypothyroidism
	  Hyperlipidaemia
	
	Biliary stasis
	Biliary tract obstruction
	  Fasting
	  Parenteral hyperalimentation
	
	Inflammation
	  Cholecystitis

vitamin K, will not be properly absorbed and the production of vitamin-K-dependent clotting factors will be impaired.

Biliary colic, which is caused by spasms of the biliary ducts as they attempt to dislodge stones, can cause one of the most severe pains experienced. The pain often *radiates through to the back under the scapula and to the right shoulder.* The pain can result in prostration. Of patients with gallstones, 20% to 50% are asymptomatic and 18% have biliary pain.

Stones may lodge anywhere along the biliary tract (Fig. 24-2). If they lodge in the small bile ducts, hepatic duct, or common bile duct (choledocholithiasis), the stones obstruct bile flow, serum bilirubin levels are elevated, and the patient becomes jaundiced. Obstruction of the common bile duct prevents bile from getting to the GI tract and clay-coloured (greyish-white) stools will result. Stones may also cause pressure and subsequent necrosis and infection of the walls of the biliary ducts. Occasionally a stone, because of its location, blocks the entrance of pancreatic fluid and bile into the duodenum. This condition is difficult to differentiate from obstruction caused by malignancy. Cholelithiasis may precede or follow cholecystitis. Complications are similar to those for cholecystitis.

Cholecystitis may be acute or chronic and is usually associated with gallstones or other obstructions of the biliary tract system. In acute cholecystitis, the gallbladder is usually very enlarged and resembles a distended sac. Inflammation occurs, and the wall of the gallbladder becomes thickened and oedematous. The inflammation results in leukocytosis (increased production of white blood cells) and fever. Impaired circulation, oedema, and distension of the gallbladder produce ischaemia, which can lead to necrosis

Table 24-1 Biliary tract disorders

Disorder	Signs and symptoms	Therapy
Cholecystitis	History of intolerance of fatty foods, gaseous eructations after meals, flatus, diarrhoea, abdominal distension Nausea, vomiting Pain: right upper quadrant, referred to right scapula Fever, tachycardia Leukocytosis	Conservative: NBM, nasogastric intubation, IV infusions, pethidine hydrochloride, spasmolytics, anticholinergics (chronic condition), antibiotics for acute episode, surgery
Cholelithiasis Choledocholithiasis	As for cholecystitis Biliary colic: intense spasmodic pain with diaphoresis, tachycardia and prostration Jaundice, greyish-white stools Elevated serum bilirubin Prolonged prothrombin time	First pain control; stabilize haemodynamically; surgery; endoscopic retrieval of stones; shock wave lithotripsy; chemidissolution of stones
Carcinoma	Jaundice, weight loss, pain, right upper quadrant mass	Pain control; surgery for comfort

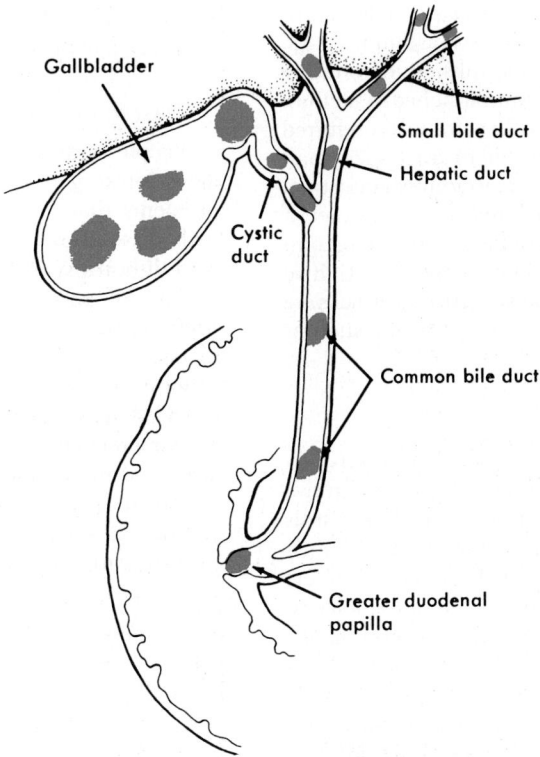

Fig. 24-2   Common sites of gallstones.

and gangrene. Perforation of the gallbladder may occur, leading to biliary peritonitis, pancreatitis, and fistula formation. Bacterial invasion can lead to empyema of the gallbladder, ductal cholangitis, abscess formation, and sepsis.

Chronic cholecystitis may produce a variety of structural changes whether or not stones are present. The structural changes are not the result of an infectious process but are related to a diseased gallbladder wall with inefficient emptying. Chronic cholecystitis is caused by chemical or mechanical irritation from stones causing pressure on the mucosa or from biliary stasis. Eventually, because of destruction of the mucosa, outpouchings of the epithelium may form. Bacteria and other irritants may become trapped in these outpouchings, which may maintain a chronic inflammatory process.

Several acute attacks of moderate severity usually precede the chronic form of the disease. People with chronic disease may not be as ill as those with acute disease and therefore may not seek medical attention until they experience pain from biliary obstruction or develop jaundice. (See Chapter 22 for a discussion of jaundice.)

CARCINOMA OF THE BILIARY SYSTEM

Cancer can occur anywhere in the biliary system. Unfortunately, at present no method of early diagnosis exists. Identification is often made during surgery. Jaundice may be the first sign and indicates that the lesion has developed sufficiently to obstruct bile passage at some point. Spread by direct extension to the liver resulting in hepatic dysfunction or to the peritoneal surface resulting in peritonitis may be the initial manifestation. The prognosis is usually one of rapid deterioration with death ensuing within a few months. Surgery is only done for palliation. Drainage of the biliary tract or surgical bypass of the area of obstruction can improve the patient's comfort. (See Chapter 9 for a general discussion of cancer.)

TREATMENT OF BILIARY TRACT DISEASE

Conservative management

A variety of treatment measures are used in biliary tract disease (see Table 24-1). Conservative treatment of acute cholecystitis/cholelithiasis usually will effect improvement within 1-7 days. Food is witheld until acute symptoms subside. If vomiting persists, a nasogastric tube is inserted and attached to suction. Pethidine hydrochloride may be given for pain and is preferred because its spasmogenic effect on the biliary tract is less than occurs with opiates. Antispasmodics may diminish intestinal and biliary spasms. When food is tolerated, a reducing diet (if appropriate) and careful avoidance of fat usually are recommended until definitive treatment is implemented. Definitive treatment will be recommended because recurrent attacks are common and may result in more severe problems such as pancreatitis.

Surgery

After stabilization of the patient's physical status, diagnostic tests are initiated to determine the best definitive treatment. The most common treatment for cholecystitis and cholelithiasis is laparoscopic cholecystectomy (LC) using a laser or cautery to remove the gallbladder. LC offers several advantages over the common abdominal cholecystectomy including: (1) less invasive and thus less chance of wound infection or respiratory impairment, shorter healing time, and shorter recuperative time; (2) no unsightly scar; and (3) less pain and thus much more rapid return to normal activities. Importantly, the mortality and morbidity associated with LC is no greater than that associated with the traditional cholecystectomy, which is very low. Most patients are discharged on the day of surgery or on the first postoperative day.

LC involves preprocedure preparation of the patient similar to any patient having abdominal surgery, including nil-by-mouth after midnight, an enema to reduce the mass of the colon, and an antibiotic given with any premedications for anaesthesia. In the operating theatre, the patient receives a general anaesthetic, has a nasogastric tube and foley catheter inserted, and has intravenous fluids started.

The surgery is carried out using video monitors and instrumentation through four cannulas introduced by trocars into the peritoneal cavity via four small (5 mm to 10 mm) incisions. These incisions are made at the umbilicus, midline in the epigastric region and in the right upper quadrant at the midclavicular line and at the anterior axillary line. After the first incision is made at the umbilicus, carbon dioxide is introduced to insufflate the abdominal cavity, which allows for the insertion of the instruments. The carbon dioxide is removed at the end of the surgery.

An LC is not the surgery of choice for everyone. People who have had extensive abdominal surgery may have too many adhesions to allow for this procedure. Gallstones within the common bile duct cannot be removed with this procedure. Of course, people who cannot tolerate general anaesthesia cannot be treated with this procedure. Potential complications of the procedure include injury to the hepatic or common bile duct, injury to the bowel, wound infection, abdominal abscess formation, and retained stones in the common bile duct.

The alternative surgical approach to LC is removal of the gallbladder through an abdominal incision. An abdominal incision may be used for other types of surgery on the gallbladder or duct system. Other types of surgical procedures that may be carried out are defined in Box 24-2.

Dissolution agents and gallstone lithotripsy

People with gallbladder problems who are not candidates for surgery because of the presence of other health problems that make anaesthesia too risky may be treated with dissolution agents or shock wave lithotripsy. Shock wave lithotripsy and dissolution therapy are currently used in 10% of patients with cholelithiasis.[11] Gallstone lithotripsy is still being implemented under strictly defined protocols.

Chenodeoxycholic acid and ursodeoxycholic acid (UDCA) now are being used to dissolve small (≤20 mm in diameter) cholesterol stones. These compounds are bile acids and increase cholesterol solubility. The drugs, which are taken daily for up to 2 years, can cause elevated hepatic enzymes and diarrhoea. Also, gallstones can reoccur after the drugs are discontinued.

24-2 | **Surgeries of the biliary tract**

Cholecystectomy
Removal of gallbladder

Cholecystostomy
Creation of an opening into gallbladder for drainage

Choledochotomy
Incision into common bile duct

Choledocholithotomy
Incision into common bile duct to remove a stone

Choledochoduodenostomy
Anastomosis of common bile duct with duodenum

Choledochojejunostomy
Anastomosis of common bile duct with jejunum

Cholecystogastrostomy
Anastomosis of gallbladder with stomach

Lithotripsy involves the use of shock waves to disintegrate gallstones. Shock waves are applied to the gallstones located in the gallbladder or common and hepatic bile duct, which are located by use of ultrasound. The shock waves are usually passed through a water medium, although some machines are "dry" lithotripters and use liquid couplers contained by membranes between the shock wave source and the patient's skin.[2] Approximately 1500 shocks are delivered over 1 to 2 hours. The fragments of the disintegrated stones are excreted through the common bile duct into the small intestines.

Biliary drainage

External biliary drainage is used in empyema, for fistula, when chronic decompression of the biliary tract is required, and often after abdominal cholecystectomy when the common bile duct has been explored. Drainage is provided by a catheter inserted into the gallbladder (cholecystostomy) or by a T-tube inserted into the common bile duct (choledochostomy). Usually stab wounds are used to bring these tubes through the skin.

The T-tube is inserted to maintain patency of the common bile duct and to ensure drainage of bile out of the body until oedema in the common duct has subsided enough for bile to drain into the duodenum normally. (For some patients with extensive ductal disease, the T-tube may be used for long periods of time.) Cholangiograms are commonly performed in the operating room to ensure patency of the common bile duct; radiopaque dye is inserted through the T-tube.

When a T-tube is used after exploration of the common bile duct, at first the entire output of bile (normally 500 to 1000 ml/day) may flow through the T-tube, but within several days most of the bile will be flowing into the duodenum. If bile is not flowing out the tube or into the duodenum, it can be assumed that drainage is obstructed and that bile is being forced back into the common bile duct into the liver. The patient is observed closely for jaundice, particularly in the sclerae.

Before the T-tube is removed, the patency of the common bile duct must be assessed. The tube is clamped for variable intervals and the patient monitored for signs of distress. If distress occurs, the tube is unclamped immediately and the doctor is informed. A cholangiogram is usually performed to confirm patency of the duct before the tube is removed. After removal of the T-tube, the patient may have chills and fever caused by oedema and a local reaction to the bile; these symptoms usually subside within 24 hours.

Pain control

Pain control is a need of all people with biliary tract disease before definitive treatment. Analgesics such as pethidine will be needed to control the pain from biliary colic adequately and should be freely administered. Measures to decrease nausea and vomiting, such as maintenance of an NBM status or dietary fat restriction, will be necessary.

Pain control remains a need in the posttreatment period regardless of the treatment, although pain is much less after laparoscopic cholecystectomy. For the patient who has an abdominal cholecystectomy, pain remains a problem for up to 6 weeks. Immediately after surgery injectable analgesics are necessary. After the person is ambulating well and eating well, oral analgesics are usually satisfactory. For patients who had lithotripsy treatment, pain may continue for some time until the disintegrated stones are passed into the duodenum. Pain control is necessary to allow for adequate ambulation, deep breathing, and nutritional intake after definitive treatment.

Dressings, such as those present after abdominal surgical treatment of biliary tract disease, are monitored for moisture, which is uncomfortable and increases the risk of infection. Moist dressings are changed immediately. Additionally, great care is taken to avoid tension on biliary drainage tubes, another source of discomfort.

Teaching

The time available for preoperative or prelithotripsy teaching is often limited because patients may be acutely ill and undergoing diagnostic procedures and treatments to prepare them for surgery or lithotripsy within a short time. Or, conversely, the patient scheduled for elective surgery or lithotripsy may come to the hospital the morning of treatment 1 to 2 hours before the treatment. The nurse must be prepared to give essential information in the brief period that is available, as well as to address the patient's expressed concerns.

Important teaching points for patients with chronic biliary system disorders are summarized in Box 24-3.

DISORDERS OF THE PANCREAS

Acute and chronic pancreatitis and benign and malignant tumours are the major problems of the pancreas. Table 24-2 summarizes the signs, symptoms, and medical therapy for these problems.

PANCREATITIS

Pancreatitis is a serious inflammatory disorder of the pancreas that can be *acute* or *chronic*. Acute pancreatitis can occur as a single episode or as recurrent attacks (recurrent acute pancreatitis). The unique morphological feature of acute or recurrent acute pancreatitis is that, except in cases of alcohol-induced pancreatitis, the pancreas returns to normal after successful treatment.[31]

In chronic pancreatitis permanent and progressive destruction of the pancreas occurs, with normal tissue being replaced by fibrous tissue. Chronic pancreatitis can eventually lead to chronic insufficiency of pancreatic hormones (insulin).

Aetiology/Epidemiology

The causes of pancreatitis are numerous. Biliary disease is a common cause of acute pancreatitis. Many times in acute pancreatitis the cause is unknown. The principal cause of chronic pancreatitis in adults in Britain is smoking.[39] A major cause in children is cystic fibrosis; approximately 85% of patients with cystic fibrosis have impaired pancreatic exocrine function.[12] See Box 24-4 for a summary of causes of pancreatitis.

Patient Teaching 24-3

The patient with a chronic biliary system disorder

Dietary restrictions
  Low-fat diet if fat is poorly tolerated
  Low-calorie diet if weight reduction is necessary
Drug therapy, if appropriate
  Medication: importance in preventing recurrence of symptoms
  Medications: when and how to use
Dressings or drainage tube
  Biliary drainage: expected amount
  Dressing change or emptying of drainage bag: how to do and frequency
  Dressings: need to keep dry and skin clean (soap and water is sufficient by time of discharge); a daily shower may be permitted
  Dressing change: technique and availability of supplies
  Signs to report to doctor: excessive drainage, leakage, obstruction (jaundice, greyish-white stools)
Follow-up care
  Signs and symptoms to report to health care provider (pain, fever, jaundice, dark urine, greyish-white stools, pruritus, tube dislodgement)
  Follow-up care: plans

Pathophysiology

Although many causes of pancreatitis are known, the manner in which they result in acute inflammation is unknown. The currently favoured pathological factor leading to the acute inflammation is *autodigestion*. This theory proposes that proteolytic enzymes, particularly trypsinogen, are activated within the pancreas itself. Once activated to trypsin, trypsinogen can activate itself and other enzymes. The activated proteolytic enzymes digest pancreatic and surrounding tissues and cellular membranes. This autodigestion results in oedema, interstitial haemorrhage, vascular drainage, coagulation necrosis, fat necrosis, and parenchymal cell necrosis. The injured tissue releases histamine and bradykinin, which increase vascular permeability, cause vasodilation, and cause more oedema. The initiation of activation of the proteolytic enzymes is thought to result from reflux of bile into the pancreatic duct, obstruction of the pancreatic duct or ampulla of vater, ischaemia, anorexia, trauma, endotoxins, and exotoxins.

Regardless of the cause, the acute inflammatory process and autodigestion result in a spectrum of physiological alterations that can cause mild to very critical events. Pain may result from distension of the pancreatic capsule, from obstruction of bile flow caused by compression of the common bile duct, and from peritoneal irritation. The pain may radiate to the back, flanks, and substernal area and may be more intense when the person is lying supine. Difficulty in breathing may accompany the severe pain. Ascites and ileus distend the abdomen and lead to hypoventilation. Vomiting at first relieves pain, but continued vomiting worsens it. The patient often assumes a flexed posture to relieve pain.

Fluid and electrolyte abnormalities result from vomiting, local oedema, ascites, or calcium precipitation into the inflamed pancreas. Hypovolaemic shock may ensue if fluid loss is severe. Shallow respirations may reflect metabolic alkalosis (induced by loss of gastric contents), limited diaphragmatic excursion, or ascites. Decreased breath sounds may be the result of atelectasis or pleural effusion. Crackles may be present.

Multiple complications can occur as a result of acute pancreatitis. These complications can affect all systems. Box 24-5 lists some of the major complications.

Acute pancreatitis may be divided into three stages, oedematous or interstitial, haemorrhagic, and necrotizing. The majority of patients (80% to 90%) with acute pancreatitis recover without any residual dysfunction. The mortality rate is approximately 10%.[5] The occurrence of the following factors increases the risk of death from acute pancreatitis:

1. Hypotension
2. Need for massive fluid and colloid replacement
3. Respiratory failure associated with adult respiratory distress syndrome
4. Hypocalcaemia

The organ destruction that occurs in chronic pancreatitis is caused by the same factors as those described for acute pancreatitis, that is, autodigestion. In chronic pancreatitis caused by alcohol, the pancreatic juices secreted contain decreased bicarbonate, increased protein, and a decreased amount of substances that inhibit trypsin activation.[26] In addition, the pancreatic juices of people with chronic pancreatitis may be altered in other ways that allow for calcium precipitation. The changes described above would allow for formation of protein plugs that block the pancreatic ducts and precipitate autodigestion, inflam-

24-4

Causes of pancreatitis

Excessive alcohol consumption
Biliary tract disease
Postoperative—abdominal or nonabdominal surgery
Postretrograde cholangiopancreatography
Cystic fibrosis
Blunt abdominal trauma
Metabolic problems (increased serum calcium (hyperparathyroidism and postrenal transplant patients) hypertriglyceridaemia)
Cancer of pancreas
Infections (especially viral)
Connective tissue disease with vasculitis such as systemic lupus erythematosus
Drugs (antihypertensives, diuretics, antimicrobials, immunosuppressives, and oral contraceptives)
Intestinal diseases such as regional enteritis and penetrating duodenal ulcers
Malnutrition

Adapted from Toskes PP, Greenberger NJ: Acute and chronic pancreatitis, *Disease-a-Month* 29:5-81, 1983; and Toskes PP: Recurrent acute pancreatitis, *Hosp Pract* 20:85-88, 90-92, 1985.

2. Fluid status returns to normal and is maintained at normal as evidenced by weight, intake and output, vital signs, and skin turgor.
3. Gradually increases participation in self-care activities.
4. States goal and methods of treating substance abuse.
5. Has access to supportive services for long-term excessive alcohol comsumption or hospice services when prognosis for pancreatic carcinoma is poor.
6. Expresses less apathy and identifies one example of improvement in situation.
7. Takes replacement enzymes with bland food.
8. Explains how to implement medical regimen and other self-care needs on discharge.

Implementation

Assistance with achievement of therapeutic goals

Acute pancreatitis

Medical treatment is directed towards (1) decreasing secretions of the pancreas, (2) resting the pancreas, (3) preventing and treating complications (see Box 24-5), and (4) controlling pain.

Rest of the pancreas during the acute phase is achieved by measures that reduce stimulation of the exocrine secretions such as the following:

1. Nil-by-mouth (NBM) status
2. Nasogastric suction
3. Histamine$_2$ receptor blockers
4. Antacids

These measures decrease stimulation of the vagus nerve, and thus decrease secretion of hydrochloric acid, and decrease secretion of the pancreatic enzymes and fluid and electrolyte secretions stimulated by secretin, gastrin, and CCK. Antibiotics are not usually administered in the oedematous stage or in the absence of complications.

Pain relief is usually achieved with pethidine hydrochloride rather than morphine or codeine, because it is less spasmogenic on the sphincter of Oddi. Some patients find that pain is decreased if they assume a sitting position with the trunk flexed or lie on their sides with their knees drawn up to the abdomen.

The following nursing interventions are used depending on the presence or extent of fluid and electrolyte deficit and the presence of complications of acute pancreatitis:

1. Maintain intravenous fluid replacement (blood, albumin, plasma, fluids) and electrolytes as ordered.
2. Monitor vital signs and central venous pressure every 1 to 4 hours, or even more frequently if necessary.
3. Monitor intake and output every 1 to 4 hours.
4. Administer vasopressors and other measures for shock.
5. Maintain patency of the gastrointestinal tube.
6. Monitor for elevated glucose levels, Chvostek's and Trousseau's signs, and increasing abdominal girth.
7. Encourage deep breathing.
8. Administer as prescribed for complications: insulin, calcium, antibiotics, vitamin K.

As soon as the acute attack passes, oral fluids and foods are started.

Chronic pancreatitis

Therapy for the acute attack of chronic pancreatitis includes the therapies discussed above (NBM, nasogastric suction, antacids, and other medications, and IV fluids). In addition, as the acute attack subsides, medical attention will turn to confirming the diagnosis, to treating the malabsorption, and, in some instances, to surgery. Pancreatic enzyme replacement drugs contain amylase, lipase, and trypsin. They are taken at mealtimes to aid digestion and to facilitate the absorption of nutrients and fat-soluble vitamins. The patient should observe stools for steatorrhoea, which should decrease when fat intake is lowered and enzymes improve absorption.

Surgery

An exploratory laparotomy may be performed in acute pancreatitis when a diagnosis cannot be established and the possibility of general peritonitis, perforation of an organ, or a bowel obstruction cannot be excluded. If biliary obstruction is present, a surgical or endoscopic procedure may be done to divert or increase bile flow at the sphincter of Oddi and thereby reduce regurgitation of bile into the pancreatic duct.

For the treatment of pseudocysts the surgeon may employ external drainage, construct anastomoses between the pancreas and gastrointestinal tract (for example, pancreatojejunostomy), or resect part or all of the pancreas.

Exploratory surgery is often necessary to diagnose pancreatic tumours. Various techniques may be used to treat pancreatic tumours or to relieve pancreatic duct obstruction. Procedures to relieve obstructive jaundice are sometimes helpful in providing comfort (cholecystostomy, choledochojejunostomy). Often malignant tumours of the pancreas are inoperable by the time diagnosis is made.

Pancreatoduodenal resection (Whipple's procedure) is sometimes done when the carcinoma is localized with no evidence of metastasis. Whipple's procedure involves resection of the antrum of the stomach, duodenum, varying amounts of pancreas, and often the gallbladder. Anastomoses are constructed between the stomach, common bile duct and pancreatic ducts, and the jejunum. Malabsorption syndrome follows total pancreatectomy (protein, fat, iron, calcium, phosphate, vitamin B_{12} deficiencies occur), as does carbohydrate intolerance.

The patient with extensive pancreatic surgery or disease may have a prolonged postoperative course. Malnourishment, postoperative complications (haemorrhage, fistulas, anastomotic leak, infection) and metabolic derangements may occur. Haemorrhagic and hypovolaemic shock can lead to renal failure. Wound care must be meticulous. Drains are usually employed, and dressings should be inspected frequently and changed as often as necessary to maintain dryness. If a pancreatic fistula develops, severe tissue breakdown can occur from digestion of skin and underlying tissues by the pancreatic enzymes. Measurement of biliary or pancreatic drainage is carefully recorded.

Interventions to achieve patient outcomes

The patient with acute pancreatitis may be acutely ill and require intensive care. The priorities of care are controlling pain, managing fluids and electrolytes, and monitoring for complications. The patient with chronic pancreatitis and pancreatic tumours needs care to control pain, nutritional support, and help dealing with the potential hopelessness.[37,38] The person with chronic pancreatitis often needs help to deal with substance abuse. All patients have teaching needs.

Controlling discomfort

Control of pain is a major priority. Pethidine hydrochloride, 75 to 100 mg every 3 to 4 hours, may be necessary to reduce pain. As stated in the preceding section, some patients find that the pain is decreased if they assume a sitting position with the trunk flexed or a side-lying, knee-chest position with their knees drawn up to the abdomen.

The measures used to rest the pancreas (NBM status, nasogastric suctioning, and medications) will also assist with pain control by decreasing the continual autodigestive process and associated oedema and inflammation. In addition, the nurse should help the patient initiate relaxation techniques (deep breathing, imagery, and distraction techniques such as music, TV, and sewing) to help with pain control (see Chapters 5 and 8). These measures should be introduced after the patient has adequate pain control from the analgesic. If the patient is highly distressed, these techniques are not easily used. Comfort measures such as backrubs and purposeful touch are important and should be implemented.

Maintaining fluid and electrolyte balance

As soon as the patient is admitted, the nurse should institute monitoring related to fluid and electrolyte status, cardiac output, and renal status. This is a critical need. Monitoring includes intake and output; vital signs; daily weights; daily electrolytes; and blood urea nitrogen (BUN), creatinine, and haemodynamic measurements as necessary. An indwelling catheter may be necessary in acute pancreatitis because decreased renal function can occur in association with the hypotension and shock. Monitoring parameters and frequency of monitoring depend on the stability of the patient's condition. Fluids, electrolytes, colloids, or blood are given as necessary. The nurse is responsible for administering these and for monitoring the patient's response to them. Frequent adjustments in therapy may be necessary in relation to the patient's response to fluid therapy. If the patient develops shock, all the care described in Chapter 7 will be necessary.

Providing self-care

During the acute phase of the illness the patient will need assistance with all care. Dehydration and potential malnutrition make the patient particularly prone to skin breakdown.

Promoting healthy lifestyle patterns

If unhealthy lifestyle patterns such as excessive alcohol consumption are indicated as a cause of pancreatitis, the nurse must work with the patient on this problem. This care will be instituted after the patient is stabilized, but it must be introduced before the patient leaves the hospital.

Counselling

Patients with chronic pancreatitis and their families require much support. Long-term illness, physical deterioration, and chronic pain combined with alcohol, and, sometimes, narcotic misuse often result in apathy and hopelessness. These factors and the patient's affect or behaviour may evoke the same feelings of apathy and hopeless-

---

The Elderly with Biliary or Pancreatic Problems

Assessment

Assess elderly person for changes in ability to tolerate dietary fats; pancreatic secretions decrease with age.

Assess acutely ill elderly patients, especially after surgery, for signs of pancreatitis.

Intervention

Teach elderly people to avoid overweight and to exercise regularly within their capabilities to help decrease gallstone formation.

Teach people to report changes in ability to tolerate dietary fats and any sudden unrelieved abdominal pain suggestive of gallstones or pancreatitis.

Assist people who have gradual development of dietary fat intolerance to plan a low-fat diet.

Common disorders in elderly

Cholelithiasis
Cholecystitis
Pancreatitis after surgery or major organ failure

---

ness in health care providers.

The nurse who has developed self-awareness about perceptions and the responses evoked by apathetic patients may be more able to encourage hopefulness in patient interactions. Patients can be helped to maintain or develop hope by nurses who do the following:

1. Promote self-esteem.
2. Make referrals for treatment of substance abuse.
3. Reassure that pain can be controlled by prescribed measures.

Promoting nutrition

The patient is NBM and often has a nasogastric tube in place during the acute phase of the illness. Institution and maintenance of NBM status is a major intervention. Good oral hygiene is necessary to decrease discomfort from the NBM status and from the nasogastric tube. When the acute symptoms decrease (3 to 5 days), oral fluids and food are restarted. The patient is started on clear liquids and then advanced to a low-fat, bland diet, distributed over five to six small feedings daily. When refeeding starts, the patient is observed carefully for pain, nausea, and vomiting, all of which indicate continuing inflammation. If these occur, the doctor is notified and the methods described previously for inhibition of pancreatic activity are reinstituted. If food is restricted for long periods, parenteral hyperalimentation may be necessary. After discharge from the hospital, patients are advised to avoid alcohol and other gastric stimulants, such as caffeine, and to remain on a low-fat, bland diet with several small feedings daily. The patient needs to know how to take the pancreatic enzyme supplements. The dietitian may need to work with the patient to help plan an appropriate diet.

24-6

Patient Teaching

The patient with pancreatic disorders

After pancreatic surgery
  Self-care as to dressings, tubes, medications
  Need for low-fat, high-calorie diet, as appropriate
  Need for continued medical follow-up care
After pancreatitis
  Prevention of further attacks (avoidance of alcohol, narcotics, and abdominal injury; medical care when ill)
  Reporting symptoms indicating relapse or complications
    Pain
    Nausea and vomiting
    Abdominal distension
    Steatorrhoea
    Polyuria, polydipsia, polyphagia
    Weight loss
    Fever
  Maintaining low-fat, bland diet with several small feedings per day and vitamin supplements
  Avoiding rich foods to keep pancreatic secretions at a minimum
  Continuing medication therapy (pancreatic enzymes, bile salts, oral hypoglycaemic agents, or insulin)—scheduling, rationale, dose, side effects
  Need for continued medical follow-up care
Pain management
  Avoidance of pain stimulants
  Timing of food and enzyme replacements
  Use of antacids, histamine$_2$ receptor blockers

Teaching the patient

Teaching the patient and significant others is ongoing. At the beginning of hospitalization, the patient and significant others need basic instructions about the disease, the diagnostic tests, and the treatment. Because of the pain and the distress it causes and because of potential fluid status and cardiovascular instability, the patient and family experience tremendous stress and anxiety. Therefore explanations and instructions should be brief and as simple as possible and may need to be repeated. Support and continuity of care are also instituted to help decrease anxiety. Long-term education is directed towards prevention of future attacks by avoiding alcohol, maintaining a nutritious diet, and continuing medications as prescribed. The patient must report immediately any recurrence of signs and symptoms. Follow-up care is explained in detail. See Box 24-6 for summary of priority teaching points.

Evaluation

The expected patient outcomes serve as the basis for evaluating the extent to which patient status was improved. Questions to ask may include the following:

1. Was discomfort relieved?
2. Was detection and treatment of complications prompt?
3. Did serum amylase return to normal?
4. Were self-care needs met?

5. Were patient and family referred to appropriate supportive services?
6. Did the patient identify examples of improvement?
7. Was patient adequately prepared to manage the treatment regimen at home?

SUMMARY

1. The incidence of cholelithiasis and cholecystitis increases with age.
2. In the elderly, pancreatitis after surgery occurs more frequently.
3. Prevention of excessive alcohol consumption is a major way to decrease the occurrence of pancreatitis.
4. Cholecystitis (often associated with cholelithiasis) can be an acute or chronic inflammatory process.
5. In cholecystitis conservative treatment (NBM, pain control, intravenous fluids) may allow later elective surgery.
6. Laparoscopic cholecystectomy is the treatment of choice for cholelithiasis.
7. Nursing priorities for the patient having an LC are teaching and control of pain.
8. Nursing priorities for patients having abdominal cholecystectomies include measures to prevent RLL complications, to control pain, and to promote wound healing and biliary tube drainage.
9. Acute pancreatitis involves autodigestion of pancreatic tissue. Treatment includes measures to reduce pancreatic secretions (NBM, nasogastric drainage, H$_2$ receptor blockers, antacids).
10. Acute attacks of pancreatitis may be seen in relapsing acute pancreatitis or in chronic pancreatitis.
11. Chronic pancreatitis is characterized by permanent structure changes, diminished exocrine and endocrine secretions, malnourishment, and the development of pseudocysts.
12. Pancreatic surgery may be used in patients with pseudocysts and other complications of pancreatitis and in patients with pancreatic tumours or biliary obstruction.
13. Pain control is very complex in chronic pancreatitis.

STUDY QUESTIONS

- How would you explain the differences between laparoscopic and abdominal cholecystectomy to a patient as you counsel him or her?
- How do the needs differ in a patient with acute pancreatitis as compared with the patient with chronic pancreatitis?
- How would you explain to a patient's family why pain is sometimes so severe in biliary disease? In pancreatitis?

REFERENCES AND SELECTED READINGS

1.* Adinaro D: Liver failure and pancreatitis: fluid and electrolyte concerns, *Nurs Clin North Am* 22(4):843–852, 1987.
2. Adwers JR: Clinical trials of gallstone lithotripsy, *Hosp Pract* 24(7):83–90, 1989.
3.* Bagg AM: Whipple's procedure: nursing guidelines, *Crit Care Nurse* 8(5):34–45, 1988.
4.* Birdsall C, Fiore-Lopez N: How do you manage pancreatic sump tubes, *Am J Nurs* 87:770–771, 1987.

5.* Blake RL: Acute pancreatitis, *Prim Care* 15:187–199, 1988.

6. Bradley EL: Complications of chronic pancreatitis, *Surg Clin North Am* 69:481–497, 1989.

6a.* Brown A: Acute pancreatitis: pathophysiology, nursing diagnoses, and collaborative problems, *Focus Crit Care* 18:121–130, 1991.

7. Crist D, Cameron JL: The current management of acute pancreatitis, *Adv Surg* 20:69–124, 1987.

8. DiMagno EP: Early diagnosis of chronic pancreatitis and pancreatic cancer, *Med Clin North Am* 72:979–992, 1988.

9. Fain JA, Amato-Vealey E: Acute pancreatitis: a gastrointestinal emergency, *Crit Care Nurse* 8(5):47–63m, 1988.

9a.* Farha GJ, Beamer L: New options for treating gallstone disease, *Am Fam Physician* 44:1295–1304, 1991.

10. Frazee RC, et al: Open versus laparoscopic cholecystectomy, *Ann Surg* 213:651–653, 1991.

11. Glassman JA: *Biliary tract surgery: tactics and techniques.* New York, 1989, Macmillan Publishing.

12. Greenberger NJ: Chronic pancreatitis and exocrine insufficiency, *Hosp Pract* 20(1A):33–38, 40–45, 1985.

12a.* Greifzus, Dest V: When the diagnoses is pancreatic cancer, *RN* 22(9):38–45, 1991.

13.* Haicken BN: Laser laparoscopic cholecystectomy in the ambulatory setting, *J Post Anesth Nurs* 6(1):33–39, 1991.

14. Jeffres C: Complications of acute pancreatitis, *Crit Care Nurse* 9(4):38–46, 1989.

15.* Jurf JB, Clements L, Llorente J: Cholecystectomy made easier, *Am J Nurs* 90(12):38–39, 1990.

16. Lancaster S, Biaro-Marshall D: Gallstone lithotripsy, *Am J Nurs* 88:1629–1630, 1988.

17.* Marta MR: Endoscopic retrograde cholangeopancreatography: its role in diagnosis and treatment, *Focus on Crit Care* 14(5):62–63, 1987.

18.* Munn NE: When the bile duct is blocked, *RN* 20:50–57, 1989.

19.* Nurses Clinical Library: *Gastrointestinal disorders,* Springhouse, Pa, Nursing '85 Books, 1985, Springhouse.

20. Potts JR: Acute pancreatitis, *Surg Clin North Am* 68:281–299, 1988.

20a. Richards K: Lasers in general surgery, *Nurs Clin North Am* 25:667–671, 1990.

21. Rottenberg R: An update of pancreatic cancer, *Patient Care* 20(3):144–146, 151, 154–156, 158, 162, 1986.

22. Rowland GA, Marks DA, Torres W: The new gallstone destroyers and dissolvers, *Am J Nurs* 89:1473–1478, 1989.

23. Sabesin S: Countering the danger of acute pancreatitis, *Emerg Med* 19(17):71–73, 81–83, 87–89, 91–92, 95–96, 1987.

24. Sleisenger MH, Fordtran JS, editors: *Gastrointestinal disease: pathophysiology, diagnosis, management,* ed 4, Philadelphia, 1989, WB Saunders.

25. Southern Surgeon Club: A prospective analysis of 1518 laparoscopic cholecystectomies, *N Engl J Med* 324:1073–1078, 1991.

26. Steer ML: Classification and pathogenesis of pancreatitis, *Surg Clin North Am* 69:467–480, 1989.

27. Swazuk KJ, Mueller BG, Daly CJ: Laser cholecystomy: A perioperative nursing view, *AORN J* 50:998–1001, 1004–1005, 1989.

28. Tilkian SM, Conover MB, Tilkian AG: *Clinical complications of laboratory tests,* ed 4, St Louis, 1987, Mosby–Year Book.

29. Toskes PP: Diagnosis of chronic pancreatitis and exocrine insufficiency, *Hosp Pract* 20(10):97–100, 102–103, 107–108, 1985.

30. Toskes PP: Recurrent acute pancreatitis, *Hosp Pract* 20(7):85–88, 90–92, 1985.

30a. Wolfe BM, Gardiner B, Frey CF: Laparoscopic cholicystectomy, a remarkable development, *JAMA* 265:1573–1574, 1991.

31. Wyngaarden JB, Smith LH, editors: *Cecil textbook of medicine,* ed 18, Philadelphia, 1988, WB Saunders.

32. Dougherty WM: Serum bilirubin, *Nurs* '82 (11):138–139, 1982.

33. Kelber MB: Pancreatic enzymes: deciphering diagnostic studies, *Nurs* '82 12(12):65–67, 1982.

34.* Knudsen F: Gastrointestinal and metabolic problems in older adults. In Steffle B, editor: *Handbook of gerontological nursing,* New York, 1984, Van Nostrand Reinhold.

35.* Taylor DL: Gallstones: physiology, signs and symptoms, *Nurs 83* 13(6):44–45, 1983.

36.* Taylor DL: Jaundice: physiology, signs and symptoms, *Nurs 83* 13(8):52–54, 1983.

37. Herth, K: The relationship between level of hope and the level of coping response and other variables in patients with cancer. *Oncology Nursing Forum.*

38. El-Gamel, V: Usefulness of hope assessment in the oncology unit. *Journal Cancer Care,* October 1993.

39. Lidingham, JPP, Warrel, DA: *Oxford Textbook of Medicine,* Chpt. 12:164, 1984.

FURTHER READING

Herlihy B: Hepatic and biliary systems—physiology review, *Critical Care Nurse* 4(1):104–105 1984.

Kelber MB: Pancreatic enzymes—deciphering diagnostic studies, *Nursing* 12(12):65–67 1982.

Smith J, Davies B: An inside view—endoscopic retrograde cholangiopancreatography (ERCP), *Nursing Mirror* 157(22):30–33 1983.

*Suggested for student reading.

25

The Patient with Urinary Problems

Roberta Stokes
H. Fred Farley

After studying this chapter, the learner should be able to:

- Describe interventions for urinary retention and urinary incontinence.
- Describe the causes and methods of prevention of urinary tract infections (UTI).
- Explain pathophysiological differences among, signs and symptoms of, and therapeutic modalities and nursing interventions for glomerular disorders.
- Describe the pathophysiology of obstructive urinary disorders.
- Describe the pathophysiology and interventions for renal calculi.
- Compare different approaches to prostatectomy and the related nursing interventions.
- Describe the care of the person undergoing surgery of the urinary tract.
- Differentiate between acute and chronic renal failure, including pathophysiology, signs and symptoms, medical therapy, and nursing interventions.
- Explain the physiological principles of dialysis and the types of renal replacement therapies and related care.

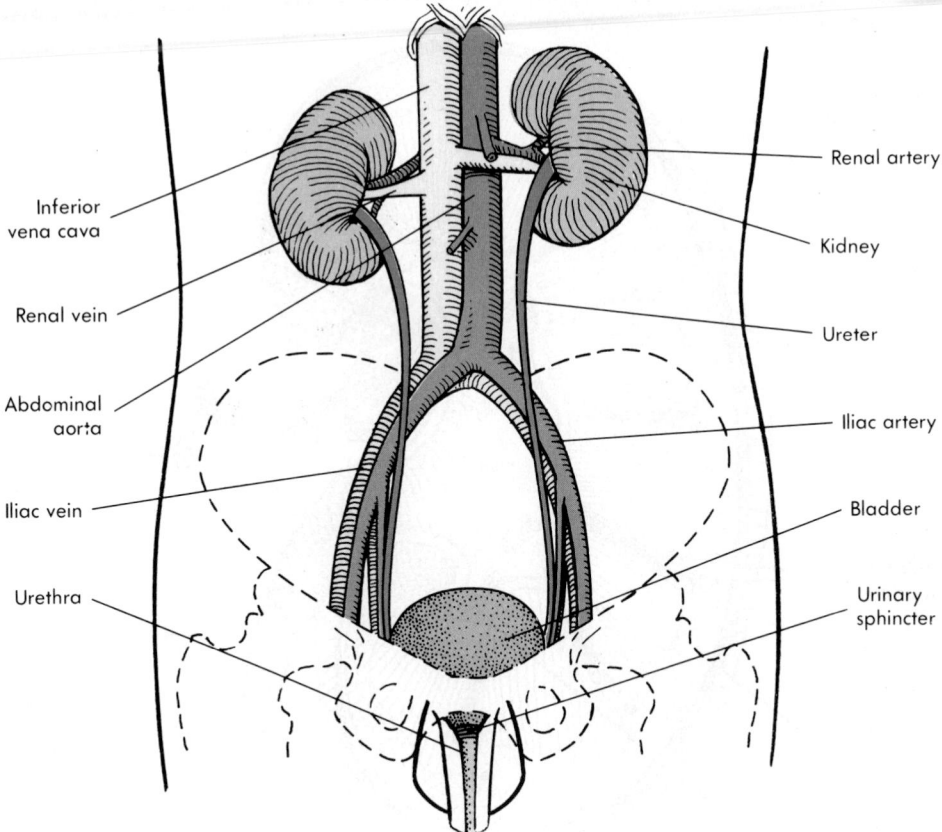

Fig. 25-1   Kidneys and other structures of urinary system.

The maintenance of *homeostasis*, defined as the state of the dynamic equilibrium of the internal environment, is essential for life. The body must regulate blood pressure, acid-base balance, hormonopoiesis (hormone production), fluid volume, and electrolyte composition. Moreover, the body must have a mechanism for eliminating the end products of metabolism.

The kidneys and other structures of the urinary system play major roles in the regulation of the internal environment. Some of the urinary disorders discussed in this chapter may lead to destruction of renal tissue, with subsequent alterations in fluid and electrolyte balance, excretion of body wastes, and regulation of body processes.

This chapter begins with a brief review of the major concepts relating to anatomy and physiology of the urinary system. (For a more intensive review, the reader is referred to a physiology text.) The next part of the chapter describes major urinary disorders, some of which may lead to renal failure. The last part of the chapter discusses renal failure, both acute and chronic, and includes renal replacement therapies.

ANATOMY AND PHYSIOLOGY

The urinary system consists primarily of the kidneys, ureters, bladder, and urethra (Fig. 25-1). Although the prostate gland is primarily a male reproductive organ, it is discussed in this chapter because enlargement or infection of the prostate affects the urinary tract.

Upper Urinary Tract

Kidney anatomy

The kidneys are vital organs for maintaining homeostasis. They have the important task of regulating the composition and volume of the plasma which, in turn, produces similar changes in the interstitial fluid. The kidneys receive about 1 L/min or 25% of the total cardiac output of 4 to 5 L/min. The entire plasma volume is filtered approximately 60 times every 24 hours (or 1200 ml/min). This enables the kidneys to regulate the components of plasma precisely.

Gross structure of the kidney

The kidneys are paired, retroperitoneal, bean-shaped organs located just above the waistline on either side of the vertebral column. The right kidney is usually lower because the right lobe of the liver lies above it. The upper border of the left kidney is protected by the eleventh and twelfth ribs. Each kidney is encased in a hard fibrous capsule (Fig. 25-2) that contains pain receptors. Perirenal fat cushions the kidneys and helps hold them in place. Both the capsule and perirenal fat tend to limit bleeding when the kidney is injured. An adrenal gland is located atop each kidney.

The outer layer, the *cortex*, contains the glomeruli, proximal and distal convoluted tubules, the first portion of the loops of Henle, and the collecting tubules. The inner layer, the *medulla*, contains conical masses or pyramids formed by the loops of Henle and the collecting tubules.

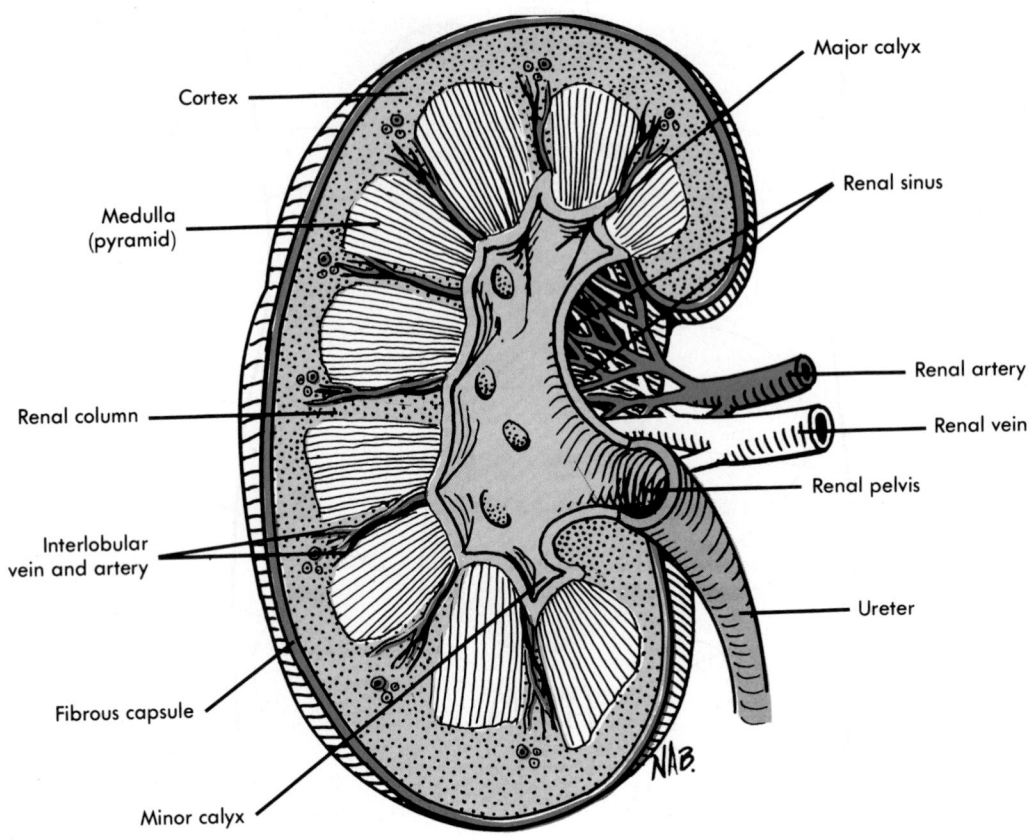

Fig. 25-2 Frontal section of kidney.

The nephron

Types of nephrons

The nephron is the basic functional unit of the kidney (Fig. 25-3). Each kidney contains approximately one million of these units. Because of its ability to compensate, about 75% to 80% of the nephron can be destroyed without causing harmful effects.

There are two types of nephrons, cortical and juxtamedullary. *Cortical* nephrons are located in the outer two thirds of the cortex and have a high-pressure peritubular capillary network. This network arises from the efferent arteriole and surrounds the proximal and distal convoluted tubules and loops of Henle. This is where filtration occurs and urine is formed. The cortical nephrons also have a low-pressure capillary network that is nutritive, supplies blood to the rest of the nephron, and allows for reabsorption from the tubule back into the blood.

Juxtamedullary nephrons have a more complex vasculature. The efferent arteriole of juxtamedullary nephrons also branches into a second peritubular capillary network that surrounds the proximal and distal tubules of these nephrons. However, this capillary network is located in the deep cortex.

A series of hairpin loops called *vasa recta,* located in the medulla, wrap around and run parallel to the long thin loops of Henle. The vasa recta branch into capillary networks around the loops of Henle and the collecting ducts of both types of nephrons. The presence of the vasa recta results in increased resistance in juxtamedullary nephrons. This resistance leads to a higher filtration rate and less blood flow. Vasa recta also act as a countercurrent exchanger, preventing the interstitial gradient from being dispersed. This action contributes significantly to the kidney's ability to concentrate urine.[53]

Juxtaglomerular apparatus

The juxtaglomerular apparatus is a combination of specialized cells located near the glomerulus at the junction of the afferent and efferent arterioles. Juxtaglomerular cells contain granules of inactive renin. The juxtaglomerular apparatus is believed to secrete renin and to play a role in both autoregulation of the glomerular filtration and renal control of extracellular fluid volume through the renin-angiotensin-aldosterone system.[53]

Flow of blood and urine

The nephron contains two types of microscopic structures, those for blood flow and those for urine flow.

Blood flow

Blood flow through the kidneys begins in the *renal artery,* which arises from the abdominal aorta. Blood then flows through increasingly smaller arteries: the *interlobar, arcuate,* and *interlobular* arteries. The interlobar arteries divide into the *afferent arterioles* located in the cortex. These arterioles subdivide into a tuft of capillaries or glomeruli,

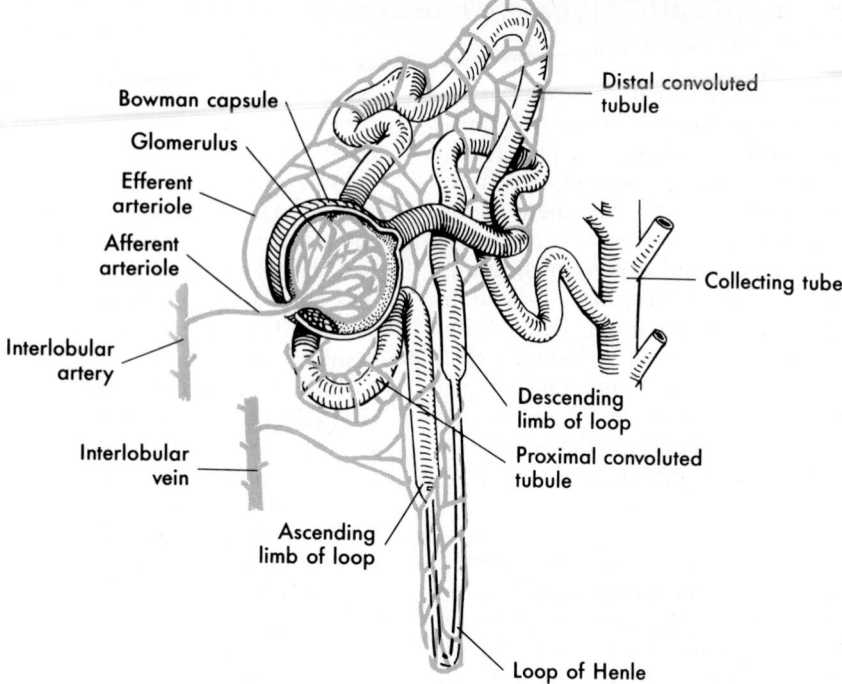

Fig. 25-3 Nephron.

which are finely coiled within Bowman's capsule. The distal ends of the glomeruli are connected to *efferent arterioles*, which divide to form peritubular capillaries that surround the tubules (as described earlier); this allows material to be selectively transferred between the tubules and peritubular capillary network. After passing through the capillaries, blood returns to the *venules*, and then to the *renal vein*, which leaves the kidney through the hilum and joins the inferior vena cava.

Urine flow

Urine is filtered from the glomerulus into Bowman's capsule. From there it flows through a long tubule subdivided into the proximal convoluted tubule, loop of Henle, distal convoluted tubule, and collecting tubule (see Fig. 25-3). The latter joins other collecting tubules. Urine empties through papillary ducts into the calyces (see Fig. 25-2) and into the renal pelvis. Urine then flows down the ureter into the urinary bladder and is excreted through the urethra via the urinary meatus.

Renal Physiology

The functions of the kidney are summarized in Box 25-1. These functions, accomplished during the formation of urine, are described in succeeding paragraphs.

Urine formation

Glomerular filtration

The first process involved in urine formation is called *glomerular filtration*. It is defined as the movement of water and select substances through the glomerular capillaries into Bowman's capsule.

The glomerular filtrate arising from the glomerular capillaries approximates 180 L/day. The amount of glomerular filtrate in a given time period is called the *glomerular filtration rate* (GFR). The GFR in an average-sized man is approximately 125 ml/min (7.5 L/hr). The average GFR in a woman is about 10% less. The same forces that affect fluid transport between vascular and interstitial spaces in other parts of the body (see Chapter 6) also affect filtration in the glomerular capsule. The GFR is affected by

25-1	Major functions of the kidneys	
	Urine formation	Glomerular filtration, tubular reabsorption and secretion
	Fluid and electrolyte control	Maintain correct balance of fluid and electrolytes within a normal range by excretion, secretion, and reabsorption
	Acid-base balance	Maintain pH at normal range by directly excreting H^+ ions and forming bicarbonate for buffering
	Excretion of waste products	Direct removal of metabolic waste products contained in the glomerular filtrate
	Blood pressure regulation	Regulate blood pressure by controlling circulating volume and renin secretion
	RBC production	Erythropoietin secreted by kidneys stimulates bone marrow to produce RBCs
	Regulation of calcium-phosphate metabolism	Vitamin D activation regulated by kidneys

changes in hydrostatic pressure. Such changes can be caused by (1) diminished renal perfusion from hypovolaemia, (2) occlusion of the glomeruli from diabetic nephropathy, (3) alteration in the plasma protein concentration from hypoproteinaemia, (4) alterations of the basement membrane from an autoimmune disorder, and (5) arteriolar constriction from sympathetic stimulation or medication.

The blood supply to the kidneys is basic to the formation of glomerular filtrate, or beginning urine, and to the nutrition and respiration requirement of kidney cells. Severe and prolonged problems with maintaining cardiac output and renal perfusion have profound effects on the formation of urine and the viability of the cells responsible for maintaining consistency in the internal environment.

Tubular phase

The second process in urine formation involves the selective alteration and reduction of the glomerular filtrate. When blood enters the glomerular capillaries at a pressure not less than 60 to 70 mm Hg, an ultrafiltrate of plasma is formed. This *ultrafiltrate* (primitive urine) contains approximately the same concentration of the elements of plasma minus the proteins. The ultrafiltrate then passes through the tubular system and is modified into actual urine. During this process, there is a constant movement of particles and fluid between the tubule lumen, interstitium, and peritubular capillaries. The ultrafiltrate is altered by the processes of reabsorption, secretion or both. *Reabsorption* is the transport of substances that the body needs, such as sodium, chloride, potassium, bicarbonate, and water from the tubular lumen into the interstitium and blood. *Secretion* is the transport of substances not needed by the body from the blood and interstitium into the tubule lumen.

Fluid and electrolyte control

Were it not for some conserving mechanism in the kidneys, a person would be depleted of fluid and salts within 3 to 4 minutes. The *proximal convoluted tubule* reabsorbs up to 85% to 90% of water in the ultrafiltrate; up to 80% of filtered sodium; and the majority of filtered potassium, bicarbonate, chloride, phosphate, glucose, and protein.

Dehydration would still occur if the body did not have an additional mechanism within the kidneys to conserve filtered water. This mechanism allows urine to be concentrated to less than 1% of the daily filtered volume. The kidneys can vary the amount of fluid excreted so precisely that intake over that required for normal fluid balance is excreted and intake under that required for normal fluid balance leads to further concentration of the urine. The mechanisms responsible for this increased urine concentrating ability and precision in excreting appropriate urine volume exist in the loop of Henle and the distal convoluted and collecting tubules. The *loop of Henle* reaches into the medullary portion of the kidney, which is highly hypertonic in comparison to the filtrate. In the *descending* portion of the loop, sodium diffuses into the filtrate as the tubule passes deeper into the medullary area, and water moves out of the primitive urine in response to the high sodium concentration. The result is a reduction in volume of the glomerular filtrate and a dramatic increase in its osmolality. In the *ascending* limb of the loop of Henle, sodium is reabsorbed into the interstitium, but the loop is impermea-ble to the movement of water either into or out of the tubule. The primitive urine now presented to the *distal convoluted* and *collecting tubules* is greatly reduced in volume but hypotonic because of the reabsorption of sodium. The influence of antidiuretic hormone (ADH) on these last two segments of the tubule allows water to be reabsorbed into the interstitium in an amount compatible with maintenance of proper fluid balance. The reabsorption of water from the forming urine increases osmolality and results in the excretion of a hypertonic urine.

Electrolyte balance is achieved mainly in the distal convoluted and collecting tubule portions of the nephron. As with fluid, the major conservation site for electrolytes is the *proximal convoluted tubule* where the vast majority of all filtered electrolytes are reabsorbed, thus preventing rapid depletion of these substances. The precise regulation of body electrolyte composition occurs in the distal tubular segments. Depending on the concentrations of electrolytes presented to the tubular cells in the primitive urine and the concentrations of these substances in the interstitium, tubular cells secrete or further reabsorb electrolytes into the urine (Table 25-1).

Regulation of acid-base balance

The kidney maintains the blood at the slightly alkaline pH of 7.35 to 7.45. The alkalinity of blood is controlled by the rate at which bicarbonate ions are excreted from the body and by the rate at which bicarbonate ions are restored to the buffering system. The secretion of hydrogen ions is accomplished by the cells of the proximal and distal convoluted tubule and the thick portion of the loop of Henle. Secretion of hydrogen ions is accompanied by the restoration of bicarbonate ions.

The most abundant buffer in the extracellular fluid is the sodium bicarbonate-carbonic acid system (see Chapter 7). Remember that strong acids react with sodium bicarbonate and convert into a weak acid (carbonic acid). Carbonic acid then dissociates into carbon dioxide and water. The carbon dioxide is eliminated by the lungs. During the process one mole of bicarbonate is lost from the extracellular fluid for each mole of acid reacting with the buffer system. The buffering system is replenished by the kidney.

Two processes result in the restoration of bicarbonate: regeneration and reabsorption. For every filtered bicarbonate ion that combines with a hydrogen ion, a filtered sodium ion is reabsorbed along with a bicarbonate ion. Bicarbonate ions are also formed when carbon dioxide combines with water in the tubular cell. The net result is excretion of hydrogen ions with the return of bicarbonate to the peritubular capillaries.

Excretion of waste products

Metabolic wastes are excreted in the glomerular filtrate. Creatinine is little modified in its passage through the nephron; creatinine contained in the glomerular filtrate is excreted unchanged in the urine. Other wastes, such as urea, are excreted unchanged in the glomerular filtrate but undergo reabsorption during passage through the nephron. The amount of waste material excreted in urine in such an instance is only a fraction of that originally contained in the glomerular filtrate.

Table 25-1   Fluid and electrolyte control by kidney

Site	Function	Effect	Physiological basis
Glomerulus	Filtration of water and electrolytes	Beginning of urine formation	Hydrostatic pressure
Proximal convoluted tubules	Reabsorption of large amounts of water, sodium, potassium, bicarbonate, chloride, phosphate	Conservation of fluid and electrolytes	Reabsorption by active and passive transport Bicarbonate reabsorption controlled by acid-base imbalance
Loop of Henle Descending limb	Diffusion of sodium into tubule Reabsorption of water	Reduction in urine volume; urine is hypertonic	Medulla of kidney is hypertonic
Ascending limb	Reabsorption of sodium	Urine becomes hypotonic	Water remains in loop because membrane is impermeable to water
Distal convoluted tubule and collecting tubule	Reabsorption of water Secretion of potassium, hydrogen and ammonia ions as needed Reabsorption of sodium	Fluid and electrolyte control depending on body needs	Water is reabsorbed as needed by effect of ADH Extra potassium is secreted Hydrogen and ammonia ions are secreted, depending on acid-base imbalances Sodium is reabsorbed by effect of aldosterone

Excretion of drugs by the kidneys occurs through both filtration at the glomerular level and secretion into the urine by distal tubular cells. Penicillin is an example of a drug secreted by tubular cells.

Blood pressure regulation

Renal regulation of blood pressure is controlled by the renin-angiotensin-aldosterone system. *Renin* is a hormone released by the juxtaglomerular apparatus (adjoining the glomerulus) in response to sodium depletion, renal artery hypoperfusion, or stimulation of the renal nerves through the sympathetic pathways. *Angiotensinogen,* which is produced in the liver, is activated to *angiotensin I* in the presence of renin. An enzyme in the lungs converts angiotensin I to the active form, *angiotensin II.* Angiotensin II is a powerful *vasoconstrictor* that also stimulates the release of aldosterone by the adrenal glands. *Aldosterone* increases sodium reabsorption by the kidney; water follows the sodium, leading to an increase in blood volume. A low GFR, seen with numerous kidney diseases (such as glomerulonephritis, nephrotic syndrome, polycystic disease, renal trauma, renal failure) usually leads to hypertension by activation of the renin-angiotensin-aldosterone system. (See Chapter 18 for a discussion of hypertension.)

Stimulation of red blood cell production

Red blood cell (RBC) production is primarily controlled by the kidneys. *Erythropoietin* is a hormone that is secreted by the kidneys. Erythropoietin stimulates bone marrow to produce RBCs. People with chronic renal failure often have serum hematocrit values of 18% to 30% (normal values are 42% to 47%). This decrease in haematocrit values is the result of decreased secretion of erythropoietin from the diseased kidneys compounded by bone marrow toxicity, decreased life span of RBCs and increased bleeding, all of which are associated with the altered metabolic state present in chronic renal failure.

Regulation of calcium-phosphorus metabolism

Calcium-phosphorus metabolism is controlled by the kidneys. Most of the reabsorption of calcium (65%–70%) occurs at the proximal tubule with the rest occurring at the loop of Henle (20%–25%) and the distal tubule (10%). The amount of calcium reabsorption is primarily determined by parathyroid hormone (PTH) and vitamin D.

Vitamin D (cholecalciferol), which is classified as a hormone, facilitates intestinal absorption of calcium. Vitamin D itself is not the active substance; instead, vitamin D precursors must undergo a series of metabolic changes to be converted to 1,25 dehydroxycholecalciferol (1,25-DHHC), the biolocalally active form. Normal kidney and liver function are essential for the conversion.[22]

Lower Urinary Tract

Anatomy

The *ureters* arise as extensions of the kidney pelves and empty into the bladder in an area called the *trigone*. These small tubes are composed of smooth muscle; their function is to propel urine from the kidney into the bladder. Spasm and severe colic-type pain result from obstruction of the ureters. The *bladder*, situated behind the symphysis pubis, is a collecting bag for the urine. The mucous membrane is arranged in folds called *rugae* that, together with the elasticity of the muscular walls, can distend the bladder considerably to hold large amounts of urine. A layer of skeletal muscle encircles the base of the bladder, forming the *external urinary sphincter*. The bladder is innervated by both the sympathetic and parasympathetic nervous system, whereas the ureters receive fibres only from the sympathetic nervous system.

The *urethra* transports urine from the bladder to the external meatus. Male and female urethras differ in length and accessibility of reproductive organs. The female urethra is short (about 4 cm long), exits anterior to the vagina (see Fig. 27-1), and is separate from the reproductive organs. The male urethra (see Fig. 27-3) is 18 to 20 cm long and transports semen as well as urine. The urethra is innervated by both the sympathetic and parasympathetic nervous systems.

The *prostate gland* is a male reproductive gland about the size of a walnut that encircles the upper portion of the male urethra. It is shaped like a doughnut with the urethra passing through the "hole." When the prostate is enlarged, the urethra is squeezed, causing obstruction of urinary flow. Numerous prostatic ducts empty into the urethra. Bacteria from urinary tract infections may travel up these ducts, causing prostatic infection.

Micturition

Urine flows out the kidney pelves and is propelled through the ureters by peristaltic action. About 200 to 300 ml of urine can collect in the bladder before the urge to void is initiated. Baroreceptors in the bladder wall are triggered by the stretching of the bladder walls, which causes reflex stimulation of parasympathetic nerves to the bladder, resulting in bladder contractions. When the motor nerves to the external urinary sphincter are inhibited, the muscle relaxes, opening the sphincter and permitting urine to be expelled. Stimulation of the sphincter muscles can keep the sphincter contracted against strong bladder contractions. Voluntary control over micturition can be exerted by stimuli transmitted over descending spinal pathways from the brainstem.

Use of a large balloon (30 ml) in-dwelling catheter (such as after a transurethral resection of the prostate) can stimulate the parasympathetic nerves, causing uncomfortable bladder contractions. Pressure on the sphincter by the balloon can also create an urge to void, although the bladder has been emptied by the catheter.

Physiological Changes With Ageing

A direct relationship exists between blood supply to the kidneys and renal function. The rate of blood flow to the kidneys is about 5 to 10 times greater than that to the heart, liver, and brain. Glomerular capillary pressure, which is the force that promotes ultrafiltration, is controlled by blood flow to the kidneys. Therefore, physiological alterations in the vascular bed can lead to age-related changes in renal function.

Arteriosclerotic changes in renal arteries are the most common form of renal vascular pathology.[1] Arteriosclerotic changes occur to some extent in most normal individuals with ageing. The degree of morphological change experienced depends on the specific arteries affected and the extent of involvement.

Ageing is also known to cause predictable increases in both systolic and diastolic blood pressure.[40] This slow increase in blood pressure begins at birth and continues through adulthood. Untreated hypertension further accelerates the development of atherosclerosis, which can lead to renal failure.

Changes also occur in kidney structure and function with ageing. About 40% of glomeruli are lost by age 70. The glomerular and tubular basement membranes thicken, leading to a 46% decrease in GFR from age 20 to 90.[1] If heart failure is also present with compensatory vasodilation, renal ischaemia is increased further and the risk of renal failure is increased.

The ability to concentrate urine and sensitivity to ADH stimulation also decreases with age. Elderly people have greater difficulty eliminating heavy solute loads and are slower to conserve fluids with fluid restriction.[29] Electrolyte imbalance may occur more readily from a decreased ability to conserve sodium, excrete potassium, and form and excrete ammonia.

Urinary incontinence may occur in acutely ill elderly people who lack energy for voluntary control or who may be confused or disoriented. Stress incontinence may be noted in women with relaxed perineal muscles or in males following prostatectomy. Benign prostatic hypertrophy (p. 973) occurs in more than half of all men over age 50 and 75% of men over age 70; the enlarged prostate presses on the urethra, resulting in urinary symptoms.

PREVENTION AND HEALTH EDUCATION

Primary Prevention

Two measures can be effective in reducing the incidence of renal failure: (1) identification of individuals at risk and (2) identification and control of environmental factors that can result in renal failure. Box 25-2 summarizes conditions and substances that can result in injury to the kidneys.

Secondary Prevention

Renal dysfunction can be somewhat elusive. Renal function can be described as being on a continuum—at one end of the continuum is normal renal function, whereas at the other end is renal failure. It is when people near the point of renal failure that they begin to exhibit signs and symptoms. Two other points on this continuum are decreased renal reserve and renal insufficiency. *Decreased renal reserve* exists when renal function has diminished to the point at which additional physiological stress results in signs and symptoms. This stress could result from intercurrent illness, infection, or dietary overindulgence. Signs and symptoms of decreased renal reserve usually resolve once the stress is removed. *Renal insufficiency* is defined as the reduced capacity of the kidney to perform its functions. Renal insufficiency is generally experienced when the GFR is 20% to 40% of normal. The person with renal insufficiency typically requires symptomatic management by the doctor. It is important to follow these two points on the renal function continuum, because proper management can prevent the loss of more renal functioning and eliminate the need for more aggressive therapy. Regular physical examination, including serum chemistry evaluation can aid in the detection of changing renal status.

Box 25-2 Conditions and substances that can result in kidney damage

Inadequate perfusion

Hypovolaemia
Blood loss (surgery, trauma)
Plasma loss (burns, surgery, acute pancreatitis)
Sodium and water loss (prolonged diarrhoea or vomiting, gastrointestinal tract drainage, sustained high fever)
Cardiac failure
Myocardial infarction
Cardiac dysrhythmias
Congestive heart failure
Septic shock
Infections (untreated streptococcal throat, untreated urinary tract sepsis)
Vascular changes (diabetes mellitus, hypertension, renal artery stenosis)

Toxic substances

Solvents (carbon tetrachloride, methanol, ethylene glycol)
Heavy metals (lead, arsenic, mercury)
Antibiotics (kanamycin, gentamicin, polymyxin B, amphotericin B, colistin, neomycin, phenazopyridine)
Pesticides
Poisonous mushrooms

Box 25-3 Risk factors for diabetes and hypertension

Diabetes

Familial history
Obesity
Race
Gender (female)
Corticosteroid medications

Hypertension

High sodium intake
Familial history
Advanced age
Obesity
Stress

Box 25-4 Urinary tract infections

Primary prevention

1. Cleanse perineal area properly; a shower is more desirable than a bath.
2. Drink adequate volume of fluid, 3 to 4 L/day.
3. Void frequently during waking hours, every 2 to 3 hours during day.

Secondary prevention

1. Seek prompt medical attention for symptoms.
2. Continue with drug therapy even though symptoms abate.
3. Follow steps 1 through 3 listed above.
4. Follow-up care with repeated urine cultures is essential.

Diabetes mellitus is the most common cause of end-stage renal disease (ESRD) in Britain.[52,36a] Hypertension and glomerulonephritis follow closely. Early detection and prompt treatment of these conditions can either prevent or slow the progression of nephron damage. People at risk for developing diabetes and hypertension (Box 25-3) should be screened regularly.

Urinary tract infections (UTI) are a significant source of morbidity in Britain.[49a] These infections contribute to illness during the active stage but also can lead to the development of chronic renal failure. Although the vast majority of UTIs clear spontaneously, there remains a portion significant enough to warrant consideration as a health problem. Early detection and treatment of a UTI decrease the probability of renal complications. Box 25-4 summarizes health care practices helpful in prevention and treatment of a UTI.

Tertiary Prevention

Tertiary prevention in people with urinary disorders focuses on helping them adapt as fully as possible to limitations imposed by their illness. For example, for patients with chronic renal failure requiring dialysis, it is the domain of nursing to assist patients and their families adjust to the treatment regimen and changes in life-style.[22] Another example is assisting patients who have had urinary diversion procedures to adapt to changes in urinary patterns and body image. Overall, tertiary prevention involves preventing further urinary disability and reduced functioning.

MAJOR HEALTH PROBLEMS OF THE URINARY SYSTEM

The major health problems of the urinary system can be categorized in a number of ways. The following common disorders will be discussed in this chapter.
1. Urinary dysfunction
   a. Urinary retention
   b. Urinary incontinence
2. Urinary tract infections
   a. Pyelonephritis
   b. Lower urinary tract infection
3. Glomerular disorders
   a. Glomerulonephritis: acute, chronic
   b. Nephrotic syndrome
4. Obstructive disorders
   a. Urinary calculi
   b. Benign prostatic hypertrophy
   c. Urethral strictures
   d. Neoplasms: renal, bladder, prostate
5. Other urinary disorders
   a. Polycystic disease
   b. Vascular disorders
   c. Diabetic nephropathy
   d. Trauma

Another major health problem of the urinary system is congenital disorders. Congenital disorders include structural malformation, lack of or poor development of one or both kidneys, dysplasia, and polycystic disease. Any of these conditions can result in morbidity in adults. (For more information about congenital disorders refer to a paediatric nursing text.)

Any of the preceding disorders can lead to loss of renal function resulting in what is called *renal failure*. Renal failure is classified as (1) acute or (2) chronic. Acute and chronic renal failure are discussed at the end of this chapter.

URINARY DYSFUNCTION

URINARY RETENTION

Aetiology

Under normal conditions, a person consuming an adequate diet, including adequate fluid intake, has a urinary output approximately equal to fluid intake. Inadequate urinary output may occur either when the kidneys are not producing urine or when urine is retained in the bladder (*urinary retention*). Causes of urinary retention include urethral obstruction, decreased sensory activity to and from the bladder, surgery, medications, and muscle tension.[59] Causes of urinary retention can be categorized as either mechanical or functional (Box 25-5).

25-5	**Major causes of urinary retention**	
	Type of retention	**Cause**
	Mechanical obstruction	
		Urethral stricture
		Urinary tract malformation
		Spinal cord malformation
	Acquired	Calculus
		Inflammation
		Trauma
		Tumour
		Hyperplasia
		Pregnancy
	Functional obstruction	Neurogenic bladder dysfunction
		Ureterovesical reflux
		Decreased peristaltic activity of the ureter
		Detrusor muscle atrophy
		Anxiety, such as fear of pain after surgery
		Medications, for example anaesthetics, narcotics, sedatives, and antihistamines

Pathophysiology

A mechanical obstruction exists when urine flow is blocked. This blockage can exist anywhere within the urinary system from the collecting ducts to the urinary meatus. Most obstructions in adults are acquired. A functional obstruction exists when there is an obstruction that cannot be attributed to a mechanical problem.

A key symptom of urinary retention is inability to void. The bladder becomes distended with urine and is sometimes displaced to either side of the midline. Percussion over a full bladder produces a "kettledrum" sound. Discomfort occurs from pressure of the bladder on other organs and the person has an urge to urinate. Restlessness and diaphoresis may also occur with a full bladder.

Voiding 25 to 50 ml of urine at frequent intervals often indicates *retention with overflow*. The intravesicular pressure increases as the bladder continues to fill with urine and overcomes the sphincter's restraining capability. A small amount of urine flows out of the bladder to reduce the intravesicular pressure to the level where the sphincter can control the flow of urine once again. The patient may state that the bladder continues to feel full. The bladder fills again and the cycle is repeated. The specific gravity of the person's urine is normal or high in retention with overflow because the kidney's ability to produce urine is not impaired.

Nursing Process

Assessment

Subjective data

The patient is asked questions to provide data on the following:

1. Understanding of the disorder
2. Voiding patterns, including absence of voiding or voiding frequently in small amounts without relief of bladder distension
3. Dietary habits, including fluid intake
4. Presence of suprapubic pain
5. History of urinary problems

Objective data

Objective data should include intake and output, assessment of level of hydration, palpation for bladder distension, and visual inspection of urine for colour, clarity, sedimentation, and odour.

Nursing analysis

Nursing analyses are determined from assessment of patient data. Possible nursing problems for the person with urinary retention may include, but are not limited to, the following:

Problem	**Possible aetiologies**
Urinary retention	Obstruction, position for voiding, immobility, effects of medications (narcotics, anaesthetics, sedatives, antihistamines)
Knowledge deficit	Lack of information

Planning: expected patient outcomes

Expected patient outcomes for the person with urinary retention may include, but are not limited to, the following:

1. Voids 200 to 400 ml at each voiding.
2. Demonstrates home care of catheter to prevent infection.
3. Describes signs of retention or UTI (for in-dwelling catheter) to be reported to doctor.

Implementation

Assisting with achievement of therapeutic goals

Interventions for urinary retention are aimed at reestablishing urine flow. Some mechanical obstructions must be corrected by surgical intervention; others, such as that caused by an enlarged prostate, may require temporary urethral catheter drainage.

Promotion of micturition

If the person is having difficulty eliminating urine from the bladder in the absence of mechanical obstruction, measures that encourage voiding are attempted before catheterization is instituted. These measures may include ensuring a position that facilitates voiding (positional stimuli), running water or blowing bubbles in water (auditory stimuli), or pouring water over the perineum or placing the hands in water (tactile stimuli). Having the person sit in lukewarm water may help to relax the urinary sphincters.

Cholinergic medications, such as bethanechol chloride or distigmine, may be given to initiate voiding by stimulating the bladder detrusor muscle to contract. However, these medications must never be given if a mechanical obstruction is either present or suspected.[9] People with long-term problems may be taught to carry out intermittent catheterizations (p. 676) rather than maintaining an in-dwelling catheter.

Catheter usage and types

Assisted urinary drainage is used in a variety of clinical situations in both acute and chronic care. Major reasons for catheter drainage include the following:

1. Relieve temporary anatomic or physiological urinary obstruction.
2. Permit healing of various parts of the urinary system postoperatively.
3. Permit accurate measurement of urinary out put in severely ill patients.
4. Relieve inability to void.
5. Achieve continence.
6. Prevent retention of urine in certain types of people with neurogenic bladder dysfunction.
7. Permit irrigation to prevent obstruction of urine flow.

Reestablishment of the flow of urine is an immediate treatment goal. The type of catheter used to provide drainage in the presence of obstruction depends on the location of the blockage.

Straight catheters are used for single catheterizations. The various catheters have different uses:

1. Robinson—intermittent catheterization (ease of insertion)
2. Coudé—prostatic hypertrophy (avoid trauma to gland)
3. Whistle-tip—presence of haematuria and blood clots (less chance of blockage)
4. Filiform (thin, stiff catheter)—urethral stricture

The *Foley catheter* is the most frequently used self-retaining catheter; it is used when continuous drainage is required. The Foley catheter has a double lumen with an inflatable balloon at the distal end. The balloon is inflated with either normal saline or sterile water after it has been placed well within the bladder (Fig. 25-4). In-dwelling urethral catheters must be securely anchored to prevent accidental dislodging of the catheter (Fig. 25-5). Proper

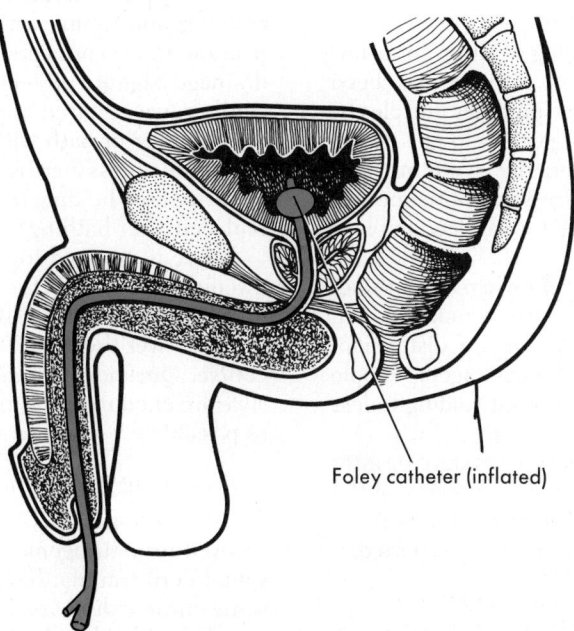

Foley catheter (inflated)

Fig. 25-4   Foley catheter in place with balloon inflated.

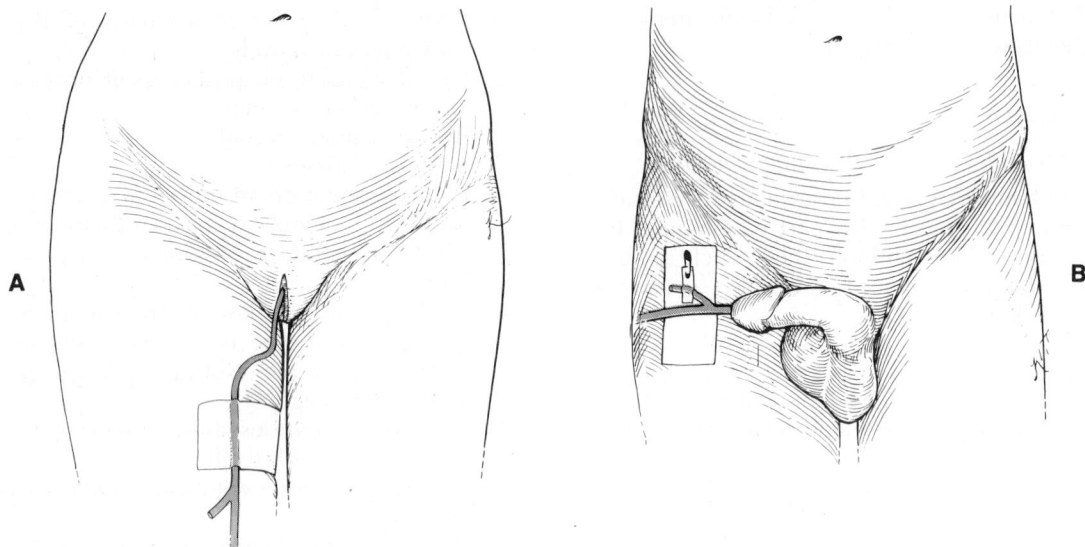

Fig. 25-5 Anchoring of Foley catheter. **A,** In female. **B,** In male. Proper anchoring prevents accidental traction that could result in injury to bladder or urethra but keeps catheter from moving in and out of urethra.

anchoring will prevent accidental traction (possible injury to the bladder or urethra) and yet keep the catheter from moving in and out of the urethra (possible irritation and infection). Guidelines for maintenance of an in-dwelling urinary drainage system are listed in Box 25-6.

Difficulties following catheter removal

It is normal to note some dribbling of urine for a few hours after an in-dwelling urethral catheter has been removed because of dilatation of the sphincter muscles by the catheter. Dribbling of urine that persists longer than a few hours is reported to the doctor; this symptom may indicate damage to the sphincters. Stress incontinence may persist for several months if the catheter has been in place for more than a few days.

Inability to initiate voiding may occur when the catheter is removed. The person is encouraged to drink fluids to stimulate the sphincters and is assessed for distension. Measures to promote voiding are encouraged. People should not go longer than 8 hours without voiding unless fluid intake has been restricted.

Cystitis (inflammation of the bladder) may develop after catheter removal because of imcomplete emptying of the bladder as muscle tone is reestablished. Any abnormalities in colour, odour, or sediment in the urine are reported.

Home care for people with in-dwelling catheters

It is not uncommon for people to be discharged to home requiring catheter drainage on a temporary or permanent basis. Ideally, frequent disconnection of the catheter and drainage tubing should be avoided. However, people at home must disconnect the tubing at night to change from a leg bag to the overnight drainage bag and reverse the procedure in the morning. To lessen the risk of contamination, the person should wash the hands and then wipe the catheter and tubing with povidone-iodine before disconnection and reconnection. The disconnected ends of the drainage bags are protected with a connector cap or with a sterile gauze secured in place with a rubber band.

A shower or bath with a catheter in place is generally permitted unless there is an unhealed surgical incision. The adhesive tape holding the catheter in place will need to be replaced after bathing.

There is no need for men or women to remove an in-dwelling catheter before intercourse, a question people may be hesitant to ask. The man can fold the in-dwelling catheter over the penis to facilitate insertion during intercourse. Questions pertaining to resumption of usual lifestyle are encouraged so the person can be as well prepared as possible for self-care at home.

Intermittent catheterization

Intermittent catheterization of the urinary bladder may be used for neurogenic bladder dysfunction secondary to spinal cord trauma, birth defects, urinary retention, and some chronic diseases. Because periodic complete emptying of the bladder eliminates residual urine (an excellent culture medium for multiplication of bacteria) and main-

Maintenance of drainage system

Action	Rationale
Never disconnect the catheter except to irrigate	Prevent introduction of bacteria
Collect urine samples by inserting a small-bore needle into the drainage port that has been cleansed with alcohol or povidone-iodine.	Maintain closed system and prevent introduction of bacteria
Never elevate drainage bag above level of the patient's bladder or cavity being drained; suspend bag from the bed frame when the patient is recumbent and from below the knee when the patient is ambulatory.	Prevent reflux of urine back into bladder; drainage bags are available with antireflux valves
Drainage bags and tubing should never be allowed to rest on the floor.	Prevent contamination of system
Observe tubing for kinks and loops.	Obstructions result in reflux of urine
Empty drainage bag into a measuring container that is used only for that particular patient; cleanse measuring container regularly.	Prevent cross-contamination of drainage system
Cultures of urine are usually ordered at regular intervals when a patient has an in-dwelling catheter.	Provides data on changing numbers and types of organism present in urine before symptoms appear
Observe collecting system daily for sedimentation and leaks.	Replace when sediment or leaks are present

tains a good blood supply to the bladder wall by avoiding high intrabladder pressures, infections are often decreased, even when only a clean technique is used.

The goals of intermittent catheterization may vary from patient to patient but are generally to prevent urinary retention and its sequelae (UTI and renal damage) and to achieve continence. The patient should know exactly what is expected of the treatment plan to elicit full cooperation.

The *hospitalized* patient with intermittent catheter drainage of the bladder may be one for whom the treatment is temporary (as in the early phases of spinal cord trauma), one who is learning the technique for home use, or one who has been using intermittent catheterization before hospital admission. Even though the clean technique is suitable for home use, sterile technique is necessary during hospitalization to decrease the possibility of hospital-acquired (nosocomial) infection when the catheterization is performed by hospital personnel. When hospitalized, the patient who customarily performs self-catheterization may continue to use clean technique if this method is used at home, but preferably a sterile catheter will be used each time or special precautions will be taken to store the reusable catheter in a closed container. Specimens for culture must be obtained by the usual sterile catheterization technique to avoid contamination of the specimen. The patient is informed about the reasons why sterile precautions are necessary in the hospital setting.

A No. 14 Lorsric, or Scott catheter is generally used for an adult. The volume of urine obtained with each catheterization is recorded to ensure that schedule adjustments can be made if necessary. The adult bladder should not be permitted to hold more than 300 ml at any time, because greater amounts lead to overdistension of the bladder with greater susceptibility to infection. The frequency of catheterization is determined by the amount of residual urine

(more than 200 ml means that more frequent catheterization is necessary). Usually such individuals will need catheterization every 4 to 6 hours. A small amount of residual urine (less than 200 ml) after voiding means that the person will only need to do self-catheterization every 8 to 12 hours. Some individuals may also have to catheterize themselves at night if they have a large output of urine during these hours. It is important to realize that the person who normally does not perform self-catheterization at night at home may need to do so during periods where the fluid intake is greater than usual, as with intravenous fluid administration.

In some instances the doctor will prescribe the frequency of catheterizations; in other instances, adjustment of the schedule may be a nursing judgment. If the nurse notes that excess volumes of urine are being obtained with a prescribed schedule, the doctor is consulted about the need to alter the schedule.

Colour, clarity, and odour of the urine are noted, and any symptoms of a UTI are reported. Periodic urine specimens are obtained and sent for culture and sensitivity. Some individuals are given long-term antibiotic therapy prophylactically.

In most cases, clean (not sterile) catheterization technique is prescribed for *home use*. Hand washing is advised before each catheterization, and the meatal area is cleansed with soap and water. After inserting the catheter and draining the bladder, the catheter is removed and washed with soap and water before being stored in a clean, closed container for the next use. The catheter is reused until it becomes either too soft or too hard to be directed properly.

Most individuals require much support during the actual teaching but very quickly become comfortable with the procedure. Initially, a mirror is used to teach women where to place the catheter. The woman should

Table 25-2   Types of incontinence

Type	Definition	Related factors
Stress	Involuntary loss of < 50 ml urine with increased abdominal pressure	Relaxed pelvic muscles associated with age, obesity, incompetent bladder outlet
Reflex	Involuntary loss of urine when a specific volume is reached, occurring at somewhat predictable intervals	Neurological impairment such as spinal cord lesion
Urge	Involuntary loss of urine occurring soon after a strong sense of urgency to void	Decreased bladder capacity, bladder infection, increased fluid intake, increased urine concentration, overdistension of bladder
Functional	Involuntary unpredictable loss of urine	Sensory, cognitive, or mobility deficits
Total	Continuous and unpredictable loss of urine	Neurological dysfunction; independent contractions of detrusor muscle as a result of surgery, trauma, or disease affecting spinal cord nerves; fistulas

learn to catheterize while sitting on the commode, using palpation to locate the urethral meatus. Men may sit or stand to catheterize themselves. It is important that men use generous amounts of lubricant to avoid urethral irritation; women generally do not require lubrication of the catheter.

If sterile catheterization technique is needed for home use, more time and practice will be required to learn good sterile technique. Careful explanation of sterilization of equipment must be provided, and planning for adapting sterile intermittent self-catheterization to the individual's usual life-style must be worked out with the person.

If teaching of self-catheterization is performed on an outpatient basis or if hospitalization is short, follow-up for adjustment of schedule and other concerns of adaptation to home routine should be provided. This may be done by the primary nurse, by the doctor, or by referral to a community nurse. Ongoing urological care with periodic urine cultures is essential.

Interventions to achieve patient outcomes

Relieving urinary retention

Provide the patient with privacy. If a bedpan is used, place the patient in a sitting position to enlist the aid of gravity and increase intraabdominal pressure; this may help stimulate the bladder sphincter. Warm the bedpan for comfort before offering it. Run water from the tap and flush the toilet; the sound of running water offers the power of suggestion and may facilitate voiding. If the patient is tense and can sit in warm water, the warmth may help relax the internal sphincter and perineal muscles. If these measures in addition to administrating cholinergic medications fail, catheterization may be indicated.

Facilitating patient learning

Specific patient teaching depends on the underlying cause of urinary retention and the need for an in-dwelling catheter or intermittent catheterization. Teaching may include the following:

1. Rationale for type of care required.
2. Use of Credé method of emptying bladder (if appropriate): place hands flat against abdomen below umbilicus; make firm downward strokes toward bladder six times, then apply direct pressure over bladder to force out urine.
3. Maintenance of adequate fluid intake to prevent UTI.
4. In-dwelling urethral catheter: maintenance of catheter patency, caring for equipment, dealing with catheter problems, procurement of supplies, need for ongoing care.
5. Intermittent catheterization: techniques, frequency, adaptation of catheterization routine to life-style, procurement of supplies, need for ongoing care.
6. Signs of retention or UTI to be reported to doctor.

Evaluation

Evaluation is based on expected patient outcomes. Questions to consider may include the following:

1. Has the person urinated at least 200 to 400 ml with each voiding? Is the bladder no longer palpable?
2. Does the patient know home care use of catheter, measures to prevent UTI, where to purchase supplies, and signs to report to doctor?

URINARY INCONTINENCE

Urinary incontinence, the involuntary expulsion of urine, may be encountered in a number of temporary and permanent conditions. Inability to control urination is a problem that frequently leads to emotional distress and can seriously impair an individual's socialization patterns if not managed either by the person or by others in a way that makes the person feel physically and emotionally comfortable and socially acceptable. Urinary incontinence occurs most frequently in people over the age of 65. Several types of incontinence have been identified (Table 25-2).

Aetiology

The five major causes of urinary incontinence and the nature of the incontinence they cause are outlined in Table 25-3.

Cerebral confusion is most common in the aged. In many instances the elderly person is incontinent because of a lack of awareness of the need to empty the bladder. This type of incontinence is often not associated with any definite pathological problem at the cerebral level. Cerebral clouding also occurs in acutely ill people, who may be so ill that cerebration is dulled. They may not be able to think or may not have the energy to exercise voluntary control. Likewise a person who is comatose is incontinent because of loss of the ability to control voluntarily the opening of the external sphincter. As soon as urine is released into the posterior urethra, the bladder contracts and empties. This is the reason why voiding sometimes occurs under anaesthesia.

Infection anywhere in the urinary tract may lead to incontinence because bacteria in the urine cause irritation of the mucosa of the bladder and stimulate the urethrobladder reflex abnormally.

Disturbance of the central nervous system pathways may occur in diseases such as cerebral embolus, cerebral haemorrhage, brain tumour, meningitis, or traumatic injury of the brain. Adequate voluntary (cortical or cerebral) control of bladder function is prevented in these situations. Urgency incontinence may be present as a result of the inability to inhibit completion of the urethrobladder reflex by the higher centres.

Disturbance of the urethrobladder reflex may result from lesions of the spinal cord or damage to peripheral nerves of the bladder. This form of incontinence may be seen in people with spinal cord malformations, injuries, or tumours, and those with compression of the cord caused by fractures of the vertebae, herniated disk, metastatic tumour, or postoperative oedema of the spinal cord. The person has a *neurogenic* bladder (see the following discussion) and may have either reflex or overflow incontinence. The person has no way of knowing when voiding is occurring.

Tissue damage to the sphincters of the bladder from instrumentation, surgery, or accidents, scarring following urethral infections, lesions involving the sphincter, or relaxation of the perineal structures may cause urinary incontinence. The latter cause of incontinence is seen occasionally following childbirth. The problem is local in nature and does not involve the nervous system.

Pathophysiology

People with urinary incontinence often present baffling management problems. Solutions require understanding of the physiological basis of incontinence.

Bladder and sphincter control are necessary to have urinary continence. Such control requires normal voluntary and involuntary muscle action coordinated by a normal urethrobladder reflex. As bladder filling occurs, the pressure within the bladder gradually increases. The detrusor muscle (the three-layered bladder wall) responds by relaxing to accommodate the greater volume. When a certain point of filling is reached, usually 150 to 200 ml of urine,

Table 25-3   Major causes of urinary incontinence

Cause of urinary incontinence	Awareness of need to void	Cortical ability to inhibit voiding	Reflex arc	Bladder response to filling	Result
	Factors involved				
Cerebral confusion	Impaired	Impaired	Intact	Normal	Uncontrolled voiding because of reflex response
Infection	Intact	Intact, but overcome by strong reflex response	Abnormally stimulated	Heightened	Voiding because of strong reflex response (urgency)
Disturbance of CNS pathways (cortical lesions)	Diminished	Impaired	Intact	Heightened	Voiding because of reflex response
Disturbance of urethrobladder reflex					
Upper motor neuron lesion	Destroyed	Destroyed	Intact but deranged	Heightened	Voiding because of reflex response
Lower motor neuron lesion	Destroyed	Destroyed	Destroyed or impaired	Diminished to absent	Distension or incomplete emptying
Tissue damage	Intact	Intact, but not functional because of poor muscle response	Intact	Normal	Loss of control of voiding because of muscular impairment

the parasympathetic stretch receptors located in the bladder wall are stimulated. The stimuli are transmitted through afferent fibres of the reflex arc to the reflex centre for micturition. Impulses are then carried through the efferent fibres of the reflex arc to the bladder, causing reflex contraction of the detrusor muscle. The internal sphincter, which is normally closed, reciprocally opens, and the urine enters the posterior urethra. Relaxation of the external sphincter and perineal muscles follows, and the bladder content is released. Completion of this reflex act can be interrupted and voiding postponed through release of inhibitory impulses from the cortical centre, which results in voluntary contraction of the external sphincter. If any part of this complex function is upset, there is apt to be urinary incontinence.

Neurogenic bladder

A neurogenic bladder may be one of two types, upper motor neurone, or lower motor neurone. The *upper motor neurone* or *automatic* bladder occurs with lesions above the S2 spinal cord level or impairment of the cerebrocortical centre. These lesions do not destroy the reflex arc for voiding (although they may derange it); they destroy the potential for cortical control to inhibit the reflex. The bladder is *hypertonic* and has a small capacity (less than 150 ml). The increased detrusor tone and increased sensitivity to small amounts of urine present in the bladder result in precipitous *reflex* voiding and the potential for vesicoureteral reflux.

Damage to nerves in the cauda equina or sacral segments of the spinal cord may cause destruction of the reflex arc by interruption of its afferent, efferent, or central components. The result is a *"lower motor neuron"* or *"flaccid"* bladder. The bladder is *hypotonic* with capacities of 500 ml or more. Overflow incontinence, retention of residual urine, and the potential for vesicoureteral reflux are problems imposed by a hypotonic bladder.

Overflow incontinence is considered to be caused by pressure exerted on the distended bladder by the abdominal muscles. Residual urine, urine remaining in the bladder after incomplete emptying, provides a medium for the growth of bacteria, and a UTI is common.

Stress incontinence

Urinary incontinence that occurs during coughing, straining, or heavy lifting is termed *stress incontinence*. It is seen primarily in women who have relaxed pelvic musculature, but it may also occur in men following prostatectomy. When bladder pressure is suddenly increased, urine enters the proximal third of the urethra then returns to the bladder when the pressure is decreased after exertion. Some of the urine escapes through the urethra. Usually the person is continent at night because bladder pressure is decreased in the recumbent position.

Nursing Process
Assessment

Subjective data

The following questions are asked when assessing incontinence:
1. Is there a total inability to control urination?
2. What is the frequency of incontinence?
3. Can anything be associated with precipitating incontinence (stress, fear, laughing, exercise)?
4. Is pain or burning present with incontinence?
5. Is there a state of awareness to void before incontinence?
6. Does dribbling occur?

Objective data

Important objective data to obtain include the following:
1. Volume of urine output
2. Characteristics of urine
3. Palpation of bladder to identify residual urine
4. Patient's level of consciousness to determine ability to cooperate
5. Patient's ability to follow directions
6. Is there a physiological reason for incontinence (for example, spinal cord injury)

Diagnostic tests

Normally the bladder contains little or no urine after voiding; however, certain disease states inhibit the bladder from emptying completely. Some common conditions in which incomplete emptying of the bladder occurs are benign prostatic hypertrophy, urethral strictures, and interruptions in bladder innervation. Urine left in the bladder after voiding is called *residual urine*.

One way to determine the amount of residual urine is to *catheterize* the person immediately after voiding. This may be ordered by the doctor on a one-time or on a repeated basis. Before catheterizing the person, the doctor is consulted regarding the plan for establishing urinary drainage. If a large amount of residual urine is suspected, the doctor may wish the catheter to be left in place in the bladder. *Residual urine volumes of 50 ml or less indicate near normal or returning bladder function.*

To avoid passing a catheter to measure residual urine volumes, X-ray examination of retained urine may be performed. In this procedure a radiopaque substance excreted by the kidneys is injected intravenously. As the dye is excreted in the urine, it passes into the bladder. A sufficient amount of urine containing the radiopaque material is allowed to accumulate in the bladder before the person is instructed to void. Immediately after voiding an X-ray film is taken. Any urine retained in the bladder will be visualized on the X-ray. This means of determining residual urine is used in conjunction with other studies requiring visualization of the urinary tract.

Cystometric examination is performed to evaluate bladder tone. In general, the examination is indicated when incontinence is present or when there is evidence of neurological dysfunction of the bladder. An in-dwelling catheter is inserted before the examination. After the person assumes a supine position, a litre bottle of normal saline or sterile distilled water and a cystometer are connected to the catheter. Fluid is instilled at a constant and specified rate; measurements of the pressure exerted on the fluid by the bladder musculature are recorded after the instillation of every 50 ml of fluid. The person is asked to report feelings of fullness, the need to void, and any urgency or discomfort. Fluid is instilled until urgency occurs or it is determined that the sensation is absent. During cystometric examination, bethanechol chloride may be administered to determine its effect on enhancing the tone of a flaccid bladder, or an anticholinergic medication may be given to assess relaxation in a hyperactive bladder. There is no specific care required after cystometric examination.

Electromyography may be used to evaluate sphincter tone and intactness of nerve pathways.

Nursing analysis

Nursing analyses are determined from assessment of patient data. Possible nursing problems for the person with urinary incontinence may include, but are not limited to, the following:

Problem	Possible aetiologies
Incontinence (specify type)	Altered environment, sensory deficit, neurological impairment, relaxed pelvic muscles, overdistension, decreased bladder capacity
Skin integrity, impaired, high risk for	Urine irritation
Body image disturbance	Loss of body functions, change in life-style, change in social involvement
Knowledge deficit	Lack of information

Planning: expected patient outcomes

Expected patient outcomes for the person with urinary incontinence may include, but are not limited to, the following:
1. Achieves optimal urinary control
2. Skin remains intact
3. Verbalizes feelings and frustrations without self-deprecating statements
4. Describes actions to control incontinence (as appropriate), measures to maintain skin integrity, and plans for follow-up care

Implementation

Assisting with achievement of therapeutic goals

Control of urinary incontinence is largely dependent on its cause. Measures include surgery, treatment of associated conditions, programmes of bladder retraining (p. 683), or the use of drainage devices.

Surgery for stress incontinence

Surgery may be indicated for severe stress incontinence. A *vesicourethropexy* (Marshall-Marchetti-Krantz operation) consists of fixation of the urethra to the fascia of the rectus muscle of the abdomen with support given to the neck of the bladder. A suprapubic incision is usually made, but a transvaginal repair may be carried out if there is scar tissue around the urethra from vaginal surgery. A urethral catheter is inserted postoperatively and maintained for 5 to 6 days. The urine may be pink, but the urethral catheter is not irrigated as a rule. It is not uncommon for difficulty in voiding to be experienced immediately after the in-dwelling catheter is removed. The woman is observed for signs of vaginal bleeding. Straining and use of Valsalva's manoeuvre should be avoided until healing has occurred, and mild laxatives may be given to prevent straining from constipation. Surgeons differ in the amount of activity permitted in the early postoperative period.

A surgical procedure that is less invasive is the *Stamey* procedure, a suspension of the bladder neck by sutures passed adjacent to the ureterovesical junctions.[13] A small incision is made above and lateral to the symphysis pubis. The needles are introduced suprapubically and the positions are checked by cystoscopy (a bulge can be noted at the junction wall) before suturing. The procedure is then repeated on the opposite side. A percutaneous suprapubic catheter is inserted following the suturing; the catheter is removed when spontaneous voiding occurs, which may take several days. There is minimal postoperative discomfort. Antibiotics are given for 2 weeks postoperatively. The patient should refrain from sexual activity until permitted (usually 1 to 2 months).

Sphincter dysfunction

Repair of a sphincter that has been cut is almost impossible. When the *external sphincter* has been damaged, the person will be incontinent on urgency. A voiding schedule can be planned so that voiding occurs before the bladder is full enough to exert sufficient pressure to open the internal sphincter involuntarily. When the *internal sphincter* is damaged, there may be no acute feeling of the need to void. Here the problem is not one of incontinence but of retention. To ensure regular emptying of the bladder, a regular voiding schedule is necessary. If both sphincters are damaged, there will be total incontinence.

Urge incontinence

Incontinence caused by urinary tract infection (UTI) is generally temporary, responding to treatment of the infection by systemic antibiotics. Specific causes of infection such as obstruction must be identified and corrected when possible. Provision must be made for adequate fluid intake of 3000 ml or more per day unless contraindicated by the person's medical condition. Because of heightened bladder sensitivity to even small amounts of urine, urgency to void demands rapid response by the nurse to the request for help to void.

The person who has a brain tumour, meningitis, or traumatic injury to the brain that prevents adequate voluntary control of bladder function and causes urgency incontinence by inhibiting cortical control over the urethrobladder reflex may also respond to a bladder retraining programme (p. 683). If the person's condition or response prohibits such a programme, a drainage device should be used.

Neurogenic bladder dysfunction

People with injuries of the spinal cord experience a transitory period of "spinal shock" in which urinary retention occurs. This is treated with continuous or intermittent catheter drainage that aims to prevent a UTI and overdistension of the bladder. Following this acute stage, further management depends on the exact nature of any residual neurogenic bladder dysfunction. People with a lesion *above the sacral segments* and who have an intact urethrobladder reflex may initiate voiding by pinching or stroking trigger areas of the thighs or suprapubic area. In people with a *lower motor neurone* lesion, the use of the *Credé method*, which consists of exerting manual pressure over the bladder, (p. 678), may be ordered to provide for more complete bladder emptying. The appropriateness of this technique must be determined by the doctor as based on the person's complete urological status. An increasing number of people with neurogenic bladder dysfunction are being taught intermittent self-catheterization using clean technique to prevent infection and manage incontinence. Maintenance of a regular schedule is stressed, and the frequency of catheterization is determined on an individual basis.

Certain medications are sometimes used alone or in conjunction with an intermittent catheterization programme in the management of incontinence related to neurogenic bladder dysfunction. Alpha adrenergic drugs such as ephedrine sulphate are used to increase urethral resistance. Anticholinergic drugs such as propantheline are prescribed to control the reflex bladder activity.

Urinary drainage for incontinence

Occasionally there are justifications for the use of an indwelling catheter for the incontinent patient. Such reasons include the need to protect a surgical incision or to permit healing of a decubitus ulcer in the area. In-dwelling catheterization, however, presents many potential dangers, such as UTI, urethritis, epididymitis, and urethral fistulas. All other means to manage incontinence should be tried before resorting to catheterization. Proper catheter management is essential.

In males, *external drainage* can be easily accomplished by applying a watertight apparatus to the penis. The following is one method. Select a condom of the correct size. Puncture a hole in the closed end of the condom with an applicator stick. Attach the punctured end of the condom to a firm rubber or plastic drainage tube with either a 33 mm ($1/8$-inch) piece of rubber tubing or a strip of adhesive tape. Before applying the condom, clean and dry the penis thoroughly and check it for oedema, skin breaks, or discolouration. Invert the condom and roll it onto the penis. There should be no roll at the top that could cause constriction. At least 2.5 cm (1 inch) of the condom should remain between the meatus and drainage tube to allow for penile erection. There should not be so much slack as to cause twisting and subsequent interference with drainage. Elastoplast is then applied over the condom and around the penis (never touching the skin). *Under no circumstances should adhesive tape be used.* The Elastoplast must not be constricting.

The external catheter should be removed daily, and the skin washed and checked. Frequent checking is necessary to determine whether oedema or irritation is present and to ensure proper drainage. This is especially important in men with loss of sensation. The external device is attached to straight drainage or to a leg bag.

For people who need external catheter drainage indefinitely, a rubber urinary appliance (sometimes called an *incontinence urinal*) may be used. There are several models available, and the one best suited to the person's needs is selected. Two appliances are recommended to allow for cleaning and drying. They should be washed with mild soap, turned inside out, and thoroughly dried before using.

Most people prefer to manage their own incontinence if they are at all able to do so. The nurse supports and encourages this, offering assistance as necessary and instruction in basic principles of skin care, equipment selection, and maintenance. The choice of management method should take into account the person's ability to manage as independently as is possible.

Implantation of an *artificial urinary sphincter* can be used to achieve continence when other methods have failed. In this procedure a hydraulically activated sphincter mechanism is placed around the urethra or bladder neck. The sphincter is made to open and close at will by squeezing one of two bulbs implanted under the skin of the labia or scrotum. Postoperative nursing care of the person with such an implant includes observation for and reporting of fever or pain on inflation of the device, swelling of the genitalia, and recurrence of incontinence. Complications of the procedure include erosion of the urethra, abscess, cellulitis, and mechanical malfunctions in the system. Men have had more success with the artificial sphincter than have women.

Interventions to achieve patient outcomes
Assisting with urinary control

Because the person who experiences incontinence may at times have bladder control, respond immediately when assistance to toilet is requested. Offer assistance to toilet shortly after each meal, a time when urination is most frequent because of ingested fluids. Lack of prompt assistance may lead to episodes of incontinence that further frustrate the person and may lead to the belief that nothing can be done. No programme of bladder retraining or management can be successful without the person's cooperation. Encourage self-care of incontinence whenever possible. Be supportive of the patient by providing a relaxed atmosphere when providing care for incontinence.

When incontinence is caused by dulled cerebration in the elderly, by confusion, or by acute illness, control can usually be established if a persistent *bladder retraining* schedule is carried out (see Box 25-7). A voiding schedule is developed and must be strictly adhered to until the person gradually relearns to recognize and react appropriately to the feeling of having to void. A successful programme of this type, leading to complete rehabilitation, or continence, requires mental competence of the individual. Otherwise someone else must always remind the person to follow the schedule. However, with proper support, bladder retraining is possible even when the incontinent person is not fully mentally competent.

People ordinarily void on awakening, before retiring, and before or after meals. If a diuretic such as coffee has been taken, it is usually necessary to void about 30 minutes later. Using this knowledge, the nurse can begin to set up a schedule for placing the person on a bedpan or taking the person to the toilet. Then if a record is kept for a few days of the times the person voids involuntarily, it is usually possible to determine the normal voiding pattern. If the schedule based on the pattern of incontinence is not successful, toileting every 1 to 2 hours should be carried out on a 24-hour basis.

During the retraining programme, *mobilization* of the individual, attention to the *position* assumed for voiding,

Bladder retraining

Establish patient's usual voiding patterns.

Plan toileting based on the patient's usual pattern; assist patient as necessary.

If no voiding pattern can be determined, plan toileting for every 1 to 2 hours.

Encourage patient to use normal toileting position.

Encourage patient to empty bladder completely.

Provide for a fluid intake of 3000 ml/day for adequate urine volume.

Schedule most fluids to be taken before 16.00.

The Elderly with Urinary Problems

Assessment

Determine urinary habits, especially if patient has any difficulty with urinary control.

Assess for mobility problems, diuretics, or mental changes that may contribute to functional (environmental) incontinence.

Assess for signs of urinary tract infections, commonly experienced by elderly women and men. Usual signs of fever and pain or burning with urination may be minimal or absent; confusion and anorexia may be the only symptoms.

Monitor kidney function when elderly undergo extensive testing that may lead to dehydration, which can compromise marginal kidney function in some elderly people.

Intervention

Refer people with incontinence to a doctor for further work-up; this condition is *not* a normal concomitant of ageing.

Give diuretics early in day so patient will not need to use toilet frequently after bedtime.

Arrange environment to facilitate toileting, such as moving furniture, using bedside commode, ensuring grab bars by the toilet (or raised seat), and keeping call light within reach.

Schedule fluid intake to match toileting time, about every 2 hours while awake.

Maintain patient's usual routines as much as possible.

Limit stimulants such as coffee and tea.

Plan for increased need for toileting if patient is receiving intravenous therapy.

Try to avoid use of urinary catheters; if catheter is necessary, use good aseptic technique to prevent urinary tract infection.

Teach patient to report to health care provider any change in the urine or presence of blood; be aware that the patient may not be able to monitor own urine if vision is diminished.

Common disorders in Elderly

Urinary incontinence
Urinary tract infections
Benign prostatic hyperplasia
Cancer of kidney, bladder, or prostate
Renal failure

and adequate *fluid intake* contribute to reduction of the possibility of infection. Complete emptying of the bladder eliminates the possibility of residual urine acting as a medium for bacterial growth; a high fluid intake provides for internal bladder irrigation.

Elderly people isolated from their families and familiar surroundings, confused by institutionalization, or suffering feelings of loss of self-esteem frequently respond well to mobilization in bladder retraining programmes. Their circulation is enhanced by the imposed mobility, their awareness is increased, and they respond to the attention given them. In instances in which nurses believe that it is easier to change bed linen than it is to establish an appropriate bladder retraining programme, a disservice is done to the individual and more work is actually created for the nurse. The person becomes subject to UTI and skin breakdown, and feelings of worthlessness are increased. For those who can be continent, incontinence is an indignity.

When possible, toileting should be carried out in surroundings that remind the person of the voiding function. Take the person to the bathroom to use the toilet; if this is not possible, a bedside commode can be an adequate substitute. A bedpan is unfamiliar and most people find using one distasteful. Many men can void into a urinal more easily if allowed to stand at the bedside. For women who must remain in bed, voiding into a bedpan can be facilitated if the head of the bed is elevated, a position more consistent with normal voiding and one that facilitates complete bladder emptying. Few people can void adequately in the supine position.

Providing adequate amounts of fluids, a minimum of 3000 ml per day, is necessary to ensure that there will be adequate amounts of urine produced and present in the bladder to stimulate the voiding reflex at the proper times. Fluids may be given at scheduled times, the largest portion being given during the day before 4 PM to decrease the frequency of voiding through the night. People on fluid restriction because of medical problems should, of course, receive no more fluids than the amount prescribed.

Maintaining skin integrity

Meticulous skin care is absolutely essential when caring for the person with urinary incontinence. Without proper cleansing, the person will be subject to skin breakdown, which, as a result of continued incontinence, is extremely difficult to heal. When a person who is incontinent also has a diminished level of consciousness, he or she should be assessed frequently to ensure dryness. A person who has been incontinent must be cleaned and dried immediately.

Low airflow beds help to control skin breakdown in immobile patients. This therapy offers some hope in the care of the bedridden incontinent person. The protective cover of the bed provides a one-way barrier that draws water away from the patient and assists in keeping the patient dry. The airflow also aids in drying the skin.

Facilitating positive body image

Encourage patient to discuss feelings and frustrations concerning incontinence and involve family members in activities when possible. Offer reassurance, encouragement, and concrete information regarding management, especially about those activities that are within the patient's control. Be realistic with the patient. If incontinence cannot be controlled, reassure patient that odour and discomfort can be controlled, such as by maintenance of good hygiene, use and frequent changes of incontinence pads, and frequent changes of undergarments as necessary.

Scheduling fluids to decrease probability of incontinence at selected times, such as social activities or when a toilet is not readily available, also helps to maintain a positive body image. Fluids can be limited before the desired times and increased at other periods of the day so that the desired 3000 ml of fluids are ingested in the 24-hour period.

Teaching patient and family

Because the patient, often with family assistance, is usually involved in control of urinary continence, teaching is an important aspect of patient care. Explanation of the rationale for activities such as toileting schedule, mobility, and fluid requirements will increase the probability of the person following through with the activities.

The patient can be taught *perineal exercises* to help control mild stress incontinence. The exercises consist of tightening and relaxing perineal and gluteal muscles and can be performed in a number of ways. Much of the problem of incontinence caused by a relaxed perineum in women can be prevented if perineal exercises are taught before and following childbirth. These exercises also may be included as part of the health teaching of any woman. Following are different methods for performing perineal exercises.

1. Tighten the perineal muscles as if to prevent voiding. Hold for a count of 10, then relax (Kegel exercises, see Chapter 27).
2. Inhale through pursed lips while tightening perineal muscles.
3. Bear down as if to have a bowel movement. Relax then tighten perineal muscles.
4. Hold a pencil in the fold between the buttock and thigh.
5. Sit on toilet with knees held wide apart. Start and stop the urinary stream.

Additional teaching includes care of any drainage systems, measures to maintain skin integrity, and signs and symptoms of urinary tract infection (frequency, dysuria) that should be reported to the doctor.

Evaluation

Evaluation is based on expected patient outcomes. Questions to consider may include the following:

1. Is the patient achieving optimal urinary control?
2. Is the patient's skin free of any excoriation?
3. Is the patient making comments that suggest a more positive body image?
4. Can the patient describe maintenance of any necessary equipment, bladder retraining or how to do perineal exercises (if appropriate), measures to maintain skin integrity, and plans for follow-up care?

URINARY TRACT INFECTION

Aetiology/Epidemiology

Urinary tract infection (UTI) is a significant source of morbidity in Britain and plays a significant role in the development of chronic renal failure. Infection occurs in both acute and chronic stages in all portions of the urinary tract. Females appear more predisposed to UTI than males. Factors postulated in their higher infection rates include a shorter urethra that is closer to the rectum and the lack of the prostatic fluid protection that is present in the male. Two per cent of the British female population between ages 15 and 24 years suffer UTIs. The incidence increases 1-2% every decade and by 55-64 years, 10% of the female population suffers urinary tract infections.[20a] Incidence of infection in females increases directly with sexual activity and with ageing. Pregnancy does not seem to increase infection rates, although spontaneous clearing of infections is decreased during pregnancy, and there is a higher incidence of acute kidney infections progressing upward from the lower urinary tract.

Factors contributing to UTI are summarized in Table 25-4. Structural and functional abnormalities of the urinary tract, obstruction of the flow of urine, and impaired bladder innervation promote UTI. Mechanisms involved include stasis of urine, which provides a culture medium for bacteria, reflux of infected urine higher into the urinary tract, and increasing hydrostatic pressure.

Urinary tract infections may occur in the upper portion of the urinary tract (pyelonephritis) or in the lower urinary tract (cystitis, urethritis). Most infections in the lower urinary tract result from gram-negative organisms, such as *Escherichia coli, Klebsiella, Proteus, Enterobacter, Pseudomonas,* or *Serratia,* that originate in the person's own intestinal tract and ascend through the urethra to the bladder. *Staphylococcus saprophyticus* is a gram-positive

Table 25-4 Risk factors associated with development of UTI

Risk factor	Common examples
Female	Short urethra
Structural abnormality	Strictures
	Incompetent ureterovesical junction anomalies
Obstruction	Tumours
	Prostatic hypertrophy
	Calculi
	Iatrogenic causes
Impaired bladder innervation	Congenital spinal cord malformation
	Spinal cord injury
	Multiple sclerosis
Chronic disease	Gout
	Diabetes mellitus
	Hypertension
	Sickle cell disease
	Chronic renal disease
Instrumentation	Catheterization
	Diagnostic procedures

organism that appears to affect young women, particularly in summer and autumn. The yeast *Candida albicans* tends to affect people who are debilitated by other disease or who are taking immunosuppressive medications. *Candida* found in the urine is significant because this organism is associated with sepsis and death.

Escherichia coli is the most common organism identified with pyelonephritis. Acute pyelonephritis is usually caused by bacterial infection but may also develop as a result of seeding of bacteria from the bloodstream. Chronic pyelonephritis also results from a bacterial infection; however, other factors such as urinary reflux and urinary tract obstruction also play a part.

Prevention
Primary prevention

Three considerations are important in preventing infection of the urinary tract: (1) preventing or minimizing morbidity that can accompany these infections, (2) preventing recurrence of the infection, and (3) preventing renal damage from untreated or inadequately treated ascending infection. Certain chronic health problems predispose people to UTI by changing the metabolism of tissues, creating extrarenal obstructions, and altering the function and structure of kidney tissue. Common among these health problems are diabetes mellitus, gout, hypertension, polycystic kidney disease, and glomerulonephritis. Control of these disorders decreases the potential for UTI.

Instrumentation of the urinary tract is associated with high rates of infection. Catheterization, even when performed without breaks in asepsis, results in significant infection of the bladder. *Nosocomial infections* account for a sizeable percentage of all UTIs. Drug-resistant strains of *Staphylococcus* and *Pseudomonas,* along with various other organisms commonly found in hospitals, are frequently involved in nosocomial UTIs. Prevention and control of all urinary infections can be influenced most significantly by lowering this nosocomial infection rate.

Primary prevention of UTI also includes teaching females the importance of wiping the perineal area from front to back to minimize the risk of introducing faecal flora into the urinary tract. Uncircumcised males should clean the glans of the penis daily to reduce the risk of accumulation of bacteria under the foreskin.

Secondary prevention

Although the great majority of noncomplicated urinary infections are asymptomatic and clear spontaneously, there remains a portion significant enough to warrant consideration as a health problem. There is no controversy among those practising preventive health care regarding the question of the need for screening of asymptomatic infections; however, there exists difficulty in identifying the specific risk groups in which the detection and treatment of these infections yield significant improvement in the person's health. As health care becomes more oriented towards prevention, specific target populations will be better defined and the number of screening programmes for asymptomatic UTI will increase.

Anyone with symptoms of dysuria, cloudy urine, or frequent small voidings should be examined for UTI and treated appropriately to prevent extension of a lower UTI into the kidney. People complaining of fever and costovertebral tenderness should be encouraged to seek medical attention for early treatment of pyelonephritis, thus preventing further kidney damage.

Pathophysiology
Pyelonephritis

Infection usually begins in the lower urinary tract and ascends into the kidneys. After the bacteria reach the kidney, they begin to multiply in the medullary interstitial tissue and renal tubules. As infection develops, an inflammatory exudate accumulates in the interstitium. The renal tubules become necrotic and the renal cortex may also become inflamed. The glomerular capillaries, however, are usually spared from the inflammatory process. Pockets of infection (renal abscess) develop and are distributed throughout the renal medulla or the entire kidney. After the acute inflammation subsides, healing begins through the formation of scar tissue.[43]

The clinical manifestations of acute pyelonephritis are those of inflammation and range from no symptoms to a sudden onset of fever, chills, costovertebral (flank) pain, and suprapubic tenderness (Table 25-5). Because acute pyelonephritis may cause symptoms similar to cystitis, it is extremely difficult to identify renal involvement solely on the basis of symptoms. Differentiation between upper and lower UTIs is essential for therapeutic management.[43]

Chronic pyelonephritis destroys renal tissue permanently through repeated inflammation and scarring. The process of developing chronic renal failure from repeated kidney infections occurs over a number of years or after several extensive and fulminant infections. Pyelonephritis represents a common original diagnosis of all people with chronic renal failure.

Lower urinary tract infection

Whenever stasis of urine occurs, such as with incomplete emptying of the bladder, renal calculi, or genitourinary obstructions, the bacteria have a greater opportunity to grow and a more alkaline media, which favours their growth and multiplication.

UTI occurs primarily when host resistance is impaired. The major factors in preventing a UTI are tissue integrity and blood supply. A break in the surface of the mucous membrane lining permits the bacteria to invade the tissue and cause infection. Breaks in tissue integrity result from erosions caused by tips of in-dwelling catheters or rough-edged renal stones, from neoplasms, or from invasion of the tissue by parasites such as *Schistosoma*. In the bladder, blood supply to the tissues can be compromised when the pressure within the bladder is markedly increased, as may occur with overdistension of the bladder, contracture of the bladder neck, or obstruction of the urethra by an enlarged prostate, metastatic growth, or urethral stricture.

The symptoms that bring the patient to medical attention typically include urinary urgency, burning on urination (dysuria), and slight to gross haematuria. Most people, however, are asymptomatic or minimally symptomatic, the infection being identified only on routine examination of the urine. Bacteriuria and positive urine cultures serve as

<u>REVIEW</u>

Table 25-5   Urinary tract infections

Disorder	Signs and symptoms	Medical therapy
Pyelonephritis	Sudden fever, chills Costovertebral tenderness Leukocytosis WBCs in urine	Antibiotics Bed rest for acute episode Hydration
Cystitis/urethritis (lower UTI)	Urgency Frequency Dysuria Suprapubic discomfort Cloudy urine with WBCs	Antibiotics Hydration
Prostatitis	Fever Chills Low back pain Perineal pain Urgency Frequency Dysuria Tender prostate Urethral discharge	Antibiotics Bed rest for acute episodes Sexual abstention Analgesics Stool softeners Sitz baths

the basis for diagnosing a lower UTI. Growth of a single pathogen in excess of 1×10^5 organisms/ml of urine in a properly obtained and stored midstream specimen indicates infection.

Nursing Process
Assessment
Subjective data

Specific questions are directed at eliciting presence of abnormal findings. *Dysuria* is often described as "burning with urination" and is usually associated with *frequency* and *urgency* (see Box 25-8) when a UTI is present. Ask the patient about the approximate amount of urine at each voiding: small amounts may be caused by infection whereas large amounts may be the result of increased fluid intake or a diuretic. Frequency associated with suprapubic discom-

fort and sense of fullness is more likely to be caused by retention with overflow (p. 674). *Nocturia* may accompany frequency; if present, ask the number of times this occurs per night, amount of fluid taken over 24 hours (especially during the evening), and if this is a change from the usual pattern.

Pain resulting from urinary disorders is located in different areas depending on the organ involved. Pain from the kidney is usually experienced in the flank over the kidney site in the back between the twelfth rib and the iliac crest (costovertebral angle). Pain from the ureters may begin over the kidney area but then radiates to the front along the course of the ureter and down into the groin. Pain from the bladder is usually suprapubic.

Additional data seen with pyelonephritis include history of chills and fever, nausea or vomiting, and fatigue and anorexia.

Table 25-6   Urinalysis

Test	Normal	Abnormal
Colour	Amber-yellow	Red indicates haematuria (possible urinary obstruction, renal calculi, tumour, renal failure)
Clarity	Clear	Cloudy: debris, bacterial sediment (urinary infection)
pH	4.6–8 (average 6)	Alkaline on standing or with UTI Increased acidity with renal tubular acidosis
Specific gravity	1.010–1.025	Usually reflects fluid intake; the less the fluid intake, the higher the specific gravity If specific gravity remains low (1.010–1.014), renal disease is suspected
Protein	less than 100 mg/24 hr	Proteinuria may occur with high-protein diet and exercise (particularly prolonged) Seen in renal disease
Sugar	0	Glycosuria occurs after a high intake of sugar or with diabetes mellitus
Ketones	0	Ketonuria occurs with starvation and diabetic ketoacidosis
Red blood cells	0–4	Injury to kidney tissue (see haematuria)
White blood cells	0–5	Urinary tract infection (UTI)
Casts	0	UTI, renal disease

25-8	Urinary symptoms	
	Dysuria	Painful urination
	Frequency	Voiding at frequent intervals
	Urgency	Need to void immediately
	Hesitancy	Difficulty initiating voiding
	Nocturia	Awakening at night with need to void

Objective data

Assess body temperature for fever because fever is indicative of infection. Although fever caused by pyelonephritis can spike to high temperatures, this may not occur in older people. Inspect the urine for colour and clarity, which can indicate the presence of bacteria. The urine will generally be cloudy from precipitate of phosphate salts in an alkaline urine or from bacterial growth. A urinary or vaginal discharge may also give the urine a cloudy appearance.

Diagnostic tests
Urinalysis

Ideally, the urine specimen is collected from the first voiding of the day. This sample is preferable because it is concentrated and abnormal constituents are more likely to be present. Cleansing the meatus before collecting the specimen decreases the likelihood of external contamination; mild soap followed by water or a special antiseptic solution may be used. About 50 to 100 ml of urine is sufficient to determine specific gravity in addition to microscopic analysis (see Table 25-6). WBCs, bacteria, and pus may be identified with UTI. Protein may be noted with pyelonephritis, especially with chronic infection. If the urine cannot be analyzed immediately, the specimen must be refrigerated to retard bacterial growth.

Urine culture

Urine cultures are used to confirm suspected infections, to identify causative organisms, and to determine appropriate antimicrobial therapy. Cultures are also obtained for periodic screening of urine when the threat of UTI persists.

A sample of urine that has been properly collected and stored is considered to be normal if it contains 10,000 or fewer organisms per millilitre. Organisms of this magnitude are the result of normal urethral flora and do not signify UTI. A UTI is diagnosed when bacterial counts in a properly collected and stored sample reach *100,000 or more organisms per millilitre* and the organisms are of one or very largely one bacterial type.[47] Contamination of the urine specimen during collection is most likely when bacterial counts include predominant colonies of *Staphylococcus, Streptococcus,* and diphtheroids, when two or more organisms contribute significantly to the total bacterial count, or when repeated cultures yield differing results. All these results indicate a need to repeat the culture, with particular attention to the collection of the specimen and to its handling.

Specimens for urine culture may be obtained either by catheterization or by midstream voiding. It should be made clear, however, that *urethral catheterization should never be used routinely in collecting urine for culture because of the risk of introducing additional bacteria into the bladder.* Catheterization may be necessary to obtain a sterile urine specimen when the person is unable to void after being adequately hydrated or if the person is incontinent of urine. When a catheter is passed, meticulous attention is given to nontraumatic aseptic technique. After urine flow from the catheter is established, 5 to 10 ml of urine should be collected directly into a sterile specimen container. Care must be taken to ensure that the rim and the inside of the container are not touched by the catheter or by the hands. If a culture tube with a cotton plug is used as specimen container, care must be taken to keep the tube upright to prevent moistening the cotton and thereby contaminating the specimen. Cultures may also be ordered on the urine taken from the renal pelvis during ureteral catheterization or when ureterostomy or nephrostomy tubes are in place.

In collecting a voided specimen for culture, the nurse must decide if the patient is capable of independently obtaining the specimen or if nursing or medical personnel will need to collect a midstream specimen. Most people who are ambulatory and are given precise and unhurried directions will be able to collect their own midstream urine specimen.

The first voided specimen of the day should be used whenever possible because bacteria will be more numerous. If the specimen is not cultured immediately, refrigeration is mandatory to prevent growth of organisms in the specimen.

Other tests

A noninvasive technique used in localizing the *precise* site of infection involves determining the presence of antibody-coated bacteria (ACB) in the urine of patients with UTI. The existence of ACB in urine correlates closely with the incidence of upper UTI; people with lower UTI do not show ACB in their urine. *Blood cultures* may also be necessary to identify the source of infection.

Renal function tests may be performed to determine the effect of kidney infection on renal function. If renal damage is extensive with chronic pyelonephritis, blood urea and serum creatinine will be elevated. *Radiological examinations* and *renal biopsy* (p. 690) may be required to make a differential diagnosis in chronic pyelonephritis.

A more extensive urological workup, including intravenous pyelogram (IVP) and voiding cystogram, may be performed for men and young children after a repeated or even first UTI, or when infection does not abate. This workup is performed on women when infection occurs repeatedly or cannot be cleared up with treatment. The rationale for this extensive workup is that a UTI is not common in men and young children and that a significant portion of infections in these populations involve abnormality of the urinary tract.

Nursing analysis

Nursing analyses are determined from assessment of patient data. Possible problems for the person with UTI may include, but are not limited to, the following:

Problem	Possible aetiologies
Infection, high risk for	Catheterization, alkaline urine
Pain: costovertebral, suprapubic, perineal	Urinary tract infection
Knowledge deficit	Lack of information

Planning: expected patient outcomes

Expected patient outcomes for the patient with UTI may include, but are not limited to, the following:
1. Further infection has been avoided.
2. Verbalizes relief of symptoms.
3. States feeling comfortable.
4. Describes antibiotic regimen, need for high fluid intake, symptoms to report to doctor, and plan for follow-up care as indicated.

Implementation

Assisting with achievement of therapeutic goals
Monitoring

Monitor the vital signs of a person with pyelonephritis every 4 hours; chills and fever associated with hypotension and tachycardia can be indicative of sepsis and bacteraemic shock. Report increased flank or suprapubic pain, or foul-smelling or cloudy urine to the doctor immediately.

Administering antibiotics

Medications commonly used in the treatment of UTI include antibiotics such as ciprofloxacin and co-trimoxazole. Administer antibiotics on time as prescribed to maintain adequate blood levels. If given intravenously, have prescribed antibiotic serum levels drawn at the correct times to ensure reliable results. Most antibiotics are measured at peak levels (30-60 minutes after infusion) and trough levels (30-60 minutes before the next dose).

Maintaining hydration

Encourage fluid intake of at least 3000 ml/day unless contraindicated by oliguria or other symptoms of renal failure. Increased fluids dilute the urine, which (1) prevents crystallization of sulphonamides, (2) provides a continual flow of urine to discourage urine stasis with multiplication of bacteria, (3) helps wash away ascending bacteria, and (4) lessens dysuria.

Interventions to achieve patient outcomes
Preventing further infection

Use urinary catheterization *only* when mandatory. If needed, use meticulous sterile technique during insertion and irrigation. Follow guidelines for maintaining drainage (p. 677) to prevent reflux of urine. Provide perineal care at least every shift and as needed. Offer the patient cranberry, plum, or prune juices, which acidify the urine; bacteria do not grow in an acidic medium.

Promoting comfort

Medicate as prescribed for flank or suprapubic pain. Sitz baths may provide some relief from urethritis. Back massages often provide short-term relief. High fluid intake can help relieve the urinary "burning" feeling of a lower UTI.

Facilitating patient learning

Patient teaching is important and includes the following:
1. Take the antibiotics for the prescribed period, even after symptoms abate; infection may still be present even if asymptomatic. The course of antibiotic therapy may extend over weeks.
2. Report for urine cultures as instructed (usually 2 weeks after drug therapy is discontinued and possibly every month thereafter for several months).
3. Maintain a fluid intake of at least 3 L/day.
4. Monitor urinary output and report decreased output (may indicate decreased renal function).
5. Report signs of recurrence to doctor (flank pain, chills, and fever for pyelonephritis; dysuria, frequency, and urgency for lower UTI).

Evaluation

Evaluation is based on expected patient outcomes. Questions to consider may include the following:
1. Has further infection been avoided?
2. Is the patient free of fever and pain?
3. Can the patient explain the reason for a fluid intake of at least 3000 ml/day and describe plans to follow this?
4. Can the patient describe the antibiotic regimen, need to continue taking the medication, and report for follow-up urine cultures?

GLOMERULAR DISORDERS

Glomerular disorders, which are a group of diseases that result from injury to the glomeruli, are termed *glomerulonephritis*. The glomerulus plays an essential role in the functioning of the kidneys; therefore, any injury to the glomerulus is likely to result in some change in renal functioning.

There are several different diseases of the glomerulus resulting in a number of classification systems to assist in defining glomerulonephritis[1]. For purposes of discussion, in this chapter glomerulonephritis is discussed as either

---

25-9

Classification of glomerular diseases

Primary glomerulonephritis

Acute diffuse proliferative glomerulonephritis
Rapidly progressive glomerulonephritis
Membranous glomerulonephritis
Minimal change disease
Membranoproliferative glomerulonephritis
Chronic glomerulonephritis

Secondary to systemic diseases

Systemic lupus erythematosus
Goodpasture's disease
Wegener's granulomatosis
Bacterial endocarditis
Diabetes mellitus

<u>REVIEW</u>

Table 25-7   Glomerular disorders

Disorder	Signs and symptoms	Urine characteristics	Medical therapy
Acute glomerulonephritis	Headache, malaise, facial oedema, mild fever, flank pain, oliguria, shortness of breath, elevated blood urea and creatinine	Protein 1-3+, casts, blood	No specific therapy; antibiotics for residual streptococcus, bed rest, dietary protein and sodium restriction as needed
Chronic glomerulonephritis	Usually asymptomatic initially, hypertension; may progress to renal failure	Albumin, casts, blood	No specific therapy; treatment for exacerbation of acute episodes
Nephrotic syndrome	Massive oedema with anorexia, fatigue, shortness of breath, hypoalbuminaemia, hyperlipidaemia	Large amount of protein, casts	No specific therapy; bed rest and corticosteroids for severe oedema

acute or chronic; the nephrotic syndrome is described as a component of glomerulonephritis. Table 25-7 provides a summary of the major glomerular disorders, including aetiology, signs and symptoms, and medical therapy.

ACUTE GLOMERULONEPHRITIS
Aetiology/Epidemiology

Glomerulonephritis (GN) is a disease that affects the glomeruli of both kidneys. Aetiological factors are many and varied; they include immunological reactions (lupus erythematosus, streptococcal infection), vascular injury (hypertension), metabolic disease (diabetes mellitus), and disseminated intravascular coagulation (DIC). Glomerulonephritis exists in acute, latent, and chronic forms. The most common form of *acute glomerulonephritis* occurs 1 to 2 weeks after a streptococcal infection. Common sites of infection include the throat (tonsillitis, strep throat) and the skin (impetigo).

School-aged children and adolescents are most likely to develop the illness. The prognosis of acute poststreptococcal glomerulonephritis (APSGN) is generally good; however, some patients develop chronic GN and end-stage renal disease, requiring dialysis or transplantation.[22]

Pathophysiology

Normal glomerular membranes consist of three types of cells: epithelium, basement membrane, and endothelium. Any or all three of these cells may be affected by glomerulonephritis. Acute glomerulonephritis is the result of an antigen-antibody reaction with glomerular tissue that produces swelling and death to capillary cells. The antigen-antibody reaction activates the complement pathway, resulting in chemotaxis of polymorphonuclear (PMN) leukocytes with release of lysosomal enzymes that attack the glomerular basement membrane (GBM). (Leukocytosis is a common symptom.) The response in the GBM is an

increase in the three types of glomerular cells. The various disease entities tend to attack specific cells, therefore, differential diagnosis is usually made by renal biopsy. The ability to make a differential diagnosis has been greatly aided by the tremendous increase in knowledge about the immune system.

Signs and symptoms reflect *damage to the glomeruli* with leaking into urine by protein (proteinuria) and red cells (haematuria). As the disease process continues, scarring occurs, leading to *decreased glomerular filtration* producing oliguria and retention of water, sodium, and nitrogenous wastes (increased blood urea and serum creatinine level). This results in fluid overloading, oedema, and azotaemia as noted by shortness of breath, oedema, hypertension, headache, weakness, and anorexia. Elevated antistreptolysis O (ASO) titres are encountered in APSGN; however, no relationship exists between the rise in ASO titre and the incidence or severity of APSGN.[43]

Nursing Process
Assessment
Subjective data

The patient with acute glomerulonephritis is likely to present with some signs and symptoms of renal failure, and should be assessed for changes in voiding patterns and presence of headaches and flank pain. The patient may complain of recent flulike symptoms and a sore throat.

Objective data

Objective data include evaluation of the extent of fluid retention and characteristics of the urine, as a baseline for ongoing assessment and evaluation:
1. Breath sounds, for signs of rales (crackles)
2. Oedema of legs, sacrum, periorbital areas
3. Body weight: weigh daily for increase
4. Blood pressure, for elevations
5. Urine, for signs of increased blood, cloudiness, casts, increased specific gravity

Diagnostic tests

The most important immediate diagnostic test is urinalysis to determine presence of proteinuria, haematuria, and cellular debris. Blood urea and serum creatinine are obtained to determine renal function. Immunological tests such as antigen-antibody titres, immunoelectrophoresis and ASO may be obtained.

A composite urine for creatinine clearance and protein can also provide important information.

Renal biopsy

The differential diagnosis for glomerulonephritis can often be difficult to establish. A renal biopsy may be necessary to assist in diagnosis and establishing a definitive treatment plan. The biopsy can be performed either through a skin puncture (closed biopsy) or through an incision (open biopsy). The use of a fluoroscopic guided needle biopsy now allows for most renal biopsies to be obtained by the closed method.

Inherent in taking a biopsy specimen of this vascular tissue is the potential threat of haemorrhage. Throughout the procedure, care is taken to prevent and to detect early loss of blood. Before biopsy is performed, a thorough medical evaluation with particular attention to detection of any abnormality in bleeding or coagulation time is carried out. The patient's blood is usually typed and cross-matched with 2 units of blood; the blood is held for the patient until any threat of bleeding has passed.

An open biopsy carries less risk of haemorrhage and provides better visualization of the kidney; however, the risk of infection is increased, and a longer period of recovery is required.

Preprocedure care. Preparation before biopsy includes discussing the procedure with the patient. Topics covered include the necessity for the examination, the procedure itself, the care to be anticipated, and any questions of concern to the patient. The preparation of the patient is shared by the doctor and nurse. It is necessary to have the patient sign a consent before having the biopsy performed. The biopsy may be carried out in the radiology department, or in the operating theatre.

Procedure. Before *percutaneous (closed) biopsy,* the patient is taken to the radiology department for localization of the kidney by a plain film, a dye contrast film, or fluoroscopic location. The position of the kidney in relation to body landmarks is marked on the skin in ink. The lower pole of the kidney is located for biopsy site because it contains the lowest number of large vessels. Sedation is usually not required except for children or adults who are restless and unable to relax sufficiently to follow necessary instructions during the test. The patient is placed prone over a sandbag or firm pillow and an additional soft pillow. The body is bent at the level of the diaphragm, with the shoulders on the bed and the spine in straight alignment. The doctor identifies the location for biopsy, and a local anaesthetic agent is injected. As the biopsy is being taken, the patient is instructed to hold his or her breath. Pain may be felt in the kidney region as the tissue sample is taken. The needle is withdrawn immediately, and direct pressure is applied to the site for 20 minutes. A pressure bandage is then applied.

Postprocedure care. After the procedure the patient is turned supine and is kept flat and motionless for 4 hours. One small pillow may be used under the head. Coughing and other activity that increases abdominal venous pressure is to be avoided during this time. Blood pressure and pulse are taken each 15 minutes for 1 hour, every 30 minutes during the next hour, and every hour for an additional 2 to 3 hours to assess for haemorrhage. The patient should remain in bed for at least 24 hours following the procedure.

Liberal intake of fluids is encouraged to help maintain a dilute urine and prevent intrarenal clot formation. Serial urine specimens should be obtained to evaluate haematuria.[22] Bed rest is maintained until the urine is clear. Initially, the urine is likely to demonstrate blood, but this rarely continues after a 24-hour period.

Complications include persistent haematuria, perirenal or intrarenal arteriovenous fistula, aneurysm, and laceration of organs or blood vessels adjacent to the biopsied kidney.[22]

Nursing analysis

Nursing analyses are determined from assessment of patient data. Possible nursing problems for the person with acute glomerulonephritis may include, but are not limited to, the following:

Problem	Possible aetiologies
Fluid volume excess	Compromised regulatory mechanism, excess fluid intake, excess sodium intake
Infection, high risk for	Decreased immune response
Knowledge deficit	Lack of information

Planning: expected patient outcomes

Expected patient outcomes for the patient with acute glomerulonephritis may include, but are not limited to, the following:

1. Maintains fluid balance as near normal as possible.
2. Maintains stable weight from day to day.
3. Maintains vital signs close to normal limits.
4. Does not acquire any infection.
5. Describes nature of illness, therapeutic regimen, signs and symptoms indicating medical attention, and need for follow-up care.

Implementation

Assisting with achievement of therapeutic goals

The care of the person with acute glomerulonephritis can be complex because of the overall ramifications of the disease.

Control of infection

Persistent infection is treated promptly to help further decrease antigen-antibody complex formation. People with poststreptococcal glomerulonephritis are given a prophylactic antibiotic; the drug of choice is a penicillin. Rationale for this therapy is based on preventing further infections that could reactivate the nephritis. Prophylactic therapy may be continued for months after the acute phase of illness.

Activity

Bed rest is instituted until clinical signs disappear; this may involve a period of several months. Ambulation is allowed when blood sedimentation rates and blood pressure are normal and oedema abates. If ambulation causes an increase in proteinuria or haematuria, bed rest is reinstituted. Because the period of bed rest may be long and the patient usually does not feel ill, the nurse may need to continue reinforcing the importance of bed rest and assist in planning diversionary activities. When bed rest is reinstituted after periods of ambulation, the patient may become depressed. Helping the patient to express concerns and feelings can serve as a basis for helping to make realistic plans about the illness and its sequelae.

Maintenance of fluid balance

Oedema and fluid overloading are anticipated and treated initially with dietary sodium restrictions. Remember that water follows sodium; restricting sodium decreases fluid retention. The amount of restriction depends on the severity of fluid retention, and it is maintained until dependent oedema and circulatory overload are no longer a problem. Diuretics are generally reserved for managing severe fluid overload and pulmonary oedema. The nurse is constantly alert for signs of fluid overload. Blood pressure elevation is treated with antihypertensive drugs only after fluid control has proved unsuccessful in controlling hypertension. Dietary protein is reduced only when blood urea and creatinine levels are elevated. The diet should contain sufficient carbohydrate to prevent catabolism and thus maintain nitrogen balance.

Interventions to achieve patient outcomes
Preventing fluid volume excess

Keep strict records of fluid intake and output. Calculate the difference between fluid intake loss and determine the net fluid change.[43] Fluid restrictions must be maintained.

It is important to weigh the patient at least daily. Use a metric scale, if possible, because it is easier to calculate fluid changes. Balance the scale before each use and weigh the patient at the same time each day with the same clothing. Teach the patient how to obtain a correct weight, if necessary.

Take vital signs at least twice daily, including apical pulse. Listen for presence of a dysrhythmia. Assess for neck vein distension indicating fluid overload and congestive heart failure. Assess for periorbital, pretibial, pedal, and sacral oedema. Measure oedematous legs.

Administer diuretics when prescribed. Evaluate their efficacy and monitor for complications such as hypokalaemia. Monitor the serum potassium levels closely, especially for those diuretics that eliminate potassium (see Chapter 17).

Preventing infection

Exposure to any infection must be avoided because even mild infections may reactivate nephritis. The patient must avoid contact with any people with upper respiratory infections (URI). The patient should know to seek prompt medical treatment for sore throats and URIs. Cultures should be obtained and, when indicated, appropriate antibiotics should be prescribed.

Facilitating patient learning

Because of the long-term nature of glomerulonephritis, patient teaching is important. Proteinuria, haematuria, and cellular debris may exist microscopically even when other symptoms subside. Although fatigue may be present, these people usually feel well; therefore, they often must be convinced of the need to continue prescribed treatment and to return for follow-up care. Teaching includes the following:

1. Nature of the illness and effect of diet and fluids on fluid balance and sodium retention.
2. Diet teaching regarding prescribed sodium and fluid restrictions (provide written information regarding sodium content of foods, as necessary).
3. Medication regimen (dose, frequency, side effects, need to continue as per doctor's instructions).
4. Need to pace activities with rest if fatigue is present.
5. Avoidance of trauma and infection (may exacerbate the illness).
6. Signs and symptoms indicating need for medical attention (haematuria, headache, oedema, hypertension).
7. Importance of follow-up health care.

Evaluation

Evaluation is based on expected patient outcomes. Questions to consider may include the following:

1. Are signs of fluid retention decreased?
2. Is the patient eating a balanced diet according to prescribed guidelines (low salt, sufficient carbohydrate)?
3. Has the patient been following prescribed fluid restrictions?
4. Are there any signs of other infections?
5. Does the patient know the nature of the illness, therapeutic regimen, and need for follow-up health care?

CHRONIC GLOMERULONEPHRITIS

Aetiology/Epidemiology

Although chronic glomerulonephritis (CGN) may follow the acute disease, the majority of people give no history of the disease. In most instances no evidence of predisposing infection can be found. The course of chronic glomerulonephritis is extremely varied. Some people with minimal impairment in renal function continue to feel well and show little progression of disease. With other individuals the progression of renal deterioration may be slow but steady and end in renal failure. In still other individuals the progression of disease is rapid.

Pathophysiology

CGN is characterized by slow progressive destruction (sclerosis) of glomeruli and gradual loss of renal function. The glomeruli have varying degrees of hypercellularity and become sclerosed (hardened) as the disease progresses. This results in decreased renal function and increased presentation of signs and symptoms of renal failure. The kidneys decrease in size; eventually there is tubular atrophy, chronic interstitial inflammation, and arteriosclerosis. The underlying pathophysiological changes are the immune responses described for acute glomerulonephritis.

Various symptoms of *failing renal function,* none of which may seem severe, may lead the person to seek health care. There may be a slow onset of recurrent dependent *oedema,* or there may be mild *headache,* especially in the morning. *Dyspnoea on exertion* or difficulty sleeping in a flat position may be noted. *Blurring of vision* may lead the patient to an ophthalmologist, who may be the first to suspect chronic renal disease based on ocular vascular changes. Occasionally, chronic nephritis is discovered during routine physical examination or may be discovered by a school nurse who observes marked visual changes and lassitude in a student. Early in the disease urinalysis shows the presence of albumin, casts, and blood. At this point renal function tests may be normal. The ability of the kidneys to regulate the internal environment will begin to decrease as more and more glomeruli become scarred and the amount of functional renal tissue is reduced. Finally, when few intact nephrons remain, haematuria and proteinuria decrease, the specific gravity of the urine becomes fixed, and the nonprotein nitrogen level in the blood increases. Although the process is insidious and slow, CGN eventually results in end-stage renal disease. This may take 10 to 15 years.

Nursing Process
Assessment
Subjective data

General questions to ask include: (1) Have you experienced shortness of breath, headaches, weakness, or anorexia? (2) Have you noticed any change in your pattern of urination, either frequency or volume? and (3) Do you recall a recent infection of symptoms of a virus? It is also important to determine if there is a history of renal problems in the past.

Objective data

It is important to establish baseline vital signs including temperature, pulse, respirations, and blood pressure. Vital signs are assessed frequently, at least every 6 hours, until stable. The patient is assessed daily for oedema. Daily weighing is one of the best means of assessing the patient's fluid status. Intake and output should be assessed at least every 8 hours until stable. The urine is assessed for colour, clarity, specific gravity, and odour.

Diagnostic tests

Urinalysis is essential to determine the presence of proteinuria, haematuria, and cellular debris. Blood urea and serum creatinine are obtained to determine renal function. Immunological tests such as antigen-antibody titres and immunoelectrophoresis may also be obtained. A composite urine for creatinine clearance and total protein can also provide important data about renal function. Renal biopsy may be necessary to make the differential diagnosis.

Nursing analysis

Nursing analyses are determined from assessment of patient data. Possible nursing problems for the person with chronic glomerulonephritis may include, but are not limited to, the following:

Problem	Possible aetiologies
Activity intolerance	Generalized weakness, electrolyte imbalance
Knowledge deficit	Lack of exposure/recall

Planning: expected patient outcomes

Expected patient outcomes for the patient with chronic glomerulonephritis may include, but are not limited to the following:
1. Maintains bed rest as prescribed.
2. Obtains adequate rest.
3. Resumes usual activities within tolerance when permitted.
4. Describes medication and dietary regimen and need for follow-up care.

Implementation
Assisting with achievement of therapeutic goals

No specific therapy exists to arrest or reverse the disease process. With some forms of CGN, steroids and cytotoxic agents may be attempted, although results of these therapies in arresting disease are not well documented. Treatment of renal failure begins when the illness destroys so much kidney tissue that the individual's kidneys are no longer able to control the internal environment independently.

With any exacerbation of haematuria, hypertension, and oedema, the person is put to bed, and treatment similar to that for acute glomerulonephritis is instituted. Signs of pulmonary oedema and congestive heart failure (resulting from fluid retention) are monitored. Treatment is symptomatic and supportive.

Interventions to achieve patient outcomes
Promoting activity tolerance

During the period of enforced bed rest, assist the patient with ADL as necessary. Coordinate assessments and interventions to minimize interruptions and maximize rest. Place objects well within the patient's reach to avoid undue exertion. Provide bed exercises within the prescribed activity limitations to promote muscle strength and tone. After bed rest is no longer necessary, establish a progressive but gradual activity regimen that will help increase physical endurance.

Facilitating patient learning

The teaching for the patient with chronic glomerulonephritis is the same as for acute glomerulonephritis (p. 691). Care involves teaching the patient to live healthfully, to avoid infections, to eat a balanced diet with moderate sodium intake if prescribed, to appropriately administer medication, and to maintain follow-up health care visits and report to the doctor any exacerbations in signs and symptoms.

Women with CGN who become pregnant appear to be susceptible to toxaemia and to spontaneous abortion. The woman who has had nephritis of any nature should be urged to see a doctor if she plans on pregnancy. When pregnancy does occur, she should remain under close health supervision.

The person also needs to know what resources are available in the community to assist with chronic renal disease. The National Kidney Federation* may be able to provide information and locate resources.

Evaluation

Evaluation is based on expected patient outcomes. Questions to consider may include the following:

1. Has the patient participated in bed activities within activity prescription without expressing fatigue?
2. Did the patient resume usual ADL when permitted without fatigue?
3. Can the patient describe health regimen and need for follow-up care?

NEPHROTIC SYNDROME
Aetiology

Nephrotic syndrome is not a single disease entity but a constellation of symptoms. In nephrotic syndrome there is damage to the glomeruli and quantities of protein are lost in the urine. This condition has been associated with allergic reactions (insect bites, pollen, acute glomerulonephritis), infections (herpes zoster), systemic disease (diabetes mellitus, sickle cell disease, amyloidosis), circulatory problems (severe congestive heart failure, chronic constrictive pericarditis), selected drugs and chemicals, and pregnancy. Known glomerular disease is the most common precipitating event in adults; in children the syndrome appears frequently with no evidence of a causative factor. In approximately 25% of children and 50% to 75% of adults who develop nephrosis the disease progresses to renal failure within 5 years.[43] In other individuals (particularly children) there may be remissions or nephrosis may exist in a chronic form. Other than treating the underlying illness, little can be done to prevent a recurrence of nephrosis.

Pathophysiology

The initial change in nephrotic syndrome is a derangement of cells in the glomerular basement membrane, resulting in increased membrane porosity with loss of large amounts of protein into the urine (proteinuria). As protein continues to be excreted, serum albumin is decreased (hypoalbuminaemia), thus decreasing the serum osmotic pressure. The capillary hydrostatic fluid (push) pressure in all body tissues becomes greater than the capillary osmotic (pull) pressure, and generalized oedema results. As fluid is lost into the tissues, the plasma volume decreases, stimulating secretion of aldosterone to retain more sodium and water and decreasing the glomerular filtration rate to retain water. This additional fluid also passes out of the capillaries into the tissue, leading to even greater oedema. Altered renal function and development of symptoms of renal failure occur as a result of progressing glomerulo-nephritis. Loss of appetite and fatigue are common. Women usually have amenorrhoea or other disturbances in their reproductive cycle.

In many instances of nephrotic syndrome, there is an elevation of serum total lipids, cholesterol, phospholipids, and triglycerides.[56] The low-density lipoproteins (see Chapter 17) are usually increased. The mechanism that causes the disturbance in lipid metabolism is not clear.[43]

Nursing Process
Assessment
Subjective data

The patient with nephrotic syndrome displays the signs and symptoms of acute glomerulonephritis (p.689). General questions for the patient with nephrotic syndrome include the following:

1. Have there been changes in voiding patterns?
2. Is the person experiencing headaches or nausea?
3. Has appetite changed? Any anorexia?
4. Is fatigue present?

Objective data

The patient with nephrotic syndrome is assessed for signs of fluid retention and infection:

1. Oedema: amount, location, degree of pitting
2. Intake and output: monitored every 8 hours until stable
3. Daily weights and abdominal girths
4. Condition of skin: assess frequently as severe oedema may lead to skin breakdown
5. Respiratory status: monitored at least each shift (as renal failure progresses, pulmonary oedema may develop)
6. Signs and symptoms of infection

Diagnostic tests

The diagnosis of nephrotic syndrome is made on the basis of proteinuria, hypoalbuminaemia, and hyperlipidaemia. It is essential that serum albumin, cholesterol, and triglycerides be obtained. Urinalyses and a composite urine specimen (p. 687) for total protein are collected. A renal biopsy is sometimes used as a means of definitive diagnosis.

Nursing analysis

Nursing analyses are determined from assessment of patient data. Nursing problems for the person with nephrotic syndrome may include, but are not limited to, the following:

Problem	Possible aetiologies
Nutrition, altered, less than body require ments	Anorexia, oedema
	Decreased nutrition, immobility, oedema
Infection, high risk for	Lack of exposure/recall
Knowledge deficit	

Planning: expected patient outcomes

Expected patient outcomes for the person with nephrotic syndrome may include, but are not limited to, the following:

1. Eats a diet high in protein and calories and low in sodium.
2. Weight remains stable.
3. Skin remains intact.

---

*National Kidney Federation, 6 Stanley St., Worksop, Nottinghamshire, S81 7HX

4. Follows prescribed measures when infection occurs.
5. Describes dietary and drug therapy and symptoms requiring immediate attention.

Implementation

Assisting with achievement of therapeutic goals

Treatment of nephrotic syndrome is directed towards reducing albuminuria, controlling oedema, and promoting general health. Corticosteroids may be useful in controlling the illness, but the response to them will vary from remission of nephrosis to no response. Prednisolone is the steroid most frequently prescribed. The diet should contain normal to increased amounts of protein (1 g/kg body weight per day) and be high in calories. Periodic determination of proteinuria and measures of renal function enable the doctor to monitor response to treatment and level of kidney function.

To control oedema, sodium intake is reduced and diuretics may be employed to increase excretion of fluid. When diuretics are administered over prolonged periods, hypokalaemia usually results. Potassium may be supplemented through dietary intake. Medication supplements should be initiated only after attempts to increase serum potassium through dietary means have failed. Close monitoring of oral and parenteral fluid is necessary. Bed rest is usually ordered when oedema is severe; however, immobility is contraindicated for prolonged periods.

Interventions to achieve patient outcomes

Promoting nutrition

Appetite may be diminished as a result of fluid retention. Sodium intake is restricted, which further reduces palatability of foods and leads to a decreased nutritional intake. Use measures to promote food intake (Chapter 4). Develop a diet plan together with the patient, family, and dietitian to include foods the patient likes. The diet should be high in calories to provide energy, low in sodium to reduce fluid retention, and contain the maximum allowable protein that can be tolerated by the kidney, yet replace lost protein. Whenever possible, the protein should be of high biological value (lean meat, fish, poultry, and dairy products).

Offer oral hygiene at regular intervals. Good mouth care can help to reduce the unpleasant metallic taste and breath odour that is partially responsible for the anorexia of renal failure.

Preventing infection

People with nephrosis need to direct particular attention towards preventing infection, because body defences are impaired by urinary protein losses. When infection is suspected, it is important to attend to the problem immediately. Obtain specimens for culture and sensitivity according to established protocols. Administer antibiotics at prescribed times to maintain blood levels. Inform the patient of the importance of prescribed medications and the need to take all the antibiotic as directed.

Oedematous tissue is particularly susceptible to injury and infection. During periods of severe oedema, meticulous skin care is essential to prevent skin breakdown. As oedema increases, the patient becomes increasingly uncomfortable. Careful positioning and frequent changes in position may increase comfort while also protecting the skin. If the scrotum becomes very oedematous, a sling to support it not only provides comfort but also aids in reducing swelling (see Chapter 27).

Facilitating patient learning

As the patient begins to convalesce, the teaching plan includes the following:
1. Medication regimen: type, dosage, side effects, and need to finish antibiotic prescription (as appropriate)
2. Nutrition teaching
3. Self-assessment of fluid status: weight, presence of oedema
4. Signs and symptoms requiring immediate attention (increase in oedema, fatigue, headache, infection)
5. Need for follow-up care.

Evaluation

Evaluation is based on expected patient outcomes. Questions to consider may include the following:
1. Is the person eating the prescribed diet in sufficient quantities?
2. Has weight remained stable?
3. Is skin intact without signs of infection?
4. Can the person describe dietary and drug therapy and symptoms requiring follow-up?

OBSTRUCTIVE DISORDERS

Obstructive disorders are a significant source of morbidity. Obstruction of the urinary tract can occur in any portion of the urinary tract from the urinary calyces to the meatus. The signs and symptoms that a person displays are usually characteristic of the location and extent of the obstruction. Box 25-10 summarizes the locations and major causes of the common urinary tract obstructions.

Obstruction of the urinary tract produces pathophysiological changes leading to symptoms of obstruction. Therapy consists of reestablishing drainage and relieving the acute discomfort. In the following pages, the pathophysiology of and therapy for urinary obstruction will be discussed. Several major causes of urinary obstruction are then described in more detail; these topics include the following:
1. Urinary calculi
2. Benign prostatic hypertrophy
3. Urethral strictures
4. Neoplasms: renal, bladder, prostate

Pathophysiology of Urinary Obstruction: Hydronephrosis

Obstruction of any part of the urinary system from the kidney to the urethra will generate pressure that may cause functional and anatomical damage to the renal parenchyma. When any part of the urinary tract is obstructed, urine collects behind the obstruction producing a dilation of the structure. Muscles of the affected areas contract in an effort to push the urine around the obstruction. Partial obstruction may produce slow dilation of structures above the obstruction without functional impairment. As the

Location and causes of urinary tract obstruction	
Location	**Major causes**
Kidney	Calculi
	Ptosis
	Polycystic disease
Ureteral ob-	Calculi
struction	Trauma
	Nephroptosis ("floating" or "dropped" kidney)
	Enlarged lymph nodes
	Lymphosarcoma
	Reticulum cell sarcoma
	Hodgkin's disease
Lower uri-	Bladder neoplasm
nary tract	Urethral strictures
	Trauma
	Chronic inflammation
	Calculi
	Tumours
	Benign prostatic hypertrophy (BPH)

25-10

obstruction increases, however, pressure builds up in the tubular system behind the obstruction causing a backflow of urine and dilation of the ureter (*hydroureter*). The urine backup eventually reaches the kidney, causing dilation of the kidney pelvis (*hydronephrosis*). Pressure buildup in the renal pelvis leads to destruction of kidney tissue and eventual renal failure.

With obstruction urine flow is decreased even to the point of stagnation. This stagnant urine provides a good culture medium for bacterial growth, and rarely is obstruction seen without some infection. The specific effects that occur with obstruction depend on the location of the obstruction, the extent of obstruction (partial or complete), and the duration. Obstruction in the *lower* urinary tract causes bladder distension. If this is prolonged, muscle fibres become hypertrophied and *diverticuli* (herniated sacs of bladder mucosa) develop between the hypertrophied muscle bands. Because the diverticulum holds stagnant urine, infection often occurs, and bladder stones may form.

Obstruction of the *upper* urinary tract leads even more quickly to hydronephrosis because of the small size of the ureters and kidney pelvis. Increased pressure causes partial ischaemia of arteries between the renal cortex and medulla and dilation of the renal tubules leading to tubular damage. Stasis of urine in the dilated pelvis predisposes to infection and calculi, which add to the renal damage. Some urine can flow back up the renal tubule into the veins and lymphatics as a compensatory mechanism to prevent kidney damage. The unaffected kidney then takes on increased elimination of waste products. With prolonged obstruction the unaffected kidney hypertrophies and may function as effectively alone as both kidneys did before the obstruction. Obstruction of both kidneys leads to renal failure.

Hydronephrosis can occur without any symptoms as long as kidney function is adequate and urine can drain. An acute upper urinary tract obstruction will cause pain, nausea, vomiting, local tenderness, spasm of the abdominal muscles, and a mass in the kidney region. The pain is caused by the stretching of the tissues and by hyperperistalsis. Because the amount of pain is proportional to the rate of stretching, a slowly developing hydronephrosis may cause only a dull flank pain, whereas a sudden blockage of the ureter such as may occur from a stone causes a severe stabbing (colicky) pain in the flank or abdomen. The pain may radiate to the genitalia and thigh and is caused by the increased peristaltic action of the smooth muscle of the ureter in an effort to dislodge the obstruction and force urine past it.

The nausea and vomiting frequently associated with acute ureteral obstruction are caused by a reflex reaction to the pain and will usually be relieved as soon as pain is relieved. A markedly dilated kidney, however, may press on the stomach causing continued GI symptoms. If the renal function has been seriously impaired, nausea and vomiting may be symptoms of impending uraemia.

When the bladder is distended from lower urinary tract obstruction, the person will experience lower abdominal discomfort and a feeling of the need to void although voiding may not be possible. The bladder may be palpated above the symphysis pubis. With partial obstruction such as by benign prostatic hypertrophy the patient first complains of increasing urinary frequency because the bladder fails to empty completely at each voiding and therefore refills more quickly to the amount that causes the urge to void (usually 250 to 500 ml). Nocturia may also be present.

Therapy for Urinary Obstruction

The person with a sudden obstruction is usually acutely ill and may have severe colic but will not be able to remain in bed until the pain has been relieved. It is not unusual to see a person with acute renal colic walking the floor doubled up and vomiting. Narcotics such as morphine and pethidine and antispasmodic drugs such as propantheline are usually necessary to relieve severe colicky pain. After narcotics have been given, the patient will be dizzy and must be protected from injury. As the pain eases, the patient can usually be made relatively comfortable in bed. As soon as the nausea subsides large amounts of fluids are urged.

If a *ureter* becomes obstructed, a catheter must be placed directly into the renal pelvis. This prevents renal damage that otherwise would occur as pressure in the kidney increases because of continued urine formation. When there is complete obstruction of a ureter, a *nephrostomy* or *pyelostomy* tube may be inserted surgically into the renal pelvis. The surgical incision is located laterally and posteriorly in the kidney region. Catheters used as nephrostomy or pyelostomy tubes are usually of the Pezzer (mushroom) or Malecot (batwing) types. An alternate form of drainage for a ureteral obstruction is the surgical placement of a ureterostomy tube (a whistle-tip or many-eyed Robinson catheter, No. 6 or No. 8 Fr) that is passed through an incision in the upper outer quadrant of the abdomen into the ureter above the obstruction. The catheter is then passed through the ureter to the renal pelvis.

If the ureter is unobstructed or partially obstructed, the *renal pelvis* may be drained by a ureteral catheter, which is passed up the ureter to the renal pelvis by a cystoscope. Ureteral catheterization is performed before gynaecological and lower abdominal surgery when there is danger of not recognizing and accidentally injuring the ureter during the operation. Ureteral catheterization is also used after surgery involving the ureters to prevent stricture as the ureter heals. When used for this purpose, the catheter is referred to as a *splinting catheter*. Whether it is expected to drain urine will depend on its relation to other catheters used.

Adequate anchorage of nephrostomy catheters must be provided to prevent accidental dislodgement and trauma to the tissues in which they lie. The openings made for these tubes are essentially fistulas that rapidly decrease in size on removal of the catheter. Even 30 minutes after removal of this type of catheter it is often impossible to reinsert a similar-sized tube. When a catheter is inserted during surgery, it is usually sutured in place. In this case, additional anchorage consists of affixing the tube to the skin with adhesive tape after the skin has been cleansed. When the tube is not sutured in place, it should be anchored to the skin at *two points* using adhesive—with some slack in the tubing between the anchor points.

Free drainage of catheters leading to the renal pelvis is of the utmost importance. Because the normal renal pelvis has only a 5- to 8-ml capacity, great pressure can be exerted on renal structures even when these catheters are obstructed for only a few minutes. Care must be taken to prevent kinking of the tubes while the patient is in the side-lying position in bed.

In some cases nephrostomy tubes may be left in place for several months, with the patient returning to the hospital later for their removal. Occasionally, the nephrostomy tube serves as a form of urinary diversion for long-term use. The person at home with a catheter draining the kidney pelvis must know how to obtain medical assistance quickly should the catheter become obstructed or dislodged.

When obstruction occurs below the *bladder,* constant drainage must be provided to prevent renal damage, which may occur because of inadequate emptying of the lower urinary system. One means of providing drainage is by the use of a *cystostomy* tube (usually a Foley, Malecot, or Pezzer catheter), which is placed directly into the bladder through a suprapubic incision. This method is usually used when the urethra is completely obstructed or when the prolonged use of a urethral catheter is to be avoided in a male patient. During some operative procedures both a cystostomy tube and a small urethral catheter will be inserted to drain the bladder. Both catheters must be monitored for patency. If patency is assured, it is not necessary to record the output from each catheter separately, because both tubes drain the bladder. The catheters will not necessarily drain equal amounts of urine. As is true with nephrostomy and ureteral catheters, secure anchorage of these catheters.

URINARY CALCULI
Aetiology/Epidemiology

Urinary stones, which are termed *urolithiasis* ("lith" refers to stones), may develop at any level in the urinary system, but are most commonly found within the kidney (nephrolithiasis). Fig. 25-6 illustrates the most common locations of urolithiasis. Supersaturation of urine is believed to be the major cause of urinary calculi. When concentrations of the stone-forming substance exceeds its solubility in urine, stone growth can occur. No demonstrable cause can be found for over half of the urinary stones that occur (idiopathic). A major predisposition is urinary tract infection. Other factors are listed in Box 25-11.

It is estimated that 28 of every 100,000 of Britons will develop urolithiasis. About one third of the individuals who have recurrent upper urinary tract calculi will eventually need to have the affected kidney removed.[40a]

Prevention

Measures can be taken to decrease the potential for renal stones in people at high risk. Adequate hydration (intake of 2500 ml/day or more unless contraindicated) will help to prevent urinary stasis that can lead not only to stone formation but also to a UTI. People restricted to bed should be encouraged to turn and move frequently, exercising their arms if the legs are immobilized. Changing the body position of a bedfast patient by sitting up in a wheelchair (if permitted) can help to prevent urinary stasis. Even with exercises and the use of a wheelchair, however, paraplegics and quadriplegics often develop urinary calculi. *People with in-dwelling catheters need scrupulous aseptic technique in catheter care to prevent infection and require adequate hydration and good catheter drainage to wash away minerals that can be deposited at the tip of the catheter.*

25-11	**Renal calculus composition and contributing factors**	
	Composition of stone	**Factors contributing to stone formation**
	Calcium (oxalate and phosphate)	Hyperphosphaturia and/or hypercalciuria resulting from: Hyperparathyroidism Vitamin D intoxication Multiple myeloma Immobilization Severe bone disease Renal tubular acidosis Prolonged intake of steroids
	Uric acid	High purine diet Gout
	Cystine	Cystinuria resulting from genetic disorder of amino-acid metabolism

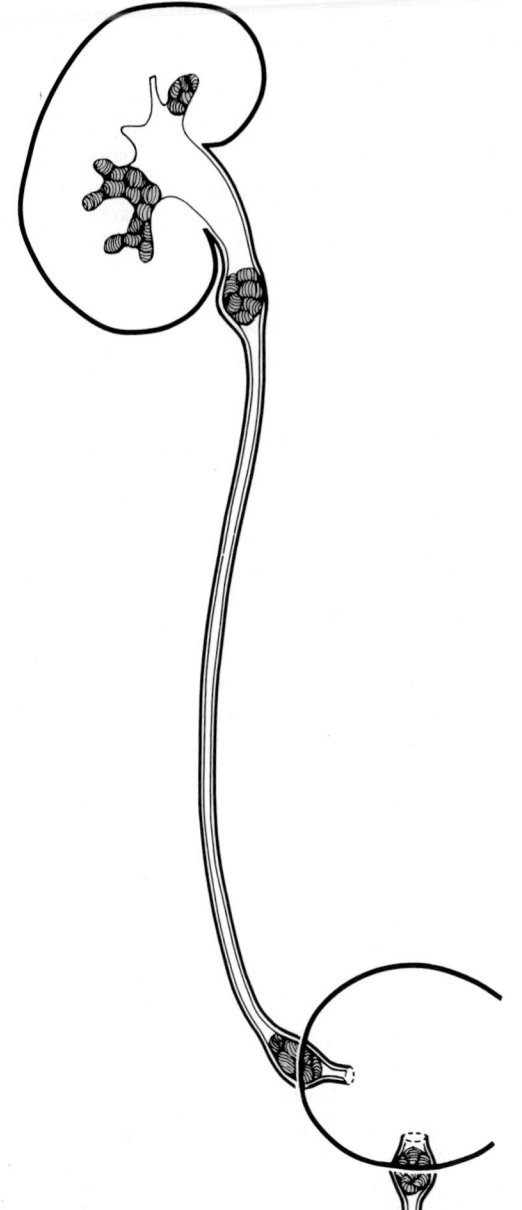

Fig. 25-6   Common locations of renal calculus formation.

People at risk for developing calcium oxalate or phosphate or magnesium ammonium phosphate stones may be placed on an acid ash diet to promote excretion of an acid urine.

Pathophysiology

Urinary calculi result in obstruction of the urinary tract; the obstruction may be partial or complete. Complete obstruction leads to *hydronephrosis* with its associated signs and symptoms.

The pathophysiological processes associated with urinary stones tend to be mechanical in nature. Urinary calculi (stones) are crystallizations of minerals around an organic matrix such as pus, blood, devitalized tissue, tumours, or urates. The mineral composition of renal calculi varies. About three fourths of stones are calcium and oxalates; other stones are calcium phosphate, uric acid, and cystine.

Increased concentration of urine solutes, resulting from low fluid intake, as well as increased organic matter from urinary tract infections or urinary stasis, may provide the nidus for stone formation. In addition, infection increases the alkalinity of the urine (by the production of ammonia), resulting in precipitation of calcium phosphate and magnesium ammonium phosphate.

Nursing Process
Assessment
Subjective data

Pain (*renal colic*) is the primary symptom in an acute episode of renal calculi. The location of the pain depends on the location of the stone. If the stone is in the pelvis of the kidney, the pain is caused by hydronephrosis and is more dull and constant in character, occurring primarily in the costovertebral angle. As the stone moves along the ureter, the pain can be excruciating and is intermittent in character. It is caused by spasm of the ureter and anoxia of the wall of the ureter from the pressure of the stone. Pain follows the anterior course of the ureter down to the suprapubic area and radiates to the external genitalia. Often a stone is "silent" causing no symptoms for years; this is especially true of very large renal stones. Extremely small smooth stones may be passed without the person's awareness. Nausea and vomiting often accompany renal colic.

Objective data

The urine is monitored for the presence of blood. *Gross haematuria* may occur if the stone has rough edges, and microhaematuria is usually present. Whenever a stone is suspected, all urine is strained to determine the presence of stones that are frequently passed during voiding. Patterns of urination are also noted because frequency or voiding in small amounts may be experienced. The acidity or alkalinity of the urine can be determined with pH paper.

Diagnostic tests

Urinalysis, to determine the urine pH, presence of casts, crystals, and blood cells, and urine culture, to identify UTI, are performed. A 24-hour urine collection is made to measure calcium oxalate, phosphorus, and uric acid levels. A nitroprusside urine test may be performed to check the presence of cystine.

Blood urea and serum creatinine tests are important to determine the level of renal function. Because urinary stones are frequently composed of calcium, phosphorus, and uric acid, these serum levels are usually obtained.

Calcium stones are radiopaque and can be noted with a KUB (kidney, ureter, bladder) X-ray examination; uric acid stones usually cannot be seen in radiographic studies. An intravenous pyelogram (IVP) may also be obtained. IVP may demonstrate dilation of the ureter above an obstructing stone. Very small stones, however, may be washed away during radiographic studies. Ultrasound of the kidneys may also be ordered to detect hydronephrosis.

Nursing analysis

Nursing analyses are determined from assessment of patient data. Possible nursing problems for the person with urinary calculi may include, but are not limited to, the following:

Problem	Possible aetiologies
Pain	Visceral inflammation
Knowledge deficit	Lack of exposure/recall

Planning: expected patient outcomes

Expected patient outcomes for the patient with urinary calculi may include, but are not limited to, the following:

1. Describes feeling more comfortable.
2. Describes measures to prevent urinary calculi recurrence and symptoms of recurrence to be reported.

Implementation

Assisting with achievement of therapeutic goals

About 90% of urinary calculi are passed spontaneously. Therefore, *the urine of all patients with relatively small stones should be strained.* Urine can be strained easily by placing two opened 4-inch × 8-inch gauze sponges over a funnel. The urine from each voiding is strained, and one needs to watch closely for the stone because it may be no bigger than the head of a pin and the patient may not realize that it has been passed.

Stones smaller than 5 mm have a good chance of being passed. If there is no infection or obstruction, the stone may be left in the ureter for several months. The person is observed closely but permitted to carry out usual activities. A person who is up and about is more likely to pass a stone than one who is in bed. Fluids should be taken freely (3000 ml/day or more) to promote passage of the stone and prevent infection.

Patients frequently have two or three attacks of acute renal colic before the stone passes. This is probably because the stone gets lodged at a narrow point in the ureter, causing temporary obstruction. The ureters are normally narrower at the ureteropelvic and ureterovesical junctions and at the point where they pass over the iliac crest into the pelvis. If the stone is to pass along the ureter by peristaltic action, the patient will have some pain. The patient is involved in determining when pain medication is needed.

If the stone fails to pass, one or two ureteral catheters may be passed through a cystoscope up the ureter and left in place for 24 hours. The catheters dilatate the ureter, and when they are removed the stone may pass into the bladder.

If there are *signs of infection,* an attempt is made to pass a ureteral catheter past the stone into the renal pelvis. If such an attempt is successful, the catheter is left as a drain, because pyelonephritis will quickly follow if adequate urinary drainage is not reestablished. When there is a catheter in each ureter, each catheter is labelled and should drain into a separate drainage bag. Check the catheters frequently to see that they are draining. Patients with ureteral catheters are usually confined to bed to prevent possible dislodgement of the catheters.

If the stone has passed to the lower third of the *ureter,* it can sometimes be removed by *manipulation.* Special catheters with expanding baskets and loops are passed through the cystoscope, and an attempt is made to "snare" the stone. This procedure is performed with the patient under anaesthesia. The aftercare of a patient on whom manipulation has been carried out is the same as that following cystoscopy. Watch for any signs suggestive of peritonitis or a decreased urinary output because the ureter occasionally is perforated during manipulation.

Bladder stones may be crushed with a lithotrite (stone crusher) that is passed transurethrally. This procedure is known as a *litholapaxy.* Following bladder stone removal, the bladder may be irrigated (intermittently or constantly) with an acid solution such as magnesium and sodium citrate to counteract the alkalinity caused by the infection and to help wash out the remaining particles of stone.

Percutaneous nephrolithotomy

Until the early 1980s surgery was usually required to remove a urinary stone. Percutaneous nephrolithotomy (endourology) is now a common method for urinary stone removal. A small nephrostomy tract is made through a skin incision over the kidney region. An endoscope is then passed through the tract and a snare basket is used to retrieve the calculi. If the calculi cannot be removed, ultrasonic lithotripsy (breaking up of the stone by ultrasound) is used. If infection is present, the area may be irrigated with an acidifier. Local anaesthesia may be used and recovery is rapid. The person may experience renal colic pain postoperatively, which is usually relieved with pethidine. There may be copious drainage of urine or serous fluid from the tract for 3 to 4 days postoperatively. Dressings are changed frequently to prevent infection and aid in patient comfort. A 2-week course of antibiotics is prescribed after surgery. Complications are rare but may include haemorrhage or sepsis; the patient should report signs of urinary bleeding, pain, or unexplained fever to the doctor immediately.

Extracorporeal shock wave lithotripsy

Extracorporeal shock wave lithotripsy (ESWL) is another recent development in the treatment of urinary stones. It is usually accomplished by submerging the patient in a large tub of warm water and aiming ultrasonic waves over the area of the urinary calculi. The water bath is used to allow the passage of shock waves into the body. Repeated firing of the ultrasonic waves results in the disintegration of the calculi. It may require more than 1500 shock waves to break up a large stone. The small particles pass spontaneously over 2 to 5 days. Because the procedure is uncomfortable general, regional, or local anaesthesia may be used. Aiming the sound waves is best accomplished when the patient is able to control both breathing and movement while in the water bath.

A newer method of ESWL omits the water bath. A membrane coupling device is applied to the skin over the kidney.[47] Because this approach requires less energy, intravenous sedation may be all that is necessary.

The patient may experience renal colic pain for several days after ESWL when passing the stone fragments. Pain is controlled by narcotic analgesics. Occasionally, urinary obstruction may occur as a result of stone fragments blocking urine flow. The patient is instructed to observe the volume of urine output for several days following discharge. Flank pain may indicate urinary retention. When these symptoms occur, the patient should contact the doctor immediately.

Open surgical removal of urinary calculi

Open surgery to remove renal calculi is performed less often since the advent of percutaneous nephrolithotomy and ESWL. The stone may be removed through the renal pelvis (pyelolithotomy), through the renal tissue (nephrolithotomy), or directly into a ureter. Large bladder stones may be removed through a suprapubic incision. Care of the patient undergoing urological surgery is discussed below.

Long-term care

People who have recurrent urinary calculi benefit from ongoing prophylactic therapy, which is determined by the type of stone being produced. *All* people with recurrent renal stones should drink fluids in sufficient quantity to produce very dilute urine and nocturia (unless contraindicated as with CHF). This may amount to a daily intake of up to 4 L of fluid. The purpose of the increased fluid intake is to rinse away any precipitates that can serve as a nidus for stone formation.

Any underlying identifiable cause of calciuria is treated to prevent recurrence of calcium stones. Hydrochlorothiazide (HCTZ) in doses of 50 mg twice a day may be prescribed for people with hypercalciuria to decrease urinary excretion of calcium. People receiving HCTZ therapy must be monitored carefully for signs of electrolyte imbalances, especially hypokalaemia.

As previously stated, more than 50% of calcium stones are idiopathic. Foods high in calcium are sometimes restricted, but a very low-calcium diet is usually unsatisfactory because it is unpalatable. The solubility of oxalate salts is not pH dependent; therefore manipulation of pH is not useful. Sodium or potassium phosphate, 1.5 to 2 g/day, may be prescribed to decrease levels of urinary calcium.

Phosphate calculi develop in alkaline urine; thus their prevention depends on keeping the urine acid and preventing a UTI. Medications such as ascorbic acid or ammonium chloride may be given for a time to increase urine acidity.

Prophylaxis for *uric acid* stones consists of alkalinizing the urine by the administration of sodium-potassium citrate solution sufficient to maintain a urine pH of 6 to 6.5. Allopurinol may be prescribed to inhibit synthesis of uric acid.

Interventions to achieve patient outcomes

Alleviating pain

Assess and document the quality, location, intensity, and duration of the pain. Administer prescribed narcotics and antispasmodics and evaluate and document the response. Provide warm blankets, heating pad (if prescribed) to affected area, or warm baths to increase regional circulation and relax tense muscles. Back rubs are especially helpful for a postoperative patient who was in a lithotomy position during surgery. Because renal colic pain is especially excruciating, other measures to help reduce pain (Chapter 8) may be tried, but may not be very successful.

Notify the doctor of a sudden cessation of pain. This can signal the passage of a stone. Strain all urine for solid matter and send fragments or stones to the laboratory for analysis, as instructed.

Facilitating patient learning

Teaching focuses on methods to prevent recurrence of urinary calculi and symptoms of recurrence to be reported to the doctor.
1. Methods to prevent UTI (which may lead to stasis and deposition of crystals leading to stone development):
   a. Drink at least 3000 ml of fluids each day.
   b. Avoid situations that lead to urinary stasis whenever possible (such as long periods of inactivity).
   c. Practise good perineal hygiene.
2. Dietary prescriptions, including a variety of menus that include necessary dietary restrictions (acid or alkaline ash diets).
3. Prescribed medication regimen: names, dosages, side effects.
4. Need to report signs and symptoms of calculi recurrence (flank pain or pain radiating down into the groin).

Evaluation

Evaluation is based on expected patient outcomes. Questions to consider may include the following:
1. Does the patient have signs and symptoms of flank pain or pain radiating down into groin?
2. Has the medication been effective in relieving the patient's pain?
3. Can the patient describe measures to prevent recurrence of urinary calculi and signs of recurrence to be reported to doctor?

UROLOGICAL SURGERY

Surgery of the urinary tract may be performed for various reasons, such as renal calculi, tumours, multiple cysts, trauma, congenital defects, "floating" kidney (nephroptosis), or renal hypertension. The types of surgeries are described in Table 25-8.

Preoperative Care

General preoperative preparation for surgery (Chapter 14) is appropriate for the urology patient. Patient concerns may be focused not only on the diagnosis but also on possible changes in urinary elimination. For many patients, interruption in urinary elimination is temporary. If one kidney is removed, adequate waste removal can be maintained by the remaining kidney or by even less than half of one kidney remaining functional. The remaining kidney may grow to handle the extra load.

Partial removal of the bladder will decrease capacity of the bladder to about 60 ml immediately postoperatively, but the elastic tissue of the bladder will regenerate so that the person is able to retain from 200 to 400 ml of urine within several months. If the entire bladder is removed, diversion of the urinary tract is necessary.

Instructions in effective deep breathing exercises are crucial after kidney surgery because of the high flank incision interfering with ventilation.

Postoperative Care

The basic needs of the patient requiring urological surgery are the same as those of any other surgical patient. Special

Table 25-8 Types of urological surgery

Site	Surgery	Description
Kidney	Nephrectomy	Removal of a kidney
	Partial nephrectomy	Removal of part of a kidney
	Pyelolithotomy	Incision into renal pelvis for removal of calculi
	Nephrolithotomy	Incision into kidney parenchyma for removal of calculi
	Nephropexy	Fixation of a floating kidney
	Pyeloplasty	Plastic repair of ureteropelvic junction
Ureters	Ureterolithotomy	Incision into ureters for removal of calculi
	Ureterectomy	Excision of a ureter
	Ureterostomy	Creation of a new outlet for a ureter
Bladder	Cystectomy	Removal of the bladder
	Segmental bladder resection	Partial removal of the bladder

emphasis is placed on promotion of ventilation and adequate urinary output, prevention of distension and haemorrhage, and attention to drainage tubes and dressing (see Box 25-12).

Promoting ventilation

Surgery of the kidney or upper ureters usually involves a flank incision that can influence respiratory status. Because the incision is directly below the diaphragm, deep breathing is painful and the patient is reluctant to take deep breaths. Splinting of the chest is common, and therefore atelectasis or other respiratory complications must be guarded against. In addition, because of the placement of the incision there is a greater incisional pull every time the person moves, as compared with an abdominal incision. The patient is often reluctant to turn in bed or to get up to ambulate. Most patients will be more comfortable turning themselves if they are given time, side rails to hold onto, and encouragement. Incisional pain usually requires a narcotic every 3 to 4 hours for 24 to 48 hours after surgery. Turning, ambulation, and deep breathing exercises can be planned so that these activities occur at the time the analgesic has the greatest effect. Patients may lie on the affected side unless a nephrostomy tube is in place. Even then they can be tilted to the affected side with pillows placed at the back for support. Ascertain that the tube is not kinked and that there is no traction on it.

Promoting adequate urinary output

Monitor urinary output carefully for several days postoperatively to ascertain adequate renal functioning and drainage. The output should be at least 50 ml/hour, preferably greater, to prevent urinary stasis and subsequent infection. A urinary output of 20 to 30 ml/hour in a patient with satisfactory fluid intake (at least 1200 ml/day) and in the absence of signs of urinary retention is reported imme-

diately to the doctor. Urinary output includes drainage from nephrostomy or cystostomy tubes, urethral or ureteral catheters, and an estimate from urine-soaked dressings. Daily weights are compared with the preoperative weight and with each other to identify fluid retention.

Relieving distension

Following kidney surgery most patients have some abdominal distension that may result in part from pressure on the stomach and intestinal tract during surgery. Patients who have had renal colic before surgery frequently develop paralytic ileus postoperatively. This condition may be related to the reflex GI tract symptoms caused by postoperative pain. Because of the problem of abdominal distension following renal surgery, food and fluids by mouth are often restricted 24 to 48 hours postoperatively. By the fourth postoperative day most patients tolerate a regular diet. Fluids are then usually forced to 3000 ml/day.

Preventing haemorrhage

Haemorrhage may follow such operative procedures as prostatectomy, nephrolithotomy, or nephrectomy. It occurs most often when the highly vascular parenchyma of the kidney has been incised. The bleeding may occur on the day of surgery, or it may occur 8 to 12 days postoperatively, during the period when tissue sloughing normally occurs with healing. The presence of bright red blood on the dressing or in the urine is reported immediately to the doctor. The patient is observed for signs of shock. Because many patients with urological disease have hypertension, the blood pressure may be relatively high but still represent a marked drop for the individual. Comparisons should therefore be made with baseline data.

If haemorrhage occurs, a pressure dressing is applied over the incision while the doctor's arrival is awaited. Measures to prevent shock are instituted. Several litres of sterile saline solution for irrigation should be available.

Changing dressings

There may be large amounts of urinary drainage following urological surgery, except after nephrectomy. The drainage may be pink or dark red but should not be bright red. If the surgery involves a flank incision, drainage is usually the heaviest on the posterior edge of the dressing because of gravity flow. It is important therefore to turn the patient on the side opposite the surgery to examine the posterior edge of the dressing. When a suprapubic incision is present, drainage is heaviest on the side and in the inguinal region.

The dressings are usually held in place by straps and must be changed frequently. Urinary drainage irritates the skin, has an unpleasant odour, and leads to discomfort. If a drain is present, the end of the drain should be placed over dressings, then covered with additional dressings to absorb the drainage. If a drainage tube is present, presence of large amounts of drainage on the dressing with little drainage coming from the tube indicates blockage of the tube. If a large amount of drainage is present, a disposable drainage bag used for urinary stomas may be applied over the drainage site.

The patient following urological surgery

Promote ventilation:
  Encourage breathing exercises.
  Encourage frequent self-turning in bed.
  Encourage ambulation.
Monitor output and maintain patency of urinary
  catheters.
Prevent complications:
  Change wet dressings to protect skin.
  Restrict food and oral fluids if paralytic ileus is
    present.
  Encourage fluids to 3000 or more ml/day
    when permitted.
  Monitor for bright red blood on dressing or in
    urine.

A catheter is usually inserted during surgery to drain urine from the operative area and permit healing to occur. Different types of drainage tubes may be inserted, and each tube is connected to a separate drainage system. It is important to know the purpose of the catheter and the area to be drained.

BENIGN PROSTATIC HYPERTROPHY

Aetiology/Epidemiology

Benign prostatic hypertrophy (BPH) is an adenomatous enlargement of the prostate gland. More than half of all men over 50 years of age and 75% of men over 70 have some symptoms of prostatic enlargement. The cause is not known but appears to be related to changing hormone levels that are experienced during the ageing process.

Pathophysiology

The prostate is an encapsulated gland, weighing about 20 g, that encircles the male urethra below the bladder neck. The signs and symptoms associated with BPH are the result of the enlargement of the prostate causing a partial or complete obstruction of the lower urinary tract.

One of the early symptoms of benign prostatic hypertrophy is *nocturia* (awakening at night to void) and urinary *frequency* in general. The man notices that the urinary stream is smaller and more difficult to start (*hesitancy*). The bladder muscle must contract more forcibly to push the urine past the partial obstruction, and the overworked muscles hypertrophy. Stagnant urine is held in trabeculae, or cellules, formed by sagging of the atonic mucous membranes between hypertrophied muscle bands. The bladder will not empty completely at each voiding (residual urine). This urine becomes alkaline from stasis and is a fertile medium for bacterial growth. The man will then complain of symptoms of cystitis (frequency, urgency), and bladder stones may occur. Some men develop haematuria from rupture of blood vessels that have become overstretched. Destruction of renal function can eventually occur from back pressure up the ureter to the kidney. Acute urinary retention is not uncommon.

Assessment
Subjective data

The most frequent and disturbing symptoms of BPH include dysuria and nocturia. The man is asked about urinary patterns, including the presence of frequency, hesitancy, dribbling, number of times he must get up at night to void, and the force of the urinary stream. *Hesitancy* refers to difficulty in initiating voiding that is often accompanied by a decrease in the force and flow of the urinary stream. The man is asked if he has to strain to start or maintain the urinary flow.

Because urinary tract infection may occur as a result of stasis of urine, the man is assessed for chills and pain or burning on urination.

Objective data

Patterns and amounts of urination are noted. The bladder is distended and, when percussed, elicits a "kettle drum" sound.

Diagnostic tests

Urinalysis is performed to determine the presence of casts, crystals, and blood cells, and a urine culture is obtained to assess for infection. Blood urea and serum creatinine tests are important to determine the level of renal function. An IVP is usually obtained to evaluate the functions and structure of the kidneys and urinary tract.

Enlargement of the lateral lobes of the prostate gland may be palpated by digital rectal examination. Enlargement of the middle lobe is diagnosed by signs of partial obstruction of the urethra, and the obstruction and bladder trabeculae are visualized by cystoscopy.

Cystoscopy

Cystoscopy is the direct examination of the bladder using an instrument called a *cystoscope*. The cystoscope relies on a flexible optical fibre to provide illumination into the urinary tract. The instrument is attached to the illuminating source then slowly passed through the urinary tract, thus enabling direct visualization of the urethra, ureteral orifices, and bladder.

Preprocedure care

Fluids are forced for several hours before the procedure. This ensures a continuous flow of urine, in the event that specimens need to be collected, and aids in preventing multiplication of bacteria that may be introduced during the procedure. If X-rays are to be taken during the procedure, bowel preparation may be ordered.

Method

If the patient is relatively comfortable and relaxed, the cystoscope can be passed with little discomfort, provided there is no obstruction in the urethra. A local anaesthetic such as lignocaine may be instilled into the urethra before insertion of the cystoscope. Any discomfort felt during this procedure is the result of contraction or spasm of the bladder sphincters; this can be decreased through deep-breathing exercises and general relaxation on the part of the patient. A sedative such as diazepam may be given to the anxious patient. General anaesthesia is required when the patient is overly apprehensive or when much manipulation is anticipated. In these instances, anaesthesia reduces the possibility of trauma to the urethra or perforation of the bladder caused by sudden vigorous movement of the patient during the examination.

When the patient is awake, passing the instrument will be followed immediately by a strong desire to void. This occurs as a result of the pressure the instrument exerts against the internal sphincter. During the examination the bladder is distended with distilled water to make visualization more effective. As the bladder becomes increasingly distended, the urge to void increases.

During cystoscopy a number of tests may be performed on the urinary system. *Cystography* involves the injection of a radiopaque dye or air as a contrast medium to visualize the bladder and determine its size, shape, and any irregularities. Bladder capacity may be measured through instillation of distilled water. A *voiding cystourethrogram* can reveal reflux of urine into the ureters on voiding, a bladder malfunction that can lead to pyelonephritis.

Ureteral catheterization (with a nylon, radiopaque, No. 4 to 6 Fr catheter) can be performed through the cystoscope. The catheter is inserted into the ureteral opening in the bladder, into the ureter, and into the renal pelvis. This procedure may involve one or both ureters. It is performed (1) when culture and analysis of urine from individual kidneys is required; (2) when tests of renal function are to be performed on the kidneys separately; and (3) when visualization of the urinary tract is desired and intravenous pyelogram visualization has been inadequate, obstruction is present, or sensitivity to intravenous radiopaque material is noted.

Postprocedure care

Care should be taken that the patient does not stand or walk alone immediately after cystoscopy. Blood that has drained from the legs while the patient is in the lithotomy position will flow back into the vessels of the feet and legs as the person stands. Accidents caused by dizziness and fainting can occur from the sudden change in distribution of blood.

Three complications of cystoscopy that need to be monitored are bleeding, perforation of the bladder, and spread of infection throughout the urinary tract or into the bloodstream (sepsis). Observation for frank bleeding (pink-tinged urine is normal) is necessary. Monitor urinary output and voiding pattern to detect obstruction, and increase fluid intake to prevent stasis. Administer mild analgesics for discomfort, and provide warmth if the patient complains of being chilly. Monitor vital signs as necessary.

Interventions

If urinary retention is present, the man is catheterized to relieve the retention. If the obstruction is severe, an indwelling catheter is inserted. Urinary tract infection is treated with antibiotics. Surgery is the primary treatment for BPH. During surgery the capsule of the prostate gland is left intact, and the adenomatous soft tissue is removed by one of four surgical routes: transurethral, suprapubic, retropubic, or perineal (Table 25-9).

Two newer approaches include *balloon dilatation* of the prostate under endoscopy, and *transurethral incision of the prostate* (TUIP) at the bladder neck. These measures break the prostatic capsule and allow for decompression of the prostate.[54]

Table 25-9 Comparison of types of prostatic surgery

	Transurethral resection	Suprapubic resection	Retropubic resection	Perineal resection	Total perineal resection
Reason for surgery	Enlargement of medial lobe surrounding urethra	Extremely large mass of obstructing tissue	Large mass located high in pelvic area	Large mass located low in pelvic area	Cancer of prostate gland
Location of incision	No incision; removal by way of urethra	Low midline abdominal incision through bladder to prostate gland	Low midline abdominal incision into prostate gland (bladder not incised)	Incision between scrotum and rectum	Large perineal incision between scrotum and rectum
Drainage tubes	Three-way Foley catheter with 30-ml bag in urethra, constant irrigation for 24 hr	Cystotomy tube or drain through incision; Foley catheter with 30-ml bag in urethra	Foley catheter with 30-ml bag in urethra, constant irrigation for 24 hr	Foley catheter with 30-ml bag in urethra	Foley catheter with 30-ml bag in urethra; drain in incision
Bladder spasms	Yes	Yes	Few	Few	Few
Dressing	None	Abdominal dressing easily soaked with urinary drainage	Abdominal dressing; no urinary drainage	Perineal dressing; no urinary drainage	Perineal dressing; urinary drainage
Complications	Haemorrhage; water intoxication; incontinence	Haemorrhage; wound infection	Haemorrhage; wound infection	Haemorrhage; wound infection	Urinary incontinence; wound infection; impotence; sterility

Transurethral prostatectomy

Transurethral prostatic resection (TURP) is performed when the major enlargement exists in the medial lobe that directly surrounds the urethra. There must be a relatively small amount of tissue requiring resection so that excessive bleeding will not occur and the time required to complete the surgery will not be prolonged. A resectoscope (an instrument similar to a cystoscope but equipped with a cutting and cauterization loop attached to electric current) is passed through the urethra. The bladder is irrigated continuously during the procedure. Tiny pieces of tissue are cut away, and the bleeding points are sealed by cauterization. A transurethral prostatectomy may be performed with the patient under general or spinal anaesthesia.

Urinary drainage

Following a TURP, a large (No. 24 Fr) three-way Foley catheter with a 30-ml balloon is usually inserted into the urethra. After the retention balloon of the catheter is inflated, the catheter is pulled down so that the bag rests in the prostatic fossa and provides haemostasis. Traction may be applied to the Foley catheter to increase pressure on the operative area to control bleeding. The large-size catheter (No. 24 Fr) is used to facilitate removal of clots from the bladder. Because the catheter retention balloon exerts pressure on the internal sphincter of the bladder, the patient continually feels the urge to void. If the catheter is draining properly, the strongest of these sensations usually passes momentarily. Attempting to void around the catheter causes the bladder muscles to contract and results in a painful "bladder spasm."

Discuss the physiology of the "need to void" with the patient preoperatively so that spasms will be seen as an expected event and not an abnormal complication. Teach the patient that the catheter produces the sensation of fullness and that *not* straining to pass urine around the catheter and drinking large amounts of fluids reduces irritation and spasm. Narcotics are given to lessen the pain sensation; antispasmodics are prescribed to relieve bladder spasms. As the nerve endings become fatigued, the frequency and severity of spasms decrease, usually in 24 to 48 hours.

The bladder is constantly irrigated initially by a three-way drip with normal saline or other prescribed solution. The purpose of constant irrigation is to keep the bladder free of clots that would block urinary drainage. Constant bladder irrigation is usually discontinued after 24 hours if no clots are draining from the bladder. The catheter may then be irrigated manually as necessary.

The patient may not be able to void after removal of the catheter because of urethral oedema, and the catheter may have to be reinserted. There may also be some urinary incontinence after catheter removal because the internal and external sphincters, which lie above and below the prostate gland, may have been disturbed during surgery. Continence usually returns. The time, amount, and control of voiding is recorded until normal urinary elimination patterns return.

Complications

Persistent bladder discomfort, bladder spasms, or failure of a catheter to drain properly usually signifies one of several serious complications that require immediate medical attention: (1) haemorrhage and clot retention, (2) catheter displacement, or (3) unsuspected *bladder perforation* during surgery as evidenced by severe abdominal pain.

Bleeding may result from a full bladder causing pressure on the outside of the prostatic fossa, "milking" the bleeding vessels. Straining to have a bowel movement may also cause prostatic haemorrhage, as can enemas, rectal tubes, and rectal thermometers, all of which are avoided for about a week postoperatively. About 2 weeks after TURP, when desiccated tissue is sloughed out, there may be a secondary haemorrhage. Instruct the patient to report any bleeding to the doctor.

Patients now rarely develop *water intoxication* as a result of excessive irrigating solution being absorbed into the venous sinusoids during surgery, but it may occur. Cerebral oedema may result, and patient confusion and agitation may be the first signs of this condition.

Suprapubic prostatectomy

The alternate methods of prostatectomy are open operations. In the *suprapubic resection* the prostate gland is removed from the urethra by way of the bladder; this type of resection is performed when a large mass of tissue must be resected. The usual method of draining urine following surgery is illustrated in Fig. 25-7, A. There will be some type of haemostatic agent placed in the prostatic fossa and urine will be drained by Foley catheter or cystotomy tube or both.

Haemorrhage is a possible complication, and the precautions are the same as those taken following TURP. Because there is some oozing of blood from the prostatic fossa, continuous bladder irrigations are usually ordered for the first 24 hours.

Cystotomy tubes are usually removed 3 to 4 days postoperatively; urethral catheters generally remain until the suprapubic wound is healed. After the urethral catheter has been removed, the nursing care of the patient is similar to that for the patient undergoing transurethral resection. If the suprapubic wound should reopen and drain, a urethral catheter is usually reinserted.

Retropubic prostatectomy

In a retropubic prostatectomy a low abdominal incision similar to that used for suprapubic prostatectomy is made, but the bladder is not opened. Rather, it is retracted and the adenomatous prostatic tissue is removed through an incision in the anterior prostatic capsule (Fig. 25-7, B).

Sphincter muscles are seldom damaged by retropubic prostatectomy, and there is no urine fistula. A large Foley catheter is inserted postoperatively, but bladder spasms are not usually a problem. When the Foley catheter is removed, the patient seldom has difficulty voiding. Haemorrhage from the prostatic fossa and wound infection may complicate the surgery; therefore, precautions to prevent bleeding as discussed under TURP are taken. There should be no urinary drainage on the abdominal dressing. If urinary drainage on the abdominal dressing, purulent drainage,

Nursing Care Plan

Man with transurethral resection prostatectomy for benign prostatic hypertrophy

DATA: M. S. is a 72-year-old retired car mechanic. He had been in his usual state of good health until about 4 months ago when he stated to develop nocturia. Several weeks later he noted difficulty initiating voiding. He also noted mild dribbling after voiding. On physical examination his doctor noted moderate enlargement of his prostate. He is being admitted for cystoscopy and possible TURP. His vital signs are stable. He is married and states that his wife provides him support at home. He lives in a two-storey, single-family home.

The nursing history obtained on admission identified the following:
1. He has not been hospitalized before.
2. He does not take any medications.
3. He enjoys outdoor activities and exercises daily by walking 2 to 3 miles.
4. His expectations are that he will have the procedure and return to his normal life-style within a few days.
5. His wife is in constant attendance and tends to answer any questions that are asked of the patient.

Collaborative nursing actions include those to monitor for postoperative complications, including bleeding and dysuria. Specific nursing actions include monitoring the following:
1. Signs and symptoms of haemorrhage: haematuria; increased pulse; decreased blood pressure; restlessness; cool, moist skin
2. Inability to void once urinary catheter is removed

Nursing analysis: Urinary retention, high risk for: related to obstruction secondary to TURP

Expected patient outcomes	Nursing interventions	Rationale
Retention of urine does not occur	Monitor urinary output and characteristics	Detect retention early
	Maintain constant bladder irrigation as prescribed during first 24 hours	Prevent clots from obstructing urine flow
	Maintain patency of in-dwelling urinary catheter by irrigating	Prevent clots from obstructing catheter
	Encourage high fluid intake (2500 to 3000 ml/day)	Promote urinary flow
	After catheter is removed, continue to monitor for signs of retention	Detect retention early

Nursing analysis: Pain: related to bladder spasm

Expected patient outcomes	Nursing interventions	Rationale
Mr S. states feeling more comfortable	Teach Mr. S. not to try to void around catheter	Reduce likelihood of spasm
	Monitor for pain at regular intervals for 48 hours to identify early signs of bladder spasm	Identify presence of spasms so that medication may be administered
	Give prescribed medications (analgesics, antispasmodics)	Relieve pain
	Tell Mr. S. spasms will decrease in intensity and frequency within 24 to 48 hours	Decreased anxiety will decrease pain

Nursing analysis: Injury, high risk for: haemorrhage or infection related to surgery

Expected patient outcomes	Nursing interventions	Rationale
Infection does not occur Bleeding is minimized	Monitor vital signs, report signs of shock or fever	Prevent shock before it occurs
	Monitor appearance of urine for persistent bright red colour rather than expected dark red beyond first few hours postoperatively	Urine should change from cherry pink to amber in the first 2 to 3 postoperative days

Nursing analysis: Injury, high risk for: haemorrhage or infection related to surgery—cont'd

Expected patient outcomes	Nursing interventions	Rationale
	Teach Mr. S. to avoid Valsalva manoeuvre	May initiate prostatic bleeding during initial postoperative period because of pressure
	Avoid use of rectal thermometers, rectal examinations, or enemas for at least 1 week	May initiate prostatic bleeding
	Maintain strict asepsis of urinary drainage system, irrigate only when necessary	Minimize potential of introducing organisms that could cause infection
	Encourage high fluid intake to 3000 ml/day	Increase urinary output that will reduce potential of infection

Nursing analysis: Incontinence, stress or urge: related to catheter removal following surgery

Expected patient outcomes	Nursing interventions	Rationale
Mr. S. achieves urinary control	Assess Mr. S. for dribbling after catheter is removed	Detect incontinence
	If dribbling occurs:	
	a. Tell Mr. S. this is common occurrence and continence will return	Patient needs to be reassured this is normal
	b. Teach perineal exercises	Assist in bladder control

Nursing analysis: Sexual dysfunction: high risk for, related to TURP

Expected patient outcomes	Nursing interventions	Rationale
Sexual functioning is maintained	Give Mr. S. opportunity to discuss feelings about effects of prostatectomy on sexual intercourse	This is a difficult subject for many patients to raise
	Provide information as necessary	Lack of knowledge may create anxiety and lead to sexual dysfunction
	a. Probable return of previous level of functioning	
	b. Occurrence of retrograde ejaculation (urine may have a milky appearance)	
	Avoid sexual intercourse for 3 to 4 weeks after surgery	Bleeding and discomfort may occur

Nursing analysis: Knowledge deficit: related to TURP

Expected patient outcomes	Nursing interventions	Rationale
Mr. S. describes activity restrictions and need for medical follow-up	Teach Mr. S.:	May initiate bleeding
	a. Avoidance of heavy activities for 3 to 4 weeks (check with doctor regarding resumption of long walks)	
	b. Avoidance of straining at stool for 4 to 6 weeks; use of stool softeners or laxatives as necessary	Straining may initiate bleeding; stool softeners will reduce the need to strain at stool
	c. Fluid maintenance of at least 2500 ml to 3000 ml/day	Will reduce potential of infection and clot formation
	d. Instructions for medical follow-up	Follow-up is essential to ensure no complications have developed

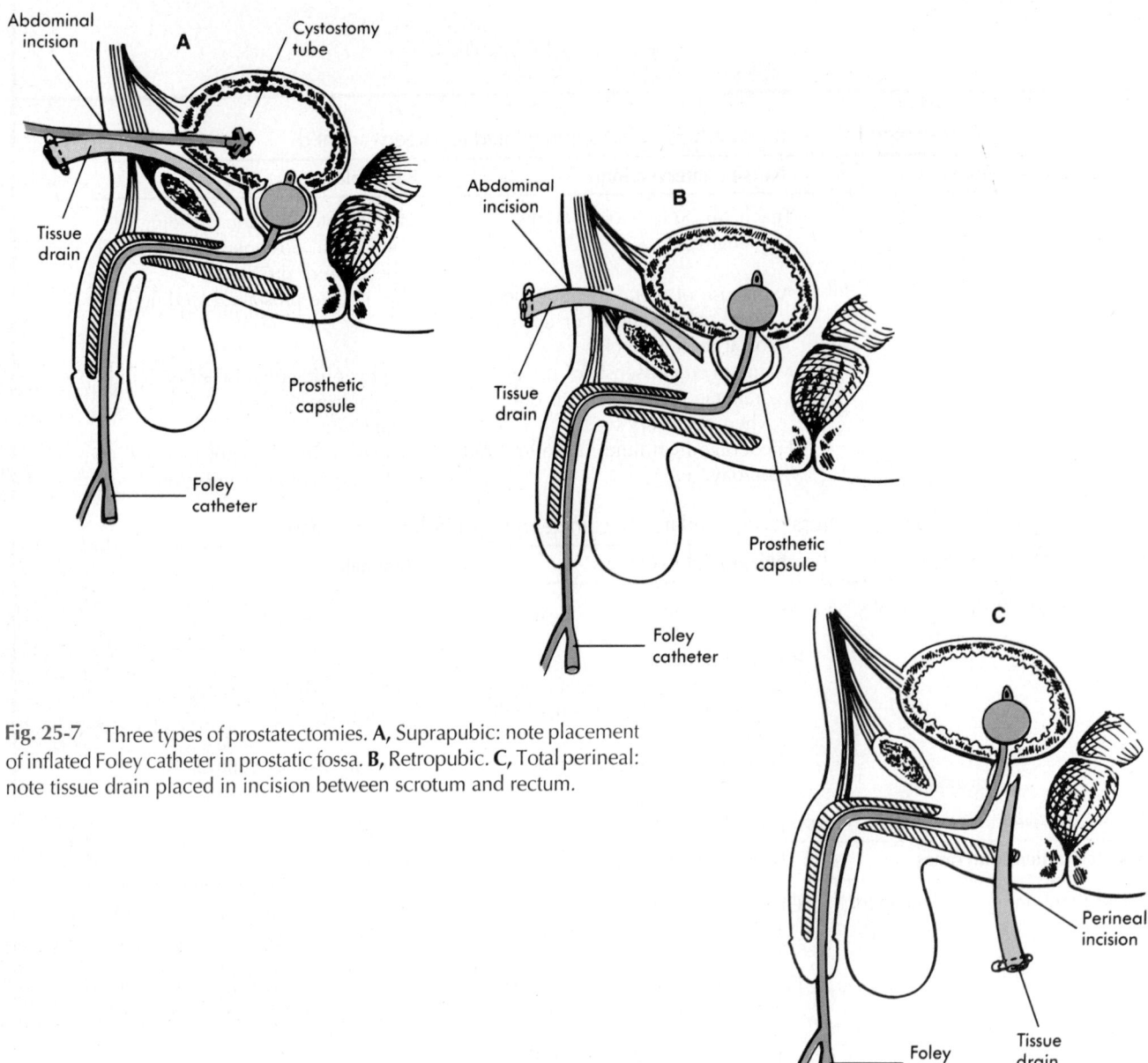

Fig. 25-7   Three types of prostatectomies. **A,** Suprapubic: note placement of inflated Foley catheter in prostatic fossa. **B,** Retropubic. **C,** Total perineal: note tissue drain placed in incision between scrotum and rectum.

fever, or increased pain with ambulation occurs, notify the doctor because these symptoms may indicate deep wound infection or pelvic abscess.

Perineal prostatectomy

The perineal approach is used primarily for confirmed or suspected cancer of the prostate (Fig. 25-7, C). The incision is made between the scrotum and rectum. In addition to removal of the adenomatous prostate tissue, adjacent tissue may be excised when cancer is confirmed. Preoperative and postoperative care is similar to that given a patient having radical perineal surgery.

Postoperative counselling and teaching

Common to all patients undergoing prostatectomy are concerns regarding *sexual functioning* and the *ability to be continent of urine.* The nurse may need to provide an opportunity during interactions with the patient to promote expressions of these concerns by the patient. Impotence may occur physiologically if the perineal nerves are cut during a radical perineal prostatectomy, not with the other types of prostatectomies. If the man believes that the surgery will or may produce impotence, however, this may occur because of psychological influences. Temporary urinary incontinence frequently follows transurethral or suprapubic prostatectomy. Most men have some difficulty with continence after any type of prostatectomy. The patient should understand that this is normal for a period after surgery, and he should be taught perineal exercises to hasten recovery of control over voiding.

The following points should be included in preparing the patient for discharge from the hospital: (1) Vigorous exercises, heavy lifting, and sexual intercourse should be avoided for about 3 weeks after returning home. (2) Driving during this period is also not advised. (3) Straining with defecation should be avoided; stool softeners or mild cathartics may be prescribed as home-going medication. (4) Fluids are encouraged to prevent stasis and infection and to keep stools soft. (5) The patient is instructed to notify his GP should his urinary stream diminish. The urinary stream also will be checked on the patient's postoperative visit to the hospital. This is important because urethral mucosa in the prostatic area is destroyed during surgery and strictures may form with healing.

URETHRAL STRICTURES

A urethral stricture is a narrowing or constriction of the lumen of the urethra. Urethral strictures can be congenital or acquired. Congenital urethral strictures can occur in isolation or in combination with other urinary tract anomalies. Acquired urethral stricture can result from trauma secondary to accident or instrumentation, infection, muscular spasm, or pressure from the outside, by adjacent structures, or by growing tumours. Urethral strictures occur more often in men than women, primarily because of the length of the urethra.

Urethral strictures are repaired by transurethral visual urethrotomy or by urethroplasty with end-to-end anastomosis or with an inlay graft. Care of the person after transurethral visual urethrotomy is similar to that after a TURP (p. 703). The urethroplasty is open surgical repair through a lower abdominal approach; the care of the patient is similar to that following other urological surgeries (p. 699).

NEOPLASMS

Neoplasms of the urinary system are a significant source of morbidity. The major neoplasms are found in the kidney and bladder. Cancer of the prostate causes urinary problems by pressure on the urethra, leading to obstruction (Table 25-10). Tumours growing anywhere within the abdominal cavity can result in renal involvement through metastasis or invasion, or by pressure of the tumour creating urinary obstruction. Urinary diversion (p. 709) may be required in treating urinary neoplasms.

RENAL NEOPLASMS

Malignant renal tumours, primarily adenocarcinomas, account for 1.6% of cancers in men and 1% in women (OPCS 1986). Small benign renal tumours (adenomas) may occur without causing significant damage or symptoms. Renal cell carcinomas rarely occur before the age of 40 years, are more commonly seen in the 50-to 70-year age range, and occur twice as often in men as in women.[47]

Haematuria is the most frequent symptom of renal cell carcinoma. Unfortunately, the haematuria is often intermittent, lessening the person's concern and causing procrastination in seeking medical care. Any person with hae-

maturia should have a complete urological examination, because it is only by immediate investigation of the first signs of haematuria that there is any hope of cure. Other symptoms may include dull flank pain, flank mass, weight loss, fever, hypercalcaemia, increased sedimentation rate, and polycythaemia. Hypertension may result from stimulation of the renin-angiotensin system.

An IVP may show a distortion of renal outline suggesting a kidney tumour. Small tumours in the parenchyma may not be apparent on a routine pyelogram but may be identified by ultrasound or CT scan. A CT scan is also useful in differentiating between renal cell carcinoma and renal cyst. Angiography may also be performed to differentiate a cyst from a tumour.

Unless the patient is a poor surgical risk or has extensive metastases, the diseased kidney is removed (*nephrectomy*) through a transabdominal, thoracoabdominal, or retroperitoneal approach. The first two approaches are preferred to secure the renal artery and vein and prevent any spread of malignant cells. (See p. 699 for care of the patient requiring urological surgery.)

Following surgery for a malignant tumour that is radiosensitive, the patient may be given a course of X-ray therapy. Hospitalization may not be necessary during this time. Chemotherapy has not yet proved of value in the treatment of renal cell carcinomas. The survival rate after therapy depends on the extent of metastasis. The 10-year survival rate is very low, especially because many people do not seek initial treatment until the disease is far advanced.

TUMOURS OF THE BLADDER

Aetiology/Epidemiology

The most common site of cancer in the urinary tract is the bladder. It occurs four times more often in men than women, and more often in people over the age of 50. Bladder cancer occurs twice as often in *smokers* than nonsmokers.[3,6a] Other risk factors include aniline dye and schistosomiasis.

Pathophysiology

Almost half of bladder tumours involve the trigone of the bladder, and most of the remainder are found on the posterior and lateral walls. Tumours range from small benign papillomas to large invasive carcinomas. Most of the neoplasms begin as papillomas; therefore, all bladder papillomas are considered premalignant and are removed when identified. Squamous cell carcinoma occurs less frequently and has a poorer prognosis.

Grades I (well differentiated) and II (medially differentiated) bladder tumours are usually superficial, while grades III (poorly differentiated) and IV (anaplastic) tumours are usually invasive. Bladder cancers are *staged* according to the depth of invasiveness:

Stage O:	Mucosa
State A:	Submucosa
Stage B:	Muscle
State C:	Perivesical fat
State D:	Lymph nodes

<u>REVIEW</u>

Table 25-10   Tumours of the urinary tract

Site	Incidence	Signs and symptoms	Medical therapy
Kidney	2%	Haematuria Dull flank pain Flank mass Unexplained weight loss Fever Polycythaemia	Nephrectomy Radiation
Bladder	5%	Intermittent haematuria Anaemia Cystitis Suprapubic pain RBCs, WBCs, and bacteria in 　urine	Transurethral fulguration or excision of small papillomas Segmental or total cystectomy Intravesicular chemotherapy if the bladder is not removed Palliative chemotherapy
Prostate	20%	Urethral obstruction Low-back pain Haematuria Anaemia	Radical resection of prostate Radiation Hormonal therapy

Painless *haematuria* is the first symptom in the majority of bladder tumours. It is usually intermittent, and the individual may fail to seek treatment. Painless haematuria occurs also in nonmalignant urinary tract disease and in cancer of the kidney; therefore, any haematuria should be investigated. Cystitis may be the first symptom of a bladder tumour because the tumour may act as a foreign body in the bladder. Renal failure from obstruction of the ureters sometimes is the reason given for seeking medical care. Vesicovaginal fistulas may occur before other symptoms develop. The last two conditions indicate a poor prognosis because usually the tumour has infiltrated widely.

Diagnostic tests

Cytology examination of the urine may identify malignant cells before the lesion can be visualized by cystoscopy. The diagnosis is established by cystoscopic visualization of the bladder with biopsy. Clinical determination of the invasiveness of the tumour is important in establishing a therapeutic regimen and in predicting the prognosis. Any patient who has had a papilloma removed should have a cystoscopic examination every 3 months for 2 years and then at less frequent intervals if there is no evidence of a new lesion. The necessity for frequent examination should be fully explained by the urologist, and the explanation should be reinforced by the nurse. Emphasize the need for repeated cystoscopies because papillomas tend to recur without symptoms until they are far advanced tumours.

Interventions

Surgery

Small tumours with minimal tissue layer involvement may be adequately treated with transurethral fulguration or excision. A Foley catheter may or may not be inserted after surgery. Nd:YAG-lasers may be used for low-grade tumours. The urine may be pink tinged, but gross bleeding is unusual. Burning on urination may be relieved by forcing fluids and applying heat over the bladder region by means of a heating pad.

If the tumour involves the dome of the bladder, a *segmental resection* of the bladder (p. 700) may be carried out. Over half of the bladder may be resected. A *cystectomy*, or complete removal of the bladder, usually is performed only when the disease appears curable. Complete removal of the bladder requires permanent urinary diversion (p. 709).

Radiation

External cobalt radiation of large invasive tumours may be given before surgery to retard tumour growth. Supervoltage irradiation can be given when the patient physically cannot tolerate surgery. Radiation is not curative and has little value in patient management if the tumour is deemed inoperable. Internal radiation is rarely used since the introduction of better methods of external radiation.

Chemotherapy

Chemotherapy is primarily palliative. Thiotepa may be instilled into the bladder as a topical treatment. The patient is dehydrated 8 to 12 hours before thiotepa treatment, and the drug remains in the bladder for 2 hours.

CANCER OF THE PROSTATE

The prostate gland is the second most common site of cancer among men. There is a familial tendency for the disease. Prostate cancer is responsible for 9% of all deaths from cancer in men in Britain.[53a] It rarely occurs before age 50 and the incidence increases with age. The younger the man at the age of onset, the more lethal is the disease. Although cancer may start anywhere within the prostate gland and may be multifocal in origin, it usually arises in the peripheral lobes resulting in a palpable nodule. Early detection of nodules on palpation can lead to early treatment and improve the prognosis significantly. For this reason all men over age 40 should have regular rectal examinations.

Prostate specific antigen (PSA) is elevated in the serum of about 60% of men with prostate cancer and serves as a tumour marker.[47] It is not a useful tool for prostate cancer screening, because up to 30% of men with BPH can have false-positive levels and 30% of men with prostatic cancer can have false-negative levels.[54] However, the PSA serum level drops sharply with complete response to treatment, which makes it helpful for determining effectiveness of therapy. Prostatic biopsy is performed for palpable prostate nodules.

Prostate cancer usually begins with changes in voiding patterns, including frequency, urgency, and nocturia because of the enlarged gland pressing on the urethra. Complete urethral obstruction can develop. Haematuria can occur resulting in anaemia. Treatment is surgery or radiation.

Total Prostatectomy

Total prostatectomy is usually curative in patients in whom a diagnosis of prostatic cancer is made before local extension of the cancer or distant metastasis. The entire prostate gland, including the capsule and adjacent tissue, is removed. The remaining urethra is then anastomosed to the bladder neck. The perineal approach is the favoured approach, but a retropubic route may also be used (see p. 703). Because the internal and external sphincters of the bladder lie close to the prostate gland, urinary incontinence may occur in about 4% of patients after prostatectomy.

Preoperative care

If a perineal approach is planned, the patient is given a bowel preparation similar to that for bowel surgery (Chapter 24) and only clear fluids the day before surgery to prevent faecal contamination of the operative site. Postoperatively, when food is permitted, a low-residue diet may be given until the wound has healed.

Total prostatectomy results in physiological sexual dysfunction from disruption of genital innervation in 20% of men.[54] Most of these patients lose emission, ejaculation, and erectile potency. Both the man and his sexual partner are alerted to the potential for sexual dysfunction before surgery, but it can be stressed that 80% will not experience sexual difficulties.

Postoperative care

The patient returns from surgery with an in-dwelling urethral catheter. A large amount of urinary drainage on the dressing for a number of hours is not unusual. This can be managed by use of an ostomy bag around the dressing. Urinary drainage should decrease rapidly. There should not be the amount of bleeding that follows other prostatic surgery.

Because the catheter is not being used for haemostasis, the patient usually has few bladder spasms. The catheter is used both for urinary drainage and as a splint for the urethral anastomosis; therefore, care is taken that it does not become dislodged or blocked. The risk of blockage is greatest during the first hour. The catheter may be irrigated intermittently or continuously as ordered by the urologist. The catheter is usually left in the bladder for 2 to 3 weeks.

Faecal incontinence may occur after surgery as a result of relaxation of the perineal musculature. Control of the rectal sphincter usually returns readily. Return of function can be facilitated by perineal exercises (p. 684) started within a day or two after surgery and continued after rectal sphincter control returns, to strengthen bladder sphincters (unless the bladder sphincters have been permanently damaged).

The patient who experiences sexual dysfunction or incontinence after total prostatectomy is often very depressed. At times the man may have difficulty talking to his sexual partner about his concerns and the effect of his impotence on their relationship. The nurse can encourage each person to share his and her feelings separately, then gently encourage and facilitate mutual sharing by the partners.

Radiation

Radiation may be used in place of surgery, especially with older men with curative lesions or in the absence of metastasis. The 15-year results are better with surgery than radiation for patients with localized lesions. External beam radiation or interstitial radiation may be used.

Palliative therapy

Patients with metastatic disease may be given androgen therapy in the form of diethylstilbesterol (DES) or orchiectomy (removal of the testes). Luteinizing hormone-releasing hormone (LHRH) agonists may be given to suppress LH and serum testosterone.[47] Corticosteroids may be given for bone pain.

URINARY DIVERSION

Urinary diversion procedures are surgical procedures that divert the urinary flow from its normal flow patterns to a newly created opening, usually on the abdominal wall. Although urinary neoplasms are one of the major reasons for urinary diversions, these procedures may also be performed for neurogenic bladder dysfunction, chronic progressive pyelonephritis, urinary birth defects, or irreparable urinary tract trauma.

Urinary Diversion Procedures

The most common urinary diversion procedures include ureterostomy, ileal or colonic conduits, and continent urostomie (see Box 25-13). These procedures require placement of an external abdominal stoma.

A *cutaneous ureterostomy* is used when the physical condition of the patient prohibits more extensive surgery. This is usually temporary therapy followed by more extensive treatment. The ureters drain directly through the stoma; there is no reservoir. Initially the ureterostomy stoma appears pink, but it turns pale in several weeks. Stricture of the ureter at the stoma may occur and is treated with dilatation; untreated strictures can result in hydronephrosis from urine backup. UTI is also a common complication.

The *ileal conduit (ileal loop)* is the most common permanent urinary diversion. A section of the ileum is resected with the mesentery and blood supply intact, and the ileum itself is then anastomosed (Fig. 25-8). The ureters are excised from the bladder and anastomosed to one end of the

25-13

Types of urinary diversions

Cutaneous ureterostomy
Ureters excised from bladder and brought out
  through skin in one or two stomas.

Conduit urostomies
Ureters drain into reservoir; urine flows freely
  through reservoir and out through stoma into a
  drainage bag
  Ileal conduit (ileal loop): a section of ileum is
    used to form a reservoir (Fig. 25-8)
  Colonic conduit: a section of the colon is used
    for the conduit reservoir

Continent urostomies
Ureters drain into a reservoir that has a valved
  stoma; stoma is catheterized to remove urine
  (drainage bag not required)
  Kock continent ileal reservoir: reservoir is
    formed from loops of small intestine (Fig. 25-9)
  Caecoileal continent urinary reservoir (Indiana
    pouch): reservoir formed from portion of
    large intestine and ileum

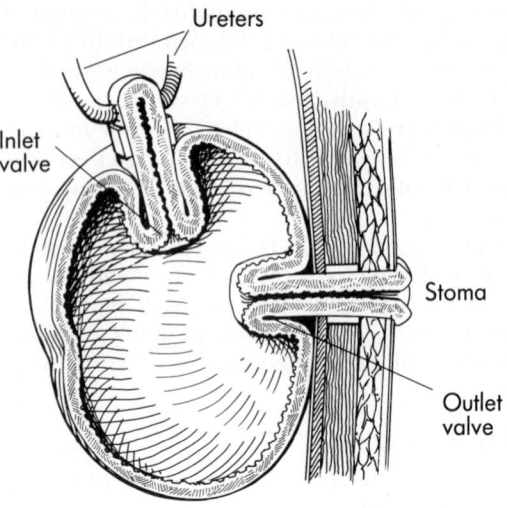

Fig. 25-9   Kock continent ileal urinary reservoir.

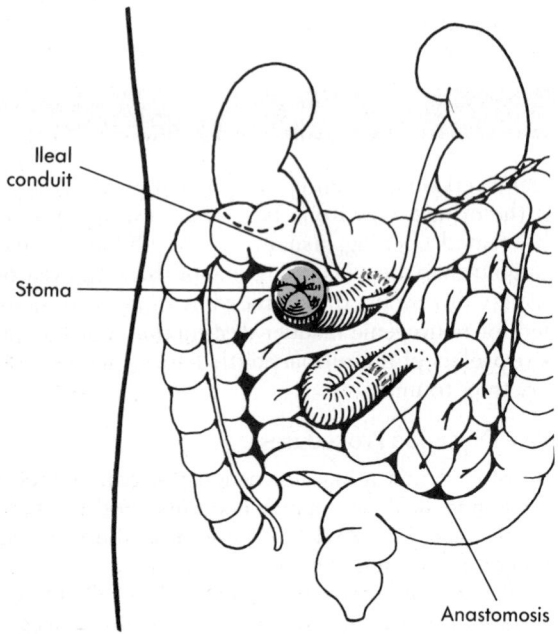

Fig. 25-8   Ileal conduit or ileal loop.

resected ileal portion; that end is then sutured closed to
form a pouch that serves as a conduit reservoir. The open
end of the resected ileal portion is then brought through the
abdominal wall to the skin to create a stoma. The urinary
bladder may be left intact or resected, depending on the
reason for the diversion. The *colonic conduit* is preferred by
some surgeons because it has been shown to reduce the
incidence of urinary reflux in some people.[6]

Continent urostomies, which are newer procedures,
differ from the ileal and colonic conduits by formation of a
"valved" stoma (Fig. 25-9). The urine remains in the
reservoir until removed by catheter; thus an external drainage bag is not required.

In the ileal and colonic conduits and continent
urostomies, the stoma should initially be bright red in
colour. Complications include haemorrhage, infection,
separation of the anastomosis, and paralytic ileus. Proce-
dural complications include leakage at the ureteral
anastomosis, obstruction of the ureter, mucocutaneous
separation, and stoma necrosis. UTI and stomal problems
may occur subsequently.

Preoperative Care

Changes in body image can be a significant effect of any
procedure that leads to the formation of a stoma, therefore,
it is important to prepare the patient appropriately for the
surgery. Individuals who have been well informed about
the surgery do better both in the immediate postoperative
period and in the long term. The person's questions must
be answered honestly and completely. The goals for
preoperative teaching must reflect the individual patient's
needs. Not every patient will want to see a stoma model or
urinary pouches before surgery; however, certain basic
information must be conveyed. The person should be able
to describe the surgical procedure and expected outcomes.

The person is instructed concerning the appearance of
the stoma. Anatomical charts, models, and simple drawings
are ways of explaining the placement of the stoma. It is
stressed that work, hobbies, physical activities, diet, and
clothing should not change significantly after surgery.

A patient who is willing may be given an opportunity to
handle a urostomy appliance to dispel any misconceptions.
Patients can be reassured that stoma care will be provided
immediately after surgery and that they will be assisted in
mastering self-care before hospital discharge.

When the nurse perceives that it is appropriate, a visit from a person who has mastered the care of a urostomy can be reassuring to the patient. Many local cancer societies have volunteers available to provide this support. Preoperative preparation for ureterostomy is similar to that for other bowel procedures (Chapter 23).

Location of the stoma on the abdomen depends on the procedure. Ideally, the determination of the exact location of the stoma is made before surgery and includes an evaluation of the person's body when lying, sitting, and standing. The reason for this careful evaluation is to ensure that the location of the stoma allows for a smooth, even skin surface surrounding the stoma, for optimal adherence of the appliance. Many hospitals have access to a Clinical Nurse Specialist in Stoma Care, who can tailor resources and information to the patient's needs.

Postoperative Care
Immediate care

Following a *cutaneous ureterostomy*, the patient generally returns from surgery with catheters (stents) inserted through the ureters to drain the renal pelves. The stents are usually left in place for 7 to 14 days. Patency of the catheters must be maintained because hydronephrosis can ensue rapidly if obstruction occurs.

After an *ileal* or *colonic conduit*, stents are usually left in place in the stoma for 7 to 10 days to promote urinary drainage. The person with a *continent urostomy* will usually have a catheter in the stoma sutured in place to allow drainage from the reservoir. Another drain tube may be placed into the pelvic area. These catheters prevent overdistension of the reservoir that may cause anastomosis leakage. A nasogastric tube with suction is also used for 2 to 3 days postoperatively to allow for the return of effective intestinal peristalsis and healing of the intestinal anastomosis. Nothing is permitted by mouth until the return of bowel sounds or passing of flatus; the diet is then gradually advanced from small amounts of fluids to a normal diet.

During the immediate postoperative period, urinary output is monitored closely; decreased urinary output could signal obstruction of urinary drainage or complications such as dehydration or renal failure. Urine is tested for presence of blood. Blood in the urine is expected in the immediate postoperative period; however, it should clear within the first few postoperative days.

The abdominal incision is assessed daily for healing and signs and symptoms of infection. Care of the abdominal incision is sometimes complicated by the leakage of urine into it; this complication is minimized by using appropriate drainage bags postoperatively.

Skin care

In any type of urinary diversion care must be taken to prevent urine leakage onto the surrounding skin and the abdominal incision. For the ureterostomy and the conduit procedures, a transparent pouch is placed around the stoma in the operating room. This allows visualization of the stoma, catheter or stents, and stoma sutures. Any evidence of grey or black discolouration, indicating stomal necrosis, is reported to the surgeon. The pouch is changed in 24 to 48 hours postoperatively to allow for better visualization and assessment of the stoma and peristomal skin.

In the early postoperative period, the pouch is positioned to drain to the side of the bed, facilitating drainage and emptying of the pouch. The urostomy pouch has a valve at the bottom that permits emptying. Drainage tubing and a collection bag can be attached to the valve of the pouch to allow continuous drainage in the postoperative period.

The skin is examined closely whenever the pouch is changed or if signs of skin problems are noted. Teach the patient to take action to correct problems that occur.

Use and care of pouches

The stomal oedema begins to subside within 7 days, but the stoma continues to decrease gradually in size for the next 6 to 8 weeks. The patient should be taught how to measure the stoma before going home, and how to adjust the pouch size to accommodate the smaller stoma. Too large an opening is a frequent cause of skin problems for people with an ileal or colon conduit. Too small an opening in the pouch may restrict circulation or cause trauma to the stoma.

Several types of pouches are available. All have two things in common: a pouch to collect the urine and an outlet or valve at the bottom for easy emptying every 3 to 4 hours. The basic types of pouches are (1) permanent pouches that can be washed and reused, (2) semidisposable pouches that fit onto a permanent disk or faceplate, and (3) one-piece or two-piece disposable pouches that are discarded after use. All adhere to the body with some form of adhesive to form a watertight seal. The type of pouch selected depends upon the patient's preference, body build, and special needs, such as physical or visual impairment. The enterostomal therapist can assist in the assessment and selection of the appropriate pouch for the patient.

Most people can wear a pouch for 3 to 5 days between changes. An interval longer than 7 days should be discouraged because of potential odour, crystallization problems, or risk of infection. An appropriate schedule that eliminates leakage and provides the best skin protection needs to be determined based on patient adaptation.

Proper cleaning of reusable equipment is essential for odour control, general hygiene, and prevention of stomal complications. Manufacturers include cleaning instructions with their equipment. The following are the principles for proper cleaning of reusable urinary appliances:
1. Clean equipment promptly.
2. Use adhesive remover as necessary to remove residue.
3. Avoid soaking equipment for prolonged periods of time (20 to 30 minutes in soap and water is sufficient). Longer soaking speeds deterioration of many appliances.
4. For odour problems, soak appliances in half-strength vinegar water for an additional 20 to 30 minutes.

Patient teaching

A teaching plan for the person with a urinary diversion includes the following:
1. Nature of the urinary diversion
2. Assessment of stoma appearance and changes that require medical attention
3. Methods to protect the skin
4. Use and care of pouches
5. Signs and symptoms of UTI
6. Community resources to obtain supplies and for ongoing support
7. Need for follow-up care

OTHER URINARY DISORDERS

Several disorders of the urinary tract do not fit into the classifications discussed thus far. These disorders, polycystic disease, vascular disorders, diabetic nephropathy, and trauma are discussed in this section.

POLYCYSTIC DISEASE
Aetiology/Epidemiology

Polycystic disease is an inherited defect that involves the kidneys bilaterally. It is categorized into two groups, infantile and adult. The infant usually develops symptoms and dies within a few months after birth. In adults, the disease is inherited as an autosomal dominant trait, and affects about 1 of every 500 adults. Symptoms usually develop between the ages of 20 to 50. It is evenly distributed between the sexes and accounts for 5% to 8% of adults with end-stage renal disease (ESRD), which is usually reached 10 to 15 years after symptoms arise.

There is no preventive care for polycystic disease. However, early detection and medical care can prevent and control infection of the diseased kidneys and retard the development of ESRD.

Pathophysiology

The kidneys are usually enlarged and filled with cysts. In adults, the collecting tubules are usually involved. At first only segments of the nephrons are cystic, but gradually the cysts increase in number and size. As the cysts enlarge, they distort the calyces and pelves and compress surrounding tissue causing ischaemia. Both kidneys can become large, grossly appear to be full of variously sized bubbles, and feel bumpy. The cysts can be filled with tubular fluid (urine), serous fluid, blood, or a combination of fluids.

Signs and symptoms relate to loss of tubular function and tissue destruction (haematuria, calculi, polyuria, proteinuria, and hypertension) and increased kidney size (abdominal fullness and palpable abdominal mass). Also, the kidneys often become infected and lose their ability to concentrate urine or regulate sodium. Patients with polycystic kidney disease are not as anaemic as other patients with ESRD because the site of erythropoietin production is not affected. Therefore, the energy level of these patients may be slightly higher than that of other patients with ESRD.

Patients with polycystic kidney disease usually continue to excrete a variable amount of urine, even though its quality is poor as a result of a gradual loss of tubular function. These patients do not retain as much fluid as an anuric patient with ESRD and can actually become volume depleted.

Nursing Process
Assessment
Subjective data

The patient is questioned about the presence and extent of discomfort and pain in the flank. Colicky pain may be experienced when clots are passed down the ureter. Symptoms of uraemia may be present when renal function has deteriorated to the point of end-stage renal disease. Fever, chills, and general malaise may be experienced by the patient. The patient may express concerns about the failing kidney.

Objective data

Monitor urine for blood. Monitor vital signs and report repeated elevations of blood pressure. On physical examination, the enlarged kidneys appear as large palpable abdominal masses.

Diagnostic tests

Serum and urine electrolytes and creatinine clearance tests provide accurate data about renal function. A urine culture is obtained to determine the presence of UTI. Although a retrograde pyelograph and KUB can give valuable data about the size of the kidneys, the intravenous pyelogram (IVP) (p. 697) is most often used to confirm the diagnosis.

Nursing analysis

Nursing analyses are determined from assessment of patient data. Possible nursing problems for the person with polycystic disease may include, but are not limited to, the following:

Problem	Possible aetiologies
Pain	Renal inflammation
Grieving, anticipatory	Loss of renal function
Coping, ineffective individual	Situational crisis, personal vulnerability
Knowledge deficit	Unfamiliarity with information sources

Planning: expected patient outcomes

Expected patient outcomes for the patient with polycystic disease may include, but are not limited to, the following:
1. States feeling more comfortable.
2. Verbalizes feelings about potential loss of renal function and shares feelings with family members.
3. Uses other support systems as appropriate.
4. States symptoms of infection and haematuria to report to doctor, and plans for follow-up care.

Implementation
Assisting with achievement of therapeutic goals

Interventions for the patient with polycystic disease centre largely on preventing infection and bleeding. Infection is difficult to eradicate in people with polycystic kidneys, and when infection is uncontrolled it leads to further destruction of kidney tissue. Frequent culture of the urine is performed and instrumentation and catheterization of the urinary tract are avoided whenever possible. Antibiotic therapy is often instituted. When antibiotics are ordered, they should be given on time and on a regular schedule to ensure adequate blood levels. Monitor the patient's urinary output closely.

Interventions to achieve patient outcomes
Promoting comfort

Analgesic drugs may be necessary to control flank pain associated with enlarged kidneys. When bleeding from ruptured cysts becomes severe enough to turn the urine from pink to red, bed rest is usually instituted. At these times, the patient will require assistance with ADL. Otherwise, independence in ADL should be encouraged.

Facilitating anticipatory grieving

Approaches to helping patients during grieving are discussed in Chapter 11. Offer the patient opportunities to explore and communicate feelings regarding anticipated loss of renal function. Provide an open and supportive environment for both patient and family or significant others. Anticipate tears, anger, and regressive behaviour and explain to family that the patient's behaviour is not directed at them personally. Provide an atmosphere of trust and concern. Explore the need to restructure short- and long-term goals. Provide opportunities for patient and family to discuss these concerns alone.

Assisting with coping

The emotional overtones of this illness can be severe for both the individual and the family. Challenges exist in helping the person deal with an illness on an individual basis when relatives have died of the same disease and children have not yet developed symptoms. Counselling regarding family health care and the individual's role in passing on a potentially fatal disease to children will, at times, be required. Assist patient to find supportive people, such as family or friends, clergy, and support groups.

Facilitating patient learning

The patient should know how to perform the following:
1. Monitor for signs of infection and haematuria (fever, increased flank pain, blood in urine) and report signs to doctor.
2. Monitor urinary output and report changes to doctor.
3. Report for diagnostic tests as instructed to identify early signs of kidney tissue destruction.
4. Take antibiotics as instructed.
5. Report to doctor for follow-up care as instructed.

Evaluation

Evaluation is based on expected patient outcomes. Questions to consider include the following:
1. Is the patient comfortable?
2. Have patient and family had opportunities to verbalize and share feelings regarding anticipated loss of renal function?
3. Has patient identified appropriate sources of support, such as clergy and support groups?
4. Does patient know signs of infection and haematuria to report to doctor?
5. Does patient state plans for follow-up care?

VASCULAR DISORDERS

Renal diseases resulting from vascular disorders are caused by one of two processes: *renal artery stenosis,* which is a narrowing of the main renal artery, or *nephrosclerosis,* which is sclerosis of renal arterioles. *Diabetic nephropathy* is also a vascular disorder that occurs as diabetes progresses.

Renal Artery Stenosis
Aetiology/epidemiology

Stenosis of the renal arteries is usually classified as either arteriosclerosis or fibromuscular dysplasia. Atheromatous plaques may produce narrowing of the renal artery or arteries at the origin, main trunk, or one of the main branches. It is more common in men, especially those over age 50, and in patients with diabetes mellitus. Fibromuscular dysplasia involves the layers of the renal arteries and their branches. It occurs more commonly in young women. The end result of the stenosis is narrowing of the lumen of the arteries supplying the kidneys. Obstruction of the renal arteries can also be caused by aneurysms, thromboses, and emboli.

Pathophysiology

Renal stenosis results in a major reduction in circulation to the kidneys. This change in perfusion causes increased secretion of renin and activation of the renin-angiotensin-aldosterone system (Chapter 18). The end result is accelerated hypertension, which, if left untreated, leads to further pathological changes in the kidneys. These changes include nephrosclerosis.

The signs of renal artery stenosis are:
1. Hypertension
2. Disparity in size of kidneys
3. Delayed appearance of contrast medium in renal arteriograph
4. Hyperconcentration of contrast medium in calyceal system on IVP.
5. Lesion evidenced on renal arteriograph.

Interventions

Medical treatment includes vigorous antihypertensive therapy to control blood pressure. When a well-defined lesion exists in the renal artery, vascular surgery may be performed to remove the affected area.

Nursing interventions are the same as those for hypertension (Chapter 18). The patient should know the importance of medical follow-up for identification of renal insufficiency.

Nephrosclerosis
Aetiology

Renal disease associated with hypertension is called *nephrosclerosis. Benign nephrosclerosis* is associated with chronic, mild, or moderate hypertension and slowly developing renal insufficiency. *Malignant nephrosclerosis* is associated with marked hypertension, diastolic pressure greater than 140 mm Hg, rapidly developing renal failure, headaches, blurred vision, and congestive heart failure.

Pathophysiology

The renal vasculature is affected in *benign* nephrosclerosis. The renal arterial vessels show thickening and narrowing of their lumens and some glomerular capillaries are sclerosed and collapsed. Renal blood flow can be reduced as a result of these vascular changes. The renal tubules can also be affected, resulting in tubular atrophy.

Signs and symptoms are usually mild and include mild proteinuria from glomerular damage. Nocturia may occur from moderate loss of tubular concentrating ability. There may be casts in the urine from tubular injury. Although the renal insufficiency is relatively mild, these patients are at risk for acute renal failure.

In *malignant* nephrosclerosis, the major changes are necrosis and thickening of the arterioles and glomerular capillaries and diffuse tubular loss and atrophy. There is gross haematuria with red cell casts, heavy proteinuria, and elevated plasma creatinine. Malignant nephrosclerosis is a medical emergency, and the high blood pressure must be lowered to prevent permanent renal damage as well as damage to other vital organs.

Interventions

Treatment of both benign and malignant nephrosclerosis is directed towards early detection and treatment of hypertension. Antihypertensive therapy is initiated.

For hypertensive emergencies, potent vasodilators such as sodium nitroprusside are used. These intravenous medications usually act rapidly. Sodium nitroprusside is given as a continuous intravenous drip, monitored by the nurse. It is titrated on the basis of patient response, as prescribed. Monitor the patient continuously for headache, hypotension, muscle twitching, tachycardia, restlessness, and retrosternal or abdominal pain.

When significant renal damage exists, stabilizing the person's current level of renal function or slowing deterioration of renal tissue is the treatment goal. Control of hypertension is continued, and management of end-stage disease and uraemic symptoms provides for comfort and increased independence in daily living, although renal function may not improve.

DIABETIC NEPHROPATHY

Diabetic nephropathy is the leading cause of end-stage renal disease (ESRD). Approximately 30% of patients who begin treatment for ESRD are diabetic, and 50% with type I diabetes develop renal failure within 15 to 18 years of disease onset.

Diffuse glomerulosclerosis is the most common lesion seen in the kidneys of patients who have had diabetes for more than 2 years. There is glomerular basement thickening and mesangial cell proliferation. Although the cause is unknown, it is thought that it may be secondary to complement-mediated tissue injury.

Spherical masses called Kimmelstiel-Wilson lesions are observed in about 50% of patients and are thought to arise from the thickened capillary wall of the glomerulus. As nodule size increases, the adjacent capillaries are compressed until the entire glomerulus becomes ischaemic. Progressive diabetic nephropathy is characterized by proteinuria leading to nephrotic syndrome (p. 693) and finally ESRD. Dialysis is of limited value but renal transplantation shows promising results.

TRAUMA TO THE URINARY TRACT

Assessing intactness of the urinary tract structures must be a part of the evaluation of any person with traumatic injury to the lower trunk. Injuries that are particularly conducive to urinary tract damage include fractures of the pelvis and sharp blows to the abdomen or flanks.

Trauma of the Lower Urinary Tract

Pelvic fractures may result in *bladder perforation* and *ureteral* and *urethral tearing*. After bladder perforation or ureteral or urethral injury, urinary output may be scant or absent, the urine may be bloody, and symptoms of peritonitis may appear. Treatment is directed towards stabilizing the patient and surgically repairing the perforation or laceration. After stabilizing the patient, a cystotomy may be performed to provide urinary drainage when the injury involves the bladder or urethra. When the ureters are involved, splinting catheters may be required. When injury is extreme, urinary diversion may be required (p. 709). The immediate treatment goal is to provide for adequate urinary drainage to prevent damage to the kidneys.

Kidney Trauma

A sharp blow to the body, particularly to the lower back or flanks, may result in contusion, tearing, or rupture of a kidney (Fig. 25-10). Signs and symptoms of trauma to the kidneys include frank bleeding from the urinary meatus, haematuria, pain, and tenderness of the upper abdominal quadrant and flank on the involved side. Signs of shock may be present if haemorrhage is extensive. Treatment includes controlling bleeding, preventing shock, and promoting drainage of the urinary tract. Vital signs, fluid balance, and haematocrit levels are monitored to assess haemostasis. Complaints of pain may indicate development of ureteral colic, signifying obstruction of the ureter by a clot. Surgical intervention is required to control severe haemorrhage; spontaneous healing of the kidney is otherwise permitted. Nephrostomy with catheter placement may be required to permit adequate urinary drainage. Bed rest is maintained until gross haematuria clears; thereafter, activity is progressed according to continued absence of haematuria. In the presence of extensive damage a nephrectomy may be required.

A kidney may become loosened and "float" or become displaced (*nephroptosis*). If symptoms of obstruction occur in the presence of nephroptosis, the kidney may be sutured to its anatomic site (*nephropexy*) to eliminate kinking of the ureter. Postoperatively, the patient is positioned with hips elevated to prevent tension on the suture line.

RENAL FAILURE

Renal failure is the inability of the kidneys to function. *It is a state of total or nearly total loss of the kidneys' ability to excrete waste products, to maintain fluid and electrolyte balance (including acid-base balance), and to control blood pressure.* The person in renal failure cannot independently sustain life.

Renal failure may be acute in onset or may develop slowly and progressively over several years. When renal failure occurs suddenly, such as within a few days, biochemical changes are often dramatic and the patient has little time to adjust to these changes. The patient becomes very ill and usually requires care in a critical care unit.

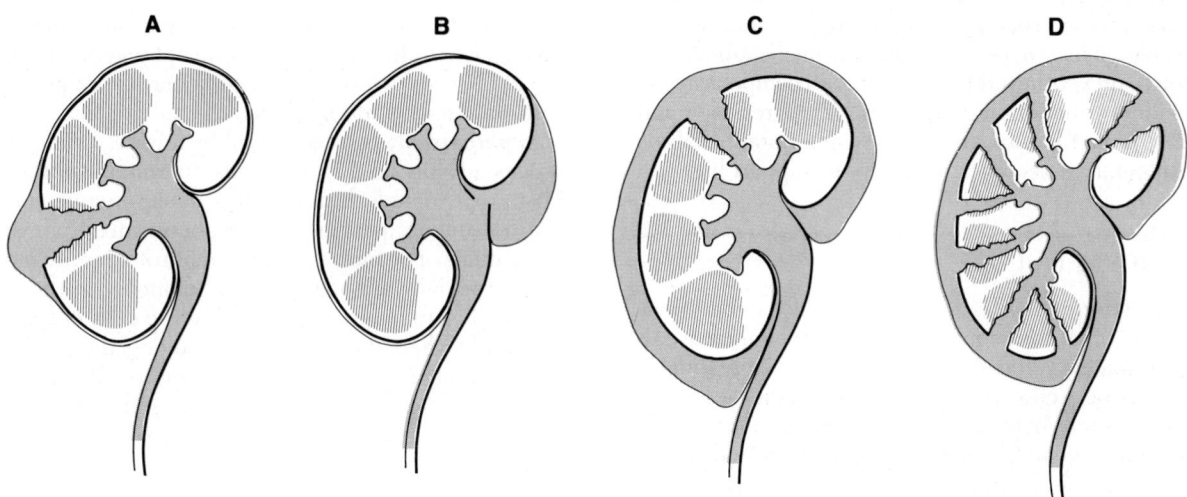

Fig. 25-10   Four degrees of renal trauma. **A,** Urine is extravasating from split in renal parenchyma but confined under renal capsule. **B,** Urine is extravasating through tear in renal pelvis. **C,** Urine is extravasating through rent in kidney and capsule and surrounds kidney and renal pelvis. **D,** Kidney is shattered and urine is extravasating in all areas. (From Winter CC, Morel A: *Nursing care of patients with urologic diseases,* ed 4, St Louis, 1977, Mosby–Year Book.)

Table 25-11   Common causes of acute renal failure

Classification	Causes: conditions or substances
Prerenal ARF	
Hypoperfusion	Haemorrhage, dehydration, burns, diarrhoea, vomiting, third spacing, cirrhosis, peritonitis, nephrotic syndrome, renal artery/vein thrombosis or stenosis, renal infarction, diuretic abuse
Vasodilation	Sepsis and anaphylaxis
Decreased cardiac output	Cardiogenic shock, dysrhythmias, severe congestive heart failure, pericardial tamponade, acute pulmonary embolism
Intrarenal ARF	
Glomerular damage	Acute poststreptoccal glomerulonephritis and SLE, Goodpasture's syndrome, bacterial endocarditis
Vascular disease	Polyarteritis nodosa, periarteritis, vasculitis, hypersensitivity angiitis, scleroderma, hypertension
Other disease	Insterstitial nephritis, papillary necrosis, acute pyelonephritis, allergic nephritis, hypercalcaemia, uric acid nephropathy, kidney myeloma
Ischaemia (ATN)	Hypovolaemia, cardiogenic shock, severe prolonged ARF
	Circulation to kidney interrupted less than 30 minutes (surgical cross-clamping above renal arteries)
	Procurement of cadaver kidneys for transplantation
Nephrotoxicity (ATN)	Heavy metals and ions: mercuric chloride, copper sulphate, gold
	Organic solvents: carbon tetrachloride, ethylene glycol
	Antibiotics: aminoglycosides (gentamicin, kanamycin, amikacin). Other antimicrobials: vancomycin, amphotericin, tetracycline, some cephalosporins
	Analgesics: phenacetin, paracetamol, NSAIDs (ibuprofen)
	Immunosuppressive agent: cyclosporin
	Chemotherapeutic agents: cisplatin, methotrexate, carmustine, lomustine, mitomycin, bleomycin, cyclophosphamide
	Radiological contrast media: iodine-based dyes
Postrenal ARF	
Obstruction	Ureteral: fibrosis, calculi, crystals, clots, accidental ligation
	Bladder: neoplasms
	Urethral: stricture, prostatic hypertrophy

When renal failure occurs as the end result of a chronic kidney illness in which kidney tissue is destroyed progressively over the course of several months or years, control of symptoms and preservation of functional abilities are achieveable goals. Dietary adjustment, medications, and attention to preventing additional illnesses compensate for loss of kidney function in early stages of progressing renal failure. As renal function continues to deteriorate, dialysis or transplantation becomes necessary to support life.

ACUTE RENAL FAILURE

Acute renal failure (ARF) is defined as a sudden impairment or decline in renal function associated with an increase in the serum concentration of urea (*azotaemia*) and creatinine. It is often associated with *oliguria* (urine output less than 400 ml/24 hours), hyperkalaemia, and sodium retention. ARF is often reversible; however, prolonged episodes may lead to irreversible kidney failure, which requires either dialysis or transplantation.

Aetiology

Acute renal failure generally follows an identifiable trauma that is either toxic or ischaemic in nature. The health of the individual before the insult is usually good to adequate. Conditions that can precipitate acute renal failure include the following:

1. Ischaemia
2. Nephrotoxicity
3. Acute glomerular disease
4. Acute severe kidney infection
5. Bilateral occlusion of the renal arteries
6. Mechanical obstructions of the urinary tract
7. Haemoglobinaemia and myoglobinaemia

All these conditions can lead to massive and rapid destruction of kidney tissue. ARF has been organized into three classifications depending upon the aetiology or physiological location of the renal insult: prerenal, intrarenal, and postrenal ARF (see Table 25-11).

Prerenal acute renal failure

Prerenal factors are directly related to *hypoperfusion* states (decreased amount of blood flow to the kidneys). Conditions that result in decreased cardiac output, vasodilation, or decreased circulating blood volume can result in decreased blood flow to the kidneys.

Intrarenal acute renal failure

Intrarenal (parenchymal) ARF results from injury to renal tissue. It is typically associated with intrarenal ischaemia, toxins, or prolonged prerenal ARF. Damage may be to the glomerulus, or more commonly to the tubular system. ARF resulting from tubular damage is termed *acute tubular necrosis* (ATN). Ischaemia or nephrotoxicity are the two most common conditions that cause ATN.

Ischaemic kidney injury occurs when kidney perfusion is obliterated or reduced below a mean arterial pressure of 60 or 70 mm Hg in the afferent arteriole. Below this critical level the ability of the afferent and efferent arterioles to maintain glomerular filtration is lost. As a result, the glomerular filtration rate decreases. Ischaemia also occurs when kidney circulation is interrupted for longer than 30 minutes. Prolonged or severe prerenal ARF is a common cause of ATN. Ischaemic injuries damage not only the tubular epithelial cells but also the basement membrane cells, which, unlike tubular cells, do not regenerate. Therefore, ATN resulting from ischaemia may cause permanent nephron damage and irreversible renal failure.

Nephrotoxicity can be caused by a wide variety of substances (Table 25-11) injurious to renal tubules. The substances include heavy metals, ions, organic solvents, contrast media, pesticides, poisonous mushrooms, and medications. The most common nephrotoxins are medications, especially aminoglycosides belonging to the antibiotic group. Aminoglycosides bind to the cells of the proximal tubule where they have a very prolonged half-life. This causes damage to the tubules, leading to ARF. The basement membrane cells are not damaged; therefore, the chances of reversibility of ATN resulting from nephrotoxicity are good.

Postrenal acute renal failure

Postrenal ARF usually results from *obstruction* to the outflow of urine from the renal calyces to the urethral meatus. For renal failure to develop the obstruction must be bilateral below the level of the bladder or unilateral in the person with only one functioning kidney. Postrenal ARF is frequently reversible; however, prolonged obstruction may result in intrarenal damage and irreversible renal failure.

Pathophysiology

The course of acute renal failure is usually characterized by an initial oliguric phase followed in a number of days to a few weeks by a diuretic period. Major problems during the *oliguric* phase include inability to excrete fluid loads, to regulate electrolytes, and to excrete metabolic waste materials (Table 25-12). During the *diuretic* phase large amounts of fluid and electrolytes are lost.

Oliguric phase

The oliguric phase of ARF is the period during which the patient's urinary volume is less than 400 ml in 24 hours. It usually lasts 1 to 2 weeks. If the oliguric phase is prolonged beyond 2 weeks, the prognosis for recovery decreases.

Inability to excrete fluid loads

Because of the decreased kidney function, fluids are retained in the body, resulting in fluid overload and oedema (Chapter 6). When fluid overload is excessive, congestive heart failure and pulmonary oedema may occur. Hypertension accompanies acute renal failure when the person is hypervolaemic, although this is usually not a finding when fluid balance is controlled.

Inability to excrete fluid loads leads to decreased urinary output. Either *oliguria* (urinary output below 100 ml in 24 hours) or *anuria* may be present, although oliguria is more common. Classically, the patient in acute renal failure shows a fall in urinary output within 1 to 2 days to between 50 and 400 ml in 24 hours. The urine *specific gravity is low* (1.010), and the osmolality of the urine approaches that of

Table 25-12   Symptoms caused by physiological changes in acute renal failure

Symptoms	Physiological effects	Findings
Oliguric phase		
Nausea, vomiting, drowsiness, confusion, coma, GI bleeding, asterixis, pericarditis	Inability to excrete metabolic wastes	Increased blood urea and creatinine levels
Nausea, vomiting, cardiac dysrhythmias, Kussmaul's breathing, drowsiness, confusion, coma	Inability to regulate electrolytes	Hyperkalaemia, hyponatraemia, acidosis
Oedema; congestive heart failure; pulmonary oedema; hypertension	Inability to excrete fluid loads	Fluid overload, hypervolaemia
Diuretic phase		
Urinary output of up to 4 to 5 L/day, postural hypotension, tachycardia	Increased production of urine	Hypovolaemia, loss of sodium and potassium in urine
Increasing mental alertness and activity	Slowly increasing excretion of metabolic wastes	Initially, high blood urea (fluid loss greater than solute loss), gradual return of blood urea to normal

the person's serum (280-320 mOsm/kg). Specific gravity and urine osmolality remain within this fixed range and reflect tubular damage with loss of concentrating ability.

Electrolyte imbalances

The three major electrolyte problems are hyperkalaemia, hyponatraemia, and acidosis.

Potassium imbalance. In the normal individual the potassium ion is exchanged in the distal convoluted tubule of the nephron for either sodium or hydrogen ions; for the healthy person there is no mechanism in the body to conserve the potassium ion. However, in the individual with acute renal failure in whom a large number of tubular cells are no longer functional, no mechanism exists to remove potassium from the body. *Hyperkalaemia* is said to exist when the serum concentration of this ion reaches a level of 5.5 mol/L or higher. Serum concentrations of 7 to 10 mol/L can be quickly reached in acute renal failure and are incompatible with normal cardiac function and life.

In monitoring for signs of potassium toxicity, electrocardiography and laboratory determinations of serum potassium are the most reliable indicators. Rarely does the patient become symptomatic, and pulse changes must not be relied on to indicate the degree of rise of potassium in the patient's system.

Sodium imbalance. *Hyponatraemia* in acute renal failure most commonly develops with overhydration of the patient. The oliguric patient cannot excrete large volumes of urine; when the administration of sodium-free or low-sodium intravenous or oral fluids continues in such an individual, the serum is diluted and the serum concentration of sodium falls.

In this situation hyponatraemia is accompanied or caused by hypervolaemia. In the very acutely ill, the situation commonly occurs when the patient receives numerous drugs and fluids in an attempt to treat coexisting life-threatening problems. When the volume of drugs and

fluids cannot be reduced to a safe level, dialysis is required to remove the excess fluid and restore sodium balance.

Signs and symptoms of hyponatraemia include warm, moist, flushed skin; muscle weakness, muscle twitching; and behavioural changes involving confusion, delirium, coma, and convulsions. Serum sodium concentrations will be below 130 mol/L. The haematocrit and haemoglobin values fall suddenly without evidence of bleeding; this is caused by haemodilution.

Increases in total body content of sodium also occur in acute renal failure. This commonly occurs when the patient is receiving medications high in sodium content and excess sodium in the diet. Oedema and increasing blood pressure indicate retention of sodium and fluids even though the serum sodium concentration is normal or below normal.

Metabolic acidosis. Acidosis develops when hydrogen ion secretion and bicarbonate ion production diminish in the tubular cells. The pH of the blood decreases, the carbon dioxide content decreases, and central nervous system symptoms of drowsiness progressing to stupor and coma may appear. Although the lungs are unable to compensate totally for the increasing acid load, they help determine the rate at which acidosis develops and the frequency or need for dialysis. In compensating for increased metabolic acid loads, the lungs attempt to excrete more carbon dioxide. Kussmaul's breathing is noted.

Inability to excrete metabolic wastes

Decreased kidney function alters the body's ability to get rid of metabolic waste materials, producing typical signs and symptoms referred to as *uraemia*. Blood urea and serum creatinine values rise sharply. In the person who has already sustained illness and trauma, blood urea values may increase at a rate of 30 mg/100 ml/day. Signs and symptoms include neurological manifestations such as confusion, convulsions, coma, and asterixis. GI bleeding may result from uraemic gastritis or colitis. Serum uric acid and phosphate levels also rise. Decreased cellular immunity causes an increased tendency for infections to develop. Bruising and bleeding result from changes in blood coagulation factors. Pericarditis (Chapter 17) is thought to develop as a result of pericardial irritation from uraemic toxins.

Diuretic phase

The diuretic phase begins when the 24-hour urine volume exceeds 400 ml and ends when blood urea and serum creatinine levels begin to fall. Increased output indicates that the damaged nephrons are healing and are able to begin excreting urine. At first daily urine volume increases slowly, although within 1 to 2 days diuresis up to or exceeding 4 to 5 L/day may occur. Although fluid can be excreted, the kidneys are not yet healed. Often there is inability to excrete proportional amounts of waste materials, and blood urea may rise or remain elevated as urine volume increases. At times excessive excretion of sodium and potassium occurs during diuresis. Complete recovery of renal function is slow and requires anywhere from days to several months. Return of the renal function to normal or near-normal levels is evidenced when the kidney can both conserve and dilute urine and when serum electrolytes and nonprotein nitrogen levels become normal.

Prognosis

Recovery from an episode of ARF depends on the underlying illness, condition of patient, and careful supportive management given during the period of kidney shutdown. The leading cause of death is infection, such as of the urinary tract, lungs, and peritoneum. Infection develops in approximately 80% of patients with ARF. The incidence of GI bleeding, the second most frequent cause of death, is about 25%. Mortality from fluid overload and acidosis has been reduced as a result of dialysis and other forms of therapy. There is potential for recovery of renal function in patients who survive the acute episode of tubular insufficiency. Although kidney tissue may regenerate more completely after toxic injury than ischaemia, both forms usually show return to normal or near-normal renal function.

For those in whom acute renal failure has been caused by glomerular disease or severe infection of kidney tissue, the prognosis may not be as favourable. Return of renal function is determined by the extent of scarring and obliteration of functional renal tissue that has occurred during the acute episode of kidney failure. A significant number of adults who develop acute glomerulonephritis show some decrease in renal function, which may remain at a level at which biochemical abnormalities are not produced, or may progress to a chronic form of renal failure.

Prevention and Health Education
Primary prevention

The most important nursing intervention associated with ARF is primary prevention. The incidence of ARF can be reduced through identification and observation of individuals at risk for ARF, control of environmental factors, a thorough understanding of the pathophysiology of ARF, strategic planning of nursing interventions, and continued evaluation of those interventions. It is important for nurses to monitor urinary output and laboratory values of patient receiving antibiotics (especially aminoglycosides) and cyclosporin.

The greatest incidence of ARF occurs in people who have undergone major trauma, extensive burns, aortic surgery, massive blood loss, or severe myocardial infarction. ARF also frequently occurs in patients with sepsis and in those having abnormal intravascular coagulation, such as DIC, because these acutely ill people are prime candidates for inadequate kidney perfusion. Frequent monitoring of urinary output and detection of excessive fluid losses helps to identify instances of inadequate renal perfusion before renal failure develops.

Significant factors in preventive care for the general population include control of nephrotoxic drugs, increased medical supervision of people with sore throats and upper respiratory tract infections, and increased case finding and treatment of individuals with bacteriuria and obstructive disease of the urinary system. Attempts to control the distribution and identification of nephrotoxic drugs and chemicals is largely accomplished through the Department of Health and Home Office. Identification of nephrotoxic drugs and chemicals, enforced labelling of these substances, and drug dispensing by prescription only are examples of these agencies' attempts to promote public health. Proper labelling and storage of potentially toxic drugs and chemicals in the home can reduce further the number of accidental ingestions of nephrotoxic substances.

Secondary prevention

Early detection and prompt diagnosis is essential to prevent permanent damage to renal tissue. Encourage people who complain of persistent symptoms to seek prompt medical evaluation. All possible measures to optimize patient survival can be taken if the patient's condition is diagnosed early in the course of ARF.

Medical Therapy for Acute Renal Failure

Before the early 1980s there were basically three treatment options for ARF: conservative management, haemodialysis (HD), and peritoneal dialysis (PD). Conservative management with pharmacology and diet therapy still remains the primary approach to stabilize the patient with ARF. This approach, however, may be ineffective in some situations. Therefore, HD (p. 731) and PD (p. 734) have been the standard aggressive therapies for invasive intervention.

Haemodialysis is often a difficult procedure to perform when the patient is haemodynamically unstable, has bleeding complications, or needs more than a prescribed 3- to 4-hour treatment to correct underlying fluid overload, acid-base imbalance, and uraemia associated with ARF. For many years clinicians have had to use aggressive HD once or twice daily because of threatening conditions that must be reversed immediately, such as hyperkalaemia, severe acidosis, or pulmonary oedema.

Although peritoneal dialysis is considered less taxing than HD, it may be problematic in the critically ill patient. History of abdominal surgery, abdominal trauma, certain diseases, or lack of surgical support for catheter placement may eliminate PD as an option of ARF management.

In 1982, the U.S. FDA approved a safer, gentler modality for the management of ARF called *continuous renal replacement therapy* (CRRT), which is now the invasive intervention of choice for the critically ill ARF patient and used now in Britain. HD and PD continue to be used to treat ARF, but whenever possible they are reserved for haemodynamically stable patients or those with end-stage renal disease.

Continuous renal replacement therapy

CRRT provides continuous (8-24 hours or more) *ultrafiltration* (filtration as a result of hydrostatic pressure) of extracellular fluid and clearance of uraemic toxins. This technique uses a highly porous, extracorporeal haemofilter that is perfused continuously by blood flowing from the cannulation of a large artery and returning through a large vein. The goal of CRRT is to remove fluid from the patient either by gravity drain system or by a suction-assisted fluid collection system. The removed fluid contains dissolved noncellular components of the patient's plasma, such as urea, creatinine, and electrolytes.

There are three variants of CRRT: slow continuous ultrafiltration (SCUF), continuous arteriovenous haemofiltration (CAVH), and continuous arteriovenous haemofiltration dialysis (CAVHD).[42] *SCUF* provides a slow ultrafiltration that decreases the patient's fluid volume over several hours to days of therapy. No fluid replacement is prescribed, and solutes such as creatinine and urea are minimally removed. SCUF is usually used for patients with congestive heart failure or myocardial infarction accompanied with low renal perfusion secondary to decreased cardiac output.[42]

CAVH is often the preferred therapy when a patient's clinical status requires moderate fluid removal and solute clearance. The ultrafiltration rate ranges from 500 to 800 ml/hour. However, a haemodynamically compromised patient cannot tolerate aggressive fluid shifts, so fluid replacement is administered by means of continuous infusion. The replacement fluid amount is based on the hourly net fluid loss goal of 50 to 400 ml/hour. CAVH is also prescribed when the serum chemistries are high, especially potassium and urea, or when the serum bicarbonate is low, which indicates metabolic acidosis. Replacement fluids may be standard fluids, such as lactated Ringer's solution or normal saline. However, solutions used most often include half-normal saline with calcium gluceptate or chloride, or quarter-normal saline with two ampules of sodium bicarbonate.[42]

CAVHD is used when the patient's volume status is excessive and the uraemia is severe. With CAVHD, either peritoneal dialysate (hypertonic dialyzing fluid) or a custom dialysate is infused countercurrent to the patient's blood flow through a *haemofilter*. The countercurrent flow increases the diffusibility toxins from the patient's uraemic plasma. The dextrose contained in the dialysate enhances fluid removal by the osmotic effect across the semipermeable membrane of the haemofilter. CAVHD is different from standard HD in that the flow rate of the dialysate is reduced, which is better tolerated by the critically ill ARF patient.

Nursing Process
Assessment
Subjective data

Assessment should include questions that ascertain the following:

1. Voiding patterns, including any recent changes
2. Unexplained weight gain
3. Presence of nausea and anorexia
4. Family history of renal disease
5. Recent history of flulike symptoms
6. Presence of nephrotoxins, including those in environment, at work, and in medications
7. Preexisting diseases, especially cardiac disorders, vascular disease, urinary diseases, and systemic conditions (such as diabetes mellitus and SLE) known to affect renal function
8. Recent surgeries or acute illnesses

Objective data

Objective data must include the measurement of fluid intake and urine output in a 24-hour period. Daily weighings are essential because they provide the best measure of fluid status. Blood pressure, including postural changes, is measured frequently until stable, and the pulse rate and rhythm are also recorded. Fluid status is assessed by observing for skin turgor and peripheral oedema and auscultating breath sounds. The person is assessed for the presence of halitosis that can result from acidosis and from ammonia secretion. The person is observed carefully for any changes in mental status.

Diagnostic tests

Diagnostic tests include urinalysis and creatinine urinary clearance to monitor changes in kidney function. Serum creatinine and blood urea are also obtained. Blood chemistries must be followed closely to ensure that the person is maintaining homeostasis. Specific tests used to assist in making the diagnosis and identifying the cause of acute renal failure include KUB, IVP, cystoscopy, and renal ultrasound. In some cases a renal biopsy may be performed to provide the differential diagnosis.

When oliguria or rising serum creatinine and blood ureas values are noted, the doctor must determine whether the decreased output and decreased renal function are the results of inadequate renal perfusion or of frank renal failure. This distinction directs treatment. In instances of poor kidney perfusion, restoring circulating volume by adding fluids and otherwise increasing cardiac output prevents the death of kidney tissue and subsequent renal failure. In contrast, the treatment of true renal failure is supportive and is based on careful balance of input and output of fluid, electrolytes, and wastes.

In addition to the urine sodium concentration as a diagnostic sign, the doctor may wish to challenge the patient's ability to excrete fluid. In this instance usually 100 to 500 ml of fluid is given as rapidly as possible intravenously. A poorly perfused but intact kidney should respond with increased urinary output. During this treatment the patient must be closely monitored for signs and symptoms of congestive heart failure and pulmonary oedema. The kidney in acute failure will be unable to produce a greater urine flow in response to this fluid challenge. The doctor may give frusemide, 40 to 80 mg intravenously, in an attempt to produce a greater flow of urine. The test may be repeated if there is no response to the initial trial, although subsequent attempts to produce urine in this manner are contraindicated.

Nursing analysis

Nursing analyses are determined from assessment of patient data. Possible nursing problems for the person with acute renal failure may include, but are not limited to, the following:

Problem	Possible aetiologies
Injury, high risk for	Sensorimotor deficits, lack of awareness of environmental hazards, bleeding tendency
Infection, high risk for	Urinary stasis, decreased immune response
Nutrition, altered: less than body requirements	Anorexia, nausea, and vomiting
Coping, ineffective individual	Changes in health status, situational crisis
Knowledge deficit	Cognitive limitations, lack of interest in learning, unfamiliarity with informational sources

Planning: expected patient outcomes

Expected patient outcomes for the person with acute renal failure may include, but are not limited to, the following:

1. Does not become injured or sustain bleeding.
2. Displays no signs of infection.
3. Eats prescribed diet.
4. Describes alternative ways of coping.
5. Describes nature of illness, diet therapy, signs to report to doctor, and plans for follow-up care.

Implementation

Assisting with achievement of therapeutic goals
Oliguric phase

During the oliguric phase of acute renal failure, development of hyperkalaemia, severe acidosis, severe fluid overload and pulmonary oedema, infection, convulsions, or pericarditis indicate need for immediate intervention. Nursing care of the patient with ARF in the oliguric phase is summarized in Box 25-14.

Control and excretion of metabolic waste buildup. Because the patient's ability to excrete metabolic wastes (nonprotein nitrogen products and acids) cannot keep pace with production of these substances, alternative routes of excretion and control over production of these materials must be found. Means available to accomplish this include providing carbohydrate to spare protein stores, preventing additional tissue trauma, and increasing excretion of wastes through the lungs and through dialysis.

Decreasing the production of metabolic wastes can be influenced through dietary means. Calories in the form of carbohydrates and fats provide energy and spare body

---

Guidelines for Care   25-14

The patient in oliguric phase of acute renal failure

Control and excretion of metabolic waste buildup
  Provide carbohydrate to spare protein stores
  Prevent additional trauma
  Give pulmonary hygiene to prevent atelactasis
Maintain fluid and electrolyte balance
  Maintain fluid restrictions
  Keep accurate records of intake and output
  Weigh patient daily
  Monitor vital signs frequently, including postural signs
  Assess patient's fluid status
  Administer phosphate-binding medications as prescribed
  Monitor serum electrolytes
Maintain nutrition
  Monitor intravenous fluids
  Take measures to relieve nausea (antiemetics, comfort measures)
  Give fluids in frequent small amounts, when permitted
  Provide a diet high in carbohydrates during protein restrictions
  Provide a diet low in potassium during hyperkalaemia and high in potassium during hypokalaemia
Prevent injury
  Assess orientation; orientate confused patient
  Maintain bed rest during acute phase
  When patient is ambulatory, assess motor skills and monitor ambulation
  Protect patient from bleeding; instruct patient to use soft toothbrush, administer stool softeners, perform guaiac tests on stools and emesis
Prevent infection
  Assess for signs and symptoms of infection
  Maintain strict asepsis for any intrusive procedures
  Provide pulmonary hygiene
  Protect skin when patient is on bed rest
  Turn weak or immobile patient frequently
  Protect patient from others with infections

---

protein stores, thus decreasing nonprotein nitrogen production. The body recycles urea to synthesize amino acids for protein building so that some regeneration of tissues can occur even though protein intake is curtailed.

In compensating for increased metabolic acid loads, the lungs attempt to excrete more carbon dioxide. To maximize this pathway for acid excretion, pulmonary hygiene should be carried out. Preventing atelectasis and maintaining maximal lung expansion are goals of nursing care.

Control of fluids. The oliguric or anuric patient is unable to excrete more than minimal amounts of fluid. Nursing care is directed towards three broad objectives: (1) monitoring for signs of fluid overload, (2) maintaining the patient's energy expenditure at a level compatible with the individual's state of health, and (3) controlling or helping the patient to control fluid intake.

All observations regarding the patient's state of hydration need to be recorded so that hour-to-hour and day-to-day comparisons can be made. Any finding indicating retention of fluids is reported to the physician. Oedema can first be noted in dependent areas such as the feet and legs, in the presacral area, and around the eyes. The patient is observed carefully for signs of pulmonary oedema and congestive heart failure. Central venous or arterial monitoring lines will help to provide data for short-term comparisons in managing the fluid balance of the critically ill person. Accurate recording of intake and output is extremely important as are daily weight records.

The patient in renal failure is unable to excrete fluid loads, and much energy is expended just to maintain current functional status. Positioning and activity are determined daily based on assessment of the energy level and ability to ventilate adequately.

Controlling fluid intake is essential when the ability to excrete fluid is limited. All fluid (parenteral and oral) must total only slightly more than daily output if severe overhydration is to be avoided. When the patient is neither to gain nor lose additional body fluid, the doctor will calculate the patient's fluid replacement using the following as a guide: intake will approximate 500 ml/day plus urinary output and adjustments for additional fluid lost through fever, diarrhoea, and wound drainage. Fortunately, when sodium intake is controlled, extreme thirst does not develop.

Devices that allow 50 to 150 ml of fluid to be isolated from the main intravenous solution container and drip chambers that allow precise control of fluids through administration of smaller drops of fluid are added safety measures when giving fluids parenterally to anuric or oliguric individuals. Accuracy in fluid balance records is essential. For the patient who is unable to take medications with small amounts of fluid, medications may be given in soft foods.

Interventions for hyperkalaemia. Interventions to control the rise of serum potassium and to prevent cardiac arrest include those that (1) decrease the intake of potassium, (2) protect the cardiovascular system, and (3) assist in removal of potassium from the body by nonrenal means.

Decreasing the intake of potassium is achieved by administering intravenous feedings or a diet in which the potassium content is very low or absent. All fluids and drugs that the patient receives intravenously should be checked for potassium content. Some medications (for example, most penicillin preparations) contain large amounts of this ion.

Protecting the cardiovascular system from high levels of extracellular potassium (K^+) *is essential.* When high K^+ levels occur and the patient is exhibiting cardiovascular effects, renal dialysis is required. Because it takes several hours to get the dialysis treatment under way and for the K^+ to be reduced to safe levels, other therapy is instituted. Hypertonic glucose (25%) may be given with 1 unit of insulin per 2 g of glucose. Over a 30-minute period, 200 to 300 ml of fluid is given to promote the movement of K^+ back into the cells. This lowers the serum K^+ level and reduces cardiac instability resulting from the high serum K^+ levels. The K^+ levels will begin to fall in 1 hour and will remain lowered for 4 to 6 hours.[15] In addition to hypertonic glucose, calcium gluconate may be given intravenously to reduce the irritability of cardiac cells caused by the hyperkalaemia.

To *promote the excretion of potassium* from the body when the kidneys are nonfunctional, an exchange resin such as polystyrene sulphonate resins may be ordered for the patient as a temporary measure before a dialysis treatment when (1) the serum K^+ level is high and rising rapidly; (2) the serum K^+ level is rising, although at a controlled rate, and other metabolic disturbances do not necessitate dialysis; or (3) control of a rising serum K^+ is required before a patient's transfer to an acute-care area where dialysis can be provided. This drug reduces serum potassium by exchanging calcium or sodium for potassium ions in the intestinal tract. It can be administered orally, through a nasogastric tube, or by enema. The medication is given orally when the patient's condition permits; oral daily dose is 15 g 3-4 times a day. When administered in enema form, the usual dose is 30 g of exchange resin for each enema retained for 9 hours. It may be repeated daily or as necessary to lower serum potassium. Typically, polystyrene sulphonate resins induce an osmotic fluid shift into the bowel producing diarrhoea, which helps to expel the medication, additional K^+, and additional fluid from the GI tract. If spontaneous bowel movements do not occur, a laxative or cleansing enema can be given to ensure the elimination of potassium from the bowel.

Diuretic phase

Medical therapy during the diuretic phase is symptomatic. Electrolyte imbalances are likely to persist and are treated as in the oliguric phase. When polyuria is present, dehydration can become a problem and fluid replacement then becomes necessary. Assess patient for adequate hydration. Detection of fluid losses and electrolyte imbalances (sodium and potassium) continue to be important. Assess for changes in mental status indicative of low serum sodium levels. Monitor for hypokalaemia (serum potassium less than 3.5 mmol/L, muscle weakness, and constipation). Encourage early ambulation and independence in ADL as tolerated. Place patient in a room with a bathroom nearby or provide a bedside commode to avoid fatigue from frequent voiding.

Interventions to achieve patient outcomes
Preventing injury

The confused, agitated, or restless patient must be protected from injury. Keep siderails elevated at all times and pad them if necessary. To allay patient anxiety, explain the rationale for the mental status change (electrolyte or acid/base imbalance, uraemia). Offer reassurance and support. Accompany an ambulatory patient to the bathroom and monitor closely to prevent accidents. Reorientate patient to person, place, and time at regular intervals. Facilitate orientation by placing a calendar, television, or radio, and familiar objects nearby. Involve family members in the reorientation process.

Bleeding may occur from changes in blood coagulation factors. Use measures to prevent bleeding (see Box 25-14). Further information on protection from bleeding can be found in Chapter 19. Use meticulous skin care to prevent skin breakdown from oedema.

Preventing infection

Preventing infections and tissue breakdown decreases production of metabolic wastes. Aseptic technique should be rigorously pursued in all treatments performed on the patient. In-dwelling lines and catheters are a common source of infection and are to be avoided when possible. *The patient should be isolated from anyone with an infection, including other patients, health care personnel, and visitors.* Detecting existent infections early so that treatment can be instituted promptly decreases tissue breakdown. When the patient is extremely weak and immobile, frequent turning and repositioning to prevent bed sores must be performed. Skin care for patients with oedematous tissues should include observation and prevention of pressure and trauma; these tissues are particularly prone to breakdown.

Pruritus commonly occurs and may lead to skin lesions from scratching. Measures to relieve pruritus include bathing patient every day (or more often if necessary). Administer prescribed antipruritics.

Maintaining adequate nutrition

Most people in acute renal failure are too ill to tolerate oral feedings either initially or for sustained periods. Some patients who are able to tolerate fluids orally find that eating food compounds their nausea as a result of an altered biochemical environment and accompanying GI tract irritation. Intravenous hypertonic glucose in amounts of 100 g/day or more provides a temporary source of energy that slows the burning of the body's own protein stores. Main-taining a positive nitrogen balance is not feasible when the patient is severely ill or nauseated. During this period, administer antiemetics as prescribed. Rinsing the mouth frequently helps to keep lips and mouth moist. Use meticulous mouth care to protect teeth and mucous membranes.

When the patient can tolerate oral fluids, provide fluids frequently in small amounts; soft drinks are often tolerated better than other fluids. When oral feedings are started, dietary protein and potassium are restricted unless dialysis has been initiated. In dialysis cases, controlled amounts of protein and potassium are allowed to increase protein available for tissue building and to increase the palatability of the diet. Foods high in carbohydrate and fat are encouraged. A total intake of 2000 calories per day is desired but often not achieved because of anorexia.

Avoid giving the hyperkalaemic patient potassium-rich foods, such as bananas, potatoes, chocolate, and nuts. Conversely, encourage the hypokalaemic patient to eat these foods. In both situations, monitor the patient closely and administer medications (either an exchange resin or potassium supplement) as indicated. As potassium levels become normalized in the diuretic phase, a more normal diet is permitted. Protein restrictions are continued until blood urea and serum creatinine levels decline.

Facilitating coping

The person with ARF faces the reality of renal failure at a time when energy resources for coping are at a low level. Encourage development of a nurse-patient relationship that assists the patient in expressing perceptions of illness. When patient begins to feel stronger during the diuretic phase, assist him or her to explore various coping methods (see Chapter 5). Involve significant others in patient care. Promote patient independence when patient begins to feel better.

Table 25-13   States of chronic renal failure

Stage	Clinical features
Stage I Decreased renal reserve	Residual renal function 40% to 75% of normal Asymptomatic: normal blood urea and serum creatinine levels Excretory and regulatory renal functions are intact Homeostasis is maintained At least 50% to 60% loss of renal tissue required before signs are evident; no symptoms are evident until loss of renal tissue is at least 80%
Stage II Renal insufficiency	Residual renal function 20% to 40% of normal Decreased glomerular filtration rate, solute clearances, ability to concentrate urine, and hormone secretion Symptoms: rising blood urea and serum creatinine, mild azotaemia, polyuria, nocturia, and anaemia Signs and symptoms can become more severe if kidneys are stressed, such as with fluid volume depletion or exposure to a nephrotoxic substance Decreased ability to maintain homeostasis
Stage III End-stage renal disease (ESRD)	Residual renal function less than 15% of normal Excretory, regulatory, and hormonal renal functions severely impaired Unable to maintain homeostasis (fluid, electrolyte, and pH imbalances) Markedly elevated blood urea and serum creatinine, anaemia, hyperphosphataemia, hypocalcaemia, metabolic acidosis, hyperuricaemia, hyperkalaemia, fluid overload (usually oliguric with urine osmolality similar to plasma osmolality) Uraemic syndrome develops; all body systems are affected from renal failure Last stage of progressive chronic renal failure

Facilitating patient learning

During the diuretic phase, the patient is usually ready for learning about kidney disease and measures to prevent recurrence of renal failure. Teaching includes the following:

1. Cause of renal failure and problems with recurrent failures.
2. Identification of preventable environmental or health factors contributing to the illness (such as hypertension, nephrotoxic drugs).
3. Prescribed dietary and medication regimen.
4. Explanation of risk of hypokalaemia and reportable symptoms.
5. Signs and symptoms of infection and of returning renal failure to be reported to the doctor.
6. Need for ongoing follow-up care.

Evaluation

Evaluation is based on expected patient outcomes. Questions to consider may include the following:

1. Is the patient free of injury and infection?
2. Is the patient orientated to person, time, and place?
3. Has the patient's potassium level returned to normal range?
4. Is the patient eating a well-balanced diet?
5. Is the patient coping with the illness?
6. Does the patient know the nature of the illness, dietary and medication regimen, reportable symptoms, and need for follow-up care?

CHRONIC RENAL FAILURE

Chronic renal failure (CRF) exists when the kidneys are no longer capable of maintaining an internal environment consistent with life and when return of function is not anticipated. For the majority of individuals the transition from health to a state of chronic or permanent disease is a slow one extending over a number of years (Table 25-13). Recurrent infections and exacerbations of nephritis, obstruction of the urinary tract, and destruction of vessels from diabetes and long-standing hypertension lead to scarring of kidney tissue and progressive loss of renal function. Some individuals, however, develop total irreversible loss of renal function acutely; such loss of renal function usually develops in a matter of a few hours or days and follows a direct traumatic insult to the kidneys.

Prognosis

The individual with CRF can to some extent control and manage the symptoms of the disease. Although renal function that has been lost as a result of destruction of kidney tissue cannot be recovered, the life of the person can be maintained by limiting the intake of substances that require renal excretion and by providing alternative routes of excretion for waste products and electrolytes. By adhering to a prescribed management routine, albeit quite strict and demanding, life may be sustained. For some individuals medication and diet therapy alone may control uraemic symptoms; other individuals may require dialysis or transplantation to control the symptoms of their disease.

Prevention and Health Education

Primary prevention

Obstruction and infection of the urinary tract and hypertensive disease are common and often asymptomatic causes of renal damage and renal failure. A significant reduction in the incidence of renal failure can be affected through increasing attention to general health promotion. Yearly health checks in which blood pressure is determined, urinalysis is performed, and the person is questioned about dysuria or pain in the urinary tract assist in early detection of diseases that may lead to renal failure.

Secondary prevention

General health maintenance can reduce the number of individuals progressing from renal insufficiency into frank renal failure. Care is aimed towards adequately treating medical problems and closely supervising the person's health status in times of stress (infection, pregnancy).

Aetiology

CRF can be caused by a variety of conditions, including renal disorders (glomerular, tubular, infection, obstruction) and systemic diseases (see Box 25-15).[22]

Pathophysiology and Clinical Manifestations

During chronic renal failure, some of the nephrons (including the glomerulus and tubules) are thought to remain intact while others are destroyed (intact nephron hypothesis). The intact nephrons hypertrophy and produce an increased volume of filtrate with increased tubular reabsorption in spite of a decreased GFR. This adaptive method permits the kidney to function until about 75% of the nephrons become destroyed. The solute load then becomes greater than can be reabsorbed, producing an osmotic diuresis with polyuria and thirst. Eventually, as more nephrons are damaged, oliguria occurs with retention of waste products.

The point at which the patient becomes obviously symptomatic and displays signs of typical renal failure occurs when approximately 80% to 90% of renal function has been lost. At this level of renal function, creatinine clearance values will fall to 15 ml/minute or less.

The symptoms of uraemia usually develop so slowly that the patient and family often do not recall the time of onset of the illness. Common symptoms include the following:

1. Early symptoms—lethargy, headaches, physical and mental fatigue, weight loss, irritability, depression.
2. Later symptoms—anorexia, persistent nausea and vomiting, shortness of breath on either mild or no exertion, and pitting oedema; pruritus may be absent, mild, or severe.

As renal function deteriorates, *all organ systems are affected* (see Table 25-14). Every aspect of the patient's physical, social, and psychological functioning is affected by the disease.

Integumentary system

Patients with end-stage renal disease (ESRD) have a characteristic yellowish, grey-bronze skin hue from retained pigments[53] and an underlying pallor from anaemia. The patient usually complains of dry skin and pruritus

25-15	**Causes of chronic renal failure**

Congenital or developmental disorders
    Malformations of urinary tract
    Medullary cystic disease
    Polycystic kidney disease
    Hereditary glomerulonephritis with deafness
Glomerulonephritis
    Glomerulopathies
        Diffuse: involves all glomeruli
        Focal: involves some glomeruli
        Segmental: involves portions of individual
            glomeruli
        Membranous: glomerular capillary wall
            thickens
        Proliferative: number of glomerular cells in-
            creased
        Acute: changes occur over days or weeks
        Chronic: changes occur over months or
            years.
    Acute streptococcal glomerulonephritis
Tubular disorders
    Renal tubular disorders
    Fanconi syndrome
    Heavy metal poisoning (lead, mercury)
Renal neoplasms: benign, malignant, Wilms'
    tumour
Infectious renal diseases: pyelonephritis, renal tu-
    berculosis
Obstructive renal disorders: nephrolithiasis, retro-
    peritoneal fibrosis
Renal disorders and systemic disorders
    Diabetic nephropathy
    Diabetes insipidus
    Primary hyperparathyroidism
    Hepatorenal syndrome
    Gout
    Amyloidosis
    Scleroderma
    Goodpasture's syndrome
    Systemic lupus erythematosus
    Nephrotic syndrome
    Hypertensive nephropathy
Renal problems in pregnancy

caused by the depressive effect of the uraemic toxins on the oil and sweat glands and calcium or phosphate deposition on the skin surface. Uraemic frost, a white dustlike material, is rarely seen today, because dialysis is usually initiated promptly for treatment of severe azotaemia.[22]

As a result of protein wasting, the patient's nails are brittle, thin, and easily broken; ridges are typically visible on the nail surface. The hair tends to be coarse and dry and may fall out easily.

Cardiovascular system

Five major cardiovascular conditions occurring with CRF include hypertension, accelerated atherosclerosis, myocardial dysfunction, pericarditis, and hyperkalaemia.

Hypertension. Hypertension is the most common cardiovascular problem observed in CRF. It results chiefly from sodium and water retention and from malfunction of the renin-angiotensin system. Sodium and water retention occur when the kidneys lose their ability to filter and excrete salt and water. The patient with CRF often produces excessive amounts of renin.[53] Renin is converted to angiotensin II, which is a potent vasoconstrictor and a substance that stimulates aldosterone secretion. Both peripheral vasoconstriction and aldosterone elevate blood pressure. Normally an increase in blood pressure reduces renin production; however, in CRF, renin is often produced despite an elevated blood pressure. Angiotensin-converting enzyme (ACE) inhibitors, such as captopril, inhibit the conversion of angiotensin I to angiotensin II, thus reducing the effects of chronic renin secretion in the ESRD patient.[11]

Accelerated atherosclerosis. Patients with CRF have an increased incidence of atherosclerosis. The reasons for this are not well understood. Hyperlipidaemia, commonly seen in this patient population, is a possible contributing factor.[11]

Myocardial dysfunction. Left ventricular hypertrophy with CRF is often a result of hypertension, atherosclerosis, and anaemia. Excessive myocardial hypertrophy decreases myocardial contractility because there is insufficient blood supply for the increased muscle mass. Additionally, fluid overload may cause congestive heart failure in a patient whose myocardial function is compromised.

Hyperkalaemia. Hyperkalaemia is a life-threatening complication of renal failure (p. 717). High serum potassium levels change the balance between intracellular and extracellular potassium. The membrane potential is altered, affecting the electrical activity of the heart. Potentially lethal cardiac dysrhythmias may result in cardiac arrest and death.[11]

Pericarditis. Pericarditis is a frequent cardiovascular complication of CRF. If it is not treated, it may lead to haemorrhagic pericardial effusion and cardiac tamponade (see Chapter 17). The pericardium may become inflamed by uraemic toxins, bacteria, or viruses. Signs include a pericardial friction rub (from harsh rubbing of pericardial layers), low-grade fever, hypotension, and chest pain. The heart may become significantly compressed by pleural effusion between the pericardial layers (cardiac tamponade), requiring pericardial fenestration or pericardiectomy to maintain cardiac output and prevent death.[11]

Respiratory system

Respiratory problems in CRF include pulmonary oedema, pleural effusions, uraemic pleuritis, and a condition referred to as *uraemic lung* or *uraemic pneumonitis*. The sputum is tenacious and the cough reflex is depressed. Susceptibility to infection is increased because of the reduction in pulmonary macrophage activity that occurs in uraemia. A superimposed bacterial infection in the "wet" uraemic lung is common. The respiratory system tries to compensate for the metabolic acidosis by increasing the respiratory rate (Kussmaul's respirations) to eliminate carbon dioxide in an effort to decrease the carbonic acid concentration of the body.[11]

Table 25-14 Manifestations of chronic renal failure

System	Manifestation	Aetiology
Integumentary		
Skin	Yellow, grey, bronze pigmentation	Retained pigments
	Pallor	Anaemia
	Dryness, scaliness	Decreased size of sweat glands and activity of oil glands
	Pruritus	Dry skin, phosphate crystals
Nails	Thin, brittle	Protein wasting
Hair	Dry	Decreased oil gland activity
	Coarse	Protein wasting
Cardiovascular	Hypertension	Fluid overload, sodium/water retention
	Accelerated atherosclerosis	Hyperlipidaemia
	Myocardial dysfunction	Left ventricular hypertrophy
	Congestive heart failure	Fluid overload, hypertension
	Hyperkalaemia	Decreased excretion of potassium by kidney
	Pericarditis	Uraemic toxins in pericardial fluid; increased pericardial membrane permeability
Respiratory	Uraemic lung or pneumonitis	Decreased macrophage activity
	Pulmonary oedema	Fluid overload
	Uraemic pleuritis, pleural effusion	Increased permeability of pleural membrane because of uraemic toxins
	Kussmaul's respirations	Compensatory mechanism for metabolic acidosis
Neuromuscular	Somnolence, confusion, coma	Fluid/electrolyte and acid/base imbalance, uraemic toxins
	Peripheral neuropathy "restless leg" and "burning feet" syndromes	Decreased nerve conduction, both motor and sensory, because of uraemic toxins
Gastrointestinal		
Oral cavity	Halitosis, stomatitis	Urea converted to ammonia by saliva
Stomach	Anorexia, nausea, vomiting	Decomposition of urea in stomach releases ammonia, which produces small ulcerations and bleeding
Bowel	Diarrhoea	Hypermotility from electrolyte imbalance, particularly hyperkalaemia
	Constipation	Hypomotility from electrolyte imbalance, particularly hypokalaemia; decreased fluid intake; decreased bulk in diet and decreased activity
Hematopoietic	Anaemia	Decreased erythropoietin secretion; loss of RBCs through GI tract and decreased RBC survival time; uraemic toxins interfering with folic acid activity
	Platelet dysfunction	Decreased cell surface adhesiveness
	Susceptibility to infection	Decreased neutrophil phagocytosis and chemotaxis
Metabolic	Carbohydrate intolerance	Decreased sensitivity to insulin in peripheral tissues; decreased production of insulin
	Hyperlipidaemia	Increased production of serum triglycerides; increased liver output of glycerides from increased insulin levels; reduction in lipase activity
	Protein wasting	Accumulation of end products of protein metabolism with decreased renal function; decreased protein intake
Skeletal	Hypocalcaemia	Decreased GI reabsorption because of decreased renal conversion of vitamin D; response to elevated serum phosphatase
	Hyperphosphataemia	Decreased renal excretion
	Metastatic calcifications	Deposition of calcium phosphate crystals in soft tissue and other structures
	Bone dissolution and demineralization	Secondary hyperparathyroidism
Reproductive	Diminished fertility, changes in menstruation	Hormonal changes because of uraemic toxins

Neuromuscular system

Changes in mental functioning are a profound result of CRF. Patients may exhibit confusion, decreased memory, short attention span, and inability to think clearly. Somnolence, stupor, coma, and seizures may also occur in severe cases. These changes are related to fluid/electrolyte and acid-base imbalances and uraemic toxin accumulation. Also as a result of the latter a slowing of peripheral nerve conduction occurs, which leads to peripheral neuropathy. Symptoms include bilateral paraesthesia and a burning sensation beginning in the toes and spreading up the legs. Painful leg cramps, and crawling, prickling, and itching sensations of the legs develop, usually at night. This syndrome is often relieved by movement and thus is called "restless leg" syndrome. Symptoms of "burning feet" syndrome may also occur and include bilateral painful, burning, prickling, and tingling sensations in the feet. If dialysis is initiated before motor nerve dysfunction develops, these neuropathic changes may be prevented.[11]

Gastrointestinal system

The accumulated uraemic toxins and ammonia resulting from the decomposition of urea are irritating to the mucosal lining of the GI tract. These irritants cause anorexia, nausea, and vomiting, which interfere with nutrition. If the patient cannot ingest an adequate amount of calories, catabolism occurs to provide the necessary energy, further accelerating and aggravating the uraemia.[11]

In the oral cavity small painful ulcerations occur (stomatitis). Often the patient experiences the taste of blood as a result of the mouth lesions. In addition, as urea decomposes, it emits a distinctive odour that resembles urine. This causes halitosis, which is not only foul smelling but also alters the patient's taste sensations. These changes in the oral cavity further impede nutritional intake.

The gastric mucosa also becomes irritated by the decomposing urea, causing small gastric ulcerations. Bleeding that results from these ulcerations and from increased capillary fragility produced by the uraemic toxins is usually manifested as slow GI oozing rather than full GI bleeding.

Bowel function is rarely normal. Hyperkalaemia is frequently accompanied by hypermotility and diarrhoea. Hypokalaemia produces hypomotility and constipation. In addition, decreased fluid intake, activity level, and dietary bulk, and ingestion of phosphate binders serve to aggravate the constipation.

Haematopoietic system

The three major haematopoietic manifestations of CRF are anaemia, platelet dysfunction, and increased susceptibility to infection.

Anaemia. Anaemia, one of the most debilitating effects of CRF, is caused by the following: (1) decreased erythropoietin secretion by the dysfunctional kidneys, (2) loss of RBCs through the GI tract or haemodialysis, (3) decreased RBC survival time from the effect of uraemic toxins, (4) production of crenated cells by the hypertonic serum resulting from action of uraemic toxins, and (5) decreased folic acid activity because of interference of

the uraemic toxins. Recombinant human erythropoietin, EPO, plays a critical role in regulating erythropoiesis; the patient treated with this hormone has increased haemoglobin levels, decreased need for transfusions, and less fatigue.

Platelet dysfunction. The uraemic toxins adversely change the surface of the platelets, decreasing adhesiveness or aggregation capabilities, which results in bleeding. Bruises and petechiae are often seen on the skin. The patient is also at increased risk for bleeding as a result of platelet dysfunction.

Metabolic dysfunction

The three aspects of endocrine dysfunction in CRF are carbohydrate intolerance, hyperlipidaemia, and protein imbalance.

Carbohydrate intolerance. Carbohydrate intolerance in CRF results from an insensitivity of peripheral tissues to insulin, delayed production of insulin by the pancreas, and an increased half-life of insulin. The serum insulin level is often elevated in uraemia because of slowed insulin degradation by the kidney; however, the insulin cannot be effective because of peripheral resistance. These changes do not typically result in hyperglycaemia or ketoacidosis. Adequate insulin is released to prevent these conditions in most instances.[22]

Hyperlipidaemia. Serum triglyceride levels are elevated in uraemia because of increased production and decreased removal of triglycerides. The increased production is related to the peripheral resistance to insulin, and to elevated serum insulin, which cause an increased output of glycerides by the liver. Reduction in activity of the enzyme lipoprotein lipase contributes to the abnormality.[22]

Protein imbalance. There is an accumulation of end products of protein metabolism with decreased renal function, as evidenced by an elevated blood urea.

Skeletal system

Calcium, phosphorus, vitamin D, the parathyroid glands, the skeletal system, and the kidneys exist in an intricate and balanced relationship; renal failure inevitably disrupts this balance. Individuals with renal failure will develop one or more of the following problems: hyperphosphataemia, hypocalcaemia, hyperparathyroidism, inadequate vitamin D metabolism, osteodystrophies, or metastatic calcifications. Abnormalities of calcium, phosphorus, or vitamin D metabolism are among the earliest changes to occur with progressive loss of renal function. Early recognition and treatment can prevent the significant damage to the skeletal system that can result from these imbalances.[11]

Reproductive system

Multiple problems related to sexual and reproductive functioning occur in the patient with renal failure. The causes are multifactorial and include hormonal abnormalities, psychological problems, anaemia, antihypertensive medications, and malnutrition. Dialysis may result in some improvement. Transplantation often results in normalization of sexual functioning.[11]

Testosterone is markedly decreased in males and ovarian hormone secretion is suppressed in females. There appears to be end-organ resistance to follicular-stimulating hormone in both sexes. These changes can result in decreased spermatogenesis in males, and amenorrhoea and infertility in females.[11]

Nursing Process
Assessment
Subjective data

The nursing assessment of the patient in chronic renal failure is extremely complex, particularly because of the multisystem involvement and chronicity of the disorder. Subjective data to be collected include the following:

1. Perception of illness
   a. Reason for coming to the hospital initially
   b. Understanding of proposed plan of care
   c. Expectations of results of therapy
2. History of past illness
   a. Illnesses associated with renal disease
   b. Other illnesses and hospitalizations
   c. Medication regimen
   d. Other therapies
3. Activity
   a. Ability to ambulate, climb stairs, and get in and out of a chair
   b. Presence of bone pain
   c. Fatigue: presence, extent
   d. Usual daytime activities
   e. Recent employment history
   f. Recreational interests
4. Rest and sleep
   a. Nightly sleeping pattern
   b. Activities that induce sleep at night
   c. Daytime napping pattern
   d. Presence and extent of pruritus
5. Nutrition
   a. Present dietary prescription and ability to follow diet
   b. Daily eating patterns
   c. Fluid intake in 24 hours
   d. Impediments to eating (anorexia, nausea and vomiting, bad taste in mouth)
6. Elimination
   a. Frequency and difficulties with urination
   b. Usual amount voided in 24 hours
   c. Colour of urine
   d. History of UTI
   e. Usual bowel habits and use of laxatives or enemas
   f. Occurrence of diarrhoea or constipation
7. Reproductive system
   a. Menstrual pattern (females)
   b. Recent changes in sexual functioning
   c. Concerns about reproductive or sexual functioning
8. Social
   a. People living at home; relationships
   b. Support people called upon for help
   c. Type of dwelling and presence of stairs
9. Psychological: other concerns

25-16

Monitoring parameters for the person with chronic renal failure

1. Intake and output every 8 hours
2. Fluid excess: palpating for oedema, auscultating breath sounds, checking blood pressure (lying and standing) at least every 8 hours, daily weight records
3. Cardiac rhythms every 8 hours
4. Level of consciousness every 8 hours
5. Signs of electrolyte imbalances
6. Presence of fatigue and shortness of breath
7. Signs of GI bleeding (bleeding gums, guaiac-positive stools)
8. Presence of pruritus and evidences of skin excoriations
9. Presence of discomfort: muscle cramping, headaches, ocular irritations
10. Insomnia
11. Anorexia, bad taste in mouth, daily dietary intake
12. Signs of infection

Objective data

Objective data to be collected for the patient with chronic renal failure includes the following:

1. Height and weight
2. Vital signs: temperature, pulse (radial, apical, peripheral), respirations and breath sounds (adventitious sounds, friction rub), blood pressure (lying and standing), heart sounds.
3. Signs of fluid retention: oedema (peripheral, periorbital), neck vein distension, obvious difficulty with breathing, cough with frothy sputum
4. Status of vascular access for dialysis (if present)
5. Neuromuscular difficulties
   a. Muscle tone and strength, symmetry
   b. Weakness or loss of function in extremities
   c. Balance
   d. Loss of sensation, tremors
   e. Senses: vision, touch, taste/smell
   f. Ability to speak
   g. Orientation
   h. Level of alertness and responsiveness
6. Skin: colour, turgor, temperature, lesions, condition of nails
7. Urine: colour, specific gravity.

Once the initial data are obtained, they must be continuously updated. All subsequent assessments are determined by the medical regimen and nursing interventions. Some areas of ongoing assessment are listed in Box 25-16.

Diagnostic tests

A wide variety of diagnostic tests is required once the diagnosis has been made. Many tests will be required to confirm the initial diagnosis. As renal failure progresses, the person will continue to have blood chemistries monitored to ensure that treatment is adequate. Serial creatinine clearance, serum creatinine, and blood urea are monitored.

Nursing analysis

Nursing analyses are determined from assessment of patient data. Possible nursing problems for the person with chronic renal failure may include, but are not limited to, the following:

Problem	Possible aetiologies
Fluid volume excess	Compromised regulatory mechanism
Nutrition, altered: less than body requirements	Electrolyte imbalances, protein imbalance, anorexia, bad taste in mouth
Oral mucous membrane, altered	Decomposing urea
Infection, high risk for	Compromised immune response
Injury, high risk for	Neurological changes, bleeding potential, hyperkalaemia
Skin integrity, impaired, high risk for	Pruritus, dry scaly skin
Fatigue	Uraemia, anaemia, insomnia
Pain: muscle cramps, ocular irritation	Uraemic toxins
Coping, ineffective, individual	Situational crisis
Knowledge deficit	Lack of exposure, cognition limitations

Planning: expected patient outcomes

Expected outcomes for the patient with chronic renal failure may include, but are not limited to, the following:

1. Does not show signs of additional fluid retention.
2. Eats a balanced diet within prescribed limits.
3. States mouth feels comfortable and bad taste is lessened.
4. Does not show signs of infection.
5. Does not incur any injury.
6. Is free of skin lesions.
7. States feeling more rested and less fatigued.
8. States muscles and eyes are not uncomfortable.
9. Describes feelings about illness and plans for activities that facilitate social interactions.
10. Develops trusting relationship with health care professionals.
11. Describes nature of CRF, rationale for therapy, therapeutic regimens, and need for follow-up care.

Implementation

Assisting with achievement of therapeutic goals

The treatment goals for the person with CRF are listed in Box 25-17. Conservative therapy consists of controlling fluid, sodium, and protein intake. Medications are given to control hypertension, decrease serum phosphate, replace calcium, manage congestive heart failure, decrease potential for GI irritation, and control anaemia.

Medications

When kidney function is impaired, drugs are not excreted effectively, thus their effects may be prolonged. People with CRF must therefore be monitored closely for signs of side effects of toxicity. These patients must have the necessary information to monitor themselves at home. Because hypertension commonly occurs with CRF, antihypertensive drugs may be prescribed (Chapter 18).

Measures to decrease hyperphosphataemia help to protect the bones and kidney from further damage. Medications such as calcium carbonate and aluminium hydroxide bind phosphorus in the intestinal tract and allow it to be eliminated. These drugs should be taken at meals to bind the phosphates in the food. The drugs should not be taken with other medications because they also bind drugs in the intestinal tract.

The major electrolyte requiring replacement in a patient with renal failure is *calcium*. Calcium requires vitamin D for absorption; therefore it is not sufficient to administer calcium preparations alone. The active form of *vitamin D* must be given in order for the calcium to be absorbed, either alfacalcidol or calcitriol.[22] Examples of calcium supplements include those used for hyperphosphataemia as well as calcium gluconate and calcium lactate.

Cardiac glycosides are used to manage congestive heart failure that often occurs. Examples include digoxin and digitoxin; digoxin is the preferred because of its greater margin of safety.

Diuretic agents are prescribed to increase the formation of urine and enhance the excretion of fluids and solutes. The major contribution of diuretics lies in their ability to potentiate the effect of the antihypertensive agents. Frusemide, bumetanide, metolazone, and spironolactone are commonly used.

Histamine H_2 receptor antagonists, such as ranitidine or cimetidine, are used to decrease the potential of gastric irritation, ulceration, and bleeding occurring secondary to renal failure.

Anaemia is treated with recombinant human erythropoietin, EPO (p. 726) and an *iron supplement.* Transfusions are avoided unless the patient has been refractory to EPO or iron therapy or has experienced significant blood loss, because transfusions depress the patient's stimulus to RBC production, and may cause transfusion reactions.

Vitamin supplements frequently given patients with CRF include the B complex vitamins, vitamin C, folic acid, and vitamin B6. These vitamins are water soluble and are lost during haemodialysis. It may be appropriate to administer vitamin K to the patient receiving antibiotics.

Interventions to achieve patient outcomes
Promoting fluid balance

It is important to adhere to the fluid prescriptions. Fluid intake must be sufficient to maintain renal function without producing diuresis or fluid retention. The patient needs to understand the effects of excessive or inadequate fluid intake and signs indicating fluid retention or dehydration in order to maintain the fluid prescriptions both during hospitalization and at home. During hospitalization, monitor the patient's fluid intake and output carefully. Weigh the patient daily at the same time of day and wearing the same clothes.

Facilitating nutrition

Although severely restricted *sodium* diets are *not* now usually prescribed, most people with CRF require some salt restrictions. If a no-added salt (NAS) diet is prescribed, a normal diet is followed except that no extra salt is added to prepared foods, and obviously salted foods are omitted. For more restricted diets, the specific amount of sodium permitted is prescribed; the dietitian can be especially helpful to patients in planning meals that meet the sodium restriction. *Salt substitutes should be avoided* by all people with CRF because these substitutes contain large amounts of potassium.

Potassium intake may need to be restricted. If severe hyperkalaemia is present, measures to remove the excess serum potassium must be taken (p. 721). If hyperphosphataemia is present, dietary restriction of *phosphates* will be necessary. Food high in phosphorus include meat, poultry, fish, eggs, milk and cheese, and legumes.

Protein intake is reduced to decrease azotaemia, acidosis, and hyperkalaemia, and to relieve distressing GI symptoms. Some protein is needed to help maintain nitrogen balance. The preferred proteins are those of high biological value that contain more essential amino acids, such as fish, poultry, eggs, milk. A newer approach to protein replacement that promotes positive nitrogen balance is the use of mixtures of essential amino acids and ketoacid analogues. *Carbohydrates* are encouraged to provide energy without placing an undue load on the kidneys.

Because the patient is frequently anorexic and may have a bad taste in the mouth, it requires creativity on the part of nurse and family to encourage the patient to eat the prescribed diet (see Chapter 4). Decreased salivary flow and ammonia from breakdown of urea can lead to irritation of the oral mucous membranes. Provide *oral hygiene* several times a day, especially before meals. Mouth care can help remove the taste of blood and urea. Lip emollients can help keep lips moist.

Preventing infection

Patients with CRF are at greater risk for infection than the general population because of decreased neutrophil phagocytosis and chemotaxis. Prevention and control of infection is similar to that for acute renal failure (p. 722). Inform the patient to avoid exposure to individuals with known infections and to avoid extreme fatigue, which lowers body resistance. Encourage the patient to seek medical attention for early signs of infection.

Promoting safety and maintaining skin integrity

Significant rises in serum potassium can be averted by preventing tissue breakdown. Potassium is largely an intracellular cation, and extensive tissue damage can liberate a lethal amount of this ion into the system of the patient with CRF. Oedema also adds to poor nutrition of the skin. Carry out measures to prevent undue pressure on the skin. Because uraemia retards wound healing, instruct patient to monitor scratches for evidence of infection.

Most people with end-stage renal disease develop pruritus. Patients say that itching is of a deep sensation. Factors that appear to exacerbate the itching include increasing levels of serum phosphorus, dry skin, and warm moist heat. Itching is largely symptomatic, and measures that are effective in controlling it vary. Keeping the skin moist and supple through use of lotions and bath oils, controlling the room temperature during sleep to prevent excessive warmth, and bathing with a vinegar solution are measures that, used

---

25-17

Treatment goals for the person with chronic renal failure

1. Stabilization of the internal environment as demonstrated by the following:
   a. Mental alertness, attention span, and appropriate interaction with the environment
   b. Absence or control of peripheral oedema, absence of pulmonary oedema
   c. Control of electrolyte balance:

Sodium	125–145 mEq/L
Potassium	3–6 mEq/L
Bicarbonate	>15 mEq/L
Calcium	9–11 mg/dl
Phosphate	3–5mg/dl

   d. Serum albumin   >2g/dl
   e. Control of protein catabolism and protein breakdown products

Blood urea	<100 mg/dl
Creatinine	<15 mg/dl
Uric acid	<12 mg/dl

   f. Absence of joint inflammation and pain
2. Infection and abnormal bleeding are not present.
3. Blood pressure is controlled at less than 160/100 mm Hg sitting, less than 30 mm Hg postural change on standing.
4. Anorexia, nausea, and pruritus are absent or controlled.
5. Intercurrent illness is resolved or controlled (heart failure, infection, dehydration).
6. There is no toxicity from inadequately excreted medication.
7. Nutrient intake is sufficient to maintain positive nitrogen balance.
8. Fluid restrictions are maintained.
9. Adjustment to life-style changes is adaptive.
10. Coping mechanisms are appropriate.
11. Trusting relationship is established between patient and nurse.

---

alone or in combination, may provide some relief from itching. Antipruritic medications may be prescribed. Injury to the skin from vigorous scratching may lead to skin infections. Fingernails can be trimmed closely, and a soft cloth rather than the fingernails should be used to scratch the skin.

Mild soaps should be used to avoid excessive skin dryness. Pruritus often decreases with a reduction in uraemia and improved phosphorus control. Encourage the use of phosphate binders and the reduction of dietary phosphorus if elevated phosphorus is a problem.

GI bleeding needs to be diminished when possible. Urea is broken down to ammonia by the action of intestinal bacteria. Because ammonia is a mucosal irritant, ulcers and bleeding can occur. Administer prescribed antacids (every 2 to 4 hours) and H_2 receptor antagonists to prevent bleeding. Suggest that the patient use a soft toothbrush to decrease bleeding of the gums. Instruct the patient to look for and report signs of melaena.

Neurological changes can also lead to injuries from decreasing patient alertness or vision, or from muscle weakness. Assess the patient's awareness of the environment. At times the person may need to be helped in limiting activities to a level commensurate with mental processes and level of awareness. Individuals caring for the patient need to be aware of the possibility of seizure activity and take appropriate precautions. Correction of abnormal body chemistries will help to decrease the potential for injury.

Promoting rest

Fatigue is a common complaint of people with CRF because of the effects of uraemia, anaemia, and recurring thoughts concerning the disease state and resultant changes in life-style. Treatment for uraemia and anaemia will help to decrease fatigue. Plans for daily activities should include provision of rest periods. Naps are best taken early in the day; late naps interfere with the quality of sleep. Measures to promote sleep are appropriate.

Promoting comfort

Muscle cramping in the lower extremities and hands may be temporarily relieved by heat and massage in some people. *Ocular irritation* in CRF is caused by hyperphosphataemia leading to calcium deposits in the conjunctiva, which cause burning and watering of the eyes. Hypromellose (artificial tears) placed in the conjunctival sac every few hours helps to reduce irritation.

Facilitating coping

Numerous alterations in life-style, group membership, and feelings regarding the self occur for the patient with CRF. The numerous physical changes that occur often make it difficult to carry on activities that were once normally pursued. Chronic fatigue may make it impossible for the patient to continue to be employed. Because the patient is often tired and not feeling well, it may be difficult to plan in advance for social events. The former roles of the sick member of the family must often be taken on by another. When roles cannot easily be changed or assumed by other members of the family, serious threats to the organization of the family group occur. Physical appearance also changes and is of much concern to most people. As uraemia progresses, the individual often becomes thin and weaker and appears sallow. Thoughts concerning death and the quality of life are common.

Denial often becomes a chief defence mechanism for the patient. With it the individual can periodically forget the constant threat to life. The use of this mental mechanism for the person with CRF can be quite appropriate as long as it is not manifested by maladaptive or harmful behaviour. Inappropriate uses of denial involve continuous dietary indiscretion and failure to take prescribed medications.

Patients with chronic renal failure need the hope and encouragement that with treatment discomfort will be lessened and they will be allowed to pursue what seems most productive and important to them. Hope should not be focused on cure, but on learning to manage a new style of life. In managing the changes that occur as a result of CRF, patients should be encouraged to be as independent and as active as possible. They should be taught to manage the treatment and should be given the responsibility of doing so. Nursing care should be provided as part of the team approach that assists patients in identifying problems and resources to meet them, and helps patients and their families adjust to the changes in their life-style.

Facilitating patient learning

To promote self-care, every aspect of health care promotion pertaining to end-stage renal disease must be conveyed to the patient and significant others who may be participating in care (see Box 25-18). Education about *medications*, concerning prescribed, over-the-counter, and folk medicines, is carried out with the patient. The use of popular medications that are sold without prescription must be discouraged. All medications should be prescribed by the doctor. Aspirin may be hazardous because it is normally excreted by the kidneys and may rapidly build to toxic levels and prolong bleeding time. Many cold preparations contain large amounts of sodium. Remembering to take prescribed medications can be a problem for the patient who may have many pills to take each day, especially if the person is confused. Correlating pill-taking times with major activities of the day or use of mechanical devices to separate the daily allotment of pills may be helpful. Patient teaching includes the following:

1. Nature of chronic renal failure
2. Diet regimen, including fluid restrictions
3. Medication regimen, including action, dosage, frequency, and side effects
4. Relationships between diet, fluid restriction, medication, and blood chemistries
5. Relationships between symptoms and their causes
6. Need for rest periods, and need to pace activities to prevent fatigue
7. Availability of community resources
8. Symptoms that must be reported to the doctor (changes in urinary output, oedema, weight gain, dyspnoea, infection, behavioural changes)
9. Need for continued medical follow-up

Evaluation

Evaluation is based on expected patient outcomes. Questions to consider include the following:

1. Is the patient following the required fluid and diet prescription?
2. Does the patient state that mouth feels comfortable and bad taste is lessened?
3. Have infection and injury been prevented?
4. Has skin integrity been maintained?
5. Does the person describe feeling more comfortable and less fatigued?
6. Has the patient planned for activities to facilitate social interactions and developed a trusting relationship with health care professionals?
7. Can the person describe the nature of CRF, rationale for therapy, therapeutic regimen, and symptoms to be reported?

The patient with chronic renal failure

Administer prescribed medication (antihypertensives, calcium products, vitamin D preparations, cardiac glycosides, diuretics, histamine H$_2$ receptor antagonists, EPO, iron supplements, and vitamin supplements).

Encourage the person to remain within prescribed fluid restrictions.

Encourage a diet high in carbohydrates within the prescribed limits of sodium, potassium, phosphorus, and protein.

Administer phosphate-binding agent with meals, as prescribed.

Provide oral hygiene at frequent intervals, especially before meals.

Protect the patient from infection.

Assess the environment and protect the patient from injury.

Provide rest periods to decrease fatigue.

Use measures to decrease pruritus, muscle cramping, and eye irritation.

Provide patient with opportunities to discuss feelings about chronicity of disease.

Provide counselling if denial interferes with therapy.

Encourage hope by helping the patient learn how to manage the new life-style.

Teach the patient about the nature of CRF, rationale for therapy, therapeutic regimens, and need for follow-up care.

RENAL REPLACEMENT THERAPIES
Dialysis

Dialysis involves the movement of fluid and particles across a semipermeable membrane. It is a treatment that can help restore normal fluid and electrolyte balance, control acid-base balance, and remove waste and toxic material from the body. It can sustain life successfully in both acute and chronic renal failure where substitution for or augmentation of normal renal function is needed. Specifically, dialysis is used to remove excessive amounts of drugs and toxins in poisoning of both an intentional and accidental nature, to correct serious electrolyte and acid-base imbalances, to maintain kidney function when renal shutdown occurs as a result of transfusion reactions, to temporarily replace renal function in people with acute renal failure of various origins, and to permanently substitute for loss of renal function in people with chronic end-stage renal disease.

Physiological principles of dialysis

Dialysis is based on three principles: diffusion, osmosis, and ultrafiltration (Fig. 25-11). *Diffusion* involves the movement of *particles* from an area of greater concentration to an area of lesser concentration. In the body this usually occurs across a semipermeable membrane. Diffusion is involved in the clearance of solute from the patient's body in both haemodialysis and peritoneal dialysis. Diffusion results in the movement of urea, creatinine, and uric acid from the patient's blood into the dialysate solution.

This solution contains fewer particles to be removed from the bloodstream and higher concentrations of particles to be added to the blood (Fig. 25-12). Because the dialysate contains no protein waste products, the concentration of these substances in the blood will decrease because of random movement of the particles across the semipermeable membrane into the dialysate. The same principle applies to the movement of potassium ions. Although the concentration of red blood cells and protein is high in blood, these molecules are quite large and do not diffuse through the membrane pores; hence they are not lost from the blood.

Osmosis involves the movement of *fluid* across a semipermeable membrane from an area of lesser to an area of greater concentration of particles. Osmosis is responsible for movement of extra fluid from the patient, particularly in peritoneal dialysis. Fig. 25-12 shows that glucose has been added to the dialysate to make its particle concentration greater than that of the patient's blood. Fluid will then move through the pores of the membrane from the patient's blood to the dialysate.

Ultrafiltration involves the movement of fluid across a semipermeable membrane as a result of an artificially created pressure gradient. Ultrafiltration is more efficient than osmosis for removal of fluid and is used in haemodialysis for this purpose. During dialysis, osmosis and diffusion or ultrafiltration and diffusion occur simultaneously.

Haemodialysis
Procedure

Haemodialysis involves shunting the patient's blood from the body through a dialyzer in which diffusion and ultrafiltration occur and back into the patient's circulation. To perform haemodialysis there must be access to the patient's blood, a mechanism to transport the blood to and from the dialyzer, and a dialyzer (area in which the exchange of fluid electrolytes and waste products occurs). Presently there are five major means for gaining access to the patient's bloodstream. These include the following:

1. Arteriovenous fistula (Fig. 25-13, A)
2. Arteriovenous graft (Fig. 25-13, B)
3. External arteriovenous shunt (Fig. 25-13, C)
4. Femoral vein catheterization (Fig. 25-13, D)
5. Subclavian vein catheterization (Fig. 25-13, E)

Many people expect to leave the dialysis treatment with a feeling of well-being. Few people feel this way; most experience some minor discomfort that diminishes within several hours after dialysis. The greatest feeling of well-being seems to occur the day after dialysis.

Dialysis for an acute problem may be carried out daily or as often as the condition of the patient warrants. Haemodialysis for chronic renal failure is usually performed two or three times a week.

Nursing care of the patient during haemodialysis should centre around (1) monitoring the physical status of the patient before and during dialysis for evidence of physiological imbalance and change, (2) comfort and safety needs of the patient, and (3) helping the patient to understand and adjust to the care and changes in life-style. This latter objective involves educating the person as to the

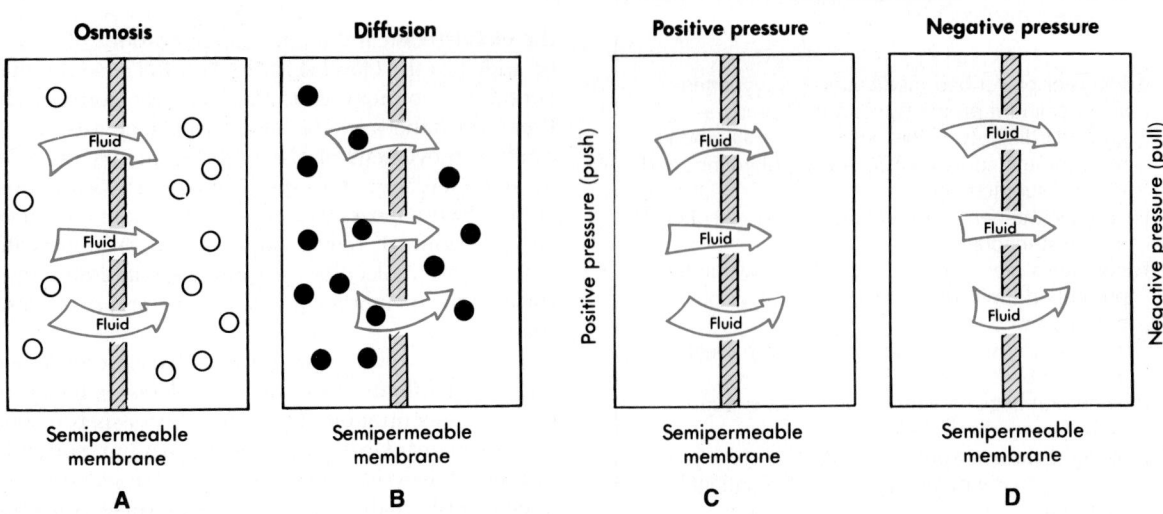

Fig. 25-11 Dialysis is based on principles of **A**, osmosis, and **B**, diffusion and ultrafiltration. Ultrafiltration occurs when either **C**, positive pressure or **D**, negative pressure is placed on the system. Ultrafiltration can be maximized by exerting both positive and negative pressure on system simultaneously.

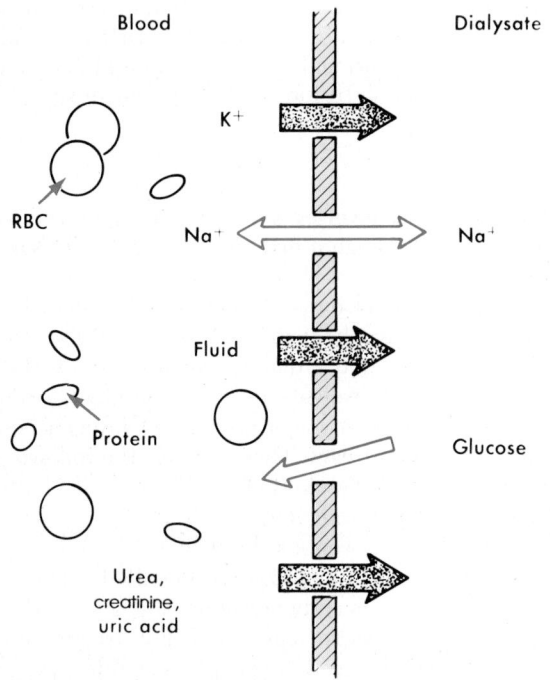

Fig. 25-12 Osmosis and diffusion in dialysis. Net movement of major particles and fluid is illustrated.

specifics of the treatment programme (diet and medications in particular) and how these relate to altered kidney function. The patient is encouraged to express concerns and feelings, and attempts must be made to help the individual work through these feelings. If dialysis is performed at home, the patient and back-up person must be able to institute all the care described.

The environment must provide protection from conditions that would promote infection. Because there is the potential for blood spills as a result of the treatment, all equipment must be easy to clean. Great care must also be taken to dispose properly all soiled articles to prevent cross-contamination between patients.

Because the patient spends a great deal of time at the dialysis centre, the environment should be warm and inviting. Activities should be available to assist the patient in using the time on dialysis as fully as possible. Art and music therapy both provide effective and productive diversion.

Predialysis care

When possible before the procedure, patients should have an opportunity to become familiar with the dialysis unit. They should be given an explanation of what will happen and what will be expected of them during the treatment. Patients often want to know (1) what types of pain will be experienced during the treatment, (2) how long and how often the dialysis will be, (3) what they should feel like during and after the treatment, (4) what they will be allowed to do during dialysis, and (5) if family members may be present during the therapy. Monitoring activities include the following:

1. Record current weight and compare to patient's dry weight (estimated weight with no excess fluid and near normal blood pressure).
2. Obtain baseline vital signs.
3. Assess patient for fluid overload (pedal oedema, periorbital oedema, neck vein distension, adventitious breath sounds).
4. Assess vascular access for patency and infection.

A blood sample is drawn to determine the level of electrolytes and waste products, and the patient's physical status is assessed.

Patients should be told that they may experience some headache and nausea during the treatment and for a few hours afterward. Headache and nausea result from change

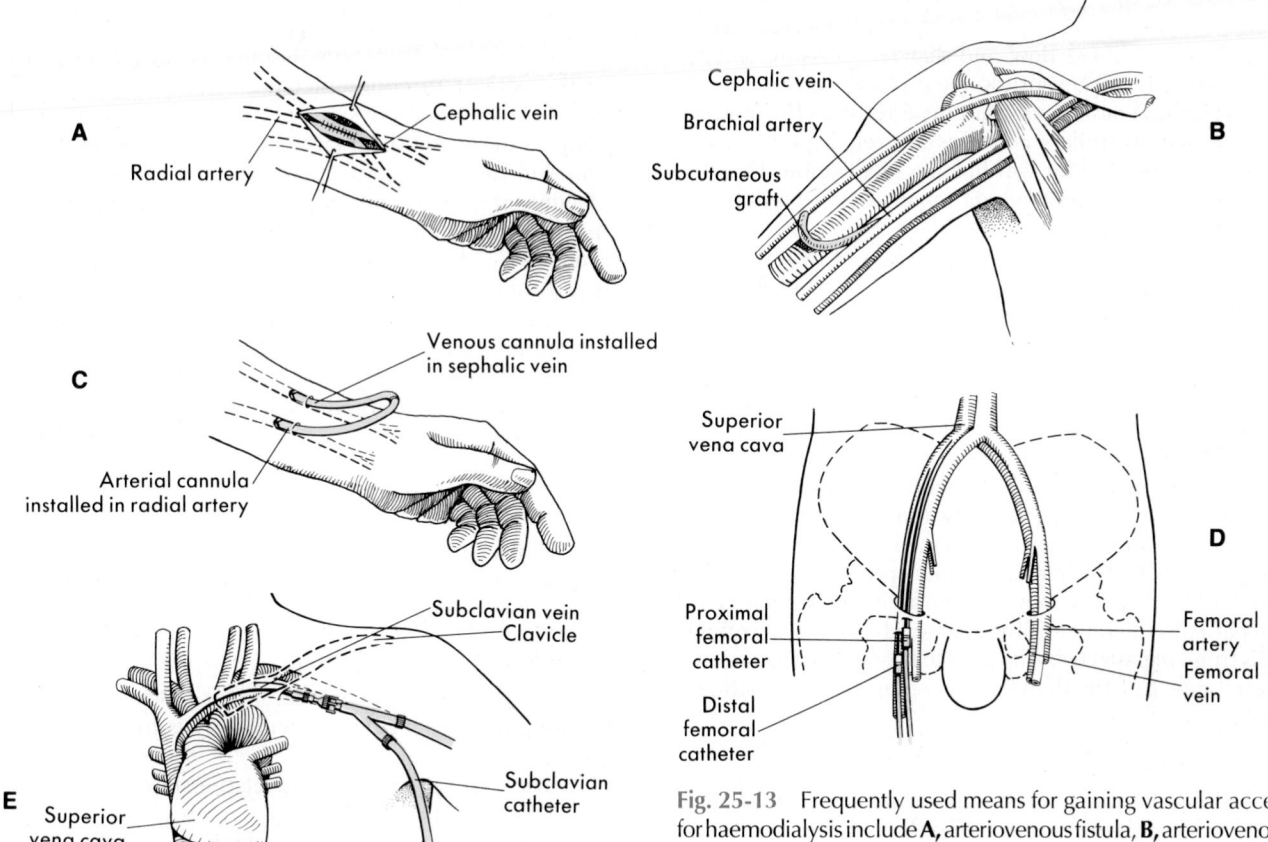

Fig. 25-13   Frequently used means for gaining vascular access for haemodialysis include **A,** arteriovenous fistula, **B,** arteriovenous graft, **C,** external arteriovenous shunt, **D,** femoral vein catheterization, and **E,** subclavian vein catheterization.

in fluid, acid-base, and waste balance during dialysis. The symptoms should never be extreme, and relief should be attained from rest and sleep, mild analgesics, or antiemetics. Postural hypotension may also occur following dialysis; it is transitory in nature and caused by a relative depletion of intravascular volume secondary to fluid removal. The hypotension may produce dizziness and faintness. Relief should be obtained within a few hours with rest. The patient is assured that all of these symptoms will abate and that frequent monitoring during the procedure will help to control the degree of change that occurs during dialysis and the development of these symptoms.

Care during haemodialysis

When the patient has an external shunt used for temporary situations only, no pain should be experienced during initiation of dialysis. However, pain of a moderate degree may be present when venipuncture is performed in an arteriovenous fistula. A local anaesthetic is used in most dialysis centres before insertion of the needles.

Nursing care includes measures to increase the patient's physical comfort. Lying relatively immobile for even a few hours can produce pressure over bony prominences and general restlessness. Changing the patient's position increases tolerance to limited movement. Mouth care is required if the patient is nauseated and vomiting. Because an arm is generally kept immobile during dialysis, the patient may need help with activities requiring the use of both hands.

Activity during dialysis is largely a matter of individual preference. Some people sleep throughout their treatment; others read or carry on various activities.

Eating during dialysis is largely a matter of individual preference. Some individuals may become quite hungry, whereas for others the smell of food causes nausea. Patients may ask that they be allowed to eat foods not generally allowed during dialysis. Practice indicates that either allowing or discouraging eating freely during dialysis is a matter of individual unit philosophy. Because of the frequency of nausea, vomiting, and disequilibrium many patients experience during haemodialysis, it may be best to discourage eating to decrease the potential of aspiration.

Hypovolaemia

Most physical problems that occur during dialysis are related to hypotension from removal of fluid and disequilibrium from a rapid reduction in extracellular electrolytes and wastes. Hypovolaemia and shock can occur during dialysis as a result of rapid removal of *fluid* from the intravascular compartment. Because this can occur faster than reequilibration of intracellular and intravascular volume relationships, the person may appear oedematous and yet exhibit signs of shock. Signs and symptoms that indicate that the intravascular volume is being rapidly depleted are anxiety, restlessness, dizziness, nausea and vomiting, diaphoresis, tachycardia, and hypotension. Activities to prevent hypovolaemia include the following:

1. Check blood pressure and pulse every 30 to 60 minutes (more frequently if signs of shock present); blood pressure should show only a slight increase.

2. Monitor blood flow and dialyzer pressure settings carefully to prevent too-rapid blood flow.
3. Withhold rapid-acting antihypertensives the morning of dialysis (unless person is severely hypertensive).
4. Evaluate need for withholding medications that predispose to hypovolaemia (analgesics, tranquillizers, hypnotics).

In treating a patient who shows signs of hypovolaemia, initial nursing measures include placing the head of the bed in a flat position, and raising the patient's feet. Administration of normal saline solution may be necessary to restore blood pressure. Throughout a hypotensive episode vital signs, level of consciousness, and any complaints offered are closely monitored. Vomiting frequently accompanies hypotension. Because of arm immobility, it may be difficult for the patient to clear the mouth if vomiting should occur. The patient is helped to a safe position so that aspiration is avoided.

When the weight losses of several dialysis treatments are correlated with the patient's blood pressure, pulse, and other indications of hypovolaemia, an individual pattern of the patient's tolerance to fluid removal can be determined. This trend or pattern can be used to help adjust the rate and overall effect of the dialysis in keeping with the patient's physiological tolerance.

Disequilibrium phenomenon

A disequilibrium phenomenon occurs for many dialysis patients towards the end of or after dialysis. Disequilibrium results when excess *solutes* are cleared from the blood more rapidly than they can diffuse from the body's cells (particularly those of the central nervous system) into the vascular compartment. Hence, disequilibrium exists in the concentration of solute inside and outside the cells. Because particle content is greater inside the cells, water is taken in and oedema results. Intracellular pH changes are also present. To some degree this process occurs with all patients with each dialysis procedure and helps to explain why patients do not feel their best immediately after treatment. *Severe disequilibrium,* or *disequilibrium phenomenon,* is most likely to be seen in the person whose blood chemistry values are exceptionally high before dialysis. Signs and symptoms of disequilibrium include *headache, restlessness, mental confusion,* and *nausea* and *vomiting.* Severe disequilibrium may result in convulsions, especially in children when blood urea levels exceed the concentration of 100 mg/ml.

Treatment includes anticipation of severe disequilibrium. Often when a patient is beginning dialysis treatments, the procedures are kept short and may be spaced more frequently than normal during the first week. This allows solute to be cleared from the body without producing the extremely wide swings in body chemistry that would result in severe disequilibrium. Keeping the patient quiet, reducing environmental discomfort such as temperature extremes and bright lights, and closely supervising the patient to ensure physical safety are nursing care requirements. Mild analgesics may help to relieve headache. If disequilibrium becomes severe and the patient is still on dialysis, the therapy may be discontinued.

Blood loss

To prevent the patient's blood from clotting as it flows through the dialyzer, heparin is administered. Epoprostenol may also be used. Protamine sulphate is not generally given to the patient to counteract the effect of heparin. The patient is watched for signs of bleeding anywhere in the body. At the end of the treatment when dialysis needles are removed from the fistula, manual pressure is held until bleeding or oozing ceases. Pressure dressings are applied to the puncture sites. The sites are observed at frequent intervals to detect haemorrhage or oozing. During and shortly after dialysis, treatments that cause tissue trauma such as venepuncture or intramuscular injections should not be performed. The patient who has had recent surgery, dental extractions, or recent trauma to soft tissues will have clotting times monitored frequently during dialysis to prevent haemorrhage. These patients need to be closely observed for signs of bleeding.

Postdialysis care

Following dialysis, the person's weight is recorded again to determine the amount of fluid loss during treatment and postural vital signs are assessed.

Facilitating patient learning

A sample teaching plan is described in Box 25-19. Major teaching points specific to haemodialysis include the following:

1. The process of dialysis and relationship to the person's own body needs.
2. Care of the vascular access, including monitoring for complications (absent thrill or bruit over artery indicating no blood flow, constriction of fistula, infection, haemorrhage).
3. Where to obtain care if complications occur.
4. Common complications of haemodialysis.
5. Changes in medication schedule required before and after dialysis treatments.
6. Ways to schedule dialysis treatments for minimal interference with life-style.
7. Alternative modes of treatment for end-stage renal disease.

Peritoneal dialysis

In peritoneal dialysis the dialyzing fluid is instilled into the peritoneal cavity and the peritoneum becomes the dialyzing membrane. In comparison with haemodialysis treatments, which last 3 to 6 hours, peritoneal dialysis is maintained continuously for up to 36 hours. This is repeated each week and is called *intermittent peritoneal dialysis.* The procedure, once instituted, is largely a nursing responsibility. Peritoneal dialysis is used in treating acute as well as chronic renal failure. It can be performed in the hospital or at home.

The major advantages of peritoneal dialysis include the following:

1. The procedure provides a steady state of blood chemistries.
2. Any location can be used, and machinery is not needed.
3. The process can be easily taught to patient or family.
4. Few dietary restrictions are required; because of the loss of protein across the peritoneal membrane into the dialysate, the patient is usually placed on a high-protein diet.

25-19

Patient Teaching

The patient on haemodialysis

Orientation to haemodialysis and visit to the unit when appropriate
Nature of renal failure
    Normal kidney function
    Kidney failure specific to patient's pathophysiology (types, causes)
Dietary reinforcement, including rationale: restriction of protein, potassium, sodium, and fluids, and increase in calories
Review of medication regimen
    Purpose of each prescribed medication
    Common side effects
    Dosage and times of each medication
    Prescription filling procedure
Care of vascular access (if appropriate)
    Procedure for assessing presence of thrills and bruits and who to notify if these signs are absent
    Guarding against constriction of fistula (such as sleeping on affected arm or wearing tight clothing)
    Hygiene and removing dressing after dialysis
    Signs and symptoms of infection
    Measures to control haemorrhage should it develop when away from dialysis unit
Haemodialysis process
    Principles of dialysis (teach on basis of patient's learning level)
    Sequence of activities during haemodialysis
    Common sights and sounds of dialysis unit
    Common complications and their treatments: hypotension, nausea, vomiting, cramping
Laboratory data: types, meaning, and effects of haemodialysis, diet, and medications on each value
Alternative modes of treatment of ESRD: dedicated haemodialysis centres, home dialysis, peritoneal dialysis, kidney transplantation

5. The patient has more control over daily life.
6. The procedure can be used for people who are haemodynamically unstable.

Preprocedure care

Weight, blood pressure, and pulse are recorded before the procedure is initiated. These values serve as baseline information to assess changes in the patient's condition. For people undergoing insertion of a peritoneal catheter before dialysis, assessment should be made of their knowledge of the procedure and their anxiety level. A mild sedative may help the severely anxious person to better tolerate the insertion of the catheter. It is important that these patients void just before catheter insertion; this decompresses the bladder and prevents accidental puncture during catheter placement.

Care during peritoneal dialysis

The patient undergoing acute peritoneal dialysis may be confined to bed during the treatment as a result of general fatigue and the constant fluid exchanges that take place. Comfort measures and diversionary activities should be of high priority. During the dialysis, the patient is able to turn from side to side and move about in bed as desired as long as the catheter remains undisturbed. The patient is provided assistance with hygiene care as needed. If peritoneal dialysis is carried out at home, the patient and a backup person need to be able to do all steps of the procedure to ensure that therapy is not interrupted when the patient is too ill to perform dialysis alone.

Nursing activities during peritoneal dialysis include the following:
1. Maintain strict aseptic technique to prevent infection.
2. Monitor vital signs frequently.
3. Maintain strict intake and output records.
4. Assess catheter site for signs of infection.
5. Assess patient for oedema.
6. During cycles maintain accurate record of each cycle, including the following:
    a. Type of dialysate
    b. Amount of dialysate infused
    c. Amount of dialysate recovered
    d. Time dialysate was left in-dwelling
    e. Characteristics of returned dialysate (effluent); samples for microbiology

Complications of peritoneal dialysis

Complications most commonly associated with peritoneal dialysis include hypotension and hypovolaemia, inadequate drainage of fluid from the peritoneal space, pain, atelectasis, respiratory distress, and peritonitis. As with haemodialysis, *hypotension* is most likely to result from rapid removal of fluid from the intravascular space. In addition to checking vital signs and observing the patient's behaviour, records of fluid balance are crucial in determining the amount of fluid that has been removed. The net gain or loss of fluid from the abdomen should be determined at the completion of each cycle. To decrease the amount of fluid that is being removed from the vascular space, the doctor may decrease the hypertonicity of the dialysate and may increase the rate at which fluid is administered through an intravenous line.

Drainage of fluid from the abdomen can be slow or impossible to start. Generally, this problem results when the tip of the catheter has become lodged against abdominal tissues. It may also result from plugging of the catheter with blood or fibrin that has accumulated as a result of tissue trauma. A small amount of heparin may be added to the dialysate to decrease the chance of a clot forming in the catheter. When the dialysate does not drain freely from the abdomen, the patient should stand or turn from side to side in an attempt to reposition the catheter in the peritoneal cavity. If the flow of the dialysate does not increase, the doctor is called to irrigate the catheter or reposition it.

Severe *pain* should not be experienced during peritoneal dialysis. Moderate levels of pain are often experienced as fluid is instilled and withdrawn from the peritoneal cavity. Lignocaine may be instilled with the dialysate in an attempt to control the patient's discomfort. Mild analgesics may be ordered for administration at 3- to 4-hour intervals during the procedure.

When the patient is markedly overhydrated and shows evidence of congestive failure and pulmonary oedema, *respiratory difficulty* may be encountered as the dialyzing fluid infuses. The quality and rate of respiration should be closely observed. The head of the bed can be raised to decrease the pressure of the dialysate on the diaphragm. The amount of dialyzing fluid used for each cycle may be decreased when respiratory distress becomes prolonged and severe. The patient, although encouraged to eat while being dialyzed, may find that this increases respiratory difficulty. To help overcome additional pressure created by a full stomach, frequent small meals may be provided.

Peritonitis is an ever-present threat during peritoneal dialysis. Aseptic technique must be rigidly maintained during insertion of the catheter and throughout the procedure. Care should be taken to avoid contaminating the solution or the tubing when dialysate solution is hung. Cultures of the dialysate fluid are performed routinely to ensure continued attention to asepsis and to identify organisms if peritonitis should develop subsequently. The patient should be observed for signs of peritonitis. These include an elevated temperature, tenderness or pain of the abdomen, and cloudy effluent. In more severe cases, the patient may have fever, nausea, vomiting, chills, and diarrhoea.[16]

Other approaches to peritoneal dialysis

Several advances in the management of patients with chronic end-stage renal disease have led to two variations of peritoneal dialysis. These technologies emphasize home- and self-dialysis. *Continuous ambulatory peritoneal dialysis* (CAPD) is one development that is leading to safe self-dialysis that is practical and relatively inexpensive when compared to haemodialysis and that promotes patient independence. Basically, CAPD involves continuous contact of dialysate with the peritoneal membrane. Approximately 2 L of dialysate are maintained interperitoneally and exchanged by the patient through a permanent peritoneal catheter 4 to 5 times a day.[22] No special equipment is required for the exchanges, and the patient can therefore lead a fairly normal life-style. Exchanges can take place at home or at work by connecting an empty bag to the catheter and opening a clamp to allow drainage. A full dialysate bag is then instilled and the patient has completed an exchange.

The second method is *continuous cyclic peritoneal dialysis* (CCPD). CCPD differs from CAPD in that a machine known as a *cycler* is used to instill and drain dialysate from the patient. The machine has a series of clamps that are controlled by timers. The timers open and close the clamps in sequence to allow for instillation and drainage of dialysate from the patient. The cycle times for patients with chronic renal failure generally allow for the patient to be dialyzed in 6 to 8 hours. A patient can therefore connect up to the cycler at bedtime, set the machine, and be dialyzed while sleeping. A number of alarms are built into the cycler to protect the patient from such malfunctions as dialysate that is too hot or cold, long or short dwell times, improper return of fluid, and changes in catheter pressures. The greatest advantage of CAPD and CCPD over other forms of dialysis is that both offer patients unprecedented freedom in managing their own care.

Facilitating patient learning

The teaching requirements for the patient undergoing peritoneal dialysis are consistent with the teaching plan for haemodialysis. However, the patient will need to be instructed in the specifics of the process of peritoneal dialysis. If CAPD is planned, training should be accomplished in a dialysis unit that is equipped to assist the patient in dealing with home care.

Kidney Transplantation

Kidney transplantation is performed to prolong the life of a person with chronic renal failure. It is not a cure for CRF but rather an ongoing therapy with its own side effects and potential complications. Kidneys may be obtained from cadavers (preferred approach) or from related donors.

During surgery the transplanted kidney is placed in the iliac fossa. Generally, the peritoneal cavity is not entered. The patient's own kidneys are not disturbed unless they are infected or are the cause of significant hypertension, in which case the recipient undergoes bilateral nephrectomy before or after transplant surgery. The recipient's kidneys are left intact whenever possible to maintain erythropoietin production, blood pressure control, and prostaglandin synthesis and metabolism. The donor ureter is used to the extent that is possible. If long enough, the donor ureter is connected to the bladder in such a way as to prevent reflux of urine. If the ureter is short, a ureteroureterostomy may be performed.

SUMMARY

1. The kidneys are essential for the following reasons:
   a. Regulate electrolytes
   b. Eliminate wastes
   c. Regulate fluid volume
   d. Maintain acid-base balance
   e. Regulate blood pressure
   f. Stimulate production of RBCs
   g. Regulate calcium-phosphate metabolism
2. The kidneys regulate blood pressure by controlling fluid volume as well as mediating the renin-angiotensin-aldosterone system.
3. Diabetes mellitus (diabetic nephropathy) is the leading cause of end-stage renal disease.
4. Hypertension is another leading cause of renal disease that could be minimized by early detection and adequate treatment.
5. Urinary retention can result in hydronephrosis that leads to permanent damage to the kidneys.
6. Control of urinary incontinence is largely dependent on its cause. Accurate diagnosis of the cause of the incontinence is therefore essential before a programme to reestablish continence is developed.
7. The clinical manifestations of the nephrotic syndrome include the following:
   a. Severe generalized oedema
   b. Pronounced proteinuria
   c. Hyperalbuminaemia
   d. Hyperlipidaemia

The presence of these findings defines nephrotic syndrome.

8. Obstruction of any part of the urinary system from the kidney to the urinary meatus may lead to hydronephrosis and may cause functional and anatomic damage to the renal parenchyma.

9. Lithotripsy is fast becoming the treatment of choice for renal stones because of its noninvasive nature and the short recovery period.

10. A transurethral prostatectomy is the treatment of choice for prostatic hypertrophy but can only be employed if there is a relatively small amount of tissue to be removed; otherwise bleeding can be excessive.

11. An essential component of the preoperative teaching plan for the patient about to undergo any urostomy surgery is preparation for the presence of the ostomy and a drainage appliance.

12. Major components of the treatment of a patient with polycystic disease are prevention, early detection, and treatment of any infections that develop so that renal function can be preserved.

13. Causes of acute renal failure may be prerenal (hypofusion, vasodilation, decreased cardiac output), intrarenal (damage to kidney tissue, primarily ischaemia or nephrotoxicity), or postrenal (lower urinary tract obstruction).

14. The oliguric phase of ARF is characterized by inability to excrete fluid loads (oliguria), hyperkalaemia, hyponatraemia, metabolic acidosis, and uraemia. In the diuretic phase there is excessive diuresis with loss of sodium and potassium.

15. Nursing care during the oliguric phase includes controlling the buildup of metabolic waste, maintaining fluid and electrolyte balance and nutrition, and preventing injury and infection. During the diuretic phase, monitoring fluids and electrolytes continues, coping is facilitated, and patient teaching is instituted.

16. The three stages of chronic renal failure are decreased renal reserve, renal insufficiency, and end-stage renal disease.

17. ARF and CRF can be treated by conservative medical management, haemodialysis, or peritoneal dialysis and its variations. Continuous renal replacement therapy is an option for the patient who is critically ill with ARF. Kidney transplantation may be considered with end-stage renal disease.

18. Nursing interventions for CRF include administering medications, promoting fluid balance and nutrition, preventing infection and injury, maintaining skin integrity, promoting rest and comfort, facilitating coping, and teaching the patient.

19. Dialysis involves movement of fluid and particles across a semipermeable membrane by diffusion, osmosis, and ultrafiltration. Haemodialysis involves shunting the patient's blood through a dialyzer to exchange fluids, electrolytes, and waste materials. With peritoneal dialysis, the peritoneum becomes the dialyzing membrane.

20. Kidney transplantation is not a cure for renal failure but rather an ongoing therapy with its own side effects and potential complications.

STUDY QUESTIONS

- What are the major causes of urinary incontinence? What measures can the patient take to reduce incontinence? How would you go about planning a bladder retraining programme?
- What are the differences between upper and lower urinary tract infections in terms of causative organisms, clinical manifestations, and treatment? Why is it important to stress prevention of UTIs to patients who are at risk for infection?
- What is the effect of obstruction of urinary flow from the kidneys? How would you explain this to the patient? What conditions can cause urinary obstruction?
- In what ways do the four types of prostatectomy surgeries differ? How would patient teaching differ for each type?
- How do acute and chronic renal failure differ in terms of course of the disease, outcomes, medical management, and nursing interventions?

REFERENCES AND SELECTED READINGS

1. Abuelo IG: *Renal pathophysiology: the essentials,* Baltimore, 1988, Williams & Wilkins.
2.* Alt B, Balduf R, Thompson E: When a vascular access site complicates care, *RN* 49(10):36-39, 1986.
3. American Cancer Society: *Cancer facts and figures—1991,* Atlanta, 1991, The Society.
3a.* Baer CL, Lancaster LE: Acute renal failure, *CCNQ* 14(4):1-21, 1992.
4.* Barat M: Correcting electrolyte imbalances, *RN* 50(2):30-33, 1987.
5.* Bristoll S, et al: The mythical danger of rapid urinary drainage, *Am J Nurs* 89:344-345, 1989.
6.* Brogna L, Lakaszawski ML: The continent urostomy, *Am J Nurs* 86:160-163, 1986.
6a. Cartwright RA, Adib R, Appleyard I: Cigarette smoking and bladder cancer. Epidemiological enquiry in West Yorkshire. *J Epidemiology of Community Health* (37) 256, 1983.
7.* Chambers J: Save your diabetic patient from early kidney damage, *Nursing 85* 15(5):58-63, 1985.
8. Chambers JK: Fluid and electrolyte problems in renal and urologic disorders, *Nurs Clin North Am* 22:815-826, 1987.
9. Clark JB, Queener SF, Karb VB: *Pharmacologic basis of nursing practice,* ed 3, St Louis, 1990, Mosby–Year Book.
10.* Conti MT, Eutropius L: Preventing UTIs: what works? *Am J Nurs* 87:307-309, 1987.
11. Crandall BI: *Chronic renal failure.* In Ulrich BT: *Nephrology nursing: concepts and strategies,* Norwalk, Conn, 1989, Appleton & Lange.
12. Eschback JW, Adamson JS: Recombinant human erythropoietin: implications for nephrology, *Am J Kidney Dis* 11:203-209, 1988.
13. Fowler JE, Crowley JL: Stress urinary incontinence: endoscopic suspension of the vesical neck, *AORN J* 45:922-933, 1987.
14. Gillenwater JY: *The 1991 year book of urology,* St Louis, 1991, Mosby–Year Book.
15. Goldberger E: *A primer of water, electrolyte and acid-base syndromes,* ed 7, Philadelphia, 1986, Lea & Febiger.
16. Graham-Macaluso MM: Complications of peritoneal dialysis: nursing care plans to document teaching *ANNA J* 18(5):479-483, 1991.
17. Guyton AC: *Textbook of medical physiology,* ed 8, Philadelphia, 1991, WB Saunders.
18.* Harwood C: Pulverizing kidney stones: what you should know about lithotripsy, *RN* 48(7):32-37, 1985.
19. Jacobson JR: *The principles and practice of nephrology,* St Louis, 1990, Mosby–Year Book.
20.* Kadas N: Reducing fluid overload without dialysis, *RN* 49(5):27-31, 1986.
20a. Kass EH: Asymptomatic infection of the urinary tract, *Trans Ass Am Physician* 69, 56, 1956.

* Recomended for student reading.

21. Klake S, Schreener G, Ichikawa I: The progression of renal disease, *N Engl J Med* 318(25):1657-1665, 1988.

22. Lancaster LE: *Core curriculum for nephrology nursing:* 1991 edition, Pitman, NJ, 1990, American Nephrology Nurses Association.

23. Leadbetter GW, Gillenwater JY: Contempo 1991: Urology, *JAMA* 265(23):3175-3176, 1991.

24. Levinsky NG, Rettig RA: The medicare end-stage renal disease program, *N Engl J Med* 324(16):1143-1148, 1991.

25. Lu I: Incontinence stress index: measuring psychological impact, *J Gerontol Nurs* 3(7):18–25, 1987.

26.* Martin JP: Transrectal ultrasound: a new screening test for prostate cancer, *Am J Nurs* 91(2):69, 1991.

27. Massry SG: Contempo 1991: Nephrology, *JAMA* 265 (23):3135-3137, 1991.

28. McCormick KA, Scheve AA, Leahy E: Nursing management of urinary incontinence in geriatric inpatients, *Nurs Clin North Am* 23:231-264, 1988.

29. Metheney N: *Fluid and electrolyte balance: nursing considerations*, Philadelphia, 1987, JB Lippincott.

30. Moriarity MB: The NIH puts the spotlight on incontinence, *RN* 52(3):44-45, 1989.

31. Newman D, Smith D: Incontinence: the problem patients won't talk about, *RN* 52(3):42-43, 1989.

32. Newman DK, et al: Restoring urinary continence, *Am J Nurs* 91(1):28-34, 1991.

33.* Niel JV: What's wrong with this peristomal skin, *Am J Nurs* 91(12):44-45, 1991.

34. Nolph K, Linblad A, Novak J: Continuous ambulatory peritoneal dialysis, *N Engl J Med* 318(24):1595-1599, 1988.

35.* Norris MK: Dialysis disequilibrium syndrome, *Nursing* 19(4):33, 1989.

36.* Palmer MH: Incontinence: the magnitude of the problem, *Nurs Clin North Am* 23:139-158, 1988.

36a. *Oxford Textbook of Medicine.*

37.* Percutaneous lithotripsy for renal calculi, *Am J Nurs* 85:772-773, 1985.

38.* Petillo MH: The patient with a urinary stoma: nursing management and patient education, *Nurs Clin North Am* 22:263-280, 1987.

39.* Plawecki HM, et al: Chronic renal failure, *J Gerontol Nurs* 13(12):14-17, 1987.

40. Porth C: *Pathophysiology*, ed 3, Philadelphia, 1990, JB Lippincott.

40a. Power C, Baker JP, Blackwick NJ: Incidence of renal stones in 18 British towns—A collaborative study, *BJ Urol* (59):105, 1987.

41. Prevention and treatment of kidney stones. (Kidney Stone Consensus Conference), *JAMA* 260:977-981,1988.

42. Price CA: Continuous renal replacement therapy: the treatment of choice for acute renal failure, *ANNA J* 18(3):239-244, 1991.

43. Richard C: *Comprehensive nephrology nursing*, Boston, 1986, Little, Brown & Co.

44. Rowland RG, Mitchell ME, Bihrle R: Alternative techniques for a continent urinary reservoir, *Urol Clin North Am* 14(4):797-804, 1987.

45.* Ruge CA: Shock (wave) treatment for kidney stones, *Am J Nurs* 86:400-401, 1986.

46. Schrier R: *Renal and electrolyte disorders*, ed 3, Boston, 1986, Little, Brown & Co.

47. Schroeder SA et al: *Current medical diagnoses and treatment*, ed 30, Norwalk, Conn, 1991, Appleton & Lange.

48.* Smith DAJ: Continent restoration in the homebound patient, *Nurs Clin North Am* 23:207-218, 1988.

49.* Solomon J: Does renal failure mean sexual failure? *RN* 49(8):41-43, 1986.

49a. Stamey TA: Recurrent UTI—An overview of management treatment, *Rev Infect Dis* 9, Supp 2:5195, 1987.

50.* Strangio L: Believe it or not: peritoneal dialysis made easy, *Nursing 88* 18(1):43-46, 1988.

51. Tanagho EA, McAninch JW: *Smith's general urology*, ed 13, Norwalk, Conn, 1991, Appleton & Lange.

51a.* Tootla J, Easterling AD: Current options in bladder cancer management, *RN* 55(4):42-49, 1992.

52. Trusler LA: Simultaneous kidney-pancreas transplantation, *ANNA J* 18(5):487-491, 1991.

53. Ulrich BT: *Nephrology nursing: concepts and strategies*, Norwalk, Conn, 1989, Appleton & Lange.

53a. Waterhouse JA, Muir C, Shanmugarstnam K: Cancer incidence in five continents, *4 IARC, Lyon; IRAC Scientific publication No 42*.

54. Way LW: *Surgical diagnosis and treatment*, ed 9, Norwalk, Conn, 1991, Appleton & Lange.

55. Williams SR: *Essentials of nutrition and diet therapy*, ed 5, St Louis, 1990, Mosby–Year Book.

55a.* Willis D: Taming the overgrown prostate, *Am J Nurs* 92(2):34-40, 1992.

56.* Wiseman K: Nephrotic syndrome: Pathophysiology and treatment, *ANNA J* 18(5):473-474, 1991.

57. Hadley E, et al: Bladder training and related therapies for urinary incontinence in older people. Proceedings of the National Institute of Aging workshop, Bethesda, Md, April 26-27, 1983.

58. Lancaster L: *The patient with end-stage renal disease*, ed 2, New York, 1984, John Wiley & Sons.

59. McConnell MF, Zimmerman MF: *Care of patients with urologic problems*, Philadelphia, 1983, JB Lippincott.

60. *Blandy* Lecture notes in urology. Oxford, 1992, Blackwell Scientific Publications.

FURTHER READING

Kidd PA: Action STAT! Ruptured bladder, *Nursing* 19(1):33 Jan 1989.

Lowthian P: Preventing trauma... in-dwelling urethral catheters, *Nursing Times* 85(21):73-75, May 24-30, 1989.

Randles J: An alternative to urinary conduit, *Nursing Standard* 6(46):33-36, Aug 5-11, 1992.

Weiskittell P, Sommers MS: The patient with lower urinary tract trauma, *Critical Care Nurse* 9(1):53-66, Jan, 1989.

Sexual and Reproductive Problems

Unit Nine

Sexuality in Health and Illness

Nancy Fugate Woods
Donald D. Kautz

After studying this chapter, the learner should be able to:

- Describe physiological changes that occur during the phases of human sexual response.
- Describe changes in sexuality that occur with ageing.
- Appreciate the variety of sexual expression.
- Identify ways in which illness and environment affect sexuality.
- Relate types of alterations in sexual health and appropriate nursing interventions.
- Describe methods of prevention of sexual problems.
- State approaches that facilitate assessment of sexual health.
- Describe nursing interventions for people with alterations of sexual health.

This chapter discusses content basic to considering sexual concerns of medical-surgical patients. Content includes the relationship of sexuality to health and to illness; sexual concerns, difficulties, and dysfunctions; prerequisites for nursing intervention (including awareness of own value system); nursing assessment; and roles of the nurse in providing sexual health care.

It is difficult to estimate how many nurses include sexual assessments as a routine part of their practice, but it is believed that many yet do not do so. In one study, nurses stated they believed (1) discussing sexual issues was not a priority, (2) most hospitalized patients were too ill to discuss sexual concerns, (3) talking about sex would make the patients anxious, and (4) most patients had only minor sexual concerns.[27] However, several studies have shown that 75% to 85% of patients wanted to discuss sexual concerns yet would not initiate the discussion. These patients indicated that they felt it was the nurse's responsibility to initiate the subject. Some health problems discussed in this text have been found to create sexual problems. It is currently estimated, for example, that 50% of all men with diabetes experience difficulties attaining erections.[23] Thus at least one out of every two men with diabetes may have sexual problems. Nurses can include a 5-minute to 10-minute assessment of sexuality as a routine part of their care and can assist patients to prevent or overcome sexual problems that are a result of or exist concurrently with their illness.

SEXUALITY AND HEALTH

Human sexuality is not merely a biological phenomenon, but one that pervades the total person. A complex interrelationship exists among biological, psychological, and sociocultural aspects of our sexuality. The very complexity of human nature makes it difficult to define sexuality, much less sexual health. Nevertheless, the recognition of the importance of sexuality as a component of health has led the World Health Organization to suggest the following definition:[78]

> Sexual health is the integration of the somatic, emotional, intellectual, and social aspects of sexual being, in ways that are positively enriching and that enhance personality, communication, and love.

Sexual function, sexual self-concept, and sexual roles and relationships are important dimensions of sexual health. *Sexual function* refers to the ability of an individual

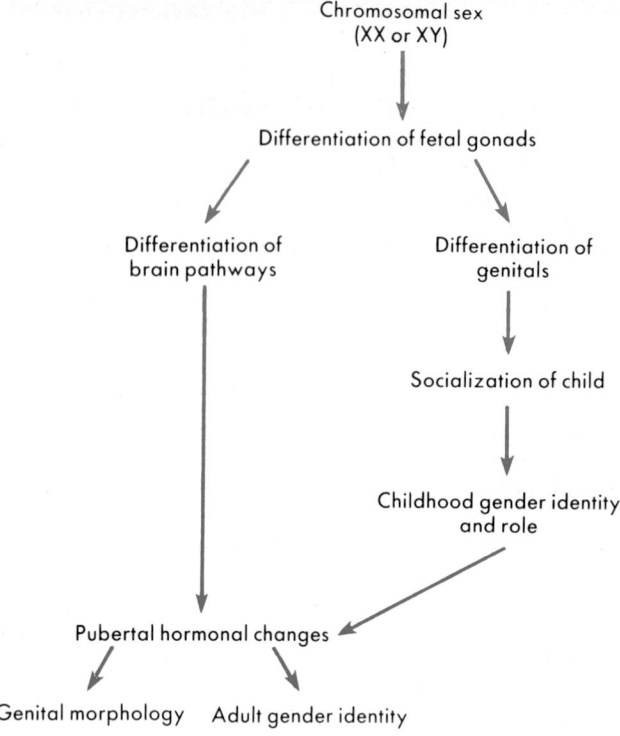

Fig. 26-1 Evolution of sexuality.

to give and receive sexual pleasure. *Sexual self-concept* refers to the image one has of oneself as a man or a woman and the evaluation of that image as masculine or feminine. Sexual self-concept includes body image and the evaluation of one's body and self within the context of the culture. *Sexual relationships* are the interpersonal relationships in which one's sexuality is shared with another.

Evolution of Human Sexuality

The evolution of our sexuality illustrates the complexity and interrelationship of the dimensions of our sexuality. From the moment of conception a variety of factors come into play to influence our sexuality, not only as children but also as adults. In early embryonic life the X or Y chromosome from the paternal sperm sets in motion a process analogous to a relay race; that is, each component has control of the process for a time, eventually yielding control to another[74] (Fig. 26-1). The chromosomes tag the undifferentiated fetal gonads as male or female, thus setting in motion another process by which hormonal secretions of the testes in turn affect not only the appearance of the genitals but also pathways in the brain.

The appearance of the infant's genitals at birth initiates another series of events, those primarily dependent on socialization of the child. The behaviour of other people during infancy and early childhood and the appearance of the child's external genitals are instrumental in the evolution of childhood gender identity and role (Box 26-1). In fact, gender identity seems to be well established by the time a person is 18 months of age. At puberty, biological influences again come to the fore as hormones influence the genital structure and eroticism.

26-1	Definition of terms	
	Biological sex	Female or male
	Gender identity	Person sees self as man or woman
	Gender role	Outward manifestations of masculinity or femininity

Table 26-1 Significant developmental experience related to sexual function, sexual self-concept, and sexual relationships

	Sexual function	Sexual self-concept	Sexual role-relationship
Infancy	Orgasmic potential present Erectile function present	Gender identity reinforced Association of sexuality and good–bad Distinction between self and others	
Childhood	Genital pleasuring and explanation Engages in sensual activity (e.g., hugging)	Core gender identity solidified (by age 3)	Sex role differences learned Discrimination between male and female role models Learns sexual vocabulary
Preschool	Sex play Exploration of own body and those of playmates Self-pleasuring (masturbation)		Learns about sex roles Parental attachment and identification
School age		Curiosity about sex Sexual fears and fantasies Interest in aspects of sexual development Self-awareness as sexual being	Same-sex friends
Adolescent, prepubertal	Menarche Seminal emissions	Concerns about body image	Same-sex sexual experiences as part of friendship
Early adolescence	Awkwardness in first sexual encounter (50% not sexually active) Masturbation, petting	Sexual thoughts, fantasies Anxiety over inadequacy, lack of partner, virginity	Beginning appropriate sex friendships Dating Learning
Late adolescence	May or may not be sexually active	Responsibility for sexual activity	Learning intimacy in relationship Sex role behaviours, lifestyles explained
Young adult	Experimentation with sexual positions, expression Explanation of techniques	Responsibility for sexual health, e.g., contraception, STD prevention Development of adult sexual value system, tolerance for others	Learning to give and receive pleasure Long-term commitment to relationship
Middle adult	Adaptation to altered sexual function, e.g., vaginal dryness of menopause, slower erections	Accept body image changes related to ageing	Adjustment of relationship as roles change
Late adult	Slower sexual function	Accept slowed sexual response cycle without ending sexual aspects of relationship	Develop new ways for sharing sexual pleasure and intimacy with ageing Adaptation to loss of partner or illness of partner

From Woods NF: Human sexuality, an overview. In Mitchell PH et al: *AANN's neuroscience nursing: phenomena and practice,* Norwalk, Conn, 1988, Appleton & Lange.

Thus from conception we are all sexual beings subject to multiple influences throughout life. If the previous processes proceed without interference, the person's biological sex is congruent with gender identity and gender role.

This complex set of biological and psychosocial variables begun at conception has a pervasive influence on the remainder of our lives. The biological component of sexuality (sexual function or expression) constantly interacts with the psychological components (gender identity, thoughts, and feelings), as well as with social factors (such as sanctioned role, mores, and folklore regulating sexual expression). Such complexity mandates a holistic approach to conceptualizing a person's sexual problems and concerns.

Sexual development continues throughout the life span, with each component of sexuality being influenced by biological development as well as sociocultural forces. Some of the significant developmental experiences related to sexual function, sexual self-concept, and sexual relationships are outlined in Table 26-1.

Physiological Aspects of Human Sexuality
Phases of the human sexual response

Masters and Johnson, pioneers in the scientific study of the physiological aspects of sexual behaviour, demonstrated that sexual response is a cyclic phenomenon consisting of four phases[71] (Box 26-2). The physiological changes seen during human sexual response (Table 26-2) depend on two main principles: myotonia and vasocongestion. It is through the congestion of pelvic blood vessels and involuntary muscular contractions in the pelvic organs and other parts of the body that changes supportive of orgasmic experience are attained.

Excitement phase

The excitement phase is the initial component of the cycle. It develops from sexually arousing stimuli such as touch. An increase in sexual tension is observed during this phase. Vasocongestive changes are seen in the external genitals and the breast in both women and men. In addition, a sex flush, which looks like a red, maculopapular rash, appears over the chest in some people. An increase in both the heart rate and blood pressure is evident, paralleling the level of sexual excitement.

Plateau

The plateau phase is a consolidation period during which sexual tension becomes intensified. Vasocongestion continues. The uterus continues to elevate in the pelvis, which creates a tenting effect in the innermost portion of the vagina. The sex flush continues to spread, sometimes involving the neck, face, and arms. Hyperventilation occurs in both sexes, along with heart rates of 100 to 175 beats per minute. There is elevation of systolic blood pressure (20 to 60 mm Hg for women, 20 to 80 mm Hg for men) and diastolic blood pressure (10 to 20 mm Hg for women, 10 to 40 mm Hg for men).

Orgasm

Orgasm, the involuntary climax of sexual tension, involves only a small portion of the sexual response cycle. The climactic release of sexual tension is evident in contractions throughout the body. Uterine contractions are also noted in women with orgasm, much like those characteristic of labour.

Resolution

During the resolution phase, the changes involving the blood vessels, sexual organs, and muscular tension are reversed. The uterus and testes return to their normal positions. Cardiovascular and respiratory rates quickly return to normal. Occasionally, a thin film of perspiration may appear over the entire body. Women may at this time begin another sexual response cycle immediately; men have an obligatory period during which they cannot be restimulated to higher levels of sexual tension.

Triphasic concept of human sexual response

Kaplan[66] has suggested a triphasic concept of human sexual response. She delineates three phases—desire, excitement, and orgasm—that are related components of sexual response but are governed by separate neurophysiological systems. This notion is useful for understanding not only the physiology of sexual response, but also the consequences of pathophysiological conditions, the aetiology of sexual dysfunction, and appropriate therapies.

Desire phase

The desire phase refers to the experience of a sexual appetite or drive produced by the activation of a neural system in the brain. Sexual desire is experienced as sensations that move the person to seek sexual experiences. It is likely that the sexual centres of the brain have either neural or chemical connections with the pleasure and pain centres of the brain. The pleasure centres are stimulated when we have sex, which accounts for the pleasurable quality of sexual behaviour. On the other hand, the pain centres can inhibit the sexual system. Some people suggest that the pleasure centre is stimulated by release of endorphins in sexual behaviour. If a sexual object or situation produces pain, then it will cease to evoke desire.

Testosterone is important in mediating sexual desire in both men and women. Luteinizing hormone and the neurotransmitters serotonin (s-hydroxytryptamine) and dopamine also may be important in mediating sexual desire. Bonding to another person and love are powerful

	Phases of the human sexual response	
26-2	**Phase**	**Description**
	Excitement	Increase in sexual tension evidenced by swelling of genitalia and vaginal lubrication
	Plateau	Intensification of sexual tension with more pronounced genital swelling
	Orgasm	Involuntary climax and release of sexual tension evidenced by muscle contraction
	Resolution	Dissipation of muscle tension and swelling

stimuli to sexual desire. Many stimuli seem to be capable of evoking sexual desire, such as sight, smell, and other sensory cues, and some of these are conditioned by culture. Fear and pain, however, are potent inhibitors.

The connections between the sex centre and other parts of the brain also make it possible for people to "turn off" sexual desire when other stimuli are more important or when it is not to the individual's advantage to pursue sexual activity. Hypoactive desire and inhibited sexual desire are common problems of the sexual desire phase.

Excitement phase

The excitement phase is similar to the excitement and plateau phases described by Masters and Johnson and is produced by reflex vasodilation of the genital blood vessels. This vasodilation causes the genitalia to swell and changes their shape to adapt to their reproductive function. The vasocongestion is primarily a parasympathetically mediated response, and an intense sympathetic response such as that produced by fear and anxiety can instantly lead to loss of erection. It is believed that erection is governed by two spinal reflex centres. The thoracolumbar centre (psychogenic) appears to respond more to psychic stimuli, whereas the sacral centre is stimulated from tactile input to the genitalia. It is believed that the spinal reflex centres and the higher neural connections are analogous in men and women. Disorders of the excitement phase include difficulty in attaining or maintaining erection in men and difficulty with swelling and lubrication in women.

Orgasm phase

The orgasm phase corresponds to orgasm as described by Masters and Johnson. It is also a genital reflex governed by spinal neural centres, but it consists of reflex contractions of certain genital muscles. Disorders of the orgasm phase include inadequate ejaculatory control (premature ejaculation), retrograde ejaculation in men, and orgasmic dysfunction in women. Other disorders include painful intercourse and sexual phobias.

Requirements for sexual response

The requirements for the physiological sexual response include intact sexual organs, adequate vasculature to support the vasocongestive changes, functional innervation of the genital organs, and the appropriate hormonal milieu.[58] The changes of myotonia and vasocongestion are thought to be mediated by the autonomic nervous system. Perception of the sexual experience at cortical levels requires intact sensory pathways from the genitals and other peripheral structures to the cortex. The capacity to stimulate oneself or a partner sexually depends on the presence of intact motor pathways from higher centres to the effector muscles involved. It should also be noted that thoughts and feelings or visual, auditory, and olfactory-gustatory stimuli alone may result in arousal to orgasmic experience even in the absence of tactile perception.

Adequate hormonal milieu, with appropriate hormonal release, influences both the structure and function of the genitals; for example, the decreased oestrogen levels during menopause are believed to be responsible for a decreased amount of vaginal lubrication. Finally, the presence of intact genital structures is usually thought to be a requisite for sexual response, but substitution of prosthetic devices for sexual organs is an option. Although each of these components is important in sexual response, it is possible for humans to have profound sexual pleasure even when one or more of these is absent.

Sexuality and Ageing

Changes in sexual function become accentuated during middle age (see Box 26-3), although their onset is gradual and they probably begin long before they are perceived.

Table 26-2   Sex organ changes during sexual response

Phase	Changes in female	Changes in male
Excitement	Vaginal lubrication Vagina becomes longer and wider Uterus begins to elevate in pelvis Clitoris becomes longer and wider Labia minora extend outward Nipples enlarge, areolae become engorged, breast size increases	Penis becomes erect Scrotal sac tenses Testes begin to rise towards perineum Nipples enlarge
Plateau	Clitoris retracts Labia and outer part of vagina (orgasmic platform) become congested Uterus continues to rise in pelvis	Diameter of penis continues to increase Testes increase in size 50% and elevate close to perineum
Orgasm	Orgasmic platform contracts rapidly (throbbing sensation) Uterine contractions Rectal sphincter contractions	Expulsive contraction along entire urethra to expel semen Internal bladder sphincter contractions (prevent semen from entering bladder) Rectal sphincter contractions
Resolution	Vasocongestion decreases rapidly from vagina/labia and slowly from clitoris and breasts Uterus descends to usual position	Rapid loss of penis size to 1 to 1.5 times usual size Slower resolution of penis size to usual size Testes descend into scrotum

26-3	Factors that influence sexual interest and activity in middle and old age	
	Women	**Men**
	Marital status: availability of a partner	Past sexual experience
	Age	Age
	Enjoyment of sex in earlier years	Objective and subjective health ratings
		Social class

Men need more time to attain an erection, and once attained, it is likely to be less full than in earlier years. The testes elevate more slowly with sexual excitement, and vasocongestive changes in the scrotum and testes are less noticeable. With prolongation of the plateau phase, middle-aged men actually achieve much better control over ejaculation than they had as young adults.

Orgasm is perceived as happening more quickly, and feelings of ejaculatory inevitability may disappear entirely. Resolution of sexual tension becomes more rapid with age, and the obligatory refractory period (a period during which the man cannot be restimulated to orgasm) becomes longer. With ageing, men actually gain better control of ejaculation, and because of reduced ejaculatory demand, they may be satisfied not to ejaculate with each intercourse.[25]

In women, menopausal changes may lead to delay in production of vaginal lubrication and diminished expansion of the vaginal barrel. Changes in external genitals and the breasts are apparent. The woman's orgasmic experience becomes shorter, and resolution occurs more rapidly.[25]

Studies of healthy ageing individuals indicate that a decline in overall interest and activity is seen with age. However, men from each age range tend to report greater interest and activity than women in each respective age range. Several factors can influence sexual interest and activity in middle and old age. Level of sexual activity in youth appears to be related to that in older years.[40,43,54]

As men age, an interest-activity gap appears; that is, they desire more sexual activity than they are able to experience. This gap grows as men age; however, it remains small for women. Women without a socially acceptable partner may adaptively inhibit their sexual interest. The wider interest-activity gap for men may reflect their socialization to express more interest in sex. Other social factors, such as the role loss associated with children leaving the parents' home and retirement, are likely to influence the older person's sexual interests.

In spite of these changes, many older adults remain sexually active. Kaplan[25] estimates that 50% of healthy people over age 60 remain sexually active. However, there is a tendency among health professionals to ignore sexuality in the aged, possibly because of two reasons. First, health professionals may assume that older people would be too embarrassed to discuss sexual concerns. In response to a caution that the nursing assessment was going to include some potentially embarrassing questions regarding sexual-

ity, one 70-year-old woman responded, "My dear, I've been having sex longer than you've been alive; you're not going to embarrass me." Second, health professionals may assume that older people would not be interested. Yet, in their study of women with heart disease, Baggs and Karsh[4] found that all of the separated and divorced women wanted to be asked about sexual activity, as did 76% of widows, including their oldest participant, age 88. These examples illustrate the need to conduct sexual assessments with people of all ages, regardless of marital status.

In addition, most older adults have chronic illnesses. Diabetes, hypertension, arthritis, heart disease, and chronic obstructive lung disease are examples of chronic illnesses prevalent in older adults and known to cause sexual problems. Some older people maintain sexual interest and activity in spite of physiological changes, whereas others do not.[35]

Recent Changes in Societal View of Sexuality

Most people who write about sexuality agree there has been a sexual revolution in most western countries. Many believe this revolution began in the 1960s, but the beginning can probably be traced to publications by Kinsey and his associates on sexuality in the human male and female in 1948[67] and 1953.[68] In D'Emilio's and Freedman's recent history of sexuality in America,[15] they postulate that the combination of the gay rights movement, the women's movement, the US Supreme Court legalization of abortion, relaxation of the ban on pornography, and the availability of the birth control pill created an atmosphere that drastically changed the way sexuality was viewed. Magazines, television, and other media portrayed a societal consensus that sexuality was good, sexual expression was a right of every individual, and "if it feels good, do it." It is important to remember that not everyone thought this way, but the media message was strong. During this time, nursing texts began to include chapters on sexuality; in 1979, the first edition of Phipps, Long, and Woods *Medical-Surgical Nursing* included a chapter on sexuality.

Several political and social events occurred in the 1980s, however, that have changed this view of sexuality. Teenage pregnancy rates rose; AIDS incidence increased. Both these issues have been targeted, by the Department of Health, for action during the 1990s and into the next century.[13a]

The 1990s are likely to bring even more changes. The government in the United Kingdom and the U.S. Congress continued to debate the issues of the legality and timing of abortion, funding or permitting exhibition of sexually explicit art, and the status of sex education in the schools. Another issue, also discussed in Britain, was the routine testing of health care workers for HIV infection. Those in favour of this practice believe that the public has a right to know; those against it believe that the risk of a health care provider transmitting HIV to a patient is extremely low.

Differing viewpoints exist within nursing as well. For example, some nurses believe that nurses should include an assessment of every patient's knowledge of safe sex practices, whereas others believe that this is inappropriate for the majority of patients. Nurses are encouraged to keep an open mind, to consider both sides of issues related to sexuality, and to recognize that patients may have different opinions.

Variations in Sexual Expression

Sexual behaviour is a product of society and culture and our biology. Each culture has a set of norms that prescribes which behaviours are sexual and which are acceptable. In cross-cultural comparisons of sexual behaviour, a wide variety of sexual expression is found. In Western society, sex is frequently equated with penis-in-vagina intercourse. Yet a wide range of behaviours exists encompassing sexual meaning (for example, talking, sharing thoughts and feelings, or just touching another person). This wide range of behaviours causes us to question what is "normal." Yet normal can refer to prevalence of a behaviour, optimal function, a statistical distribution, or fashionable or socially acceptable behaviour. Comfort[63] suggests that as professionals we not restrict our definition of normal to what we, personally, admit to enjoying. Instead he recommends that we consider the following questions:

1. What does the behaviour mean to the individual?
2. Does the behaviour enrich or impoverish the sexual life of the individual and those people with whom sexual relations are shared?
3. Is the behaviour tolerable to society?

Variation in sexual behaviour is bounded only by one's imagination and to some extent by the culture. Different types of sexual expression are described in Box 26-4.

Sexual intercourse may be restricted to marriage or to a similar relationship in some societies. In others, there may be legitimized extramarital rights, and in some, premarital sexual freedom is encouraged. The position for intercourse varies between cultures and within cultures. Usually the position assumed for intercourse reflects other aspects of the culture; for example, in cultures where families sleep in the same quarters, often side-to-side positions are used to afford some privacy from other occupants of the room.

Culture also dictates whether the woman plays an active or passive role in sexual activity and the duration of the act of intercourse. Precopulatory stimulation may be brief or lengthy, and the type used, such as kissing, painful acts, and manipulation of the breasts or genitals, varies with the culture. Sexual frequency may also be governed by norms, and in some cultures is prohibited during menses, lactation, or pregnancy, or before hunts or battles.

Heterosexuality is the most prevalent form of sexual expression among adults of known societies, but it is rarely the only type of sexual behaviour in which humans engage. Homosexual behaviour is found in most species of mammals; in humans it is most common among adolescents and males. Since "normal" sexual response may be determined by cultural norms as well as physiological, phylogenetic, legal, statistical, moral, and social standards, it is impossible to state a hard and fast definition of what constitutes the "normal state."

Homosexuality

Homosexuality is the most common sexual variation, yet it is poorly understood by health professionals. It has been

26-4	Sexual variations*	
	Heterosexuality	Choice of adult sexual partner of opposite sex
	Homosexuality	Choice of adult sexual partner of same sex
	Bisexuality	Choice of adult sexual partners of same and opposite sex
	Transvestism	Sexual satisfaction achieved by dressing in clothing of opposite sex
	Incest	Sexual relations with close relative, for example, child
	Zoophilia	Choice of sexual object is an animal
	Fetishism	Sexual object is an inanimate object
	Voyeurism	Sexual satisfaction achieved by watching others
	Exhibitionism	Sexual satisfaction achieved by exposing genitals
	Sadism	Sexual satisfaction achieved by inflicting pain
	Masochism	Sexual satisfaction achieved by receiving pain

* In the United Kingdom, some of these variations are unlawful.

viewed as an illness, a criminal offence, and a lifestyle in Western society. In the United States, the American Psychiatric Association has removed homosexuality from the "illness" classification; however, the social climate remains less liberated. Although many in society still seem to subscribe to the definition of homosexuality as an illness, most homosexuals do not classify themselves as ill. The association of HIV infection and AIDS with homosexual and bisexual men has contributed to the perception of homosexuality as an illness.

Kinsey[67,68] estimated that 13% of women and 37% of men had had at least one homosexual experience leading to orgasm. The extent to which these people engaged in homosexual behaviour varied greatly. Thus Kinsey suggested that a continuum existed on which the two poles represented exclusive heterosexuality (0) and homosexuality (6), and the five remaining categories (1 through 5) represented a combination of the two. Individuals in categories 1 and 5 had predominant heterosexual or homosexual orientations. Those in categories 2 and 4 still had a clear preference for heterosexual or homosexual relations, but retained an active interest in the other form. Category 3 represented people who had equal heterosexual and homosexual interests.

In the United States the Institute for Sex Research[62] conducted a large-scale study of the sexual dimensions of homosexual experience in the San Francisco Bay area. Although the authors of the report are careful to point out that their results may not mirror the entire homosexual population, the study did include men and women, both white and black. Results revealed that homosexuality encompasses more than the person's sexual tendencies. Although there was variability on the homosexual-heterosexual continuum for both male and female homosexuals, there was more heterosexuality in the feelings and behaviours of homosexual women than men.

Most of the homosexual men and women were relatively covert about their homosexuality. The mother and siblings were more likely to be aware of the individual's homosexuality than other family members. Families were more likely to be aware of the person's homosexuality than other members of society. In most cases friends, employers, and colleagues were aware of the person's homosexuality.

Homosexual men or women could not be stereotyped as sexually hyperactive or inactive; instead, the amount of activity varied with each individual. Public cruising (purposeful search for a sexual partner) was infrequent among lesbians. Of those homosexuals involved in public cruising, most conducted their sexual activity in their own homes.

Gay bars were the most popular cruising locales.

Homosexual men had many more sexual partners than did lesbians. There seemed to be more emphasis placed on sexual activity among males. This may be a function of lesbians' preference for relationships based more on emotions than on sex, or it may merely be a function of the problems male homosexuals have in meeting partners. For both male and female homosexuals, a relatively steady relationship with a love partner was a meaningful event.

The male homosexual subculture seemed to place more emphasis on youth than did women. Social prestige did not seem to be a major determinant in sexual appeal.

A variety of sexual techniques was used. Male homosexuals most frequently employed fellatio, hand-genital stimulation, and anal intercourse. Female homosexuals most frequently engaged in masturbation with their partners and in cunnilingus. Men and women both specified receiving oral-genital sex as a preferred technique.

Sexual problems encountered included difficulty in meeting a suitable sexual partner, maintaining affection for the partner, and meeting the other's sexual request. There was a lower incidence of these problems among lesbians. Almost two thirds of the male homosexuals had at some time contracted a sexually transmitted disease from homosexual sex, but only one of the lesbians had done so. More women than men had considered stopping their homosexuality, but only a minority in each case had done so. At interview, more men than women regretted their homosexuality.

About 20% of the homosexual males had been married, and more than 33% of the white lesbians and almost 50% of the black lesbians had been married once. They did not perceive their homosexuality as having a particular effect on their children.

Homosexual men and women seemed to have more friends than their heterosexual counterparts. Their friends included both homosexuals and heterosexuals. Lesbians were more involved in activities outside the home or with others than were homosexual males. Men were more likely than women to have had social difficulties, but few had been arrested because of their homosexuality.

When homosexual respondents were compared with their heterosexual counterparts in terms of adult psychological adjustment, it appeared that the dysfunctional and asexual homosexuals were less well off than those in the heterosexual group. However, homosexual adults who have come to terms with their homosexuality are no more distressed psychologically than heterosexual men and women.[62] Thus therapists would do well to consider why a person's homosexuality is problematic and examine ways to enhance the person's life rather than direct therapy at changing the person's sexual orientation.

Sexual Practices and HIV Infection/AIDS

The increased incidence of AIDS has led to frank and open discussion of sexual practices. Many publications, newspapers, and magazines have published discussions of sexual practices linked with HIV infection.

Although AIDS is a disease of heterosexual as well as homosexual and bisexual men, the onset of the AIDS epidemic has had a profound effect on the sexual lifestyles of

---

26-5

Risk of HIV infection from sex practices

No risk (no exchange of HIV-infected body fluids)

Analingus with barrier
Body-to-body rubbing
Cunnilingus with barrier
Erotic bathing/showering
Exhibitionism
Fellatio with condom
Kissing (dry/wet)
Massage, touch
Mutual/solo masturbation
Nibbling/biting (with no blood)
Nipple stimulation
Nonmucosal body licking/kissing
Sadomasochistic activity with no blood drawn
Unshared sex toys

Low risk (exchange of HIV-infected body fluids may occur)

Analingus without barrier
Cunnilingus without barrier (higher risk during menstruation)
Fellatio without condom without ejaculation
Ingestion of urine or faeces
Penile-vaginal/rectal intercourse with condom (risk of leakage)
Sadomasochistic activity with blood drawn but precautions used

High risk (exchange of HIV-infected body fluids)

Coitus interruptus without condom
Penile-vaginal/rectal intercourse without condom
Shared sex toys

Modified from Chateauvert M, Duffie A, Gilmore N: HIV antibody testing: counselling guidelines from the Canadian Medical Association, *Patient Educ Counsel* 18:35-49, 1991.

homosexual men. Two sexual practices that have been found to increase the risk of HIV infection are unprotected anal intercourse and sex with multiple partners. Before the onset of AIDS, these practices were common in homosexual and bisexual men. In efforts to reduce the incidence of HIV infection, particularly in homosexual and bisexual men, campaigns to teach safer sex practices have been instituted. In addition to these educational programmes, anonymous testing for HIV infection is offered. Professionals who care for people with AIDS agree that these preventive programmes have been effective with the general population of gay men, and that these men now practise safe sex. Some people, however, still continue to place themselves at risk.[49] This may be because some gay men may not perceive themselves as being at risk.[69] In Britain, health promotion has changed at-risk behaviours in older gay men but younger gay men continue to indulge in risk behaviours.

These data illustrate the need for nurses working in all settings to have a basic understanding of safe sex practices to answer patients' questions and for health teaching. The guidelines in Box 26-5 rank sexual activities by risk, ranging from no risk to high risk for HIV infection; these recommendations are for all people, regardless of sexual orientation. (For additional information regarding HIV infection, see Chapter 13.)

SEXUALITY AND ILLNESS

People today seem to be more comfortable in expressing their concerns about their sexual health than has previously been the case. As a result of this increased comfort, nurses are increasingly expected to provide accurate information about sexuality and health, as well as to listen with comfort and understanding to the sexual concerns patients describe. Although many people can openly describe their problems, others are too embarrassed or lack the vocabulary necessary to do so. For this reason it is important that nurses have a frame of reference to help them identify people at risk for sexual problems or concerns.

There are many ways in which illness may affect sexuality and sexual function. Illness may influence sexuality through changes in body structure or function, use of certain medications, or alteration in the person's body image.

Changes in Body Structure

Changes in the structure of the nervous system, circulatory system, or genital organs may result in sexual health problems. Many examples of these structural changes and the probable mechanism by which they interfere with sexual health are given in Table 26-3. Anatomical disruptions are probably best exemplified by the spinal cord-injured per-

Table 26-3   Changes in body structure and sexual health

System	Probable mechanism of interference
Central and peripheral nervous systems	
Spinal cord injury	Disrupts integrity of peripheral nerves and spinal cord reflexes involved in sexual response (for example, erection)
Spinal cord tumours	
Herniated disc	
Multiple sclerosis	
Spina bifida	
Motor neurone disease	
Tumours of frontal or temporal lobes	May interfere with function of centres controlling sexual drive
Cerebrovascular accident	
Trauma to frontal or temporal lobes	
Cardiovascular system	
Thrombus formation in vessels of penis	May interfere with blood supply to penis, thus interfering with erection
Leriche's syndrome	
Sickle cell disorders	
Leukaemia	
Trauma to vasculature supplying sexual organs	
Reproductive/sexual system	
Prostatectomy	May destroy nerve supply, interfering with sensory and motor aspects of sexual response
Abdominal perineal resection	
Lumbar sympathectomy	May result in disturbed ejaculation
Rhizotomy	May result in impotence, as well as disturbed ejaculation
Absence of penis or penile injury	Precludes or discourages penetration
Amputation of penis	
Imperforate hymen	
Congenital absence of vagina	
Pelvic exenteration	
Vulvectomy or removal of vagina	
Obstetric trauma or poor episiotomy	Leaves gaping vaginal opening or painful scarring, thus discouraging intercourse
Damage to pubococcygeus muscle	

son who has sustained irreversible damage to neural pathways that interferes with some methods of sexual function (Chapter 29).

Changes in Body Function

Many illnesses alter physiological processes essential to the sexual response, including nervous transmission, vasocongestion, hormonal metabolism myotonia, and perception of pleasurable sensation. Table 26-4 illustrates some illnesses that have the potential to interfere with sexual response and the hypothesized mechanisms by which they affect sexual response.

In general, it appears that the extent of a physiological disorder and its chronicity determine relative frequency of sexual problems. Women with diabetes have a higher rate of difficulty with lubrication than do nondiabetic women, particularly women who have been diabetic for 6 years or longer and who have neuropathy.[28,51] This relationship between chronicity and dysfunction is also observed in men with diabetes. A high incidence of problems with erection, however, is found among men with diabetes during the first year after diagnosis. It is believed in this instance that the lack of diabetic control (physiological derangement) is responsible for the sexual dysfunction.[31] For chronic illnesses as a group, it is easy to hypothesize a relationship between perception of health status, degree of fatigue, metabolic derangements, altered roles, fear of dying, and the demands of a chronic illness on the partner and changes in the sexual relationship.

Although some medical-surgical conditions do not interfere directly with sexual functions, their perceived seriousness or the presence of symptoms discourages people from engaging in their usual sexual practices. One very common example is associated with cardiac disease, more specifically myocardial infarction. Although marital sex probably does not demand a great energy expenditure, many people are fearful of attempting intercourse after having a heart attack. One study of married men who had had myocardial infarctions demonstrated that heart rates with orgasm were much lower in this group than among the younger group studied by Masters and Johnson.[64] An active physical conditioning programme did produce significant improvements in the frequency and quality of sexual activity for men who had had a myocardial infarction. This energy expenditure associated with sex seemed to be better tolerated by those who exercised regularly.

Table 26-4   Influence of changes in body function on sexual health

Physiological interferences	Hypothesized mechanism of action	Physiological interferences	Hypothesized mechanism of action
Systemic diseases			
Pulmonary disease	Debility, pain, and	Trauma to penis	
Renal disease	depression probably	Vaginal infections	
Malignancies	interfere with sexual	Senile vaginitis	
Infections	desire and expression	Vulvitis	
Degenerative diseases		Leukoplakia	
Some cardiovascular diseases		Bartholin's cyst	
		Allergic response to toiletries	
Metabolic disruptions			
Cirrhosis	Hepatic problems in men	Vaginitis after radiation ther-	Local irritability, damage
Glandular fever	result in oestrogen	apy	to genitalia, and con-
Hepatitis	buildup from inability	Pelvic inflammatory disease	sequent interference
	of liver to conjugate	Fibroadenomas	with reflex mecha-
	oestrogens; similar	Endometriosis	nisms involved in
	processes occur in	Uterine prolapse	erection and ejacula-
	women along with	Anal fissures, haemorrhoids	tion
	general debility	Pelvic masses	
Hypothyroidism	By depression of CNS	Ovarian cysts	
Addison's disease	function, general debili-	Prostatitis	
Hypogonadism	tation, and depres-	Urethritis	
Hypopituitarism	sion, libido may be		
Acromegaly	decreased, and im-		
Feminizing tumours	paired erectile abilities		
Cushing's disease	in men may result		
Diabetes mellitus		**Medical or surgical castration**	
		Orchiectomy	Lowered androgen levels
Diseases of the genitalia		Radiation therapy	depress libido and
Priapism	Each of these problems	Oophorectomy, adrenalec-	lead to impotence, re-
Peyronie's disease	involves damage to	tomy	tarded ejaculation, or
Balanitis	genital organs, which		impaired sexual re-
Phimosis	may result in painful		sponsiveness
Genital herpes	intercourse		

Modified from Kaplan HS: *The new sex therapy*, New York, 1974, Quadrangle Press.

In general, the literature indicates that the postmyocardial infarction patient may return to regular sexual activity provided there are no symptoms of congestive heart failure. However, certain conditions that increase energy expenditure during intercourse are to be avoided. These include having intercourse shortly after a meal or soon after alcohol consumption, because both increase the heart rate and metabolic demands. Extremes in temperatures and anxiety-provoking or secretive situations should also be avoided. The energy expenditure in climbing two flights of stairs appears to produce a greater increase in heart rate than does orgasm.[42]

Effects of Pharmacological Agents

Pharmacological agents that may affect sexual drive as well as performance are listed in Table 26-5. The relationship between extent of physiological problems and degree of sexual dysfunction may be demonstrated by pharmacologically induced changes. For example, alcohol induces transiently positive changes; in small doses it initially promotes relaxation and release of inhibitions, as do other psychoactive drugs. However, in larger doses, alcohol has negative effects on sexual function, leading to central nervous system depression and interference with motor activity.

Several categories of drugs have demonstrably negative effects on sexual function. These include antihypertensives, antidepressants, antihistamines, antispasmodics, sedatives, tranquillizers, alcohol, some sex hormone preparations, and some narcotics and psychoactive drugs.

Patients who take medications that have negative effects on sexual function should be informed that there may be alternative medications. For example, those who are taking the antidepressant Amoxapine (Asendin) might not experience sexual dysfunction with Imipramine (Tofranil). Those taking one antihypertensive may experience less sexual side effects with another. Thus nurses should recommend that patients talk to their doctor about sexual side effects, to see if an alternative drug is available.[53]

Pharmacological agents are now being used as one option to treat erectile dysfunction. Pharmacological erection programmes (PEP) are offered by urologists who specialize in the treatment of impotence. As a part of an extensive educational programme, men are taught to self-inject the penis with doses of vasoactive drugs in order to

Table 26-5   Drug effects on human sexual behaviour

Drug or drug category	Effect	Probable mechanism of action
Oral contraceptives	Positive	Permits separation of sexual activity from concern about conception
Antihypertensives Clonidine Guanethidine Methyldopa Propranolol Trimethaphan	Negative	Peripheral blockade of nervous innervation of sex glands
Antidepressants Amitriptyline Desipramine Imipramine Nortriptyline Phenelzine sulphate Protriptyline Tranylcypromine sulphate	Negative	Central depression; peripheral blockade of nervous innervation of sex glands
Antihistamines Chlorpheniramine Diphenhydramine Promethazine	Negative	Blockade of parasympathetic nervous innervation of sex glands
Antispasmodics Glycopyrrolate Poldine	Negative	Ganglionic blockade of nervous innervation of sex glands
Sedatives and tranquillizers Benperidol Chlordiazepoxide Chlorpromazine Chlorprothixene Diazepam Haloperidol Lorazepam Phenoxybenzamine Prochlorperazine Thioridazine	Negative and positive	Central sedation; blockade of autonomic innervation of sex glands; suppression of hypothalamic and pituitary function Tranquillization and relaxation

Continued.

Table 26-5 Drug effects on human sexual behaviour - cont'd

Drug or drug category	Effect	Probable mechanism of action
Alcohol	Negative	Central depression; suppression of motor activity; diuresis
	Transiently positive	Release of inhibitions; relaxation
Barbiturates	Negative	Central depression; suppression of motor activity; hypnosis
Diuretics	Negative	Diuresis
Bendrofluazide		
Chlorthiazide		
Spironolactone		
Sex hormone preparations	Negative	Antiandrogenic effects on sexual function; loss of libido; decreased potency
Cyproterone acetate		
Finasteride		
Nandrolone		
Methadone	Negative	Suppresses secondary sex organ function in men
Potassium nitrate	Questionable	Diuresis
Cantharis	Negative	Irritation and inflammation of genitourinary tract; systemic poisoning
Yohimbine	Questionable	Stimulation of lower spinal nerve centres
Strychnine	Questionable	Stimulation of neuraxis; priapism
Narcotics and psychoactive drugs	Negative	Central depression; decreased libido and impaired potency
Amphetamines		
Cocaine		
Heroin	Transiently positive	Release of inhibitions; increased suggestibility; relaxation
LSD		
Marijuana		
Methadone		
Morphine		
Levodopa	Questionable	Improvement of well-being
Amyl nitrite	Questionable	Vasodilation of genitourinary tract; smooth muscle relaxation
Caffeine	Questionable	Central nervous system stimulant
Vitamin E	Questionable	Supports fertility in laboratory animals
Selenium	Questionable	Supports fertility in laboratory animals
Lithium carbonate	Questionable	Produces broad endocrine changes; diuresis
Clomiphene citrate	Questionable	Stimulates gonadotropic hormones; enhances expectations of achieving pregnancy
Bromocriptine	Questionable	Stimulates gonadotropic hormones
Cimetidine	Negative	Unknown
Clofibrate	Questionable	Unknown
Disulfram	None by itself; negative with alcohol	Blocks alcohol metabolism; produces aldehyde syndrome

achieve an erection that lasts from 30 to 40 minutes and is sufficiently hard to permit intercourse. Papaverine HCl, used alone or in combination with phentolamine mesylate, are used. These agents affect only the ability to get an erection; they do not affect orgasm or ejaculation. PEP programmes are widely used by men with impotence from diabetes, hypertension, pelvic trauma, and arteriosclerosis who want to continue intercourse and do not wish to have a penile implant.[57]

Body Image Changes

The extent to which distortion of body image influences sexuality often depends on the perceptions of two people: oneself and partner. Multiple variables may influence the body image of a woman who has had a mastectomy. Although one might suspect that the extent of surgery and pain in the operative area would be most important, the value she assigned to her breasts, her preoperative body image, and social factors such as the quality of her preoperative sexual relationship are also influential. In one study the quality of the relationship the woman had with her husband before the surgery was the most important determinant of her return to sexual functioning after surgery.[77]

The visibility of a defect plays an important role in sexual adaptation. Visibility of a disability seems to be just as disruptive of marital and family relations as it is of other social relationships.[79]

Finally, the meaning and significance one attaches to the changed body part may interfere with sexual behaviour. The amputee who views the loss as castration, the woman who sees her hysterectomy as a neutering surgery, and the person who equates an ostomy with loss of adult control are likely to experience problems with self-image and, in turn, sexual adjustment. Thus both society's perception of the person and the individual's concept of self can interfere with sexual health. Some common health problems resulting in body image change are listed in Box 26-6.

Several authorities believe that the interpersonal components of sexual problems are of primary importance. They advise that both partners be involved in the treatment of sexual problems.

Environmental Restrictions

Environmental factors such as privacy, competing stimuli, and segregation interfere with sexual expression. Institutionalization rarely affords sufficient privacy for sexual expression. Many institutions segregate people on the basis of sex. For whatever reason this may be done, the act of segregation may elicit a range of adaptation, including masturbation, homosexual activity, or withdrawal from human warmth. Often these adaptive behaviours are punished, and those who resort to them are stigmatized. In some institutions staff members may assume an in loco parentis stance, treating even ageing people as if they required protection from their sexual desires.

SEXUAL CONCERNS, DIFFICULTIES, AND DYSFUNCTIONS

People have a variety of sexual problems ranging from concerns about sexual phenomena to alterations in sexual health. Each type of problem usually is the consequence of antecedents, and each requires somewhat different therapeutic approaches.

Sexual Concerns

Sexual concerns constitute a source of worry, dissatisfaction, or discomfort but do not produce difficulty in sexual function, profound problems in the sexual relationship, or a greatly altered sexual self-concept. Sexual concerns arise because of misinformation or lack of information, conflicting values, difficulty communicating about sexual issues, and anxiety or guilt about sexual phenomena.

These concerns are usually amenable to sex education strategies, such as permission giving, provision of limited information, values clarification exercises, rehearsal of communication, validation of normality, and provision of anticipatory guidance.

Sexual Difficulties

Sexual difficulties create discomfort in the sexual relationship, may occasionally interfere with sexual function, and sometimes may challenge the person's sexual self-image. Sexual difficulties include the following:

1. Inability to relax
2. Disinterest in sexual activity
3. Sexual dissatisfaction
4. Inability to please or be pleased by a partner
5. Disagreement about when to engage in sexual behaviour

26-6

Some health problems resulting in body image changes that may raise sexual concerns

Surgically induced
Mastectomy
Ostomy
Hysterectomy
Amputation of limb or limbs
Vulvectomy

Traumatically induced
Burns
Lacerations, scarring
Amputations
Pelvic irradiation

Others
Dermatological disorders
Obesity
Congenital anomalies of sexual organs (for example, absence of penis, hypospadias)
Unusual breast size, including immaturity or hypertrophy.

These difficulties are amenable to counselling approaches, including relaxation training, exploration of alternatives in the sexual repertoire, provision of specific suggestions, and training in communication skills.

Alterations in Sexual Health

Contemporary systems for classification of *sexual dysfunction* include desire phase, arousal phase, and orgasm phase dysfunctions, coital pain, and dissatisfaction with sexual frequency.[66] Although this schema addresses the functional dimension of sexual health, it does not address the dimensions of self-concept and relationships. The following paragraphs describe alterations in sexual function, sexual self-concept, and sexual relationships as a basis for a diagnostic taxonomy for nursing practice.

Alterations in sexual function
Alterations in sexual desire

Alterations in sexual desire include low sexual desire and sexual aversion. Low sexual desire reflects lack of interest in sex. Low frequency of self-stimulation and activity with a partner and diminished desire for sexual activity, incidence of fantasy, erotic dreams, or seeking erotic stimulation define this alteration. Low sexual desire and aversion are part of a continuum on which aversion includes a clearly negative response to the idea of sex.

Physiological and psychosocial factors contribute to alterations in sexual desire. Depression, severe stress, certain pharmacological agents, low androgen levels, and certain illnesses can interfere with sexual desire. Pharmacological agents such as narcotics, sedatives, and alcohol, centrally acting antihypertensives (such as methyldopa), and testosterone antagonists are associated with low sexual desire.

Illness-associated malaise, thought processes, and fear and anger produced by interpersonal conflicts, as well as concerns about intimacy or sexual self-concept, can also inhibit sexual desire. Anxiety and guilt linked to childhood experiences such as sexual abuse, pressure to have sex, and repeated unpleasant experiences may also interfere with sexual desire. Common problems in nursing practice include the following:

Low sexual desire related to chronic pain, medication regimen, partner's poor health and inability to have intercourse, or depression

Sexual aversion related to rape trauma

Therapies for low sexual desire and sexual aversion relate to underlying causes when this can be determined. When low sexual desire is related to chronic pain, the strategies may include identification of positions of maximum comfort and alternative stimulation that does not intensify pain. Sexual aversion typically is treated in the context of intensive sex therapy or psychotherapy.[66]

Alterations in sexual arousal/excitement

Many alterations in sexual arousal exist for men and include decreased subjective arousal, difficulty attaining an erection, difficulty maintaining an erection, and decreased subjective arousal combined with difficulty in some aspect of attaining or maintaining an erection. Alterations in women's sexual arousal include decreased physiological arousal and decreased physiological subjective arousal. Diminished vasocongestion is a symptom of diminished physiological arousal, whereas loss of erotic sensation is a symptom of diminished subjective arousal.[66]

Alterations in sexual arousal typically reflect body-mind-social interaction. Transient episodes of alterations in arousal are common. Pharmacological agents such as certain antihypertensives, sedatives, and tranquillizers may interfere with physiological sexual arousal in both men and women. Diseases affecting vascular function, such as diabetes, can impair vasocongestion.[53] As people age, vasocongestive responses to sexual stimuli and vaginal lubrication appear more slowly, and the response may be less intense than in younger years. Anxieties about sexual performance and fear of failure are commonly associated with alterations in sexual arousal.

Alterations in sexual arousal commonly encountered in nursing practice include the following:

Decreased vasocongestion and vaginal lubrication related to diabetic neuropathy

Decreased vaginal lubrication related to anxiety about pain with intercourse

Difficulty attaining an erection related to a medication

Difficulty maintaining an erection related to fear of failure.[76]

Strategies for treating alterations in sexual arousal include reducing anxiety about the problem and correcting or transcending the physiological problems if possible. Anxiety can be reduced through desensitization exercises in which the person is instructed to use erotic imagery to approximate sexual situations evoking anxiety.

Structuring sexual encounters so they are not demanding is a second strategy. Exercises that emphasize pleasure rather than pressure to perform often begin by refocusing the person's attention on sensual aspects of touch without genital touching for a period of time. After the person has pleasure in sensual experiences without anxiety, sexual activity is gradually reintroduced.

Physiological problems can sometimes be modified to restore sexual function. Drug regimens can be modified and strategies can be introduced to people to amplify erotic sensations in parts of their bodies not affected by disease. A penile prosthesis may be implanted in men as a method of treatment for organic erectile dysfunction.

Alterations in orgasm

Alterations in orgasm in men include problems with ejaculation and orgasm and with the perception of pleasure associated with orgasm. Ejaculatory problems include premature ejaculation and inhibited ejaculation. *Premature ejaculation* occurs when men ejaculate too rapidly for their own or a partner's pleasure. Often men with premature ejaculation do not perceive erotic sensations that occur before orgasm and progress rapidly from very low to very high levels of arousal. Anxiety about sex is common, and many men have learned to make their sexual encounters quick. *Inhibited ejaculation*, sometimes referred to as retarded ejaculation, implies the inability to ejaculate during sexual activity or the need for an extended period of time to ejaculate, even with adequate stimulation. Inhibited ejaculation is often associated with anger or lack of trust. Physiological alterations and medications can interfere with ejaculation.[67,76]

Alterations in orgasm for women include *anorgasmia*, a global inability to have orgasm, and situational anorgasmia, the inability to have orgasm in certain situations. Anorgasmia with intercourse is common. Inadequate stimulation, self-observation, and fear of loss of control over sexual or aggressive impulses often produce these alterations.

Both physiological and psychosocial mechanisms can produce orgasm phase alterations. Because a person has a physiological problem does not justify attributing the alteration to the disease; instead, an emotional or cognitive process may be involved.

Therapeutic strategies for anorgasmia include structuring situations for sexual activity that reduce anxiety. Distraction from self-observation through the use of fantasy and imagery along with self-pleasuring exercises often reduce anxiety sufficiently to enhance awareness of erotic sensation and orgasm.

Strategies for premature ejaculation include the use of the start-stop techniques, in which stimulation is withdrawn intermittently, or the source of stimulation is stopped intermittently to increase awareness of erotic sensations and to increase tolerance of pleasure associated with arousal. Retarded ejaculation is treated with a combination of relaxation and stimulation techniques, and these are sometimes enhanced by the use of imagery.

Pain with coitus

Vaginismus is a relatively rare sexual problem characterized by an involuntary, conditioned spasm of the vaginal outlet, thus causing it to shut tightly. This problem precludes sexual intercourse, but vaginismic women may be orgasmic with alternative methods of sexual stimulation.

Dyspareunia, or painful intercourse, may be attributable to a number of factors ranging from a full lower bowel to feelings of aversion towards sexual intercourse. It is sometimes felt by women with steroid alterations, for example, the postpartum mother and postmenopausal women.

Alterations in sexual self-concept

An individual's sexual self-concept can be changed dramatically because of developmental transitions or health-related events. In response to surgery or injury that produces changed body image or in response to taking on the identity of a disease, sexual self-concept may change. Embarrassment and shame associated with bodily changes can produce anxiety about sexual relationships.

Problems commonly associated with alteration in sexual self-concept include the following:

Altered sexual self-concept related to identification with an illness

Anxiety about sexual encounters related to changed body image (for example, after ostomy surgery)

Anxiety about sexual encounters related to feelings of inadequacy as a man or woman

Altered sexual self-concept related to a partner's lack of acceptance of change in one's body

Strategies for enhancing sexual self-concept include those directed at accepting and transcending alterations in body image, transcending the sick role, obtaining support from a partner, and enhancing perception of one's sexual self-concept as positive.

Alterations in sexual relationships

Sexual relationships can be changed by developmental transitions and changes in health status. Value conflicts about sexual activity, difficulty communicating about sexual issues, dissatisfaction with sexual frequency, a partner's inability to provide sexual stimulation, inability to please a partner, and conflicts about the timing of sexual activity may all occur as people experience ill health.

Some examples of problems related to alterations in sexual relationships include the following:

Value conflicts related to using alternative forms of sexual expression required by the illness, by partner's inability to reconcile roles as carer/lover, by partner's lack of acceptable sexual outlet, or by partner's inability to provide sexual stimulation because of reduced mobility

Adjustment, impaired sexual related to dissatisfaction with decreased sexual frequency

Strategies for promoting healthy sexual relationships include facilitating involvement that is mutually acceptable to both partners. Communicating clearly and comfortably about concerns and problems, negotiating mutually acceptable solutions to conflicts, obtaining adequate information about the consequences of health problems for sexuality, and clarifying sexual values can enhance the quality of sexual relationships.

Gender Disorders

Although many gender disorders exist, they are encountered less often in nursing practice than the problems discussed earlier.

Transsexualism refers to the condition of people who are convinced that they are "trapped in the body of the wrong sex." This gender identity problem may be encountered in some medical-surgical situations. Transsexuals believe that they belong to the opposite sex and desire the body, appearance, and social status of the opposite sex. Many actually live in the role of the opposite sex before treatment. Male-to-female transsexuals are usually treated initially with hormonal therapy, and later surgical revision of the genitals is performed. The surgery involves removal of the male genitals and revision of the scrotal and neighbouring tissue to resemble the female genitals. Usually the surgery is cosmetically successful, and an artificial but functional vagina can be created. These women are, of course, sterile, since they have neither ovaries nor uterus.

The female-to-male transsexual has a less cosmetically effective and functional surgical transformation. In a series of procedures, the breasts and vulva are revised and a phallus is created. Hormonal therapy is also used to effect the transformation. Often the creation of the penis requires extensive grafting and surgical revision, and the female-to-male transformation is consequently more difficult and usually less satisfactory. After the transformation these men are also sterile.

Both men and women electing transsexual surgery require considerable emotional support. They usually have careful psychological assessments before and after the surgery. Because of their cultural conditioning, nurses sometimes find it difficult to relate appropriately to the transsexual. Often it is necessary to analyze one's attitudes and values carefully to be accepting of these patients.

Transsexualism should not be confused with *tranvestism,* the act of dressing in the clothing of the opposite sex. Additionally, transsexuals are not homosexuals.

Hermaphroditism is a congenital condition in which the reproductive structures appear ambiguous. Early life experiences seem to have profound effect on our gender identities. It is important, therefore, that sexual assignment be correctly established early in life to prevent gender confusion later.

NURSING PRACTICE
Prerequisites for Intervention

Three prerequisites are important before practitioners can help individuals with their sexual problems:

1. A knowledge base
2. Awareness of own value system
3. Ability to communicate genuinely and therapeutically with patients

Knowledge base

The knowledge base that is required is listed in Box 26-7. Without such knowledge the nurse has no basis for the interpretation of patients' concerns and thus no basis for intervening.

Awareness of own value system

In addition to an adequate knowledge base, an awareness of one's own value system, including the biases and beliefs about appropriate and inappropriate sexual behaviour, is

26-7	Knowledge base prerequisite for addressing sexual concerns

Understanding of sexual response
Knowledge of the variety of sexual behaviours that exist in our society and their prevalence
Understanding of the types of sexual dysfunctions
Awareness of the relationship between age, life events, pathological conditions, behavioural problems, pharmaceutical agents, and sexual function

26-8	Principles that facilitate obtaining a sexual history	
	Action	**Effect**
	1. Obtain sexual history early in nurse–patient relationship	Legitimizes sexuality as part of health. Provides permission for patient to discuss sexual concerns
	2. Avoid overreaction or underreaction to patient's comments	Facilitates truthful data gathering
	3. Use language patient understands	Facilitates accurate data gathering
	4. Move from less sensitive to more sensitive areas	Facilitates patient-nurse comfort
	5. Terminate sexual history by inquiring if patient has additional questions or concerns	Conveys a willingness by nurse to further explore sexual matters

also important. Unless professionals can accept their own sexuality and are comfortable with their own behaviour, it is difficult to convey comfort to others. Self-acceptance is seen as prerequisite to the development of a nonjudgmental and tolerant approach. Just as individuals have belief systems related to sexual phenomena, so do professionals. This does not imply that the sex educators or counsellors must condone every variety of sexual activity. Rather, it is essential that they be aware of their own feelings and values and attempt to keep them in perspective by acknowledging them. This assists them in maintaining a supportive climate that encourages sharing of feeling by patients and simultaneously permits professionals to acknowledge the validity of their own beliefs.

Furthermore, there may be some issues about which the professional has such strong beliefs that these values would interfere with effective intervention. An example encountered in practice is the health professional whose basic conviction is that homosexuality is an illness or deviation rather than a variation in sexual expression or orientation. No matter how extensive the professional's training, knowledge base, and therapy skills, such a strong basic belief is likely to interfere greatly with the ability to relate objectively to a homosexual's sexual problems. Often professionals need to acknowledge their inability to deal with sexual problems because of their own value systems. Topics likely to elicit biases among health professionals include abortion, alternative lifestyles, and sexual variations.

One strategy that may be helpful in discussing sexual topics is to practise presenting opposing viewpoints on a sexual issue. For example, being able to discuss both pro-choice and pro-life stands on abortion may facilitate discussing other topics in a nonjudgmental manner.

Therapeutic communication

Finally, the professional needs to be able to communicate genuinely and therapeutically with patients. Often this involves using the person's own language, which may be different from that of the health professional. Without the ability to interact accurately and empathetically with individuals, the most sophisticated knowledge base and objective attitudes are of little benefit.

Nurses frequently encounter behavioural problems that involve the individual's sexuality. One common problem is the patient who acts out sexually, for example, by making inappropriate sexual gestures, using explicit sexual language, or exposing the sexual organs. Two general principles are helpful in coping with such a situation:

1. Analyze what meaning this behaviour might have for the patient.
2. Assert the right as a human being to establish limits that protect the nurse's integrity.

In responding to a patient who has exhibited sexual behaviour that is deemed inappropriate, one can analyze why the behaviour occurs and share this observation with the patient. Is the patient attempting to gain control in a situation in which he or she has little or no control? Is the patient trying to obtain validation of his masculinity or her femininity? Is the patient unaware that the behaviour has sexual overtones or is making the nurse uncomfortable?

Nurses have the right to establish limits with patients to protect their own integrity. Violation of certain body boundaries, for example, touching the breasts or buttocks of the nurse or exposing one's genitals, is not behaviour that nurses must tolerate to be "accepting of patients." Nurses' responses, however, can address three important points:

1. The inferred meaning of the behaviour can be shared— "I know you feel helpless at the moment. . ."
2. The boundary can be established—"That's not acceptable behaviour."
3. The patient's sexuality can be validated—"You're a good looking man, but that's just not acceptable behaviour."

Some patients cannot respond appropriately to these strategies, and in some instances the nurse may need to believe that not working with this patient is permissible.

Assessment
Sexual history

Many health care providers may not be experienced in eliciting a sexual history and at first may be uneasy. No doubt this uneasiness is conditioned by social prohibitions about discussing intimate matters such as sexual experiences or behaviour. However, health professionals are expected to be informed, willing to discuss sexual matters openly with patients, and prepared to educate and counsel them appropriately. Nurses who are hesitant to deal with sexual matters with patients are helped by working through their own feelings about sex and sexual matters. Seeking counsel from other nurses or health professionals who are comfortable with the topic is often helpful. Some nurses may find it helpful to attend a workshop on sexuality for nurses.

Although there is no single approach to taking a sexual history, application of certain principles facilitates both the patient's and the nurse's comfort. Absolute requirements for history taking include the following:

1. Provision of privacy, such as in a closed room
2. An atmosphere of trust between patient and nurse, such as assurance of confidentiality for the patient
3. Comfort on the part of nurses with their own sexuality

Some principles for promoting patient-nurse comfort are listed in Box 26-8. The sexual history itself may be therapeutic. Within the context of obtaining the data, the nurse can provide permission for the patient to discuss concerns, provide limited information or suggestions, or validate the normality and acceptability of the patient's concerns and practices.

It may be necessary for both patient and nurse to define their terms. Colloquial terms may be unfamiliar to the nurse, and highly technical language may be confusing to the patient. The nurse may need to become familiar with some commonly used colloquial terms to be sure of what the patient is reporting.

The technique of moving from less sensitive to more sensitive areas paves the way for both the patient and nurse. For example, the nurse may explore a woman's sexual role before discussing her ability to have orgasm, her menstrual history before her experience with sexual variations, and her personal experiences with sex education before her actual sexual experiences. In all of these situations, the decision to pursue the topics depends on the cues presented by the patient that sexual concerns are present.

Brief sexual assessment

A brief assessment can be incorporated in the nursing history by means of three questions (see Box 26-9). The first of these questions deals with the person's role, the next with the affective-cognitive elements of sexuality, and the last with biological aspects of sexual function. The questions may be modified to deal with illness, hospitalization, life events, or any other relevant entity that may influence or interfere with sexual health.

The questions may also be adapted to elicit the patient's expectations of changes resulting from procedures or hospitalization that he or she is about to experience. These brief items invite the patient to explore sexual concerns. Often it is unnecessary for the nurse to ask the second and third questions, because many patients proceed to state their concerns about masculinity, femininity, and sexual functioning without further prompting.

26-9

Brief sexual history

1. Has your (illness, pregnancy, or hospitalization) interfered with your being a (husband, wife, father, mother)?
2. Has your (abortion, heart attack, etc.) changed the way you see yourself as a (woman, man)?
3. Has your (colostomy, hysterectomy, etc.) changed your ability to function sexually (or your sex life)?

26-10

Selection of self-help and other organizations offering support and information about sexuality

British Diabetic Association
Ileostomy Association of Great Britain and Ireland
Multiple Sclerosis Society of Great Britain and Northern Ireland
SPOD (Association to promote the sexual and personal relationships of people with disabilities)

Roles of the Nurse in Providing Sexual Health Care

Nurses may intervene with sexual problems among patient populations through four strategies: educating patient groups likely to have sexual concerns, providing anticipatory guidance throughout the life cycle, promoting a milieu conducive to sexual health, and validating normality about sexual concerns.

Providing patient education

Several self-help groups and other organizations publish easy-to-read pamphlets which include sexuality (see Box 26-10). These pamphlets may be free or can often be purchased for a nominal fee and given to patients. Most pamphlets can be obtained directly from the organization or local branches. Many self-help groups offer the opportunity to discuss the effects of the illness or surgery upon sexuality.

Nurses can also write their own pamphlets for patients. Although this requires some effort, it may provide additional incentive for staff to address sexuality. Once developed, these pamphlets can be made available to others.

Nurses can also assist patients by providing specific information relating to conditions conducive to optimal sexual functioning, specific approaches to sexuality for patients with certain diseases or surgeries, and directives for coping with some sexual dysfunctions. One specific suggestion often incorporated in sexual education is that a couple having difficulties with intercourse abstain for a specified period. This admonition is designed to reduce the "pressure to perform" perceived by a member of the dysfunctional couple.

Patients with ostomies, who often have concerns about appliance leakage during intercourse, can be given specific suggestions (see Box 23-19 in Chapter 23).

Nurses can offer some simple directives for coping with specific sexual dysfunction. The man whose problem is premature ejaculation can be taught to use the squeeze technique or the partner may learn to apply it. The technique consists of applying pressure over the coronal ridge of the glans, exerting enough pressure for 3 to 4 seconds to relieve the feeling of ejaculatory inevitability during intercourse. The squeeze technique is used three to four times during one session of intercourse. Often the technique must be used several times over a 2-week to 3-week period to produce results. (For additional information consult reference 56.)

Another area of health promotion is in the correct use of condoms. For condoms to be effective in preventing the spread of STDs and AIDS, the guidelines produced by the CDC in the United States should be followed (see Chapter 27).

Patient education implies more than mere dissemination of information. Just as nurses learn to examine their own values and to communicate with others, patients may also need assistance in exploring the attitudes and values that shape their sexual behaviour and in developing the ability to communicate comfortably about sexual phenomena. Thus providing accurate information about sex and sexuality is not synonymous with education for a healthy sexuality.

Providing anticipatory guidance

Nurses are often in strategic positions to provide anticipatory guidance at sensitive points in the life cycle. Adolescence and middle age are two life periods during which anxiety about sexuality is likely to surface. By informing individuals about the usual changes experienced at these points (for example, nocturnal emissions or concerns about masturbation in adolescents or worry about effects of menopause on the ability to function sexually among middle-aged people), nurses can assist individuals to cope realistically with major changes in their bodies. Adults with young children can also benefit from anticipatory guidance regarding their children's sexuality. Many books and leaflets are available to assist parents in anticipating sexual concerns of their children. However, the chance to discuss concerns is often of great value.

Anticipatory guidance can also be given to patients who have been admitted to the hospital, to assist them with sexual concerns that are likely to arise when they return home. For example, a woman who has a mastectomy can be advised that she may not feel like having sex until her incision heals. Both she and her partner may have concerns about how her body will look. She will be given information about specially designed bras and breast prostheses (see Chapter 28). Finally, she may benefit from being advised that friends and family will be curious about how she looks, and she may find them staring at her breasts. One woman confided that while attending church services a few weeks after her mastectomy, she was shocked at the number of people, including the minister, who stared at her breasts when talking with her. While she was aware that these people had a natural curiosity, she was not prepared for their reaction. While the nurse cannot prevent this reaction from occurring, the patient can be assisted to think through how she will handle this situation if and when she experiences it.

Promoting a milieu conducive to sexual health

The first step in promoting a milieu conducive to sexual health is to give patients permission to ask about intimacy and sexual concerns. By including sexuality as a routine part of a comprehensive nursing assessment, the nurse is saying, "It's okay to talk about sensitive issues."

Another approach is providing time for privacy and intimacy for patients and their partners while in the hospital or other health care setting. Patients and families experience tremendous crises during hospitalizations and often need time alone to help each other cope effectively. A young man who had recently become a quadriplegic in a motor vehicle accident became very anxious at night in the intensive care unit. The nursing staff became concerned that his anxiety might prevent him from being weaned from the ventilator. His girl friend also became extremely anxious at night and was having difficulty sleeping in the waiting room knowing he was anxious in the ICU. The staff elected in this situation to allow her to sleep with him in the ICU bed. This anxiety-reducing intervention benefited the patient, his partner, and the staff, and he was weaned from the ventilator within a few days.

Other approaches include minimizing guilt felt in conjunction with sexual thoughts, feelings, and behaviour. This may be accomplished by assisting people in examining objectively the consequences of their activities within a reality-oriented framework. Reduction of performance anxiety (for example, concern about how well one is able to function) can be facilitated by helping individuals understand the relationship between being attentive to their own performance and losing touch with their sexual feelings. "Spectatoring" refers to the habit of watching oneself or a partner perform. Just as in athletics, one cannot be both spectator and performer without minimizing the effectiveness of the performance.

Often individuals need to be advised to modify their environments to reduce competing stimuli. Use of anxiety-provoking settings or those settings prone to interruption may establish dysfunctional patterns. The relationship between anxiety and orgasmic dysfunction and premature ejaculation has been well established.

Finally, maintenance of good general health facilitates optimal sexual functioning. Fatigue, pain, and malaise are stimuli that compete with sexual pleasure.

Validating normality

Validating normality is a function that nearly all health professionals perform but sometimes undervalue. Often the focus is on finding out what is wrong, what the pathophysiological process is, and what therapy to prescribe to correct the malfunction. Often family members approach health professionals to find out whether they are normal, acceptable, and not perverted. They seek out the health professional for validation of their sexual normality. People may be concerned about their thoughts, fantasies, dreams, and feelings, as well as overt sexual behaviour. In the process of validating normality, nurses often help patients exchange labels. Often labels bearing negative connotations such as "dirty," "perverted," or "abnormal" are exchanged for labels such as "healthy" and "okay."[61] Although most sexual acts could be considered normal in some sense, patients do need to be made aware of the consequences of their behaviour. The health professional cannot ignore patients' ethical codes or the legal code.

One situation sometimes encountered in nursing practice is the adolescent questioning whether it is "normal" not to be sexually active. For example, a young woman came to a clinic requesting a prescription for an oral contraceptive. The doctor who saw her did a pelvic examination and gave her the prescription. The nurse, who had been with her during the examination, noted that she was quite anxious about the procedure and was very hesitant to leave the examining room. After pursuing the reason for her obvious discomfort with the situation, the nurse found that the woman was seeking a prescription at her boyfriend's insistence; furthermore, she was *not* convinced that she wanted to become sexually active, but she feared that the relationship would end if she did not meet the young man's demands. She wanted some reassurance that she was "normal" for having these reservations and that *not* being sexually active was okay.

Another occasion for validating normal sexual attitudes is during the physical examination. Many nurses who perform pelvic examinations make these an educational experience for their patients. At the beginning of the examination, the examiner asks the woman whether she would like a mirror so that she can watch the examination as it is being performed. As the examiner inspects the external genitals, it is possible to identify the anatomical parts, pointing out how healthy the genitals appear. The examiner using a lighted speculum can identify the woman's internal pelvic structures. For many women, this is the first time they have been able to see their external genitals, to say nothing of their cervices and other internal structures.

Families often encounter disabling diseases or injuries that interfere with usual forms of sexual expression. Couples may ask nurses to validate the normality or health of the adaptations they make, such as the exploration of new types of sexual expression.

Using sexual information to promote health in other areas

Addressing sexual concerns may promote the adoption of other health habits by patients. For example, nurses teach patients with chronic obstructive pulmonary disease to maintain optimal levels of endurance with low levels of exercise, stopping smoking, using pursed lip and abdominal breathing techniques, and complying with medications and breathing treatments. All of these activities not only serve to stabilize the disease and increase the ability to perform ADLs, but they also can potentially increase their sexual performance. In addition, the nurse can suggest these patients wear their nasal oxygen cannula and use proper breathing techniques during lovemaking.

26-11

Common sexual concerns of patients with strokes and their partners

Changes that occur with sexual function

Interferences with desire: A patient who is aphasic will have difficulty communicating sexual feelings and desires. Both partners may fear lack of ability to perform and so may not initiate sex. If sex is not initiated, there is no proof of erectile dysfunction or vaginal dryness.

Interferences with excitement and orgasm: Most people are "sexually conditioned" to use only certain positions or certain sex acts. After a stroke a couple may need to try other "unusual" positions to be successful.

Changes in sexual self-concept

Depression, dementia, and emotional lability are all common to stroke. Depression severely reduces desire, which then can make the depression worse. Stroke survivors may have perceptual problems and not realize how disabled they are, which interferes with forming realistic expectations about sex and intimacy. Dementia interferes with understanding what is happening. Emotional lability is very difficult to deal with during sex; making love while crying or laughing uncontrollably is not very romantic.

Changes in sexual roles and relationships

If the person who had the stroke needs some physical care, this will change the roles of each person in the relationship. One of the most common concerns of spouses is the "loss" of part of their partner and whether the spouse will be the "same person I've been married to for the last 40 years." The partner of a person with dementia may have ethical concerns about whether the stroke survivor can continue to consent to participate in a sexual relationship. People who have strokes who have not been involved in relationships for a long time due to death of a spouse may respond inappropriately to "intimate" touching as part of routine nursing care by the staff.

Recommendations and nursing interventions

Always ask if patients have sexual concerns, no matter how old they are. Encourage the expression of feelings of both partners. Patients have reported an overwhelming need for information that was completely ignored by health professionals.[39] Recommend making slow changes in sexual activities, spending time talking with their spouse, just being together, and not trying to have sex too quickly after hospital discharge. Recommend they try different coital positions. A man who is hemiplegic will probably not be able to support himself in a superior position, and thus the couple may need to try a side-lying or other position for intercourse.[8,33,39]

Sexual concerns may motivate self-care. A woman with multiple sclerosis (MS) sought out community services to assist her in learning to perform her own intermittent catheterization for bladder management. Even though her MS had caused visual problems, poor hand and wrist strength, and paraplegia, the community nurse and occupational therapist were able to teach her to catheterize herself with the use of a "cock up" wrist splint, "labia spreader," lighted magnifying mirror, hard rubber catheters, and a urinal. The patient expressed her gratitude that her husband would no longer need to perform this activity for her.

Burgener and Logan[8] report that a 64-year-old male with a stroke described his distress at his wife's helping him to toilet. This distress affected his sexual self-concept, as well as his relationship with his wife. The nurse assisted him to become independent in toileting, and he became confident in resuming a more sexual relationship, rather than a patient-carer relationship, with his wife.

Putting It All Together

This chapter has outlined some skills and knowledge useful for nurses in addressing sexual concerns. Box 26-11 illustrates some typical sexual concerns of stroke patients and their partners, and interventions the nurse can use to prevent or assist to overcome sexual problems.

SUMMARY

1. Human sexuality is a complex of interrelating biological and psychosocial variables that begin at conception and continue through life; components include biological (sexual function or expression), psychological (gender identity, thoughts, and feelings), and social factors (such as sanctioned role, mores, and folklore regulating sexual expression).
2. The physiological phases of human sexual response may be divided into four categories (excitement, plateau, orgasm, resolution) or three categories (desire, excitement, orgasm).
3. The excitement and plateau phases are characterized by vasocongestion of pelvic blood vessels leading to swelling of genitalia and by vaginal lubrication, the orgasm phase by myotonia (involuntary muscle contractions in the pelvic organs and other parts of the body), and the resolution phase by muscle relaxation and return of normal blood flow.
4. Although generally a decline in overall interest and sexual activity is seen with age, many people continue with an active sexual life into old age; the level of activity appears related to the extent of sexual activity during youth.
5. Sexual expression varies and includes heterosexuality, homosexuality, bisexuality, transvestism, incest, zoophilia, fetishism, voyeurism, exhibitionism, sadism, and masochism; social norms influence expected sexual expressions.
6. Illness may affect sexuality and sexual function through changes in body structure, changes in body functions, effects of pharmacological agents, body image changes,

or environmental restrictions (privacy, competing stimuli, partner segregation).

7. Sexual concerns and difficulties generally do not produce profound problems in sexual response although they may temporarily interfere with sexual functioning; sexual concerns and difficulties are usually amenable to sex education and counselling.
8. Alterations in sexual health include alterations in sexual function (desire, arousal, orgasm), in sexual self-concept, and in sexual relationships.
9. Alterations in sexual desire include low sexual desire and sexual aversion. Therapy is directed towards underlying causes; intensive sex therapy or psychotherapy is often required for sexual aversion.
10. Alterations in sexual arousal reflect body-mind-social interaction and may result from drugs, diseases affecting vascular function, age, and anxiety about sexual performance. Transient episodes of alteration in arousal are common. Therapies include anxietyreducing approaches and exercises that emphasize pleasure rather than pressure to perform.
11. Alterations in orgasm include ejaculatory problems in men and anorgasmia in women; both physiological and psychological mechanisms can produce orgasm phase alterations. Therapies include anxiety-reducing strategies for anorgasmia and relaxation-stimulation techniques for ejaculatory problems.
12. Alterations in sexual self-concept may result from disease or injury. Therapies include strategies towards accepting and transcending body image changes, transcending the sick role, obtaining partner support, and enhancing a positive self-concept.
13. Alterations in sexual relationships during illness result from value conflicts about sexual activity, problems with communication, or difficulties in sexual functioning. Therapies include promoting communication and providing education to resolve conflicts and promote sexuality.
14. Nursing interventions for people with sexual concerns, sexual difficulties, and alterations in sexual response include awareness of the nurse's own value system, therapeutic communication, prevention of sexual problems through education, anticipatory guidance, and promotion of a milieu conducive to sexual health.

STUDY QUESTIONS

- What instances in your own life shaped some of your feelings about yourself as female or male?
- What nursing behaviours would increase your comfort in describing your own sexual history?
- Examine your beliefs about homosexuality. In what ways might your beliefs help or hinder working with homosexual patients who have sexual concerns?
- Examine the list of diseases in Table 30-4 and the list of medications in Table 30-5. Have any of these conditions existed for patients for whom you have provided care recently? How might their sexual response have been affected? Did they express any concerns about their sexuality or sexual response? Discuss the nursing care that could have been offered.

REFERENCES AND SELECTED READINGS

1.* Allen M: A holistic view of sexuality and the aged, *Holistic Nurs Pract* 1(4):76-83, 1987.
2. Andersen BL, LeGrand J: Body image for women: conceptualization, assessment, and a test of its importance to sexual dysfunction and medical illness, *J Sex Research* 28:457-477, 1991.
3.* Bachers E: Sexual dysfunction after treatment for genitourinary cancers, *Semin Oncol Nurs* 1(1):18-24, 1985.
4.* Baggs J, Karch AM: Sexual counseling of women with coronary heart disease, *Heart Lung* 16:154-159, 1987.
5. Bernhard L: Sexuality expectations and outcomes in women having hysterectomies, *Chart* 83(10):11-15, 1986.
6.* Bernhard L, Dan A: Redefining sexuality from women's own experiences, *Nurs Clin North Am* 21:125-136, 1986.
7. Brink P: Cultural aspects of sexuality, *Holistic Nurs Pract* 1(4):12-20, 1987.
8. Burgener S, Logan G: Sexuality concerns of the post-stroke patient, *Rehab Nurs* 14:178-181, 195, 1989.
9.* Campbell M: Sexual dysfunction in the COPD patient, *DCCN* 6(2):70-74, 1987.
10. Chateauvert M, Duffie A, Gilmore N: HIV antibody testing: counselling guidelines from the Canadian Medical Association, *Pat Educ Council* 18:35-49, 1986.
11. Cochran SK, Peplau LA: Sexual risk reduction behaviors among young heterosexual adults, *Soc Sci Med* 33:25-36, 1991.
12.* Cohen J: Sexual counseling of the patient following myocardial infarction, *Crit Care Nurse* 6(6):18-29, 1986.
13.* Cooley M, et al: Sexual and reproductive issues for women with Hodgkin's disease: overview of issues, *CA Nurs* 9:188-193, 1986.
13a. Department of Health, *Health of the Nation: A strategy for health in England. Presented to parliament by the Secretary of State for Health*, London, 1992, HMSO.
14. Donlou J, et al: Psychosocial aspects of AIDS and AIDS-related complex: a pilot study, *J Psychosoc Oncol* 3(2):39-55, 1985.
15. D'Emilio J, Freedman EB: *Intimate matters, a history of sexuality in America,* New York, 1988, Harper & Row.
16.* Fischman S, et al: Changes in sexual relationships in postpartum couples, *JOGNN* 15(1):58-63, 1986.
17. Fogel CI, Lauver D: *Sexual health promotion,* Philadelphia, 1990, WB Saunders.
18.* Frank-Stromberg M: Sexuality and the elderly cancer patient, *Semin Oncol Nurs* 1(1):49-55, 1985.
19. Friend R: Sexual identity and human diversity: implications for nursing practice, *Holistic Nurs Pract* 1(4):21-41, 1987.
20. Gloeckner M: Perceptions of sexuality after ostomy surgery, *J Enterost Ther* 18:36-38, 1991.
21.* Grunbert K: Sexual rehabilitation of the cancer patient undergoing ostomy surgery, *J Enterost Ther* 13:148-152, 1986.
22.* Heinrick K: Effective response to sexual harassment, *Nurs Outlook* 35(2):70-72, 1987.
23. Kaiser FE: Sexuality and impotence in the aging man, *Clin Geriatr Med* 7:63-72, 1991.
24. Kansky J: Sexuality of widows: a study of the sexual practices of widows during the first fourteen months of bereavement, *J Sex Marital Ther* 12:307-321, 1986.
25. Kaplan HS: Sex, intimacy, and the aging process, *J Am Acad Psychoanal* 18:185-205, 1990.
26.* Katzin L: Chronic illness and sexuality, *Am J Nurs* 90(1):55-59, 1990.
27. Kautz DD, Dickey CA, Stevens MN: Using research to identify why nurses do not meet established sexuality nursing care standards, *J Nurs Qual Assur* 4(3):69-73, 1990.
28. Koch PB, Young EW: Diabetes and female sexuality: a review of the literature, *Health Care Women Int* 9:251-262, 1988.
29.* Kus R: Sex, AIDS, and gay American men, *Holistic Nurs Pract* 1(4):42-51, 1987.
30.* Lamb M: Sexual dysfunction in the gynecologic oncology patient, *Semin Oncol Nurs* 1(1):9-17, 1985.
31. Leese DL: An overview of urologic complications in diabetes mellitus, *Urol Nurs* 11:17-20, 1991.

32. Lichtenberg PA, Strzepek DM: Assessments of institutionalized dementia patients competencies to participate in intimate relationships, *Gerontologist* 30:117-120, 1990.
33. Litz BT, Zeiss AM, Davies HD: Sexual concerns of male spouses of female Alzheimer's disease patients, *Gerontologist* 30:113-116, 1990.
34. Lloyd EE, Toth LL, Perkash I: Vacuum tumescence: an option for spinal cord injured males with erectile dysfunction, *SCI Nurs* 6:25-28, 1989.
35. LoPiccolo J: Counseling and therapy for sexual problems in the elderly, *Clin Geriatr Med* 7:161-179, 1991.
36.* MacElveen-Hoehn P: Understanding sexuality in progressive cancer, *Semin Oncol Nurs* 1(1):56-62, 1985.
37. Mason DR: Erectile dysfunctions: assessment and care, *Nurse Pract* 14:23-24, 1989.
38. Mason JO, McGinnis JM: Healthy people 2000: an overview of the national health promotion and disease prevention objectives, *Pub Health Rep* 105:441-446, 1989.
39. McCormick GP, Riffer DJ, Thompson MM: Coital positioning for stroke afflicted couples, *Rehab Nurs* 11(2):17-19, 1986.
40. McCracken AL: Sexual practice by elders: the forgotten aspect of functional health, *Sex Marital Ther* 14:13-18, 1988.
41. McCusker J, et al: Responses to the AIDS epidemic among homosexually active men: factors associated with preventive behaviour, *Pat Educ Council* 13:15-30, 1989.
42.* McCann ME: Sexual healing after heart attack, *Am J Nurs* 89:1133-1140, 1989.
43. Mulligan T, Palguta RF: Sexual interest, activity, and satisfaction among male nursing home residents, *Arch Sex Behav* 20:199-204, 1991.
44.* Papadoupolous C, et al: Sexual activity after coronary bypass surgery, *Chest* 90:681-685, 1986.
45. Penkower L, et al: Behavioral, health and psychosocial factors and risk for HIV infection among sexually active homosexual men: the Multicenter AIDS Cohort Study, *Am J Pub Health* 81:194-196, 1990.
46.* Persaud D: Assessing sexual functions of the adult with traumatic quadriplegia, *J Neurosurg Nurs* 18(1):11-12, 1986.
47.* Price J: Promoting sexual wellness in head-injured patients, *Rehab Nurs* 10(6):12-13, 1989.
48.* Schain W: Breast cancer surgeries and psychosexual sequelae: implications for remediation, *Semin Oncol Nurs* 1:200-205, 1985.
49. Schechter MT, et al: Patterns of sexual behaviour and condom use in a cohort of homosexual men, *Am J Pub Health* 78:1535-1538, 1988.
50. Siegel K, et al: Factors distinguishing homosexual males practicing risky and safer sex, *Soc Sci Med* 28:561-569, 1989.
51. Slob AK, et al: Sexuality and psychophysiological functioning in women with diabetes mellitus, *J Sex Marital Ther* 16:59-69, 1990.
52. Smedley G: Addressing sexuality in the elderly, *Rehab Nurs* 16:9-11, 1991.
53. Steele D: Drugs causing sexual dysfunction and their alternatives: a reference tool, *Urol Nurs* 9:10-12, 1989.
54. Turner BF, Adams CG: Reported change in preferred sexual activity over the adult years, *J Sex Res* 25:289-303, 1991.
55. Waterhouse J, et al: Development of the sexual adjustment questionnaire: impact of cancer and surgery, *Oncol Nurs Forum* 13(3):53-59, 1986.
56. Williams CB: Controlling premature ejaculation: patient guide, *Med Asp Hum Sexual* 25(3):15-16, 1991.
57. Williams L: Pharmacologic erection programs: a treatment option of erectile dysfunction, *Rehab Nurs* 14:264-268, 1989.
58.* Woods NF: Toward a holistic perspective of human sexuality: alteration in sexual health and nursing diagnoses, *Holistic Nurs Pract* 1(4):1-11, 1987.
59. Woods NF: Human sexuality: an overview. In Mitchell PH, et al: *AANN's neuroscience nursing: phenomena and practice,* Norwalk, Conn, 1988, Appleton & Lange.
60. Zapka JG, et al: HIV antibody test result knowledge, risk perceptions and behavior among homosexually active men, *Pat Educ Council* 18:9-17, 1991.
61. Annon J: *The behavioral treatment of sexual problems,* Honolulu, 1974, Enabling Systems.
62. Bell A, Weinberg M: *Homosexualities,* New York, 1978, Simon & Schuster.
63. Comfort A: The normal in sexual behavior: an ethnological point of view, *J Sex Ed Ther* 2:1-7, 1975.
64. Hellerstein H, Friedman FH: Sexual activity and the postcoronary patient, *Arch Intern Med* 125:987-999, 1970.
65. Kaplan HS: *Disorders of sexual desire and other new concepts and techniques in sex therapy,* New York, 1979, Simon & Schuster.
66. Kaplan HS: *The new sex therapy,* New York, 1974, Brunner/Mazel.
67. Kinsey AC, Pomeroy WB, Martin CW: *Sexual behavior in the human male,* Philadelphia, 1948, WB Saunders.

*Recommended for student reading.

68. Kinsey AC, et al: *Sexual behavior in the human female,* Philadelphia, 1953, WB Saunders.

69. Larson J: *Heart rate and blood pressure responses of coronary artery disease patients during sexual activity and a two-stair climbing test,* Master's thesis, Seattle, 1978, University of Washington.

70. Masters W, Johnson V: *Homosexuality in perspective,* Boston, 1979, Little, Brown.

71. Masters W, Johnson V: *Human sexual response,* Boston, 1966, Little, Brown.

72. Masters W, Johnson V: *Human sexual inadequacy,* Boston, 1970, Little, Brown.

73. Mims F: A model to promote sexual health, *Nurs Outlook* 26:121, 1978.

74. Money J, Ehrhardt A: *Man and woman, boy and girl,* Baltimore, 1972, The Johns Hopkins University Press.

75. Rubin A, Babbott D: Impotence and diabetes mellitus, *JAMA* 168:498-500, 1958.

76.* Woods NF: *Human sexuality in health and illness,* ed 3, St Louis, 1984, Mosby–Year Book.

77. Woods NF, Earp JA: Women with cured breast cancer: a description of women's experiences four years after mastectomy, *Nurs Res* 27:279-285, 1978.

78. World Health Organization: *Education and treatment in human sexuality: the training of health professionals,* Tech Rep Series, No 572, Geneva, 1975, The Organization.

79. Zahn MA: Incapacity, impotence, and invisible impairment: their effects upon interpersonal relations, *J Health Soc Behav* 14:115-123, 1973.

80. Zalar MK: Role preparation for nurses in human sexual functioning, *Nurs Clin North Am* 17:351-363, 1982.

FURTHER READING

Ainslie S: Sexuality and the cancer sufferer, *Nursing Mirror,* 159(10):38-40, 1984.

Bancroft J: *Human sexuality and its problems,* Edinburgh, 1983, Churchill Livingstone.

Donohoe G: Sensitivity can break the taboo. Female sexual problems and treatment approaches, *Professional Nurse* 7(5):304-308, 1992.

Glover J: *Human sexuality in nursing care,* Kent, 1985, Croom Helm.

Irwin R: critical re-evaluation can overcome discrimination. Providing equal standards of care for homosexual patients, *Professional Nurse* 7(7):435-438, 1992.

Janes G: An open approach to minimise the effect. Sexuality and renal patients, *Professional Nurse* 6(2):69-71, 1990.

Platzer H: Sexual orientation: improving care, *Nursing Standard* 4(38):38-39, 1990.

Savage J: *Nurses, gender and sexuality,* London, 1987, Heinemann.

Savage J: Sexuality: an uninvited guest, *Nursing Times* 85(5):25-28, 1989.

Webb C: *Sexuality, nursing and health,* Chichester, 1985, Wiley.

Webb C, Askham J: Nurses' knowledge and attitudes about sexuality in healthcare—a review of the literature, *Nurse Education today* 7:75-87, 1987.

27

The Patient with Reproductive Problems

Barbara C. Long
Greer Glazer

After studying this chapter, the learner should be able to:

- Describe the primary and secondary prevention for genital infections and malignancies.
- Carry out health teaching regarding menstruation and menopause and alterations in sexual functioning.
- Describe approaches used for sterilization and infertility.
- Differentiate types and effects of inflammatory and structural disorders of the reproductive tract in females and males.
- Identify the incidence and therapeutic approaches for cancer of the reproductive tract in females and males.
- Plan nursing care for people undergoing surgery of the reproductive tract.
- Describe the transmission, prevention and control of sexuality transmitted diseases.
- Describe the transmission, prevention and control of sexually transmited diseases.
- List the causative agent, incubation period, signs and symptoms, medical therapy, and long-term effects of gonorrhoea, syphilis, herpes genitalis and chlamydial infection.

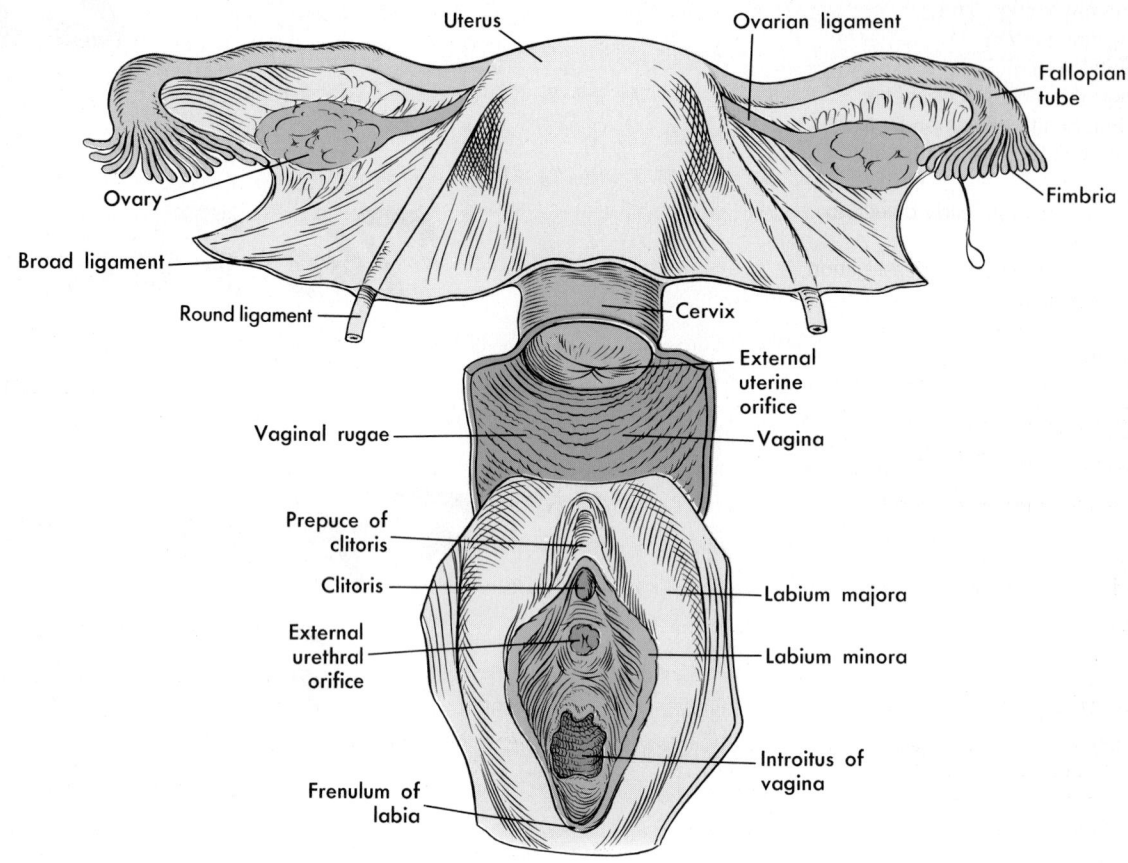

Fig. 27-1 Female internal organs of reproduction. Major ligaments are shown.

Nurses and lay people have become more enlightened about the prevention of problems of the reproductive system. This increased awareness has led many people to initiate requests for information about or treatment of reproductive system problems. Although men and women are better informed today about matters relating to reproductive health, many neglect preventive measures and ignore signs or symptoms of illness because of embarrassment and the special significance that they attach to the reproductive organs.

In spite of advances in medicine, nursing, science, and technology, diseases and disorders of the genital system continue to threaten the lives and the physical and emotional health of men and women, sometimes needlessly. Many of these problems are preventable; many of them can be treated and cured.

ANATOMY AND PHYSIOLOGY
Female Genital System
External structures

The external genitalia, or vulva, of the female consist primarily of the labia majora, labia minora, and clitoris (Fig. 27-1). Two glands are located in this area: Skene's glands (paraurethral), opening into the urethral orifice, and Bartholin's glands, situated at each side of the vaginal opening near the base of the labia. These glands are common sites of infection.

Internal organs

The female internal reproductive organs, consisting of the vagina, uterus, uterine fallopian tubes, and ovaries, are shown in Fig. 27-1. These organs are located within the cavity of the true pelvis unless their size is increased by disease or pregnancy.

Vagina

The vagina leads from the external structures to the uterus. The length of the vaginal canal varies, and the posterior wall is longer than the anterior wall. The uterine cervix protrudes into the upper vagina, creating recesses (fornices) around the margins of the cervix.

The vagina is lined with pink mucous membrane arranged in folds called *rugae*. Physiological events such as pregnancy and pathological conditions such as infections often alter the colour of the vaginal mucosa because of congestion with blood. The membrane is lubricated by vaginal secretions that are normally acidic during the years of ovarian function; neutral or alkaline secretions are normally found in postmenopausal women. An alkaline medium promotes growth of bacteria.

Uterus

The uterus consists of three portions: the fundus (upper crest), the main body (corpus), and the neck (cervix). In adult females the position of the uterus may vary. It is usually anteverted (tipped forward) and slightly anteflexed (bent forward at an angle), but it may also be retroverted, retroflexed, or in midposition. During menopause the uterus decreases in size.

The uterus has three functional layers: parametrium or outer layer, myometrium or middle muscular layer, and endometrium or mucous membrane lining. The outer surface of the uterus is covered by the peritoneum. Reflection of the peritoneum posteriorly between the uterus and rectum creates a space known as the *pouch of Douglas*. This space is a common entry site for endoscopy or for surgical drainage of the peritoneal cavity.

Uterine tubes

The uterine or *fallopian* tubes are two narrow muscular canals 8 to 14 cm long. They extend outward from the uterine corpus near the fundus (Fig. 27-1). The uterine tubes serve as a site for union of the sperm and ovum and transport of the fertilized ovum to the uterus. Strictures of the fallopian tubes prevent passage of the ovum.

Ovaries

The ovaries are endocrine glands as well as reproductive organs. Their functions are to store follicles, to produce mature ova, and to produce and secrete oestrogen, progesterone, and androgens. Ovarian functions are readily disturbed by acute and chronic diseases. These functions can also be altered or interrupted by surgery, radiation, and the ingestion of drugs such as oral contraceptives. After menopause the ovaries undergo rapid regressive changes and decrease in size.

Endocrine functions

The major hormones produced by the ovaries are oestrogen and progesterone. *Oestrogen* is the hormone responsible for the development of secondary sex characteristics at the time of puberty. After puberty the primary function of oestrogen is to cause development of the endometrium in preparation for implantation of a fertilized ovum. Oestrogen causes the retention of calcium and phosphorus and thus promotes bone growth. After menopause the decline of oestrogen levels may account for some of the symptoms that sometimes occur, such as hot flushes, osteoporosis (loss of calcium from bone), and vaginal atrophy. *Progesterone* enhances the action of oestrogen on the endometrium. It also prevents muscular contractions of the myometrium as an aid for maintaining pregnancy should the ovum become implanted.

Secretion of ovarian hormones is cyclic, with each cycle requiring an average of 28 days. Unless stimulated by pituitary hormones, however, the ovaries do not fulfil their hormone-secreting and ovum-producing functions.

The phases of the menstrual cycle are illustrated in Fig. 27-2 and described in Box 27-1. The secretory (luteal) phase is the least variable part of the menstrual cycle. Irregular menstrual cycles are most frequently related to longer or shorter menstrual or proliferative (follicular) phases.

On the day of ovulation, about 25% of women experience pain in the lower abdomen on the side of ovulation. This pain (mittelschmerz) is probably a result of peritoneal irritation from follicular fluid or blood released from the ovary with the ovum. This sign rarely occurs with every

---

27-1

Menstrual cycle

Menstrual phase (menstruation): Day 1 to day 4
Oestrogen and progesterone withdrawn before onset of menstrual flow
Shedding of endometrial lining

Proliferative (follicular) phase: Day 5 to day 14
Regrowth of endometrial tissue
Secretion of follicle-stimulating hormone (FSH) by the pituitary gland
Development in ovary of a mature graafian follicle containing a mature ovum
Secretion of increasing amounts of *oestrogen* by graafian follicle
Suppression of FSH when oestrogen level becomes high, leading to secretion of luteinizing hormone (LH) by pituitary gland

Secretory (luteal) phase: Day 15 to days 25/28
Rupture of graafian follicle releasing ovum (ovulation) starts the secretory phase
Movement of ovum through fallopian tube to uterus
Formation of corpus luteum at site of ruptured graafian follicle
Production of *progesterone* by corpus luteum
Stimulation by progesterone of endometrial cell growth
Significant decrease in progesterone level if implantation does not occur; menstrual phase then begins again

---

cycle and is therefore an unreliable indicator of ovulation. If the pain occurs on the right side and is severe, it may be mistaken for appendicitis.

Male Genital System

The male reproductive organs and associated structures are shown in Fig. 27-3. The male reproductive organs produce sperm, suspend the sperm in a liquid, and deliver the sperm into the vagina to fertilize an ovum. Another important function is secretion of male hormones, the androgens. Sperm are produced in the testes and are conveyed through the vas (ductus) deferens to the urethra. Semen consists of sperm with fluids from the seminal vesicles and the prostate gland. The prostate gland is important clinically because of its affinity for congestive, inflammatory, hyperplastic, and malignant disease. Because the prostate gland encircles the urethra, even benign enlargement (hypertrophy) may lead to obstruction of the urethra.

The male hormone *testosterone* is produced by the interstitial cells of the testes and is responsible for development of the genitalia during puberty and for maintaining the genitalia in a functional state during life. Androgenic hormones are also responsible for the development of secondary sex characteristics including growth of body hair and thickening of the vocal cords. Testosterone secretion is closely related to pituitary gland function, and the rate of secretion is determined by levels of luteinizing hormone (LH) in the blood. Secretion of testosterone decreases slowly with age.

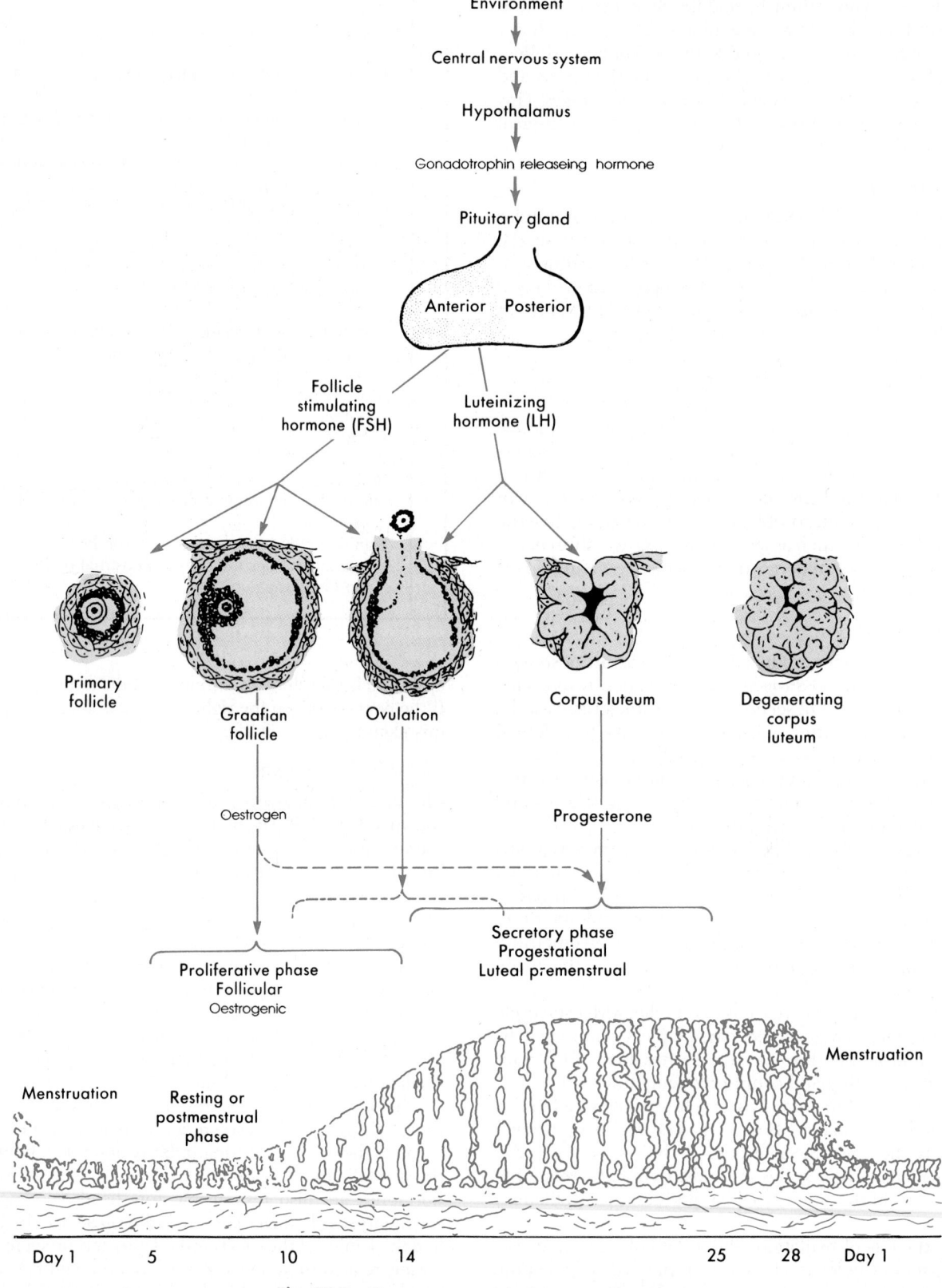

Fig. 27-2 Hormone control of menstrual cycle.

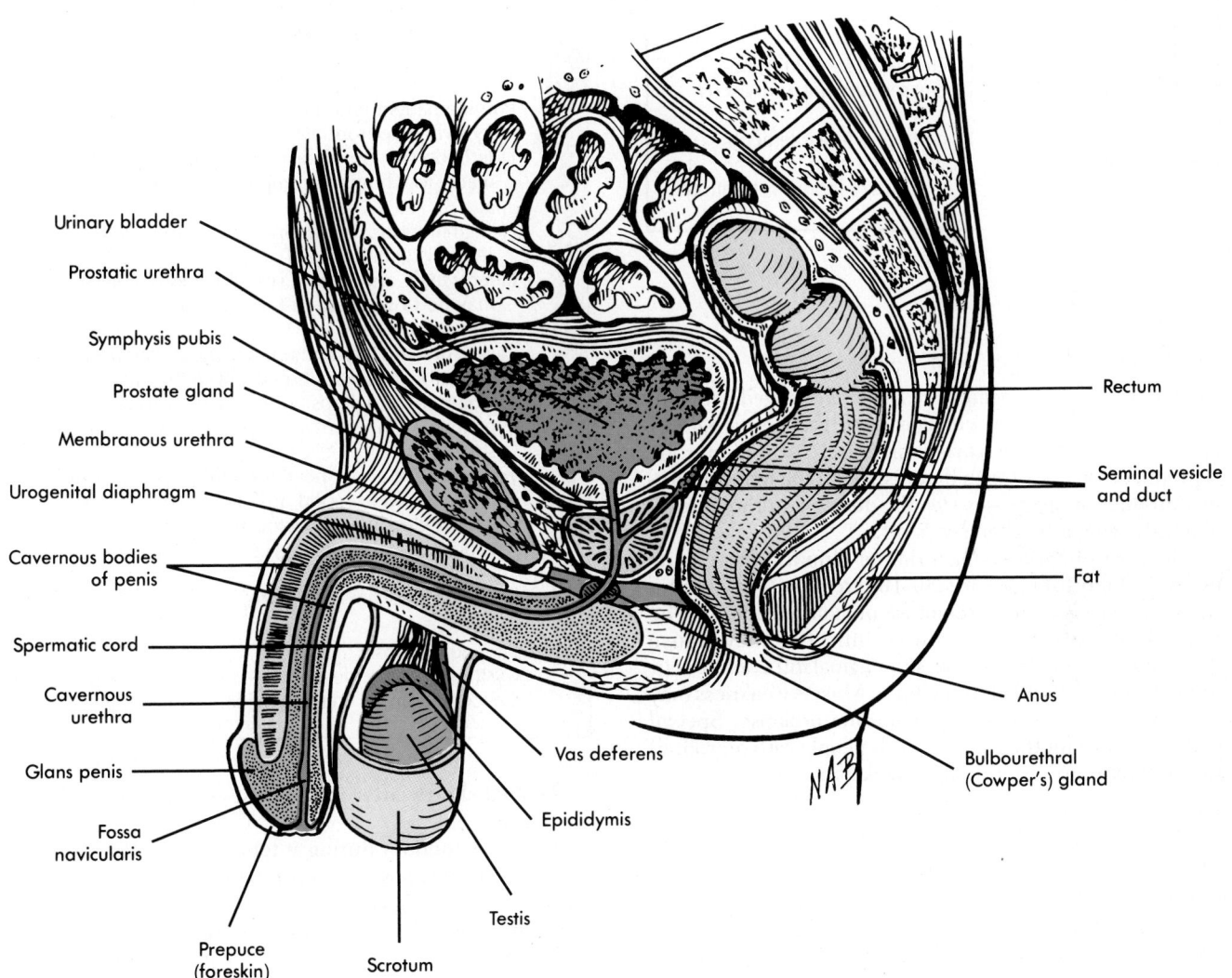

Urinary bladder

Prostatic urethra

Symphysis pubis

Prostate gland

Membranous urethra

Urogenital diaphragm

Cavernous bodies
of penis

Spermatic cord

Cavernous
urethra

Glans penis

Fossa
navicularis

Prepuce
(foreskin)

Scrotum

Testis

Epididymis

Vas deferens

Rectum

Seminal vesicle
and duct

Fat

Anus

Bulbourethral
(Cowper's) gland

NAB

Fig. 27-3   Male organs of reproduction.

27-2	**Physiological changes in reproductive tract with ageing**
	Female
	Uterus — Decreased size
	Ovaries — Atrophy, with decreased size
	Vagina — Decreased width and length
	Vaginal entrance (introitus) narrowed
	Vaginal secretions decrease and become more alkaline
	Male
	Testes — Decreased size and firmness
	Seminal fluid — Decreased amount and viscosity
	Prostate gland — Hypertrophy (enlargement)
	Penile erection — Slower, decreased frequency of involuntary morning erections

Physiological Changes With Ageing

Menopause, which occurs in the middle-aged woman, results in physiological changes from the hormonal decrease (Box 27-2). When ovulation ceases, no progesterone is produced and oestrogen diminishes. In the male, androgen production decreases steadily during adulthood until about the age of 60 then levels off.

The physiological changes do not diminish the elderly person's ability to engage in sexual intercourse (see Chapter 26) but may lead to discomfort or complications. The vaginal dryness and narrowed introitus may cause dyspareunia (painful intercourse). Vaginal infections occur more readily in the alkaline medium. Muscle weakness may lead to cystocele, rectocele, or uterine prolapse. Special considerations for the care of elderly people with reproductive problems are listed in the special box.

PREVENTION AND HEALTH EDUCATION
Primary prevention: Prevention of Infection

Vaginal infections may result from the presence of large numbers of invading organisms or from decreased resistance to infection. Those women in whom the natural barriers to infection are at a minimum (low oestrogen levels, thinness of the vaginal epithelium, or reduced acidity of the vagina) are at greatest risk (Box 27-3).

Large numbers of organisms may invade the vagina or urethra from inadequate personal hygiene, from another person during sexual intercourse, or from use of unclean toilet articles. Decreased resistance to infection may result from vaginal secretions becoming more alkaline, providing a more suitable medium for bacterial growth. Vaginal fungal infections may be a side effect of drugs such as the antibiotics or oral contraceptives. Preventive measures include the following:

1. Wipe from front to back (female) after bowel movements

The Elderly with Sexuality and Reproductive Problems

Assessment

Determine meaning of sexuality to patient; age does not imply loss of sexuality.

Assess for problems engaging in sexual intercourse because of disability or disease.

Determine frequency of regular gynaecological examination in elderly women; some women are not ware that these examinations should be continued after menopause.

Assess for signs of vaginitis (vaginal pruritus and discharge).

Assess for signs of cystocele or rectocele (urinary incontinence, low back pain).

Intervention

Provide patient with information regarding sexuality, when appropriate.

Elderly do not lose their need for affection, intimacy, touching, or companionship as they age.

A vaginal lubricant is helpful for women with senile vaginitis.

Elderly male and female sexual responsiveness may be slower, but just as enjoyable as for younger adults.

Past sexual activity and enjoyment are the best indicators of sexual behaviour in the elderly.

Changes in sexual positions may be helpful for patients with arthritis, myocardial infarction, stroke, and other disabilities.

Teach patient about need for annual pelvic examinations and to report any signs of postmenopausal bleeding to doctor (possible uterine cancer).

Common disorders in elderly

Vaginitis
Uterine prolapse
Cystocele, rectocele
Cancer of cervix, uterus, vagina, prostate, penis

2. Void shortly after intercourse to wash away organisms
3. Use a condom during intercourse if either partner has been exposed to a genital infection
4. Recognize signs of infection in sexual partners and urge them to seek medical attention
5. Abstain from intercourse if one partner has a genital infection
6. Avoid douching (which may alter vaginal pH) unless advised by a doctor for treatment
7. Seek immediate medical attention for early signs of vaginal infection (abnormal vaginal discharge, vaginal itching), especially in people at high risk.

Secondary Prevention: Early Detection of Cancer

Dramatically decreased rates of death from cancer are associated with early detection and treatment. People at high risk for cancer of the cervix include women who were sexually active at an early age and those with multiple sex partners. Sexually transmitted diseases (STDs) that are associated with cervical cancer include human

Risk factors for vaginal infections

Ageing
Diabetes
Pregnancy
Malnutrition
Inadequate perineal hygiene
Excessive douching
Use of vaginal inserts
Oral contraceptives
Broad-spectrum antibiotics
Intercourse with infected partner

Risk factors for uterine cancer

Cancer of the cervix

First sexual intercourse at early age
Multiple sexual partners
Cigarette smoking
Certain STDs

Cancer of the endometrium

History of infertility
Failure of ovulation
Prolonged oestrogen therapy without added progestogen
Late menopause
Combination of diabetes, high blood pressure, and obesity

Examinations for prevention of uterine cancer generally recommended

1. After three or more consecutive annual Pap tests with normal findings, test may be performed less frequently at discretion of the doctor.
2. More frequent Pap tests for people at high risk
3. Endometrial tissue sample at menopause for people at high risk for endometrial cancer

Patient Teaching

Menstruation

Knowledge of the physiological process
Factors that may alter the menstrual cycle: stress, fatigue, exercise, acute and chronic illness, changes in climate or working hours, pregnancy
Personal hygiene
  Wear pads during early period of heavy flow
  Change tampons frequently to decrease risk of toxic shock syndrome
  Consult a doctor if tampons cause discomfort
  Take a daily bath for comfort (warm bath may relieve slight pelvic discomfort)
Exercise
  Exercise is not contraindicated and may help prevent discomfort
  Modify exercise if fatigue occurs
Diet
  Restrict salt intake if fluid retention is present
  Consult a doctor if fluid retention persists after menstruation
Discomfort (dysmenorrhoea)
  For mild discomfort take aspirin, paracetamol, or ibuprofen, apply warmth, rest
  For prolonged severe discomfort, consult a doctor.

papillomavirus (HPV) and *Herpesvirus hominis* type 2 (HVH-2). High-risk factors for endometrial cancer include early problems with menstruation or ovulation or late menopause, lack of progesterone with prolonged oestrogen therapy, and obesity[1] (Box 27-4).

The decline in deaths from cervical cancer is primarily the result of increased use of the Papanicolaou (Pap) smear for mass screening, combined with more frequent and more thorough gynaecological examinations. Cancer of the cervix is easier to detect through Pap smear than is cancer of the endometrium.

Health teaching for prevention of uterine cancer includes regular pelvic examinations that include a Pap smear. General recommendations to detect cancer early are listed in Box 27-5.

Health Teaching Related to Menstruation and Menopause

Menstruation

Menstruation occurs on an average of every 28 days; the normal range is 26 to 34 days. The menstrual flow usually lasts for 3 to 7 days (average 4 days). Normally 30 to 180 ml (average 50 ml) of menstrual fluid is lost during the period. One half to three fourths of the fluid is blood, and the remainder is mucus, fragments of endometrial cells, and desquamated vaginal epithelium.

Normally menstrual fluid does not clot unless it is retained in the uterus or vagina for a prolonged time. It is believed that the endometrium produces an anticoagulant that prevents clotting of blood in the uterus. An occasional very small clot may occur during the first 24 hours, and this is probably a particle of endometrial tissue. Large clots or pus in the menstrual flow are never normal.

During pregnancy menstruation ceases, and then returns within 6 to 8 weeks after delivery, although lactation suppresses the menses for varying periods of time. Unless disease occurs, the menstrual periods recur during adult life until menopause.

Menstruation is a manifestation of normal body function and should be treated as such. The "period" and "monthly period" are accurate terms to use if the woman does not wish to say "menstruating." Terms such as "being sick," "on the rag," or "having the curse" are to be avoided because of their negative connotation. Suggestions for health teaching related to menstruation are listed in Box 27-6.

Table 27-1 Activities to modify PMS discomfort

PMS symptoms	Activity
Behavioural changes	Increase intake of foods rich in vitamin B$_6$ (yeast, wheat germ, whole-grain cereals, liver, legumes); decrease dairy products intake; increase outdoor exercise
Water and sodium retention	Restrict salt intake; restrict intake of coffee, tea, cola, chocolate; increase intake of foods rich in vitamin B$_6$ (see above)
Increased appetite, (especially for sweets), headache, fatigue	Restrict free sugar, sodium, and animal fat intake; substitute complex carbohydrates for simple sugars
Depression	Increase intake of green leafy vegetables, legumes, and whole-grain cereals (high in B vitamins)

Adapted from Abraham G: Nutritional factors in the etiology of the premenstrual tension syndrome, *J Reprod Med* 28:446-464, 1983.

To become knowledgeable about the patterns of their menstrual cycles, women are encouraged to keep a written record. Establishing this habit makes it possible to predict the onset of the next menstrual period and to determine the range of cycles and duration of flow. Should it be necessary to seek the attention of a health professional for any reason, it is helpful to know the date of onset of the last menstrual period (LMP).

Premenstrual syndrome

Premenstrual syndrome (PMS), which occurs in approximately 10% of all menstruating women, is the presence of symptoms in the premenstruum or early menstruation with the absence of postmenstrual symptoms. Identical symptoms must occur in three consecutive cycles to confirm a diagnosis of PMS. Symptoms vary considerably among women and may include behavioural changes (tension, irritability, mood swings, anxiety, crying, depression, insomnia), fatigue, signs of water and sodium retention (oedema, weight gain, breast enlargement and tenderness, and abdominal bloating), palpitations, increased appetite, headache, and backache.[27] The cause is unknown although many factors have been suggested.

The nurse can assist women with PMS by acknowledging the existence of the syndrome and its attendant symptoms, which may be severe for some women. Encourage women to keep a menstrual symptom calendar to document the cyclic nature of the symptoms.[27]

Simple measures to relieve PMS symptoms include dietary changes, not smoking and drinking, and participating in planned exercise. A diet high in complex carbohydrates, moderate in protein, and low in refined sugar and sodium should be eaten, especially during the premenstrual interval. The consumption of caffeine (in tea, coffee, caffeine-containing beverages), chocolate, and alcohol, and smoking should be reduced or eliminated. Regular exercise

---

27-7

Causes of dysmenorrhoea

Primary dysmenorrhoea
High concentration of uterine prostaglandins

Secondary dysmenorrhoea
Pelvic inflammatory disease
Endometriosis
Malpositioned uterus
Cervical stenosis

---

three to four times a week for 30 minutes is encouraged, especially during the premenstrual interval. Because fatigue may exaggerate PMS symptoms, adequate rest, sleep, and relaxation are helpful. Additional activities are listed in Table 27-1.

Dysmenorrhoea

Although menstruation is a normal physiological process, some women experience varying degrees of discomfort (menstrual cramps). Dysmenorrhoea is the greatest single cause of absenteeism by women from school or work. Dysmenorrhoea may result from various causes (Box 27-7). An intrauterine device (IUD) may also cause menstrual discomfort. Primary dysmenorrhoea often disappears after pregnancy or by age 25.

Women who are consistently unable to engage in usual activities because of pain associated with menstruation should be urged to seek health care for diagnosis and treatment of any existing secondary dysmenorrhoea.

Treatment of secondary dysmenorrhoea is aimed at the organic cause. Surgical and pharmacological interventions may be appropriate depending on the severity and type of pathology. If the uterus is found to be in an abnormal position and can be manually returned to a normal position, a pessary may be inserted for a trial period to learn whether malposition is the cause of dysmenorrhoea. Dilatation of the cervical canal is done when a cervical stricture is found and thought to be the cause of dysmenorrhoea.

If no organic cause of dysmenorrhoea can be found, the woman is advised to try rest, moderate exercise, and avoidance of constipation. Local application of heat and mild analgesics are usually prescribed. Aspirin is a prostaglandin antagonist. Heat causes vasodilation of blood vessels, thereby increasing the blood flow and relieving ischaemia, increasing elimination of the menstrual flow, and decreasing muscle hypertonus.

Because prostaglandins cause uterine contractions, medications that usually give the best relief of discomfort are the prostaglandin inhibitors. These drugs include ibuprofen, mefenamic acid, naproxen, and fenoprofen. Ibuprofen can be obtained without a prescription. These drugs are effective when started at the onset of bleeding. Encourage taking prostaglandin inhibitors with milk or food to prevent side effects. Oral contraceptives have also been used to suppress ovulation by inhibiting prostaglandin levels.

Other measures that may be explored include systematic relaxation, exercise, muscle toning, massage, effleurage, breathing techniques, manual pressure on the abdomen, and orgasm. Biofeedback and autogenic training have also been used. Positive attitudes towards menstruation and alternative interventions from which to select the most useful interventions are helpful for the woman experiencing dysmenorrhoea.

Menopause

The *climacteric* is the transitional phase between reproductive and nonreproductive ability. Menopause is said to have occurred when there has been no menstrual flow for 1 year (although some women have periods even after 1 year of amenorrhoea). During the climacteric, which usually lasts for 12 to 18 months, there is a gradual decline in ovarian function. The ovaries gradually cease to produce ova and oestrogen, and as a result the menses become scanty, irregular, and further apart, until they stop altogether.

Natural menopause may occur between 35 and 60 years of age (average age 51 years). Cigarette smoking and living at high altitudes are associated with early menopause.

Menopause may be artificially induced by such procedures as irradiation of the ovaries, surgical removal of both ovaries, or hysterectomy. Each of these has one common consequence, namely, cessation of menstruation. However, surgical removal or irradiation of the ovaries results in menopause with all its physiological changes, whereas ovaries left intact after hysterectomy will continue to function provided the age of climacteric has not yet been reached.

Physiological factors in menopause

Physiological changes in the genital organs as a result of loss of hormonal functioning are listed in Box 27-2, p. 768. Because sexual functioning does not depend on the release of ova or hormones, women can enjoy sexual activity during the climacteric and after the menopause.

Many women go through the climacteric with little awareness of its occurrence. Some women, however, experience *hot flushes*, which are felt as waves of warmth accompanied by flushing of the skin, especially the face, neck, and arms, and perspiration. The hot flush is the perception of the spread of heat from an anatomic point of origin on the body to other areas of the body. Hot flushes may be so mild that they are hardly noticed or so severe that they produce distress. Hormone-replacement therapy (HRT) may be prescribed in severe cases. During oestrogen therapy women should be seen at least every 6 months for examination because of increased risk of endometrial cancer and for review of menopausal symptoms. The examination should include the breasts and reproductive organs, Pap smear, and blood pressure.

Vaginal changes (vaginal dryness, burning, itching, and occasional bleeding after menopause) result from thinning of the vaginal mucosa because of decreased oestrogen. Vaginal infections occur more frequently because vaginal secretions are more alkaline. Oestrogen therapy helps decrease vaginal difficulties.

Skeletal changes may also occur from lack of oestrogen. About 25% of postmenopausal women develop *osteoporosis* characterized by decreased bone mineral content and bone calcium. Osteoporotic problems include back pain, de-

---

Patient Teaching   27-8

Menopause

Knowledge about menopause
  Cessation of ovarian function with cessation of menstruation over 12 to 18 months
  Changes in reproductive ability
    Conception still possible during the period of change
      Contraception should be used for 1 year after last menstrual period
      Rhythm method unreliable contraceptive method during this period
    Ability to conceive ceases when menopause completed
  Sexual ability still present
  Physical symptoms vary from mild to severe; oestrogen therapy may be given to relieve severe symptoms (hormone-replacement therapy)
Promotion of health and physical appearance
  Moderate exercise to maintain muscle tone and help prevent osteoporosis
  Dietary control to prevent weight gain
  Calcium supplement or HRT to prevent osteoporosis
  Activities that encourage self-esteem and interest outside of self
  Peer support groups during menopause, if necessary
Prevention of discomfort
  Relief of vasomotor reactions (hot flushes)
    Moderation of factors identified by the person as exacerbating hot flushes (excitement, alcoholic beverages, heavy eating, excessive clothing, impairment of heat loss in hot weather)
  Vitamin E or B complex vitamins
  Prevention of dyspareunia (painful intercourse): local application of lubricant or vaginal cream
  Relief of vaginal itching: vitamin E or oestrogen therapy

---

creased height and mobility, and fractures of the spine, arm, upper femur, and ribs (Chapter 32). A significant factor in the development of osteoporosis is a low calcium/high phosphorus imbalance. Many women ingest inadequate amounts of calcium; an intake of 1200 mg of calcium daily is desirable (1500 mg for postmenopausal women). For absorption of calcium, 400 IU of vitamin D a day is needed. Hormone replacement therapy is protective against osteoporosis for as long as it is administered.

Counselling and teaching

Most women have heard of the "change of life." The negative image of menopause is reinforced by the media, books, health professionals, and the general public. Depending on the climate in which they were reared and on their own changes in attitude towards normal functions of the reproductive organs, women may feel more or less free to discuss menopause and their feelings and concerns during this period of life. Because many problems related to the reproductive organs occur in this age group, and because it is important for mental health that women be helped to make menopause as comfortable as possible, it is important for nurses to identify women who can profit from interventions.

Feelings of depression and uselessness may occur, particularly among women who have been highly invested in the maternal role. Peer support groups may be very helpful in these situations.

Education regarding menopause should precede its onset (Box 27-8). Women approaching menopause, regardless of whether it is an event of normal ageing or is artificially induced, need to know what menopause is, why it occurs, the effects menopause has on reproductive and sexual ability, what can be done to make menopause more comfortable, and those symptoms that require medical attention.

INTERFERENCES WITH REPRODUCTION

The ability to have children may be modified either to prevent conception or to terminate a pregnancy (Box 27-9). Some people are unable to procreate. The topics of contraception and abortion are covered in maternity nursing texts and are not repeated here.

Sterilization

Voluntary sterilization has become increasingly acceptable to both men and women as a method of preventing pregnancy. It is the most commonly used method of fertility control for married couples older than 30 years. Sterilization may also be performed in selected instances where pregnancy would create risks to the health or life of the woman or infant (for example, heart disease, severe diabetes, probable genetic defects to the infant).

Because sterilization may be a permanent method of contraception, it is absolutely necessary to obtain voluntary, informed consent.

Methods of sterilization

Methods of sterilization are described in Table 27-2. The abdominal approaches are favoured by some gynaecolo-

gists because they are familiar with the female pelvic anatomy as viewed from the abdomen and because the fallopian tubes are free and suspended in this position, which makes them easy to see, manipulate, and ligate or cauterize. The vaginal approach is favoured by some gynaecologists and women because of the absence of a visible scar, ease of peritoneal entry, and rapid postoperative recovery; however, because of its higher complication rate, it is less frequently used today.

Successful sterilization (conception prevented) is dependent on the technique used and the surgeon's experience in performing the procedure. The main causes of failure in the female are recanalization of the fallopian tube, erroneous ligation, and pregnancy resulting from tuboperitoneal fistula. In the male spontaneous recanalization (reanastomosis) may occur; the cause is unknown but duplication of the vas deferens has occasionally been noted.

Effects of sterilization
Physiological effects

Although tubal sterilization usually terminates a woman's ability to bear children, ovarian hormones and menstrual functioning are not altered and artificial menopause is not induced. Ability to derive satisfaction from sexual intercourse should not be impaired, and some women may experience greater enjoyment from intercourse free from fear of pregnancy.

Because vasectomy interrupts the continuity of the vas deferens, sperm are prevented from being ejaculated with other components of the semen. However, sperm are still produced and the ejaculate is not noticeably diminished in amount. Residual fertility lasting for a variable period is present because of sperm in the semen beyond the point of occlusion of the vas. Sperm *gradually* disappear from the ejaculate; thus conception is possible in the immediate postoperative period. Semen analysis will determine when sperm have finally disappeared.

27-9

Interferences with reproduction

Contraception Process of temporary prevention of impregnation or conception

Sterilization Process of making an individual incapable of reproducing, either permanently or until the process is reversed

Abortion Termination of a pregnacy before the fetus is viable

Infertility Inability to achieve a pregnancy within a stipulated time (at least 1 year) of unprotected sexual intercourse.

27-10

General informed consent guidelines relating to sterilization

Choice is made by patient, without pressures
Benefits and risks of sterilization are described:
  Benefits: permanent, no further costs or decision making.
  Risks: usual surgical risks, possibility of future pregnancy (not 100% effective).
Alternative contraceptive methods are described.
Patient is encouraged to ask questions.
Patient may decide not to undergo sterilization without penalty.
Explanations are given about the entire sterilization procedure, and possible side effects (effects on hormones, weight changes, menstrual changes, sexual response).
Written instruction and risk factors are explained to patient.
Written consent to the procedure is signed by patient.
After consent, counselling may precede the sterilization.

Psychological effects

Men and women who elect sterilization seem to have little or no regret after surgery if they understand what to expect during and after the procedure and are able to express their feelings and have questions answered before the procedure. People with preexisting emotional problems have reported depression, loss of self-esteem, guilt, and difficulty in sexual adjustment after surgery.

Preoperative care

Preoperative counselling is indicated to identify men and women before surgery who may later have strong regrets and emotional problems. One aim of counselling before surgery is to confirm that the decision for sterilization is made as objectively as possible. Previous experience with other methods of contraception can be explored and reasons for dissatisfaction with the methods determined. There may be lack of knowledge about contraceptive methods, and with adequate information the couple might choose a means other than sterilization. Young people and those who are unhappy about pregnancies or who have marital problems are poor candidates for sterilization because they may change their minds at a later date. The discussion of sterilization methods should be based on the informed consent guidelines (Box 27-10).

Postoperative care

Many sterilization procedures are performed on an outpatient basis, and the patient can be discharged when the effects of general anaesthesia have worn off and vital signs are stable. If the patient expresses feelings of guilt or regret about having been sterilized, a review of the reasons for sterilization and positive effect on sexual relationships may

need to be repeated. Teaching guidelines following a sterilization procedure are described in Box 27-11.

Sterilization reversal

Requests for reversal of previous sterilization may be made because of divorce and remarriage, death of children or

---

Patient Teaching   27-11

The patient who has had a sterilization procedure

Woman
Rest for 24 to 48 hours after procedure
No heavy lifting or strenuous exercise for 1 week
Abstain from sexual intercourse
　Abdominal method: until wound is healed and no discomfort is present
　Vaginal method: 1 week
Report to doctor signs of fever, persistent abdominal pain, or bleeding from incision

Man
Apply ice to scrotum, take warm baths for minor discomfort and swelling
Wear scrotal support for 48 hours
Rest for 48 hours after procedure
No heavy lifting or strenuous exercise for 1 week
Abstain from sexual intercourse for 3 days
Use an alternative method of contraception until the doctor reports semen no longer contains sperm
Report to the doctor signs of fever, persistent scrotal pain, or profuse incisional bleeding

---

Table 27-2   Methods of sterilization

Method	Description	Comments
Female		
Tubal sterilization		
Abdominal		
Minilaparotomy	Ligation or cutting of fallopian tubes under direct vision through small abdominal incision	Local or general anaesthesia Complications: wound infection, haematoma, bladder injury Advantages: good chance for sterility reversal
Laparoscopy	Electrocoagulation and sectioning of segment of fallopian tubes by laparoscopy through small abdominal incision	Local or general anaesthesia Advantages: minimal discomfort, short procedure
Vaginal		
Culpotomy	Ligation or cutting of fallopian tube through small incision in pouch of Douglas	Local, spinal, or general anaesthesia Higher complication rate than laparoscopy (infection, haemorrhage)
Culdoscopy	Electrocoagulation of segment of fallopian tubes by culdoscope through small incision in pouch of Douglas	Local anaesthesia Higher complication rate than laparoscopy
Male		
Vasectomy	Removal of a segment of vas deferens through small incision in scrotum	Local anaesthesia Complications rare Bruising, mild oedema, and mild discomfort common

27-12	**Causes of infertility**	
	Disorder	**Effect**
	Female	
	Obstructions of fallopian tubes	Interfere with transport of ovum
	Diseases of body or cervix of uterus	Inhibit passage of active sperm
	Hormonal deficiencies	Inhibit release of ovum
		Inhibit development of endometrium for implantation
	Male	
	Obstruction of vas deferens	Interfere with transport of sperm
	Diseases of testes, undescended testes, hormonal deficiencies	Inhibit development of sperm
	Sperm-bound immunoglobulins	Inhibit sperm penetration of ovum

change in economic status, as well as for other reasons. The chances of reversing the effects of sterilization are improving as a result of refinement of microsurgical techniques.

Reconstruction of the fallopian tubes involves an end-to-end anastomosis of the ligated or dissected tubes. Success of restoration of tubal function is partly dependent on the original surgery performed, especially regarding the length of the tubal portion excised. Ligation of the tubes produces adhesions that must be dissected away to the point of tubal patency; this reduces the amount of remaining tubal structure. Also the length of the fallopian tube remaining after reconstruction may play a role in permitting adequate time for the fertilized ovum to undergo maturational changes in preparation for implantation. Reports of success after microsurgical reversal are reported to be 40% to 75%.[22]

In the male, reconstruction consists in attempting to rejoin the severed ends of the vas deferens (vasovasostomy). Success is measured by the presence of sperm in the semen after reconstruction. Reports of success in restoring fertility range from 29% to 85%.[22]

Infertility

It has been estimated that 10% to 15% of all couples in Britain are infertile. Approximately 50% of couples who undergo assessment and treatment for infertility are likely to conceive. Although infertility is most often attributed to women, in about 50% of infertile marriages the man is infertile.[22,37a]

The fertility of a couple is affected by coital frequency and the age of the man and the woman. Increased coital frequency enhances fertility. Frequent ejaculation improves sperm motility unless ejaculation is excessive, which results in depletion of available sperm. Fertility peaks at age 24 years in women and age 25 years in men.

Cause and prevention

There are many causes of infertility in men and women (Box 27-12). Some are preventable or correctable, others are not. There is no known cause in 10% to 20% of infertility cases.

One of the most common preventable causes of infertility in women is infection of the pelvic organs (PID),

especially as a result of gonorrhoea and chlamydia, which cause obstruction of the fallopian tubes. Such serious consequences are preventable through prophylactic use of a penicillin for women exposed to gonorrhoea and through early diagnosis and treatment of all vaginal and cervical infections. Gonococcal cultures should be obtained every 6 months for women with multiple partners. If infection is present and the woman has an IUD, the device should be removed. Barrier contraceptives reduce the risk for infections and PID.

Many of the ovarian and hormonal problems that cause infertility produce symptoms such as menstrual irregularities and ill health before a problem with conception is ever recognized. Many of these problems can be managed with hormone therapy, provided women seek help at an early age or as soon as deviations are noticed. Birth control pills should be avoided by women who have not established normal menses.

In males, bilateral undescended testes (cryptorchidism) should be corrected surgically before puberty. The incidence of testicular cancer in undescended testes is 30% to 50% higher than in descended testes.[58] In later life cryptorchidism may produce sterility because of failure of the testes to develop their sperm-producing function, even if the condition is surgically corrected. Destruction of testicular tissue by infectious processes can be prevented through prompt treatment when symptoms first appear.

Assessment

It is important that couples who wish to have children seek medical advice if they are unsuccessful after about a year of trying to achieve pregnancy. Infertility evaluation often requires a long time.

Attempts to correct infertility are based on data obtained through a detailed history and physical examination as well as from laboratory tests and clinical studies. A sexual history is taken and sexual practices are reviewed. Suggestions about sexual intercourse are given if this seems to be the problem. The couple should attempt to be at the first interview together because they share responsibility for infertility, information is needed by both partners, and this may be their first opportunity to confront their feelings about being infertile.

27-13

Examination for infertility	
Tests	**Data obtained**
Male	
Multiple semen examination	Determine presence, number, and motility of sperm
Testicular biopsy if sperm count low or absent	Presence of sperm indicates obstruction of vas deferens
Female	
Basal body temperature chart	Determine that ovulation is occurring
Postcoital test of cervical secretions	Measure ability of sperm to penetrate cervical mucus and remain active, and quality of the mucus
Endometrial biopsy, serum progesterone and oestradiol levels, laparoscopic inspection of ovaries	Determine whether ovulation is occurring (if in question)
Laparoscopy	Determine patency of fallopian tubes
Hysterosalpingography (X-ray after insertion of contrast medium)	Determine patency of uterus and fallopian tubes
Hormonal tests for males and females	Determine whether the problem is hormonal

Examination of the man

Many doctors prefer to carry out examination of the man first, because it is more easily accomplished and less time consuming. Stricture and varicoceles (dilated veins of the spermatic cords) may be corrected by surgery.

If sperm count and motility of sperm are low, vitamins may be prescribed along with a well-balanced diet, rest, and moderate exercise. A lack of vitamins A and E in the diet may cause some atrophy of the sperm-producing structures. The couple is advised to have intercourse every other day during the fertile period (usually 12 to 16 days before the beginning of the next menstrual period). When the man is completely aspermatic, conception is impossible, and the couple should be counselled regarding the alternatives available to them.

Examination of the woman

If the man is found to be fertile, examination of the woman is carried out (Box 27-13). If sperm are being destroyed by vaginal and cervical secretions, smears from these sites are studied. If the secretions are too acid or too alkaline, medicated douches may be prescribed. A douche with sodium bicarbonate (15 ml to 1 L water) performed just before intercourse has been found to increase the motility of sperm in many cases. Tubal strictures or obstructions are sometimes repaired by microsurgery. Underlying metabolic diseases are corrected if possible.

Coping with infertility

Couples who wish to have children but find themselves unable to do so experience immeasurable emotional distress. Feelings of inadequacy are common, as are anger and guilt. The infertile couple must confront feelings about lack of control, self-image, self-esteem, and sexuality. Couples who are informed that they will never be able to have children experience a life crisis with all of its ramifications, and they have a strong need to grieve. Those who are told that they are a normal and fertile couple, but for whom pregnancy does not result despite months or years of tests, studies, examinations, and advice, commonly have feelings of frustration alternating with hope.

All these couples require emotional support, including encouragement to grieve, to express their anger and other feelings in order to regain objectivity and to avoid premature decisions and actions about alternatives. The urgent need for such support is reflected in the emergence of support groups organized by infertile individuals and couples.

Alternative infertility approaches

Among the alternatives available to infertile couples are adoption, remaining childless, artificial insemination, in vitro fertilization, and surrogate motherhood.

Artificial insemination is the placement of a few drops of donor semen in the cervicovaginal, intracervical, or intrauterine (more painful) area. It is simple, safe, inexpensive, and highly successful. The major indication for artificial insemination is male infertility. Previous loss of children because of Rh or ABO incompatibility or severe hereditary defects transmitted by the man are other indications. Therefore, artificial insemination is not reserved exclusively for infertile couples.

Artificial insemination is homologous (AIH) when the partner's semen is used and heterologous (AID) when donor semen is used. Criteria for donor selection is based on semen analysis as well as on a complete history and physical examination. Donor candidates with venereal disease, diabetes, hepatitis, blood diseases, prostatic infection, AIDS, and a family history of hereditary disorders are excluded. Fertility of donors must be proved by semen analysis.

In vitro fertilization (IVF) involves recovering one or more of the woman's ova from her ovarian follicles through laparoscopy and fertilizing the ova with the partner's sperm in a petri dish. If fertilization and cleavage occur, the resulting embryos are transferred into the woman's uterus about 48 hours after the ova retrieval has taken place. This procedure is indicated for women with complete blockage of the fallopian tubes, for oligospermia of the male, for immunological causes of infertility, and for unexplained infertility. The chance of a successful pregnancy is about 20% per IVF attempt, so the odds are very much against any one couple achieving a pregnancy.

Gamete intrafallopian transfer (GIFT) consists of aspirating oocytes from follicles by laparoscopy or minilaparotomy, or by vaginal aspiration. The oocyte is mixed with washed sperm and then placed in the fallopian tube by laparoscopy or minilaparotomy. The preembryo

travels to the uterus for implantation 4 days after ovulation on a natural timetable. Higher pregnancy rates have been obtained with GIFT than with IVG.

Zygote intrafallopian transfer (ZIFT) consists of aspirating oocytes transvaginally guided by ultrasound, mixing the oocytes with sperm, then placing the fertilized ova (zygotes) in the uterine end of the fallopian tube.

Surrogate mothers are women who contract to conceive by artificial insemination and give the baby to the semen donor after delivery. There are many social, moral, psychological, and legal implications surrounding this approach.

MAJOR HEALTH PROBLEMS OF THE REPRODUCTIVE SYSTEM

The major problems of the reproductive system include inflammation, structural disorders, tumours, and sexually transmitted diseases. The first three types of disorders are discussed separately in this chapter for women and men because of the inherent anatomical differences. Sexually transmitted diseases are discussed in the Infection Unit. The various disorders that fall within the cited categories are as follows:

1. Female disorders.
   a. Inflammatory disorders: vaginitis, cervicitis, pelvic inflammatory disease, toxic shock syndrome
   b. Structural disorders: relaxed vaginal outlet, uterine displacement, uterine prolapse, fistulas
   c. Tumours: ovarian tumours and cysts, endometriosis, uterine fibroid tumours, cervical polyps, and cancer of the cervix, endometrium, and ovary
2. Male disorders
   a. Inflammatory disorders: urethritis, prostatitis, epididymitis, orchitis
   b. Structural disorders: hydrocele, spermatocele, varicocele, torsion of spermatic cord
   c. Tumours: cancer of the testes, prostate gland, penis

INFLAMMATORY DISORDERS IN WOMEN

Types of Inflammatory Disorders

Inflammations of the female reproductive tract are seen most commonly in the vagina, cervix, or fallopian tubes and adjacent areas (Table 27-3). Many of these infections can be prevented (p. 768).

Aetiology and Pathophysiology
Vulva and vagina

Normally the vagina is protected from infection by its pH and the presence of *Döderlein's bacilli*. If the vaginal pH is altered, if the invading organisms are numerous, or if the women's resistance is decreased by ageing, malnutrition, stress, or disease, the risk of infection is increased. Fungal organisms grow best in an acid pH less than 4.7, whereas *Trichomonas* and organisms causing nonspecific vaginitis thrive in a pH greater than 5 (more alkaline).

Organisms causing infection of the vulva and vagina are most often introduced from outside sources such as clothing, hands, douche nozzles, or other contaminated articles or during intercourse. In sexually active women reinfection may occur after treatment unless their sexual partners are also successfully treated.

Women of menopausal and postmenopausal age often develop vaginitis (sometimes referred to as *atrophic* or *senile vaginitis*). Increased alkalinity of the vaginal secretions is a contributing cause, and the pyogenic bacterial invasion of the thin vaginal mucosa produces symptoms of burning, pruritus, and *leukorrhoea* (whitish-yellow vaginal discharge).

Inflammation may also occur in Bartholin's glands or less frequently in Skene's glands. The infection is usually unilateral but may be bilateral. With infection the duct from the gland becomes partially or completely obstructed, resulting in severe redness, enlargement of the gland, and oedema of the surrounding tissues. The area becomes tender, and walking may become painful. The usual result of the infectious process is an abscess. Occasionally, acute bartholinitis subsides, leaving fibrotic or scar tissue. When this occurs, a Bartholin's cyst develops. The cyst may vary in size, from a few centimetres in diameter to the size of a hen's egg and is mobile. Pain occurs with large cysts and with infection.

Cervix

Cervicitis, infection of the cervix, is the most common gynaecological disorder, affecting more than half of all women. There are two forms of cervicitis, acute and chronic, of which the chronic is the most frequent. Cervicitis usually progresses from the acute to the chronic form if not treated and it may go undetected for a long time. In fact, the cervix may heal and appear quite healthy after the disease has spread upward. This condition presents few symptoms, and those symptoms that occur do not ordinarily lead women to seek medical attention. If the vaginal discharge is slight, the women may not become concerned.

Cervicitis may follow childbirth or abortion or it may be caused by infection of a cervical laceration or erosion. In untreated cervicitis the tissues are constantly irritated, and there is some evidence that this irritation predisposes to cancer.

REVIEW

Table 27-3   Inflammatory disorders of the female reproductive tract

Disorder	Causative organisms	Signs and symptoms	Medical therapy
Vulvitis/vaginitis	*Candida, Trichomonas, Gardnerella*, coliform bacteria, *Gonococcus*, herpes simplex	Itching of vulva or vagina, vaginal discharge, dyspareunia	Antifungal agents, antibiotics (oral, topical), warm baths
Cervicitis	*Gonococcus, Chlamydia*, Streptococcus, Staphylococcus, herpes virus	Mucopurulent discharge, red, oedematous cervix, low back pain	Antibiotics, cauterization of cervix (if eroded)
Pelvic inflammatory disease (salpingitis)	*Gonococcus, Chlamydia*, coliform bacteria, *Streptococcus, Mycoplasm*, anaerobic bacteria	Severe abdominal pain, lower abdominal cramps, intermenstrual spotting, dyspareunia, fever and chills, malaise, nausea and vomiting, foul-smelling purulent vaginal discharge	Cefoxitin with doxycycline, tetracycline; rest; heat to abdomen, analgesics, sexual abstinence until recovery
Toxic shock syndrome	Toxin from *Staphylococcus aureus*	High fever, vomiting, watery diarrhoea, sore throat, myalgia, erythematous rash with desquamation; if severe, impaired renal, hepatic, cardiopulmonary function	Antibiotics, rapid hydration, supportive therapy for septic shock

Fallopian tubes

Inflammation of the fallopian tubes, *salpingitis*, may be local or more often may spread to the ovaries, pelvic peritoneum, pelvic veins, or pelvic connective tissue. This widespread inflammation is termed *pelvic inflammatory disease* (PID). The pathogens may invade the pelvic organs during sexual intercourse, childbirth or the postpartum period, or after abortion. Risk factors for PID include young age at first sexual intercourse, multiple sex partners, high frequency of sexual intercourse, and use of IUDs.[7] Contraceptive barrier methods *decrease* the risk of PID.

Pathogenic organisms are usually introduced from outside the body and pass up the cervical canal into the uterus. They seem to cause little trouble in the uterus but pass into the pelvis by way of the fallopian tubes, through thrombosed uterine veins, or through the lymphatics of the uterus (Fig. 27-4). The invaded structures become host to an acute or chronic inflammatory process.

Many of the pathogens causing PID lodge in the fallopian tubes. Purulent material collects in the tubes, adhesions form, strictures may occur, and sterility is a frequent result. Adhesions resulting from inflammation may cause such distress that complete removal of the uterus, fallopian tubes, and ovaries is necessary. Although generalized peritonitis can occur, the infection usually remains confined to the lower abdomen and pelvis. A severe inflammatory process may lead to dehydration, electrolyte imbalances, and prostration.

Toxic shock syndrome

Toxic shock syndrome (TSS), although not exclusively a reproductive disorder, occurs most commonly in menstruating females, especially among those using superabsorbent tampons. These tampons provide a milieu favourable to bacterial growth because they can contain a large amount

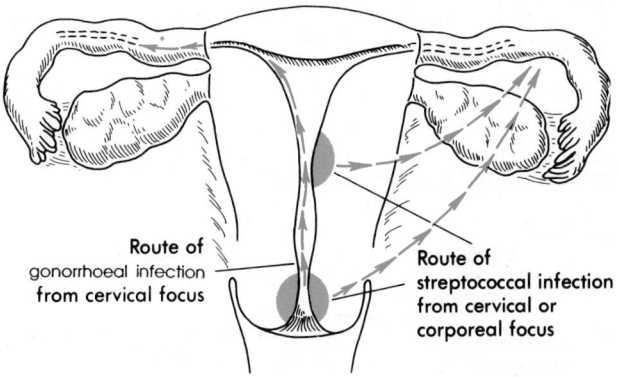

Route of gonorrhoeal infection from cervical focus

Route of streptococcal infection from cervical or corporeal focus

Fig. 27-4   Two chief routes of pelvic infection. (From Novak ER, Jones GH, Kones HW Jr: *Novak's textbook of gynecology*, ed 9, Baltimore, 1975, Williams & Wilkins.)

of menstrual blood and may be left in place more than 6 hours. Women at increased risk for TSS are those who insert tampons with their fingers instead of the applicator, and those who have a chronic vaginal infection or herpes genitalis. TSS has been associated with toxins produced by *Staphylococcus aureus* that result in sepsis. Septic shock is discussed in Chapter 7.

Nursing Process
Assessment

Subjective data
Itching

Itching is a major symptom of vulvular or vaginal infection. The itching may result from irritation from the vaginal discharge or from end products of the inflammatory response. The degree of itching experienced is monitored for signs of decreasing intensity as the inflammation subsides. Itching is most intense with *Trichomonas* infections.

Causes of vulvar or vaginal itching other than infection include epithelial changes seen with menopause, high urinary sugar content as in diabetes mellitus, pediculosis pubis, scabies, allergies, pinworms, or cancer of the vulva. With severe pruritus there are usually excoriations of the skin caused by scratching, and secondary infection may result. Dysuria may occur as a consequence of local irritation of the urinary meatus.

Pain

Pain is primarily a symptom of PID. In *acute* PID there is usually severe cramping lower abdominal pain; in chronic PID the pain is typically dull and aching and may be located in the lower back as well as the lower abdomen. Occasionally women have been thought neurotic because of ongoing reports of the diffuse pain, only to have chronic PID diagnosed later.

Objective data

Vaginal discharge is a major finding in most inflammations of the female genital tract. The *character* and *amount* of the discharge are monitored because these differ depending on the type and severity of the disorder (Box 27-14). Normally, many women have a scant, thin, whitish vaginal discharge, primarily at the time of ovulation.

Nursing analysis

Nursing analyses are determined from assessment of patient data. Possible nursing analyses for the woman with a gynaecological inflammation may include, but are not limited to, the following:

Analysis	Possible aetiologies
Pain: itching	Inflammation, vaginal discharge
Sexual dysfunction: dyspareunia	Vaginal inflammation, discomfort from PID
Knowledge deficit	Lack of exposure/recall, information misinterpretation

Planning: expected patient outcomes

Expected patient outcomes for the woman with a gynaecological inflammation may include, but are not limited to, the following:

1. States feeling more comfortable.
2. Describes how infections of the reproductive organs occur and spread.
3. Describes potentially undesirable effects of infections of the reproductive tract.
4. States signs that indicate improvement or lack of response to therapy.
5. Describes methods to prevent infection of sexual partner and reinfection of self.
6. Describes plans for sexual abstinence until inflammation subsides.
7. States that intercourse is no longer painful.

Implementation

Usual methods for medical therapy are given in Table 27-3. Some alternative therapies developed by women are included in Table 27-4.

Assisting with achievement of therapeutic goals
Medications

The major types of prescribed medications are antibiotic, antifungal, or amoebicidal agents (Box 27-15). The medications should be used by the patient for the prescribed number of days. They may be prescribed to be taken orally, used topically, or as a pessary (to be placed in the vagina) or tampon.

Supportive therapy

Patients with severe PID are usually hospitalized for intensive therapy. They are usually placed on bed rest in a supported sitting position to provide dependent drainage so that abscesses will not form high in the abdomen where they might rupture and cause generalized peritonitis. Fluids are given intravenously to correct dehydration and acidosis.

Table 27-4 Alternative therapies for vaginitis

Infection	Intervention	Dosage	Administration
Candida (Monilia)	Gentian violet	Few drops/qt water 0.25% to 2% (over-the-counter drug)	Douche or local application
	Vinegar (white)	1 tbsp/1 pt water	Douche every day for 5 to 7 days; twice daily for 2 days
	Acidophilus culture	2 tbsp/1 pt water	Douche twice daily
	Acidophilus yogurt	1 application to labia hourly	
	Plain yogurt	and as needed for symptom relief	
Trichomonas	1 handful chapparel chamomile	Steep in 1 qt water for 20 min	Douche 2 to 3 times/wk for 2 wk
Nonspecific vaginitis	Vinegar douche	5 tbsp/2 qt water	Every other day for 1 week
	Salt (sea)	1 tbsp/1 qt water	Every other day for 1 wk
	1 tsp goldenseal and 1 clove minced garlic	Steep in 1 qt boiling water	Douche every day for 1 wk
	1 tsp goldenseal	Steep in 1 pt water; strain	Douche every day for 1 wk

From Fogel CI, Woods NF: *Health care of women: a nursing perspective*, St Louis, 1981, Mosby–Year Book.

27-14	Types of vaginal discharges with inflammation

Inflammation	Discharge
Vaginitis	
Candida	White, curdlike, cheesy, sweetish odour
Trichomonas	Yellow to green, frothy, foul odour, copious
Gardnerella	Greyish white, fishy or foul odour, scanty
Cervicitis	Whitish yellow (mucopurulent), amount varies

27-15	Drugs commonly prescribed for inflammations of the female reproductive tract

Drugs	Route
Antibiotic	
Ampicillin	Oral
Fluconazole	Oral
Tetracycline	Oral
Antifungal	
Clotrimazole	Vaginal, topical
Micronazole	Vaginal, topical
Nystantin	Vaginal, topical, oral
Amoebicidal	
Metronidazole	Oral
Tinidazole	Oral

Surgical procedures

Surgical intervention may be necessary in selected instances as described below.

Incision and drainage of abscess. An abscess of a Bartholin's gland may need to be incised and drained (I & D). After I&D a small amount of purulent drainage tinged with blood is expected, but any active, bright red bleeding should be reported to the gynaecologist. Relief from pain occurs almost immediately after I&D. The woman may experience soreness or mild pain for about a day. Warm baths serve the purpose of cleansing and giving comfort. Warm water can be used to cleanse the involved area after each voiding or bowel movement.

Cauterization of cervix. When cervical lacerations or erosions are present, the area is usually cauterized. Silver nitrate sticks may be used to remove very small lesions. For larger areas requiring cauterization, an electric or thermal cautery unit is used. The woman is informed that a small, lubricated sheet of lead will be placed against the skin under the lumbar areas as a safety device for grounding electrical charges and that there will be slight bleeding, which will be controlled by a tampon or packing inserted by the doctor.

The odour of burning tissue when cautery is used is distressing to some patients. They are told to expect an odour but that the odour is insignificant and that the procedure is over quickly. Slight discomfort may be experienced.

Instructions for follow-up care vary, but usually include the following:
1. Leave the tampon or packing in place as long as the doctor advises (usually 8 to 24 hours).
2. Report to the doctor if bleeding is excessive (more than occurs during a normal menses).
3. Do not douche or have sexual relations until the next visit to the gynaecologist unless specific instructions have been given for resumption of intercourse.
4. An unpleasant discharge caused by sloughing of destroyed cells may appear 4 to 5 days after cauterization; frequent warm baths will help this condition.

Removal of reproductive organs. If a tubal abscess develops with PID, a salpingectomy (removal of the fallopian tubes) may be necessary. In severe chronic PID more reproductive organs may also need to be removed. Surgery of the reproductive tract is discussed on p. 785.

Interventions to achieve patient outcomes
Assisting with comfort

Itching is the primary discomfort with inflammations of the vulva and vagina. Frequent bathing may be helpful. Soothing lotions may be prescribed. Vinegar douches that decrease the alkalinity of the vagina may also relieve the pruritus.

Pain is the primary discomfort with PID. Heat (a warm, hot water bottle or electric heating pad) applied to the abdomen may promote circulation and comfort. Analgesics are often necessary to relieve the pain.

27-16	Patient Teaching	The woman with an inflammation of the reproductive tract

Knowledge of spread of infection and its effects
Application of vaginal medication
1. Wash hands before and after procedure
2. Lie on back for 10 minutes after insertion to facilitate distribution of medication in vagina
3. Do not douche after insertion of medication
4. Wear a minipad
Sexual intercourse
    Abstain, if possible, to prevent discomfort and spread of infection to partner
    If abstention not feasible, advise male to use a condom
If repeated infections have occurred:
    Use an alternative brand of birth control pill or alternative method of control
    Use only clean equipment if douches are used
    Restrict frequency of sexual intercourse
    Encourage sexual partner(s) to seek medical attention
Report signs of further infection (increased vaginal discharge, bleeding, pain, fever).

Dyspareunia (discomfort with intercourse) may be present as a result of inflammation. Abstinence is advised until the inflammation subsides.

Counselling and teaching

Women with PID are usually of childbearing age. If severe or chronic PID is present, infertility may result from adhesions in the fallopian tubes or from removal of reproductive organs. The woman needs opportunities to identify her feelings regarding potential or actual infertility. Many women with inflammations of the reproductive tract can be treated on an ambulatory basis. Women who are hospitalized will require further therapy at home. The woman needs to know the nature of the inflammation, how to apply vaginal medications, and how to prevent reinfection (Box 27-16).

Evaluation

Evaluation is based on expected patient outcomes. Questions to consider may include the following:

1. Does the patient state that she feels more comfortable including during intercourse?
2. Can the patient describe how infections of the reproductive organs occur and spread?
3. Can the patient describe potentially undesirable effects of infections of the reproductive tract?
4. Can the patient state signs that indicate improvement or lack of response to therapy?
5. Can the patient describe methods to prevent infection of her sexual partner?
6. Does the patient describe plans for sexual abstinence until inflammation subsides?

STRUCTURAL DISORDERS IN WOMEN
Types of Structural Disorders

Women may experience problems with relaxation of the vaginal outlet, displacement or prolapse of the uterus, or fistulas that may develop between the bladder or rectum and the vagina (Table 27.5).

Aetiology and Pathophysiology

Most of the structural problems of the reproductive tract experienced by women result primarily from stretching and weakening of the ligaments supporting the uterus or of the muscles of the perineum. Structural problems rarely occur in nulligravidas. When the pelvic-supporting tissues are *relaxed*, the urinary bladder may sag below the uterus and

press against the vaginal wall (*cystocele*) (Fig. 27-5). This leads to stress incontinence (see Chapter 25). Similarly the posterior vaginal wall may weaken and the rectum may herniate into the vagina (*rectocele*). The weakened rectal wall predisposes to constipation and haemorrhoids. Causes of cystocele and rectocele include unrepaired childbirth lacerations, loss of pelvic muscle tone from repeated pregnancies, or congenital weakness.

The uterus itself may be *displaced*, either flexed forward (anteflexion) or backward (retroflexion) or tilted backward (retroversion) (Fig. 27-6). A displaced uterus may be congenital or may be caused by PID, endometriosis, pregnancy, pelvic tumours, or trauma. In addition the uterus may lose its support because of childbirth injuries or muscle relaxation due to age, and descend (*prolapse*) into the vaginal canal. With complete uterine prolapse, the cervix protrudes beyond the vaginal orifice. Cystoceles, rectoceles, and uterine prolapse are more commonly seen in older women.

Fistulas are abnormal passageways between two organs. *Vesicovaginal fistulas* are openings between the bladder and vagina and lead to leakage of urine through the vagina. Because the vagina does not have a sphincter, urinary incontinence results. *Rectovaginal fistulas* which are less common, are passageways between the rectum and vagina. These lead to faecal incontinence and uncontrollable flatus expulsion. Causes of fistulas include radiation of the cervix, gynaecological surgery, or trauma during childbirth. Both types of fistulas may close spontaneously but frequently need to be repaired surgically. If so, 4 to 6 months are required for the inflammation to subside before surgery can be attempted.

Nursing Process
Assessment

Women with structural disorders of the reproductive tract often experience low-grade discomfort in the pelvic area and back. In addition, problem with urinary or faecal control may be present. Data to be collected if incontinence is present include the following:

1. Extent of incontinence
2. Pattern of incontinence: incontinence from a cystocele is intermittent, occurring most during stress (such as laughing or crying); incontinence from fistulas is continual seeping
3. Usual methods of coping (for example, use of pads, plastic pants, avoidance of fluids before social occasions)
4. Feelings regarding incontinence

REVIEW
Table 27-5   Structural problems of the female reproductive tract

Disorder	Signs and symptoms	Medical therapy
Relaxed vaginal outlet	Dragging pain in back of pelvis, stress incontinence, constipation, haemorrhoids	Plastic surgery
Uterine displacement	May be asymptomatic; dysmenorrhoea, backache	Postural exercises, vaginal pessary
Uterine prolapse	Bearing down sensation, backache	Vaginal pessary, hysterectomy
Fistulas	Vaginal leakage of urine, gas, or faeces	Surgical removal of fistula (fistulectomy)

Nursing analysis

Nursing analysis are determined from assessment of patient data. Possible nursing analyses for the woman with a gynaecological structural disorder may include, but are not limited to, the following:

Analysis	Possible aetiologies
Pain: backache	Vaginal or uterine structural disorder
Incontinence, stress	Relaxed pelvic muscles
Knowledge deficit	Lack of information

Planning: expected patient outcomes

Expected patient outcomes for the woman with a gynaecological structural disorder may include, but are not limited to, the following:

1. States feeling comfortable.
2. Performs self-care measures to remain continent.
3. Describes care following surgery.

Implementation

Assisting with achievement of therapeutic goals

If symptoms interfere with the woman's ability to function effectively, the primary medical therapies are the use of a *pessary* (plastic ring inserted to support the uterus [Fig. 27-7]), or *surgery* to repair weakened muscles and walls or fistulas (Box 27-17).

Preoperative care

If the rectum is involved, preoperative laxatives and enemas are usually given to reduce bowel contents. Clear liquids are given 24 hours before surgery.

Postoperative care

Repair may be accomplished vaginally or through a suprapubic incision. In the latter method, a suprapubic tube may be inserted and maintained for several days to permit healing (see Chapter 25). An indwelling urethral

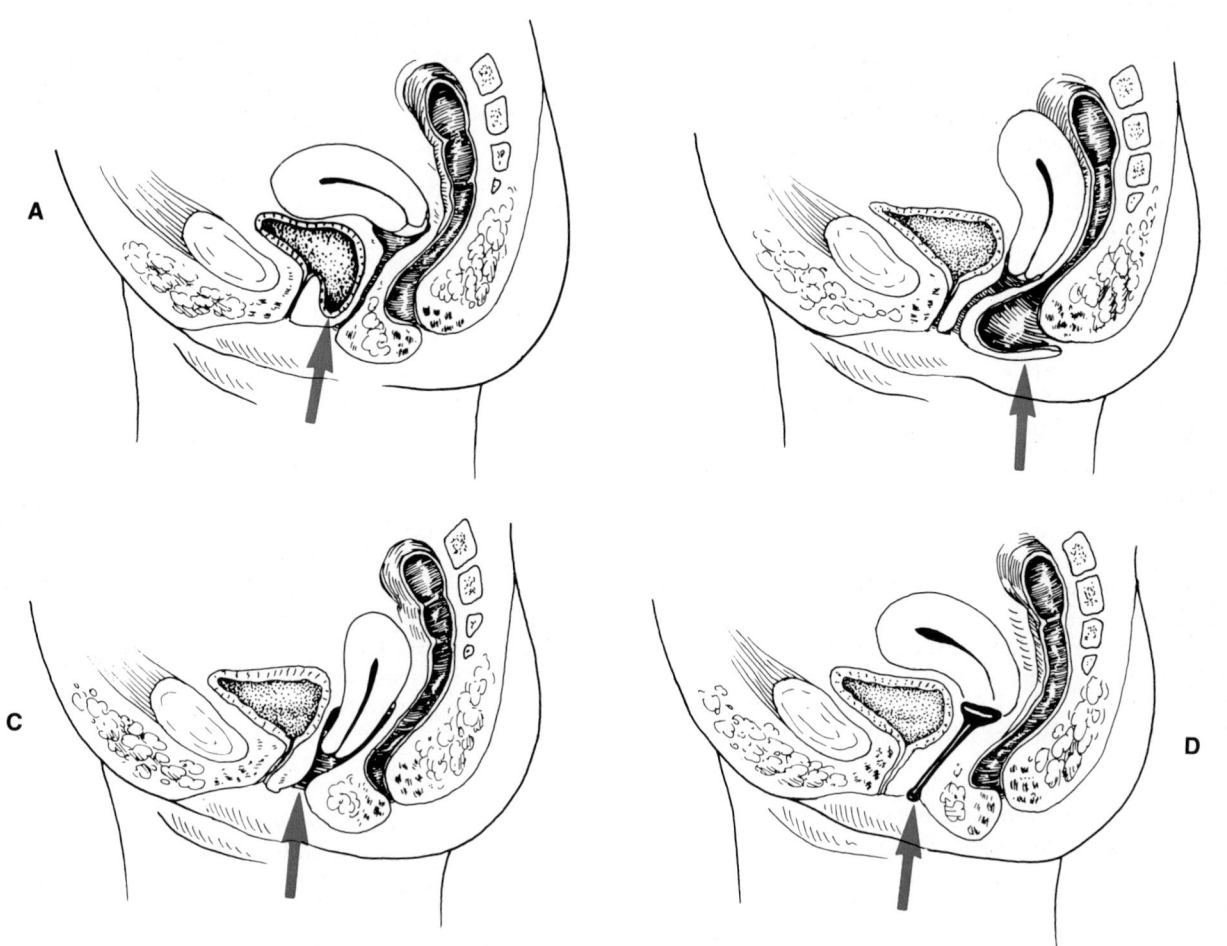

Fig. 27-5 Abnormalities of vagina. **A,** Cystocele: downward displacement of bladder towards vaginal orifice. **B,** Rectocele: pouching of rectum into posterior wall of vagina. **C,** Prolapse of uterus into vaginal canal. **D,** Stem pessary in place to maintain normal anatomical position of uterus.

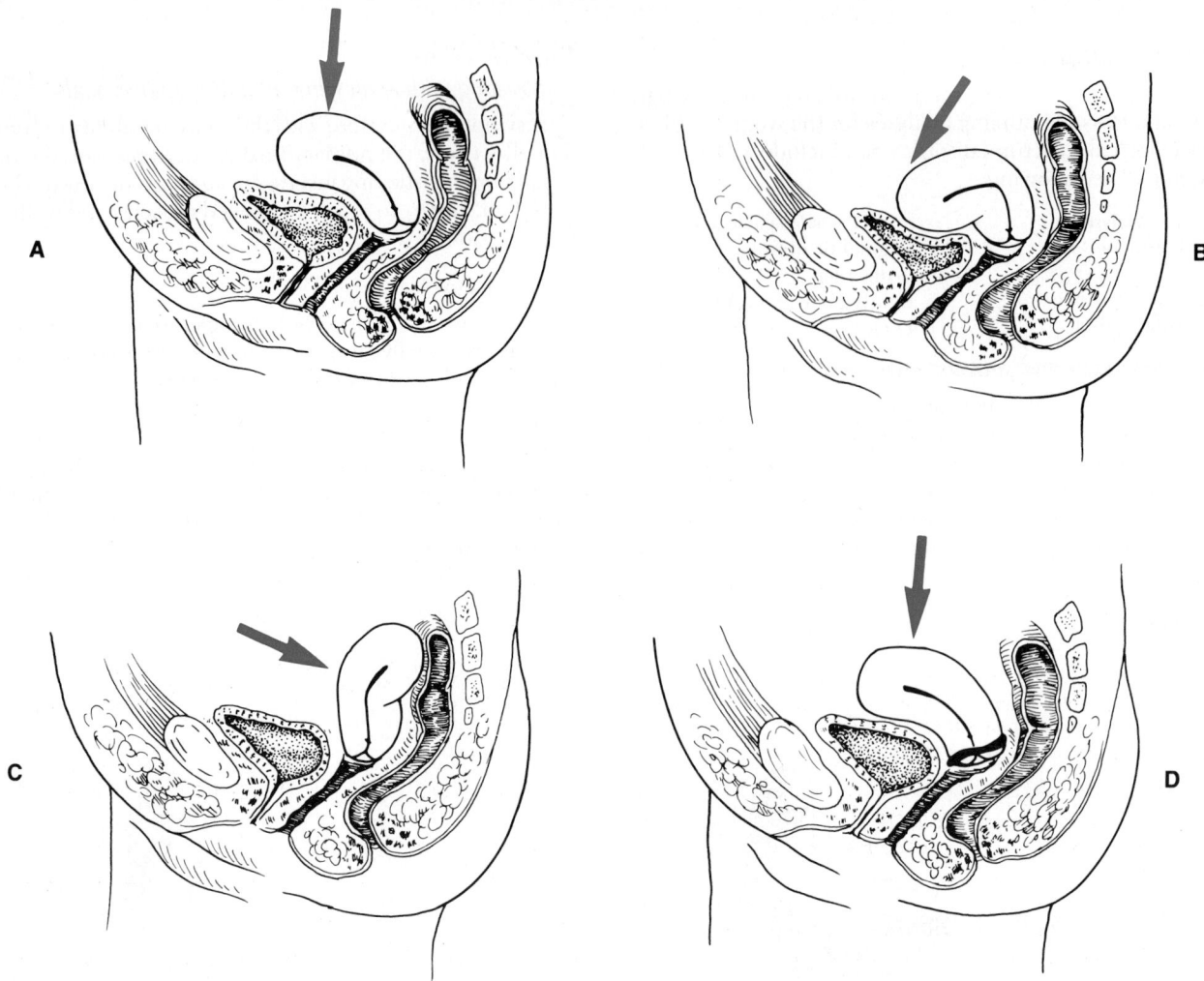

Fig. 27-6 Normal and abnormal positions of uterus. **A,** Normal anatomical position of uterus in relation to adjacent structures. **B,** Anterior displacement of uterus. **C,** Retroversion (backward displacement) of uterus. **D,** Normal anatomical position of uterus maintained by use of rubber S-shaped pessary.

catheter is inserted after anterior colporrhaphy to keep the bladder empty and to allow oedema to subside to prevent pressure on the incision.

After surgery involving the rectum, laxatives may be given to prevent strain on the incision. Care of the patient after rectal surgery is described in Chapter 23.

Prevention of infection is effected by good perineal care after voiding or defecation. A heat lamp at the perineal area may be used for comfort and to promote healing.

Interventions to achieve patient outcomes
Assisting with comfort and ADL

Pain from structural disorders is usually minimal. Nonsalicylate analgesics usually provide comfort.

Psychological discomfort related to incontinence is usually more of a problem. The woman can be helped to explore her feelings about the incontinence and possible effects on social life and sexual functioning. Before surgery is planned, alternative methods of keeping dry can be explored. For a vesicovaginal fistula, a menstrual rubber cap (Tassette) may be attached to a catheter and leg bag

urinal. For stress incontinence, menstrual pads or padded plastic pants may be helpful.

Dribbling of faecal matter into the vagina from the rectovaginal fistula is particularly distressing and may be temporarily lessened by a high enema; this is useful before social situations. Constipating diets to decrease faecal leakage are not useful because they eventually cause pressure that may aggravate the condition and increase the size of the fistula.

Counselling and teaching

Kegel exercises can be learned by women to help prevent stress incontinence and prolapse of the uterus, bladder, or rectum. The Kegel muscle is a major support muscle for the pelvic floor. The muscle surrounds the urethra, vagina, and rectum; it may be felt by placing a finger along the upper vagina wall while tightening the perineum. Because the muscle may lose tone if not exercised, women are encouraged to do Kegel exercises 100 times a day for life. Kegel exercises consist of tightening the perineum (as if to prevent voiding) and holding the contraction for a count of 10, then relaxing; it is repeated 100 times.[23]

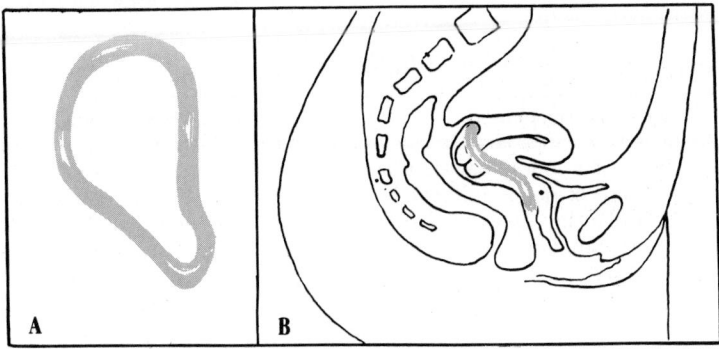

Fig. 27-7   **A**, Albert Smith pessary. **B**, Pessary in place to hold posterior vaginal fornix, and with it attached cervix, will backward and upward in pelvis. (From Beacham DW, Beacham WD: Synopsis of gynecology, ed 10, St. Louis, 1982, Mosby–Year Book.)

Preoperative and postoperative teaching include the following:

1. Preoperative
   a. Do Kegel exercises as instructed.
   b. Do pelvic exercises to assist in repositioning of uterus:
      (1) Knee-chest position for 5 minutes three times a day
      (2) Lie on abdomen 2 hours a day
   c. Seek medical consultation for symptoms of lower abdominal pain or incontinence.
2. Postoperative
   a. Use douches or mild laxatives as prescribed (gently inserting douche nozzle).
   b. Avoid heavy lifting, prolonged standing, or sexual intercourse until permitted (usually about 6 weeks).
   c. Expect loss of vaginal sensation for several months (normal response).
   d. Avoid enemas after rectal surgery until healing is complete. Report signs of infection or increased pain to the doctor.

Evaluation

Evaluation is based on expected patient outcomes. Questions to consider may include the following:
   1. Does the woman feel more comfortable?
   2. Does she have better control of her incontinence?
   3. Does she know what to do after she goes home?

BENIGN TUMOURS IN WOMEN
Types of Tumours

Many different types of benign neoplasms affect the female reproductive tract. The more common sites for these tumours are the ovaries or myometrium of the uterus (Table 27-6).

Ovarian tumours

Most ovarian tumours are benign and are often asymptomatic. There are numerous types depending on the site and tissue involved. Ovarian cysts occur frequently. Simple cysts are thin-walled structures containing serous fluid and often occur during menopause. Corpus luteum cysts result

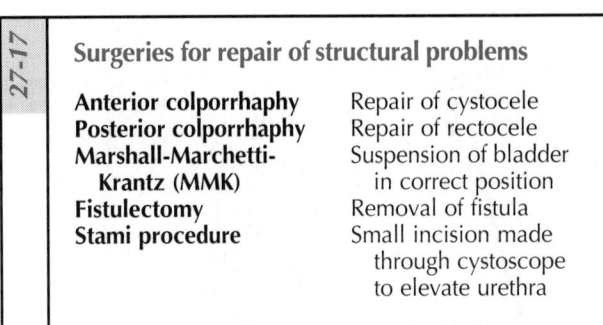

27-17	**Surgeries for repair of structural problems**	
	Anterior colporrhaphy	Repair of cystocele
	Posterior colporrhaphy	Repair of rectocele
	Marshall-Marchetti-Krantz (MMK)	Suspension of bladder in correct position
	Fistulectomy	Removal of fistula
	Stami procedure	Small incision made through cystoscope to elevate urethra

from an exaggeration of the process of formation and resorption of the corpus luteum. Follicle cysts arise during the evolution or involution of the graafian follicle. Cysts do not become malignant. Severe pain may result if a cyst becomes twisted on its pedicle, and the symptoms may resemble appendicitis.

Polycystic ovarian disease (Stein-Leventhal) is characterized by enlargement of the ovaries, with numerous cystic follicles encased in a fibrotic capsule. Effects of these tumours are often not noted unless there is compression of a neighbouring organ or blood supply, a menstrual disorder, or infertility.

Endometriosis

Endometriosis is a condition in which endometrial cells that normally line the uterus are seeded throughout the pelvis and occasionally extend to as distant a location as the umbilicus (Fig. 27-8). With each menstrual period the endometrial cells are stimulated by the ovarian hormones and bleed into the surrounding areas, causing an inflammation. Subsequent adhesions may be so severe that pelvic organs become fused together, occasionally causing a stricture of the bowel or interference with bladder function. Encased blood may lead to palpable tumour masses, which often occur on the ovary and are known as *chocolate cysts*. Occasionally these cysts rupture and spread endometrial cells still farther throughout the pelvis.

Endometriosis begins with dysmenorrhoea, then progresses to pain felt several days before menstruation.

Table 27-6   Benign tumours of the female reproductive tract

Type	Signs and symptoms	Medical therapy
Ovarian tumours and cysts	Increased abdominal size; fatigue; sense of pelvic fullness	Ovarian cystectomy Oophorectomy
Endometriosis	Pain that increases in severity during menstruation, dyspareunia, irregular menstrual cycles	Antiovulation drugs (progestogens, danazol), analgesics Surgery: younger than 35 years, resection of lesions; older than 35 years, total hysterectomy, salpingectomy, oophorectomy
Uterine fibroid tumours	Menorrhagia, low back pain, dysmenorrhoea, constipation, irregular enlarged uterus	Small tumours; no treatment Severe symptoms or rapidly growing tumours: myomectomy or hysterectomy
Cervical polyps	Leukorrhoea, abnormal vaginal bleeding	Surgical removal (polypectomy)

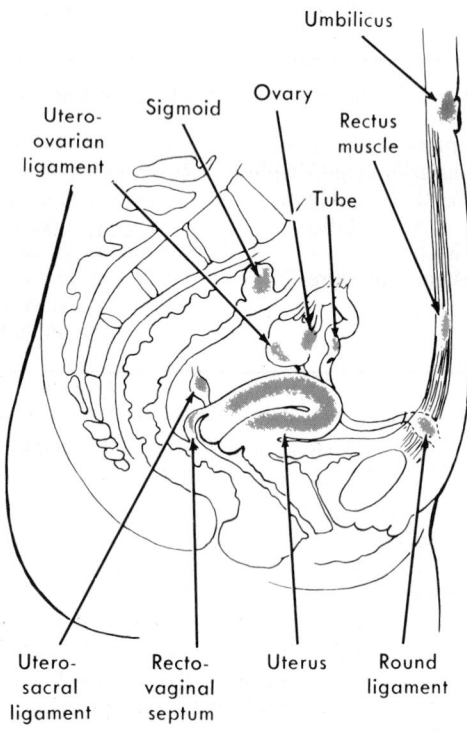

Fig. 27-8   Sites of endometrial implants.

Rupture of a large endometrial cyst produces a severe peritoneal reaction requiring surgery.[58] Approximately half of the women with endometriosis are infertile, and endometriosis is sometimes first detected when a woman complains of inability to conceive.

If the woman is young and wants children, the treatment for endometriosis is usually as conservative as possible. Pregnancy is beneficial, because menstruation ceases during this time. If a young woman has endometriosis, she and her husband usually are advised to have their family early, because the fertility rate is low, sterility caused by adhesions may occur, and a hysterectomy may have to be done within a reasonable period of time. Nursing the infant is also recommended because it delays the onset of menstrua-

tion after delivery. Menopause stops the progress of this condition.

Uterine fibroid tumours

Fibroid tumours are the most common tumours of the female genital tract. They are discrete benign tumours of the uterine muscle and connective tissue. The sizes of myomas are variable. Most are found in the body of the uterus (corporeal) but some occur in the cervix or may involve the broad ligament. Submucous tumours may impinge on the blood vessels of the endometrium and produce bleeding. As they grow larger they may impinge on the opposite uterine wall and distort the cavity of the uterus. In some instances submucous tumours develop pedicles and may protrude through the vagina or cervix, resulting in infection or ulcerations.

Fibroid tumours of the uterus tend to disappear spontaneously with menopause. They rarely become malignant. Infertility may result from a myoma that obstructs or distorts the uterus or fallopian tubes. Myoma in the body of the uterus may cause spontaneous abortions, and those near the cervical opening may make the delivery of a baby difficult and may contribute to haemorrhage postpartally. Myomectomy is the procedure of choice during childbearing years.

Cervical polyps

Cervical polyps form when an area of the mucosa proliferates. These growths are usually visible at the cervical os as bright red, vascular, fragile areas. They are most often pedunculated and appear to protrude from the cervical canal. Polyps may occur singly or in clusters.

Because of the vascularity of the polyp, bleeding is a common symptom. The bleeding is small in amount and occurs between menstrual periods and closely resembles that of early cancer of the cervix. Especially characteristic is the contact bleeding produced by coitus, douching, or vaginal examination.

The pedicle by which the polyp is attached is usually quite small, and the polyp can easily be removed by twisting the pedicle at its base or by biopsy. Tissue examination of removed polyps is essential because epidermoid cancer arises from cervical polyps in a small percentage of cases.

Surgery of the Reproductive Tract

Minor surgical procedures are performed primarily for diagnostic purposes. Major surgery involves removal of one or more reproductive organs (Box 27-18). Most major surgeries require hospitalization. Laparoscopically Assisted Vaginal Hysterectomy (LAVH) is a newer procedure; the uterus is detached laparoscopically then removed vaginally. The patient is scheduled to undergo surgery early in the morning and then goes home late the same day.

Minor procedures
Preoperative care

Dilatation and curettage (D and C) is the standard procedure for investigating any irregular bleeding. In addition it may be performed to correct a cervical stricture or to treat dysmenorrhoea. Cervical biopsy and conization of the cervix are done to test for the presence of malignancy. All these procedures may be performed as ambulatory surgery. Cervical biopsy does not require anaesthesia, whereas local or general anaesthesia may be used for D and C or conization. The usual preoperative preparation is given; shaving is rarely required.

Postoperative care

Monitoring vaginal bleeding

Bleeding is monitored every 15 minutes for 2 hours and then as necessary thereafter. The blood loss is best recorded in estimated millilitres. A blood loss of at least 60 ml is required to saturate a perineal pad. It is important to record each pad change as well as blood loss. Any excessive bleeding is reported to the doctor. More blood is lost by conization of the cervix than with the other procedures, and oozing may be controlled by packing inserted at the time of surgery.

Promoting comfort

Mild abdominal cramping may be experienced postoperatively. Mild analgesics such as codeine and nonsalicylate analgesics are usually ordered to relieve pain. Abdominal pain after D and C that is continuous, sharp, and not relieved by analgesics should be reported immediately to the surgeon; this type of pain may indicate perforation of the uterus.

Teaching the patient

1. If vaginal packing is in place, remove when instructed (usually 8 to 24 hours).
2. Do not douche or wear tampons until instructed.
3. Report the following to the surgeon:
   a. Soaking 3 or 4 pads a day with bright red blood
   b. Excessive pain
   c. Temperature greater than 38° C (100° F)
4. Resume sexual intercourse as instructed (usually when the woman feels comfortable)
5. Resume normal activities as instructed (usually in 1 week)
6. Avoid vigorous exercise for 3 to 4 weeks.

27-18

Surgeries of the female reproductive tract

Minor procedures

Dilatation and curettage (D and C)
  Dilatation of the cervix and scraping of uterine walls
Cervical biopsy
  Punch biopsy of the cervix
Conization of cervix
  Removal of cone-shaped portion of cervix

Major procedures

Oophorectomy
  Removal of ovaries
Salpingectomy
  Removal of fallopian tubes
Hysterectomy (vaginal, abdominal)
  Removal of uterus, either through the vagina or abdomen
Radical hysterectomy
  Removal of uterus, upper vagina, and parametrium
Pelvic exenteration
  Removal of pelvic viscera (bladder, rectosigmoid) and all reproductive organs

---

Major procedures
Preoperative care

Preparation of the patient for gynaecological surgery is similar to that for major abdominal surgery. Function of other systems within the pelvis (urinary, intestinal) is evaluated, particularly if there are any symptoms of dysfunction.

Psychological preparation

Removal of reproductive organs can significantly affect the woman emotionally, and time may be needed to help her adjust to the proposed changes. The reproductive organs are a major component of "womanhood," and loss of these organs creates a change in body image. Many women see menstrual functioning as a symbol of femininity; therefore, with sudden cessation of menstruation some women state feelings of being "less of a woman." Partners may also be dealing with disturbed feelings.

Feelings of sexuality in terms of sexual relations are also threatened. Some women worry that sexual relations may be hindered or be less satisfactory. In actuality, many women find that sexual relations after hysterectomy are enhanced because fear of pregnancy has been removed. Except in rare instances of pelvic exenteration, sexual intercourse is possible after healing has occurred.

Women who experience some difficulties in adjusting may be those of childbearing age and those at menopause. The latter are still adjusting to life's changes and may be at a crisis period in their life. The nurse's role is to help the woman and her partner explore feelings and to correct myths or misunderstandings before surgery to facilitate an easier recovery.

A woman undergoing major gynaecological surgery

Preoperative care

1. Identify patient's understanding of planned surgical procedure and correct misunderstandings
2. Encourage and support self-exploration of feelings related to proposed surgery
3. Provide support stockings for people at high risk for thromboembolism
4. Teach breathing and leg exercises

Postoperative care

1. Monitor
   a. Fluid and electrolyte balance
   b. Breath sounds and respiratory excursion
   c. Abdominal distension
   d. Pain in abdomen
   e. Pain in thighs
   f. Dressing
   g. Signs of urinary tract infection
2. Encourage breathing exercises every 2 to 4 hours until patient becomes active
3. Provide urinary drainage
   a. Maintain patency of indwelling urinary catheter
   b. When catheter is removed, monitor for leakage of urine in vagina (sign of urinary fistula)
4. Provide pain medication (see Chapter 8)
5. For wind pains, apply heat (warm hot water bottle, electric heating pad) to abdomen, encourage ambulation, try a rectal tube
6. Prevent thrombophlebitis
   a. Teach patient to avoid sharp flexion of knee or thighs; no pillows under knees
   b. Continue support stockings for patients at high risk
   c. Encourage leg exercises every hour while awake until ambulating freely
   d. Lower head of bed to flat position for a short time every 2 hours for 24 hours, then every 4 hours until ambulating freely
   e. Encourage walking, increasing distance
   f. Encourage deep breathing (enhances venous return)
7. Continue providing emotional support
8. Teach patient
   a. Resume home activities gradually
   b. Avoid douches or tampons until instructed by doctor
   c. Avoid heavy lifting (over 20 lbs) or vigorous activity (tends to cause pelvic blood congestion) for 6 weeks
   d. Resume driving in 3 to 4 weeks as desired
   e. Resume preoperative sexual activities such as cuddling or closeness immediately; sexual intercourse in 6 weeks.
   f. Report immediately to doctor any signs of thromboembolism

Physiological preparation

Close proximity of the urinary tract and bowel to the reproductive organs requires measures to prevent infection. Preoperative measures are also taken to prevent postoperative thromboembolism:

1. Antibiotics to treat or prevent infection
2. Bowel preparation if bowel will be involved
   a. Mechanical cleansing (laxatives, enemas) or oral bowel cleansing solution (see Chapter 23)
   b. Liquid diet for 24 hours
3. Medicated douches if risk of infection is high
4. People at high risk for thrombophlebitis (varicose veins, obesity, diabetes mellitus, history of venous thrombosis or pulmonary embolus)
   a. Low-dose heparin
   b. Support stockings
   c. Discontinuation of oral contraceptives 3 to 4 weeks preoperatively.

Postoperative care

General care of the patient after major gynaecological surgery is essentially the same as that after abdominal surgery. Measures to prevent respiratory complications are important. Fluid and electrolyte balance is monitored carefully.

Preventing thromboembolism

Thrombophlebitis and pulmonary embolism are major postoperative complications after pelvic surgery as a result of venous stasis in the major pelvic veins. Symptoms may be absent until signs of pulmonary embolism occur (chest pain, haemoptysis) 1 week later. Because the involved veins are usually deep in the thigh, the only local symptoms may be pain and swelling in the thigh and a positive Homan's sign (pain with dorsiflexion of foot). Preventive activities are described in Box 27-19.

Promoting urinary function

Urinary *retention* is a common occurrence after gynaecological surgery as a result of handling of the bladder during surgery. An indwelling urinary catheter is usually inserted for at least 24 hours postoperatively until muscle function returns. Urinary *fistula* may result despite careful surgical technique. It is identified by leakage of urine through the vagina. Many such fistulas close spontaneously.

Promoting gastrointestinal function

Gastrointestinal function usually returns 24 to 72 hours after surgery, depending on the extent of handling of the intestines. Persistent nausea and vomiting with severe abdominal distension may indicate ileus, and all oral intake is stopped and a nasogastric tube is inserted. Most patients, however, have return of function. Abdominal distension with abdominal cramping may result from collection of wind in the sluggish bowel. Ambulation and heat encourage expulsion of the wind (see Chapter 23).

Counselling and teaching

Postoperatively, many women feel depressed for several days. The patient often is unable to explain why she is

Table 27-7   Cancer of the female reproductive tract (United States)

Site	Incidence	Usual age (yr)	Signs and symptoms	Medical therapy
Cervix	2.5%	30 to 50	Early: may be asymptomatic, vaginal discharge, spotting between menses Late: dark, foul vaginal discharge, pain	Conization of cervix for cancer in situ in young women; hysterectomy, radiation (internal, external)
Endometrium	6%	50 to 70	Early: postmenopausal bleeding Late: uterine enlargement, pain	Hysterectomy and bilateral salpingo-oophorectomy, radiation (internal, external), progestin for metastases
Ovary	4%	All ages	Early: asymptomatic Late: ascites, oedema of legs, pain	Salpingo-oophorectomy; hysterectomy may also be necessary; chemotherapy, radiation

depressed and crying. Grieflike responses to loss of a body part may appear as they do after loss of other body parts. Feelings of guilt, shame, and remorse are common. Encouraging the woman to continue activities associated with being feminine, such as using makeup, arranging her hair, and wearing her own clothing, often helps her regain her feminine perspective. During this time she needs understanding and empathic care. Partners may need help in understanding the woman's need for reassurance of continued love and affection. Postoperative teaching includes home care, resumption of activities, and follow-up care (Box 27-19).

Operative Endoscopy

Surgery may also be performed in some instances through a laparoscope. Examples of operative endoscopy are ovarian cyst enucleation, oophorectomy, salpingectomy, endocoagulation of endometriotic implants, and enucleation of myomas or extrauterine fibromas. Recovery after operative endoscopy is longer than incisional surgery because of longer duration of anaesthesia and greater manipulation. Women require the same nursing interventions as those for major gynaecological surgery. There is a higher incidence of postoperative bleeding and bowel and urinary problems.

CANCER IN WOMEN
Epidemiology

Malignancies in the female reproductive tract occur primarily in the uterus (cervix and endometrium) and in the ovaries (Table 27-7); they may also occur, although less frequently, in the vagina or vulva. Mortality from cancer of the reproductive tract now ranks fourth to cancer of the breast, lung, and colorectum in females in England and Wales.[27a]

The death rate from cancer of the *cervix* has fallen steadily over the past 40 years. This decline has been attributed to early detection through annual examinations (including a Papanicolaou smear) and improved surgical and radiotherapeutic techniques. Cancer of the cervix identified and treated early at the preinvasive stage is 100% curable, thus *early detection* (p. 769) *is vitally important.* The incidence of *endometrial* cancer is not decreasing sig-

nificantly partly because it is primarily a disease of postmenopausal women and women are living longer.

Because cancer of the *ovary* is asymptomatic in the early stages, it is often far advanced before diagnosis is made. The only effective means of ensuring early diagnosis is a pelvic examination every 6 months, including careful ovarian palpation, and surgical exploration of any questionable ovarian growth. The Pap test does *not* reveal ovarian cancer.

Pathophysiology
Cancer of the cervix

Most cervical cancers are squamous carcinomas that arise in the intraepithelial layers (preinvasive stage or carcinoma in situ). This stage is classified as cervical intraepithelial neoplasia (CIN). Predisposing factors include human papillomavirus (HPV) (Chapter 27), early sexual activity, multiple partners, and chronic inflammation. It usually takes 2 to 10 years for squamous cell carcinoma to become invasive beyond the basement membrane. Spread usually occurs by direct extension or by means of the lymph system. Therapy depends on the stage (extent of spread) (Table 27-8).

Cancer of the endometrium

Cancer of the endometrium is primarily a slow-growing adenocarcinoma. Because it occurs mostly in postmenopausal women, oestrogen stimulation unopposed by progesterone is thought to be implicated. Prolonged use of oestrogen without added progestogen during menopause increases the risk of endometrial cancer. Cancer of the endometrium is usually diagnosed when the postmenopausal woman seeks medical care for vaginal bleeding.

Cancer of the ovary

Ovarian cancer causes more than twice as many deaths as cancer of the uterus because the patient with ovarian cancer may be asymptomatic until the cancer is far advanced. The pathophysiology of ovarian cancer is complex, and there is a great variety of tumours. The ovaries may be a site of metastasis from the gastrointestinal tract, breast, pancreas, or kidneys. The risk for ovarian cancer increases with age.

Table 27-8 Stages of cancer of female reproductive tract

Stage	Cervix	Endometrium	Ovary
0	Confined to epithelium (CIN)	Confined to epithelium	–
I	Confined to cervix	Confined to corpus	Confined to ovary
II	Extends outside cervix but does not involve pelvic wall or lower third of vagina	Involves corpus and cervix	Involves ovaries with pelvic extension
III	Involves pelvic wall and lower third of vagina	Involves pelvic and vaginal wall (but not bladder or rectum)	Intraperitoneal metastases
IV	Involves bladder, rectum, or metastatic spread	Involves bladder, rectum, or metastatic spread	Involves metastatic spread

---

27-20

Guidelines for Pap tests

1. Schedule Pap tests:
   a. Premenopausal: first half of menstrual cycle before ovulation
   b. Postmenopausal, not taking combined hormone therapy: at any time
   c. Postmenopausal, taking combined hormone therapy: at first part of cycle (*not* when taking progesterone)
2. Avoid douching, coitus, tampons, or vaginal medications for 48 hours before examination.
3. Slight vaginal bleeding (spotting) may occur after the examination; excessive bleeding should be reported.

Diagnostic Tests
Pelvic examinations

Pelvic examinations are useful for visualization of changes in the vulva, vagina, and cervix; for palpation of internal organs, especially the ovaries and surface of the uterus; and for obtaining Pap smears.

Women are advised to avoid douching and applying any vaginal preparation (medicinal or deodorant) for at least 24 hours before examination. They should void immediately before the examination, because an empty bladder makes palpation of the pelvic organs easier, decreases patient discomfort, and eliminates possible distortion of the position of pelvic organs caused by a full bladder. The technique for performing pelvic examinations is described in most physical examination texts.

After the pelvic examination a woman may need assistance in removing her legs from the stirrups and getting down from the table. Elderly women merit careful assistance after the pelvic examination because unnatural positions, such as the knee-chest and lithotomy positions, may alter the normal circulation of blood sufficiently to cause faintness.

Papanicolaou (Pap) test

The Pap test is a cytology test that makes it possible to detect abnormal cells, not all of which are cancerous. However, the Pap test has made it possible through routine use to detect precancerous conditions and cancer of the cervix early enough to make treatment of these conditions almost 100% successful. For detection of atypical cells, the Pap test is 95% accurate. False-negative reports are most frequently the result of an inadequate sample or improper technique. Guidelines for Pap tests are listed in Box 27-20.

The Pap test involves microscopic examination of cells collected from the vaginal pool, exocervix, and endocervical canal. Samples of cells are obtained by using a cytology brush, applicator, spatula, or vaginal irrigation. Secretions containing exfoliated cells are preferably obtained from the cervix or external os. The secretions are collected, smeared on the slide, and immediately fixed with cytological spray or liquid. The slide may also be placed in a 95% alcohol fixative for 15 to 30 minutes, then allowed to dry.[20] The slides are labelled and sent to the laboratory.

Women who have had subtotal hysterectomy in which the cervical stump was left intact should continue to have regular Pap testing.

Obtaining endometrial cells for study

The Pap test is not ideal for detecting endometrial cancer, although samples may be obtained by cervical aspiration when performing a Pap test. Less than half of women with uterine cancer have an abnormal Pap test result at the time of routine Pap test screening. Probably the main reason the Pap test is inadequate is that cells rarely exfoliate from the endometrium in the early stages of uterine cancer.

One method of obtaining endometrial cells for study is by *vacuum curettage*. The procedure and apparatus used for vacuum curettage are similar to those used in suction curettage for performing an abortion, except that the curette is much thinner. With the patient under general anaesthesia, the cervix is dilated and the suction tip is inserted through the cervix into the uterus. Suction is applied and the entire uterine cavity is suctioned to secure specimens. Vacuum curettage is considered to be at least as good as conventional endometrial biopsy for diagnosing endometrial cancer.

An *endometrial biopsy* is performed by presenting a small curette into the uterus and obtaining several strips of endometrial tissue. The specimens are taken from several sites of the uterine cavity to increase the chances of obtaining malignant cells. For diagnosis of endometrial cancer, the biopsy method is considered to be about 90% accurate.

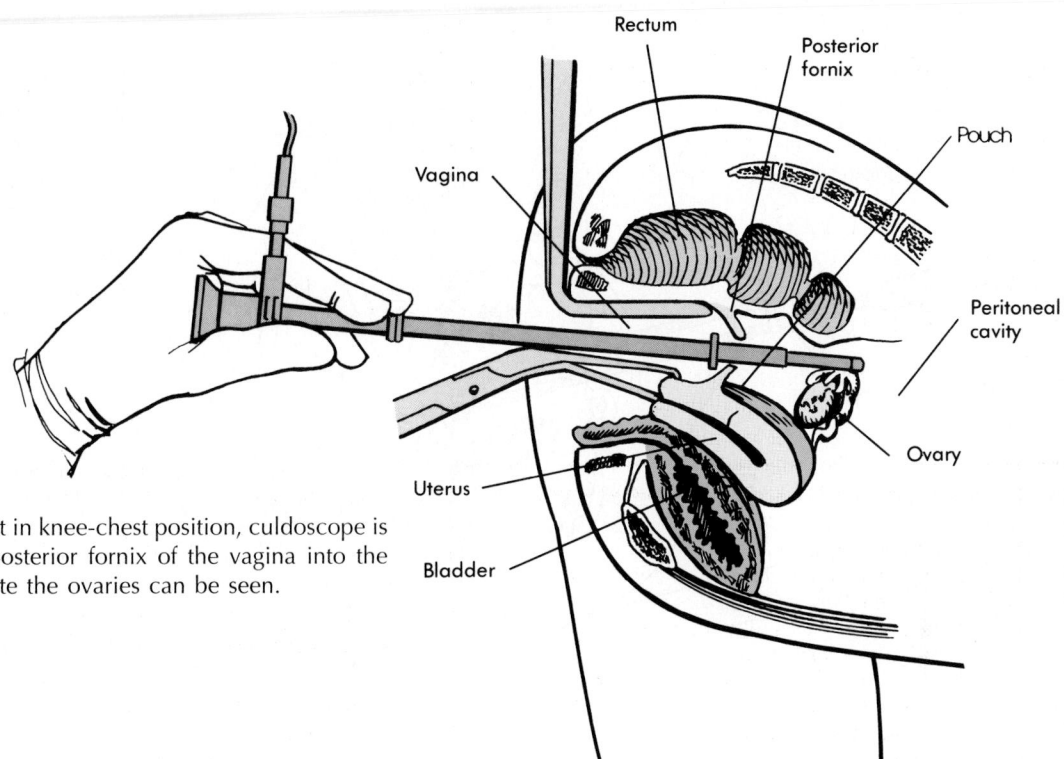

Fig. 27-9   With patient in knee-chest position, culdoscope is inserted through the posterior fornix of the vagina into the pouch of Douglas. Note the ovaries can be seen.

> ## 27-21   Endoscopic procedures for visualization of pelvic organs
>
> **Colposcopy**
> Visualization of vagina and cervix under low-power magnification
>
> **Culdoscopy**
> Insertion of a culdoscope through posterior vaginal vault into the pouch of Douglas for visualization of fallopian tubes and ovaries (Fig. 27-9)
>
> **Hysteroscopy**
> Insertion of a hysteroscope through the cervix for visualization of inside of the uterus
>
> **Laparoscopy**
> Insertion of a laparoscope (under local anaesthesia) through small incision in abdominal wall (inferior margin of umbilicus), which is insufflated with carbon dioxide; permits visualization of all pelvic organs (Fig. 27-10)

Endoscopy

The pelvic organs and surrounding tissues can be directly visualized by endoscopy. Endoscopic procedures include colposcopy, culdoscopy (Fig. 27-9), peritoneoscopy (laparoscopy), and hysteroscopy (Box 27-21). The most common procedure is the laparoscopy (Fig. 27-10). Depending on the organs and structures inspected, these methods are valuable for determining the cause of abnormal bleeding, in evaluating the stage of malignancies, and for inspecting organs for size, shape, and position.

Most of the procedures used for visualizing the pelvic organs can be performed on an outpatient basis; this allows the gynaecologist to schedule the procedure at the appropriate time of the menstrual cycle.

Maintaining asepsis throughout any of the endoscopic procedures is important in preventing infection. Air may enter the abdominal cavity during the procedures and cause discomfort; a prone position with a pillow under the abdomen may increase comfort. Douching and intercourse should be avoided for about 1 week following a culdoscopy. Complications such as haemorrhage and infection are rare, but women should be cautioned to report fever or pain in the lower abdomen.

Other diagnostic approaches

Ultrasound has become a useful diagnostic tool for gynaecological problems. It can be used to locate pelvic masses, displaced IUDs, and ectopic pregnancies. Uterine fibroids can be located and measured. *Computed tomography* (CT) and *magnetic resonance imaging* (MRI) provide better indirect visualization of masses and affected lymph nodes, especially in obese women and those with abdominal distension.

Treatment Modalities
Surgery

Total abdominal hysterectomy (TAH) with or without bilateral salpingo-oophorectomy (BSO) is the most common treatment for gynaecological cancer (Box 27-18, p. 785). A

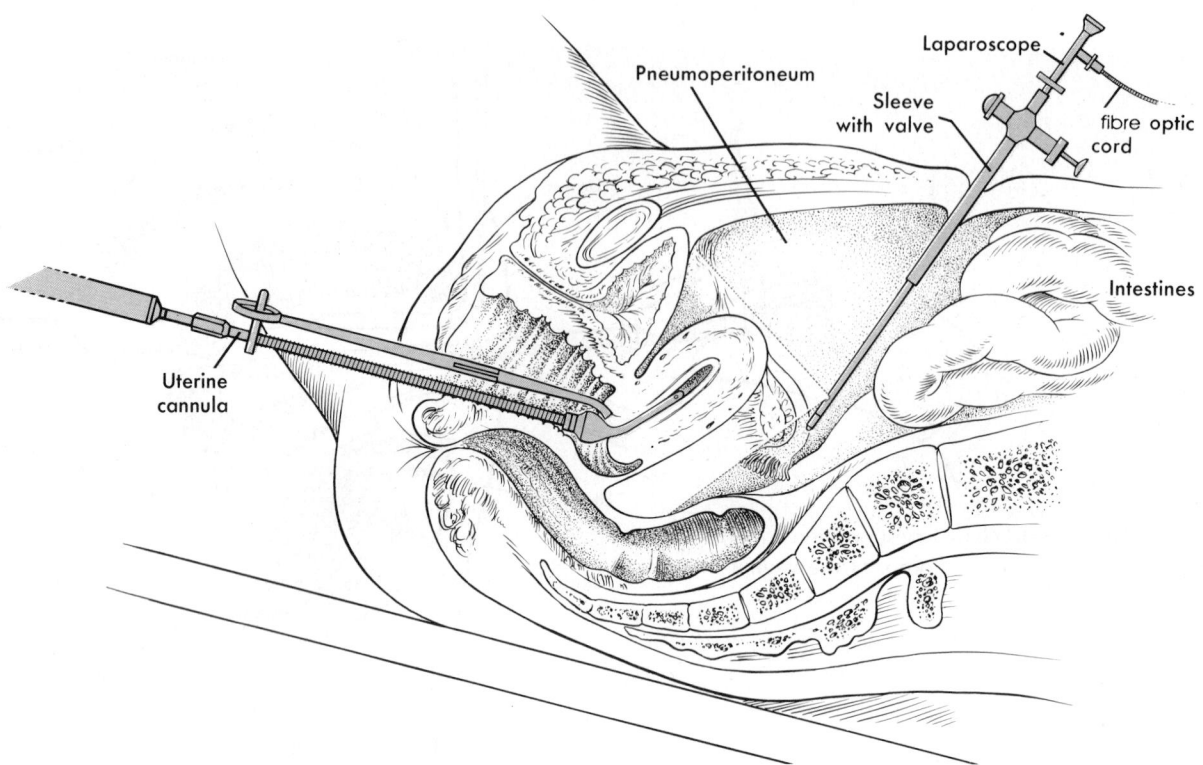

Fig. 27-10 Schema of gynaecological laparoscopy. (From Cohen MF: *Laparoscopy, culdoscopy and gynecography: techniques and atlas,* vol 1, Philadelphia, 1970, WB Saunders.)

unilateral *salpingo-oophorectomy* may be performed for women of childbearing age who have stage I ovarian cancer. The woman with cancer not only experiences the same feelings associated with loss of her reproductive organs as other women but at the same time faces the concerns related to cancer (Chapter 9). Anxiety is commonly experienced, and the woman requires considerable empathy and emotional support as she works through her feelings.

Radical hysterectomy (Box 27-18, p. 785) may be recommended for stage II cervical or endometrial cancer. Radical hysterectomy usually requires a longer hospitalization than TAH. Retroperitoneal drains are inserted and connected to low-pressure suction. The drains are removed when drainage is less than 50 ml/day (usually in 3 to 5 days). Because the bladder is usually atonic as a result of nerve damage, either an indwelling or suprapubic catheter is required for 2 to 3 weeks. The woman is taught care of the catheter before hospital discharge. The catheter is removed when the woman can void with less than 100 ml of residual urine. Additional care of the patient with hysterectomy is discussed on p. 786.

Pelvic exenteration (Box 27-18) may be performed for selected patients with recurrent or persistent cancer of the cervix. The procedure is done only when there is no lymphatic involvement and there is chance of cure. Nursing care includes care following hysterectomy as well as care following abdominoperineal bowel resection (Chapter 23) and urinary diversion (Chapter 25). Because of the great extent of the surgery, the woman may be overwhelmed

psychologically. She usually experiences changes in body image, sexual relations, and social life-style, in addition to dealing with the fears pertaining to cancer recurrence and death. Both the woman and her partner need ongoing supportive nursing care.

Radiotherapy

Intracervical, intrauterine, or external whole pelvic irradiation may be given preoperatively to shrink the tumour to facilitate safety of the operation. Radiation may also be used as adjunct therapy postoperatively. Guidelines for radiation therapy are described in Chapter 9. Premenopausal women who receive pelvic irradiation will lose their ovarian function.

Radiation of the pelvic organs may create problems in sexual functioning, including lack of libido, marked pain or discomfort with intercourse, and feelings of a narrow or shortened vagina. These problems may add to the woman's feelings of sexual inadequacy from interferences with reproductive function.

Intracavitary implant

Radium or cesium may be inserted through a tandem placed in the uterine cavity (Figs. 27-11 and 27-12). During an intracavitary implant, it is important that all normal tissues remain in their natural position. Gauze packing is usually inserted into the vagina to push both the rectum and the bladder away from the area being irradiated. A urinary catheter is inserted before therapy to prevent bladder

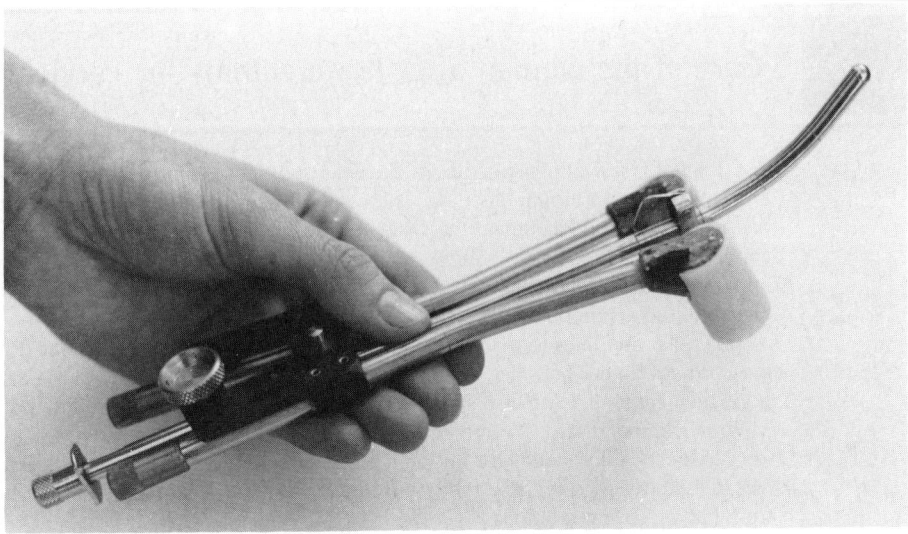

Fig. 27-11   Assembled configuration of tandem and colpostat before placement.

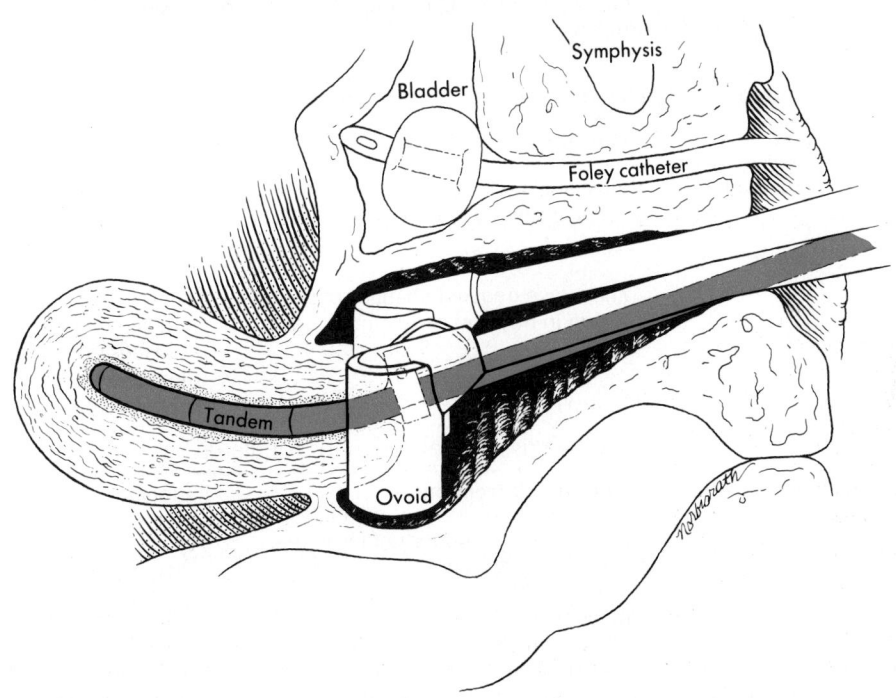

Fig. 27-12   Placement of tandem and colpostat before vaginal packing.

distension. Low-residue diet and cleansing enemas are given before therapy, and the enema is repeated after therapy to prevent bowel distension.

Nursing care consists of the following guidelines:
1. Keep patient flat in bed; may turn side to side
2. Provide analgesics for severe uterine contractions from dilatation of cervix
3. Provide good perineal care; there will be foul-smelling vaginal discharge from cell destruction; a room deodorizer is helpful
4. Encourage fluids to 3000 ml/day to maintain urinary adequacy
5. Follow general guidelines for internal radiation (Chapter 9)
6. Plan care that includes measures to decrease social isolation.

Radiation sickness may result as a systemic reaction to the breakdown and reabsorption of cell proteins. Local reaction may include cystitis and proctitis. Vaginal discharge will continue for some time after termination of therapy, and the patient may need to take douches for as long as the odour and vaginal discharge persist. Some vaginal bleeding may occur for 1 to 3 months after irradiation of the cervix. The woman who is at home should report

Nursing Care Plan

Care of the woman after hysterectomy for cervical cancer

DATA: Mrs. C., age 42, saw her gynaecologist 2 weeks ago because of bleeding between periods and occasional postcoital bleeding. The result of her Pap smear 5 years previously had been negative. The Pap smear this time was positive and a cervical biopsy confirmed cancer of the cervix, stage I. She was admitted yesterday for a total hysterectomy.

Admission notes indicate that Mrs. C. is married and has two teenagers, a boy and a girl. Her husband accompanied her to the hospital and appeared to be supportive. Mrs.C. is a bank teller and likes to read, knit, and watch TV. She has varicose veins but states these do not bother her. Her preoperative concerns centred mainly on the cancer: "I hope they get it all." She also stated, "Well, at least I hadn't planned any more children. My boy joked and said, 'You're going to be neutered like our cat was!' I wonder how it feels to be so-called neutered. I hope it won't affect my sex life." The nurse explored Mrs. C.'s knowledge of the surgery and explained that the surgery would not prevent her from having sexual relations.

Mrs. C. returned from the recovery room alert with an IV running and stable vital signs. The dressing was dry. She had an order for morphine sulphate (MS) 10 mg 1M q3h PRN. Monitoring activities included checking vital signs, breath sounds, urinary output, fluid intake, and dressing checks.

Nursing analysis: Pain, abdominal, related to abdominal incision

Expected patient outcomes	Nursing interventions	Rationale
Mrs. C. states feeling more comfortable	Give analgesic on a regular basis for first 24 hr, then as necessary	Giving the analgesic regularly will prevent severe pain and thus be more effective; morphine sulphate (MS) also reduces anxiety
	Encourage frequent changes of position in bed and early ambulation	Activity decreases pain by increasing circulation and reducing muscle tension; ambulation will also encourage peristalsis, decreasing possibility of gas pains

Nursing analysis: Change of body image: high risk for, related to loss of uterus

Expected patient outcomes	Nursing interventions	Rationale
Mrs. C. verbalizes concerns about loss of uterus	Provide Mrs. C. opportunities to express feelings and concerns about loss of uterus	Mrs. C. may feel fear to talk about her feelings if opportunities are provided
	Be empathetic about Mrs. C.'s feelings, which may include grief, guilt, shame or remorse	Feelings associated with grief may also be expressed when grieving over loss of a body part
Mrs. C. demonstrates interest in her personal appearance	Encourage Mrs. C. to continue activities associated with femininity, such as fixing hair, using makeup, wearing own apparel	Feelings of femininity will emphasize "feminine" rather than "neuter," and that she herself has not changed
Mrs. C. verbalizes plans to resume former activities	Help Mrs. C. make plans for resumption of former activities	If life pattern is not changed, her thoughts about her body changes may diminish

Nursing analysis: Constipation: high risk for, related to pelvic surgery

Expected patient outcomes	Nursing interventions	Rationale
Stool is soft and formed	Monitor stool characteristics and frequency	Peristalsis may be decreased from handling of pelvic viscera
	Encourage oral fluids when permitted	Hydration will promote a soft stool
	Encourage ambulation	Ambulation promotes peristalsis

Nursing analysis: Urinary elimination, altered patterns related to pelvic surgery

Expected patient outcomes	Nursing interventions	Rationale
Mrs. C. voids insufficient quantities	Monitor urinary output until she voids sufficiently Monitor for distension above symphysis pubis and for lower abdominal discomfort other than incisional pain	Handling of bladder during pelvic surgery may decrease bladder muscle tone, leading to urinary retention (Mrs. C. did not have an indwelling catheter)

Nursing analysis: Tissue perfusion: altered peripheral, high rish for, related to pelvic venaus stasis from surgery

Expected patient outcomes	Nursing interventions	Rationale
No leg or thigh pain occurs	Monitor discomfort in legs/thighs	Early detection will ensure early treatment of thrombophlebitis
	Encourage leg exercises and frequent turning in bed until ambulating well	Exercises promote venous return (muscle pumps)
	Avoid use of knee gatch or pillows under knees; encourage Mrs. C. to keep knees flat when in bed	Pressure on popliteal veins or sharp knee flexion may increase venous stasis
	Encourage to lie completely flat in bed for short periods q2hr for 24 hr then q4hr until ambulating well	Lying flat for periods of time will help blood return from the pelvic veins
	Encourage ambulation	Ambulation promotes venous return (muscle pumps)
	Provide antiembolic stockings	Mrs. C. is at higher risk for thrombophlebitis because of varicose veins (sluggish circulation) and sedentary life pattern

Nursing analysis: Knowledge deficit, related to surgery

Expected patient outcomes	Nursing interventions	Rationale
Mrs. C. describes self-care	Teach Mrs. C. When activities can be resumed (see text)	Activities are resumed gradually to permit healing; heavy activities are avoided for 6-8 weeks
	Signs of thrombophebitis to be monitored and reported	Thrombophlebitis may occur 7-10 days postoperatively, after patient goes home
	Signs of vaginal bleeding to be reported	Bleeding could indicate impaired healing
	Need for medical follow-up	To ensure that metastasis has not occurred
	Reinforce the preoperative explanations of the surgery and effect on sexual relationships	Preoperative anxiety may have decreased her awareness; hysterectomy does not interfere with satisfactory sexual relationships
	Find out what she has told her daughter about regular Pap smears	Regular Pap smears enhance early detection of cervical cancer
	Suggest she use support hose in her job as bank teller	Preventive measure for thrombophlebitis because of her varicose veins

Table 27-9 Inflammatory disorders of the male reproductive tract

Disorder	Causative organisms	Signs and symptoms	Medical therapy
Urethritis	*Chlamydia trachomatis*, urea-plasma, urealyticum	Urgency, frequency, and burning with urination, purulent urethral discharge	Antibiotics
Prostatitis	*Chlamydia trachomatis, Neisseria gonorrhoeae*	Perineal pain, fever, dysuria, urethral discharge	Antibiotics, rest, hydration, analgesics, stool softener, warm baths
Epididymitis	Same as for prostatitis	Sudden scrotal pain, scrotal oedema	Antibiotics, injection of procaine around spermatic cord, bed rest with scrotal elevation, analgesics
Orchitis	Pyogenic bacteria, gonoccoci	Same as for epididymitis; nausea and vomiting, pain radiating to inguinal canal	Same as for epididymitis

persistent rectal irritation to the doctor. The patient is usually discharged from the hospital within a day or two after the applicators are removed, but may return for another course of radiation.

Complications to watch for after radiation of the uterus are vesicovaginal fistulas, ureterovaginal fistulas, cystitis, phlebitis, and haemorrhage. Each is caused by the radiation or by extension of the disease process. The patient is urged to report even minor symptoms to her doctor.

Chemotherapy

Chemotherapy has not significantly improved cancer of the uterus and therefore is rarely used in this situation. Chemotherapy is used more often for cancer of the ovaries. Combinations of drugs such as cisplatin, doxorubicin, and cyclophosphamide may be given. The drugs are not curative, but some long-term remissions may result.[58] If cancer of the ovaries has spread to peritoneal surfaces throughout the abdomen, a more effective method of giving chemotherapy is by the intraperitoneal route. Higher drug concentrations can be given than by the intravascular route.[10]

INFLAMMATORY DISORDERS IN MEN

Nonspecific pyogenic organisms as well as specific organisms such as the gonococci and tubercle bacilli may cause stubborn infection of the male reproductive system. Urethritis, prostatitis, epididymitis, and orchitis are the most common infections (Table 27-9). Infecting organisms may reach the genital tract by direct spread through the urethra, or they may be borne by blood or lymph.

Aetiology and Pathophysiology
Prostatitis

Prostatitis is commonly associated with urethritis. It may be acute or chronic; recurrent episodes of acute prostatitis may cause fibrotic tissue to form. The fibrosis causes a hardening of the prostate gland that may initially be confused with carcinoma. In the granulomatous form of prostatitis, the enlargement may take 3 to 6 months to resolve.

Epididymitis

Epididymitis is one of the most common inflammations of the male reproductive system. It is frequently a complication of gonorrhoea or the first indication of tuberculosis of the genitourinary tract. It may follow instrumentation or prostatectomy.

Traumatic or chemical epididymitis is a sterile inflammation caused by direct injury or reflux of urine down the vas deferens. The chemical form is frequently seen in military recruits during basic training as a result of straining with a full bladder, which causes urinary reflux.

Bilateral epididymitis usually causes sterility. Untreated epididymitis leads rather rapidly to necrosis of testicular tissue and septicaemia, which can be fatal.

Orchitis

When mumps are contracted after puberty, approximately 18% of the cases are complicated by orchitis (inflammation of the testes). Orchitis may also be caused by bacteria, trauma, or surgical manipulation, or it may follow septicaemia or tuberculosis. Usually both testes are involved, and if it is bilateral, sterility often results. Sterility does not occur with unilateral involvement.

Prevention

Because urethral infection spreads so readily to the genital organs, men should not be catheterized unless it is absolutely necessary. Some trauma to the urethral mucosa is likely to accompany catheterization or the passage of instruments, such as a cystoscope, because of the length and curvature of the male urethra. The distal part of the urethra is not sterile, and trauma makes the urethra susceptible to attack from bacteria. Fluids should be given liberally after passage of instruments through the urethra.

Any postpubertal male who is exposed to mumps usually is given normal immunoglobulin immediately unless he has already had the disease. If there is any doubt about exposure, normal immunoglobulin usually is given. Although it may not prevent mumps, the disease is likely to be less severe, with less likelihood of orchitis developing and subsequent sterility.

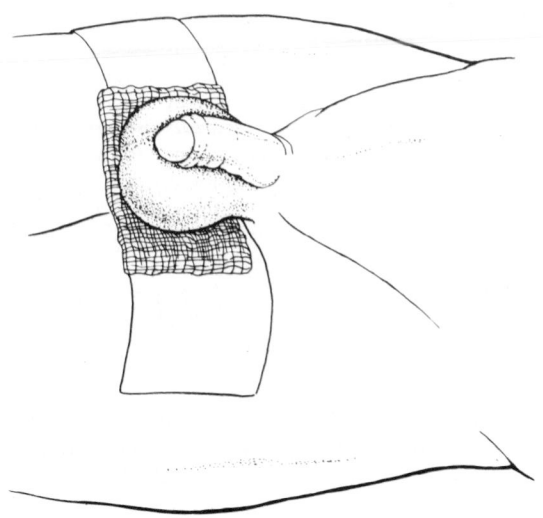

Fig. 27-13   Bellevue bridge.

Diagnostic Tests

The site of the infection will influence treatment. The doctor may obtain segmented bacteriological localization cultures to make the determination. Four sterile culture tubes are used for collection. The patient must be well hydrated, have a full bladder, and be able to cooperate.

1. The first 5 to 10 ml of a voiding is collected.
2. After approximately 200 ml have been voided, a 5 to 10 ml midstream specimen is collected.
3. The patient is asked to stop voiding, and the prostate gland is massaged rectally until prostatic secretions are collected.
4. The next 5 to 10 ml of urine are collected, and the bladder is then emptied.
5. If not cultured immediately, the specimens are refrigerated and taken to the laboratory for culture within 4 hours.

Intervention
Assisting with comfort

Mild to moderate discomfort may be experienced by the man with an inflammation of the genital tract. *Heat* may be applied for prostatitis, but is *contraindicated for epididymitis or orchitis* because of possible destruction of sperm cells. *Cold* is applied in the latter cases for relief of swelling and discomfort. If an ice cap is used, it should be placed under the scrotum and should be removed for short intervals every hour to prevent ice burns. A plastic glove may be filled with crushed ice and placed with the palm of the glove under the scrotum; the fingers provide cold to the sides.

Swelling and discomfort of the scrotum can also be relieved by elevation of the scrotum, either on a folded towel or with adhesive strapping known as a Bellevue bridge (Fig. 27-13).

Counselling and teaching

Female nurses must be particularly sensitive to the reaction and feelings of male patients who have diseases of the reproductive system. The patient may feel more comfortable discussing his problems with a male nurse. However,

27-22	Male reproductive disorders that may affect sexual functioning
Sterility	**Impotence**
Bilateral epididymitis	Radical prostatectomy
Severe bilateral orchitis	External radiation of
Torsion of testes	pelvic floor
	Total penectomy

it is incumbent on all nurses to provide a comfortable environment in which these patients can verbalize their concerns and feelings.

Patient comments with subtle sexual connotations may reveal concerns the patient has regarding his sexuality, and he often must be given permission to discuss these concerns. The patient may "try out" his sexuality on a female nurse. Rejections from her may be perceived by the patient as less threatening than rejection by a loved one would be.

Certain reproductive disorders in the male are accompanied by a high incidence of sexual dysfunction. The patient may be worrying needlessly about possible sterility (inability to conceive a child) or impotence (inability to have an erection). If the patient does have a condition in which the incidence of sexual dysfunction is high, the nurse needs to know the specific patient situation, because these dysfunctions do not always occur in each disorder (Box 27-22).

Teaching includes the need to continue antibiotic therapy for the prescribed length of time (which may be lengthy in chronic prostatitis).

STRUCTURAL DISORDERS IN MEN

Structural disorders of the testes and scrotum that may occur in males include hydrocele, spermatocele, varicocele, or torsion of the spermatic cord (Box 27-23). Immediate medical attention should be sought for any swelling of the scrotum or the testes within it. Any acute swelling of sudden onset must be considered twisting (torsion) of the spermatic cord until proved otherwise.

Hydrocele is treated by aspiration of the fluid and injection of a sclerosing drug. Usually no therapy is needed for *spermatocele*, although aspiration or surgical excision may be done. *Varicocele* is often seen in men with low fertility. Ligation of the spermatic vein has been shown to improve semen quality.

Torsion of the spermatic cord interrupts the blood supply, leading to ischaemia and severe pain that is not relieved and may be aggravated by scrotal elevation. Absence of pain indicates infarction and necrosis. *Immediate surgery* is necessary and the infarcted testis is removed to minimize an immune reaction to antigenic sperm that may cause infertility.[58] The contralateral testis is usually fixed prophylactically to the scrotal wall (orchiopexy) to prevent torsion of its spermatic cord with subsequent infertility.

Body image disturbances may include fears of castration, loss of masculinity, sterility, and impotence. The possibility of these fears being justified depends on the degree of insult to the testis and the functioning of the remaining testicle.

Table 27-10 Cancer of the male reproductive tract

Site	Usual age (yr)	Signs and symptoms	Medical therapy
Testes	18 to 35	Painless enlarged testis, gynaecomastia	Surgery: orchiectomy; radiation, chemotherapy
Prostate gland	>60	Urethral obstruction, low back pain, anaemia	Surgery: radical resection of prostate gland, radiation, hormonal therapy
Penis	40 to 60	Nodular growth on foreskin, fatigue, weight loss	Laser surgery, radiation, surgery (partial or total penectomy), chemotherapy

---

27-23

Structural disorders of testes and scrotum

Hydrocele
Benign nontender collection of clear amber fluid within the outer covering of the testes, leading to scrotal swelling

Spermatocele
Benign nontender cystic mass attached to epididymis containing milky fluid and sperm

Varicocele
Dilation of spermatic vein, primarily on left side (because of increased retrograde pressure of left renal vein)

Torsion of spermatic cord
Kinking and twisting of spermatic cord and artery

TUMOURS IN MEN

Tumours of the male reproductive tract are usually malignant. The more common tumours involve the testes, prostate gland, and penis (Table 27-10).

Pathophysiology
Cancer of the testes

Cancer of the testes accounts for less than 1% of all cancers[21a] and is the most common malignancy in men between the ages of 18 and 35 years and is the second most common cause of death from cancer in this age group. The most common type of testicular cancers is seminomas (75%), which usually spread slowly through the lymphatics. Embryonal tumours invade the spermatic cord and metastasize early to the lungs.[51]

Removal of the testis, with examination of the nodes, is indicated for testicular cancers. *Biopsy of the testis is contraindicated* because of the highly metastatic character of testicular carcinoma. The prognosis following treatment of seminomas is good: 95% for Stage I (confined to testicle), 70% to 90% for Stage II (metastasis to retroperitoneal nodes), and 50% to 70% for Stage III (distal metastases).

Cancer of the prostate gland

The prostate gland is the third most common site of cancer among men (following lung and bowel cancers); it is responsible for 7% of all deaths from cancer in men. It rarely occurs before the age of 60 years, incidence increases with age, and there is an increased familial risk. (Prostatic cancer is discussed in Chapter 25).

Cancer of the penis

The incidence of penile cancer is highly dependent on hygienic standards as well as cultural and religious practices. It almost never occurs in a male who was circumcised at birth. Circumcision after puberty does not decrease the risk of cancer when compared with the incidence among uncircumcised males. Circumcision removes the prepuce, or foreskin, which provides a haven for bacteria. The bacteria act on desquamated cells producing smegma, which is irritating to the tissue of the glans penis and the prepuce. This chronic irritation is considered to be carcinogenic. Trauma and sexually transmitted diseases are felt to be coincidental to penile cancer rather than causative. Most penile malignancies are squamous cell carcinomas. The lesion may cause erosion through the prepuce with a foul odour and discharge.

Prevention and Health Education

Regular testicular self-examination (TSE) is recommended to detect cancer of the testes in its early stages when it is most likely to be localized and most curable. *All young men should be taught testicular self-examination* (Box 27-24). By performing TSE routinely, each man can get to know what is normal for him and more readily identify any lumps or abnormalities. Any swelling that is not normal should be examined by a doctor. Nine of ten testicular cancers are detected by the patient or his sexual partner.

Diagnostic Tests

The prostate can be palpated by digital examination. A newer screening tool is transrectal ultrasound. Because prostatic tissue is rich in acid phosphatase, there is usually an increase in serum acid phosphatase with cancer of the prostate. Diagnosis of cancer of the prostate gland is confirmed by *prostatic biopsy*. If the transrectal route is used for biopsy, no bowel preparation is required. There is no discomfort because the prostate has no nerves. Vital signs are monitored for possible haemorrhage because of the high vascularity of the gland. Bleeding may be from the urethra or the bladder and may be internal. The man is observed for fever, acute urinary retention, rectal bleeding, and pain or swelling of the scrotum.

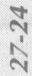

Testicular self-examination (TSE)

Perform TSE after a bath or shower when scrotum
   is warm and most relaxed
Grasp testis with both hands and palpate gently
   between thumb and fingers (Fig. 31-14)
The testis should feel smooth, egg-shaped, and
   firm to touch
The epididymis, found behind the testis, should
   feel like a soft tube

27-24

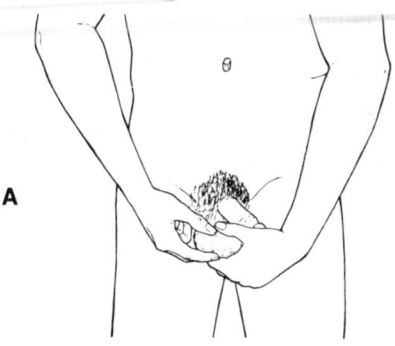

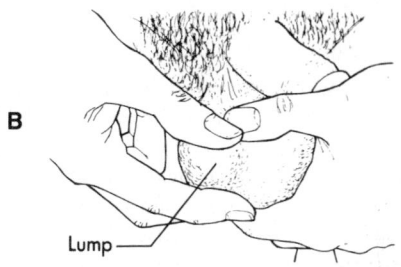

Fig. 27-14   Testicular self-examination. **A,** Grasp testis with both hands; palpate gently between thumb and fingers. **B,** Abnormal lumps or irregularities are reported to the doctor. (Modified from Fred Hutchinson Cancer Research Cancer Control Program: Self testicular exam, Seattle, 1980, Cancer Control Program.)

Surgery

Surgery of the prostate gland is discussed in Chapter 25.

Surgery of the testicle

Orchiectomy consists of en bloc excision of the spermatic cord, the contents of the inguinal canal, and the testis with the tunica attached. The adjacent area is explored for metastases.

Preoperative care

In addition to usual preoperative care, psychological preparation for surgery is important. The man will usually be concerned about the effects of castration. *Unilateral* removal of a testis will *not* demasculinize him or cause sterility. Prostheses are available to replace the removed testis.

Postoperative care
Activity

Bed rest may be instituted for 24 to 48 hours after extensive removal of tissue, but ambulation usually is begun within 12 hours after surgery. Leg exercises are important if bed rest is to be maintained. The scrotum is elevated on a rolled towel, or the man may wear an athletic supporter while in bed. An athletic supporter or tight undershorts should be worn for support when the patient is ambulating.

Postoperative complications

The two major problems after scrotal surgery are oedema and intrascrotal haemorrhage. Oedema may be controlled by ice bags for the first 12 hours and a compression dressing for 3 to 5 days. Ice is best applied by filling a rubber glove with crushed ice. Signs of haemorrhage or complaints of increasing discomfort are reported to the doctor.

Teaching

1. Avoid prolonged standing, which increases scrotal oedema.
2. Wear athletic supporter or tight undershorts until healing is complete.
3. Take 20-minute tub baths three times per day for 1 week after discharge.
4. Avoid heavy lifting for 4 to 6 weeks.

Penile surgery

Small noninvasive tumours may be removed by laser surgery. Large lesions without deep infiltration require partial penectomy, removing the penis at a point 2 cm beyond the tumour.[58] The remaining penis must be long enough for the man to void standing, direct the stream, and not void on himself. If this is possible, sexual function will probably be retained. Large deep infiltrating tumours require total penectomy with perineal urethrostomy (the urethra is redirected to an opening between the scrotum and the anus). Sexual counselling is indicated for the man with a total penectomy. Some men with urethrostomy have experienced orgasm and ejaculation following stimulation of the perineal, scrotal, and testicular regions. Counselling may also be helpful for the partner.

Radiation

Testicular seminomas respond to radiotherapy whereas nonseminomas do not. External beam radiation is given to the abdomen following orchiectomy.

Although the normal testis is shielded during external radiation of an involved testis, it does receive radiation scattered from the abdomen. A period of 70 days is required to determine whether spermatogenesis has been affected. Spermatogenesis may be decreased for 7 months to 5 years or more. Although genetic defects are possible after irradiation, there is currently no evidence to cause serious concern. Genetic counselling may be helpful for those couples desiring children.

Radiation for *prostatic* cancer may be delivered by external beam or by implant. The testes are shielded during external radiation. Erectile dysfunction may occur. Iodine-125 retropubic prostatic implantation may be used initially or after failure of external radiation therapy. Complications of iodine-125 implantation include blood loss from multiple needle punctures during implantation, deep vein thrombosis, pulmonary emboli, haematomas, and abscesses. Potency is retained.

Small noninfiltrating *penile* tumours can be treated with external beam radiation. Nodal radiation is not as effective as surgery.

Chemotherapy

Chemotherapy is given following *orchiectomy* for those patients with metastases. Combination chemotherapy with cisplatin, vinblastine, and bleomycin is effective. For *prostatic* or *penile* cancer, chemotherapy is given only for palliative effect with deep distant metastasis.

Hormone Therapy

Oestrogen therapy may be used for advanced prostatic cancer when metastasis has occurred, especially to the bone. Bilateral orchiectomy to eliminate androgen may be combined with oestrogen therapy. Oestrogen may also be given prophylactically following surgery or radiation therapy. In males, oestrogen frequently causes gynaecomastia (enlargement of the breasts), loss of libido, arrest of spermatogenesis, and testicular atrophy.

Oestrogen helps to decrease pain and reduce tumour size. The use of hormone therapy provides a longer symptom-free period but makes palliation more difficult when symptoms recur. If endocrine therapy is delayed, symptoms recur earlier but longer palliation is possible.

SEXUALLY TRANSMITTED DISEASES

AETIOLOGY/EPIDEMIOLOGY

Sexually transmitted diseases (STDs) are diseases that usually are or can be transmitted from one person to another with heterosexual or homosexual intercourse or intimate contact with the genitalia, mouth, or rectum. In Britain, only three conditions are classified as venereal: syphilis, gonorrhoea, and chancroid (very rare in the United Kingdom). The term *venereal* has medicolegal implications, and new cases are notifiable by law. Nonvenereal STDs are also monitored but statistics may be inaccurate where reporting does not occur or where people (probably less than 10%) seek treatment outside the National Health Service. In the 1980s several diseases were added to the list of STDs. These include *Chlamydia trachomatis,* genital herpes, human papillomavirus (HPV), genital mycoplasmas, cytomegalovirus, hepatitis B, vaginitis, enteric infections, and ectoparasitic disease.[14a]

Early in the 1980s the human immunodeficiency virus (HIV) was identified and AIDS emerged as a major STD. Because of its profound effect on the immune system, Chapter 13 is devoted to the discussion of AIDS.

The diseases classified as STDs and their causative organisms are listed in Box 27-25. Because of improved laboratory and epidemiological methods, the prevalence, modes of transmission, and clinical consequences of these newer STDs are better understood than in earlier decades. In addition, many of the newly recognized STDs have become epidemic or hyperendemic as a consequence of

27-25	Sexually transmitted diseases	
	Type of organism	**Disease**
	Bacteria	Gonorrhoea, chancroid, granuloma inguinale, *Gardnerella vaginalis*
	Spirochaete	Syphilis
	Chlamydia	Nongonococcal urethritis, epididymitis, cervicitis, pelvic inflammatory disease, lymphogranuloma venereum
	Virus	Herpes genitalis, hepatitis B, cytomegalovirus, AIDS, genital warts
	Protozoa	Trichomoniasis
	Yeast	Candidiasis
	Parasites	Pediculosis pubis, scabies

changing sexual behavioural patterns. Not only has the incidence of many STDs increased, but for agents with multiple modes of transmission (for example, hepatitis B virus (HBV), enteric pathogens), the proportion of infections that are transmitted sexually has also increased. In addition to the immediate consequences of STDs there are the recognized effects on maternal and infant morbidity, as well as on human reproduction and fertility.

It is a legal requirement that each case of syphilis and gonorrhoea is reported to the appropriate community medical officer. Reporting of other STDs, for example herpes, candidiasis, trichomoniasis, warts, granuloma inguinale, is also important in determining trends and planning services. As already stated, the true incidence of STDs is not known because of variable reporting requirements and also because some cases are not reported by the clinicians who treat them; for example trichomoniasis and candidiasis are not usually reported, even when they are sexually transmitted.

During 1990 there were 168,000 new cases of STDs seen in genitourinary medicine clinics in the United Kingdom, and many of these were in people under 30 years.

In addition to the immediate consequences of STDs there are serious complications, most of which have the greatest impact on women and children. The most serious complications are pelvic inflammatory disease (PID), sterility, ectopic pregnancy, blindness, cancer associated with the HPV, fetal and infant deaths, birth defects, and learning difficulties.

SEXUAL TRANSMISSION

The STDs are contagious diseases spread almost exclusively by contact during sexual intercourse; that is, when mucous membrane surfaces come in contact during genital, oral, or anal sexual activity. Because the causative organisms survive only very briefly outside a warm, moist environment, there is almost no way to contract STDs from toilet seats, towels, or bed linens. Although STDs are not usually transmitted in public toilets, conditions caused by fungi, bacteria, and lice can be transmitted from water in unclean toilet bowls. Women using a conventional toilet expose the vaginal and anal area to pathogens that can be introduced by the splashback of contaminated toilet water.

There are some notable exceptions to sexual transmission. During pregnancy the foetus may become infected in utero by placental transmission, and the infant may acquire congenital syphilis or be stillborn. Infants of mothers with gonorrhoea may contract infections of the eyes (ophthalmia neonatorum) during birth, and unless treated, this can lead to permanent blindness.

Prevention and Health Education

Prevention and control measures for STDs include three levels of prevention. *Primary prevention* is directed at preventing the disease. This includes educating noninfected people so that they can take responsibility for their own health and not expose themselves to an infected person; identification and treatment of exposed people who are asymptomatic; interviewing people with infection for identification of contacts; examination and preventive treatment of contacts; educational programmes for the public; and active involvement of professionals in programmes of control. The goal of these efforts includes eradication of the reservoir of disease in the population. *Secondary prevention* is directed towards prevention of complications. *Tertiary prevention* focuses on the following: (1) prevention of complications, (2) supporting and counselling infected people to receive treatment, and (3) asking infected people to notify their sexual partners so that they can be examined and treated if infected.

Partner notification (contact investigation)

In the prevention and control of STDs, especially gonorrhoea, emphasis was once placed on interviewing for information regarding sexual contacts. The named contacts were sought out for examination and treatment. Lay people knowledgeable about the required reporting to the local health department of some of the diseases were very hesitant to name their sexual contacts. Young people often feared that their parents and the parents of the sexual partner would find out about their infection. Minors need to know that they can probably obtain treatment without parental consent. Presently genitourinary medicine clinics and family doctors are permitted to treat minors for STDs without obtaining parental consent. People also may perceive reporting of STDs as a threat from an official agency and may hesitate to name their contacts out of a sense of protection if they do not know that no punishment is involved.

Interviewing the patient for contacts is done at the time of the initial visit in the event that the patient does not return for follow-up. It is probably best that this interview takes place after the patient is examined, the type of infection is determined, and the treatment is prescribed. If assessment is accompanied by information giving, the person should be better informed about STDs and how they are treated, and be more willing and able to give information about sexual contacts.

Interviewing for contacts involves two aspects. The patient is first asked to name sexual contacts. Second, the patient is interviewed for "cluster suspects," who are friends or acquaintances who may have been exposed to the same contacts, or who have symptoms of an STD.

Because one focus of STD control is increasing self-referrals, the patient is asked to inform known contacts (partner notification) and cluster suspects to come in for examination and treatment. Confidentiality is stressed. There is reason to believe that patients do not name all their contacts at the time of the first interview and that a reinterview will usually result in additional names of contacts. Because of the understandable reluctance of many people to name their sexual contacts, the patient may be given the responsibility of informing the contacts and advising them of their need for treatment. (The contacts are not named, but instead cards that permit both examination and treatment without identification may be given to the contacts by the patient.) Local health departments cooperate in locating, examining, and treating these contacts as necessary.

Whenever possible, the contacts of the infected person are located and advised to have an examination and tests as soon as possible. If the sexual partner(s) does not have symptoms of infection at the time of the first examination, treatment is instituted to abort infection. Giving preventive treatment to named contacts who have no clinical evidence of infection has gained popularity and acceptance in recent years, and there are indications that this same approach is being used more often in the management of patients having the "minor" STDs.

Nursing Process
Assessment
Subjective data

The following information is collected from a person suspected of having an STD:
1. Exposure to STD contact including HIV.
2. STD history, treatment.
3. Sexual orientation: "Have you been having sex with men, women, or both?".
4. Timing of last sexual activity.
5. Number of sexual partners in the past two months.
6. Women are questioned about:
   a. Vaginal discharge
   b. Vulvar itching
   c. Dysuria
   d. Urinary urgency
   e. Lower abdominal pain
   f. Rectal symptoms
   g. Sore throat
   h. Genital lesions
   i. Skin rashes or itching
   j. Menstrual periods.
7. Heterosexual men are questioned about:
   a. Urethral discharge
   b. Dysuria
   c. Genital lesions
   d. Skin rashes
   e. Itching
   f. Testicular pain
   g. Sore throat.

8. Homosexual or bisexual men are asked the same questions as heterosexual men plus the following:
   a. Rectal symptoms such as pain, bleeding, discharge, and diarrhoea.
9. If hepatitis is also suspected, the person is questioned about:
   a. Dark-coloured urine
   b. Clay-coloured stools
   c. Fatigue
   d. Jaundice.

Objective data

Objective data include the following:
1. Inspection and palpation of the integumentary system, reproductive system, and anorectal area.
2. Examination for women includes the following:
   a. Inspection of skin of lower abdomen, inguinal area, hands, palms, and forearms
   b. Inspection of pubic hair for lice and mites
   c. Inspection and palpation of external genitalia, including perineum and anus
   d. Speculum examination of vagina and cervix
   e. Bimanual pelvic examination
   f. Palpation for inguinal and femoral lymphadenopathy
   g. Inspection of mouth and throat, including tonsils.
3. Examination of heterosexual men includes the following:
   a. Inspection of the skin and pubic hair
   b. Inspection of the penis, including the meatus, with retraction of the foreskin and "milking" of the urethra
   c. Palpation of the scrotum.
4. Examination of homosexual or bisexual men is the same as for heterosexual men plus the following:
   a. Inspection of the mouth, throat including the tonsils, and anorectal area
   b. Proctoscopic examination if there are rectal symptoms.

Diagnostic tests

Specific diagnostic tests are used to establish the diagnosis of each of these diseases. Diagnostic tests will be discussed under the specific disease later in this chapter.

Nursing analysis

Problems are determined from analysis of patient data. Possible problems for the person with an STD may include, but are not limited to, the following:

Problems	Possible aetiologies
Knowledge deficit	Lack of exposure/recall, information misinterpretation, lack of familiarity with information sources about STDs
Health maintenance, altered	Lack of knowledge, cultural practices, lack of material resources

Planning: expected patient outcomes

Expected patient outcomes for the person with an STD may include, but are not limited to, the following:

1. Person and/or partner can explain the aetiology and factors contributing to the STD.
2. Person and/or partner can state the name, dosage, and timing of administration of drug therapy, as well as its possible side effects.
3. Person and/or partner can explain the need for adherence to the entire treatment regimen.
4. Person and/or partner can state the reasons for abstaining from sexual activity during the infectious stages of the STD.
5. Person and/or partner can state effects of the STD on the reproductive system of oneself and one's partner.
6. Person and/or partner can state indications for seeking immediate healthcare if signs and symptoms reappear.
7. Person and/or partner can explain necessity for treatment of sexual partner or partners.
8. Person and/or partner can accept the occurrence of the STD.
9. Person and/or partner can explain how to prevent the transmission of STDs by using safer sex practices including the type of condom to use, when and how to apply it, and how to remove it.

Implementation

Assisting with achievement of therapeutic goals

Medical therapy for each STD will be discussed under the specific diseases.

Interventions to achieve patient outcomes
Facilitating learning

The nurse's first responsibility in STD control is to educate patients who have a sexually transmitted infection or may develop one. Nurses must be knowledgeable about the diseases most prevalent, the signs and symptoms, methods used in diagnosis, treatments used, and where individuals can obtain help and information. They can also influence the knowledge and attitudes of their colleagues and peers towards an STD and its control. Nurses can exert influence in the community by taking an active role in programmes of education. Perhaps the best way to reduce the risk of an STD is for people who are sexually active to know their sexual partners. Sexual activity with different partners increases the risk of infection.

Preventive measures such as washing or showering with soap and water and using a condom are recommended but are no guarantee against STDs. Good laundry and personal hygiene practices also may help reduce risk.

Before nurses can be effective in working with patients who have STDs, they must confront their own feelings and attitudes about such diseases. The patient is often young, fearful of pain, and unaccustomed to surroundings in a clinic or doctor's surgery. Young patients especially fear that their families and friends may learn they have an STD.

Once the diagnosis, tentative or conclusive, is made, focus should first be placed on obtaining a cure and preventing complications and reinfection. Many lay people know that the treatment for syphilis and gonorrhoea is penicillin, but they may not be fully informed about this and other aspects of treatment. Because some of the diseases respond to penicillin or other antibiotics, many people believe that all genital infections can be cured easily, and this is not so. Some people believe that antibiotics not only cure an infection but that they produce immunity against reinfection too. People receiving an antibiotic or other medications for STDs must be informed of the action of the drug, its duration of effectiveness, side effects, chances of cure, and the need for follow-up. They need to be advised that treatment failures do occur and that reinfection rates are high. Return visits should be encouraged whenever possible, because adequacy of treatment of all of the STDs is evaluated best by laboratory analysis for the specific organism.

Providing social and emotional support

Many patients focus on how the diseases are spread rather than on the consequences of having an infection. For single people, contracting an STD and securing help means they must admit to sexual activity, and some of them may feel guilty. Their self-esteem may be threatened by what has happened to them. Patients with an STD have not only a physical problem, but a social, emotional, and perhaps economic problem as well. They need constructive and comprehensive help. The nurse who is successful in working with people with an STD is one who can create an atmosphere of trust in which the person feels free to discuss all aspects of the problem.

People who seek help recognize they have a problem; they want to get better and stay well. Because of this they are highly motivated to do what is necessary, receptive to information and advice, and attentive when advice is given. Nurses can take advantage of the patient's readiness to learn and motivation to improve and maintain health.

Promoting self-care

People treated for sexually transmitted infections need information about self-care. To understand their therapy and to responsibly engage in self-care, they must be informed about the sexual nature of the infection, how it is transmitted, and the *possibility of reinfection and infection of their sexual partner or partners*. The patient needs to know that it is important for sexual partners to be checked for signs of infection, to be advised of what the signs are, and to have a culture for asymptomatic infection. Patients should be advised to abstain from intercourse until cured. *It also should be stressed that condoms should be used to prevent infection or reinfection, if people persist in engaging in intercourse even when advised not to.*

Teaching about hygiene and personal health practices is beneficial in reducing the chances of secondary infection, recurrence, and infections of various types in the future. Frequent bathing and hand washing are indicated. It is known that many of the organisms that cause STDs are destroyed by soap and water. All women should be informed that, for personal cleanliness, douching at any time is *not* advisable, because this may disturb the vaginal and cervical environments and predispose the woman to infection. Rarely, if douching is prescribed by the doctor, the patient should be instructed in the procedure.

If the lesions are present on body surfaces, the patient should be instructed in their care. Unless contraindicated, a hot bath is taken two to three times a day; and lesions are kept as dry as possible between baths. Men and women should be advised to wear cotton underwear, and women should be advised to avoid wearing tights, because they tend to trap moisture and prevent circulation of air to the genitalia. Unless they are specifically prescribed as local medications, the patient should not apply any lotion, cream, or ointment to any of the lesions associated with an STD.

Self-examination is important for sexually active people, especially those with more than one partner. Inspecting skin, mouth, genitals, and perianal areas for lesions and discharges is recommended. In addition, people can learn to inspect their partners casually during the initial period of lovemaking to identify any signs of STDs. Urinating after sexual activity can be helpful in cleansing the urethra of organisms.

Promoting healthy sexual attitudes

Opportunities for promoting healthy attitudes about sexual activity and STDs frequently arise. These topics are approached tactfully and with consideration of the patient's feelings. Adolescents especially require an approach that indicates understanding balanced with the ability to help them set limits. They need to understand that they are responsible for their own bodies and they do not have to give in to sexual pressures. It is well documented, however, that the strongest influence on teenagers comes from their peer group. For this reason, discussion with groups of teenagers about their sexual responsibilities may be helpful. In the climate of the 1990s there should be no doubt that abstinence is the only absolute way to prevent STDs. If a teenager elects to be sexually active, he or she needs to understand that the consequences of unprotected sex may include unwanted pregnancy and an STD. Monogamous relationships and the proper use of condoms should be stressed for those who are sexually active.

Evaluation

Evaluation is based on the expected patient outcomes. Questions to be asked include the person's and/or partner's ability to do the following:

1. State the factors that contributed to the present infection with the STD (multiple sexual partners; not using a condom).
2. State the drug therapy to be followed, including name of drug, dosage, timing of administration, and side effects.
3. Explain why the therapy must be taken without interruption (to prevent resistant strains of organisms from developing).
4. State why he or she should not engage in sexual activity while the STD is infectious.
5. State effects of STDs that may develop in the reproductive system of either partner.
6. State signs and symptoms (fever, pain, discharge) that indicate need for immediate healthcare.
7. Verbalize understanding of the necessity of treatment for his or her sexual partner or partners.

8. Verbalize that she or he has an STD and identify ways to prevent further STD infections.
9. Explain what is meant by practising "safer sex", including what type of condom to use, when and how to apply it, and how to remove it.

GONORRHOEA

Aetiology, Epidemiology, and Pathophysiology

The incidence of gonorrhoea in the United Kingdom decreased dramatically in the 1980s (Fig. 27-15). However, the proportion of antibiotic-resistant gonoccocal organisms in the United Kingdom increased from 0.3% in 1980 to 1.3% in 1987; the peak year was 1984 with 2.3% (Fig. 27-16). Clinically significant resistance to the three widely used classes of drugs—the penicillins, the tetracyclines, and the aminoglycosides—has been reported.[38] In addition, women have few, if any, signs or symptoms of gonorrhoea and thus are often not diagnosed.

Young adults 20 to 24 years of age are at highest risk of acquiring gonorrhoea, with the next highest rates found among teenagers 15 to 19 years of age. In fact, 1 of every 30 teenagers in this age group will acquire gonorrhoea each year.

It is estimated that the total cost of gonorrhoea in the United Kingdom is very large each year. Women and their offspring suffer the major physical, emotional, and economic burden. Pelvic inflammatory disease occurs in 10 to 20% of women with gonorrhoea; and even when treated, these women are likely to suffer from recurrent salpingitis, ectopic pregnancy, infertility, and menstrual abnormalities and may face surgical removal of the pelvic organs, as well as fetal loss.

Many cases of PID are diagnosed and treated yearly; in 1985 more than 16,000 cases were admitted to hospital in England and Wales (a five-fold increase in 20 years).

Asymptomatic people, or those with few symptoms, are an important reservoir for infection, because they usually

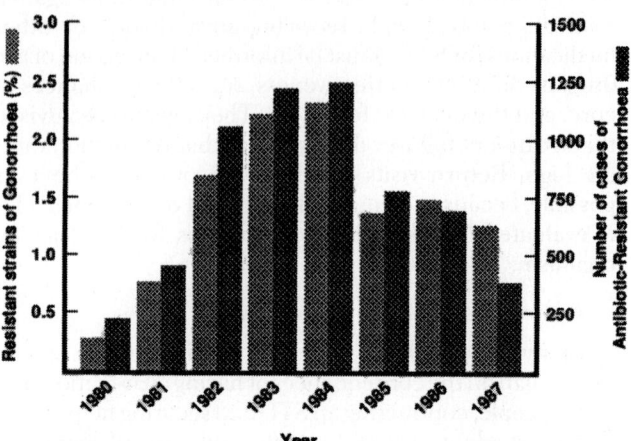

Fig. 27-16   Percentage and numbers of antibiotic-resistant strains of gonorrhoea in the United Kingdom, 1980 to 1987.

remain untreated. As many as 10 to 40% of gonorrhoeal infections in men are asymptomatic, and in women as many as 80% of infections are asymptomatic. Homosexual men can harbour reservoirs of anorectal and pharyngeal infections.

Gonorrhoea, often referred to as *GC* or *the clap* by lay people, is caused by N. *gonorrhoeae*. Gonorrhoea is of great concern because people with it often have another STD such as chlamydia or HIV. They also have a high reinfection rate and serious residual effects. The incubation period is 3 to 30 days in men and three days to an indefinite period in women.

Prevention and Health Education

Prevention of gonorrhoea and its complications can be achieved in three stages. The *first* and most crucial *stage, primary prevention*, is prevention of the disease. The *second stage, secondary prevention*, involves prevention of compli-

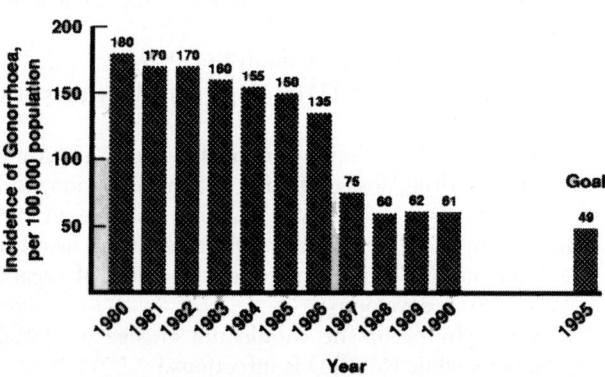

Fig. 27-15   Incidence of gonorrhoea in the United Kingdom, 1980 to 1990, per 100,000 population (15–64). The goal for 1995 is 49 cases per 100,000. (Department of Health: The Health of the Nation. A strategy for Health in England. Presented to Parliament by the Secretary of State for Health, London, 1992, HMSO.)

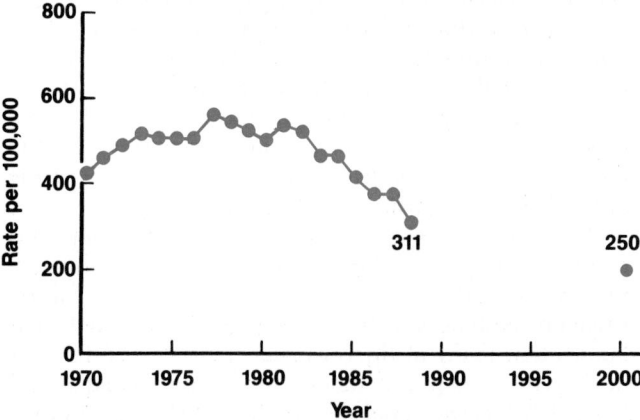

Fig. 27-17   Cases of pelvic inflammatory disease per 100,000 women in the US. The number 250 per 100,000 is the goal for the year 2000. (From US Department of Health and Human Services: *Healthy people 2000: national health promotion and disease prevention objectives,* Washington, DC, 1990, US Government Printing Office.)

cations of the disease, such as PID. The *third stage, tertiary prevention*, is reversal of the damage caused by the disease, such as by tubal reconstruction.

Early treatment of infected people is the most effective method to prevent new infection of sexual partners. Mechanical barrier methods such as condoms used with spermicides may reduce, but not prevent gonorrhoea.[33a] Education to acquaint people with the symptoms of gonorrhoea, the efficacy of condoms, and the availability of diagnostic and treatment resources is also important. Early detection through partner notification and screening can reduce the serious complications of gonorrhoea. There is no effective vaccine for gonorrhoea, although clinical trials have been attempted.[33a]

Signs and Symptoms

The most common signs and symptoms are listed in Box 27-26.

Diagnostic tests

Gonorrhoeal infection may be suspected on the basis of history, symptoms, and clinical evidence obtained by physical examination. However, *identification of the organism is necessary to confirm the diagnosis* and to rule out other problems. In men the diagnosis is confirmed by Gram-stained smear of the discharge from the penis. Culture of the discharge from the penis is usually reserved for those whose smears are negative in the presence of strong clinical evidence.

Gram-stained cervical smears are inadequate for diagnosing gonorrhoea in women. These smears are negative in about 50% of women having gonorrhoea and are falsely positive in some cases. Therefore, cultures from the cervix,

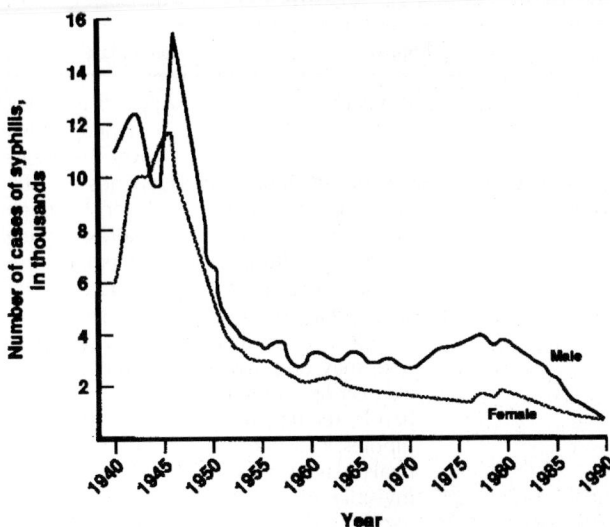

Fig. 27-18 Incidence of syphilis (all stages) in the United Kingdom, 1940 to 1990, in thousands.

urethra, throat, and anus are usually taken. Because of the great length of time required to obtain reports of cultures for gonorrhoea, treatment is usually begun on a presumptive basis.

Treatment

Therapy for gonorrhoea presents a greater problem than for syphilis, because the gonococcus tends to develop resistance to antibiotics. Several drug regimens are in use. Emphasis is on single-dose treatment because it avoids the need for follow-up and patient cooperation.

A recommended treatment regimen is as follows:
1. Amoxycillin 2–3 g as a single dose in combination with probenecid 1 g; alternatives to amoxycillin include its esters such as bacampicillin and pivampicillin.
2. Alternative therapy includes spectinomycin 2g intramuscularly once, ciprofloxacin 500mg orally once, or acrosoxacin 300mg orally once.

Spectinomycin is recommended for the treatment of people with resistant strains of *N. gonorrhoeae*.

SYPHILIS

Epidemiology, Aetiology, and Pathophysiology

The incidence of syphilis is now at a very low level in the United Kingdom (Fig. 27-18). In 1990 there were around 2,000 new cases of syphilis in the United Kingdom.

Syphilis is caused by a spirochaete, *Treponema pallidum*, that gains entry into the body through either the mucous membrane or skin during intercourse. The organism is readily destroyed by physical and chemical agents, including heat, drying, and mild disinfectants such as soap and water.

The incubation period for syphilis is usually three weeks. However, symptoms can appear as early as nine days or as long as three months after exposure, which is the case for rectal infections in homosexual men.

27-26	**Signs and symptoms of gonorrhoea**

Heterosexual men
1. Urethritis—often first symptom
2. Severe dysuria—especially with first voiding in morning
3. Purulent discharge from urethra
4. Swelling of the penis and balanitis—rare symptoms

Homosexual and bisexual men
1. Rectal gonorrhoea is common—usually asymptomatic and discovered by rectal culture
2. Pharyngeal gonorrhoea— usually asymptomatic

Women
Women rarely have early, distressing symptoms such as men have. When symptoms are present, they include the following:
1. Slight purulent vaginal discharge
2. Vague feeling of fullness in pelvis
3. Discomfort or aching in abdomen
4. If bladder is involved—burning, frequency, and urgency, which usually cause the person to seek medical attention
The first three symptoms are so slight that they may be ignored by the person.

Table 27-11   Stages of syphilis

	Primary	Secondary	Latent	Late
Duration	2–8 weeks	Appears 2–4 weeks after chancre appears; extends over 2–4 years	5–20 years	Terminal if not treated
Signs and symptoms	Hard sore or pimple on vulva or penis that breaks and forms painless, draining chancre; may be a single chancre or groups of more than one; may be present also on lips, tongue, hands, rectum, or nipples; chancre heals leaving almost invisible scar	Depends on site; low-grade fever, headache, anorexia, weight loss, anaemia, sore throat, hoarseness, reddened and sore eyes, jaundice with or without hepatitis, aching of joints, muscles, long bones; sores on body or generalized fine rash; condylomata accuminata (venereal warts) on rectum or genitalia	No clinical signs	Tumour-like mass, (gumma), on any area of body; damage to heart valves and blood vessels; meningitis; paralysis; lack of coordination; paraesis; insomnia; confusion; delusions; impaired judgement; slurred speech
Communicability	Exudates from lesions and chancre are highly contagious	Exudates from lesions highly contagious; blood contains organisms	Contagious for about 2 years; not contagious to others after that; blood contains organisms; may be transmitted placentally to fetus	Noncontagious; spinal fluid may contain organisms

Signs and Symptoms

The signs and symptoms of the four stages of syphilis are listed in Table 27-11. If syphilis is adequately diagnosed and treated during the primary stage, the other stages can be prevented.

Assessment

The subjective and objective data to be collected from a person suspected of having any STD are discussed on p. 799.

Diagnostic tests

Syphilis is most often diagnosed by standard serological tests. Massive screening programmes in the past made serological diagnosis of syphilis very common. Mass screening with the Venereal Disease Research Laboratory (VDRL) test is no longer practised except in high-risk populations, on pregnant women, and on blood donated for transfusion. Dark-field microscopic examination of tissue scrapings from lesions or material obtained by aspiration of regional lymph nodes also reveals the presence of the spirochaete, especially during the primary and secondary stages. A presumptive diagnosis is made on the basis of suspicious lesions, positive serological tests, known exposure to infection, and involvement of regional lymph nodes. False-positive VDRL reactions are common among people previously treated for syphilis, but fluorescent treponemal antibody (FTA) and absorption (ABS) tests are more specific (Table 27-12). Also, *once a VDRL test is positive, it remains so and is not useful for identifying reinfection.*

Table 27-12   Serological tests for syphilis (STSs)

Type	Description	Examples	Comments
Flocculation	Antibody–antigen reaction produces a precipitation (flocculation)	VDRL RPR	Used primarily for screening; performed in standard laboratories
Complement fixation	Complement is used up in antigen–antibody reaction (fixed); haemolysis occurs	Reiter (Wasserman outdated)	Nonspecific; used less frequently; performed in standard laboratories
Fluorescent antibody	Antigen of killed *Treponema pallidum* is labelled with a fluorescent dye	FTA FTA-ABS	More specific than flocculation or complement-fixation test; differentiates false-positive from true syphilis-positive results; performed in special laboratories
Treponema pallidum immobilization	Serum is mixed with live *Treponema pallidum;* presence of antibody decreases organism mobility	TPI	Most sensitive test; performed only at a specialist laboratory

Treatment

Syphilis can be successfully treated at any stage of the disease, although treatment may have to be more prolonged in latent and late syphilis. Even though syphilis can be cured in late stages, the damage to the body is much more difficult to manage.

Because penicillin continues to be effective in the treatment of syphilis, it remains the drug of choice. All types of penicillin are effective, but procaine penicillin is preferred because it is long-acting and can be given in a limited number of injections.

Syphilis is treated with intramuscular procaine penicillin 1.2 g for 10–15 days; procaine penicillin may be used in combination with benzylpenicillin. When the use of penicillin is contraindicated because of drug sensitivity, doxycycline 200mg orally daily for two weeks or tetracycline 500mg orally four times a day for two weeks is given. For people who cannot take tetracycline, erythromycin 500mg four times a day for two weeks may be given. Compliance with any oral treatment regimen can be difficult, especially when the person is a chronic drug misuser and engages in other high-risk behaviours. The patient will need follow-up reminders to take the drug as prescribed.

If there is a question of whether or not the person is allergic to penicillin, penicillin skin tests and desensitization should be considered (see Chapter 34).[26a]

Pregnant women with penicillin sensitivity pose problems for treatment. In the large dosage required to treat syphilis, tetracycline produces mottling and staining of fetal teeth and possible abnormal bone formation. If given the usual adult dose, inadequate placental transfer of tetracycline is likely, and congenital syphilis would probably develop. Erythromycin in a dose of 30g over a period of 15 days seems to be the best alternative treatment for pregnant women with syphilis. Neurosyphilis is treated with intravenous penicillin. Sexual partners are treated with procaine penicillin.

CHLAMYDIAL INFECTION

Aetiology/Epidemiology

Chlamydia trachomatis is caused by the Gram-negative obligate, *C. trachomatis*. It is recognized as the most commonly reported STD in the United Kingdom. In England and Wales, where nongonococcal urethritis (about half the cases of which are caused by *C. trachomatis*) is a reportable disease, the incidence has nearly doubled in the last decade.[49a]

Chlamydial infections are responsible for about 20 to 30% of diagnosed PID cases, and it is estimated that many thousands of women each year become involuntarily sterilized and suffer ectopic pregnancies as a result of this organism. Chlamydial infections can be transmitted to infants during delivery, causing conjunctivitis and pneumonia in many.

Chlamydia is highest in young, promiscuous, indigent, unmarried women who live in the inner city and in those who have had a history of an STD.

Table 27-13 *Chlamydia trachomatis* infections

Males	Females	Infants
Transmission		
Males ⟷	Females →	Infants
Infections		
Urethritis	Cervicitis	Conjuctivitis
Postgonococcal urethritis	Urethritis	Pneumonia
Proctitis	Proctitis	Asymptomatic pharyngeal carriage
Conjuctivitis	Conjuctivitis	Asymptomatic gastrointestinal carriage
Pharyngitis	Pharyngitis	
Subclinical lymphogranuloma venereum	Subclinical lymphogranuloma venereum	
Complications		
Epididymitis	Salpingitis	
Prostatitis	Endometritis	
Reiter's syndrome	Perihepatitis	
Sterility	Ectopic pregnancy	
Rectal strictures*	Infertility	
	Vulvar/rectal carcinoma*	
	Rectal stricture*	

From Centers for Disease Control, Chlamydia Trachomatis Infections, Policy Guidelines for Prevention and Control, MMWR (suppl) 35:54, 1985.
*Associated with lymphogranuloma venereum.

Pathophysiology

Chlamydia trachomatis is a parasite that has specific requirements for adenosine triphosphate (ATP) and amino acids. There are two stages in the life cycle of the organism. In *stage 1*, the *infective stage*, the *elementary body attaches* to the host cell and is ingested by phagocytosis. In *stage 2*, the *elementary body undergoes metamorphosis* to become a *reticulate or initial body*. This is the *metabolic phase* of the life cycle. The initial body duplicates by binary fission and changes into the elementary body. The host cell, which contains the elementary bodies, undergoes lysis, liberating infectious organisms that are capable of reinfecting new cells.[89]

It is estimated that between 20 and 40% of sexually active women have been exposed to the bacterium and have antibody titers to *C. trachomatis*.[89] Table 27-13 shows how the infection can be transmitted between male and female sexual partners and from females to infants. It also lists the various ways the disease is manifested in males, females, and infants.

Signs and symptoms

The clinical clues used to diagnose chlamydia in women are presented in Box 27-25, p. 806. Men usually have non-specific urethritis or may seek treatment for epididymitis. However, up to 80% of women and 25% of men may be asymptomatic.

27-25

Clinical clues used to diagnose chlamydia in women

Purulent discharge
Endocervical mucous
Bleeding after intercourse
Bleeding between periods
Vague lower abdominal pain
Cervical atypia (not normal)
Infertility
C. trachomatis should be looked for when there is premature rupture of amniotic membranes

Data from Faro S: *Chlamydia trachomatis* infection. In Rakel RE, editor: *Conn's current therapy,* Philadelphia, 1991, WB Saunders.

Diagnostic tests

Chlamydia trachomatis infection may be diagnosed by traditional tissue culture or by one of the new rapid tests listed below.

1. Enzyme immunoassay (EIA) (chlamydiazime or test patch (Abbott)).
2. Direct immunofluorescence—several of which are commercially available.
3. If none of the above are available, a tentative diagnosis can be made by microscopic examination of an endocervical specimen.

Medications

1. Doxycycline 100mg orally twice a day for seven days or
2. Tetracycline 500mg orally four times a day for seven days
3. During pregnancy, erythromycin 500mg orally four times a day for seven days or
4. Erythromycin ethyl succinate 400 to 800mg orally four times a day for seven days.

Because neonatal infection rates of infants of untreated women approach 50%, all women diagnosed during pregnancy should receive treatment. Their sexual partners must be treated simultaneously, otherwise the women can be reinfected. The follow-up culture should be performed 7 to 14 days after treatment is completed.[8a]

Patients with PID being treated with cephalosporin must also be given an agent effective against chlamydia, such as doxycycline or erythromycin.

HUMAN PAPILLOMAVIRUS (GENITAL WARTS)

Aetiology, Epidemiology, and Pathophysiology

Genital warts caused by the HPV are important because of their possible role in the development of cervical cancer. In 1987 there were 8,400 cases of genital warts in the United Kingdom. Genital warts occur in or around the vulva, vagina, cervix, perineum, anal canal, urethra, and glans penis. They enlarge during pregnancy and may cause haemorrhage or obstruction during delivery. The disease is most common in adolescent girls and young women. The HPV can remain dormant for decades before recurrences appear.

Diagnosis

Diagnosis is made by clinical appearance or histological examination.

Treatment

Cryotherapy is recommended as the treatment of choice. Podophyllum, which was previously recommended, is less effective and is toxic if applied to a wide area at one time. It still may be used in a 15% solution in compound benzoin tincture to treat one or two lesions. Neither treatment cures the disease.

HERPES GENITALIS

Aetiology, Epidemiology, and Pathophysiology

Herpes genitalis (genital herpes, HSV-2) is caused by infection with Herpes simplex virus type 2 (HSV-2). Herpes genitalis was the most important STD of the 1970s. Its chronicity, frequent recurrences, and difficult treatment and prevention distinguish it from other STDs. In 1990 there were in excess of 20,000 new cases of herpes in the United Kingdom.[45a] Its peak incidence parallels the young age groups affected by other STDs. Once acquired, herpes genitalis is a lifelong disease and carries with it not only intense and recurrent discomfort, but also anxieties about future childbearing, malignancy, and sexual function. In early pregnancy, women infected with herpes have an increased chance of miscarriage. Because genital herpetic lesions endanger the fetus during delivery, caesarean delivery is often necessary. Genital herpes has also been associated with cervical cancer. It is now generally accepted that HSV-2 is spread by sexual contact.

The incubation period is three to seven days. The primary lesion appears as a vesicle on the external genitalia in men; often in the rectum in homosexual men; and on the vagina, cervix, or external genitalia in women. These lesions often ulcerate, especially when located on moist surfaces. Following primary herpes, the virus persists in a *latent* or *unrecognized* form in most patients. It is believed that latent infections are localized in the ganglia of sensory nerves to the genitalia. When the host factors favour it, the *latent infection* becomes clinically apparent as *recurrent herpes*.

Signs and symptoms

The common signs and symptoms of primary herpetic infection are the following:

1. Local inflammation
2. Pain
3. Enlargement of inguinal lymph nodes
4. Generalized signs of infection
   a. Photophobia
   b. Headache
   c. Flu-like symptoms.

Although primary herpetic lesions begin as single or multiple reddish papules that then develop into clear, fluid-filled vesicles, once they rupture they form ulcerations that may fuse with other lesions to form large ulcerated areas. The disease tends to be more extensive in women than in men. In some women cervical infection accompanies the external lesions, and in certain cases it may be the only infected site. Cervical involvement may be mild or severe with extensive ulceration and pus. Genital lesions often worsen during the first 10 to 15 days but usually heal within three to four weeks. These symptoms usually lead the individual to seek medical attention.

Vaginal discharge is common among women, and discharge from the urethra is usual in men having primary infections. Urinary tract involvement may occur and is reflected in symptoms of dysuria or urinary retention. The lesions can cause severe pain, requiring hospitalization for parenteral analgesia. Subclinical infections in which patients are unaware of any problem occur in only about 10% of the cases of genital herpes. Unfortunately, about 75% of all patients have at least one recurrence. Fortunately, recurrent infections are usually milder and of shorter duration than primary infections and usually produce local rather than systemic reaction. The patient experiencing a recurrent infection often has prodromal signs of paraesthesia and burning at the site where the lesion will erupt. Factors known to predispose to recurrent infection include fever, emotional upsets, premenstrual states, and overexposure to heat and sunshine. Although the mode of recurrent infection is not clear, it has been theorized that during primary infection the virus ascends sensory nerve sheaths, localizing in corresponding nerve ganglia, and that when the environment becomes favourable, the virus is reactivated. Recurrent herpes usually begins with abnormal sensation or itching of a localized genital area. Lesions of recurrent infections usually occur at the site of the primary infection. Herpes encephalitis may also occur.

Diagnostic tests

Diagnosis of herpes genitalis is made by isolation of the virus from specimens obtained from lesions. Cervical smears or fluid from the vesicles collected in transport medium demonstrates cellular characteristics of viruses.

Treatment

Treatment for genital herpes has most often been symptomatic, because there is no known cure for the disease. Acyclovir appears capable of inhibiting the replication of herpetic viruses *in vitro*; in clinical trials with patients who had antibodies against herpes simplex viruses, acyclovir prevented active herpes infections. Acyclovir ointment, 5%, is recommended for genital herpes. The ointment is applied to cover all lesions every four hours, five times a day for 5 to 10 days. The acyclovir treatment reduces viral shedding and the duration of the disease in patients with primary initial infections who are treated early before the onset of symptoms. It does not prevent recurrences. There is no effective treatment to prevent recurrences or to shorten their duration.

Symptomatic treatment consists of using hydrogen peroxide and soap and water to cleanse the lesions. The involved areas are blown dry with a hair dryer, and the skin is then dusted with cornflour. Women are advised to use a mirror and speculum to examine the vulva, vagina, and cervix for hidden lesions.

HEPATITIS B

Aetiology/epidemiology

In the United Kingdom, hepatitis B is frequently transmitted by sexual contact. People at high risk for sexual transmission of HBV include homosexual/bisexual men, heterosexual men and women with multiple sex partners, and sexual partners of injecting drug users.

Aetiology is established by serological testing. Most people with acute viral hepatitis are asymptomatic. Because there is no specific treatment for HBV, emphasis is placed on prevention.

Prevention and Health Education
Primary prevention

Vaccination is recommended for all the people identified above as being at high risk. In addition, residents of correctional or long-term care facilities, people seeking treatment for STDs, and prostitutes should be vaccinated. Vaccination is also recommended for healthcare workers because of the possibility of needle-sticks.

Secondary prevention

It is recommended that *postexposure prophylactic treatment* with hepatitis B immune globulin (HBIG) should be considered in the following situations: sexual contact with a person who has active hepatitis B or who contracts hepatitis B, and sexual contact with a hepatitis B carrier (blood test positive for hepatitis B surface antigen: HBsAg). The prophylactic treatment should be given within 14 days of sexual contact.

Because pregnant women can transmit HBV to their infants at delivery, HBIG and hepatitis B vaccine is given to the infant after birth. All pregnant women should be screened during their first obstetric visit for the presence of HBsAg. If they are HBsAg positive, their newborns should be given HBIG as soon as possible after birth and subsequently immunized with hepatitis B vaccine. The HBIG is also given to healthcare workers who suffer a needle-stick. For more information about hepatitis see Chapter 22.

SUMMARY

1. Premenstrual syndrome (PMS) consists of behavioural changes, fluid retention, fatigue, headache, backache, or increased appetite, which occurs repeatedly in many women before and during menstruation.
2. Dysmenorrhoea is a common cause of absenteeism from work or school. Interventions include prostaglandin inhibitors, rest, heat applications, and moderate exercise.
3. Methods of sterilization include tubal ligation in the female and vasectomy in the male; although sterilization may be reversed in some cases, this is not always successful.
4. Infertility may result from obstructed fallopian tubes or vas deferens, from uterine or testicular disorders, or from hormonal deficiencies. Couples who are assessed as infertile need support in coping with the infertility

and in examining alternative strategies (remain childless, adopt, artificial insemination, in vitro fertilization, GIFT, ZIFT, and mother surrogate).

5. Genital infections occur most often in females with low oestrogen levels, who are malnourished, who have alkaline vaginal secretions, or who have been exposed to large numbers of organisms. Good personal hygiene, protection from infected sexual partners, and avoidance of unprescribed douching can help to prevent genital infections.

6. Pelvic inflammatory disease (PID) is a widespread inflammation of female pelvic organs; spread is up the genital tract. Chronic PID may cause adhesions requiring removal of some of the organs.

7. In the male, the common genital inflammatory disorders are urethritis, prostatitis, epididymitis (most common), and orchitis. Bilateral epididymitis usually causes sterility.

8. Common *benign* genital tumours in the female include ovarian cysts and tumours, uterine fibroid tumours, cervical polyps, and endometriosis (seeding of endometrial cells in the pelvis). Cervical polyps are removed for biopsy. Uterine fibroid tumours are removed only when growth is rapid or when size is causing other difficulties.

9. Removal of the uterus (hysterectomy) ends menstruation but does not lead to menopausal symptoms if the ovaries are left intact.

10. The most common genital cancer in females is cancer of the endometrium, occurring primarily in postmenopausal women. However, ovarian cancer causes more deaths than uterine cancer. The incidence of cancer of the cervix has decreased because of better screening by means of Pap smears.

11. Women should have a Pap test at least every 3 years after two initial negative tests 1 year apart. People at high risk for cervical cancer (early sexual activity, multiple sex partners) should have more frequent Pap tests.

12. Most genital cancers in males are prostatic cancers occurring primarily in men over age 60. Young men have a higher incidence of cancer of the testes, that can be detected early by testes self-examination (TSE).

13. The term *STDs* refers to diseases that are usually transmitted by heterosexual or homosexual intercourse.

14. The three venereal diseases are gonorrhoea, syphilis, and chancroid.

15. A major concern in the treatment of gonorrhoea is the increased resistance of the organism to penicillin and other antibiotics.

16. Gonorrhoea in women is often asymptomatic and is only diagnosed when complications such as salpingitis occur.

17. Herpes genitalis is a lifelong disease with no cure. It can be transmitted to the fetus during delivery and thus caesarean delivery is often recommended.

18. Treatment for herpes genitalis is symptomatic, and topical acyclovir applied to the lesions reduces viral shedding and the duration of disease. It does not prevent recurrences.

19. *Chlamydia trachomatis* infections are recognized as the most prevalent STD in the United Kingdom.

20. Condylomata accuminata (genital warts) is caused by the papillomavirus; it is most common in adolescent girls and young women.

21. Genital warts are of particular concern because they can undergo malignant changes after a latent period of 5 to 40 years.

22. In the United Kingdom, hepatitis B is often transmitted by sexual contact.

23. It is recommended that all people at high risk for hepatitis B be vaccinated. This includes healthcare workers because of the possibility of needle-sticks.

STUDY QUESTIONS

• What are the similarities and differences between genital inflammations in women and in men in terms of method of infection, types of organisms, and usual therapy? What is a serious side effect of PID and of bilateral orchitis?

• Compare the incidences of the different types of genital cancers in both sexes. Which cancers occur more frequently? Why are cervical cancers identified earlier than ovarian cancers? What effect does this have?

• Why do body image disturbances occur frequently after genital surgery in women and men? What implications does this have for nursing?

• What services are available in your community for detection and treatment of STDs?

• In what form are human sexuality and prevention of STDs taught in your local schools?

• Describe the nurse's role in working with people with a newly diagnosed STD.

REFERENCES AND SELECTED READINGS

1. American Cancer Society, *Cancer facts and figures,* 1991, Atlanta, 1991, The Society.

2. Barbo DM, editor: Symposium on the postmenopausal woman, *Med Clin North Am* 71(1):1-148, 1987.

3.* Berger PH et al: Radical hysterectomy: treatment for ad-vanced cervical carcinoma, *AORN J* 52:1212-1218, 1990.

4.* Boarini JH, Bryant RA, Ingang SF: Fistula management, *Semin Oncol Nurs* 2:287-292, 1986.

5. Boyd AS: Varicoceles and male infertility, *Am Fam Physician* 37:252-258, 1988.

6.* Cashavelly BJ: Cervical dysplasia: an overview of current concepts in epidemiology, diagnosis, and treatment, *Cancer Nurs* 10:199-206, 1987.

7. Centers for Disease Control: Pelvic inflammatory disease: guidelines for prevention and management, *MMWR* 40(RR-5):1-25, 1991.

8. Chamorro T: Cancer of the vulva and vagina, *Semin Oncol Nurs* 6(3):198-205, 1990.

8a. Faro S: *Chlamydia trachomatis* infection. In Rakel RE *Conn's current therapy 1991,* Philadelphia, 1991, WB Saunders, pp 1012-1014.

9. Davis DC, Dearman CN: Coping strategies of infertile women, *J Obstet Gynecol Neonatal Nurs* 20(3):221-227, 1991.

10.* Doane LS, Fischer LM, McDonald TW: How to give peritoneal chemotherapy, *Am J Nurs* 90(4):58-64, 1990.

11. Dodek OI: The infertile couple, *Am Fam Physician* 38:101-112, 1988.

12.* Dulaney PE, Crawford VC, Turner G: A comprehensive education and support program for women experiencing hysterectomies, *J Obstet Gynecol Neonatal Nurs* 19(4):319-325, 1990.

13. Eriksson JH, Walczak JR: Ovarian cancer, *Semin Oncol Nurs* 6(3):214-227, 1990.

14. Feldman JE: Ovarian failure and cancer treatment: incidence and interventions for the premenopausal woman, *Oncol Nurs Forum* 16:651-657, 1989.

14a. *Healthy People 2000: National health promotion and disease prevention objectives*, U.S. Dept. of Health and Human Services, Public Health Service, Washington, DC, 1990.

15.* Fehring RJ: Methods used to self-predict ovulation: a comparative study, *J Obstet Gynecol Neonatal Nurs* 19(3):233-237, 1990.

16.* Fehring RJ: New technology in natural family planning, *J Obstet Gynecol Neonatal Nurs* 20(3):199-205, 1991.

17. Frank DI: Factors related to decisions about infertility treatment, *J Obstet Gynecol Neonatal Nurs* 19(2):162-167, 1990.

18.* Frank EP: What are nurses doing to help PMS patients? *Am J Nurs* 86:136-140, 1986.

19. Fullerton JT: Papanicolaou smear: an update on classifi-cation and management, *J Am Acad Nurse Pract* 1(3): 84-90, 1989.

20.* Ginsberg CK: Exfoliative cytologic screening: the Papanicolaou test, *J Obstet Gynecol Neonatal Nurs* 20(1):39-46, 1991.

21.* Hampton BG: Nursing management of a patient follow-ing pelvic exenteration, *Semin Oncol Nurs* 2:275-286,1986.

21a. Hancook B, Bradshaw JD: *Lecture notes on clinical oncology*, London, 1992, Blackwell Scientific Publications Ltd.

22. Hatcher RA et al: *Contraceptive technology 1988-1989*, ed 14, New York,1989, Irvington.

23.* Henderson JS, Taylor KH: Age as a variable in an exercise program for the treatment of simple urinary stress incontinence, *J Obstet Gynecol Neonatal Nurs* 13:266-272, 1987.

24.* Higgs DJ: The patient with testicular cancer: nursing management of chemotherapy, *Oncol Nurs Forum* 17(2):243-249, 1990.

25.* Hubbard JL, Holcombe JK: Cancer of the endometrium, *Semin Oncol Nurs* 6(3):206-213, 1990.

26.* Jenkins B: Patients' report of sexual changes after treat-ment of gynecologic cancer, *Oncol Nurs Forum* 15(3):349-354, 1988.

26a. Noble RC: *Syphilis*. In Rakel RE: *Conn's current therapy, 1991*, Philadelphia, 1991, WB Saunders Co, pp 685-688.

27. Keye WR: Premenstrual symptoms: evaluation and treatment, *Compr Ther* 14:19-26, 1988.

27a. King Edward's Hospital Fund for London: *The Nation's Health: A Strategy for the 1990's*, London, 1991, The King's Fund Centre.

28. Kirkpatrick MK, Brewer JA, Stocks B: Efficacy of self-care measures for perimenstrual syndrome (PMS), *J Adv Nurs* 15:281-285, 1990.

29.* Lamb MA: Psychosexual issues: the woman with gynecologic cancer, *Semin Oncol Nurs* 6(3):237-243, 1990.

30.* Lasater SJ: Testicular cancer: a perioperative challenge, *AORN J* 51(2):513-523, 1990.

31. Lavy G: Hysteroscopy as a diagnostic aid, *Obstet Gynecol Clin North Am* 15:61-72, 1988.

32.* Lincoln R, Roberts R: Continence issues in acute care, *Nurs Clin North Am* 24(3):741-754, 1990.

33.* Lindow KB: Premenstrual syndrome: family impact and nursing implications, *J Obstet Gynecol Neonatal Nurs* 20(2):135-138, 1991.

33a. Smith CE, McAllister CK: *Gonorrhea*. In Rakel RE: *Conn's current therapy 1991*, Philadelphia, 1991, WB Saunders.

34. Lindsay R: The menopause: sex, steroids, and osteoporosis, *Clin Obstet Gynec* 95:963-972, 1987.

35.* Martin FL: When the solution is a prosthesis, *RN* 53(3):32-35, 1990.

36.* Martin JP: Transrectal ultrasound: a new screening tool for prostate cancer, *Am J Nurs* 91(2):69, 1991.

37.* McKeon VA: Cruel myths and clinical facts about menopause, *RN* 52(6):52-59, 1989.

37a. McOwen J. *Practice of Medicine 14th edition*, 1984, Churchill Livingstone.

38.* Menken J, Trussell J, Larsen V: Age and infertility, *Science* 233:1389-1394, 1986.

38a. US Department of Health and Human Services, Public Health Service: Antibiotic-resistant strains of *Neisseria gonorrhoeae*: policy guidelines, *MMWR* 36(5S):1S-18S, 1987.

39.* Milne BJ: Couples' experience with in vitro fertilization, *J Obstet Gynecol Neonatal Nurs* 17:347-351, 1988.

40.* Moore J: Vaginal hysterectomy: its success as an outpatient procedure, *AORN J* 48(6):1114-1120, 1988.

40a.* Moore S et al: Nerve sparing prostatectomy, *Am J Nurs* 92(4):59-64, 1992.

41.* Nolte S, Hanjani P: Intraepithelial neoplasia of the lower genital tract, *Semin Oncol Nurs* 6(3):181-189, 1990.

42. O'Laughlin KM: Changes in bladder function in the woman undergoing radical hysterectomy for cervical cancer, *J Obstet Gynecol Neonatal Nurs* 15:380-385, 1986.

43.* Pace-Owen S: Gamete intrafallopian transfer (GIFT), *J Obstet Gynecol Neonatal Nurs* 18:93-97, 1989.

44. Persinger C: Carcinoma of the penis, *J Urol Nurs* 7(2):398-407, 1988.

45. Pernoll ML, Benson RC: *Current obstetric and gynecologic diagnosis and treatment*, ed 7, Norwalk, Conn, 1991, Appleton & Lange.

45a.* US Public Health Service, 1989 STD treatment guidelines, *MMWR* (suppl) 38(8):Sept 1, 1989.

46.* Reznichek CG, Reznichek R: The problem most men won't talk about: impotence, *RN* 54(3):28-32, 1990.

47.* Rubin D: Gynecologic cancer: cervical, vulvular and vaginal malignancies, *RN* 50(5):56-63, 1987. 46.* Reznichek CG, Reznichek R: The problem most men won't talk about: impotence, *RN* 54(3):28-32, 1990.

48.* Rubin D: Gynecologic cancer: uterine and ovarian malignancies, *RN* 50(6):52-57, 1987.

49. Sampselle CM: Changes in pelvic muscle strength and stress urinary incontinence associated with childbirth, *J Obstet Gynecol Neonatal Nurs* 19(5):371-377, 1990.

49a. Darrow WW: Changes in sexual behavior and venereal disease, *Clin Obstet Gynecol* 18:255-267, 1975.

50. Schover LR et al: Sexual dysfunction and treatment for early stage cervical cancer, *Cancer* 63(1):204-212, 1989.

51. Schroeder SA et al: *Current medical diagnosis and treatment*, ed 30, Norwalk, Conn, 1991, Appleton & Lange.

52.* Secor RMC: Bacterial vaginosis: a comprehensive review, *Nurs Clin North Am* 23:865-875, 1988.

53. Shattuck JC: Pelvic inflammatory disease: education for maintaining fertility, *Nurs Clin North Am* 23(4):899-906, 1988.

54. Speroff L, Glass RH, Kase N: *Clinical gynecologic endocrinology and infertility*, ed 4, Baltimore, 1989, Williams & Wilkins.

55.* Thompson LJ: Cancer of the cervix, *Semin Oncol Nurs* 6(3):190-197, 1990.

56.* Tinkle MB: Genital human papillomavirus infection: a growing health risk, *J Obstet Gynecol Neonatal Nurs* 19(6):501-507, 1990.

57. Velduis JD: Management of amenorrhea, *Hosp Pract* 23(11A):40-56, 1988.

58. Way L: *Current surgical diagnosis and treatment*, ed 9, Norwalk, Conn, 1991, Appleton & Lange.

59. Yoder LH: The epidemiology of ovarian cancer: a review, *Oncol Nurs Forum* 17(3):411-415, 1990.

60.* Zion AB: Resources for infertile couples, *J Obstet Gynecol Neonatal Nurs* 17:255-258, 1988.

FURTHER READING

Adler MW: *ABC of sexually transmitted diseases*, ed 2, London, 1990, British Medical Journal Publications.

Barton SE, Taylor-Robinson D, Harris JRW: Female prostitutes and sexually transmitted diseases, *Br J Hosp Med* 7:34-45, 1987.

Beardsley J: Education to undermine a taboo. Understanding herpes simplex virus, *Professional Nurse* 8(5):322-328, 1993.

Cameron S, Peacock W, Trotter G: Reaching out, *Nurs Times* 89 (7):34-36, 1993.

Csonka GW, Oates JK: *Sexually transmitted diseases. A text book of genitourinary medicine*, London, 1990, Bailliere Tindall.

Gould D: Assessing menstrual cycle function, *Nursing Standard* 6(23):24-7, Feb 26-Mar 3, 1992.

Ratliff DR: Nursing management of vaginal fistulas, *Oncology Nursing Forum*, 18(3):601-2, April, 1991.

Riedmann GL: The fertility history card: clinical use in improving contraceptive efficacy, *J Nurse-Midwifery* 33(1): 15-24, Jan-Feb, 1988.

Thin RN: *Lecture notes on sexually transmitted diseases*, Oxford, 1989, Blackwell Scientific Publications.

Von Hagens G, Romrell L, Ross M, Tiedmann K: *The visible human body: An atlas of sectional anatomy*, London, 1991, Lea and Febiger.

---

*Recommended for student reading.

28

The Patient with Problems of the Breast

Barbara C. Long

After studying this chapter, the learner should be able to:

- Evaluate breast self-examination (guidelines, techniques).
- Differentiate between benign and malignant breast disorders.
- Describe the pathophysiology and interventions for women with benign breast disorders.
- Explain the risk factors and pathophysiology of breast cancer.
- Describe the types of surgery for breast cancer, most common procedures, and postoperative care.
- Describe types of breast reconstruction and required care.

Guidelines for breast self-examination

1. Perform BSE regularly each month
   a. Premenopausal women: 7 to 8 days after conclusion of the menstrual period
   b. Postmenopausal women: at a set time each month (such as the first day of the month)
2. Use a systematic approach (one of the three listed here)
   a. Palpate in concentric circles beginning at outer rim of breast tissue and move towards nipple
   b. Divide breast into quadrants and examine area in each quadrant from outer perimeter towards nipple
   c. Palpate inner half then outer half of breast
3. Examine the entire breast tissue, including the tail (Fig. 28-1) and the nipple
4. Carry out examination in both the horizontal and vertical body positions (Fig. 28-2)
5. Use the flat parts of the fingers for palpation

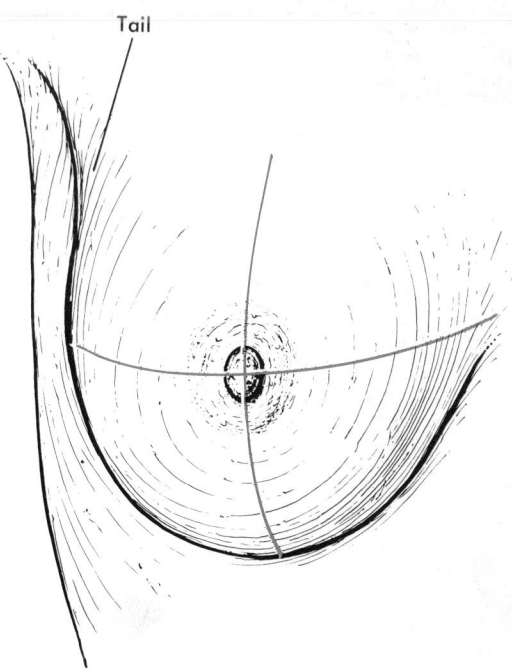

Tail

Fig. 28-1   Breast mass includes "tail" that extends from upper, outer quadrant towards axilla. (From Malasanos L, et al: *Health assessment*, ed 4, St Louis, 1990, Mosby–Year Book.)

The breasts are associated with feelings of sexuality and are an integral component of sexual behaviour. The development of the breasts in the female adolescent indicates her approaching womanhood and emphasizes her femininity. The breast, especially the nipples, which are erectile tissue, are erogenous areas in sexual activity. The advertising media emphasize the desirability of the female breast; femininity is typified by a fashion model's breasts, whereas masculinity is typified by the flat, expansive chest of the lifeguard. Diseases of the breast, therefore, evoke varied feelings and cause fears and concerns that influence the practice of breast self-examination or the seeking of diagnostic and therapeutic care.

ANATOMY AND PHYSIOLOGY

The breasts lie over the pectoralis muscles of the chest. Each breast is composed of 12 to 20 lobes of glandular tissue separated by connective tissue. The lobes are held in place by suspensory ligaments connected both to the skin and to the underlying fascia. The milk gland ducts in each lobe join to form a larger duct that terminates in a small hole in the nipple. The glandular tissue is surrounded by fat that determines the size of the breasts. Lymphatic drainage of the breasts is primarily to the axillary nodes but some lymph also drains towards substernal and diaphragmatic nodes.

The breasts are associated functionally with the reproductive system as an organ for milk production in the postpartum woman. The female sex hormones influence the development of the breasts and the production of milk.

Physiological Changes With Ageing

As fat decreases and tissue atrophies with age, the breasts generally become smaller and hang more loosely. The nipples become smaller and flatter. The breasts may feel more granular with palpation.

PREVENTION AND HEALTH EDUCATION
Primary Prevention: Avoidance of Common Breast Problems
Premenstrual breast discomfort

Tenderness, discomfort, and swelling of the breasts before menstruation are normal functional changes in the breasts that respond to monthly cyclical changes in oestrogen and progesterone. Water retention contributes to the swelling. Women who experience some of these problems can be taught to reduce dietary salt intake during the immediate premenstrual period. Increased physical activity during this time will improve cardiovascular dynamics and help reduce the tight, puffy feeling.

Breast discomfort during physical activity

Bras provide support for the breasts and help prevent sagging and pulling on the underlying muscles. All but small-breasted women may find physical activity uncomfortable unless a bra is worn. A *jogbra*, which does not contain metal clips or fasteners and which has seams on the outside of the fabric away from the skin, may provide greater comfort for physical activity.

Secondary Prevention: Early Detection of Malignancy
Examination of the breast

Mortality from breast cancer can be prevented in many instances through early diagnosis and treatment. It is generally recommended that examination of the breast occurs as follows:

1. Monthly breast self-examination by *all* women over 20 years of age

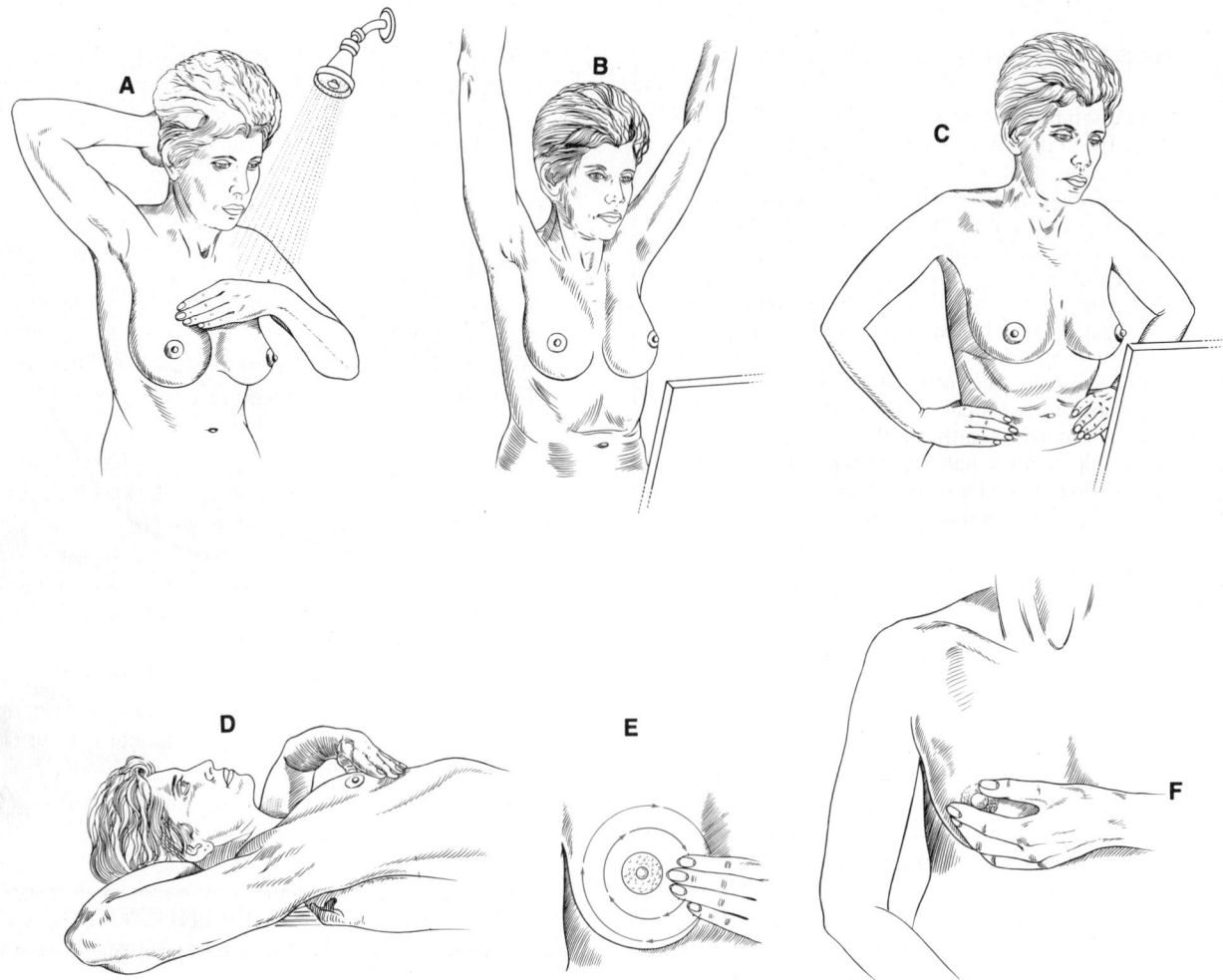

Fig. 28-2   Breast self-examination. **A,** Examine breasts during bath or shower, since flat fingers glide easily over wet skin. Use right hand to examine left breast and vice versa. **B,** Sit or stand before a mirror. Inspect breasts with hands at sides, then raised overhead. Look for changes in contour or dimpling of skin. **C,** Place hands on hips and press down firmly to flex chest muscles. **D,** Lie down with one hand under head and pillow or folded towel under the scapula. **E,** Palpate that breast with other hand using concentric circle method. It usually takes three circles to cover all breast tissue. Include the tail of the breast and the axilla. Repeat with other breast. **F,** End in a sitting position. Palpate the areola areas of both breasts, and inspect and squeeze nipples to check for discharge.

2. Women at high risk before age 50: mammography yearly; breast examination by a doctor every 2 years
3. Women 20 to 40
   a. One baseline mammogram on post menopausal women
   b. Breast examination by a doctor every 3 years
4. Women 40 to 49: breast examination by a doctor and mammography every 1 to 2 years (the newest recommendations are mammography yearly after age 40)
5. Women over 50: breast examination by a doctor and mammography yearly

Studies have shown that the groups of women who are least likely to have regular breast examinations by a doctor are elderly, poorly educated, low-income, and black. Some of the reasons are as follows:

Lack of knowledge
Low priority set on preventive measures
Fear of finding a tumour
Concern over possibility of breast removal
Fear of death
Possible life changes if breast cancer is found
Embarrassment
Examination is considered too trivial for a busy doctor

Most breast cancers (about 90%) are discovered by self-examination. Breast cancer is usually curable when discovered early and treated immediately. All women, beginning at high school age, should know how to carry out breast self-examination.

Breast self-examination (BSE)

Nurses working in the hospital or community settings have the responsibility of teaching women how to examine their breasts and of explaining why it is necessary. Patients can be asked during the admission history if they practise BSE, and necessary instructions can be given when feasible.

Women need to have opportunities to *practise* doing BSE while receiving feedback from the nurse on correct technique and interpretation of any palpable findings. Practice makes women feel more confident about doing BSE, and they are then more apt to practise BSE on a regular basis. Guidelines for BSE are listed in Box 28-1.

When working with groups of women, arrangements can be made with Family Health Service Associations (FHSA) for showing movies developed for the general public describing the traditional method of self-examination. Models of breasts are available for women to practise palpation of lumps.

Some women have engorgement of the breast premenstrually, and the breasts normally may have a lumpy consistency at this time. The condition usually disappears a few days after the onset of menstruation.

DIAGNOSTIC TESTS FOR BREAST EVALUATION
Radiographs
Mammography

Mammography is an X-ray examination of the breast used to detect early lesions before they are palpable (Fig. 28-3). Mammography is about 90% accurate in detecting early breast cancer. It does have limitations, particularly in the penetration of dense breasts as in adolescents, young nulliparous women, or women with large breasts. A *low-energy*

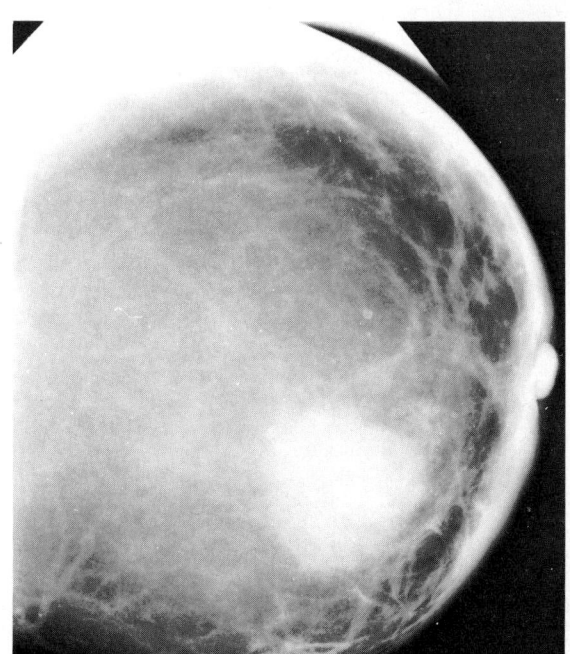

Fig. 28-3   Mammogram of patient with area of density indicating carcinoma. (From Cramer LN, Lapoyowker MS: *Applied anatomy of the female breast: surgical, radiographic, and thermographic.* In Masters FW, Lewis JR Jr: *Symposium of aesthetic surgery of the face, eyelid, and breast,* vol 4, St Louis, 1972, Mosby–Year Book.)

X-ray beam is used to delineate the breast structures; this radiation dose is acceptable for use in frequent reexaminations. During the examination the breast is pressed firmly against the film holder, causing momentary mild discomfort, and several films are taken of each breast.

Xeroradiography

Xeroradiography is similar to mammography except that an aluminium plate with an electrically charged selenium layer is used in place of the familiar black and white mammogram X-ray film. The resulting film is blue and white (Fig. 28-4). Xeroradiography is thought to provide sharper contrast of blood vessel patterns and tissue densities.

Ultrasonography

Ultrasound may be helpful in detecting lesions in the dense breasts of young women. Although ultrasound can differentiate the presence of a cystic mass, it does not indicate calcium deposits or tissue configurations, facts considered important in the diagnosis of malignant tumours. Ultrasound is used primarily to differentiate solid and cystic masses and to locate cysts that are difficult to palpate before needle aspiration.

Aspiration

Aspiration of an identified soft breast mass may be performed if a cyst is suspected. A large-bore needle is inserted into the mass and the contents withdrawn and sent to the laboratory for cytological studies. Cysts usually contain a brownish-greenish fluid. The only discomfort is associated with insertion of the needle. If cytology tests are positive, a biopsy is performed. If the tests are negative and there are characteristics of cystic disease, no further tests are performed. If there are some doubts, despite the negative results, further radiographical studies may be performed.

Breast Biopsy

Biopsy is the only way to determine conclusively whether a tumour is benign or malignant. Most lesions (80%) are found to be benign.

The procedure is usually performed with a patient under local or general anaesthesia in an ambulatory surgical suite. An incision is made and a portion of the mass (or the entire mass if it is very small) is removed and sent to the laboratory for examination. Following the procedure the patient may experience mild discomfort. Results will be available immediately if a frozen section is done, or within 48 to 72 hours.

Sometimes the small lesion size makes location of the lesion difficult or uncertain when biopsy is attempted. Therefore, to locate areas for surgical biopsy, a small methylene blue dye mark is made within the area of the breast using a syringe and needle during mammographic monitoring (needle localization). This is done in the X-ray department a few hours before the surgical biopsy, and the mark is made while the patient is under local anaesthesia. No colour disfiguration is apparent on the breast surface as a result of this procedure, but the mark ensures that the biopsy tissue corresponds to the site identified by

mammogram. This procedure requires preinstruction to the patient and support in the X-ray department.

Breast lesions may be benign or malignant. Although benign lesions are more common, cancer of the breast is a major type of cancer in women and requires much more nursing care. Therefore, cancer of the breast is discussed in more detail. Breast disorders occur primarily in women, but *they can also occur in men*.

BENIGN BREAST DISORDERS

The major benign breast disorders are fibrocystic in nature (mammary dysplasia, cysts), benign tumours (fibroadenomas), or infections (mastitis with or without breast abscess) (Table 28-1). The most common disease of the breast is mammary dysplasia.

Pathophysiology

Benign breast disorders are usually characterized by one or more movable breast masses, often seen bilaterally (Fig. 28-5). The nodularity may be discrete or diffuse. If tenderness is present, it usually occurs or is increased premenstrually. Any nipple discharge, which may be clear, green, or brownish (but not bloody), is usually spontaneous, especially just before menstruation. Women who take oral contraceptives may experience some nipple discharge that ceases when the pill is discontinued.

Males may have overdevelopment of breast tissue (gynaecomastia) as a result of oestrogen production during puberty or older age, adrenal or gonadal tumours, or certain drugs, for example, amphetamines, antidepressants (tricyclic), antihypertensive agents, antineoplastic agents, cimetidine, diazepam, digitalis, oestrogen, human chorionic gonadotropin, isoniazid, and phenothiazines.

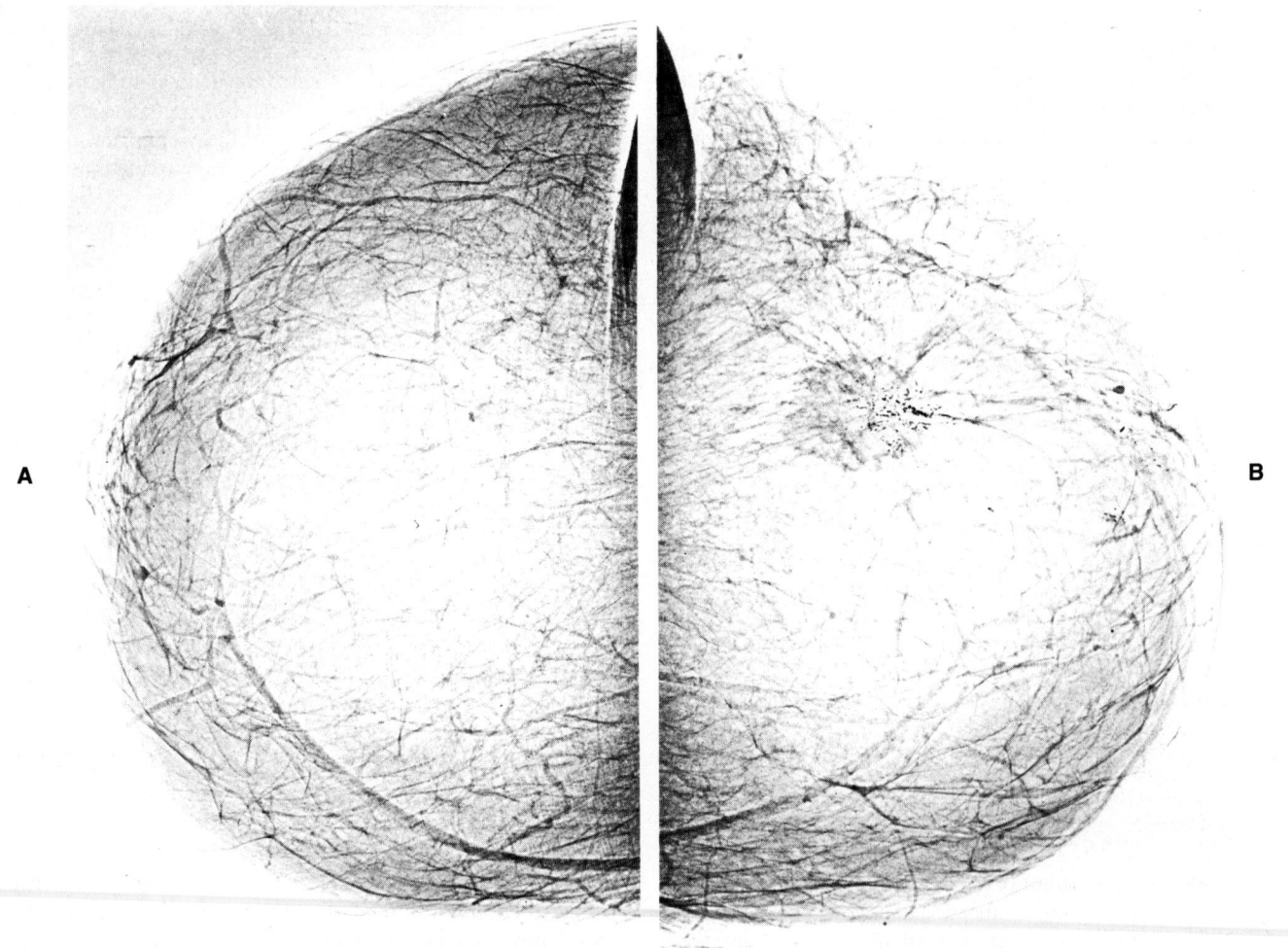

Fig. 28-4 Xeroradiographs. **A,** Normal left breast. **B,** Right breast shows mass with spiculated margins characteristic of neoplasm. (Courtesy University Hospitals of Cleveland, Ohio.)

<u>REVIEW</u>
Table 28-1   Benign breast disorders

Disorder	Characteristics	Signs and symptoms	Medical therapy
Mammary dysplasia (fibrocystic disease)	Refers to several cystic nodular disorders of the breast that become painful during menstruation; seen mostly in women age 30 to 50; oestrogen hormone a causative factor	Painful, often multiple and bilateral soft masses in breast; may increase in size or remain the same	Aspiration of probable cyst; biopsy of doubtful cyst to confirm diagnosis; yearly mammograms; intermittent diuretics for premenstrual breast engorgement; symptomatic pain relief
Fibroadenoma	Fibroplastic tumours commonly seen in young women under age 25	Firm, round, freely movable, nontender mass in breast	Surgical excision with patient under local anaesthesia on outpatient basis
Mastitis	Inflammation of breast, usually from cracked or infected nipples	Pain, redness, swelling of breast, fever	Systemic antibiotics; incision and drainage if an abscess forms; symptomatic pain relief

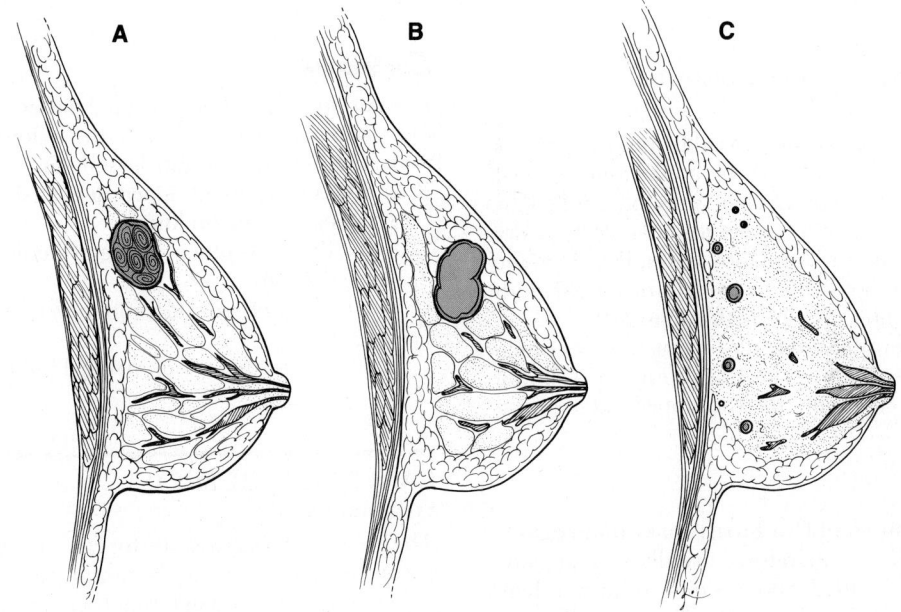

Fig. 28-5   Benign breast disorders. **A,** Fibroadenoma. **B,** Cyst. **C,** Adenosis (mammary dysplasia).

Nursing Process
Assessment

Data are collected concerning the person's feelings and knowledge about the disorder, including the following:

1. Concerns about the mass
2. Knowledge of benign versus malignant tumours
3. Knowledge regarding breast self-examination
4. Presence of discomfort

Nursing analysis

Nursing analyses are determined from assessment of patient data. Possible nursing problems for the person with a benign breast disorder may include, but are not limited to, the following:

Problem	Possible aetiologies
Pain	Breast disorder
Anxiety	Fear of cancer
Knowledge deficit	Lack of information/recall, information misinterpretation

Planning: expected patient outcomes

Expected patient outcomes for the person with a benign breast disorder may include, but are not limited to, the following:

1. Reports breasts feel more comfortable.
2. Signs of anxiety are decreased.
3. Demonstrates correct technique for BSE.
4. Describes:

Table 28-2   Differences between benign and malignant breast masses

Benign	Malignant
Usually bilateral; may be unilateral	Unilateral
Found often in outer quadrants but may occur anywhere	Found most often in upper outer quadrant and tail or in central nipple portion
Single or multiple	Usually single
Well-circumscribed	Irregular
Soft or firm	Firm
Movable	Nonmovable
Usually have cyclic tenderness; may be nontender	Nontender
No skin changes	Later findings: skin thickened; dimpling
	Very late: ulceration
No palpable lymph nodes	Palpable lymph nodes except in early period
No nipple retraction; discharge usually bilateral, serous, or greenish	Nipple retraction; discharge usually unilateral and may be bloody

a. Difference between benign and malignant breast disease
b. Plans to do monthly BSE
c. Plans for yearly medical follow-up

Implementation

Interventions to achieve patient outcomes
Assisting with comfort

Breast discomfort may be decreased by mild analgesics (such as aspirin or paracetamol), by application of heat or cold, or by breast support. Heat may be applied by application of a warm damp washcloth covered by a dry towel and heating pad or warm hot water bottle. Some women experience relief from an ice bag or a washcloth wrung out in cold water (especially for mastitis).

Wearing a firm bra both day and night may also help to relieve breast discomfort. The bra should fit well and give good support, especially for the upper outer breast quadrant.[65]

Reducing anxiety

Most women who identify a breast mass immediately think of cancer and are, therefore, usually very anxious until the diagnosis is verified. Spouses or significant others may also experience anxiety. Even after being told that the condition is benign, some women continue to have some anxiety. *Mild* anxiety is useful as this acts as a stimulus for continuing medical follow-up.

The woman who is moderately or severely anxious needs an opportunity to express her concerns to an empathic listener. As the anxiety decreases, the woman is better able to deal with any discomfort and continue her usual activities.

Facilitating learning

The risk of breast cancer in women with mammary dysplasia is twice that for women in general. It is *very important*, therefore, that these women know how to perform accurate breast self-examination and how to recognize masses that differ from the masses of their dysplasia (Table 28-2). More frequent medical follow-up than that specified for asymptomatic people is indicated.

The role of methylxanthines in the reduction of symptoms in benign breast disorders is controversial. Omission of coffee, tea, and chocolate from the diet may help some people and is worth a try.

Evaluation

Evaluation is based on expected patient outcomes. Questions to consider may include the following:
1. Is breast discomfort lessened?
2. Does the patient appear less anxious?
3. Does the person know:
   a. The difference between benign and malignant disease?
   b. The method and frequency of breast self-examination?
   c. The frequency of medical follow-up?

CANCER OF THE BREAST
Epidemiology

The breast is the leading site for cancer in women but is now second to lung cancer in the number of deaths from cancer in women. It is estimated that there are 18,000 new cases of breast disease in England and Wales each year, with 1 in 16 women affected at some time in their life by the disease, and this probability increases with age.[70] The incidence of breast cancer has been increasing in Britain at about 3% per year since 1980; some of this increase is believed to result from early detection during screening programmes.[1] Mortality rates have remained about the same, 50% at 5 yrs and 32% at 10 yrs.[10a]

Numerous risk factors have been identified for breast cancer (see Box 28-2). A major factor that places the woman at risk is a long uninterrupted time period of cyclic hormone changes, that is, early menarche, late menopause, and no pregnancy. Epidemiological studies have supported the hypothesis that high fat consumption is positively associated with a higher incidence of breast cancer.[5] It must be noted, however, that 75% of women with breast cancer are *not* in the high risk group; therefore *all* women should be considered at risk for breast cancer.

Table 28-3 TNM classification of breast cancers

Stage	Tumour size	Nodal involvement	Metastasis
I	Less than 2 cm (T1)	None (N0)	None (M0)
II	Less than 5 cm (T1 or T2)	Movable axillary nodes (N1)	None (M0)
III	Greater than 5 cm with invasion of skin or attached to chest wall	Movable or fixed axillary nodes (N1 or N2)	None (M0)
IV	Any size (any T)	Any nodes (any N)	Yes (M1)

28-2

High-risk factors associated with breast cancer

Sex	Female (99% in women)
Age	80% are over age 35; mean and median age is 60
Familial history	Mother/sister, especially with premenopausal or bilateral breast cancer
Menstrual history	Menarche before age 11; menopause after age 50
Pregnancy	First live birth after age 30; or nullipara
Medical history	Primary breast cancer (risk increased 7 times for a second primary breast cancer); uterine endometrial cancer; mammary dysplasia
Diet	High fat intake

Pathophysiology

Breast cancer is not one disease but many, depending on the tissue of the breast involved, its oestrogen dependency, and the age of onset. Most breast tumours at the time of diagnosis are infiltrating tumours of the ducts. About 6% to 8% are invasive lobular, and 4% to 6% are noninvasive.

Malignant breast tumours differ from benign tumours (Table 28-2). They are usually solitary, irregularly shaped, firm, nontender, nonmobile masses with a tendency to adhere to the pectoralis muscles and to the skin, causing retraction or dimpling of the skin. The skin may become thickened, giving it an "orange peel" effect. Involvement of the lymph nodes is present in about two thirds of the women at the time of diagnosis. Even when the lymph nodes are negative, it is believed that micrometastasis is present. Favoured sites for metastasis are the lungs, bone, liver, brain, adrenal glands, and ovaries.

Breast cancers are classified using the TNM classification (described in Chapter 9). *T* refers to tumour size, *N* to nodal involvement, and *M* to metastasis. The classification of breast cancer (Table 28-3 and Fig. 28-6) serves as a basis for prognosis and direction for treatment.

The stage of breast cancer is the most reliable indicator of prognosis. Stage I tumours have 75% to 90% cure rate with the accepted forms of therapy.[65] Stage III tumours are more poorly differentiated and have a high rate of recurrence. Patients with negative hormone receptors and neg- ative lymph nodes have a higher recurrence rate than patients with positive hormone receptors and negative lymph nodes.

Medical Therapy

Because two thirds of patients with breast cancer eventually show metastasis, breast cancer is now considered to be a *systemic* rather than a local disease.[65] Even when the lymph nodes are negative it is thought that micrometastasis has already occurred by the time of diagnosis. Medical therapy, therefore, has now changed from primarily local therapy (surgery of the breast) to include additional therapies (radiation, chemotherapy, hormone therapy).

Surgery of the breast

Eighty to ninety percent of breast cancers are operable. The type of surgery depends on the extent of the growth and patient choice. Because breast cancer is being identified at earlier stages than in the past (as a result of BSE and mammography screening), surgical procedures are less radical than in the past. The two most commonly used procedures are lumpectomy with axillary dissection and modified radical mastectomy.

Lumpectomy

Lumpectomy is a type of segmental mastectomy in which only the tumour and a margin of surrounding clear tissue are removed, not the entire breast (as in mastectomy). *Cryolumpectomy* consists of freezing and thawing the tumour several times before removing it. *Quadrantectomy* is another form of segmental mastectomy in which the quadrant of the breast in which the tumour is located is removed. In most instances, axillary nodes are dissected through a separate incision to examine the nodes for metastasis, to determine further treatment, and as a preventive method for spread of metastasis.

Lumpectomies are an option when the tumour is small (less than 4 cm) and can be totally removed. When lumpectomy is combined with a course of radiation, the long-term results are similar to those following a modified radical mastectomy. Although the breast is not removed, breast appearance does change because of loss of tissue through biopsy and surgery, and from skin changes with radiation. Hospital stays generally average 1 to 2 days.

Modified radical mastectomy

The entire breast tissue, axillary lymph nodes, and fascia underlying the breast are removed with a modified

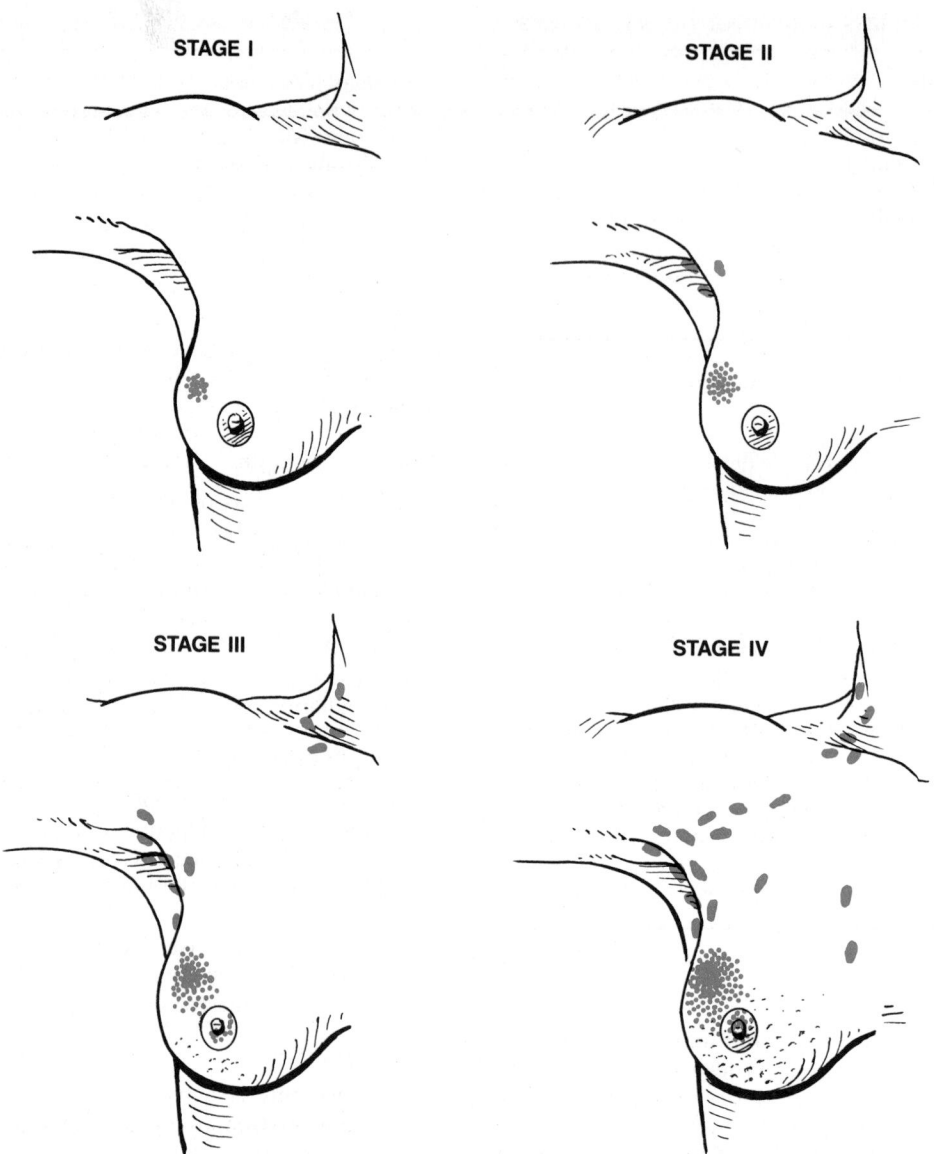

Fig. 28-6 Stages of breast cancer. Note that in Stage I the tumour is small and there is no nodal involvement. As the tumour progresses to Stage IV, tumour size increases, nodal involvement is more extensive, and the skin finally dimples.

radical mastectomy. The pectoralis major muscle remains intact. Because the majority of breast cancers are ductal and the ducts lead to the nipple, the nipple is removed, but as much skin as possible is retained. Following removal of early cancers, breast reconstruction (p. 828) may be done at this time if the patient so desires. Hospital stays generally average 3 to 5 days, but may be longer if reconstruction has been done.

Radiation therapy

Radiation therapy alone, without surgery, is not an effective therapy for breast cancer. Radiation may be used with far advanced cancer to contain the tumour before surgery. After lumpectomy, radiation is very useful to prevent recurrence. The entire breast is radiated 5 days a week for

5 weeks, followed by a boost to the tumour bed, either by external beam therapy or by interstitial implants (brachytherapy). For *brachytherapy*, a hospital stay of 2 to 3 days is necessary. Hollow catheters are placed (with the patient under anaesthesia) in parallel rows under the skin over the affected breast area. The patient then returns to a single room on the ward, where radioactive strands are threaded by the doctor into the tubes and fastened with "buttons". If Iodine-125 is used, a low-energy radioisotope, a thin rubberized lead shield, is placed over the dressing to minimize radiation exposure; more extensive shielding is necessary if Iridium-192 is used.[41] There is generally little discomfort except a dull aching sensation that can be relieved by analgesics. The implant is usually removed in 24 hours. Except for a pulling sensation, there is little

discomfort with removal. The patient should not shower while the implant is in place. Radiation of the breast tissue continues for several weeks and may cause some mild discomfort. (Care of the patient with internal radiation is discussed in Chapter 9.)

Adjuvant therapy

Because micrometastases occur even in patients with normal axillary nodes, the European Breast Cancer Treatment collaborative group recently showed clear evidence that adjuvant therapy (hormonal) enhanced 10-year survival.[70] All patients are now being evaluated after surgery and appropriate adjuvant therapy is being recommended.

Hormonal therapy, usually tamoxifen, is recommended for women with positive hormone receptors, except for the premenopausal woman with positive lymph nodes. *Chemotherapy* is recommended for all women with negative hormone receptors and for the premenopausal woman with positive lymph nodes and positive oestrogen receptors. Combined chemotherapy, especially CMF (cyclophosphamide, methotrexate, fluorouracil) is more effective than single drugs.[65]

Every patient is considered individually. Factors in deciding therapy include risk of recurrence and benefits of therapy as compared with side effects. Tamoxifen is usually well tolerated. Side effects may include hot flushes, vaginal discharge or dryness, and loss of menstrual cycles in premenopausal women. With chemotherapy, most women experience mild weight gain, nausea, mild fatigue, hair thinning or loss, loss of menstrual cycles (in premenopausal women), and decreases in WBC and RBC counts. Some women experience vomiting, total hair loss, infection, and stomatitis. During chemotherapy, women are encouraged to eat well, get sufficient sleep, drink plenty of liquids (to help prevent side effects of cyclophosphamide), remain involved, and report signs of illness or stomatitis. In general, chemotherapy is well tolerated by most women.

A new approach for the patient with *advanced* breast cancer is high-dose chemotherapy with autologous bone marrow transplantation (ABMT). Bone marrow is removed before chemotherapy, purged of any remnants of cancer, then reintroduced after chemotherapy to regenerate new bone marrow. This procedure results in higher frequency of complete remissions in patients with metastatic breast cancer, and may keep some patients disease-free for extended periods of time.

Nursing Process
Assessment

If a malignant breast tumour is suspected or diagnosed as such, the following *subjective data* are obtained as a baseline for planning:
1. Concerns about the diagnosis and forthcoming therapy
2. Feelings and thoughts about sexuality and the relationship of the breast to these feelings
3. Thoughts about feelings of the sex partner (if appropriate) concerning the forthcoming potential therapy options
4. Future goals, life expectancies, zest for living, and actual or perceived responsibility to others
5. Usual coping mechanisms
6. Family relationships and the existence and availability of support people

7. Knowledge about BSE (for examination of other breast)

If possible, data are obtained from the sex partner (if appropriate) regarding attitudes about the forthcoming therapy. This identifies possible conflicts in perceptions, the degree of support that can be anticipated from the sex partner, and the potential effects of the partner's feelings on the woman's adaptation and relationships.

Objective data include observations about the woman's behaviour and vital signs, which might indicate signs of high anxiety.

Nursing analysis

Nursing analyses are determined from assessment of patient data. Possible nursing problems for the person with breast cancer may include, but are not limited to, the following:

Problem	Possible aetiologies
Decisional conflict (treatment options)	Unclear values, lack of information, support system deficit
Anxiety	Fear of surgery, cancer, removal of breast, change in family relationships; decision making about surgery
Altered body image or self-esteem	Loss of breast, difficulty making decisions
Infection, high risk for	Loss of skin intactness, decreased immune response (node removal)
Mobility, impaired physical	Restricted shoulder movement
Pain	Incision, loss of breast tissue
Fatigue	Surgery, adjuvant therapy
Coping, ineffective individual	Fear of cancer recurrence, death
Sexuality patterns, altered	Loss of breast
Knowledge deficit	Lack or misinterpretation of information

Planning expected patient outcomes

Expected patient outcomes for the patient with cancer of the breast may include, but are not limited to, the following:
1. Participates in making decisions concerning therapy, as possible.
2. Demonstrates signs of decreased anxiety.
3. Demonstrates femininity, such as by applying make-up, fixing hair, putting on own nightgown.
4. Incision does not become infected.
5. Participates in arm exercises.
6. States feeling more comfortable.
7. Rests between activities.
8. Looks at incision.
9. Interacts with others appropriately, especially with spouse or significant other.
10. Describes:
    a. Plans for breast prosthesis (if appropriate)
    b. Ways to prevent infection and oedema in affected arm
    c. Plans for monthly BSE
    d. Personal and community support resources, as needed

Implementation

Interventions to achieve patient outcomes

Because surgery is the primary therapeutic approach for patients with breast cancer, nursing care focuses on preoperative and postoperative care. Care of the patient following mastectomy is summarized in Box 28-3. Patients having lumpectomy and axillary node dissection require similar care except for the type of exercises and not requiring information on breast prostheses.

Preoperative care

Assisting the patient with decision making

Patients report that the period from the time of tumour identification until surgery is one of high anxiety. Making decisions when anxiety is high is very difficult. Providing necessary information and support can facilitate the decision-making process.

When the diagnostic work is completed and the tumour has been classified, the doctor, often after consulting the hospital tumour management team (medical, surgical, and radiation oncologists) and plastic surgeon, discusses and proposes treatment options. The patient and spouse/friend are involved at this point in the treatment decision plan. If the malignancy is in stage I or II, the woman usually has several options for therapy that offer her a comparable prognosis. The choices are usually lumpectomy with radiation, or mastectomy. Information about cancer treatment can be obtained from the British Association of Cancer United Patients.* Women may be influenced by magazine articles and may need help in acquiring accurate information and in sorting out what is best for them from their standpoint. She is the one making the final decision and it should be an educated decision. Female nurses have the advantage of facilitating decision making because of their expertise as health professionals while taking into consideration the subjective hesitations of the woman. The nurse can help the woman work through the steps of the decision-making process. Providing structure for the process can help decrease the anxiety about making a "wrong" decision.

For the patient with stage III cancer there are fewer options and greater consequences. Mastectomy is generally the treatment of choice from a medical standpoint. The woman may feel a sense of *powerlessness* at this point. Letting her make decisions about other aspects of her life and activities of daily living, when possible, helps her hold onto a sense of control of her life.

Women having a mastectomy usually have the option of choosing immediate or delayed breast reconstruction (p. 828). This information often helps to decrease the concerns of the woman who fears deformity from loss of a breast and may facilitate making the decision regarding therapy.

Assisting with coping with preoperative anxiety

The preoperative period has been reported by patients as a time of high anxiety. After finding the lump, the first

---

*BACUP, 15-19 Britton Street, London, SW3 3TZ

Guidelines for Care   **28-3**

The patient who has had a mastectomy

Preoperative care

1. Help patient explore feelings about loss of breast and fears related to cancer
2. Provide simple explanations; repeat as necessary
3. Teach patient:
   a. Expectation of catheter to drain wound
   b. Need for postoperative exercises

Postoperative care

1. Give immediate care
   a. Place patient in supported sitting position
   b. Wound care:
      (1) If Haemovac suction is used, empty when half full to maintain suction
      (2) Check dressing and bed for signs of drainage
   c. Elevate arm on pillow
   d. Monitor circulation of arm on affected side; report signs of swelling and numbness of lower arm or inability to move fingers
   e. Avoid blood pressure readings, blood testing, IVs, or injections in affected arm
   f. Teach patient to sit up in bed by *pushing* up on elbow of *unaffected* side, rather than pulling up with arm
   g. Encourage deep breathing exercises
   h. Give analgesics for comfort
2. Encourage postmastectomy arm exercises
   a. Start gentle exercises early (see p. 824)
   b. Start special mastectomy exercises (see p. 824) when prescribed
3. Encourage rest periods; monitor for fatigue
4. Provide emotional support
   a. Continue to help patient explore feelings
   b. Prepare patient in advance concerning size of incision and be with her, if possible, when she looks at incision
   c. Encourage patient to identify feelings about resuming sexual activities (if appropriate) and to discuss these feelings with sexual partner
5. Teach patient
   a. Wear a bra padded with a soft fluffy filling or temporary soft prosthesis until incision is healed (if appropriate)
   b. Substitute a regular breast prosthesis later
   c. Avoid clothing that constricts the underarm
   d. Avoid injections, blood drawing, and blood pressure measurements in affected arm
   e. Report symptoms indicating a need for immediate medical attention:
      (1) Oedema of affected arm
      (2) Redness of infection of scar
      (3) Breakdown of scar tissue
      (4) Mass in other breast or axillae
   f. Plan to do monthly breast self-examination on remaining breast

concern is whether or not it is malignant. Couples often have to wait a few days after the biopsy for the report and they describe this waiting period as being very difficult. The major concern of the woman after receiving the diagnosis is *survival*; this includes the extent of the cancer, fear of recurrence, and worry about a shortened life span.[49] Other concerns include ability to return to previous life style, concerns about children, coping ability, treatments, and appearance.[49]

The nurse provides opportunities for the woman to explore her feelings. Simple explanations with repetition may decrease fears of the unknown. If the woman does not fully comprehend the doctor's explanation, the nurse can repeat the explanation and report this to the doctor, who in turn can talk with the woman again and clarify any misconceptions, alleviating needless anxiety. Because attention span, memory, and perception are limited when anxiety levels are high, it is helpful if the nurse can be present when information is given the patient. The nurse can then repeat, reinforce, or clarify the information.

The Breast Care and Mastectomy Association* actively encourages and supports professionals to develop local support services for their patients with breast disease, by sending out their workers to the professional to discuss the needs of the area and population they serve. Volunteer visiting programmes may also be developed where there is no immediate service from a Breast care nurse specialist. This assures the woman that she will receive practical help from someone who has made a satisfactory adjustment to the same operation. Although most of the patient visits by the volunteer occur during the postoperative period, preoperative visits can be requested and may be very helpful to some women.

Spouses also report feelings of stress and anxiety in the preoperative period, both during the diagnostic period and on the day of surgery.[49] Nurses having contact with spouses can provide the same support given the woman.

Promoting self-esteem

Because much emphasis is placed on the breast as a symbol of attractiveness, the thought of losing a breast becomes almost intolerable to many women. This is particularly true of those who depend largely on physical attractiveness to hold the esteem of others and to secure gratification of their emotional needs. Psychologists have pointed out that there is a symbolic connection between the breasts and motherhood that is severely threatened when a breast must be removed. In addition, cancer of the breast often occurs at menopause or soon after when some women feel that they have lost much of their sexual attractiveness. Surgical removal of the breast may save a woman's life, but it also may make her feel less feminine.

The woman may be coping with feelings of "being less than a woman," disfigurement, sexual acceptance, or social isolation. Although these feelings are experienced more often by the woman who will have a mastectomy, some of the same feelings occur even when only part of the breast is removed. Some women preoperatively have been unable to discuss their concerns and feelings with those close to them, including their spouse. The nurse can help the

patient express feelings and understand what breast surgery means to her as a person. It may be helpful to assist the woman to share her concerns about sexual acceptance with her spouse/significant other. The woman who is having breast surgery, be it a lumpectomy or a mastectomy, has a special need to feel understood and accepted by all people who are providing care.

Preoperative teaching

Preoperative teaching includes the following information if a mastectomy or lumpectomy with axillary dissection is planned:
1. A catheter attached to suction will be used to drain the incision.
2. The arm on the affected side will be elevated.
3. Sitting up and turning in bed should be done by *pushing* up on the unaffected side rather than pulling, to prevent strain on the incision.
4. Postoperative exercises will be started early.

Postoperative care
Preventing infection of incision

Following the completion of surgery and closure, a stab wound may be made and a catheter inserted and attached immediately to a low, constant suction, such as with a Haemovac or other low suction system. The purpose of the catheter is to remove blood and serum that may collect under the skin that would prevent healing and predispose the tissue to infection. There is usually no drainage from around the incision when a catheter is draining correctly. The catheter is usually removed within 3 to 5 days or when the amount of drainage is less than 5 to 10 ml in 24 hours.

The dressing is checked often for the first few hours to detect haemorrhage or excessive serous oozing. The bedclothes under the patient must be examined for blood that may flow down from the surgical site. Any evidence of bleeding is reported to the surgeon. After 24 hours, the incision may be left covered or uncovered. Because the incision is not healed by the time of hospital discharge, the patient is taught signs and symptoms of infection to be reported immediately to the doctor.

Facilitating shoulder range of motion

When the patient returns from surgery, after axillary nodes have been removed, she is placed in a supported sitting position to decrease venous oozing. The arm is elevated to enhance circulation and prevent oedema. The pillows are arranged so that the hand is higher than the arm and the arm is above the level of the right atrium. *No blood pressure readings, injections, or blood testing* should be done on the *affected* arm because of the risk of circulatory impairment or infection (to prevent lymphoedema). A sign or tape should be placed on this side of the bed with this message.

Exercises are essential to prevent shortening of muscles, stiffness, and contracture of the shoulder girdle, and to preserve muscle tone so that the affected arm can be used without limitations. To prevent additional deformities, exercises should be bilateral ones with the patient using both arms simultaneously. The time to start specific postoperative exercises depends on the extent of the operation.

*BACUP, 15-19 Britton Street, London, SW3 3TZ

Nursing Care Plan	**Patient following mastectomy for cancer**

DATA: Mrs. L., age 35, discovered a lump in her right breast quite accidentally while bathing. She is not familiar with breast self-examination. Mammography and a breast biopsy confirmed the diagnosis of cancer. In a conference with the surgeon and plastic surgeon, Mrs. L. elected to have a modified radical mastectomy with consideration of breast reconstruction in 6 months.

Mrs. L. was very quiet during the admission procedure. The primary nurse talked with her the evening before surgery, and Mrs. L. stated that her major concern was "whether they would get it all." She is glad to know that breast reconstruction can be done in the near future because she doesn't think she wants to go through life with a deformed chest. She also said her husband had supported the surgery, and they both feel it will not affect their relationship. Mr. L. accompanied his wife to the hospital for admission and spent the evening with her. Her mother is caring for their 3- and 6-year-old daughters while Mrs. L. is in hospital.

After surgery, Mrs L. returned to the division with intravenous fluids and wound catheter attached to a Haemovac suction. Vital signs were stable.

Collaborative nursing actions included monitoring the dressing and catheter for wound drainage and observing the arm for signs of enlargement (lymphoedema). Medical orders included keeping her right arm elevated on pillows to prevent lymphoedema. A sign was placed on her bedS reminding others to avoid blood pressure readings, starting IVs, and injections, or taking blood samples from Mrs. L.'s right arm.

Nursing analysis: Pain: related to surgical incision

Expected patient outcomes	Nursing interventions	Rationale
States feeling more comfortable	Give prescribed narcotic on a regular basis for first 24 hr; then re-evaluate	Expected incisional pain is better controlled if not allowed to become severe; Mrs. L. will participate in exercises earlier if comfortable
	Encourage deep breathing exercises every 2-4 hr	Narcotic will ease discomfort from deep breathing; these exercises will prevent lung problems that would increase Mrs. L.'s discomfort

Nursing analysis: Mobility, impaired physical: related to shoulder immobility

Expected patient outcomes	Nursing interventions	Rationale
Participates early with arm exercises	Demonstrate early exercises (keep instructions simple) Visit Mrs. L. every 2 hours to provide encouragement	Because of discomfort and narcotic, Mrs. L. may have difficulty concentrating
	Explain rationale for exercises to Mr. L. so he can encourage Mrs. L.	Exercises will help prevent stiffness and contractures of shoulder from disuse

Nursing analysis: Change in body image: related to loss of breast

Expected patient outcomes	Nursing interventions	Rationale
Begins to look at incision and to talk about loss of breast	Spend planned time talking with Mrs. L. Give Mrs. L. opportunities to talk about her feelings Don't push Mrs. L. but listen to what she says Observe for signs of her touching dressing and use this as an opening to discuss Mrs. L.'s thoughts about her surgery Check with Mrs. L.'s surgeon about a volunteer visitor and then explain the programme Encourage Mrs. L. to put on makeup and wear her own clothes as soon as possible	Mrs. L. may need to deny her feelings initially As Mrs. L. begins to think about her surgery, she may need reassurance that the nurse is interested and willing to listen to her concerns Interacting with someone who has been through the experience is often helpful in adjustment Mrs. L. may need reassurance of her femininity

Nursing analysis: Knowledge deficit: related to lack of information

Expected patient outcomes	Nursing interventions	Rationale
States plans to do BSE regularly on other breast and to teach her daughters when older	Teach BSE: demonstration with return demonstration	Women who have a chance to practise BSE under supervision are more confident about doing BSE
	Explain high risk of daughters for breast cancer and need for continued monitoring	Mother's breast cancer is a high risk factor for daughters
States plans to continue exercises until full shoulder ROM returns	Demonstrate exercises to be done later; give Mrs. L. booklet from BCMA with instructions	Seeing and returning a demonstration and having written for reference will promote follow up of the activity
States plans for rest periods at home	Explain reason for expected fatigue after surgery and help Mrs. L. to plan her day to include rest periods	Care of young children is tiring and Mrs. L. still needs additional ennergy for healing; rest will give her additional energy for coping
Identifies where to obtain breast prostheses, if needed	Encourage visit by a volunteer; if not, discuss types of prostheses and where to obtain them	Mrs. L. may postpone reconstructive surgery or may want to use a soft prosthesis before surgery
Describes symptoms to be reported to the doctor	Instruct Mrs. L. to report signs of arm oedema, redness or infection of incision, or any mass in other breast	Lymphoedema and incisional breakdown are better treated if identified early; Mrs. L. is at a high risk for cancer in other breast
States ways to prevent oedema and infection	Discuss ways to prevent infection and oedema of right arm	Mrs. L. is at risk for infection and oedema of right arm because right axillary lymph nodes were removed

---

28-4

Postmastectomy arm exercises

Exercise: climbing the wall
1. Stand facing wall with toes 6-12 inches from wall.
2. Bend elbows and place palms of hands against wall at shoulder level.
3. Move both hands parallel to each other up the wall as far as possible until incisional pull or pain occurs.
4. Move both hands down to starting position.
5. Goal is complete extension with elbow straight.
6. Activities that use the same action: reaching top shelves, hanging out clothes, washing windows, hanging curtains, setting hair.

Exercise: elbow pull-in
1. Extend arms sideways to shoulder level.
2. Clasp hands behind neck.
3. Pull elbows forward until they touch.
4. Return to position 2.
5. Unclasp hands and extend arms sideways at shoulder level.
6. Lower arms to side.

Exercise: back scratch
1. Place hand of unoperated side on hip for balance.
2. Bend elbow of affected arm, placing back of hand on small of back.
3. Work hand up the back slowly until fingers reach opposite shoulder blade.
4. Lower arm and straighten both arms.

Exercise: rope pull
1. Attach a rope over a shower rod, hook, or over top of an open door.
2. Sit on a chair (with door between legs if using a door) and grasp each end of rope.
3. Alternately pull on each end, raising affected arm to a point of incisional pull or pain.
4. The goal is to raise the affected arm almost directly overhead.

28-5

Postlumpectomy arm exercises[54]

Straight arm raising: while lying flat, raise arm straight back along side of head
Elbow push: while lying flat, place hands behind neck and push elbows back against surface
Shoulder rotation: raise shoulders and rotate in a forward direction
Fist clenching: while sitting, raise arm forward level with shoulder, then clench and unclench fist
Climbing wall: see Box 32-4

The patient is encouraged under close supervision to exercise each day more and more to the limits of incisional pulling and pain. A specific exercise schedule planned by nurse and patient together is imperative. It is an important aspect of nursing care for the patient.

Continuing exercises after mastectomy are recommended by the Breast Care and Mastectomy Association (BCMA) (see Box 28-4). Exercises are begun with 5 repetitions, working up to a maximum of 20 repetitions unless otherwise specified. The woman is instructed to move slowly and rest when pain occurs. With exercise, full range of motion will return; that is, both arms can be extended equally high above the head. This will not be achieved for 2 to 3 months; therefore, the patient must learn and be motivated in the hospital so she will continue to exercise at home on a regular basis. Exercises to help regain full range of motion after *lumpectomy* are described in Box 28-5.

Promoting comfort

Pain in the operated area may be referred to the affected arm or shoulder. Sensations of numbness and tingling over the chest that are painful may cause the patient to take short, shallow breaths in the early postoperative period. She is kept comfortable with analgesics, and a deep breathing routine is started. Each chest excursion may painfully discourage compliance, and the patient may need considerable encouragement.

Phantom symptoms of the missing breast occur in those women who had painful breasts or nipples before the surgery. This can be very disconcerting to the woman, and reassurance may be needed that these sensations will eventually disappear.

Promoting rest

The body requires increased energy for healing and for coping with the grief over the loss of the breast. *Fatigue* occurs not only in the early postoperative period but often for up to 6 weeks after surgery. The woman needs to know that this is a normal reaction and that she should plan for rest periods.

Patients with advanced breast cancer usually experience *asthenia*, a combination of physical and mental fatigue. These patients need to know that this sense of fatigue is normal and that rest periods should be planned before and after activities. Support by family and friends in facilitating rest is helpful.

Slings are usually avoided. Gentle exercises started early in the postoperative course help to decrease muscle tension as well as to regain muscle function more quickly.

Early exercises for postmastectomy patient

Surgical day	Flex and extend fingers; pronate and supinate forearm
First postoperative day	Squeeze rubber ball
As soon as tolerated	Brush teeth and hair

The patient must know what motion is intended in each exercise, such as shoulder abduction. For example, the patient may brush her hair with the arm on the affected side, but she may lower her head and hunch her shoulders in such a way that she does not get normal use of the shoulder girdle. The whole intent of the exercise may, therefore, be lost.

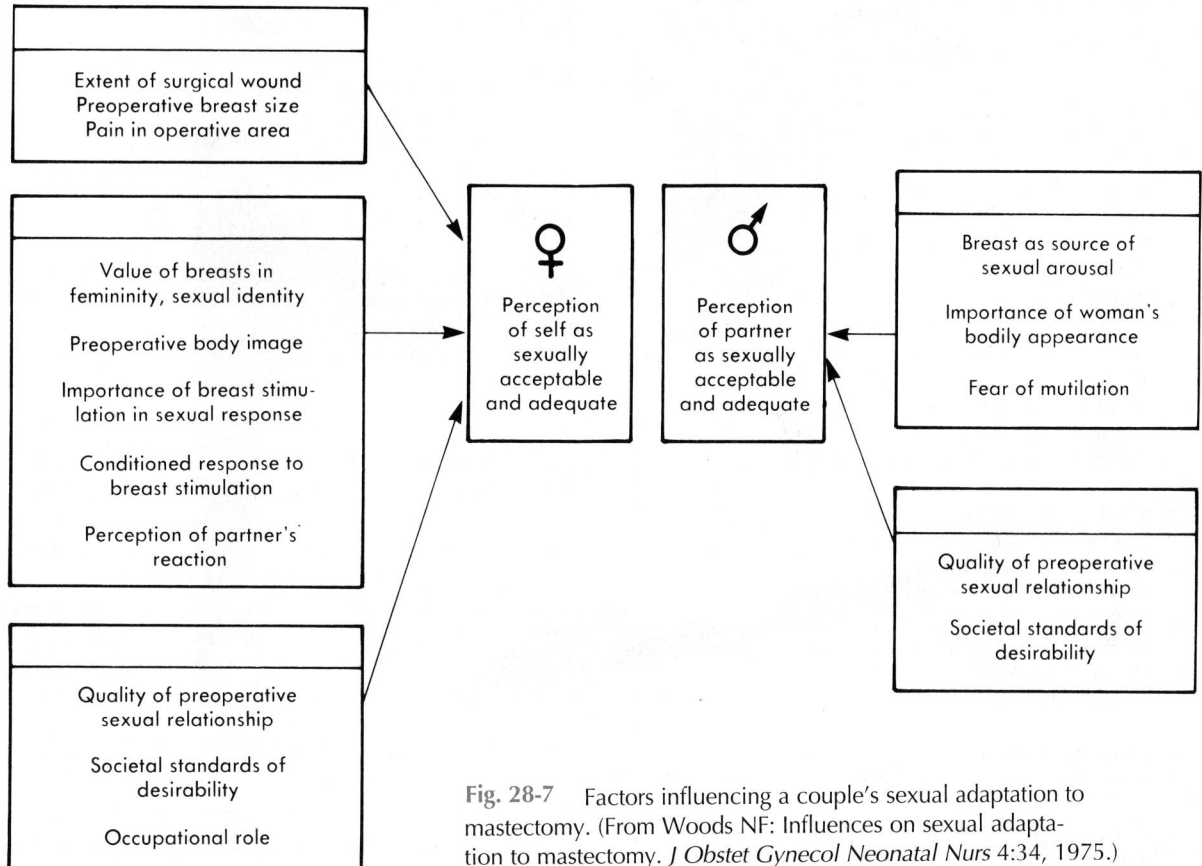

Fig. 28-7   Factors influencing a couple's sexual adaptation to mastectomy. (From Woods NF: Influences on sexual adaptation to mastectomy. *J Obstet Gynecol Neonatal Nurs* 4:34, 1975.)

Facilitating coping

After surgery, denial of the changes in body image may take the form of the woman speaking about "the cancer" and "the mastectomy" but never dealing with her loss or her fears on an emotional level. Denial here is a conservation of energy. If she is to express herself on an emotional level, she must have someone who is capable and responsible to support her according to *her* need. If she does not receive this professional assistance, the impact of her loss occurs at a later date when support systems may not be available.

Not looking at the dressing or incision can be expected initially from both the patient and spouse. The incision is large, and the feeling experienced by most women is that of mutilation. Postponing looking at the incision delays the impact of the realization that the breast is indeed gone. Preparing the woman in advance concerning the appearance of the incision is helpful, but she still needs considerable support when viewing the incision and her new image. She is usually physically capable when she feels stronger and begins to respond socially to others. She is encouraged to look at the incision several times before discharge from the hospital while health professionals are available for support.

Feelings of anger and resentment may occur and, if present, frequently are projected onto female staff or friends. Families may also express anger or anxiety and may complain without cause about the care the patient is receiving. Feelings of decreased self-worth and self-esteem on the part of the patient plus increased dependency needs often produce depression.

The feeling of being isolated and alone during this experience can be helped by interaction with others who have had the same experience. They hold the potential of motivating the patient, extending hope, and providing visible evidence that femininity, personality, and activity can be retained. They can be good resource people as the patient moves from the hospital to the community. Often whether the patient has the opportunity to use this resource depends on a nurse initiating the contact.

Patients often experience periods of depression for weeks to months after breast surgery, especially after mastectomy. Emotions are more labile and the woman may cry more easily. It is helpful for her to know in advance that this may occur. She may have difficulty sleeping or concentrating if she is still acutely grieving with little recognition or little support. She usually will be unable to express her needs; significant others can be told of her continuing need for support and patience and can help to extend the kind of support needed. Women who have *immediate* breast reconstruction generally have fewer episodes of depression.

Facilitating sexual adaptation

Woods[69] has identified a number of factors that can influence sexual adaptation following mastectomy (Fig. 28-7). Women with very small or very large breasts may have long-unresolved feelings about breast size and may also experience more difficulty in obtaining a satisfactory breast prosthesis. They may perceive the surgery as mutilating, and withdraw from the sexual relationship, fearing rejection from their partner. Women who felt sexually inad-

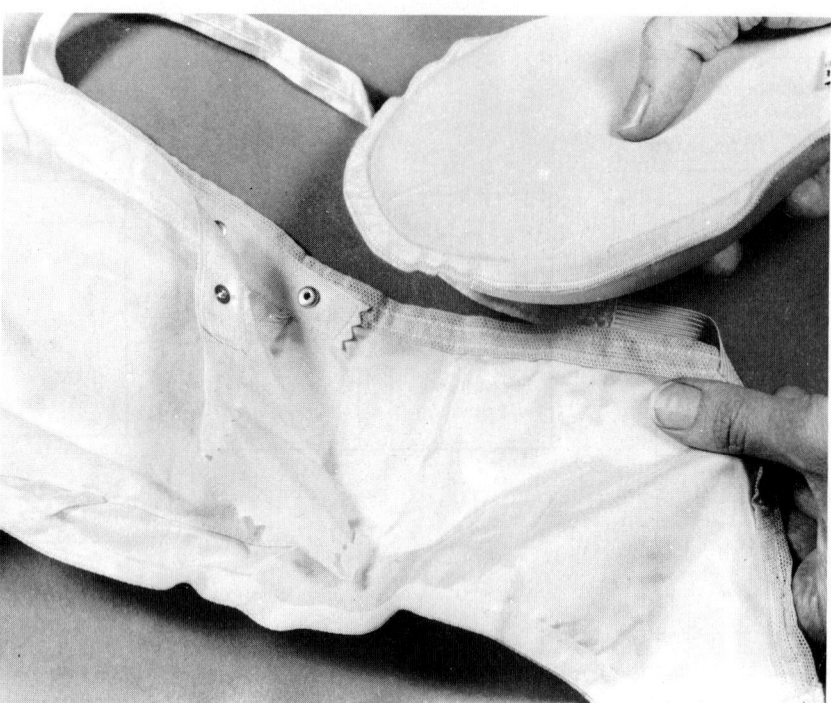

Inner pocket can be made in patient's own bra that holds padding or prosthesis securely. Note that snaps simplify removal of padding.
Fig. 28-8

equate before surgery may find these feelings enhanced postoperatively and use the surgery as a reason for withdrawing from sexual relationships.

The nurse can initiate a discussion with the patient concerning her thoughts and feelings about return to sexual activity (if appropriate) and can encourage the patient to talk about her concerns with her sexual partner. Sexual and marital counselling is helpful for couples who are unable to communicate their feelings openly with each other.

Facilitating learning
Breast prosthesis

Unless a breast reconstruction has been done immediately following breast removal, information about breast prostheses is given to the patient whenever she asks about them or appears interested. A breast care nurse is a good resource person for current information and suggestions concerning prostheses and clothing. A volunteer may accompany the patient as she shops for her first prosthesis, serving as a support person. Breast prostheses are not fitted until at least 6 weeks postoperatively or until the incision has healed and is no longer tender.

Until the incision is well healed, the woman is advised to wear one of her own bras, which can be lightly padded with a soft, fluffy filling (Fig. 28-8) or a temporary soft prosthesis that will not shift and embarrass her. Opaque, loose-hanging gowns are usually most acceptable to the patient.

Breast prostheses vary in type and weight (Figs. 28-9 and 28-10). Women want prostheses to make them look symmetric and *feel* bilaterally weighted. Even small-breasted women will change posture if weighting is

not balanced. Firm, moulded prostheses have a disadvantage of remaining elevated when the woman is lying supine, whereas fluid types have a more natural look.

Preventing infection in affected arm

When axillary nodes are removed the affected arm is more susceptible to infection because of decreased lymph drainage. Instructions to the patient to prevent infection include the following:
1. Avoid injections and blood drawing in the affected arm.
2. Wear a thimble when sewing.
3. Use a soft cloth to push back cuticles.
4. Shave affected axilla with an electric razor with a narrow head to reduce nicks or scratches.
5. Wear gloves when gardening or using strong detergents.
6. Use insect repellent to avoid stings or bites.
7. Avoid burns and sunburns.
8. Wash cuts well on affected arm, apply an antiseptic cream, and cover with a sterile dressing. Check often for signs of infection.
9. Consult the doctor if infection of the affected arm occurs; treatment is antibiotics, heat, rest, and elevation of the arm.

Preventing lymphoedema

Many patients develop a slight oedema of the affected upper arm that disappears within a week. A few patients, however, develop severe oedema that persists, that may become permanent, and that is caused by surgical interruption of lymph channels when the axillary nodes are dissected. The incidence is

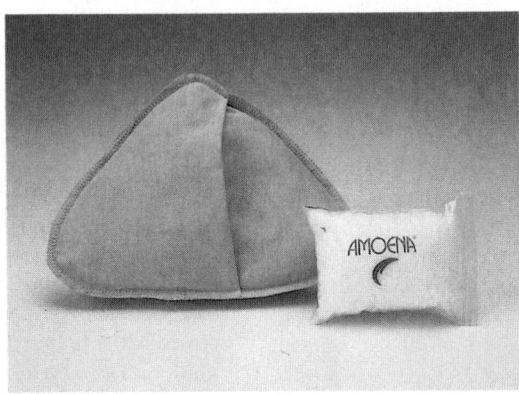

Fig. 28-9   Cotton-covered, fibrefill breast prothesis. (Courtesy AMOENA (UK) Ltd, Hampshire.)

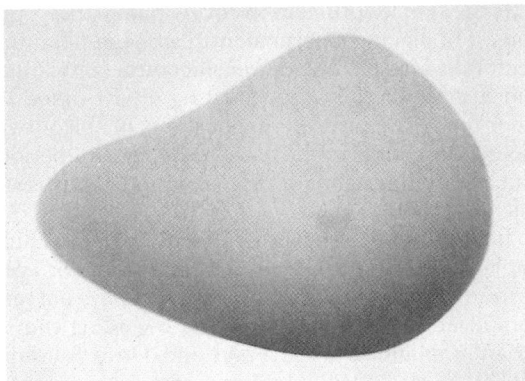

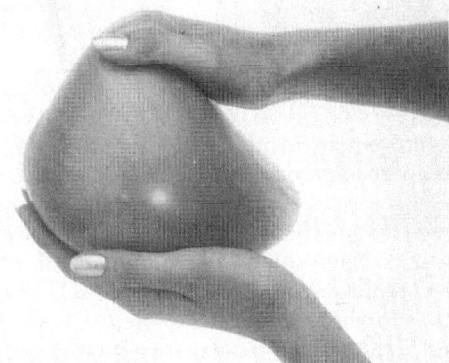

Fig. 28-10   Silicone-filled breast prostheses. (Courtesy AMOENA (UK) Ltd, Hampshire.)

greater in people who are obese, develop infections, or are subjected to radiation. Some surgeons order an elastic sleeve (similar to an elastic stocking) that should extend from the wrist to the shoulder. It may be removed when the patient is in bed.

Measures to help prevent oedema include:

1. Avoid blood pressure measurements in affected arm.
2. Avoid injuries and infection of affected arm.
3. Wear clothing that does not restrict the underarm or wrists (avoid elastic cuffs).
4. Wear watch and bracelets on unaffected arm.
5. Carry heavy packages or handbags using unaffected arm.
6. Consult the doctor if oedema occurs.

Early identification of recurrence

Over half of breast cancer recurrences are seen within the first 3 years and another 20% within the next 2 years. Therefore, the woman needs to carry out SBE on the remaining breast tissue and opposite breast *regularly* every month. Ask the woman to demonstrate BSE and teach her any aspects that she is not performing correctly. If the woman has daughters, they are at increased risk for breast cancer and need to practise BSE regularly also. Encourage the patient to carry out follow-up visits to the doctor as instructed and to have yearly mammograms.

Use of community resources

After patients return home from the hospital, they often feel isolated and alone. Many women find it helpful to attend support groups for breast cancer patients or for cancer patients in general. If additional information about therapy is desired, the patient can contact societies that offer information on breast cancer. Local hospitals may also provide local support groups for people with cancer.

Evaluation

Evaluation is based on expected patient outcomes. Questions to consider when evaluating the care of women who have had therapy for breast cancer may include the following:

1. Did the patient participate in making decisions concerning therapy?

2. Does the patient appears less anxious?
3. Has the patient had an opportunity to discuss her feelings and begin dealing with the change in her body image?
4. Does the patient know ways to prevent infection and oedema of the arm?
5. Has the patient been exercising during her hospital stay, and does she know the home exercises?
6. Does the patient state that she feels more comfortable?
7. Is the patient aware that she will tire easily for at least 6 weeks after therapy is completed and needs to plan rest periods?
8. Has the patient identified people to turn to for support when she feels depressed or needs help?
9. Is the patient interacting with others, especially her spouse or partner, appropriately?
10. Does the patient know where to obtain a breast prosthesis, if appropriate?
11. Can the patient perform breast self-examinations, and does she plan to carry them out monthly?
12. Is the patient aware of the need for yearly follow-up by a doctor?

BREAST RECONSTRUCTION

Since 1980 improvement in plastic surgery techniques have made breast reconstruction a viable alternative to breast prostheses for many women. There is no evidence that breast reconstruction changes the course of the disease or masks recurrence.[65] For some women, however, breast reconstruction is not essential to their positive self-image and self-esteem, femininity, or sexual experience. Some do not want the added surgery and accompanying anaesthesia, the cost in terms of time, or the pain. Other women consider breast reconstruction necessary for their self-esteem and continuing relationships with others. Breast reconstruction is contraindicated when there is an aggressive tumour, a probability that metastasis has occurred, or a concern about adequate healing.

The benefits of breast reconstruction include avoidance of an external prosthesis that has potential for slipping, greater choice of clothing (including lower necklines), and loss of self-consciousness about appearance. Women say they feel better about themselves and experience fewer periods of depression following breast reconstruction.

The *original* nipple is no longer "saved" because there is always a question about the possible spread of cancer cells into the nipple. Creation of a new areola and nipple is performed as ambulatory surgery at a later date. The areola is formed by free grafting of tissue, either from part of the other areola (if it is large) or from skin of the upper thigh just below the pubic hair. The nipple is more difficult to fashion; the more common approach is to create folds of tissue with local skin and fat flap grafts.

Timing of breast reconstruction

Breast reconstruction can be performed immediately after surgery or at a later time. An increasing number of women are electing immediate reconstruction; this may prolong the initial hospitalization, but eliminates the need for a second hospitalization and contributes to self-esteem from the beginning.

The decision for reconstruction should be made in combination with the surgeon, plastic surgeon, and patient. The goal of reconstruction is a breast mound and nipple-areola complex that is similar to the remaining breast. The new breast will not have the exact contours of the natural breast; it is generally a little rounder and flatter and will not sag. The opposite breast can be altered to match the reconstructed breast.

Types of breast reconstruction

The two major approaches to breast reconstruction are the submuscular insertion of an *implant* to provide breast form or a *muscle flap graft* (Table 28-4). The implant is used when the pectoralis major muscle is intact and there is good skin cover. Muscle flap grafts are used when muscle and skin are inadequate; the grafts may be obtained from the back (latissimus muscle) or from the abdomen.

Breast implant

If the skin is sufficient to cover an implant, surgery may consist of placing a permanent silicone implant under the pectoralis muscle. The newer silicone gel implants are soft and flexible, better approximating breast tissue than the older models. Possible complications of silicone implants include infection in the early postoperative period, deflation, a hard round breast, false mammography results, and silicone leaks.

It has also been suggested that the silicone filling or the implant covering can lead to autoimmune or connective tissue disease. Although most surgeries have not resulted in complications, differing opinions regarding the safety of breast implants led the Food and Drug Administration (FDA) in early 1992 to issue some recommendations. Breast implants were permitted following breast cancer surgery (because of the offsetting positive contributions to recovery), but a moratorium was imposed on breast implants solely for cosmetic purposes until data establishing safety could be provided.

If the skin covering the breast is tight, the skin can be stretched (like stretching of the abdomen during pregnancy) by gradually expanding the area below the skin. An all-saline sac or a combination saline/silicone gel sac is implanted under the muscle; the sac is then slowly expanded over a 3-month period by adding saline by injection into a receiving port placed subcutaneously below the axilla. When the desired volume has been achieved, the temporary sac is surgically removed and the permanent silicone implant is inserted into the enlarged space, or the injection port is removed from the permanent implant. The woman will experience minimal discomfort with this procedure.

The woman is asked not to smoke for at least 1 week before surgery because complications occur more frequently among smokers.[9] Postoperative teaching includes the following:

1. Report signs of drainage, fever, or other signs of infection.
2. Wear a bra continuously until healing occurs to maintain the implant position and alignment.

Table 28-4 Types of reconstruction breast surgery

Surgery	Description	Comments
Implants		
Silicone implant	Implant inserted into a pocket beneath the pectoralis major muscle	Simplest procedure but may lead to complications Short hospital stay Requires ample residual skin Result is less symmetric than in other surgeries No ptosis
Tissue expansion	Temporary or permanent expandable bag inserted in submuscular pocket; bag is expanded slowly over time by saline injections in subcutaneous port	Common procedure Short hospital stay Useful following modified radical mastectomy if enough tissue present Requires frequent office visits
Flap grafts		
Abdominothoracic	Flap graft advanced from area below breast	Longer hospital stay Provides better breast detailing than implants More prominent abdominal scar
Latissimus dorsi	Flap graft advanced from latissimus dorsi muscle (lateral upper back)	Longer hospital stay Useful following radical surgery when tissue lacking Implants may be needed Horizontal back scar
Transabdominal	Flap graft using rectus abdominus muscle tunnelled from lower abdomen to breast area	Longer hospital stay Useful following radical surgery when tissue lacking Horizontal scar on lower abdomen Removes some abdominal fat (lipectomy)

3. Avoid raising arms (such as to wash hair or reach cupboards) for 1 to 3 weeks, as instructed.
4. Avoid hard pushing movements, for 1 to 3 weeks in order to avoid separation of the pectoralis muscle where the implant has been inserted and to avoid pulling out the sutures.
5. Avoid heavy lifting for 6 weeks.

Latissimus dorsi flap graft

A latissimus dorsi graft is a free flap graft in which an "island" of latissimus muscle, fat, and skin (Fig. 28-11) is transferred to the breast area where it provides adequate cover for an implant. Care of the patient with a flap graft is discussed in Chapter 34.

Transabdominal island flap

The transabdominal island flap (TAIF) method creates a breast that better approximates breast tissue than the silicone implant. TAIF surgery involves transferring a section of abdominal skin and fat and part of the rectus abdominis muscle to the breast area by tunnelling under the skin. The tissue is then shaped as a new breast.

TAIF involves more extensive surgery than the implant procedure and usually requires a week-long hospital stay. Following surgery, the patient will experience abdominal discomfort, tightness, and paresthesia. The abdomen will be flatter (tummy tuck) but the waistline may be temporarily larger.[29] Possible complications after TAIF surgery include haematoma/seroma, infection, or flap necrosis in the early postoperative period. Fat necrosis is identified by the appearance of a local indurated area. Hernias and abdominal-wall weakness may occur later.

Preoperatively, a liquid diet is prescribed for 24 hours to aid bowel decompression, which is necessary for a relaxed abdominal wall. Postoperative care includes the following:
1. Position patient with head elevated and knees flexed, to prevent pull on abdominal incisions.
2. Monitor and empty suction drains from breast and abdomen every 30 minutes for 24 hours; notify the surgeon if drainage is less than 50 ml/hr.
3. Monitor colour and temperature of new breast tissue (it should be paler and cooler than surrounding tissue but not mottled or cold).
4. Give prescribed isoxsuprine and oxygen by nasal cannula to aid flap oxygenation.
5. If nausea is present, give prescribed antiemetic to prevent pull on abdominal incision from vomiting.
6. Clean umbilicus and tape over incision with cotton swab saturated with antiseptic to prevent infection.
7. Suggest patient ambulate during first week by leaning slightly forward with knees flexed, to ease pull on abdominal incisions.
8. Teach the patient to do the following;
   a. Avoid raising arms above shoulder level for 4 weeks.
   b. Avoid heavy lifting for 6 weeks.

The regional breast care centres can provide information about breast reconstruction, and may be able to put individuals in touch with volunteers who have undergone breast reconstruction themselves.

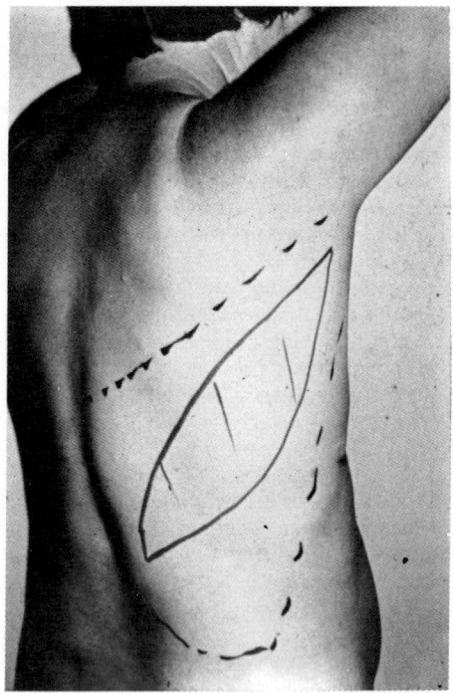

Fig. 28-11 Free latissimus flap. Flap has been outlined on patient before removal. (From Meeker MH, Rothrock JC: *Alexander's care of the patient in surgery*, ed 9, St Louis, 1990, Mosby–Year Book.)

METASTATIC DISEASE

Metastasis from the breast is primarily by way of the intramammary lymphatics to regional nodes and then to systemic dissemination. Spread may also be from the primary mass to extension of local structures (skin, ribs). As stated earlier, the most common metastases are to bone, lung, liver, and brain. Bone metastases have a better prognosis whereas multiple sites of metastases and short disease-free intervals have a worse prognosis.[25]

Treatment is primarily palliative and includes radiation, hormone therapy, and chemotherapy. Hormone therapy may include ablation of the ovaries or tamoxifen. Chemotherapy with autologous bone marrow transplantation is now being used. The care of the patient with advanced cancer is discussed in Chapter 9.

SUMMARY

1. A baseline mammogram should be obtained by all post-menopausal women. It should be obtained earlier in women with a family history of breast disease, or in those who have previously had breast disease before the menopause.
2. Most breast cancers are discovered by BSE; therefore, BSE should be performed by all women over age 20.
3. Lumps from benign breast disorders are usually seen bilaterally and are discrete, tender, and freely movable. Lumps from malignant tumours are usually solitary, irregularly shaped, nontender, and nonmobile.

4. Common benign breast disorders include fibrocystic disease, fibroadenomas, and mastitis.
5. Breast discomfort from benign breast lesions may be decreased by mild analgesics, heat or cold, or by breast support.
6. Radiological tests for breast cancer include mammography and xeroradiography. The only way to determine conclusively whether a tumour is malignant is by breast biopsy.
7. High-risk factors for breast cancer are a mother or sister with breast cancer (especially premenopausal), menarche before age 11, menopause after age 50, or first live birth after age 30; however, *all* women are considered at risk.
8. The most common surgical procedures for stages I and II are lumpectomy with axillary dissection and radiation, and modified radical mastectomy. The choice is made by patient and spouse based on the surgeon's recommendations.
9. Adjuvant therapy is recommended to prevent recurrence. Chemotherapeutic regimens are more effective for premenopausal women, whereas hormonal therapy for oestrogen receptor-positive tumours is more effective in postmenopausal women.
10. Loss of a breast is a traumatic experience for many women and may lead to feelings of decreased femininity and self-worth. Women need considerable support during this time.
11. Breast Care and Mastectomy Association consists of specially trained volunteers who can provide support and information to women having mastectomies.
12. Shoulder exercises following a mastectomy are started early and continued until the shoulder regains full movement.
13. Breast prostheses of various types may be purchased to wear in a bra after the incision has healed.
14. Lymphoedema (swelling of the upper arm) may result after axillary node removal because of interference with lymphatic drainage. Elevating the arm after surgery and starting exercises early can help to prevent lymphoedema.
15. Infection of affected arm may be prevented by avoiding trauma and bites, and treating all lesions early.
16. New advances in breast reconstruction have made this an option for many women who are not satisfied with a breast prosthesis. Types of breast reconstruction include a breast implant, latissimus dorsi flap, and a transabdominal island flap.

STUDY QUESTIONS

- What are some reasons why many women do not practise BSE? What implications does this have for patient teaching?
- What are the factors that can influence the type of surgery selected by women with stage I or II breast cancer?
- Mrs. Smith has stage III breast cancer. She has just read an article about lumpectomy with radiation and says she

does not understand why the surgeon said this would be ineffective for her. How would you reply?
- Ms. Jones asks you why she needs radiation after her lumpectomy when a friend of hers had her breast removed without needing radiation. How would you reply?
- What screening and support resources are available in your community for people with breast cancer?

REFERENCES AND SELECTED READINGS

1. American Cancer Society: *Cancer facts and figures: 1991,* New York, 1991, The Society.
2. American Cancer Society, Reach to Recovery: *Exercises after mastectomy, patient guide,* New York, 1983, The Society.
3.* Brown-Daniels CJ, Blasdell A: Early breast cancer: adjuvant drug therapy, *Am J Nurs* 90(11):32-33, 1990.
4. Bruera E et al: Asthenia in breast cancer, *Am J Nurs* 89(5):737-741, 1989.
5. Butrum RR, Clifford CK, Lanza E: NCI dietary guidelines: rationale, *Am J Clin Nutr* 48:888-895, 1988.
6.* Cawley M, Kostic J, Cappello C: Informational and psychosocial needs of women choosing conservative surgery/primary radiation for early stage breast cancer, *Cancer Nurs* 13(2):90-94, 1990.
7.* Chavez A: Conservation surgery with radiotherapy: an alternative in breast cancer, *Semin Oncol Nurs* 1:195-199, 1985.
8. Clark JC et al: Reintegration and maintenance of employees with breast cancer in the workplace, *AAOHN J* 37(5):186-196, 1989.
9. Cohen IK, Turner D: Immediate breast reconstruction with tissue expanders, *Clin Plast Surg* 14:491-498, 1987.
10. Culver J et al: Implementing the American Cancer Society Breast Cancer Awareness program in the workplace, *AAOHN J* 37(5):166-170, 1989.
10a. Cuschieri A, Wright PSG: *Essential Surgical Practice,* Bristol, 1982.
11.* d'Angelo TM, Gorrell CR: Breast reconstruction using tissue expanders, *Oncol Nurs Forum* 16(1):23-27, 1989.
12.* Dietrick-Gallagher M et al: Teaching patients to care for drains after breast surgery for malignancy, *Oncol Nurs Forum* 16(2):263-265, 1989.
13.* Dinner M, Coleman C: Breast reconstruction: use of autogenous tissue, *AORN J* 42:490-496, 1985.
14. Ediken S: Mammography and palpable cancer of the breast, *Cancer* 61:263-265, 1988.
15.* Eich SJ: Promising early breast cancer treatment without mastectomy, *Cancer Nurs* 8:51-58, 1985.
16.* Ellerhorst-Ryan JM et al: Evaluating benign breast disease, *Nurs Pract* 13:13-29, 1988.
17.* Ellerhorst-Ryan JM: Breast cancer: saving lives through early detection, *Ohio Nurses Rev* 64(3):8-9, 1989.
17a. FDA nears decision on breast implants, *Am J Nurs* 92(1):11-12, 1992.
18.* Feather BL, Lanigan C: Looking good after your mastectomy, *Am J Nurs* 87:1048-1049, 1987.
19. Feather BL, Wainstock JM: Perceptions of postmastectomy patients, part I: The relationships between social support and network providers; part II: Social support and attitudes towards mastectomy, *Cancer Nurs* 12(5):293-300, 301-309, 1989.
20.* Fernsler JI: Employee counseling with respect to lifestyles, life events, and breast cancer risks, *AAOHN J* 37(5):158-164, 1989.
21. Fowble B et al: *Treatment of breast cancer,* St Louis, 1991, Mosby–Year Book.
22.* Fox K: Ellen's going home: can she manage without you? Preparing your postmastectomy patient for discharge, *Nursing 89* 19(5):80-81, 1989.
23.* Greitzu S: Breast cancer: the risks and options, *RN* 49(10):26-32, 1986.
24.* Gottschalk LA, Hoigaard-Martin J: The emotional impact of mastectomy, *Psychiatry Res* 17:153-167, 1986.
25. Harris JR et al: *Breast diseases,* ed 2, Philadelphia, 1991, JB Lippincott.
26. Hellman S et al: *Cancer of the breast.* In DeVita V: *Cancer: principles and practices of oncology,* ed 3, Philadelphia, 1989, JB Lippincott.
27. Hery M et al: Conservative treatment (chemotherapy/radiotherapy) of locally advanced breast cancer, *Cancer* 57:1744-1749, 1986.
28. Holmberg K et al: Psychosocial adjustment after mastectomy and breast-conserving treatment, *Cancer* 64:969-974, 1989.
29.* Hutcheson HA: TAIF: new option for breast reconstruction, *Nurs 86* 16(2):52-53, 1986.
30.* Hutcheson HA: Breast reconstruction using abdominal tissues: a nursing diagnosis approach. *Plast Surg Nurs* 7(1):11-16, 1987.
31.* Jussak PF: Male breast cancer, *Innovations Oncol Nurs* 2(1):1-5, 1986.
32.* Knobf MT: Primary breast cancer: physical consequences and rehabilitation, *Semin Oncol Nurs* 1:214-224, 1985.
33.* Knobf MT: Early-stage breast cancer: the options, *Am J Nurs* 90(11):28-30, 1990.
34. Leffall LD: Breast cancer in black women, *Cancer* 31:4-6, 1987.
35. Levitt SH: Primary treatment of early breast cancer with conservation surgery and radiation therapy, *Cancer* 55:2140-2148, 1985.
36.* Lewis RM, Ellison ES, Woods NF: The impact of breast cancer on the family, *Semin Oncol Nurs* 1:206-213, 1985.
37. Lippmann ME, Lichter AS, Danforth DN: *Diagnosis and management of breast cancer,* Philadelphia, 1988, WB Saunders.
38. Love RR et al: Side effects and emotional distress during cancer chemotherapy, *Cancer* 63:604-612, 1989.
39. Love SM: Fibrocystic diseases, *Patient Care* 24(7):65-82, 1990.
40.* Mach E: Most breast lumps aren't cancer, *RN* 53(12):20-23, 1990.
41.* Mast DE, Mood DW: Preparing patient with breast cancer for brachytherapy, *Oncol Nurs Forum* 17(2):267-270, 1990.
42. McGee RF, White CH: Helping employees and families cope with breast cancer treatment, *AAOHN J* 37(5):178-185, 1989.
43.* McKann CF: The changing role of surgery in the treatment of breast cancer, *Semin Oncol Nurs* 1:176-180, 1985.
44.* Morra ME: Breast self-examination today: an overview of its use and its value, *Semin Oncol Nurs* 1:170-175, 1985.
45.* Nash JA: Breast cancer: screening detection and diagnosis, *Semin Oncol Nurs* 1:163-169, 1985.
46. National Cancer Institute: *Clinical alert,* Bethesda, Md, May 16, 1988, The Institute.
47.* Nielsen BB, East D: Advances in breast cancer: implications for nursing care, *Nurs Clin North Am* 25(2):365-375, 1990.
48.* Northouse LL: A longitudinal study of the adjustment of patients and husbands to breast cancer, *Oncol Nurs Forum* 6(4):511-516, 1989.
49.* Northouse LL: The impact of breast cancer on patients and husbands, *Cancer Nurs* 12(5):276-284, 1989.
50.* Norwood SL: Fibrocystic breast disease: an update and review, *J Obstet Gynecol Neonatal Nurs* 19(2):116-121, 1990.
51. Owen P et al: Facilitating adherence to ACS and NCI guidelines for breast cancer screening, *AAOHN J* 37(5):153-157, 194-196, 1989.
52. *Radiation therapy and you: a guide to self-help during treatment,* No 80-2227, Washington, DC, 1985, National Institutes of Health.
53.* Relfsnider E: Educating women about benign breast disease, *AAOHN J* 38(3):121-126, 1990.
54.* Rush DL, Kloppenborg EM: Don't underestimate the lumpectomy patient's needs, *RN* 53(3):58-65, 1990.
55.* Sawyer RF: Breast self-examination: hospital-based nurses aren't assessing their clients, *Oncol Nurs Forum* 13(5):44-48, 1986.
56.* Schain WS: Breast cancer surgeries and psychosexual sequelae: implications for remediation, *Semin Oncol Nurs* 1:200-205, 1985.
57.* Schain WS: The sexual and intimate consequences of breast cancer treatment, *Cancer* 38:154-161, 1988.
58. Schroeder SA et al: *Current medical diagnosis and treatment,* ed 30, Norwalk, Conn, 1991, Appleton & Lange.
59.* Solomon J: The good news about breast reconstruction, *RN* 49(11):47-48, 1986.
60. Systemic sclerosis following breast implants, *Nurses Drug Alert* 13(11):86-87, 1989.
61. Taplin S et al: Breast cancer risk and participation in mammographic screening, *Am J Pub Health* 79:1494-1497, 1989.
62. Tackenberg JN: Cryolumpectomy: another option for breast cancer, *Nursing 90* 20(5):32J, 32L, 1990.

* Recommended for student reading

63.* Vogel CL: Systemic therapy for breast cancer, *Semin Oncol Nurs* 1:188-194, 1985.

64.* Ward S et al: Factors women take into account when deciding upon type of surgery for breast cancer, *Cancer Nurs* 12(6):344-351, 1989.

65. Way LW: Current surgical diagnosis and treatment, ed 9, Norwalk, Conn, 1991, Appleton & Lange.

66.* Wellisch DK: The psychologic impact of breast cancer on relationships, *Semin Oncol Nurs* 1:195-199, 1985.

67. Willis MA et al: Interagency collaboration: teaching breast self-examination to black women, *Oncol Nurs Forum* 16:171-177, 1989.

68.* Zenmore R, Shepel LF: Effects of breast cancer and mastectomy on emotional support and adjustment, *Soc Sci Med* 28:19-27, 1989.

69. Woods NF: Influences on sexual adaptation to mastectomy, *J Obstet Gynecol Neonatal Nurs* 4:33-37, 1975.

70. The European Breast Cancer Treatment collaborative group report on adjuvant therapy, cited *Lancet* Jan 1992.

FURTHER READING

Aspinall VA: An effective way to reduce mortality—screening for malignant breast disease, *Professional Nurse* 283-287, Feb 1991.

Hollinworth H: Comfort of strangers, *Nursing Times* 88(40):38-40, Sep 30-Oct 6 1992.

McKinney B: Empowering your patients to do self-breast exams, *J Practical Nursing* 42(4):15-8, Dec 1992.

McLuckie A: Anxiety and the patient for breast biopsy, *British Journal of Theatre Nursing* 2(4):13-5, Jul 1992.

Rowley T: An emotional scar...mastectomy, *Nursing Times* 85(22):35-8, May 31-Jun 6 1989.

Toughill EH: Sexual counseling for the mastectomy patient, *Occupational Health Nursing* 32(8):416-8, August 1984.

Problems of Cognition, Sensation, and Motion

Unit Ten

29

The Patient with Neurological Problems

Elizabeth Schenk

After studying this chapter, the learner should be able to:

- Explain the difference in types of neurones and how they transmit impulses.
- Explain three components of the neurological assessment.
- Explain the importance of primary, secondary, and tertiary prevention of problems of the nervous system.
- State five symptoms of raised intracranial pressure.
- List five nursing actions to decrease intracranial pressure.
- Explain the pathophysiology involved in two degenerative diseases and three infection-related diseases of the nervous system.
- Define cerebrovascular accident, cerebral thrombosis, cerebral embolism, transient ischaemic attack, and cerebral haemorrhage.
- State two complications of brain surgery and their treatment.

ANATOMY AND PHYSIOLOGY

The application of the nursing process to patients with neurological problems requires knowledge of the structure and function of the nervous system. The nervous system works as an electrical conductance system. It coordinates and controls all activities of the body. These activities can be divided into the following four kinds of functions:

1. Receiving information (stimuli) from the internal and external environment over sensory (afferent) pathways
2. Communicating information between distant parts of the body (periphery) and the central nervous system
3. Computing or processing the information received at various reflex (spinal cord) and conscious (higher brain) levels to determine responses appropriate to existing situations
4. Transmitting information rapidly over varied motor (efferent) pathways to organs for body action control or modification

Neuroglia cells

While the basic structural and functional unit of the nervous system is the neurone, *neuroglia cells* serve as an adjunct. Neuroglia cells make up almost half of the microscopic structures of the spinal cord and brain. They provide nourishment, support, and protection for the neurones.

Neurone

The basic structural and functional unit of the nervous system is the *neurone*. It is a highly specialized and differentiated cell, but it has all the basic biological and biochemical properties of other body cells. The single neurone acts as a miniature nervous system and has properties specific for its electrical function. Its specialized properties are excitation and electrical-chemical conduction. The neurone consists of a *cell body* (soma, or perikaryon) with two extensions: *dendrites*, which receive information from axon terminals at special sites called *synapses*, and *axons*, which transmit information away from the cell body to adjacent neurones (Fig.29-1). A cell membrane encloses the outer boundary of the soma, dendrite, and axon (Fig. 29-1).

Neurones can be classified according to structure and function. Structurally, the divisions include the number of processes. *Unipolar neurones* have only one process or pole; the general sensory neurone is an example of a unipolar neurone. The *bipolar neurone* contains two poles: one dendrite and one axon. These neurones are found in the rods and cones of the retina, the mucous membrane of the nose, and other special sensory areas. The multipolar neurone consists of one axon and one or more dendrites.

Neurones may also be classified by the length of the axon. *Golgi type I neurones* are large and have long axons. They make up the long fibre tracts of the spinal cord, cerebellum, and cerebral cortex. *Golgi type II cells* are smaller cells that are found in the brain and spinal cord. They have short axons that branch repeatedly. The purpose of these neurones is to establish complex circuits in the nervous system.

Neurones are functionally known as *afferent, internuncial,* or *efferent*. Afferent neurones are sensory neurones that conduct impulses from the periphery *to* the central nervous system. Internuncial neurones are found in the central nervous system and assist in impulse conduction. Efferent or motor neurones transmit impulses *from* the central nervous system to the periphery.

Neurones are grouped in chains in the peripheral nervous system to form *nerves*. These collections are called *fibre tracts* in the central nervous system.

Collections of neurones are connected in complex ways. The connection determines what each collection of neurones is capable of doing. The neurones are organized into circuits, some of which are simple and made up of relatively few neurones and others that are very complicated. A single neurone may be a part of several different neurological circuits and thus may have a role in several functions.

Many of the important functional properties of the neurone lie within the *cell membrane*. The membrane is permeable to oxygen, carbon dioxide, and certain inorganic ions, and it is impermeable to organic compounds (proteins) and other inorganic ions. This characteristic of the membrane is called *differential permeability*.

The neurone also can be characterized by the property of *excitability*. Excitability means that the resting potential of neurones is unstable under certain conditions, as when the membrane of the neurone is stimulated. This unstable condition gives rise to *action potentials*. Action potentials can only arise from excitable cells. All nervous system functions occur from the phenomenon of the action potential.

Action Potential

Two phases occur within the action potential—*depolarization* (positive state) and *repolarization* (return to the more normal resting potential). When resting, the nerve fibre is charged, with the inside of the cell membrane negatively charged in relation to the outside. A high concentration of sodium exists extracellularly, and a high concentration of potassium exists intracellularly. When the nerve fibre is stimulated, there is an influx of sodium and a loss of intracellular potassium by diffusion. The cell becomes positive, and the action potential (depolarization) occurs. After depolarization, the ion flow is reversed and the membrane is returned to its resting state. During depolarization and part of the repolarization process, there is a time interval called the *absolute refractory period*. During this time the nerve cannot be restimulated. This prevents repetitive excitation of the nerve.

When an action potential is generated it proceeds automatically to completion regardless of the type of stimulus that started the depolarization. This means that a strong stimulus does not cause a larger action potential. The action potential also spreads over the entire membrane without a decrease in velocity. The velocity is related to the size of the axon (velocity is higher with a larger diameter) and whether myelin is present.

Myelin is an excellent insulator of axons. The myelin sheath is deposited around the axons by Schwann's cells, and this layer may be as thick as the axon itself. Myelin prevents almost all ion flow across the axon and its membrane. However, at distances of approximately 1 mm, the sheath is interrupted by *nodes of Ranvier*. At these small, uninsulated areas, ions can flow easily between the extracellular fluid and the axon (Fig. 29-3).

The presence of myelin causes such fibres to be called *large fibres*; those without myelin are called *small fibres*. Large fibres have a greater conduction velocity because (1) the jumping effect allows depolarization to proceed quickly and (2) energy is conserved, because only the nodes depolarize. Large fibres appear white because of the myelin; the *white matter* of the nervous system is made up of myelinated fibres.

Many action potentials of neurones originate in a receptor neurone where internal and external stimuli are normally received. A receptor is like a transducer and can change one form of energy into another form. A receptor, however, responds or depolarizes to *only one* type of stimulus. For example, the retina of the eye responds only

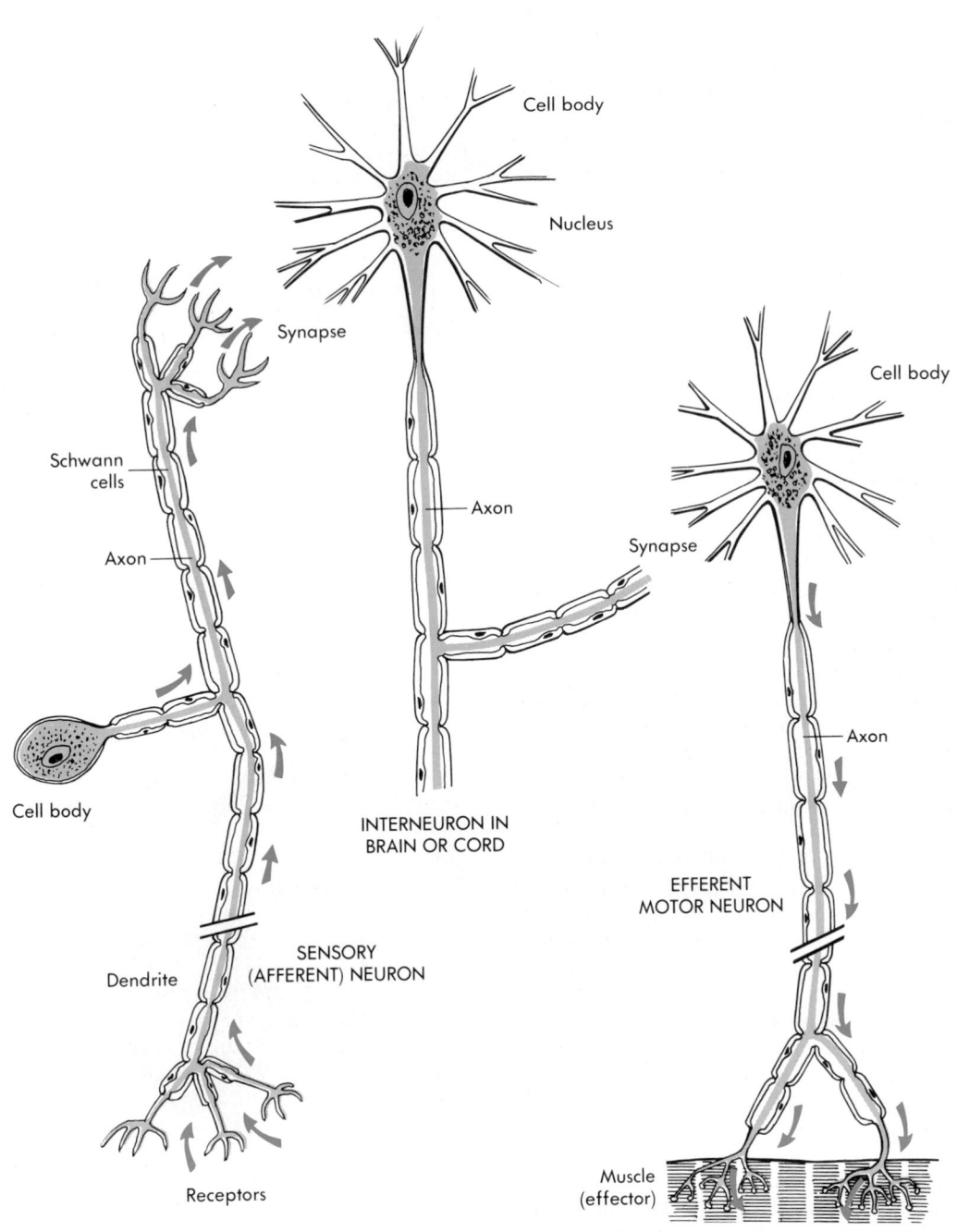

Fig. 29-1 Diagram of neurones showing the cell body (soma), dendrites, and axon. Direction of impulse conduction indicated by arrows.

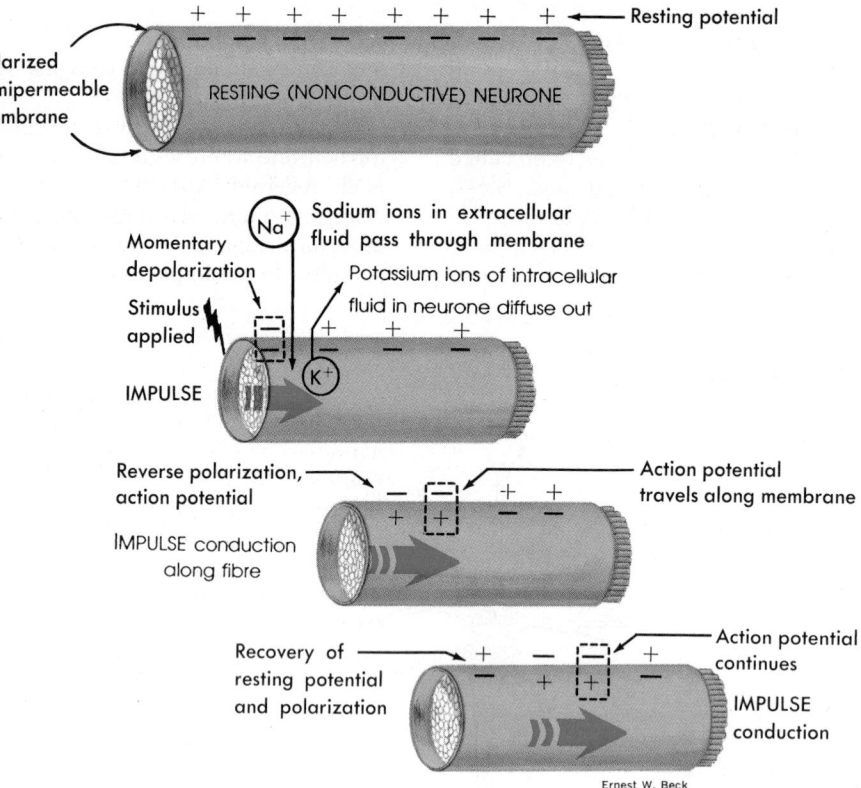

Fig. 29-2 Upper diagram represents polarized state of membrane of nerve fibre when it is not conducting impulses. Lower diagrams represent nerve impulse conduction: a self-propagating wave of negativity or action potential travels along membrane. (From Thibodeau GA: *Anthony's textbook of anatomy and physiology*, ed 13, St Louis, 1990, Mosby–Year Book.)

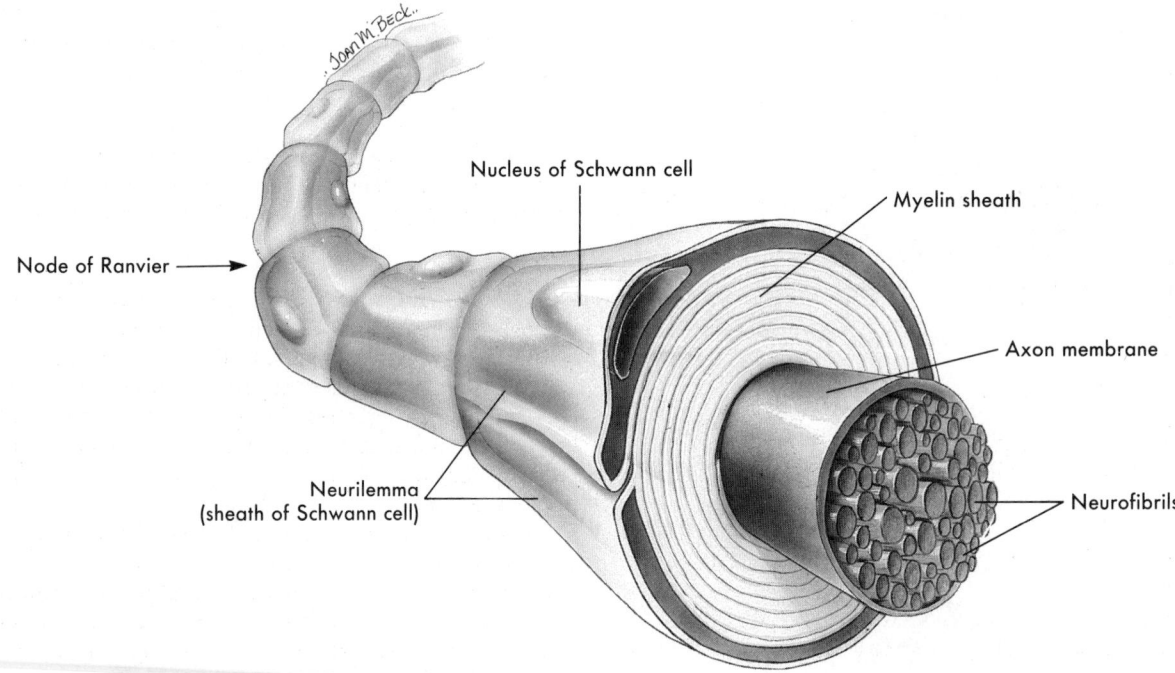

Fig. 29-3 Diagram of a nerve fibre and its coverings. This myelinated axon is located outside the central nervous system. Myelin is produced by the concentric layers of the Schwann cell. The neurilemma is the outer sheath of the Schwann cell and is indented by successive nodes of Ranvier. (From Christensen BL, Kockrow EO: *Foundations of nursing*, St Louis, 1991, Mosby–Year Book.)

to the stimulus of light, which is converted to electrical energy and travels over the optic nerves to the visual cortices for perception.

Synapses

Neurones make contact with one another at sites called *synapses*. Transmission occurring across a synapse is a chemical process that occurs because of the release of neurotransmitters. The synapse consists of the *presynaptic terminal*, the *synaptic cleft*, and the *postsynaptic membrane*. Three types of interneuronal synapses occur. When the axon of one neurone synapses with the cell body of another neurone, it is called *axosomatic*. *Axodendritic* synapses occur between the axon of one neurone and the dendrites of another. Finally, *axoaxonic* synapses occur when one axon connects with another axon.

The end of the axon contains a chemical substance that is released by the action potential. The substance diffuses across the synapse to the adjacent cell membrane. *Synaptic transmission* is both *excitatory* and *inhibitory* in nature. Excitatory neurotransmitters react with receptor sites on the postsynaptic membrane to enhance permeability to sodium, chloride, and potassium ions. Inhibitory neurotransmitters decrease the postsynaptic membrane permeability to sodium while increasing the permeability to potassium and chloride ions. The membrane becomes *hyperpolarized*. The amount of neurotransmitter released depends on the amount and speed of impulses stimulating the presynaptic terminal. Whether a neurone fires depends on the sum of the excitatory and inhibitory inputs.

At least 30 different neurotransmitters can affect transmission of an impulse at the synapse.

These actions include the following:

1. Acetylcholine—plays role in speeding impulse transmission
2. Noradrenaline—maintains arousal (awakening from a deep sleep, dreaming, and regulation of mood)
3. Dopamine—involves gross subconscious movement of the skeletal muscles and character of emotional responses
4. Serotonin (5-hydroxytryptamine)—induces sleep, affects sensory perception, controls temperature, and has a role in controlling mood

In the past few years another group of chemical messengers, known as *neuropeptides*, has been discovered. Some of these function as neurotransmitters themselves, but most often they increase or decrease the response of the other neurotransmitters. In 1975 *enkephalins* were discovered; they act as a natural painkiller. Enkephalins are thought to inhibit pain impulses and bind with the same receptors in the brain with which chemicals such as morphine bind.

Chemical endorphins have been isolated in the pituitary. They are thought to suppress pain and are linked with memory, learning, and sexual activity.

Chemicals allowing excitatory transmission are *acetylcholine*, *noradrenaline*, *dopamine*, and *serotonin*. Those inhibiting transmissions are *gamma aminobutyric acid* (GABA) in brain tissue and *glycine* in the spinal cord.

Divisions of the Nervous System

Macroscopically, the nervous system has two major divisions. These are the *central nervous system* and the *peripheral nervous system* (Fig. 33-8).

Central nervous system

The central nervous system (CNS) is made up of collections of neurones and their connections into the brain and spinal cord. All the basic informational processes occur within the CNS. Areas of the brain and spinal cord are distinguished where cell bodies are concentrated into *nuclei* and groups of axons run in *tracts* that interconnect the parts. Collections of neurones are connected in complex ways. The connections determine the capability of each collection of neurones. The brain and spinal cord are structurally continuous. The brain is housed in the skull and the spinal cord in the vertebral column.

Skull

Surrounding the brain is the skull, a bony structure that encloses and protects it. The skull is divided into two primary sections: the *cranium* and the *bones of the face*. Only the former will be discussed here.

The cranium is made up of eight bones that are joined by a series of fixed joints called *sutures*. The bones are made up of three layers that are called the *outer table*, the *diploe*, and the *inner table*. The outer and inner table are solid, whereas the diploe is spongy. The inner table forms an inner cavity that is divided as follows:

1. Anterior fossa—contains frontal lobes
2. Middle fossa—contains temporal, parietal, and occipital lobes
3. Posterior fossa—contains brainstem and cerebellum

The *foramen magnum* is a large oval shaped opening at the base of the skull. It is at this level that the spinal cord and brain connect.

Brain

The brain weighs about 1300–1400 g and is divided grossly into the following three main areas: (1) the cerebrum, (2) the brainstem, and (3) the cerebellum.

Cerebrum

The cerebrum of each hemisphere (right and left) is composed of the following four major lobes: the *frontal*, *parietal*, *temporal*, and *occipital*. The cerebrum is the largest part of the brain and is covered on the outside by the cerebral cortex, which is about 6 mm thick and contains several billion neurones. It receives and analyzes all impulses, controls voluntary movement, and stores knowledge of all impulses received.

The cerebrum is longitudinally divided into right and left hemispheres. The major folds of the cortex divide each hemisphere into four lobes. Each cerebral lobe, named for the overlying cranial bone, carries out specific functions such as general sensation, perception, special senses, and speech (Fig. 24-9).

Deep within the cerebrum are the *basal nuclei*. These are masses of grey matter (cell bodies) and include the caudate nucleus, putamen, and globus pallidus. The basal nuclei function as part of the extrapyramidal system and control postural adjustment and fine voluntary movements, especially those of the hands and lower extremities.

One function of the cerebrum deserves special mention—that of speech. Speech is a function of the dominant hemisphere, which is on the left side of the brain for all right-handed people and most left-handed people. The two identified speech centres are Broca's area and Wernicke's area. *Broca's area* is in the frontal lobe adjacent to the motor cortex and controls verbal, expressive speech. *Wernicke's area* is in the posterior part of the temporal lobe and may extend to adjacent parts of the parietal lobe. It is responsible for reception and understanding of language. An area in the frontal lobe governs ability to write words, and an area in the occipital lobe controls ability to understand written material. The specific functions of the cerebral cortexes are listed in Box 29-1.

Brainstem

The *brainstem* lies deep in the centre of the hemisphere and connects with the spinal cord at the level of the medulla. It carries all nerve fibres passing between the brain hemisphere and the spinal cord; additionally, all cranial nerves except cranial nerve I arise from it. Several structures are contained in the brainstem. These include the diencephalon, the midbrain, the pons, and the medulla oblongata. The diencephalon is often called the innerbrain because it lies directly beneath the cerebrum. It contains the thalamus and the hypothalamus. The thalamus, an oval structure with two lobes, is approximately 2.5 cm (1 inch) in diameter; it composes four fifths of the diencephalon. The thalamus serves as a relay station for some sensory impulses while interpreting other sensory messages, such as pain, light touch, and pressure.

The *hypothalamus*, which lies below the thalamus, plays a vital role in the *control of body temperature, fluid balance, appetite,* and *certain emotions,* such as *fear, pleasure,* and *pain.* Both the sympathetic and parasympathetic divisions of the autonomic nervous system are under the control of the hypothalamus, as is the pituitary gland. Thus the hypothalamus influences the heartbeat, the contraction and relaxation of the walls of blood vessels, and hormone secretion.

The specific functions of each of the structures that are located in the brainstem are listed in Box 29-2.

Of special importance is the core of tissue that extends throughout the entire brainstem called the *reticular formation* or the *reticular activating system* (RAS). This interconnecting network of cells is the integrating centre for respiration, cardiac function, motor systems, and states of consciousness. Stimulating these cells leads to wakefulness, and decreasing stimulation results in sleepiness (as in anoxia caused by increased intracranial pressure).

Cerebellum

The cerebellum is located below the posterior cerebrum and is about one fifth the size of the cerebrum. It has two lateral hemispheres and a medial part called the *vermis.* It controls skeletal muscles to produce coordinated movement, equilibrium, and erect posture. It acts with the cerebrum to coordinate muscle activity and produce skilled movement. Voluntary movements can proceed without the cerebellum, but they are clumsy and incoordinated (as in *asynergia* and *cerebellar ataxia*). The cerebellum receives both sensory and motor impulses, and it can detect errors in muscle synergy and adjust muscular control within the body.

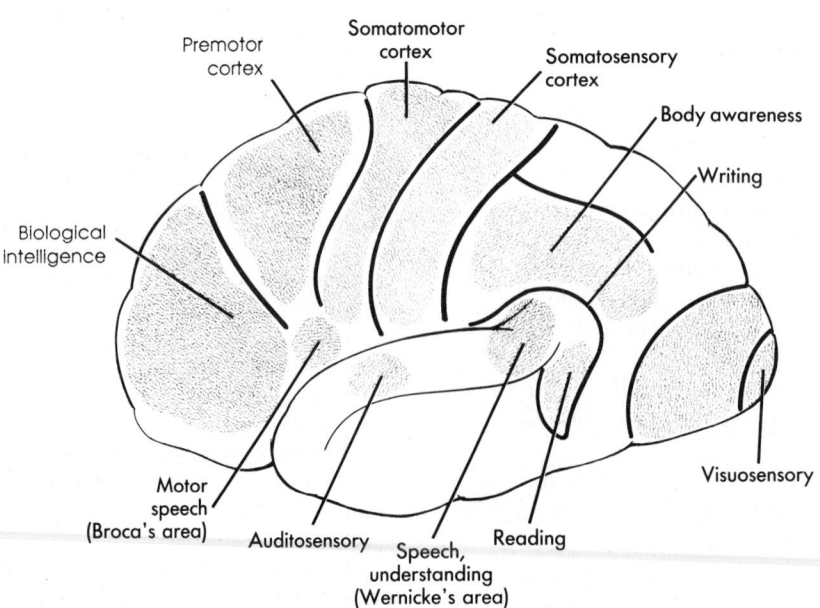

Fig. 29-4   Lateral view of the cerebrum, showing the lobes.

29-1 Specific functions of cerebral cortexes

Frontal cortex	Conceptualization
	Abstraction
	Judgment formation
	Motor ability
	Ability to write words
	Higher level centres for autonomic functions
Parietal cortex	Highest integrative and coordinating centre for perception and interpretation of sensory information
	Ability to recognize body parts
	Left versus right
	Motor movement
Temporal cortex	Memory storage
	Auditory integration
	Hearing
Occipital cortex	Visual centre
	Understanding of written material

receptors from the periphery. The grey matter also contains internuncial neurones that send impulses from one level to another, from the dorsal to ventral horns, and from one lateral half of the spinal cord to the other. The ascending pathways transmit sensory information from receptors in the periphery to the spinal cord and brain. The descending pathways transmit impulses from the brain to the motor neurones in the spinal cord (*upper motor neurones*) or to the peripheral nervous system (*lower motor neurones*).

The spinal cord is also the site of reflex pathways. Reflexes do not require relay to the brain level for action—they are an example of the simplest neural circuit. A reflex action consists of a specific stereotyped motor response to an adequate sensory stimulus. The response may involve skeletal muscle movement. A reflex may involve only one spinal cord level, or it may involve more spinal cord levels (segmental reflex). One example of the simple reflex arc is the knee jerk (Fig. 29-5).

Circulation of the brain and spinal cord

The arterial system of the brain includes the larger conducting arteries and the penetrating smaller vessels that enter the brain at right angles after branching off from the conducting vessels. The smaller vessels supply nutrients to the neurones. The conducting arteries and the areas they supply include the following:

Spinal vertebrae

The vertebral column is divided into these five regions: *cervical, thoracic, lumbar, sacral,* and *coccygeal*. The total number of vertebrae is 33 and is divided as follows:
1. 7 cervical
2. 12 thoracic
3. 5 lumbar
4. 5 sacral vertebrae fused to form the sacrum
5. 3 to 5 fused bones forming the coccyx

Each vertebra is separated from those above and below by *cartilage* and *fibrous tissue* called *intervertebral discs*. The *vertebral foramen* is the centre of the spinal cord and is part of the vertebral canal containing the spinal cord and spinal meninges. Muscles and ligaments are attached to the vertebrae at the vertebral processes.

Spinal cord

The spinal cord is the downward continuation of the medulla oblongata. It is 45 to 48 cm (17 to 18 inches) long and extends from the brainstem to the second lumbar vertebra. It starts at the level of the foramen magnum and ends at L2. The cord tapers in the lower thoracic region into a cone-shaped structure called the *conus medullaris*.

The spinal cord includes H-shaped central grey matter (cell bodies) surrounded by white matter composed of ascending and descending tracts. The grey matter resembles a butterfly. The front or ventral horn consists of multipolar neuronal structures such as cell bodies and dendrites that form the efferent neurones of the ventral roots and the spinal nerves. The dorsal horn contains cell bodies and dendrites of afferent neurones and sensory

29-2 Brainstem functions

Diencephalon

Receives sensory impulses (pain, temperature, and touch)
Acts as relay station
Controls pain threshold
Acts in synthesis of ADH and oxytocin
Helps maintain wakeful state
Controls temperature
Generates emotional response

Pons

Pneumotaxic centre (rhythmicity of respirations)
Connection between medulla, midbrain, and cerebellum
Origin of cranial nerves V, VI, VII, and VIII

Midbrain

Motor movement
Relay of impulses
Postural reflex patterns
Auditory reflexes
Righting reflex
Some control of vision
Origin of cranial nerves III and IV

Medulla oblongata

Cardiac, vasomotor, and respiratory centre
Centre for cough, swallowing, and hiccuping
Role in reticular activating system
Origin of cranial nerves IX, X, XI, and XII

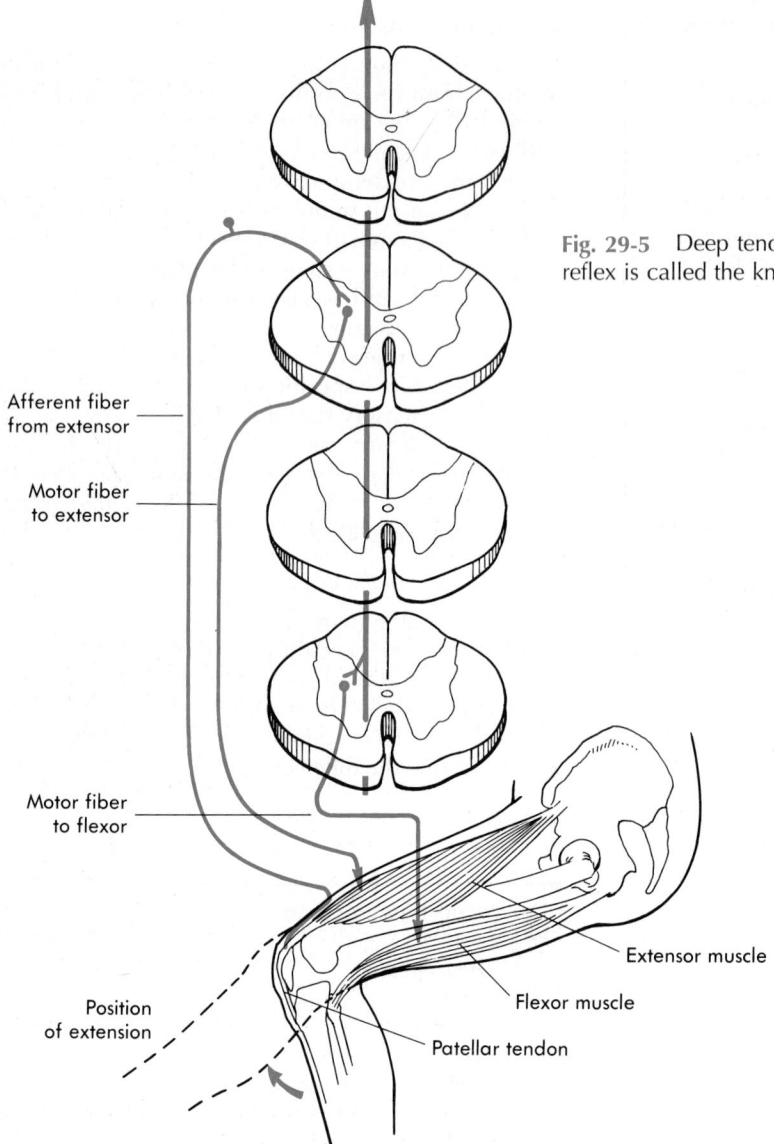

Fig. 29-5 Deep tendon reflex that demonstrates the reflex arc. This reflex is called the knee jerk or patellar tendon reflex.

Afferent fiber
from extensor

Motor fiber
to extensor

Motor fiber
to flexor

Position
of extension

Extensor muscle

Flexor muscle

Patellar tendon

1. Internal carotid arteries—80% of blood supply
   a. Anterior cerebral arteries
   (1) Medial surface of the frontal and parietal lobes
   (2) Basal nuclei
   (3) Portions of the internal capsule and corpus callosum
   b. Middle cerebral arteries
   (1) Lateral surfaces of parietal, frontal, and temporal lobes
   (2) Precentral (motor) gyri
   (3) Postcentral (sensory) gyri
2. Vertebral arteries—20% of blood supply
   a. Basilar artery
   (1) Brainstem
   (2) Cerebellum
   b. Posterior cerebral arteries
   (1) Portions of temporal and occipital lobes
   (2) Vestibular organs
   (3) Cochlear apparatus

The posterior cerebral artery connects to the middle cerebral artery by the posterior communicating branches. The anterior cerebral arteries connect through the anterior communicating branches. The purpose of this connection in the circle of Willis is to ensure circulation in case of a problem in any of the four main arteries. Branches of cerebral arteries reach all parts of the brain.

Circulation to the brain has several unique characteristics. Systemic circulation favours the CNS overall, balancing parts to assure a constant supply of nutrients (glucose and oxygen) to the brain. The brain is also able to change its blood flow to respond to changes in blood pressure. In the presence of increasing blood pressure, cerebral vessels constrict, whereas they dilate when blood pressure falls. Vasodilation also occurs with elevated carbon dioxide content, hypoxia, and an elevated hydrogen ion concentration.

Cerebral veins have no valves. All veins of the brain terminate in sinuses created by the dura mater. They empty into the superior vena cava via the jugular vein.

The blood supply to the spinal cord comes from the spinal artery and two radicular arteries. The spinal artery arises from the vertebral arteries, whereas the radicular arteries arise from the aorta.

Blood-brain barrier

The blood-brain barrier is a physiological mechanism that aids in maintaining the homeostasis of the brain through selective permeability. Normally, substances enter the blood by way of capillaries into the cerebrospinal fluid or by the capillaries into the extracellular fluid. The barrier is permeable to O_2, CO_2, and water. It is slightly permeable to electrolytes but is impermeable to fixed acids and bases and most drugs.

Cerebrospinal fluid (CSF)

Cerebrospinal fluid (CSF) is found in the ventricles of the brain, in the central canal of the spinal cord, and in the subarachnoid space. It serves as a fluid cushion for the tissue of the nervous system and helps support the weight of the brain. Cerebrospinal fluid is formed in the vessels of the choroid plexus. In a 24-hour period the choroid plexus secretes approximately 500 to 570 ml of CSF. However, only 125 to 150 ml is circulating at any one time. After circulating around the brain and spinal cord, the fluid returns to the brain and is absorbed from the subarachnoid space through the arachnoid villi. The cerebrospinal fluid then enters the venous system and follows the pathway through the jugular vein to the superior vena cava into the systemic circulation.

29-3	Normal characteristics of cerebrospinal fluid (CSF)	
	Specific gravity	1.007
	pH	7.35 to 7.45
	Chloride	120 to 130 mmol/L
	Glucose	2.5–4.0 mmol/L
	Pressure	50 to 200 mm water
	Total volume	80 to 200 ml (15 ml in ventricles)
	Total protein	150–450 mg/L (lumbar) 100–250 mg/L (cisternal) 50–150 mg/L (ventricular)
	Gamma globulin	6% to 13% of total protein
	Cell count	
	RBC	none
	WBC	0–5 0–10 cells (all lymphocytes and monocytes)

Normally there are up to 8 lymphocytes/ml of spinal fluid. An increase in the number of cells may indicate an infection, such as tuberculosis or a viral infection. Bacterial infections such as tuberculous meningitis often lower the blood sugar level, as well as the chloride levels. Spinal fluid protein is increased in the presence of degenerative disease and/or brain tumour. Blood in the spinal fluid indicates haemorrhage from somewhere in the ventricular system. See Box 33-3 for normal characteristics of CSF.

Ventricles

The ventricular system is made up of four cavities. The two lateral ventricles are found within each cerebral hemisphere and are the largest cavities. They are separated by a thin layer called the *septum pellucidum*. Each of the lateral ventricles communicates with the central ventricle, which communicates with the fourth ventricle. Parts of the lateral, third, and fourth ventricles are lined with a dense layer of capillaries called the *choroid plexus*.

Meninges

The coverings of the nervous tissue in the brain and spinal cord are called the meninges. These coverings help support, protect, and nourish the vital tissues below. The outermost is the *dura mater*. It is a very tough membrane with two layers. One of these meningeal layers sends four processes deep into the brain. These processes form fibrous compartments for protection of the brain. The *arachnoid* is a delicate membrane that lies beneath the dura and closely covers the brain. Projections called *arachnoid villi* extend into the overlying dura. The innermost of the meninges is the *pia mater*, which is a vascular membrane with many minute plexuses of blood vessels. The same three meninges are also found in the spinal cord.

Three potential spaces are associated with the meninges. These include the following:
1. Extradural (external to the dura)
2. Subdural (between the dura and the arachnoid)
3. Subarachnoid (between the arachnoid and the pia mater.

Peripheral nervous system

The peripheral nervous system (PNS) is basically a set of common channels located outside the CNS. *Peripheral nerves are individual nerves or bundles of nerves that are motor sensory, or "mixed"* (both sensory and motor fibres). The peripheral nervous system consists of *12 pairs of cranial nerves,* which carry impulses to and from the brain, and *31 pairs of spinal nerves,* which carry impulses to and from the spinal cord. Each spinal nerve innervates a specific part of the body for sensation; these parts are called *dermatomes.* Several spinal nerves may also join together to form a complex network of nerve fibres called plexuses.

Peripheral nerves that transmit information towards the CNS are *afferent* or sensory in nature, and peripheral nerves that transmit information away from the CNS are *efferent* or motor in nature. In the peripheral nervous system the motor and sensory nerves usually travel together but separate at the cord level into a *posterior* or *sensory root* and an *anterior* or *motor root.*

The peripheral nervous system is divided into the *somatic* and *autonomic nervous systems.* The somatic nervous

Table 29-1 Parasympathetic and sympathetic nervous system influence

Organ system	Parasympathetic influence	Sympathetic influence
Heart	Decreases rate	Increases rate
Blood vessels	Dilates visceral and brain vessels	Constricts
Lung	Constricts bronchi	Dilates bronchi
Gastrointestinal	Increases peristalsis	Decreases peristalsis
Anal sphincter	Opens	Closes
Urinary	Contracts bladder	Relaxes bladder
	Opens sphincter	Closes sphincter
Eye	Constricts pupil	Dilates pupil
	Accommodates for near vision	Accommodates for far vision
Skin	Not applicable	"Goose flesh"
Gastric and salivary secretions	Increases	Decreases
Liver	Not applicable	Stimulates glycogen production
Adrenal medulla	Not applicable	Stimulates production of adrenaline

system innervates skeletal (striated) muscles. Fibres of axons liberate the neurotransmitter *acetylcholine* at the skeletal muscle cells; this produces an action potential and movement.

Autonomic nervous system

Body functions regulated by the autonomic nervous system include those of the *cardiovascular, respiratory,* and *endocrine systems.* Regulatory efforts have the goal of preserving homeostasis. Fibres of the autonomic nervous system synapse once after leaving the CNS at a site called the *ganglion.* The neurotransmitter is *acetylcholine.* The autonomic nervous system can be subdivided into the *sympathetic nervous system* and the *parasympathetic nervous system.* The sympathetic system functions to maintain homeostasis and to provide defence against stressors. During stress, sympathetic responses include an *increase* in blood pressure and heart rate and *vasoconstriction* of peripheral blood vessels. The parasympathetic system conserves and restores regulatory functions (see Table 29-1).

Sensory System Pathways

Stimulation of receptor neurones in the body is the first step in sensation. These receptor neurones provide the brain with information about the internal and external environments. The general sensory system includes the following:
1. Receptor neurones, which respond to specific stimuli
2. Posterior roots of the peripheral or afferent sensory nerves, which carry nerve impulses (action potentials) towards the CNS
3. Ascending or sensory tracts within the spinal cord and brain
4. Sensory area of the cerebral cortex, in which stimuli are perceived and interpreted

From the receptor neurone, the sensory impulse travels to the spinal cord along the afferent fibres of the nerve involved. These fibres enter the spinal cord through the posterior root and proceed along either the *spinothalamic tracts* or the *posterior columns.* The pathway followed is specific to the sensation.

Motor System Pathways

After sensation has been perceived by the brain, corrective action or response is initiated. This action is conveyed by the descending motor pathways, which include the *corticospinal (pyramidal) tracts,* the *extrapyramidal system,* and the *cerebellar system.* The corticospinal system is primarily concerned with skilled, voluntary movement of skeletal muscle. Fibres that combine to form the corticospinal tracts arise from the upper motor neurones, which are located in most areas of the cerebral cortex.

After fibres leave the cerebral cortex they travel to the medulla, in which the majority of fibres *decussate* (cross over) to the opposite side. These fibres eventually synapse with the anterior horn cells, which are in the spinal cord and the motor nuclei in the brainstem. These cells are the *lower motor neurones* and the final communication pathway with muscles via the *myoneural junction* (Fig. 29-6).

The *extrapyramidal tracts* provide *separate pathways* between the *cortex,* the *basal nuclei,* the *brainstem,* and the *spinal cord.* These include all descending motor pathways other than the corticospinal tracts, and they are named for their points of origin and termination. Generally, the extrapyramidal tracts help maintain muscle tone and control of gross autonomic skeletal muscle movement.

Visceral efferent pathways from the spinal cord control the action of involuntary or smooth muscles located within the walls of hollow organs, tubes, the heart, and glands.

Effectors

Effectors are cells of the body that "do something." They interact with the internal and external environments in some way and carry out the commands of the nervous system. The two classes of effectors are muscles and glands. They are both transducers and are capable of converting one form of energy into another. *Effectors,* like nerve tissue, are *excitable tissues* and are *able to generate action potentials.* The nervous system controls muscles and glands by directly turning them on or by altering the level of spontaneous activity.

Physiological Changes With Ageing

Studies have shown that the nervous system does change with ageing. The effect of these changes is variable. The brain itself significantly *decreases in weight* with ageing, along with a substantial loss of neurones. Those cells not destroyed undergo structural changes. Brain cells are lost

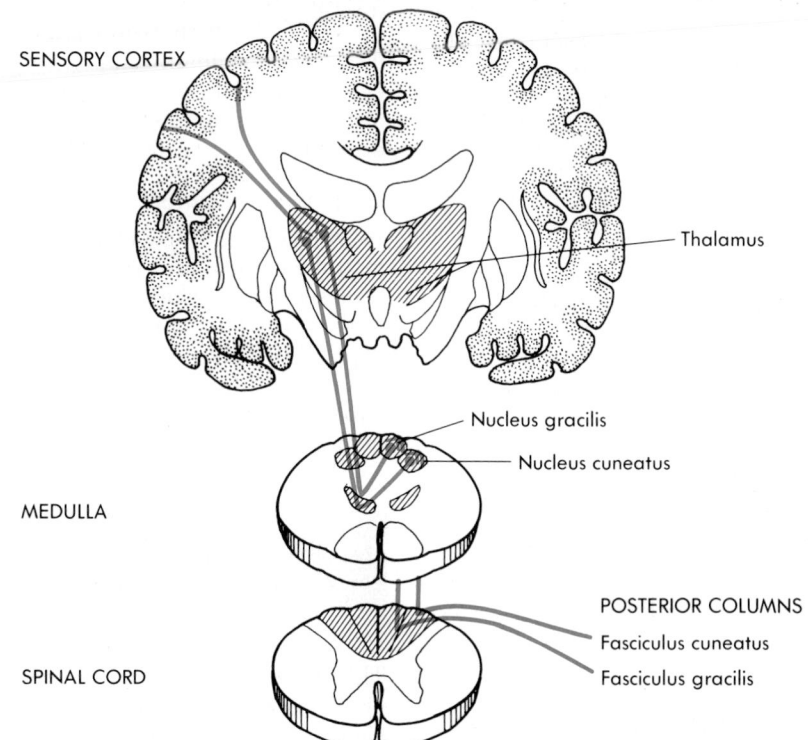

SENSORY CORTEX

Thalamus

Nucleus gracilis

Nucleus cuneatus

MEDULLA

POSTERIOR COLUMNS

Fasciculus cuneatus

Fasciculus gracilis

SPINAL CORD

Fig. 29-6   Pathways for fine touch, deep touch and pressure, vibration, and proprioception. Note how stimuli entering through dorsal route (posterior) travel on same side as posterior columns to medulla where they cross to opposite side, ascend to thalamus, and end in somasthetic area where perception occurs.

at a rate of 1% a year after 50 years of age.[30] The loss is inconsistent, so that some parts of the brain lose cells at a faster rate. The cortex generally loses cells at a faster rate than the brainstem. There may be a general decline in interconnections of dendrites. Also senile plaques and neurofibrillary plaques, as well as the age pigment lipofuscin, are found in neuronal cells. In addition, there is a significant *reduction of cerebral blood flow, a decrease in brain metabolism, and a decrease in oxygen utilization.*

The aged may also experience an altered *sleep/wakefulness ratio* and a *decreased ability to regulate body temperature.* These suggest changes in the function of the hypothalamus in the ageing.

The control of the autonomic nervous system over various functions of the body is unpredictable and labile in the elderly, but some changes do occur. Additionally, sensory and motor conduction *decreases in velocity of nerve impulses* occur with ageing, sensory conduction decreasing faster than motor. This occurs especially in peripheral nerves and more often in females. In the spinal cord the blood supply to the white matter has been found to be decreased, leading to diminished reflexes in the lower (distal) extremities.

It is important for the nurse to realize that normal changes that occur with ageing in the nervous system cannot be equated with senility, Alzheimer's disease, or organic brain disease. These conditions occur in a small number of older people, and many aged people reach advanced ages without any deterioration in the ability to think.

PREVENTION AND HEALTH EDUCATION

Problems that occur in the nervous system can have devastating results. These results often have impact on almost every body system and produce changes that are chronic and debilitating. Problems in other body systems, if discovered and treated in a timely fashion, can have much more satisfactory results than those in the nervous system.

Primary Prevention: Prevention of Disease

Many of the problems of the nervous system have no known cause and thus cannot be prevented. For other problems, however, preventive measures can be emphasized. Neurological problems can be divided into several main categories in terms of prevention as follows.

Problems resulting from vascular disease

Neurovascular diseases can at times be prevented, or their results can at least be minimized. Many of the cerebrovascular diseases are thought to occur more frequently as a result of the presence of certain risk factors. These same factors also increase the risk of cardiac disease:

1. Cigarette smoking
2. Hypertension
3. Hypercholesteraemia
4. Obesity
5. Stress-related occupations and a hectic pace of life

Problems resulting from metastasis

Cigarette smoking has been identified as a major cause of lung cancer. This is significant to the nervous system because neoplasms of the lung often metastasize to the brain. In fact, a significant number of lung malignancies are discovered after signs and symptoms of brain metastasis occur.

Problems resulting from trauma

Some actions can play an important role in preventing head injuries and spinal cord injuries. Factors that can influence the outcome include the following:
1. Use of seat belts in motor vehicles
2. Use of helmets while riding motorcycles, bicycles and horses
3. Practice of firearm safety—keeping guns correctly
4. Minimal use of drugs and alcohol
5. Not driving after drinking or taking drugs
6. Safe use of motor vehicles—no showing off or speeding
7. Use of precautions while swimming and especially not diving into shallow water

Problems resulting from infections

Neurological diseases resulting from infections can sometimes be prevented. Because ear or sinus infections can be a source of brain abscess or meningitis, it is important that these infections be treated. Also, because several of the neurological diseases related to infections are spread through sexual contacts, such as AIDS and syphilis, the practice of safe sex is important. This may include abstinence, monogamy, or the use of latex condoms.

Secondary Prevention: Early Detection

Early detection of neurological diseases often is difficult. Many initial symptoms are so vague that it is easy to deny or minimize their importance. Also, some changes may occur over such a long period of time that adaptation to them occurs. Certain *warning symptoms* can be found in such vague patterns that patients may be thought at first to be suffering from hysteria. The symptoms that are significant include the following:
1. Headaches that first occur after middle age or change in character, especially ones that are worse in the morning or awaken a person from sleep
2. Clumsiness or loss of function in an extremity
3. Changes in visual acuity
4. Any new or worsened seizure activity
5. Numbness or tingling in one or more extremities
6. Pain that is neurological in nature
7. Galactorrhoea
8. Cessation of menses
9. Personality changes

Tertiary Prevention: Prevention of Complications

It is important to mention the issue of tertiary prevention for the patient with neurological dysfunction. Unfortunately, many of these patients are *prone to iatrogenic complications*, as well as *functional disabilities*. These occur secondary to the neurological problems and include contractures, decubiti, and eye damage, as well as other hazards of immobility.[102] It is extremely important for the nurse working with neurologically impaired patients to be aware of rehabilitative concepts and apply them in nursing care. Many patients with neurological dysfunctions may also benefit from formal inpatient rehabilitative care after an acute hospitalization.

Looking to the Future

In the United Kingdom the Department of Health has identified stroke as a key area for action.[18b] Targets have been set which include reducing deaths from stroke by 40% in those aged under 65 and those aged 65–74 by the year 2000.[18b] In Britain over 1% of people over 65 suffer a stroke each year.[50a] Some 12% of deaths in England are due to stroke and 5% of these occur in people under 65 years of age.[18a]

COMMON NEUROLOGICAL MANIFESTATIONS

The practice of neurological nursing is concerned with problems of the nervous system that have a variety of causes. Whatever the cause, various symptoms occur, at times related to both organic and functional causes. Because of the nature of the anatomy and physiology of the nervous system, *organic lesions or trauma result in clinical manifestations related to the site affected, regardless of the underlying pathological condition.* Other manifestations result not from the damaged site itself, but from other parts of the nervous system that are affected by the damaged site. One example of this is a lack of control or regulation. The nurse must realize that patients with neurological problems may have to make significant changes in lifestyle and adaptation. The psyche and the body are one in the person; often there is no clear-cut distinction of symptoms. A person is an open system in which many subsystems interplay.

In this section, we will discuss neurological manifestations resulting from alterations in neurological function and structure that are common to many pathological conditions. A brief review of neurological assessment is helpful in this discussion.

NEUROLOGICAL ASSESSMENT

Complete neurological assessment is usually performed in phases and depends on the condition of the patient and the urgency in collecting the data. It includes a history and neurological examination.

Neurological examination of the conscious adult includes physical examination of the following:
1. Mental status
   a. Level of consciousness
   b. Orientation
   c. Mood and behaviour
   d. Knowledge
   e. Vocabulary
   f. Memory

Table 29-2　Commonly used states of awareness and associated behaviours

	State				
	Conscious-aware		**Semiconscious-semicomatose**		**Unconscious-comatose**	
Level	Alert	Confused	Obtunded, drowsy	Stupor	Light coma	Deep coma
Behaviours	Normal activity	Poor coordination	Sleepy	Apathetic	Not oriented to	Absence of
	Aware, mentally	Delirium	Very short atten-	Slow moving	time, place or	response to
	functional	Hallucinations	tion span	Blank expression	person	even the
		Restlessness	Ready arousal	Drooping head	Response is only	most pain-
		Excitable	Responds appro-	Staring	by grimace or	ful stimuli
		May be combat-	priately when	Arousal only to	withdrawing	
		ive	aroused	vigorous stim-	limb from	
		Short attention	Ability to respond	uli	pain	
		span	verbally	Incomplete	Primitive and	
		Inappropriate ac-	Fends off painful	arousal to	disorganized	
		tions and judg-	stimuli with	painful stimuli	response to	
		ments	purposeful	No verbal re-	painful stimuli	
		Decreased aware-	movement	sponse or		
		ness		moaning		
		Disorientation		Response to ver-		
				bal communi-		
				cation is in-		
				consistent and		
				vague		

*From Phipps W and others: Medical-surgical nursing, ed 4, St Louis, 1991, Mosby-Year Book.

2. Cranial nerve function
3. Language and speech
4. Meningeal signs
5. Sensory status
   a. Touch
   b. Pain
   c. Temperature
   d. Proprioception
6. Motor status
   a. Gait and stance
   b. Muscle strength
   c. Muscle tone
   d. Coordination
   e. Involuntary movements
   f. Muscle stretch reflexes

More detailed descriptions of selected portions of the examination will be covered in specific parts of this chapter. The reader is also referred to a neurological nursing text for additional information.

In clinical settings, it is not feasible or essential to completely repeat the total neurological exam during the shift-to-shift assessment of the patient. In many settings, such as intensive care units, the neurological checks are performed every hour. Certain features have been identified as most important and should be emphasized when one is doing these checks. Generally these include the following:

1. Orientation
2. Level of consciousness (Table 29-2)
3. Ability to speak
4. Muscle strength
5. Involuntary movements
6. Any abnormal posturing

29-4

Glasgow Coma Scale (GCS)

	Stimuli	Score
Eyes open	Spontaneously	4
	To speech	3
	To pain	2
	None	1
Best verbal response	Oriented	5
	Confused (disorientated)	4
	Inappropriate words (monosyllabic response)	3
	Incomprehensible	2
	None	1
Best motor response	Obeys commands	5
	Localizes to pain	4
	Flexes to pain	2
	None	1

N.B. There is a modified GCS where the best motor response has been further divided (see figure 33-23). Some authorities also use different wording for best verbal response—see brackets.[84a]

GLASGOW COMA SCALE

One way to standardize observations of patients is the Glasgow Coma Scale. It was developed in 1974 and consists of assessment of three parts of the neurological assessment.

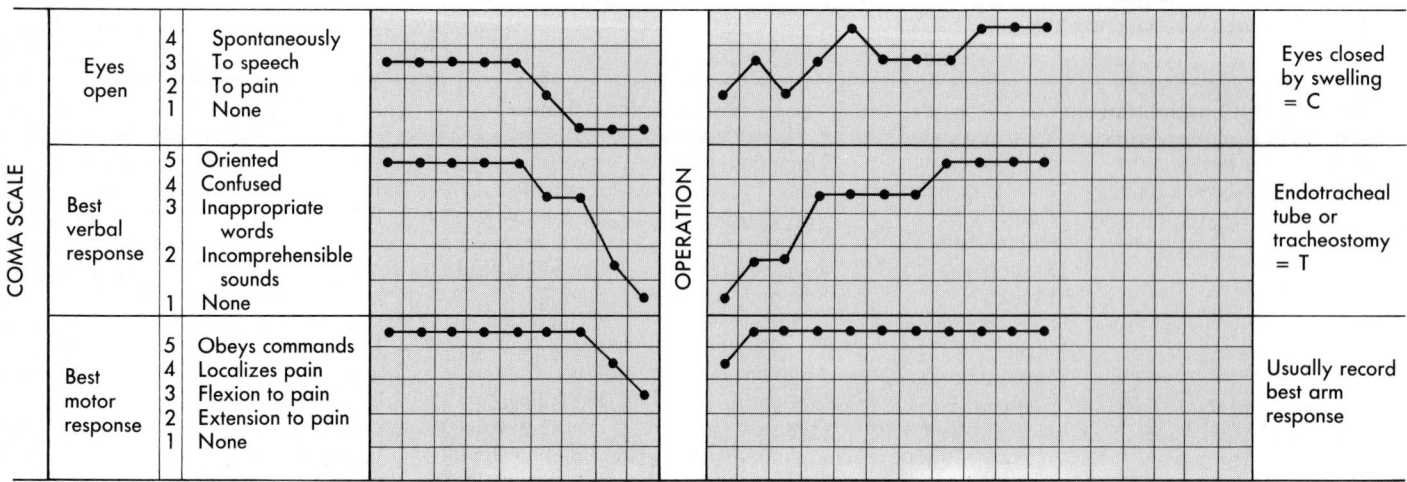

Fig. 29-7   Glasgow Coma Scale, demonstrating measurement of level of consciousness. Notice change in patient's condition just before and after surgery.

These include the following:
1. Eye opening
2. Best motor response
3. Best verbal response

The stronger the stimulus needed to obtain a response, the lower the score assigned to the part (see Box 29-4). The number value assigned to each parameter is added to yield an objective score. The score for normal persons who are not neurologically impaired is 14. The lowest possible score is 3. Any score of 7 or less is commonly accepted as a definition of coma (Fig. 29-7).

HEADACHE

Headache is a common symptom experienced by many patients. It can result from many pathological processes, and its significance also is variable. *The source of recurring headache should be determined through careful physical examination with appropriate neurological assessment.* People have been known to self-treat headaches for months, believing them to be nothing to worry about, only to learn later that the pain was caused by a more serious problem such as a brain tumour. Because of the site of some tumours in the brain, headache may be the only symptom for many months.

Pathophysiology

Headache may have many causes. Some of these are as follows:
1. Expanding brain masses such as neoplasms
2. Intracranial bleeding
3. Inflammation of the meninges as in meningitis
4. Other infections of the brain and spinal cord
5. Head trauma
6. Cerebral hypoxia
7. Dilation of the cerebral blood vessels
8. Psychological factors such as stress
9. Systemic disease including eye, ear, and sinus problems.
10. Allergies

The exact pathophysiology of head pain is not known. Although the skull and brain tissues are not capable of sensory pain, pain arises from the scalp and its blood vessels and muscles, from the dura mater and its venous sinuses, from the blood vessels at the base of the brain, and from some cervical cranial nerves. Blood vessels dilate and become congested with blood. Headaches are divided into the following three categories:
1. Vascular
   a. Migraine
   b. Cluster
   c. Hypertensive
2. Tension
   a. Psychogenic problems (tension or stress)
   b. Medical problems (cervical arthritis)
3. Traction-inflammatory
   a. Infection
   b. Intracranial or extracranial
   c. Occlusive vascular structures
   d. Arteritis

Efforts have been made to make the classification of headache more meaningful for the neuroscience nurse.[84] See Table 29-3 for details about and comparison of three specific types of headache.

Nursing Process
Assessment

Both subjective and objective data are important in determining more about the cause and nature of the headache.

Subjective data

1. Patient's understanding of headache and possible causes
2. Awareness of any precipitating factors such as stress
3. Measures that relieve symptoms, including medications
4. Location, frequency, pattern, and character of head pain, including site of return, time of day, and intervals between headaches
5. Initial onset of headache

6. Presence of any prodromal symptoms
7. Presence of associated symptoms
8. Family history of headaches (especially important with migraine)
9. Situations that make headache worse
10. Presence of allergies

Objective data

1. Behaviour: signs indicating stress or anxiety or pain
2. Change in ability to carry on daily activities
3. Abnormalities on physical assessment part of neurological examination
4. Temperature
5. Sinus drainage

Information about the patient's understanding of the nature and precipitating factors is helpful for planning necessary teaching. It is not unusual for the patient to manifest little objective data in the presence of subjective complaints.

Headache pain may be made worse by stress or tension. Knowledge of the patient's perception of the effect of stress on the symptoms is important in planning for measures that relieve or reduce effects of stress.

Migraine headaches are unusual in that there are *prodromal signs* and *symptoms* that occur before the acute attack. These may include the following:

1. Visual field defects
2. Confusion
3. Paraesthesias
4. Paralysis in rare cases

During the actual attack, signs and symptoms may include nausea, vomiting, sensitivity to light, chilliness, fatigue, irritability, sweating, oedema, and other autonomic signs.

In assessing headache several key points are considered. These include the following:

1. Localized type of head pain is usually associated with migraine headaches or an organic disorder.
2. Generalized headache is usually related to psychological causes or the presence of increased intracranial pressure.
3. Migraine headaches may change from one side of the head to the other but affect only one side of head at one time.
4. Headaches that occur with increased intracranial pressure usually are present on awakening and may awaken the person from sleep.
5. Sinus headaches typically occur early in the morning and increase in intensity as the day progresses.
6. Many headaches are related to stress.
7. Pain described as dull, nagging, aggravating, and ever present often occurs with psychogenic headaches.
8. Organically caused pain tends to be constant and progressive in nature.
9. Migraine headaches may be associated with menstruation.
10. Headaches may be precipitated by eating foods containing monosodium glutamate, sodium nitrate, or tyramine, as well as by alcohol.
11. A family history of headache is important, especially with migraine headaches.
12. Sleeping too long, fasting, or inhaling toxic fumes in work situations with inadequate ventilation can cause headaches.

Table 29-3 Comparison of migraine, cluster, and tension headaches

Type	Onset	Frequency	Duration	Nature	Prodromal symptoms/ associated symptoms	Treatment
Migraine headaches	Occur at any age Strongly hereditary More common in women than men	Episodic, tend to occur with stress or life crisis May occur with menstruation	Hours to days	Occur slowly; pain becomes severe, with one side of head affected more than other	Prodromal: visual field defects, confusion, paraesthesias Associated: nausea, vomiting, chills, fatigue, irritability, sweating, oedema	Ergotamine tartrate Methysergide maleate Beta blockers Nonnarcotic analgesics Relaxation techniques Application of heat or cold Avoidance of dietary tyramine, nitrate, and glucconate
Cluster headaches	Early adulthood; precipitated by alcohol or nitrates More common in men	Episodes clustered together in quick succession for few days or weeks with remissions that last for months	Few minutes to few hours	Pain intense: throbbing, deep, often unilateral; begin in infraorbital region and spread to head and neck	Prodromal: uncommon Associated: flushing, tearing of eyes, nasal stuffiness, sweating swelling of temporal vessels	Narcotic analgesics during acute phase, often intramuscularly Nonnarcotic analgesics Relaxation techniques
Tension headaches (muscle contraction)	Often in adolescence; related to tension or anxiety No family history	Episodic; vary with stress	Variable, can be constant	Dull, constant, uncommon aggravating pain, vary in intensity; usually bilateral and involve neck and shoulders; pain may be poorly defined	Prodromal: uncommon Associated: sustained contraction of head and neck muscles	Amitriptyline

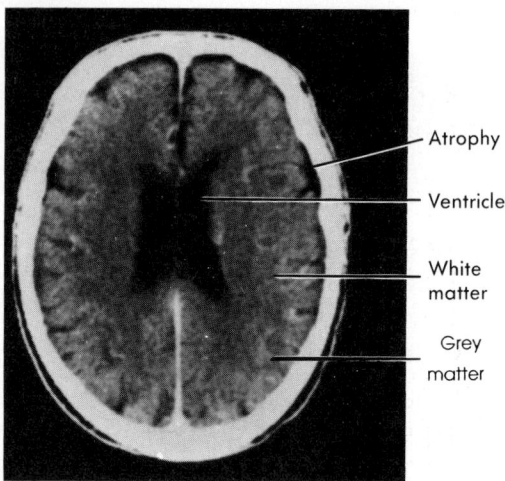

Atrophy

Ventricle

White matter

Grey matter

Fig. 29-8 CT scan printouts. CT brain scan differentiates between grey and white brain matter. (From Ballinger PW: *Merrill's atlas of radiographic positions and radiologic procedures*, ed 7, St Louis, 1991, Mosby–Year Book.)

13. Oral contraceptives may make migraine headaches worse.
14. Any secondary gains that patients receive from headaches must be assessed.

Diagnostic tests

It is important to evaluate headaches that are not slight and transient. Usual testing includes a neurological examination, including a CT scan. The CT or EMI scan is becoming more available as a way to easily and safely detect abnormalities in the CNS (Fig. 29-8). It has replaced many invasive and painful procedures that neurological patients previously were subjected to during diagnosis. See Box 29-5

The MRI scan may also be performed.[69] See Box 29-6 for information. Another scan that is similar to the CT and the MRI is the PET (positron emission tomography) scan (see Box 29-7). In this scan the patient receives an injection of deoxyglucose with radioactive fluorine. The head is scanned and a colour composite picture is obtained. Various shades of colours indicate levels of glucose metabolism.

A lumbar puncture may also be performed. A lumbar puncture is not done, however, if there is evidence of raised intracranial pressure or if a brain tumour is suspected, because the quick reduction in pressure produced by removal of the spinal fluid may cause brain herniation. In this situation a CT scan must be done first. Box 29-8 outlines the procedure for lumbar puncture (see Fig. 29-9.

At times, because of anatomical abnormalities or other causes, a lumbar puncture may not be possible. At these times a cisternal puncture may be attempted. The cisternal puncture is made between the first cervical vertebra and the base of the skull (Fig. 29-10) (see Box 29-9).

Other tests that may be done include a brain scan (Fig. 29-11) and plain skull films (see Box 29-10 for preparation for brain scan).

The skull x-ray films will demonstrate bony abnormality as well as congenital changes, but will not yield the information that more sophisticated procedures do.

29-5 | **Computed tomography (EMI, CT, or CAT scan)**

Purpose

Detection of cerebral and spinal cord pathology using a technique of scanning without radioisotopes

Preparation of patient

1. No special physical preparation
2. Patient teaching
   a. Explain procedure
   b. Time: Approximately 20 to 30 minutes for CT scan without contrast medium; 60 minutes if scans with and without contrast medium are done
   c. Sensation: Procedure is painless, except for slight discomfort when IV is started for injection of contrast medium. Also, there is some discomfort in lying still and possible feelings of claustrophobia as a result of head being positioned in head holder
   d. Patient must maintain motionless position until scan is completed
      If contrast medium is used, history of allergy to iodine (seafood) is determined before medium is given

Procedure

1. Patient lies supine with the head positioned within a rubber head holder to prevent air gaps between the machine and scalp.
2. Head is scanned in two planes simultaneously and at various angles. Each image is a specific layer of brain tissue.
3. The computer calculates tissue absorption in contiguous layers of brain tissue and displays a printout. Selected photographs of the printouts are taken.
4. Tumour densities are compared with the normal brain tissue. (Tumours, infarctions, bone displacement, and the ventricles are well visualized.)
5. If a contrast study is desired, the patient receives the contrast medium and the scanning process is repeated.

After procedure

1. No adverse effects except the risk of transient raised intracranial pressure in patients with masses or other brain pathology.
2. Plan period of rest as needed for the patient.

Nursing analysis

Problem	Possible aetiologies
Sleep pattern disturbance	Pain/discomfort, anxiety
Anxiety	Threat/change in health status/role functioning/situational/maturational crisis
Pain	Headache
Coping, ineffective individual	

29-6   Magnetic resonance imaging (MRI)

Purpose

Detection of cerebral and spinal cord pathology using a technique of scanning using magnetic forces to image body structures

Preparation of patient

1. No special physical preparation
2. Patient teaching
   a. Explain procedure
   b. Time: approximately 45 to 60 minutes
   c. Sensation: Procedure is painless, except for discomfort in lying still and possible feelings of claustrophobia as a result of head being positioned in head holder
   d. Patient must maintain motionless position until scan is completed
   e. Machine makes different noises during procedure that could startle patient
   f. Because scan involves a magnetic force, patient should remove all credit cards, watches, or other metal from clothing before entering scan room
3. Patient should be questioned about presence of metal in body (orthopaedic appliances, aneurysm clips, pacemakers)

Procedure

1. Patient lies supine with the head positioned in a head holder.
2. Machine slowly scans parts of the brain or spinal cord. Images appear on a monitoring screen.
3. Magnetic field is used to measure the activity of the tissues.

After procedure

1. No adverse effects

29-7   Positron emission tomography (PET scan)

Purpose

Detection of cerebral and spinal cord pathology using radiactive fluorine

Preparation of patient

1. No special physical preparation
2. Patient teaching
   a. Explain procedure
   b. Time: Approximately 45 minutes
   c. Sensation: Procedure is painless, except for slight discomfort when fluorine is injected; also, there is some discomfort in lying still
   d. Patient must remain motionless until the scan is completed

Procedure

1. Patient is injected with or inhales radioactive fluorine
2. Patient lies supine with head immobilized
3. Head is scanned
4. A colour composite picture is obtained. Various shades of colours indicates level of glucose metabolism

After procedure

1. No adverse effects
2. Patient may need period of rest

Problems are determined from analysis of patient data. Possible problems for the person with headache may include, but are not limited to, the following:

Problem	Situational crises
Knowledge deficit	Possible aetiologies
	Lack of exposure, information misinterpretation, cognitive limitation
Self-care deficit	Pain/discomfort, depression

Planning: expected patient outcomes

Expected patient outcomes for the person with headache may include, but are not limited to, the following:

1. Patient can demonstrate prescribed relaxation techniques.
2. Anxiety is decreased.
3. Headache pain is decreased.
4. Patient can carry out ADL with minimal difficulty.
5. Patient demonstrates improved coping mechanisms.
6. Patient can explain prescribed medication (dosage, action, side effects, and frequency).
7. Patient can explain the importance of continuing medical supervision for chronic headache.
8. Patient can identify any factors that trigger headache.
9. Patient can explain the danger of continued use of over-the-counter drugs for chronic, recurring headache.
10. Patient is able to sleep at least 6 hours per night.

Implementation

Assisting with achievement of therapeutic goals

Medications

Treatment for headache often includes the use of selected medications. These will be described in terms of their use for migraine, cluster, and tension headaches.

Migraine headaches. Management of migraine comprises treatment of acute episodes and prophylaxis to prevent attacks. Agents that provoke attacks, such as cheese, chocolate and alcohol, should be eliminated if possible. Acute episodes may respond to paracetamol or aspirin, although they are commonly insufficient. Ergotamine tartrate may be used orally, sublingually, rectally, or by inhalation. It is essential not to exceed the recommended dose of 6 to 8 mg per attack and 12 mg per week, because serious side-effects may develop. Various combination preparations are available, which contain these agents with antiemetics or caffeine. Sumatriptan, a serotonin antagonist, may also be used.

Clonidine, methysergide and pizotifen may be used in the prevention of migraine. Beta blockers such as propranolol

29-8 Lumbar puncture

Purpose

To obtain cerebrospinal fluid (CSF) for examination or relief of pressure.

Preparation of patient

1. A consent form may be signed by patient or family member.
2. Occasionally sedation is given before procedure.
3. Patient teaching
   a. Explain procedure
   b. Time: approximately 10 to 15 minutes
   c. Sensation: slight pain and pressure may be felt as the dura is entered. A sharp shooting pain down one leg may be felt, caused by the needle coming close to a nerve.
   d. Other: Remind patient to lie still and not to move suddenly.

Procedure

1. Patient is usually positioned on the side with both knees and head flexed at an acute angle to allow maximum lumbar flexion and separation of interspinous spaces. Occasionally patients may be positioned sitting up and leaning over the bedside table.
2. Local anaesthetic is usually used to anaesthetize the lumbar area.
3. Under strict aseptic technique the needle is inserted below the level of the spinal cord at the L4-L5 or L5-S1 interspace (Fig. 29-8).
4. Inner needle is removed to allow drainage and measurement of spinal fluid.
5. Level of fluid column in manometer used to measure pressure is read.
6. Fluid is collected for various tests or to relieve pressure. Occasionally the first specimen of spinal fluid contains blood from slight bleeding at the site of puncture. This specimen should not be sent for cell count.
7. *Queckenstedt's test* may be performed to test for subarachnoid block. The jugular veins are compressed for 10 seconds, first on one side, then on the other side, and then on both sides at the same time. Any change in spinal fluid pressure during the compression is noted.
8. Needle is withdrawn.

After procedure

1. Patient lies flat in bed for several hours. Caution patient not to lift head.
2. Site of puncture should be observed for any leakage of CSF.
3. Headache is fairly common and is thought to be caused by the loss of spinal fluid through the dura mater. The sharpness and size of the needle, the skill of the doctor, whether the patient lies flat, and the patient's emotional state may determine whether a headache occurs.
4. Headaches are usually treated with bed rest, analgesics, and ice applied to the head.

29-9 Cisternal puncture

Purpose

To obtain CSF for examination, or for instillation of contrast medium for diagnostic studies

Preparation of patient

1. A consent form may be signed.
2. Back of patient's neck may be shaved.
3. Procedure is performed in the patient's bed or in treatment room.
4. Patient is positioned on their side at the edge of the bed or treatment table with the head bent forward.
5. Patient teaching
   a. Same as for lumbar puncture.
   b. Procedure may be more frightening to the patient because of the close proximity of the procedure to the brain.

Procedure

1. Same as for lumbar puncture except for different site (between C1 and base of skull).
2. Head of patient should be held firmly during procedure so it does not rotate.

After procedure

1. Patient observed immediately for dyspnoea, apnoea, or cyanosis.
2. Headache occurs less frequently than with lumbar puncture.

and metoprolol are also effective agents. Other agents that may be used include amitriptyline, cyproheptadine, nifedipine and verapamil.

Cluster headaches. Because the pain associated with cluster headaches is so severe, narcotic analgesics are often prescribed during the acute attack. Often these must be administered intramuscularly for optimal relief.

Patients with cluster headaches usually feel fine between attacks, so no analgesia is needed during these times.

Tension headaches. The nonnarcotic analgesics are often prescribed for tension headaches. These include paracetamol and aspirin. Narcotic analgesics such as codeine may be prescribed along with diazepam for relief of tension. It is far better, however, to counsel the patient to develop other ways to relieve the headache.

Interventions to achieve patient outcomes

Promoting rest and relaxation

Because stress and emotional upsets may precipitate some headaches and make others worse, measures are taken to facilitate relaxation and rest. Relaxation techniques (Chapter 8), planned sleeping hours, and rest periods as needed may prove helpful. Because alcohol has been found to be significant in causing cluster headaches,

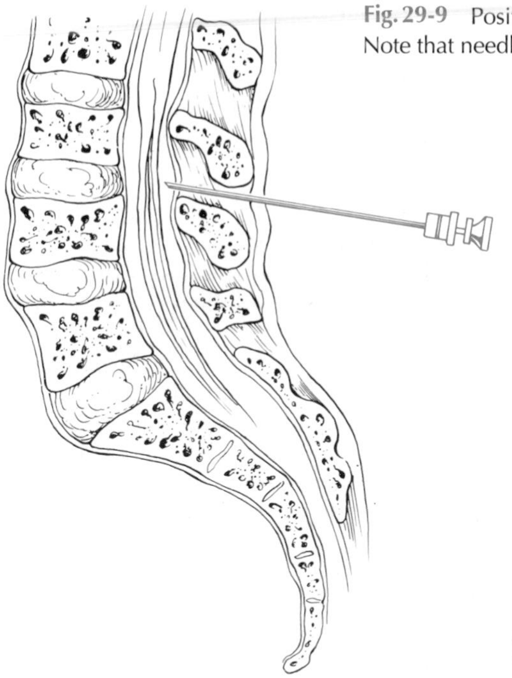

Fig. 29-9 Position and angle of needle when lumbar puncture is performed. Note that needle is in fourth lumbar interspace below level of spinal cord.

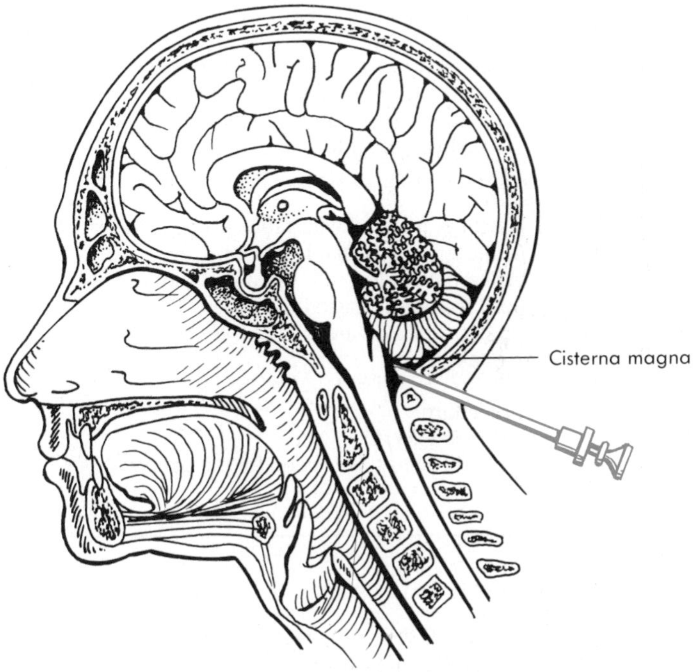

Cisterna magna

Fig. 29-10 Cisternal puncture. Position of needle when cisternal puncture is performed. Note needle length and short bevel.

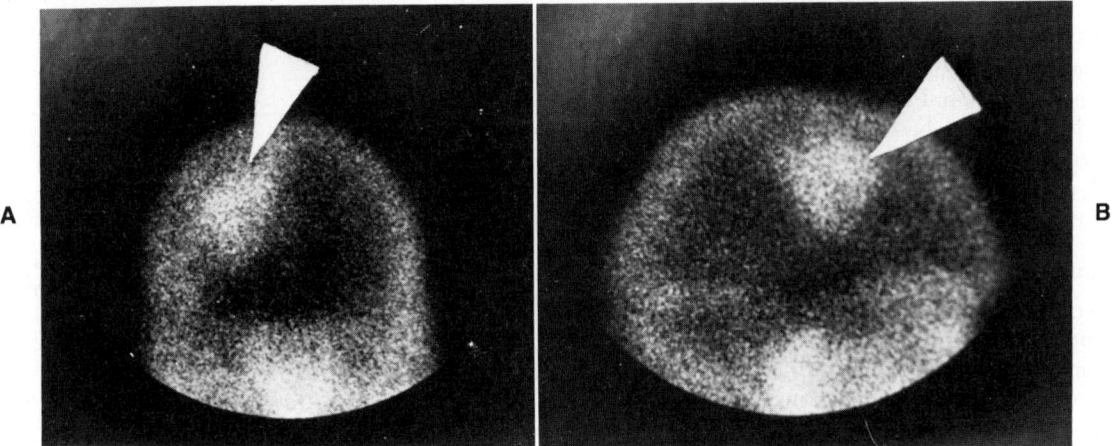

Fig. 29-11 Brain scans. **A,** Anteroposterior view. **B,** Lateral view. White pointers indicate tumour seen in both views. (From Pagana KD, Pagana TJ: *Diagnostic testing and nursing implications: a case study approach*, ed 3, St Louis, 1990, Mosby–Year Book.)

Brain scan

Purpose
Detection of cerebral pathology using radio
active isotopes and a scanner

Preparation of patient
1. No physical preparation of patient
2. Patient teaching
   a. Explain procedure.
   b. Time: approximately 45 minutes for the
      actual scan
   c. Sensation: minimal discomfort associated
      with the IV administration of radio-
      active isotope. Some patients may find
      it uncomfortable to lie still for the scan.

Procedure
1. Patient is injected with radioisotope
   (sodium pertechnetate Tc 99m)
2. While patient lies still, usually in supine position, scanner is passed over head. This picks
   up concentrated areas of uptake. Several scans
   are taken.

After procedure
1. No adverse effects.
2. Plan period of rest as needed for the patient.

it should not be used as a way to relieve tension.

Some patients who have tension headaches have found
relaxation by regular physical exercise to be helpful.

Decreasing anxiety

Patients with chronic headaches may respond to psychotherapy. It may be used to help the patient develop
awareness of stressors, as well as to deal with feelings about
being the victim of headache pain.

Assisting with comfort and ADL

Other treatments that have been found to be helpful
with headache include cold packs applied to the forehead
or base of the brain. Pressure applied to the temporal and
carotid arteries may be helpful depending on the cause of
the headache. Patients who are having migraine headaches, especially, may be most comfortable lying in a dark
room with minimal auditory stimulation.

Identifying triggering factors

Discovery of triggering factors associated with severe
recurring headaches will need to be made through ongoing
assessment of the person's personality, habits, and ADL.
Clues may be obtained from seeking information about the
person's goals and aspirations, work habits, family relationships, coping mechanisms, and relaxation patterns. The
person may be asked to keep a diary of activities and the
occurrence of headaches, as well as the nature of the
headaches and how they were treated.

Triggering factors may include the following:
1. Fatigue
2. Alcohol
3. Stress
4. Climatic changes
5. Hunger
6. Menstruation
7. Allergies

Facilitating learning

Teaching is an important part of nursing care of the
patient with head pain. Box 29-11 lists appropriate teaching activities.

It may be helpful to educate the patient about foods that
may cause headaches or make them worse. These include
those containing tyramine, nitrates, or glutamate. For
example, monosodium glutamate (MSG) is often used in
Chinese cooking. Other foods that may provoke headaches
are included in the following list:
1. Vinegar
2. Chocolate
3. Yoghurt
4. Alcohol
5. Fermented or marinated foods
6. Ripened cheese
7. Herring
8. Cured meats
9. Excessive caffeine
10. Pork

Evaluation

Evaluation of headaches is based on the expected patient
outcomes and should be done in conjunction with the
patient. Questions to consider may include the following:
1. Is the patient able to sleep?
2. Has the patient's anxiety decreased?
3. Is pain decreased?
4. Is the patient functioning optimally?
5. Does the patient demonstrate improved coping mechanisms?
6. Is the use of medication within medical guidelines?
7. Is the patient following medical advice?
8. Is the patient keeping follow-up appointments?

The patient with headache

1. Avoid factors found to trigger or increase
   headache.
2. Use relaxation measures (such as biofeedback)
   when emotional tension is present.
3. Maintain regular sleep patterns.
4. Take medications as ordered—be aware of
   their side effects and report these to doctor.
5. Follow up with medical care as indicated.
6. Allow others to assist with activities during
   headaches.
7. Structure home and work environment to keep
   stressors at a reasonable level.

29-12

Site of problem and resulting neurological pain

Site of problem	Results	Characteristics of pain
Peripheral cutaneous nerves	Pain usually limited to anatomical area supplied by affected nerve or nerves	Often described as burning sensation, but can be described as sharp or dull and aching Pain may be constant or permanent Often described as severe Also called local pain
Root pain	Limited to dermatomes supplied by affected sensory nerve roots (pain from lesion arising from deep somatic and visceral stimulus may radiate beyond dermatomes) (Fig. 29-8)	Aggravated by anything that causes direct or indirect movement of spinal cord (sneezing, coughing, or straining)
Central lesion within thalamus	Pain confined to contralateral side of body	Pain described as burning, pulling, and swelling Often aggravated by emotional stress and fatigue Influenced by cutaneous stimulation
Central spinothalamic tract	Pain sensation distributed to level of tract involved Hemisection of spinal cord produces loss of pain and temperature sensation on contralateral side at a level one or two segments below injury	May be similar to thalamic pain, but less disturbing

29-13

Types of pain sensation

Paraesthesia	Abnormal sensation
Hyperalgesia	Increased pain sensation
Hypoalgesia	Decreased pain sensation
Analgesia	Blocked pain sensation
Dysaesthesia	Pain sensation caused by stimulus that normally would not be painful
Referred pain	Pain that occurs in a site other than its origin
Causalgia	Intense, continuous, burning pain
Local pain	Occurring as a result of direct stimulation of pain receptors

NEUROLOGICAL PAIN

Pathophysiology

Neurological pain other than headache is commonly seen in nursing. It is sometimes difficult to distinguish between pain produced by lesions within the nervous system that cause objective sensory abnormalities and peripherally produced, somatic pain in a distant organ (see Box 29-12). Although in practice pain may be viewed from the standpoint of neural transmission, the transmission of pain impulses is not fully understood. Neurological pain may arise from lesions involving peripheral cutaneous nerves, the sensory nerve roots, the thalamus, and the central pain tract (spinothalamic) at some level. Pain receptors are not adaptable. Pain impulses continue at the same rate as long as the stimulus is present. They are specific for pain only. Pain receptors can be activated by the following:

1. Cellular damage
2. Certain chemicals such as histamine
3. Heat
4. Ischaemia
5. Muscle spasms
6. Sensations of heat, cold, and itching that go beyond a specific level of intensity

Pain that is described as unbearable and does not respond to treatment is classified as *intractable*. It is chronic and often disabling.

Nursing Process
Assessment

Both subjective and objective data are important to assess in the patient with neurological pain. Again, it should be remembered that pain is highly subjective, and there may not be a great deal of objective data to accompany the subjective complaints.

Subjective data

1. Patient's understanding of the pain
2. Any precipitating factors
3. Measures that relieve symptoms, including medica
   tion
4. Site, frequency, and nature of pain
5. Usual coping patterns when under stress
6. Presence of associated symptoms
7. Measures that make pain worse

Objective data

1. Behaviour: signs indicating pain or stress
2. Change in ability to carry out ADL
3. Muscle weakness or wasting
4. Vasomotor responses (flushing, for example)
5. Spinal reflexes and sensory examination

The quality of pain and its distribution are important factors to assess. Pain may vary from mild to excruciating. Terms with which the nurse should be familiar include those listed in Box 29-13.

As stated earlier, neurological pain may arise from lesions involving peripheral cutaneous nerves, the sensory nerve roots (posterior), the thalamus, and the central pain tract. Each of these sources produces characteristic pain.

Diagnostic tests

It is extremely difficult to evaluate pain objectively. Electrical stimulation may be attempted to define the pain

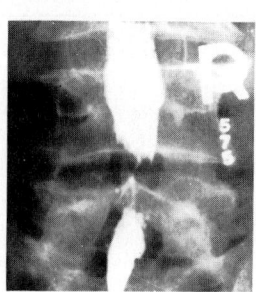

Fig. 29-12 Myelogram showing almost complete block in interspace between fourth and fifth lumber vertebrae. (From Moseley HF, editor: *Textbook of surgery*, ed 3, St Louis, 1959, Mosby–Year Book.)

to a greater extent. The person with intractable pain may undergo psychological testing as part of the diagnosis. Tests to rule out causes of the pain may be indicated, including the myelogram (see Box 29-14). This is commonly done when back pain is present (Fig. 29-12).

Nursing analysis

Problems are determined from analysis of patient data. Possible problems for the person with neurological pain may include, but are not limited to, the following:

33-14

Myelogram

Purpose
To identify lesions in the intradural or extradural compartments of the spinal canal by observing the flow of radiopaque dye through the subarachnoid space.

Preparation of patient
1. Consent form is signed.
2. If iotrolan is to be used the patient should not take the following drugs for 48 hours before the test:
   a. Neuroleptics
   b. Antidepressants
3. Lower extremity strength and sensation should be assessed for baseline.
5. Patient teaching
   a. Explain procedure.
   b. Time procedure takes.
   c. Sensation: slight pain and pressure may be felt as dura is entered. Some patients find varied positions they must assume during procedure uncomfortable.

Procedure
1. Patient is usually positioned on the side with both knees and head flexed at an acute angle to allow maximum lumbar flexion and separation of interspinous spaces. Cisternal puncture may also be done.

2. Local anaesthetic may be used to anaesthetize the puncture site.
3. Under strict aseptic technique needle is inserted.
4. Inner needle is removed to allow drainage, measurement of pressure, and collection of specimens.
5. Dye is instilled and needle removed.
6. Patient is turned to varied positions to visualize the spinal cord while radiological films are taken.

After procedure
1. Bed rest for 24 hours
2. Headache is fairly common.
3. Strength and sensation of lower extremities should be assessed.
4. Patient's head and thorax must remain elevated 30° to 50° for at least 6 hours.
5. Fluids are encouraged.
6. Common side effects include nausea, vomiting, and seizures.
7. Site of puncture should be assessed for leakage of CSF.
8. Avoid drugs previously listed—they lower seizure threshold. (When nausea occurs after a myelogram, non-neuroleptic antiemetics may be used.)

Problem	Possible aetiologies
Anxiety	Threat/change in health status
Coping, ineffective individual	Chronic physical/psychosocial disability Pain/discomfort
Sleep pattern disturbance	Pain/discomfort
Mobility, impaired physical	Pain/discomfort
Self-care deficit	Lack of exposure/recall, information misinterpretation
Knowledge deficit	

Planning: expected patient outcomes

Expected patient outcomes for the person with neurological pain may include, but are not limited to, the following:

1. Patient demonstrates minimal anxiety.
2. Patient demonstrates improved coping mechanisms.
3. Patient demonstrates good management of sleep and rest patterns.
4. Patient explains the relationship between pain and emotional upsets.
5. Patient's pain is decreased.
6. Patient demonstrates physical methods including proper positioning that can be used for pain control.
7. Patient demonstrates minimal difficulty in carrying out ADL.
8. Patient has minimal restrictions in physical mobility.
9. Patient demonstrates ability to maintain home.
10. Patient states the plan for follow-up care.
11. Patient explains medications to be taken, including dosage, action, side effects, and frequency.

Implementation

Assisting with achievement of therapeutic goals

Medications

Treatment for patients with neurological pain may include the use of medications. These often include the nonnarcotic analgesics—paracetamol, ibuprofen and aspirin. Narcotic analgesics such as codeine may be prescribed along with diazepam or amitriptyline hydrochloride. The emphasis should be on helping the patient learn other measures to control pain.

Nonsurgical methods of pain relief

Neurological pain has been found to respond to other methods of pain control. These include transcutaneous electrical nerve stimulators (TENS) and spinal cord stimulators. Both use electrodes applied near the site of pain or on or around the spine. The goal is to modify the sensory input by blocking or changing the painful sensation with a stimulus that is perceived to be less painful or nonpainful.

Acupuncture has also been used to treat patients with neurological pain. See Chapter 8 for a further explanation of these procedures.

Nerve block

A nerve block involves the injection of a substance such as a local anaesthetic or alcohol or phenol close enough to a nerve to block the conduction of impulses. It is used to treat chronic pain that may result from trigeminal neuralgia, cancer, or peripheral vascular disease.

Surgery

In cases of intractable pain that does not respond to medical and nursing actions, surgery may be necessary to reduce or abolish pain. Neurosurgical procedures that may be done include the following:

1. Neurectomy—interruption of the peripheral or cranial nerve supplying a specific part of the body. The nerve fibres to the affected area are severed from the cord. Fibres controlling movement and position sense are also interrupted. Cannot be used to control pain in the lower extremities.
2. Rhizotomy—resection of a posterior nerve root just before it enters the spinal cord. Cannot be used with pain in the lower extremities because position sense is lost. Involves a laminectomy.
3. Cordotomy—pain pathways in spinothalamic tract (anterior and lateral aspect of the cord) on the side opposite the cord are severed. This results in a wide sense of analgesia, while other sensory and motor functions are preserved. In a percutaneous cordotomy, a spinal needle is inserted laterally between C1 and C2. A wire electrode is inserted into the lateral cord, and a lesion is made to destroy ascending pain fibres.

These procedures all have potential complications that must be considered before the decision is made to do surgery. For example, with cordotomy, the patient may expect to have problems with postural hypotension, temperature sensation, and possibly bladder and motor function. Also, patients may have a temporary paralysis or leg weakness and loss of bowel and bladder control that results from oedema of the cord. Usually this disappears in several weeks.[104]

Interventions to achieve patient outcomes

Promoting rest and relaxation

As with headache, stress and emotional upsets may precipitate neurological pain or make it worse. Rest and relaxation should be facilitated. Relaxation techniques, planned sleeping hours, and rest periods throughout the day may be helpful. Relaxation techniques used include biofeedback and meditation.

Some patients with pain, especially pain defined as intractable, may respond well to psychotherapy. It can help the patient develop awareness of stressors and how they influence the perception of pain.

Assisting with mobility and ADL

A patient having neurological pain may be extremely uncomfortable. The nurse should help the patient attain a position of comfort. For example, the patient with root pain should avoid movements that cause direct or indirect movement of the spinal cord. Significant nursing activities include the following:

1. Patient should not lie in a horizontal plane for long periods, as this causes tension or traction on the thoracic and sacral nerve roots.

The patient with neurological pain

1. Avoid factors that increase pain
2. Use relaxation measures such as biofeedback and meditation when emotional tension is present
3. Maintain regular rest and sleep pattern
4. Take medication as prescribed
5. Be aware of physical methods of controlling pain (such as positioning) and use them
6. Follow up with medical care as indicated
7. Structure home and work environment to keep stressors at a minimum

2. Sitting may help to relieve tension on the nerve roots.
3. When moving a person with root pain, sharp flexion of the neck and extension of the legs should be avoided as much as possible.
4. Straining during bowel movements can intensify pain—stool softeners are often indicated.

The identification of any triggering factors of neurological pain is important. This can be done by a thorough assessment of personality, habits, and ADL. The person may be asked to keep a diary of ADL and the occurrence of the pain.

Facilitating learning

Teaching is an important part of nursing care for the patient with neurological pain. Appropriate teaching activities are listed in Box 29-15.

Evaluation

Evaluation of the patient with peripheral nerve or intractable neurological pain considers how the person is functioning in spite of the pain. Questions to consider may include the following:

1. Is the patient showing little anxiety and good coping strategies?
2. Is the patient sleeping at least 6 hours a night?
3. Is the patient using physical methods to control the pain in a correct way?
4. Is the patient able to carry on normal ADL?
5. Is the patient's mobility improved?
6. Is the patient able to manage home maintenance activities?
7. Is the patient following up with appointments?
8. Is the use of medications within guidelines?
9. Is the patient cooperating with medical advice?
10. Is the patient's pain improved?

RAISED INTRACRANIAL PRESSURE

Pathophysiology

Raised intracranial pressure (ICP) is a complex manifestation that is the consequence of multiple neurological conditions. It often occurs suddenly and requires surgical intervention.

The contents of the skull, or cranial contents, are brain tissue, vascular tissue, and cerebrospinal fluid. The brain makes up 80% of the intracranial content, blood volume makes up 10% and the cerebrospinal fluid makes up the remaining 10%. Any increase in the volume of one of the cranial contents results in increased intracranial pressure, because the cranial vault is rigid, closed, and nonexpandable. Specific causes of raised ICP are listed in Box 29-16.

An increase in any one of the cranial contents is usually accompanied by a reciprocal change in the volume of one of the others. Brain tissue cannot expand without serious effects in the flow and amount of cerebrospinal fluid and cerebral circulation. Space-occupying lesions displace and distort the brain and vascular tissues as pressure increases. The buildup of pressure may occur slowly (days or weeks) or rapidly, depending on the cause. At first, one hemisphere of the brain will be more involved, but eventually both hemispheres will be affected.

As the pressure increases within the cranial cavity, it is at first compensated for by venous compression and cerebrospinal displacement. As the pressure continues to rise, the cerebral blood flow decreases and inadequate perfusion occurs. This inadequate perfusion initiates a vicious circle causing the Pco_2 to increase and the Pco_2 and the pH to fall. These changes cause vasodilation and cerebral oedema. The oedema further increases the intracranial pressure, causing increased compression of neural tissue and an even greater increase in intracranial pressure.

When the pressure exceeds the brain's ability to compensate, pressure is exerted on surrounding structures where the pressure is lower. This movement of pressure is called *supratentorial shift* and can result in two kinds of herniation. *Central* or *transtentorial herniation* is the downward displacement of the cerebral hemispheres through the tentorial notch. This compresses the diencephalon and brainstem. The other type of herniation is called *uncal herniation* and occurs when expanding masses in the middle fossa or temporal lobe shift over the lateral edge of

Causes of raised intracranial pressure

Space-occupying lesions that increase tissue volume

Cerebral contusions
Haematomas
Infarctions
Abscesses
Intracranial tumours

Cerebrospinal problems

Increase in production of cerebrospinal fluid
Blockage in ventricular system
Decreased absorption of cerebrospinal fluid

Cerebral oedema

Use of contrast dye that changes homeostasis of brain
Overhydration with hypotonic solution
After effects of trauma to brain

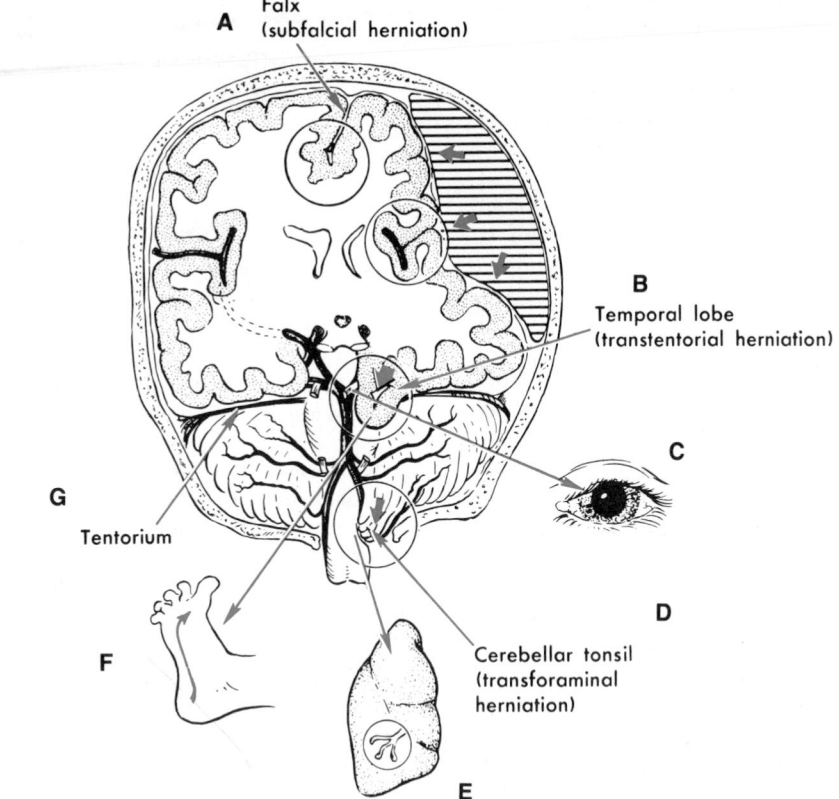

A
Falx
(subfalcial herniation)

B
Temporal lobe
(transtentorial herniation)

C

G

Tentorium

D

F

Cerebellar tonsil
(transforaminal
herniation)

E

Fig. 29-13   Consequences of raised intracranial pressure. Expanding temporoparietal epidural haematoma with medial and downward pressure has produced subfalcial, transtentorial, and transforaminal internal herniations. Note distortion of falx, *A*, bulging of medial temporal lobe at tentorial edge, *B*, and herniation of cerebellar tonsil with descending pressure on brainsteam, *D*. Also note how major blood vessels are collapsed in encircled areas. Some consequential effects of continuing and/or expanding pressure on neural structure with alterations in body functions are detailed: *C*, homolateral dilation and fixation of pupil with ptosis of eyelid; *E*, life-threatening respiratory arrest through indirect effects on respiratory centres in brainstem; *F*, contralateral Babinski sign showing extension of view of brainstem. (Modified from an original painting by Frank H Netter, MD; from Clinical symposia. Copyright by Ciba Pharmaceutical Co, Division of Ciba-Geigy Corp, Summit, NJ. All rights reserved.)

the tentorium, pushing the uncus towards the midline. As a result of herniation, the brainstem is compressed at variable levels, which in turn compresses the vasomotor centre, the posterior cerebral artery, the oculomotor nerve, the corticospinal nerve pathway, and the fibres of the ascending reticular activating system (Fig. 29-13). The life-sustaining mechanisms of consciousness, blood pressure, pulse, respiration, and temperature regulation fail.

Nursing Process
Assessment

Subjective data

1. Patient's understanding of condition
2. Presence of visual changes: diplopia or blurred vision
3. Ability to think
4. Presence of pain, especially headache
5. Ability to carry on daily activities
6. Presence of nausea

Objective data

1. Level of consciousness
2. Pupillary signs
3. Vital signs
4. Focal motor or sensory signs
5. Presence of vomiting or hiccuping
6. Eye changes including papilloedema
7. Speech patterns

The detection of increased intracranial pressure must occur early when it is still reversible and before the stage of decompensation. The ability to make accurate observations, to interpret observations intelligently, and to record observations carefully is the most important part of nursing care for patients with increased intracranial pressure.

Level of consciousness

A decreasing level of consciousness is an early sign of increased intracranial pressure. *Any change in the level of consciousness is one of the most important observations for the nurse to make, report,* and *record.* Restlessness, disorientation, and lethargy may be the first signs seen.

The observations are recorded in terms of *behaviours* and *symptoms* and not in terms of labels. Flow sheets that document neurological changes in an objective way are helpful, especially when frequent neurological observations are being done.

The Glasgow Coma Scale is another way to document the neurological patient's condition.[98] See p. 847 for a description of this tool. A description of levels of consciousness is presented in Box 29-17.

Pupillary signs

Pupil responses are controlled by cranial nerve III (the oculomotor nerve). This nerve carries sensory, motor, and parasympathetic fibres, as well as sympathetic fibres. As the brain herniates, the oculomotor nerve is compressed by the herniating tissue, the pupilloconstrictor fibres in the top part of the nerve being the first affected. The ipsilateral pupil (when the lesion is in one hemisphere) remains dilated and is incapable of constricting. The pupil appears larger than that of the affected side and does not react to light. As cerebral pressure increases and both hemispheres are affected, bilateral pupil dilation and fixation occur—the pupil may respond to light slowly. Dilating pupils are a sign of impending tentorial herniation. When pupils dilate or change in ability to react, the doctor should be notified immediately. A pupil that is fixed and dilated is sometimes referred to as a "blown pupil" and is an ominous sign[49] (Fig. 29-14).

Visual disturbances

Another sign of raised intracranial pressure that occurs fairly early is some type of visual disturbance. These may

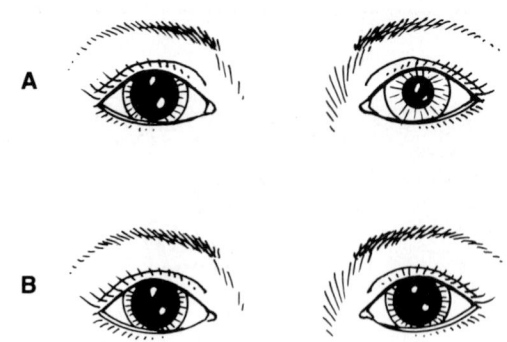

Fig. 29-14 **A,** Unequal pupils, also called anisocoria. **B,** Dilated and fixed pupils, indicative of severe neurological deficit.

include *diplopia* or *blurring* or *decreased visual acuity.* Diplopia usually results from paralysis or weakness of one of the muscles that controls eye movement.

Vomiting usually occurs in patients who have lesions below the tentorium. This vomiting usually occurs without the presence of nausea.

Blood pressure and pulse

The effect of raised intracranial pressure on pulse and blood pressure is variable. Compensatory changes occur in the cerebral vasculature relative to hypoxia. Herniation, however, causes ischaemia of the vasomotor centre. This excites the vasoconstrictor fibres, causing the systolic blood pressure to rise. If the intracranial pressure continues to increase, blood pressure may fall, especially the diastolic blood pressure. An increased systolic blood pressure followed by a sharp drop in blood pressure is often seen as the patient's condition deteriorates.

Pressure in the vasomotor centre also increases the transmission of parasympathetic impulses through the vagus nerve to the heart; as a result the pulse rate slows. Slowing of the pulse rate in conjunction with a rising systolic blood pressure is a significant observation that should be reported. For consistency, blood pressure and pulse should be taken in the same arm.

A widened pulse pressure, increased systolic blood pressure, and bradycardia are together referred to as *Cushing's response.* It is considered an important diagnostic characteristic of late-stage raised intracranial pressure.[3]

It is important to assess the trend of blood pressure and pulse. Indications of Cushing's response should be reported immediately.

Headaches

The patient with raised intracranial pressure (RIP) may complain of a headache. It is thought to result from *venous congestion* and the *tension in the intracranial blood vessels* as the cerebral pressure rises. The location and duration of the headache should be elicited from the patient. Headache that occurs with raised intracranial pressure usually increases in intensity with coughing, straining at stool, or stooping. *Headache is usually present in the early morning* and *may awaken* the *patient from sleep.*

It is important to realize that patients do not always complain of headache. Even if they do, the complaints may

29-17	**Levels of consciousness**	
	Alert	Responds appropriately to auditory, tactile, and visual stimuli
	Loss of ability to abstract	Inattentiveness, slowed thinking, difficult to arouse
	Confusion	Disorientation, inability to follow simple commands
	Stupor	Responds to verbal commands with moaning or groaning, if at all
	Semicomatose	Loss of ability to cooperate, responds only to pain—response may range from purposeful to decerebrate or decorticate
	Comatose	Loss of ability to respond to any external stimuli and loss of all brain functions[16]

29-18	**Classic signs of early raised intracranial pressure** Restlessness, disorientation, or lethargy Headache Contralateral hemiparesis Vital signs relatively stable Pupils dilated ipsilaterally Blurring of vision, decreased visual acuity, or diplopia Vomiting usually not present Normal temperature

be vague and uncertain (see Box 29-18 for signs of RIP). As the intracranial pressure increases, the headache usually becomes worse.

Respiration

Herniation produces respiratory dysrhythmias that are variable and related to the level of the brainstem compression or failure. The breathing pattern may be deep and stertorous or periodic (Cheyne-Stokes) respirations. See Table 29-4 for description of respiratory patterns. Another breathing pattern found with raised intracranial pressure is *ataxic breathing*. This is an irregular and unpredictable breathing pattern with random shallow and deep breaths and occasional pauses. This type of breathing is seen in patients with medullary damage.[29] As intracranial pressure increases to fatal levels, respiratory paralysis occurs. The beginning of periods of apnoea is significant. It is important to remember that the patient with a decreased level of consciousness will require assistance in keeping the airway clear. People with acute raised intracranial pressure require supplemental oxygen to prevent hypoxia, which can further increase intracranial pressure.

Controlled mechanical hyperventilation may be used to lower intracranial pressure. Increasing the tidal volume setting on a ventilator lowers the $Paco_2$ to a significant degree. During hyperventilation, arterial blood gases and tidal volumes are monitored. This type of therapy should not be used for more than 48 hours because the brain may adapt to the lower $PaCO_2$ levels, leading to local ischaemia. The patient must be weaned from the hyperventilation because an abrupt stop may lead to swelling of the brain.

Temperature

Failure of the thermoregulatory centre because of compression occurs later with raised intracranial pressure and gives rise to high, uncontrolled temperatures. Hyperthermia must be controlled because it increases the metabolism of brain tissue.

Focal motor and sensory symptoms

Compression of the *upper motor neurone pathway* (corticospinal tract) *interrupts transmission* of *impulses* to the *lower motor neurone*, and *progressive muscle weakness* occurs. This often begins with the presence of drift and may progress to hemiparesis and hemiplegia. *Drift* is tested by asking the patient to close the eyes and extend the arms straight out in front for about 30 seconds. If one arm is weakened, it will drift downward without the patient being aware of it. Testing of the lower extremities includes the ability to push and pull against the tester, the ability to dorsiflex and plantar flex the feet, and the ability to do straight leg raises.

The presence of the *Babinski sign, hyperreflexia,* and *rigidity* are *additional signs of decreased motor function.* Seizures may occur. Herniation of the upper part of the brainstem produces *decerebrate rigidity* (fixed posture with arms, legs, and trunk extended and with flexion of the palms and plantar joints) or decorticate rigidity (fixed posture with flexion of the arm, wrist, and fingers, with adduction of the arm and extensors and internal rotation of the legs) (see Fig. 29-15). The worsening of existing motor defects is significant, and such signs should be reported to the doctor.

Papilloedema

The *blind spot* of the retina measures the size and shape of the optic papilla or optic disc. As intracranial pressure

---

Table 29-4   Altered respiratory patterns in coma

Respiratory pattern	Characteristics	Indications
Cheyne-Stokes	Periods of hyperventilation that gradually diminish to apnoea of variable duration; respirations then resume and gradually build up to hyperventilation	Bilateral deep hemispheric and basal nuclei dysfunction; the upper brainstem may be involved
Central neurogenic hyperventilation (CNHV)	Continuous rapid and deep respirations at a rate of 25/min	Systemic acidosis and hypoxaemia should be excluded; has no segmental localizing influence; increasing regularity correlates with increasing depth of coma
Apneustic breathing	Prolonged inspiratory phase followed by apnoea (inspiratory cramp)	Indicates lower pontine damage
Cluster breathing	Closely grouped respirations followed by apnoea	Indicates lower pontine damage
Ataxic breathing	Chaotic respirations	Indicates damage to medullary centres; can precede respiratory arrest
Gasping breathing	Characterized by gasps followed by apnoea of variable duration	Indicates damage to medullary centres; can precede respiratory arrest
Depressed breathing	Shallow, slow, and ineffective breathing	Usually caused by medullary depression

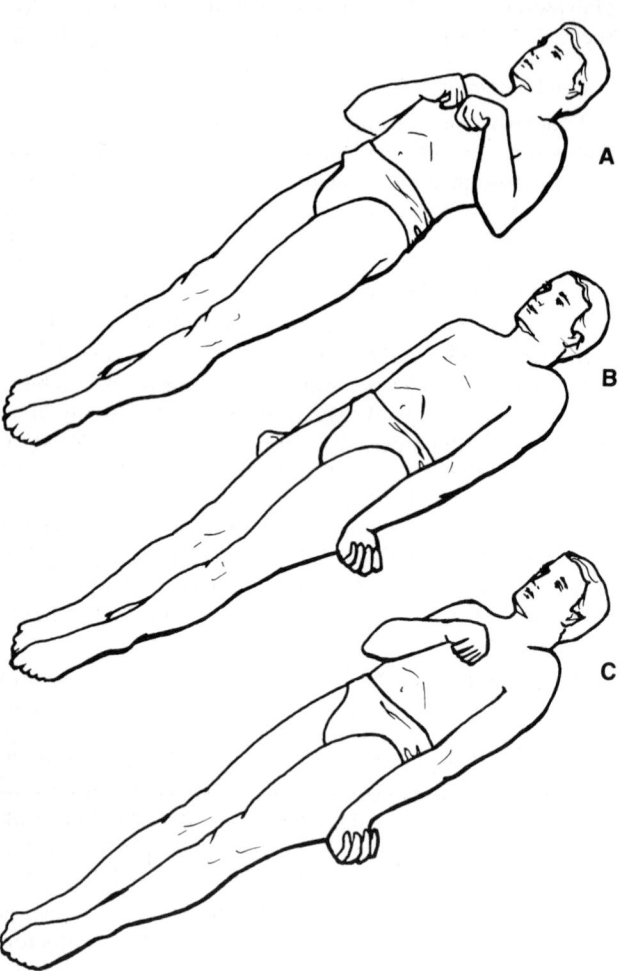

Fig. 29-15 Decorticate and decerbrate responses. **A,** Decorticate response. Flexion of arms, wrists, and fingers with adduction in upper extremities. Extension, internal rotation, and plantar flexion in lower extremities. **B,** Decerebrate response. All four extremities in rigid extension, with hyperpronation of forearms and plantar extension of feet. **C,** Decorticate response on right side of body and decerebrate response on left side of body. (From Zschoche D: *Mosby's comprehensive review of critical care,* ed 3, St Louis, 1985, Mosby–Year Book.)

increases, the pressure is transmitted to the eyes through the cerebrospinal fluid and to the optic disc. Because the meninges of the brain reflect out around the eyeball, they permit the direct transmission of pressure along the spaces through the cerebrospinal fluid. As the optic disc swells, the retina is also compressed. The damaged retina cannot detect light rays. Visual acuity is lessened as the blind spot enlarges.

Papilloedema is also referred to as choked disc, which is caused by the engorgement of the retinal veins.

Vomiting

Projectile vomiting may be associated with raised intracranial pressure. The significance of vomiting and its

frequency and character must be associated with other clinical signs.

Hiccuping

Compression of the vagus nerve (cranial nerve X) causes spasmodic contraction of the diaphragm. This compression occurs as brainstem herniation occurs. *Hiccuping in a patient who is at risk for raised intracranial pressure or who has other symptoms should be reported to the doctor immediately.*

Diagnostic tests

The diagnosis of raised intracranial pressure can be made with the CT scan, which can show actual structural herniation and shifting of the brain. The displacement of the brain to the right or left occurs at a relatively late stage of raised intracranial pressure. Most of the time, however, *acute raised intracranial pressure is a medical emergency,* and there is little time for diagnostic tests. The diagnosis must be made on the basis of observation and neurological testing. Although the frequency of "neuro obs" is often ordered by the doctor, the nurse should use judgment to decide whether more frequent assessments and recordings are indicated. The presence of even subtle changes may be very significant.

In some postoperative or critically ill patients internal measuring devices are used to diagnose raised intracranial pressure. One of the most common requires the placement of a hollow screw through the skull into the subarachnoid space. The screw is attached to a Luer-Lok, which is connected to a transducer and oscilloscope for continuous monitoring. The transducer is fastened level with the screw for accurate readings. A manometer may be attached for intermittent readings, or constant monitoring is available with the monitor.

It has become evident that the traditional *clinical signs of raised intracranial pressure do not always correlate with the actual pressure changes as seen on the monitor.* Many of the classic signs of increased pressure do not appear until the pressure has reached extremely high levels, and the chance to reverse the rising pressure and prevent permanent brain damage has already passed.

Nursing analysis

Problems are determined from analysis of patient data. Possible problems for the person with raised intracranial pressure may include, but are not limited to, the following:

Problem	Possible aetiologies
Injury, high risk for	Sensory/motor deficits
Sensory/perceptual alteration	Altered sensory reception/transmission/integration
Mobility, impaired physical	Neuromuscular impairment
Pain	Raised intracranial pressure
Tissue perfusion, altered cerebral	Decreased cerebral blood flow
Airway clearance, ineffective	Perceptual/cognitive impairment
Breathing pattern, ineffective	Neuromuscular impairment
Hyperthermia	Illness/trauma

Planning: expected patient outcomes

Expected patient outcomes for the person with raised intracranial pressure may include, but are not limited to, the following:

1. Patient does not have an injury resulting from trauma.
2. Patient has minimal problems as a result of sensory-perceptual alterations.
3. Patient maintains optimal levels of mobility.
4. Patient has minimal pain.
5. Cerebral tissue pressure is adequate.
6. Cerebral oedema is reduced.
7. Patient's airway is patent.
8. Patient's breathing pattern is effective.
9. Patient's temperature returns to normal.

Implementation

Assisting with achievement of therapeutic goals

The prevention of raised intracranial pressure may not be possible, but prevention of further rises in pressure and resulting damage to brain tissue is crucial. The detection of early signs is important to prevent irreversible effects.

The medical treatment of patients with raised intracranial pressure depends on the cause of the pressure. For example, if it is caused by an intracranial tumour, the tumour is removed surgically (p. 913). If surgery is not possible (or not indicated), efforts are made to reduce the pressure through the use of drug therapy or direct physical measures.

Mechanical decompression

Rapidly rising intracranial pressure is often relieved by mechanical decompression. This may include a craniotomy, in which a bone flap is removed and then replaced or a craniectomy, in which the bone flap is removed and not replaced. This latter procedure is commonly performed to decompress the brain when pressure is high.

Other means of decompression may include continuous ventricular drainage or drainage of any subdural haematoma.

Medications

The three types of drugs usually administered to patients with raised intracranial pressure are *osmotic diuretics, corticosteroids,* and *anticonvulsants.* Osmotic diuretics are also referred to as *hyperosmolar drugs.* They draw water from the oedematous brain tissue. Fluid is also drawn from uninjured tissue and can lead to fluid and electrolyte imbalance. The traditional osmotic diuretic is mannitol in a 20% solution. The usual dose is 1 g/kg of body weight administered over 30 to 60 minutes. It starts to reduce raised intracranial pressure within 15 minutes and its effects last for 4 to 6 hours. It is important for the patient receiving this drug to have a Foley catheter in place because of the large amounts of urine that usually are produced. Glycerol is another osmotic diuretic that is sometimes given, but it has the disadvantage of causing rebound swelling of brain tissue and must be given orally.

The corticosteroid most likely to be given is dexamethasone. An antacid may be given with it. Monitoring blood glucose levels is important because steroids can affect carbohydrate metabolism and glucose utilization.

Anticonvulsants are given to prevent seizures. Phenytoin is the most commonly prescribed drug. It can be given intravenously but is not recommended to be given intramuscularly.

Narcotics and other drugs that cause respiratory depression are avoided.

Internal monitoring devices

Internal monitoring devices are being used more frequently to diagnose and monitor raised intracranial pressure. *Three basic monitoring systems* are used. These include the following:

1. *Ventricular catheter*—consists of cannula that is implanted through burr holes into the anterior horn of the lateral ventricle of the nondominant cerebral hemisphere. The catheter is connected to a transducer and recording device.
2. *Subarachnoid bolt or screw*—one of earliest methods. It is inserted through skull into the subdural or subarachnoid space. The screw is attached to a transducer and oscilloscope so that continuous monitoring may be done.
3. *Epidural sensory*—placement of a fibreoptic sensor in the epidural space through a burr hole in the skull. The sensor cable is connected to the monitor.

Monitoring produces pressure waves that can be evaluated to indicate pathology.[50]

Interventions to achieve patient outcomes

Preventing injury

Numerous nursing activities are geared towards providing a safe environment for the patient with raised intracranial pressure. The patient may have altered sensory/perceptual reception and this can lead to increased confusion and agitation. The nurse should be aware that the *patient is at risk for seizures* and take necessary precautions.

Promoting mobility

Any patient at risk is discouraged from doing isometric exercises. Passive range of motion exercises are appropriate and will not increase systemic blood pressure because they are not resistive. Spacing of nursing activities is important in maintaining lower pressure levels.[3,10,61,101]

Maintaining comfort

The patient with increased intracranial pressure may experience headache. Narcotics and other drugs that cause respiratory depression are avoided. The use of cool cloths may help headache pain. The patient may be sensitive to light and noise. If this occurs, keeping the patient in a darkened, quiet environment may help ease discomfort.

Maintaining cerebral perfusion

Conservative measures to reduce venous volume may be implemented. The head of the bed is elevated to 30 to 45 degrees to promote venous return, and the neck is kept in a neutral position. Positioning to avoid flexion of the hips, waist, and neck is important. Rotation of the head, especially to the right, has been found to increase intracranial pressure. Nursing care is planned to cause the least distress to the patient. Care is grouped to allow adequate rest. Keeping the patient comfortable will help in maintaining cerebral blood flow.

Fluid intake may also be restricted. When osmotic diuretics are administered, urine output must be carefully monitored. An indwelling catheter is often used. The Valsalva manoeuvre is eliminated to the extent it is possible because it causes increased intrathoracic pressure, which indirectly increases intracranial pressure. This includes not allowing the patient to become constipated or to strain during defecation.

Maintaining effective respirations

Suctioning should be performed only when necessary (and then with the patient well preoxygenated) because it causes coughing and gagging. Suctioning should not be performed at the same time as other procedures that could cause raised intracranial pressure.

Oxygen therapy via mask or cannula is administered to improve brain oxygenation. Endotracheal intubation may be necessary. With the use of controlled ventilation, the P_{CO_2} can be lowered to below normal, which causes a slightly alkaline pH. The decrease in the P_{CO_2} and the increase in the pH will decrease vasodilation and thereby decrease intracranial pressure.

Lignocaine may be given via an IV line or an endotracheal tube to suppress the cough reflex if cough is a problem.

Preventing hyperthermia

A hypothermia blanket may be necessary to control the patient's body temperature. Increased temperature may lead to accelerated brain damage. Care must be taken when using the blanket not to bring the patient's temperature down too quickly or to leave the blanket on for too long a period of time. The temperature of a neurologically impaired patient will tend to continue to decrease after the blanket is turned off.[23]

Evaluation

Evaluation of the patient with raised intracranial pressure includes frequent observations to evaluate neurological status. Questions to consider may include the following:

1. Is the patient's safety monitored and in good control?
2. Is the patient experiencing minimal problems as a result of sensory-perceptual alterations?
3. Is the patient maintaining optimal levels of mobility?
4. Is the patient's pain minimal?
5. Are signs and symptoms of raised intracranial pressure decreased?
6. Are nursing measures being spaced in a way to avoid further increases in intracranial pressure?
7. Is effective respiration occurring?
8. Is the patient's temperature maintained?
9. Is fluid intake limited and is careful measuring of intake and output occurring?
10. Are the patient and family being supported, and is the patient being kept as comfortable as possible?

ALTERATIONS IN MUSCLE TONE AND MOTOR FUNCTION

Pathophysiology

Motor function disturbances are the *most commonly encountered neurological symptoms*. Because the nervous system is designed primarily for the movement of the body in space and of the various parts in relation to each other, damage to it often causes serious problems in mobility. A loss of function, either motor or sensory, is called *paralysis*. A lesser degree of paralysis is called *paresis*. Damage to sensory pathways that are concerned with motor function may occur at the same time as the loss of motor function.

Injury or disease of motor neurones results in *alterations of muscle strength, tone,* and *reflex activity*. The specific clinical manifestations differ according to whether the lesion involves an upper motor neurone or a lower motor neurone (Fig. 29-16).

Lower motor neurone signs

The lower motor neurones (LMNs) consist of a large anterior horn cell located in the grey matter of the spinal cord. They are also found in the motor cranial nuclei of the brainstem. This anterior horn cell, in conjunction with the anterior spinal nerve and the peripheral nerve involved, forms a motor unit that affects skeletal muscle activity (voluntary and reflex). When a lesion selectively involves some part of the lower motor neurone, the results include the following:

1. Flaccid muscle weakness or paralysis
2. Loss of reflex activity
3. Loss of muscle tone
4. Atrophy confined to the involved muscle or muscles

The degree of muscle weakness is directly related to the extent and severity of the lesion.

The involved muscles become *flaccid* because the motor unit has been damaged and normal reflex activity has been interrupted. This flaccidity also is manifested in *hypotonia* and *hyporeflexia* and/or *areflexia* (reduced or absent muscle stretch reflexes). This interruption of the motor unit results in localized muscle atrophy or wasting. This atrophy also increases with nonuse of the muscle. In some LMN lesions, the affected muscle exhibits small localized, spontaneous, and involuntary contractions called *fasciculations*.

Upper motor neurone signs

Upper motor neurones (UMNs) originate in the motor strip of the cerebral cortex and in multiple brainstem nuclei. These axons then pass through the brainstem, decussate (cross) in the medulla, and descend in the spinal cord via the corticospinal tracts. These fibres synapse with LMNs in the spinal cord. The collective working of both the UMN and LMN is essential for fine, orderly, and smooth muscle movements.

When a UMN lesion is rostral to the medulla, as in a cerebrovascular accident, deficits will occur contralateral to the lesion and will result in *hemiplegia*. The distribution or degree of paralysis is not always equal within hemiplegic distribution. The following are upper motor neurone signs:

1. Paresis or paralysis of voluntary muscle tone and spasticity
2. Hyperreflexia
3. Late atrophy from disuse
4. Increased muscle tone

Initially, the muscles affected by an upper motor lesion are *flaccid (hypotonic)* and *hyporeflexic*. Gradually, and with variability, the reflex arcs become increasingly hyperreactive. Then paresis, or paralysis of voluntary muscle movement, occurs with increased tone and spasticity. The spasticity is characterized by *increased resistance* to

Patient Teaching   29-21

The patient with motor or sensory dysfunction

1. Always brake wheelchair when transferring patient
2. Check condition of affected eye frequently
3. Be aware of placement of affected extremities before movement
4. Protect paralyzed limbs from injury
5. Ask patient to wear shoes (*not* slippers) that fit well for ambulating or transferring

Skin care
1. Regular inspection of skin surfaces, using mirror or other device
2. Need to turn frequently
3. Weight shifts
4. No use of heating pads, hot water bottles, or excessively hot water for bathing

Activity needs
1. Range of movements
2. Proper positioning
3. Frequent changes in position

Medications
1. Use of medication, side effects, dosage, and timing
2. Reporting of side effects to doctor
3. Importance of not combining medication with other mood-altering drugs or alcohol

Nutrition-diet
1. Foods that can be easily tolerated
2. Measures to decrease swallowing difficulty
3. Use of special appliances to assist with eating

ADL
1. Teaching techniques of bathing, grooming, dressing
2. Importance of having meaningful recreational activities
3. Bowel and bladder care

Other teaching
1. Importance of good fluid intake
2. Follow-up care—where to procure equipment, supplies
3. Methods for relieving feelings of frustration

5. Are the joints freely moveable?
6. Is the patient receiving adequate nutrition?
7. Is the patient swallowing without difficulty?
8. Is the patient's fluid intake adequate?
9. Does the patient assume control of bowel and bladder programme?
10. Is the patient as independent in ADLs as possible?
11. Does the patient verbalize a positive self-concept?
12. Can the patient state plans for follow-up care?
13. Does the patient verbalize knowledge of the medication regimen?

ALTERATIONS IN SENSORY FUNCTION

Pathophysiology

The presence of a lesion anywhere within the sensory system pathway, from the receptor to the sensory cortex, alters the transmission or perception of sensory information. The parietal lobe cortex is of major importance in interpretation of sensation with the exception of sight, hearing, smell, taste, and thermoregulation. Loss, decrease, or increase in sensation of pain, temperature, touch, and proprioception, singly or in combination, results in difficulty in daily living. Because these sensations normally help the person to be aware of alterations in the internal and external environments, any alteration in sensation lessens the ability to be completely and accurately protected.

One specific loss is that of *proprioception*, or *the ability to know the position of the body and its parts without looking directly at the part*. Lack of control of body temperature, or *hyperthermia*, is another dysfunction and occurs as a result of malfunction in the thermoregulatory centre in the brain, such as that which occurs after brain surgery near the hypothalamus or from head injury.

Fig. 29-18 presents common patterns of sensory loss. A cerebral lesion results in various alterations in sensation contralateral to the lesion. This distribution results because all sensory fibres have decussated (crossed) before reacting the sensory cortex of the cerebrum. On the other hand, transection of the spinal cord results in total bilateral sensory loss distal to the lesion, because all pathways have been severed. The characteristic distribution of deficits with Brown-Sequard syndrome is ipsilateral (same side) loss of proprioception and vibratory sense and contralateral (opposite side) loss of pain, temperature, and crude touch sensation.

Nursing Process
Assessment

The sensory examination is the most difficult part of the neurological examination. Subjective data are collected as follows.
Subjective data
1. Patient's understanding of the sensory disturbance
2. Measures that relieve symptoms, including medications
3. Site of sensory abnormality
4. Onset of sensory problem

Evaluation

Evaluation of the patient with motor dysfunction is made based on the perception of the patient and measurement against the defined patient outcomes. Questions to consider may include the following:
1. Does the patient remain free of traumatic injury?
2. Is the patient's skin intact?
3. Is the patient doing skin checks or asking staff to do them?
4. Is the patient knowledgeable about range of movements?

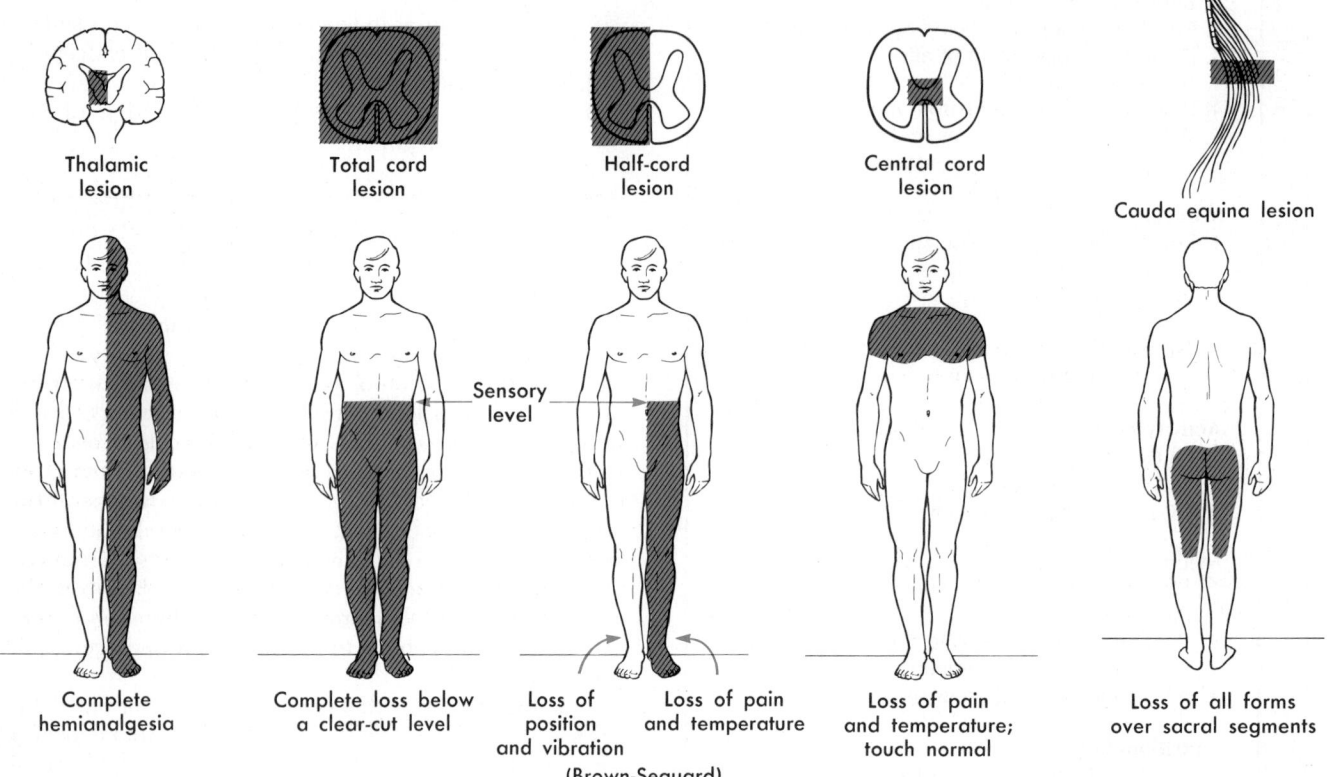

Fig. 29-18   Common patterns of sensory abnormality. Upper diagrams show site of lesion; lower diagrams show distribution of corresponding sensory loss. (Modified from Bickerstaff, ER: *Neurology for nurses,* ed 2, London, 1971, English Universities Press Ltd, and Hodder & Stoughton, Ltd.)

5. Presence of associated symptoms
6. Alteration in sensation
   a. Pain
   b. Touch
   c. Temperature
   d. Proprioception
   e. Stereognosis

Nursing analysis

Problems are determined from analysis of patient data. Possible problems for the person with sensory dysfunction may include all those listed under Alterations in Muscle Tone and Motor Function (p. 866), with the addition of the following:

Problem	Possible aetiologies
Sensory/perceptual alteration	Altered sensory reception/ transmission/ integration

Planning: expected patient outcomes

Expected patient outcomes for the person with sensory dysfunction may include, but are not limited to, the expected patient outcomes listed under Alterations in Muscle Tone and Motor Function (p. 866), as well as the following:

1. Patient can demonstrate how to compensate for each sensory deficit or loss.
2. Patient can explain safety factors needed in ADLs to protect against injury.
3. Patient can demonstrate how to inspect the affected body parts for injury.
4. Patient can state signs and symptoms that would indicate worsening of the condition and the need to seek medical assistance.
5. Patient demonstrates minimal anxiety.
6. Patient's discomfort or pain is minimal.

Implementation

Interventions to achieve patient outcomes

Facilitating learning

The most important nursing intervention for the patient with sensory dysfunction is teaching the person and family protective measures in relation to the sensory deficit or alteration (see Box 29-21). Teaching the person to use noninvolved senses to an increased extent helps to avoid injuries. For example, teaching the person with hypoaesthesia (lessened touch) to visually inspect involved body parts regularly will help to prevent injuries.

Evaluation

Evaluation of the patient with sensory dysfunction involves the patient and family. Questions to consider may include those listed under Alterations in Muscle Tone and Motor Function (p. 869), as well as the following:

1. Is the patient carrying out ADL in a safe manner?
2. Is the patient successfully compensating for sensory deficits?
3. Is the patient inspecting affected body parts for injury?
4. Can the patient state signs and symptoms that indicate the need to notify the doctor?
5. Is the patient free of pain or discomfort?

MAJOR HEALTH PROBLEMS OF THE NEUROLOGICAL SYSTEM

Functioning of the neurological system can be interrupted for a variety of reasons. These include the following:

1. Interference with impulses because of conduction of impulses
2. Interference because of degenerative changes
3. Interference because of vascular problems
4. Interference because of infection
5. Interference because of trauma
6. Interference because of tumours

Some common neurological disorders are listed in Box 29-22.

INTERFERENCE WITH FUNCTION BECAUSE OF PROBLEMS WITH CONDUCTION OF IMPLUSES

EPILEPSY OR SEIZURES

Epilepsy (convulsive disorder) is one of the oldest diseases known to humans. (For purposes of this text the terms *epilepsy, seizure disorder,* and *convulsive disorder* will be used interchangeably.) Seizures occur in all races and affect males and females equally. There is no apparent geographic distribution. Epilepsy can begin at any age, but in many the onset is before the age 20. The incidence is about 1 in every 200 to 300 people, but accurate figures are hard to estimate. Many of these are children.

There are numerous ways to classify seizures. One common way is the International Classification of Epileptic Seizures. In this classification, seizures are identified as partial (beginning locally), generalized (bilaterally symmetric and with no local onset), unilateral, or unclassified. Another way to classify seizures is based on the clinical features of the attack. The five groups in this type of classification are the following:

1. Grand mal (major or generalized)
2. Petit mal
3. Psychomotor
4. Jacksonian and focal
5. Miscellaneous (myoclonic, akinetic)

Table 29-5 shows the characteristics of each type of seizure.

Pathophysiology

Epilepsy may be defined as a transitory disturbance in consciousness or in motor, sensory, or autonomic function with or without loss of consciousness. It is associated with sudden, excessive, and disorderly electrical discharges in the neurones of the brain that result in the sudden, violent, involuntary contraction of a group of muscles. The patterns or forms of seizures vary and depend on the area of the brain from which the seizure arises. The pattern is stereotyped in the individual, although variations may occur with progression of cerebral lesions (Fig. 29-19).

29-22	**Health problems of the neurological system**

1. *Interference with function because of problems with conduction of impulses*
   a. Epilepsy or seizures
   b. Myasthenia gravis
2. *Interference with function because of degenerative diseases*
   a. Multiple sclerosis
   b. Parkinson's disease
   c. Motor neurone disease (MND)
   d. Alzheimer's disease
   e. Neurofibromatosis
3. *Interference with function because of vascular conditions*
   a. Cerebrovascular accident (CVA)
   b. Intracerebral haemorrhage
4. *Interference with function because of infection/inflammation*
   a. Meningitis
   b. Encephalitis
   c. Brain abscess
   d. Poliomyelitis
   e. Guillain-Barré syndrome
   f. Neurosyphilis
   g. AIDS
5. *Interference with function because of trauma*
   a. Craniocerebral
   b. Spinal cord
   c. Peripheral nerve
6. *Interference with function because of tumours*
   a. Intracranial
   b. Intraspinal

Table 29-5 Characteristics of seizures

Type of seizure	Aetiology	Characteristics	Clinical signs	Aura	Postictal period
Grand mal	Most common	Generalized, characterized by loss of consciousness for several minutes	Aura Cry Loss of consciousness The fall Tonic-clinicmovements Incontinence	Present Flashing lights Smells Spots before eyes Dizziness	Present Need for sleep 1 to 2 hrs Headache common
Petit mal	Usually occur during childhood and adolescence Frequency decreases as child gets older	Sudden impairment in or loss of consciousness with little or no tonic-clonic movement Occurs without warning Has tendency to appear a few hours after arising or when person is quiet	Sudden vacant facial expression with eye focused straight ahead All motor activity ceases except perhaps for slight symmetric twitching about eyelids Possible loss of muscle tone Consciousness returns	Not present	Not present
Psychomotor	Occur at any age	Sudden change in awareness associated with complex distortion of feeling and thinking and partially coordinated motor activity Longer than petit mal	Behaves as if partially conscious Often appears intoxicated May do antisocial things such as exposing self or carrying out violent acts Autonomic complaints may occur Chest pain Respiratory distress Tachycardia Gastrointestinal distress Urinary incontinence	Present Complex hallucinations or illusions	Present Confusion Amnesia Need for sleep
Jacksonian-focal	Occur almost entirely in patients with structural brain disase	Depend on site of focus May or may not be progressive	Commonly begin in hand, foot, or face May end in grand mal seizure	Present Numbness Tingling Crawling feeling	Present
Myoclonic	May antedate grand mal by months or years	May be very mild or may have rapid, forceful movements	Sudden involuntary contraction of muscle group, usually in extremities or trunk No loss of consciousness	Not present	Not present
Akinetic	Not common	Peculiar generalized tonelessness	Person falls in flaccid state Unconscious for minute or two	Rarely present	Not present

Seizures can involve essentially all parts of the brain at once, as in the generalized type, or only a minute focal spot. In the first type, the excessive neuronal discharges are thought to originate in the brainstem portion of the reticular activating system; these then spread throughout the CNS including the cortex and the deeper parts of the brain. The process may last from a few seconds to as long as 3 to 5 minutes, or it may stop immediately, as in a *petit mal seizure*. Stoppage of a seizure is thought to result from fatigue of the neurones involved in precipitating the seizure or by inhibition of certain structures within the brain. The excessive neuronal discharges may result in a *tonic convulsion*, with the contraction of all muscles at once, or a *clonic convulsion*, with alternate contraction and relaxation of opposing muscle groups. This gives the characteristic jerking movements of the body. Seizures are followed by inhibition of cerebral function with a variable length. This is called the *postictal period*.

When recurrent generalized seizure activity occurs at such frequency that full consciousness is not regained

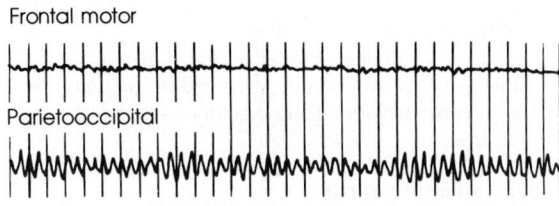

Frontal motor

Parietooccipital

Normal adult, 10/sec. activity in occipital area.

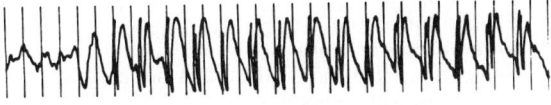

Absent attacks (petit mal seizures).
Synchronous 3/sec. spikes and waves.

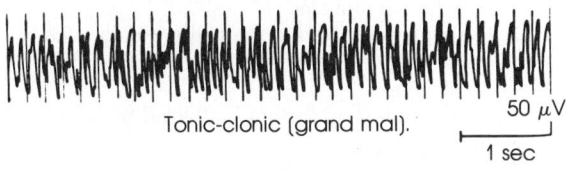

Tonic-clonic (grand mal).

50 μV

1 sec

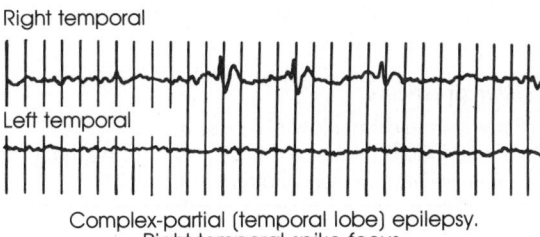

Right temporal

Left temporal

Complex-partial (temporal lobe) epilepsy.
Right temporal spike focus.

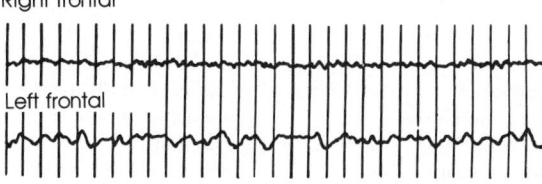

Right frontal

Left frontal

Brain tumour. Left frontal slow wave focus.

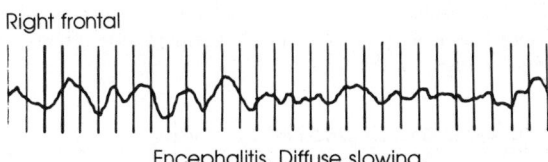

Right frontal

Encephalitis. Diffuse slowing.

Fig. 29-19   Tracings of electroencephalogram. The normal tracing is demonstrated as are several pathological states.

between seizures, it is called *status epilepticus*. This is a medical emergency and requires intensive medical and nursing care to prevent death from brain damage secondary to prolonged hypoxia and exhaustion.

Seizures occur in many childhood and adult illnesses. Causes include the following:

1. Cerebral anoxia
2. Hypoglycaemia
3. Disturbance of calcium balance
4. Other electrolyte imbalances
5. Disturbance in hydration
6. Injection of drugs and poisons with convulsive activity
7. Numerous metabolic disturbances and disorders
8. Infections that cause high temperature elevations
9. Generalized inflammatory processes
10. Degenerative tissue disorders
11. Hysteria

In many patients with epilepsy, a localized organic lesion serves as the focus for the abnormal neuronal discharges from the damaged brain tissue. These organic lesions include the following:

1. Neoplasms
2. Inflamed areas or abscesses
3. Sclerosis
4. Vascular formations or haematomas
5. Congenital malformations
6. Trauma
7. Other space-occupying lesions

Nursing Process
Assessment

Assessment of both subjective and objective data is important in the patient who is having a seizure (see Box 29-23).

Subjective data

1. Patient's understanding of the seizure disorder and what might be causing it
2. Awareness of precipitating factors
3. Presence of an aura
4. Postictal feelings
5. Presence of amnesia

An *aura* is defined as the set of symptoms that occurs before the seizure. An aura occurs in about 50% of all patients with *grand mal seizures* and usually includes a change in sensation or a change in affect. The exact character of the aura varies from person to person but may include numbness, flashing lights, dizziness, tingling of the arm, smells, or spots before the eyes. The patient may not be able to describe the aura precisely, but it gives conclusive evidence of the impending seizure and allows the patient to seek privacy and safety before it occurs.

During the postictal phase the individual is groggy and acts in a confused way. Complaints of headache or muscular pain are common. A deep sleep usually follows. During this phase the pupils may remain dilated and plantar reflexes may be abnormal. After a variable period of time the patient awakens and is frequently unaware of the occurrence of the seizure. A dull headache and depression are common.

29-23

Observations to be made about a person having a seizure

Aura

Presence or absence; nature if present; ability of patient to describe it (somatic, visceral, psychic)

Cry

Presence or absence

Onset

Site of initial body movements; deviation of head and eyes; chewing and salivation; posture of body; sensory changes

Tonic and clonic phases

Movements of body as to progression; skin colour and airway; pupillary changes; incontinence; duration of each phase

Relaxation (sleep)

Duration and behaviour

Postictal phase

Duration; general behaviour; ability to remember anything about the seizure; orientation; pupillary changes; headache; injuries present

Duration of seizure

Length from aura to relaxation phase

Level of consciousness

Length of unconsciousness if present

Presence of injury

Injury to mouth, lips, tongue, or soft tissues from seizure
Injury to extremities

29-24

Electroencephalogram (EEG)

Purpose

To provide evidence of focal or diffuse disturbances of brain function produced by organic lesions by measuring the electrical activity of the brain (Fig. 29-19).

Preparation of patient

No special preparation beforehand
Patient is encouraged to be quiet and rest before the procedure
Scalp and hair should be clean
Patient teaching
  Explain procedure
  Time: 1 hour or more
  Sensation: not painful—electrodes are applied to scalp with collodion

Procedure

1. Patient usually sits in a comfortable chair or lies on a couch with eyes closed. Testing is done in a special room where outside electrical activity is eliminated
2. Electrodes are fixed to the scalp, usually with collodion, in a set pattern to cover all scalp areas
3. The basic resting rhythm is affected by opening the eyes or altering attention
4. Recordings can be made while the patient is asleep or when sleep deprived
5. Comparisons are made of different patterns of the recordings

After procedure

Patient should be allowed to rest if tired
Patient should be assisted if necessary in washing hair and removing collodion from scalp

---

Objective data

1. Number of seizures occurring within a specific time
2. Behaviour: signs of stress or fatigue
3. Character of seizure
4. Injuries sustained

Diagnostic tests

By far the most common test used to evaluate seizure disorders is the electroencephalogram (EEG) (see Box 29-24). It is safe and noninvasive and allows for more specific diagnosis.

Nursing analysis

Problems are determined from analysis of patient data. Possible problems for the person with seizures may include, but are not limited to, the following:

Problem	Possible aetiologies
Anxiety	Threat/change in health status
Adjustment, impaired	Disability requiring change in lifestyle
Coping, ineffective individual	Situational crisis of diagnosis
Social isolation	Alteration in behaviour during seizures
Oral mucous membrane, altered	Treatment with phenytoin
Injury, high risk for	Seizures
Knowledge deficit	Lack of exposure/recall
Noncompliance with medications	Treatment side effects

Planning: expected patient outcomes

Expected patient outcomes for the person with seizures may include, but are not limited to, the following:

1. Seizures are reduced or at least do not increase in severity or number.

Table 29-6   Some anticonvulsants used to prevent seizures

Drug	Use related to seizure type	Average daily dose	Toxic effects
Phenytoin	Grand mal, focal, psychomotor	0.3–0.6 g (divided dose)	Ataxia, vomiting, nystagmus, drowsiness, rash, fever, gum hypertrophy, lymphadenopathy
Phenobarbitone	Grand mal, focal, psychomotor (adjunctive)	60–100 mg at night	Drowsiness, rash
Primidone	Grand mal, focal, psychomotor	Up to 1.5 g	Drowsiness, ataxia
Ethosuximide	Petit mal, psychomotor, myo-clonic, akinetic	1–1.5 g	Drowsiness, nausea, agranulocytosis
Diazepam	Status epilepticus, mixed	10–20 mg	Drowsiness, ataxia
Carbamazepine	Grandmal, psychomotor	0.8–1.2 g	Rash, drowsiness, ataxia
Sodium valproate	Petit mal, absence of seizures	1–2 g	Nausea, vomiting, indigestion, sedation, emotional disturbance, weakness, altered blood coagulation
Clonazepam	Petit mal, akinetic, myoclconic	4–8 mg	Grand mal seizures, drowsiness, ataxia, hypotension, respiratory depression

2. Patient shows a low level of anxiety.
3. Patient shows social participation.
4. Patient remains free of traumatic injury.
5. Patient can describe medication to be taken, including action, side effects, toxic effects, and dosage timing.
6. Patient can explain the importance of avoiding alcohol while taking anticonvulsant drugs.
7. Patient explains how to use available community resources.
8. Patient and significant other can explain the necessary measures to carry out if a seizure does occur.
9. Patient can explain the importance of taking medication regularly even when the seizures are controlled.
10. Patient wears medical alert tag.
11. Patient demonstrates a patent airway.

Implementation

Assisting with achievement of therapeutic goals

Medications

Treatment of patients with a seizure disorder almost always includes the use of one or more of the anticonvulsant drugs (see Table 29-6). Other anticonvulsants that are used in the treatment of epilepsy include methylphenobarbitone, clobazam, acetazolamide and the newer agents, lamotrigine and vigabatrin. In status epilepticus, chlormethiazole, lorazepam and paraldehyde may also be used. The choice of medications depends on the type of seizure. Anticonvulsant medications act generally on the cerebral cortex and are not selective in acting on the part of the brain involved in abnormal neuronal discharges.

The dosages of anticonvulsant drugs are difficult to establish and regulate because of the high incidence of side effects and the toxicity of the drugs. The drug of choice is introduced in an average therapeutic dose, and the dose is increased until seizure control is reached. If toxicity is reached before control of the seizures, the dose is decreased to the previous nontoxic or tolerated dose. Additional secondary drugs may be introduced at this time to aid in seizure control.

Failure to take the prescribed medication or to take an adequate dose is often the cause of failure in treatment. Tests to determine the blood level of the anticonvulsant are helpful in providing an accurate check on the therapeutic and toxic levels of the medications taken.

Surgical treatment

Surgical treatment of seizures is very rare but it may be used in some cases in which medical therapy is not effective. *Cortical resection* is one surgical approach. It involves removal of the brain tissue in which the focus of electrical discharge is located. The localization of tissue must occur in a part of the brain that is easily accessible to surgery and that can be removed without leaving the person with a serious disability.

Another surgical approach involves *stereotactic* procedures using electrical stimulation. This technique is used to interrupt the pathways of seizure activity, to destroy the foci, or to alter the actions of the cortical nerve cells.

Interventions to achieve patient outcomes

Promoting adjustment and socialization

Because most people with seizures do not have symptoms between attacks and because a majority of seizures can be controlled by medication, the person with seizures should be encouraged to lead as normal a life as possible. Until seizures are controlled, however, the person should avoid dangerous activities such as driving a car, working on or about machinery, or swimming. Once the person has achieved seizure control for a significant period and has learned the importance of taking the medication regularly

Nursing actions during a seizure

1. Never leave the person alone.
2. If patient is in upright position, lower to floor or bed and move adjacent articles and equipment away to prevent injury.
3. Loosen constricting clothing, especially around the neck.
4. Turn head to one side to aid with airway.
5. No effort should be made to restrain the person manually or with restraints.
6. On no account is any object put between the teeth.
7. Pad cot sides if the patient is confined to bed or has seizures during sleep. Pillows should not be used for padding because of danger of suffocation.
8. Accurate observations should be made and recorded.

Patient Teaching 29-26

The patient with a seizure disorder

1. Use of medication, including side effects, dose, timing; reporting side effects to doctor
2. Importance of avoiding the use of alcohol with anticonvulsants
3. Safety measures to avoid injury in case of seizures
4. Good oral hygiene if patient is taking phenytoin
5. Importance of adequate rest and diet
6. Importance of taking medication even when free of seizures
7. Community resources
8. Restrictions concerning driving
9. Importance of follow-up care
10. Importance of verbalizing feelings
11. Need to avoid excessive stress
12. Importance of wearing medical alert bracelet
13. Importance of not overprotecting self
14. Avoiding certain occupations and leisure activities.

and avoiding alcoholic beverages, these restrictions can be relaxed. Maintaining adequate rest and nutritional intake is also important. Family members need to be assisted to discuss their attitudes and feelings about the individual's illness.

The issue of driving a car is one that often poses a problem. Epilepsy does impose driver limitations. Usually a period of time without seizures must elapse before the person is eligible to drive and then only if seizures are completely controlled. The drug-therapy is also considered when driving becomes an issue.

Promoting good oral hygiene

The patient who is taking phenytoin is especially prone to developing gingival hyperplasia. Good mouth care, utilizing a soft toothbrush, is essential. The teeth should be brushed in a gentle fashion to prevent excessive bleeding. Regular visits to the dentist are important.

Preventing injury

The primary goals of the nurse and family caring for a patient having a seizure are protection from injury and observation and recording of the seizure activity. Specific actions are listed in Box 29-25.

Facilitating learning

Teaching is an important part of the care of the patient with seizures. This includes the patient, as well as members of the family, who should learn to care for the person during and after a seizure. Involvement of the family or significant other during the hospitalization is essential. One of the more important things for the family to learn is the need to be calm and accept the family member's seizures.

Teaching for the patient with a seizure disorder includes the actions defined in Box 29-26.

Evaluation

As with other conditions, evaluation of the patient experiencing seizures is made using the feelings and input of the patient. Questions to consider may include the following:

1. Is the number of seizures decreased?
2. Is the patient verbalizing feelings?
3. Is the patient socializing with others?
4. Is the patient refraining from dangerous activity?
5. Can the patient explain daily routine that includes adequate rest?
6. Is the patient able to identify available community resources?
7. Is follow-up care occurring as prescribed?
8. Is the patient wearing a medical alert bracelet?
9. Is the patient taking the medication as prescribed?
10. Are blood levels of the prescribed anticonvulsants within normal limits?
11. Is the patient coping well?
12. Is the patient receiving regular dental care?

MYASTHENIA GRAVIS

Myasthenia gravis is a neuromuscular disease that affects the lower motor neurones and muscles. Excessive fatigue occurs along with weakness of muscles, especially those involved with the face, eyes, larynx, and pharynx and the process of respiration. The fatigue and weakness worsens with exercise and is improved with rest. It affects about 1 in 20,000 people.

The cause of myasthenia is unknown, although it is thought to be an autoimmune disease. It characteristically starts between the ages of 20 and 30 or in late middle age. In younger peolpe, women are affected more than men, but in older people men are affected to a greater extent. Familial occurrence is rare.[68]

Pathophysiology

No structural change in the muscle or nerve is observed in cases of myasthenia gravis. Nerve impulses fail to pass to muscles at the myoneural junction. It is not known specifically why the motor nerve impulses fail to pass to the muscle and cause it not to contract. This is believed to be caused by a *decrease in the release of acetylcholine* from the presynaptic terminals or a *blockage of or a reduction in the number of postsynaptic membrane receptor sites*. It is known that circulating antibodies to the acetylcholine receptor (AChR) are present and are believed to cause the myasthenic weakness.

About 10% of patients with myasthenia have been found to have a thymoma, and nearly 70% have changes in the cellular structure of the thymus gland (usually hyperplasia). The role of the thymus gland in the pathophysiology of myasthenia gravis is unclear.

In severe cases, the respiratory muscles and bulbar cranial nerve may be involved, leading to severe respiratory infection and possible death. However, sensation is not lost and the involved muscles usually do not atrophy.

Diagnostic tests

Diagnosis of myasthenia gravis is partially made on the basis of EMGs that rule out other muscle disorders. A specific diagnostic test that is used is the edrophonium chloride test. Edrophonium is a very short-acting anticholinesterase drug. The procedure for the test is as follows:

1. Edrophonium and normal saline are drawn up in separate syringes.
2. Each is injected intravenously separately.
3. It is important that the patient not be aware which solution is being given.
4. Increased strength in a predetermined muscle group with the administration of edrophonium is a positive test.

The results occur in 30 seconds to 1 minute and usually last only a few minutes.

A chest X-ray examination or CT scan of the chest may be done to determine the presence of a thymoma. The curare test may be done if all other tests are normal or questionable. Because curare causes respiratory paralysis, equipment and personnel to intubate the patient should be available. The curare test may be definitive when other tests are not.[68]

Nursing Process

Implementation

Medical management

Medications that are used in myasthenia gravis are neostigmine, distigmine and pyridostigmine. These drugs block the action of cholinesterase at the myoneural junction and allow acetylcholine to act. Atropine or other anticholinergic agents that block the effects of acetylcholine can be used to treat the side effects of these drugs. Treatment is planned so that the patient receives the drug in the amount tolerated without side effects and yet is able to carry out activities essential for normal living. Usually, the patient is allowed to adjust the dosage. Corticosteroids such as prednisolone are sometimes used as an adjunct to other drug therapy.

It is often difficult to distinguish between *myasthenic crisis* (too little drug) and *cholinergic crisis* (too much drug), because both conditions cause severe muscle weakness. Administering edrophonium intravenously differentiates between the two conditions. A positive test (increase in strength) indicates underdosage of the drug. An increase in weakness is a sign of overdosage.

Nursing interventions

Maintaining an effective airway

Respiratory complications are common for the patient with myasthenia gravis, and for this reason they are usually advised not to live alone. They are also cautioned to avoid crowds or other circumstances where infections are common. Upper respiratory infections are seen because patients may not have the energy needed to cough effectively and may develop pneumonia or airway obstruction. Aspiration is common. Many patients have airway equipment at home.

During acute episodes of the disease, the following are important:

1. Tracheostomy set at bedside, because respiratory status may change rapidly
2. Serial determinations of vital capacity, minute volumes, and tidal volumes
3. Suction as necessary
4. Nasogastric tube if swallowing is too dangerous (patient will not be able to cough to indicate if tube is in trachea, so careful assessment of the position of tube is important)
5. With severe impairment in respiratory function, the patient will probably require endotracheal intubation and ventilator assistance (see Chapter 16 for further discussion of the patient on mechanical ventilation)

Maintaining activity

Patients with severe symptoms of myasthenia gravis may be too weak to do anything for themselves. The nurse may have to turn and position the patient in addition to doing most of the other ADL. It is important to remember that the patient with myasthenia gravis will remain alert and will often be very frightened. Psychological support and reassurance are essential.

Facilitating learning

The patient with myasthenia gravis often has a great deal of control over his/her medication schedule and can do much to prevent respiratory problems. A well-informed patient is more likely to stay healthy.

INTERFERENCE WITH FUNCTION BECAUSE OF DEGENERATIVE DISEASES

The term *degenerative diseases* is used to refer to neurological diseases in which there is a premature senescence of nerve cells, there is a known or suspected metabolic disturbance, or the cause of the disease is unknown. Included in this section are five such diseases. They are the following:

Table 29-7 Comparison of degenerative neurological diseases

Disease	Pathological signs	Effect	Medical treatment
Multiple sclerosis	Multiple foci (patches) of nerve degeneration throughout the brain and spinal cord	Demyelination causes nerve impulses to be interrupted (blocked) or distorted (slowed)	No specific treatment Symptomatic treatment Judicious use of ACTH or corticosteroids
Parkinson's disease	Destruction of nerve cells of basal nuclei of brain	Decreased dopamine (neurotransmitter substance with anticholinergic effect)	Anticholinergic drugs Levodopa Carbidopa-levodopa Surgery in selected cases
Alzheimer's disease	Degeneration of neurofibrils and presence of plaque in brain	Destruction of neurones leading to impairments in intellectual functioning	No specific treatment Symptomatic and supportive care

1. Multiple sclerosis (MS)
2. Parkinson's disease (PD)
3. Motor neurone disease (MND)
4. Alzheimer's disease
5. Neurofibromatosis (Von Recklinghausen's disease)
See Table 29-7 for a comparison of MS, PD and Alzheimers disease.

Another degenerative disease is syringomyelia. This is a destruction of the grey and then white matter of the spinal cord that occurs as a result of the development of *syrinxes* (cysts filled with CSF). As a result, nerve pathways in the spinal cord are destroyed and nerve impulses are interrupted. This disease will not be discussed in further detail, but the nurse should be aware of it.

MULTIPLE SCLEROSIS

Aetiology/Epidemiology

Multiple sclerosis is a common degenerative neurological disease. It affects around 1 in 2000 people in the United Kingdom. The cause remains unknown despite research. Several hypotheses have been advanced as to the cause:

1. Genetic—it has been found that relatives of people with multiple sclerosis have a much higher incidence of the disease than the general population. Several studies have demonstrated an increased incidence of multiple sclerosis among siblings and even distant relatives. A person with an identical twin with the disease has a 20% risk of having the disease.[106]
2. Epidemiological—the disease is rare between the equator and latitudes 30 to 35° north and south.[106] When they move to another region, they retain the same risk.
3. Viral—the serum and cerebrospinal fluid of patients with multiple sclerosis has been found to contain antibodies to many viruses, including measles, mumps, herpes simplex, and influenza.
4. Immunological—most people with multiple sclerosis have been found to have abnormalities of the spinal fluid indicative of autoimmune disease.

The onset of symptoms usually occurs between the ages of 20 and 40. The course of the disease is estimated to be 12 to 25 years. Females are more likely to be affected by multiple sclerosis than males. There has been no evidence to suggest a sexual mode of transmission.

Pathophysiology

Multiple foci of demyelination are distributed randomly in the white matter of the brainstem, spinal cord, optic nerves, and cerebrum. During the demyelination process (primary degeneration), the myelin sheath and the sheath cells are destroyed, but there is early sparing of the axon cylinder. The outer myelin sheath destruction causes interruption or distortion of the impulse so that it is slowed or blocked. There is evidence of partial healing in areas of degeneration, which accounts for the transitory nature of early symptoms. In later stages the degeneration may extend to grey areas of the cord and limit healing. Although the outer surface of the brain appears normal, brain weight may be decreased and the ventricles may be enlarged.

Because of the wide distribution of areas of degeneration, the variety of signs and symptoms in multiple sclerosis is greater than in other neurological diseases. It is a chronic, remitting, and relapsing disease. The majority of people recover from their early episodes, with remissions lasting for a year or more. Exacerbations of multiple sclerosis may be aggravated or precipitated by fatigue, chilling, and emotional disturbances. In rare cases the disease may terminate in death within a few years of onset.

Nursing Process
Assessment

Early symptoms of multiple sclerosis are usually transitory. Many people may be considered neurotic because of the wide variety and temporary nature of symptoms and the emotional instability produced by the disease. Subjective symptoms are important in making the diagnosis.

Subjective data

1. Patient's understanding of disease
2. Presence of eye problems
   a. Diplopia
   b. Scotomas (spots before the eyes)
   c. Blindness
3. Presence of weakness or numbness of part of the body such as hand
4. Presence of unusual fatigue
5. Presence of tremor
6. Presence of emotional instability
7. Presence of bowel and bladder problems
8. Presence of impotence in men

9. Loss of joint sensation and proprioception
10. Presence of vertigo

Objective data

1. Documented abnormalities in neurological testing
   a. Nystagmus
   b. Scanning speech
   c. Muscle weakness and spasms
   d. Changes in coordination
   e. Spastic ataxic gait
2. Behaviour: presence of euphoria, emotional, lability, mild depression
3. Urinary incontinence, frequency, or retention
4. Difficulty in swallowing
5. Intentional tremors of upper extremities

It is suspected that the presence of euphoria is caused by patient's attempts to reassure themselves that their condition is not serious. Motor signs associated with multiple sclerosis have UMN characteristics. Pain is not a common symptom.

Diagnostic tests

Examination of the cerebrospinal fluid usually shows elevated gamma globulin level and an increased white blood cell count. An electroimmunodiffusion determination is done. A CT scan may demonstrate enlargement of the ventricles. Cerebral atrophy is present in advanced disease.

Even in early stages of multiple sclerosis, abnormal visual and brainstem evoked potentials are present. The visual evoked response will show optic atrophy in the majority of cases. Evoked potentials are electrical measurements of physiological maturation of the human nervous system. They provide information about the primary sensory areas of the cortex.

Nursing analysis

Problems are determined from analysis of patient data. Possible problems for the person with multiple sclerosis may include, but are not limited to, the following:

Problem	Possible aetiologies
Incontinence, total or urge	Neurological dysfunction
Incontinence, bowel	Neuromuscular impairment
Nutrition, altered: less than body requirements or more than body requirements	Chewing or swallowing difficulties
Skin integrity, impaired, actual or high risk for	Immobility, mechanical forces
Activity intolerance	Generalized weakness
Mobility, impaired physical	Neuromuscular impairment
Self-care deficit: feeding, bathing/hygiene, dressing/grooming, toileting	Neuromuscular impairment
Pain	Immobility, spasticity
Adjustment, impaired	Disability requiring change in lifestyle
Knowledge deficit	Lack of information about MS

Planning: expected patient outcomes

Expected patient outcomes for the person with multiple sclerosis may include, but are not limited to, the following:

1. Patient has minimal complications because of urinary incontinence.
2. Patient remains free of infection.
3. Patient's bowel patterns are continent to the degree possible, and complications of any incontinence or constipation are minimal.
4. Patient maintains adequate nutrition.
5. Patient's skin is intact.
6. Patient maintains optimal mobility.
7. Patient has minimal deficits in self-care activities.
8. Patient has minimal discomfort.
9. Patient verbalizes a positive self-concept.
10. Patient demonstrates minimal anxiety.
11. Patient/family can verbalize knowledge of disease.
12. Patient can explain the action, side effects, and toxic effects of prescribed medications.
13. Patient can state plans for follow-up care.
14. Patient can state how to secure community help.

Implementation

Assisting with the achievement of therapeutic goals
Medications

At present there is no specific treatment for multiple sclerosis. Favourable results seem to occur with the use of adrenocorticotrophic hormone (ACTH) and the corticosteroids. Their efficacy remains controversial. Some doctors prefer oral prednisolone or intramuscular or oral dexamethasone. ACTH may be given intramuscularly or intravenously. The effects of ACTH and the steroids on the demyelinating process is unknown. It is known from testing that (1) nothing is gained from long-term treatment, and (2) some gain is possible from taking high doses of steroids at the start of an exacerbation, because the episode then seems to resolve more rapidly.

Interventions to achieve patient outcomes
Preventing bladder problems

Urinary frequency and urgency may respond to timed doses of propantheline bromide. Prevention of urinary tract infection remains a problem, and such infections are a major cause of death. Cholinergic drugs such as bethanechol may be helpful for the patient with atonic bladder. Oxybutynin chloride (Ditropan) is used to treat neurogenic bladder. It acts by exerting a direct antispasmodic effect on smooth muscles. Some patients are given prophylactic doses of medications such as co-trimoxazole or nitrofurantoin. Cystometric studies can be helpful in defining the specific bladder problem.[76a]

The patient should be encouraged to drink adequate fluids.

Preventing bowel complications

Constipation is common for patients who have multiple sclerosis. It is important that the diet include foods high in fibre, as well as adequate fluids. The use of prune juice may be helpful, as well as stool softeners that are prescribed by the doctor. Laxatives should be used judiciously, so as not to cause dependence on them.

Nursing Research 29-27

Buelow J: A correlation study of disabilities, stressors and coping methods in victims of multiple sclerosis, *J Neurosci Nurs* 23(4):247–252, 1991.

Patients admitted to the hospital for an exacerbation of their multiple sclerosis were asked to identify the stressors in their daily lives. These 20 patients were also asked to identify the copying mechanisms they used to deal with the stressors. The Bathel scale was used to measure the overall stress, with the overall mean stress score for the 20 patients of 1.49 on a scale of 1 to 3. The most stressful items identified were feeling tired, inability to walk, and uncertainty about the future. The most common coping theme was self-reliance. Coping mechanism used more frequently included a sense of humour and trying to learn more. No relationship was found between the degree of disability and stressors. A negative correlation was found between depression and optimistic coping. Uncertainty about the future and fatalistic coping were positively correlated.

Patient Teaching 29-28

The patient with multiple sclerosis

1. Use of medications, including side effects, dose, timing; importance of reporting side effects to doctor
2. Importance of good fluid intake
3. Importance of spacing activities so that time is left for relaxation and fun activities
4. Range of movement exercises, as well as other exercises
5. Good, balanced diet
6. Emotional reactions of people with multiple sclerosis
7. Safety factors to prevent injury
8. Positioning for prevention of decubiti
9. Importance of skin inspection
10. Importance of avoiding temperature extremes
11. Community resources and how to obtain them
12. Disease process
13. Compensatory techniques for visual problems

If bowel incontinence is a problem, assessment of the patient's usual bowel habits is important. A bowel training protocol may be instituted. See Chapter 23 for further discussion of this topic.

Maintaining adequate nutrition

A well-balanced diet with plenty of high-vitamin foods is important. Obesity should be avoided because it makes it more difficult for the patient to manoeuvre and to meet daily needs. High-fibre foods and prune juice may help reduce constipation.

Preventing skin breakdown

Many people with multiple sclerosis have motor involvement that prevents them from moving about freely and changing position readily. Also, they may have sensory disturbances that affect how they sense pressure. As a result, decubiti can easily develop. Patients must be taught the importance of turning at least every 2 to 3 hours. Other devices such as air mattresses or special beds may also be helpful.

Promoting activity and mobility

People with multiple sclerosis should have a daily routine for rest and activity. They are usually advised to exercise regularly but never to the point of extreme fatigue. During an acute exacerbation, patients are often kept as quiet as possible, bed rest is maintained, and all activities are limited.

One side of the body is usually affected more than the other. The patient may learn to stabilize the gait by leaning towards the uninvolved side. Having the foot slap forward in taking a step may sometimes be overcome by putting the heel down in a pronounced fashion and rolling the weight forward on the side of the foot.

The judicious use of passive and active exercises, when the person is not in acute exacerbation, can be useful in maintaining function. Drugs such as diazepam and dantrolene sodium, as well as baclofen, have been used to prevent spasticity.

Effort is made to maintain activity and work or education as long as possible. Patients can be helped to plan their activities so that they may continue to function even when the disease is well advanced.

Controlling the environment

Hot baths should be avoided because the heat can increase weakness in the person with multiple sclerosis. Travelling in hot weather should be carefully planned to prevent travel during the warmest part of the day.

Promoting adjustment

People with multiple sclerosis need a peaceful, relaxed environment. They may have slowness of speech and slowness in the ability to respond. Members of the family may need help in understanding this problem and meeting it calmly. The person may have sudden explosive emotional outbursts of crying or laughing. Box 29-27 discusses a research study of persons with multiple sclerosis.

Facilitating learning

Teaching is important for both the patient with multiple sclerosis and his/her significant others. In late stages of the disease all functions of care usually have to be assumed by someone other than the patient. Teaching needs are listed in Box 29-28.

Evaluation

Evaluation should include the patient and caregivers. Questions to consider may include the following:

1. Is the patient infection free?
2. Is elimination occurring without difficulty?
3. Is patient able to maintain weight at a desired level?
4. Is the skin free of pressure sores?
5. Is an exercise programme being followed?
6. Can daily functions be accomplished?
7. Is discomfort kept to a minimum?
8. Does the patient verbalize a positive adjustment?
9. Is the patient's anxiety minimal?
10. Is the patient taking medication as ordered?
11. Can the patient explain the use of the medication?
12. Is the patient reporting for follow-up care?
13. Can the patient explain how community agencies may be of assistance?

PARKINSON'S DISEASE

Epidemiology

Parkinson's disease is one of the more common diseases of the nervous system. It is also referred to as idiopathic Parkinson's and paralysis agitans. The disease was first described in 1817 by James Parkinson. It affects both men and women in their middle and late years (50 to 70 years old). The mean age at onset is 60 years of age, and the prevalence of the disease increases with age. It has been increasing as a cause of mortality in the elderly in the past 20 years.[40] The incidence is about 500 per 100,000 population. It affects all races and classes of people. The course of Parkinson's disease varies from person to person.

The cause of Parkinson's disease includes viral, toxic, vascular, and genetic aetiologies, as well as some unknown factors. The characteristic symptoms are also sometimes found in arteriosclerotic patients, leading some to believe that arteriosclerosis may be a causative factor. Drug-induced parkinsonian syndromes occur with drugs that interfere with the synthesis or storage of dopamine or interfere with the striatal dopamine receptors. These drugs include the following:
1. Phenothiazines
2. Butyrophenones (e.g., haloperidol)

Pathophysiology

The pathological process that occurs with Parkinson's disease is basically a *depigmentation* of the *substantia nigra of the basal nuclei*. The loss of neurones in the substantia is severe. Also, selective depletion of dopamine occurs and can be correlated with the degree of striatal degeneration. Without dopamine inhibitory influence is lost and excitatory mechanisms are unopposed.

Nursing Process
Assessment

Like many of the other neurological diseases, Parkinson's disease starts with subtle symptoms and progresses slowly. The person may not be able to recall the onset of symptoms.

Subjective data

1. Patient's understanding of disease
2. Complaints of fatigue
3. Presence of incoordination
4. Defects in judgment and emotional instability
5. Heat insensitivity

Objective data

1. Presence of tremor (pill-rolling motion of the fingers or resting tremor)
2. Muscular response to movement (bradykinesia)
3. Postural reflexes
4. Appearance of face (masklike facies)
5. Presence of drooling
6. Shuffling gait
7. Trunk forward extension
8. Sensory testing
9. Inability to carry out daily activities
10. Presence of dementia (in about 30% of cases)
11. Presence of constipation, sometimes severe
12. Abnormal swallowing
13. Presence of scaly erythematous eruptions of skin, particularly near the ears and eyebrows and in scalp and nasolabial folds

The tremor is the outstanding sign of Parkinson's disease. Two other frequent signs are muscular weakness with rigidity and loss of postural reflexes. It is essentially a problem of motion. Muscle rigidity prevents normal response and results in characteristic changes. These changes include a masklike appearance of the face and slowed, monotonous speech; drooling; shuffling gait that is propulsive and may not be able to be stopped until an obstruction is met; and moist and oily skin.

Diagnostic tests

No test is diagnostic of Parkinson's disease. The clinical examination and history, along with the response of the patient to administration of medication used to treat Parkinson's disease, confirms the diagnosis.

If there is a history of chronic dementia, the CT scan may show cerebral atrophy. The EEG may show minimal slowing, or it may be normal. Upper GI studies may show delayed emptying of the stomach and hypomotility.

Nursing analysis

The list of problems for Parkinson's disease is the same as for multiple sclerosis (p. 879)

Planning: expected patient outcomes

The expected patient outcomes for Parkinson's disease are the same as for multiple sclerosis (p. 879).

Implementation
Assisting with achievement of therapeutic goals
Medications

Treatment for Parkinson's disease is palliative and symptomatic and depends on pharmacological manipulation of the disease. The severity of symptoms and the presence of associated disease processes determine the drugs to be used. Particular drugs and their characteristics can be found in Table 29-8. These drugs have had a dramatic effect on the course of the disease. With proper medications many of the symptoms never develop.

After prolonged treatment with some of the drugs, there may be an increased appearance of side effects as well as a decrease in the effectiveness of the medication. It has been found helpful to admit some patients to the hospital for a *drug holiday,* during which all medications are withdrawn

Table 29-8   Medications used in Parkinson's disease

Medication	Action/effects	Side effects	Comments
Anticholinergic drugs Benzhexol Methixene Benztropine Orphenoctine Procyclidine Procyclidine Biperiden	Some degree of CNS anticholinergic action, but incapable of restoring striatal balance	Central and peripheral cholinergic actions Blurring of vision Dryness of mouth and throat Constipation Urinary retention or urgency Ataxia Dysarthria Mental disturbances	Optimal results depend on dosage that provides compromise between improvement and development of side effects
Levodopa Co-benaldopa	Assists in restoring striatal dopamine deficiency	Kidney, liver damage Nausea, vomiting	Side effects common Co-benaldopa contains levodopa and benseraide
Amantadine hydrochloride	Acts by blocking the reuptake and storage of catecholamines and allowing accumulation of dopamine in extracellular or synaptic sites	Mental confusion Visual disturbances Seizures	May not be effective for longer than 3 months
Lysuride Bromocriptine	Stimulates remaining dopamine receptors	Nausea, vomiting, headache, fatigue, drowsiness, hypotension, psychotic reactions	Usually for patients in whom levodopa is insufficient or not tolerated
Pergolide	Stimulates dopamine receptors (D_2)	Hallucinations, confusion, dyskinesia, nausea, dyspepsia, insomnia, double vision, hypotension, drowsiness	
Seligiline	Monoamine oxidase-B inhibitor	Hypotension, nausea, vomiting, confusion, agitation	Usually used in severe cases with levodopa

for a period of time. The medications are then restarted, and often much smaller doses are able to produce favourable results. *This type of drug holiday must take place in the hospital.* Complications such as aspiration pneumonia can occur because immobility, rigidity, and other symptoms will return when the drugs are withdrawn.[18]

Surgery

A surgical procedure has been used with some success in the treatment of selected patients with Parkinson's disease. It includes destroying portions of the globus pallidus (to relieve rigidity) or the thalmus (to relieve tremor) in the brain by stereotactic methods through the use of cautery, removal, or injection of alcohol. Operative techniques involving cooling or freezing with liquid nitrogen have been attempted with good results in selected cases. Medications used to control rigidity and tremor are discontinued several days preoperatively so that symptoms will be at their maximum during the surgery. Preoperative and postoperative care are the same as for the patient undergoing cranial surgery and will be discussed later in this chapter. Many patients cannot be treated surgically. Results seem best in younger patients with unilateral involvement following other diseases and who have marked tremor and rigidity.

A relatively new and still experimental treatment for Parkinson's disease is the adrenal medullary transplant. In this procedure tissue from the adrenal medulla is placed in contact with the substantia nigra with the hope of restoring the balance of dopamine and acetylcholine. The procedure is difficult because the patient undergoes three major surgeries at the same time: (1) stereotactic localization of the caudate nucleus, (2) craniotomy, and (3) laparotomy for the adrenalectomy. Results so far have been somewhat encouraging.[18]

Another new treatment approach for Parkinson's disease involves human foetal dopamine cell transplants. Beginning studies suggest that this procedure may be more effective than adrenal medullary transplants. The subject of using foetal tissue, however, is filled with controversy.[25a]

Interventions to achieve patient outcomes

Maintaining elimination

The patient with Parkinson's disease may feel urgency and hesitancy in voiding. Measures appropriate for the patient with multiple sclerosis also apply to those with Parkinson's disease. Fluids are forced to at least 2000 ml per day. Acidification of urine is encouraged. Medications such as methenamine mandelate may be prescribed.

Chronic constipation may be a real concern. The patient should be on a diet high in residue and fibre. Fluids are encouraged and stool softeners, suppositories, and prune juice are often helpful. Mild cathartics such as milk of magnesia are used if other measures are not helpful.

Maintaining adequate nutrition

Feeding the patient becomes a real problem when the disease is far advanced because of the danger of aspiration; aspiration pneumonia may be fatal. Unless the disease is well controlled by medication, drooling can be a problem and increases with general excitement. Clothes should be protected by appropriate measures. When patients are dressed, garments with generous pockets for tissues will help them be less conspicuous and more comfortable.

Promoting activity and mobility

Special attention should be paid to posture. Lying on a firm bed without a pillow may help to prevent the spine from bending forward. Lying in the prone position also helps. Holding the hands folded behind the back when walking may help to keep the spine erect and prevent the arms from falling stiffly at the sides. The tremor is often less apparent when people are sitting in an armchair, because they can grip the arms of the chair and partially control the tremor in their hands and arms.

Facilitating learning

Teaching is important for the carer and the patient with Parkinson's disease. The teaching is the same as that for the patient with multiple sclerosis (p. 880).

Evaluation

The evaluation of the care of the patient with Parkinson's disease is based on the expected patient outcomes and is the same as for the patient with multiple sclerosis (p. 880).

ALZHEIMER'S DISEASE

Alzheimer's disease is a degenerative disorder that affects the cells of the brain and causes impairment of intellectual functioning. It is recognized as the *most common cause of dementia in the older adult*. It affects men and women equally. Most newly diagnosed people are in late middle age, but the disease has been documented in some people as young as 40 years old.

One of the difficulties in making a definitive diagnosis of Alzheimer's disease is that evidence is often obtained only from a post-mortem examination.

Pathophysiology

The changes in the brains of patients with Alzheimer's disease are visible in the cerebral cortex. The first change is the presence of microscopic plaques found in brain tissue. These plaques consist of a core surrounded by strands of fibrelike material. In addition, there is degeneration of some of the small fibres (neurofibrils) that run through the body of the nerve cells. These changes were first discovered in 1907 by the German neurologist Alzheimer.[24]

Nursing Process
Assessment

Subjective data

1. Patient's understanding of disease
2. Mental status part of neurological examination
3. Onset of symptoms

Objective data

1. Inability to carry on ADL
2. Behaviour: evidence of agitation, restlessness
3. Presence of incontinence

The patient with Alzheimer's disease goes through three rather distinct stages. These stages are described in Box 29-29.

The diagnosis of Alzheimer's disease is made after ruling out conditions in which there is memory loss. These include the following diseases:

1. Pernicious anaemia
2. Drug reactions
3. Hormonal imbalances
4. Depression
5. Drug or alcohol misuse
6. Brain tumour
7. Chronic meningitis
8. Head trauma
9. Pick's disease
10. Parkinson's disease with dementia

The signs and symptoms of Alzheimer's disease occur progressively, but the rate at which they occur varies between individuals. In a few cases, the decline may be very rapid, but in most cases deterioration is gradual. Cause of death is often pneumonia or other infections.

One author cites *four* stages involved with Alzheimer's disease.[24]

Stage 1—mild memory lapses, difficulty with attention span, little interest in immediate surroundings or personal affairs

Stage 2—obvious short-term memory lapses, great hesitancy in verbal responses with confabulation to hide memory problems, disoriented to time, frequent losses of objects

Stage 3—disintegration of personality; disoriented to self, time, and place; apraxia; wandering behaviour

Stage 4—terminal stage with severe physical and mental deterioration, incontinence, loss of ability to communicate, no recognition of family or self, swallowing problems

Diagnostic tests

No diagnostic test is specific for Alzheimer's disease. A CT scan is used to rule out other abnormalities. Often neuropsychological testing can reveal characteristic changes in the ability to think. A family history of Alzheimer's aids in the diagnosis.

Nursing analysis

The possible problems for the patient with Alzheimer's disease are the same as for the patient with multiple sclerosis (p. 879), with the following additions:

Problem	Possible aetiologies
Injury, high risk for	Sensory/motor deficits
Sleep pattern disturbance	Confusion
Violence, high risk for:	Sensory-perceptual
self-directed or	alterations
directed at others	

The violence that sometimes occurs in the patient with Alzheimer's disease occurs most often when the patient does not understand what is happening or what nursing care is being done. It is not an intentional harmful act, but an effort to avoid that which is not understood.

Clinical stages of Alzheimer's disease

Stage one

Mild mental impairment
Forgetfulness
Impairment in judgement
Decrease in initiative
Lack of spontaneity

Stage two

Confusion
Agitation
Irritability
Extreme restlessness
Incontinence of urine and faeces
Need for constant supervision

Stage three

Total inability to care for self
Inability to communicate
Total incontinence

Planning: expected patient outcomes

The expected outcomes for the patient with Alzheimer's disease are the same as those for the patient with multiple sclerosis with the addition of:

1. Injury and violence are avoided.
2. Accommodations are made to manage sleep pattern disturbances.

One difference between the two diseases is that in many cases the person with Alzheimer's disease is mentally incompetent, so that the caregiver needs to have major involvement in planning for the outcomes. The patient may not be able to have real input into them.

Implementation

Assisting with achievement of therapeutic goals

No treatment can cure, reverse, or stop the progression of Alzheimer's disease. Nursing care is directed towards maintaining nutrition, continence, hydration, and safety. Emotional support of both the patient and family is important. Appropriate drugs can sometimes be used to lessen anxiety, agitation, and unpredictable behaviour.

Interventions to achieve patient outcomes

Preventing injury

One large area for intervention concerns safety. Because of forgetfulness, patients with this condition often do dangerous things. This includes walking outside without appropriate clothing, turning on cookers, getting lost, and setting things on fire. The family must make plans to protect the patient from these hazards. This includes removing controls from the cooker at night, double-locking all doors and windows, and keeping the person under supervision at all times.

Adapting to sleep pattern disturbances

One very frustrating part of Alzheimer's disease is that many of the patients sleep for only short periods of time and are awake most of the night. This problem must be solved if the carer is to get any rest.

Preventing violence

The violence that sometimes occurs in the patient with Alzheimer's disease occurs most often when the patient does not understand what is happening or what nursing care is being given. It is not an intentional harmful act but an act to avoid that which is not understood.

Efforts to control this violence centre most often on controlling the environment. It is important to approach the patient with calmness and unhurried motions. Excessive stimulation is kept to a minimum. Routines should not be changed unless absolutely necessary. *Medications should be used only when all other approaches have failed.*

Evaluation

Evaluation of the patient with Alzheimer's disease focuses on the patient outcomes. Refer to the evaluation section for multiple sclerosis for appropriate questions to ask (p. 880). Additional questions to consider may include the following:

1. Is the patient safely carrying out daily activities?
2. Has violence been avoided?
3. Is carer getting sufficient rest?
4. Patient can verbalize knowledge of the disease and symptoms to watch for.
5. Patient has minimal discomfort.

INTERFERENCE WITH FUNCTION BECAUSE OF VASCULAR CONDITIONS

Interference with function because of vascular conditions is common in neurological nursing. In this section of the chapter the following two conditions will be discussed:

1. Cerebrovascular accident
2. Intracranial haemorrhage

CEREBROVASCULAR ACCIDENT

Cerebrovascular accident (CVA) is the most common disease of the nervous system and is ranked as the third leading cause of death in the United Kingdom.[18a] In 1989 there were approximately 63,400 deaths due to stroke in England.[18a] Men are more likely to be affected than women. Figures for England show that during 1989 there were 350 per 100,000 males ged 65-74 who died from a stroke compared with 270 per 100,000 females.[18a] Stroke affects people in all age groups, but the greatest number occurs in older adults over 75. In this section, the term *cerebrovascular accident* (CVA) will be discussed as a general term. Most neurologists and neurosurgeons, however, refer more specifically to the cause of the CVA. These causes are as follows:

Pathophysiology

The brain is very dependent on oxygen and has no reserve oxygen supply. When anoxia occurs, as in CVA, cerebral metabolism is promptly altered, and cell death and permanent damage can occur within 3 to 10 minutes. Any condition that alters cerebral perfusion will cause hypoxia or anoxia. Hypoxia first leads to cerebral ischaemia. Short-term ischaemia (less than 10 to 15 minutes) causes temporary deficits but no permanent deficits. Long-term ischaemia causes permanent cell death and results in cerebral infarction, with accompanying cerebral oedema.

The type of permanent focal deficits will depend on the area of the brain that has been affected. The area of the brain affected depends on which cerebral vessels are involved. The vessel most commonly affected is the middle cerebral artery; the second most commonly affected is the internal carotid artery. Permanent focal deficits may be unknown when the patient is first seen because of generalized cerebral ischaemia that may later resolve.

Cerebral thrombosis

Thrombosis is the most common cause of a CVA, and the *most common cause* of *cerebral thrombosis* is *atherosclerosis*. Additional disease processes commonly found with thrombi are hypotension and other types of vascular injury such as arteritis. CVA secondary to thrombosis is seen most often in the 60- to 90-year-old group. Thrombi usually occur in larger vessels and are associated with damage to the vessel wall at the point where the occlusion occurs. The internal carotid arteries are a common source of thrombi.

The onset of symptoms of CVA secondary to thrombosis tends to occur during sleep or soon after arising. This is thought to be related to the fact that elderly people have decreased sympathetic activity, and recumbency causes a lowering of blood pressure, which can lead to brain ischaemia. These people often also have postural hypotension and poor reflex response to changes in position. Neurological signs and symptoms very frequently worsen for the first 48 hours after thrombosis.

Cerebral embolism

Embolism is the second most common cause of CVA. Patients who have CVAs secondary to embolism are usually younger, and most commonly the emboli originate from a thrombus in the heart (mural thrombi). The myocardial thrombus is most commonly caused by rheumatic heart disease with mitral stenosis and atrial fibrillation.

Emboli usually affect small vessels and are commonly found at points of bifurcation where the vessels narrow. They most frequently occur in the middle cerebral artery. Another type of emboli is called septic and originates from bacterial endocarditis.

Transient ischaemic attack

The term *transient ischaemic attack (TIA)* refers to transient cerebral ischaemia with temporary episodes of neurological dysfunction. The neurological dysfunction can be profound with complete loss of consciousness and loss of all sensory and motor function, or there may only be focal

---

29-30

Conditions causing CVA

Thrombosis
Atherosclerosis in intracranial and extracranial arteries
Adjacency to intracerebral haemorrhage
Arteritis caused by collagen (autoimmune) disease or bacterial or arteritis
Hypercoagulability such as in polycythaemia
Cerebral venous thromboses

Embolism
Valves damaged by rheumatic heart disease (RHD)
Myocardial infarction
Atrial fibrillation (this arrhythmia causes variable emptying of left ventricle; blood pools, and small clots form, and then at times the ventricle will be emptied completely with release of small emboli)
Bacterial endocarditis and nonbacterial endocarditis causing clots to form on endocardium

Haemorrhage
Hypertensive intracerebral haemorrhage
Subarachnoid haemorrhage
Rupture of aneurysm
Arteriovenous malformation
Hypocoagulation (as in patients with blood dyscrasias)

Generalized hypoxia
Severe hypotension, cardiopulmonary arrest, or severe depression in cardiac output caused by arrhythmias

Localized hypoxia
Cerebral artery spasm associated with subarachnoid haemorrhage
Cerebral artery vasoconstriction associated with migraine headaches

1. Thrombosis
2. Embolism
3. Haemorrhage (discussed on p. 890)

The medical and nursing care may differ for each, depending on the specific cause (see Box 29-30). *Stroke* is another term used when referring to CVA; clinically, stroke refers to the sudden and dramatic development of focal neurological deficits.

CVAs can be precipitated by many underlying factors and are frequently associated with other chronic diseases that cause vascular problems. These include heart disease, hypertension, kidney disease, peripheral vascular disease, and diabetes mellitus. Other risk factors for stroke include obesity, high serum cholesterol, cigarette smoking, stress, and a sedentary lifestyle. Women who use oral contraceptives are also at increased risk. The presence of more than one risk factor increases the risk of stroke and hemiplegia. See Box 29-31 for comparison of right and left hemiplegia.

29-31	Comparisons of left and right hemiplegia		
		Left hemiplegia	**Right hemiplegia**
	Language	Usually intact	Receptive or expressive aphasia in varying degrees
	Speech	Dysarthria	Dysarthria
	Sensation	Left sensory loss Left homonymous hemianopsia	Right sensory loss Right homonymous hemianopsia
	Perception	Decreased awareness of left side of body Other perceptual problems	Normal awareness of right side of body
	Movement	Left-sided paralysis or paresis Apraxia	Right-sided paralysis or paresis Less often apraxic
	Behaviour	Impaired judgment Increased emotional lability	Judgment intact Increased emotional lability
	Memory	Deficit of new spatial information	Deficit of new language information

deficits. *The most common deficit is contralateral weakness of lower face, hands, arms, and legs, transient dysphasia, and some sensory impairment.* Ischaemic attacks may occur over days, weeks, or months—between attacks the neurological examination is normal. *TIAs most commonly precede cerebral thrombotic attacks.* They can be caused by any of the causes of CVA.

The *major importance of TIAs is that they warn the patient and health care professional of the existence of an underlying pathological condition.* At least one third of patients who have TIAs will have a CVA in 2 to 5 years. A person with a TIA needs to be aggressively assessed to determine if preventive measures can be taken.

Nursing Process
Assessment
Subjective data

1. Patient's understanding of disease or symptoms
2. Characteristics of onset of symptoms
3. Presence of headache—nature and location
4. Any sensory deficit
5. Visual ability—presence of diplopia, blurred vision
6. Ability to think clearly
7. Any other concomitant symptom

Objective data

1. Motor strength—paresis or plegia is common
2. Change in level of consciousness, including unconsciousness
3. Signs of increased intracranial pressure
4. Respiratory status
5. Ability to verbalize—presence of aphasia

The exact clinical picture varies depending on the area of the brain affected. The most common focal signs and symptoms are caused by disruption of flow through the midcerebral artery. These symptoms include the following:

1. Contralateral paralysis or paresis
2. Contralateral sensory loss
3. Sensory and motor loss most noticeable in face, neck, and upper extremities
4. Dysphasia or aphasia; occurs if dominant hemi sphere is affected (left hemisphere in right-handed people and most left-handed people)
5. Spatial-perceptual problems, changes in judgment and behaviour, neglect of paralyzed side, and inability to recognize paralyzed extremity as own (*anosognosia*) if nondominant hemisphere is affected
6. Contralateral *homonymous hemianopsia*

Aphasia is a disorder of language caused by damage to the speech-controlling areas of the brain. It includes all ares of language, including speech, reading, writing, and understanding.[42,88,89] These abnormalities can occur in a variety of ways as follows:

1. *Sensory aphasia*—inability to comprehend spoken word (also called receptive aphasia)
2. *Motor aphasia*—inability to use the symbols of speech (also called expressive aphasia)
3. *Global aphasia*—inability to understand the spoken word, as well as to speak[88,89]

Diagnostic tests

A lumbar puncture (p. 852) is usually performed and may reveal increased spinal fluid pressure. If the CVA is caused by haemorrhage, blood will be present in the spinal fluid. The CT scan may show an area of decreased density. The MRI scan will visualize this pathology also. A brain scan can demonstrate diminished perfusion.

After TIAs, a cerebral angiogram may be used to discover blocked or occluded vessels. In some cases a digital subtraction angiogram (DSA) is used instead.

Nursing analysis

Problems are determined from analysis of patient data. Possible problems for the person with a stroke may include, but are not limited to, the following:

Problem	Possible aetiologies
Mobility, impaired physical	Perceptual/cognitive impairment
Nutrition, altered: less than body require-ments	Chewing or swallowing difficulties
Swallowing, impaired	Neuromuscular impairment
Activity intolerance	Generalized weakness
Incontinence, bowel	Neuromuscular impairment
Incontinence, urge or total	Neurological dysfunction/disease
Disuse syndrome, high risk for	Immobility, weakness
Injury, potential for	Sensory/motor deficits
Adjustment, impaired	Disability requiring change in lifestyle
Sensory/perceptual alteration	Altered sensory reception/transmission/integration
Self-care deficit: feeding, bathing/hygiene,dressing/grooming, toileting	Neuromuscular impairment
Communication, impaired verbal	Aphasia
Knowledge deficit	Lack of exposure/recall

Planning: expected patient outcomes

Expected patient outcomes for the person who has had a stroke may include, but are not limited to, the following:

1. Patient's skin is intact.
2. Patient can explain the importance of frequent position changes and can demonstrate such positioning
3. Patient or carer can demonstrate exercises to maintain function.
4. Patient can maintain an adequate nutritional status.
5. Patient's swallowing is intact.
6. Patient has minimal complications as a result of incontinence.
7. Patient's continence is improved.
8. Patient remains free of traumatic injury.
9. Patient verbalizes minimal anxiety.
10. Patient has minimal problems because of altered verbal communication.
11. Patient develops alternative means of communication.
12. Patient safely compensates for visual field defects, perceptual, motor, and sensory losses.
13. Patient shows optimal ability to manage activities of daily living and home maintenance.
14. Patient or carer can explain medication regimen—side effects, times, doses, and route.
15. Patient can state plans for follow-up care.
16. Patient has an effective breathing pattern.
17. Patient has minimal discomfort.

Implementation

Assisting with achievement of therapeutic goals: care in the initial phase

Goals in the initial phase are directed towards survival needs and preventing further brain damage. Care must take into account that some patients may be unconscious. Neurological assessment is performed at regular intervals to detect changes in status, as well as any complications. Any indication of rising intracranial pressure should be reported at once. Drugs to reduce intracranial pressure, such as dexamethasone may be given. The patient may have an intracranial monitoring device in place. See p. 863 for a description of these devices.

The use of anticoagulants is controversial. In an attempt to prevent further thrombosis or emboli, heparin may be given if it is certain that the cause of the CVA is cerebral thrombosis or emboli and not cerebral haemorrhage.

Interventions to achieve patient outcomes: care in the acute phase

Goals for care in the acute phase are directed towards preventing complications from the original CVA, from the immobility and dependence it causes, and from the loss of function caused by focal deficits.

Promoting mobility

Because the CVA frequently results in some paralysis, refer to p. 867 for a discussion of the care of the person with loss of motor function.

Maintaining adequate nutrition

Fluids may be restricted for the first few days after a CVA in an effort to prevent oedema of the brain. In patients who are comatose or who have swallowing difficulties, it may be necessary to use intravenous fluids, or a nasogastric tube may be inserted and tube feedings started. When patients are more alert, food and fluids are offered in small amounts. Returning as soon as possible to a normal diet and a normal fluid intake is desirable.

Promoting activity

Rest and quiet are important even if the CVA has not been serious enough to cause complete loss of consciousness. The length of time the patient remains in bed depends on the type of CVA and the judgment of the doctor in regard to early mobilization.

Prevention of joint deformity is initiated during the acute stage. This includes positioning of affected limbs in anatomical position and a full range of exercises. There should be a regular programme for turning the patient to avoid the danger of circulatory stasis, hypostatic pneumonia, and decubitus ulcers.

Maintaining elimination

Urinary output should be noted carefully and recorded for several days after a CVA. Retention of urine may occur, but it is more likely that the patient will be incontinent. If urinary incontinence occurs, the patient should be told that control of elimination should improve day by day. Offering a bedpan or urinal immediately after meals and at other regular intervals is a start to bladder training. A retention catheter may be used for the first several days. In the male patient who is not retaining urine, an external device may be very helpful.

Faecal incontinence also is a fairly common occurrence after a CVA. Some patients develop constipation, and impaction can develop rapidly. Elimination must be noted carefully because diarrhoea may develop in the presence of an impaction, thus causing it to go unnoticed. Suppositories such as bisacodyl may be prescribed, along with stool softeners. Retention enemas are sometimes given when impactions occur. The patient must be cautioned not to strain at the stool (valsalva manoeuvre). The patient also usually needs assistance in getting on and off the bedpan. Cot sides that can be held onto while turning or a trapeze that can be reached with the unaffected arm and hand will help the patient move independently.

Interventions to achieve patient outcomes: care in the rehabilitation phase

The greatest challenge for the nurse in care of the patient who has had a CVA comes after the patient is past the point of danger, because then the long, slow process of learning to use whatever abilities remain or can be relearned must be faced. Also, adjustments to limitations must be faced and made if meaningful life is to continue.

The nurse is an important member of the rehabilitation team. Three nursing goals are:

1. Prevention of further impairment
2. Maintenance of existing abilities
3. Restoration of as much function as possible

Knowledge of the physical arrangements for after-hospital care is important in setting priorities and planning care.

Promoting return of function

Return of motor impulses and movement in involved extremities occurs in stages. These stages can last from hours to months. Recovery may also halt at a specific stage and progress no further. Brunnstrom has defined these recovery stages in degrees of *synergy*. *Synergy has been defined as muscles acting together as a bound unit in stereotyped movement patterns.* See Box 29-32 for these stages.

Return of motor function and impulses is significant for the future use of the affected part but presents new problems. Muscles that draw the limbs towards the midline become very active, and the arm may be held tightly adducted against the body. The affected lower limb may be held inward and adducted to, or even beyond, the midline. Muscles that draw the limbs into flexion are also stimulated, with the result that the heel is lifted off the ground, the heel cord shortens, and the knee becomes bent. In the arm, flexor muscles draw the elbow into the bent position, the wrist is flexed, and fingers are curled in palmar flexion.

Persistent nursing efforts must be directed towards prevention of further impairment. It is important that no part of the body remains in a position of flexion long enough for the occurrence of muscle shortening and joint changes that might interfere with free joint action. Appropriate interventions include the following:

1. Passive exercise—stimulates circulation and may help to reestablish neuromuscular pathways
2. Active exercise started as soon as possible
3. Attention to the unaffected limbs to maintain strength—includes keeping unaffected leg in position of slight internal rotation
4. Early ambulation—facilitates vasomotor tone and has positive psychological effects on the patient and family members

The *Bobath technique* is a treatment approach designed to normalize muscle tone. This is accomplished by providing as many sensations of normal muscle tone, posture, and

29-32	Recovery stages	
	Flaccidity	No voluntary motion, lack of muscle tone
	Partial synergy	Muscle tone develops and muscles contract either voluntarily or with spasticity. Patient can move extremities in part of synergy pattern.
	Synergy	Spasticity moderate to severe. Patient can move joints through all or most of synergy pattern.
	Breaking out of synergy	Spasticity decreased. Patient can perform combinations of movements that are out of synergy.
	Partially isolated	Less influence of spasticity. Movement combinations are less like stereotyped patterns.
	Isolated	Near normal movement with good control of voluntary movement and little spasticity

movement as possible. The *goal of the treatment* is to *redirect short-term memory towards an appreciation of normal movement of the paralyzed side by incorporating techniques of weight bearing, counter-rotation,* and *protraction of the shoulder girdle and pelvis.* The reader is referred to a rehabilitation nursing text for further description of this technique.

Preventing injury

When patients begin to move about and try to help themselves, they may have several problems that can affect their ability to proceed. This predisposes them to injuries. They may have loss of position sense, so that it is awkward for them to handle their bodies normally, even when they have the muscular coordination to do so. They may have dizziness, spatial-perceptual deficits, diplopia, and alteration of skin sensations. They may also have to work harder to receive a normal amount of air on inhalation because the involved side of the chest does not expand easily.

Facilitating emotional adjustment

If the patient who has had a CVA survives the first few days, consciousness usually returns, and some of the paralysis may disappear. It is then that great understanding is needed to help the patient accept his or her limitations. Using quiet assurance, a nurse can help the patient feel that progress towards recovery and self-sufficiency has begun and will continue.

The patient who has sustained a CVA may be overly emotional, and this reaction, combined with the fear and frustration on becoming aware of his or her condition, may be upsetting to the family. Crying for no apparent reason is common in these patients. Family, staff, and sometimes other patients need reassurance that they are not the cause of the patient's crying.

Facilitating communication

The role of the nurse is very important in dealing with the patient with an impairment in verbal communication. A number of principles have been found to be helpful in working with the aphasic patient. The first is to make communication statements as simple as possible. This includes introducing one idea at a time and using short sentences with common words. It is important to limit choices given to the patient and allowing ample time for response.

The patient should be commended for positive steps. The nurse should avoid correcting errors that will discourage the patient from making further attempts to communicate. It is important for the nurse not to talk down to the patient or to treat the patient like a child. Frustration on the part of the patient should be accepted as part of the problem. It is not unusual for the patient to be able to sing songs or to verbalize other automatic speech. This may include swearing.

When attempting to communicate with an aphasic patient, the environment should be as free of distractions as possible. The patient should be comfortable. The nurse should not communicate a sense of urgency or impatience if at all possible—this only worsens communication problems. Stress felt by the patient will decrease the ability to talk. For patients who can manage its use, a communication board is helpful. These boards include either the alphabet or pictures of common objects. The patient can point to the item that is needed or can spell out the necessary word.

For patients with receptive problems, the nurse should be sure that the patient comprehends what is needed. This may include demonstrations of functions to the patient. The family of the patient with aphasia should be educated about the problem and encouraged to interact with the patient.

Maintaining perceptual ability

After a stroke, people may have difficulty relating to themselves and their environment. After the acute stage, mixing with other patients is advocated, because the sensory input from others is helpful. *Hemianopsia*, or decreased visual field, occurs commonly. Approaching patients from the side of intact vision and teaching them to scan with their eyes will help make them more aware of stimuli and help prevent injury. Diminished awareness or denial of the affected side (*anosognosia*) can occur and can be a safety hazard. This possibility should be considered when the patient runs into objects or allows the affected arm or leg to drag behind.

Promoting activities of daily living

The patient is evaluated regarding his or her ability to carry out the usual ADL and is assisted by the occupational therapist or nurse in becoming independent in each activity to the extent possible. Rehabilitation in this way is essentially a teaching-learning process in which the patient is actively involved. Many aids are available through the health service or commercially.

Facilitating learning

The teaching for a patient with CVA is the same as that for the patient with an alteration in motor function (p. 869).

Evaluation

See p. 869 for the evaluation questions for the patient with an alteration in motor function and p. 871 for evaluation questions for the patient with an alteration in sensory function. In addition to those questions, questions to consider for the patient with CVA may include the following:

1. Can the patient explain the importance of frequent position changes and demonstrate various positions?
2. Is the patient's continence improved, and have minimal complications resulted from incontinence?
3. Has the patient developed alternative means of communication?

Surgery

After the patient's condition is stable (with a CVA), or after one or more TIAs, surgery may be used for selected patients. If the symptoms are associated with an atherosclerotic lesion in the extracranial system (internal carotid artery or common carotid artery), a carotid endarterectomy may be performed.

A carotid endarterectomy involves the clearing out of the diseased vessel under either local or general anaesthesia. *Postoperative care* includes the following:

1. Close attention to neurological signs (changes in strength, mentation, speech, and level of consciousness)
2. Observation for bleeding in the incisional area
3. Observation for swelling of the neck or complaints of dysphagia
4. Availability of tracheostomy tray in case of severe respiratory distress

Revascularization procedures are now possible with the use of stereoscopic microscopes. Commonly, the superficial temporal artery is anastomosed to an artery within the brain such as the midcerebral artery. Other vessels can be used. The purpose is to provide for greater blood flow. The surgery usually does not resolve any permanent deficits, but it may prevent further problems. The *care of the patient preoperatively and postoperatively* is similar to that for any patient with cranial surgery, but it also includes the following:

1. Checking for pulse in anastomosed vessel
   a. Doppler
   b. Gentle palpation
2. Keeping graft areas free of pressure
   a. Eyeglass frames bent out so as not to occlude vessel
   b. No other restricting bands around head

The patient will have a postoperative angiogram to assess the patency of the vessel.[56]

INTRACRANIAL HAEMORRHAGE

Intracerebral or intracranial haemorrhages include bleeding into the subarachnoid space or into the brain tissue itself. These haemorrhages cause damage to the brain by destroying and replacing brain tissue. Nursing and medical treatment of a patient with an aneurysm and intracranial haemorrhage can be significantly different from that of a patient with a CVA.

The Elderly with Neurological Problems

Assessment

1. Assess for changes in cognitive function, such as confusion , disorientation, changes in judgment, and difficulty in concentration, abstract thinking, and problem-solving.
2. Monitor for new onset of confusion. Many factors can affect mental status of hospital ized elderly, such as medications, dehydration, pain, need to toilet, or strange equipment.
3. Assess availability of home support persons.

Intervention

1. Provide cues to help maintain orientation; with each contact, remind patient who you are, the time of day, and procedure or routines that will be occurring.
2. Orient the person to unfamiliar equipment, tubings, or changes in the environment.
3. Decrease chances of sensory deprivation by making certain eyeglasses and hearing aids are functioning and properly fitted.
4. Provide opportunities for problem-solving; include person in all aspects of decisions regarding treatments and procedures, no matter what the cognitive ability.
5. Keep structured, familiar routines as much as possible (such as bathing, eating, physiotherapy, nighttime rituals).
6. Teach significant others approaches to facilitate patient orientation. If spouse is providing home care, provide resources for obtaining assistance with care and for ÷time off÷ periods for spouse.

Common disorders in elderly
Transient ischaemic attacks
Cardiovascular accidents
Parkinson's disease
Alzheimer's disease

Intracranial haemorrhages are the third most common cause of CVAs. The peak incidence of aneurysms is in the 35- to 60-year-old age group. Women are affected slightly more often than men. A ruptured cerebral aneurysm is the most common cause of subarachnoid haemorrhage not related to trauma. Bleeding may be from a vessel on the surface of the brain, and the bleeding may be limited to the subarachnoid space. Bleeding from a vessel in the brain substance may form a cerebral haematoma and extend through the brain tissue to the ventricles.

The most common causes of cerebral haemorrhage are as follows:

1. Berry aneurysms—usually congenital defects
2. Fusiform aneurysms—from atherosclerosis
3. Mycotic aneurysms—from necrotic vasculitis and septicemboli
4. Arteriovenous malformations—tangled, interconnected vessels that allow blood to pass directly from the artery to the vein[70]
5. Rupture of cerebral arterioles—from hypertension, which causes thickening and degeneration

Pathophysiology

Any of the causes listed can result in subarachnoid haemorrhage, intracerebral haemorrhage, or combination of the two. The most common site for berry aneurysms is the anterior portion of the Circle of Willis at the junction of the internal carotid and posterior communicating arteries. Multiple aneurysms are found in many people.

Aneurysmal rupture occurs when a small hole occurs in a part of the aneurysm. The haemorrhage spreads rapidly, producing localized changes and irritation to the cerebral vessels. The bleeding is usually halted by the formation of a plug consisting of fibrin-platelets and by tissue compression. Within 3 weeks the haemorrhage begins to undergo resorption. Recurrent rupture is a serious risk 7 to 10 days after the initial haemorrhage. The rupture of a vessel causes disruption of the blood flow to a selected area, focal ischaemic changes, and infarction of brain tissue. In addition, the sudden release of blood has the effect of a concussion, and unconsciousness occurs. It also causes a rapid rise in cerebrospinal fluid pressure with displacement of the brain. Bleeding into brain tissue itself can cause damage by dissecting the brain along the fibre tracts. In addition, haemorrhage may produce a filling of the ventricular system or produce a haematoma that distorts brain tissue.

Blood itself is a noxious agent, and as it is haemolyzed it irritates the blood vessels, the meninges, and the brain. The presence of the blood and the release of vasoactive substances promote arterial spasms, which can further decrease cerebral perfusion. This arterial spasm, or vasospasm, usually occurs from 4 to 10 days after the haemorrhage and causes constriction or narrowing of the cerebral arteries. These vasospasms are serious complications: They can cause focal neurological decline, ischaemia of the brain, and infarction.

About 50% of the patients with rupture of an aneurysm recover from the initial episode, but at least 50% of these people will have recurrences of haemorrhage if untreated. Recurrence may occur within 2 weeks, and the danger of death increases with each bleeding episode.

Nursing Process
Assessment

The assessment for intracerebral haemorrhage includes the factors identified in the subjective and objective assessment for the patient who has had a CVA. Symptoms of an intracranial haemorrhage include the following:

1. Sudden, explosive headache
2. Photophobia
3. Neck rigidity
4. Nausea and vomiting
5. Loss of consciousness
6. Convulsions
7. Respiratory distress
8. Shock

Nursing analysis

Possible problems for the patient with an intracerebral haemorrhage are the same as for the patient who has had a CVA (p. 886) with the addition of:

The patient with an intracranial haemorrhage

1. Use gentleness in moving patient.
2. Keep room darkened.
3. Keep patient resting in bed—head of bed is usually elevated 30 degrees. Occasionally the patient is allowed up to use the toilet.
4. Give patient no ice water.
5. Initiate a bowel programme to prevent constipation and straining at stool.
6. Allow few visitors.
7. Decrease stimuli in room—no TV or radio in severe cases.
8. Take no rectal temperatures.
9. Encourage patient to seek assistance for change in position.

Problem	Possible aetiologies
Tissue perfusion, altered cerebral	Decreased cerebral blood flow

Planning: expected patient outcomes

In addition to those patient outcomes defined for the patient with a CVA (p. 887), these additional outcomes are important:

1. Patient does not develop signs of raised intracranial pressure.
2. Patient does not develop complications from the immobility.
3. Patient can explain the need for surgery and relevant factors.
4. Patient can explain any restrictions in activity.

Implementation

Assisting with the achievement of therapeutic goals

The immediate treatment for intracranial haemorrhage is to keep the person absolutely quiet to prevent additional bleeding. An antifibrinolytic agent may be used to break up the clot. Other nursing actions to be used may include those listed in Box 29-33.

Surgery

The only satisfactory treatment for aneurysm is surgery. Surgery is not usually performed to repair arteriovenous anomalies or hypertensive vascular disease. If an intracerebral haematoma has formed, it may be evacuated after the patient's condition is stable. Before surgery can be performed, angiography must be performed to determine location of the aneurysm. The time after the acute rupture until the surgery is performed varies with the person, their age, the intensity and kind of symptoms present, and the judgment of the surgeon to determine when surgery will be recommended. (See Box 29-34 for postoperative care of the patient with intracranial surgery).

Surgery consists of a craniotomy and location of the aneurysm. When found, the aneurysm may be obliterated by ligation at its neck with the application of a silver clip. If the base of the aneurysm is too large for ligation to be practical, it may be coated with a liquid, adherent, plastic substance that hardens to form a firm support about the weakened vessel wall or it may be wrapped.[70] If the

Postoperative care of the patient with intracranial surgery

1. Assess neurological status including ability to move, level of orientation, and alertness and pupil checks.
2. Assess degree and character of drainage.
   a. Amount of drainage and bleeding should be minimal.
   b. Initial head dressing can be reinforced as necessary.
   c. Often incision is left open to air after first several days.
3. Promoting mobility
   a. Turning to either side is permitted exceptwhen large brain tumours have been re-moved. If this is the case, patient is not turned to affected side as gravity may cause displacement of brain structures.
   b. For supratentorial surgery, the head of the bed is elevated at least 30 degrees.
   c. If infratentorial surgery was performed, the bed is flat or elevated only slightly and a small pillow is placed under the nape of the neck. Neck flexion is avoided.
   d. Early ambulation is encouraged to prevent complications of bed rest. Observe carefully for signs of postural hypotension and raise head of bed gradually; patient should always sit before standing.
4. Promoting decreased intracranial pressure
   a. Space nursing activities to allow patient to rest between them.
   b. Coughing and vomiting should be avoided.
   c. Suctioning should be done only as necessary, and then gently and cautiously.
5. Protecting safety of patient
   a. Use of mittens; make sure fingers are separated and fingers are placed around large roll. Change mittens at least daily—exercise hand at this time.
   b. Keep cot sides up at all times.
6. Promoting electrolyte balance
   a. Accurate intake and output with measurement of specific gravity. Frequent testing for sugar and acetone if patient is taking steroids.
   b. Resumption of diet as soon as possible; assess for difficulty in swallowing or absence of gag reflex.
   c. Monitor electrolytes for evidence of abnormalities.
7. Promoting comfort
   a. Medicate for comfort with codeine sulphate or nonnarcotic analgesic.
   b. Ice cap to head for headache may be helpful.

aneurysm has not ruptured but has produced symptoms, attempts may be made to produce thrombosis by use of an electrical current and other means.

The patient with intracranial haemorrhage

1. Importance of following activity restrictions
2. Importance of keeping as free of stress as possible
3. Very specific teaching about what activities are restricted
4. Use of medication and what it does
5. Information about preoperative and postoperative care will be useful

1. Is the patient's neurological status stable?
2. Does the patient verbalize understanding of surgery planned?
3. Is the patient cooperating with the activity restrictions?
4. Does the patient verbalize understanding of the restrictions?
5. Is the patient relatively calm?

INTERFERENCE WITH FUNCTION BECAUSE OF INFECTION/ INFLAMMATION

Interference with function because of infection/inflammation is a fairly common occurrence. Specific conditions to discuss include the following:

1. Meningitis
2. Encephalitis
3. Brain abscess
4. Poliomyelitis
5. Guillain-Barré syndrome (polyneuritis)
6. Neurosyphilis
7. Herpes zoster
8. Acquired immunodeficiency syndrome (AIDS)

Because these conditions contain many common characteristics, they will be discussed together.

The nervous system may be attacked by a variety of organisms and viruses and may suffer from toxins of bacteria and viruses. These toxins reach the nervous system through a variety of routes. Untreated chronic otitis media and mastoiditis, chronic sinusitis, and fracture in any bone adjacent to the meninges may be the source of infection. Some organisms such as the tubercle bacillus reach the nervous system by means of the blood or lymphatic system. Meningitis can occur as a complication of an invasive procedure such as a lumbar puncture. The exact route of some other organisms is not known.

The goal of this immobility is to prevent raised intracranial pressure. Nursing actions to prevent problems of immobility need to be initiated. The reader is referred to the section concerning motor problems (p. 864).

Other procedures

Not all aneurysms can be treated surgically at the site of the lesion. If surgery is not feasible, the common carotid artery in the neck may be completely or partially obliterated to lessen the flow of blood to the site of the aneurysm and reduce the chances of haemorrhage. This is contingent on whether sufficient blood can be supplied from collateral vessels to preserve brain function. The procedure usually is performed in stages over several days. A clamp (Silverstone or Salibi) with a detachable screw stem that can be tightened gradually is used. Usually the surgeon adjusts it each day, and the nurse assesses the patient closely and is instructed to release the clamp at once if there is evidence of inadequate blood supply, as shown by decreased neurological status. Immediate removal of the clamps may prevent irreversible complications such as hemiplegia, aphasia, and loss of consciousness. If complete occlusion can be tolerated, the vessel may be permanently ligated. Serial embolizations of blood vessels that "feed" the aneurysm may also be performed via the femoral or axillary route. The procedure is similar to a cerebral angiogram, and the postoperative care is the same. Thrombus formation with resultant cerebral embolism may complicate the patient's postoperative course after any surgery for a cerebral aneurysm.

Interventions to achieve patient outcomes

Facilitating learning

If the patient with an intracranial haemorrhage has neurological deficits consistent with a CVA, the teaching is the same. Additionally, the points listed in Box 29-35 are important.

Evaluation

In addition to the questions that should be considered in the evaluation of a patient who has had a CVA, questions to consider when evaluating a patient with intracranial haemorrhage may include the following:

MENINGITIS

Aetiology and Pathophysiology

Meningitis is an acute infection of the meninges. It is usually caused by one of the following organisms:

1. Pneumococci
2. Meningococci
3. Staphylococci
4. Streptococci
5. *Haemophilus influenzae*
6. Aseptic agents (usually viral)

The effect of the bacteria or other organisms in the subarachnoid space is an inflammatory reaction in the pia, arachnoid, and CSF. Pus accumulates in these areas. The bacteria or its toxin, if not treated in a timely manner, may injure cranial and spinal nerves and other structures. In addition, the purulent material that occurs may obstruct the flow of CSF, resulting in hydrocephalus. The longer the infectious process occurs before it is treated, the more complications and neurological sequelae that can occur.

Meningitis can be classed as bacterial or aseptic. The term *aseptic meningitis* was introduced in 1925 and was first thought to refer to a specific disease. It is now recognized as a complex of symptoms that result from many infective agents, the majority of which are viral. *Herpes simplex* is an example of a virus that can cause aseptic meningitis. Any other pathogenic organism, such as the tubercle bacillus, that gains access to the subarachnoid spaces can also cause meningitis. In the United States the incidence of bacterial meningitis is higher in autumn and winter when upper respiratory tract infections are common. Children are more often affected than adults because of frequent colds and ear infections.

Pathological changes that occur include any or all of the following:

1. Hyperaemia of the meningeal vessels
2. Oedema of brain tissue
3. Raised intracranial pressure
4. Generalized inflammatory reaction with exudation of white blood cells into the subarachnoid spaces
5. Associated hydrocephalus caused by exudate blocking the small passage between the ventricles

Nursing Process
Assessment

Subjective and objective assessment are important in any patient with an infection of the nervous system. This assessment includes characteristics that are common to all the infections/inflammations discussed in this section.

Subjective data

1. Patient's understanding of process and possible causes
2. Any history of infection such as upper respiratory infections
3. Measures that relieve symptoms
4. Presence of discomfort, including headache or stiff neck
5. Initial onset of symptoms
6. Presence of difficulty in thinking
7. Presence of muscle weakness, soreness, or incoordination

Objective data

1. Behaviour: signs indicating discomfort or disorientation
2. Change in ability to carry out daily activities
3. Abnormalities on physical assessment part of neurological examination
4. Elevated temperature
5. Presence of vomiting
6. Pulse and blood pressure
7. Increased respirations
8. Abnormal CT results
9. Meningeal irritation
10. Evidence of presence of seizures

The onset of meningitis is usually sudden and characterized by severe headache, stiffness of the neck, irritability, malaise, and restlessness. Nausea, vomiting, delirium, and complete disorientation develop quickly. Temperature, pulse rate, and respirations are increased. Two pathological signs that occur with meningitis are the following:

1. *Kernig's sign*—the inability of the patient to extend the legs completely without extreme pain
2. *Brudzinski's sign*—flexion of the hip and knee

Diagnostic tests

Most of the infections affecting the nervous system can be diagnosed by examining the cerebrospinal fluid. A CT scan and EEG may also be used. These prodecures were discussed earlier in this chapter.

Nursing analysis

Problems are determined from analysis of patient data. Possible problems for the person with meningitis may include, but are not limited to those for a patient who has had a CVA (p. 886) or motor dysfunction (p. 866).

Planning: expected patient outcomes

Expected patient outcomes for the person with meningitis may include, but are not limited to, those for a patient who has had a CVA (p. 887) or motor dysfunction (p. 866).

Implementation
Assisting with achievement of therapeutic goals

Treatment of meningitis consists of massive doses of the antibiotic or antibiotics specific for the causative organism. Treatment with multiple antibiotics is common. Culture and sensitivity studies demonstrate the most effective antibiotic. Usually a course of at least 10 days of parenteral administration is needed. The antibiotic may also be given directly into the spinal canal (intrathecally). Hyperosmolar agents or steroids may be necessary to decrease cerebral oedema. Anticonvulsants may be given to prevent seizures.

Nursing care for the patient with meningitis includes the following:

1. General care given a critically ill patient
2. Darkened room, with noise kept to a minimum, because sensory stimulation can cause seizures
3. Careful neurological observations at frequent intervals
4. Padded cot sides

Residual damage from meningitis includes deafness, blindness, paralysis, and learning difficulties. These complications are usually the result of chronic arachnoiditis. Hydrocephalus may also develop, requiring a shunting procedure.

Isolation of the patient depends on the causative organism. Check the infection control protocols of your institution for specific guidelines.

Evaluation

Evaluation of the patient with meningitis includes those points considered in the evaluation of the person with a CVA (p. 889).

If the patient has motor dysfunction, appropriate evaluation questions can be found on p. 871.

ENCEPHALITIS

Aetiology and Pathophysiology

Encephalitis is an inflammation of the brain tissues and its covering. Occasionally, the meninges of the spinal cord are also involved. It can have a variety of causes, including the following:

1. Syphilis
2. Exogenous poisoning such as that which follows the ingestion of lead or arsenic or inhalation of carbon monoxide.
3. Reaction to toxins produced by infections such as typhoid fever, measles, and chickenpox
4. Reaction to vaccination
5. Various viruses, including arbovirus (those transferred by biting arthropod to humans)

Encephalitis caused by a virus and occurring in epidemic form was common during the early part of the 20th century. Viral encephalitis was also called *sleeping sickness*, a term still used by lay-people. The demonstration that viruses can affect the central nervous system after a prolonged incubation period has resulted in considerable search for viral agents in many chronic neurological diseases.

Nursing Process
Assessment

The subjective and objective data for encephalitis are the same as for meningitis (p. 893). The onset of encephalitis is often abrupt, with a high fever, headache, meningeal signs, nuchal rigidity, and vomiting. Drowsiness or coma and focal or generalized convulsions usually develop within 24 to 48 hours after onset of symptoms. Focal neurological signs develop, such as hemiplegia and cranial nerve palsies. There are typical findings in the CSF. Mortality may be as high as 60%.

Nursing analysis

The reader is referred to the problems in the discussion of CVA on p. 890.

Implementation

Nursing care consists of symptomatic or supportive care and careful observation. Any change in appearance or behaviour should be reported because the progress of this disease sometimes is extremely rapid. Bed rest is advocated. If disorientation is present, the patient must be attended constantly. During the time when temperature is increased, tepid sponging or other hypothermia methods are used.

No specific medical treatment for this disease is available. No isolation is necessary because encephalitis is not transmitted from person to person. Prevention of arboviral infections includes destruction of larvae and elimination of breeding places such as pools of stagnant water. Control includes avoiding bites of the mosquito or tick vectors.

Evaluation

Evaluation includes those questions listed under the evaluation section of CVA on p. 889.

BRAIN ABSCESS

The frequency of abscesses in the areas of the brain is site specific, with most found in the cerebrum (75%) and cerebellum (25%). Some abscesses, as many as 20%, have multiple foci. Of patients with brain abscesses, 30% to 60%

may die and those surviving may have different types of residual deficits, including paralysis and seizures.

A brain abscess is almost always secondary to a foci of infection somewhere else in the body, such as extension of chronic middle ear, sinus, or mastoid infections. The bacteria gain access to the cranial vault directly through bone, through the dura mater, across the subarachnoid and subdural spaces, or along venous routes. Common sites of the primary infection include the following:

1. Ear
2. Sinus or mastoid
3. Lung
4. Heart
5. Pelvic organs
6. Teeth
7. Skin

The three most common organisms involved are the streptococci, staphylococci, and pneumococci. Brain abscesses are most common in older children and young adults but may be seen at any age.

Complications from ear infections account for almost 50% of all brain abscesses. These abscesses are often found in the frontal lobe. Abscesses originating from infections in the frontal, ethmoid, and sphenoid sinuses are also found in the frontal lobe. The sphenoid sinuses may also seed into the temporal lobe. If the abscess is disseminated through the blood stream, the abscesses are multiplied and found in the white matter. Penetrating head injuries, compound fractures, and osteomyelitis of the skull lead to the formation of brain abscesses.

Pathophysiology

The first stage of brain abscess is characterized by local oedema, hyperaemia, infiltration by leukocytes, and softening of the parenchyma. Septic thromboses of some vessels occur, and the surrounding brain tissue becomes necrotic and oedematous. Days to weeks after the beginning stages, there is a process of central liquefaction and necrosis of brain tissue with the formation of a cystic wall of pus. This becomes encased by a wall that is thinner on the ventral side with a predisposition to rupture. If rupture occurs, the infection extends through the entire brain, leading to meningitis.

Nursing Process
Assessment

The questions to ask in collecting data from the patient with a brain abscess are the same as for the patient with meningitis (p. 893). With a brain abscess, there may be a history of infection. The most common symptom is a constant or intermittent headache that is not relieved by medication and that is increased by straining (see Box 29-36 for other symptoms).

The evolution of symptoms is variable. In some patients there may be a rapid progression of symptoms ending in death, whereas in others the course is more benign. Generally, however, the mortality is high with brain abscess, and residual disability often results.

Symptoms of brain abscess

1. Constant and severe headache
2. Drowsiness
3. Confusion
4. Mental slowness
5. Focal or generalized seizures
6. Fever with bradycardia
7. Signs and symptoms of raised intracranial pressure
8. Nuchal rigidity

Diagnostic tests

The diagnosis of brain abscess is made primarily on the basis of the history and examination of the CSF. EEG changes are present (significant slowing at the site of the abscess), and there will be areas of increased uptake on the CT scan. The brain scan is able to locate abscesses that are over 1 cm in size. Arteriography can be helpful in locating temporal lobe abscesses or cerebellar abscesses. The lumbar puncture is contraindicated when intracranial pressure is raised because of the danger of causing herniation of the brain.

Nursing analysis

The problems and the expected patient outcomes are the same for the patient with brain abscess as for the patient with a CVA (p. 887).

Implementation

Assisting with the achievement of therapeutic goals

Nursing care consists of administering the appropriate antibiotics, often for extended periods of time. Combined antibiotics along with broad-spectrum antibiotics may be used. Antibiotics that are used include a penicillin and chloramphenicol. If anaerobic bacteria have been identified, metronidazole (Flagyl) may be used. Agents to reduce intracranial pressure may be necessary. Ongoing assessment for signs and symptoms of increased intracranial pressure is important. These patients often must undergo long hospitalizations and periods of treatment; as a result, they may need a great deal of psychological support.

Surgical treatment consists of aspiration or complete excision and evacuation of the abscess. The method of evacuation depends on the site and accessibility.

Evaluation

For the evaluation of a patient with a brain abscess, consider the evaluation questions listed for the patient with a CVA (p. 889).

POLIOMYELITIS

Poliomyelitis is an acute febrile disease caused by poliomyelitis virus types 1, 2, and 3. Paralysis is more common with type 1. With discovery of the Salk vaccine, its wide use since 1956, and the availability of the Sabin vaccine, this disease has become rare. At one time it was a serious crippler of children and young adults.

Pathophysiology

The incubation period for poliomyelitis is from 7 to 21 days. The virus attacks the anterior horn cells of the spinal cord where the motor pathways are located and may cause motor paralysis. Sensory perception is not affected, because posterior horn cells are not attacked. Poliomyelitis sometimes takes a somewhat different form and attacks primarily the medulla and basal structures of the brain, including the cranial nerves. This is called *bulbar paralysis*. If the medulla is involved, the patient will need respiratory assistance.

GUILLAIN-BARRÉ SYNDROME (POLYNEURITIS)

Guillain-Barré syndrome is also known as *acute inflammatory polyradiculoneuropathy* and *postinfectious polyneuritis*. It is often serious because of the extent to which the nervous system is involved. It involves an acute type of peripheral nerve syndrome resulting in widespread inflammation and demyelination of the peripheral nervous system. The disease affects people of all ages and is seen equally in men and women. The cause is unknown, but it is thought to be either a viral agent or the result of an autoimmune reaction.

Pathophysiology

In Guillain-Barré syndrome, patchy demyelination occurs in peripheral nerves, nerve roots, root ganglia, and spinal cord. Axons are generally spared so recovery may occur early, although they may be affected in severe cases.

Variations in the pattern of onset of weakness occur, as well as in the rate of progression of symptoms. The progression may stop at any point. If cranial nerves VII, IX, and X are involved, the patient may have difficulty in swallowing, speaking, and breathing. The vital centres in the medulla may be affected.

The pathophysiology also is related to infiltration of the peripheral nervous system with mononuclear cells. It is thought that sensitized lymphocytes have a part in the demyelination because more than half of the individuals affected have had a nonspecific infection 10 to 14 days before the onset of the disease.

Symmetric muscle weakness and lower motor neurone paralysis (flaccidity) are present with Guillain-Barré syndrome. The paralysis usually starts in the lower extremities and moves upward to include the thorax, upper extremities, and face. Paraesthesias may occur. Respiratory failure is possible if the intercostal muscles are affected; without mechanical ventilation, mortality is 10% to 20%. Autonomic symptoms, such as fluctuating blood pressure, also occur. The bowel and bladder are rarely affected.

Of the people suffering from Guillain-Barré syndrome, 85% will regain complete function. The recovery period is variable, ranging from weeks to years. Those not recovering completely will have some degree of permanent neurological deficit. Generally, recovery from the disease occurs in the *reverse order* of how paralysis or weakness occurred.

Nursing Process

Assessment

Subjective data

1. Patient's understanding of the disease
2. History of an infection in recent past
3. Initial onset of symptoms and nature of symptoms
4. Presence of muscle weakness

Objective data

1. Abnormalities found in the physical assessment part of the neurological examination
2. Presence of increased temperature
3. Presence of muscle weakness
4. Abnormalities found with arterial blood gases
5. Presence of dyspnoea
6. Blood pressure abnormalities

Nursing analysis

See section on the patient with a CVA (p. 887).

Planning: expected patient outcomes

See section on the patient with a CVA (p. 887).

Implementation

Assisting with achievement of therapeutic goals

A priority goal is the maintenance of respiratory function. Close monitoring of respiratory function is necessary. Observation should include serial measurements of the patient's vital capacity, tidal volume, and minute volume. Patients who develop respiratory failure require mechanical ventilation and may require tracheostomy. Arterial blood gas monitoring is common. The patient may also require nutritional maintenance intravenously or through a nasogastric tube. If the patient has severe paralysis and is expected to have a long recovery period, a gastrostomy tube may be inserted. Special eye care is important to prevent corneal damage.

Adrenocortical steroids are used at times to treat symptoms. Convalescence may require many months. Attention to the prevention of iatrogenic complications, such as contracture, decubitus ulcers, muscle atrophy, and loss of range of motion, is imperative to allow complete recovery.

Evaluation

The questions listed under Evaluation for the patient with a CVA (p. 889) also apply to the patient with Guillain-Barré syndrome.

HERPES ZOSTER

Herpes zoster (Varicella zoster), also known as *shingles*, is a common disease, occurring at higher rates among the old and patients with lymphomas, cancer, and Hodgkin's disease.

Aetiology and pathophysiology

The causative organism is the varicella virus, similar to the one that causes herpes simplex. It may occur as a result of a reactivation of the viral infection that lies dormant in the ganglion after a primary case of chickenpox. It is not communicable, except to people who have not had chickenpox. An acute inflammatory reaction takes place in the spinal or cranial sensory ganglions, the posterior grey matter of the cord, and the meninges.

The rash seen in herpes zoster consists of a vesicular, cutaneous eruption within a dermatome. It may be preceded by severe itching, pain in the area, fever, and malaise. Segmental weakness and atrophy may exist in the same area as the sensory changes. A small percentage of patients first seek medical attention for ophthalmic herpes, with the rash and pain occurring along the distribution of the trigeminal nerve.

Nursing process

Assessment

Subjective data

1. Complaints of pain
2. Any sensory changes
3. Complaints of malaise
4. Complaints of itching

Objective data

1. Fever
2. Presence of rash…vesicular cutaneous eruption within a dermatome
3. Presence of weakness or atrophy in the area of sensory changes

Nursing analysis

Problems are determined from analysis of patient data. Possible problems for the person with herpes zoster may include, but are not limited to, the following:

Problem	Possible aetiologies
Infection, high risk for	Decreased immune response
Knowledge deficit	Lack of exposure/recall
Pain	Nerve root inflammation
Skin integrity, altered, actual or high risk for	Irritation from the rash of herpes zoster

Planning: expected patient outcomes

Expected patient outcomes for the person with herpes may include but are not limited to the following:

1. Patient remains infection free.
2. Patient can explain prescribed medication (dosage, action, side effects, and frequency).
3. Patient has minimal discomfort.
4. Patient is able to sleep at least 6 hours per night.
5. Patient's skin integrity improves.

Implementation

Assisting with the achievement of therapeutic goals

Treatment for herpes zoster consists mainly of supportive care with medication for control of pain. Acyclovir may be used in some cases. The pain may persist for some time after the rash disappears. Some people have pain along the affected nerve root for 1 to 2 years after the initial infection.

Phenytoin and carbamazerine may be helpful for control of persistent pain. Steroid therapy started early in the disease course is believed to shorten the course but is not recommended for patients with suppressed immune responses.

A newer treatment for post-herpetic pain is capsaicin cream. It may be used after the lesions have healed and applied 3-4 times daily.

Interventions to achieve patient outcomes

Preventing infection

Isolation may be necessary for staff who have not had chickenpox. This is especially true for the pregnant employee. Also, patients with malignancies, lymphomas, or Hodgkin's disease who have not had chickenpox should be protected from exposure to the patient.

Because the virus is spread by direct contact and airborne routes, strict isolation is often necessary, at least until drainage from any lesions stops. The protective measures are listed in Box 29-37.

Facilitating learning

It is important to educate the patient about the risk of spreading herpes zoster to others. The importance of good hand washing is stressed. The prescribed medications should be reviewed with the patient as to dosage, action, side effects, and timing for administration.

Evaluation

Evaluation of the patient with herpes zoster includes the following questions:

1. Is the patient free of infection?
2. Is the patient able to state the required medications including dosage, side effects, times, and expected results?
3. Is the patient having minimal pain?
4. Is the patient's rash improving?

INTERFERENCE WITH FUNCTION BECAUSE OF TRAUMA

Interference with neurological function can occur as a result of trauma. Parts of the nervous system commonly subjected to trauma include the craniocerebrum, the spinal cord, and the peripheral nerves. Traumatic lesions usually result from direct physical force or from sustained compression.

CRANIOCEREBRAL TRAUMA

Craniocerebral trauma, or head injury, causes death or serious disability in people of all ages. Head injury is a major cause of serious neurological deficit and is a significant cause of death and disability in younger age groups.

29-37	**Isolation measures for patient with herpes zoster**

1. Private room with private toilet facilities
2. Gown, masks, and gloves required of caregivers
3. Strict hand washing
4. Linen handled as isolation linen
5. Double-bagging of dressings
6. Disposable dishes if possible
7. Transport patients only as necessary
8. Isolation procedure for visitors

Brain injury causes more deaths than does injury to any other organ. Causes of head injury include motor vehicle accidents, falls, industrial accidents, assaults, and sports-related accidents. Legislation requiring the use of seat belts in motor vehicles (cars must have front seat belts and where belts are fitted for rear seat passengers they must be used), and crash helmets for motorcyclists has made a significant contribution to reducing the incidence of serious head injury.

Pathophysiology

Craniocerebral trauma may result in injury to the scalp, skull, and brain tissues, either singly or collectively. Some of the variables that may modify the extent of the injury to the head include the following:

1. Location and direction of the impact
2. Rate of the energy transfer
3. Surface area of the energy transfer
4. Status of the head at the time of the impact

Injuries vary from minor scalp wounds to concussions and open fractures of the skull with severe damage to the brain. The amount of obvious damage is not indicative of the seriousness of the trouble. General effects of moderate to severe head injury include *cerebral oedema, sensory and motor deficits,* and *raised intracranial pressure.* Later damage can occur as a result of *brain herniation, cerebral ischaemia,* and *hypoxaemia.*

Injuries to the brain can result from direct or indirect trauma to the head. Indirect trauma is caused by *tension strains* and shearing forces transmitted to the head by stretching of the neck. Direct trauma occurs when the head is directly injured. This results in *acceleration-deceleration* with *cavitation* (release of dissolved gases from the CSF, blood, or brain tissue). The release of gases damages nervous tissue. Direct trauma also results in rotation of the skull and its contents. These forces can occur at the same time or in succession and can damage the brain by compression, shearing, or tension.

Acceleration injuries occur when the head is struck by a moving object and set in motion. As a result of acceleration forces, *bruising* or *contusion* of the occipital and frontal lobes, brainstem, and cerebellum may occur.

Deceleration injuries occur when the head strikes a solid immovable object with a rapid deceleration of the skull. The brain decelerates more slowly.

29-38	**Damage to brain tissue caused by trauma**			
		Characteristics	**Structural alteration**	**Effects**
	Concussion	Characterized by immediate and transitory impairment of neuro-logical function caused by me-chanical force	No	May be loss of consciousness that is instant or delayed—usually reversi-ble
	Contusion	Likened to bruising with extravasa-tion of blood cells	Yes	Injury may be at site of impact (coup) or at opposite site (contrecoup) Often damage to cortex
	Laceration	Tearing of tissues caused by sharp fragment or shearing force	Yes	Haemorrhage is serious complication

Acceleration-deceleration movements that occur with lateral flexion, hyperflexion, hyperextension, and turning cause the cerebrum to rotate about the brainstem, resulting in *shearing, stretching,* and *distortion of neural tissue.* The stretching or tension causes fracture of the axons.

Head injuries can be *open* or *closed.* Open head injuries result from skull fractures or penetrating wounds. The amount of injury with this type of wound is determined by the velocity, mass, shape, and direction of the impact. Usually there is some type of skull fracture. These include:

1. Linear—simple break in bone
2. Comminuted—two or more common breaks that divide the bone into more than two fragments
3. Depressed—one forced below the line of normal contour
4. Compound—can be linear, comminuted, or depressed

Fractures at the base of the skull are usually serious because of their location. When one is sustained, vital centres, cranial nerves, and nerve pathways may be perma-nently damaged. Trauma and the resulting oedema may obstruct cerebrospinal fluid flow directly or indirectly, with resultant raised intracranial pressure. If the injury has caused a direct communication between the cranial cavity and the middle ear or the sinuses, meningitis or a brain abscess may develop. Bleeding from the nose and ears suggests a basal fracture. Serosanguineous drainage from these orifices may contain cerebrospinal fluid and should be noted.

Closed head injuries include concussions, contusions, and lacerations. See Box 29-38 for a comparison of these injuries.

The effect of a blow on the cranium to the brain tissues within the skull is one of sudden movement. This effect can be likened to what happens as one stops suddenly when moving quickly with an open dish of fluid—some of the fluid spills. The only difference is that instead of spilling in the closed cavity, the brain tissue strikes the bony covering forcibly. A contusion or laceration directly below the site of the cranial impact is called a *coup* lesion. A lesion opposite the impact site is called *contrecoup,* which occurs when the brain hits the cranium on the opposite side of the blow. Damage to the brain tissues may include concussion, contusion, or laceration.

Lacerations of the scalp bleed profusely because of its large blood supply. Haemorrhage resulting from craniocerebral trauma may occur at the following sites:

1. Scalp
2. Epidural
3. Subdural
4. Intracerebral
5. Intraventricular

Two of these, *epidural* and *subdural haematomas,* re-quire careful and continuous observation by the nurse and pose special problems to the patient with a head injury. Epidural haematomas form as blood collects rapidly be-tween the dura and skull. Bleeding in this area is commonly caused by laceration of the middle meningeal artery, which is capable of producing rapid clot formation. Common sites for bleeding include sites of basal and temporal skull fractures. If lethargy or unconsciousness develops after the patient regains consciousness, an epidural haematoma may be suspected. Bleeding needs to be controlled promptly and the blood removed.

A subdural haematoma forms as venous blood collects below the dural surface. Because the bleeding is under venous pressure, the haematoma formation is relatively slow. The clot formation will, however, cause pressure on the brain surface and may eventually displace brain tissue. If the expanding clot is not evacuated it can cause raised intracranial pressure with compression of vital areas. The focal neurological signs of clot formation are related to the site of the clot. If a patient who has been conscious for several days to weeks after a head injury becomes unconscious or develops neurological symptoms, a *subdural haematoma* should be suspected. Subdural haematomas can be classed as follows:

1. Acute—occurs within 24 to 48 hours
2. Subacute—occurs within 48 hours to 2 weeks
3. Chronic—can occur weeks or months after the injury. These occur most commonly in the 60-70 year age range. At times, the cause of haematoma is uncertain.

Intracerebral haemorrhage usually occurs in the frontal or temporal regions.

Most deaths from head injury are from cerebral oedema caused by damage rather than the actual primary destruction of vital centres. Brain oedema is a major cause of raised intracranial pressure. Along with the swelling, local and systemic disturbances in circulation occur with resulting anoxia. The brain damage may be severe and not related to the demonstrated structural damage.

Nursing Process
Assessment

Subjective data

1. Patient's understanding of injury and resulting pathology—also patient's ability to understand
2. Information about nature of the injury-how it happened
3. Presence of headache, nausea, or vomiting
4. Presence of diplopia or other visual problems
5. Unusual sensations (paraesthesias, ringing in ears)
6. History of bleeding from ear, nose, eye, or mouth
7. History of loss of consciousness
8. Use of alcohol or drugs
9. Time of most recent food intake

Objective data

1. Respiratory status (presence of patent airway, need for suctioning, need for intubation and mechanical ventilation)
2. Arterial blood gases
3. Level of consciousness and alertness
4. Pupils: size, equality, reactivity
5. Orientation
6. Motor status
7. Vital signs
8. Presence of bleeding
9. Presence of vomiting
10. Speech patterns—abnormalities
11. Presence of raised intracranial pressure

Because many people with head injury, especially from motor vehicle accidents, have sustained other injuries, the intrathoracic and intraabdominal areas are checked carefully and the limbs are examined for fractures and injuries to nerves or arteries.

Diagnostic tests

Diagnostic tests performed for patients with head injury include skull X-ray films, CT scan, MRI, and possibly cerebral angiography. These procedures were described earlier in this chapter. Other diagnostic tests such as skull and chest films rule out other injuries.

Nursing analysis

Problems are determined from analysis of patient data. Possible problems for the person with craniocerebral trauma may include, but are not limited to, the following:

Problem	Possible aetiologies
Tissue perfusion, altered cerebral	Decreased arterial cerebral blood flow
Airway clearance, ineffective	Perceptual/cognitive impairment
Breathing pattern, ineffective	Neuromuscular impairment
Injury, high risk for	Sensory/motor deficits
Thermoregulation, ineffective	Trauma/illness
Infection, high risk for	Decreased nutrition
Incontinence, bowel	Neuromuscular impairment
Incontinence, urge or total	Neurological dysfunction
Coping, ineffective individual	Situational crises
Activity intolerance	
Mobility, impaired physical	Immobility, generalized weakness
Self-care deficit: feeding, bathing/hygiene, dressing/grooming, toileting	Neuromuscular impairment
	Neuromuscular impairment
Skin integrity, impaired, actual or high risk for	Pressure, immobility
Knowledge deficit	Lack of exposure or recall

Planning: expected patient outcomes

Expected patient outcomes for the patient with craniocerebral trauma may include, but are not limited to, the following:

1. Cerebral oedema is decreased.
2. Patient can maintain a patent airway.
3. Patient can maintain an effective breathing pattern.
4. Patient remains free of injury.
5. Patient's temperature remains normal.
6. Patient remains free of infection.
7. Patient has minimal complications as a result of incontinence.
8. Patient has regular bowel movements without diarrhoea or constipation.
9. Patient regains bowel and bladder continence if able.
10. Patient demonstrates increased independence.
11. Patient maintains optimal mobility and activity.
12. Patient has minimal deficits in ADL.
13. Patient's skin remains intact.
14. Patient can explain and demonstrate prescribed therapy to follow at home.
15. Patient can explain homegoing medication regimen (side effects, desired effects, time, dose, and route) to be followed at home.

Implementation

Assisting with the achievement of therapeutic goals
Medications

Medications are used to reduce cerebral oedema and raised intracranial pressure, which are common problems in patients with head injuries. These medications include the following:

1. Osmotic diuretics that penetrate the brain slowly such as 20% mannitol
2. Dexamethasone

If the patient is receiving mannitol and is not alert, a Foley catheter should be inserted to enable accurate accounting of output. Large amounts of urine can be anticipated.

Electrolyte imbalance

Careful monitoring of electrolytes is necessary. Several types of imbalance may occur with a head injury including the following:

1. Natriuresis (increased urinary excretion of sodium)
2. Inappropriate ADH syndrome (increased plasma levels of ADH, serum hyponatraemia, and hypotonicity)
3. Hypernatraemia
4. Cerebral sodium retention
5. Elevated plasma cortisol levels

Interventions to achieve patient outcomes

Immediate care is directed towards lifesaving measures and the maintenance of normal body function until the time when recovery is assured. The major aims of medical and nursing management are as follows:

1. To be constantly alert for changes in the patient's condition, especially changes that indicate any increase in intracranial pressure
2. To sustain the patient's vital functions until recovery allows the functions to resume
3. To manage complications that will be life threatening and interfere with full recovery

Promoting effective airway clearance and breathing patterns and improved cerebral perfusion

It is extremely important to maintain a patent airway and ensure adequate oxygenation. Anoxia with a buildup of carbon dioxide can produce cerebral hypoxia and subsequent cerebral oedema, which can lead to altered cerebral perfusion. It is important to assess the ability to clear the airway. Blood or mucus from injuries may block the airway, or the patient may have vomited and suctioning may be necessary. Inability to clear the airway can lead to airway obstruction, as well as aspiration pneumonia. Oxygen should be given to the patient with a head injury, and if the patient cannot clear the airway an endotracheal tube is inserted. Arterial blood gas levels are checked frequently to determine whether respiratory exchange is adequate. Suctioning should be done as necessary.

Preventing injury

The patient should be kept as quiet as possible. No vigorous effort should be made to "clean the patient up" during the first few hours after the accident. Cot sides should always be on the bed because restlessness may come on suddenly or convulsions may occur. The head of the bed is usually elevated 30 degrees. Restlessness may be caused by the need for a change of position, pain, or the need to empty the bladder. Codeine or other analgesics that do not depress the respiratory system are used for pain control. Anticonvulsants may be given to prevent seizures.

Maintaining thermal regulation

The blood pressure, pulse, and respiratory rate are taken frequently until they have stabilized and remain within safe limits. A sudden sharp rise in temperature, which may go to 42° C or higher, and a sudden drop in blood pressure indicate that the regulatory mechanisms have lost control. The prognosis is poor. Measures are used to reduce temperature to normal because hyperthermia increases brain metabolism, resulting in brain damage. These measures include the following:

1. Administration of aspirin
2. Tepid sponging
3. Ice bags to the groin and axilla
4. Reducing temperature of patient's room
5. Electrically controlled cooling mattress

Preventing infection

The patient's ears and nose are checked carefully for signs of blood and serous drainage, which would indicate that the meninges have been torn and that spinal fluid is escaping. No attempt should be made to clean out the orifices. Loose sterile cotton wool may be placed in the outer openings only. This procedure is performed with caution so that the cotton does not act as a plug to interfere with the free flow of fluid. The cotton should be changed whenever it becomes moist. If there is evidence of drainage of CSF from the nose, the patient should not cough, sneeze, or blow the nose. These activities may enable air to enter the cranial cavity where it may increase symptoms of raised intracranial pressure. If there is question about whether drainage from the nose is CSF, it can be tested for the presence of sugar, which is normally found in CSF.

Meningitis is a possible complication when communication with the nose and ears occurs. With basal skull fracture, antibiotics are commonly used because of the high rate of infection after this type of fracture.

Maintaining elimination

The patient's intake and output should be carefully measured and recorded. The specific gravity of the urine is also measured and can yield clues to electrolyte imbalance. In acute situations these measurements are repeated hourly.

The urinary output should be approximately 0.6 to 1 ml/ kg of body weight/hour. If osmotic diuretics have been given, this amount will be greater. An indwelling catheter may be necessary; if so, catheter care to prevent infection should be used (see Chapter 29 for details). The person with cranial trauma should also be assessed for symptoms of diabetes insipidus, a common occurrence.

Bowel evacuation is not encouraged for several days after a head injury. Mild bulk laxatives, bisacodyl suppositories, or retention enemas may be used. A stool softener is often prescribed, and the patient is taught not to strain at stool. When the patient is receiving dexamethasone or other steroids, it is important to check the stool for the presence of occult blood. This will also give a clue to the presence of stress ulcers, which are somewhat common after head injury. The ulcers are apparently caused by autonomic imbalances associated with the injury. Cimetidine and antacids may be given if the patient with a closed head injury is receiving steroids.

Supporting coping ability

It is not uncommon that the patient with a head injury manifests loss of memory and loss of initiative. Behavioural problems associated with lack of judgment and restlessness may also occur. These patients need firm but gentle care, with specific guidelines for what behaviour is allowed. It is not helpful to argue with the patient. It may be helpful to redirect their attention to another subject or task. Memory aids such as a log book or written plan can be very useful in assisting with reorientation. The patient and family need to have gains in functioning pointed out, as it is easy to become frustrated and depressed when progress is slow.[52]

Promoting activity and mobility

The length of convalescence will depend on the amount of brain damage and how rapid the recovery has been. Patients are usually urged to resume normal activity as soon as possible. Headache and dizziness may be present for some time after a head injury. Some people require intensive and lengthy rehabilitation in a rehabilitation centre. Many brain-injured patients recover physically but have behavioural and psychological problems that make it difficult for them to function completely independently.[52,64]

Some patients are left with serious deficits including hemiplegia. They will need to be taught compensatory techniques so that they can perform self-care measures. The nursing care of these patients is described in the section on patients who have had a stroke (p. 888).

Maintaining skin integrity

Patients who have experienced craniocerebral trauma may be prone to develop skin problems. The care for the patient who has motor difficulties or is comatose is the same as for the patient with paralysis. The reader is referred to p. 867 for a discussion of maintaining skin integrity.

Facilitating learning

Patients with head injury may be seen in an accident and emergency department but not admitted to the hospital. These patients need teaching about observations for complications. A sample set of instructions is found in Box 29-39.

Teaching for the patient with a head injury who is left with deficits severe enough to require extended rehabilitation is similar to that for the patient with a motor problem. See p. 869 for a description of this teaching. In addition, the following points are important:

1. Causes of raised intracranial pressure
2. Factors that can increase or decrease intracranial pressure
   a. No sneezing
   b. No heavy lifting, bending, or straining
   c. No straining at stool
3. Signs and symptoms to report to the doctor

It is essential that the family be present at the teaching sessions.

Evaluation

Evaluation of the patient with a head injury is based on the expected patient outcomes. Questions to consider may include the following:

1. Are there symptoms of raised intracranial pressure?
2. Does the patient have a patent airway and effective breathing pattern?
3. Is the patient able to swallow safely and maintain an adequate diet?
4. Is the patient practicing safety techniques?
5. Is the patient afebrile?
6. Has infection been avoided?
7. Is the patient continent of bowel and bladder?
8. Is the patient demonstrating a positive self concept?
9. Is the patient compensating for sensory-perceptual difficulties?
10. Is the patient functioning in a socially acceptable way?

29-39 | **Instructions for the patient with a head injury**

Patient should be awakened periodically through the first 24 hours to be sure he or she can wake up easily.

Also, for the first 24 to 48 hours, the family should watch carefully for the following warning signs:

1. Vomiting—often with force behind it
2. Unusual sleepiness, dizziness, and loss of balance or falling
3. Complaint of seeing two of everything or blurry objects, jerking movement of the eyes
4. Bleeding or discharge from nose or ears
5. A slight headache may be expected; however, if it gets worse and the patient complains of feeling even worse when moving about, it should be reported
6. Convulsions (fits)—any twitching or movements of arms or legs that the patient is not able to stop
7. Any behaviour or symptom that is not normal for the individual

Call a doctor at once if any of these signs are observed by the family.

Call either your family doctor or the emergency services.

Courtesy Department of Nursing, University Hospitals of Cleveland, Cleveland, Ohio.

---

11. Is the patient's mobility functioning at optimal levels?
12. Does the patient have minimal difficulties in carrying out ADL?
13. Is the patient's skin intact?
14. Is the patient able to verbalize follow-up care and discharge regimen?
15. Is the patient taking medication accurately?

SPINAL CORD TRAUMA

Spinal cord injury from accidents is a common and increasing cause of serious disability and death in the United Kingdom. It has been estimated that 30-40,000 people in the United Kingdom are paralyzed as a result of spinal cord injury or disease and that 700 more are paralyzed every year (Source—Spinal Injuries Association). Most persons involved with spinal cord injuries are males between the ages of 18 and 25. Road traffic accidents, accidents at home and work, and sports injuries are major causes of spinal cord injuries. The largest number of spinal cord injuries are caused by vehicular accidents.

The most common sites of injury are the lower cervical region and the junction of the thoracic and lumbar region.

Pathophysiology

The spinal cord may be damaged by lesions arising outside the cord or by lesions within the cord itself. The latter are

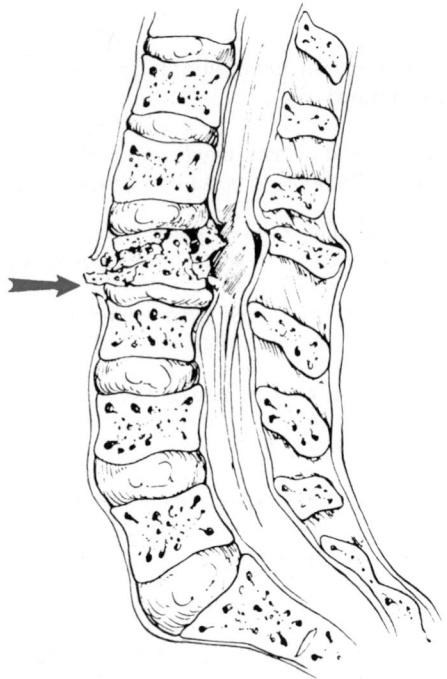

Fig. 29-20 Damage to spinal cord and distortion of adjacent structures that may occur in traumatic injuries to spine.

a less common cause and are usually the result of tumours. Trauma to the spinal cord can result in *concussion, contusion, laceration, complete* or *partial transection, haemorrhage,* or loss of blood supply to a part of the cord (Fig. 29-20).

The soft tissue of the spinal cord is protected by the vertebral column. This column can be injured by various mechanisms, including the following:

1. Hyperextension—also called whiplash. These occur most often in the cervical region and result from the forces of acceleration-deceleration and the reduction of diameter of the spinal cord.
2. Hyperflexion—results in overstretching, compression and deformity of the spinal cord.
3. Vertical compression—primarily occurs in the area of T12 to L2. Injuries result from a force applied downward from the cranium that often results in a burst vertebra.
4. Rotation injury—can involve all parts of the vertebrae.

Injuries that occur to the vertebrae include the following types:

1. Simple fracture—single break affecting the spinous or transverse process of the vertebra. The spinal cord is not usually compressed and the alignment of the vertebrae is not altered.
2. Compressed or wedged fracture—occurs when the vertebral body is compressed anteriorly. Cord compression may be present.
3. Comminuted or burst fractures—vertebral body shatters into many fragments, any of which may injure the cord.
4. Dislocation of vertebrae—may result in nonalignment of vertebral column with injury to the spinal cord. Partial dislocation is called subluxation.

Severe traumatic lesions of the spinal cord may result in total transection of the spinal cord or a tearing of the cord from side to side at a particular level, with a complete loss

of spinal cord functions. This total transection is also referred to as a "complete cord injury." With the complete injury all voluntary movement below the level of the lesion is lost. A partial transection or "incomplete injury" involves a partial transection or injury of the cord. Quadriplegics are patients who sustain injuries to one of the eight cervical segments of the spinal cord. Paraplegics are those whose lesions are confined to the thoracic, lumbar, or sacral regions of the spinal cord. The symptoms of incomplete injuries can vary depending on the nature of the injury and the resultant syndrome. Resultant syndromes can include the following:

1. Anterior cord syndrome
2. Central cord syndrome
3. Brown-Séquard syndrome
4. Herniated disc syndrome

The *anterior cord syndrome* most often results from a *flexion injury* to the *cervical vertebrae. It is the most common type of cord syndrome* and *damages the anterior spinal artery, as well as the spinal cord.* Upper and lower motor function is lost. The *central cord syndrome* results from *flexion or hyperextension injuries.* There is resultant compression of the anterior horn cells and oedema of the central spinal cord, causing mixed upper and lower motor neurone loss and spasticity below the level of the injury. Usually more impairment occurs in the upper extremities.

Another syndrome is the *Brown-Séquard syndrome*, which results from *rotation-flexion injuries where subluxation or dislocation of the fracture fragments occurs.* There is ipsilateral paresis, loss of proprioception, and contralateral loss of pain and temperature sensation.

The last syndrome is the *herniated disc syndrome*, which is very common. In this syndrome, there is *displacement of discs with the escape of cartilage.* It occurs spontaneously or in response to activity or slight injury.

All of these injuries are more common in older people because of degenerative changes with ageing. The lower lumbar and lumbosacral areas are affected most often.[8]

Spinal shock

Initially, in most spinal cord injuries there is a period of flaccid paralysis and a complete loss of reflexes below the level of the lesion. Sensory and autonomic functions are also lost. This is called spinal or neural shock, or areflexia, and it is a transitory event. Spinal shock results from the loss of inhibition of the descending tracts. During this period persons may require temporary respiratory assistance until recovery begins.

Within hours, days, or weeks the involved muscles gradually become spastic and hyperreflexic with the characteristic signs of an upper motor leurone lesion. These changes are thought to represent the release of the muscle stretch reflexes from the inhibitory influence of the damaged pyramidal tract, resulting in hyperactive responses.

The amount of disability that results from spinal cord injury depends on the level of injury. See Box 29-40 for specifics of muscle function after spinal cord injury.

Voiding Urine

The centre for micturition is located in the conus medullaris (S2-S4) and is linked to the detrusor muscle of the bladder by parasympathetic sensory and motor fibres that

	Muscle function after spinal cord injury		
29-40	**Spinal cord injury**	**Muscle function remaining**	**Muscle function lost**
	Cervical above C4	None	All, including respiration
	C5	Neck	Arms
		Scapular elevation	Chest
			All below chest
	C6-C7	Neck	Some arm, fingers
		Some chest movement	Some chest
		Some arm movement	All below chest
	Thoracic	Neck	Trunk
		Arms (full)	All below chest
		Some chest	
	Lumbosacral	Neck	Legs
		Arms	
		Chest	
		Trunk	

run in the pelvic nerves. Spinal cord injuries that occur at levels above the conus result in a bladder that is capable of emptying itself reflexly or involuntarily after the spinal shock phase. The bladder is hypertonic and it is variously known as an "upper motor neurone bladder" and "reflex neurogenic bladder." The emptying occurs spontaneously or automatically. The patient has no control over the act of micturition. Voiding may occur at intervals of 3 to 4 hours; there may be frequency, urgency, and incontinence. The reflex arc is intact in this type of bladder. When the cord lesion is at or below the micturition centre, the centre or the sacral nerve roots are destroyed; the reflex arc is no longer intact. This type of bladder condition is known as a "lower motor neurone bladder" or an "autonomous neurogenic bladder." Contractions of the bladder muscle are the result of impulses transmitted through a mechanism within the bladder wall but are not of sufficient strength or duration to empty the bladder. Abdominal straining or manual compression is necessary for this to happen. *Retention of urine and infection are common complications.*

Autonomic dysreflexia

One complication of spinal cord injury that is extremely important to understand is *autonomic dysreflexia*, or hyperreflexia. It occurs in patients with cord lesions above the sixth thoracic vertebra and most commonly in patients with cervical injuries. Autonomic dysreflexia occurs as a result of abnormal cardiovascular response to stimulation of the sympathetic division of the autonomic nervous system. The clinical signs include the following:

1. Bradycardia
2. Paroxysmal hypertension
3. Sweating
4. "Goose flesh"
5. Severe headache
6. Nasal stuffiness

Patients tend to develop individual symptoms of this condition and are soon able to recognize them.
The most common cause is visceral distension, which can include a distended bladder or impacted rectum. *It is a*

medical emergency that requires immediate treatment, because it can lead to cerebrovascular accident, blindness, or death. Treatment is discussed later in this chapter (p. 906).

Sexual function

In most cases, men experience impotence, decreased sensation, and difficulties with ejaculation. Impairment of fertility is common. The act of erection is under the control of sensory and parasympathetic fibres, while ejaculation requires sympathetic and parasympathetic innervation. Lesions above S2 leave the parasympathetic reflex area intact; patients may be able to have an erection, but ejaculation is not usually possible. Lesions in the S2 to S4 area usually prevent erection and ejaculation. The higher the level of injury, the more likely a man with complete cord injury is able to perform sexually. The experience of orgasm is described as different from before the injury. Women with spinal cord injury are able to continue to perform sexually, although perception of sexual pleasure is usually altered.

Nursing Process
Assessment

Assessment of the patient with spinal cord injury includes both subjective and objective data.

Subjective data

1. Patient's understanding of injury and resulting deficit
2. Information about nature of injury—how it happened
3. Reports shortness of breath
4. Unusual sensations (paraesthesias, and so on)
5. History of loss of consciousness
6. Presence of pain
7. Absence of sensation—sensory level

Objective data

1. Respiratory status
2. Level of alertness and consciousness
3. Orientation
4. Pupil size, equality, and reactivity

5. Proper alignment of body in neutral alignment
6. Motor strength
7. Temperature, blood pressure, and pulse
8. Skin integrity
9. Bowel and bladder status and distention
10. Presence of other injuries

As with the patient with a head injury, the patient with spinal cord injury should be assessed carefully for the presence of other injuries, primarily fractures or head injury.

Diagnostic tests

It is most important to first detect if there has been any cervical vertebra fracture or displacement. X-ray films are always taken to detect any fracture-dislocations. These often occur before the patient is moved from the backboard or stretcher. A spinal tap or myelography may also be used to detect blockage. It can be carried out also without moving the patient if the dye is injected at the junction between the first cervical vertebra and the base of the skull. CT scanning may also be very helpful in ruling out spinal cord injury. The MRI can detect spinal cord compression and oedema. These procedures were discussed earlier in this chapter.

Nursing analysis

Problems are determined from analysis of patient data. Possible problems for the person with spinal cord injury may include, but are not limited to, the following:

Problem	Possible aetiologies
Infection, high risk for	Spinal cord injury
Injury, high risk for	Sensory/motor deficits
Mobility, impaired physical	Neuromuscular impairment
Activity intolerance	Immobility
Urinary retention	Inability to initiate stream of urine
Incontinence, reflex or total	Neurological impairment
Incontinence, bowel	Neuromuscular impairment
Dysreflexia	Distended bladder, impacted rectum
Breathing pattern, ineffective	Neuromuscular impairment
Skin integrity, impaired, actual or high risk for	Immobility
Coping, ineffective individual	Situational crisis
Knowledge deficit	Lack of exposure/recall
Self-care deficit: feeding, bathing/hygiene, dressing/grooming, toileting	Neuromuscular impairment
Adjustment, impaired	Disability requiring change in lifestyle
Sexual dysfunction	Physiological limitations

Planning: expected patient outcomes

Expected patient outcomes for the patient with spinal cord injury may include, but are not limited to, the following:
1. Patient remains infection free.
2. Patient remains free of further injury.
3. Patient's function is preserved to the extent possible with no increase in the level of injury.
4. Patient demonstrates an optimal level of mobility.
5. Patient can demonstrate exercises to maintain function.
6. Patient can explain importance of frequent position changes, including the use of the prone position and weight shifts in the wheelchair.
7. Patient demonstrates minimal complications of bowel and bladder incontinence.
8. Patient evacuates bowel on a regular plan without diarrhoea or constipation.
9. Patient can carry out or direct own bowel and bladder programme, including possible intermittent catheterization and use of suppositories and digital stimulation.
10. Patient can explain autonomic dysreflexia, characteristic symptoms, and the actions to be taken when it occurs.
11. Patient's airway is maintained.
12. Patient maintains an effective breathing pattern.
13. Patient remains free of respiratory complications.
14. Patient can explain the need for assisted coughing if required and ask caregiver to demonstrate.
15. Patient's skin is intact.
16. Patient can do skin inspection or direct others in the inspection of the skin.
17. Patient verbalizes a positive self-concept.
18. Patient is able to direct own care and his involvement in plan of care.
19. Patient demonstrates optimal coping skills.
20. Patient makes a reasonable choice for living arrangements.
21. Patient has minimal limitations in ADL.
22. Patient can explain the medication regimen (side effects, desired effects, time, dose, and route).
23. Patient can explain plans for follow-up care.
24. Patient can explain how to obtain community resources, including the Disablement Resettlement Officer.
25. Patient remains sexually active, if so desired.

Implementation

Assisting with achievement of therapeutic goals

Immediate stage

Cervical injuries. Immediate care after spinal cord injury is directed toward realignment of the cervical bony column in the presence of demonstrated fractures or dislocations. These measures include the following:
1. Simple immobilization
2. Skeletal traction
   a. Crutchfield tongs
   b. Halo traction
   c. Stryker or Foster frame
3. Surgery for spinal decompression

It is important to maintain strict body alignment, with the body kept straight and the head flat. Sandbags may be used to maintain alignment.

With Crutchfield tongs it is important to check the traction and orthopaedic frame frequently (usually every 4 hours). The tongs should be secure, and the weights should hang freely. The sites where the tongs enter the head are cleansed with appropriate solution, and povidine-iodine solution is applied. Usually this is done every shift. When halo traction is used it is also important to check the pin sites and cleanse them as described previously. The traction is attached to a fibreglass body jacket, which should be checked for proper fit. The nurse should be able to insert a finger between the cast and the skin. If the nurse cannot insert a finger, the cast is too tight and the doctor should be notified.

With the use of a frame (Foster or Stryker), it is important to check pressure areas before and after the patient is turned. At least two persons should turn the patient, and all bolts on the frame should be tightened securely before turning. Padding may be used for comfort, but care must taken to maintain body alignment. It is important to assess the patient for any respiratory or cardiovascular difficulty when on the frame.

Often surgical decompression is not performed until after a period of skeletal traction. This allows the patient's condition to stabilize and some initial swelling of the cord to subside. The beginning spontaneous healing of the fracture site provides more stability. With the introduction of the anterior surgical approach to the cervical spinal column, surgical intervention is safer and can be attempted earlier in the hospitalization. The primary advantage of the anterior surgical approach is that it provides immediate stabilization of the spinal cord by techniques of interbody cervical fusion and the direct removal of any extruded disc materials.

Intubation and respiratory assistance may be required in the immediate stage after upper cervical cord injury. Any patient with a cord lesion at the C4 level probably will require permanent ventilatory support. Careful monitoring of blood gas levels and regular pulmonary toilet are essential.

Thoracic and lumbar injuries. Less immediate attention to thoracic and lumbar fracture immobilization is necessary for the patient with limited neurological deficits. The patient is often treated with bed rest, hyperextension, and bracing. Stabilization of the spine may occur early in the recovery course or may be delayed until some healing has occurred.

Medications. The use of corticosteroids for the prevention and alleviation of spinal cord oedema is widespread. It is believed that the steroids assist in the reestablishment of membrane stability and in the control of central nervous tissue stability.

Intermediate stage

Throughout all stages of hospitalization of the patient with a spinal cord injury, nursing and medical interventions are directed towards restoration of structural or body integrity. All efforts are taken to ensure that the following occur:

1. Contractures do not develop.
2. Range of movements is maintained to the greatest degree possible.
3. Muscle tone is consistent with pathological condition.
4. Bowel and bladder function are maintained.
5. Skin is intact.

The reader is referred to the section on care of the patient with a motor dysfunction (p. 867). Most of the care described there applies to the patient with a spinal cord injury. Additional care is described below.

Position and movement. In addition to frequent positioning, the patient with a spinal cord injury is usually placed on a bed with a firm surface or on a specially designed bed that maintains support of the spine.

Early mobilization of the patient is important. When patients, especially quadriplegics, begin to sit up, it may be necessary to wrap their legs with elastic wraps to encourage venous return. Slowly increasing the angle of sitting is essential to prevent hypotension. For this reason a newly quadriplegic patient should use a recliner wheelchair until he or she is able to sit at a 90-degree angle for several hours.

Before the patient is permitted to be up after a spinal injury, a brace may be prescribed. All braces and corsets must be custom made; the cost depends on the type of material used. The brace or corset should be applied before the patient gets out of bed. Some patients are placed in a halo brace. The patient should wear a thin, knitted undershirt next to the skin to keep the brace clean and to protect the skin. For some paraplegics, leg braces may permit them to stand and ambulate. Many find, however, that the effort to walk is not justified.

Urinary elimination. Because there is no sensation of needing to void in the patient with spinal cord injury, distension occurs easily. Usually a Foley catheter is inserted initially. Later, bladder training is started. Measures important in this training can be found in Chapter 25.

The presence of an indwelling catheter makes the patient highly susceptible to urinary infection, which can include bladder or kidney infections. These are major causes of death in patients with spinal cord injury, so it is imperative that infection be avoided, if at all possible. The best means of preventing infection is maintenance of fluid intake (3 to 4 L day) and meticulous aseptic technique. Prophylactic antibiotic therapy such as nitrofurantoin or co-trimoxazole will usually be prescribed.

Autonomic dysreflexia is one complication associated with urinary elimination in the patient with spinal cord injury. It is a medical emergency, and the nurse should be aware of the actions to take in preventing and alleviating the symptoms. The care required with the presence of symptoms is outlined in Box 29-41.

Bowel elimination. Patients are started on a bowel programme early in the recovery period. At first, bisacodyl suppositories are given at regular intervals—usually every other night. This is followed by digital stimulation to further stimulate peristalsis. The goal is to eliminate the need for the suppositories. Other aids to bowel programmes are the use of adequate fluids, stool softeners, and prune juice.

<table>
<tr><td>

29-41

Guidelines for Care

The patient with autonomic dysreflexia

1. Place patient in sitting position to decrease blood pressure.
2. Check patency of catheter for kinking. If catheter is blocked, insert new catheter immediately.
3. Check rectum for impaction.
4. If it is necessary to remove impaction, a local anaesthetic should be instilled in the rectum.
5. Send urine for culture if no other cause is found; urinary infection can lead to symptoms of autonomic dysreflexia.
6. Administer ganglionic blocking agent such as trimetaphan or a vasodilator such as sodium nitroprusside if conservative measures are not effective.

</td><td>

29-42

Sexual functioning in patients with spinal cord injury

1. Reflexogenic erections occur not only as a result of stimulation of the genitalia, but also as a result of stimulation of "trigger points."
   a. Stroking the thigh
   b. Stimulating the rectum with a finger
   c. Manipulating the catheter
2. Male patients with catheters can either remove the catheter just before sexual activity or turn it back on the penis where it provides extra support.
3. Bowels should be emptied before intercourse to prevent incontinence.
4. Female patients who have a catheter can keep it in place if desired.
5. Female patients should realize that they maintain the ability to conceive—birth control should be practised if pregnancy is not desired.

</td></tr>
</table>

Respiratory function. Generally, patients with cervical injuries below C4 are able to breathe without ventilatory support. However, they do not have normal control of chest muscles or the diaphragm, which makes them prone to respiratory complications. Care of the patient may include use of the inspirometer to increase tidal volume. Other breathing exercises may also be prescribed. The patient may require assisted coughing in which the carer exerts upward and inward pressure on the fleshy part of the abdomen just below the diaphragm while the patient attempts to cough. This action is similar to the Heimlich manoeuvre but less force is used. The patient should also be encouraged to avoid situations where respiratory infections may be transmitted. Respiratory infections are often the cause of death in patients with spinal cord injury, especially those with high cervical injury.

If a patient is ventilator dependent, attempts are made to have the patient use a portable ventilator, which allows for mobility. Diaphragmatic pacemakers may be inserted. This is still an uncommon procedure, but it has been effective in allowing patients time off the ventilator.

Skin integrity. Another problem that occurs with spinal cord injury is decubitus ulcers. Every effort should be made to avoid skin breakdown, which is a major cause of morbidity in the patient with spinal cord injury.

Facilitating learning

Teaching of the patient with spinal cord injury encompasses all of the points covered in teaching the patient with a motor dysfunction and sensory dysfunction (Box 29-20, p. 869). In addition, the patient needs assistance in learning about the effects of the injury on sexual functioning (see Box 29-42). The important thought to keep in mind is that most patients with a cooperative partner are able to engage in a satisfying sexual relationship. The limitation depends on the site of the lesion and whether the cord injury is complete or incomplete. Generally, the higher the lesion, the more normal sexual function is likely to be. Males with sacral lesions are the only patients with spinal cord injured

who are not able to have erection and ejaculation. Education of the patient in the area of sexual function includes the points outlined here.

Evaluation

Evaluation is based on expected patient outcomes. When evaluating the care of the patient with spinal cord injury, questions to consider may include the following:

1. Is the patient free of injury and has further injury been avoided?
2. Does the patient demonstrate an optimal level of mobility and exercises to maintain function?
3. Can patient explain the importance of frequent position changes?
4. Does the patient assume control of bowel and bladder programme?
5. Is the patient's airway maintained?
6. Does the patient maintain an effective breathing pattern?
7. Does the patient remain free of respiratory complications?
8. Can the patient explain the need for assisted coughing if required and can carer demonstrate it?
9. Is the patient's skin intact?
10. Is the patient doing skin checks or asking staff to do them?
11. Does the patient verbalize a positive self-concept?
12. Is the patient directing and involved in own plan of care?
13. Does patient demonstrate optimal coping skills?
14. Has patient made a reasonable choice for living arrangements?
15. Is the patient as independent in ADL as possible?
16. Can patient explain medication regimen, plans for follow-up care, and how to use community resources?
17. Does the patient remain sexually active, if desired?

PERIPHERAL NERVE TRAUMA

The peripheral nerves that lie outside the brain and spinal cord include the cranial nerves and spinal nerves and their branches and plexuses. *The disorders involving the peripheral nerves are similar to those that affect the central nervous system and are the result of traumatic, degenerative, vascular, inflammatory, neoplastic, and metabolic causes.* Important terms are listed in Box 29-43.

Traumatic causes of peripheral nerve injuries include gunshot and knife wounds, fragmented fracture wounds, and surgical transections, as in denervation surgery and amputation. They result in stretching, laceration, and compression of the peripheral nerve. The degree of injury is variable. Recovery is also variable—axons of peripheral nerves are capable of regeneration under favourable conditions.

Pathophysiology

After trauma (or disease) the axon undergoes secondary or *wallerian degeneration* distal to the lesion and for several segments proximal. The axon and myelin sheath degenerate and undergo fragmentation. The fragmented particles are completely ingested within several weeks; the axis cylinder remains. Schwann's cells and fibroblasts begin to proliferate, covering the degenerated fibres. During the regenerattive phase, new axoplasm forms at the proximal edge of the injury and the regenerating fibres now grow distally and enter the empty neurolemmal sheath, which has in the meantime proliferated. Myelin then forms around the regenerated axon. When a nerve has been severely damaged and fibrous tissue is abundant, regeneration is interfered with by a tangled mass known as a *traumatic neuroma*; they may have to be removed surgically.

Nursing Process
Assessment

Assessment includes both subjective and objective data.

Subjective data

1. Patient's understanding of condition
2. Alteration in sensation
   a. Pain
   b. Touch
   c. Temperature
   d. Proprioception
3. Site of sensory problems
4. Onset of problem
5. Presence of associated symptoms

Objective data

1. Presence of motor alterations.
2. The clinical signs and symptoms resulting from peripheral nerve lesions depend on the exact location of the lesion and the specific function of the involved nerve or nerves. Because peripheral nerves contain both sensory and motor components, there may be deficits in both components distal to the site. Alterations will occur in pain, touch, temperature, proprioception, and stereognosis. Motor alteration

29-43	Common terminology with peripheral nerve trauma	
	Neuropathies	Noninflammatory disorders
	Mononeuropathy	Disorder affecting one peripheral nerve
	Polyneuropathy	Disorder involving multiple nerves
	Neuritis	Inflammatory disorder
	Neuralgia	Painful nerve disorder

includes *lower motor neurone signs* such as *flaccid paralysis* and *muscle wasting in the muscles innervated by the affected nerves.*

Nursing analysis

The problems and expected patient outcomes are the same as those for the patient who has sensory (p. 870) or motor dysfunction (p. 866).

Planning: expected patient outcomes

See Expected Patient Outcomes for Alterations in Muscle Tone and Motor Function (p. 866) and Alterations in Sensory Function (p. 870).

Implementation

Nursing care is specific on the areas of the body affected by the sensory and motor deficits. Plans for care include measures found in the section on motor dysfunction and sensory dysfunction. Promotion of good health habits in general assists in the creation of conditions favourable to nerve regeneration.

Evaluation

The evaluation for the patient with peripheral nerve dysfunction is the same as for the patient with motor (p. 869) and sensory problems (p. 871).

TRIGEMINAL NEURALGIA

Trigeminal neuralgia is one specific kind of peripheral nerve problem. It is also called *tic doloreaux*. It usually affects people in middle or late adulthood and is slightly more common in women.

Assessment

Assessment is basically the same as for any patient with peripheral nerve trauma. Trigeminal neuralgia is characterized by excruciating, burning pain that radiates along one or more of the three divisions of the fifth cranial nerve (Fig. 29-21). The second and third divisions are most commonly affected. The pain typically only extends to the midline of the face and head, because this is the extent of the tissue supplied by the offending nerve. There are areas along the

<table>
<tr><td>

29-44

Postoperative concerns for the patient with trigeminal neuralgia

1. Preservation of eye function (if the upper branch is completely severed the corneal reflex is lost)
   a. Eye shield to prevent dust or lint from getting into the cornea
   b. Avoidance of contact with eye while bathing
   c. Eye baths with methylcellulose solution
   d. Inspection of eye several times a day
2. Promoting mouth function (lower branch of fifth cranial nerve)
   a. Avoidance of hot food
   b. Food should be placed in unaffected side of mouth
   c. Mouth care after each meal
3. Safety concerns
   a. Electric razor should be used for shaving

</td><td>

29-45

Comfort measures for patients with tic doloreaux

1. Keep room free of draughts
2. Avoid walking briskly to bedside of patient
3. Place bed out of traffic area to prevent jarring of bed
4. Avoid touching the patient's face
5. Patients should not be urged to wash or shave the affected area or to comb the hair
6. Avoid hot or cold liquids that trigger pain
7. Diet may have to be pureed and lukewarm and taken through straw

</td></tr>
</table>

course of the nerve known as trigger points, and the slightest stimulation of these areas may initiate pain. People with trigeminal neuralgia try desperately to avoid triggering them.

Implementation

Assisting with the achievement of therapeutic goals

Medication

Carbamazepine is the drug of choice for the treatment of trigeminal neuralgia pain. Drugs such as nicotinic acid, thiamine, analgesics, and even cobra venom have been tried with little success. Absolute alcohol may be injected into the peripheral branches of the trigeminal nerve. This provides relief for weeks to months.[1]

Surgery

Permanent relief of pain is obtained only by surgery that consists of either inserting a fine needle through the cheek and injecting an alcohol solution or by surgical resection of the sensory root of the trigeminal nerve. This is not always successful. Preoperative care includes the following:
1. Measures of comfort
2. Allowing patient to voice questions or concerns
3. Teaching about procedure and what to expect
Postoperative care includes the measures listed in Box 29-44.

Within 24 hours after a fifth nerve resection, many patients develop herpes simplex (cold sores) about the lips. Usually the lesions heal in about a week.

Interventions to achieve patient outcomes

Maintaining comfort and ADL

It is not uncommon for patients with trigeminal neuralgia not to have eaten properly for some time, because eating causes pain. They may be undernourished and dehydrated. They may not have washed or shaved or combed the hair for some time. Oral hygiene often has been neglected.

Measures to increase comfort preoperatively or of patients being treated nonsurgically are found in Box 29-45.

Facilitating learning

Teaching for the patient with trigeminal neuralgia is found in Box 29-46.

BELL'S PALSY (PERIPHERAL FACIAL PARALYSIS)

Pathophysiology

Bell's palsy is thought to be caused by an inflammatory process involving the facial nerve (VII) anywhere from the nucleus in the brain to the periphery. Other theories of causation include local ischaemia and oedema or emotional trauma with resultant vasoconstriction. Any of the three branches of the facial nerve may be affected. The disorder can be unilateral or bilateral. Most patients (80%) recover spontaneously over a period of a few weeks, although recovery may take as long as a year.

Assessment

Subjective and objective data are the same as for the patient with peripheral nerve trauma (p. 907). With Bell's palsy there is usually an abrupt onset of numbness or a feeling of stiffness or drawing sensation of the face. *Unilateral weakness of the facial muscles usually occurs*, resulting in *inability to wrinkle the forehead, close the eyelid, pucker the lips,* or *retract the mouth on that side.* The *face appears asymmetric with drooping of the mouth and cheek.*

Other symptoms that may occur with Bell's palsy include the following:
1. Loss of taste
2. Reduction in saliva on affected side
3. Pain behind the ear
4. Ringing in ear or other hearing loss

Nursing analysis

See appropriate section in the discussion of the patient with peripheral nerve trauma (p. 907).

Implementation

There is *no specific therapy for Bell's palsy.* Electrical stimulation or warm moist heat along the course of the

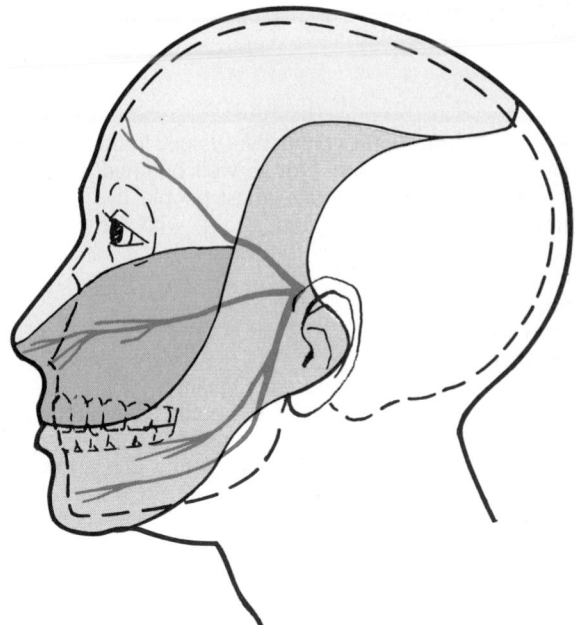

Fig. 29-21   Pathway of trigeminal nerve and facial areas innervated by each of the three main divisions of this nerve.

nerve may help. Steroids given early in the course may speed recovery. Protection of the eyes when the eyelid does not close is important. Massage of the affected areas is sometimes recommended. Exercises may be prescribed for 5 minutes three times a day. These include wrinkling the brow and forehead, closing the eyes, and puffing out the cheeks.

INTERFERENCE WITH FUNCTION BECAUSE OF TUMOURS

INTRACRANIAL TUMOURS

Pathophysiology
Intracranial tumours include both benign and metastatic lesions. All areas and structures of the brain can be affected. Primary intracranial tumours, or neoplasms, arise from the intrinsic cells of brain tissues and the pituitary and pineal glands. Secondary or metastatic tumours are also a frequent contributing type of intracranial tumour. The prognosis for patients with an intracranial tumour depends on early diagnosis and treatment because as the tumour grows it exerts pressure on vital centres and causes brain damage and death. Although approximately one half of all tumours are benign, they may also cause death by exerting pressure on vital centres.

Brain tumours are named for the tissues from which they arise. The more frequently encountered ones are described in Table 29-9. The brain, in addition, is also a frequent site for secondary tumours from other organs.

The symptoms of intracranial tumours result from both local and general effects of the tumour. Locally, the effects are from infiltration, invasion, and destruction of brain tissues at a particular site. Direct pressure is also exerted on

nerve structures, causing degeneration and interference with local circulation. Local oedema develops, and intracranial pressure increases. The raised intracranial pressure is then transmitted throughout the brain and the ventricular system. Eventually, the ventricular system is distorted and displaced sufficiently to cause partial ventricular obstruction (Fig. 29-22). Papilloedema results from the general effects of the raised intracranial pressure. Death is usually from brainstem compression resulting from herniation.

Nursing Process
Assessment
It is important to assess both subjective and objective data in the patient with an intracranial tumour. Box 29-47 on p. 911 contains a comparison of the symptoms of tumours in specific brain lobes.

Subjective data
1. Patient's understanding of diagnosis
2. Changes in personality or judgment
3. Presence of abnormal sensations (paraesthesia or anaesthesia)
4. Visual problems—loss of visual acuity or diplopia
5. Complaints of unusual odours (often accompanies tumours of temporal lobe)
6. Presence of headache
7. Hearing loss
8. Inability to carry on daily activities

Objective data
1. Motor strength
2. Gait
3. Level of alertness and consciousness
4. Orientation
5. Pupils: size, equality, and reactivity
6. Vital signs
7. Fundoscopic examination for evidence of papilloedema
8. Presence of seizures
9. Speech abnormalities
10. Cranial nerve abnormalities
11. Symptoms of increased intracranial pressure
Seizures occurring for the first time after middle age are very suggestive of a brain tumour in the cerebrum or its

Table 29-9   Types of brain tumours

Type	Incidence	Pathology
Glioma	Accounts for 50% of brain tumours	Arises in any part of the brain connective tissue. Infiltrates primarily the cerebral hemisphere tissue. Not so well outlined as to be incised completely. Grows rapidly—most people live months to years. Tumours assigned grade from 1 to 4, with 4 the most malignant. Different gliomas are as follows: 1. Astrocytomas 2. Oligodendrogliomas 3. Ependymomas 4. Medulloblastoma 5. Glioblastoma multiforme—most malignant
Meningioma	13% to 18% of all primary tumours in intracranial cavity	Arise from the meningeal coverings of the brain. They are usually benign but may undergo malignant changes. Usually encapsulated, and surgical cure is possible. Recurrence is possible.
Pituitary tumour	Occurs in all age groups but more often in women	Arise from a varied number of tissues. Surgical approach is usually successful. Recurrence is possible.
Neuroma (schwannoma, neurofibroma)	Acoustic neuroma is most common	Arises from Schwann's cells inside the auditory meatus on the vestibular portion of cranial nerve VIII. Usually benign but may undergo cellular change and become malignant. Will regrow if not completely excised. Surgical resection is often difficult because of location.
Metastatic tumours	From 2% to 20% of all patients with cancer have metastasis to the brain	Cancer cells spread to the brain via the circulatory system. Surgical resection is very difficult; even with treatment prognosis is very poor. Survival beyond a year or two is uncommon.

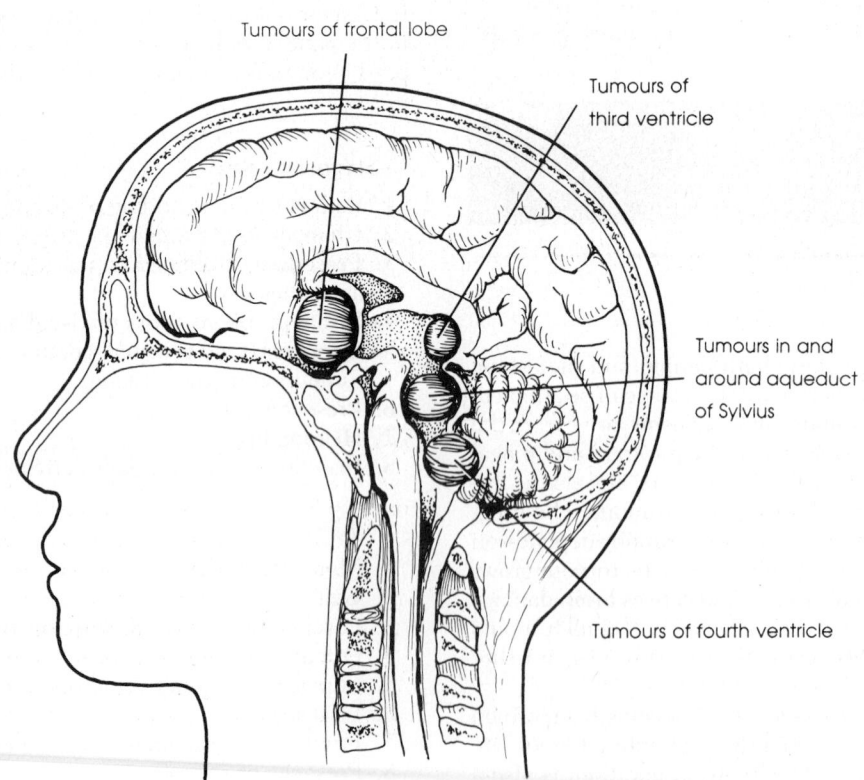

Fig. 29-22   Sites of brain tumours adjacent to ventricular system. Note how developing tumour at varied sites with extension distorts, compresses, and obstructs ventricular system at some point so that increased intracranial pressure occurs early. (From Yahr WD: *Hosp Med* 9:8, 1973.)

Comparison of symptoms of tumours found in specific brain lobes	
Area of the brain	**Symptoms**
Frontal lobe	Personality disturbances (range from subtle personality changes to frank psychotic behaviour)
	Inappropriate affect
	Indifference of bodily functions
Precentral gyrus	Jacksonian seizures
Occipital lobe	Visual disturbances preceding convulsions
Temporal lobe	Olfactory, visual, or gustatory hallucinations
	Psychomotor seizures with automatic behaviour
Parietal lobe	Inability to replicate pictures
	Loss of right-left discrimination

29-47

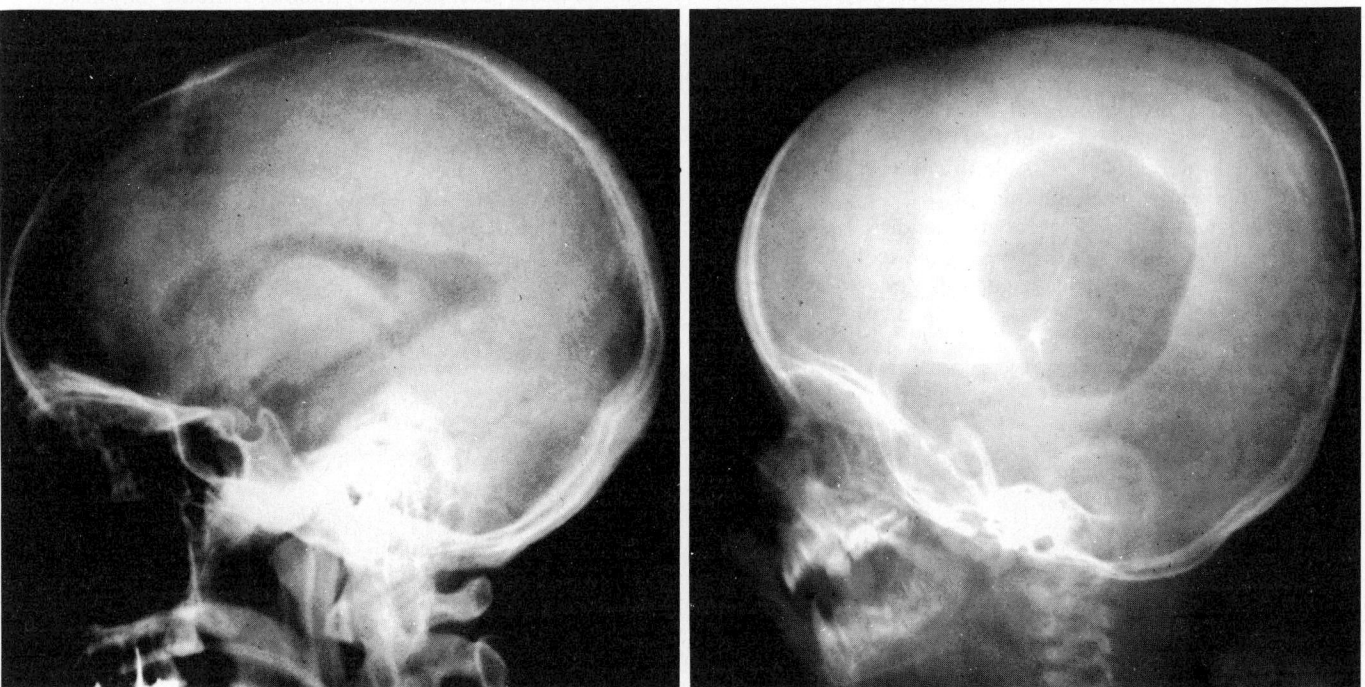

A

B

Fig. 29-23 Pneumoencephalogram. **A,** Lateral view showing outline of normal ventricle. **B,** Lateral view showing marked distention of ventricle with cerebrospinal fluid (caused by hydrocephalus).

coverings. Intracranial tumours occurring within the cerebral lobes present disturbances that can be related to the function of the specific part of the brain.

Signs and symptoms of raised intracranial pressure resulting from intracranial tumours usually occur after localized signs and symptoms have been present for varying periods. See the previous discussion of raised intracranial pressure (p. 858). Headache is at first transitory and later becomes constant; it increases in intensity with straining, coughing, stooping, and change of position. The headache is present in the morning and often awakens the person from sleep. Nausea and vomiting usually occur as the headache increases.

Diagnostic tests

No one procedure is entirely diagnostic of brain tumours, but the CT scan is often the basis of the diagnosis.

Other tests that may be used include the brain scan and the EEG. These are discussed on p. 854 and p. 873. Another test that is used less frequently since the introduction of the CT scanner is the pneumoencephalogram (Fig. 29-23).

Other tests that may be helpful in locating the tumour are *arteriography* or *ventriculography*. The ventriculogram is used when the suggested diagnosis is such that a spinal or lumbar puncture is contraindicated because of the presence of raised intracranial pressure. Fig. 29-24 shows an aneurysm found on a cerebral angiogram.

Nursing analysis

Problems are determined from analysis of patient data. The problems for the patient with an intercranial tumour are the same as for the patient with raised intracranial pressure (p. 862) or motor dysfunction (p. 866).

Planning: expected patient outcomes

Expected patient outcomes for the person with an intracranial tumour may include, but are not limited to those found in the sections for raised intracranial pressure (p. 863) and motor dysfunction (p. 870).

Implementation

Assisting with the achievement of therapeutic goals

The general methods of treatment for intracranial tumours include surgical removal when feasible, radiotherapy, and chemotherapy. The choice of therapy is determined by the tumour type and site of the tumour. A combination of methods is often necessary.

When gliomas are located in areas that are not critical to vital functions, they are usually removed surgically. Most gliomas, however, infiltrate and are difficult to completely excise and treat. Surgery is often combined with radiotherapy and chemotherapy. When the tumour is located in a more critical area where removal would leave the patient with impaired function, a biopsy of the tumour is performed, it is "debrided" if possible, and the patient is treated with radiotherapy or chemotherapy.

Meningiomas are commonly treated by complete excision of the tumour (and overlying bone if infiltrated), because they are usually located in areas that permit removal. Meningiomas are often encapsulated, which aids in their removal.

Surgery

Intracranial surgery is commonly used for all types of pathological conditions of the brain, including the relief of raised intracranial pressure and removal of tumours.

A surgical opening through the skull is known as *craniotomy*. It is a basic preparatory procedure for intracranial surgery. A series of burr holes is made first, and then the bone between the holes is cut with a Gigli saw to permit removal of the bone. Bone is then removed in such a way that it can be replaced if desired. Brain surgery may be performed with the patient under hypothermia to lessen bleeding during the procedure. Drugs to treat hypotension may be used, such as noradrenaline. Patients may also be placed in a barbiturate coma during the surgery and for several days after it to lessen brain activity, metabolism, and oxygen needs. This may help to prevent worsening of deficits because of hypoxia.

When the brain lesion is in the supratentorium (above the tentorium or in the cerebrum), the incision is usually made behind the hairline. When the incision is into the infratentorium (below the tentorium or in the brainstem and cerebellum), it is made slightly above the nape of the neck.

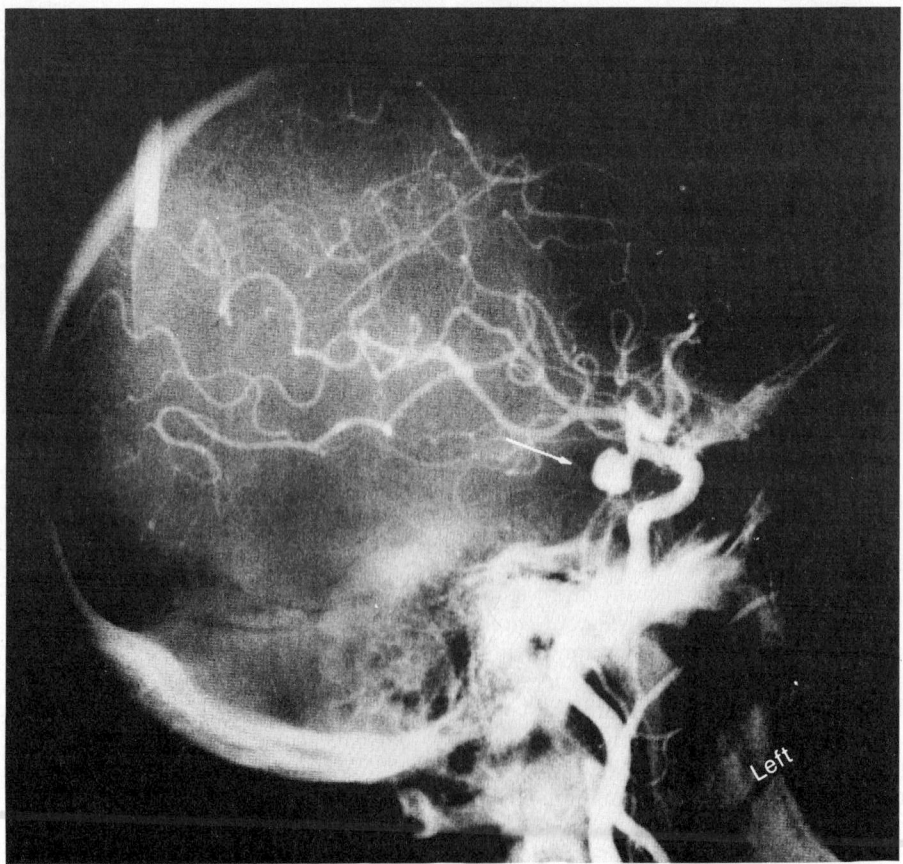

Fig. 29-24 Cerebral angiography showing location of aneurysm at posterior communicating artery. (From Tortorici M: *Fundamentals of angiography*, St Louis, 1982, Mosby–Year Book.)

29-48   **Preoperative care of the patient undergoing intracranial surgery**

1. Baseline data of neurological and physiological status should be recorded.
2. Patient and family should be encouraged to verbalize fears.
3. Treatments and procedures are explained fully, even if unsure whether patient understands.
4. If head is shaved, it is usually done in the operating theatre.
5. Antiseptic shampoo may be ordered night before surgery and may be repeated in morning.
6. If hair is shaved, it is saved and given to patient or family.
7. Prepare family for appearance of patient after surgery.
   a. Head dressing
   b. Oedema and ecchymosis of face common
   c. Temporary decreased mental status (possible).

Guidelines for Care

29-49   **Postoperative care of the patient after a shunting procedure**

1. Monitoring
   a. Assess neurological status frequently for any decrease in mental status.
   b. Observe for symptoms of subdural haematoma, one of the possible side effects of the surgery.
   c. Monitor for symptoms of overdrainage, as evidenced by headache, especially when patient is sitting upright or standing.
   d. Assess degree and character of drainage.
   (1) Amount of drainage and bleeding should be minimal.
   (2) Reinforce dressing as needed.
   (3) Often incisional areas are left open to air after several days.
2. Maintain gastrointestinal status
   a. Check frequently for signs of paralytic ileus, because the manipulation of the bowel that occurs with the placement of the peritoneal part of the shunt can predispose the patient to this.
   b. Patient is usually kept NBM for first day, and then clear liquids are started.
   c. Regular diet is resumed as soon as good bowel sounds are present and patient tolerates liquids.
3. Maintaining comfort
   a. Patient may need more frequent pain medication because of involvement of abdominal area.
   b. Keep pressure off incisional sites.
4. Promoting mobility
   a. Turning to either side is permitted.
   b. Raise head of bed gradually when mobilizing patient.
   c. Patient is encouraged to ambulate as much as possible to encourage adaptation to decreased intracranial pressure.

After craniotomy and removal of the bone, an incision is made into the meninges and the tumour is removed or other cranial surgery performed. The removed bone is carefully saved or preserved and may be replaced at the end of the surgery if there is no indication of infection or raised intracranial pressure. If it is not replaced, a bone prosthesis may later be placed over the deficit. *The removal of part of the skull without replacement is called craniectomy. Cranioplasty is the repair of a cranial defect through use of a substitute bone material such as plastic or methylmethacrylate cement.*

Tumours involving the pituitary gland that do not extend outside the sella turcica are usually removed using a transsphenoidal approach. After the surgery, packing is placed inside the nose and remains for 3 to 4 days. A muscle graft from the thigh is used to close the defect in the dura. With this type of surgery, recovery is relatively rapid and the patient has no loss of hair or external cranial incision.

Preoperative preparation of both the patient and family is important. They both are usually very threatened by the prospect of brain surgery. Specific fears may be related to those of a permanent change in appearance, dependency, or both. Preoperative care includes the points listed in Box 29-48.

During the postoperative period the patient is observed regularly for signs of raised intracranial pressure. The frequency of making and recording specific observations depends on the patient's condition. A device to measure intracranial pressure is often inserted during the surgery. Any change in the patient's vital signs, state of consciousness, pupillary response, or ability to move muscles is reported at once. Restlessness, often secondary to tissue hypoxia, may be the first warning of raised intracranial pressure. See p. 858 for specifics about intracranial pressure.

Postoperative care is determined by the patient's condition. Most patients spend at least 1 or 2 nights in an intensive care unit, where arterial monitoring and close nursing observation is possible. Other details of postoperative care are found in the section on intracerebral haematomas.

Hydrocephalus

Occasionally a catheter is placed in a ventricle of the brain to drain excess spinal fluid and to prevent hydrocephalus and raised intracranial pressure. The catheter is usually attached to a drainage system. *The tubing and drainage receptacle should be sterile, and care must be taken to prevent kinking of the tubing.* If drainage seems to have stopped, the neurosurgeon should be notified. At times, the nurse may adjust the level of the drainage device to facilitate drainage, using specific parameters ordered by the neurosurgeon. For example the neurosurgeon may order that the patient should drain 30 ml every 4 hours. The catheter is usually left in place for 24 to 48 hours and then is removed by the surgeon.

Hydrocephalus of a more permanent nature also occurs in the presence of intracranial tumours and is manifested by symptoms of raised intracranial pressure. Hydrocephalus can be communicating or noncommunicating. In communicating hydrocephalus an obstruction exists outside the ventricular system. The ventricles contain an excessive amount of CSF because fluid is not adequately absorbed from the cerebral subdural space. In noncommunicating, or intraventricular hydrocephalus CSF is accumulated secondary to a blockage of the normal flow at some point in the ventricular system. The cerebral ventricle proximal to the blockage then dilates.

Treatment consists of a shunting procedure. The different types of shunt procedures are named for their point of origin and termination and include the following:
1. Cyst to peritoneal
2. Lumbar-peritoneal
3. Ventricular-jugular
4. Ventricular-peritoneal

In this type of surgery excessive CSF is shunted away from the central nervous system and into either the peritoneal cavity (where it is absorbed) or the jugular vein. At times a Ryckham reservoir is placed through a burr hole into the ventricle. This device can easily be palpated through the skin. Some of the shunts have an on-off valve, as well as a part that may be pumped to facilitate drainage. Valves that are inserted can be set for a specific pressure with some control over the amount of fluid drained.

Preoperative care is the same as for any patient having intracranial surgery. Key points of postoperative care are listed in Box 29-49.

Normal pressure hydrocephalus does not result in intracranial pressure. People with normal pressure hydrocephalus have dilated ventricles with normal tissue mass and a normal intracranial pressure. The cause of normal pressure hydrocephalus is unknown.

Radiation therapy and chemotherapy

In some patients with intracranial tumours surgery may not be possible or indicated. In these cases radiation therapy and/or chemotherapy may be used. They are also used at times after intracranial surgery. See Chapter 9 for the care of the patient undergoing these treatments.

Hyperthermia

The use of heat may be combined with chemotherapy. Often, cancer cells have been found to be heat sensitive. The hyperthermia catheter is inserted percutaneously under a stereotactic approach guided by CT. The area is then heated to 40.5° to 42°C for a period of time. Side effects that may occur during treatment are seizures or an embolus.

Interventions to achieve patient outcomes
Maintaining comfort and ADL

Some patients who have had cranial surgery will have residual physical and mental limitations. The patient may have hemiplegia, aphasia, and personality changes. The rehabilitative care and planning are the same as for other patients with chronic and permanent neurological disease (see sections on the patient with motor dysfunction and the patient with a CVA). Regardless of the eventual prognosis and the diagnosis of the tumour, each patient should be helped to be as independent as possible for as long as possible.

Evaluation

Evaluation of the patient with an intracranial tumour involves both the patient and the family. It is based on the expected patient outcomes. The reader is referred to the sections concerning increased intercranial pressure (p. 864) and motor dysfunction (p. 869) for appropriate questions to consider.

INTRAVERTEBRAL TUMOURS

Pathophysiology

The pathological condition that results from spinal cord tumours is caused by spinal cord destruction and infiltrates, displacement and compression of the cord, and disruption of the blood supply or CSF circulation. The severity of symptoms depends on the degree of compression and the speed with which it develops. Adaption can occur with slow-growing tumours. Eighty-five percent of spinal cord tumours are benign.

Primary neoplastic tumours occur *either extramedullary* (outside the cord) or *intramedullary* (within the cord). Secondary or metastatic tumours may also involve the spinal cord, its coverings, and the vertebrae.

Extramedullary tumours of the *intradural type* may at first cause *subjective nerve root pain*. With tumour growth there will be motor and sensory deficits related to the level of the root and spinal cord involvement. As the tumour enlarges, it compresses the cord. Eventually, the patient loses all motor and sensory function below the level of the tumour.

An intramedullary tumour, beginning within the spinal cord, often initially appears as a central cord syndrome including segmental loss of pain and temperature function. In addition, anterior horn cell function is often lost, especially in the hands. Most of the central long tracts next to the grey matter become dysfunctional. Loss of pain and temperature sensations and motor weakness are gradual, progressive, and descending. Caudal motor and sensory functions are the last to be lost, including loss of bowel and bladder function.

Assessment

The subjective and objective data for the patient with an intravertebral tumour are the same as for the patient with spinal cord injury (p. 903).

Implementation

Assisting with the achievement of therapeutic goals
Surgery

A spinal decompression is commonly used even when complete removal of the tumour is not considered possible. As much of the tumour as possible (and possibly bone) is removed to reduce the obstruction for a time. It can be performed at any level of the vertebral column and may include several vertebrae. The operation is sometimes palliative. Care of the patient undergoing spinal decompression is found in the section on spinal cord injury (p. 905).

Interventions to achieve patient outcomes

Maintaining comfort and ADL

Convalescent care and rehabilitation depend entirely on the type of tumour and whether it has been successfully removed. The decompression operation may give relief of symptoms for months and sometimes for years. If the tumour is a slow-growing one, radiation therapy may be given while the patient is in the hospital and continued after discharge.

Evaluation

The evaluation of the care of the patient with an intravertebral tumour is the same as for the patient with a motor dysfunction (p. 869) or spinal cord injury (p. 906).

SUMMARY

1. Normal changes that occur in the nervous system cannot be equated with senility, Alzheimer's disease, or organic brain disease.
2. The Glasgow Coma Scale is one tool that is useful in standardizing observations of neurological patients.
3. The source of headache should be determined through careful assessment because it may be a symptom of serious neurological pathology.
4. The CT scan is an important diagnostic tool in the assessment of brain pathology.
5. The lumbar puncture is not done if there is a question of raised intracranial pressure because the puncture may result in brain herniation.
6. It is extremely difficult to evaluate neurological pain objectively.
7. Any increase in the volume of one of the cranial contents (brain tissue, vascular tissue, and cerebrospinal fluid) results in raised intracranial pressure because the cranial vault is rigid, closed, and nonexpandable.
8. Classic signs of raised intracranial pressure include restlessness, disorientation, headache, contralateral hemiparesis, an ipsilaterally dilated pupil, and visual changes that include blurring of vision or diplopia.
9. Nursing care measures can significantly influence intracranial pressure.
10. Lower motor neurone (LMN) lesions result in flaccid muscle weakness, loss of reflex activity, loss of muscle tone, and atrophy confined to the involved muscles.
11. Upper motor neurone (UMN) lesions result in spasticity and paresis of voluntary muscle tone, hyperreflexia, late atrophy from disuse, and increased muscle tone.
12. Epilepsy is a transitory disturbance in consciousness or in motor, sensory, or autonomic functions with or without loss of consciousness caused by sudden, excessive, and disorderly electrical discharges of the brain.
13. The aura is a set of symptoms that occurs before a seizure and varies from person to person.
14. No object should ever be put in the mouth of a person having a seizure.
15. Respiratory complications are common in patients with myasthenia gravis.
16. Early symptoms of multiple sclerosis are usually transitory.
17. The use of adrenocorticotrophic hormone (ACTH) and corticosteroids has shown favourable results in the management of multiple sclerosis.
18. Drug-induced parkinsonian syndromes occur with drugs that interfere with the synthesis or storage of dopamine or interfere with the striatal dopamine receptors.
19. Alzheimer's disease is a degenerative disorder, usually of older adults, that affects the cells of the brain and causes impairment of intellectual functioning.
20. Cerebrovascular accident (CVA) is the most common disease of the nervous system and can be caused by thrombus, embolus, or haemorrhage.
21. General effects of moderate to severe head injury include cerebral oedema, sensory and motor deficits, and raised intracranial pressure.
22. Injuries to the brain result from direct or indirect trauma to the head.
23. Direct trauma to the head causes acceleration-deceleration injuries.
24. Contusion or laceration directly below the site of the cranial impact is called a coup lesion, whereas one opposite the impact site is called a contrecoup injury.
25. Subdural haematomas can occur from hours to months after the initial head injury.
26. Many patients with head injury may recover physically, but they will have behavioural and psychological problems that make it difficult for them to function completely independently.
27. The amount of disability that results from spinal cord injury depends on the level of injury.
28. Autonomic dysreflexia is a complication of spinal cord injury that occurs as a result of abnormal cardiovascular response to stimulation of the sympathetic division of the autonomic nervous system and is considered a medical emergency.
29. The symptoms of intracranial tumours result from both local and general effects of the tumour.
30. Raised intracranial pressure is one of the most common complications of intracranial surgery.
31. Hydrocephalus may occur after intracranial surgery; it can be treated with a shunt.
32. The pathological conditions that result from spinal cord tumours are caused by spinal cord destruction and infiltrates, displacement and compression of the cord, and disruption of the blood supply or CSF circulation.

STUDY QUESTIONS

- Explain how medical and nursing treatment varies with patients suffering from a cerebrovascular accident depending on the cause.
- What nursing interventions would be helpful in facilitating the adjustment of a young spinal-cord-injured patient?
- What nursing interventions can increase intracranial pressure?

- How would you assist a patient with apraxia with dressing?
- A mother wants to shelter her teenage son with epilepsy. How would you work with this overprotective mother?

REFERENCES AND SELECTED READINGS

1. Adler R: Trigeminal glycerol chaemoneurolysis: nursing implications, *J Neurosci Nurs* 21:337-341, 1989.
2. Ake J, Perlstein L: AIDS: impact on neuroscience nursing practice, *J Neurosci Nurs* 19:300-304, 1987.
3.* Andrus C: Intracranial pressure: diagnosis and nursing management, *Neurosci Nurs* 23:85-92, 1991.
4.* Arsenault L: Selected postoperative complications of cranial surgery, *J Neurosurg Nurs* 17:155-163, 1985.
5.* Aumick J: Head trauma: guidelines for care, *RN* 54(4):27-31, 1991.
6. Baggerly J: Epidural catheters for pain management: the nurse's role, *J Neurosci Nurs* 18:290-295, 1986.
6a.* Barker E, Moore K: Neurological assessment, *RN* 55(4):28-35, 1992.
7.* Barker E: Action stat SCI, *Nurs 90* 20(11):33, 1990.
8.* Barker E, Higgins R: Managing a suspected SCI, *Nurs 89* 19(3):52-59, 1989.
9. Beckham M, Rudy R: Acquired immunodeficiency syndrome: impact and implications for the neurological system, *J Neurosci Nurs* 18:5-10, 1986.
10.* Boortz-Marz R: Factors affecting intracranial pressure: a descriptive study, *J Neurosurg Nurs* 17:89-94, 1985.
11. Boss B: The neuroanatomical and neurophysiological basis of learning, *J Neurosci Nurs* 18:256-264, 1986.
12.* Buelow J: A correlational study of disabilities, stressors and coping methods in victims of multiple sclerosis, *J Neurosci Nurs* 23:247-252, 1991.
13. Campbell C: Acoustic neuroma: nursing implications related to surgical management, *J Neurosci Nurs* 23:50-56, 1991.
14. Christ M, Hohloch F: *Gerontologic nursing: a study and learning tool,* Springhouse, Pa, 1988, Springhouse Publishing.
15. Cooper P: *Head injury,* Baltimore, 1986, Williams and Wilkins.
16. Daly B: *Intensive care nursing,* ed 2, Garden City, NY, 1985, Medical Exam Publishing.
17.* Davenport-Fortune P, Dunnum L: Professional nursing care of the patient with increased intracranial pressure: planned or "hit or miss," *J Neurosurg Nurs* 17:367-370, 1985.
18.* Delgado J, Billo J: Care of the patient with Parkinson's disease: surgical and nursing interventions, *J Neurosci Nurs* 20:142-150, 1988.
18a. Department of Health, *Health of the Nation: a consultative document for health in England. Presented to parliament by the Secretary of State for Health,* London, 1991, HMSO.
18b. Department of Health, *Health of the Nation: A strategy for health in England. Presented to parliament by the Secretary of State for Health,* London, 1992, HMSO.
19. Dittmar S: Rehabilitation nursing: process and application, St Louis, 1989, Mosby-Year Book.
20. Edwards D et al: Hyperthermia treatment for malignant astrocytomas: nursing implications, *J Neurosci Nurs* 23:34-38, 1991.
21. Emich-Herring B, Wood P: A team approach to neurological based swallowing disorders, *Rehab Nurs* 15:242-247, 1990.
22. Ferido T, Habel M: Spasticity in head trauma and CVA patients: etiology and management, *J Neurosci Nurs* 20:17-22, 1988.
23. Fickel V: Acoustic neuroma: postoperative deficits and the role of the neuroscience nurse, *J Neurosci Nurs* 23:57-60, 1991.
24.* Finocchiaro D, Hersfeld S: Understanding Alzheimers disease, *AJN* 90(9):56-60, 1990.
25. Flaskerud J: *AIDS-HIV infection: a reference guide for nursing professionals,* Philadelphia, 1988, WB Saunders.
25a. Fletcher S: Innovative treatment or ethical headache? Fetal transplantation in Parkinson's disease, *Professional Nurse* 7(9):592-595, 1992.
26.* Fode N: Subarachnoid haemorrhage from ruptured intracranial aneurysm, *AJN* 88:673-680, 1988.
27.* Franges E, Beideman M: Infections related to intracranial pressure monitoring, *J Neurosci Nurs* 20:94-103, 1988.
28.* Friedman D: Taking the scare out of caring for seizure patients, *Nurs 88* 18(2):52-60, 1988.
29. George M: Neuromuscular respiratory failure: what the nurse knows may make the difference, *J Neurosci Nurs* 20:110-117, 1988.

30. Gioiella E, Bevil C: *Nursing care of the aging client: promoting healthy adaptation,* Norwalk, Conn, 1985, Appleton-Century-Crofts.
31. Grabbe L, Brown L: Identifying neurological complications of AIDS, *Nurs89* 19(5):66-73, 1989.
32. Gryfinski J: Intramedullary spinal cord abscesses, *J Neurosci Nurs* 20:34-38, 1988.
33.* Haight K: What you should know about epidural analgesia, *Nurs 87* 17(9):58-59, 1987.
33a.* Hall G: This hospital patient has Alzheimer's, *Amer J Nurs* 91(10):45-52, 1991.
34. Hansberry J et al: Managing chronic pain with a permanent epidural catheter, *Nurs 90*(10):53-57, 1990.
34a.* Hickey J: Myasthenic crisis...your assessment counts, *RN* 54(5):54-59, 1991.
35. Hickey J: *The clinical practice of neurological and neurosurgical nursing,* ed 2, Philadelphia, 1986, JB Lippincott.
36. Hinkle J: Nursing care of the patient with minor head injury, *J Neurosci Nurs* 20:8-16, 1988.
37. Hodges K, Root L: Surgical management of intractable seizure disorder, *J Neurosci Nurs* 23:93-100, 1991.
38.* Jess L: Investigating impaired mental status: an assessment guide you can use, *Nurs 88* 18(6):42-50, 1988.
39. Jones A et al: Side effects following metrizamide myelography and lumbar laminectomy, *J Neurosci Nurs* 19:90-94, 1987.
40. Joynt R: Neurology, *JAMA* 265:3134-3135, 1990.
41. Kalbach L: Unilateral neglect: mechanism and nursing care, *J Neurosci Nurs* 23:125-129, 1991.
42. Keller C et al: Psychological responses to aphasia: theoretical considerations and nursing implications, *J Neurosci Nurs* 21:290-294, 1989.
43. Kim T: Hope as a method of coping in amyotrophic lateral sclerosis, *J Neurosci Nurs* 21:342-347, 1989.
44. Kirk E, Bradford L: Effects of alcohol on the CNS: implications for the neuroscience nurse, *J Neurosci Nurs* 19:326-335, 1987.
45.* Konikow N: Alterations in movement: nursing assessment and implications, *J Neurosurg Nurs* 17:61-65, 1985.
46. Krause E et al: Radiosurgery: a nursing perspective, *J Neurosci Nurs* 23:24-28, 1991.
47. Lamb C, Barbaro N: Neurosurgical approaches to the management of chronic pain syndrome, *Orthop Nurs* 6(1):23-29, 1987.
48.* Larsen P: Psychosocial adjustment in MS, *Rehabili Nurs* 15:242-247, 1990.
49. Lord-Feroli K, Maguire-McGinley M: Toward a more objective approach to pupil assessment, *J Neurosurg Nurs* 17:309-312, 1985.
50. Luchka S: Working with ICP monitors, *RN* 54(3):34-37, 1991.
50a. Macleod J, Edwards C, Bouchier I: *Davidson's principles and practice of medicine,* ed 15, Edinburgh, 1987, Churchill Livingstone.
51. Maher M, Strong S: Organ donation: a nursing perspective, *J Neurosci Nurs* 21:357-361, 1989.
52.* Mahon D, Elger C: Analysis of posttraumatic syndrome following head injury, *J Neurosci Nurs* 21:382-384, 1989.
53.* Mauser G: Neuromuscular respiratory failure—what the nurse knows makes a difference, *J Neurosci Nurs* 20:110-117, 1988.
54.* McBride E, DiStefano K: Explaining diagnostic tests for MS, *Nurs 88* 18(2):68-72, 1988.
55. McCaffery M, Beebe A: Giving narcotics for pain: a problem solver handbook, *Nurs 89* 19(10)L161-168, 1989.
56. Mitchell S, Yates R: Extracranial/intracranial bypass surgery, *J Neurosurg Nurs* 17:288-292, 1985.
57.* Mocsny N: Slow virus diseases of the central nervous system, *Rehab Nurs* 14(3):130-132, 1989.
57a.* Morgan S: A passage through paralysis, *Amer J Nurs* 92(4):54-58, 1992.
58.* Muswaswes M: Increased intracranial pressure and its systemic effects, *J Neurosurg Nurs* 20:217-222, 1988.
59. Nikas D: Critical aspects of head trauma, *Crit Care Nurs Q* 10(1):19-44, 1987.
59a.* North B et al: Living in a halo, *Amer J Nurs* 92(4):54-58, 1992.
60.* Olson E et al: The hazards of immobility, *Am J Nurs* 90(3):43-48, 1990.
61. Palmer M, Wyness M: Positioning and handling: important considerations in the care of the severely head-injured patient, *J Neurosci Nurs* 20:42-49, 1988.
62. Perlstein L, Ake J: AIDS: an overview for the neuroscience nurse, *J Neurosci Nurs* 19:296-299, 1987.
63.* Pettibone K: Management of spasticity in spinal cord injury: nursing concerns, *J Neurosci Nurs* 20:217-222, 1988.
64. Plylar P: Management of the agitated and aggressive head injury patient in an acute hospital setting, *J Neurosci Nurs* 21:353-356, 1989.

*Recommended for student reading.

65.* Pollack-Latham C: Intracranial pressure monitoring: Part II. Patient care, *Crit Care Nurs* 7(6):53, 1987.

66. Price M, DeVroom H: A quick and easy guide to neurological assessment, *J Neurosurg Nurs* 17:313-320, 1985.

66a.* Purath J: Assessing headache pain, 54(10):26-31, 1991.

67. Raney D: Malignant spinal cord tumors: a review and case presentation, *J Neurosci Nurs* 23:44-49, 1991.

68.* Rhynsburger J: How to fight Myasthenia's fatigue, *AJN* 89:337-341, 1989.

69. Rudy E: Magnetic resonance imagery: new horizons in diagnostic testing, *J Neurosurg Nurs* 17:331-337, 1985.

70. Rutledge B: Aneurysm wrapping: principles applicable to the neuroscience nurse, *J Neurosci Nurs* 21:370-375, 1989.

71. Santilli N, Sierzant T: Advances in the treatment of epilepsy, *J Neurosci Nurs* 19:144-157, 1987.

72.* Schaefer S: Relieving pain—analgesic guide, *Am J Nurs* 88:815-827, 1988.

73.* Scherer A: How HIV attacks the CNS, *AJN* 90(5):66-71, 1990.

74. Selcher D: Helping your patients dress for success, *RN* 43-45, 1991. August.

75. Sherburne E: A rehabilitation protocol for the neuroscience intensive care unit, *J Neurosci Nurs* 18(3):140-145, 1986.

76.* Sherman D: Managing an acute HI, *Nurs 90* 20(4):46-51, 1990.

76a. Snyder M: ed A guide to neurological and neurosurgical nursing, ed 2, New York, 1991, Delmar Publishers.

77. Stevens S, Becker K: A simple, step-by-step approach to neurological assessment-art 1, *Nurs 88* 18(9)53-61, 1988.

78. Stevens S, Becker K: A simple, step-by-step approach to neurological assessment…part 2, *Nurs 88* 18(10)51-58, 1988.

79. Stone N: Amyotrophic lateral sclerosis: a challenge for constant adaptation, *J Neurosci Nurs* 19:166-173, 1987.

80.* Sullivan J: Neurological assessment, *Nurs Clin North Am* 25:795-809, 1990.

81. Tosch P: Patients' recollection of their posttraumatic coma, *J Neurosci Nurs* 20:223-228, 1988.

82. Turner H et al: Comparison of nurse and computer recording of ICP in head injured patients, *J Neurosci Nurs* 20:236-239, 1988.

83. U.S. Dept. of Health and Human Services: *Healthy people: national health prevention disease prevention objectives,* Public Health Service, Washington, DC 1990.

84. Whitney C, Daroff R: An approach to migraines, *J Neurosci Nurs* 20:284-289, 1988.

84a. Watson M, Horn S, Curl J: Searching for signs of revival. Uses and abuses of the Glasgow coma scale, *Professional Nurse* 7(10):670-674, 1992.

85.* Whitney F: Relationship of laterality of stroke and emotional and functional outcome, *J Neurosci Nurs* 19:158-165, 1987.

86. Wilton L: Thalamic pain syndrome, *J Neurosci Nurs* 21:362-365, 1989.

87. Ballenger M: The neurological system and level of consciousness, *Emergency* 16:52-55, 1984.

88. Boss B: Dysphasia, dyspraxia, and dysarthria: distinguishing features, part I, *J Neurosurg Nurs* 16:151-160, 194, 1984.

89. Boss B: Dysphasia, dyspraxia, and dysarthria: distinguishing features, part II, *J Neurosurg Nurs* 16:211-216, 1984.

90. Brunnstrom S: *Movement therapy in hemiplegia,* New York, 1970, Harper and Row, Publishers.

91.* Burnside J: Alzheimer's disease: an overview, *J Gerontol Nurs* 5:14-20, 1979.

92. Byers V, Gendell H: Using metrizamide for lumbar myelography: adverse reactions and nursing implications, *J Neurosurg Nurs* 14:315-317, 1982.

93. Carlson C: Psychological aspects of neurological disability, *Nurs Clin North Am* 15:309-320, 1980.

94. Chui L, Bhatt K: Autonomic dysreflexia, *Rehab Nurs* 8:16-20, 1983.

95.* Hart G: Strokes causing left versus right hemiplegia: different effects and nursing implications, *Geriatr Nurs* 4:39-43, 1983.

96. Hendrickson S: Psychological care of the patient with neurological dysfunction, *J Neurosurg Nurs* 16:202-207, 1984.

97. Hummelbard AB et al: Prognostic value of brainstem auditory evoked potentials in head injury, *J Neurosurg Nurs* 16:181-187, 1984.

98.* Jones S: Glasgow coma scale, *Am J Nurs* 79:1551-1554, 1979.

99. King R et al: Symposium on rehabilitative nursing: rehabilitation of the patient with a spinal cord injury, *Nurs Clin North Am* 15:225-243, 1980.

100. Malkmus D et al: *Rehabilitation of the head injured adult-comprehensive cognitive management,* Downey, Calif, 1980, Professional Staff Association of Ranchos Los Amigos Hospital.

101.* Mitchell P et al: Moving the patient in bed: effects on increased intracranial pressure, *Nurs Res* 30(4):212-218, 1981.

102. Olson E et al: The hazards of immobility, *Am J Nurs* 67:779-797, 1967.

103.* Ozuna J, Friez P: Effects of enteral tube feedings on serum phenytoin levels, *J Neurosurg Nurs* 16:289-290, 1984.

104. Terzian M: Neurosurgical intervention for the management of chronic intractable pain, *Top Clin Nurs* 1:75-88, 1980.

105. Warren J, Peck E: Factors which influence neuropsychological recovery from severe head injury, *J Neurosurg Nurs* 16:248-252, 1984.

106. Wintrobe M et al: Harrison's principles of internal medicine, New York, 1970, McGraw Hill.

107.* Young M: A bedside guide to understanding the signs of increased intracranial pressure, *Nurs 81* 11(2):59-62, 1981.

FURTHER READING

Abley C: Learning to live with Parkinson's. A teaching programme to boost patient understanding, *Professional Nurse* 6(8):458-461, 1991.

Action for Research into Multiple Sclerosis, *Why a diet rich in essential fatty acid?,* London, 1986, ARMS.

Adams T: HIV-related dementia, *Nursing Times* 84(3):45-46, 1988.

Banks SA: Multiple sclerosis—the unpredictable enemy, *Professional Nurse* 5(1):576-580, 1990.

Banks SA: Consider the mind as well as the body. Nursing care and support in multiple sclerosis, *Professional Nurse* 6(1):9-16, 1990.

Minardi HA: When the brain is the target: support in neurological manifestations of HIV/Aids, Professional Nurse 5(6):298-302, 1990.

Rose, V: Understanding motor neurone disease, *Professional Nurse* 7(12):784-786, 1992.

Ross Russell RW, Wiles CM: *Integrated clinical science: neurology,* London, 1985, Heinemann.

Woodward S, Roberts J: Fostering a change in policy. HIV, Aids and the neuroscience nurse, *Professional Nurse* 9(6):359-361, 1993.

30

The Patient with Eye Problems

Wilma J. Phipps

After studying this chapter, the learner should be able to:

- Describe measurement and alterations in visual acuity and types of corrective lenses.
- Identify eye safety measures.
- Identify nursing interventions for the newly blind person.
- Describe major eye inflammations and appropriate nursing interventions.
- Compare the nature of cataracts, glaucoma, and retinal detachment and appropriate interventions for each.
- Write a nursing care plan for an 80-year-old woman having cataract surgery in a Day Surgery Unit.

ANATOMY AND PHYSIOLOGY
Accessory Eye Structures

The eye is protected from dirt and foreign bodies by the eyebrow, eyelashes, and eyelids. The *conjunctiva* is a thin membrane that lines the eyelids (palpebral conjunctiva) and most of the anterior portion of the eye (bulbar conjunctiva) except for the pupil. The palpebral conjunctiva folds back on itself where it joins the bulbar conjunctiva, forming a saclike recess (conjunctival sac). Although the conjunctiva is transparent, the palpebral portion appears pink, reflecting the underlying blood vessels. Small blood vessels may be noted in the bulbar conjunctiva over the sclera of the eye. The conjunctiva protects the eye and prevents it from drying. Inflammation of the conjunctiva (conjunctivitis, p. 928) gives a reddened appearance to the eye.

The *lacrimal gland* is located above and lateral to the eyeball (Fig. 30-1). Lacrimal fluid (tears) is secreted by the lacrimal gland. The tears provide moisture to lubricate the cornea; excessive secretion drains into the lacrimal sac, on the nasal side of the eye, and through the nasolacrimal ducts into the nose. Eye medications that are dropped into the inner canthus rather than the conjunctival sac drain out into the nose and thus lose their effectiveness on the eye.

Eyeball
Layers of the eye

The eyeball is composed of three coats or layers of tissue: the sclera, the choroid, and the retina (Fig. 30-2). The tough outer coat, or *sclera*, is opaque (white) but becomes transparent anteriorly over the iris and pupil to form the *cornea*. The middle layer, the *choroid*, contains blood vessels and is modified anteriorly into the ciliary body, which is attached to the suspensory ligament and to the iris. The inner coat, the *retina*, which does not have an anterior portion, contains the photoreceptors (rods and cones). These photoreceptors synapse in the retina with bipolar neurones and then with ganglion neurones, and these become the fibres of the optic nerve. The cones, which are less numerous than the rods, are found mostly near the centre of the retina and are considered to be the receptors for bright daylight and colour vision. The rods, found mostly in the periphery of the retina, are receptors for dim or night vision. Rods contain rhodopsin, a photosensitive protein that becomes rapidly depleted in bright light. The slow regeneration of rhodopsin, which is dependent on the presence of vitamin A, explains the time needed for the eyes to adjust from bright to dim light. Vitamin A deficiency affects night vision.

Chambers of the eye

The interior of the eyeball is divided into two cavities, the anterior and the posterior. The *anterior cavity*, in front of the lens, is further subdivided into two *chambers, an anterior chamber (between the cornea and the iris) and a posterior chamber (between the iris and the lens).* The anterior cavity is filled with a clear liquid, the aqueous humor, which is produced in the ciliary body, drains into the posterior chamber, passes through the pupil into the anterior chamber, and drains out the canal of Schlemm at the junction of the iris and cornea (anterior chamber angle). Obstruction of this drainage leads to glaucoma (p. 935). The *posterior cavity* of the eye is filled with a clear gelatinous

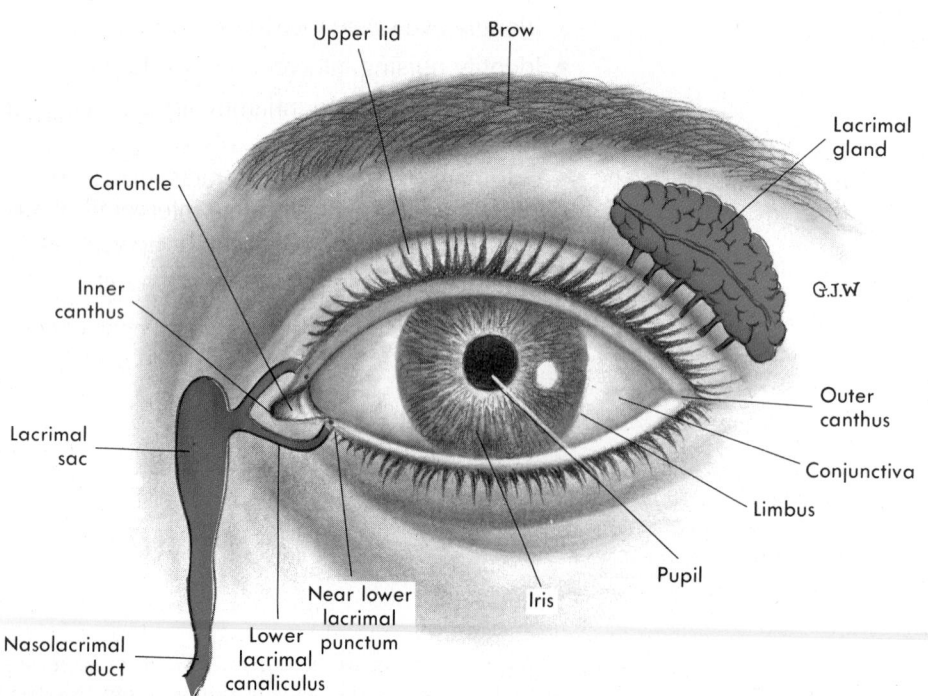

Fig. 30-1   External eye structures. (From Thompson JM, et al: *Clinical nursing*, St Louis, 1986, Mosby–Year book.)

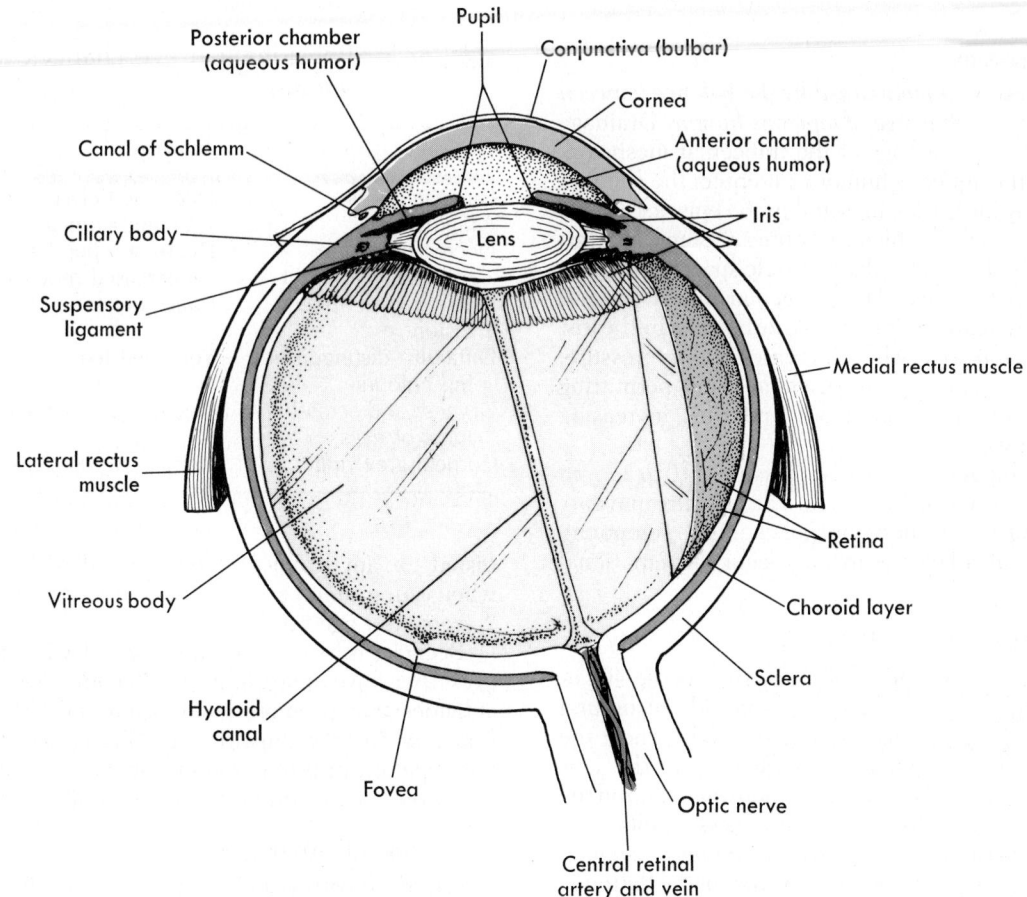

Pupil

Posterior chamber
(aqueous humor)

Conjunctiva (bulbar)

Cornea

Canal of Schlemm

Anterior chamber
(aqueous humor)

Ciliary body

Lens

Iris

Suspensory
ligament

Medial rectus muscle

Lateral rectus
muscle

Vitreous body

Retina

Choroid layer

Hyaloid
canal

Sclera

Fovea

Optic nerve

Central retinal
artery and vein

Fig. 30-2   Horizontal section through left eyeball.

substance, the vitreous humor, which helps maintain eye body. If vitreous humor is removed, the eye collapses.

Iris and lens

The iris is a coloured, ring-shaped membrane containing involuntary dilator and sphincter muscles that control pupillary size. The pupil is the space in the centre of the iris. The size of the pupil varies in response to light intensity and to focusing from far to near objects (accommodation) to en-hance visual acuity; the pupil constricts with bright lights or for near vision. The pupil also responds to autonomic nervous stimulation; pupils dilate with stress to permit more light to enter to see better during the "fight or flight" response.

The lens of the eye is a crystalline, transparent biconvex structure behind the iris, separating the anterior and posterior chambers. The lens is composed of epithelial cells and is covered by an elastic membrane (capsule). It is held in place by fibres from the ciliary body. Because of its elasticity, the lens can change shape, becoming more or less convex. The more convex the lens, the greater the refraction (see below). If the lens becomes cloudy and opaque, it is called a *cataract* (p. 933).

Muscles of the eye

Eye muscles are of two types, extrinsic and intrinsic. The extrinsic voluntary muscles outside the eyeball control extraocular movement. The intrinsic involuntary muscles within the eye are the ciliary body, which controls the shape of the lens, and the iris, which controls pupil size.

Physiology of Vision

Light rays entering the eye bend (refraction) as they pass over the curved surfaces of the cornea and through various structures of the eye (cornea, aqueous humor, lens, vitreous humor), which have different densities, to focus on the retina. *When light rays do not focus on the retina, it is called a refractive error.*

The eyes adjust (accommodation) so as to see objects at various distances by flattening or thickening of the lens. Near vision requires contraction of the ciliary body, which decreases the distance between the edges of the ciliary body, thus relaxing the suspensory ligament attached to the lens. The lens then bulges to bend the light ray more acutely so that the rays focus on the retina. Continual close vision may produce eye strain through constant contraction of the ciliary muscle; this can be relieved by frequent shifting of the eyes to distant objects. Accommodation is also facilitated by changing the size of the pupil. With near vision the iris constricts the pupil to force light rays to pass through the shortened but thicker lens.

Light rays are absorbed by the photoreceptors on the retina and are changed to electrical activity to transmit the image to the cortex. The fibres of the optic nerve (cranial nerve II) divide at the optic chiasm, the medial portion of each nerve crosses to the opposite side, and the impulses are then transmitted to the visual cortex (see Fig. 30-5). *Bilateral vision provides depth perception.*

Intraocular Pressure

Intraocular pressure is maintained by the balance between the production and drainage of aqueous humor. Drainage can be impeded by blockage of the trabecular meshwork (which filters the aqueous humor as it enters the canal of Schlemm) or by increasing pressure in the episcleral veins into which the canal of Schlemm empties.[28] Some aqueous humor may also drain into ciliary muscle spaces, then into the suprachoroidal space. The trabecular meshwork and entrance to the canal of Schlemm can be blocked by the iris. The Valsalva manoeuvre, which increases venous pressure, increases the pressure in the episcleral veins, permitting less aqueous humor to drain out and thus increasing intraocular pressure.

The normal range of intraocular pressure is 10 to 21 mm Hg, with a mean value of 16 mm Hg. The pressure may vary up to 5 mm Hg as a result of diurnal changes. Temporary increases in intraocular pressure may occur with emotional stress.

Physiological Changes With Ageing

Visual acuity declines rapidly, often by the middle 40s or early 50s. By age 70 most people use visual aids. Structural changes occur in the retina, pupil, lens, and cornea; the retina loses cells, the pupils decrease in size, the lens becomes less elastic and may become more opaque, and the cornea flattens (Table 30-1). Farsightedness results from the decreased elasticity of the lens (*presbyopia*). *Astigmatism* may occur from the irregular curvature of the flattened cornea. *The smaller pupil permits less light to reach the retina and, in addition to a decrease in rhodopsin in the rods, night vision is decreased. Older people, therefore, require more light for seeing objects,* especially for near vision, than do younger people. The lens also yellows with age, leading to increased difficulty distinguishing among colours, especially at the blue end of the spectrum.

Peripheral vision decreases with age. It is uncertain, however, which of the above factors leads to this problem.

Secretions of the eye also decrease with age. Fewer tears are produced and those that are produced tend to evaporate more quickly, producing a feeling of scratchiness or dryness of the eyes. Artificial tears may be required. Tearing may occur, despite the decreased quantity, if the tear ducts become blocked. Aqueous production is diminished, but because the anterior chamber becomes smaller, a relatively stable intraocular pressure is maintained.[10] Older people, however, have an increased chance of developing glaucoma from increased pressure in the anterior chamber (p. 935).

A common eye change noted in older people is a hazy grey ring around the periphery of the cornea resulting from fat deposits.

PREVENTION AND HEALTH EDUCATION

Vision is one of the most important senses. It orients us to the world around us. It provides pleasure through beautiful sights. It provides data to promote safety and effective interaction with others. Vision also contributes to our self-concept and feeling of personal worth and well-being. People should therefore be encouraged to have their eyes

Table 30-1   Physiological eye changes with ageing

Problem	Aetiology
Farsightedness	Decreased elasticity of lens
Astigmatism	Flattened cornea
Decreased vision, especially at night	Decreased pupil size, decreased rhodopsin
Decreased peripheral vision	Cause unknown
Difficulty distinguishing colours	Yellowed lens
Dryness and scratchiness of eyes	Decreased tear production
Corneal grey ring	Corneal fat deposits

tested for any problems encountered with visual acuity when young, about every 5 years as a young adult, and every 2 years after age 40.

Because nurses come into contact with people of all ages, they have opportunities to become involved in many activities that promote good vision and help to prevent injury or further impairment. This is accomplished by participation in promotion of visual acuity, promotion of safety measures, and detection of possible eye disorders.

Promotion of visual acuity

Interference with visual acuity may result from refractive errors or disturbances in visual fields.

Refractive errors

Bending of the light ray (refraction) depends on the shape and condition of the eye. If the anteroposterior dimension of the eye is abnormally long, the light rays will focus in front of the retina (*myopia*). Conversely, if the anteroposterior dimension is abnormally short, the rays will focus behind the retina (*hypermetropia*) (Fig. 30-3). As noted earlier, decreased elasticity of the lens occurring with age (presbyopia) also produces hypermetropia. The curvature of the cornea may also be asymmetric or irregular so that rays in the horizontal and vertical planes do not focus at the same point (astigmatism). *Refractive errors account for the largest number of impairments of good vision.*

Measurement of visual acuity

Distance vision is usually determined by use of a Snellen chart (Fig. 30-4). The person sits or stands 6 m (20 feet) from the chart, covers one eye with a piece of stiff paper or a plastic occluder, and reads the line specified by the examiner. The eyes are tested with and without distance lenses. Some experts recommend that the right eye be tested first, followed by the left eye. Adhering to this procedure ensures that recording errors will not be made.

Visual acuity is expressed as a fraction; a reading of 6/6 is considered normal. The upper figure refers to the distance at which the person can read the chart, and the lower figure indicates the distance at which a normal eye can read the line. For example, if an individual is able to read at 6 m only the line that should be readable at 24 m, he or she has 6/24 vision in the eye tested.

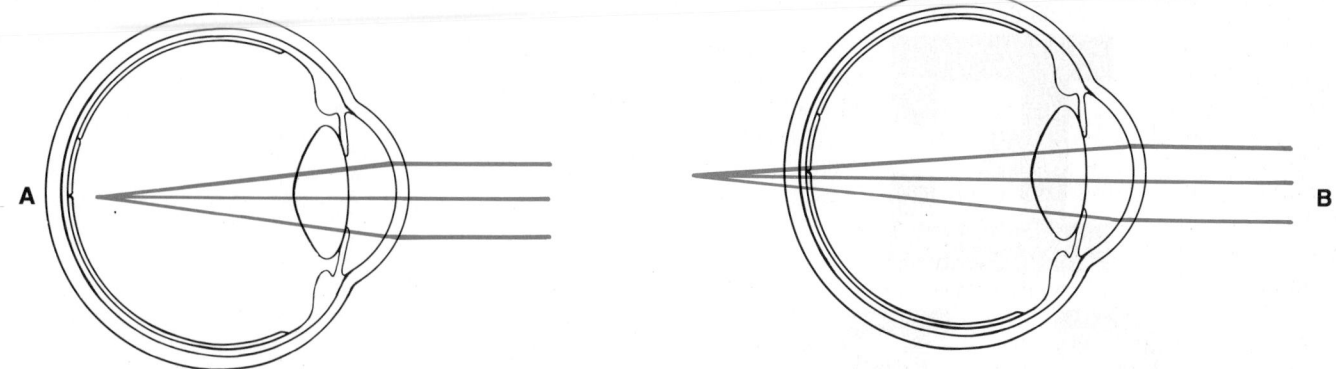

Fig. 30-3   A, Myopia (nearsightedness); image is focused in front of retina. **B,** Hypermetropia (farsightedness); image is focused behind retina.

30-1	**Terms describing visual acuity**	
	Accommodation	Ability to adjust for far and near objects
	Emmetropia	Normal eyesight; light rays focus on retina
	Ametropia	Refractive error; light rays do not focus on retina
	Myopia	Nearsightedness; light rays focus in front of retina (Fig. 30-3)
	Hypermetropia	Farsightedness; light rays focus behind retina
	Presbyopia	Hypermetropia from loss of lens elasticity because of age
	Astigmatism	Irregular curvature of cornea; light rays do not focus at same point

Near vision is tested by reading small print, such as news-print, held 35 cm (14 in) from the eye. Any person with vision less than 6/9 in either eye is referred to an ophthalmologist, ophthalmic optician or optometrist for further testing.

Some terms related to acuity are defined in Box 30-1.

Visual fields

The visual field is that portion of the environment that the eye can perceive. The field of vision thus includes peripheral or indirect vision. Normality depends on intactness of all parts of the visual pathways of the eye. Lesions of the retina, optic pathways, and central nervous system affect sections of the field of vision. *Damage to the optic disc (retina) or to the optic nerve anterior to the optic chiasm, as seen with glaucoma, affects only the field of the involved eye* (Fig. 30-5, *B1*). Lesions at the chiasm or posterior to it produce bilateral visual field defects of a wide variety. For example, a pituitary gland tumour compressing the optic chiasm damages the crossing fibres from the nasal retina and classically causes *bitemporal hemianopsia,* or the *loss of vision in the temporal halves of each eye* (Fig. 30-5, *B2*). *Loss of vision in the corresponding halves of both visual fields produces homonymous hemianopsia* (Fig. 30-5, *B3*) and can be further designated as right or left. For example, patients with *right cerebrovascular accidents often experience hemianopsia with left field loss.*

Measurement of visual fields

Visual fields can be tested by various means. One method (*confrontation test*) is to ask the person *to cover one eye and focus on a point directly ahead.* An object, such as *a pencil,* is *placed peripherally beyond the person's vision,* then *advanced centrally until the person first indicates that the object is seen.* Normally, the *person should see about 60 degrees nasally, 90 degrees temporally, 50 degrees superiorly,* and *70 degrees inferiorly.*

Types of lenses

Lenses may be worn as glasses or contact lenses. Glasses may have one focus (for near or far vision), *bifocal* (upper part for distance, lower part for near vision) or *trifocal* (for distance, intermediate, and near vision).

Contact lenses are usually chosen for cosmetic reasons or for sports activities because they do not fog or break easily. People who have lenses removed because of cataracts (but without lens implants) achieve better vision with contact lenses than with glasses. Some industrial occupations prohibit use of contact lenses because of irritation of the cornea by dirt or dust trapped under the lens.

Contact lenses are small corrective lenses made of different types of ground plastic worn over the cornea of the eye or between the cornea and sclera (scleral lens). The *lenses may be of various types: rigid, gas permeable (rigid), soft, or extended-wear (soft).* The rigid lenses are commonly used because they are cheaper and easier to maintain; they cannot be worn for long periods (usually not over 12 to 24 hours).

The disadvantages of soft-type lenses may include a higher initial cost and more frequent replacement. They are also more difficult to clean and maintain. The use of extended-wear soft contact lenses is increasing. Although some of these lenses can be left in place for as long as a

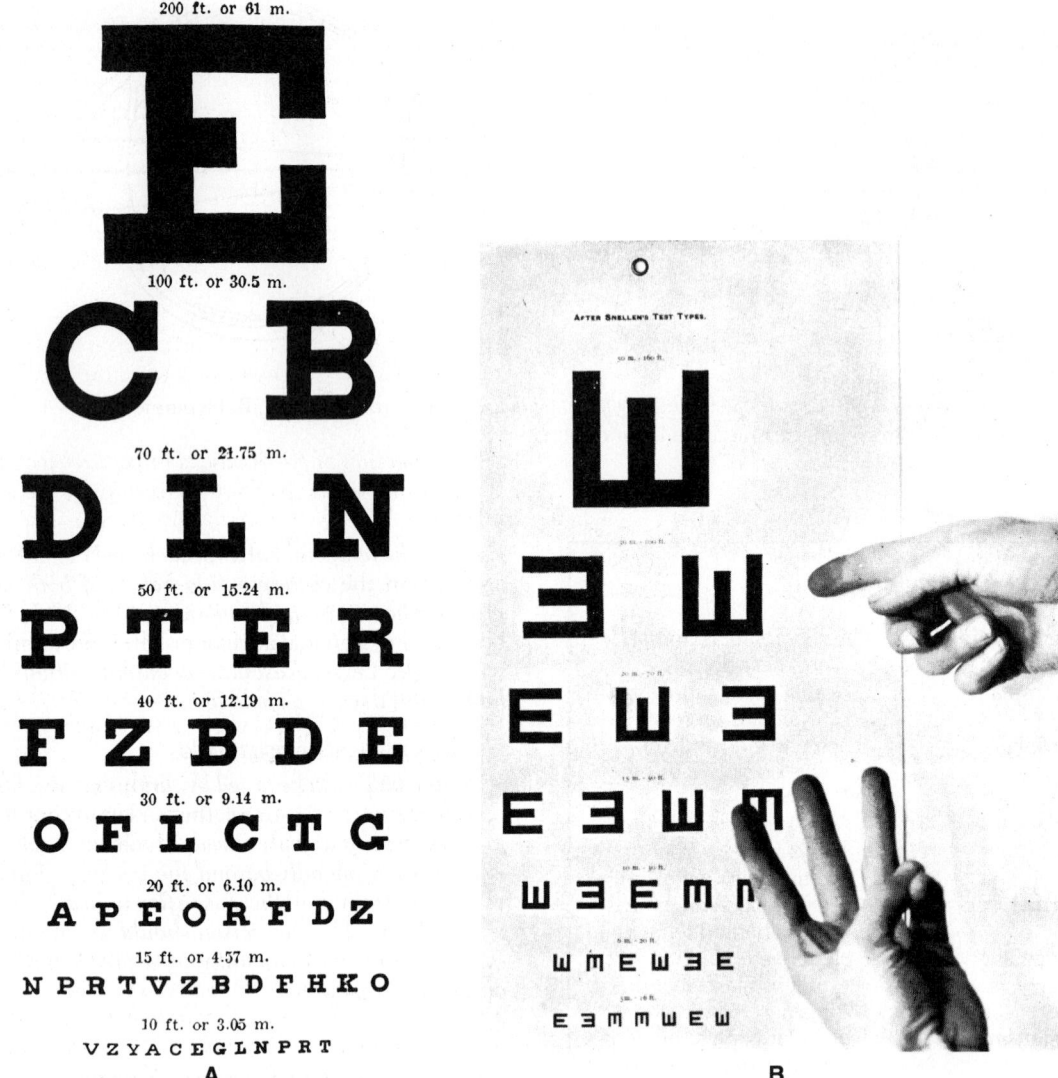

Fig. 30-4 **A,** Snellen chart used in testing vision. **B,** Modified Snellen chart, called "E" game, for testing vision of small children and people unfamiliar with English alphabet.

month, the current trend is to limit wear to 1 week before removal for cleaning and disinfection. People who use extended-wear lenses must be educated and prepared for the extra care required for these lenses. Scleral lenses are more difficult to wear than corneal lenses and are less frequently prescribed.

Newer contact lenses with the optical qualities of the rigid lenses and the comfort of the soft are now available. Because of their special properties, along with specially developed contact lens solutions, some of the complications associated with both the rigid and soft lenses can be avoided.

Contact lenses are inserted after being cleaned thoroughly and immersed in a wetting agent. Conjunctival secretions provide the lubrication needed for the lenses to be worn in comfort. The lenses are held in place by capillary attraction and by the upper lid. *If the person is injured or unconscious, the nurse removes the contact lenses.* Lenses are stored separately in special containers, labelled left or right lens. Soft lenses are kept wet at all times with special solution or sterile saline solution.

Lenses should not be worn longer than the prescribed length of time. Overwearing can cause oedema and abrasion of the cornea. All contact lenses can cause problems; most problems are minor and can be managed by changes in routine or lenses. However, problems should not be ignored, because they may lead to or be indicative of more serious problems.

Primary Prevention

Promoting eye safety

Everyone should know how to protect their eyes from injury. Many people keep unused eye medications and then use them for self-treatment at a later date. This is hazardous because it not only may lead to eye injury but may delay

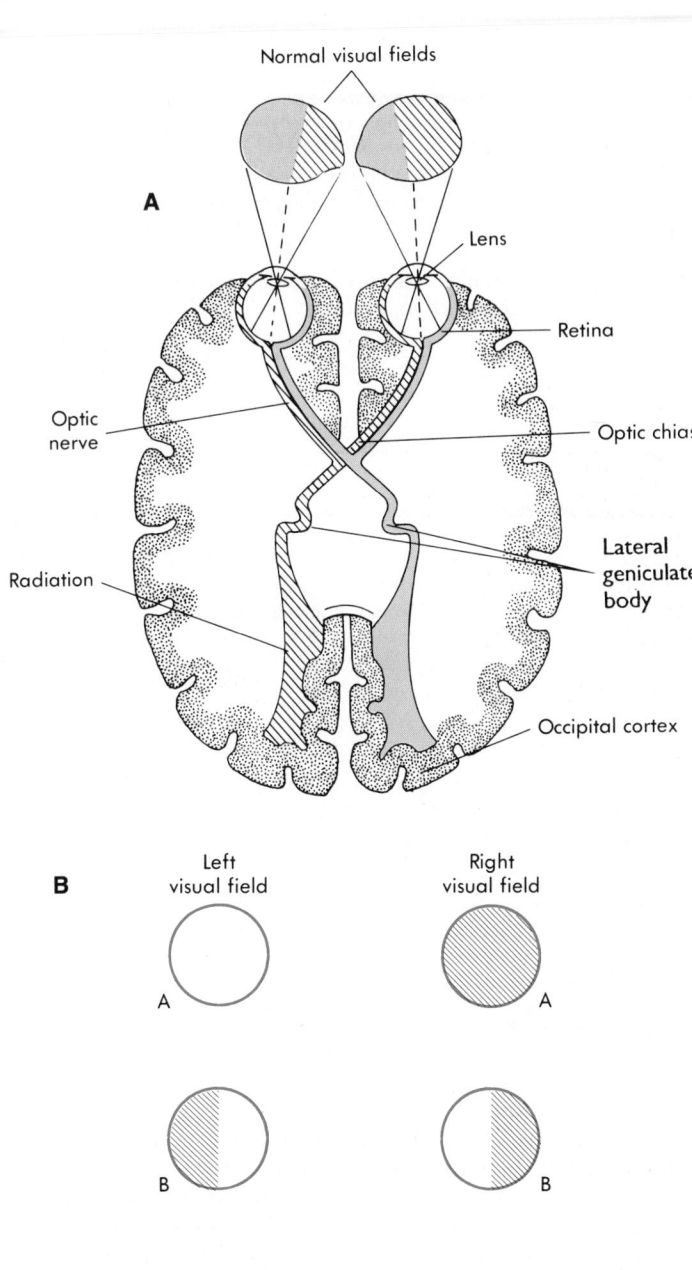

Fig. 34-5 **A,** Visual pathways showing partial decussation at optic chiasm. Normal visual fields show reversal of light rays from the temporal and nasal sides to receptors in the retina. **B,** Abnormal visual fields. *A,* Normal left field of vision with loss of vision in right field as a result of complete lesion of right optic nerve. *B,* Loss of vision in temporal half of both fields as a result of lesion of optic chiasm. This is called bi-temporal hemianopsia. *C,* Loss of vision in nasal field of right eye and temporal field of left eye caused by lesion of the right optic tract. This is called homonymous hemianopsia.

necessary treatment. Ophthalmic drugs may deteriorate, become more concentrated from evaporation of liquid, or become contaminated with bacteria or fungi.

Many thousands of people suffer eye injuries each year. These range from fairly minor to those severe enough to result in total loss of vision. Injuries may be work-related or occur in the home, garden and during sporting activities. Nine out of 10 eye injuries could have been prevented if safety practices and protective eyewear had been used.[20]

Preventive goggles and break-resistant corrective lenses should be worn by people who engage in very active physical activities such as sports and selected occupations. Prompt and appropriate care of an injured eye may prevent serious vision impairment or loss of the eye (Table 30-2).

Secondary Prevention

Early detection of eye disease is imperative for protection of vision. Inflammations of the eye are more easily detected than other eye disorders; the person usually complains of discomfort, and redness and discharge are easily observed. Glaucoma is the greatest threat to vision in older people; the permanent vision loss it causes is preventable if the condition is identified early. Mass screening programmes for glaucoma detection have been instituted in many communities, and everyone is urged to participate. All people with symptoms suggestive of eye disease (Table 30-3) are urged to seek medical assistance.

Diseases of other parts of the body may also affect the eye (Table 30-4). Early detection and treatment of these diseases can help to prevent loss of vision.

VISUAL IMPAIRMENT: BLINDNESS

Vision is essential to most employment and necessary in countless experiences that make life enjoyable and meaningful. In the United Kingdom there are over a million people, of all ages, who have some form of visual impairment. According to the Royal National Institute for the Blind about 1 in 60 of the population is either blind or partially sighted.

In developing countries there is a high incidence of blindness from preventable causes such as malnutrition and eye infections. The visually impaired population includes not only those who are certified blind. There are many people who, although unable to see well enough to read a newspaper, have vision better than 6/60. Also, there are people who are monocularly blind, with a small proportion having a defective but not blind second eye. Most people in this visually impaired but not certified blind population are between the ages of 25 and 64. Many people over the age of 65 have some form of visual impairment: blindness in both eyes or inability to read newsprint even with eyeglasses.

Although there has been a reduction of blindness in developed countries from infections and certain diseases and injuries, *blindness from diseases that occur most frequently among older people,* including *diabetic retinopathy, glaucoma, cataract,* and *retinal degeneration, has increased.* It is likely that the incidence of blindness will continue to increase because of the steady growth in the number of people aged 65 and older.

Table 30-2 First aid for eye injuries

Injury	Interventions
Burns: chemical, flame	Flush eye immediately for 15 minutes with cool water or any available nontoxic liquid; seek medical assistance
Loose substance on conjunctiva: dirt, with water if insects	Lift upper lid over lower lid to dislodge substance, produce tearing; irrigate eye necessary; do not rub eye; obtain medical assistance if above interventions fail
Contact injury: contusion, ecchymosis, laceration	Apply cold compresses if no laceration present; cover eye if laceration present; seek medical assistance
Penetrating objects	Do not remove object; place protective shield over eye (e.g., paper cup); cover uninjured eye to prevent excess movement of injured eye; seek medical assistance

Table 30-3 Symptoms suggestive of eye disease

Symptom	Eye disease
Conjunctival redness	Conjunctivitis, blepharitis, stye
Crusting discharge	Conjunctivitis, blepharitis, stye
Ocular pain	Foreign body, stye, acute lid infection, glaucoma, keratitis, uveitis
Foreign body sensation ("something in eye")	Foreign body, corneal erosion, blepharitis, chronic conjunctivitis
Blepharospasm	Keratitis, corneal ulcer
Multiple spots ("floaters")	Retinal detachment, intraocular haemorrhage, diabetic retinopathy
Photophobia	Uveitis, keratitis, glaucoma, corneal abrasions
Vision changes	
Blurred vision	Refractive error, cataract, glaucoma, uveitis, retinal detachment
Double vision	Strabismus
Halos around lights	Glaucoma
Blind spots	Haemorrhage, choroiditis
Sudden vision loss	Central retinal artery or vein occlusion

Impaired Vision

Vision impairment ranges from refractive errors correctable with lenses to total blindness, in which the person may not even be able to perceive light. For legal purposes blindness is defined very precisely in order to determine eligibility for assistance of various kinds (see Box 30-2). *Although many nonseeing people now prefer to be called visually handicapped, the term blindness is still in common usage.*

Responses to Loss of Vision
Impact of visual loss

People who are born blind or develop blindness very early in life and who are brought up as if they could see, and are neither overprotected or rejected, frequently are self-confident people able to lead active productive lives.

Loss of vision may affect self-esteem and the ability to interact with others and with the environment. The adult who becomes blind fairly rapidly usually has greater difficulty adjusting to the handicap. The impairment may cause a decrease in self-confidence and self-concept. Communication with others is affected, and a sense of isolation may develop. Familiar hobbies that require vision, such as reading, sewing, or crafts, may no longer be possible. Even listening to television creates problems when gaps in sound occur. Mobility or ability to carry out activities of daily living may be restricted or at least modified. Career options,

job opportunities, and financial security may be affected. Blindness may influence the person's ability to remain independent, to feel socially adequate, or to feel that he or she is a contributing member of society.

Limitations in the range and variety of experiences are related to the fact that a person who cannot see must use touch and kinesthetic experience to gain knowledge of the world. Objects too large or too small to handle are not perceivable. Many blind people feel that the restriction in mobility resulting from blindness is its most serious effect. Blind people cannot move about as quickly, as securely, or as easily as sighted people. These individuals need to rely on canes, guide dogs or other people, particularly when they are in unfamiliar areas.

Coping with visual loss

After a person has been told that blindness will result, there is a *normal reaction* described as *a period of mourning for the "dead" eyes. Grief and mourning over the loss of vision can cause emotional reactions such as denial, anger, guilt, resentment, hopelessness, loneliness, and depression.* These strong emotional feelings interfere with the blind person's ability to plan new ways of accomplishing tasks of living.

Fluctuating vision, a common occurrence for many visually impaired people, *leads to frustration and difficulties*

Table 30-4 Eye manifestations of systemic disorders

Disorder	Effect on eye
Diabetes mellitus	Senile cataracts occur earlier and progress more rapidly
	Diabetic retinopathy; retinal changes lead to decreased vision
	Vitrious haemorrhages
	Retinal detachment
Persistent systemic hypertension	Retinal haemorrhage, retinal oedema, and retinal exudate lead to loss of sight
Cerebral vascular accident	Loss of sight in one half of visual field (hemianopsia)
	Emboli may occlude retinal vessel
Demyelinating neurological disorders (multiple sclerosis)	Nerve damage to eye
Raised intracranial pressure	Papilloedema (swelling of optic disc)
Nutritional disorders	
Lack of vitamin A and B	Changes in conjunctiva, cornea, and retina
	Tears reduced
	Eyes and lids become reddened and inflamed
	Night blindness
Excess of vitamin A	Retinal damage
AIDS	Cytomegalovirus (CMV) retinitis

in planning or implementing tasks. Fears and uncertainties about the progression of visual impairment can lead to concern about the ability to cope with further deterioration of vision or the necessity of preparing for the future.

The ability to cope with the loss depends on the extent and duration of the handicap, the age at which it occurs, how the people has successfully coped in the past, and the presence of available support systems (family and friends).

Over time, people with visual losses appear to be able to compensate for their deficit by an increase in sensitivity of the other senses. For example, *many blind people compensate by increasing auditory acuity, tactile acuity, sense of smell, or kinesthetic awareness.*

Role of the Nurse in Working With the Newly Blind

Counselling

Newly blind people who are trying to cope need an opportunity to talk about their feelings, concerns, and anxieties about the future. Once they have identified these feelings and concerns, they can be helped to identify their strengths and resources and to consider different approaches to dealing with tasks of everyday living. Alternate forms of recreation and pleasurable activities can also be explored. For example, the person who enjoyed reading may be interested in learning Braille or listening to "talking books."

Some people need assistance in developing a new self-image. It is not unusual for the person to reject initially any aids that officially identify them as "blind," such as the white cane. Patience is required; it sometimes takes a long time to change self-image.

People who become blind do not develop impaired hearing or intelligence, yet some sighted people insist on speaking loudly. Communication should be as it would be for a sighted person (see Box 30-3).

30-2

Criteria for certification of blindness/partial sight

In the United Kingdom visual impairment is divided into two categories - blindness and partial sight.

Visual acuity is tested using a Snellen's type chart with the person wearing their corrective lenses. Account is taken of restriction in the person's visual field.

Blindness
Blindness is further subdivided into three groups
1. Visual acuity less than 3/60 Snellen
2. Visual acuity of 3/60 but less than 6/60 Snellen with severe visual field restriction
3. Visual acuity of 6/60 or more with severe visual field restriction

Partial sight
1. Visual acuity of 3/60 but less than 6/60 Snellen without visual field restriction
2. Visual acuity up to 6/24 Snellen with moderate restriction of the visual field, loss of the crystalline lens or opacities
3. Visual acuity of 6/18 Snellen or more with severe restriction of the visual field

The actual criteria for certification are very complex and readers requiring more specific information are advised to consult the guidance notes produced for consultant ophthalmologists to assist in completing form BD8 (1990) (HMSO).

People with impaired vision can be helped considerably by retraining for suitable occupations and the legislation which covers the employment of people with disabilities.

30-3

Guidelines for communicating with blind people

1. Talk in a normal tone of voice.
2. Do not try to avoid common phrases in speech, such as "See what I mean?"
3. Introduce yourself with each contact (unless you are well-known to the person).
4. Explain why you are in the room.
5. Announce when you are leaving the room so the blind person is not put in the position of talking to someone who is no longer there.

30-4

Facilitating independence in ADL for blind people

Place clothing in specific locations in drawers or cupboards to facilitate clothing selection.

Keep furniture in specific places to facilitate mobility.

Encourage use of cane when walking in unfamiliar areas.

When assisting a blind person in walking, let the person take *your* arm.

Provide descriptions of food on plate in terms of a clock face, for example, "The peas are at 7 o'clock."

Provide privacy while the newly blind person is learning to cope with eating unless they ask that someone stay.

Assisting with ADL

Given time, most blind people develop ways of coping with activities of daily living (ADL) (see Box 30-4). One elderly blind lady was able to take her many medications accurately by devising a system using rubber bands and strings around the medication bottles to provide clues as to when they were to be taken.

Referring to community services

Many services are provided for people with severe visual impairment (certified blind or partially sighted) by central government, local authorities and the voluntary organizations. The health professional can refer these people and their families to a social worker familiar with services and facilities available in their home area. Community nurses often have this information readily available. *Services to visually impaired people include mobility training, personal counselling, vocational rehabilitation, relearning independent self-care, special education, benefits and financial assistance in some instances.* "Talking books" and other tapes are available from public libraries, as well as from organizations for the blind.

Some organizations for the blind loan tape players to blind people. They post tapes or records, Braille and Moon publications and large print books. All Braille and Moon publications are carried post free.

Government Assistance

Being certified blind entitles a person to certain benefits, e.g. tax allowance, employment assistance, social security benefits and a reduction in the cost of a television licence. Not all of these are offered to those who are partially sighted. Local authorities keep a voluntary register of people with visual impairment which helps to ensure that individuals obtain those services to which they are entitled.

MAJOR HEALTH PROBLEMS OF THE EYE

The most common disorders of the eye in adults include the following:
1. Inflammatory disorders of the eyelid, conjunctiva, cornea, choroid, ciliary body, and iris
2. Cataracts: opaqueness of the lens
3. Glaucoma: increased intraocular pressure
4. Retinal detachment
Each of these is discussed in this chapter.

INFLAMMATORY EYE DISORDERS

Inflammations and infections may occur in any of the eye structures (Table 30-5), and *account for more than half of eye disorders.*

Aetiology and Pathophysiology

Most eye inflammations are caused by microorganisms, mechanical irritation, or sensitivity to some substance. Fortunately, a large percentage of inflammations are self-limiting, with no permanent scars. Severe corneal inflammation or ulceration can damage the cornea, causing visual impairment. Complications from uveitis can lead to formation of adhesions, secondary glaucoma, and loss of vision.

The *most common eye inflammations* are *styes and conjunctivitis.* Styes are relatively mild infections of the follicle of an eyelash or gland at the lid margins. Staphylococci are often the infecting organisms. These infections tend to occur in crops because the infecting organism spreads from one hair follicle to another. Poor hygiene and excessive use of cosmetics may be contributing causes. People should be taught not to squeeze styes because the infection may spread and cause cellulitis of the lids.

Conjunctivitis is the most common eye disease and may be acute or chronic. Acute bacterial conjunctivitis is usually transmitted by direct contact; the person touches the eyes following finger contact with contaminated objects such as towels or tissues. The *most common infecting organisms are staphylococci* and *adenoviruses.* Simple conjunctivitis is usually self-limiting.

Infection by *Chlamydia trachomatis* leads to *trachoma,* a form of conjunctivitis that is rare in the United Kingdom, but is the leading cause of blindness worldwide, particularly in low-income people living in the dry, hot Mediterranean countries, Africa and the Far East. Following the acute conjunctivitis stage in trachoma, the eyelids become scarred, and granulations form on the inner surface

REVIEW

Table 30-5   Inflammatory disorders of the eye

Disorder	Description	Signs and symptoms	Medical therapy
Hordeolum (stye)	Staphylococcal infection of gland at eyelid margin	Localized abscess at base of eyelash, oedema of lid, pain	Hot compresses to hasten pointing of abscess, topical antibiotic
Chalazion	Cyst from obstruction of sebaceous gland at eyelid margin	Initial oedema and discomfort; later, painless mass in lid	Warm compresses and topical antibiotic initially; surgical removal if large and pressing on cornea
Blepharitis	Inflammation of lid margins, usually by staphylococci	Itching, redness, lid pain, lacrimation, photophobia; crusting ulceration; lids become glued together during sleep	Warm compresses followed by chloramphenicol or fusidic acid eye ointment; steroid eye drops may be prescribed
Conjunctivitis (pink eye)	Inflammation of conjunctiva by viruses, bacteria (highly infectious), chlamydia, allergy, trauma (sunburn)	Redness of conjunctiva, lid oedema, crusting discharge on lids and cornea of eye; itching with allergies	Cleansing of lids and lashes, warm compresses; topical antibiotics; steroid eye drops for allergies (contraindicated for herpes simplex virus); no eye patch
Keratitis	Inflammation of cornea by bacteria, herpes simplex virus, allergies, vitamin A deficiency	Severe eye pain, photophobia, tearing, blepharospasm, loss of vision if uncontrolled	Warm compresses; topical antibiotics for bacterial infections; atropine sulphate; idoxuridine or acyclovir for herpes simplex; eye patch, rest; corneal grafting if cornea injured
Corneal ulcer	Necrosis of corneal tissue from trauma, inflammation; may be superficial or may penetrate deeper tissue	Pain and blepharospasms may occur; ulcer may be outlined by fluorescein dye	Superficial ulcer; antibiotic eye drops, eye patch Deep ulcer: topical and systemic antibiotics, atropine sulphate, warm compresses, eye patch; cauterization; corneal transplant if necessary
Uveitis	Inflammation of iris and ciliary body (anterior) or choroid (posterior); the cause is often unknown	*Anterior:* eye pain, photophobia, lacrimation, blurred vision, small pupil *Posterior:* blurring, decreased vision, mild eye discomfort	Hyoscine or atropine to dilate pupil (rests pupil, prevents adhesions), moist eye compresses, corticosteroids

of the lids and invade the cornea. The entire cornea may eventually become involved with subsequent loss of vision. Secondary bacterial infection is common. Trachomas can be arrested in the early stages with topical and oral tetracycline. Hygienic measures are important in the prevention and treatment of trachoma. Corneal scarring may require corneal transplantation.

Allergic conjunctivitis is commonly associated with hay fever. It is usually chronic and recurrent.

Nursing Process
Assessment
Subjective data

People with inflammations of the eye may complain of itching, pain (mild to severe), lacrimation, sensitivity to light (photophobia), or spasms of the eyelids (blepharospasms).

Objective data

The external structures of the eye are routinely inspected during the physical examination. *Inflammations are identified by the presence of redness, oedema of the lids, and pus or discharge from the eye.* When *considerable discharge is present, the lids may become stuck together during sleep.*

Corneal ulcers may be identified by instilling sterile fluorescein, a yellow-green harmless dye. Because fluorescein harbours the growth of microorganisms such as *Pseudomonas,* only a new, unopened bottle should be used. Also available are *single-use fluorescein-impregnated paper strips that are gently touched to the inside of the lower lid.* The ulcer is then assessed by shining a penlight obliquely across the eye from the side. If pain and blepharospasm interfere with examination, a drop of anaesthetic such as 0.5% amethocaine can be used.

30-5

Guidelines for Care

Care of the patient with an eye inflammation

1. Wash hands
2. Apply warm moist compresses as prescribed for healing and to decrease pain.
3. Irrigate eye, if prescribed, to remove discharge.
4. Administer prescribed eye medications.
5. Use eye pads only for inflammations without infection.
6. Dim bright lights if photophobia is present.
7. Give prescribed analgesics for pain.
8. Prevent spread of infection by:
   a. Using separate medication bottles or tubes for each eye if infection is present.
   b. Washing hands before and after touching eye.
   c. Using face cloths and face towels only once if infection is present.

30-7

Guidelines for Care

Eye irrigation

1. Wash hands.
2. Place patient lying towards side to be irrigated to prevent fluid from flowing into other eye.
3. A plastic squeeze bottle is used unless very large amounts of fluid are needed.
4. Direct the irrigating fluid along the conjunctiva from the *inner* to the outer canthus.
5. Avoid directing a forceful stream onto the eyeball.
6. Avoid touching any eye structures with irrigation equipment.
7. A piece of gauze may be wrapped around the index finger to raise upper lid for better cleaning if heavy discharge is present.
8. Place a kidney dish at side of face to collect irrigating fluid. An alternative is to collect the solution in a folded towel held at the side of the face.

30-6

Guidelines for Care

Application of warm moist eye compresses

1. Use sterile technique when infection or ulceration is present; clean technique may be used for allergic reactions.
2. Use separate equipment for bilateral eye infections.
3. Wash hands before treating each eye.
4. Temperature of compresses should not exceed 49°C (120° F).
5. Change compresses frequently over 10 to 20 minutes.
6. Do not exert pressure on eyeball.
7. Sterile yellow soft paraffin may be used on skin *around* eyes, if desired, to protect skin.
8. If sterility is not necessary, moist heat may be applied by means of a clean face flannel.

1. Patient states pain is decreased.
2. Infection does not spread to opposite eye.
3. The patient can:
   a. State name, dosage, and frequency of eye medication to be taken and the need to discard unused ophthalmic medications after therapy.
   b. Describe method and frequency of eye compresses to be used.
   c. Describe measures to prevent spread of infection to the uninvolved eye and to others in the household.
4. If corneal grafting has been performed, the person can:
   a. Describe the medication programme.
   b. Describe activities and movements to be avoided.
   c. Describe the need for medical follow-up.

Implementation

Nursing interventions for the person with an eye inflammation consist primarily of giving eye treatments and medications to hasten healing and decrease pain, and helping prevent the spread of infection (see Box 30-5).

Assisting with achievement of therapeutic goals
Eye compresses

Warm moist compresses help relieve pain, promote healing, and help to cleanse the eye, which is normally cleansed by tears. Treatment is repeated two to four times a day.

Cold moist saline compresses may be ordered to prevent or control oedema and severe itching of the eyes and to help control bleeding immediately after eye injury. A small basin of sterile solution may be placed in a bowl of chipped ice at the bedside. *Sterile forceps are used to wring out and apply the compress. If the compress does not need to be sterile, a face flannel or compress may be placed on pieces of ice in a basin.* A rubber glove or small plastic bag packed with finely chipped ice may be applied to the eye and requires fewer compress changes.

Nursing analysis

Problems are determined from analysis of patient data. Possible problems for the person with an eye inflammation may include, but are not limited to, the following:

Problem	Possible aetiologies
Pain	Oedema of the eye, secretions, photophobia
Infection, high risk for infection of nonaffected eye	Lack of information about how eye infections are spread
Knowledge deficit	Lack of exposure to information

Planning: expected patient outcomes

Expected patient outcomes for the person with an eye inflammation may include, but are not limited to, the following:

Table 30-6 Types of ophthalmic drugs

Type	Action	Uses
Mydriatic	Dilates pupil	Examination of interior of eye Prevents adhesions of iris with cornea in eye inflammations
Cycloplegic	Dilates pupil Paralyzes ciliary muscle and iris	Decreases pain and photophobia and provides rest in inflammations of iris and ciliary body and diseases of cornea Eye examinations
Miotic	Contracts pupil Permits better drainage of intraocular fluid Decreases intraocular pressure	Glaucoma Acute glaucoma Eye surgery
Secretory inhibitor	Decreases production of intraocular fluid	Glaucoma
Topical anaesthetic	Decreases sensation (pain)	Surgery, treatments Eye inflammations
Topical antibiotic	Antiinfective	Eye inflammations
Steroid	Antiinflammatory	Eye inflammations and allergic reactions

Eye irrigation

Irrigation is used to remove secretions, discharge, foreign bodies, and chemical irritants from the eye (see Box 30-7). Physiological saline solution or lactated Ringer's solution is commonly used because these isotonic solutions do not remove the electrolytes necessary for normal eye action. If only a small amount of fluid is needed, sterile cottonwool balls may be used to drip fluid into the eye.

Eye pads

Eye pads are contraindicated in general eye infections because they enhance bacterial growth. They may be used for photophobia when the inflammation is *not* caused by bacteria and to protect the eye when corneal ulceration is present.

Eye medications

Accuracy and safety in the administration of eye medications is essential to prevent irreparable damage to the eye. The correct eye to receive the medication must be identified. Labels must be checked carefully, and all medications with labels that are smeared or obliterated are discarded. Solutions that have changed colour, are cloudy, contain sediment, or are outdated are also discarded. Elderly people are particularly susceptible to side effects of medications.

Ophthalmic medications may be instilled as eyedrop solutions or applied as an ointment.

All patients should have their own bottles of eyedrops or tubes of ointment to prevent cross-infection. If an eye infection is being treated with an antibiotic and the same drug is being given prophylactically in the other eye, separate bottles or tubes are used for each eye.

Different types of drugs are used for treatment of eye diseases (Table 30-6). The most commonly used drugs for eye inflammations are antibiotic, steroid, and cycloplegic drugs (Tables 30-7 and 30-8).

Drugs applied topically to the eye can be absorbed and may cause systemic side effects. To avoid undesired systemic reactions, care should be taken with topically applied medications to give exactly what is ordered and no more.

Corneal surgery

When the cornea is so damaged from corneal inflammation (keratitis) or from a corneal ulcer, corneal transplantation (keratoplasty) may be performed. Corneal grafts are taken from healthy donor eyes, preferably from young donors (ages 25 to 35) who have died from an acute disease or from injury.[28] The corneas need to be obtained within 5 hours of death. Until recently, the donor cornea had to be transplanted within 24 to 48 hours. Newer corneal preservation media make it possible to use the cornea up to 7 or more days after the death of the donor. By adding insulin and growth factors to the preservation media, it is hoped that the number of endothelial cells transplanted will increase; this should increase the chance of graft success.[4] Another advantage of this new medium is that the increased time of preservation allows the corneal transplant to be planned in advance by the usual surgical team, which increases the chance of a successful outcome.[4]

People wishing to donate their eyes for use in keratoplasty can make their wishes known to relatives and ensure that the correct forms are completed and mention made in any will made. Nurses need to be alert to situations where corneas may be obtained and to offer the suggestion to the family of a recently deceased person.

Either total or partial replacement of the cornea may be performed (Fig. 30-6). The total penetrating graft is the most frequently used type and is the most effective. A second transplant may be performed if the first is unsuccessful.

Keratoplasty may be *performed* with *local or general anaesthesia* or *a combination of both*. The new cornea is sutured in place, and an antibiotic is injected subconjunctivally. An eye shield is applied, remains in place until the day after surgery, and is reapplied at night

Table 30-7 Mydriatic and cycloplegic drugs

Drug	Maximal effect	Duration
Mydriatic action (dilates pupil)		
Phenylephrine	20 min	3 hr
Adrenaline	3 to 5 min	–
Cycloplegic and mydriatic action (dilates pupil; paralyzes ciliary muscle and iris)		
Atropine sulphate	30 to 120 min	2 wks
Cyclopentolate	15 to 45 min	2 days
Homatropine	10 to 90 min	2 to 3 days
Hyoscine hydrobromide	15 to 45 min	5 to 7 days
Tropicamide	20 to 35 min	4 to 6 hrs

Table 30-8 Other ophthalmic drugs

Ophthalmic drug	Use and effect
Antiinfectives	
Polymyxin B, neomycin, gromicidin	Antibiotic agents may be given for acute inflammatory con-
Neomycin sulphate	junctivitis, styes, eyelid infections, keratitis, and uveitis;
Gentamycin sulphate	idoxuridine and acyclovir are antiviral, especially for herpes
Chloramphenicol	simplex eye infections
Tetracycline hydrochloride	
Chlortetracycline hydrochloride	
Sulphacetamide sodium	
Norfloxacin	
Idoxuridine (Herplex, Dendrid, Stoxil)	
Acyclovir (Zovirax)	
Adrenocorticoids	
Betamethasone	Topical ophthalmic steroid therapy is indicated for allergic
Dexamethasone	conjunctivitis, nonpyogenic eye inflammations, and for
Fluorometholone	eye trauma (burns, foreign body penetration); chronic
Hydrocortisone	therapy may cause increased intraocular pressure, suscepti-
Prednisolone	bility to fungus infections, glaucoma, and cataracts
Tears substitutes	
Hydroxyethylcellulose	Artificial tears provide lubrication when tears are deficient
Hypromellose	(age, heredity, connective tissue disorders, environment);
	also used for lubrication with contact lenes and artificial
	eyes

to prevent inadvertent injury during sleep. Postoperative care of the person having eye surgery is discussed on p. 934. Glasses may be worn during the day to protect the eye and the patient can expect that some vision will be restored immediately. Vision continues to improve over the next 6 to 12 months.

Corneal grafts heal very slowly because of the lack of blood vessels in the cornea. The patient is advised to avoid bending, lifting, or straining for 1 month to prevent increased intraocular pressure or suture strain; strenuous activities should be avoided for 3 months.

The graft is never totally integrated into the eye; therefore, the person must check his or her eye for the remainder of life for signs of rejection (redness, photosensitivity, pain, vision loss).[37] Any symptoms that persist or increase in severity in a 24-hour period are reported to the doctor.

Interventions to achieve patient outcomes
Assisting with comfort

Pain from eye inflammations can be reduced by applying warm moist compresses several times each day and by instilling prescribed eyedrops (particularly cycloplegic drugs, which put the iris and ciliary body at rest). If photophobia creates discomfort, the patient's room is kept semi-dark. Avoid using overhead lights that would shine in the patient's eye when he or she is lying in bed. Mild analgesics such as aspirin or paracetamol usually suffice, but if pain is severe (as may occur with uveitis) a narcotic may be required.

Preventing spread of infection

When a highly infectious eye condition, such as acute bacterial conjunctivitis, is present, precautions need to be

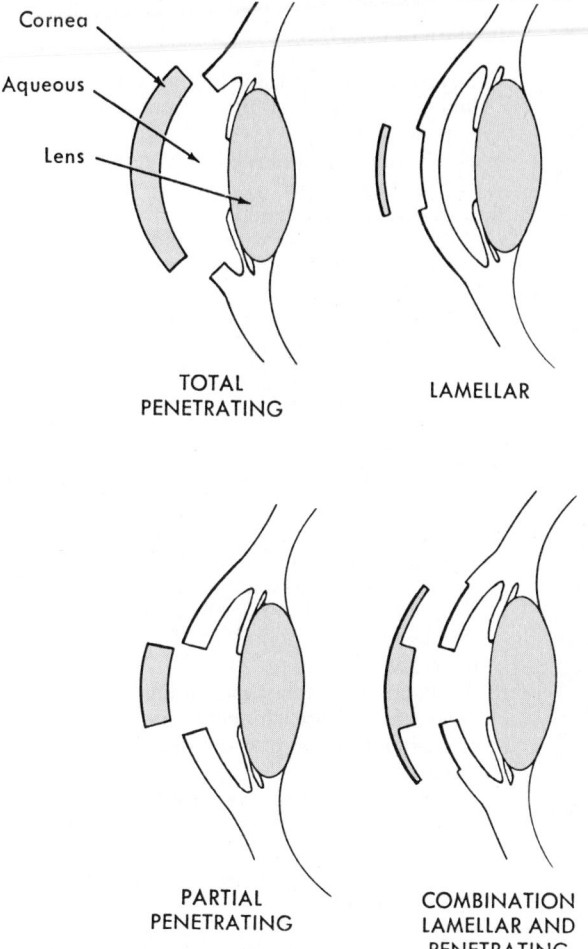

Cornea

Aqueous

Lens

TOTAL PENETRATING

LAMELLAR

PARTIAL PENETRATING

COMBINATION LAMELLAR AND PENETRATING

Fig. 30-6   Types of corneal grafts now being used. Note that in lamellar graft, defect does not penetrate entire thickness of cornea.

taken to prevent the spread of infection to others. Individual flannels and towels should be used and discarded after each use. Hands should be washed before and after any contact with the infected eye.

Facilitating learning

The patient needs to be taught how to care for the inflamed eye and how to prevent further episodes of inflammation. Teaching includes instruction about medications and their proper use.

Evaluation

When providing care for the patient with an eye inflammation or infection, questions to consider may include the following:

1. Is the patient comfortable?
2. Is the uninvolved eye free of signs of infection?
3. Does the patient know how to carry out prescribed treatments after discharge?
4. If corneal surgery has been performed, does the patient know about activity limitations and need for continued medical follow-up?

CATARACT
Aetiology and Epidemiology

A cataract is a clouding or opacity of the lens that leads to gradual painless blurring of vision and eventual loss of sight. The most common cause of cataract formation is ageing (senile cataract). By 80 years of age, about 85% of people have some clouding of the lens. These *senile cataracts are the most common cause of blindness in the elderly*. Other causes of cataract include trauma, other eye diseases (for example, uveitis), systemic diseases (diabetes mellitus), or congenital defects (either hereditary or as a result of antenatal viral infections such as German measles).

Pathophysiology

The lens of the eye is normally transparent, so that light rays can pass through. Biochemical changes may occur within the lens, or trauma may cause fibre changes that cause the lens to become cloudy and finally opaque, thus blocking the light rays from reaching the retina. A *mature cataract is a developed cataract that separates easily from the lens capsule*. It was previously thought that a cataract had to be mature ("ripe") before it could be extracted. Now cataracts are removed whenever the decreased vision interferes with the person's activities of daily living. Cataracts may develop in both eyes, such as with senile cataracts, but usually they do not develop at the same time.

Assessment

Subjective data and *objective data* include the following: Acquired cataracts, either from ageing or disease, usually develop gradually. The predominant symptom is progressive loss of vision; the degree of loss depends on the location and extent of the opacity. People with an opacity in the centre portion of the lens can generally see better in dim light, when the pupil is dilated. The person with presbyopia may find that reading without glasses is possible in the early stages because of resulting myopia. People who wear glasses may clean them frequently thinking that dirty glasses are the reason they cannot see as well as usual. In fact, this is a common complaint for which the elderly may seek medical assistance.

If the cataract results from trauma, blurring of vision may be immediate.

Cataract surgery

Surgery is the only method for treating cataracts, although only a small percentage of senile cataracts progress to the point where surgery is required. The decision to remove the cataract depends on the degree of visual impairment, general health, and the use made of the eyes.

Because surgery is usually indicated only for advanced cataracts, elderly people may believe that they should wait until vision loss is far advanced before consulting an ophthalmologist. Delaying medical examination of the eye can lead to permanent vision loss if there is glaucoma, either alone or in combination with cataracts.

Cataract surgery has changed in recent years as a result of the use of the operating microscope, better instrumentation, improved suture material, and refinement of the intraocular lens.[38] Even patients who are in their nineties can often be operated on with good results. Between 90% and 95% of all cataract operations are successful. Cataracts are usually removed under local anaesthesia. The most popular method of cataract removal is the extracapsular cataract extraction. In this method, only the anterior portion of the lens capsule plus the capsule contents are removed. *Phacoemulsification using ultrasonic vibrations is used to break up the lens, which is then aspirated in small pieces.*

Cataracts can also be removed within their capsule (intracapsular extraction). In this method a freezing *(cryo)* probe that adheres to the surface of lens is used to extract the cataract.

Preoperative care

Preparation of the eye includes instillation of eyedrops, such as a mydriatic/cycloplegic and a local anaesthetic (e.g. cocaine) on the day of surgery. A tranquillizer or mild sedative may also be prescribed. If a topical anaesthetic is given before surgery, the eye can be protected by an eye pad or glasses.

Intraoperative care

Some eye surgery is now being performed as day case surgery except when complications are present preoperatively. Local anaesthesia is used for most of the procedures in adults; a general anaesthetic (such as thiopentone) may be used briefly for initial eye injections and incision. Because the pupil is widely dilated during surgery, the patient can see only light but not the surgeon's actions. The patient's head is positioned so as to avoid movement during surgery.

Postoperative care

The *goals of postoperative care* are to *prevent* (1) *increased intraocular pressure,* (2) *stress on the suture line,* (3) *haemorrhage into the anterior chamber,* and (4) *infection.* When intraocular pressure (IOP) is increased, pressure is placed on the suture line and bleeding may occur. Anterior flexion of the head not only increases IOP but also may cause anterior synechia (adhesion of the iris to the cornea) because of decreased fluid in the anterior chamber and inflammation from the trauma of surgery. Thus activities that increase IOP, such as straining and leaning over, are contraindicated after surgery because a sudden increase in pressure places stress on the suture line. Protection (eye shield, glasses) of the eye prevents injury. Infection is prevented by the correct use of eye drops and eye pads; topical antibiotics may be given prophylactically.

Specific instructions regarding activities to avoid, eye drops to be instilled, and symptoms to be reported are provided to the patient by the surgeon and nurse. The instructions may include those listed in Box 30-8.

Corrective lenses
Intraocular lens

Cataract surgery now involves intraocular lens implantation at the time of surgery.[38] The intraocular lens provides binocular vision and better optical results than external lenses. It restores vision to near 6/6. There are different styles of lenses, but all the lenses consist primarily of two

---

30-8

Patient Teaching

The patient following eye surgery

1. Sleep on unaffected side for the prescribed time (3 to 4 weeks) to prevent pressure on operated eye.
2. Wash hands before instilling eyedrops or changing eye pad.
3. If an eye pad is required:
   a. Use two oval eye pads, to provide snug, but gentle pressure to prevent blinking against resistance
   b. Apply tape (paper or silk) diagonally from above nose to lower cheek.
4. Apply metal eye shield at night or when having a nap to protect eye.
5. Use glasses indoors and sunglasses with side sections outdoors to protect eyes from foreign substances and ultraviolet light until healing occurs.
6. Avoid rubbing or pressing on the eye (creates pressure and may dislodge sutures).
7. Avoid showers and shampooing hair (soap may irritate eye) for specified period as instructed; the time period differs from 1 day to up to 2 weeks.
8. Avoid bending at the waist or lifting heavy objects for at least 1 month to prevent increased intraocular pressure or adhesions of the iris.
   a. To pick up objects from floor, kneel while keeping head erect.
   b. To put on stockings or to tie shoes, sit and raise foot to reach hand while keeping head erect.
   c. Long pick-up gadgets can facilitate picking up small objects from the floor without having to bend over.
9. Avoid straining with bowel movements or with other activities and avoid violent coughing (increases intraocular pressure).
10. Limit reading (back and forth movement may loosen stitches); television viewing is usually permitted.
11. Report signs of swelling, discharge, or pain to doctor (may indicate infection or haemorrhage).

---

parts: the lens (usually made of polymethylmethacrylate), and the attached flexible loops to hold the lens in position. *The lenses may be implanted in the anterior chamber in front of the iris or in the posterior chamber behind the iris. The posterior lens implant, suitable for an extracapsular lens extraction, is used in the majority of patients.*

External lenses

If an intraocular lens is not inserted during surgery, the person must wear an external lens (Table 30-9). Cataract glasses are the least desirable but are used if the person cannot use contact lenses. Loss of depth perception and some peripheral vision make walking difficult. The final pair of glasses is not prescribed until vision has stabilized several months after surgery.

Contact lenses correct some of the problems encountered with cataract glasses but not entirely.[28] The extended-wear soft contact lens (p. 923) is commonly used. Interruption of the nerve supply to the cornea from surgery usually facilitates the wearing of a contact lens.[28] People with rheumatoid arthritis, hemiplegia, parkinsonism, or Alzheimer's disease may have difficulty inserting and maintaining contact lenses.

GLAUCOMA
Aetiology and Epidemiology

Glaucoma is a group of eye disorders characterized by increased intraocular pressure (IOP) and loss of vision (Fig. 30-7). *It is a leading cause of irreversible blindness in the United Kingdom.* The incidence of glaucoma is increasing as the number of older people increases. About 2% of people over the age of 40 years are thought to be affected by glaucoma in the United Kingdom.

Glaucoma may be either primary or secondary to other eye disorders. *Primary glaucoma* has a *genetic predisposition. Primary open-angle glaucoma (the most common form) is six to eight times more common in Blacks than in Whites.* Because early signs may be absent in some forms of glaucoma, *many people are unaware that they have glaucoma until loss of vision occurs.*

In addition to age and race, other risk factors include diabetes, myopia, and a family history of glaucoma. Early diagnosis and treatment are essential to prevent loss of vision.

Pathophysiology

IOP is maintained by ongoing production and drainage of aqueous humor in the anterior cavity (p. 922). Glaucoma results when there is interference with the outflow of aqueous humor, leading to a higher-than-normal IOP (normal range is 10 to 22 mm Hg). The pressure may vary as much as 5 mm Hg as a result of diurnal changes. *If the pressure remains elevated, eye damage occurs.* The *optic nerve degenerates* at its origin (has a "cupping" appearance), and the *ganglionic and nerve cells of the retina degenerate. These changes produce loss of vision, first peripheral vision, then eventual blindness if the condition is untreated.*

The two major types of glaucoma are primary in origin, open-angle and angle-closure (closed-angle). *Secondary glaucomas may result from eye disorders that block aqueous outflow or increase vitreous pressure (lens changes, uveitis, melanoma of the uveal tract), eye trauma or surgery, or long-term topical steroid therapy.*

Open-angle glaucoma

Most glaucomas (90% to 95%) are *primary open-angle glaucomas.* Both eyes are involved. *The onset is insidious and the disorder is slowly progressive. It is termed open-angle because the aqueous humor has open access to the trabecular meshwork.* However, drainage is impeded by degenerative changes in the trabecular meshwork, canal of Schlemm,

---

The Elderly with Eye Problems

Assessment

Assess all older patients for problems with distance and close vision, seeing in dim light, colour perception, and glare.

Check on availability and cleanliness of vision aids.

Interventions

Obtain low-vision aids for visually impaired older patients: large-print instructional materials, magnifying glasses, and talking books.

Set up meal tray according to clock face and instruct patient accordingly.

Provide plenty of light during meals, toileting, and ambulation because vision of elderly is decreased in dim light.

Alert all staff about patient's visual impairment.

Provide nonambiguous large-type signs at eye level with important instructions and names; for example, TOILET.

Common disorders in elderly

Cataracts
Glaucoma
Diabetic retinopathy

Table 30-9   Corrective lenses after cataract surgery

Type	Advantages	Disadvantages
Lens implant	Cannot be lost or broken Better binocular vision No handling required	Possible complications: vitreous loss, inflammation
Contact lenses	Better visual correction than glasses Better cosmetic appearance Better binocular vision if only one lens removed	Awkward for some elderly people to manage Easy to lose Difficult adjustment for some people May cause irritation
Cataract glasses	More acceptable to some elderly people No physical complications	Magnify objects by 25%; objects appear closer than they actually are Distort peripheral images and colours Heavy lenses May cause visual distortion if poorly positioned

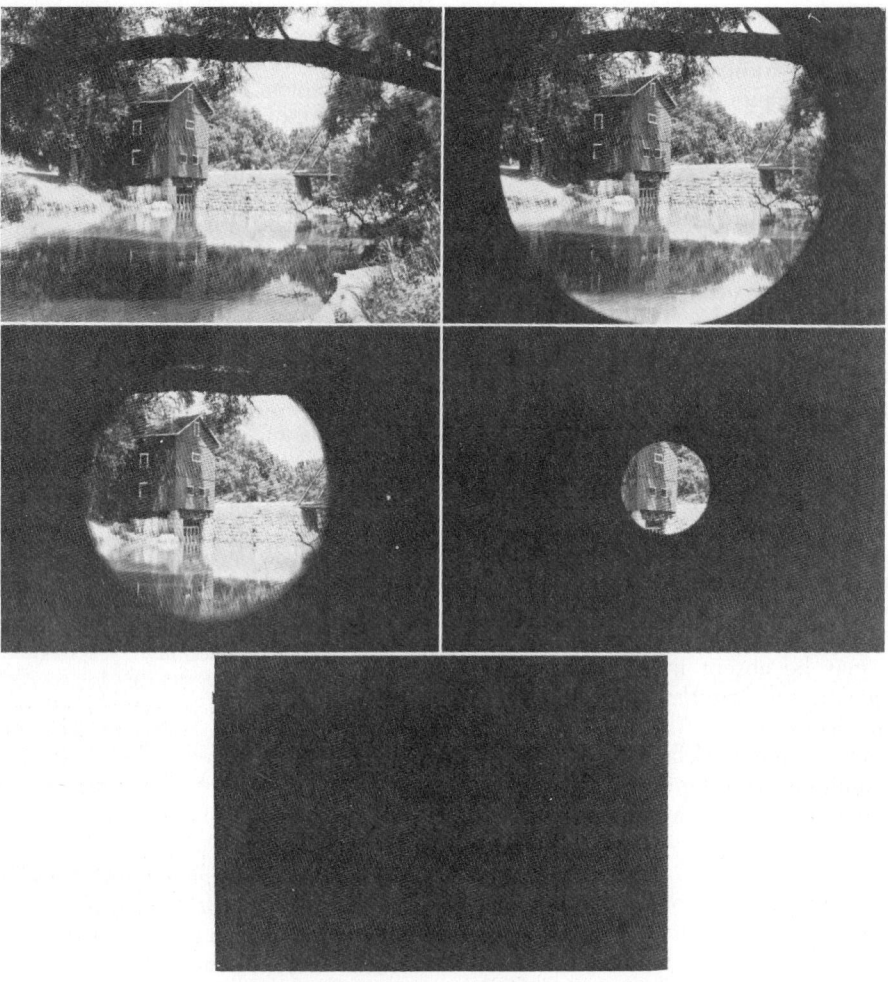

Fig. 30-7   Gradual loss of sight from glaucoma so insidiously destroys vision that person is unaware of impending blindness until extensive and irreversible damage is already present. (From Saunders WH, et al: *Nursing care in eye, ear, nose, and throat disorders*, ed 4, St Louis, 1979, Mosby–Year Book.)

and adjacent canals.[38] Degenerative changes in the optic nerve may also occur. Early signs are usually absent, but the disorder can be diagnosed by the increased IOP and the normal anterior chamber angle. The pressure may eventually lead to dull eye pain (Table 30-10).

Angle-closure (closed-angle) glaucoma

Closed-angle glaucoma usually occurs as an acute episode, although it may be subacute or chronic. It is termed angle-closure because the anterior chamber is anatomically narrow allowing the iris to be pushed forward, adhering to the trabecular meshwork and impeding aqueous humor flow to the canal of Schlemm. The forward movement of the iris may result from increased vitreous pressure, buildup of fluid in the posterior chamber, or thickening of the lens with age. Intraocular pressure is normal when the angle is narrow but open and the drainage is not blocked. Symptoms result from sudden closure, with an increase in IOP, and include severe eye pain, blurred vision, and halos seen around lights. The adhered iris produces a dilated pupil. If untreated, a blind painful eye results.

Nursing Process
Assessment

Subjective data

Subjective data include the following:
1. Assess discomfort
   a. Eye pain: dull, severe
   b. Headache: severity
   c. Nausea and vomiting
2. Assess report of halos around lights

Objective data

Objective data include the following:
1. Vision: note changes
   a. Visual acuity: Snellen chart if available, reading distant signs, close reading
   b. Visual fields: confrontation test (p. 923)

Diagnostic tests

Intraocular pressure is measured by means of *tonometry.* In an ophthalmology clinic, an applanation tonometer is generally used. With the use of a slit lamp, a small area of

Table 30-10 Types of glaucoma

Type	Characteristic	Signs and symptoms	Medical therapy
Primary			
Open-angle (chronic, simple)	Most common type (90%) Usually caused by obstruction in trabecular meshwork	Frequently no signs or symptoms in early stages Slow loss of vision Peripheral vision lost before central Tunnel vision Persistent dull eye pain Difficulty adjusting to darkness failure to detect colour changes Later: headache, pain, blurred vision, halos around lights	Medical: miotics, beta-blockers, carbonic anhydrase inhibitors Surgical: trabeculectomy, trabeculoplasty
Angle-closure (narrow-angle, acute)	Outflow impaired as result of narrowing or closing of angle between iris and cornea Intermittent attacks, pressure normal when angle open; if persistent, acute ocular emergency	Acute: severe prostrating pain, decreased vision, pupil enlarged and fixed, coloured halos around lights, eye red, steamy cornea Permanent blindness if marked increase in IOP for 24-48 hours	Medical: osmotic diuretics, carbonic anhydrase inhibitors, miotics Surgical: peripheral iridectomy, iridotomy
Congenital	Abnormal development of filtration angle Can occur secondary to other systemic eye disorders Rare (0.05%)	Enlargement of eye, lacrimation, photophobia, blepharospasm	Goniotomy (incision into region of trabecular meshwork) Trabeculotomy
Secondary	Can result from ocular inflammation, blood vessel changes, trauma	May be similar to open-angle and angle-closure, depending on cause	Directed at cause as well as at decreasing IOP

the cornea is flattened to counterbalance a spring-loaded measuring device that measures the pressure. A less accurate direct method, but useful because the instrument is cheaper and portable, is the Schiøtz tonometer. The eye is anaesthetized and the tonometer is placed directly on the cornea. The amount of indentation that the instrument plunger makes on the cornea is measured on the attached scale. Noncontact tonometers measure IOP by deformation of light reflex from the cornea from a puff of air.[28] Readings greater than 24 mm Hg may suggest glaucoma.

The anterior chamber angle can be visualized using a contact lens and special lens (*gonioscopy*). This technique distinguishes open-angle from closed-angle glaucoma. Visualization of the optic disc by ophthalmoscopy will show cupping of the disc; visual field testing may show decreased peripheral vision.

Nursing analysis

Problems are determined from analysis of patient data. Possible problems for the person with glaucoma may include, but are not limited to, the following:

Problem	Possible aetiologies
Health maintenance, altered	Impairment in vision, difficulty in doing ADL independently
Knowledge deficit about glaucoma	Unfamiliarity with information resources
Pain	Increased IOP
Sensory/perceptual alteration: visual	Altered sensory reception/transmission

Planning: expected patient outcomes

Expected patient outcomes for the person with glaucoma may include, but are not limited to, the following:

1. Vision is not decreased further.
2. Patient is able to perform ADL more independently.
3. Patient can state recognition of lifetime need for eye medication.
4. Patient can state name, dosage, frequency, and side effects of prescribed eye medications.
5. Patient can describe measures to prevent complications.
6. Patient can list signs or symptoms indicating need to report immediately to ophthalmologist.
7. Patient states discomfort is decreased.
8. Patient can walk independently.

Implementation

Assisting with achievement of therapeutic goals
Medications

It is vital in the control of glaucoma that eye medications be given as prescribed. The purpose of pharmacological therapy is to keep the pupil constricted to permit better drainage of the aqueous humor and to decrease the amount of aqueous humor produced.

Pilocarpine is the miotic drug of choice in the treatment of open-angle glaucoma. Pilocarpine may be given in solution (eye drops) or by modified-release delivery system (Ocusert). The Ocusert is placed in the upper or lower conjunctival sac, preferably at night so the miotic effect reaches a stable level by morning; the effect lasts for 1 week. Miotics frequently decrease vision for 1 to 2 hours after instillation and may cause eye spasms in younger people.

Beta-adrenergic blocking agents can be used alone or in combination with other drugs, and include tetaxolol, carteolol, levobunolol, metipranolol and timoptol. Pressing the lacrimal duct for 1 minute after insertion of eye drops helps to prevent rapid systemic side effects.

In severe acute conditions, osmotic agents are given to lower the IOP by drawing fluid from the eye. If the oral osmotic agent is ineffective or produces nausea, mannitol is given intravenously.

Mydriatics and cycloplegic agents are *contraindicated* in people with glaucoma because these drugs may further restrict drainage of aqueous humor.

Surgery

Surgical intervention is indicated when conservative treatment fails to control the IOP. Two common procedures are trabeculoplasty and trabeculectomy. *Trabeculoplasty is the application of a laser beam (argon) on the trabecular meshwork. This produces a nonpenetrating thermal burn that changes the configuration of the meshwork and leads to increased outflow of aqueous humor. Trabeculectomy is a filtering procedure in which an opening or fistula is made at the limbus under a partial-thickness scleral flap.* The new opening circumvents the obstruction and aqueous humor flows into the subconjunctival spaces.

Trabeculectomy usually requires overnight hospitalization. *Trabeculoplasty,* however, is frequently performed as a day case, and the person usually remains for 3 to 4 hours following the procedure so that the IOP can be checked. A complication of the procedure is a sudden rise in the IOP immediately after surgery. It takes 4 to 8 weeks to see if the procedure is effective. However, glaucoma medications usually must be continued.

Postoperative care

Nursing care for the patient following *trabeculectomy* includes:
1. Routine postanaesthesia care
2. Protection of operative eye with patch, shield, positioning patient on back or unoperative side, and safety measures such as cot sides
3. Maintaining comfort in the operative eye
4. Assessment, as appropriate, of the IOP, appearance of the bleb, and anterior chamber depth
5. Administration of medications such as a cycloplegic, a mydriatic, and a combination antibiotic and steroid

Interventions to achieve patient outcomes
Monitoring health maintenance

As the patient adjusts to visual changes, he or she may need assistance with activities of daily living. The patient will also need to learn how to modify his or her daily activities so that they can be performed safely and independently.

Assisting with comfort

Pain usually decreases as the IOP decreases. Analgesics may be prescribed. Cold eye compresses may be helpful for painful eye spasms.

Facilitating learning

Glaucoma is a chronic condition, and the patient with newly diagnosed glaucoma needs assistance in understanding and learning to live with the disease. Despite explanations from the doctor, the person frequently hopes that an operation will provide a cure, that no further treatment will be necessary, and perhaps that the lost sight will be restored. *It should be explained that lost vision cannot be restored but that further loss can usually be prevented and normal activities can be pursued if the person continues medical care.* There usually is no restriction on the use of the eyes (see Box 30-9 for teaching guidelines).

Evaluation

Evaluation is based on the expected patient outcomes. Questions to ask include the following:
1. Can the patient perform ADL independently?
2. Does the patient know the chronic nature of the disease and treatment?
3. Does the patient understand the need for lifetime eye medication?
4. Can the patient state name, dosage and so on of prescribed medications?
5. Can the patient describe how to avoid complications?
6. Can the patient state signs and symptoms that need to be reported to the ophthalmologist?
7. Is the patient comfortable?
8. Can the patient walk independently?

30-9

Patient Teaching

The patient with glaucoma

1. Medical follow-up and eye medication will be required for the rest of life.
2. Eye drops *must* be continued as long as prescribed, even in the absence of symptoms
   a. Blurred vision decreases with prolonged use
   b. Avoid driving for 1 to 2 hours after administration of miotics.
3. To prevent complications:
   a. Press lacrimal duct for 1 minute after eye drop insertion to prevent rapid systemic absorption
   b. Keep reserve bottle of eye drops at home
   c. Carry eye drops on person (not in luggage) when travelling.
   d. Carry card or wear Medic-Alert bracelet identifying glaucoma and the eye drops solution prescribed.
4. Bright lights and darkness are not harmful.
5. There is no apparent relationship between vascular hypertension and ocular hypertension.
6. Report any reappearance of symptoms immediately to ophthalmologist.
7. If admitted to hospital for a different medical condition, alert the staff of continued need for prescribed eye drops.
8. Avoid the use of mydriatic or cycloplegic drugs (for example, atropine) that dilate the pupils.

Person with open-angle glaucoma

DATA: Mr. M. is a 76-year-old man with a history of open-angle glaucoma. His peripheral vision is markedly decreased. He was admitted for prostate surgery, but his primary nurse elicited the following information during the admission history: he has prescribed eye drops (pilocarpine 1% 4 times/day, timolol 0.5% twice daily) that he uses periodically. He states the drops blur his vision. He knows that his "eye pressure is high" but says he thinks it's getting better because his eyes don't bother him. His wife notes that he bumps into objects more frequently.

Nursing analysis: Knowledge deficit: related to lack of recall and misinterpretation of information

Expected patient outcomes	Nursing interventions	Rationale
Mr. M. describes chronic nature of glaucoma and need for continued treatment	Ask Mr. M. to explain understanding of glaucoma: What it is Result if untreated Symptoms to be reported Need for medical follow-up	Start teaching at Mr. M.'s level of knowledge. Because glaucoma is a chronic condition, he needs to know the effects of nontreatment (painful blind eye) and how to prevent it
Mr. M. states symptoms requiring reporting to doctor	Teach him about glaucoma and need for lifetime eye medication	
Mr. M. or wife demonstrates correct instillation of eye drops	Ask him or wife to demonstrate instilling eye drops; correct his technique as necessary	If his vision is decreasing, he may be having difficulty instilling his eyedrops and wife will do it for him

Nursing analysis: Noncompliance with medications: related to drug side effects and lack of knowledge about need for lifetime medication

Expected patient outcomes	Nursing interventions	Rationale
Mr. M. states plans to use eye drops at correct times	Explore other reasons for not using eye drops	Mr. M. may have difficulty reading the labels or remembering
	Ask Mr. M.'s wife to bring in the eye drop bottles and role play with him use of bottles and how to remember to use the eye drops	Role playing will help to identify problems he may be having reading the labels
	Enlist him and his wife in developing a plan to help remember how and when to take the eye drops (such as after meals and at bedtime)	Mrs. M. participation in planning ensures greater probability of carrying out plan; connecting of carrying out plan; connecting the eye drops with an activity helps the person remember
	Explain relationship of blurred vision with pilocarpine; suggest he consult doctor and not plan specific activities for about 1 hr after instilling eye drops	Blurred vision is a side effect of pilocarpine; it usually improves in 1 to 2 hrs

Nursing analysis: Injury, high risk for: related to decreased peripheral vision

Expected patient outcomes	Nursing interventions	Rationale
Mr. M. describes measures to prevent injury	Explain nature of decreased peripheral vision and relate it to bumping into objects	Knowledge of rationale may increase probability of actions to prevent injury
	Suggest Mr. M. turn head to see each side	Increases field of vision
	Suggest couple consider clearing wider walk areas in living quarters	Reducing clutter will decrease chance of falls, and injury caused by bumping into things
	Suggest that Mr. M. consider the whole question of driving	Loss of peripheral vision makes Mr. M. less aware of vehicles approaching from side

RETINAL DETACHMENT
Aetiology and Pathophysiology

The retina is the part of the eye that perceives light; it coordinates and transmits impulses from receptor nerve cells to the optic nerve. It consists of two layers. Retinal detachment occurs when the two retinal layers separate as a result of accumulation of fluid or traction produced by contraction of the vitreous body. As the detachment extends and becomes complete, blindness results. Myopic degeneration, trauma, and aphakia (absence of the crystalline lens) are the most frequent causes of retinal detachment. Detachment may follow sudden severe physical exertion, especially in people who are debilitated. Most often, however, there is no apparent cause. Retinal detachment may occur suddenly or develop slowly.

Nursing Process
Assessment

Subjective and *objective* data include the following: The person first notices flashes of light, followed by floating spots before the eye and progressive loss of vision. The floating spots are blood and retinal cells that are freed at the time of the tear and cast shadows on the retina as they seem to drift about the eye. The area of visual loss depends entirely on the location of the detachment. Usually there is a superior retinal detachment and inferior visual loss. When the detachment is extensive and occurs quickly, the patient may have the sensation that a curtain has been drawn before the eyes. The diagnosis is confirmed by ophthalmoscopic appearance of the retina.

Ongoing nursing assessment includes the patient's subjective statements concerning changes in vision and observations related to signs of anxiety. The person with both eyes covered is assessed for ability to carry out activities of daily living.

Nursing analysis

Problems are determined from analysis of patient data. Possible problems for the person with retinal detachment may include, but are not limited to, the following:

Problem	Possible aetiologies
Anxiety	Threat of loss of vision, threat to self-concept, threat of change in role functioning
Injury, high risk for	Sensory deficit, lack of awareness of environmental hazards
Knowledge deficit regarding condition, surgery, preoperative and postoperative care, and self care at home	Lack of experience with retinal detachment and its treatment
Pain	Inflammation, increased IOP
Sensory/perceptual alteration, visual	Altered sensory reception/transmission

Planning: expected patient outcomes

Expected patient outcomes for the person with retinal detachment may include, but are not limited to, the following:

1. Anxiety is decreased.
2. No further vision loss occurs.
3. No injuries occur.
4. Patient can describe
   a. Correct use of eye medications
   b. Signs and symptoms indicating further retinal detachment and for immediate medical care
   c. Plans for dealing with limitation of activity.
5. Patient states pain is absent or improved.
6. Patient adjusts to alteration in vision by walking independently.

Implementation preoperatively
Assisting with achievement of therapeutic goals
Promoting eye rest

Immediate care for the person with detachment of the retina includes keeping the eye at rest and in position to prevent further detachment until surgery can be performed to repair the detachment. Bed rest with monocular or bilateral eye patches is usually prescribed. The head is positioned so the retinal hole is in the most dependent position (gravity may help prevent the first retinal layer from pulling further away from the second coat).

Although most surgeons do not use binocular patches, some do patch both eyes preoperatively and for 2 or 3 days postoperatively. Safety precautions, such as cot sides, are essential if binocular patching is used. Call signals are placed within easy patient reach. Activities that facilitate communication with blind people are employed.

Providing emotional support

Anxiety frequently results from concern over possible loss of vision and feelings about having eyes bandaged. Generally, the person has lost vision rapidly and is afraid of losing more vision. Patients need an opportunity to discuss their concerns. Although the promise of restoration of vision cannot be made, it can be comforting to the person to know that with care most retinal detachments can be repaired by surgery.

Retinal surgery

Intraoperative care. Surgery may be performed under either local or general anaesthesia. Cyclopentolate or phenylephrine is used to keep the pupils widely dilated so that tears in the retina may be identified during the operation. The surgical procedure may include draining the fluid from the subretinal space so that the retina returns to its normal position, thereby closing the opening in the retina. To drain the fluid from the subretinal space, the sclera and choroid are perforated at the time of the operation.

The retinal breaks are sealed off by various methods that produce an inflammatory reaction (*chorioretinitis*) in the area of the tear so that adhesions will form between the edges of the break and the underlying choroid to obliterate the opening. When the retinal tears are small or of recent origin, diathermy may be applied through the sclera with needlepoint electrodes to produce the inflammatory process. An intense beam of visible light directed to the area by means of an elaborate ophthalmoscope may be used to close a retinal tear when the retina is not elevated (*photocoagulation*). The *laser beam* is used by some surgeons as a source of intense energy to produce chorioretinitis. Subfreezing temperatures (-40° to -60° C) may be applied to the surface of the sclera in the area of the hole to produce the inflammatory reaction (cryo-therapy). Nitrous oxide or carbon dioxide under pressure, flowing through a tube attached to a delicate instrument, is used to produce these low temperatures.

For some retinal detachments, *scleral buckling* procedures are used. In this procedure, the sclera and choroid are indented (buckled) towards the retinal break. Buckling is accomplished by placing silicone of various shapes and sizes in the region of the break. In addition an encircling tape of silicone can be placed around the entire eye. By these procedures, the choroid is pushed into contact with the retinal tear during healing, and vitreous adhesions that have exerted traction, or pull, on the retinal break are relaxed as the size of the scleral shell is decreased.

Postoperative care. The postoperative care for the person with retinal detachment includes the following:
1. Position and ambulate the patient as ordered.
2. Assist with activities of daily living, as required.
3. Administer eye medications as ordered (mydriatics, cycloplegics, and combination steroid/antibiotic).
4. Apply cold compresses as ordered to reduce swelling and promote comfort.
5. Implement safety measures such as cot sides.
6. Instruct the patient to avoid jerking motions of the head (sneezing, coughing, vomiting).
   a. Administer antiemetics, as required.
   b. Administer cough medication, as required.

Implementation postoperatively
Interventions to achieve patient outcomes
Promoting safety

As mentioned earlier, most surgeons do not patch both eyes (binocular), some do patch both eyes preoperatively and for 2 or 3 days postoperatively. Safety precautions such as cot sides are essential if binocular patching is used. Call signals need to be kept within reach. Explanation of the immediate environment is also indicated. Everyone entering the room of the patient with both eyes patched should call out the patient's name to announce their presence and introduce themselves. Failure to do so can make the patient very anxious because he or she can usually sense that someone is in the room though they can't see them.

Facilitating coping

Patients are usually anxious and apprehensive when admitted to the hospital. Generally there has been a rapid loss of vision, and patients fear losing more vision. Restoration of sight will depend on the extent and duration of the detachment and the success of the surgery. Opportunity to discuss concerns needs to be provided. The nurse caring for the patient should plan time to sit down and listen to the patient's concerns. Nurses can do much to allay apprehension by answering questions honestly and instilling realistic hope.

Facilitating learning

Patient teaching for people with retinal detachment includes:
1. Report to ophthalmologist any signs of redetachment (increase in floaters, flashes of light, decreased vision).
2. Use appropriate techniques for administration of eye medications.
3. Limit activities to sedentary work for 1 to 2 weeks.
4. Check with doctor about resumption of activities such as active sports or heavy lifting.
5. Discuss plan for medical follow-up (appointment with ophthalmologist and so on).

Evaluation

Evaluation is based on expected patient outcomes. Questions to consider may include the following:
1. Has patient had opportunities to express concerns?
2. Has further detachment been avoided?
3. Has injury been avoided?
4. Does patient know expectations after discharge?
5. Is patient comfortable?
6. Is the patient able to move about independently?

SUMMARY

1. Eye safety measures include early medical care of eye problems, avoidance of use of previously prescribed eye medications, protecting eyes against foreign objects or bright lights, and removing nonembedded foreign objects immediately by rinsing with water or by carefully removing from the conjunctival sac.
2. Activities for the newly blind person consist of facilitating their independence in ADL and providing counselling to facilitate coping.
3. Inflammation of the eye can occur in the external structures, cornea, and uvea (iris, ciliary body, and choroid); the most common inflammations are styes and conjunctivitis.
4. Treatments for eye inflammations include eye compresses, eye irrigations, and ophthalmic antibiotics (steroids may be given for allergic but not pyogenic inflammations).
5. If the cornea becomes damaged, corneal grafts (keratoplasty) may be performed using donor corneal tissue.
6. A cataract is an opacity of the lens. A cataract that interferes with vision may be removed either extracapsularly (leaving the posterior capsule intact) or intracapsularly (lens and entire capsule). Many people now have an intraocular lens implanted at the time of surgery.
7. Much eye surgery is performed as day surgery. Preoperative care includes insertion of mydriatic or cycloplegic (dilates pupil and relaxes ciliary muscle) and local anaesthetic eye drops.
8. Postoperative care centres on preventing increased IOP, stress on the suture line, haemorrhage into the anterior chamber, and infection.
9. The characteristic sign of glaucoma is increased IOP. Most glaucomas are of the primary open-angle type in

which aqueous outflow is blocked because of degenerative changes in the trabecular meshwork, canal of Schlemm, and adjacent channels; the disorder is insidious in onset, slowly progressive, and usually lacks symptoms in the early stage.

10. Closed-angle glaucoma occurs in a person with a narrow anterior chamber when the iris falls forward, blocking entrance to aqueous fluid outflow; it is often sudden in onset and requires immediate medical attention; symptoms include severe eye pain, blurred vision, and halos seen around lights.

11. People with glaucoma require continued treatment for life to prevent buildup of IOP; lost vision cannot be restored.

12. Retinal detachment results when the two retinal layers separate, interfering with vision; symptoms include flashes of light, floating spots before the eye, and progressive loss of vision. People with retinal detachment require immediate medical treatment.

13. Surgery is performed to return the retina to its original position and adhere the first layer to the bottom layer by means of an inflammatory process. Postoperative care includes avoiding jerking movements of the head and limiting exertional activities until healing has occurred; eye drops are required during this period to rest the eye and prevent infection.

STUDY QUESTIONS

- Examine the drug chart of a patient with an eye problem. Explain the rationale for the drug therapy.
- Write a care plan for a patient with limited vision. How would a care plan for a person who has recent loss of vision compare with that of a person blinded from childhood?
- Consider bandaging your eyes for one day and carry out all your usual activities. What problems did you encounter? What did you find helpful?
- Describe how you would respond to a person who says, "I don't see as well as I used to. I don't have to go to an optician; he'll only tell me I need glasses, and I already have a pair."
- What services and facilities are available to people in your community who have limited vision? How are these financed?
- Pretend for 2 days that you have had eye surgery and are instructed not to bend at the waist or lift any heavy objects or to strain with any activity. What problems did you encounter? Now consider that your knees are crippled with arthritis: how would that affect an activity such as putting on tights, given the same restrictions?

REFERENCES AND SELECTED READINGS

1. American Foundation for the Blind: *directory of services for the blind and visually impaired in the US*, ed 23, New York, 1988, The Foundation.
2. Arentsen JJ: The dry eye, *J Ophthal Nurs Technol* 6:134-137, 1987.
3. Bentz LN: Caring for and communicating with blind and visually impaired persons, *J Visual Impair Blindness* 81:472-481, 1987.
4. Binder PS: Ophthalmology, *JAMA* 265(23):3143-3144, 1991.
5. Bishop VE: Visually handicapped people and the law, *J Visual Impair Blindness* 81:53-58, 1987.
6. Bocking H et al: Artificial eyes, *Nurs Times* 86(8):40-41, 1990.
7.* Boruchoff SA: Ophthalmic surgery: risks and benefits, *Emerg Med* 19(11):59-62, 1987.
8.* Boyd-Monk H: Eye trauma in the workplace, *AAOHN J* 38(10):487-491, 1990.
9. Boyd-Monk H, Steinmetz CG: *Nursing care of the eye*, Norwalk, Conn, 1987, Appleton & Lange.
10.* Boyd-Monk H, Starita RJ: Surgical intervention to stop glaucoma, *JONT*, 4(3):12-15, 1985.
11. Capeno D et al: The elderly patient with cataracts, *Hosp Pract* 22(3):19-24, 1987.
12.* Carver JA: Cataract care made plain, *Am J Nurs* 87:626-630, 1987.
13. Contact lens allergy: the new conjunctivitis, *Am J Nurs* 87:11-12, 1987.
14. Danyluk AW, Paton D: Diagnosis and management of glaucoma, *Clin Symp* 43(4):2-32, 1991.
15.* DeBlase R et al: Postintraocular lens implants, *Geriatr Nurs* 9(6):342-343, 1988.
16.* Ehrenberg M: Blindness prevention, *AAOHN J* 35-243-245, 1987.
17. Frank A, Werfel N: ECCE with pharmacoemulsion, *J Ophthalmic Nurs Technol* 5:103-105, 1986.
18. Gottsch JD et al: Cataracts: diagnosis and treatment, *Hosp Med* (suppl) 23(4):21-29, 1987.
19. Hamrick S et al: Therapeutic ultrasound, *AORN J* 47:950-960, 1988.
20. Healthy People 2000 National Health Promotion and Disease Prevention Objectives, U.S. Department of Health and Human Services, Public Health Service, Washington D.C., 1990.
21. Javitt JC et al: Undertreatment of glaucoma among black Americans, *N Engl J Med* 325(20):1418-1422, 1991.
22. Karb VK, Queener SF, Freeman JB: *Handbook of drugs for nursing practice*, St Louis, 1989, Mosby–Year Book.
23. Lawlor MC: Common ocular injuries and disorders, *J Emerg Nurs* 15(1):36-43, 1989.
24.* Lent-Wunderlich E et al: Helping your patient through eye surgery, *RN* 49(6):43-47, 1986.
25. Lindstrom RL: Advances in corneal transplantation, *N Engl J Med* 315(1):57-59, 1986.
26. Mason G et al: Postanesthesia care of the ophthalmic patient, *J Post Anesth Nurs* 1:23-25, 1986.
27.* Misuse of steroid eye medications, Nurses' Drug Alert, *Am J Nurs* 87:71-1987.
28. Newell F: *Ophthalmology: principles and practice*, ed 7, St. Louis, 1992, Mosby–Year Book.
29. Nowell P: Lasers in ophthalmology, *Nurs Clin J North Am* 25(3):635-643, 1990.
30. Pasby T: Eye injuries in sports, *J Ophthalmic Nurs Technol* 8:99-101, 1989.
31. Seddon JM: The differential burden of blindness in the United States, *N Engl J Med* 325(20):1440-1442, 1991.
32. Shingleton JF: Eye injuries, *N Engl J Med* 325(6):408-413, 1991.
33.* Smith S: Day-care cataract surgery: the patient's perspective, *J Ophthalmic Nurs Technol* 6(2):50-56, 1987.
34. Soll DB et al: Drugs and glaucoma, *Am Fam Physician* 34(1):181-185, 1986.
35. Spencer RE: Transitions, being blind in a sighted world, *J Ophthalmic Nurs Technol* 7:220-222, 1988.
36. Traynar M: Day care eye surgery, *Nurs Time* 86(39):54-56, 1990.
37.* Tooke MC, Elders J, Johnson DE: Corneal transplantation, *Am J Nurs* 86:685-687, 1986.
38. Vaughan D, Asbury T: *General ophthalmology*, ed 11, Los Altos, Calif, 1986, Lange Medical Publications.

FURTHER READING

Burns E, Mulley GP: Practical problems with eye-drops among elderly ophthalmology outpatients, *Age and Ageing* 21 (3):168-170, 1992.
Dobree JH, Boulter E: *Blindness and visual handicap: The facts*, Oxford, 1982, Oxford University Press.
Dobson F, Dobson M: Eye Contact, *Nursing Times* 89(30):26-29, 1993.
Smith H: Day-Release Cataracts, *Nursing Times* 89(39):29-33, 1993.

*Suggested for student reading.

31

The Patient with Ear Problems

Wilma J. Phipps

After studying this chapter, the learner should be able to:

- Describe the mechanics of sound waves and hearing.
- Describe measures to prevent hearing loss.
- Describe the pathophysiology and nursing requirements for people with ear infections.
- Describe the pathophysiology and care of the person with a balance disorder.
- Describe care of the person having ear surgery.
- Differentiate between conductive and sensorineural hearing loss.
- Describe methods of assessment for conductive and sensorineural hearing loss.
- Describe methods of aural rehabilitation and communication with hearing impaired people.

The ear is the organ of hearing and equilibrium. Sound reaches the inner ear where it is converted to neural activity and transmitted to the brain for interpretation. Interference with this process leads to impaired hearing. In addition, structures in the inner ear maintain an individual's sense of equilibrium; interference with this mechanism leads to vertigo, producing dizziness and loss of balance.

The root word for the ear is *oto-*, such as in *otology* (science of the ear) or *otosclerosis* ("hardening of the ear"). In some instances the second "o" is dropped, such as in *otitis* (inflammation of the ear).

Nurses are involved primarily in prevention and detection of hearing and vestibular disorders. In addition, nurses participate in health teaching for hearing-impaired people, in facilitating communication when hearing-impaired people are hospitalized, and in providing care for persons receiving treatment for disorders of the ear.

ANATOMY AND PHYSIOLOGY

The ears are normally placed on each side of the head at eye level; an imaginary line parallel to the floor can be drawn from the outer canthus of the eye to the top of the outer ear. A lower placed ear may indicate chromosomal or congenital renal abnormalities. The ears are located in the temporal bone, which provides protection for the organs of hearing and equilibrium. Each ear is divided into the following parts: the external ear, the middle ear and mastoid, and the inner ear.

External Ear

The external ear consists of two parts, the pinna (auricle) and the external auditory canal. The *pinna* is composed primarily of cartilage and skin with little subcutaneous fat except for the lobule (lower tip). The external ear is innervated by cranial nerve V (trigeminal), a branch of cranial nerve X (vagus), and cervical nerves.

The ear canal provides a channel along which sound travels to the eardrum. The canal is an S-shaped curve about 2.5 cm (1 inch) long through the temporal bone in an inward, forward, and downward slope in an adult. There are constrictions in the canal close to the midpoint and the eardrum. The canal and outer ear drum are covered by thin sensitive skin. Numerous fine hairs protect the canal from foreign debris, and sebaceous glands in the distal third of the canal provide cerumen (wax) for lubrication.

The *tympanic membrane* (eardrum) separates the external ear from the middle ear. The eardrum is a thin, tough, translucent membrane, nearly oval in shape and directed obliquely downward. The malleus ossicle of the middle ear generally can be seen through the membrane. The tympanic membrane protects the middle ear and vibrates with incoming sound waves for hearing.

Middle Ear

The middle ear lies directly behind the eardrum and is a small air-filled space located in the petrous portion of the temporal bone (towards the face). It contains the ossicles, oval and round windows, and the pharyngotympanic tube

(eustachian or auditory tube) (Fig. 35-1). The *ossicles* are three movable small bones that transverse the middle ear; these three bones are called the *malleus* (hammer), *incus* (anvil), and *stapes* (stirrup) because of their shapes. The malleus is attached at one end to the tympanic membrane and at the other end to the incus. The incus is connected to the *stapes which is fixed in the oval window*. The stapes is in direct contact with the perilymph of the inner ear. The ossicles mechanically transmit sound vibrations to the fluid in the inner ear. The *oval window* is not a true window because it is covered by the footplate of the stapes. The *round window* located beneath the oval window provides an exit for sound vibrations from the inner ear.

The pharyngotympanic tube is a channel extending from the middle ear into the nasopharynx. It allows air to enter and leave the middle ear to equalize pressure on both sides of the eardrum. Swallowing or yawning can move air in and out of the middle ear to change air pressure in the middle ear. Portions of the facial nerves that control movement of the face and supply taste to the tongue are located in the middle ear.

The *mastoid* portion of the temporal bone is located posterior to the external ear and includes the mastoid air cells and mastoid antrum (cavity) that connects to the middle ear. Because of this direct connection infection of the middle ear may lead to mastoiditis. The mastoid process is a conical-shaped portion of mastoid bone that protrudes behind the lower portion of the pinna. The mastoid assists the middle ear in adjusting to pressure changes and lightens the mastoid bone.

Inner Ear

The inner ear (labyrinth) contains both the organs for hearing (cochlea) and the organs of balance (semicircular canals and vestibule) (Fig. 31-2). The bony labyrinth is a rigid capsule. The membranous labyrinth (consisting of three semicircular canals, vestibule, and cochlea) lies within the bony labyrinth but does not completely fill it. Position and balance are maintained by the semicircular canals (rotational movement) and by the membranous utricle and saccule in the vestibule (linear movements).

Two separate fluids are found in the labyrinth, the *perilymph* between the bony and membranous laybrinths and the *endolymph* within the membranous labyrinth. The endolymph is in a contained closed system; the perilymphatic spaces connect to the subarachnoid space containing cerebrospinal fluid.

The *cochlea* is a spiralling bony tube resembling a snail shell. The tube is separated into two compartments by a membranous tube called the *cochlear duct*, which contains endolymph and the organ of Corti. The two compartments of the cochlea contain perilymph; the upper compartment (scala vestibuli) leads from the oval window of the middle ear to the apex of the cochlea, and the lower compartment (scala tympani) from the apex of the cochlea to the round window to permit the sound vibrations to escape.

The organ of hearing, the *organ of Corti*, lies on the basilar membrane of the cochlear duct for its entire length. The organ of Corti has thousands of tiny "hair cells" that project into the endolymph; these hair cells are the most fragile elements in the inner ear and are crucial for hearing.

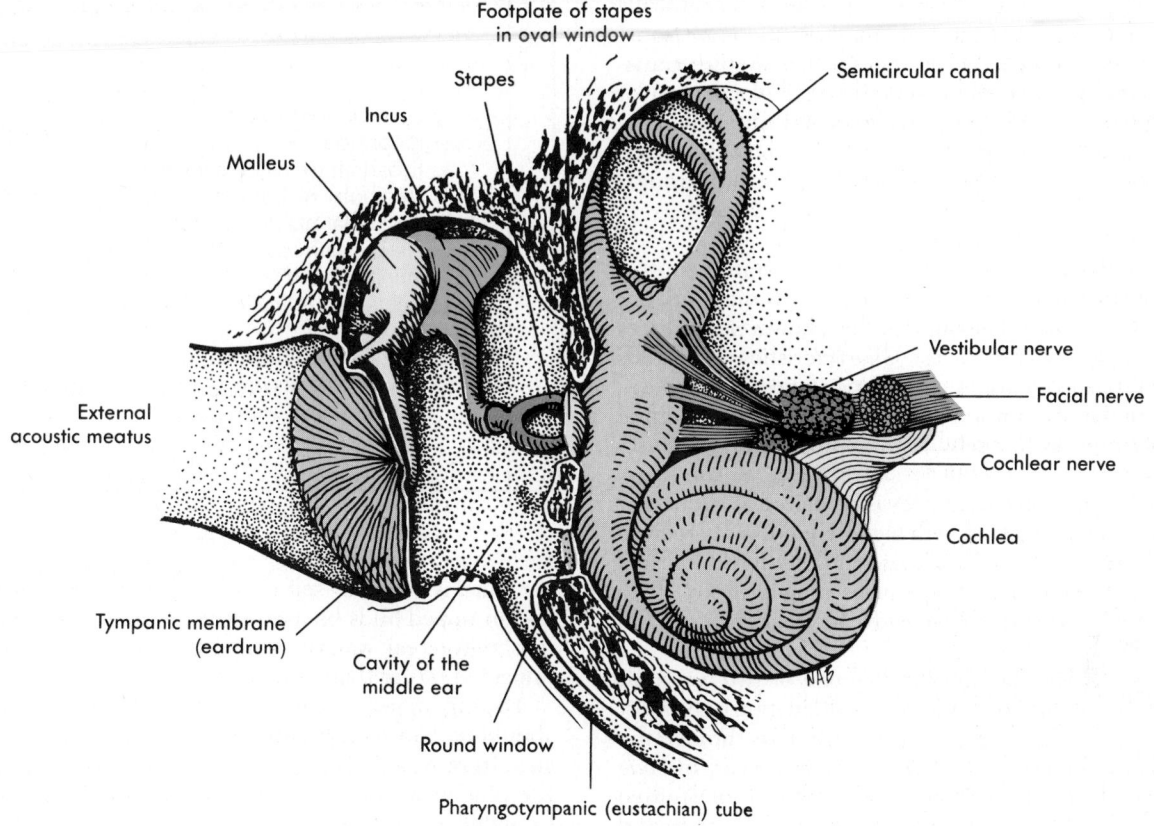

Fig. 31-1   Structures of the ear.

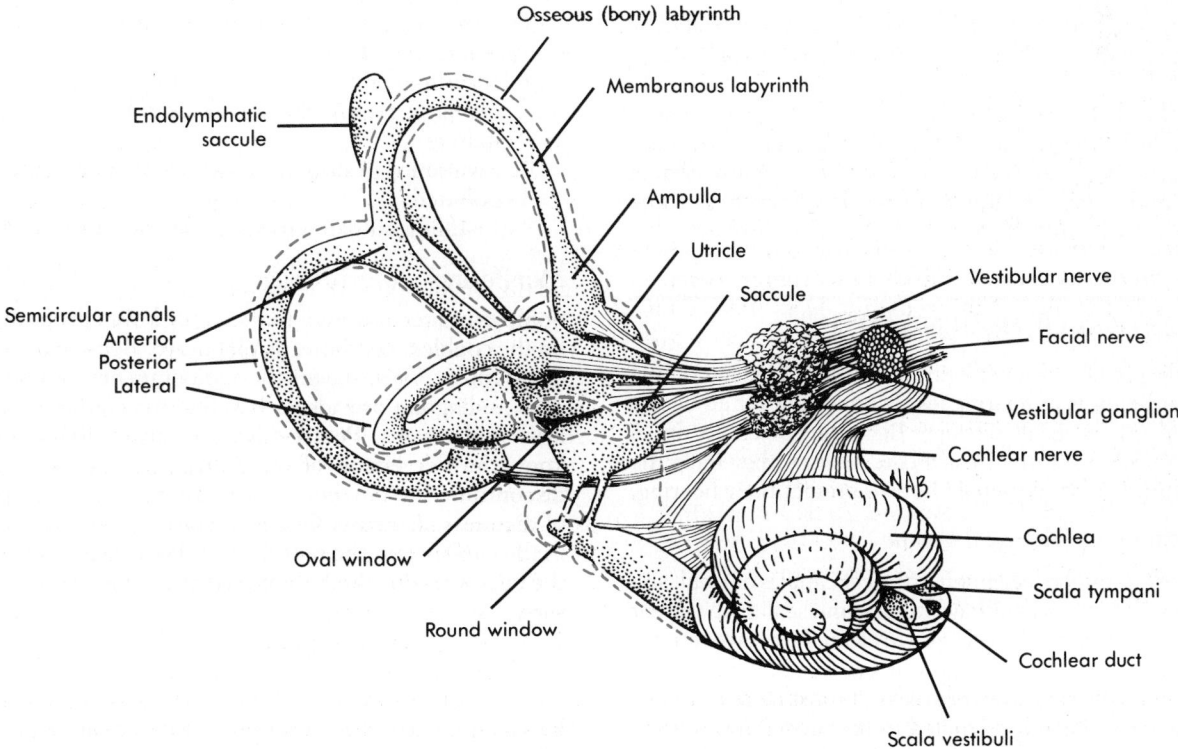

Fig. 31-2   Structures of the inner ear.

Sound waves enter the cochlear duct and mechanically bend the hair cells. Mechanical sound vibrations are transformed into electrochemical impulses that are then transmitted along the cranial nerve VIII (vestibulocochlear or acoustic nerve) to the temporal cortex of the brain and are interpreted as meaningful sound. Destruction of the vestibulocochlear nerve by a tumour leads to loss of hearing.

Sound Waves and Hearing

Sound is a form of energy generated by a vibrating source. Pure tones such as those generated by a tuning fork are simple sound waves. The human voice, however, produces more complex sound waves. Characteristics of sounds include intensity, loudness, frequency, and pitch.

Speech that is comfortably loud to a person with normal hearing ranges in intensity from approximately 40 to 65 decibels.

A sound with a low frequency is perceived as a tone low in pitch, whereas a sound with high frequency is perceived as a high-pitched tone. A child or young adult with normal hearing can often hear frequencies ranging from 20 to 20,000 Hz. Hearing is most sensitive for frequencies of 500 to 4000 Hz.

Sound reaches the inner ear by one of two ways: air conduction or bone conduction. Air conduction is the most sensitive. In air conduction sound waves pass through the ear canal to the ossicular chain to the inner ear. In *bone conduction* hearing is caused by sound being transmitted through the bones of the skull to the inner ear. Sound energy is transformed in the inner ear into neural energy and is then "decoded" and interpreted by the brain as sound.

Statokinetic System (Equilibrium)

Subjective orientation of the body in space is controlled by a complicated system that includes the structures listed in Box 31-1.

Of the structures listed in Box 31-1, the *end organ of equilibrium consists of* (1) the semicircular canals and utricle, (2) the vestibular division of the eighth cranial nerve, and (3) the vestibular nuclei. Together these three structures are referred to as the *statokinetic system.*[6]

PREVENTION OF HEARING LOSS

Hearing problems may begin at any age. Understanding the many causes of hearing loss is important for all health team members in all settings. Because nurses occupy a unique position in the health care system, they have the opportunity to teach people how to protect their hearing.

Preventing Ear Disease/Trauma

A certain amount of cerumen in the ear canal is normal, and people who have no wax have itching and scaling in the ear canal. Usually it is not necessary to clean the ears to remove wax. Occasionally, when the wax becomes impacted and causes pain or temporary deafness, it must be removed by the doctor or person instructed in the procedure.

The outer ear may be washed with soap and water during bathing, although this is often unnecessary as the

---

31-1

Structures involved in subjective orientation of the body in space[6]

1. Eye and eye muscles
2. Proprioceptive system
* 3. Labyrinth (semicircular canals) and utricle
* 4. Vestibular division of the eight cranial nerve
* 5. Vestibular nuclei and the brainstem
6. Neural pathways from vestibular nuclei to midbrain and temporal lobe
7. Central coordination mechanisms in the cerebellum
8. Vestibular spinal tract (posterior columns)
9. Afferent fibres coming from muscles and joints via the vestibular tract

*Make up end organ of equilibrium

---

ear canal is generally self-cleaning. On no account should cotton-tipped buds be used to clean the ears, particularly in children; ear wax is commonly pushed in further and impacted rather than removed.

During upper respiratory tract infections, the nose should be blown with both nostrils open. Excessive pressure from nose blowing can force infected secretions up the pharyngotympanic tube into the middle ear, leading to middle ear infection.

People having ear pain, swelling, drainage, prolonged feelings of blocked ears, or decreased hearing are referred to a doctor for treatment. *Chronic problems such as perforated ear drums and necrotic ossicles may result from inattention to early signs of ear disorders.*

The following activities may lead to ear infection or trauma and should be *avoided*:

1. Inserting foreign objects into the ear (such as a hard object to remove wax or to scratch the ear canal if itching)
2. Swimming in stagnant water or in water identified as polluted
3. Instilling outdated medicated solutions into the ear

Monitoring Ototoxic Drugs

Some drugs are ototoxic; that is, they have adverse effects on the cochlea, vestibule, or VIII nerve. Before an ototoxic drug is prescribed a diagnostic audiogram may be obtained. This audiogram provides a baseline for comparison with later audiograms. People taking ototoxic drugs need to know the side effects of these drugs so that they can be discontinued before they cause loss of hearing. If symptoms of dizziness, decreased hearing acuity, or tinnitus (ringing in the ears) occur, the next dose of the drug is omitted and the doctor is consulted. Audiometric testing may be necessary.

Monitoring Noise Pollution

A major cause of hearing loss is occupational exposure to hazardous noise levels. Exposure to *industrial noise* levels greater than 85 to 90 db for months or years causes cochlear damage. Nurses working in industry can help prevent deafness caused by noise of high intensity by teaching employees why they should wear earplugs or other protective ear devices. Courses are available to familiarize nurses with industrial hearing conservation requirements.

The Health and Safety Executive has established acceptable levels of noise in work environments. *Unprotected* exposure to noise levels in excess of 90 db over an 8-hour day is considered excessive and should be avoided.

If *proximity to the high noise level cannot be avoided, ear protectors or earplugs should be worn*. The earplugs are inserted into the external auditory canal and can reduce the noise reaching the middle ear by 10 to 30 db. Usually standard plugs are effective, but custom-made plugs moulded to the person's ear canal may be obtained. *If the noise level is extremely high (sound levels may reach 140 db or higher), individuals are not adequately protected with earplugs alone and must wear specially made ear muffs*. Ear muffs are commonly used by airport workers exposed to the noise of jet airplanes.

In people between the ages of 35 and 65, hearing loss is most commonly noise induced. Many millions of people are at increased risk because of occupational exposure to hazardous noise levels (factory, maintenance, and farm workers). In younger people, noise from amplified music and motorcycles can affect high-frequency hearing. It is important to educate people so that they understand that noise-induced hearing loss is often preventable and that once hearing is lost it cannot be regained.

Environmental exposure to noise in the workplace is monitored by the Occupational Health Departments and the Health and Safety Executive which sets acceptable levels of noise pollution. In occupations where excessive or prolonged noise is likely to occur, it is necessary to do regular audiometric testing of noise-exposed workers.

One in four workers exposed to 90 db and over for a working lifetime will develop a hearing impairment. Workers exposed to industrial noise may not show a hearing loss for as many as 10 years after initial exposure. The hearing loss results from progressive destruction of sensory cells in the ear. Once damaged, these cells can neither repair themselves nor be medically restored. Noise-induced hearing loss becomes more severe with continued exposure to noise.[10] In England, Scotland and Wales it is estimated that some 7.5 million (17%) adults have some hearing impairment.[17a] This may range from mild loss of hearing to total deafness. For the enormous number of people involved the impact of hearing loss on their ability to work, learn, communicate and enjoy life is a very significant consideration.

MAJOR HEALTH PROBLEMS OF THE EAR

Ear disorders may occur in any part of the ear. The more common ear disorders are discussed in this chapter under three headings because of the commonalities in the required care. Disorders included in each category are as follows:

1. Infections of the external/middle ear
   a. External otitis (otitis externa)
   b. Otitis media: serous, purulent (acute, chronic)
   c. Chronic mastoiditis
2. Disorders affecting balance
   a. Labyrinthitis
   b. Ménière's disease
   c. Acoustic neuroma
3. Disorders affecting hearing
   a. Conductive hearing loss: otosclerosis
   b. Sensorineural hearing loss
   c. Presbycusis

INFECTIONS OF THE EXTERNAL/MIDDLE EAR

The most common disorders of the external and middle ear are infections (Table 31-1). Although many of these infections occur in children, they may also occur in adults.

Aetiology and Pathophysiology

Organisms may enter the external ear by way of the external orifice or the middle ear via the pharyngotympanic tube, resulting in infections. Infection of the labyrinth (inner ear) may result from extension of middle ear infections, but the effect is primarily on balance (See Box 31-1).

Infections of the external ear, *external otitis*, are primarily bacterial (staphylococci or gram-negative organisms) or fungal. A form of seborrhoeic dermatitis (Chapter 34) may result from extensive use of objects such as earphones. Infection develops in the skin lining the ear canal, and swelling and debris may lead to closure of the canal. Furuncles (boils) may also develop. Pain results from pressure on the sensitive skin lining and can be severe because there is no room for expansion in the bony canal. *Activities leading to water retention in the ear such as swimming, especially in contaminated water, promote external otitis.*

Infection of the middle ear, *otitis media*, is the most common disorder of the middle ear. The infection may be serous or purulent and acute or chronic. *Serous otitis media develops from collection of sterile serum in the middle ear when the pharyngotympanic tube becomes blocked because of previous infection or allergy. Purulent otitis media* develops from bacterial infection and may be acute or chronic. Chronic infection may spread into the mastoid (chronic mastoiditis) or cause necrosis of the tympanic membrane or ossicles, leading to hearing loss. Acute mastoiditis is rare because of antibiotic treatment of acute otitis media. With chronic mastoiditis, a *cholesteatoma* (benign growth) may develop. It is a skin-lined sac with debris and is often infected. The cholesteatoma may recur when removed.

Nursing Process
Assessment

A person with an ear infection is usually diagnosed and treated as an outpatient. *Early detection and treatment are important to prevent development of chronic infections with subsequent loss of hearing.*

Subjective data

The major symptoms of external and middle ear infections are *pain* and *loss of hearing*, and data are collected about the onset, duration, and severity of these symptoms. *Pain results from pressure on the sensitive skin lining the external canal or pressure on the eardrum from fluid buildup in the middle ear.* Loss of hearing is the result of a blocked external canal or fluid in the middle ear that interferes with passage of sound waves. People with ear infections should be questioned about their knowledge of preventive measures.

Objective data

The external ear is inspected for signs of drainage, either serous or purulent. The auricle is also inspected for signs of redness, scaliness, and crusting. When assessing the external ear, manipulation of the ear is important. If the patient complains of pain when any part of the ear is palpated, a *furuncle*, *lesion*, or some kind of inflammatory process of *the ear canal* is *suspected.* Water in the ear canal from showering or swimming may aggravate the symptoms.

When an otoscopic (auriscopic) examination is performed, care must be taken not to cause the person unnecessary pain. A furuncle may be close to the opening of the canal, causing increased pain from the pressure of the speculum.

Otoscopic (auriscopic) examination of the external ear canal and eardrum

The eardrum is important in physical assessment of the ear because it serves as a translucent window through which disease processes in the middle ear can be inferred. The normal tympanic membrane has a wide range of coloured hues, the most common being pearly grey. Located in the membrane or seen through it are certain landmarks. For visualization of the external ear canal and eardrum, an otoscope (auriscope) is used; it has an ear piece (speculum) that can be placed into the ear canal, has illumination to visualize the eardrum, and may have magnification for a more accurate assessment. Otoscopy is performed by persons (including nurses) who are specially instructed in the use of an otoscope (auriscope).

Operating microscopic examination

The binocular-operating microscope is found in many ear, nose and throat departments. The speculum holds open the outermost portion of the external ear canal and allows the passage of both light and instruments. The appropriate speculum size for adults is from 4 to 7 mm in diameter. The microscope provides the examiner with excellent illumination, increased depth perception, and three-dimensional vision. Most operating microscopes allow changes in magnification to be made. Some nurses may be trained in the use of the microscope to distinguish normal from abnormal, remove cerumen, and suction drainage.

Nursing analysis

Problems are determined from analysis of patient data. Possible problems for the person with an external ear infection may include, but are not limited to, the following:

REVIEW
Table 31-1   Infections of the external/middle ear

Disorder	Description	Signs and symptoms	Medical therapy
External otitis	Inflammation of the external ear; may be acute or chronic	Pain with movement of auricle, redness, scaling, itching, swelling, watery discharge, crusting of external ear	Cleaning to remove debris; antibiotic drops or ointment, systemic antibiotics if necessary
Serous otitis media ("glue ear")	Collection of sterile serum in middle ear; may be acute or chronic	Sense of fullness in ear, hearing loss, low-pitched tinnitus, earache	Removal of pharyngotympanic obstruction by aspiration or insertion of tubes (grommets) for drainage
Acute purulent otitis media	Infection of middle ear, usually by pneumococci, streptococci, staphylococci, or *Haemophilus influenzae*	Sense of fullness in ear, severe throbbing pain, hearing loss, tinnitus, fever	Antibiotics. If severe, bed rest, analgesics, nasal vasoconstrictors. Myringotomy if necessary
Chronic otitis media	Chronic inflammation of middle ear; sequela of acute otitis media	Deafness, occasional pain, dizziness, chronic discharge from ear	Local debridement; topical and systemic antibiotics; mastoidectomy and tympanoplasty may be necessary
Chronic mastoiditis	Spread of infection into mastoid from repeated otitis media	Middle ear drainage	Mastoid irrigation; antibiotics; may need mastoidectomy

Problem	Possible aetiologies
Pain	Pathophysiological ear pain caused by infection, inflammation, and swelling
Knowledge deficit about problem	Lack of exposure to information: unfamiliarity with information sources.
Sensory/perceptual alteration, auditory	Decreased hearing caused by debris and infection in ear canal

Planning: expected patient outcomes

Expected patient outcomes for the person with an external ear problem may include, but are not limited to, the following:
1. The patient states discomfort in the ear is decreased.
2. The patient can describe measures for prevention of external ear problems.
3. The patient can describe symptoms requiring medical attention.
4. The patient demonstrates correct technique in application of eardrops and ear ointment.
5. The patient is prepared for the possibility of minor surgery.
6. The patient's hearing is improved.

Implementation

Assisting with achievement of therapeutic goals

Manipulation of the ear during treatments requires gentle handling to maintain comfort. Cross-contamination is prevented by good medical asepsis, including washing hands before and after treatments.

Ear wash

A solution of boric acid (which can be obtained at the chemist) may be used to clean the external ear and provide a drying effect. Ear wash is contra-indicated if the eardrum is perforated. A small (50 ml) syringe is used to instil the fluid, and the solution is warmed to body temperature to prevent discomfort or dizziness. The person places the affected ear upward. The pinna is pulled up, back, and out, and the tip of the syringe is placed in the ear canal. The warmed solution is pumped repeatedly in and out of the canal. The patient then leans over and lets extra solution run out into a small basin or a folded towel. An ear wash is usually prescribed to be used twice a day until the ear stops draining. Dryness is checked by inserting a cotton-tipped applicator into the ear canal (no farther than the cotton tip).

Ear irrigation (syringing)

The ear may be irrigated to remove wax, drainage, or debris. A larger amount of solution is used than for an ear wash. *Irrigations are avoided if the eardrum is perforated (causes further inflammation).* Tap water is generally used. A large syringe is used, but the technique for insertion of the syringe tip is similar to an ear wash. The person's clothes are protected with a plastic cape, and a kidney-dish is placed below the ear to catch the solution. The fluid is directed in a steady stream along the upper wall of the ear canal.

Ear wicks

Ear wicks are used to promote drainage or for instillation of eardrops if the external canal is occluded. A bayonet forcep is used to insert the wick gently into the ear canal. Commercially prepared wicks or a single piece of ¼-inch gauze about 2 cm long may be used.

Eardrops

Antibiotics and antiinflammatory agents may be prescribed locally as eardrops, especially for external otitis.

Ear ointment

Use a cotton-tipped applicator to apply ear ointment. Insert the applicator no farther than the cotton end, and use a new one for each application. Allergic reactions to the medication can occur. Itching, redness, or a feeling of fullness in the ear are common symptoms of allergy.

Surgery

Surgery may be performed on the eardrum to relieve fluid pressure or to repair a perforation. If it is desirable to keep the eardrum open for fluid drainage, transtympanic tubes (grommets) can be inserted in a myringotomy incision; the tubes usually drop out by themselves in several months. Surgery of the ear is performed under high power magnification. If mastoidectomy is indicated, a simple procedure is preferred, if possible, as this maintains hearing. Tympanoplasty may follow mastoidectomy if the ossicles are removed. Care of the person after ear surgery is described on p. 952.

Interventions to achieve patient outcomes

Assisting with comfort

Because ear pain results from the fluid exudate of the inflammatory process, pain usually begins to subside with adequate antibiotic therapy and drainage measures. Analgesics may be helpful. External heat such as a warmed towel may be comforting to some patients.

Monitoring hearing

The patient's hearing is assessed before and after surgery.

Facilitating learning

Ear infections may recur and become chronic; therefore, people with ear infections need to know how to prevent chronic infection. Teaching includes prevention of further infection, care of the infected ear, and signs requiring further medical attention.

Evaluation

Evaluation is based on expected patient outcomes. Questions to consider may include the following:
1. Is the patient comfortable?
2. Can the patient describe care required at home?
3. Can the patient describe measures to prevent recurring infection?

DISORDERS OF BALANCE
Pathophysiology

Disturbance of the function of the *statokinetic system* (semicircular canals, vestibular portion of the eighth cranial nerve, and vestibular nuclei) results in a subjective sensation of whirling or spinning or of being propelled or

REVIEW
Table 31-2   Disorders affecting balance

Disorder	Signs and symptoms	Medical therapy
Suppurative labyrinthitis	Severe, whirling vertigo Tinnitus Sensorineural hearing loss *Results in:* total hearing loss and non-functional labyrinth	Hospitalization High-dose antibiotics IV Drugs to treat symptoms, such as antiemetics and antihistamine drugs
Acute toxic labyrinthitis	Whirling vertigo reaching its maximum in 24 hours Nausea and vomiting Incapacity for 3-5 days Any movement of the head causes whirling vertigo No hearing loss	Bed rest in supine position until symptoms abate Avoid movement of head Reassurance that attack will subside in 3-5 days
Ménière's disease	Triad of: 1. Attacks of whirling vertigo 2. Tinnitus 3. Fluctuating sensorineural hearing loss	Low-salt diet (1.5 g/day) Drug therapy 1. Diuretics 2. Peripheral vestibular suppressant: betahistine, cyclizine 3. CNS vestibular suppressant: diazepam 4. Antiemetic: antihistamines 5. Anticholinergic: hyoscine
Acoustic neuroma	First symptom is tinnitus, hearing loss may not occur for months or years Hearing loss, usually to high-frequency sounds Unsteadiness if tumour is large. Vertigo is unusual but may occur. Facial paralysis if seventh and eighth cranial nerves are compressed into internal auditory canal	Diagnosis: MRI will detect early tumours lying within internal auditory canal and is the best diagnostic tool Treatment: Surgical removal of the neuroma

tilted in space. These sensations of true whirling or motion of the body are called *systematized vertigo*. Three of the conditions causing vertigo—labyrinthitis, Ménière's disease, and acoustic neuroma—are disorders of the inner ear involving the *statokinetic system*[6] (see p. 946).

Labyrinthitis is the most common cause of *vertigo*. There are two major types of labyrinthitis, *suppurative* and *acute toxic* (Table 31-2). Suppurative labyrinthitis is caused by an invasion of the internal ear by infection. Acute toxic labyrinthitis is caused by acute febrile illnesses such as pneumonia, cholecystitis, or influenza; toxic reactions to drugs; overindulgence in alcohol; food or drug allergy; or extreme fatigue. Hearing loss usually does not accompany acute toxic labyrinthitis, but total hearing loss and a non-functioning labyrinth are the results of suppurative labyrinthitis. *If the suppurative type of labyrinthitis is inadequately treated with antibiotics or if the diagnosis is delayed, meningitis can result.* Certain drugs, especially streptomycin, are toxic to the eighth cranial nerve and can destroy the vestibular portion of the nerve.

Ménière's disease is thought to be caused by an over-production of endolymph in the middle ear. This is why the disease is classified as endolymphatic hydrops, although it is most commonly called Ménière's disease.

Whirling vertigo, in which the body seems to be whirl-

ing when the eyes are closed or the environment seems to be turning when the eyes are open, is found in Ménière's disease. Any sensation of movement, up and down or side to side, suggests that the statokinetic system is involved.[6] A triad of symptoms is seen in Ménière's disease. In addition to attacks of whirling vertigo, tinnitus and fluctuating sensorineural hearing loss occur.

Early in the disease one or two symptoms may occur without the third. In two thirds of patients, vertigo is the primary symptom. The diagnosis of Ménière's disease is *not made until all three symptoms are present.*

Ménière's disease is most common in people between the ages of 30 and 50. Hearing loss is present initially in only one ear. However, 25% to 40% of patients develop bilateral hydrops resulting in deafness in both ears. The therapy for Ménière's disease is outlined in Table 31-2. Surgical treatment may become necessary when medical therapy has failed to relieve the severe attacks of vertigo. Less than 10% of patients require surgery. Several surgical procedures can be used, but none of them is considered the "perfect" surgical therapy for Ménière's disease.[6]

The person with Ménière's disease usually has recurrent attacks at varying intervals. During an attack, the person is unable to sit or walk and must lie with the head absolutely still to prevent further vertigo. In *most cases, loss of hearing is progressive until deafness results in that ear. There is no cure for the disease, but control is possible.*

An *acoustic neuroma* is a slow-growing, benign tumour of the vestibular portion of cranial nerve VIII causing signs and symptoms listed in Table 35-4. The neuroma can be removed easily without side effects if identified early. If allowed to grow, however, it encroaches on the brain and more extensive surgery is necessary with loss of hearing.

Nursing Process
Assessment
Subjective and objective data

When the examiner is attempting to evaluate vertigo, six basic questions should be asked[6]:

1. Does the patient experience true whirling? The direction and character of the motion are not important, but whether the patient feels that he or she is in motion.
2. What is the pattern of dizziness? Are there paroxysmal attacks with intervals of no attacks? Onset, course, severity, duration, time of day, and relationship to menstrual cycles, occupation, and trauma should be determined.
3. Are there associated symptoms such as nausea and vomiting? If nausea and vomiting accompany vertigo and there is absence of signs of CNS disease, the cause is usually labyrinthine disease.
4. Is there hearing loss or tinnitus? When either accompanies dizziness, it helps to localize the disorder.
5. Is there history of motion sickness or vestibular sensitivity? When the patient has no history of motion sickness and experiences true whirling vertigo, this indicates significant vestibular abnormalities. Patients who have motion sickness require a less severe ocular, proprioceptive, or vestibular abnormality to elicit symptoms of vertigo.
6. What is the drug history? This is very important because so many classifications of drugs can cause symptoms of dizziness. See Box 31-2.

Subjective data are collected initially from a patient subject to vertigo. Data include knowledge of the disorder, patterns of the episodes (frequency, duration), accompanying symptoms, and safety measures taken. Because of the discomfort of vertigo, many people fear the attacks; therefore the person's feelings concerning the vertigo are explored. Initial *objective data* include an assessment of the person's hearing ability (p. 953) because of the close relationship between balance and hearing in the inner ear.

During an attack of vertigo, the following additional data are collected:

1. Onset and duration of the attack.
2. Presence of nystagmus (involuntary jerky movements of the eyes); note if nystagmus occurs in one eye or both eyes and the rapidity of the movement.
3. Reports of tinnitus (ranges from buzzing sounds to painful, loud ringing noises).
4. Colour and moisture of skin (pallor and diaphoresis from an autonomic nervous system response).
5. Occurrence of vomiting (also an autonomic nervous system response).

31-2	**Classes of drugs causing vertigo**
	Antibiotics
	Anticonvulsants
	Antihistamines
	Antihypertensives
	Antiinflammatories
	Diuretics
	Muscle relaxants
	Sedatives
	Tranquillizers

Diagnostic tests

Specific diagnostic tests include *electronystagmography* (ENG) and a caloric stimulation test. ENG is a test used to measure nystagmus. It records the position and movement of the eyeball by recording the changes in the electrical field around the eye when there is a change in position of the eye. Electrodes are placed on the face around the eye; no discomfort is involved.

In the *caloric stimulation test*, cold water or air is irrigated in the external auditory canal. When the vestibular portion of the eighth cranial nerve is intact, labyrinthine function is normal, and the person experiences vertigo and nystagmus. In labyrinthine disorders, the response is hyperactive or absent.

Audiometric testing (p. 957) is performed to identify concurrent hearing loss. With many labyrinthine disorders, the test initially reveals low-tone sensorineural hearing loss. Neurological opinion is usually obtained to rule out neurological disease.

Nursing Analysis

Problems are determined from analysis of patient data. Possible problems for the person with a balance disorder may include, but are not limited to, the following:

Problem	Possible aetiologies
Injury, high risk for	Loss of balance during attack of vertigo
Sensory/perceptual alteration: auditory	Inner ear disorder
Anxiety	Concern about future attacks
Knowledge deficit	Lack of exposure/recall, information misinterpretation of information

Planning: expected patient outcomes

Expected patient outcomes for the person with a balance disorder may include, but are not limited to, the following:

1. Injury from loss of balance does not occur
2. Attacks of vertigo and tinnitus occur less frequently
3. Patient states he or she is less anxious about an attack of vertigo
4. The person describes:
   a. The nature of the disorder
   b. Circumstances that precipitate an attack and what to do when an attack occurs
   c. Safety precautions to take
   d. Prescribed medication regimen
   e. Symptoms requiring medical intervention

Implementation

Assisting with achievement of therapeutic goals
Medications

Most people with a vertiginous disorder receive therapy on an outpatient basis. Medications may be prescribed to decrease the incidence or severity of the vertigo and consist primarily of *antihistamines*, such as cyclizine. A *diuretic* such as hydrochlorodiazide may be prescribed to help decrease fluid volume of the endolymph. A *low-salt diet* (1.5 gm/day) is usually prescribed for the same reason as a diuretic.

Surgery of the ear

Types of surgery. Surgery may be performed for Ménière's disease if the attacks are incapacitating and cannot be controlled by medication. About 5% to 10% of people with the disorder require surgery.

Surgery is required for removal of acoustic neuromas. A translabyrinthine or mastoidectomy approach is preferred, although a suboccipital approach may be needed. Very large tumours may require resection of the facial nerve.

Preoperative care. Ear surgery is often performed with local anaesthesia, with the person receiving sedation to relieve anxiety and provide relaxation. The following instructions are given about what to expect in the postoperative period:

1. Minor earache can be expected, but pain is not usually a problem
2. Hearing is decreased because of the ear packing
3. Noises such as crackles or pops may be heard
4. Swelling of the ear will occur
5. Extent of postoperative vertigo depends on the nature of the procedure (more extensive with inner ear surgery)

Postoperative care

1. Position patient with operative ear uppermost for 4 hours after surgery
2. Medicate as necessary for discomfort or vertigo
3. Keep cot side up when patient is in bed (when vertigo is present)
4. Supervise patient during ambulation if vertigo/dizziness is present
5. Monitor patient for:
   a. Changes in hearing, tinnitus, or vertigo
   b. Headache
   c. Bleeding (rare)
   d. Signs of facial paralysis if extensive inner ear surgery is performed (asymmetry when frowning, smiling, closing eye, baring teeth, or blowing through lips)
6. Instruct patient to keep mouth open if sneezing or coughing and to blow nose gently one side at a time, if necessary (prevents increased middle ear pressure and transmission of organisms into the middle ear)
7. Reassure patient that improvement in hearing may not be immediate because of oedema and packing in ear.

Most ear surgeries require only a cotton ball in the ear after surgery because only small amounts of serosanguineous drainage are expected. Dressings may be used for surgeries other than transcanal approaches. Hospital stays range from 1 to 4 days. Guidelines for patient teaching are listed in Box 31-3.

Interventions to achieve patient outcomes
Promoting comfort and safety

During an attack of vertigo, the person either feels as though the room is spinning around or that he or she is spinning in a stationary room. To prevent falling and to decrease the vertigo sensation, the person has to lie down, avoiding all head movements that aggravate the spinning sensation. If tinnitus is severe, the person may cover the ears in an attempt to lessen the sound. Measures must be taken to protect the person from falling at the onset of the attack. The acute manifestations may last from 1 to 3 hours.[21] After an attack the person is exhausted and requires rest and sleep.

Measures that help reduce vertigo or dizziness include the following:

1. Stand directly in front of person when speaking so person does not have to turn head
2. Encourage person to move *slowly*
3. Avoid bright, glaring lights
4. If bed rest is prescribed:
   a. Assist with ADL as needed
   b. Keep cot side up
5. Assist with ambulation as needed to prevent falls
6. If vertigo occurs when person is ambulating, have person lie down immediately and hold head still.

Supporting coping

The threat of vertigo usually leads to anxiety. The person may dread the experience of an attack or may be embarrassed by the concurrent side-effects such as vomiting. Give the person opportunities to explore feelings and concerns. Anxiety may be decreased by awareness of measures to decrease vertigo occurrences or to minimize the effects.

Facilitating learning

Teaching for the patient with vertigo includes the nature of the disorder, actions to take during an attack, measures to prevent injury, the prescribed medication regimen, and symptoms requiring medical attention (see Box 31-4).

Evaluation

Evaluation is based on the identified patient outcomes. Questions to consider may include the following:

1. Has injury from falls been prevented?
2. Does the patient ask for assistance in ambulating if dizziness is present or if vertigo is imminent?
3. Have signs of anxiety decreased?
4. Does the patient know the nature of the disorder, the medication regimen, and what to do if an attack occurs?
5. Does the patient plan for ongoing medical supervision?

Patient Teaching

The patient after ear surgery

1. Change dressing in ear daily as prescribed
2. Open mouth when sneezing or coughing and try not to sneeze or blow nose for 1 week. If must blow nose, blow gently one side at a time (to prevent increased ear pressure and infection)
3. Keep ear dry for 6 weeks (to prevent infection)
   a. Do not wash hair for 1 week
   b. Protect ear when outdoors using two pieces of cotton (use petroleum jelly on outer ball)
   c. Protect ear with shower cap when bathing
4. Wear ear protectors as necessary for exposure to loud noises
5. Follow activity guidelines
   a. No physical activity for 1 week or until deep external packing is removed
   b. No exercises or active sports for 3 weeks
   c. Return to work in 1 week (3 weeks for strenuous work)
6. Avoid exposure to people with upper respiratory tract infections
7. Avoid flying for at least 1 week (to prevent effects of pressure changes)

Patient Teaching

The patient with vertigo

1. Nature of the disorder
   a. Physiological basis for the vertigo
   b. Avoidance of any known precipitating factors
   c. Rationale for a low-salt diet
2. Actions to take during an attack
   a. Lie down immediately and call for help if necessary at the first sign of an attack
   b. If driving when an attack occurs, pull over immediately to the curb
   c. Lie immobile and hold head in one position until vertigo lessens
3. Ask for assistance when ambulating if dizzy
4. Take prescribed medications as instructed, even if no recent attacks have occurred; check with doctor before discontinuing any medication
5. Symptoms requiring medical attention: changes in symptoms or nature of attacks

HEARING LOSS

Most ear disorders interfere with hearing to a lesser or greater extent. Inflammations may plug the ear canal or fill the middle ear with fluid, interfering with transmission of sound waves. If the ossicles become fixed, they are less able to transmit the sound vibrations. Inner ear disorders also interfere with the sound vibrations reaching the organ of Corti. Growth of acoustic neuromas places pressure on the cochlear division of the eighth cranial nerve.

Implications of Impaired Hearing

As already stated there are about 7.5 million adults in Great Britain with some form of hearing impairment.[17a] Most of these have mild or moderate hearing loss—7.2 million, with only some 0.3 million affected by severe or profound hearing loss.[17a] The vast majority (75%) of hearing impaired people are aged 60 or over.[17a] People with hearing impairments may have less desirable jobs and lower incomes than those without hearing impairments.

Hearing is as important as speech in our daily lives. Sound helps keep us in touch with reality and our environment; it adds aesthetic pleasure, as well as warnings of danger, to our world. The sense of hearing is critical to normal development and maintenance of speech. Infants learn to speak by imitating others and listening to the sounds they make in relationship to the sounds of others. Congenitally deaf people lack aural stimulation, which affects their development of speech and conceptual ability. This severe handicap can affect both personality development and responses on intelligence tests.

As hearing diminishes, the effect of not understanding others and not being understood may make people withdraw from social situations, and they may become anxious and insecure. Fear of inadequacy and inferiority may make them suspicious and depressed. When hearing is completely gone, they may find the silent world almost intolerable.

People who are hard of hearing or deaf are not easily recognized; they appear quite normal. When they fail to respond or respond inappropriately to oral communication, their actions are interpreted as slow or odd, and the speaker may withdraw. This withdrawal response of others may be perceived as rejection by the aurally handicapped person and may further increase isolation and withdrawal. The person who is hard of hearing or deaf may experience varying degrees of stress, depending on personality, the extent and type of loss, the age at onset of loss, and the reaction of family and friends to the loss of hearing.

Older adults with hearing impairment may suffer from reduced interpersonal communication, social isolation, depression, reduced mobility, and exacerbation of coexisting psychiatric conditions.[10] Employment legislation should improve the job opportunities for those with hearing impairment. Recent advances in communication technology also allows the deaf person to function more easily in the workplace.

Classification of Hearing Loss
Conductive hearing loss

Any interference with conduction of sound impulses through the *external ear canal*, the *eardrum*, or the *middle ear produces a conductive hearing loss*. The inner ear is not involved and sound amplification will reach the inner ear. Causes of conductive hearing loss are listed in Box 31-5.

The external auditory canal can be obstructed by cerumen, foreign bodies in the canal, tumours, and swelling from infection. The most common cause is impacted cerumen.

Damage to the eardrum and middle ear can be caused by thickening (tympanosclerosis), scarring, perforation, or retraction of the ear drum. In the middle ear, hearing loss

Nursing Care Plan

Person with Ménière's disease

DATA: Mrs. B. is a 59-year-old schoolteacher. During the past 6 months, she has had three attacks of "whirling in space" or vertigo, fluctuating hearing in the left ear, noise or tinnitus in the left ear, nausea and vomiting, and a sense of fullness or pressure in the left ear. Two attacks have occurred during class, and one attack occurred at home, where she lives alone. Embarrassment, fear, anxiety, and uncertainty are some of her feelings. Mrs. B. was referred to the ear, nose and throat department where diagnostic tests were performed.

These tests included an audiogram, tympanometry, electronystagmography, electrocochleography, a nursing assessment, and physical examination. A diagnosis of Ménière's disease was made. A 1500 mg sodium-restricted diet, hydrochlorothiazide orally every day, labyrinthine compensatory exercises, and nicotinic acid 100 mg 3 times a day were prescribed to control the incapacitating attacks of vertigo.

Nursing analysis: Anxiety related to effects of disorder

Expected patient outcomes	Nursing interventions	Rationale
Signs of anxiety are decreased	Encourage Mrs. B. to explore concerns about decreased hearing and effects of dizziness attacks and to take action in relation to the concern Explore Mrs. B.'s knowledge of the disorder and correct misunderstandings Encourage realistic hope about expected hearing ability as described by doctor Refer Mrs. B. to necessary support services, such as social worker or audiologist	Expressing concerns and receiving realistic counselling and support reduce helplessness and apprehension

Nursing analysis: Sensory perception, alteration in vestibular, auditory

Expected patient outcomes	Nursing interventions	Rationale
Mrs. B describes actions to avoid dizziness Mrs. B. interacts with others accurately	Help Mrs. B. identify avoidable actions that precipitate dizziness attacks Encourage Mrs. B. to move slowly and not turn head suddenly when dizziness is present If tinnitus is distressing, increase background noises such as music If hearing is decreased: 1. Use measures to facilitate communication with hearing impaired (see text) 2. Refer Mrs. B. to audiologist, if appropriate	Understanding cause of dizziness and measures to reduce it may lessen occurrence

Nursing analysis:: Injury, high risk for, trauma related to dizziness

Expected patient outcomes	Nursing interventions	Rationale
Injury does not occur	Keep cot side up when Mrs. B. is dizzy and in bed Assist with ambulation as needed Encourage Mrs. B. to sit or lie down and to remain immobile if signs of dizziness occur Teach Mrs. B. to stop car at side of road and turn ignition off immediately at first signs of dizziness while driving	Knowledge of safety measures reduces possibility of injuries

Nursing analysis: Self-care deficit, high risk for

Expected patient outcomes	Nursing interventions	Rationale
ADL needs are met Mrs. B. functions as independently as condition permits	Provide desired foods and fluids if nausea is present Assist with hygiene as needed while encouraging independence; place washing things so that Mrs. B. does not have to turn head Provide sufficient time for ADL so Mrs. B. can move slowly	Assistance with ADL makes it possible for Mrs. B. to function independently and feel in control of situation

Nursing analysis: Coping, ineffective individual

Expected patient outcomes	Nursing interventions	Rationale
Mrs. B. identifies coping pattern and resultant effects Mrs. B. describes alternative coping behaviours	Make decisions regarding safety of Mrs. B. and others when patient is unable to do so Assist Mrs. B. to identify usual coping behaviours and the consequences of the behaviours Assist Mrs. B. to identify personal strengths Teach Mrs. B. alternative coping behaviours	Support and understanding by caregivers improve coping. Discussing possible coping behaviours assists Mrs. B. to choose behaviours that are most functional for her

Nursing analysis: Knowledge deficit about pathophysiology of Ménière's disease related to lack of exposure to information

Expected patient outcomes	Nursing interventions	Rationale
Mrs. B. describes nature of disorder, therapy, and safety measures	Teach Mrs. B. about the disorder, therapy, and need for medical follow-up (see text) Teach Mrs. B. ways to protect self from injury and to prevent dizziness attacks when possible	Need for information regarding disease increases learning, which assists Mrs. B. to care for self and to live as independently as possible

31-5

Causes of specific types of hearing loss

Conductive hearing loss—occurs when sound cannot reach cochlea

Obstruction of the external ear canal by ceru
 men, foreign body, etc.
Tympanic membrane perforation
Serous otitis media
Adhesive otitis
Ossicular discontinuity—trauma, infection, cho-
 lesteatoma
Tympanosclerosis
Otoscierosis
Ossicular fixation

Sensorineural hearing loss—occurs when cochlea or eighth cranial nerve is damaged

Presbycusis
Occupational hearing loss (noise-induced)
Head trauma
Drug toxicity—ototoxic drugs
Endolymphatic hydrops (Ménière's disease)
Tumour—neuroma of eighth cranial nerve
Perilymphatic leak

From DeWeese DD, Saunders WH: *Textbook of otolaryngology,* ed 7, St Louis, Mosby–Year Book, 1988.

is caused by the presence of liquid (pus, serum, or blood), absence or increase in mobility of the ossicles (tympanosclerosis or otosclerosis), adhesions, tumours, or dislocated or absent ossicles (congenital or acquired).[6]

Otosclerosis is the most common cause of conductive hearing loss in people between the ages of 15 and 50 years. It is a hereditary condition of unknown cause. Women are affected more than men. Hearing loss may first be noticed in the late teens or early twenties. It may progress more rapidly during or after pregnancy, but no causal relationship has been established for this. If cochlear function is normal or near normal, the hearing loss can be improved by microsurgery with a stapedectomy and replacement with a prosthesis or by a stapedotomy alone.[6]

Sensorineural hearing loss

Sensorineural hearing loss results from damage to the cochlea or the eighth cranial nerve. It can be present at birth (hereditary deafness) or develop later in life. The hearing loss may result from a known disorder (see Box 31-5), it can be a functional hearing loss (no organic cause), or it may be the result of ageing (presbycusis). Hearing loss may fluctuate initially, but further progressive hearing loss oc-curs. Most disorders of the inner ear produce some hearing loss, and a characteristic of severe loss is the inability to discriminate words. Amplification of sounds often causes sound distortion and increases the hearing problem.

Cohlear implants are now available for people with complete hearing loss. An external device consisting of a small computer changes spoken words to electrical impulses. The impulses are transmitted across the skin to an im-

planted coil that carries the impulses to an electrode inserted through the round window into the cochlea. Single channel implants are available, but newer multi-channel implants that increase speech discrimination are being employed.

Other types of hearing loss

Mixed hearing loss is a combination of both sensorineural and conductive hearing loss. Both elements of air and bone conduction hearing loss occur.

Central hearing loss is a form of sensorineural hearing loss resulting from some type of damage to the brain's auditory pathways or auditory centre, such as with a cerebral vascular accident. Sounds may be conducted normally through the ear to the neural pathways, but the person is deaf.

Presbycusis is the term used to describe hearing loss associated with ageing. The degenerative changes in this type of hearing loss are similar to the degenerative changes occurring in other body tissues. In many cases, there is atrophy of the ganglion cells in the cochlea or changes in the basilar membrane. Presbycusis accounts for the majority of neurosensory hearing loss in the elderly. There are three major characteristics of presbycusis: (1) gradual progressive development, (2) loss of higher frequencies, manifested by loss of discrimination in noise, and (3) a narrow range of tolerance to sound intensity. There is no treatment for presbycusis, but hearing can be improved by hearing aids.[6]

Presbycusis becomes increasingly common after age 50. It is reported in 23% of people between ages 65 and 74, 33% of people aged 75 to 84, and 48% of people 85 and older. These figures are believed to underestimate the number of people affected. When the older person also has a visual problem, it impairs his or her ability to use visual cues for speech-reading and further exacerbates the hearing impairment.[10]

Nursing Process
Assessment

The extent of assessment of auditory acuity by nurses depends on the nurse's preparation and focus of care. All nurses, however, should be prepared to carry out an inspection of the outer ear and at least a gross assessment of hearing ability for all people entering a health care setting, regardless of the presenting problem. Gross assessment of hearing may be accomplished by evaluating the logical sequences of replies the patient makes during the admission history. One method is to turn one's head away from the individual when asking a simple question that cannot be answered by a yes or no response.

Subjective data

If the person has been identified as having hearing loss, the following data are obtained:

1. Onset, nature and progression of the hearing loss
2. Noticed differences in hearing in right or left ear
3. Family history of hearing loss
4. Presence of other ear symptoms: pressure or pain in ears (middle ear), or ringing in ears or dizziness (inner ear)

Behavioural clues indicating difficult hearing

Any adult who

Is irritable, hostile, hypersensitive in interpersonal relations

Has difficulty in hearing upper frequency consonants

Complains about people mumbling

Turns up the volume on television

Asks for frequent repetition and answers questions inappropriately

Loses sense of humour; becomes grim

Leans forward to hear better; face serious and strained

Shuns large- and small-group audience situations

May appear aloof and "stuck-up"

Complains of ringing in the ears

Has an unusually soft or loud voice

Repeatedly states, "What did you say?"

---

5. History of head trauma or exposure to noise (past, present)
6. Current medications with known ototoxic effects
7. Any neurological symptoms, including visual or speech disorders

Objective data

The person who begins to have difficulty hearing usually demonstrates some behavioural clues indicating that hearing is decreased (see Box 31-6). People who exhibit any of these behavioural clues should have their ears examined by an otolaryngologist, who will perform a complete evaluation.

Auditory acuity

Each ear must be tested separately to estimate the hearing. One of the patient's ears is occluded with a finger. While standing 1 to 2 feet away, the nurse whispers two-syllable numbers softly towards the unoccluded ear, and the patient is asked to repeat the numbers. The intensity of the nurse's voice can be increased from a soft, medium, or loud whisper to a soft, medium, or loud voice. If the nurse suspects that the patient is speech-reading, the nurse's face should be turned away. The patient is asked if hearing is better in one ear than in the other ear. If the auditory acuity is different, the ear that hears better should be tested first. Then noise is produced in the better-hearing ear by rapidly but gently moving the finger in the patient's ear canal while testing the other ear.

A watch tick can also be used to test hearing. However, a watch tick is a higher-pitched sound and less relevant to functional hearing than the voice test.

The tuning fork also provides a general estimate of hearing loss. The three major tuning fork tests date from the nineteenth century and are named after their originators: Weber, Rinne, and Schwabach.

Weber test. The tuning fork is set into vibration by striking the tines on the examiner's knuckles or knee. The rounded tip of the handle is placed on the patient's forehead or teeth. Placement on the teeth (even if the patient has false teeth) is generally more reliable. The patient is asked whether the tone is heard in the middle of the head, the right ear, or the left ear. The Weber test is useful in cases of unilateral loss.

Rinne test. The vibrating tuning fork is shifted between two positions: against the mastoid bone (bone conduction) and 2 inches from the opening of the ear canal (air conduction). As the position is changed, the patient is asked to indicate which tone is louder (in front of the ear or behind the ear) or is asked to indicate when one of the tones is no longer heard. The Rinne test is useful to differentiate between conductive and sensorineural hearing losses.

With conductive hearing loss, the pathways of normal sound conduction are blocked. However, vibrations against the mastoid bone can bypass the obstruction; therefore bone conduction lasts longer than air conduction. With sensorineural hearing loss, the acoustic nerve has decreased ability to perceive vibrations from either route: therefore normal patterns are reported by the patient.

Schwabach test. This test is also used to differentiate between a conductive and sensorineural hearing loss. The Schwabach test compares the hearing of the examiner (who must have normal hearing) with the patient. However, the Rinne test has replaced this test.

These aforementioned tests can be performed at the bedside by the nurse to give some indication of the amount of hearing. More elaborate and specific hearing tests are performed in a soundproof room.

Audiometric testing

Functional examination for sensitivity (ability to hear sounds) and for speech discrimination (ability to distinguish different speech sounds) is done by audiometry. The graph of the hearing levels of both of these is called an *audiogram. Hearing threshold is defined as the lowest intensity of sound at which an auditory stimulus can be heard.*

Audiologists (specialists in administering hearing tests) have developed audiometric tests to determine not only whether a hearing loss is present, but also the frequency of the loss, how well the person can understand speech, and whether the problem site is in the middle ear (conductive loss), or inner ear or auditory nerve system (sensorineural loss).

Pure-tone audiometry must be performed in a specially constructed soundproof booth for best results. To test the sound intensity by air conduction, people wear earphones and are instructed to signal (usually with a finger) when they first hear the tone and when they no longer hear it. The middle frequencies are tested first, and the operator alternately increases and decreases the intensity of the sound until the dial setting is found at which the person being tested can just perceive sound (threshold). In audiometric testing the frequencies 125, 250, 500, 1000, 2000, 4000, and 8000 Hz are commonly employed to assess the hearing sensitivity of an individual.

Hearing loss is identified as the number of decibels reached before the person hears the sound for each specific frequency. Zero loudness is calibrated for that sound barely heard by a person with normal hearing. Up to 20 db loss is considered to be within the normal range.

Nursing Analysis

Problems are determined from analysis of patient data. Possible problems for the hard-of-hearing person may include, but are not limited to, the following:

Problem	Possible aetiologies
Sensory/perceptual alteration: auditory	Altered sensory transmission from loss of hearing
Knowledge deficit	Lack of exposure/recall, information misinterpretation about hearing
Coping, ineffective individual	Situational crises, personal vulnerability

Planning: expected patient outcomes

Expected patient outcomes for the person who is hard of hearing may include, but are not limited to, the following:
1. Patient indicates by facial expression, gestures, or answers that oral communications are heard
2. Patient can explain:
   a. The basis for the hearing loss and any appropriate therapy
   b. Care of hearing aid, if appropriate.
   c. Available community resources
3. Patient exhibits coping ability by actively seeking aural rehabilitation appropriate to level of hearing loss

Implementation

Interventions to achieve patient outcomes

Activities for the hearing impaired person include facilitation of communication and aural rehabilitation. It is not uncommon for people who are beginning to lose their hearing to deny that changes are occurring and that an evaluation of hearing and follow-up of rehabilitative methods are important. Much support and encouragement to explore methods to improve hearing may be necessary.

Facilitating communication

Specific actions to facilitate hearing or lip-reading for people with impaired hearing are listed in Box 31-7.

Additional activities can be used if the person is hospitalized. Patients are helped to use visual cues by placing them in a bed where they can observe activity and anticipate others approaching them. They will be easily startled if people suddenly enter the unit if the vision is obscured. Because hearing-impaired people are often sensitive to light changes, they can easily be awakened by turning on a light. Many patients feel less isolated if the nurse touches them lightly on the arm to gain attention and wakes them by touching them on the arm. Special efforts must be made to communicate information about hospital routines and diagnostic tests.

Promoting aural rehabilitation

If hearing loss is irreversible or not amenable to surgical intervention or if the person elects not to have surgery, aural

---

31-7

Facilitating communication for people with impaired hearing

1. Get the person's attention by raising an arm or hand.
2. Stand with a light on your face; this helps the person lip read. Do not stand with your back against a window.
3. Face the person when speaking.
4. Speak clearly, but do not overaccentuate words.
5. Speak in a normal tone; do not shout. Shouting overemploys normal speaking movements and may cause distortion and be too loud for the person with sensorineural damage. If the person has conductive loss only, sometimes making the voice louder without shouting is helpful.
6. If the person does not seem to understand what is said, express it differently. Some words are difficult to "see" in lip reading, such as *white* or *red*.
7. Move close to the person and toward the better ear if the person does not hear you.
8. Write out proper names or any statement that you are not sure was understood.
9. Do not smile, eat, or cover the mouth when talking to a person with limited hearing.
10. Observe for inattention that may indicate tiredness or lack of understanding.
11. Use phrases to convey meaning rather than one-word answers. State the major topic of the discussion first and then give details.
12. Do not show annoyance by careless facial expression. Persons who are hard of hearing depend more on visual clues for acceptance.
13. Encourage the use of a hearing aid if the person has one; allow the person to adjust it before speaking.
14. If in a group, repeat important statements and avoid asides to others in the group.
15. Avoid the use of the intercommunication system as this may distort sound and cause poor communication.
16. Do not avoid conversation with a person who has hearing loss.

Modified from Conover M, Cober J: *Nurs Clin North Am* 5:497, 1970.

---

rehabilitation may increase communication. The purpose of aural rehabilitation is to maximize the hearing-impaired person's communication skills.

The auditory sense is our primary mode of communication, and rehabilitation is directed towards teaching the person more effective use of the senses of vision, touch, and vibration plus maximizing the use of any remaining hearing ability. Rehabilitation is affected by the person's background and by the severity of impairment. As with other forms of rehabilitation, success depends on the degree of the patient's motivation.

Types of aural rehabilitation. Aural rehabilitation includes *auditory training, lip reading, speech training, sign language,* and the *use of hearing aids.* The use of instruments and training are involved. *Auditory training* is an approach to enhance listening skills. The hearing-impaired person is initially exposed to gross differences in sound and then gradually "fine tuned" so that subtle differences in discrimination of two similar sounds can be made. The primary purpose of auditory training exercises is to help the person concentrate on the speaker. For some people, only gross differences between sounds may be recognized.

Speech reading is the current term used for lip reading and is an important means of communication. Speech training is the process of understanding vocal communication by the integration of lip movements with facial expressions, gestures, environmental clues, and conversation contexts. Lip reading is very difficult, however, without auditory cues. Many movements for speech are very rapid, many sounds are very similar (b, m, p), and certain sounds of any language are invisible (the h in English). The hearing-impaired person must guess at a high percentage of the words. Knowledge of this fact alone will help the nurse be more understanding of the person who is lip (speech) reading.

Because of reduced auditory feedback (the inability of hearing-impaired people to monitor their own speech), the clearness, pitch quality, or rate of their speech may deteriorate. These abnormal effects alter the efficiency of communication and reduce the intelligibility of speech. *The goal of speech training is to conserve, develop, or prevent deterioration of speech skills.*

Sign language is a useful aid for hearing-impaired individuals and many thousands of people now use British Sign Language (estimated 50,000 to 55,000).[17a]

Hearing aids. Hearing aids are instruments made up of miniature parts working together as a system to amplify sound in a controlled manner. They are used by both hard-of-hearing people (slight or moderate hearing loss) and deaf people (severe or profound hearing loss). *Hearing aids make sound louder* but *do not improve the ability to hear.* Therefore people with decreased discrimination (the ability to understand what is spoken) benefit less from a hearing aid. Appropriate aural rehabilitation will ensure successful adjustment of most problems. The hearing aid amplifies all background noises such as hospital machinery, footsteps, and department store noises, as well as speech. These noises may mask conversation or confuse the hearing-impaired person, especially the elderly.

Types of hearing aids. Hearing aids vary according to size and location to be worn. Regardless of the type of aid, the hearing aid consists of the following parts:

1. Microphone to receive sound waves from the air and change sounds into electrical signals
2. Amplifier to increase the strength of electrical signals
3. Battery to provide the electrical energy needed to operate the hearing aid
4. Receiver (loudspeaker) to change the electrical signals back into sound waves

---

The Elderly with Ear Problems

Assessment
1. Assess all elderly for hearing loss of high-pitched sounds, sensitivity to background noise, loss of sibilant consonants, and use of hearing aids.
2. Assess function of hearing aid and identify availability of extra batteries.

Intervention
1. Modify communication skills when speaking to person with hearing impairment:
   a. Face person with light on your face.
   b. Get person's attention. Touch lightly on arm, if necessary.
   c. Speak slowly and distinctly but do not exaggerate lip movements.
   d. Use short phrases and punctuate with body language.
   e. Be aware that vision may also be diminished.
2. Alert all personnel that patient is hard of hearing.
3. Try to obtain pocket amplifier for patient if hearing aid is not available.
4. Determine if patient sees otologist regularly so that ears are checked for wax.

Common disorders in elderly
Presbycusis

On all types of hearing aids but the body-worn type, all four components are housed in one small case. The louder sounds are then directed into the ear through a custom-fitted earmould.

Assisting the person with a hearing aid. The person with a hearing aid should know how to care for the aid and what to do if the aid does not work. The nurse must also have a basic knowledge of the hearing aid to assist the person unable or unwilling to care for the aid when ill. The person is encouraged to use the hearing aid and to store it safely in its case when it is not in use.

People who are reluctant to wear their hearing aids (often for cosmetic reasons) need counselling about the benefits of wearing the aid and the improvements in their ability to speak more distinctly. The aid may also serve to notify others to speak more distinctly. When a person with a hearing aid is hospitalized, it is important to encourage use of the aid during hospitalization and its safe storage when not in use.

Assistive hearing devices. Other types of technologies are available to assist the hearing-impaired or deaf people who do not have hearing aids. One type of assistive hearing device is a hand-held amplifier attached to headphones. The speaker holds the amplifier when communicating with the hearing-impaired person wearing the headphones.

Special amplifiers can also be placed in telephones to magnify the sound for hearing-impaired people; these amplifiers are obtained from the telephone company.

Implantable hearing devices. Three types of implanted hearing devices are either available for use or in the investigation stage. They are *cochlear implants, bone hearing devices,* and *semi-implantable hearing devices.*

Cochlear implants for those patients with no hearing at all are currently available. This device incorporates a small computer that changes the spoken word to electrical impulses. The impulses are transmitted across the skin to an implanted coil that carries the impulse to the hearing nerve endings in the cochlea by an electrode introduced through the round windows. The best of the cochlear implants use multichannels and are able to return about half of the patient's hearing and understanding. Cochlear implants are available for both children and adults.

In some cases of hearing loss, sound can be transmitted through the skull to the inner ear. Patients with a conductive hearing loss can use a device in which the receiver is implanted under the skin into the skull. The external device transmits the sound through the skin. This device is worn above the ear and not in the ear canal.

Patients who already use a hearing aid will gain the most from the implantable device. Clinical research has shown that a magnet implanted in the middle ear can be stimulated by an ear canal driver that changes sound to a magnetic force. This system eliminates several bothersome problems of hearing aids, such as feedback and difficulties with hearing in noisy environments. A semiimplantable hearing device is the first step to a totally implantable device that would eliminate any external device. However, many challenges have yet to be met before a workable device is available.

Referring to special services

Special services for people with a hearing loss are offered by audiology clinics in hospitals. Central and local government also provide certain services for those who are hearing impaired, e.g. special education for deaf children. National organizations available to give information and counselling include the following:

1. British Deaf Association; provides regional and local branches. It concentrates on people deaf from birth and those who became hearing impaired as children, although it functions to help all deaf people. It provides education through courses and conferences and supports the use of British Sign Language.
2. British Tinnitus Association; part of the RNID which serves to help those affected by tinnitus and raise awareness of this disabling condition.
3. National Deaf Children's Society; provides support to parents through numerous self-help groups. Offers information and advice on all areas affecting the education and welfare of hearing impaired children.
4. Royal National Intitute for Deaf People (RNID); concerned with helping all hearing impaired people. Also involved in work to prevent deafness and minimize its effects on the individual. It provides an information service, various specialist units, and a library.

Evaluation

Evaluation is based on expected patient outcomes. Questions to consider may include the following:

1. Does the person respond appropriately during interactions?
2. Does the person know (1) the nature of the disorder, (2) care of the hearing aid (if worn), and (3) where to seek appropriate assistance?
3. Has the person obtained appropriate aural rehabilitation?

SUMMARY

1. Sound reaches the inner ear by air conduction through the ear canal and ossicles of the middle ear and by bone conduction through the skull bones to the inner ear. In the cochlea of the inner ear the sound waves are transformed into neural energy and transmitted to the brain for interpretation.
2. Balance is affected by changes in the inner ear involving the semicircular canals, the eighth cranial nerve, and the vestibular nuclei.
3. Disorders that plug the outer ear, add fluid to the middle ear, make the ossicles unmovable, destroy the hair cells of the organ of Corti, or interfere with nerve stimulus transmission over the vestibulocochlear nerve will lead to decreased hearing.
4. Hearing can be preserved by preventing infection or trauma of the ear, by using ototoxic drugs with caution and seeking medical attention if symptoms occur, and by preventing frequent exposure to loud noises (or using ear protection for constant loud noises).
5. Ear infections are the most common disorders of the external and middle ears; pain results from pressure by fluid buildup within the enclosed spaces.
6. Serous otitis media ("glue ear") develops from collection of serous fluid in the middle ear when the pharyngotympanic tube becomes blocked. Purulent otitis media develops from bacteria entering the middle ear through the pharyngotympanic tube; pus collects in the middle ear.
7. Ear infections are treated with antibiotics, given by eardrops, by ear ointments, or systemically. Treatments to remove drainage may include ear wash, ear irrigation, or surgery of the eardrum.
8. The person with an ear infection should avoid getting water in the ear (care during showering and shampooing and avoiding swimming).
9. Vertigo is the primary symptom of disorders (such as labyrinthitis, Ménière's disease, acoustic neuroma) affecting the statokinetic system. Tinnitus (ringing in the ears) often accompanies vertigo. Potential for injury is a major problem for the person with vertigo.
10. The uncomfortable sensation of vertigo can be minimized by lying down and holding the head absolutely still.
11. Most ear surgeries are microsurgeries performed through the ear canal. After surgery, hearing will be temporarily decreased because of the swelling and ear packing; crackling noises may be heard. The patient is instructed postoperatively to avoid actions that may increase intraaural pressure or that may lead to infection.

12. Conductive hearing loss, a problem of decreased amplification, is the result of problems of the external or middle ear; it responds well to aural rehabilitation. Otosclerosis (immobility of the ossicles) produces conductive hearing loss.

13. Sensorineural hearing loss results from interference with hearing in the inner ear or neural pathways; it may result from a known disorder or be idiopathic.

14. Presbycusis (hearing loss resulting from ageing) is a form of sensorineural hearing loss. The hearing loss is primarily that of sound discrimination, and amplification may further distort the sound.

15. Aural rehabilitation includes the use of hearing aids or other assistive hearing devices, auditory training (improving listening skills), speech-reading (lipreading), use of sign language, or speech training (improving speech clarity).

REFERENCES AND SELECTED READINGS

1. Alberti PW, Ruben RJ, editors: *Otologic medicine and surgery,* vol 1, New York, 1988, Churchill Livingstone.

2. Alberti PW, Ruben RJ, editors: *Otologic medicine and surgery,* vol 2, New York, 1988, Churchill Livingstone.

3. Bates B: *A guide to physical examination,* ed 4, Philadelphia, 1987, JB Lippincott.

4. Bulechek GM, McCloskey JC: *Nursing interventions, treatments for nursing diagnosis,* Philadelphia, 1985, WB Saunders.

5.* DeBlase R, Kucler M: Assistive hearing device aids patient-staff communication, *Geriatr Nurs* 6:223-224, 1985.

6. DeWeese DD, Saunders WH: *Textbook of otolaryngology,* ed 7, St Louis, Mosby–Year Book, 1988.

7. Fairbanks DNF: *Antimicrobial therapy in otolaryngology—head neck surgery,* ed 5, Washington, DC, 1989, AAO-HNS Foundation.

8. Fountain D: Hearing aids and their care, *Geriatr Nurs Home Care* 7(2)12-14, 1987.

9. Gardner G: Ménière's disease. In Rakel RE, editor: *Conn's current therapy 1990,* Philadelphia, 1990, WB Saunders.

10. Healthy People 2000: *National health promotion and disease prevention objectives,* US Dept of Health and Human Services, Public Health Services, Washington, DC, 1990, Government Printing Office.

11.* Jackson J: Don't shout nurse!: hearing problems in the elderly, *Geriatr Nurs* (Oxford) 6(3):12-13, 1986.

12. Lee JC: Deafness: the next ten years, *J Rehab* 51(4):79-83, 1985.

13.* Levene B: Sorry nurse, I can hear you but I can't understand you, *Nurs 85* (Oxford) 2(41):1221-1225, 1985.

14. Mitchell VL: Cochlear implantation: a nursing perspective, *J Soc Otorhinolaryngol Head Neck Nurs* 5(2):11-15, 1987.

15. Reiner A: *Manual of patient care standards,* Rockville, Md, 1988, Aspen Publishers.

16. Plan of the National Institute on Deafness and Other Communication Disorders, Bethesda, Md, 1989, Institute of Health.

17. Riley MAK: *Nursing care of the client with ear, nose and throat disorders,* New York, 1987, Springer Publishing.

17a. Royal National Institute for Deaf People: *Factsheet—Statistics Relating to Deafness,* London, 1992, Information Services Division RNID.

18.* Rubin W: Noise-induced deafness: major environmental problem, *Hosp Med* 23(7):19-21, 25-27, 1987.

19. Serra AM, Bailey CM, Jackson P: *Ear, nose and throat nursing,* England, 1986, Blackwell Scientific Publications.

20. Tortora ML: Noise-induced hearing loss: prevention in the work environment, *AAOHN J* 35:271-273, 1987.

21. Wolfson RJ, et al: Vertigo, *Clin Sympt* 38(6):2-32, 1986.

22. Becker G, Nadler G: The aged deaf: integration of a disabled group into an agency serving elderly people, *Gerontologist* 20:214-221, 1980.

23.* Koch KJ: The deaf and hard of hearing: some hints, *Nurs Times* 77(32):Suppl 19-20, 1981.

*Recommended for student reading.

FURTHER READING

Bull PD: *Lecture Notes on Diseases of the Ear, Nose and Throat,* ed 6, Oxford, 1985, Blackwell Scientific Publications.

Freeland A: *Deafness: The Facts,* Oxford, 1989, Oxford Medical Publications.

The Patient with Musculoskeletal Disorders

Wilma J. Phipps

After studying this chapter, the learner should be able to:

- Describe three measures to prevent musculoskeletal dysfunction.
- Describe four conservative health measures for people with joint and muscle disorders.
- Describe the pathophysiological changes and therapy for rheumatoid arthritis, systemic lupus erythematosus (SLE), degenerative joint disorders, and scoliosis.
- Describe the nursing care of the patient undergoing a total hip or total knee replacement.
- Discuss the care of the patient undergoing spinal fusion.
- Identify different types of fractures and their treatment.
- Explain the pathophysiology of bone healing.
- Describe problems that may occur with immobilization.
- Describe care of the patient after closed and open reduction of hip fractures (including cast care and traction).

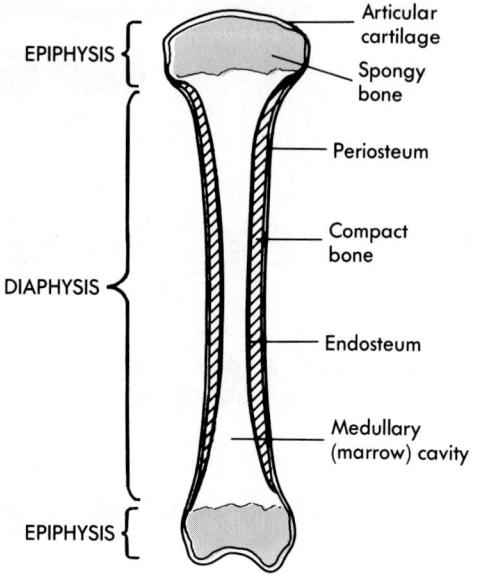

Fig. 32-1   Structure of long bone as seen in longitudinal section.

ANATOMY AND PHYSIOLOGY

Among the characteristics that distinguish man as a species is the ability to maintain an erect posture and to move about. The individual's posture and movements depend on the proper functioning of the musculoskeletal system. The *musculoskeletal system* is composed of bones, muscles, cartilage, ligaments, tendons, fascia, bursae, and joints.

Components of the Musculoskeletal System

Bones

Bones are composed of both living cells and nonliving intracellular material. They are derived from embryonic hyaline cartilage that undergoes *osteogenesis* to become bone. This process is accomplished by cells called *osteoblasts*. The hard quality of the bone is the result of the deposits of calcium salts.

The functions of the bones are as follows:
1. *Support* body tissues and provide the skeletal framework of the body
2. *Protect* body organs (for example, the bony casing of the skull protects the brain)
3. Provide for *movement* (muscles are attached for contraction and motion)
4. Be a *storehouse* for mineral salts (for example, calcium)
5. Provide for *haematopoiesis* (formation of red blood cells in red bone marrow)

Bones are classified into four groups according to their shape:
1. *Long bones* (femur, humerus) consist of a shaft and two epiphyses (see Fig. 32-1). The shaft is formed mainly of *compact* bone tissue. The epiphyses are formed from spongy (cancellous or trabecular) bone. Trabecular bone provides strength to bone while reducing its weight.
2. *Short bones* (carpals) are irregularly shaped and have

an inner core of *cancellous* (spongy) bone with an outer layer of compact bone.
3. *Flat bones* (skull) consist of two outer plates of compact bone with an inner layer of cancellous bone.
4. *Irregular bones* (vertebrae) are similar to short bones.

Muscles

Muscles are divided into three major groups, with the principal function to contract and produce movement of parts of the body or of the entire body. The grouping of muscles is as follows:
1. *Skeletal (striated)* muscle: found in the skeletal system; provides controlled movement, maintains posture, and produces heat
2. *Visceral (smooth)* muscle: found in the digestive tract, urinary tract, and blood vessels; innervated by the autonomic nervous system; contractions not under voluntary control
3. *Cardiac* muscle; found only in the heart; contractions not under voluntary control

Skeletal muscles are organs; they vary in size and shape from long and thin to broad and flat, or they may form bulky masses. Skeletal muscles contract only if they are stimulated. The energy for muscle contraction is supplied by the breakdown of adenosine triphosphate (ATP) and the action of calcium. Muscle fibres that are adequately oxygenated will contract more forcefully than those not adequately oxygenated.

Movements are produced by muscles pulling on bones that serve as levers and joints that serve as fulcrums.

Skeletal muscle is highly vascular. During muscle contraction chemical changes occur, resulting in the formation of waste products. Muscle fatigue and pain result when insufficient oxygen is delivered to the muscle and when waste products are not removed.

Cartilage

Cartilage is composed of fibres embedded in a firm gel. It is strong but flexible, and it is avascular. Nutrients reach the cartilage cells by the process of diffusion through the gel from capillaries located in the *perichondrium* (fibrous covering of the cartilage) or, in the case of articular cartilage, through the synovial fluid. The number of collagenous fibres found in the cartilage will determine its type: fibrous, hyaline, or elastic. *Fibrous* (or fibrocartilage) has the most fibres and therefore the greatest tensile strength. Fibrocartilage composes the intervertebral disks. *Articular* (hyaline) cartilage—smooth, white, shiny, and resilient—covers the articular surfaces of the bone and serves as a cushion. *Elastic* cartilage has the fewest fibres and may be found in areas such as the external ear.

Ligaments

Ligaments are *bands of dense fibrous connective tissue* that are flexible and tough. They connect the articular ends of bones and provide stability. Examples are the medial and lateral collateral ligaments of the knee, which provide mediolateral stability to the knee joint, and the anterior and posterior cruciate ligaments within the joint capsule of the knee, which provide anteroposterior stability. Ligaments may also attach to soft tissue to suspend structures. An example of this is the suspensory ligament of the ovary that passes from the tubal end of the ovary to the peritoneum.

Tendons

Tendons are *bands of dense fibrous tissue* that form the termination of a *muscle* and serve to *attach it to a bone*. The tendon is an extension of the fibrous sheath that envelops each muscle and is continuous with the periosteum at its other end. *Tendon sheaths* are tubular structures of connective tissue that enclose certain tendons, especially in the wrist and ankle. These sheaths are lined with synovial membrane that provides lubrication for easy movement of the tendon.

Fascia

Fascia is a *sheet of loose connective tissue* that may be found directly under the skin as *superficial fascia* or as a sheet of dense, fibrous connective tissue making up the sheath of muscles, nerves, and blood vessels. The latter is known as *deep fascia*.

Bursae

Bursae are *small sacs of connective tissue* located wherever pressure is exerted over moving parts. They may, for example, occur between skin and bone, between tendons and bone, or between muscles. Bursae are lined with *synovial membrane* and contain synovial fluid. They serve as cushions between moving parts. Such a bursa, the *olecranon bursa,* is located between the olecranon process and the skin.

Joints

Movement would not be possible unless some flexibility was provided within the skeletal framework. This flexibility is provided by *joints,* or places where the bones come together. The shape of the joint determines the amount and type of movement that is possible, and the classification of joints is based on the amount of movement they allow.

Classification of joints

There are three major classes of joints:

1. *Synarthroses* or *immovable joints*: Bones connected by fibrous tissue or cartilage, such as the bones of the skull that allow no movement.
2. *Amphiarthroses* or *slightly movable joints*: Joints that allow little movement (for example, intervertebral joints). There is no joint cavity, but tissue (fibrous, cartilage, or bone) is found between the articular surfaces.
3. *Diarthroses* or *freely movable joints*: These include most joints in the body, such as the hip, knee, shoulder, and elbow. The adjacent ends of the bones are covered with hyaline cartilage and surrounded by a fibrous *joint capsule* lined with a synovial membrane that secretes synovial fluid to lubricate the joint (Fig. 32-2). Ligaments and tendons of muscles play an important part in stabilizing the joint. Movements permitted by these joints are as follows:

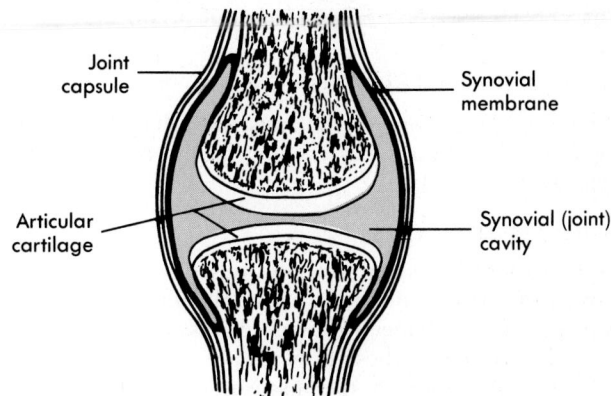

Fig. 32-2   Structure of diarthrodial joint.

a. Flexion
b. Extension
c. Adduction
d. Abduction
e. Rotation
f. Circumduction
g. Special movements, that is, supination, pronation, inversion, eversion, and protraction

Physiological Changes With Ageing

There are periods in the life span when individuals are most vulnerable to musculoskeletal changes. These changes may occur during childhood and adolescence because of rapid growth and development or from the onset of maturity to old age. Changes in musculoskeletal structure and function vary among individuals during the ageing process.

Changes that occur with ageing constitute a continuation of the decline that began in the middle years. The total number of body cells diminishes, resulting in evident connective tissue changes, decrease in the amount and elasticity of subcutaneous tissue, and loss of muscle bulk, tone, and strength. Total body fat is decreased and redistributed from the periphery to the centre of the body and especially on the abdomen. Other physiological changes are as follows.

1. There is a general decrease in stature of 6 to 10 cm from onset of maturity to old age.
2. Shoulder width decreases.
3. Flexion occurs at the knees and hips.
4. A narrowing of the intervertebral disk causes diminished size of the intervertebral and intercostal spaces.
5. The following occurrences are common:
   a. Compression fractures of the vertebrae.
   b. Increased curvature of the thoracic spine (senile kyphosis, dowager's hump, or widow's hump).
   c. Backward tilting of the head and a shortening of the neck to compensate for the kyphosis deformity.
   d. Greater arm span than height, thus giving the older person a "gangly" appearance.
   e. Unsteady gait, with changes in the muscles and motor function.

PREVENTION AND HEALTH EDUCATION

People at Risk and Risk Factors

Whatever the nature of the musculoskeletal disability, there are prevention and teaching factors that must be considered.

Nonpreventable factors

Many of the diseases that affect the musculoskeletal system have at this time an unknown cause. Rheumatoid arthritis and the diffuse connective tissue diseases are but a few examples. Although these diseases are not now preventable, complications of the diseases are preventable—contractures, atrophy, skin breakdown, and others. In these instances, prevention depends on teaching the patient about the disease process and how to employ preventive measures. These preventive measures will be covered in this chapter.

Preventable factors

Polio vaccine, screening of school-aged children for scoliosis, and screening tests for streptococcal infections with early treatment of the infection to prevent rheumatic fever are examples of preventive measures that can be employed on a community-wide basis in combating illnesses that cause musculoskeletal disability. Early attention to posture; good dietary habits; genetic counselling for individuals with sickle cell anaemia and haemophilia; teaching of good body mechanics for individuals whose jobs entail lifting or carrying heavy objects; and concern and attention to the recommendations of the Royal Society for the Prevention of Accidents, and the Department of Health, to help avoid accidents at home, on the job, and on the road are all examples of preventive measures that may be employed to decrease musculoskeletal disability within the general population.

Preventive Health Teaching

Promotion of safety

For those individuals who have limitations of motion or mobility, a variety of precautions and protective or safety devices can be employed in the hospital or the home. Examples would be grab bars that can be mounted on a wall near a bath or toilet, safety arms that fit around a toilet, and rails that fasten onto the side of a bath. These devices provide the person with both a stable place to hold onto and a point of leverage for assuming a standing or sitting position. Throw rugs and obstacles should be removed from areas used by individuals with ambulatory difficulties, and floors should not be highly waxed. Wheel chairs should have adequate locking devices, and patients who must use wheelchairs should be taught how to lock and unlock the chair. Nurses should know where in the community needed equipment can be obtained.

Prevention of muscle and joint complications

Maintenance of joint mobility

For the individual with limited motion or mobility, range of motion exercises should be carried out to prevent joint stiffness or contracture from disuse. Whenever it is possible, except in conditions where acute joint inflammation is present, range of motion exercises should be performed several times a day. *Active range of motion* is most beneficial for the patient. Encouraging patients to do as much of their own care as they are able to do within the restrictions of their disability will often satisfy active range of motion requirements.

Several precautions should be mentioned. *Passive range of motion* exercises should not be performed past the point of the complaint of pain. Particularly in individuals with pathological skeletal conditions (gross deformity, osteoporosis), fractures can result if a joint is forced through "normal" range of motion. Also, acutely inflamed, painful, or septic joints should be rested, because harm can be done by moving the joint before inflammation has subsided. The person who has pain is also likely to resist movement to avoid further pain.

Maintenance of posture

Although maintenance of good posture is important for all people, it is especially important for the patient with chronic arthritis. Poor posture exerts further strain on already damaged joints and not only may cause pain and fatigue but predisposes to increased deformity.

The person who must remain in bed for a long period of time in traction or in a cast should be in a bed with a firm mattress, and a bed board should be placed under the mattress. A firm bed lessens pain by preventing motion and consequent pull on painful joints and helps to keep the spine in good alignment. Boards should be long enough and wide enough to rest firmly on the main side and end rails of the bed, not on the bedsprings. The person with arthritis should either use no pillow or should use one small pillow that fits well down under the shoulder so that forward flexion of the cervical spine is not encouraged. Knees should not be flexed on pillows, and all patients who must be confined to bed most of the day should lie prone with a pillow under the abdomen for a part of each day to relieve supine pressure areas (inferior scapular areas, sacrum, coccyx, and ischial tuberosities).

Careful positioning with *trochanter rolls* (rolled towels or bath blankets to brace an extremity in the desired position), supportive pillows, attention to avoiding extreme flexion of joints, and care to avoid compressing nerves or arteries (the result of which can be neurological or circulatory compromise) are all important considerations for both skin care and general maintenance of the patient.

The unaffected foot (or feet) should rest against a footboard at least part of the day. This helps to maintain the foot in a neutral position for a more normal walking position, prevents the weight of bedclothes from contributing to foot-drop, and provides a firm surface against which the patient can do resistive foot exercises. Patients should be taught to check the position of their lower limbs when at rest. If their problem is nonneurological, they should "toe in" to prevent external rotation contracture of the hip and pronation of the foot. These complications cause serious difficulty when walking is resumed.

For the general public, it should be remembered that *poor posture* throughout life may contribute to *hypertrophic arthritis*. Moulding the pelvis correctly with a posterior pelvic tilt will help prevent increased curvature of the lower back with its resultant strain on muscles and joints. Holding the head up with the chin in takes a great deal of strain from the joints of the upper spine. It is surprising how many older people can benefit from posture improvement even though damage may date from childhood. Nurses should teach patients good body mechanics to prevent muscle strain that could pull a joint out of alignment just enough for musculoskeletal changes to develop or to cause symptoms.

Teaching the person with joint and muscle disorders

The following are *conservative measures* for individuals with joint and muscle disorders. They can be *restorative, preventive*, or *analgesic in nature*.

Activity

Because many musculoskeletal disorders are problems of activity limitation, teaching is directed towards improving activity. Absolute rest of a limb, joint, or part of the body may be ordered to prevent further tissue destruction and pain. As symptoms subside, activity will be gradually increased.

The patient needs to recognize that clues such as pain, tiredness, and progressive loss of dexterity indicate a need for rest. The most frequent indicator that a joint has been overused or misused as in increase in pain or fatigue. Joint *protection techniques* that can be helpful, particularly for chronic inflammatory joint disorders, are as follows:

1. *Energy conservation techniques*: Examples are sliding rather than lifting objects and moving dishes, utensils, or equipment on a trolley rather than carrying them.
2. *Avoiding positions of possible deformity*: Because flexor muscles are stronger than extensor muscles, joints tend to become deformed in a position of flexion. For example, avoid sitting for long periods, keeping the knees or elbows bent to avoid pain, and twisting motions to turn doorknobs or remove a lid.
3. *Learning to avoid holding muscles or joints in one position for a long time*:
   a. Activities need to be varied (as just mentioned)
   b. Active range of motion exercises are encouraged.
4. *Learning to use the strongest joints for activities*:
   a. Use good posture when sitting and standing.
   b. Work at a comfortable height.
   c. Stoop and use the knees and not the back when lifting objects.

Assistive, supportive, and safety devices

Although the occupational therapist may recommend specific assistive devices and teach the patient how to use them, the nurse needs to understand the need for them and encourage their use in self-care activities.

Supportive devices or ambulatory aids (walkers, canes, crutches) permit part of the patient's weight to be transferred to the upper extremities. The physiotherapist determines the specific device that is needed. Physiotherapists generally select and teach the person how to use ambulatory devices. However, nurses may be called on to do this teaching. They must, in any case, know how to supervise the patient who uses ambulatory aids. The most common gait patterns that may be used with a walker, cane, or crutches are the *three-point gait*, the *two-point gait*, and the *four-point gait*. These gait patterns are covered in Chapter 18.

Examples of *safety devices* used include the following:
1. Grab bars around toilets, baths, and showers
2. Elevated toilet seats
3. Skid-proof mats or adhesive strips on bathroom floors
4. Hand rails along hallways and staircases
5. Nonskid wax applied to floors

Use of heat and cold

1. Moist heat is often used for relaxation of muscles and for sedative and analgesic effects.
2. Cold is often used to reduce or prevent swelling after trauma and to reduce pain and stiffness in some cases.
3. Precautions when using heat or cold:
   a. Apply with care to patient with decreased sensation.
   b. Check skin frequently for evidence of redness or burning.
   c. Moist compresses must be left on for 15 to 20 minutes to achieve maximal effectiveness.
   d. Dry heat must have a control device to maintain the heat at a low level.
   e. Do not use heat on joints that are or may be *infected*.
   f. Ice packs must be wrapped in towelling to protect the skin.

Splinting and bracing

Splints and braces (orthoses) are used to stabilize or support a joint to protect it from improper use or external trauma.

1. *Spring-loaded braces* are designed to oppose the action of unparalysed muscles and to act as partial functional substitutes for the paralyzed muscles.
2. *Resting splints* are designed to maintain a limb or joint in a functional position while permitting the muscles around the joint to relax (Fig. 32-3). They are used by the patient with rheumatoid arthritis to decrease muscle spasms that contribute to joint deformity.
3. *Functional splints* maintain the joint or limb in a usable position such as in the case of a drop wrist or foot-drop (Fig. 32-4).
4. *Dynamic splints* permit assisted exercise to joints, particularly after surgery to finger joints.

Special considerations for splinting and bracing include the following:
1. Corrective shoes may be ordered for the feet to provide support and safety. These should be Oxford type with laces.
2. Observations of the patient's skin should be made after an orthosis has been worn, even for short periods, for areas of skin irritation. Adjustment may be needed by the *orthotist* (brace maker).
3. Patients must learn how to apply and remove braces or splints and how to care for them.
   a. Metal braces should be stored upright.
   b. Splints of moulded materials should be stored away from sources of heat.
   c. Leather materials should be treated with Neatsfoot

Compound or other leather preservative to prevent drying and cracking.

4. The brace should be adjusted if there is a change in weight (loss or gain).

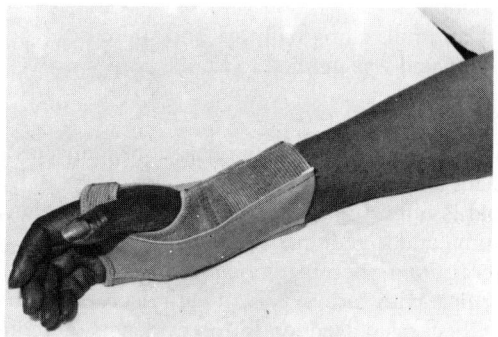

Fig. 32-3   Resting splints.

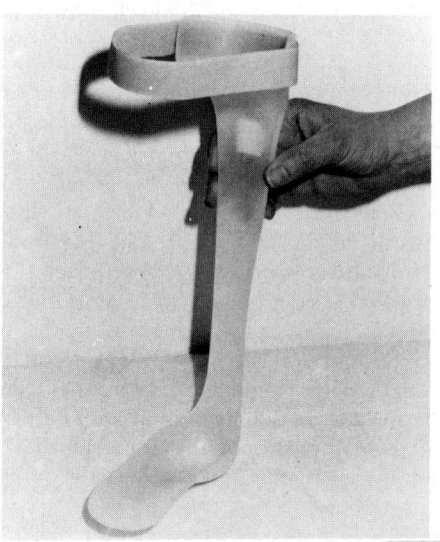

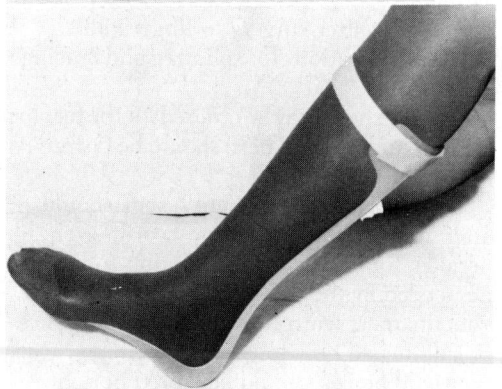

Fig. 32-4   Functional splints.

Positioning and transfer

Principles of positioning can be found in most fundamentals of nursing texts. However, because pain accompanies nearly all musculoskeletal problems, preventing or minimizing pain must be taken into consideration when positioning the patient. Nurses should be aware that patients in the acute stages of their disorders require the greatest care and gentleness when they must be moved. *Fear of pain often causes irritability and can lead to muscular resistance, which increases pain.* Care must be taken not to jar the bed. Heavy bedclothes over painful extremities may cause added pain. If bed cradles are used to support linen, caution must be taken not to accidentally bump an involved part of the body when adjusting or removing the cradle. Placing a very painful joint or extremity on a pillow or pillows to move it can reduce pain. Moving patients off the bed using a pull sheet or a roller board also facilitates comfort through the move. Frequently, patients prefer to move themselves rather than risk pain from having someone else move them; when it is safe for the patient to do so, the nurse should permit it.

If the patient must use a wheelchair, it should be adjusted to fit that individual. No wheelchair should be purchased for permanent use by a patient unless someone knowledgeable about wheelchairs, preferably a physiotherapist, has evaluated the patient and determined what special equipment is needed. Chairs poorly fitted to the patient's needs can be unsafe and encourage poor posture.

FOCUS ON THE FUTURE

Goals for the Year 2000

Limitation in major activity

The annual report of the Chief Medical Officer for 1990, revealed an average 11% of men and 15% of women in Britain had some limitations to performing major activities[16a], such as working or keeping house, or were limited in the amount or kind of major activity they could perform.

The WHO goal for the year 2000 is to reduce the proportion of people who experience limitation in major activity caused by chronic conditions.

Among noninstitutionalized people 65 and older, the chronic conditions most frequently indicated as the main reason for need for assistance with home management of activities or activities of daily living were arthritis, heart disease, lung disease, gastro-intestinal and back problems.[16a] In addition, people reporting limitations in activity were more likely to have multiple health problems.[81]

Back pain accounts for the greatest loss of work hours in the U.K., and at least 80% of the population will experience back pain at some time in their lives.[7a] To address this problem, the current emphasis is on prevention. Interventions to prevent low back injury include education, physical conditioning, weight loss, teaching people to squat and bend from the knees when lifting, and in some instances environmental redesign of certain work tasks may be indicated. Strength and endurance training and maintaining a high level of physical fitness are measures that have been shown to prevent back injuries.

Studies of back pain in nurses have revealed that back injuries result from the accumulation of general postural stress, such as patient handling.[7a] Guidelines for avoiding back strain at work are provided in *Back Pain in Nurses* by the Ergonomics Research Unit of the Robens Institute at the University of Surrey[71a] and in *The Guide to the Handling of Patients* by the National Back Pain Association and the Royal College of Nursing.[63a]

CARING FOR PEOPLE

The 1989 white paper "Caring for People" proposed changes in services for people with disabilities. The changes proposed were intended to:

* Enable people to live as normal a life as possible, in their own homes, or in a homely environment in the local community.

* Provide the right amount of care and support to help people achieve maximum possible independence by acquiring or reacquiring basic living skills, to help them reach their full potential.

* Give people a greater individual say in how they live their lives and the services they need to help them do so.[75a]

Areas for target include: employment, public services such as bus and rail transportation, public accommodations, and telecommunication services. The Disabled Persons Employment Act of 1945 forbids discrimination in hiring or promotion against a qualified person with a disability. Public places such as restaurants, hotels, and retail stores have to remove physical barriers such as steps. This means adding ramps, assuring that doorways are wide enough to accommodate wheelchairs, and providing accessible toilet facilities with grab bars in toilet stalls. Additionally, kerbs have to have cut-aways to accommodate wheelchairs, and handicapped parking spaces must be provided.

Unless one has a mobility problem it is hard to appreciate how barriers can interfere with a person's independence. Nurses, in particular, should be sensitive to the needs of those with disabilities and should survey public accommodations in their communities for their accessibility to the handicapped. If barriers exist, these should be brought to the attention of those in charge of the facility.

MAJOR HEALTH PROBLEMS OF THE MUSCULOSKELETAL SYSTEM

The disorders and injuries of the musculoskeletal system are vast in scope. They range from those that cause the patient minor discomfort and inconvenience to those that are life threatening. Among the more troublesome are the inflammatory or rheumatic diseases. These diseases, though they may involve many systems, very often have an arthritic component. There are more than 100 arthritic diseases. Ten million men and women in Britain are affected by arthritis, and one million of those affected are under 45 years old. Arthritis also affects 50,000 children (Arthritis Care, Oct., 1993). The total economic cost of arthritis including both direct (medical care) and indirect cost (lost wages), is substantial.

Listed here are some common musculoskeletal disorders that will be covered in this chapter.

1. *Inflammatory disorders*: rheumatoid arthritis, systemic lupus erythematosus, polymyositis (dermatomyositis), ankylosing spondylitis
2. *Nonarticular rheumatism*: bursitis, carpal tunnel syndrome, Dupuytren's contracture
3. *Degenerative disorders*: degenerative joint disorders and degenerative joint disorders of the spine
4. *Restrictive disorders*: scoliosis
5. *Other disorders*: gout, bacterial arthritis
6. *Trauma*: fractures of bone and soft tissue injuries

RHEUMATOID ARTHRITIS
Aetiology/Epidemiology

Rheumatoid arthritis is a chronic systemic disease. The disease process, although most prominent as a nonsuppurative inflammation in the diarthrodial joints, may also be manifested by lesions of the vasculature, lungs, nervous system, and other major organs of the body.

Rheumatoid arthritis is more prevalent in women than

men by a ratio of 2:1 or 3:1. Usually it appears during productive years of life when career and family responsibilities are greatest. Although the cause of this disease is unknown, several theories of causation are under investigation. Areas of study include (1) immune mechanisms, such as the interaction of the IgG class of immunoglobins with the rheumatoid factor (RF) that appears to play a role in perpetuating rheumatoid inflammation; (2) metabolic factors; and (3) infection, with particular attention to viruses.

The signs and symptoms and medical therapy appear in Table 32-1.

Pathophysiology

The disease process within the joints (intraarticular) begins as an inflammation of the synovium with oedema, vascular congestion, fibrin exudate, and cellular infiltrate. The inflammatory process is set off by some sort of irritation or damage to joint tissue. This is called a "triggering" event. White blood cells rush into the area, releasing chemicals (including superoxide radicals and hydrogen peroxide) useful in destroying bacteria, but also harmful to tissue cells. Also released are prostaglandins (chemicals that mediate inflammation), leukotrienes (producers of inflammation), and digestive enzymes. Particularly damaging to joint tissue is the *enzyme collagenase* because it breaks down collagen, the main structural protein of connective tissue. *The presence of these substances within the joint attracts still more white blood cells, and in rheumatoid arthritis, the process becomes chronic. Continued inflammation leads to thickening of synovium, particularly where it joins the articular cartilage.* At these junctures, granulation tissue forms a *pannus*, or mantle, that covers the surface of the cartilage. The pannus also invades subchondral bone (bone underlying the cartilage). As the amount of granulation tissue from inflammation increases, it interferes with normal nutrition of the articular cartilage and the cartilage becomes necrotic.

REVIEW

Table 32-1   Inflammatory disorder: rheumatoid arthritis

Signs and symptoms	Medical therapy
Local	**Goals**
Generalized joint aching with stiffness and limitation in motion	Relief of pain
	Maintenance of joint function
Gradual swelling, warmth, redness, and tenderness	Prevention and correction of deformities
Changes in appearance of hands	Correction of other health problems
Fusiform or spindle-shaped swelling of fingers (Fig. 32-5, A, B)	
Swan-neck deformities of fingers	**Rest**
Ulnar deviation of the hands (Fig. 32-5, C)	Complete bed rest during acute periods; otherwise 2 to 4 hr daily; rest for joints with splints
All joints can become involved: hips, knees, wrists, elbows, shouldders, and jaw	**Physiotherapy**
	Active-assistive exercises to regular programme of active exercises to preserve function
Systemic	Moist heat packs or baths for muscle relaxing and relief of pain
Fatigue, malaise, fever, tachycardia, weakness, loss of weight, anaemia; gradual bilateral, symmetric polyarthritis of small and large joints in all extremities	**Medications**
	Table 32-2 lists medications prescribed to reduce inflammation and pain
	Surgery
	Reconstructive surgery may be necessary

The degree of erosion of the articular cartilage determines the amount of articular disability. If large areas of cartilage are destroyed, adhesions form between the joint surfaces, and fibrous or bony union (ankylosis) develops between what were previously free-moving surfaces. Destruction of cartilage and bone, in addition to some weakening of tendons and ligaments, may lead to subluxation or dislocation of joints. Invasion of the subchondral bone may cause eventual regional osteoporosis.

The early manifestations of the disease may include fever, weight loss, fatigue, and generalized aching. *Early morning stiffness* lasting a few minutes to an hour or more is characteristic. The person may describe the location of aching and stiffness in general terms as opposed to naming specific joints. *This kind of discomfort, commonly referred to as fibrositis, is poorly localized.* Such discomfort may be the patient's earliest complaint. These symptoms may be present for some time before they are replaced by more specific, or localized, problems (that is, frank articular inflammation with joint swelling, pain, redness, warmth, and tenderness). In other people, fibrositis and joint inflammation occur together at the onset. Table 32-1 summarizes signs and symptoms and medical therapy.

Nursing Process
Assessment
Subjective data

The early manifestations of rheumatoid arthritis may lead the patient to describe the location of aching and stiffness "in my arms," "in my hands," or "in my legs" as opposed to naming specific joints. This kind of discomfort is more common in the morning ("early morning stiffness") and may be present for some time before the person begins to see and feel the joint changes.

Objective data

1. Inspection and palpation: check same joints on *both sides of body* for symmetry, skin colour, size and shape, tenderness, and swelling
2. Evaluate passive range of motion of synovial joints
   a. Note any deviation from normal (limited joint movement most important)
   b. Note presence of crepitation (*crepitus*), which is an audible grating sound made by movement of bony surfaces within the joint
   c. Note pain with range of motion
3. Inspect and palpate skeletal muscles bilaterally
   a. Note atrophy, tone, and tenderness
   b. Test muscle strength by having the patient move the muscle against resistance.

Diagnostic tests

1. Serological tests
   a. Erythrocyte sedimentation rate: will be elevated
   b. Red and white blood cell count: will reveal anaemia and leukocytosis
   c. Rheumatoid factor (RF) (present in 50% to 90% of patients, depending on duration and severity of disease): serum will show presence of large antibody-like protein molecules
   d. Latex fixation test is positive
2. Radiological examinations
   a. Periarticular osteoporosis: joint surface erosion
   b. Later: narrowing of joint space, subluxation, and ankylosis
3. Joint aspiration: samples of synovial fluid from within the joint cavity will determine the presence of an aseptic inflammatory process; synovial fluid is cultured and examined microscopically. Commonly there is increased turbidity and decreased viscosity of synovial fluid.

Analysis

Nursing problems are determined from assessment of patient data. Possible nursing problems for the patient with rheumatoid arthritis may include, but are not limited to, the following:

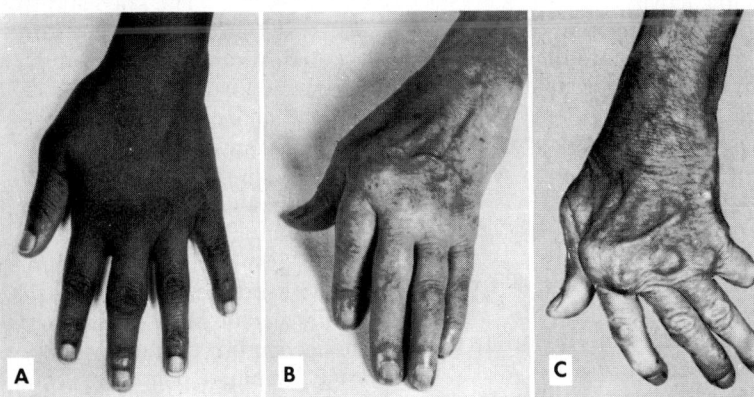

Fig. 32-5 Rheumatoid arthritis of hand. **A,** Early stage. Note fusiform swelling of proximal interphalangeal joints, especially that of middle finger. **B,** Moderate involvement. Note swelling from chronic synovitis of metacarpophalangeal joints and early ulnar rift. **C,** Advanced stage. Note marked ulnar drift and subluxation of metacarpophalangeal joints with extension of proximal interphalangeal joints and flexion of distal joints. Note also deformed position of thumb. Hand has wasted appearance. (From Brashear H, Raney R: *Handbook of orthopedic surgery,* ed 10, St Louis, 1986, Mosby–Year Book.)

Problem	Possible aetiologies
Self-care deficit; bathing/ hygiene, dressing/ grooming, toileting	Musculoskeletal impairment, inability to use certain joints/ limitations in motion
Pain, chronic: joint	Pathological changes caused by RA
Injury, high risk for	Loss of muscle strength, pain and stiffness in joints
Knowledge deficit about rheumatoid arthritis	Lack of information regarding RA or misinterpretation of information
Body image disturbance	Change in body appearance, swollen, deformed joints; change in posture

Planning: expected patient outcomes

Expected patient outcomes for the person with rheumatoid arthritis may include, but are not limited to, the following:

1. Patient demonstrates improved ability to perform ADL.
2. Patient is more comfortable; patient states joint pain is decreased.
3. Patient has improved active joint range of motion, and risk of injury is reduced.
4. Patient can explain the disease process and follow-up care including prescribed therapy (exercises, medications) and plans established for follow-up by the doctor.
5. Patient has a more positive self-concept.

Implementation

Assisting with achievement of therapeutic goals

1. Give prescribed medications on time and in prescribed doses.
2. Assist with selection of foods; assist with feeding if necessary; encourage small, frequent meals.
3. Encourage patient to maintain normal weight.

Interventions to achieve patient outcomes

Promoting mobility and preventing injury

1. *Avoid* positioning joints in such a way as to encourage contracture (for example, pillows under knees when supine, pillows forcing neck into forward flexion).
2. Encourage regular active range of motion of joints to greatest degree possible.
3. Encourage patient to assist with own ADL to greatest degree possible, with assistive aids if necessary.
4. Encourage patient to perform prescribed exercises on a regular basis.
5. Avoid injury by providing appropriate ambulatory devices and encouraging patient to wear *shoes*, not slippers, for ambulation.

Assisting with comfort and ADL

1. Assist with self-care while promoting independence as much as possible.
2. Keep patient free of pain with prescribed medications.
3. Apply heat or cold to joints as prescribed.
4. Promote frequent position changes; often patient is more comfortable changing own position.
5. Provide for adequate rest periods.
6. Encourage use of resting splints.

Facilitating learning

When teaching people about rheumatoid arthritis (and other rheumatic diseases) nurses may find it helpful to use some of the patient information that has been prepared by Arthritis Care* and written in such a way that most patients can understand and learn from them.

Patient teaching should include information about the following:[8]

---

*Arthritis Care, 6 Grosvenor Crescent, London, SW1X 7EP

1. Proper balance of rest and activity
2. Joint protection and energy conservation techniques
3. Proper use of medications—names of drugs, dosages, precautions in administration, and side effects or toxic effects
4. Plans for implementation of exercise programme prescribed by the doctor or physiotherapist
5. Proper application of heat and/or cold packs
6. Proper use of walking aids and other assistive devices
7. Safety measures to prevent injury
8. Application, appropriate use of, and care of splints, braces
9. The basics of good nutrition and the importance of avoiding weight gain
10. The importance of regular follow-up with the doctor
11. The risks of following non-medical programmes that promise a "cure"
12. Information about local arthritis support groups and programmes, services of the Arthritis Care

In teaching the patient it is helpful to understand the following biomechanical principles.

1. Using a walking stick (in the contralateral hand) can alleviate pain, and the force across a hip can be reduced by 60%.[46]
2. Arising from a chair or toilet seat may be greatly assisted by raising the level of the seat, because the highest pressures on the hip and knee joints are produced during flexion and pushing off.[46] For this reason, people with arthritis of the hip or knee can arise best from a firm (not overstuffed) chair with arms.

Promoting a positive body image

1. Compliment patient on each improvement in mobility and self-care.
2. Allow time to listen to patient's concerns about body image.
3. Encourage patient to dress self in street clothes before beginning the day's activities.
4. Encourage self-care, combing hair and shaving for men and combing hair and applying makeup for women.

Evaluation

Evaluation is based on the expected patient outcomes. Questions to be asked include the following:

1. Is the patient better able to carry out ADL?
2. Is patient comfortable?
3. Is the potential for injury lessened?
4. Can the patient explain the need for follow-up care, medications, the programme of exercises, and alternating rest and activity?
5. Does the patient exhibit a more positive attitude about body image?

Reconstructive Surgery

When rheumatoid arthritis is progressive or has caused severe joint destruction, surgery may be indicated to relieve pain and improve function.

The common types of surgery and the indications for each are outlined below.

Synovectomy. The early removal of synovial tissue to arrest the course of rheumatoid arthritis in a particular joint, to maintain joint function, and to prevent recurrent inflammation. The knee and the wrist are the joints most often subjected to this procedure.

Arthrotomy. Opening into a joint. The procedure is used to accomplish the following:

1. Explore the joint to determine the presence of a disease process
2. Drain the joint
3. Remove damaged tissue or foreign bodies within the joint
4. Most often performed on the knee

Arthrodesis. Surgical fusion of a joint. Commonly performed on knee, wrist, or ankle. The procedure is used to accomplish the following:

1. Eliminate painful motion
2. Provide stability

Arthroplasty. Resurfacing of one or both sides of a diseased joint.

1. Purposes
   a. Restore motion of the joint
   b. Relieve pain
   c. Correct deformity
2. Types
   a. Replacement of part of the joint with a prosthesis made of metal or other material such as the "cup" or "mould" arthroplasty of the hip joint.
   b. Surgical reshaping of the bones of the joint, which are then covered with soft tissue used as an interposition device.
   c. Total joint replacement where both sides of the joint are replaced by metal or polyethylene implants.

Replacement arthroplasty

Replacement arthroplasty is available for the shoulder, wrist, elbow, phalangeal joints of the fingers, hips (Fig. 32-6), knee (Fig. 32-7), and ankle. The *hip* and *knee* are the *most commonly replaced joints*. The discussion that follows will be limited to these two joints.

Rheumatoid arthritis, degenerative joint disease, and *avascular necrosis* are the *major reasons for performing total joint or replacement arthroplasty. Avascular necrosis* of the bone, or bone death, is caused by inadequate blood supply. It can be a *complication of bone fractures,* corticosteroid treatment, and systemic lupus erythematosus. Pain (even at rest), restricted motion, and gait disturbances are characteristic. Surgery in the form of total joint replacement is performed to alleviate pain and increase motion.

The knee replacement consists of a femoral and tibial component and a patellar button (Fig. 32-7). The hip prosthesis consists of an acetabular portion (cup) and a femoral component. The designs of the various prostheses vary in size of the femoral head, shape and length of the femoral shaft, and design of the acetabular component. The care of the patient undergoing total hip replacement is outlined in Box 32-1. The care of the patient undergoing total knee replacement is outlined in Box 32-2.

Replacement prosthesis may be either *cemented* (held into bone with polymethylmethacrylate) or *uncemented* (treated with a special porous coating that promotes ingrowth of new bone). The uncemented knee replacement may be held in place with short-leg "studs" placed into holes in the recipient bone.[62] The long-term survival of hip and knee replacements is discussed next.

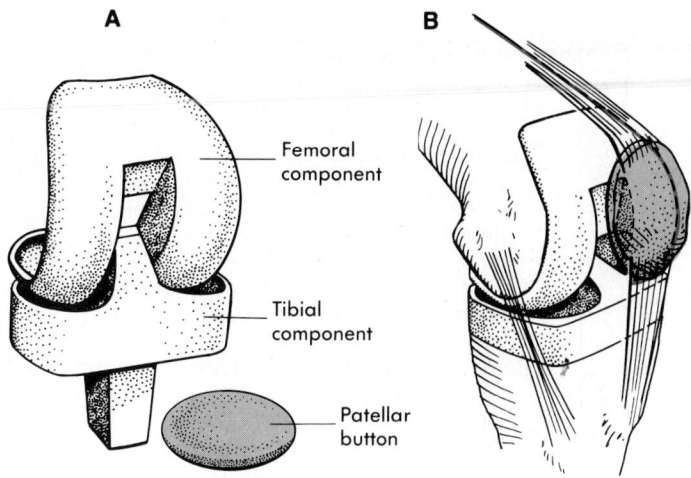

Fig. 32-7 A, Tibial and femoral components of total knee prosthesis. Patellar button, made of polyethylene, protects posterior surface of patella from friction against femoral component when knee is moved through flexion and extension. **B,** Total knee prosthesis in place.

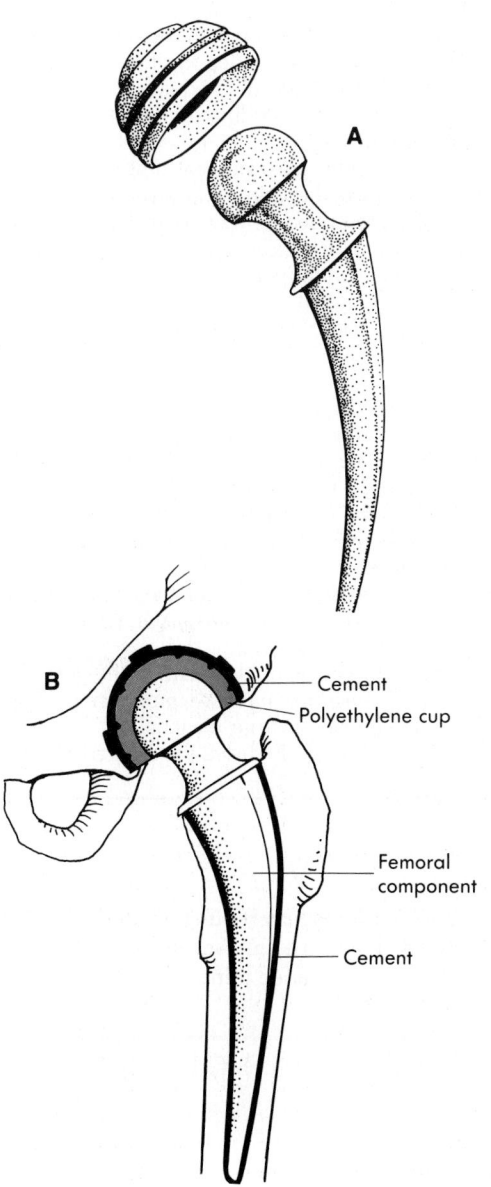

Fig. 32-6 A, Acetabular and femoral components of total hip prosthesis. **B,** Total hip prosthesis in place.

REVIEW

Table 32-2   Inflammatory disorder: systemic lupus erythematosus (SLE)

Signs and symptoms	Medical therapy
General complaints: Moderate to severe—fever, weakness, fatigue, weight loss, sensitivity to sun, erythematous rash ("butterfly" pattern over bridge of nose and cheeks)	Rest: when disease active No specific treatment; therapeutic programme is ordered for the specific problems of the patient
Polyarthralgia and arthritis with pain and swelling	Medications (Table 36-3): adrenocorticosteroid therapy to control active manifestations of SLE; salicylates for joint pains; antimalarial drugs (Chloroquine) for cutaneous lesions; cytoxic agents if other drugs fail
Polyserositis (pleurisy and pericarditis)	
Anaemia, thrombocytopaenia and renal, neurological, and cardiac abnormalities	
Alopecia (hair loss) possible during periods of active systemic disease	

Long-term survival of joint implants

Hip replacement

From the first use of replacement joints, there was concern about how long the implant would survive. In 1989, the first results were published of a 15-year follow-up of patients with hip replacement. This study reported that 78% of the implants were good or excellent and 88% were still functioning after 15 years.[60] Autopsy reports of persons who had had total hip replacement indicated that the polymethylmethacrylate, the cement used to fix the joint in place, was well tolerated. Thus polymethylmethacrylate will continue to be used to fix some, if not most, hip replacements.

The patient undergoing total hip replacement

Preoperative care

Skin care

Preparation of the skin will follow the hospital's written procedure or the surgeon's written orders.

The area must be kept free of contamination.

The patient's environment must be as free as possible from potential sources of contamination.

Reassurance and education

Patient needs to understand about the surgical procedure, postoperative care, and expectations after discharge.

Patient is to sign a consent form and have an understanding of its importance (informed consent).

Patient may have both hips replaced at one surgery.

Postoperative care

Positioning

Position will depend on the design of the prosthesis and the method of insertion.

Restrictions designed to avoid dislocation of the prosthesis usually include the following:

Flexion limited to 60 degrees for 6-10 days, then 90 degrees for 2-3 months

No adduction beyond midline for 2-3 months, therefore no sidelying on operative side. Leg is maintained in abduction when lying supine or on the nonoperative side.

No extreme internal or external rotation.

Wound care: Drains are placed in the wound to prevent formation of a haematoma.

Maintain constant suction through the self-contained vacuum.

Note amount and type of drainage. Keep area free of contamination. (Infection at the site of the prosthesis results in total failure of the surgery.)

Activity

Observe flexion restrictions when elevating head of bed.

Encourage periodic elevation and lowering of head of bed to provide motion at hip.

Instruct patient in use of overhead trapeze to shift weight and lift for bedpan, change of linen.

The patient undergoing total hip replacement—cont'd

Encourage active dorsi-plantar flexion exercise of ankles, quadriceps and gluteal setting exercises to promote venous return, prevent thrombus formation, and maintain muscle tone (see Chapter 18).

Patient may be turned to unoperative side with operative leg maintained in abduction and extension.

Begin mobilization as early as the first postoperative day, if tolerated.

Observe flexion and adduction restrictions.

Observe weight-bearing restrictions prescribed by surgeon (usually partial weight bearing assisted with walker or crutches).

Increase amount of walking each day according to patient's tolerance.

Begin sitting when patient demonstrates sufficient control of leg to sit within flexion restrictions (usually requires elevation of sitting surfaces, including use of raised toilet seat).

Medications

Prophylactic anticoagulant drugs (aspirin, low-dose heparin, or warfarin) may be prescribed to decrease risk of thrombus formation.

At first, control pain by positioning; use narcotics, gradually tapered to nonnarcotic analgesics, according to patient's tolerance. Many patients will have patient controlled analgesia (PCA).

Discharge instructions

Patient must use ambulatory aid, avoid adduction, and limit hip flexion to 90 degrees for about 2 to 3 months.

A raised toilet seat is to be obtained and used at home until flexion restrictions are removed.

Patient may need a long-handled shoe horn and reacher to facilitate ADL within flexion restriction.

Patient must be made aware of the possible lifelong need for antibiotic prophylaxis to protect the prosthesis from bacterial infection during dental work, intrusive procedures, or surgery.

Knee replacement

Research has focused on the presence and significance of wear debris, especially in the patellar component of the knee prosthesis. Because of wear debris, some orthopaedic surgeons have discontinued use of the patellar component of the knee joint.[60] Patients who have considerable wear debris may have pain and/or a squeaking of the knee with movement as the debris rubs against the underside of the patella. Such patients may require a patellectomy (removal of the patella) along with removal of the patellar component and the debris in the knee joint.

SYSTEMIC LUPUS ERYTHEMATOSUS

Aetiology/Epidemiology

Systemic lupus erythematosus (SLE) is a chronic inflammatory disease of unknown cause. It affects women, particularly adolescents and young adults, 8 to 10 times more often than men. The disease was named after its charac-

The patient undergoing total knee replacement

Preoperative care
Same as for total hip replacement.

Postoperative care
Positioning
    The operative leg(s) is (are) elevated on pillows to enhance venous return for the first 48 hours. Pillows are placed with caution not to flex the knee. Many patients have bilateral total knee replacements at one surgery.
    The patient may be turned from side to back to side.
Wound care
    Care of drains as for total hip replacement.
    Patient is assessed for systemic evidence of loss of blood (hypotension, tachycardia) if bulky compression dressing is used because it may hold large quantities of drainage before drainage becomes visible.
    Bulky dressings are removed before the patient begins active flexion.
Activity
    Passive flexion in a continuous passive motion machine (CPM) within prescribed flexion-extension limits may be started in the recovery room. Patient's leg should remain in machine as much as tolerated (up to 22 hours per day) to facilitate even healing of tissue.
    Patient is encouraged to perform active dorsiplantar flexion of the ankles, quadriceps setting, and, after the drain is removed, straight leg raising exercises.
    Patient begins active flexion exercises three to four times a day about the fifth postoperative day.
    Light weight bearing with an assistive device may be started as early as first postoperative day and increased as patient tolerates.
    Sitting in a chair with the leg(s) elevated may be started on the first postoperative day.
    Patient is encouraged to wear a resting knee extension splint (immobilizer) on the operated leg until able to demonstrate quadriceps control (independent straight leg raising).
Pain control
    Initial control of pain with narcotics, positioning; gradual decrease of medication to nonnarcotic analgesics, as patient tolerates.
    Patient is encouraged to use ice to knee(s) for 20-30 minutes before and after active flexion. Ice is very effective in reducing pain.
Discharge instructions
    Patient must observe partial weight-bearing restriction and use ambulatory aid for approximately 2 months after discharge.
    Patient should continue active flexion and straight leg raising exercises at home.
    Patient must be made aware of the possible life-long need for antibiotic prophylaxis as explained in Box 36-2.

teristic rash on the face, the erosive nature of the rash being "likened to the damage wrought by a hungry wolf."

Once thought to be relatively rare and always fatal, better techniques for recognition of the disease have demonstrated it to be fairly common, and its course can be controlled by corticosteroids. Some patients do, however, die as a result of lesions affecting major organs or from secondary infections.

The cause of the disease is unknown, although two major areas are being investigated as possible causes. One possibility is that an aberration of the immune system causes immune complexes containing antibodies to be deposited in tissue, thereby causing tissue damage; the second possibility is the presence of a viral infection caused by or resulting from some immunological abnormality. A third possibility is that both of these factors combine to produce the disease. Some drugs, notably procainamide, isoniazid, and penicillins are known to induce lupus-like syndromes.[87] The signs and symptoms and medical therapy are summarized in Table 32-2.

Pathophysiology

Pathological manifestations of the disease include the following:

1. Synovial involvement as a fibrous villous synovitis
2. Severe vasculitis with necrosis of the walls of the small arteries
3. Renal involvement with thickening of the basement membrane of the glomerular tufts and necrosis of the glomerular capillaries
4. Lymph node necrosis
5. Development of small white spots in the retina called *cytoid bodies*
6. Lesions of the nervous system

The initial manifestation of SLE is often arthritis. In many instances the joint symptoms are transient and respond to treatment. Weakness, fatigue, and weight loss may be present. The patient may complain of sensitivity to the sun, developing a rash and at times fever or arthritis on exposure to sunlight. *Erythema*, usually in a *butterfly pattern*, appears over the *cheeks and bridge of the nose.* The margins of these lesions are bright red, and the lesions may extend beyond the hairline with partial alopecia (loss of hair) above the ears. Lesions may also occur on the exposed part of the neck. Lesions spread slowly to the mucous membranes and other tissues of the body, or they may originate there. These lesions do not ulcerate but cause degeneration and atrophy of tissues.

Depending on the organs involved, the patient may have findings of glomerulonephritis, pleuritis, pericarditis, peritonitis, neuritis, or anaemia. Renal and neurological manifestations are among the more serious manifestations of the disease.

Nursing Process
Assessment

Subjective data

1. Note that patients may express vague symptoms or simply say that they are "always tired."
2. Ask patients about generalized weakness, loss of appetite, loss of weight, skin rashes, and specific joint discomfort (even at rest).

3. Identify the presence and extent of discomfort or stiffness of muscles or joints.
4. Identify the presence of sensitivity of eyes and skin to the sun.
5. Ask patients about hair loss, which occurs during acute episodes.

Objective data

1. Observe for erythema over the cheeks and bridge of the nose, above the ears, on exposed part of the neck, and over other body areas
2. Examine for loss of hair or partial loss at normal hairline
3. Check for muscle strength and range of motion of joints

Diagnostic tests

As mentioned above, many organs may be involved. Laboratory findings may be specific to the organs involved, as with proteinuria, abnormal cerebrospinal fluid, or radiological evidence of pleural reactions. A positive lupus erythematosis (LE) cell reaction and positive antinuclear antigen and immunofluorescent studies to identify the antibody responsible for LE cell reaction are helpful in making the diagnosis of the disease. Laboratory findings may also show the presence of anaemia, thrombocytopenia, leukocytosis, or leukopenia. A *skin biopsy* is taken of the rash and studied for histopathological evidence of the disorder.

Analysis

Nursing problems are determined from an assessment of patient data. Possible nursing problems for the patient with systemic lupus erythematosus may include, but are not limited to, the following:

Problem	Possible aetiologies
Activity intolerance	Fatigue/weakness, painful joints
Pain	Joint pain
Impaired skin integrity; high risk for	Altered immune system
Knowledge deficit	Lack of information, unfamiliarity with information source/not a commonly known disease
Anxiety	Change in health status; uncertainty about outcome; change in status/role/lifestyle
Altered nutrition: less than body requirements	Weakness/fatigue make eating difficult, loss of appetite

Planning: expected patient outcomes

Expected patient outcomes for the patient with systemic lupus erythematosus may include, but are not limited to, the following:

1. Patient feels less fatigue and weakness, and activity tolerance is improved.
2. Patient states feeling more comfortable and pain is under control.
3. Patient's skin is intact.
4. Patient can explain prescribed therapy and plans for follow-up care.
5. Patient appears less anxious.
6. Appetite improves, and nutrition is improved.

Implementation

Assisting with achievement of therapeutic goals

1. Medications: administer as prescribed
   a. Antiinflammatory analgesics to control arthritic pain
   b. Antimalarial drugs, particularly if rash is extensive
   c. Corticosteroids for severe neurological and renal involvement
   d. Cytotoxic agents if other drugs fail
   e. Ointments or skin creams for rash
2. Kidney dialysis or transplant for uncontrolled lupus nephritis (Chapter 25)
3. Total hip replacement for avascular necrosis consequent to high-dose steroid therapy (p. 972)

Intervention to achieve patient outcomes

Improving activity tolerance

1. Encourage planned programme of muscle strengthening and range of motion exercises.
2. Allow additional time for patient to complete activities.
3. Pace activities and provide rest periods as needed.

Assisting with comfort and ADL

1. Administer medication for pain of joints and muscles.
2. Help patient with gradual independence in ADL.
3. Provide rest periods as necessary.

Preventing skin injury

1. Protect skin when in sunlight by doing the following:
   a. Using sunscreen of at least 15 SPF whenever going out in sun.
   b. Wearing long sleeves when going out in sun.
   c. Wearing wide-brimmed hat when going out in sun.

Facilitating learning

1. The nature, course, and treatment of the disease
2. Appropriate balance of rest and activity
3. Appropriate exercise
4. How to avoid exposing skin to sunlight; for example, wearing long-sleeved blouses or dresses, slacks, broad brimmed hats, cotton gloves
5. Appropriate use of prescribed medications—dose, frequency, precautions, potential side effects
6. Application of cosmetics (hypoallergenic, approved by the doctor) to mask skin lesions, and/or wigs to mask hair loss
7. Information about lupus support groups

Providing emotional support

1. Monitor patient's anxiety level.
2. Provide time for patient to discuss fears and concern.
3. Provide realistic reassurance.
4. Refer patient to social service or another service or agency when it appears anxiety is caused by concerns that can be alleviated with appropriate assistance.

Promoting adequate nutrition

1. Encourage well-balanced diet consisting of major food groups.
2. Offer small frequent feedings that may be better tolerated than three larger meals.
3. Refer to dietitian for further help in planning meals and snacks to help increase weight.

Table 32-3   Inflammatory disorder: polymyositis(dermatomyositis)

Signs and symptoms	Medical therapy

Activities involving movement and lifting become difficult or impossible:
  Climbing stairs
  Arising from a chair
  Combing the hair
  Getting out of the bath
Weakness can lead to contractures and atrophy
Difficulty with swallowing and presence of reflux oesophagitis
Decreased peristalsis
Pulmonary function tests: may indicate impaired gas exchange, decreased vital and total lung capacity
Muscle tenderness, transitory joint pain
Dusky-red, patchy rash over elbows, dorsum of hands, knees, face, neck, shoulders (dermatomyositis)
Weight loss
	Symptomatic treatment
	Medications:
	  corticosteroids and mild analgesics
	Physiotherapy to prevent contractures, preserve muscle strength
	Frequent small meals
	Antacids for reflux oesophagitis
	May need complete bed rest with head of bed elevated on blocks
	Treatment of underlying malignancy if present

Evaluation

Evaluation is based on the expected patient outcomes. Questions to be asked include the following:

1. Can the patient explain the need for rest periods alternating with periods of activity?
2. Is the patient more comfortable?
3. Has skin integrity been maintained?
4. Can the patient explain the disorder and the need for continued follow-up care?
5. Is patient less anxious about health status and change in lifestyle?
6. Can the patient explain how to maintain adequate diet?

POLYMYOSITIS (DERMATOMYOSITIS)

Aetiology/Epidemiology

Polymyositis (dermatomyositis), an inflammatory disease involving striated (voluntary) muscle, occurs two times more frequently in women than men. The cause of the disease is unknown; however, it is thought that some reaction of the autoimmune system, perhaps triggered by a virus, is involved. The signs and symptoms and medical therapy appear in Table 32-3.

Pathophysiology

Pathological findings on histological studies of biopsied muscle vary, but the alterations found, in order of their frequency, are the following:

1. Primary degeneration of muscle fibres, either focal or extensive
2. Basophilia of some fibres with central migration of the sarcolemmal nuclei
3. Necrosis of parts or entire groups of muscle fibres
4. Inflammation of blood vessels supplying the muscles
5. Interstitial fibrosis varying in severity with the duration and, to some extent, the type of the disease
6. Variation in the cross-sectional diameter of fibres.[75]

The disease usually runs a course of exacerbations and remissions. Often it is first noted in proximal muscles, in particular the pelvic and shoulder girdles. Climbing stairs, arising from a chair, and other activities that involve lifting the body become increasingly difficult or impossible. Lifting the arms becomes progressively more difficult, and combing the hair may be impossible. Other muscles (neck flexors, the muscles of swallowing) may also become involved. Muscle pain or tenderness is present in some instances in the early stages. *The presence of a rash marks the disease as dermatomyositis.* A dusky red lesion may be found in the periorbital region, along with periorbital oedema. This dusky red rash may extend over the face, forehead, neck, upper shoulders, chest, and upper back. Lesions on the arms and legs commonly affect the extensor surfaces. These patches are sometimes scaly.

The weakness of myositis, if it persists, can lead to contractures and atrophy. Individuals with the dermatomyositis form of the disease, particularly if they are over 40 years of age, have a 40% to 50% greater chance of having evidence of a malignant neoplasm found during the first 5 years of illness than the population at large. Some physicians believe that routine yearly examinations should be performed to define or exclude the presence of neoplasms in these patients during that 5-year period.

ANKYLOSING SPONDYLITIS

Aetiology/Epidemiology

Ankylosing spondylitis is a *chronic progressive disorder affecting the joints of the hips and spine that occurs nine times more frequently in men than women, usually between the ages of 20 and 40.* The progression of the disorder usually decreases after age 50, but limitation of the spine persists. The cause of the disease is unknown, and its progression cannot be stopped by any treatment now known. There is a strong genetic link with the genetic marker HLA-B27, and it is thought that a link between the marker and some form of trigger (perhaps an infection) sets off a reaction in the immune system that leads to the inflammatory process. The HLA marker is found in about 90% of people with ankylosing spondylitis, as compared with 8% in the general population.

The signs and symptoms and medical therapy can be found in Table 32-4.

Pathophysiology

Spondylitis means inflammation of the spine. As a result of inflammation, the bones of the spine grow together, or ankylose (fuse). Inflammation usually begins around the sacroiliac joints (sacrolitis), eventually obliterating articular cartilage of the affected bones. The cartilage is replaced

REVIEW

Table 32-4 Inflammatory disorder: ankylosing spondylitis

Signs and symptoms	Medical therapy

Initial symptoms: mild with early morning stiffness and aching
Later: intermittent pain and restricted motion of the back
Extraspinal symptoms include:
  Pleuritic-like chest pain
  Achilles tendonitis
  Peripheral arthropathy (especially hips)
  Nonspecific symptoms include:
    Weight loss
    Malaise
    Fatigue
    Mood change
  "Hunchback" deformity or kyphosis at the cervicodorsal junction
	Goals of medical therapy
	  Relieve pain
	  Achieve and maintain best possible alignment of spine
	  Strengthen intraspinal muscles
	  prevent interference with breathing capacity
	Postural exercises
	Lying prone (extension) three to four times a day for 15 to 30 minutes
	Rest
	Heat
	Antiinflammatory analgesics
	  Salicylates
	  Nonsteroidal antiinflammatory agents
	  Potent antiinflammatory for short term (phenylbutazone)
	Spinal osteotomy or arthroplasty for severe symptoms

by new bony growth. Inflammation occurs where the tendon or ligament attaches to bone. The inflammatory process progresses up the spine, eventually resulting in fusion of the entire spine.

Initial symptoms may include low back pain or aching; pain and swelling of the hips, knees, or shoulders; mild fever; loss of appetite; and fatigue. Low back pain flares and subsides intermittently. Over a period of time, pain subsides and motion of the back becomes restricted. Fusion of the sacroiliac joints and spine up through the cervical vertebrae may occur over a period of 10 to 20 years; as a result, the patient may present either a "hunch-back" deformity or a kyphosis at the cervicodorsal junction. Knees are flexed as the person attempts to move the head into an upright position.

Nursing Process
Assessment

Subjective data

Many people with anklyosing spondylitis remain undiagnosed. The patient complains of low backache, stiffness, and alternating or bilateral "sciatica" that lasts for a few days at a time and subsides. They often complain that they wake up every morning in pain. Later the symptoms become more persistent and begin to include evidence of anklyosis of joints, particularly of the spine. The patient should be questioned about changes in body shape and any loss in height.

Objective data

1. Observe for pain on assuming or maintaining an erect position.
2. Examine patient's posture: patient appears bent forward at the waist, often compensating to achieve an erect position by flexing hips and knees.

3. Palpate for tenderness over the spine and sacroiliac region.
4. Note pain on motion and limitation in turning and bending upper body.

Diagnostic tests

X-rays are most helpful in delineating the disorder. Changes in the sacroiliac joints are the earliest and most diagnostic. There is blurring of the bony margins, then sclerosis, and later ankylosis. Bony growths, called *syndesmophytes*, that bridge the adjacent vertebrae give the appearance of a "bamboo spine." The presence in the serum of HLA-B27 helps to establish the diagnosis. HLA refers to the antigen (human leukocyte antigen) and B27 refers to the gene it marks.

Nursing analysis

Nursing problems are determined from assessment of patient data. Possible problems for the person with ankylosing spondylitis may include, but are not limited to, the following:

Problem	Possible aetiologies
Body image disturbance	Change in body appearance/immobility, change in lifestyle
Gas exchange, impaired	Changes in the spine and in posture change the chest cavity and decrease chest excursion
Impaired mobility	Intolerance to activity because of pain/fatigue and musculoskeletal impairment
Pain	Inflammation of the spine causing pain
Knowledge deficit	Lack of exposure to information about the disease

Planning: expected patient outcomes

Expected patient outcomes for the person with ankylosing spondylitis may include, but are not limited to, the following:
1. Patient is more accepting of change in body appearance.
2. Patient can demonstrate postural and breathing exercises to minimize interference with breathing capacity.
3. Patient is able to perform ADL with less fatigue and discomfort.
4. Patient states that pain is lessened.
5. Patient knows course of disease, prescribed therapy, and plans for follow-up care.

Implementation

Assisting with the achievement of therapeutic goals

1. Give antiinflammatory analgesics as prescribed. Indomethacin is the most commonly used NSAID.
2. Provide for rest periods alternating with activity.
3. Provide care for the patient who may have a spinal osteotomy or hip arthroplasty (p. 972).

Interventions to achieve patient outcomes

Promoting a positive body image

1. Encourage patient to express feelings about changes in body image, if able to do so.
2. Assist patient to express feelings such as anger or depression.
3. Compliment patient on each improvement in mobility.

Improving gas exchange

1. Maintain alignment of the spine
   a. Mattress should be firm.
   b. Bed board may be used.
   c. Patient should sleep flat without pillow.
   d. A back brace may be necessary for support.
2. Postural and breathing exercises
   a. Extension exercises should be performed to maintain erect posture and normal height "thinking tall" and to strengthen paraspinal muscles.
   b. Abdominal lying should be done 3 to 4 times a day for 15 to 30 minutes.
   c. Breathing exercises will help increase breathing capacity.
      (1) Perform deep breathing exercises exhaling through "pursed lips" several times a day.
      (2) Use incentive spirometer 3 times a day to increase vital capacity.

Improving mobility

1. Encourage to do prescribed exercises such as swimming and water walking.
2. Assist with exercises 3 times a day.
3. Maintain alignment of the spine as above.
   a. Firm mattress
   b. Bed board may be used
   c. Patient should sleep flat without pillow under head
   d. Back brace may be necessary for support
4. Offer back massage 3 times daily.

Assisting with comfort

1. Apply heat to painful joints.
2. Apply hydrotherapy if available 1 to 2 times daily to entire body; this is best if done just before postural and deep breathing exercises.

Facilitating learning

1. Nature and course of disease
2. Prescribed postural exercises
3. Appropriate use of prescribed medications
4. Methods of applying heat to back and hips
5. Water exercises and swimming are beneficial

Evaluation

Evaluation is based on the expected patient outcomes. Questions to be asked include the following:
1. Is the patient more accepting of changes in body appearance?
2. Is the patient able to maintain adequate breathing capacity?
3. Is the patient able to perform ADL with less discomfort?
4. Is the patient more comfortable?
5. Can the patient explain prescribed therapy and plans for follow-up care?

NONARTICULAR RHEUMATISM

Nonarticular rheumatic diseases include those disorders in which the supportive structures and structures located near the joints are inflamed, but the joints themselves are not involved except by the limitations imposed by the supportive structures. *Some of these disorders are fibrositis, tenosynovitis, Dupuytren's contracture, bursitis, and carpal tunnel syndrome.*

BURSITIS

Aetiology/Epidemiology

Bursitis is inflammation of a bursa, a small fluid-filled sac-like cavity between two articular soft tissue layers. The bursa facilitates joint movements and acts like a pad to cushion joints. The joints affected are the shoulders, elbows, hips, knees, and ankles. In some instances the inflammation of the bursa is preceded by *tendonitis*, that is, inflammation of a tendon, or by *tenosynovitis*, which is inflammation of a tendon and the tendon sheath.

Bursitis may be acute or chronic. It is usually caused by trauma, strain, and overuse of the joint with which the bursa is associated. The shoulder bursa is most often affected. The signs and symptoms and medical therapy are listed in Table 32-5.

Pathophysiology

The synovial lining of the bursal sac becomes inflamed, more fluid is secreted, and the bursa swells. Occasionally, large calcium deposits are present. The swelling is accompanied by pain and limited ability to move the associated joint or the entire extremity.

CARPAL TUNNEL SYNDROME

Aetiology/Epidemiology

Carpal tunnel syndrome is caused by pressure being exerted on the median nerve of the wrist. The condition is most common in middle-aged and often obese women and may occur as a result of trauma or of swelling of tendon sheaths caused by processes such as rheumatoid arthritis.

The person will complain of dysaesthesia, paraesthesia, and hypaesthesia of the thumb, index, and middle fingers. Complaints will usually increase when there has been forced flexion of the hand for long periods, such as when typing. The symptoms can be elicited by tapping the median nerve at the wrist (Tinel's sign). The patient may feel that the hand is swollen and may complain of clumsiness when using the hand, especially when grasping or holding onto small objects. Referred pain to the upper extremity is common. Atrophy of the thenar eminence (the padded area of the palm below the base of the thumb) may be present late in the disease.

Pathophysiology

The median nerve passes through a tunnel bounded by the carpal bones dorsally and the transverse carpal ligament volarly. Flexor tendons run through the tunnel parallel to the median nerve. Inflammation and swelling of the synovial lining of tendon sheaths narrow the space available and cause compression of the median nerve.

Treatment

The surgery involves decompression by surgical release of the transverse carpal ligament and removal of tissues that may be compressing the median nerve. Most patients are operated on in a day-care surgery setting and they go home as soon as anaesthesia wears off.

DEGENERATIVE DISORDERS

DEGENERATIVE JOINT DISEASE

Aetiology/Epidemiology

Degenerative joint disease, also known as *osteoarthritis, hypertrophic arthritis, osteoarthrosis,* or *senescent arthritis*, is an extremely common disease that is probably as old as civilization. Almost everyone past 40 years of age has hypertrophic changes in the joints. About 80% of people over age 65 show evidence of osteoarthritic changes on X-ray.[46] Although symptomatic degenerative joint disease is usually noted in the 50- to 70- year age group, it has been observed as early as age 20.

There are two forms of osteoarthritis: *primary*, for which the cause is unknown, and *secondary*, a result of trauma, infections, previous fractures, another type of arthritis (such as rheumatoid arthritis), the stress put on weight-bearing joints from long-term obesity, or the "wear and tear" on joints associated with some occupations (for example, coal mining and boxing). There may also be a

REVIEW

Table 32-5   Nonarticular rheumatism: bursitis

Signs and symptoms	Medical therapy
Deep-seated pain in area of bursa	Antiinflammatory agents are given (Table 36-2)
Pain on movement of involved extremity	Adrenocorticosteroids may be injected into bursa
Passive and active range of motion limited in adjacent joint	Rest of involved area
	Cold compresses during acute phase to help relieve discomfort
	Heat is avoided because it increases fluid exudate in the bursa during inflammatory phase
	Surgical removal of calcium deposits

genetic predisposition to the development of osteoarthritis. See Table 32-6 for signs and symptoms and medical therapy.

Prevention

1. Avoidance of obesity because of the added wear excess weight puts on joints, especially the hips and knees. For example, the knees are subject to peak impacts three to five times greater than total body weight.[46]
2. Avoidance of repeated trauma to joints.
3. Practice of techniques that protect joints in occupations that put joints at risk.

Pathophysiology

Degenerative joint disease (DJD) is a disease of the articular cartilage. Normally this cartilage is white, translucent, and smooth. When affected by the disease, it becomes yellow and opaque. Areas of cartilage soften and the surface becomes rough, frayed, and cracked. This process is thought to occur as a result of digestion of the cartilage by enzymes and alteration of the nutrition of the cartilage. Eventually the cartilage is destroyed, and the underlying subchondral bone goes through a remodelling process. *Osteophytes*, or spurs of new bone, appear at the joint margins and at the sites of attachment of supporting structures. These may break off and appear in the joint cavity as "joint mice". Unlike rheumatoid arthritis (RA), DJD affects only the joints and their surrounding tissue. It is not a systemic disease.

Healthy cartilage is 66% to 78% water, and most of its solid weight is accounted for by collagen and proteoglycans (large water-binding molecules). In osteoarthritis collagen appears unchanged, but the proteoglycan molecules are altered significantly. On microscopic examination healthy proteoglycans have the appearance of fresh Christmas trees, but in osteoarthritis proteoglycans look like scraggly trees. At present, it is not clear whether this change is a cause or a consequence of the disease.[47]

REVIEW

Table 32-6 Degenerative disorder: degenerative joint diseases (DJD)

Signs and symptoms	Medical therapy
Pain in the movable joints particularly on weight bearing	Salicylates and nonsteroidal antiinflammatory agents
Mild tenderness to aggravated pain on overuse of joint	Aspirin
	NSAIDs
	Intraarticular injection of steroids for severe pain
Joints become enlarged with loss of motion	Adjunctive analgesics (paracetamol)
Crepitation	Assistive devices to unload weight bearing from joints (walking sticks, walkers, crutches)
Changes in alignment of affected part with flexion deformity	
Stiffness after periods of rest	Rest
	Exercise
Changes in certain joints:	Joint protection
Heberden's nodes— bony protuberances on dorsal surface of distal interphalangeal joints of fingers	Surgery Arthroscopy to remove bits of broken cartilage or bone Realignment (osteotomy) Fusion (arthrodesis) Joint replacement
Bouchard's nodes— on proximal interphalangeal joints of fingers	
Coxarthrosis— a degenerative change presenting with pain in hip with weight bearing; may progress to include pain in groin and medial side of knee	
Knee involvement— varus, valgus, flexion deformity, limited range of motion	

Individuals with DJD have pain in the movable joints, particularly the large weight-bearing joints (hips, knees), and the joints of the hand. Inflammation is usually not present, and tenderness is mild; however, the joint may become enlarged. Crepitation may be present on movement, and alignment of the extremity may be changed. The patient usually has stiffness after periods of rest.

Nursing Process
Assessment
Subjective data

The person with degenerative joint disorder is usually in good health. Questions that are asked include the following:

1. When does pain occur?
2. What measures give relief?
3. What joints are involved?
4. What modifications in ADL have been made because of pain or restricted mobility?

Objective data

Because signs and symptoms are usually local, inspection and palpation are the best evaluators.

1. Affected joints may appear normal.
   a. Check for tenderness, grating, and crepitus.
   b. Palpate for enlargement or irregularity in size of joint and flexion or lateral deformities.
2. Observe the person walking. Is there a limp?
3. Evaluate range of motion of major joints.
4. Assess the vertebral column for limitation in cervical or lumbar areas.
5. Does the person have difficulty standing for periods of time or difficulty in arising from chair (particularly one without arms) after sitting for a period of time?

Diagnostic tests

1. X-ray films may be normal if pathological changes are mild.
2. Progressive changes include the following:
   a. Narrowing of joint spaces
   b. Marginal osteophyte formation
   c. *Eburnation* (sclerosis) of subchondral bone
3. Serological and synovial fluid examinations will be essentially normal

Nursing analysis

Nursing problems are determined from assessment of patient data. Possible nursing problems for the person with degenerative joint disease may include, but are not limited to, the following:

Problem	Possible aetiologies
Pain: in affected joints	Degeneration in affected joints
Impaired mobility	Musculoskeletal impairment caused by degeneration of affected joints
Activity intolerance	Restricted mobility caused by joint involvement
Self-care deficit: ADL	Pain and limited joint movement
Knowledge deficit: DJD	Lack of exposure to sources of information
Nutrition: altered, more than body requirements	Excessive intake in relation to metabolic needs

Planning: expected patient outcomes

Expected patient outcomes for the person with degenerative joint disease may include, but are not limited to, the following:

1. Patient feels more comfortable.
2. Patient is able to be more physically active.
3. Patient balances rest and activity.
4. Patient is able to perform self-care activities with less difficulty.
5. Patient is able to explain disease process, treatment measures, and plans for follow-up medical care.
6. Patient is able to state reason for achieving and maintaining normal weight.

Implementation

Interventions to achieve patient outcomes

Measures to relieve pain and discomfort and to promote mobility and increased ability to accomplish ADL are the same as those for the person who has rheumatoid arthritis (p. 972).

A recent study of the short-term, symptomatic treatment of osteoarthritis of the knee found that paracetamol was as effective as the NSAID ibuprofen in relieving symptoms. This was true when paracetamol 4000 mg/day was compared with ibuprofen 1200 mg/day and 2400 mg/day.[7] An editorial in the same issue of the *New England Journal of Medicine* points out that the publication of the article presents an opportunity to review the management of degenerative joint disease of the knee and hip, of which medication is only one component.[46]

Supporting weight loss

1. Review reasons why weight loss would improve symptoms.
2. Assess patient's motivation to lose weight.
3. Refer patient to dietitian for dietary assessment and dietary plan.
4. Compliment patient on weight loss no matter how small.
5. Make patient aware of support groups for those attempting to lose weight such as Weight Watchers.
6. Make patient aware of good exercises for people with joint disease, such as water walking, aqua-aerobics, and swimming.

Facilitating learning

The teaching plan would include the following:
1. Attention to posture
2. Weight reduction, prevention of weight gain
3. Use of ambulatory aids such as canes, crutches, or walkers to remove weight from painful joints
4. Alteration in ADL to avoid painful activities
5. Use of external measures such as local heat, prescribed exercises, and use of traction (if this is prescribed)

Evaluation

Evaluation is based on the expected patient outcomes. Questions to be asked include the following:
1. Is the patient more comfortable?
2. Is the patient able to be more physically active?
3. Is the patient able to balance rest and activity such as performing prescribed exercises independently?
4. Is the patient able to perform self-care activities with less difficulty?
5. Is the patient able to explain disease process, treatment measures, and follow-up care?
6. Can the patient discuss the reason for achieving and maintaining ideal weight?

Surgery

Surgical intervention may be necessary to remove damaged bone or cartilage from the joint, realign or change the weight-bearing surfaces of the joint, or resurface the joint. The objectives of surgery are to (1) relieve pain, (2) restore joint function (if possible), and (3) prevent disability or further progression of the disease. Surgery to the knee and hip are most common, but shoulder surgery is becoming more practical and effective. Specific surgeries are:

1. *Debridement* (usually by arthroscopic surgery or arthrotomy): See p. 972.
2. *Arthrodesis:* Through fusion of the joint, pain is relieved, joint motion is lost, but weight-bearing function is maintained. See p. 972.
3. *Osteotomy:* Bone is cut to change alignment, thereby correcting deformity in the bone or adjacent joint. The procedure corrects angulation of rotational deformities or alters the weight-bearing surface in a diseased joint. Osteotomy may be thought of as a surgical or intentional fracture, and the extremity is treated the same as after fracture with the exception that weight bearing may be started earlier. Immobilization of the extremity and nursing interventions are similar to those employed after a fracture (p. 972).
4. *Arthroplasty:* The two types of arthroplasty are:
   a. Interposition—resurfacing of one side of the joint with metal or other inert material or soft tissue such as fascia.
   b. Replacement—resurfacing of both sides of the joint with metal or polyethylene implants. Replacement implants are available for the hip (see Fig. 32-6), knee (see Fig. 32-7), shoulder, ankle, elbow, wrist, and interphalangeal joints of the fingers. Replacement prostheses may be either *cemented* (held into bone with polymethylmethacrylate) or *uncemented* (treated with a special porous coating that promotes growth of bone). Care of the patient having an arthroplasty is discussed under rheumatoid arthritis on p. 972.

DEGENERATIVE DISEASE OF THE SPINE

Degenerative disease of the spine is a common but difficult problem that merits special consideration. The signs and symptoms and medical therapy are listed in Table 32-7.

Pathophysiology

The spine has 23 intervertebral disk joints and 46 posterior facet joints (Fig. 32-8), all of which are subjected to stresses and strains in holding the human body upright and moving it about. The vertebrae in the spinal column are articulated in a series of "couplets" that are able to move through an intervertebral disk joint and two posterior facet joints. The intervertebral disks are composed of an outer layer of cartilage called the *anulus fibrosus* and an inner layer of cartilage called the *nucleus pulposus.* Several common problems arise with these structures in degenerative disease of the spine. They are the following:

1. *Herniated nucleus pulposus* (HNP) Degeneration and dehydration of the cartilage composing the anulus and the nucleus result in a loss of elasticity. As the disk loses its resiliency, a strong force exerted across it can result in herniation of the nucleus through the anulus, either posteriorly or laterally. It is commonly referred to as a "ruptured disk." This results in compression of a spinal nerve root and subsequent pain (Fig. 32-9).

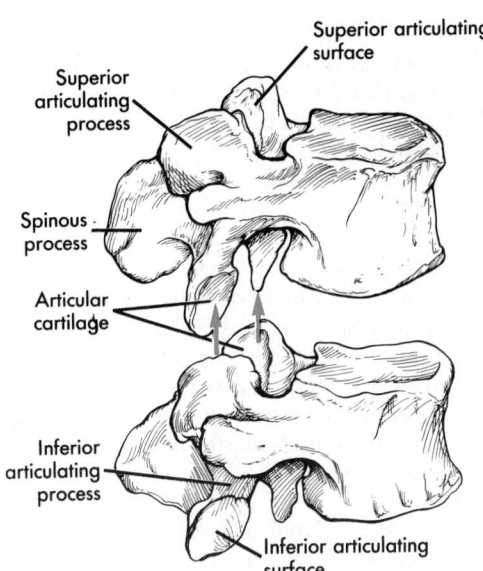

Fig. 32-8   Posterior facet joints of lumbar vertebrae. Each vertebra has four surfaces by which it articulates with its adjacent vertebrae: two on its superior aspect and two on the inferior. Superior articulating surfaces are medially located; the inferior, laterally. These joints are diarthrotic, having a joint capsule with a synovial lining.

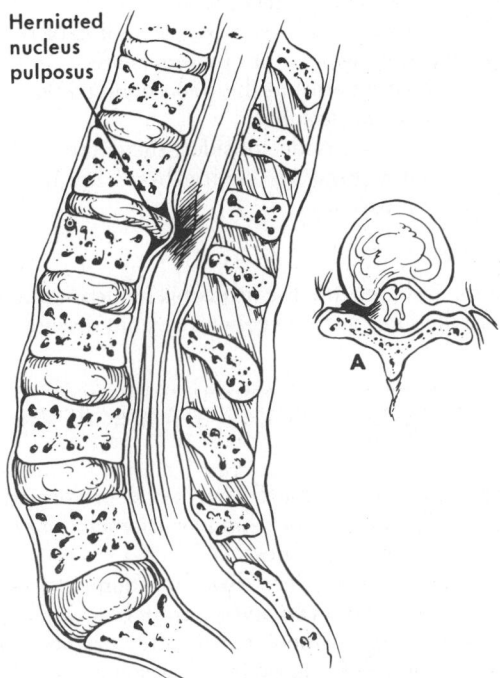

Fig. 32-9   Compression of spinal cord caused by herniation of nucleus pulposus into spinal cord. **A,** Pressure on nerves as they leave spinal canal.

2. *Osteophyte* formation along the vertebral column can cause fusion of vertebrae with consequent limitation of motion, usually in the lumbodorsal region.
3. *Spinal stenosis*, or narrowing of the intervertebral foramina at any level of the spine, creates pressure on

REVIEW

Table 32-7   Degenerative disease: degenerative joint disease of spine

Signs and symptoms	Medical therapy

Chief complaint: low back pain relieved by lying down
Occasionally pain radiates to buttocks
There may be sciatic pain radiating down leg
Pain follows overactivity
Pain aggravated by flexion of trunk, coughing, and sneezing
	Conservative
	Rest (complete or modified) depending on symptoms
	Heat
	Medications
	  Analgesics and/or antiinflammatory agents
	  Muscle relaxants (for example, diazepam)
	Traction to relieve muscle spasm
	  Bilateral Buck's traction
	  Pelvic traction
	Corset may be prescribed to support spine

nerve roots in the involved area, resulting in neurological symptoms including pain.

4. *Degenerative and/or rheumatiod involvement of the hyaline articular surfaces of the facet joints results in pain and limited motion.* Rheumatoid involvement with consequent loss of vertebral stability is particularly troublesome in the cerical spine.

The *diagnosis* of herniated disk is usally made on the basis of the history and physical examination. A history of low back pain relieved by recumbency and aggravated by flexion of the trunk, coughing, or sneezing is typical. The patient will often complain of sciatic pain radiating down the leg. Some people, after the initial injury, will have sciatic pain going down the leg but no pain in their back. Deep pressure over the interspace will usually elicit pain. Straight leg raising with the hip flexed and the knee extended (a positive Lasegue sign) will produce sciatic pain. Neurological signs and symptoms help in determining the level of the disk involved because sensory and motor changes depend on the nerve root involved. The most common sites of lumbar herniation are L3-4, L4-5, and L5-S1.

Surgery

Surgery may be necessary to relieve pressure on nerve roots and to stabilize the spine. Care of patients who are treated surgically is discusse on p. 985.

Compression of nerve roots from other causes—stenosis, vertebral instability, osteophyte formation—will also cause neurological signs and symptoms relative to the level of the nerve root(s) involved. Signs and symptoms may include the following:

1. Numbness, tingling, and/or decreased motion in one or more extremities
2. Pain
3. Weakness of one or more extremities
4. Muscle wasting in one or more extremities
5. Partial or complete loss of bowel and bladder control

Nursing Process
Assessment

Subjective data

The patient seeks help because of pain and inability to walk or to carry on normal activities. Answers to the following questions should be sought:
1. Is low back pain relieved by recumbency?
2. Is pain aggravated by flexion of the trunk, coughing, or sneezing?
3. Is there a history of injury followed by back pain?

Objective data

1. Observe movements and walking.
   a. Patient appears to guard hips and back.
   b. Patient seeks frequent position changes.
2. Straight leg raising flexing the hip with the knee extended may produce sciatic pain.
3. Palpate for tender areas and spasm of the paravertebral muscles and posterior superior iliac spine.
4. Observe relief of discomfort when patient is supine with head elevated a few degrees and knees flexed.
5. Observe for muscle atrophy; if back problem has been long-standing, changes will be seen in affected leg.

Diagnostic tests

Neurological examination

1. Neurological signs and symptoms will help in determining the level of vertebrae involved. Sensory and motor changes depend on the nerve root involved.
2. Radiological evaluation
   a. For those patients whose symptoms are of short duration, the x-ray examination may fail to reveal any abnormality.
   b. For those patients with long-standing disorders, the x-ray examination may show significant narrowing of the disk space.
   c. Myelography, valuable in localizing the lesion, is reserved for confirmation of physical findings before surgery or to exclude conditions such as tumours.
   d. CAT scanning or magnetic resonance imaging (MRI) may be used for diagnosis.

Nursing analysis and planning: expected patient outcomes

Nursing problems and expected patient outcome are similar to those for degenerative joint disease (p. 981).

Implementation

Interventions to achieve patient outcomes

For the patient being treated conservatively, the following interventions are appropriate.

Promoting comfort

1. Encourage slight elevation of head of bed and flexion of the knees (pillow under knees) when supine.
2. Roll patient onto bedpan rather than lifting onto pan.
3. Use fracture bedpan or small bedpan.
4. Apply heat as patient desires and tolerates.
5. Remove skin traction for periods of time if it causes patient discomfort.

6. Provide analgesics, antispasmodics at regular intervals as necessary.

Promoting circulation

1. Encourage patient to perform active dorsi-plantar flexion of the ankles at regular intervals.
2. Report any difficulty with brace to doctor immediately.
3. Do not drive a car during period that brace must be worn.

Facilitating learning

1. Patients should learn to turn in bed in a *logrolling* fashion to maintain good spinal alignment: *cross the arms over the chest, bend the uppermost knee to the side to which they wish to turn, and then roll over as a unit.*
2. Constipation may be a problem.
   a. Urge patient to drink 3000 ml of fluids daily.
   b. Increase amount of fibre eaten; bran and fresh fruit are helpful.
   c. Give a mild laxative if necessary.
3. If brace or corset is ordered to provide external support for the spine, explain its need and application.
4. Teach principles of body mechanics.
   a. Avoid movements and positions that cause poor alignment of the spinal column and put strain on an injured nerve.
   b. Use a straight chair, not an overstuffed one.
   c. Avoid crossing the legs at the knees.
   d. Elevate the feet but flex the knees.
   e. During acute episodes, avoid stretching of the legs, such as driving a car or climbing stairs.
   f. In picking up items off the floor, bend the knees and keep the back straight.
5. When the acute episode subsides, the doctor will order exercises designed to strengthen the back and abdominal muscles.

Evaluation

Evaluation is based on the expected patient outcomes, which are the same as for degenerative joint disease (see p. 981).

SURGERY OF THE LUMBAR, THORACIC, OR CERVICAL SPINE

A laminectomy and/or spinal fusion may be performed. The nursing care for people with lumbar, thoracic, or cervical spinal fusion is discussed next.

Care after spinal surgery (lumbar, thoracic, cervical) focuses on *positioning* and *mobility, wound care,* and *patient comfort.* Changing position in bed after *lumbar* surgery must be performed by logrolling; assistance is given as necessary, but patients can learn to do this for themselves. *Because patients tolerate sitting less well than walking or lying, sitting is avoided until the person can tolerate it.*

Thoracic spinal surgery may involve entering the chest cavity; if so, nursing care will include chest tube(s) and closed drainage as with other chest surgery (Chapter 16). Mobility restrictions are more prolonged than with lumbar surgery because the thoracic spine is more mobile; consequently, there is a greater risk of dislodging grafts through improper motion.

People with *cervical spine surgery* may *require tong* or *halo traction* (Chapter 29) or a halo brace. The person has oedema of the throat in the early postoperative period, requiring attention to the person's ability to breathe and swallow.

The care of patients undergoing spinal fusion is discussed below.

Nursing Interventions for Patients Having Surgery of the Lumbar Spine

Preoperative care

1. Instruct patient in logrolling and performance of dorsiplantar exercises
2. Instruct patient about the surgical procedure, postoperative care, and expectations at discharge

Postoperative care

1. Positioning
   a. Head of bed is kept flat.
   b. Patient is encouraged to logroll when changing position from side to back to side.
   c. Use of turning sheet is advised until patient can assist with turning.
2. Wound care: drains may be placed in wound to prevent haematoma formation.
   a. Maintain constant suction through drain if required.
   b. Maintain drain free of contamination.
   c. Inspect surgical area frequently for evidence of excess drainage or formation of haematoma (bulging of tissues surrounding surgical site).
   d. In a spinal fusion, inspect donor site (usually iliac crest) for drainage or haematoma.
3. Promoting comfort
   a. Reposition patient frequently.
   b. Narcotics are used initially; may be on patient-controlled analgesia (PCA); then nonnarcotic analgesics as patient tolerates.
   c. Use fracture bedpan or small bedpan.
4. Promoting mobility
   a. Patient with a *simple laminectomy* may be out of bed on the first day after surgery.
   b. Patient with a *laminectomy and fusion* may not be able to be out of bed for 3 to 5 days after the surgery.
   c. Two people will be required to help patient out of bed. This patient should sit as little as possible while getting up.
      (1) If the patient has a brace or corset, it is applied *before* the patient gets out of bed.
      (2) Assist patient in moving to edge of the bed before turning on side.
      (3) Instruct patient to push off the bed with the uppermost hand and lowermost elbow.
      (4) One person guides the patient's trunk, the other assists the patient's legs over the side of the bed.

   (5) The process is reversed in getting patient back in bed.
   d. Patient may walk as much as tolerated; an assistive aid such as walking stick may be necessary.
   e. Patient is encouraged to participate in ADL within prescribed limits of mobility.
5. Discharge instructions
   a. May not lift or carry anything heavier than 5 lbs (2.25 kg).
   b. May not drive car until permitted by surgeon.
   c. Should avoid twisting of the trunk.

Nursing Interventions for Patients Having Surgery of the Thoracic Spine

Preoperative care

Care is the same as for lumbar surgery.

Postoperative care

Care is the same as for lumbar surgery, with the following *additions or exceptions:*
1. Positioning
   a. Head of bed often is ordered to be elevated to 30 degrees.
2. Wound care
   a. If pleural cavity is entered, a chest tube will be inserted and must be managed after surgery (see Chapter 20).
3. Promoting comfort
   a. Assist patient in splinting chest while coughing.
4. Promoting mobility
   a. Encourage and assist patient in vigorous pulmonary care.
   b. Assist patient in maintaining bedrest for 1 week or longer with strict attention to avoidance of twisting or bending motions to prevent dislodging grafts.
   c. Discourage patient from vigorous pulling or pushing with the arms, because placing weight on them may dislodge the graft.
   d. Brace is routinely prescribed and must be applied before patient gets out of bed.
   e. Permit patient to perform whatever activities are comfortable within the limitations of the brace.
   f. Encourage participation in ADL within prescribed limits of mobility.
5. Discharge instruction
   a. Teach patient how to apply and remove the brace before getting out of bed for the first time.
   b. Teach patient to wear the brace whenever out of bed.

Nursing Interventions for Patients Having Surgery of the Cervical Spine

Preoperative Care

1. General instructions are the same as for any spine surgery.
2. If *tong* or *halo traction* or *halo brace* is to be used after surgery, familiarize patient with the apparatus before surgery by using pictures or actual tong or brace.

Postoperative care

1. Positioning
   a. Keep head of bed elevated 30 to 45 degrees, particularly if anterior surgical approach was used, to decrease swelling in throat.
   b. If patient is in a cervical brace, position is not restricted except by patient's tolerance.
   c. If patient is in cervical traction, may be turned side to back to side as tolerated.
2. Wound care
   a. Inspect surgical area, including iliac crest donor site, frequently for evidence of excess drainage or formation of haematoma.
   b. If tong or halo traction is being used, pin care may be required (see Chapter 29).
3. Promoting comfort
   a. Provide ice chips to soothe sore throat.
   b. Progress diet slowly because patient will have difficulty swallowing and will be afraid of choking. Full liquids (ice cream, custards) are often better tolerated than clear juice or broth. However, milk products may increase mucus production.
   c. Medicate with analgesics as for any spine surgery. Donor sites often cause more discomfort than cervical site.
   d. May require aerosol treatments or humidification of air to loosen mucous secretions, facilitate their removal, and make breathing more comfortable.
4. Promoting mobility
   a. If patient is in traction, encourage to perform ankle dorsi-plantar flexion exercises and quadriceps-setting 3 times daily to promote circulation, maintain leg strength.
   b. If patient is in brace, may be out of bed and walk as soon as tolerated.
   c. A walking aid may be necessary if donor site pain restricts mobility.
   d. Encourage participation in ADL to greatest extent possible.
5. Promoting safety
   a. Keep suction equipment and tracheostomy set in patient's room until swelling in throat subsides and patient is swallowing and breathing normally.
   b. Check adjustment screws and straps on brace frequently to ensure there is no loosening of the brace.
   c. When oedema decreases brace will need to be readjusted by the doctor or orthotist.
6. Discharge instruction
   a. Teach patient to wear brace at all times.
   b. Report any difficulty with brace to doctor immediately.
   c. Do not drive a car during period of time that brace must be worn.

RESTRICTIVE DISORDERS

SCOLIOSIS

Lateral deviation of the spine from the midline is known as scoliosis. The classifications of scoliosis are the following:

Congenital, acquired, idiopathic (most common), functional (postural) and structural.

Table 32-8 lists the signs and symptoms and medical therapy for scoliosis.

Prevention

Screening programmes for school-age children are effective in identifying early indications of scoliosis. Attention to good posture may be effective in preventing the disorder in both children and adults.

Aetiology

The causes of scoliosis include the following: rickets, neuromuscular disorders, vertebral disorders, idiopathic (cause unknown), and congenital.

Pathophysiology

Scoliosis may develop in localized areas of the spinal column or involve the whole spinal column. Curves may be S-shaped or C-shaped. The degree of rotation of the curve is important because it determines the amount of impingement on the rib cage. Significant cardiac and pulmonary restrictions may be imposed by curves with a large degree of rotation. The balance of the curve is also important because it affects the stability of the spine and mobility of the trunk. Significant deviations in balance of the curve affect gait patterns.

The individual may initially have slight, mild, or severe deformity. Early deformity may not be obvious except on specific examination. Deformity will increase with growth and age. In the early stages, individuals may note that clothing does not fit correctly or hang evenly. The height of the shoulders is uneven. Pain is not usually an accompanying factor. In advanced scoliosis, when the cardio-respiratory system is affected, respiration is restricted and cardiac output is decreased. The curvature of the spine is confirmed on x-ray.

Treatment

Some forms of scoliosis are not amenable to treatment with bracing or body cast; surgery may be performed to correct the scoliosis. Most commonly, lumbar fusion is performed through a posterior incision, with the bone for the graft being taken from the iliac crest. Scoliosis fusions involve internal devices such as those listed in Table 32-8.

Expected patient outcomes of surgery

1. Complications of surgery are avoided.
2. Patient is able to explain surgical procedure.
3. Patient can perform prescribed exercises correctly.
4. Patient can explain follow-up programme, including appointments with surgeon and physiotherapist.

After surgery, the patient may be immobilized in a cast that extends from neck to pelvis. The cast remains on for 6 months. The care of the patient in a cast is covered on p. 995.

The risk of postoperative pulmonary complications as a result of immobilization is high; therefore, preventive measures are important. Paralytic ileus is a common complication, and nasogastric suction is commonly em-

Table 32-8 Restrictive disorder: scoliosis

Signs and symptoms	Medical therapy

Lateral deviation of spine away from midline (in thoracic spine region)
One shoulder is higher than other
Movement of chest is restricted on deep inspiration
May complain of shortness of breath or difficulty in taking deep breath
	Early or postural scoliosis may be amenable to:
	  Postural exercise
	  Exercise combined with traction (for example, Cotrel's traction)
	In scoliosis where the curve is flexible (less than 40 degrees) and the patient is cooperative, bracing (Milwaukee brace, Risser cast, and a halofemoral or halopelvic traction) in combination with exercise may be sufficient to correct the deformity
	Corrective surgery (realignment of vertebrae and fusion) when curve exceeds 40 degrees and/or bracing has failed; usually accomplished with bone grafting and instrumentation
	  Harrington rod instrumentation—series of rods and hooks that apply compression to the posterior spinal elements
	  Dwyer instrumentation—titanium cables passed through heads of titanium screws imbedded in the vertebral bodies
	  Luque instrumentation—two L-shaped rods and a series of wires that apply transverse traction to the vertebral bodies

ployed in the first 24 to 72 hours after surgery. Patients with major *spinal procedures* also tend to retain fluid; therefore, they are *at risk for fluid overload* in the early postoperative period.

OTHER DISORDERS

GOUT

Aetiology/Epidemiology

Gout or gouty arthritis is a metabolic disorder that affects men eight to nine times more frequently than women. It can occur at any age, the peak age of onset occurring in the fifth decade. Of all people with gout, 85% have a genetic or familial tendency to develop the disease. Gout develops as a result of prolonged hyperuricaemia (elevated serum uric acid) caused by problems either in synthesizing purines or by poor renal excretion of uric acid. The signs and symptoms and medical therapy are listed in Table 32-9.

Pathophysiology

Urate crystals form in the synovial tissue, causing severe inflammation. The inflammatory process is extremely rapid, occurring over a few hours. Acute symptoms are extreme pain, swelling, and erythema of the involved joints. Typically the great toe is involved (the first metatarsophalangeal joint), but other joints, such as the heel, ankle, and knee, may also be affected. Pain is so severe that the patient may not tolerate even the weight of a sheet over the joint. Renal damage may occur, especially if recurrent uric acid stones have been present. Between attacks of gout, the patient may be asymptomatic, but repeated attacks can occur with gradually increasing frequency if the disease is untreated. Patients with gouty symptoms may develop *tophi*, or deposits of monosodium urate in their tissues. These consist of a core of monosodium urate with a surrounding inflammatory reaction. Patients with tophaceous deposits tend to have more frequent and more severe episodes of gouty arthritis.

TRAUMA TO BONE

The person who has suffered trauma to the musculoskeletal system has sustained an interruption in the integrity of one or more components of that system. *Musculoskeletal trauma is most frequently manifested as bone fracture, but it may also include injury to soft tissue, muscle, ligament, meniscus, tendon, or joint.*

FRACTURE OF BONE

Aetiology/Epidemiology

Fracture of bone usually occurs as a result of a blow to the body, a fall, or other accident. However, fracture may occur during normal activity or after a minimal injury if the bone is weakened by a disease such as primary or metastatic cancer or osteoporosis. This is called a *pathological fracture*, or a collapse of the bone. Bone may also fracture when the muscles associated with it are unable to absorb energy as they usually do. This type of fracture is called a *fatigue* or *stress fracture*. Another type of fracture occurs when a strong ligament or tendon attachment pulls a fragment of bone away from the rest of the bone. This is called an *avulsion fracture. Fracture can occur at any age, although*

REVIEW

Table 32-9   Gout

Signs and symptoms	Medical therapy
Acute: rapid onset of severe pain in inflamed joints—most frequently large toe	Medications—acute attack Colchicine (0.5) mgm—oral administration of 2- tablets initially, then 1 tablet every 2-3 hours until nausea, vomiting, or diarrhea occur, or joint symptoms subside; limit is 10 mg NSAIDs
Presence of swelling and tenderness, malaise, headache, and fever	
Chronic: always present in those who have familial tendency	
Acute exacerbations occur when not diagnosed or not treated	Absolute rest of the joint
Deposits of *tophi* (deposits of monosodium urate in tissue) most noticeable in ears), on knuckles and on great toe	*Preventative* therapy consists of reduction of the body pool of urates by one of two methods: Enhancing uric acid excretion Probenecid— 0.5 g daily for 1 week, then increased by 0.5 g weekly until serum uric acid is in normal range; max. 2 g daily Sulphinpyrazone—used for patients who do not tolerate probenecid Decreasing uric acid formation Allopurinol—100 mg a day initially, increased by 100 mg every 2-4 weeks until serum uric acid level is normal; usual dose 200-600 mg daily

older people, people with balance or mobility problems, people who work at high-risk occupations (for example, steelworkers, racing car drivers), and people with chronic degenerative or neoplastic diseases are at higher risk for injury. The signs and symptoms and immediate medical therapy are listed in Table 32-8.

Primary and Secondary Prevention

One approach to preventing fracture is to make the environment safer. Examples of measures that can be taken include the following:

1. Mounting grab bars on the wall next to a bath or toilet
2. Attaching safety arms around a toilet
3. Removing throw rugs and obstacles from areas used by individuals with locomotor problems
4. Assuring that wheelchairs have adequate locking devices

5. Teaching individuals who must use ambulatory devices and wheelchairs how to use them properly

A *second* approach is to continue to educate the public regarding the following:

1. The dangers of drinking and driving
2. The advisability of using seat belts
3. Attending to safety precautions when climbing ladders, using power tools or heavy equipment
4. Wearing recommended protective clothing (for example, steel-toed shoes, hard hats) for hazardous work at home or on the job
5. Wearing proper protective clothing while engaging in sports (for example, protective padding, well-fitting running shoes)

A *third* approach is to continue to educate women regarding the problem of *osteoporosis*. Individuals most at risk to develop osteoporosis are small-framed, nonobese, menopausal females who smoke. Contributing factors are diets low in calcium throughout life, smoking, excessive coffee intake, too much protein in the diet, and a sedentary lifestyle. Measures that can be taken to retard osteoporosis include the following:

1. Increasing calcium intake
2. Stopping smoking
3. Decreasing coffee intake
4. Decreasing excess protein in the diet
5. Engaging in regular moderate activity such as walking, bike riding, or swimming at least 3 days a week
6. Exploring with the doctor the advisability of hormone replacement at menopause

Pathophysiology and Bone Healing

A bone is said to be *fractured* or *broken* when there is an interruption in bone continuity. Commonly, a fracture is accompanied by *soft tissue* injury to surrounding tissues, that is, ligaments, muscle tendons, blood vessels, and nerves.

The classification of bone fractures is given in Box 32-3.

Immobilization of a bone that is fractured is necessary for bone healing. Immobilization takes place by the following means:

1. *Physiological splintage.* This form of splintage will occur naturally, because guarding, avoidance of use, and muscle spasm will occur as a result of pain on movement.
2. *External orthopaedic splintage.* This is accomplished with devices such as plaster casts and traction.
3. *Internal fixation.* In this method the opposing ends of the fracture are held in place by screws, plates, or rods. After immobilization is accomplished, new bone called *callus* begins to form by the following stages of growth:
   a. *Haematoma formation.* Because blood vessels are injured, bleeding occurs at the site of the fracture. The blood collects and fastens the broken ends of bones together.
   b. *Fibrin meshwork.* The haematoma becomes organized as fibroblasts invade the area, forming the fibrin meshwork. White blood cells wall off the area, localizing the inflammation.

REVIEW

Table 32-8   Fractures

Signs and symptoms	Medical therapy

Complete fracture
 	
Pain immediate and severe and aggravated by movement and pressure at site
Loss of function of injured part
Obvious gross deformity when compared with normal extremity
Loss of rigidity of injured part--motion at site of fracture
Movement produces grating sound (crepitus) of bone fragments
Soft tissue oedema—localized swelling and ecchymosis (may not be apparent for several hours or days)
Warmth over injured area resulting from increased blood flow to the area
Loss of sensation or paralysis distal to injury resulting from nerve entrapment
Signs of shock related to severe tissue injury, blood loss, or intense pain
Evidence of fracture on X-ray film
NOTE: Symptoms may be absent in linear compacted fractures.
There may be little or no swelling
Pain is present only when pressure is applied to fracture site or on use of limb or body part
	Management objectives
	
	Reduction of fracture by approximating the fracture fragments
	Maintenance of fragment in correct alignment
	Prevention of excessive loss of joint mobility and muscle tone
	
	Immediate management
	
	Provide splint before moving patient or maintain support above and below fracture site until patient can be moved and immobilization applied with splints for transportation
	Elevate extremity to minimize oedema
	Transport patient for emergency treatment
	Observe injured part at frequent intervals for local changes in colour, sensation, or temperature
	Tetanus immunization is given if compound fracture is present
	Cold applications are used to reduce haemorrhage, oedema, and pain
	Medication for pain is given
	Monitor for signs of shock—falling blood pressure, weak thready pulse, cold clammy skin, oliguria
	
	Secondary management
	Simple fracture
	
	Optimal reduction (replacing bone fragments in their correct anatomic position)
	  Manual manipulation: moving the bone fragments into position by applying traction and pressure to the distal fragment
	  Traction
	  Open reduction: surgical intervention that may incorporate use of an internal fixation device
	Immobilization
	  External fixation: cast or splint
	  Traction
	  Internal fixation: pins, plates, screws, wires, prostheses
	  Combination of the above
	Compound fracture
	
	Surgical debridement of wound to remove dirt, foreign material, devitalized tissue, and necrotic bone
	Administration of tetanus toxoid
	Culture of wound
	Packing of wound
	Treatment with antibiotics
	Observation for signs of osteomyelitis, tetanus, or gas gangrene
	Surgical closure of wound when there is no sign of infection
	Reduction of fracture
	Immobilization of fracture
	Treatment of complications is discussed in Table 32-10

c. *Invasion by osteoblasts.* The osteoblasts enter the fibrous area to help hold the union firm. Blood vessels develop, establishing a source of nutrients for building collagen. Collagen strands begin to incorporate calcium deposits.

d. *Callus formation.*
   1. Osteoblasts continue to lay the network for bone buildup.
   2. Osteoclasts destroy dead bone and help to synthesize new bone.
   3. The collagen strengthens and continues to incorporate calcium deposits.

e. *Remodelling.* In this final step, excess callus is reabsorbed and trabecular bone is laid down along lines of stress.

Factors that impede or prevent callus formation include the following:
   1. *Delayed healing or delayed union.* Delayed union occurs when the fracture does not heal within the usual time for healing.
      a. Reasons:
         (1) Callus is broken or torn apart by too much activity.

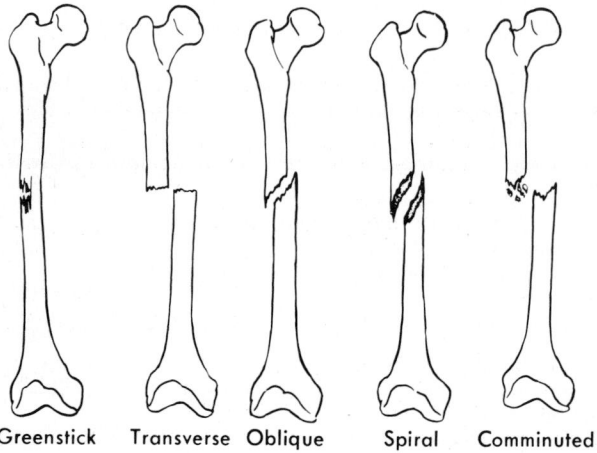

Greenstick   Transverse   Oblique   Spiral   Comminuted

Fig. 32-10   Types of fractures.

(2) Oedema at the fracture site impedes flow of nutrients to the area.
(3) Immobilization is inefficient.
(4) Infection is present at fracture site.
(5) Patient is in poor nutritional state.
b. Correction: More complete immobilization or open reduction for surgical measures.
2. *Nonunion.* Nonunion is the term used when healing does not occur even in a much longer period of time.
a. Reasons:
(1) Too much bone loss at time of injury to permit bridging of bone fragments.
(2) Bone necrosis has occurred because of lack of blood supply.
(3) Anaemia, endocrine imbalance, or other systemic conditions that interfere with the process are present.
b. Correction:
(1) Crutches may have to be used indefinitely.
(2) A brace may be worn to support the limb.
(3) Surgery may be performed to unite bone fragments with a bone graft.

Nursing Process

Assessment

Subjective data

1. Pain at site of injury
2. Loss of sensation or movement of affected part
3. Description of how trauma occurred
4. Did the person fall? In older people fracture of hip, ankle, etc., may occur first, causing the person to fall.
5. Understanding how injury sustained (may report having heard bone snap)

Objective data

1. Warmth, oedema, and/or ecchymosis over and surrounding the injured part.
2. Obvious deformity
3. Loss of normal function in the injured part—inability to bear weight
4. Immobilization device(s) applied to the injured part
5. Signs of systemic shock
6. Signs of circulatory, motor, or sensory impairment to the injured part (see Table 32-9)
7. Indicators of apprehension or fear

32-3

Classification of bone fractures

Classification according to types of fractures

Complete fracture: complete separation of the bone producing two fragments
Incomplete fracture: a partial break in the bone without separation of the bone
Simple or *closed* fracture: bone is broken; skin is intact
Compound or *open* fracture: the fracture parts extend through the skin
Fracture without displacement: bone is broken; bone fragments are in alignment in normal position
Fracture with displacement: bone fragments have separated at the point of fracture
Comminuted fracture: the bone has broken into several fragments
Impacted ("telescoped") fracture: one bone fragment is forcibly driven into another bone fragment

Classification according to line of fracture (Fig. 32-10)

Greenstick: splintering of one side of the bone (occurs most often in children with soft bones)
Transverse: break across the bone
Oblique: line of fracture at an oblique angle to the bone shaft
Spiral: line of fracture encircles the bone

Diagnostic tests

X-rays of site to determine extent of injury.

Nursing analysis

Nursing problems are determined from assessment of patient data. Possible nursing problems for the person with a fractured bone may include, but are not limited to, the following:

Problem	Possible aetiologies
Tissue perfusion, altered: peripheral	Decreased mobility, pressure, trauma
Impaired mobility	Musculoskeletal impairment, decreased strength and endurance, pain
Self-care deficit	Musculoskeletal impairment, pain/discomfort, intolerance to activity
Powerlessness	Health care environment, decreased mobility
Skin integrity, impaired, actual or high risk for	Decreased mobility, pressure, shearing forces
Infection, high risk for	Tissue trauma, surgical intervention
Nutrition, altered: less than body requirements	Fatigue, pain, chewing or swallowing difficulties
Pain	Injury to bone, injury to soft tissue at fracture site, muscle spasm, immobility, improper positioning, pressure points
Injury, high risk for	Sensory/motor deficits
Knowledge deficit: fracture	Lack of experience with fracture and how it is treated

Planning: expected patient outcomes

Expected patient outcomes for the person with a fracture may include, but are not limited to, the following:

1. Patient's skin is warm and skin and mucous membranes are pink.
2. Patient participates in a programme of progressive activity.
3. Patient is able to carry out ADL with minimal assistance.
4. Patient states he or she feels more in control of situation as mobility improves.
5. Patient's skin is intact and free of pressure ulcers.
6. Patient does not develop an infection.
7. Patient is able to maintain weight within 2–3 kg of pre-injury weight.

8. Patient states feeling more comfortable.
9. Patient does not sustain an injury.
10. Patient and/or significant other can explain the following:
    a. Nature of injury and course of treatment that must be followed to prevent injury or infection and to achieve desired result
    b. Limitations of motion and restrictions of activity to be observed and for how long
    c. How to perform or modify ADL within the limitations of activity and motion that must be observed
    d. How to care for cast, pins, or other immobilization devices, if applicable
    e. Safe use of an ambulatory or other ADL assistive device, if necessary
    f. Aseptic technique in carrying out wound care, if necessary
    g. Techniques appropriate to prevent skin breakdown, swelling, and neurocirculatory impairment
    h. Measures that can be taken for relief of pain or discomfort
    i. How to use prescribed medications
    j. Plans for follow-up care

Implementation

Interventions to achieve patient outcomes

Promoting comfort and preventing complications

The purpose of positioning is to promote comfort and prevent complications. Knowledge needed before positioning includes the following:

1. Where is the fracture?
2. What is the nature of the fracture?
3. Has the fracture been reduced?
4. What method was used to reduce the fracture?
5. What are the tolerances of the method used to reduce the fracture?
6. Is the fracture stable?
7. Has the orthopaedist requested special precautions?

After this information is obtained, positioning should be carried out with careful attention to the following:

1. Avoid altering the alignment of the fracture
2. Avoid changing the direction of the pull of traction
3. Avoid compromising the integrity of the cast
4. Avoid placing undue stress on the internal fixation device
5. Avoid changing position of patient before fracture has been reduced or splinted
6. After fracture is reduced or splinted, assist patient in changing position at *least* every 2 hours
7. Provide overhead frame and trapeze to assist patient in moving about in bed

Monitoring for neurocirculatory compromise

Monitoring for neurocirculatory compromise must be carried out every hour in the initial stages of fracture. Damage to blood vessels and/or nerves may occur at the time of the fracture or after the fracture or its reduction. Some swelling of a fractured extremity may be expected and is often well

Table 32-9 Observations for signs and symptoms of neurocirculatory impairment

Observation	Interpretation
Tissue colour white	Decreased arterial blood supply
Tissue colour blue	Venous stasis and poorly oxygenated tissue
Colour slow to return to nail bed after application of moderate pressure	Decreased arterial blood supply
Oedema	Fluid accumulating in tissues; poor venous return
Tissue cold or cool to touch	Decreased arterial blood supply
Patient unable to move parts distal to cast	Pressure on nerves innervating parts distal to cast
Patient complaint of heightened or decreased sensation or paraesthesia in part underlying or distal to cast	Pressure on nerves innervating parts underlying or distal to cast
Patient complaint of extreme pain unrelieved by elevation, analgesic, or repositioning	Pressure on nerve endings in parts underlying or distal to cast

NOTE: Comparison of tissue should be made with contralateral tissue to determine extent of deviation from normal

controlled by elevating the extremity. However, unrelieved swelling of an extremity that is in a cast or compression dressing can result in tissue damage and/or neurological impairment. *Evidence of impaired circulation or sensation must be reported to the surgeon immediately.* Frequency of neurocirculatory checks can usually be reduced if there is no evidence of compromise within 48 hours of the fracture or reduction of the fracture (See Table 32-9).

Monitoring neurocirculatory status of the injured part includes the following:

1. Palpation for warmth
2. Observation of colour
3. Application of moderate pressure to the nail bed and subsequent observation of capillary refill
4. Questioning the patient regarding pain or paraesthesias in the injured part
5. Touching the injured part to test the patient's ability to discriminate sensation
6. Observation of patient's ability to voluntarily move body part distal to fracture

Promoting mobility and self-care

Encourage the patient to do the following:

1. Move about to the greatest extent possible within the restriction of the fracture reduction and the immobilizing devices
2. Accomplish as much of own self-care as possible
3. Perform muscle toning (isometric) exercises on a regular basis: quadriceps setting, gluteal setting
4. Follow through with exercise programme (including ambulation) prescribed by the surgeon and taught by the physiotherapist.
5. Resume normal functioning for all ADL (within limits of immobilization or fixation device) as soon as possible; for example, using bedside commode or toilet instead of bedpan

Decreasing powerlessness

1. Encourage patient to express feeling about his or her injury and immobility.
2. Encourage patient to participate in planning his or her care.
3. Encourage patient to give as much of own care as possible.

4. Give the patient as much control over the daily schedule as possible.
5. Prepare patient for scheduled tests and procedures and try to avoid unexpected events.
6. Compliment the patient on even the smallest gain in being more independent.
7. Provide realistic reassurance.

Maintaining skin integrity

1. Early identification of skin areas at risk, particularly areas over bony prominences (for example, heels, sacrum, elbows, ischial tuberosities)
2. Massaging risk areas to improve blood flow
3. Regular (at least every 8 hours) inspection for signs of pressure (erythema, induration)
4. Regular turning (at least every 2 hours) within the limits of the system of fracture immobilization
5. Turning the patient with a turning sheet
6. Moving the patient from one surface to another with a pull sheet or roller board
7. Rolling the patient onto his or her side or lifting them to place them on a bedpan rather than sliding the pan under them
8. For patients who cannot be fully turned because of traction or other limiting factors, consideration should be given to using one or more of the following:
   a. Sheepskin pads
   b. Flotation pads
   c. Alternating air pressure mattress or alternating air pressure systems
   d. Foam mattress
   e. Foam heel and/or elbow pads
   f. Special beds, such as the Clinitron, or Mediscus bed
   g. Turning frames, such as the Foster or Stryker frames
9. Regular inspection of skin areas in contact with cast edges or traction apparatus and taking appropriate measures to eliminate chafing or rubbing in those areas
10. Assisting the patient with keeping skin clean and dry, especially under casts, slings, traction apparatus

Preventing infection and promoting wound healing

1. Strict attention to aseptic technique during dressing changes
2. Attention to drains to maintain their placement and patency.
3. Caring for pin site as ordered
4. Encouraging to eat a well-balanced diet

Promoting nutrition

1. Encourage patient to eat regular meals
2. Give the patient plenty of time to eat
3. Encourage self-feeding, but assist the patient or provide special assistive utensils as necessary
4. Attend to the patient's need for fibre and fluid as noted, and encourage protein intake of 150-300 g per day
5. Position the patient to facilitate comfortable intake of food and fluid.

Maintaining immobilization of the reduced fracture

The purpose of immobilization is to hold the broken bone fragments in contact with each other until healing takes place. Immobilization can be accomplished in the following ways:

1. Externally with
   a. Cast
   b. Splint
   c. Brace
   d. Cast brace
   e. Traction
2. Internally with
   a. Metal plates, pins, screws, nails
   b. Bone grafts with addition of metal plates, pins
   c. Prosthetic implants
3. Externally and internally with combinations of the above.

Assisting with comfort and ADL

Managing pain

The person with a fracture will most often have severe pain at the fracture site, pressure from oedema in damaged soft tissues adjacent to the fracture, and spasm of muscles in the fracture area. Continued pain and the muscle spasm accompanying it can put undue stress on the fracture fragments and retard efforts both to reduce and maintain reduction of the fracture. Patients who are in severe pain will resist efforts to assist them in carrying out measures designed to prevent complications. If the fracture is repaired by open reduction and internal fixation, the patient will have operative pain.

Measures the nurse can take to help reduce pain include the following:

1. During the initial stages of treatment, administer prescribed narcotic and non-narcotic analgesics in appropriate dosages at timely intervals unless patient-controlled analgesia (PCA) is being used
2. Administer prescribed drugs such as diazepam (Valium) to reduce muscle spasm
3. Apply ice compresses, as ordered, to affected part
4. Reposition the patient frequently within the restrictions of the prescribed treatment

5. Instruct the patient how to use relaxation techniques (deep breathing, imagery) to reduce tension
6. As pain subsides, negotiate with the patient a reduction in the strength and/or frequency of analgesics

It is important, in using analgesics, to try to strike a balance between having the patient comfortable enough to perform required exercises and other activities, and having the patient so overly medicated as to risk potential damage through over-extending activity or being heavily sedated. This is one advantage of PCA, which usually maintains comfort while preventing overmedication.

Preventing injury

1. Monitor the patient's movement in bed to ensure that undue stress is not put on injured part.
2. Supervise patient's exercises while in bed.
3. Monitor mobilization to ensure a safe environment.
   a. Remove unnecessary equipment from patient's room so clutter will not interfere with safe ambulation.
4. Monitor patient's use of ambulatory aid to be sure it is being used correctly and safely.

Facilitating learning

The patient and family are taught the following:

1. How bone heals and precautions taken by staff to ensure that nothing is interfering with the healing (frequent neurocirculatory checks and vital signs).
2. About how cast is applied and how it should be cared for.
3. What will be done in surgery and the types of fixation devices that may be used (pins, screws, rods, and so on).
4. About skin or skeletal traction and how it is maintained.
5. The importance of eating a diet that will assist in bone healing. Emphasis is on protein, calcium and vitamins A, B, C and D to aid in the healing process.
6. The need to maintain a fluid intake of about 3000 ml per 24 hours.
7. About the use of an ambulatory aid. The initial teaching may be by the physiotherapist, but the nurse will need to understand what has been taught so she or he can supervise the patient in use of the aid.
8. About how he or she will be gradually mobilized and the exercise programme that will need to be followed to regain full use of affected joint(s).
9. The role of the patient in his or her own recovery and rehabilitation.

Monitoring for complications

The complications of bone fractures, their mechanism, signs, onset, and treatment are listed in Table 32-10.

Evaluation

Evaluation is based on the expected patient outcomes. Questions to consider may include the following:

1. Is tissue perfusion normal (skin warm and pink)?
2. Is patient able to be up and about by self using an appropriate ambulatory aid?
3. Is patient able to be more independent in self-care?

Table 32-10   Complications of fracture

Complication	Mechanism	Signs	Onset	Treatment
Fat embolism	Pressure changes in interior of fractured bones force molecules of fat from marrow into systemic circulation, resulting in respiratory and central nervous system problems	Chest pain Pallor Dyspnoea Prostration Confusion Petechial haemorrhage of skin and conjunctivae	2-3 days after injury	Supportive measures; that is, supported sitting position, oxygen therapy, blood transfusion to relieve hypovolaemic shock, digitalization for heart failure Diuretics Bronchodilators Corticosteroids Proper immobilization and careful handling may help prevent occurrence
Ischaemic paralysis (contracture)	Arterial flow is interrupted to injured part by trauma or pressure	Coldness, pallor, cyanosis, pain, swelling distal to injury or cast	At injury or after cast application	Treatment of fracture Release of cast or constricting bandages
Osteomyelitis	Bacteria introduced through wound or from another site in body (for example, boils) Infection of marrow spaces, haversian canals, and subperiosteal space with subsequent destruction of bone by proteolytic enzymes	Hyperaemia, oedema, pain pus		Culture and sensitivity testing, antibiotics, surgical drainage, and debridement Prevention: use of aseptic technique when caring for open wound

4. Is patient more in control of situation and expressing confidence in his or her future?
5. Is patient's skin intact?
6. Is the patient free of infection?
7. Is the patient able to eat a well balanced diet?
8. Is the patient free of pain?
9. Is patient free of injury?
10. Can the patient and/or relative explain the following?
    a. Nature of injury and course of treatment
    b. Limitations of motion and restriction in activity
    c. How to modify ADL to meet prescribed limitations on motion
    d. How to care for cast, pins, and other immobilization devices
    e. How to use ambulatory aids (zimmer, crutches, walking stick) safely
    f. How to care for any wounds using aseptic technique
    g. Measures to prevent skin breakdown, swelling, and neurocirculatory impairment
    h. Measures to relieve pain or discomfort (change of position, elevation of affected part, ice packs, analgesics)
    i. How to use prescribed medications
    j. Plans for follow-up care

TREATMENT OF FRACTURES WITH EXTERNAL FIXATION DEVICES

Casts

Casts are the most common external fixation device. They are made of plaster of Paris, fibreglass, and plastic, which are available in the form of rolled bandages that are applied over the part to be immobilized in much the same manner as a bandage. *Plaster*, which has to be moistened before application, dries very slowly, is heavy, and loses its strength and integrity if it becomes wet. If a plaster cast requires revision, it generally must be removed and a new one reapplied. However, plaster is less expensive than fibreglass or plastic.

Fibreglass and *plastic* casts are also moistened before application, dry quickly, are light in weight, and may be immersed in water without losing their strength. Plastic casts may be reheated and remoulded if revision is necessary. Disadvantages include the fact that some types of fibreglass require drying under special ultraviolet lights, and people wearing fibreglass or plastic casts may suffer maceration of the skin under the cast after immersion in water unless they dry the skin throughout with a warm air dryer. Specific discussions regarding the advantages and disadvantages of various cast materials can be found in orthopaedic texts.

Before a cast is applied, the skin is cleansed and inspected for cuts or abrasions that may become infected. Skin lesions are treated with disinfectant. Normal skin may be cleaned, then wrapped with cotton padding or stockinette before cast is applied. Bony prominences are padded with sheet wadding or felt to protect them from pressure. For specific techniques of cast application, consult specialized texts.

A cast is removed by splitting it with an electric cast saw. The saw is very noisy; but if it is used properly, it will not damage the skin beneath the cast. Newer cast saws are connected to a cannister vacuum that sucks up plaster dust that results from the sawing. Skin enclosed in a cast for a period of time may be covered with an exudate of built-up

The patient in a cast

Patient education

Explain why the cast is being applied and how it will be applied

Advise the patient that the plaster cast will feel warm as it dries

Explain the extent of immobilization

Explain care of the cast and expectations after discharge

Instruct patient not to insert sharp objects (coat hangers or pencils) under the cast as these may abrade the skin and lead to infection

Handling the new cast

Support wet cast with the flat of the hands or on pillows to avoid indentations that will cause pressure on underlying skin

Place cotton blankets or other absorbent material under the cast to aid drying

Expose the cast to air as much as possible to aid drying

Turn the patient frequently to aid drying

use a cast dryer or hair dryer on a warm, not hot, setting to circulate air over the cast

Do not apply paint or varnish to the cast; plaster is a porous material that allows air to circulate to the skin

Skin care

Inspect skin at edges of cast and underlying cast for redness or irritation; apply petal-shaped strips of adhesive tape or moleskin around rough edges of cast

Remove plaster crumbs from skin with a washcloth moistened with warm water

Use creams and lotions sparingly as they may soften the skin and cause the cast to stick to the skin

Apply waterproof material around perineal area to prevent soiling of and damage to cast and irritation of the skin

Attend to patient's complaint of pain under the cast, particularly over bony prominences, as this may indicate pressure on the skin. If discomfort is not relieved by repositioning, report to doctor at once. Cast pressure may need to be relieved by cutting a window in the cast or cutting the cast in two (bivalving)

Turning—turning to any position is generally permitted as long as the integrity of the cast is not compromised and the patient is comfortable

Toileting—for a long leg or hip spica cast

Use a fracture pan with blanket roll or padding as support under the small of the back

Elevate the head of the bed, if permitted, or place the bed in reverse Trendelenburg's position

Abdominal discomfort—cast may be "windowed" (an opening cut into it) to provide relief of abdominal distention or a port for checking bladder distention

Mobilization

Weight bearing is at the discretion of the doctor, and the amount of weight bearing will be prescribed

A cast shoe or a walking heel incorporated into a lower extremity cast will permit weight bearing without damaging the cast

Prevention of neurocirculatory problems

Perform neurocirculatory checks every hr for at least 24 hours after cast application to detect difficulty from swelling or pressure of cast on nerves or vessels. Notify doctor of colour changes, alterations in sensation, or motion unrelieved by position change. Cast may need to be bivalved (cut in two) to relieve pressure

Elevate affected extremity on pillows until danger of swelling is over (usually 24–48 hours)

After mobilization of patient with lower extremity or upper extremity cast, avoid keeping extremity in dependent position for prolonged periods

After lower extremity cast is removed, encourage patient to wear elastic stocking and elevate affected leg at rest until full mobility is regained

---

secretions and dead skin. To remove this exudate, oil is applied, followed by numerous soaks and bathing with warm water. This process may take several days, but attempts to remove the exudate more rapidly may cause an uncomfortable skin irritation.

Special considerations in caring for the patient in a cast are outlined in Box 32-4.

Traction

Traction is the mechanism by which a steady pull is placed on a part or parts of the body. Traction may be used to accomplish the following:

1. Reduce a fracture
2. Maintain correct position of bone fragments during healing
3. Immobilize a limb while soft tissue healing takes place
4. Overcome muscle spasm
5. Stretch adhesions
6. Correct deformities

Countertraction is a force that counteracts the pull of traction. *Suspension* is the use of traction equipment—frames, splints, slings, ropes, pulleys, weights—to suspend a body part but not exert a "pull" on

32-5

Guidelines for Care

The patient in traction

Patient education
Explain traction in relation to fracture and surgeon's plan of treatment
Explain amount of movement permitted and how to achieve it (for example, how trapeze can be used to assist with movement)
Explain correct body positioning

Maintaining the traction
Inspect traction apparatus frequently to assure that ropes are running straight and through the middle of the pulleys; that weights are hanging free; that bedclothes, the bed, or the frame and bars on the bed are not impinging on any part of the traction apparatus
Check ropes frequently to be sure they are not frayed
Avoid releasing weights from or altering the line of pull of the traction
Avoid adding weight to the traction
Check the position of the Thomas splint frequently; if the ring has slid away from the groin, readjust the splint to its proper position without releasing traction
Avoid bumping into or jarring the bed or traction equipment
Be sure weights are securely fastened to their ropes and do not touch the floor
Avoid manipulation of pins

Skin care
Encourage the patient to turn slightly from side to side and to lift up on the trapeze to relieve pressure on the skin of the sacrum and scapulae; have the patient lift up for routine skin care.
Avoid padding the ring of the Thomas splint as this will create dampness next to the skin. Bathe the skin beneath the ring, dry it thoroughly, and powder the skin lightly
Inspect skin frequently to be sure it is not being rubbed, contused, or macerated by traction equipment; readjust splints or the extremity in the splint to free the skin from pressure
Keep skin areas around pin sites clean and dry; direct care to pin sites (that is, cleansing with cotton applicators and hydrogen peroxide or alcohol) is *controversial*, so check with patient's doctor to determine if pin care is to be done routinely and what method the doctor prefers

Toileting
Use a fracture pan with blanket roll or padding as support under the small of the back
Protect the ring of the Thomas splint with waterproof material when female patients are using the bedpan

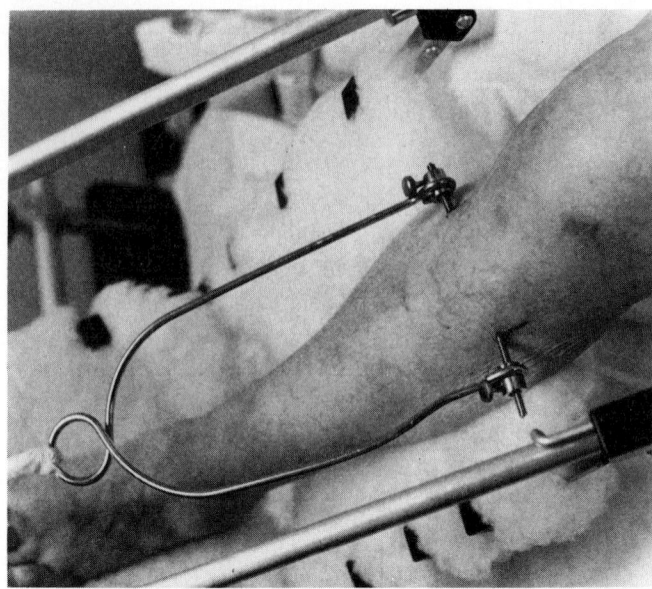

Fig. 32-11   Tibial pin traction with Steinmann pin used in treatment of a distal femoral fracture. The bow attached to the pin provides a place of attachment for the rope that holds the traction weights. The pull exerted by the weight keeps the fracture fragments aligned. Pin sites must be inspected at least daily to detect signs of pin reaction or infection.

Skin traction

Skin traction is achieved by applying wide bands of moleskin, adhesive, or commercially available devices directly to the skin and attaching weights to them. The pull of the weight is transmitted indirectly to the involved bone. Buck's extension and Russell traction are the two most common forms of skin traction used for injury to the lower extremities.

Buck's extension

Buck's extension is the simplest form of skin traction and provides for straight pull on the affected extremity. It is often used to relieve muscle spasm and to immobilize a limb temporarily; for example, after hip fracture before open reduction and internal fixation. If adhesive substances are to be used, the skin of the leg is shaved. Adhesive tape or moleskin is then placed on the lateral and medial aspects of the leg and secured with a circular gauze or elastic bandage. The adhesive material should not cover the malleoli, because skin breakdown would occur over these bony prominences. The tapes are attached to a spreader bar sufficiently wide to pull the tapes away from the malleoli. Rope is attached to the spreader, passed through a pulley on a crossbar at the foot of the bed, and suspended with weights. The maximal weight that should be applied by skin traction is 3.6 kg (8 lb). Greater amounts of weight can cause skin damage. Commercial foam rubber Buck's traction splints are also in wide use and are applied simply with Velcro straps. Contraindications to placing a patient in Buck's traction are stasis dermatitis, arteriosclerosis, allergy to adhesive tape, severe varicosities or varicose ulcers, diabetic gangrene, or marked overriding of bone fragments that would require more than 3.6 kg of weight to reduce the fracture.

that part. To suspend the part correctly and continuously, the suspension has to be balanced by weights. Suspension is often referred to as *balanced suspension*. Balanced suspension is often used in conjunction with traction.

There are two types of traction: skin traction and skeletal traction.

Russell traction

Russell traction is sometimes used because it permits the patient to move more freely in the bed and it permits flexion of the knee joint. It requires an overhead frame attached to the bed and preparation of the leg as for Buck's traction. A footplate with pulley attachments is used instead of a spreader bar. The knee is suspended in a sling to which a rope is attached. The rope is directed upward to a pulley that has been placed on the overhead frame directly above the tibial tubercle of the affected extremity. The rope is then passed downward through a pulley on a crossbar at the foot of the bed, back through a pulley on the footplate, back again to another pulley on the crossbar, and then suspended with weights. This arrangement effects a double pull from the crossbar to the footplate, so the traction is equal to approximately double the amount of weight used. Usually the foot of the bed is elevated on blocks (or the bed put in Trendelenburg position) to provide countertraction.

Russell traction is used in the treatment of intertrochanteric fracture of the femur when surgery is contraindicated. Bilateral Russell or Buck's traction may be used to treat back pain because they partially immobilize the patient and reduce muscle spasm.

Skeletal traction

Skeletal traction is traction applied directly to bone. Under local or general anaesthesia, a Kirschner wire or Steinmann pin is inserted through bone distal to the fracture (the site of insertion varies with the type of fracture) (Fig. 32-11). The pin protrudes through the skin on both sides of the extremity, and the exposed ends of the pin are covered with corks or metal protectors. Small sterile dressings are usually placed over the entry and exit sites of the pin. A metal U-shaped spreader or bow is attached to the pin, and the rope on which the traction weights are hung is tied onto the spreader. Skeletal traction can be used for fractures of the tibia, femur, humerus, and cervical spine. Skeletal traction to the cervical spine is achieved through use of tongs applied to the skull.

When a balanced suspension apparatus is used in conjunction with skin or skeletal traction, the patient is able to move about in bed more freely without disturbing the line of pull of the traction. The use of a balancing apparatus facilitates nursing measures such as bathing, skin care, and placing the bedpan. A full or half-ring Thomas splint (Fig. 32-12) is frequently used for suspension of the lower extremities. Straps of canvas, muslin, or synthetic lamb's wool are placed over the splint and secured to provide a support for the leg. The areas under the popliteal space and heel are left open to prevent pressure on these parts. If it is desirable to have the knee flexed or to permit movement of the lower leg, a Pearson attachment is clamped or fixed to the Thomas splint at the level of the knee.

Special considerations in caring for the patient in traction are described in Box 32-5.

Other Types of External Immobilization

Other devices for external immobilization of fractures include the following:

1. Braces made of rigid plastic material
2. Plaster or plastic braces that incorporate metal struts attached to pins inserted into bone (for example, a halo brace)
3. Metal struts attached to pins inserted into bone (for example, the various types of Hoffman or Charnley external fixation devices).

Devices such as the Hoffman or Charnley may be used in conjunction with plaster or alone. All of these devices provide extremely rigid fixation while allowing the patient some degree of mobility. It is quite possible for the patient in a halo brace to ambulate. The patient with an external fixator on the lower leg can be out of bed in a wheelchair, or even ambulate without bearing weight on the affected leg.

Nursing care for patients in these devices is essentially the same as for patients in casts and/or skeletal traction, with the exception that they may be mobilized earlier.

TREATMENT OF FRACTURES WITH INTERNAL FIXATION DEVICES

Open Reduction

Open surgical reduction of fractures has the advantage of allowing visualization of the fracture and surrounding tissues. It is particularly indicated when soft tissue is caught between bone fragments or when known damage to nerves or blood vessels exists. *The disadvantages of internal fixation are that it requires anaesthesia and it carries the risk of infection at the time of surgery. Internal fixation is carried out under the most vigorous aseptic conditions, and patients may receive a short course of prophylactic intravenous antibiotics after surgery.*

The internal fixation devices available include the following:

1. Plates and nails such as the Neufeld nail
2. Transfixation screws
3. Kuntschner nail (intramedullary rods)
4. Prosthetic implants such as the Austin Moore prosthesis, which are used when proximal fragment of the fracture is jeopardized

It should also be noted that *bone grafts,* either *autograft* (the patient's own bone) or *allograft* (cadaver bone), may be used either in conjunction with internal fixation devices when excessive bone is lost at the fracture site, or alone, as in spine surgery. It should also be noted that fixation with internal devices does not preclude additional fixation with external devices (casts, braces, or traction), particularly in cases of very complicated fracture or multiple trauma.

In general, the primary objective of care is to protect the fixation device until healing takes place. Metal that can fatigue and break cannot be expected to substitute for intact bone. If the fixation device breaks, healing of the fracture will be disrupted. However, mobilization of patients who have had an internal fixation is usually much faster than for those who have had external fixation. *Nursing interventions for patients with internal fixation include the following:*

1. Patient education
   a. Prepare the patient for general anaesthesia
   b. Explain the surgical procedure and general nursing care after surgery

Nursing Care Plan	**Patient with an intracapsular hip fracture, open reduction, and internal fixation with a prosthetic implant**

DATA: Mrs. W. is an 81-year-old widowed, retired secretary. This evening she tripped and fell on an icy step when leaving her niece's home. She complained of immediate, severe pain in her left hip and was unable to move her leg. An ambulance was called, and Mrs.W. was accompanied to the hospital by her niece and her niece's husband. In casualty it was noted that her left leg was shorter than her right, and it was externally rotated.

Her vital signs were stable, and the neurocirculatory status of the left leg was intact. An X-ray examination revealed an intracapsular femoral neck fracture. Intravenous fluids were started. An ECG, urinalysis, FBC, and serum electrolyte study were obtained. She was transferred to the ward with the surgeon's orders for morphine sulphate 4 to 6 mg every 3 to 4 hours as necessary for pain. Buck's extension was applied. Consent was obtained for surgical repair in the morning. Replacement of the femoral head and neck with a regular stem Austin Moore prosthesis is planned

The nursing history identified the following:
- Mrs. W. Lives alone in her own flat in a warden assisted block.
- Mrs. W. has no children but has nieces and nephews in the area who see her regularly. They assist with shopping and other errands.
- Mrs. W. would like to return to her own flat after being discharged from the hospital, but she worries that she might need help at home. Her family is considering hiring a home help.
- She takes no medications other than aspirin for occasional "stiffness" on awakening.
- She has never been hospitalized and last saw a doctor 2 years ago for "the flu."

Nursing analysis: Knowledge deficit related to lack of exposure to surgery

Expected patient outcomes	Nursing interventions (preoperative)	Rationale
Mrs. W. can explain the teaching provided by the nurse about preoperative and general postoperative care. Mrs. W. states that she is experiencing less anxiety related to fear of the unknown and/or misconceptions about surgery and the recovery period.	Assess need for instruction and provide as necessary. Provide written materials pertaining to the surgery, if available in the institution. Review preoperative instruction with Mrs. W. and family before the surgery. Evaluate Mrs. W.'s understanding of the information taught.	Information may reduce anxiety and reduce fear of the unknown.

	Nursing interventions (postoperative)	
	Collaborative nursing actions include those to identify possible complications of surgery. Immediate reporting of and treatment of early signs may prevent serious problems. Nursing actions include monitoring for the following: 1. *Neurocirculatory compromise:* Perform neurocirculatory checks hrly for the first 24-48 hr. Notify surgeon of any changes from preoperative status. 2. *Dislocation of the prosthesis:* Notify surgeon if Mrs. W. complains of sudden onset of increased pain, especially groin pain, particularly if accompanied by deformity or eternal rotation.	

Expected patient outcomes	Nursing interventions	Rationale
	3. *Impaired skin integrity and/or impaired wound healing.* Monitor pressure areas for signs of redness, monitor temperature, and assess incision for signs or symptoms of infection or excessive drainage.	
	4. *Atelectasis/respiratory infection:* Monitor breath sounds until Mrs. W. is ambulatory.	
	5. *Urinary retention:* Assess output 4 hrly.	
	6. *Constipation:* Assess bowel status each day until Mrs. W. is able to have a bowel movement.	
	7. *Fluid and electrolyte imbalance:* Monitor intake and output until Mrs. W. is taking oral fluids without difficulty, monitor IV fluid rates, and assess Mrs. W. for fluid volume excess or deficit.	
	By discharge Mrs. W. should be instructed in and be able to explain or demonstrate the following:	
	1. *Independent ambulation* on level surfaces with appropriate ambulatory aid and independent stair climbing	
	2. *Activity restrictions to be observed for approximately 2 months* or until follow-up with the surgeon, for example, limiting flexion of the affected hip to 90 degrees, avoiding adduction of the affected leg beyond midline, avoiding extreme internal and external rotation of the affected hip, and maintaining partial weight-bearing status with the walker or crutches	

Nursing Care Plan	**Patient with an intracapsular hip fracture, open reduction, and internal fixation with a prosthetic implant--cont'd**

Nursing analysis: Pain related to surgical procedure

Expected patient outcomes	Nursing interventions	Rationale
Mrs. W. states feeling comfortable. Mrs. W. is able to perform necessary postoperative routines/exercises.	Assess Mrs. W.'s pain and evaluate response to comfort measures provided. Administer prescribed analgesics (usually narcotic) at timely intervals during initial postoperative period. Teach relaxation techniques as appropriate. Use other pain relieving techniques as appropriate, for example, back rubs, repositioning. As pain decreases, use milder analgesics as prescribed.	Subjective and objective data are important in ascertaining the nature of Mrs. W.'s postoperative pain and determining its management. It is usually necessary to administer narcotics in the first 48-72 hr after surgery. Analgesics have a greater effect if they are administered before pain becomes severe. Relaxation facilitates rest and may modify the response to pain. A change in type of cutaneous stimulation may result in pain relief. Pain may be controlled by less potent analgesics (with fewer untoward side effects) as pain lessens in severity.

Nursing analysis: Impaired mobility, related to alteration in lower limb status after surgical repair of hip fracture

Expected patient outcomes	Nursing interventions	Rationale
Mrs. W. demonstrates optimal level of mobility with adaptive devices within prescribed limitations of activity by time of discharge. No injury occurs during Mrs. W.'s hospitalization.	Have Mrs. W. deep breathe and cough every 1-2 hr until fully ambulatory. Encourage Mrs. W. to perform active dorsiflexion, plantar flexion, isometric quadriceps setting and gluteal setting, and active range of motion of unaffected limbs 2 hrly until ambulatory. Determine from surgeon the limits of motion and weight bearing permitted, keeping in mind the following guidelines: 1. Hip flexion is usually limited to 90 degrees for 2-3 months. Adduction beyond midline is prohibited for 2-3 months. 2. Extreme internal or external rotation is prohibited for 2-3 months. 3. Partial weight bearing on affected body part with the aid of a Zimmer frame or crutches is usually observed for 2-3 months.	If carried out correctly and at appropriate intervals, pulmonary exercises can effectively prevent atelectasis and pneumonia. Exercising promotes venous return, prevents thrombus formation, and helps to maintain muscle tone. Restrictions on positioning are designed to avoid dislocation of the prosthesis.

Nursing analysis: Impaired mobility, related to alteration in lower limb status after surgical repair of hip fracture —cont'd

Expected patient outcomes	Nursing interventions	Rationale
	Turn Mrs. W. from back to unoperated side 2 hrly and prn. Avoid positioning patient on operative side, and observe flexion restrictions when elevating the head of the bed.	Turning and repositioning frequently promotes circulation, respiratory effort, and muscle activity.
	When turning Mrs. W., hold the operative leg in abduction; use pillows to maintain 30-degree abduction when turning is accomplished.	Prevents adduction of leg.
	Assist Mrs. W. to walk using the appropriate ambulatory aid. Begin walking the first or second postoperative day and increase the Frequency and distance of ambulation as tolerated.	Early postoperative activity, including walking, can hasten recovery and prevent postoperative complications.
	Begin sitting when Mrs. W. demonstrates sufficient control of the affected leg to sit within flexion restrictions.	Prepare Mrs. W. for discharge while assuring that Mrs. W. can sit safely within prescribed limits on flexion.
	Elevate sitting surface with pillows to keep angle of hip within preprescribed limits.	Limits hip flexion to 90 degrees.

Nursing analysis: High risk for impaired home maintenance management related to independent living situation

Expected patient outcomes	Nursing interventions	Rationale
Mrs. W. and family express satisfaction with arrangements made to facilitate self-care at home.	Discuss with Mrs. W. and family their plans for Mrs. W.'s care after discharge from the hospital. Determine with Mrs. W. what she must do for herself to return to her own home. Determine with Mrs. W. the type of equipment and services needed for return home (for example, crutches, frame, elevated toilet seat, home help, companion, physiotherapy, Meals on Wheels, and shopping services). Assess Mrs. W.'s progress at regular intervals to determine whether her functional ability will permit carrying out of the above plans. Involve appropriate department (for example, social services department) for assistance in planning, if Mrs. W. is unable to achieve functional levels consistent with the initial plan.	Adequate discharge planning will foster successful completion of rehabilitation at home or will help to identify areas in Mrs. W.'s performance of required functional abilities indicating a need for a skilled nursing facility, rehabilitation hospital, or other form of intermediate care.

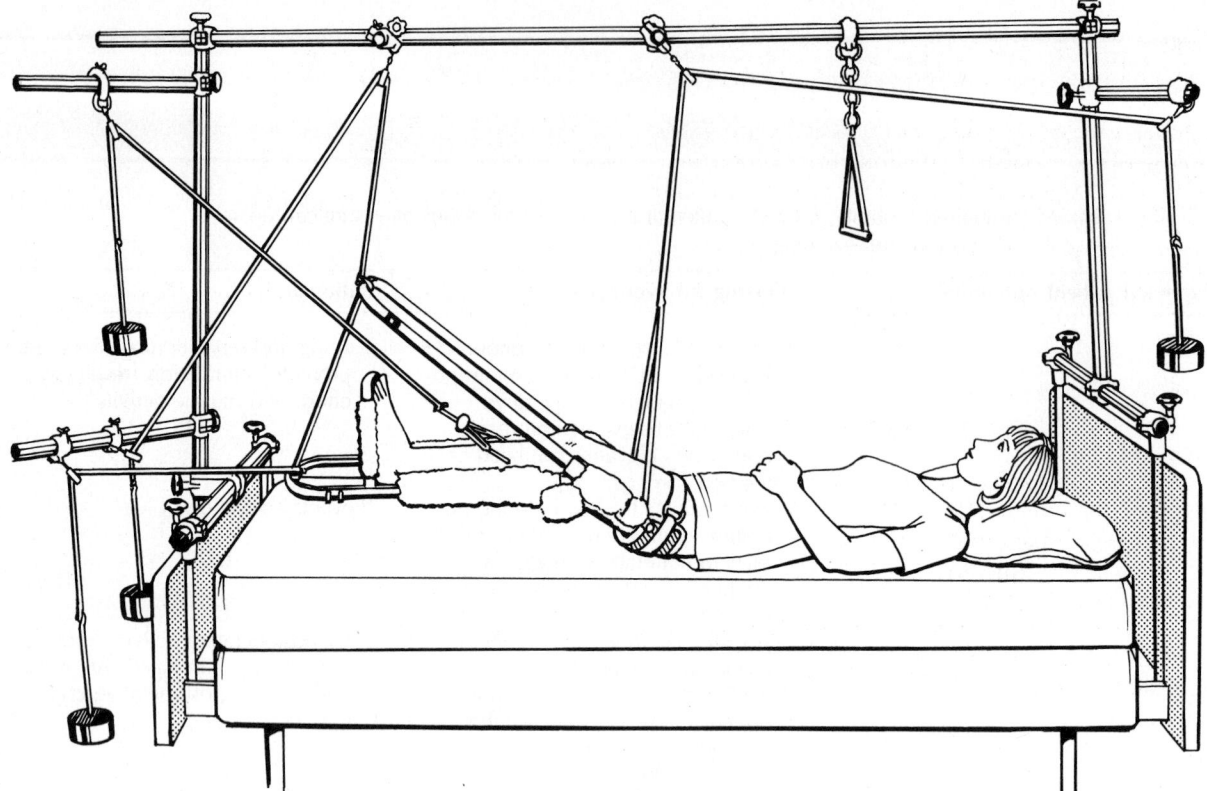

Fig. 32-12 Balanced suspension with Thomas splint and Pearson attachment. This apparatus can be used alone or, as in this case, with skeletal traction.

c. Postoperatively, explain the limits of motion and weight bearing on the affected part

2. Promoting mobility
   a. Determine, in consultation with the surgeon, the limits of motion and weight bearing permitted
   b. Assist the patient with turning within the prescribed limits
   c. Assist the patient in transferring and ambulating within the prescribed limits (may be up as early as first postoperative day)

3. Prevention of neurocirculatory problems
   a. Perform neurocirculatory checks every hour for the first 24 to 48 hours; notify surgeon of any change from preoperative status that may indicate pressure from *swelling, constriction of bandages, or damage to nerves or vessels* during surgery
   b. Maintain elevation of affected extremity

4. Maintenance of immobilization of fracture; considerations for care are the same as for patients in casts or traction (p. 995) if these devices are used

FRACTURE OF THE HIP

Aetiology/Epidemiology

Hip fractures are perhaps the most common fracture seen in the hospital. They occur more frequently in women than in men. Some factors explaining this follow:

1. Women have a wider pelvis with a tendency to coxa vara

2. Women have postmenopausal hormonal changes often accompanied by an increased incidence of osteoporosis

3. Women's life expectancy is greater than that of men

A recent study of hip fracture in women identified several factors that increase the risks of falls associated with hip fracture. These are: lower-limb dysfunction, neurological conditions, hypnotics and sedatives, and visual impairments. The authors' recommendations include the following: aggressive treatment of ocular disease and visual impairment, physiotherapy for women with mobility problems, and consideration given to discontinuing medication that affects *cognitive function.*[25]

Primary Prevention

Because most falls occur in the home and the *height of the fall* and *landing on hard surfaces increase risk of fracture,* the authors of the above study recommended several changes in the home. These include: lowering beds, installing wall-to-wall carpeting, and providing grab bars, stair rails, or other aids that would help prevent a falling person from landing on the floor.

The authors also pointed out that several studies have identified that increased body weight decreases the risk of hip fracture. Possible explanations for this are that heavier people have greater bone mass and their fatty tissue offers protection during a fall.[25]

The following is a review of the hip joint for a clearer understanding of what is involved in a fracture of this area. The hip joint is a ball-and-socket joint formed by the acetabulum, a deep round cavity in the innominate bone, and the rounded upper portion of the femur. The upper part of the femur is composed of a head, neck, greater and lesser trochanter, and shaft. The distal part of the femur ends in two condyles. The head of the femur fits into the acetabulum. The hip joint is surrounded by a fibrous capsule, ligaments, and muscles. The greater trochanter serves as a point of insertion for the abductor muscles and short rotator muscles of the hip, whereas the lesser trochanter serves as a point of insertion for the iliopsoas muscle.

Pathophysiology

Fractures of the hip may be classified into two general categories (Fig. 32-13):
1. *Intracapsular*—occurring within the hip joint and capsule; these include
   a. Subcapital fracture
   b. Transcervical fracture
   c. Basal neck fracture
2. *Extracapsular*—occurring outside the hip joint and capsule to an area 5 cm (2 in) below the lesser trochanter; these are called *intertrochanteric* fractures

The blood supply to the femoral head is of paramount importance in fractures in or about the hip joint. The blood supply to the femoral head varies with age. The chief source of blood supply to the femoral head in adults is the posterior retinacular artery. The nutrient and periosteal vessels of the femoral shaft extend into the trochanteric region and lower part of the neck.

Blood supply to the head of the femur comes up through the neck of the femur and is often disrupted in an intracapsular fracture. When blood supply is interrupted, death (*avascular necrosis*) of the femoral head may occur.

Assessment

Subjective and objective data

Signs and symptoms of hip fracture include the following:
1. Severe pain at the fracture site
2. Inability to move the leg voluntarily
3. Shortening and external rotation of the leg
4. Other signs and symptoms consistent with signs and symptoms of any fracture such as pain, bruising at site or on other places on body

Medical Management

The choice of fixation device depends on the location of the fracture, the potential for avascular necrosis of the femoral head, and the personal preference of the surgeon. An *impacted intracapsular fracture without displacement* may be treated with bedrest alone. Common choices include the following:
1. *Stable plate and screw fixation;* implies non-weight bearing status for 6 weeks to 3 months
2. *Telescoping nail fixation;* implies minimal to partial weight-bearing status for 6 weeks to 3 months
3. *Prosthetic implant*, usually Austin Moore prosthesis or Bi-Polar prosthesis, to replace femoral head and

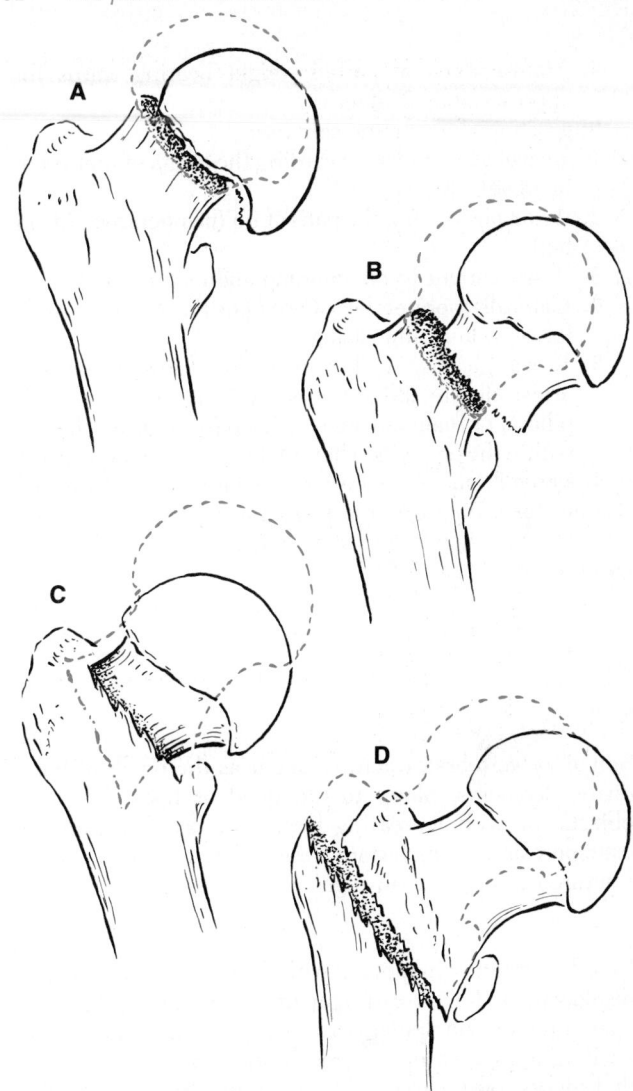

Fig. 32-13 Fractures of hip. **A,** Subcapital fracture. **B,** Transcervical fracture. **C,** Impacted fracture of base of neck. **D,** Intertrochanteric fracture.

neck; implies some position restrictions for 2 weeks to 2 months and partial weight-bearing restrictions for up to 2 months
4. *Closed reduction and external fixation* if general medical condition precludes surgery

Nursing Interventions

Nursing interventions should include those already noted for general care of patients with fractures with specific attention to interventions for people with internal fixation. Special consideration should be taken in regard to people who have had a prosthetic implant because unless they have external fixation as well, there will be specific position restrictions. These include the following:
1. Avoidance of hip flexion beyond 60 degrees for approximately 10 days
2. Avoidance of hip flexion beyond 90 degrees from the tenth day to 2 months
3. Avoidance of adduction of the affected leg beyond midline for 2 months

4. Maintenance of partial weight bearing status for approximately 2 months

Suggestions for nursing care are:

1. Instruct the patient regarding the limits of motion to be observed
2. Avoid positioning the patient on the operative side in bed
3. Assist patient in maintaining abduction of hip.
4. Carefully monitor the patient's position through transfer, standing, and sitting
5. Provide a chair with a firm, nonreclining seat and arms; elevate the sitting surface as necessary with pillows or foam cushions to keep the angle of the hip within the prescribed limits when the patient is sitting

In general, patients who have had *any* kind of internal fixation for a fractured hip should avoid elevation of the operated leg when sitting in a chair as this puts excessive strain on the fixation device.

FRACTURES OF THE SPINE

Aetiology/Epidemiology

Spinal, or vertebral, fractures occur as the result of falls, diving accidents, blows to the head or body by heavy objects, or with increasing frequency, as the result of osteoporosis and metastatic lesions of the spine. Spine fracture can occur at any age.

Pathophysiology

Vertebral fracture may occur with displacement or without displacement. If fracture fragments are displaced, they may place pressure on spinal nerves or injure the spinal cord itself. Such pressure will result in partial or complete dysfunction of the body parts innervated from the level of injury. Depending on the extent of injury to the nervous system structures, dysfunction may be permanent, partially permanent, or temporary. Fracture can occur at any level of the spine, from occiput through the sacrum.

Assessment

Subjective and objective data

Signs and symptoms of vertebral fracture include the following:

1. Pain at the site of injury
2. Partial or complete loss of mobility or sensation below the level of injury
3. Evidence of fracture/fracture dislocation on routine x-ray film, on myelography, or on high resolution CAT scans.

Medical Management

Objectives in management will be stabilization of the fracture, reduction of the fracture, and decompression (that is, removal of pressure from spinal nerves or the spinal cord).

Immediate management

1. Immobilization of the patient with backboard and cervical collar
2. Immediate transport to a hospital

Surgical management

1. Decompression of nerve structures through laminectomy (see Chapter 29) or appropriate reduction of the fracture and removal of fracture fragments
2. Reduction of the fracture through operative procedures, or in some cases, traction (for example, cervical traction through application of tongs to the skull)
3. Stabilization of the fracture with bone grafting and/or internal fixation devices such as Harrington, Jacobs, or Luque rods.
4. Maintenance of stabilization with external fixation devices such as casts, corsets, or braces as necessary

NOTE: Compression fractures of the spine may be treated with bed rest until the patient's pain subsides, then the patient is gradually mobilized, sometimes with stabilization by a corset or brace.

Nursing Interventions

Many of the nursing interventions required by the patient with spinal fracture are identical to those outlined for the patient with spinal cord injury in Chapter 29. Of special concern are interventions designed for the following purposes:

1. Maintaining the stability of the fracture fixation
   a. Pay strict attention to *logrolling* the patient for position changes.
   b. Position the patient with pillows between the legs and at the back when side lying to prevent strain on the back.
   c. Observe proper technique when turning the patient on a Stryker frame or Foster bed.
   d. Avoid elevating the head of the bed beyond the prescribed level (usually only 30 degrees and only on the surgeon's order)
   e. When the patient is to be mobilized, apply prescribed corsets or braces *before* getting the patient out of bed
2. Preventing neurocirculatory problems
   a. Perform neurocirculatory checks every hour in the first 24-48 hours after surgery; report decrease in neuromotor function to the sugeon
   b. Perform passive range of motion to involved extremities at least qid
   c. Encourage patient to actively and frequently move noninvolved extremities to the extent possible
3. Promoting comfort—in addition to usual comfort measures
   a. Reposition the patient frequently
   b. Wait a few minutes to ascertain the patient's comfort, because small adjustments may be necessary and may not be immediately recognized
4. Promoting psychological comfort
   a. Recognize that the patient may have feelings of powerlessness, anger, and/or fear about the situation, particularly if there is neuromotor deficit
   b. Encourage the patient to express such feelings
   c. Encourage the patient to take advantage of psychological and or social counselling where it is available

d. If long-term rehabilitation is indicated, prepare the patient for care in a rehabilitation setting

Other nursing interventions are similar to those for any patient who has a fracture (p. 987), including interventions for individuals in casts or traction (p. 995).

EFFECTS OF IMMOBILIZATION

People who are immobilized after a fracture may have complications related to their immobility. An outline of the effects of immobilization on the various body systems, pathophysiology, nursing assessment, and nursing interventions follows.

Cardiovascular System

Pathophysiology

The common problems associated with the cardiovascular system are as follows:

1. Increased incidence of deep vein thrombosis (DVT) and pulmonary embolus (PE)
2. Increased work load on the heart

Failure of the vessels in the legs to assume or maintain vasoconstriction results in the pooling of venous blood, decreased venous return, and diminished cardiac output.

Nursing assessment

Objective data

1. Palpate peripheral pulses.
2. Monitor blood pressure and heart rate and force.
3. Observe for signs and symptoms of DVT (pain in leg) and PE (chest pain, cough).

Nursing interventions

1. Assist patient with active and passive range of motion and isometric exercises of extremities
2. Reposition patient frequently within limitations as directed by surgeon's orders.

Respiratory System

Pathophysiology

Decreased movement, decreased stimulus to cough, and decreased depth of ventilation all contribute to the pooling of secretions in the bronchi and bronchioles.

Nursing assessment

Objective data

1. Observe for inability to cough and raise secretions.
2. Auscultate for sounds of moisture in the chest.

Nursing interventions

1. Reposition frequently within prescribed limitations.
2. Encourage active range of motion exercises of unaffected joints.
3. Prevent hypostatic pneumonia by having patient cough and deep breathe at regular intervals (at least every 2 hours). An incentive spirometer may be used 3 to 4 times daily.

Skin Integrity

Pathophysiology

Loss of skin integrity (abrasions, decubitus ulcers) is caused by friction, pressure, or tissue layers sliding on each other. The process of restricted circulation and tissue ischaemia is intensified by infection, trauma, obesity, sweating, and poor nutritional state.

Nursing assessment

Objective data

1. Observe for *areas of pressure* and *irritation,* as may occur from the plaster cast or traction equipment or from pressure on the sacrum, elbows, and heels.
2. Monitor *body temperature for elevation,* which may indicate infection.

Nursing interventions

1. Prevent decubitus ulceration by keeping skin clean and dry, especially sacrum, elbows, and heels.
2. Turn the patient as permitted to change points of pressure at frequent intervals. Some patients cannot be fully turned, for example, patients in traction. In this instance, other methods must be provided, such as the following:
   a. Flotation pads that distribute pressure equally over large skin areas.
   b. Air pressure mattresses that alternate pressures on the skin.
   c. Sheepskin pads that decrease friction, distribute pressure, and reduce moisture.
   d. Elbow and heel pads.
3. Special beds may be necessary to turn the patient from supine to prone positions. The Stryker or Foster frame permits movement in a horizontal direction to two positions—supine and prone.
4. If decubitus ulcer results, follow hospital policy for special nursing measures.

Gastrointestinal System

Pathophysiology

Constipation is the most frequent complication of immobility. The change in normal dietary habits and fluid intake, lack of activity, and having to use a bedpan are contributing factors.

Nursing assessment

Subjective and objective data

1. Ask the patient about daily bowel habits.
2. Observe appetite and foods the patient selects.
3. Monitor the fluid intake.
4. Ask the patient what is normally taken for constipation.

Nursing interventions

1. Encourage the patient to be as active as possible within the prescribed limitations (turning, moving).
2. Encourage fluid intake of 2500 to 3000 ml/day unless contraindicated.
3. Assist the patient in selecting foods that are high in roughage or fibre.
4. Give stool-softening agents and suppositories as prescribed.

Urinary System

Pathophysiology

Increased urinary calcium from bone destruction, increased urinary pH (alkaline), increased citric acid (which causes the precipitation of calcium salts), stasis of urine in the bladder, and infection can all cause urinary problems.

Nursing assessment

Subjective and objective data

1. Observe quantity of fluid intake. Ask the patient about normal fluid intake.
2. Has the patient a history of urinary problems?
3. Ask the elderly male patient about urinary problems before admission. Some men will describe hesitancy and frequency because of an enlarged prostate gland.

Nursing interventions

1. Encourage fluid intake.
2. Limit calcium intake (milk) to dietary orders.
3. Monitor urinary output and report difficulties to the doctor. (Potential is high for bladder infection and formation of renal stones.)

Musculoskeletal System

Pathophysiology

Atrophy and weakness of the muscles will occur because of disuse. Bone growth (*osteoblastic*) and bone destruction (*osteoclastic*) activity is disrupted by immobility. The osteoclastic activity takes precedence, with the result that bone matrix is destroyed and calcium is released. The end results is *osteoporosis* and renal stones.

Nursing assessment

Objective data

1. Ask patient to demonstrate prescribed exercises.
2. Ask patient to demonstrate movement of unaffected limbs.

Nursing interventions

1. Encourage active and isometric exercises of unaffected limbs.
2. Have patient demonstrate prescribed exercises.
3. Do passive exercises when patient is unable to do active movement.

SUMMARY

1. Bones have several functions. These include the following: (a) *supporting* body tissues *and* providing the *skeletal framework,* (b) *protecting* body organs, (c) *providing* for *movement,* (d) serving as a *storehouse* for mineral salts and, (e) providing for *haematopoesis.*
2. Bursae are lined with synovial membrane and serve as cushions between moving parts.
3. Joints permit the following movements:
   a. Flexion
   b. Extension
   c. Adduction
   d. Abduction
   e. Rotation
   f. Circumduction
   g. Special movements such as supination, pronation, inversion, eversion, and protraction.
4. Both heat and cold are prescribed in treating people with musculoskeletal problems, and precautions must be observed with each.
5. The cause of rheumatoid arthritis is unknown, but immune mechanisms are considered to be a strong aetiological factor.
6. The primary group of drugs used to treat rheumatoid arthritis are the nonsteroidal antiinflammatory drugs (NSAIDs).
7. Replacement arthroplasty can be used to replace a variety of joints. The most commonly replaced joints are the hip and the knee.
8. Restrictions on movement necessary to prevent dislocation of a prosthesis are prescribed by the surgeon and depend on the design of the prosthesis and method of insertion.
9. People with joint replacements will have a prescribed exercise programme, which should be followed after discharge.
10. The course of systemic lupus erythematosus (SLE) is believed to be caused by an aberration of the immune system.
11. Polymyositis (dermatomyositis) is an inflammatory disorder of striated muscles of unknown causation.
12. People with polymyositis have exacerbations and remissions of their disease.
13. Ankylosing spondylitis causes the bones of the spine to grow together, and the patient may have a "hunch-back" deformity or scoliosis.
14. Bursitis refers to inflammation of a bursa. The shoulder joint is the most commonly affected.
15. Degenerative joint disease (DJD) is also known as osteoarthritis, hypertrophic arthritis, osteoarthrosis, or senescent arthritis.
16. Prevention of DJD centres on (a) avoiding obesity, (b) avoiding repeated trauma to joints, and (c) protecting joints in occupations that put joints at risk.
17. Treatment of DJD includes agents to relieve pain, assistive devices such as a walking stick to unload weight from weight-bearing joints, rest, exercise, and surgery including arthroplasty.
18. A herniated disk is an example of a degenerative disease of the spine.
19. Sciatic pain is common in people with a herniated disk.
20. People with a herniated disk can be treated conservatively with rest, heat, analgesics, muscle relaxants, and sometimes traction to relieve muscle spasm.
21. When conservative therapy is not successful in treating a herniated disk, surgery may be necessary to relieve compression on nerve roots.
22. Scoliosis causes a visible curvature of spine when the patient leans forward from the waist.
23. Corrective surgery to realign vertebrae and fusion are used to treat scoliosis when the curve of the spine exceeds 49 degrees.
24. Treatment of gout involves preventive therapy with uricosuric agents, which either enhance uric acid excretion (probenecid) or decrease uric acid formation (allopurinol).

25. Fracture of bones is treated with immobility by splinting, bracing, casting, traction, or surgery.
26. A major complication of fracture is fat embolism, which can be life-threatening and is manifested by chest pain, pallor, dyspnoea, prostration, confusion, and petechial haemorrhage of skin and conjunctivae.
27. Monitoring for neurocirculatory status in a patient with a cast includes palpation for warmth, observation of colour, application of moderate pressure to nail bed, touching the injured part to test sensation, observing patient's ability to move body part distal to fracture, and questioning patient about pain or decreased or increased sensation distal to the cast.
28. Traction is used to reduce a fracture, maintain correct position of bone fragments during healing, immobilize a limb while soft tissue healing takes place, overcome muscle spasm, stretch adhesions, and correct deformities.
29. Maintaining traction requires that ropes run straight and through pulleys, weights hang free, and nothing impinges on any part of the traction apparatus.

STUDY QUESTIONS

- Describe the anatomic structure of bones and the purposes of the skeletal system.
- Discuss the importance of the synovial joint and the composition of the joint.
- Review the range of motion through which a joint such as the shoulder would be exercised.
- Describe the complications that may occur from immobilization of the joint; the complications that may arise from total body immobilization.
- Select a patient who has a form of "arthritis." Write a nursing care plan based on the patient's defined nursing problems.
- Outline the care of the patient immobilized in a spica hip cast.
- What precautions must be taken in the care of a patient in traction?
- What precautions must be taken in the care of a patient with a total hip replacement?

REFERENCES AND SELECTED READINGS

1.* American Nurses' Association and National Association of Orthopaedic Nurses: Orthopaedic nursing practice: process and outcome criteria for selected diagnoses, *Orthop Nurs* 6(2):11-16, 1987.
2. Anderson LP: Carpal tunnel syndrome, *Orthop Nurs* 5(4):40-41, 1986.
3.* Barden RM: Osteonecrosis of the femoral head, *Orthop Nurs* 4(4):45-51, 1985.
4. Blaha JD, Pickett JC (editors): Controversy on total knee arthroplasty, *Clin Orthop Rel Res* 192S:2-112, 1984.
5. Blake SA: Non-cemented femoral prostheses: intraoperative focus, *Orthop Nurs* 4(1):40-41, 1985.
6. Blauvelt C, Nelson F: A manual of orthopedic terminology, ed 4, St Louis, 1990, Mosby–Year Book.
7. Bradley JD et al: Comparison of an antiinflammatory dose of ibuprofen, and analgesic dose of ibuprofen, and acetaminophen in the treatment of patients with osteoarthritis of the knee, *N Engl J Med* 325(2):87-91, 1991.

7a. Braggins S: *The back: functions, malfunctions and care*, London, 1994, Mosby-Year Book Europe, Ltd.
8. Brashear HR, Ranney RB: *Handbook of orthopaedic surgery*, ed 10, St Louis, 1986, Mosby–Year Book.
9. Brooks PM, Day RO: Nonsteroidal antiinflammatory drugs-differences and similarities, *N Engl J Med*, 324(24):1716-1723, 1991.
10. Burgess S et al: Systemic lupus erythematosus and renal insufficiency, *ANNA J* 13(3):168-171, 1986.
11. Callahan J: Compartment syndrome, *Orthop Nurs* 4(4):11-18, 1985.
12.* Cochran S: Action stat! Open fracture, *Nurs 87* 17(5):33, 1987.
13.* Collier IC: Assessing functional status of the elderly, *Arth Care Res* 1(1):45-52, 1988.
14. Crocker C: Acute postoperative pain: cause and control, *Orthop Nurs* 5(2):11-16, 1986.
15. Crenshaw AH: Campbell's operative orthopaedics, ed 8, St Louis, 1992, Mosby–Year Book.
16.* Coheny MO: Porous coated femoral prosthesis: concepts and care considerations, *Orthop Nurs* 4(1):43-45, 1985.
16a. Department of Health: *On the state of the public health: the annual report of the chief medical officer of the department of health for the year 1989*. London, 1990; 25.
17.* Doheny MO, Sedlak CA: Body image considerations, for adult scoliosis patient having spinal fusion surgery, *Orthop Nurs* 6(6):18-22, 1987.
18. Enis JE: Total hip arthoplasty in the geriatric patient, *Hosp Med* (suppl) 23(4):44-48, 1987.
19. Falkenburg SA: Choosing hand splints to aid carpal tunnel syndrome recovery, *Occup Health Saf* 56(5):60-64, 1987.
20. Farrell J: Illustrated guide to orthopedic nursing, ed 3, Philadelphia, 1986, JB Lippincott.
21.* Fractured femur with internal fixation (pictorial), *Orthop Nurs* 6(2):38-41, 1987.
22. Fritzler MJ: Antinuclear antibodies in the investigation of rheumatic diseases, *Bull Rheum Dis* 35(6):1-10, 1985.
23.* Gamron R: Taking the pressure out of compartment syndrome, *Am J Nurs* 88(8):1076-1080, 1988.
24. Gardine A: Not another fractured hip, *Can Nurs* 82S(6):34-36, 1986.
25. Grisso JA, et al: Risk factors for falls as a cause of hip fracture in women, *N Engl J Med* 324S(19):1326-1331, 1991.
26.* Hansell M: Fractures and the healing process, *Orthop Nurs* 7(1):43-50, 1988.
27. Hennig LM et al: Keeping up on arthritis meds, *RN* 49(2):32-38, 1986.
28. Hines NA, Bates MS: Discharging the patient in skeletal traction, *Orthop Nurs* 6(4):21-24, 1987.
29.* Hoyt N: Infections following orthopaedic injury, *Orthop Nurs* 5(5):15-24, 1986.
30. Ignatvicius DO: Meeting the psychosocial needs of patients with rheumatoid arthritis, *Orthop Nurs* 6(3):16-21, 1987.
31. Ivey M, Clark RL: Arthroscopic debridement of the knee for septic arthritis, *Clin Orthop Rel Res* 199:201-206, 1985.
32.* Johnson J: Respiratory complications of orthopaedic injuries, *Orthop Nurs* 5(1):24-28, 1986.
33.* Johnson L: Operative management of unstable pelvic fractures, *Orthop Nurs* 8(4):21-25, 1989.
34. Jones Walton P: Effect of pin care on pin reactions in adults with extremity fracture treated with skeletal traction and external fixation, *Orthop Nurs* 7(4):29-33, 1988.
35.* Joseph N: Arthritis medications from A to Z, *Caring* 8(1):14-16, 1989.
36. Karlin L: Musculoskeletal trauma, *Emerg Care Q* 3(1):57-60, 1987.
37.* Kiem HA, Hensinger RN: Spinal deformities: scoliosis and kyphosis, *Clin Symp* 41(4):3-32, 1989.
38.* Klippel JH: Systemic lupus erythematosus, treated related complications superimposed on chronic disease, *JAMA* 263(13):1812-1815, 1990.
39.* Klippel JH, Strober S, Wofsy D: New therapies for the rheumatic disease, *Bul Rheum Dis* 38(4):1-7, 1989.
40. Koffler D: Immunology of systemic lupus erythematosus and related rheumatic diseases, *Clin Symp* 39(2):2-36, 1987.
41. Koopman WSI: Rheumatology, *JAMA* 265(23):3169-3170, 1991.
42.* Lamb K, Miller J, Hernandez M: Falls in the elderly: causes and prevention, *Orthop Nurs* 6(2):45-49, 1987.
43.* Lambert VA, et al: Coping with rheumatoid arthritis, *Nurs Clin North Am* 22:551-558, 1987.
44. Leach RE, editor: *Progress in sports medicine*, Philadelphia, 1985, JB Lippincott.
45.* Levy RN, et al: Progress in arthritis surgery: with special reference to current status of total joint arthroplasty, *Clin Orthop Related Res* 200:299-321, 1985.

* Recommended for student readings.

46.* Liang MH, Fortin P: Management of osteoarthritis of the hip and knee (an editorial), *N Engl J Med* 325(2):125-127, 1991.

47.* Liang MH: Osteoarthritis: a joint endeavor, *Harvard Health Letter,* 17(6):1-4, 1992.

48.* Liddel DR: An in-depth look at osteoporosis, *Orthop Nurs* 4S(3):23-28, 1985.

49. Lin P (editor): Posterior lumbar interbody fusion, *Clin Orthop Related Res* 193:2-132, 1985.

50. Lorish C, Richards B, Brown S: Missed medication doses in rheumatic arthritis patients: intentional and unintentional reasons, *Arth Care Res* 2(1):3-9, 1989.

51. McCarthy DJ, editor: *Arthritis and allied conditions: a textbook of rheumatology,* ed 11, Philadelphia, 1989, Lea and Febiger.

52. McGuire L: Administering analgesics: which drugs are right for your patient, *Nursing* 9020(4):34-41, April 1990.

53. Maher AB: After the emergency is over: delayed and occult injuries in the trauma patient, *Orthop Nurs* 4(2):25-27, 1985.

54.* Maher AB: Early assessment and management of musculoskeletal injuries, *Nurs Clin North Am* 21:717-727, 1986.

55. Malasanos L, et al: Health assessment, ed 4, St Louis, 1990, Mosby–Year Book.

56. Mankin HJ and Treadwell BV: Osteoarthritis: a 1987 update: *Bull Rheum Dis* 36(5):1-10, 1986.

57.* Marchette L, Marchette B: Back injury: a preventable occupational hazard, *Orthop Nurs* 4(6):25-29, 1985.

58.* Miller B: Osteoarthritis in the primary health care setting, *Orthop Nurs* 6(5):41-46, 1987.

59. Morrey BF, Kavanagh BF: Cementless joint replacement: current status and future, *Bull Rheum Dis* 39(4):1-7, 1987.

60. Morrey BF: Orthopedics, *JAMA* 265(23):3151-3152, 1991.

61.* Mourad L, Droste M: *The nursing process in the care of adults with orthopaedic conditions,* ed 2, New York, 1988, John Wiley & Sons.

62. Mourad L: *Orthopedic disorders, vol IV of Mosby's Clinical Nursing series,* St Louis, 1991, Mosby–Year Book.

63.* Mulvey MA, Sharma PK: Traumatic amputation, *RN* 54(9):26-30, 1991.

63a. National Back Pain Association/Royal College of Nursing: *The guide to the handling of patients,* ed 3, 1992.

64. National Institute of Arthritis and Musculoskeletal and Skin Disease: NIH: osteoporosis: cause, treatment, prevention, *Orthop Nurs* 5(6):29-38, 1986.

65.* Nordby EJ: A comparison of disectomy and chemonucleolysis, *Clin Orthop Related Res* 200:279-283, 1985.

66.* Nussman DS, Poole RC: Rescue and recovery in traumatic hip dislocation, *Am J Nurs* 9(11):34-38, 1991.

67. Omer G: Assessment of hand trauma, *Orthop Nurs* 4(2):29-33, 1985.

68. Osborne LJ, DiGiacomo I: Traction: a review with nursing diagnoses and interventions, *Orthop Nurs* 6(4):13-18, 1987.

69. Peters P: Successful return to work following a musculoskeletal injury, *AAOHN J* 38(6):264-270, 1990.

70. Pfeiffer CA, Wetstone SL: Health locus on control and well-being in systemic lupus erythematosus, *Arth Care Res* 1(3):131-138, 1988.

71.* Pigg J, Driscoll P, Caniff R: *Rheumatology nursing: a problem-oriented approach,* New York, 1985, John Wiley & Sons.

71a. Robens Institute Ergonomics Research Institute: *Back pain in nurses: summary and recommendations,* 1986, Robens Institute, University of Surrey.

72. Robinson JE, Marx LO: A nail-safe method, *Am J Nurs* 85(2):158-161, 1985.

73. Rodts MF: Surgical intervention for adult scoliosis, *Orthop Nurs* 6(6):11-17, 1987.

74. Schoen DC: Assessing a fractured hip, *Nurs 87* 17(3):97-98, 1987.

75. Schumacher HR: *Primer on the rheumatic diseases,* ed 9, Atlanta, 1988, Arthritis Foundation.

75a. Secretaries of State: *Caring for People, community care in the next decade and beyond.* CMND 849 HMSO 1989.

76. Sheidler V: Patient-controlled analgesia, *Curr Concepts Nurs* 1(1):13-16, 1987.

77.* Shellenbarger T: When you're asked about carpal tunnel syndrome, *RN* 54(7):40-42, 1991.

78.* Sproles KJ: Nursing care of skeletal pins: a closer look, *Orthop Nurs* 4(1):11-20, 1985.

79. Swezey RL, editor: *Straight talk on ankylosing spondylitis,* Sherman Oaks, Calif, 1985, Ankylosing Spondilitis Association.

80. Unkle D, DeLong W: Adominal trauma associated with pelvic fractures, *Orthop Nurs* 8(4):27-29, 1989.

81. United States Dept of Health and Human Services, Public Health Service, Healthy People 2000: *Health promotion and disease prevention objectives,* Washington, DC, 1990, Government Printing Office.

82.* Walsh CR, Wirth CR: Total knee arthroplasty: biomechanical and nursing considerations, *Orthop Nurs* 4(1):29-34, 1985.

83. Wick JL: The role of ergonomics in the elimination and prevention of work-related musculoskeletal problems, *Orthop Nurs* 8(1):41-42, 1989.

83a. Wise CM: *Hypeuricemia and gout.* In Rakel RE, editor: *Conn's current therapy 1991,* Philadelphia, 1991, WB Saunders.

84.* Willey T: High-tech beds and mattress overlays: a decision guide, *Am J Nurs* 89(9):1142-1145, 1989.

85.* Zubay RL: Understanding magnetic resonance imaging from a nursing perspective, *Orthop Nurs* 7(6):17-23, 1988.

86.* Cave L: Lowering the uncertainties of arthritis with nurse-led support group, *Orthop Nurs* 3(5):39-42, 1984.

87. Moskowitz RW, et al: *Osteoarthritis: diagnosis and management,* Philadelphia, 1984, WB Saunders.

88.* Olson EV (editor): The hazards of immobility, *Am J Nurs* 67:780-797, 1967.

89.* Wagner MM: Assessment of patients with multiple injuries, *Am J Nurs* 72S(10):1822-1827, 1972.

90. Department of Health: *On the State of the Public Health for the year 1990,* London, 1991, HMSO.

FURTHER READING

Booth J, Weatherley C: Anklyosing spondylitis, *Nursing Times* 82(4):28-31, 1986 Jan 22-28.

Cooper J: Food intolerance and joint symptoms, historical review and present-day application, *J Physiotherapy* 77(12):847-58, 1991.

Halverson PB, Holmes SB: Systemic lupus erythematosus: medical and nursing treatments, *Orthopaedic Nursing 1* 1(6):17-25, 1992.

Hill J: Assessing rheumatic disease, *Nursing Times* 87(4):33-5, 1991.

Hill J: Patient evaluation of a rheumatology nursing clinic, *Nursing Times* 82(27):42-3, 1986.

Loue C: Do you roll or lift?.. potential for back injury, *Nursing Times* 82(29):44-6, 1986.

Maycock J: Towards pain relief.. rheumatic disease, *Nursing Mirror.* 160(3):40-1, 1985.

O'Connor S, Wright M: An ongoing partnership in care: nursing innovations in a rehabilitation ward. *Professional Nurse* 7(6):366, 368-70.

Problems of Defence and Protection

Unit Eleven

33

The Patient with Immunological Problems

Barbara C. Long
E. Ronald Wright

After studying this chapter, the learner should be able to:

- Differentiate between B cells and T cells and their roles in the humoral and cell-mediated responces to antigens.
- Identify the immune response in immunodeficiencies, gammopathies, hypersensitivities, and autoimmunities and give examples.
- Describe methods of immunosuppression and the care of the immunodeficient person.
- Compare and contrast the four types of hypersensitivities.
- Describe the pathophysiological bases of type I hypersensitivities and related interventions.
- Describe blood transfusion and tissue transplant reactions.
- Compare autoimmune diseases based on their immunoresponse.
- Describe the transmission, prevention and control of sexually transmitted diseases.

Immunological alterations occur in a wide variety of diseases. In some disorders the immunological basis is clearcut, such as in allergic disorders and immunodeficiency diseases. In other disorders, the role of the immunological response as the causative agent is less well documented. Because immunological factors are operative in such a wide variety of disorders, much of the information about the disorders is found elsewhere in the text. This chapter describes the various categories of immune disorders and discusses in more detail those disorders not described elsewhere. HIV infection and AIDS is discussed in Chapter 13.

REVIEW OF THE IMMUNE SYSTEM

The immune system serves to protect the body from invading foreign cells and body-damaging substances. The immune system distributes through the body a variety of cells and substances that recognize and take action against invading agents. The protective body mechanisms can be divided into nonspecific and specific immune response systems.

Nonspecific Immune Response

Certain cells and proteins in the blood and tissues respond to foreign substances or to damaged self-cells in the same way, regardless of the type of invasion or cell destruction. The degree of response, however, varies in relation to the extent of damage. The outcome of the response is the *inflammatory response*.

The key cells of the nonspecific immune response are the *phagocytic* cells, including the *granulocytic white blood cells* (WBC), especially the *neutrophils*, and the monocytes. In response to tissue injury or invasion of microorganisms, WBCs are attracted to the site in response to chemical stimulation (chemotaxis). The WBCs migrate from the blood vessel into the affected tissue, where they engulf and destroy foreign materials.

Another major factor in the nonspecific response is the *complement* system. This system is composed of inactive serum proteins that, when activated in a sequential series of steps, have the ability to damage cell membranes and destroy the cell. The system can be activated by the binding of specific antibodies to foreign cell antigens, by certain bacterial cell components, or by materials released from the damaged tissues cells.

Other factors that appear in the body in response to the inflammatory response include the *acute-phase proteins*. These proteins are synthesized by the liver and multiply in the serum to provide materials that mediate the inflammatory response.

Specific Immune Response

The internal specific immune response is designed to recognize and take action against *specific* foreign molecules called *antigens (immunogens)*. The introduced antigen stimulates the production of specifically reactive molecules called *antibodies (immunoglobulins)*, or cells (*cytotoxic lymphocytes*). The immunoglobulins or cytotoxic lymphocytes bind to the antigens to inactivate or destroy the foreign agent. The system also remembers prior contact with the antigenic material and responds faster and more efficiently to subsequent contact.

Organs and tissues involved

The organs and tissues of the specific immune response system include the central organs (bone marrow and thymus) and the peripheral organs (lymph nodes, spleen, and lymphatic vessels). Within the central organs the immune response cells are synthesized and matured, whereas within the peripheral organs the mature cells are concentrated.

The *thymus serves as the control organ of the immune system*. It is the *site of differentiation of the T-cell lymphocytic* populations and through certain soluble thymic hormones *serves to regulate the overall immune system*. The activity of the thymus reaches its peak in childhood, and the organ begins to shrink in size after puberty. If the thymus is removed (thymectomy) very early in the life of an animal, a severe state of immunodeficiency is induced and T-cell mediated immunity never develops. After thymectomy, a wasting disease develops, characterized by stunted growth, diarrhoea, and death from massive infection by intestinal or respiratory tract normal flora. The B-cell function is also reduced, pointing to the cooperative effect between the two basic systems. In the adult animal the loss of the thymus creates less severe reactions, probably because of an already functional, long-lived population of T cells.

Table 33-1 Comparison of T cells and B cells

	T cells	B cells
Immune response	Cell mediated	Humorally mediated
Source	Bone marrow	Bone marrow
Site of maturation	Thymus	Bone marrow, intestinal lymphoid tissue
Storage	Medulla of regional lymph node or spleen	Cortex of regional lymph node or spleen
Functions	Destroy antigenically labelled cells	Synthesize and release immunoglobulins (antibodies)
	Release lymphokines that activate phagocytes	Form memory (B_M) cells
	Regulate T-cell function	
	Regular production of antibodies by B cells (helper T cells)	
	Prevent or modify B-cell and T-cell activity (suppressor T cells)	
	Form memory (T_M) cells	

The *lymph nodes* and *the spleen serve as the primary sites of localization of the immune response cells*. The lymph node serves to filter the lymph drained from a region of tissue. The structure of the lymph node consists of an inner medullary and paracortical region primarily populated with T cells and an outer cortex composed of clusters or germinal centres of B cells known as follicles. The spleen is structured on somewhat the same pattern, with diffusely packed T-cell areas and germinal centres of tightly packed B cells. In certain types of antigenic stimulation, either the T-cell areas or the B-cell areas will show tissue proliferation, whereas the other area remains quiescent. By the same principle, if there is a basic primary immunodeficiency of one system, the corresponding area of lymph nodes and spleen may not be populated by the normal cells (hypoplastic).

During the course of the immune response reaction, within the lymph nodes there is significant proliferation of specific cells or migration of phagocytic cells to the site, which may lead to lymph node enlargement. Enlargement of the lymph nodes in a region may be the result of infection, immune disease, intrinsic neoplasm of the lymph node, or metastatic spread of malignant cells to the node. The presence of an enlarged spleen or enlarged lymph nodes is virtually always an important clinical finding.

There are two types of specific immune responses, the *cell-mediated system*, which provides the cytotoxic lymphocytes, and the *humorally mediated system*, which provides the circulating immunoglobulins.

Cell-mediated immune response

The key cells of the cell-mediated immune response are the *T-cell lymphocytes* that are produced in the bone marrow and mature in the thymus gland. From the thymus the T cells migrate to the medulla of regional lymph nodes and spleen. Each mature immunosensitive T-cell lymphocyte is capable of responding to a specific antigenic signal. When exposed to its specific antigen, the T cell begins to divide, increasing the number of that antigenically responsive cell in the lymph node. Some of the T cells are carried by the lymph into the bloodstream to the specific antigens. The T cells then attack and destroy the antigenic molecules (cytotoxic effect). The T cells also release a number of soluble substances (lymphokines) that activate nonspecifically reactive phagocytes to attack the tissues at the site.

Other T-cell lymphocytes regulate the T-cell function and production of antibodies by the B-cell system. T-cell lymphocytes known as *helper T cells* (T_H or T_4 cells) are necessary to provide a full immunological humoral (B cell) or cell-mediated (T cell) response. Another type of T cell, known as *suppressor T cells* (T_S or T_8 cells), operates to prevent or modify the function of the two systems. Additional T cells, *memory T cells* (T_M), remember contact with the antigen and on subsequent exposure respond immediately to its presence in the body.

Humorally mediated immune response

The key cells of the humorally mediated immune response are the *B-cell lymphocytes*. These are produced in the bone marrow, but mature outside the thymus, such as in bone marrow or gut-associated lymphoid tissues. From there the B cells migrate to the cortex of regional lymph nodes and spleen.

As with T cells, the immunosensitive B cells are programmed to respond to a single antigen. When the antigen is present, the B cell begins to proliferate and differentiate into a *plasma cell*. A plasma cell is designed to synthesize and release large amounts of *immunoglobulin* (antibody) that will combine with the antigen that caused its production. These antibody molecules are released into the circulation where they become part of the gamma globulin fraction of the serum. The B cells producing the immunoglobulin remain in the lymphoid tissue and continue to synthesize additional molecules of the specific antibody. Note that this is different from the T-cell response where cytotoxic T cells are released; in this case the B cells remain, and their product is released. Thus the level of active specific antibody begins to rise in the serum fraction (*antibody titre*), as well as in the level of the gamma globulin fraction in general. These antibodies are carried by the blood and other body fluids to where they encounter their specific antigen and bind to it. Upon binding, the antibody may inactivate the antigen, precipitate it, or activate other antigen-damaging processes (such as the complement cascade) to remove the antigen.

The immunoglobulins are subdivided into different classes on the basis of molecular structure and function. The generic symbol for immunoglobulins is Ig, and each of the classes is designated by a letter of the alphabet: IgG, IgM, IgA, IgE, and IgD. The predominant immunoglobulin is IgG.

The B-cell system is similar to the T-cell system in that it is controlled by helper and suppressor T cells, forms memory (B_M) cells, and is rendered self-tolerant by the same mechanisms.

Combined immune response

Most antigens do not cause a purely humoral or purely cell-mediated response; rather, both types of response are evoked. Likewise, our protection against most harmful antigens is the result of both of these specific response systems being brought to bear on the antigen involved. In the *combined type of response, an initial perturbation occurs within the T-cell areas of the lymph node*. This becomes obvious within about 2 days after the introduction of the antigen. About 3 to 5 days later, the B-cell areas begin to proliferate.

To mount a maximal immune response, the cooperative action of the three central cell types is necessary. The macrophage serves to capture, process, and present the antigen to immunocompetent cells of both T- and B-cell ancestry. The T cells aid in the direct cell-mediated response, but a population of T cells also serves to interact with the B cell and a T-cell population controls the development of an effective immune response. A *helper T-cell* population cooperates with the B cells and T cells to enhance the activation and proliferation of the immunoglobulin synthesizing cells. The existence of the helper T cell explains the observation noted earlier in this chapter that the removal of the thymus from the neonate not only compromises the cell-mediated immune response but also significantly reduces the host's ability to mount a humoral immune response. T helper cells also mediate the normal expression of the cell-mediated immune response; therefore, the reduction or loss of this population of cells as occurs in acquired immunodeficiency syndrome (AIDS) would lead to progressive loss of immune response protection.

Another group of T cells also exerts an effect on the synthesis of circulating antibodies. *Cells known as suppressor T cells may provide a negative control function over B-cell clones and other T-cell clones, preventing the expression of an immunological response.*

Secondary immune response

As emphasized at the outset of this section, one of the touchstone characteristics of the specific response system is the ability of the system to remember prior contact with an antigen and to provide a more rapid and efficient protective reaction on subsequent contact. The *first contact between the immune response system and an antigen leads to the primary response, the events of which have been laid out in the preceding paragraphs.* When antibody synthesis is measured in a primary response, there is a significant time lag to the appearance of antibodies in the circulation. Immunoglobulins of the IgM class are the first to appear, but they maintain protective levels for only a short period. Specific IgG antibodies follow and reach protective levels within 12 to 14 days, but they too fall off fairly quickly with only this initial exposure.

When the "primed" immune response system encounters the antigen again, a *secondary response* ensues, which is more rapid, of greater intensity, and longer lasting than the primary response. This secondary response is also termed an *anamnestic response.* This "remembered" response is a characteristic of both the B- and T-cell systems. The prior contact with the antigen is stored in special memory cells of both cell lines. The memory cells respond immediately to the antigenic signal, so that the time lag between exposure to the antigen and production of protective antibody levels is greatly reduced. This phenomenon provides the basis for active immunization and "booster" doses to maintain the protective levels of immunity. In an immunized individual the memory cells elicit the rapid response in time for the immune system to overwhelm the pathogen or toxin before it can produce its damage. These memory cells are very long-living lymphocytes that are able to respond for years following their development.

Interferons

Interferons are a group of proteins produced by a wide variety of human cells, usually in response to the viral infection of the cell. When a cell is infected by a virus, the infected cell begins to make interferon almost immediately. The interferon is released into its surrounding environment where it induces uninfected cells to produce alterations that protect those cells from viral multiplication. This antiviral action is exerted before the synthesis of immunoglobulins specific for the virus reaches protective levels. The elaboration of interferons from virally infected cells continues for a few hours (up to about 24 hours) following infection, thereby playing a significant role in isolating the infective foci in many (but not all) viral infections.

Although viruses seem to be the most potent agents for the induction of interferon, production is not restricted to virus infection of cells. Other intracellular parasites such as rickettsia, bacteria, and parasites may also trigger the formation of interferon. Even bacterial and fungal extracts, as well as a variety of other materials such as double-stranded RNA, synthetic polymers, and plant extracts, may serve as signals.

Three distinct types of interferons are produced by different cell types in the human body, and each type seems to exert different protective effects. *Alpha interferon* is produced by lymphocytes and seems to have antiviral activity. *Beta interferon* is formed by fibroblasts, epithelial cells, and macrophages; it is definitely antiviral. *Gamma interferon* is produced by T-cell lymphocytes of the specific immune response system and has an immunoregulatory effect. In addition to their antiviral activities, the interferons are capable of inhibiting cell growth; therefore, they are being used widely in clinical trials as an *antitumour agent.*

Physiological Changes With Ageing

The extent of immunological changes with ageing varies among individuals depending on multiple factors, such as genetics, nutritional status, and presence of disorders that deplete the immune system. In general, however, the immune response is decreased with ageing.

The thymus gland atrophies with age. Remember that T cells mature in the thymus; therefore, the major change is a *reduction in T-cell function,* including both cytological and immunoregulatory activities. However, there is no marked change in the total number of T cells or of any T-cell subset. Although the antibody response is also variably reduced by age, this is believed to be the result of T-cell rather than B-cell changes. The resulting deficiency that develops gradually with age is one of cellular immune incompetence and is of clinical importance.[21] The contribution of age-related immunodeficiency, however, is difficult to separate from immunodeficiencies that result from underlying diseases.

The decreased immune response with age can be noted by a decreased response to skin tests by the elderly. Older people also have fewer signs and symptoms of inflammations, such as lower temperature elevations, than can be expected.

Infections occur more frequently in the elderly, even in the person with no underlying disease. Infections also tend to be more severe.[21] Common infections include influenza and pneumococcal pneumonia. Morbidity and mortality are higher than in younger people. It is because of the severity of disease commonly experienced that yearly influenza immunizations for the elderly are strongly recommended.

There is an increased *potential for cancer* associated with age. One theory for the increase is decreased immune surveillance. Another theory is that older people, by virtue of living longer, have been exposed to more carcinogens. Although tumours occur more frequently in older people, the tumours tend to grow more slowly and metastasize less frequently.[21]

MAJOR HEALTH PROBLEMS OF THE IMMUNE SYSTEM

Immunological disorders occur when the immune response malfunctions. The disorders may be a result of immune deficiencies, abnormal production of immunoglobulins, excessive response to specific antigens, or immune response to self-antigens (Table 33-2). Each of these major categories will be discussed in this chapter. The majority of immunological problems (other than the great variety of autoimmune diseases discussed throughout the text) are hypersensitivity disorders, so these disorders will be discussed in more detail.

IMMUNODEFICIENCIES

The following discussion of immunodeficiencies pertains to general immunodeficiencies. AIDS, an acquired immunodeficiency disease, is discussed in Chapter 13.

Aetiology and Pathophysiology

Protection of the host depends on an intact immune system. Interference with development of cells and tissues of the immune response leads to immunodeficient disorders. Because the cells and tissues of the immune response system develop sequentially, if a defect in that development appears, the severity of the resulting deficiency reflects the stage of development at which the abnormality arose (Fig. 33-1). Deficiencies may exist in immunoglobulin synthesis (B-cell deficiency), cellular immune functions (T-cell deficiency), or phagocyte defects.

Immunodeficiencies may be primary or secondary. Primary immunodeficiencies, those resulting from improper fetal development, are genetic disorders in children. Some primary immunoglobulin deficiencies may not become evident until the person is an adult, and these are termed *common variable immunodeficiencies* (CVI). People with CVI develop recurrent virulent infections and display a high incidence of malignancies, haematological disorders, and autoimmune diseases.

Secondary immunodeficiencies are a nonspecific depression of the immune response as a result of some interference with the immune system. These deficiencies are present to one degree or another in most of the major disease conditions experienced by people in addition to the normal response to ageing. Thus when caring for a person over the age of 60 years or with any acute disease condition, the concepts of immunodeficiency must be considered. Situations in which immunodeficiency plays a major role are listed in Box 33-1.

Major stress of any type may affect immune response as a result of increased corticosteroid production and alterations in protein metabolism. A form of immunodeficiency, immunosuppression, may result from or be deliberately created by the use of radiation, drugs, or antigens and antibodies (Table 33-3).

33-1

Disorders characterized by immunodeficiencies

Protein-energy malnutrition
Alcohol misuse
Infections (especially viral)
Cancer
Autoimmune diseases
Lymphomas (including Hodgkin's disease)
Allergies
Trauma
Transplantation (immunosuppression)

Nursing Process
Assessment

Subjective data

Subjective data to obtain from the person with immunodeficiency include the following:
1. Knowledge of the immunodeficiency
2. Knowledge of prevention of infection
3. Occurrence of recurrent infections (type)
4. Concerns related to the immunodeficiency

Recurrent viral or fungal infections are suggestive of T-cell-mediated deficiencies, whereas recurrent bacterial infections may have an underlying B-cell (immunoglobulin) deficiency.

Objective data

Objective data include monitoring for early signs of infection (fever, pain, nasal discharge, cough, and enlarged nodes). Breath sounds are monitored daily, by the doctor, for decreased sounds indicating pulmonary infection. The skin is inspected daily for lesions.

Diagnostic tests

T-cell (cellular) deficiency tests

T-cell function can be screened by delayed hypersensitivity skin testing to common antigens. Specific antigens, including purified protein derivative (PPD), *Candida* organisms, mumps antigen, streptokinase, and streptodornase, are injected intradermally. Reactions are read after 24 to 48 hours to determine hypersensitivity. The test is to determine the hypersensitivity, not the presence of disease. A person who does not react to any of these antigens is said to be *anergic*.

Sensitization with dinitrochlorobenzene (DNCB) has been used as an additional test for suspected anergic patients. DNCB is a chemical to which natural sensitivity does not occur. Following application of DNCB to the skin, contact sensitivity can be elicited after 1 to 2 weeks if T-cell function is present.

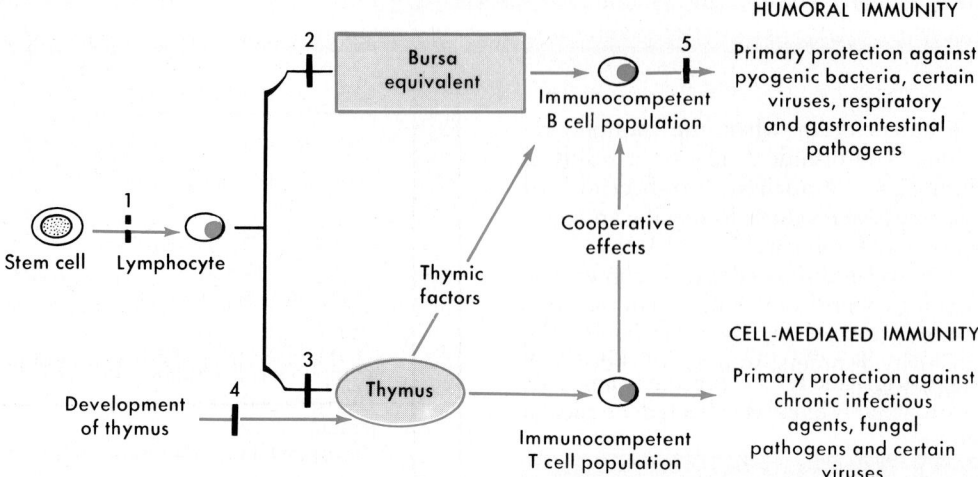

Fig. 33-1   Causes of immunodeficiencies. Abnormalities at *1* result in combined humoral and cell-mediated immunodeficiency. Blockage at *2* produces agammaglobulinaemia. Blockage at *3* or *4* results in drastic reduction of T cell-mediated function, and because of cooperative effects on B cell system some reduction in humoral response occurs. Abnormalities in synthesis of specific immunoglobulin classes are reflected by blockage at *5*. Some blockages result in complete deficiency, whereas others show up as reduction in response.

Table 33-2   Classification of immunological disorders

Category	Immune response	Examples
Immunodeficiencies	Deficiencies in the proper expression of immune response system, part of the system, or specific cells	Primary deficiencies, deficiencies associated with other diseases, acquired immunodeficiency syndrome (AIDS)
Gammopathies	Abnormal production of immunoglobulins	Multiple myeloma, hypergammaglobinaemia
Hypersensitivities	Exaggerated or inappropriate response to specific antigen	Anaphylaxis, allergies, transfusion reactions,graft rejections
Autoimmunities	Immunological attack on self-antigens	Rheumatoid arthritis, systemic lupus erythematosus (SLE), glomerulonephritis

Table 33-3   Induced immunosuppression

Method	Comments	Use
Antigen administration	Specific antigen administered in small amounts over time	Allergy desensitization
Antibody administration	Specific antibody administered to combine with antigen and block contact with immunocompetent cell	Obstetrics: prevent sensitive Rh-negative mother from responding to Rh-positive fetus during pregnancy
Monoclonal antibodies (MoAbs)	Clones of a single immunoglobulin-producing cell; react with receptors on T-cell surface preventing lysis of cells	Organ transplantation
Irradiation	Destroys lymphocytes, thus fewer cells available for immune response; total body irradiation affects haematopoietic system, gastrointestinal (GI) system, and central nervous system (CNS)	Local irradiation: renal allografts Total body irradiation: organ transplantation
Drugs	Corticosteroids impair T cell function and cause catabolism of immunoglobulins and lymphocytopenia	Diseases where immune disorder is unknown (for example, autoimmunities); tissue and organ transplantation
	Cytotoxic drugs destroy rapidly dividing immunologically stimulated cells	
	Cyclosporin acts against T helper cells and facilitates development of T suppressor cells	Organ transplantation

B-cell (humoral) deficiency tests

Plasma protein electrophoresis. The movement of colloid (protein) particles in an electrical field is called *electrophoresis*. In an applied electrical field, different proteins migrate at different rates because of their different sizes and shapes, and this property can be used to analyze plasma protein content. The plasma proteins consist of albumin and globulins, which can be further divided into alpha globulins, beta globulins, and *gamma globulins* (immunoglobulins). The serum proteins are subjected to electrophoresis in a medium that stabilizes the migration so that the proteins can be stained and examined.

Quantitative immunoglobulin test. Three of the immunoglobulins—IgG, IgA, and IgM—can be measured quantitatively, whereas IgD and IgE are present in amounts too small to measure. Venous blood is collected; no special preparation is required.

Nursing Analysis

Problems are determined from analysis of patient data. Possible problems for the person with an immunodeficiency may include, but are not limited to, the following:

Problem	Possible aetiologies
Infection, high risk for	Decreased immune response, lack of information
Knowledge deficit	Lack of exposure/recall, information misinterpretation

Planning: expected patient outcomes

Expected patient outcomes for the person with an immunodeficiency may include, but are not limited to, the following:
1. Signs of infection do not occur.
2. Describes measures to avoid infection.
3. Describes signs dictating immediate medical attention.
4. Explains the need for continued medical follow-up.

Implementation

Assisting with achievement of therapeutic goals

Replacement therapy

Specific replacement therapy may be given for primary immunodeficiencies. When B-cell deficiency is present, gamma globulin may be given at monthly intervals. Gamma globulin is a purified concentrated solution of antibodies, mostly IgG, found in normal plasma. Gamma globulin can be given intramuscularly but problems with this approach include pain at injection site, toleration of only small volumes per injection, and degradation of antibody at the injection site. *Intravenous* immunoglobulin (IVIG) is now more commonly used. Larger doses can be given with fewer side effects and less discomfort. About 3% to 12% of patients experience fever, chills, headache, myalgias, and nausea during infusion.[27] These effects can be prevented by preadministration of paracetamol, antihistamines, or hydrocortisone. The infusion is started slowly, then increased in rate if no adverse reactions occur. Vital signs are monitored, especially for a reduction in blood pressure. If changes in vital signs or other adverse reactions occur, stop the infusion, change to normal saline infusion (0.9%), and notify doctor.[41] Be prepared for anaphylaxis.

33-2

Patient Teaching

The patient with immunodeficiency

Explain immunodeficiency, that is, the inability of the body to fight infection.
Take measures to prevent infection
    Avoid people with infections (especially colds)
    Avoid bumping or breaking the skin.
    Inspect skin daily for lesions.
    Eat a balanced diet.
    Drink at least 6 glasses of fluid per day.
    Avoid becoming fatigued.
    Get a regular amount of sleep each night.
Report signs of infection to doctor immediately.
See doctor on a regular basis as instructed.

Replacement therapy for T-cell-mediated immune deficiencies is more complex. Transfer factor (extracted from lymphocytes of humans who have demonstrated delayed hypersensitivity reactions), thymosin (a thymic hormone), bone marrow transplants, and fetal thymic transplants have been used.

Interventions to achieve patient outcomes

Preventing infection

The most important factor in the care of the immunodeficient or immunosuppressed person is protection from infection. Care differs depending on whether the degree of immunosuppression is minimal, moderate, or severe:
1. Care for minimal immunosuppression
    a. Use good medical asepsis.
    b. Avoid people with infections.
    c. Remove sources where bacteria may proliferate.
    d. Avoid injections as much as possible.
    e. Maintain nutrition at optimal level (immune response is decreased by malnutrition).
    f. Maintain adequate fluid hydration (intake of more than 1500 ml/day) (hydration helps dilute effects of infection).
2. Care for moderate immunosuppression
    a. If severe leukopenia is present, place person in a single room to decrease infection potential.
    b. If person is acutely ill, give mouth care, perineal care, and pulmonary hygiene to prevent infection.
    c. Use same protective measures as for minimal immunosuppression.
3. Care for severe immunosuppression
    a. Use protective isolation by laminar air flow units (Chapter 9).
    b. Use same protective measures as for moderate immunosuppression.

Facilitating learning

People who are immunosuppressed, as well as their families, need to know the nature of immunosuppression and how to avoid infection (see Box 31-2).

Evaluation

Questions to consider may include the following:
1. Has infection been prevented during hospitalization?
2. Does the person know
   a. The nature of immunodeficiency?
   b. How to prevent and identify infection?
   c. The need for continued medical follow-up?

GAMMOPATHIES

Pathophysiology

Gammopathies, better termed *hypergammaglobulinaemias*, are elevated levels of gamma globulin in the serum. The normal synthesis of an immunoglobulin is the result of the proliferation of plasma cell differentiation of a single clone of B cells in response to an antigenic signal. In gammopathies a single clone or multiple clones of plasma cells begin to overproduce immunoglobulin product in response to inappropriate antigenic stimulation.

Monoclonal (M-type) *gammopathies* involve a single B-cell clone and are commonly referred to as *plasma cell dyscrasias*. A common monoclonal gammopathy is multiple myeloma.

Polyclonal gammopathies involve the overproduction of virtually all classes of immunoglobulins. The major causes are infectious diseases (especially chronic bacterial infections such as lung abscess and osteomyelitis), connective tissue diseases (such as SLE and rheumatoid arthritis), and chronic active liver disease. IgG and IgM are the most commonly involved immunoglobulins, and the degree of immunoglobulin level reflects the severity of the disease. The development of high levels of dysfunctional gamma globulins depresses the synthesis of normal immunoglobulins, which renders the person susceptible to infection.

MULTIPLE MYELOMA

Aetiology and Pathophysiology

Multiple myeloma is a monoclonal plasma cell malignancy seen in both men and women, occurring in middle and old age. It is characterized by widespread bone destruction, anaemia, hypercalcaemia, and hyperuricaemia. These symptoms are traced to the proliferation of plasma cell tumours from the bone marrow into the hard bone tissue, causing an erosion of the bone. Frequent recurrent infections (especially of the respiratory tract) and spontaneous pathological fractures occur because of the production of ineffective immunoglobulins, which, in turn, depress the production of normal antibodies. Renal failure may result from precipitation of urate and calcium crystals. (For additional information, see Chapter 25).

Medical Intervention

Combination chemotherapy is the major treatment. Alkylating agents, specifically melphalan and cyclophosphamide, are the drugs most commonly used.

The Elderly with Immunological Problems

Assessment
Assess nutritional status of all elderly people, especially those living alone. Good nutrition is an important factor in maintenance of the immune system.

Assess carefully elderly patients in nursing homes or those entering hospital from a nursing home for signs of infection. Risk of infection in these persons is high because of high rates of immobility from neurological or cardiovascular disorders, from high use of invasive catheters, or from malnutrition.[42]

Assess mobility status of elderly patients; immobility may lead to skin breakdown and infection.

Assess patient for changes in mental status, anorexia, claims of "feeling poorly", or comments by family members that the elderly person looks ill. These may be early signs of infection in the elderly, as compared to signs of fever and pain in the younger adult.

Intervention
Consider every elderly patient as partly immuno-deficient and take all precautions to prevent infections, especially respiratory infections.

Monitor elderly patients' responses to antibiotic therapy; the incidence of drug reactions is greater because of the older person's greater sensitivity.[42]

Monitor fluid and dietary intake to maintain fluid balance and good nutritional status; this is necessary for maintenance of the immune system.

Common disorders in older adults
Infections, especially bacteraemic pneumonia, UTI, and herpes zoster
Malignancies
Autoimmune disorders

Several weeks may elapse between the initiation of therapy and signs of improvement. Periods of remission of 6 years or more have been obtained with chemotherapy. Radiation therapy may be given for palliative treatment of localized bone pain and pathological fractures.

Supportive Nursing Care

Ambulation and adequate hydration are vitally important to prevent renal complications from the increased amounts of urates and calcium being excreted in the urine. Fluid intake should be sufficient to ensure a urinary output of a minimum of 1500 ml/24 hr. Ambulation may be difficult because of the skeletal pain and the possibility of fractures. A lightweight spinal brace and analgesics may facilitate ambulation. Be alert for neurological deficits in the lower extremities as a result of spinal cord compression.

Measures to prevent infection are instituted; they include avoidance of people with upper respiratory tract infections. Medical attention should be sought for any signs of infection, and antibiotics are often given, because infections are usually caused by Gram-positive organisms. Rest periods are planned if fatigue from anaemia is present.

Table 33-4   Summary of hypersensitivity reactions

| | Hypersensitivity type | | | |
| | Immediate (humoral) | | | Delayed (cellular) |
Property	I Anaphylactic	II Cytotoxic	III Immune complex	IV Cell mediated
Immune system mediators	IgE (IgG) bound to mast cells	IgG or IgM (+ complement)	IgG or IgM + complement	T cells, macrophages
Allergens	Exogenous antigens	Foreign cells or alteration of cell surface antigens	Soluble antigens	Infectious agent, contact allergens, foreign tissues, cancer cells
Response to intradermal skin test	Wheal and flare within 30 min, oedema	Not done	Erythema and oedema within 3 to 8 hr	Erythema and induration within 24 to 48 hr
Pathophysiological effects	Release of histamines, kinins, SRS-A from mast cells, which affect smooth muscle shock organs	Direct cytotoxic destruction of cells	Acute inflammatory reaction; primarily polymorphonuclear neutrophil leukocytes	Tissue destruction, primarily lymphocytes and macrophages
Examples	Systemic anaphylaxis, atopic allergies, hay fever, insect sting reactions	Haemolytic disease of the newborn (Rh), transfusion reactions	Serum sickness, Arthus reaction, glomerulonephritis	Tuberculin reaction, skin graft rejection, poison ivy

---

33-3

Factors influencing hypersensitivity responses

Increased responsiveness of the host
Increased amount of allergen
Nature of allergen
Entrance of allergen through appropriate site
Short time period between contacts

HYPERSENSITIVITY REACTIONS

Pathophysiology

The immune response system that has been previously sensitized is designed to provide an immediate, effective, protective reaction to subsequent encounters with the sensitizing antigen. This of course is a positive factor in the provision of immunity; however, under a given set of conditions or because of an idiotypic reactivity to a particular antigen, the response of the immune system may produce detrimental effects. This *inappropriate response* is usually manifested as a tissue-damaging overreaction to the antigen; thus it is termed *hypersensitivity* or *allergy*. The antigenic stimulants invoking the reactions are referred to as *allergens*. Hypersensitivities, then, are classic expressions of the immune system, but they take place in inappropriate sites, in excessive amounts, or with inappropriate involvement of nonspecific tissues. Whether an allergic response occurs and to what degree depends on a combination of interrelated factors (see Box 31-3).

Hypersensitivities can be broadly divided into two categories based on the components of the immune system involved in mediating the hypersensitivity reaction: humoral or immediate response (B-cell mediated) and cellular or delayed response (T-cell mediated). The humoral response can be further subdivided into type I anaphylactic, type II cytotoxic, and type III immune complex (Table 33-4). Because type I, II, and III hypersensitivities are the result of interactions involving circulating antibodies, these reactions can be transferred from a sensitized host to a nonsensitized host by serum transfer. Type IV cell-mediated sensitivities can be transferred only by lymphocyte exchange.

TYPE I HYPERSENSITIVITIES (ANAPHYLACTIC)

Aetiology

The type I hypersensitivities may take different forms depending on the type and amount of allergen and the degree of sensitization (Table 33-5). *Anaphylactic shock* is the most serious, life-threatening form and requires immediate medical intervention. Common antigens include insect bites (especially bee stings), drugs (especially penicillins and heterologous antiserum), food, pollen, and X-ray contrast media. *Urticaria (hives)* can be caused by foods, especially eggs, fish, and nuts, or drugs such as penicillins. Chronic urticaria may be caused by stress or exposure to heat or cold.

The less severe and more common forms of type I hypersensitivities are the atopic allergies, seen in about 15% of the population. *Atopy* refers to an inherited hypersensitivity. It is the tendency to become hypersensitive that is inherited, not the allergy to a specific substance. What people become hypersensitive to is determined by the allergens to which they are exposed. Common antigens include *inhalants* (pollens, mould spore, animal dander, house dust) and *contactants* (fibres in wool, furs, and nylon; plant oils; soaps; cosmetics; perfumes; hair dyes; nickel in jewellery or clothing fasteners; occupational chemicals.) Changes in temperature and stress may exacerbate symptoms.

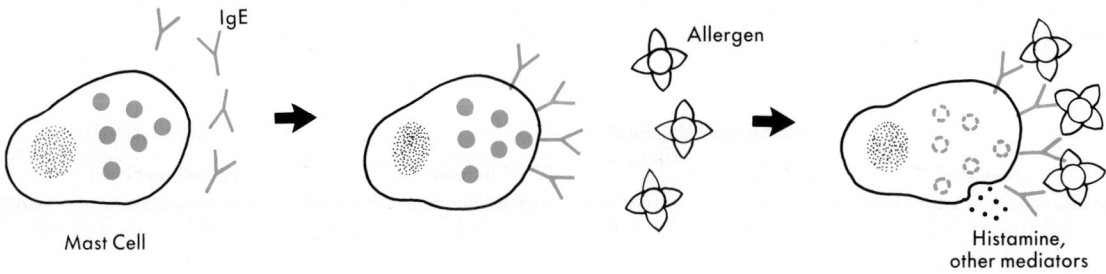

Fig. 33-2   Type I hypersensitivity. IgE binds to mast cell; allergen then binds to IgE, causing degranulation of mast cell with release of histamine and other mediators.

REVIEW

Table 33-5   Type I hypersensitivities (allergies)

Disorder	Signs and symptoms	Medical therapy
Anaphylactic shock	Initial itching and sneezing, apprehension. Oedema of face, hands, and other body parts; dyspnoea, wheezing, shock	Adrenaline intramuscularly; chlorphemiramine intravenously; aminophylline to relax bronchial spasm; tracheal intubation for tracheal oedema; control of shock
Urticaria (hives)	Skin lesions: pale pink elevated edge on an erythematous background (wheal). Pruritus	Self-limiting; adrenaline or antihistamines may be given
Atopic		
Allergic rhinitis (hay fever)	Sneezing, itching, and watery eyes, running nose	Antihistamines; sodium cromoglycate; allergic immunotherapy
Allergic asthma	Wheezing, coughing, dyspnoea	Adrenaline, bronchodilators
Atopic dermatitis	Pruritus; vesicles; oozing and crusting lesions; scaling	Wet dressings, topical steroids

Pathophysiology

Type I hypersensitivities are associated with the reactions mediated by the IgE class of immunoglobulins. The IgE immunoglobulins attach to the surface of mast cells and basophils, providing a site for allergens to bind to the cells. This causes the cell to release a variety of vasoactive substances, including histamine (Fig. 33-2).

Thus in type I reactions the detrimental symptoms are not at the site of the antigen-antibody reaction but at the site of the organs or tissues where the histamine and other mediators exert their action. If those mediators remain confined to a local area, the tissue reactions remain localized and are referred to as *local anaphylaxis*. The local hypersensitivity that most people demonstrate to an insect bite, the wheal-flare type of reaction, is the classic example of this type of reaction. The reaction may also become localized in the nose and eyes (hay fever), in the bronchial passages (allergic asthma), or in the skin (atopic dermatitis). If, however, the mediators become released systemically, the response is known as *systemic anaphylaxis*, which can produce *anaphylactic shock* (Chapter 7).

The three main effects of the vasoactive substances are the following:

1. Constricts smooth muscle such as in the bronchi, resulting in bronchial spasm
2. Increases vascular permeability, resulting in urticaria (hives) or tissue oedema
3. Increases mucous secretions, as occurs in hay fever and asthma

Symptoms depend on the type of allergy and the organ affected (Fig. 33-3) and include the following:

1. Respiratory: wheezing, sneezing, rhinitis with conjunctivitis
2. Dermal: urticaria, angiooedema, rash
3. GI: nausea, vomiting, diarrhoea
4. General symptoms: fever, malaise, joint pains, haematopoietic suppression, anaphylaxis

For type I reactions to occur, the hypersensitive individual must initially come into contact with the allergen that triggers the synthesis of specific antiallergenic IgE antibodies. This primary contact is known as a *sensitizing dose*. On subsequent contact with the allergen (termed the *shocking* or *challenging dose*), the individual exhibits the symptoms of type I sensitivity. People who are allergic to pollinating grasses will have the same symptoms no matter which grass is pollinating. If they move from one geographic area to another, they will become sensitized to whatever grasses are present in that area.

Nursing Process
Assessment

All patients should be questioned about allergies and sensitivities to drugs before drug therapy is initiated. If there is any positive history, the doctor is informed before a new drug is prescribed, and if it is given, the patient is watched closely for allergic responses.

It is usually possible to determine specific allergens to which a person is hypersensitive by taking a history that includes the following:

ALLERGY

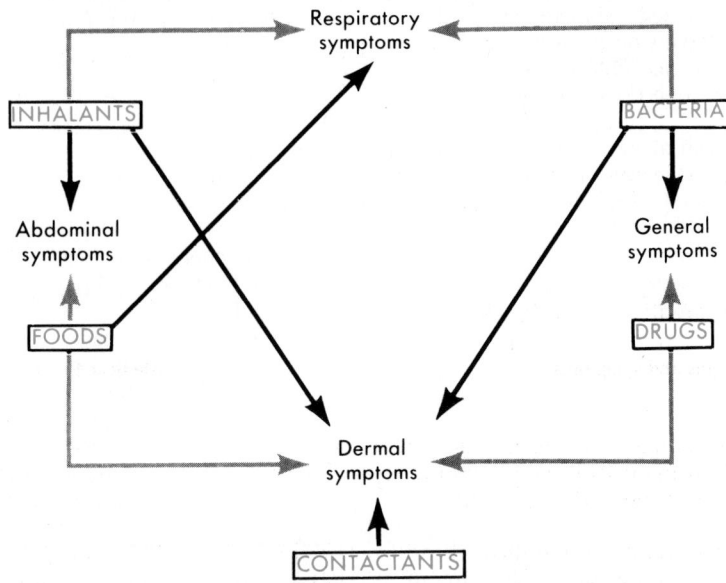

Fig. 33-3 Causes of allergic responses and symptoms produced.

1. History of allergic reactions in the past (type, frequency, perceived cause)
2. Familial history of allergies
3. Recent exposure to sensitizing substances
4. Changes in living, working, or environmental conditions
5. Characteristics of present environment (house, clothing, plants and trees, or animals)
6. Increased stress in recent past
7. Types of symptoms: respiratory, dermal, or general
8. Alleviating factors, either prescribed by a physician or self-prescribed

Diagnostic tests

Skin testing

Skin tests are often used to determine whether a person has a sensitivity to certain substances in the external environment. Several methods of testing are used (Table 33-6). Occasionally one drop of a test extract is instilled into the eye to test for sensitivity (conjunctival test). Redness of the conjunctiva and tearing will appear within 5 to 15 minutes in an allergic person. Tests for allergenic substances are usually done in a series.

Radioallergosorbent test

The radioallergosorbent test (RAST) for IgE antibodies provides the same information as skin tests. A blood sample is drawn for the test. RAST is easier to perform, more comfortable for the patient, and safer; but it is less sensitive and more costly than skin testing. RAST is especially useful for detecting IgE antibodies to occupational chemicals or potentially toxic allergens.

Use test

A person with a food allergy is asked to keep a food diary for at least a week. On the basis of this diary, suspect foods such as milk, wheat products, and eggs may be removed from the diet (elimination diet) until symptoms subside and then added one at a time in an attempt to identify the offending foods. Reaction to the use test may be immediate or over a period of time. Some people become discouraged during the testing and may need encouragement to adhere to the test plan.

Nursing Analysis

Problems are determined from analysis of patient data. Possible problems for the person with an allergy may include, but are not limited to, the following:

Problem	Possible aetiologies
Health maintenance, altered	Environmental changes, lack of knowledge
Knowledge deficit	Lack of exposure/recall, information misinterpretation

Planning: expected patient outcomes

Expected patient outcomes for the person with an allergy may include, but are not limited to, the following:
1. Demonstrates a decrease in symptoms.
2. Describes plans to alter habits or environment.
3. Describes substances that are allergenic and approaches for avoidance.
4. Describes rationale for immunotherapy and need to continue regular injections (if pertinent).

Table 33-6 Allergy skin tests

Test	Method	Time of reading	Positive signs	Use
Intradermal	Allergens are injected intradermally at spaced intervals on forearm or intrascapular area; control tests with diluent alone done concurrently	15 to 30 min	Wheal with surrounding erythema	Allergies to pollen, feathers, animal dander, dust
Scratch	Skin cleaned with alcohol and allowed to dry; skin scratched superficially (1 to 4 mm long), and extract applied to scratch	30 min	Erythema	Same as for intradermal
Patch	Sensitizing substance applied to small (1-inch) gauze square and covered with tape	48 hr	+ Erythema only ++ Erythema and papules +++ Erythema, papules, and vesicles ++++ All of above and bullae or ulceration	Allergies to clothing, detergents, perfumes, cosmetics

5. Describes need for constant availability of an anaphylaxis emergency kit for self-treatment (if anaphylaxis is a possibility).
6. Describes drug therapy to relieve symptoms.

Implementation

Assisting with achievement of therapeutic goals

Preventing anaphylactic reaction

People with a history of allergies are at high risk for developing anaphylactic reactions from drugs or animal sera. Hospitalized people who are sensitive to certain substances should be identified, and the information relayed to all staff and recorded in the medical and nursing notes. In addition, many hospitals use a special colour identification bracelet for the person who is sensitive to certain substances.

If immunization is necessary, animal sera should be avoided and another type given, if possible. When it is necessary to use animal serum, the individual should first be tested for sensitivity to the substance. An intradermal skin test preceded by a scratch or eye test is recommended. If animal sera, allergenic extracts, or contrast media containing iodide are given, resuscitation drugs, such as adrenaline, chlorpheniramine, isoprenaline, and hydrocortisone should be readily available. The patient is kept under surveillance for at least 20 minutes. Any reaction that occurs within a few minutes forewarns of an impending emergency. People with known history of anaphylactic reactions should always have ready access to an anaphylactic emergency kit containing oral antihistamine and a syringe with adrenaline for self-injection.

Therapy for anaphylaxis

At the first signs of *anaphylactic shock*, place the patient in a recumbent position and give 0.3 ml adrenaline hydrochloride (1:1000) (less for children) intramuscularly. Adrenaline causes vasoconstriction and decreases vascular permeability, thus preventing systemic spread of the aller-

---

33-4

Drugs commonly prescribed for atopic allergies

Mast cell stabilizer: cromolyn sodium (as a nasal spray, inhalation, or eye drops)
Antihistamines: chlorpheniramine, terfenadine, astemizole
Vasoconstricting agents: adrenaline, pseudephedrine
Bronchodilators: aminophylline, theophylline, terbutaline, isoprenaline, salbutamol
Corticosteroids (for severe reactions):
Oral: prednisolone
Nasal spray: beclomethasone

---

gen with more severe consequences. An antihistamine, such as chlorpheniramine, is then given; it does not reverse the effects of histamine but prevents further activation of the histamine. People outside health care settings must seek *immediate* medical attention. Corticosteroids are given to decrease the inflammatory effects of severe anaphylaxis. Aminophylline may be given for bronchospasms. Tracheal intubation may be necessary for airway maintenance. Treatments for shock, with intravenous fluids and oxygen therapy, are initiated immediately (Chapter 7).

Drug therapy for *atopic* allergies is primarily for symptom relief. Some of the common drugs are listed in Box 33-4.

Allergen immunotherapy

An attempt may be made to slowly desensitize a person by injecting small but increasingly larger doses of the allergen at regular intervals (usually 1 to 4 weeks) over a long period. This treatment may take up to 5 years. It is about 80% effective against pollens causing hay fever but is less effective against asthma or dermatitis. It is essential that the person understand that desensitization is of little value until the environment is controlled; otherwise the constant exposure to allergens will only increase antibody response.

Interventions to achieve patient outcomes

Controlling environment

People whose allergies are caused by environmental inhalants will need to avoid dust, animal dander, fungus spores, pollens, and other allergens. Methods of decreasing environmental inhalant antigens include the following:

1. House dust
   a. Use synthetic materials (avoid wool and cotton)
   b. Cover mattresses and pillows with allergy-free covers; place garments in plastic bags
   c. Avoid wool carpets or felt rugs; keep bedroom floor uncarpeted
   d. Damp dust every day; put away articles that are difficult to dust; do not shake articles
   e. Use air conditioner, if possible
   f. Change filter on warm air central heating unit or air conditioning every month during use

2. Animal dander
   a. Have no cats, dogs, or other animals with fur as pets, if possible
   b. Keep any animals with fur in outdoor enclosure
   c. Avoid furniture stuffed with feathers or horsehair
   d. Limit time with animals
3. Pollens and fungus spores
   a. Clean frequently areas of mould buildup, such as the shower and shower curtains
   b. Minimize number of indoor plants
   c. Use air conditioner, if possible; keep windows closed at night
   d. Keep car windows closed when driving
   e. Limit being outdoors between sunset and sunrise, especially when windy (highest spore and pollen counts occur between midnight and 8 am)
   f. Do not hang washing outside to dry (pollen and moulds stick to wet washing)
   g. Avoid gardening, raking leaves, mowing lawn, or being near freshly cut grass
   h. If possible, plan holidays in areas that are free of the specific allergen

Facilitating learning

The major nursing responsibility when caring for the person with an atopic allergy is teaching the patient about the nature of the disorder and the methods that can be used to avoid the allergen. The major points for teaching are summarized in Box 33-5.

Evaluation

Evaluation is based on expected patient outcomes. Questions to consider may include the following:

1. Does the person know how to avoid the specific allergens?
2. Have plans been made to decrease contact with the allergen?
3. Does the person know when to seek medical help?

TYPE II HYPERSENSITIVITIES (CYTOTOXIC)

Pathophysiology

The underlying mechanisms of type II hypersensitivities involve the direct binding of *IgG* or *IgM* immunoglobulins to an antigen on the *surface of a cell*. This antibody labelling then triggers the destruction of the cell by phagocytic attack, nonspecific lymphocytic attack, or cell lysis.

Blood Transfusion Reactions

Aetiology

The type II hypersensitivity is classically illustrated by the reactions that occur in mismatched blood transfusion reactions. Blood replacement therapy is used when there has been excessive blood loss (whole blood or blood components) or in treatment of diseases of the haematopoietic system. Replacement therapy may be whole blood or one or more of the blood components (Table 33-7). Blood transfusions are not without dangers to the recipient; therefore, the transfusion of 1 unit (500 ml) of blood for minor therapy is not recommended.

33-5

Patient Teaching

The patient with allergies

Inhalant allergy: control environment (see text).
Drug allergy
    Remind doctor of allergy when new medication is prescribed
    Read all labels of nonprescription drugs before taking a new drug
    Wear a MedicAlert bracelet indicating the known drug allergy
Food allergy
    Examine labels of new prepared foods for presence of allergen
    Avoid eating unknown foods when travelling
Contact allergy
    Use a nonallergenic soap or detergent and cosmetics and take these when travelling
    Use hypoallergenic soap if allergic to most soaps and detergents
    Coat nickel-containing jewellery or clothing fasteners with clear nail polish
    Use gloves if necessary to handle allergen (such as occupational chemicals)
Allergy to insect stings
    Avoid walking barefoot outdoors
    Avoid eating outdoors
    Keep a sting emergency medical kit readily available and know how to use it; teach its use also to significant others
All people with allergies
    Continue medical follow-up if medications are required
    Report side effects of prescribed medications
    Report severe episodes to doctor; as instructed

Table 33-7 Types of blood components

Blood component	Description	Usage	Comments
Red blood cells (RBC)			
Packed RBCs (PRBCs)	RBCs separated from plasma and platelets	Anaemia Moderate blood loss	Decreased risk of fluid overload as compared to whole blood
Washed RBCs	RBCs washed with sterile isotonic saline before transfusion	Previous allergic reactions to transfusions	Increased removal of immunoglobulins and protein
Frozen RBCs	RBCs frozen in a glycerol solution; cells are washed after thawing to remove the glycerol	Storage of rare blood type Storage of autologous blood for future use	Relatively free of leukocytes and microemboli Expensive
Leukocyte-poor RBCs	RBCs from which most leukocytes have been removed	Previous sensitivity to leukocyte antigens from prior transfusions or from pregnancy	Fewer RBCs than packed RBCs Washed leukocyte-poor RBC units have more RBCs than nonwashed
Other cellular components			
Platelets: Random donor packs	Platelets separated from RBCs by centrifuge; given in 50 ml of plasma	Thrombocytopenia Disseminated intravascular coagulation (DIC)	Plasma base is rich in coagulation factors Platelets preparations can also be packed, washed, or made leukocyte-poor
Pheresis packs	Platelets from an HLA-matched donor, separated by pheresis	Allosensitized people with thrombocytopenia	Requires specialized techniques
Granulocytes	Granular leukocytes separated by pheresis	Granulocytopenia from malignancy or chemotherapy	Allergen sensitization may occur with chills and fever
Plasma components			
Fresh frozen plasma (FFP)	Freezing of plasma within 4 hrs of collection	Clotting deficiencies Liver disease Haemophilia Defibrination	Preserves factors V, VII, VIII, IX, X and prothrombin Minimizes hepatitis risk
Factor concentrates VIII and IX	Prepared from large donor pools Heat treated to inactivate HIV	VIII: Haemophilia A IX: Haemophilia B	Increased risk of hepatitis (VIII, IX) and thromboembolism (IX) Given in small volumes
Cryoprecipitate	Precipitated material obtained from FFP when thawed	Haemophilia A Infection of burns Hypofibrinogenaemia Uraemic bleeding	Contains factors VIII, XIII, and fibrinogen

Serum albumin:
  Normal serum albumin (NSA)
  Plasma protein fraction (PPF)
	Albumin chemically processed from pooled plasma	Hypovolaemic shock
		Hypoalbuminaemia
		Burns
		Haemorrhagic shock
			No risk of hepatitis
			Does not require ABO compatibility
			Lacks clotting factors
			Hypotension may occur if PPF is given faster than 10 ml/min

Immune serum globulin	Obtained from plasma of preselected donors with specific antibodies	Hypogammaglobulinaemia Prophylaxis for hepatitis A	Given intramuscularly or intravenously

Pathophysiology

Many antigens are found on the surface of red blood cells, but in terms of potential immunological reaction the major clinically significant systems are the ABO and Rh systems.

ABO system

The four major human blood groups are listed in Box 33-6. Because type AB contains both antigens, people with type AB may receive blood from any type (Fig. 33-4). People with type O may donate blood to other types, but because both antigens are absent in type O, they may not receive another type without having a reaction.

Within the serum, individuals possess naturally occurring antibodies to the red blood cell (RBC) surface antigens of the ABO blood groups that are not present on their own RBCs. Thus a person with type A blood will possess anti-B antibodies within the serum. These antibodies, called *isohaemagglutinins,* are usually of the IgM class. The antibodies are capable of cross-reacting with the A or B antigens on the surface of the "foreign" ABO types. On transfusion, mismatched blood will be immediately coated by the isohaemagglutinins, causing agglutination of the introduced cells and the rapid lysis (breakdown) of the cells. The products released by the lysed cells are then released into the bloodstream.

Rh system

The Rh system is more complex because at least 27 different antigens are in this system. The most immunogenic is the D antigen. When the term *Rh positive* is used, the presence of antigen Rh-D is implied; *Rh negative* indicates the absence of antigen D. Approximately 85% of the Caucasian population of the United Kingdom, Western Europe and the United States has Rh-positive blood.

When the person with Rh-negative blood is first exposed to Rh-positive blood, Rh antibodies are formed. On subsequent exposures to Rh-positive blood, the Rh antibody binds to its corresponding antigen on the surface of the RBCs containing the Rh antigen. The Rh-antigen RBCs are then rapidly broken down by macrophages in the spleen with conversion of haemoglobin to bilirubin resulting in jaundice.

HLA system

Human leukocyte antigens (HLA) are found on many types of tissue cells and on blood leukocytes and platelets. The system is more complex than the RBC antigen systems, and literally thousands of combinations of the antigens can occur. Sensitization may occur through pregnancy or through exposure to platelets and white blood cells (WBCs) during transfusions. Repeated transfusions of blood cells may lead to transfusion reactions.

Prevention of transfusion reactions

Prescreening of potential blood donors is essential. In the United Kingdom, all blood is donated by volunteers, whereas in the United States some blood is still obtained from paid donors. This practice increases the risk of transfer of blood-borne infections, as these paid donors are less likely to report past or present disease or high-risk activities.

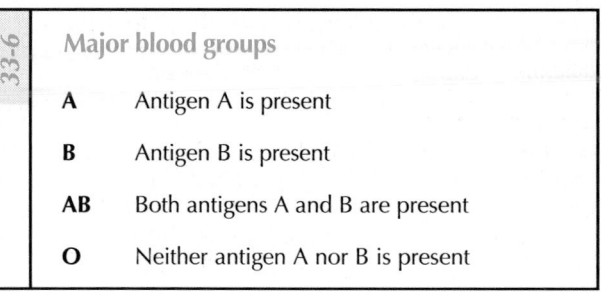

33-6	Major blood groups	
	A	Antigen A is present
	B	Antigen B is present
	AB	Both antigens A and B are present
	O	Neither antigen A nor B is present

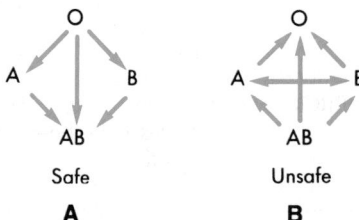

Fig. 33-4 Blood groups and the groups each can receive blood from and give blood to. **A,** Safe. **B,** Unsafe.

After the blood has been collected, the blood group and subgroups including Rh typing are identified, and the blood is tested for syphilis, hepatitis, HIV antibodies, and cytomegalovirus (CMV). The blood must be cross-matched with blood from the recipient to determine compatibility and prevent an acute haemolytic reaction. Cross-matching consists of mixing samples of the donor's blood and the recipient's blood and examining for cell clumping or haemolysis.

Most of the serious reactions that now occur during transfusions are the result of human error. Safeguards include the following:
1. Blood must be kept cold until ready to use (warm blood is a good medium for bacterial growth).
2. Blood that has remained at room temperature for more than 30 minutes should not be used or returned to refrigeration for reissue.
3. Do not transfuse a unit of blood longer than 4 hours.
4. The unit of blood must be labelled with the patient's name, and the label must be checked, by two nurses, against the patient's wristband before the blood is given.
5. All blood products should be administered through filters to prevent embolism from clots; use the correct filter for the type of blood product.
6. If blood must be warmed (rarely needed), use an in-line blood warmer with a monitoring device only (no water bath, incubator, or microwave oven) to prevent RBC haemolysis from temperatures over 38°C (100.4°F).
7. The patient must be monitored throughout the blood administration.

Complications of blood transfusions

Immunological transfusion reactions

Immunological reactions that can occur with blood transfusions include acute haemolytic, delayed haemolytic, allergic, febrile, graft versus host disease, and noncardiac pulmonary oedema (Table 33-9). The most serious reaction is the acute haemolytic reaction that occurs during ad-

Table 33-9 Immunological reactions to blood transfusions

Reaction	Cause	Mechanism	Symptoms	Occurrence	Action
Acute haemo-lytic	Recipient antibody incompatible with transfused red cells	RBCs agglutinate, rapid haemolysis Capillary plugging (type II hypersensitivity)	Lumbar pain Constriction of chest Pain in vein Fever, chills Haemoglobinuria Signs of shock	Shortly after initiation of transfusion	Stop transfusion Continue IV saline Blood unit and blood sample from patient sent to lab for immediate testing Treat for shock and renal failure
Delayed haemo-lytic	Anamnestic immune response	Slow haemolysis	Jaundice Anaemia	Days to weeks after transfusion	Monitor adequacy of urinary output and degree of anaemia
Allergic	Transfer of an antigen or a reaginic antibody from donor to recipient	Immune sensitivity to foreign serum protein (type I hypersensitivity)	Urticaria Anaphylaxis (wheezing, dyspnoea, shock)	Within 30 minutes after initiation of transfusion	Mild: give antihistamine, continue transfusion Severe: stop transfusion; give aqueous adrenaline (0.4 ml of 1: 1000 solution)
Febrile	Reaction of antigen on WBC or platelets Bacterial contamination	Leukocyte agglutination Bacterial pyrogens	Fever, chills, headaches, muscle pains	Within 30-90 min after initiation of transfusion	Stop transfusion Continue IV saline Antipyretics after ruling out haemolytic reaction Transfuse with leukocyte-poor blood or washed RBCs
Graft versus host disease	Immunodeficient person receives lymphocytes	Engraftment of donor lymphocytes, which are then "rejected"	Dermatitis Stomatitis Diarrhoea Liver dysfunction	Delayed	Steroids Azathioprine Symptomatic therapy
Noncardiac pulmonary oedema	Donor antibodies react with recipient HLA antigen	Infiltration of pulmonary bed by micro-aggregates which block blood flow	Fever, chills Urticaria Cough Orthopnoea Cyanosis Shock	During transfusion or shortly thereafter	Stop transfusion Continue IV saline Give oxygen as needed Steroids Frusemide

ministration of the first 50 ml of blood transfused. Several hours after a haemolytic reaction, the urine becomes red (port-wine urine) and the urinary output is diminished. The urine contains RBCs and albumin. This reaction is thought to be caused by the release of a toxic substance from the haemolyzed blood that causes a temporary vascular spasm in the kidneys, resulting in renal damage, and blockage of the renal tubules by the haemoglobin precipitated out in the acid urine (haemoglobinuria). If the patient receives more than 100 ml of incompatible blood, irreversible shock with complete renal failure may occur, and death may follow.

As blood cells disintegrate (lyse), large amounts of potassium are released into the bloodstream; if renal function is impaired, hyperkalaemia will develop. If this occurs, the patient may be treated with renal dialysis. Because fever is a sign of both acute haemolytic reaction and the less serious but more common febrile reaction, the transfusion is stopped until the diagnosis is made.

Nonimmunological reactions

Complications other than those of immunological origin include the following:
1. Fluid overload
   a. Occurs mostly in elderly people and those with congestive heart failure or severe anaemia (haemoglobin less than 5 g/100 mL)
   b. Can be prevented by use of packed cells and slower infusion rate for people at risk
   c. If it occurs, slow down or stop infusion (depending on severity of symptoms), administer O_2, place patient in upright position
2. Air embolism (rare now with use of IV bags rather than bottles)
   a. Results when blood is administered under air pressure following severe blood loss
   b. If occurs, place patient on left side in Trendelenburg position (diverts air away from pulmonary artery)

3. Complications of massive blood replacement (exchange of one blood volume in 24 hours)
   a. Thrombocytopaenia with abnormal bleeding (from platelet deterioration)
   b. Cardiac dysrrhythmias (from cold blood)
   c. Electrolyte level imbalances
      (1) *Hyperkalaemia* (potassium released as RBC break down)
      (2) *Hypocalcaemia* (binding of sodium citrate from donor blood with recipient's serum calcium ions)
4. Transmission of disease
   a. Hepatitis: in the United States occurs in 5% to 10% of blood transfusions; blood is screened for hepatitis B and non A, non B; hepatitis A is rarely transmitted by transfusion
   b. HIV: a rare complication; donated blood is tested but test is not 100% accurate; the number of new infections among blood product recipients has decreased; HIV is inactivated in blood products by heat treatment
   c. Syphilis and malaria: incidence is rare
   d. Cytomegalovirus: symptoms occur in about 40 days (fever, malaise, splenomegaly); the condition is benign and treatment is symptomatic
5. Transfusion haemosiderosis
   a. Defined as an iron overload from chronic transfusions for haematopoietic disorders
   b. If it occurs, RBCs are given for future transfusions to decrease number of transfusions required

Autologous blood transfusions

One method of preventing immunological blood transfusion reactions and disease transmission is by using the person's own blood for replacement. There are two approaches for using autologous blood: planned collection and autotransfusion. In *planned autologous transfusion,* blood is collected at regular intervals before the time when usage is anticipated, such as before surgery. The patient's haemoglobin level should be above 11 g/100 mL (haematocrit above 33%). The blood is then stored until needed. This method is especially useful for people with a rare blood type, for those whose religious beliefs preclude receiving donor blood, and for those undergoing planned surgeries for which blood transfusions are expected.

A different form of planned autologous transfusion is *acute normovolaemic haemodilution* in which one or two units of blood are collected from the patient immediately before surgery.[37] A concurrent intravenous administration of crystalloid or colloid solution maintains normovolaemia. The blood lost during surgery is diluted blood; the full-strength blood is then transfused after surgery.

Autotransfusion consists of collecting, filtering, and immediately reinfusing the person's own blood lost during surgery or in the Accident and Emergency department following massive trauma. The blood is suctioned into a bag and passed through a filter to remove aggregates of fibrin, RBCs, platelets, and other microaggregates. Anticoagulant is added through a volume control system. When the bag is full, it is disconnected from the system, and the blood is transfused into the patient with an administration set and a standard or a microembolic filter. Blood that has been contaminated by gastrointestinal contents or that is close to

a malignant tumour is not autotransfused.

Autotransfusion is safe and cost effective, uses warm blood, and contains more RBCs than stored blood, but platelet, fibrinogen, and clotting factors are decreased. The potential exists for nephrotoxic effect from RBC damage with release of haemoglobin.

TYPE III HYPERSENSITIVITIES (IMMUNE COMPLEX)

Pathophysiology

The type III hypersensitivities result from the union of *soluble* antigens with immunoglobulins of the IgM and IgG classes. The complexes that are formed are too small for phagocytosis, so rather than being removed by the mononuclear phagocytic system, they are deposited in body tissues. This causes an inflammatory response, usually intravascular. Immune complexes are a common factor of connective tissue (collagen) disorders, especially lupus erythematosus and rheumatoid arthritis (Chapter 32). Complexes may also be trapped in glomeruli, which results in glomerulonephritis (Chapter 25).

Serum Sickness

A type III hypersensitivity of clinical significance is serum sickness, which can develop from 1 to 3 weeks after the administration of a large amount of "foreign" serum (for example, horse serum used with some prophylactic serums N.B. very rarely used). It may also occur with the administration of certain drugs, particularly antimicrobials such as penicillins.

Itching and discomfort at the injection site are usually the first symptoms noted. These are followed by lymphadenopathy, fever, urticaria or erythematous rash, facial oedema, and joint pain. Objective signs of arthritis may be present.

Serum sickness is a self-limiting disease. Mild symptoms respond well to antihistamines, salicylates, and topical steroids. More severe symptoms may be treated with a steroid such as prednisolone, although this is rarely necessary. Adrenaline is given if an anaphylactic reaction occurs.

TYPE IV HYPERSENSITIVITIES (CELL MEDIATED)

Pathophysiology

Type IV hypersensitivities are cell mediated (delayed type) involving T cells. Antigens identified as foreign to the body can cause a reaction in two ways, by direct or by indirect action. The T lymphocyte can destroy the antigen directly by attaching itself to the antigen cell wall, breaking down the cell membrane, and causing lysis and death of the cell. This direct action approach appears to be a major factor in transplant rejections. The indirect approach consists of activating nonspecific phagocytic cells (macrophages and polymorphonuclear leukocytes) through release of lymphokines by the sensitized T lymphocytes. Cell mediated reactions occur hours to days after exposure to the antigen.

Clinical examples of type IV hypersensitivities are microbial hypersensitivity reaction, allergic contact dermatitis (Chapter 34), and tissue transplant rejection.

Microbial Hypersensitivity Reaction

An example of microbial hypersensitivity is the body's reaction to the tubercle bacillus. The body does not react initially when the bacillus invades a nonsensitized host. However, as the cell-mediated response is activated, tissue destruction (cavitation) and general toxaemia result (Chapter 16). After the initial sensitization, subsequent contact with the tubercle bacillus will elicit a hypersensitivity reaction. This is the basis of the tuberculin skin test.

Tissue Transplant Rejection

The rejection of foreign cells and tissues by the body is a beneficial function of the immune system primarily mediated by a type IV hypersensitivity. If it were not for this mechanism, the human body would be a haven for the inappropriate establishment of growth of any animal cell that penetrated the external defence mechanisms; however, this process is regarded as a disservice when it operates to prevent the positive aspects of the exchange of tissues between hosts (transplants). The antigenic determinants of the tissues that lead to transplant rejection are primarily found on the surface of cells within the transplanted tissues. These antigens are known as *human leukocyte antigens* (HLA) or histocompatibility antigens (major histocompatibility complex MHC).

Transplant tissue destruction can be prevented by immunosuppressive therapy.

AUTOIMMUNE DISEASES

Individuals sometimes respond to some of their own (self) antigens, triggering an immune response. The symptoms of such an attack are referred to as autoimmune disease or *autohypersensitivity*. Autoimmune diseases cannot be explained by a single cause. Multiple mechanisms of autoimmunity usually occur and the underlying causes are unknown.[51]

Self-reactive immunoglobulins are often associated with certain pathological states in the body but many times can also be isolated from the serum of "normal" people as well, especially in older people. The chance that the immune control mechanisms will be lost increases with age. For the most part, these self-reactions are not immunologically initiated; the causative agent lies outside the immune system, but the immune response serves as the pathogenic mechanism.

In general, the immunological *responses* in autoimmune diseases fall into three categories that correlate with three of the four hypersensitivity reactions (see Table 33-4). The three responses include the following:

1. *Type II cytotoxic humoral response* in which IgG and IgM antibodies bind to cell membranes, fix complement, and destroy the cells by lysis.
2. *Type III immune complex humoral response* in which IgG and IgM antibodies react with *serum* antigens, producing antigen-antibody complexes that are deposited in body tissues and cause an inflammatory reaction.
3. *Type IV cell-mediated response* in which cytotoxic (killer) T cells attach to cell walls, break cell membranes, and destroy the cells.

33-7

Some diseases with autoimmune aspects

Type II cytotoxic humoral response
Autoimmune haemolytic anaemia
Pernicious anaemia
Idiopathic (immune) thrombocytopenia
Grave's disease (toxic goitre)
Pemphigus vulgaris
Myasthenia gravis
Goodpasture's syndrome (glomerulonephritis)

Type III immune complex humoral response
Rheumatoid arthritis
Systemic lupus erythematosus (SLE)
Sjögren's syndrome
Poststreptococcal glomerulonephritis
Scleroderma
Ulcerative colitis

Type IV cell-mediated response
Systemic lupus erythematosus (SLE)
Multiple sclerosis
Guillain-Barré syndrome

Examples of autoimmune diseases characteristic of each of the above three categories are listed in Box 33-7. Care of people experiencing these diseases is described elsewhere in the text.

SUMMARY

1. The immune response is a biological defence mecha-nism consisting of specific responses to specific anti-gens.
2. Antigens are substances that elicit the formation of antibodies when introduced into the body; there are five different types of immunoglobulins (antibodies), each with different structures and functions.
3. The two types of cells involved in the immune response are T cells that attack foreign material directly in the body (cell-mediated immunity) and B cells that produce immunoglobulins (humoral immunity). T helper cells enhance immunoglobulin synthesis and T-cell cytotoxic activity, whereas T suppressor cells inhibit these actions.
4. Three basic mechanisms of response may be elicited when an antigen is first introduced (primary immune response): humoral response (primarily B cells), cell-mediated response (primarily T cells), or com-bined B-cell–T-cell immune response.
5. An important characteristic of the specific response system is the ability of the system to remember prior contact with an antigen (during the primary immune response) and to provide a more complete protective reaction on subsequent contact (secondary immune response). The secondary response is more rapid, of greater intensity, and longer lasting than the primary response.

6. Although immunological changes with ageing vary greatly among individuals, the immune response is decreased as evidenced by decreased T-cell function. Older people experience more severe infections (especially influenza and pneumococcal pneumonia), and have an increased potential for cancer.

7. Major health problems of the immune system may be categorized as immunodeficiencies, gammopathies, hypersensitivities, and autoimmunities.

8. Immunodeficiencies may result from deficiencies in B cells or T cells or from both cells combined. Most primary immunodeficiencies are genetic; the major secondary immunodeficiencies encountered in general practice are immunosuppression and acquired immunodeficiency syndrome (AIDS).

9. Immunosuppression may be induced by administration of antigen, specific antibodies, or monoclonal antibodies, by radiation, or by drugs (corticosteroids, cytotoxic drugs, and cyclosporin).

10. The major interventions for immunodeficiencies are replacement therapy with gamma globulin and transfer factor, and prevention of infection.

11. Gammopathies are excessive production of immunoglobulins; the most common gammopathy is multiple myeloma (an excess of plasma cells).

12. Hypersensitivity reactions are exaggerated or inappropriate responses to specific antigens (allergens).

13. Type I hypersensitivities are associated with reactions mediated by IgE immunoglobulins that are attached to mast cells; when the allergen binds to the IgE, histamine is released, producing a systemic (anaphylactic shock) or a local allergic reaction.

14. Therapy for anaphylaxis consists of adrenaline to constrict blood vessels and dilate bronchioles, counteracting the effect of histamine. Antihistamines are given to shorten the duration of anaphylaxis; corticosteroids decrease the inflammatory effects. An open airway must be maintained.

15. The most common allergens in adults are seasonal inhalants (pollens, spores, grasses), and environmental inhalants (house dust, animal dander). Patients are taught measures to avoid and control exposure to the specific antigens.

16. Type II hypersensitivities are cytotoxic reactions from the direct binding of IgG or IgM immunoglobulins to the surface of foreign cells to trigger cell destruction; an example is blood transfusion reactions.

17. The major antigens on RBCs are the AB antigens, Rh antigens, and HLA (MHC) antigens. AB blood group indicates presence of both A and B antigens; O blood group indicates absence of either antigen. Absence of an antigen produces antibodies (isohaemagglutins) that will cause agglutination of donor RBCs containing the missing antigen. Therefore, people with type O blood may donate blood to other types but may not receive another type without having a haemolytic reaction.

18. Rh-positive reactions indicate presence of antigen Rh-D; Rh-negative reactions indicate absence of antigen Rh-D.

19. Immunological reactions to blood transfusions include haemolytic (most serious), allergic, febrile, graft-versus-host disease, and noncardiac pulmonary oedema. Diseases that may be transmitted by blood transfusions include hepatitis, AIDS, syphilis, malaria, and cytomegalovirus (CMV).

20. Autologous blood transfusions consist of using the person's own blood for replacement, either by stored blood previously collected or by autotransfusion of blood from excessive bleeding.

21. Type III hypersensitivities are characterized by immune complexes formed by the union of IgM or IgG immunoglobulins with soluble antigens; the small complexes get trapped in body tissues causing an inflammatory response. An example is serum sickness that occurs after administration of a large amount of foreign serum.

22. Type IV hypersensitivities are cell-mediated (T cell) reactions, differing from the other three types, which are humoral (B cell) reactions. T cells destroy foreign antigens directly (as in transplant rejections) or they may release lymphokines to activate macrophages.

23. Autoimmune diseases are the result of an immune response to self-antigens, usually as a result of an agent outside the immune system. Immunological responses seen in autoimmune diseases may be type I, type II, or type III hypersensitivity responses.

STUDY QUESTIONS

- What are the differences between B cells and T cells in terms of origin and function? How do they relate to each other?
- How would you explain to a lay person the differences among immunodeficiencies, gammopathies, hypersensitivities, and autoimmune disease?
- Look at Fig. 33-1. Explain in your own words the immunodeficiencies that would develop at each of the five marked positions.
- A friend who gets allergic rhinitis (hayfever) is coming to visit you this summer. What advance preparations can you make to help decrease the symptoms?
- Examine the notes/chart of a patient who has received a blood transfusion. What safeguards were taken to prevent transfusion reaction? Should additional safeguards have been taken? If a reaction occurred, what actions were taken?

REFERENCES AND SELECTED READINGS

1. Anderson JA, Adkinson NF Jr: Allergic reaction to drugs and biologic agents, *JAMA* 258:2891-2899, 1987.
2.* Baron M, Tafuro PL: The extremes of age: the newborn and the elderly at increased risk for the development of infection, *Nurs Clin North Am* 20(1):181-190, 1985.
3. Barrett JT: *Textbook of immunology*, ed 5, St Louis, 1988, Mosby–Year Book.
4.* Benson ML, Benson DM: Autotransfusion is here, are you ready? *Nursing 85* 15(3):46-60, 1985.
5.* Birdsell C, Carpenter K, Considine R: How is autotransfusion done? *Am J Nurs* 88:108-111, 1988.

6.   Blansfield J: Emergency autotransfusion in hypovolemia, *Crit Care Nurs Clin North Am* 2:195-199, 1990.

7.* Bonato J: Blood transfusions: are they safe? *Crit Care Nurse* 9(7):40-45, 1989.

8.   Buckley RH: Immunodeficiency diseases, *JAMA* 258:2841-2850, 1987.

9.* Butler S: Current trends in autologous transfusion, *RN* 52(11):44-50, 1989.

10. Committee on Transfusion Practices, American Association of Blood Banks: The latest protocols for blood transfusions, *Nursing 86* 16(10):34-41, 1986.

11. Condemi JJ: The autoimmune diseases, *JAMA* 258:2920-2929, 1987.

12. Costa AJ: Anaphylactic shock: guidelines for immediate diagnosis and treatment, *Postgrad Med* 83:368-373, 1988.

13. Creticos PA, Norman PA: Immunotherapy and allergy, *JAMA* 258:2874-2880, 1987.

14. Croman LC: The relationship between nutrition, infection, and immunity, *Med Clin North Am* 69(3):519-531, 1985.

15.* Dickerson M: Anaphylaxis and anaphylactic shock, *Crit Care Nurs Q* 11:68-74, 1988.

16. DiJulio JE: Treatment of B-cell and T-cell lymphomas with monoclonal antibodies, *Semin Oncol Nurs* 4(2):102-106, 1988.

16a.* Drago SS: Banking your own blood, *Am J Nurs* 92(3):61-64, 1992.

17.* Espersen S: Nursing support of host defenses, *Crit Care Nurs Q* 9(1):51-56, 1986.

18.* Freedman S et al: Nursing considerations in the administration of blood component therapy, *Semin Oncol Nurs* 6(2):155-162, 1990.

19.* Gaunder BN: Insect bites and stings: managing allergic reactions, *Nurs Pract* 11(3):16-20, 1986.

20.* Girard NJ, Morgan RG, Orr MD: Autologous salvage of blood: perioperative nursing considerations, *AORN J* 47:492-503, 1988.

21. Graziano FM, Lemanske R Jr: *Clinical immunology,* Baltimore, 1989, Williams & Wilkins.

22.* Griffin JP: Nursing care of the critically ill immunocompromised patient, *Crit Care Nurs Q* 49(1):25-34, 1986.

23.* Gurevich I, Tafuro P: Nursing measures for the prevention of infection in the compromised host, *Nurs Clin North Am* 20(1):257-266, 1985.

24. Gurka AM: The immune system: implications for critical care, *Crit Care Nurse* 9(7):24-35, 1989.

25. Hadden JW: Immunopharmacology: immunomodulation and immunotherapy, *JAMA* 258:3005-3010, 1987.

26.* Hahn K: Monitoring a blood transfusion, *Nursing 89* 19(10):20-21, 1989.

27. Heinzel FP: Infections in patients with humoral immunodeficiency, *Hosp Pract* 24(9):99-130, 1989.

28.* Hotter AN: Wound healing and immunocompromise, *Nurs Clin North Am* 25(1):193-203, 1990.

29. Kaplan AP, Buckley RH, Mathews KP: Allergic skin disorders, *JAMA* 258:2900-2909, 1987.

30. Kaliner M, Eggleston PA, Mathews KP: Rhinitis and asthma, *JAMA* 258:2851-2873, 1987.

31. Kotwas L et al: Blood collection techniques, *Semin Oncol Nurs* 6(2):109-116, 1990.

32.* Martin E et al: Autotransfusion systems, *Crit Care Nurse* 9(7):65-73, 1989.

33.* Mennies JH et al: An overview of adult allergic disorders, *Nurs Pract* 10(6):16-23, 1985.

34. Miller DS: Intravenous immune globulin for treating primary immunodeficiency disease, *MCN* 12:244-248, 1987.

35. Minnefor AB et al: IV immune globulin efficacy and safety, *Hosp Pract* 22(10):171-183, 1987.

36. National Blood Resource Education Program's Nursing Education Working Group: Choosing blood components and equipment, *Am J Nurs* 91(6):42-46, 1991.

37. National Blood Resource Education Program's Nursing Education Working Group: Autologous transfusion, *Am J Nurs* 91(6):47-48, 1991.

38. National Blood Resource Education Program's Nursing Education Working Group: Preventing and managing transfusion reactions, *Am J Nurs* 91(6):48-50, 1991.

39. Norman PS: Immunotherapy of IgE-mediated disease, *Hosp Pract* 25(4):81-86, 1990.

40. Osserman EF, Merlin G, Butler VP: Multiple myeloma and related plasma cell dyscrasias, *JAMA* 258:2930-2937, 1987.

41.* Parsons L, Klopovich PM: Immune globulin therapy, *Semin Oncol Nurs* 6(2):136-139, 1990.

42.* Petrucci KE, Booth-Blaemire E, Watson K: Aging, immunity, and critical care nursing, *Crit Care Nurs Clin North Am* 1(4):787-795, 1989.

43.* Phillips A: Are blood transfusions really safe? *Nursing 87* 17(6):63-65, 1987.

44. Platts-Mills TAE et al: Dust mite allergy: its clinical significance, *Hosp Pract* 22(9):91-100, 1987.

45.* Pluth MN: A home care transfusion program, *Oncol Nurs Forum* 14(5):42-46, 1987.

46.* Querin JJ, Stahl LD: 12 simple sensible steps for successful blood transfusions, *Nursing 90* 20(10):68-81, 1990.

47.* Randall BJ: Reacting to anaphylaxis, *Nursing 86* 16(3):34-39, 1986.

48. Rayfield S et al: Maximizing safe blood transfusions, *Adv Clin Care* 5(5):17-19, 1990.

49.* Recking JB et al: Understanding immune system dysfunction, *Nursing 87* 17(9):34-42, 1987.

50.* Rieger PT: Monoclonal antibodies, *Am J Nurs* 87:469-473, 1987.

51. Schroeder SA et al: *Current medical diagnosis and treatment,* Norwalk, Conn, 1991, Appleton & Lange.

52.* Smith SL: Immunosuppressive drugs used in clinical practice, *Crit Care Nurs Q* 9(1):19-24, 1986.

53. Stites DP, Terr AT: *Basic and clinical immunology,* ed 7, Norwalk, Conn, 1990, Appleton & Lange.

54. Valentine MD et al: Anaphylaxis and stinging insect hypersensitivity, *JAMA* 258:2881-2885, 1987.

55. Widman FK: *An introduction to clinical immunology,* Philadelphia, 1989, FA Davis.

56. Wyngaarden JB, Smith LH: *Cecil textbook of medicine,* ed 18, Philadelphia, 1988, WB Saunders.

*Recommended for student reading.

FURTHER READING

Brozovic B, Brozovic M: *Manual of Clinical Blood Transfusion,* Edinburgh, 1986, Churchill Livingstone.

Brydon MJ: Understanding is the means to control: Management and treatment of seasonal rhinitis, *Professional Nurse* 8(10):662-666, 1992.

Cluroe S: Blood transfusions, *Nursing* 3(40):8-11, 1989.

Holgate S: *Allergy,* London, 1991, Gower Medical Publishing.

Roitt IM, Brostoff J and Male D: *Immunology,* London, 1985, Gower Medical Publishing.

The Patient with Dermatological Problems

Barbara C. Long

After studying this chapter, the learner should be able to:

- Describe the psychological effect of skin disorders.
- Differentiate skin inflammations resulting from bacteria, viruses, fungi, and parasites and appropriate therapy.
- Describe measures for relief of pruritus.
- Differentiate between contact and atopic dermatitis and methods of prevention.
- Explain the pathophysiology of psoriasis and therapeutic measures.
- Differentiate types of skin tumours and surgical interventions.
- Describe the assessment of a burns patient.
- Differentiate between the three periods of a major burn.
- Compare and contrast the different types of grafts and measures to promote healing.

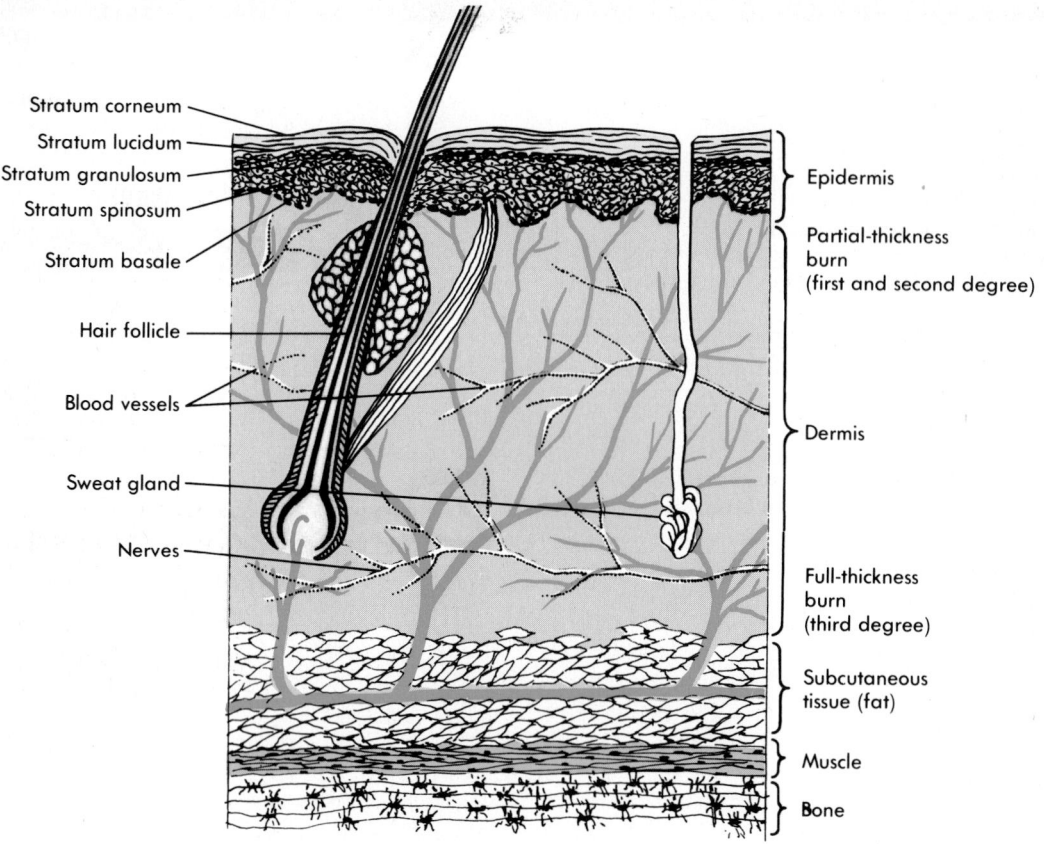

Stratum corneum
Stratum lucidum
Stratum granulosum
Stratum spinosum
Stratum basale

Hair follicle

Blood vessels

Sweat gland

Nerves

Epidermis

Partial-thickness
burn
(first and second degree)

Dermis

Full-thickness
burn
(third degree)

Subcutaneous
tissue (fat)

Muscle

Bone

Fig. 34-1   Structures of the skin and skin layers.

The skin is the largest organ of the body. It is exposed to the external environment and provides the first line of defence of the body; at the same time it is affected by changes in the internal environment. General health maintenance requires maintenance of healthy skin. Skin changes may result from environmental changes (such as heat and cold, sunlight, and lack of moisture), from systemic disorders, and from disorders of the skin itself. In this chapter the major health problems of the skin of adults and surgical correction of impairments of the skin and underlying tissue (plastic surgery) are discussed.

ANATOMY AND PHYSIOLOGY

Anatomy

The skin is composed of two main layers, the epidermis and the dermis. The *epidermis* is composed of two parts, a thin layer of closely packed dead squamous cells covering a second layer of cells containing *melanin,* which gives skin its colour. The dead cells are constantly being shed and replaced by deeper cells. Blood vessels do not reach into the epidermis (Fig. 34-1).

The second main layer, the *dermis,* is composed of bundles of collagen fibres and elastic connective tissue that act to support the epidermis. It is well supplied with nerves and blood vessels and contains the sweat glands, sebaceous glands, and hair follicles.

Below the dermis is the subcutaneous tissue, consisting of loose connective tissue and fat. It is loosely attached to underlying structures in most body areas.

Physiology

Functions of the skin include protection, heat regulation, sensory perception, secretion, and production of vitamin D (Box 34-1). Fat-soluble substances can penetrate the skin by passing through the hair follicles and sebaceous glands. Atrophic or senile skin contains fewer hair follicles; thus permeability of fat-soluble substances through skin is decreased in the elderly.

The epidermis can be weakened by scraping or stripping the surface, such as by dry razors or by removal of tape. Once the barrier has weakened, permeability to substances such as bacteria or drugs is increased. Large amounts of drugs can be absorbed by extensive denuded skin areas. Epidermis that becomes overdry may crack and lead to breaks in the surface. When the epidermis remains wet for long periods, it becomes macerated and the moisture provides a medium for bacterial growth.

Blood vessels of the skin assist in control of body temperature by constriction in cold environments to promote conservation of heat and by dilation in warm environments to promote loss of heat by radiation. Further loss of heat occurs by evaporation of perspiration from skin surfaces. These mechanisms help maintain a constant internal body temperature.

Skin Changes With Ageing

As people grow older changes occur in the skin and hair that make differentiating normal from abnormal changes more difficult. The changes result primarily from loss of subcutaneous tissue, degeneration of collagen and elastic fibres, loss of melanocytes, increased capillary fragility, decreased secretion of sweat glands, hormonal changes, and overexposure to environmental elements. The skin wrinkles and becomes looser, and spotty pigmentation develops on sun-exposed areas.

The elderly person is also more likely to have one or more chronic diseases and to be taking medications that can cause skin changes. Dry skin may cause itching and may lead to skin breakdown if scratched. Skin infections occur more readily because of increased epidermal permeability. Stasis dermatitis may result from circulatory impairment of the legs. Toenails become thicker and difficult to trim; fingernails become more brittle and develop longitudinal ridges. Body hair changes in consistency and distribution.

Types of Skin Lesions

Different types of lesions may be observed on the skin. Changes from normal skin may be in terms of colour, cell growth, presence of extra fluid, consistency, or integrity (Table 34-1). Swelling of the skin may result from the presence of fluid in or between tissue cells or from overgrowth of tissue cells (Fig. 34-2). Fluid may appear as fluid-filled sacs on the skin surface or in the tissue. *Interstitial* fluid results from increased extracellular body fluid (Chapter 6) and is termed *pitting oedema* because a finger pressed over the swollen tissue leaves a pit on the skin surface. Extra fluid *within* cells causes swelling but is not termed oedema and does not pit when pressed. Different terms are used for overgrowth of tissue cells, depending on the size of the growth. The term *tumour* refers to a growth over 2 cm and is not restricted to malignancy; tumours can also be benign.

Lesions may occur singly or in multiples. They may be discrete (separate) or they may coalesce into each other. They may occur in patches located in certain body areas or occur widely distributed in an even or uneven pattern. The use of correct medical terms when describing skin lesions facilitates communication with others.

PSYCHOLOGICAL EFFECTS OF DERMATOLOGICAL PROBLEMS

There is a certain degree of "beauty orientation" in Western culture. Cosmetics to enhance good looks are extensively used by men and women. It is no wonder that skin diseases or physical defects that detract from "good looks" produce psychological reactions.

Emotional reactions to a deformity or defect must not be underestimated. Pride in oneself, the ability to think well of oneself and to regard oneself favourably in comparison with others, is essential to the development and maintenance of a well-integrated personality. Every person with a defect or handicap, particularly if it is conspicuous to others, suffers some threat to emotional security. The extent of the emotional reaction and the amount of maladjustment that follow depend on the individual's makeup and ability to cope with emotional insults. It is not unusual for the individual to withdraw from a society that is unkind. The defect may be used to justify failure to assume responsibility or to justify striking out against an unkind society.

Skin diseases that produce marked disfigurement of visible body surfaces can therefore result in alterations in body image. Feelings of decreased worth by people with large draining lesions or with severe disfigurement are reinforced during interactions with others. Some people are repelled by the sight of severe skin diseases or may experience a threat to their own body integrity and physically withdraw to avoid interaction. Some people may experience nonverbal messages of disgust when others view their disfigurement for the first time. This is markedly poignant when those nonverbal messages are sent by significant others or by health professionals.

In working with the person with severe skin disease, the nurse first examines his or her own feelings that could be expressed nonverbally in a negative manner. The patient and family are assisted to cope with their feelings.

PREVENTION AND HEALTH EDUCATION

Prevention of dermatological conditions not only relieves the patient of discomfort but is cost effective because many skin conditions are chronic. In addition, maintenance of intact healthy skin has a positive effect on one's well-being. *Primary prevention* includes maintenance of healthy skin and avoidance of causative agents (when possible). *Secondary prevention* includes observations of skin changes and avoidance of self-treatment (Box 34-2).

MAJOR HEALTH PROBLEMS OF THE SKIN

There are numerous types of skin conditions, many of which occur only rarely. Some of the more common skin conditions discussed include the following:
1. Inflammatory skin conditions
    a. Bacterial infections: folliculitis, furuncles, and carbuncles
    b. Viral inflammations: herpes simplex, herpes zoster, warts
    c. Fungal inflammation: candidiasis, dermatophytoses
    d. Parasitic infestations: pediculosis, scabies
2. Acne
3. Dermatitis: contact, atopic, or stasis
4. Scaling papular disorders: psoriasis, pityriasis rosea, lichen planus
5. Tumours of the skin: keratoses, haemangiomas, premalignant lesions, malignant lesions

INFLAMMATORY SKIN DISORDERS

Types of Inflammatory Skin Disorders

The skin may become inflamed from bacteria, viruses, or fungal infection or by parasitic infestation.

Table 38-2 Skin lesions

Term	Description	Example
Change in colour		
Macule	Flat spot less than 1 cm	Freckle
Change in cell growth		
Papule	Raised mass less than 1 cm	Measles spot
Nodule	Raised mass 1 to 2 cm	Mole
Tumor	Raised mass over 2 cm	Epithelioma
Change involving fluid		
Vesicle	Fluid-filled sac less than 1 cm	Small blister
Bulla	Fluid-filled sac more than 1 cm	Large blister
Pustule	Pus-filled sac less than 1 cm	Acne lesion
Wheal	Circumscribed raised skin containing intracellular fluid	Hives (Urticaria)
Changes in consistence or integrity		
Plaque	Large raised surface on skin	Psoriasis
Crust	Dry exudate over a lesion	Eczema lesion
Scale	Dry exfoliation of skin cells	Psoriasis
Fissure	Crack in skin surface	Crack in corner of mouth
Ulcer	Erosion of skin surface	Decubitus ulcer
Lichenification	Leatherlike thickening of outer skin layer	Lichen planus

Bacterial skin infections

Most bacteria that normally inhabit the skin are nonpathogenic. Pathogenic bacteria that penetrate the outer skin layer may cause a superficial skin infection or superficial *folliculitis* or they may penetrate deeper, causing a deep folliculitis or a *furuncle* (Table 34-2).

Superficial folliculitis occurs most often with uncleanliness, maceration, exposure to oils and solvents, traction on the hair from tar therapy, or occlusion therapy. Furuncles and carbuncles occur most often in obese, poorly nourished, fatigued, or otherwise susceptible people with poor hygiene, in debilitated elderly people, and in people with inadequately treated diabetes mellitus.

Viral skin inflammations

Viruses may cause either simple or more serious skin inflammations (Table 34-3). One of the most common viruses found in humans is the *herpes simplex* virus (HSV). It occurs as two similar yet serologically different strands, type 1 and type 2. The type 1 virus is found primarily in lesions of the face and mouth (cold sore), eye (keratitis), and brain (encephalitis). Type 2 is associated with lesions of the genitalia that can be transmitted by sexual contact (see Chapter 27). Factors that may precipitate recurrence of herpes simplex lesions include fever, upper respiratory tract infection, exhaustion, and stress. Lesions are also more common during the menses or after direct exposure to the sun's rays. Depression of immune function may predispose to HSV infection.

Herpes zoster is caused by the same virus (varicella zoster, V-Z) that causes varicella (chickenpox). Varicella is believed to be the primary infection in a nonimmune host, whereas herpes zoster is thought to be the response in a partially immune host. Although herpes zoster is far less communicable than chickenpox, people who have not had chickenpox may develop it after exposure to the vesicular lesions of people with herpes zoster. For this reason, susceptible people should not care for patients with herpes zoster.

Herpes zoster (shingles) can be serious in any adult and may even lead to death from exhaustion in elderly debilitated people. It is one of the most drawn out and exasperating conditions found in elderly patients and leads to discouragement and demoralization. The lesions follow nerve pathways and never cross the body midline, although nerves on both sides can be affected. Although recurrence is possible, immunity usually occurs after one attack. Herpes zoster often occurs in immunocompromised people. Acyclovir, an antiviral drug, is given for herpes simplex in immunocompromised people and for people with herpes zoster. It only controls the symptoms; it does not affect the disease. Corticosteroids may be given to decrease the incidence of postherpetic neuralgia. Pain in postherpetic neuralgia can be severe and usually lasts less than 1 year, but may persist for years. *Herpetic whitlow* and *warts* are two other commonly seen viral skin inflammations (see Table 34-3).

Fungal inflammations

Fungi are larger and more complex than bacteria. They may be unicellular, such as yeast, or multicellular, such as moulds. Fungi may cause common skin disorders (Table 34-4).

Yeasts thrive in warm, moist environments such as the mouth and vagina (*candidiasis*). Problems occur when there is an overgrowth, commonly occurring with pregnancy, use of oral contraceptives, poor nutrition, antibiotic therapy, diabetes mellitus, other endocrine

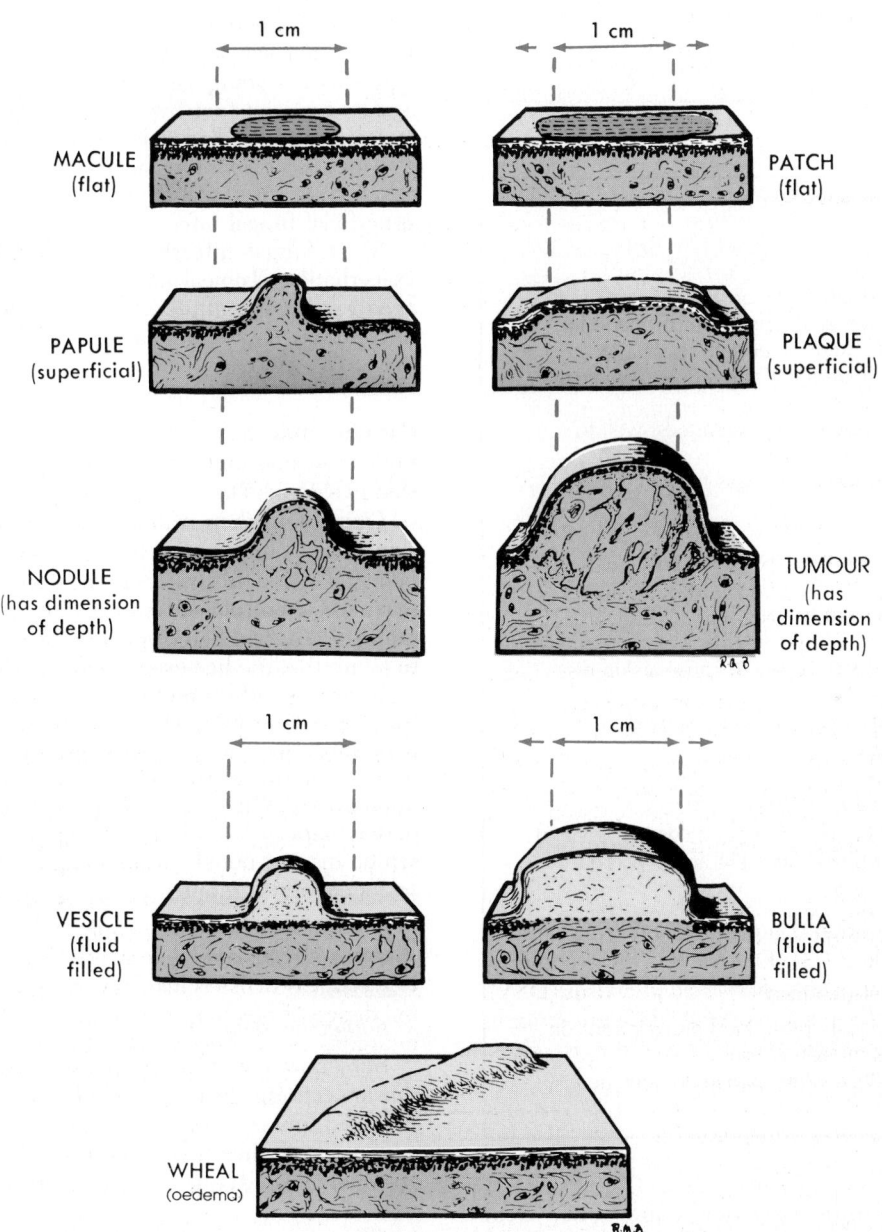

Fig. 34-2   Skin lesions. (From Stewart WD, Danto UL, Maddin S: *Dermatology: diagnosis and treatment of cutaneous disorders,* ed 4, St Louis, 1978, Mosby–Year Book.)

Functions of the skin

Protection from environment; pathogenic organisms, foreign substances, heat, rays
Heat regulation
  Conduction: transfer of heat by direct contact to other objects or air
  Convection: removal of heat by air currents on skin
  Evaporation: removal of heat by water loss from skin surface
Sensory perception: sensory receptors in skin
Excretion: removal of water and electrolytes
Production of vitamin D: effect of sunlight

Prevention of skin disorders

Maintenance of healthy skin

Avoid strong or harsh soaps or detergents.
Keep skin well hydrated; apply lubricating lotion or cream to dry areas after bathing.
Avoid scraping or stripping skin surface by dry razors or removal of tape.
Dry damp areas (such as between toes) well to prevent maceration of skin.
Wear loose clothing on hot days to permit loss of heat by evaporation.

Avoidance of causative agents

Avoid agents that cause skin disorders in most people, for example, poison ivy, excessive sunlight.
Avoid specific agents known to cause a skin disorder in self.
Use protective skin lotions when exposed to excessive sunlight.

Observation of skin changes

Note and report changes in size, colour, or general appearance of pigmented skin areas, particularly moles.
Note and report changes in size and appearance of existing skin lesions.

Avoidance of self-treatment

Do not use previously prescribed prescriptions on new and different skin lesions.
Seek medical advice when skin conditions develop.

diseases, and immunosuppressed conditions. Oral candidiasis may be the first sign of AIDS or AIDS-related complex (ARC).[29]

The more common fungal infections are the dermatophytoses (tinea). Tinea *capitis* (Fig. 34-3) (inappropriately called *ringworm of the scalp*) is transmitted readily under crowded conditions where poor hygiene exists. Minor scalp trauma facilitates implantation of the spores; hence the infection can be spread by contaminated barber's instruments, combs, or sharp brushes. Tinea *cruris* occurs frequently in men, especially those who have tinea *pedis* and those who frequently wear athletic support or tight shorts, but it is being seen more frequently in women who wear tight jeans or tights. Tinea *corporis* is seen primarily on the face, arms, or trunk, especially on exposed areas.

The most common dermatophytosis is tinea *pedis,* or athlete's foot. There are many misconceptions about prevention and treatment of athlete's foot. It is often confused with other foot eruptions, such as contact dermatitis, psoriasis, or simple intertrigo (chronic bacterial infection of the areas between the toes, or intertriginous areas). Factors that may lessen infection include wearing sandal-type shoes or going barefoot (to decrease tissue moisture) and using good foot hygiene including washing the feet frequently and drying well between the toes.

Tinea *versicolour* is caused by a different fungus than the other types of tinea. It is a common, noncontagious, superficial fungal infection.

Most fungal infections are chronic with periods of exacerbation. Topical agents that are most effective are broad-spectrum imidazoles: clotrimazole, econazole, miconazole, and ketoconazole.

Parasitic infestations

Parasites may live on the body or clothing (lice) or burrow under the skin (itch mite), causing inflammations of the skin (Table 34-5).

Lice obtain their nutrition by sucking blood from the skin. They leave their eggs on the skin surface attached to hair shafts, and this results in the transference from person to person. Control and treatment of pediculosis (lice infestation) can be hampered by people of all incomes who refuse to admit that the lice exist among family members.

Scabies is highly prevalent in areas of overcrowding. It is transmitted easily by skin to skin contact. The itch mite penetrates the skin and lays eggs; the larvae mature in 10 days and move to the skin surface, where the female is impregnated; then the cycle is repeated. The incubation period varies, but often a long period elapses before symptoms are noted. Scabies occurs among all age and socioeconomic groups.

Nursing Process
Assessment

Subjective data

Subjective data from people with inflammations of the skin are centered on the extent of *itching* and *pain*. Data are collected concerning the site, intensity, duration, and methods found to be helpful in alleviation of the discomfort. Data are also collected concerning the person's knowledge of the type of infection, measures to control spread, and prescribed treatments to be carried out at home.

Objective data

The skin is routinely assessed during physical inspection and whenever there is patient contact, such as while providing hygiene care, comfort measures, or prescribed treatments. Changes in previous lesions or occurrence of new lesions are reported and recorded.

REVIEW

Table 34-2 Bacterial skin infections

Type	Description	Signs and symptoms	Medical therapy
Folliculitis	Infections of the hair follicles, primarily by *Staphylococcus*; occurs frequently after tar or occlusive therapy	Itching of hairy areas, pustules in hair follicles; abscess may develop	Saline soaks; topical antibiotics
Furuncles (boil)	Deep folliculitis or nodule around hair follicle	Local swelling and redness; severe local pain; core turns yellow and "points" in 3 to 5 days; may rupture spontaneously	Systemic antibiotics; hot moist compresses (discontinued when drainage starts); incision and drainage; topical antibiotics after incision and drainage
Carbuncle	Cluster of furuncles		
Cellulitis	Diffuse spreading infection of skin and subcutaneous tissue, usually resulting from cocci	Area is warm, swollen, painful with poorly defined borders; fever, malaise, leukocytosis	Hot moist dressings; systemic antibiotics; rest

REVIEW

Table 34-3 Viral skin inflammations

Type	Description	Signs and symptoms	Medical therapy
Herpes simplex (cold sore)	Infection by herpes simplex virus; may occur anywhere but seen primarily on lips, mouth, genitalia	Initial burning and itching; appearance of painful, small, grouped vesicles; crust forms, healing within 10 to 14 days	Primarily symptomatic; early application of zinc sulphate solution may help;analgesics; acyclovir for immunocompromised patients
Herpes zoster (shingles)	Acute vesicular eruption by the V-Z virus along a nerve pathway	Cluster of skin vesicles along course peripheral sensory nerves; usually one side, primarily on thorax or face; crust develops and drops off in 10 to 14 days; pain, malaise, fever, may persist	Acyclovir; analgesics; rest; calamine lotion for itching; steroids to decrease incidence of Postherpetic neuralgia: analgesics
Herpetic whitlow	HSV infection of finger seen most often in health care professionals	Vesicles on finger preceded by intense itching/pain; fever, chills, and malaise may occur	Primarily symptomatic; elevation and immobilization of finger; analgesics
Warts (verruca)	Benign growths from a viral infection; plantar warts on soles of feet grow inward; anogenital warts have a cauliflower appearance	Small, circumscribed, painless, hyperkeratotic papules, usually on hands, may disappear spontaneously; pain with plantar warts; itching with anogenital warts	Removal by electrodesiccation or cryosurgery (liquid nitrogen)

Diagnostic tests

Tzanck smear

Vesicular disorders may be differentiated by a Tzanck smear. The top of the vesicle is cut and a smear taken from the base of the vesicle. Examination of the smear may identify a virus (herpes simplex or zoster) or acantholytic cells (pemphigus). The test is negative for vesicles from burns, erythema multiforme, or dermatitis herpetiforme.

KOH test

If the causative factor is believed to be a fungus, a potassium hydroxide (KOH) examination may be carried out. The lesion is scraped with a knife blade, and the scraping is placed on a slide, which is set in a KOH solution before microscopic study.

Culture

If the primary lesion is a pustule, a culture of the pustule contents may be taken to identify the causative organism. Streptococci and staphylococci are commonly seen.

Wood's light

To assist in the diagnoses of fungal infections of the hair and skin (tinea), the hair is illuminated by a special filter

REVIEW

Table 34-4 Fungal skin inflammations

Type	Description	Signs and symptoms	Medical therapy
Candidiasis (moniliasis)	Overgrowth of yeast-like fungus, primarily in mouth and vagina	Mouth; white spots like milk curd Vagina: cheesy discharge, itching	Ketoconazole orally, nystatin orally or vaginally, clotrimazole or cream
Dermatophytoses			
Tinea capitis	Fungal infection of scalp (ringworm of scalp)	Round lesion with erythema, slight scaling and some pustules around edge; temporary alopecia	Antifungal medication by shampoo or topical application
Tinea corporis	Fungal infection of nonhairy parts of body (ringworm of body)	Flat lesions with clear centres and red borders	Oral griseofulvin and topical application of antifungal medication
Tinea cruris	Fungal infection of groin	Brown to red lesion extending outward from groin, itching	Same as for tinea corporis
Tinea pedis (athlete's foot)	Fungal infection between and under toes	Cracks between toes, maceration, vesicular lesions; toenails may become thickened and discolored	Oral griseofulvin for weeks or months, antifungal topical medication
Tinea versicolour	Superficial fungal infection, mostly on trunk	Hypopigmented macules that do not tan; scaling, mild pruritis	Topical selenium sulphide; imidazole creams

REVIEW

Table 34-5 Parasitic infestations

Type	Description	Signs and symptoms	Medical therapy
Pediculosis			
Head lice	Attach to hair shaft and lay eggs (nits); transmitted by direct contact	Itching of scalp, excoriation of skin, and secondary infection from scratching	Topical application of permethrin, malathion, or phenothrin) by shampoo, lotion, or cream; combing with fine-toothed comb to remove nits
Body lice	Found in seams of underclothing; transmitted by direct contact, clothing, bed linen	Same as for head lice	Topical application of permethrin or malathion by lotion or cream
Pubic lice	Resemble tiny crabs; nits are visible in pubic hair; transmitted by sexual contact, bed linen, towels	Same as for head lice	Same as for body lice
Scabies	Female itch mite burrows under skin and lays eggs; transmitted by prolonged contact	Severe itching; wavy brownish, threadlike lines seen mostly on hands, arms, and body folds and genitalia; secondary infections	Lindane, malathion or permethrin

(Wood's filter) attached to an ultraviolet lamp. The infected hairs fluoresce a brilliant green or appear luminous under the light.

Nursing Analysis

Problems are determined from analysis of patient data. Possible problems for the person with an inflammatory skin disorder may include, but are not limited to, the following:

Problem	Possible aetiologies
Pain: itching	Skin lesions
Knowledge deficit	Lack of exposure or recall, information misinterpretation

Planning: expected patient outcomes

Expected patient outcomes for the person with an inflammatory skin disorder may include, but are not limited to, the following:

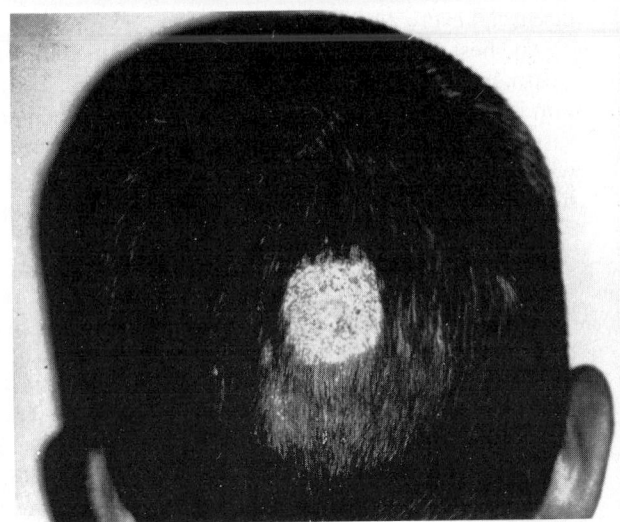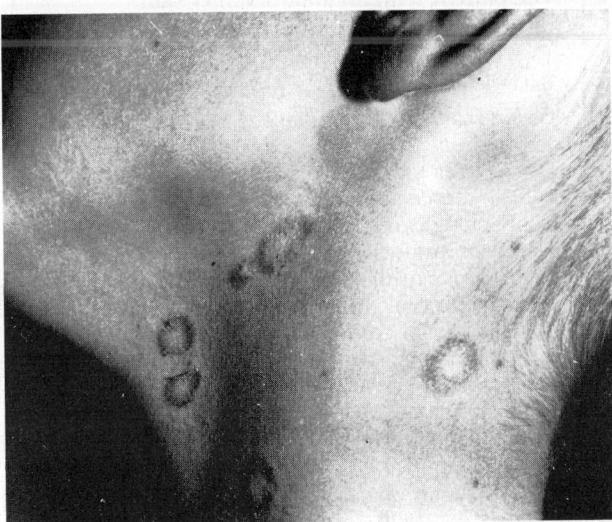

Fig. 34-3　**A,** Tinea capitis. **B,** Tinea corporis. (From Stewart WD, Danto JL, Maddin S: *Dermatology: diagnosis and treatment of cutaneous disorders,* ed 4, St Louis, 1978, Mosby–Year Book.)

1. States feeling comfortable.
2. Describes measures to prevent spread.
3. Describes prescribed treatment measures.
4. Describes plans for medical follow-up for severe inflammatory disorders.

Implementation

Assisting with achievement of therapeutic goals

Inflammatory skin disorders are treated primarily by cleaning the lesions, then applying a topical medication. If pruritus or discomfort is present, antipruritic agents or analgesics may be prescribed.

Topical medications

Topical medications can be prepared in a variety of bases. *Powders* are effective in reducing friction and moisture in intertriginous areas (between fingers and toes). The powders are first sprinkled into the hand, then applied to the skin to avoid releasing excess powder into the air and causing irritation to the mucous membrane. Powders are used sparingly to prevent caking and are not used on wet surfaces because this leads to caking. Cornstarch is *not* recommended, because it encourages growth of yeast, bacteria, and fungi.

Lotions must be shaken well because the insoluble powder may settle out. Lotions with a water or alcohol base are applied by patting gently. (Alcohol increases the cooling effect of the lotion.) A gauze pledget may be used to apply extremely thin lotions. Lotions with an oily base are applied thinly and evenly with the palm of the hand. A small area of skin is often tested to determine whether the cream or lotion will be tolerated over the entire body. The topical medication is applied to a small area, about 4 cm (1.5 in), on the person's forearm. The time and exact location of the trial are recorded, and the skin response to the trial medication is observed after 24 hours.

Ointments do not usually leave an oily residue on the skin unless they have a paraffin base. A nonporous covering such as plastic should not be used over an ointment unless so prescribed, because the heat retention may increase percutaneous absorption of the medication.

Ointments may be applied by the patient with gloved hands or with the bare palm, depending on the type of ointment used (gloves should be used by health care professionals). If a dressing is to be applied, the ointment may be spread on the dressing with a wooden spatula before application to the skin. Dithranol may be caustic to normal skin, so gloves should be worn. Coal tar is always applied in firm, long, downward strokes to prevent folliculitis, because tar is an irritant. Creams, as opposed to ointments, may be rubbed in. When ointments are applied at frequent intervals (4-6 hours), the remaining ointment is removed before more ointment is applied.

Wet dermatological dressings

Wet dressings are used frequently over various lesions for cooling, drying, antipruritic, vasoconstricting, or debriding effects. Plain tap water or physiological saline solution may be used or medications may be added. An astringent effect may be obtained with the use of aluminium acetate solution.

The type of dressing material used for a wet dressing should not have a cotton filling, because cotton leaves particles and a residue on the skin, which may cause irritation. Several layers of fine mesh gauze are ideal, and roller gauze may be used for extremities. A face mask may be designed by cutting openings for the eyes, nose, and mouth from several thicknesses of gauze. At home, muslin-

Guidelines for Care

The patient with an inflammatory skin disorder

Bacterial infections

Cleanse skin well with soap and water or with saline.
Use wet compresses to apply heat or as a medium for medication (for example, saline).
Apply prescribed antibiotic topical medication.
Elevate an extremity with cellulitis.
Teach family members how to prevent spread of staphylococcal infections:
  Avoidance of contamination from drainage
  Cleansing practices
  Disposal of contaminated articles

Viral inflammations

Assist with relief of pain and pruritus:
  Loose clothing to minimize contact
  Analgesics as prescribed
  Warm moist compresses
  Neuralgia after herpes zoster:
    Analgesics as prescribed (narcotics are usually avoided)
    Tranquillizers and sedatives as prescribed
    Other forms of pain relief measures (see Chapter 8) that might be helpful
  Calamine lotion over vesicular areas to relieve itching

Fungal inflammations

Promote dryness of affected area:
  Area dried well after washing
  Powders applied lightly to prevent maceration and caking
  Clean loose-fitting clothing for aeration
  For athlete's foot, cotton socks, changed at least daily; sandal-type shoes when possible
Promote healing:
  Give prescribed topical medication
  Teach need for continuation of treatment for prescribed time (may be weeks or months)

Parasitic infestations

Wash area well before treatment.
Remove nits with a fine-toothed comb.
Apply a *thin* layer of prescribed lotion or cream.
Shampoo, shower, or bathe thoroughly after prescribed time to remove medication.
If eyelashes are involved, remove nits and apply white soft paraffin to smother lice.
Give analgesics or antipruritic agents as necessary.
Teach prevention of spread to all family members:
  Machine wash clothing and bed linens
  Dry clothing and linens in dryer or iron after line drying
  Dry clean clothing that cannot be washed
  Treat all family members and household linens if one is infested

type cotton material such as clean old sheets may be used; the materials need not be sterilized but are washed or discarded every 24 hours.

The best effects of wet dressings are obtained by several treatment periods spaced over the waking hours. The solution is applied at room temperature to prevent the marked vasoconstriction with subsequent vasodilation that occurs with cold solutions. Although the dressings can be kept wet by adding solution, this usually leads to excessive dripping.

Interventions to achieve patient outcomes

Specific nursing interventions are summarized in Box 34-3. General nursing interventions are described below.

Promoting comfort

Pain with skin inflammations is usually minimal except in selected situations such as herpes zoster. In general, aspirin or paracetamol usually suffice as analgesics, and the application of wet dressings and topical medications usually relieves most discomfort from pain. Pruritus (itching) is a major discomfort, to one extent or another, with skin inflammations.

Pathophysiology of pruritus. Pruritus is a cutaneous symptom that provokes the desire to scratch and is an underlying symptom of many disorders. It is a modified form of pain but is less tolerable. It occurs only in the skin, certain mucous membranes, and the eyes. The areas most sensitive to itching are the nostrils, mucocutaneous junction, external ear canal, and perineum.

One of the most common causes of pruritus is dry skin, sometimes occurring as a result of excessive bathing, particularly with bubble bath, which has a drying effect.
Other causes of pruritus include the following:
Skin irritants: plastic or glass fibres, wool, plant products
Insects
Drug reactions
Psychogenic reactions
Skin diseases: inflammations, dermatitis
Infectious diseases
Systemic diseases: obstructive biliary disease (jaundice), uraemia, diabetes mellitus
Neoplasia: Hodgkin's disease, leukaemia, lymphoma
Factors that can intensify itching include vasodilation, tissue anoxia, and stasis of circulation. Pruritus leads to the motor response of scratching. People with very intense itching may excoriate the skin severely by digging deeply into the skin with their fingernails when trying to alleviate the itch. People with generalized itching may be observed to be in almost constant motion—twisting, rubbing, and scratching.

General management for relief of pruritus
1. Apply cold to cause vasoconstriction.
2. Avoid soaps and detergents with dry skin; use a bath oil.
3. Hydrate in a tepid bath followed by immediate application of an emollient lotion.

4. Use cool, light, nonrestrictive clothing or bedclothes.
5. Keep nails trimmed to avoid skin excoriation from scratching.
6. Keep the room cool (about 20° C, or 68° to 70° F) and increase the humidity (30% to 40%).

Baths and soaks

Baths or soaks to a specific part of the body are soothing and antipruritic and are an effective means of rehydrating the skin. Substances may be added to the bath for special therapeutic effects.

Facilitating learning

Prevention of spread

Bacterial infections and parasitic infestations may spread to other people, particularly caregivers and family members, if precautions are not instituted.

For *staphylococcal* infections in hospitalized patients, wound isolation procedures are instituted until drainage subsides. Hands must be washed thoroughly after contact with the patient. Gloves are usually worn when changing dressings.

It is not uncommon for entire families to have some type of staphylococcal infection after one member has had a boil. Teaching includes the following:

1. All family members should bathe and shampoo daily with bacteriostatic soap while infection lasts.
2. Razor blades are discarded after use.
3. Separate towels are used by each family member.
4. Towels are changed daily while infection lasts.
5. Contaminated wound supplies are discarded in two sealed plastic bags.

With *parasitic* infestations, all family members should take one treatment to prevent spread. Clothing, linen, and towels are washed, then dried in an automatic dryer or ironed after line drying, or are dry cleaned. Garments that have been stored for 1 month will not be infested. No special precautions are needed for other objects, because parasites do not live long away from the host.

When caring for people with *herpetic* lesions, the United States Centers for Disease Control (CDC) recommends the use of drainage and secretion precautions (see Chapter 12) until all lesions are crusted. Finger infection (herpetic whitlow, Table 34-3) may result from contact with the herpes simplex virus. To help prevent a disseminated infection, strict isolation precautions are used for protection of the immunocompromised person with a localized herpes zoster infection.

Self-help skills

Many people with skin inflammations will be carrying out treatments at home and, therefore, may need teaching about therapeutic measures. Written instructions are more likely to be followed correctly. Points to stress in teaching include the following:

1. Use medication only as prescribed.
2. Avoid harsh rubbing of the skin.
3. Avoid nonporous covering over dressing unless prescribed.
4. Dissolve completely all solid medications added to baths and soaks.
5. Apply lotions and powders in thin layers.
6. Use old clean sheets, if desired, for wet dressings.

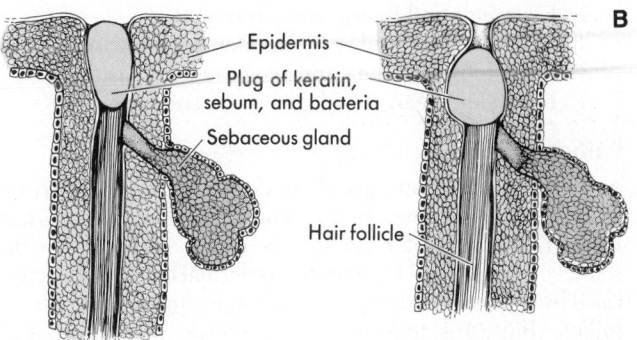

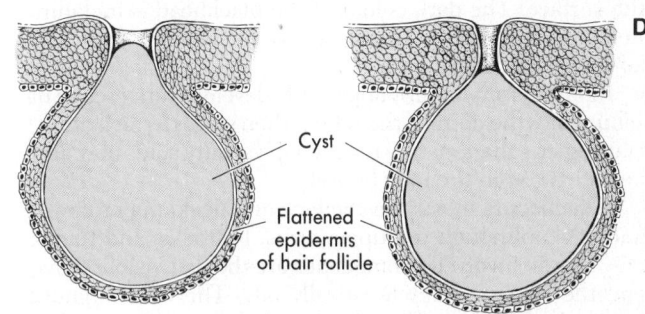

Fig. 34-4 Formation of lesions in acne vulgaris. **A,** Open comedo (blackhead), early stage. **B,** closed comedo (whitehead), early stage. **C,** Cyst formation in open comedo, advanced stage. **D,** Cyst formation in closed comedo, advanced stage. (From Parish JH: *Dermatology and skin care*, New York, 1975, McGraw-Hill.)

Evaluation

Evaluation is based on expected patient outcomes. Questions to consider may include the following:

1. Is the person comfortable?
2. Does the person know how to care for the lesions at home?

ACNE

The major form of acne is acne vulgaris seen mostly in adolescents, although it may occur in adults. A different form is acne rosacea seen in adults.

ACNE VULGARIS

Aetiology

Acne vulgaris is a common skin disorder, the cause of which is unknown but is thought to be multifactorial. Contributing factors may include free fatty acids, endocrine effects, stress, heredity, and infection. Diet and dirt are not causes of acne.[13] The disorder is more quiescent in summer because of the drying effects of the sun.

Prevention

Actions that contribute to plugging of the pilosebaceous follicles are to be avoided.

1. Keep hair and hands away from face.
2. Shampoo hair and scalp frequently.
3. Wear loose clothing and avoid tight collars.
4. Keep skin clean; avoid greasy, oil-based cosmetics.

Pathophysiology

At puberty sebaceous glands undergo enlargement from androgen stimulation. When sebum is released it passes through the follicular canal, where it is combined with sebaceous gland cell fragments, epidermal cells, and bacteria. The sebum and debris may become plugged in the hair follicle (Fig. 34-4) to form an *open comedo* (blackhead) if it is at the surface, or a *closed comedo* (whitehead) if it is below the surface. The dark colour of the blackhead is melanin, not dirt, and results from passage of melanin from the adjoining epidermal cells.

Inflammatory lesions apparently develop from escape of sebum into the dermis; the sebum then serves as an irritant, causing an inflammatory reaction. Free fatty acids may also be an irritant in the follicle itself.

Acne occurs mostly on the face and neck, upper chest, and back, although the upper arms, buttocks, and thighs may also be involved. Comedones are the first visible signs, and the skin is characteristically oily. The inflammatory lesions include papules, pustules, nodules, and cysts. Superficial lesions usually heal without scarring, whereas large lesions often result in scarring if the inflammation has involved the dermis. The typical scar resembles an old volcano (ice-pick scar); however, many other sizes and shapes may result, depending on the depth and extent of the inflammatory lesions.

Interventions

The major medical therapy for acne is drug therapy. *Systemic* therapy includes isotretinoin or antibiotics (tetracyclines, erythromycin). *Topical* therapy with tretinoin is effective. Topical antibiotics lotion or benzoyl peroxide may also be used. Commercial preparations contain benzoyl peroxide. Comedones may be removed with a comedo extractor. Disfiguring scars may be removed by dermabrasion or laser reconstruction (p. 1055).

Counselling and teaching are the major nursing therapies. Stress appears to be one of the causative factors; therefore, the person may be helped by identifying and coping with stressors (Chapter 6). Acne can be a stressor, producing facial disfigurements and sometimes leading to behaviour that is hostile, aggressive, and anxious, as well as shy and withdrawn. Psychological counselling is often desirable. Teaching the person with acne includes the following:

1. General skin care
   a. Keep skin clean; wash face two to three times daily.
   b. Use a medicated soap/cleanser or agent prescribed by doctor.
   c. Avoid vigorous rubbing of the skin (prevent further inflammation).
   d. Use cosmetics that are water based rather than cream based and avoid those that contain wax esters.
   e. Never leave cosmetics on face at night.
2. During therapy
   a. Follow the prescribed therapy even when immediate improvement is not noted for 2 to 3 weeks.
   b. Expect skin desquamation during therapy.
   c. Avoid using self-remedies during therapy.
   d. Remove cosmetics before applying topical medica-tions.
   e. Avoid exposure to direct sunlight if using tretinoin or taking tetracycline (photosensitivity).
   f. Avoid pregnancy if taking isotretinoin (possibility of birth defects).

ACNE ROSACEA

Acne rosacea is a skin condition that usually affects people over 25 years of age. The actual cause is unknown although many causative factors have been suggested. Acne rosacea begins with redness over the cheeks and nose, followed by papules, pustules, and enlargement of superficial blood vessels. Years of acne rosacea lead to an irregular, bulbous thickening of the skin of the distal part of the nose (rhinophyma), with a red-purple discolouration and dilated follicles.

Treatment includes systemic tetracycline, metronidazole, or isotretinoin. Topical therapy for papules and pustules may be prescribed: hydrocortisone cream, topical antibiotics, or benzoyl peroxide. Avoiding stimuli that cause vasodilation seems appropriate. Rhinophyma may be treated by plastic surgery.

DERMATITIS

Dermatitis, a superficial inflammation of the skin, refers to several different conditions resulting in the same type of lesions (Table 34-6). The term *eczema* is often used synonymously with dermatitis but frequently refers to the chronic type.

Aetiology and Pathophysiology

Contact dermatitis may result from irritation of the skin from the substance itself (*irritant contact dermatitis*) or from a hypersensitivity immune reaction from contact with a *specific* antigen (*allergic contact dermatitis*). The sensitizing allergen may reach the site by direct contact; by indirect contact such as transmission by animals, from one part of the body to the other, by the hands, or on clothing; or by the air such as in smoke.

Atopic dermatitis is hereditary hypersensitivity of the skin that lowers the threshold to pruritus so that minor stimuli cause intense itching. Exacerbating factors include sudden changes in temperature or humidity; exercise; psychological stress; fibres such as wool, fur, or nylon; detergents; and perfumes. There is a marked tendency towards vasoconstriction of superficial blood vessels, and the skin blanches readily. Adults with eczema often have had atopic dermatitis during infancy and adolescence.

People with atopic dermatitis are highly susceptible to viral infections, especially herpes, and to bacterial infections such as those caused by *Staphylococcus* or beta haemolytic *Streptococcus*. There is also an increased incidence of fungal infections such as tinea.

Stasis dermatitis results from decreased circulation in the legs. The cause of *seborrhoeic* dermatitis (dandruff) is

REVIEW

Table 34-6   Types of dermatitis

Type	Signs and symptoms	Medical therapy
Contact	Site and pattern of lesions depend on exposure pattern; erythema, local oedema, vesicles, then oozing, crusting and scaling; pruritus Chronic: skin becomes brownish and thickened	Weeping uninfected lesions: wet dressings with aluminium acetate solution; topical steroids; systemic corticosteroids for acute conditions
Atopic	Pruritus; lesions similar to contact dermatitis; become localized in adults to antecubital and popliteal areas, behind ears, under chin	Same as above
Stasis	Skin reddened and oedematous, pruritus, infection from excoriations with scratching	Elevation of legs; wet compresses for weeping lesions, topical corticosteroids
Seborrhoeic (dandruff)	Erythematous scaly lesions of scalp, face, ears, chest, or back	Zinc pyrithione shampoo for scalp; topical steroids for severe lesions

basically genetic and is influenced by factors such as hormones, nutrition, infection, and stress.[49]

Nursing Process

Assessment

Subjective data

When acute lesions from contact dermatitis or exacerbation of eczema occur, it is important to identify the causative factors in order to avoid further contacts or to change, if possible, any exacerbating factor. Data to collect initially include the following:

1. Knowledge of causative factors and method of contact
2. Possible contacts with irritants in the home, at work, or during recreational activities
3. History of recurrent infections (possible decreased immune response)
4. New drug prescriptions, especially penicillins or sulphonamides
5. Increase in stress noted by patient
6. Alleviating factors (doctor or self-prescribed)
7. Extent of pruritus and alleviating factors

Objective data

The lesions are inspected daily for changes and presence of infections. Observations are also made concerning the extent of scratching of the lesions by the patient.

Diagnostic tests

Hypersensitivity to specific antigens can be tested in vivo by skin tests or by the use test (Chapter 33). In skin testing, the antigens are administered to the skin either through intradermal, scratch or patch tests, or an allergen may be instilled in the eye.

Nursing Analysis

Problems are determined from analysis of patient data. Possible problems for the person with dermatitis may include, but are not limited to, the following:

Problem	Possible aetiologies
Pain: itching	Skin lesions
Knowledge deficit	Lack of exposure/recall, information misinterpretation

Planning: expected patient outcomes

Expected patient outcomes for the person with dermatitis may include, but are not limited to, the following:

1. States itching is decreased.
2. Describes:
   a. Causative agents (if known), source of the agent, and method of control
   b. Measures to prevent further contact
   c. Problems of self-treatment
   d. Treatment measures to be carried out at home

Implementation

Assisting with achievement of therapeutic goals

Weeping infected lesions respond rapidly to wet dressings with aluminium acetate solution for 20 minutes four times daily. Crusts and scales are not removed but are allowed to drop off naturally as the skin heals.

The major form of *topical* therapy consists of corticosteroid cream or ointment. Fluorinated corticosteroids may be used for localized lesions in adults but are *never used on the face*. An occlusion wrap over the steroid in adults may enhance the steroid effect but may lead to folliculitis. The occlusion wrap consists of a nonpermeable covering, such as plastic wrap, over the dressing; it is only applied when prescribed by the doctor.

Interventions to achieve patient outcomes

Promoting comfort

The focus of care is relief of the pruritus in order to break the itch-scratch cycle that leads to lesions and discomfort. Measures to promote relief of itching are described on p. 1040. Application of the wet dressings and topical steroids helps to reduce the itching. Colloidal baths may be helpful. Sedatives and tranquillizers are used judiciously to help decrease itching but not induce sleepiness.

Facilitating learning

The more the person knows about the condition and what will affect it, the better the person can prevent further contacts and enhance recovery. Teaching includes avoidance of exacerbating factors, positive effects of sunlight, and dangers of self-treatment.

Table 34-7   Types of papulosquamous disorders

Type	Characteristics	Signs and symptoms	Medical therapy
Psoriasis	Common hereditary chronic disorder; not infectious or contagious; has periods of exacerbation	Elevated, erythematous, sharply circumscribed, scaling plaques; occur mostly on scalp, elbows, and knees; mild pruritus; nails become yellowed and pitted	Wet dressings with acute flare-ups; topical steroids with occlusive wraps; PUVA therapy; coal tar therapy followed by ultra-violet light; dithranol
Pityriasis rosea	Common skin disorder in young adults, especially women; not contagious; last 6 to 8 weeks, rarely recurs	Starts with single lesion; oval, thin scaly border, yellowish centre; multiple lesions appear later; pruritus	Topical steroids; ultraviolet light, systemic steroids in severe cases
Lichen planus	Common skin disorder; may resolve in 6 to 18 months or become chronic	Shiny flat-topped papules on flexor surfaces of wrists, ankles, trunk, and mucous membranes; severe pruritus; nails become distorted	Topical steroids with occlusive wrap; intralesional or systemic steroids, PUVA therapy; isotretinoin or etretinate orally

Evaluation

Evaluation is based on expected patient outcomes. Questions to consider may include the following:

1. Is itching decreased?
2. Does the person know how to care for the skin at home and how to prevent further recurrence?

SCALING PAPULAR DISORDERS

Papulosquamous disorders are characterized by papular lesions with scaling borders. The most common of these is *psoriasis* (Table 34-7). There are no precipitating factors for psoriasis, but some people may develop exacerbations after climatic changes, stress, trauma, or infection. Pregnant women often see a remission of symptoms. *Pityriasis rosea* occurs mostly in the spring or autumn; the cause is unknown. *Lichen planus* may follow exposure to dyes, colour film developer, or gold, but usually the cause is unknown.

Pathophysiology of Psoriasis

The turnover time for normal skin is 28 days. After the cells in the basal layer of the skin divide, it normally takes them 14 days to reach the stratum corneum (outer skin layer) and an additional 14 days for the cells to be sloughed off. In psoriasis the time is accelerated to 4 to 7 days. Much of the scaling seen in psoriasis is rapid shedding of the cells; treatment is therefore based on slowing the mitotic activity.

Nursing Process
Assessment

Subjective data include the following:
1. Knowledge about the disease

2. Measures used for control at home
3. Concerns about appearance
4. Usual recreational and social activities

Objective data include observations regarding changes in the lesions.

Nursing Analysis

Problems are determined from analysis of patient data. Possible problems for the person with psoriasis may include, but are not limited to, the following:

Problem	Possible aetiologies
Body image disturbance	Change in body appearance
Knowledge deficit	Lack of exposure/recall, information misinterpretation

Planning: expected patient outcomes

Expected patient outcomes for the person with psoriasis may include, but are not limited to, the following:
1. Participates in social activities.
2. Describes:
   a. The nature of the disorder (noncurable, recurrence of symptoms).
   b. Problems with self-medication.
   c. The prescribed treatment programme.

Implementation
Assisting with achievement of therapeutic goals

Although there are several therapeutic regimens for psoriasis, the more common treatments are steroids under occlusive wraps, coal tar therapy, and PUVA therapy.

Application of occlusive wrap

Occlusive wraps are usually prescribed over topical steroid therapy for psoriasis. Plastic wrap or plastic bags may

> ### *Nursing Care Plan*   **Patient with psoriasis**
>
> DATA: Mrs. L., age 35, was referred to an outpatients clinic for a 6-day Goeckerman regimen therapy (coal tar with exposure to ultraviolet light). Mrs. L. told the nurse that she recently sent away for a new ointment that was supposed to cure her psoriasis, but the lesions began to flare up and itching increased. She also said that her husband has been urging her to go out with him more to social events, but her arms and legs have "looked so bad" that she has not wanted others to see her until she is better.
>
> *Nursing analysis:*   Body image disturbance: related to lesions on arms and legs
>
> | Expected patient outcomes | Nursing interventions | Rationale |
> | --- | --- | --- |
> | Mrs. L. states plans to go out socially with husband | Help Mrs. L. identify her positive attributes
Discuss with Mrs. L. types of clothing that could hide the more obvious lesions | Awareness of positive attributes helps to increase self-esteem
Hiding the lesions may help her feel better about herself and increase her desire to interact with others |
>
> *Nursing analysis:*   Knowledge deficit related to information misinterpretation
>
> | Expected patient outcomes | Nursing interventions | Rationale |
> | --- | --- | --- |
> | Mrs. L. describes chronicity of psoriasis and plans to follow only prescribed treatment | Review her understanding of the nature of psoriasis
Explain the lack of cure for psoriasis and problems with self-treatment
Suggest she discuss with doctor lotions or ointments to use after her present treatment when lesions itch or flare up
Review with her how to apply ointments. | Lesions may fade with treatment only to recur. Self-treatment products are often ineffective and costly

Ointment is more effective if spread in thin layer over plaques |

be used to cover large areas. The bags should not be rapidly flammable. If large areas must be covered for home therapy, a plastic exercise body suit can be worn, particularly for overnight therapy.

Coal tar therapy

Coal tar preparations may be applied as a topical medication, as a bath, or in combination with ultraviolet light (UVA). In the latter case the tar preparation is applied 12 hours before the UVA treatment. Creams and ointments are applied to the affected area for 5 minutes, then the excess is removed by patting with tissue to minimize staining. Areas treated with coal tar preparation should be protected from direct sunlight for at least 24 hours after application of the tar product. Folliculitis may result from coal tar therapy.

PUVA therapy

PUVA therapy consists of a combination of orally administered methoxsalen and long-wave ultraviolet light (UVA), hence the name. Methoxsalen is a photosensitizing agent. The person is exposed to UVA 2 hours after ingestion of the methoxsalen. Some side effects of PUVA therapy include pruritus, erythema, localized blistering, a moderate flare-up of psoriasis, and transient nausea. Because the skin remains photosensitive until methoxsalen is excreted, people receiving this treatment are warned to avoid exposure to the sun for at least 8 hours after ingestion of the medication.

Interventions to achieve patient outcomes

Counselling and teaching

Because the lesions are commonly found on visible skin areas, people with psoriasis are faced with a socially disabling disease. They may need help in identifying and coping with their feelings and with changes that may occur in their life-style. Arms and legs can be covered with clothing if the person is sensitive about appearance. Social contacts are encouraged.

Lesions may fade with treatment, only to recur eventually in the same area or elsewhere. The disease is not curable and may wax and wane continuously. People who are not aware of this may lose confidence in the doctor and seek a quick cure. Because psoriasis is so common and so stubborn in response to treatment, manufacturers of patent remedies find a lucrative field for their products among people with the disease. Self-treatment may lead to considerable expense for worthless products, increased discom-

Table 34-8 Tumours of the skin

Tumour	Description	Medical therapy
Keratoses		
Corn	Thickened skin lesion with a centre core that thickens inwardly	Corrective shoes; felt pad with a centre hole for relief of pressure
Callus	Thickened horny skin layer in circumscribed lesions often seen on plantar surface of foot	Well-fitting shoes, moleskin and padding; scraping with emery board; salicylic acid plasters
Seborrhoeic keratosis	Benign tumours; resemble large, darkened, greasy warts	Do not require treatment; may be removed by curettage and electrodesiccation or cryotherapy
Actinic keratosis (senile, solar)	Benign round or irregular tumours; red-brown to grey in colour, with a dry scaly appearance; 25% may become malignant	Removal by curettage and electrodesiccation or cryotherapy
Premalignant		
Leukoplakia	Thickened white or reddish patch on mucous membrane of mouth or vagina; may develop into invasive squamous cell carcinoma	Small lesions removed by electrodesiccation; large lesions excised
Pigmented naevi (mole)	Circumscribed pigmented papules; brown moles with hair or evenly coloured dark moles are usually benign	Excised for cosmetic reasons or if sudden change in size or colour, or bleeding
Malignant		
Squamous cell carcinoma	Malignant tumour of surface epidermis; starts as a firm module, becomes indurated with an inflammatory base; may metastasize if on lip or ear (Fig. 34-5)	Removal by surgical excision, curettage with electrodesiccation, irradiation, or chemosurgery
Basal cell carcincoma	Malignant tumour primarily over hairy areas; tumours have a translucent appearance with indurated centre; may be ulcerated with crusting; grow slowly and rarely metastasize	Same as above
Malignant melanoma	Most serious but relatively uncommon skin cancer; lesions vary in appearance and rate of growth; often have irregular pigmentation; metastasize frequently; early diagnosis leads to more favourable prognosis	Total wide excision with skin grafts to cover defects in many cases; chemotherapy, immunotherapy
Kaposi's sarcoma	Commonly seen with AIDS; discrete red, purple, or dark plaques or nodules on skin and mucous membranes; slowly progressive	Radiation therapy may be given for palliation

fort, and delay in treatment of acute episodes. People with psoriasis are encouraged to consult a dermatologist as needed.

Evaluation

Evaluation is based on expected patient outcomes. Questions to consider may include the following:

1. Is the person planning social activities with others?
2. Does the person know the nature of the disease (incurable)?
3. Does the person plan to follow medical therapy (rather than self-treatment) when exacerbation occurs?

SKIN REACTIONS FROM SYSTEMIC DISEASES

Changes in the skin may result from systemic conditions, most commonly dermatitis medicamentosa, and erythema multiforme.

DERMATITIS MEDICAMENTOSA

Skin lesions may result from toxic, metabolic, or allergic reactions to drugs. Many of the reactions are hypersensitivity immune reactions and include fever, malaise, and vasculitis

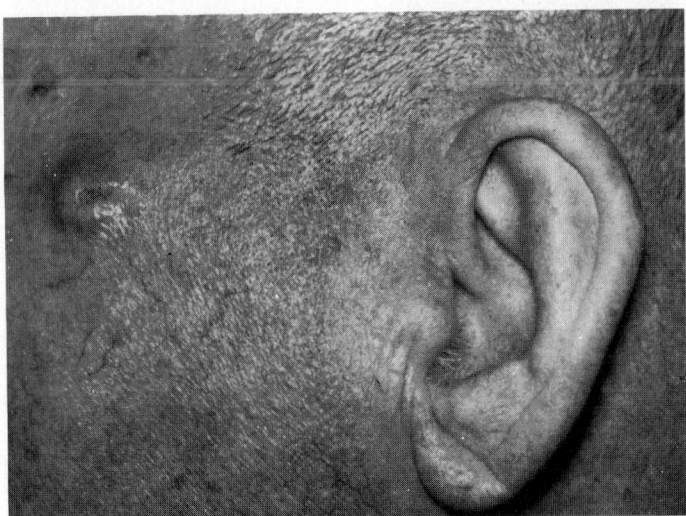

Fig. 34-5   Squamous cell carcinoma in infratemporal area, one of the commonest sites for this tumour. (From Stewart WD, Danto JL, Maddin S: *Dermatology: diagnosis and treatment of cutaneous disorders,* ed 4, St Louis, 1978, Mosby–Year Book.)

in addition to skin changes. The rash is often a bright red colour, semiconfluent, maculopapular, generalized, and bilateral. It can appear at any time, but the onset is usually sudden. Hypersensitivity occurs early when previous sensitization has taken place.

People are asked upon hospitalization if they have any allergies. For drug allergies, a sticker indicating the drug is placed on every drug prescription chart sheet to alert the doctor or nurse not to order or give the drug to the patient. Sudden skin changes in patients receiving medications are brought to the doctor's attention.

Teaching the patient may include the suggestion that the patient wear a Medic-Alert bracelet specifying the drug to which the patient is allergic so that the drug is not administered unknowingly in an emergency situation. People who are taking drugs that cause photosensitivity reactions are advised to avoid direct exposure to sunlight.

ERYTHEMA MULTIFORME

Erythema multiforme is a skin condition believed to occur secondary to an underlying systemic disease such as an infection. The skin eruption is characterized by red to purple macules, papules, and vesicles, and may be preceded by fever, chest pain, and arthralgia. The treatment is to seek out the underlying cause and eliminate it if possible.

TUMOURS OF THE SKIN

Aetiology

In the United Kingdom skin cancer (not including melanoma) accounts for 10–11% of all cases of malignant disease.

Although melanoma affects only a small number of people it is becoming more common (doubles every 10–15 years). Tumours of the skin may be benign (keratoses), premalignant, or malignant (Table 34-8).

Pathophysiology

The term *keratosis* refers to any cornification or growth of the horny layer of the skin; keratoses are benign growths. Corns and calluses result from pressure or friction from poorly fitting shoes, faulty weight-bearing, or with neuropathies such as diabetic neuropathy. Seborrhoeic keratoses are commonly seen in older people. Actinic keratoses result from exposure of the skin to radiation, primarily solar. They are noted most often on exposed skin areas of people who work outdoors and on older people. Light-skinned people are more vulnerable to skin changes from irradiation. Actinic keratoses may develop into squamous cell carcinomas.

The term *premalignant* does *not* imply that all such lesions become malignant; it does imply that the tendency to become malignant exists. Leukoplakia develop in the mucous membranes of the mouth or vagina; red patches (erythroleukoplakia) have a higher malignancy potential than white patches. External irritants, such as poorly fitting dentures, cheek biting, and pipe or cigarette smoking, appear to have an aetiological relationship to oral leukoplakia. Chronic maceration, friction, and senile atrophy may lead to leukoplakia of the vagina. Pigmented naevi are commonly seen in all people. Benign moles have an even colour.

Malignant tumours, with the exception of some tumours such as malignant melanoma, are often of less serious consequence than malignant tumours elsewhere on the body. Skin carcinomas appear mostly on exposed skin or at

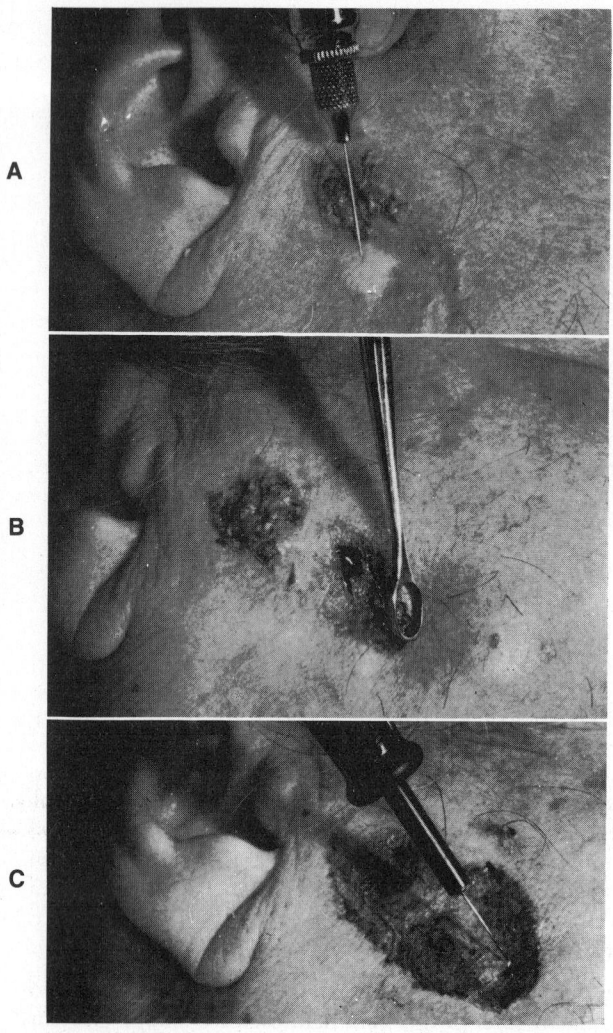

Fig. 34-6 **A,** Infiltration with local anaesthesia. **B,** Curettage. **C,** Electrodesiccation for haemostasis. (From Stewart WD, Danto JL, Maddin S: *Dermatology: diagnosis and treatment of cutaneous disorders,* ed 4, St Louis, 1978, Mosby–Year Book.)

areas of chronic irritation. Squamous cell carcinomas that develop on hair-bearing skin rarely metastasize, but lesions of the lip or ear frequently metastasize to regional lymph nodes. Basal cell carcinomas grow slowly and rarely metastasize, but untreated tumours can become locally invasive with severe tissue destruction, infection, and haemorrhage.

Prevention

Primary prevention of skin tumours includes protection of the skin from excessive solar radiation and other ultraviolet rays. Preventive measures include the following:

1. Limit sun exposure between 11 AM and and 3 PM when rays are the strongest (UV rays can pass through clouds and through 3 feet of water).
2. Wear protective clothes when in the sun, such as hats, long sleeves, long trousers, and sun glasses.
3. Use a sunscreen with a sun protection factor (SPF) of at least 15. Be sure the sunscreen protects against UVA and UVB rays.
4. Apply sunscreen over all exposed areas 15 to 20 minutes before going outdoors.
5. Avoid tanning lamps (they emit UV rays).

Secondary prevention consists of early detection of skin cancers, especially melanomas. Activities include the following:

1. Do skin self-examination monthly after a bath or shower, looking for changes in skin lesions:
   a. Stand before a mirror; examine front, back, and both sides
   b. Check forearms and upper underarms, and backs of legs (may be easier to do this while sitting)
   c. Check back of neck using a hand mirror
   d. Palpate scalp carefully; separate hair to examine any rough surfaces
2. Report the following changes to the doctor:
   a. Development of a ring of new pigment around the base of a mole
   b. Development of uneven pigmentation
   c. Sudden growth in size of a mole or tumour
   d. Loss of hair in a mole or sudden growth of hair on a nonhair-bearing mole
   e. Bleeding in a mole

Medical Therapy

Methods of therapy for skin tumour include surgery, curettage with electrodesiccation, cryosurgery, or irradiation.

Surgery

Ninety per cent of skin tumours are removed by excisional surgery. A punch biopsy may be used for identification of basal cell carcinomas. Superficial lesions can be removed by slicing off the lesion with a sharp blade. This is especially useful for removing flat lesions. *Moh's procedure* removes a malignant lesion in layers, with each layer examined under a microscope to determine where the tumour ends. This produces less loss of underlying healthy tissue.

Curettage with electrodesiccation

A spoon-shaped instrument with sharp edges is used in a downward scraping motion across a lesion (Fig. 38-6). A local anaesthetic is usually first injected around the lesion. Curettage is usually followed by electrodesiccation to stop the bleeding.

In *electrodesiccation* an electric current is used to coagulate the tissue and curtail capillary bleeding. It may also be used to cut tissue under local anaesthesia. After most electrosurgical procedures the wound is left exposed to air dry. Dressings may be used if the area is subject to frequent trauma or rubbing or if oozing is present. The wound may be wiped with 70% alcohol to hasten drying. A haemostatic nonocclusive dressing may be made by covering the wound with hydrocolloid dressing.

Cryosurgery

Cryosurgery is the rapid freezing of tissue with substances such as solid carbon dioxide or liquid nitrogen. The rapid freezing causes formation of intracellular ice, which destroys the cell membranes and produces cell dehydration. Cryosurgery is frequently used for removal of warts and keloids as well as removal of skin tumours (benign and malignant).

Although cryosurgery is not usually painful, a tingling pain occurs when the freezing substance is applied and may be uncomfortable to some people, particularly if multiple lesions are treated. Local anaesthesia may be necessary. Analgesics may be helpful during thawing.

Tissue necrosis may not be evident until 24 hours after cryosurgery. A clear or haemorrhagic bulla forms during the first day, but inflammatory reactions and bleeding are unusual. A serous exudate occurs during the first week, followed by eschar, or crust, formation. The crust drops off in 3 to 4 weeks as the underlying tissue heals. Scarring usually results. Hypopigmentation may occur because melanocytes are highly vulnerable to freezing.

Irradiation

X-ray therapy may be used in the treatment of basal cell carcinoma for selected tumours, especially when there are poorly defined margins or when the tumours are located in structures that are difficult to reconstruct, such as the eyelids or the tip of the nose.[56]

MALIGNANT MELANOMA

Melanomas differ from the other types of skin cancers because of the higher incidence of metastasis and mortality. Most deaths from skin cancer result from melanomas. As already stated the incidence of melanomas has been increasing in recent years, probably because of increased exposure to the sun. People with light skin are at increased risk for melanoma.

There are various types of melanomas. Two thirds of the melanomas are *superficial spreading* melanomas, which grow slowly and are slightly elevated, irregularly shaped, notched lesions with variations in colour (blue, black, brown, pink, grey). Less frequently seen (15%) are the *nodular* melanomas, which are blueberry shaped with variations in colour from blue-black to rose-grey. The nodular melanomas grow and metastasize more quickly than other forms. The patient's prognosis is based on the depth of invasion within the skin. The more superficial the growth the better the prognosis. Melanomas on the trunk have a poorer prognosis than those on the extremities.

Although melanomas cannot be prevented, all questionable moles should be examined by a doctor so that early treatment can be instituted if malignancy is diagnosed. Warning signals of melanoma are as follows[1]:

A Asymmetry
B Border irregularity
C Colour not uniform
D Diameter less than 6 mm

The person who has a newly diagnosed melanoma is usually very anxious and requires considerable emotional support. The nursing approach consists of empathic listening and of promoting hope without giving false reassurance. The importance of imediate therapy is stressed because it improves the prognosis. Surgery often involves a wide lesion, and skin grafting may be necessary. Regional lymph nodes are frequently dissected. Chemotherapy and immunotherapy are reserved for metastatic disease.

BURN INJURIES

Burn injuries are in many respects the worst of all tragedies an individual can experience. An intensive burn is an overwhelming insult to the patient physically and psychologically, and it is catastrophic in cost and suffering to the family involved.

Burns are caused by flame, scald, direct contact, chemicals, electrical current, and radiation. Injury is frequently a result of the victim's own actions. Eighty-one percent of the elderly population's burn injuries occur in this manner. Scald injuries are the most frequent type of injury, but flame injury is more serious.

Because of the systemic effects of the burn injury, psychological implications, and prolonged hospitalisation, comprehensive nursing care is required during the acute and long-term recovery phases.

CLASSIFICATION OF BURNS

Traditionally, burns have been classified as firs, second or third degree. A more accurate description is *partial-thickness* and *full-thickness*, which graphically describes the burn and indicates the depth and severity of the tissue injury.

Partial-thickness burs are characterised by destruction of varying depths from the epidermis (outer layer of skin to the dermis (middle layer of skin). Partial-thickness burns of the skin involve a part of the epidermis and dermis. The depth of tissue injury is described further as *superficial partial-thickness*, which *involves only the epidermis*, and *deep partial-thickness*, which *involves the entire epidermis* and *part of the dermis*. Partial-thickness burns are likely to be painful because nerve endings have been injured and exposed. They have the ability to heal because a portion of the epithelial cells has not been destroyed. During the healing phase, dryness and itching are common and are caused by increased vascularization of sebaceous glands, reduction of secretions, and decreased perspiration.

The presence of blisters often indicates a deep partial thickness injury. The blisters may increase in size as the result of continuous exudation and collection of tissue fluid.

Full-thickness burns include destruction of the epidermis and the entire dermis, as well as possible damage to the subutaneous layer, muscle, and bone. Nerve endings are destroyed, resulting in a painless wound. *Eschar, a leathery covering composed of denatured protein, may form as a result of surface dehydration.* Black networks of coagulated capillaries may be seen. Full-thickness burns require skin grafting because the destroyed tissue is unable to epithelialize. Often a deep partial-thickness burn may convert to a full-thickness burn because of infection, trauma, or decreased blood supply.

PATHOPHYSIOLOGY OF SEVERE BURNS

As a result of burns, normal skin function is diminished resulting in physiologic alterations. These include (1) *loss of protective barriers against infection*, (2) *escape of body fluids*, (3) *lack of temperature control*, (4) *destroyed sweat and sebaceous glands,* and (5) *decrease in the number of sensory receptors.* The severity of these alterations will depend on the extent of the burn and the depth to which damage has occurred.

Increased knowledge of the physiologic changes that occur during severe burns has led to the saving of many lives. There are two stages that occur *following severe burns;* the *immediate hypovolaemic stage* and *diuretic stage.*

Hypovolaemic Stage

The hypovolaemic stage begins at the time of burn injury and lasts for the first 48 to 72 hours. It is characterized by a *rapid shift of fluid from the vascular compartment into the interstitial spaces.* When tissues are burned, vasodilation, increased capillary permeability, and changes in the permeability of tissue cells in and around the burn area occur. *As a result, abnormally large amounts of extracellular fluid (ECF), sodium chloride, and protein pass through the burned area* either *to cause blister formation and local oedema* or *to escape through the open wound.*

Visible fluid loss makes up only a small part of the fluid lost from the circulating blood and other essential fluid compartments. Most of the fluid loss occurs deep in the wound, where the fluid extravasates into the deeper tissues. Burns occurring in highly vascular areas such as fluid shift than comparable burns occurring on other parts of the body. In addition, the greater the percent of injury, the greater the fluid loss. *Hypovolaemic shock* occurs, and there is a tremendous drop in blood pressure and inadequate blood flow through the kidneys, which in turn leads to further shock and anuria. Death occurs within a short time if treatment is not give promptly or is inadequate.

Respiratory distress may result from upper airways obstruction or the effects of hypovolemic shock. Upper airway obstruction is caused by inhalation of bnoxious agents or superheated air. Causing irritation of the airway, laryngeal edema, and potential obstruction.

Diuretic Stage

Return of vascular integrity begins in approximately 12 hours and rapidly progresses at 18 to 24 hours following the initial burn injury. Although full capillary integrity may not be restored for a number of days, for clinical purposes it may be considered restored at 24 hours. The diuretic stage begins at about 48 to 72 hours after the burn injury as capillary membrane integrity returns and oedema fluid shifts back from the interstitial apces into the intravascular space. Blood volume increases, leading to increased renal blood flow and diuresis unless renal damage has occurred. *Serum electrolyte* and *haematocrit levels* will be *decreased* because of *haemodilution. Fluid overload may occur as a result of the increase in intravascular volume.* The patient's vial signs, breath sounds, and urinary output are used to determine the amount of intravenous fluid replacement. Dehydration may occur if rapid urinary output depletes the intravascular reserve. A sodium deficit continues because of the loss of sodium through the burn wound and from an increase in urinary output. Hypokalaemia (lowered serum potassium) results from potassium moving back into the cells or being excreted in the urine. Protein continues to be loss from the wounds. *Metabolic acidosis remains a possibil-*

ity because of the loss of sodium bicarbonate in the urine and the increase in fat metabolism secondary to a decrease in carbohydrate intake.

Following the period of fluid shifts, the patient remains acutely ill. This period is characterised by *anaemia* and *malnutrition.* Anaemia develops from the loss of red blood cells. *Negative nitrogen balance* begins at the onset of the burn and is the result of tissue destruction, protein loss, and the stress response. It continues throughout the acute period because of continued loss of protein from the wound, tissue catabolism from immobility, and degreased protein intake. Special attention to the nutrition of the patient is important during this time. Increased metabolism from loss of water and heat from the wound, loss of fluid during diuresis, and catabolism during tissue breakdown all lead to *weight loss.*

PERIODS OF TREATMENT

Three periods of treatment can be identified in the care of the seriously burned patient. These are the *emergent,* the *acute,* and the *rehabilitative periods.*

The *emergent period* refers to the first 48 to 72 hours postburn when the patient is admitted to hospital, the severity of the injury is determined, and first aid and wound care are given. The *acute period* of treatment begins at the end of the emergent period and lasts until all of the full-thickness wounds are covered with skin grafts or partial-thickness wounds are healed. The *rehabilitation period* focuses on returning the patient to a useful place in society.

The rehabilitation of the patient actually begins during early hospitalization and is addressed throughout the hospitalization After discharge, the patient may require emotional assistance and counselling and may need to be re-admitted several times for reconstructive surgical procedures.

Comprehensive Team Approach

Comprehensive care of the burn patient can best be provided by a multidisciplinary team approach. The doctor, nurse, respiratory therapist, social workers, physiotherapist and occupational therapists, teacher and child psychologist (if a school-age child), registered dietician, religious leader and others all work together to address the needs of the patient. The *nurse's role in the team* is to *coordinate the interactions of the various disciplines* and to *incorporate the team's suggestions and approaches into an effective plan of care.*

Emergent Period

The emergent period of therapy is defined as the time required to resolve the immediate problems resulting from the burn injury. First aid measures are directed toward treating the systemic response to trauma, concurrent injuries, and the burn wound (Box 34-4).

Assessing the severity of the burn injury
Size and depth of burn

For adults, the rule of nines is used in determining the size of the burn. The percentage of body surface burned is estimated by using charts that depict anterior and posterior aspects of the body. In adults, the body is divided into areas equal to multiples of 9% (Fig 34-7). In clinical practice, the burned area is shaded in on the drawings, and the amount of body surface burned is calculated from the shaded areas. Calculations are modified for infants and children under 10 years of age because of their relatively larger head and smaller bodies (see paediatric textbooks for these figures). The depth of the burn injury is determined by appearance, colour, and sensation.

Age of victim

The severity of a burn also depends on the age of the victim. Infants under 2 years of age and adults over 60 years of age have a higher mortality than in other age groups with a similar size injury. Infants have a weak antibody response to infection and in older victims the serious burn may aggravate degenerative processes or exacerbate a pre-existing health problem.

Body part involved

The body part involved is an important factor in evaluating the severity of a burn. The anatomical part of the body burned must be considered when estimating the severity of the burn: a 3% burn of the anterior surface of the thigh will probably not be as serious as a 3% burn of the neck, face, or perineal area. Injuries that involve cosmetic and functional areas of the body require a long period of recovery because of both physical and emotional reactions to the burn injury. *A burn of the face, hands, and feet will require extensive and meticulous care. A burn of the head, neck, and chest may also involve injury to the respiratory tract and result in severe respiratory difficulty.* Burns of the perneum are difficult to manage because of the potential for contamination and infection. The *circumferential or encircling burn of a limb*, the *neck*, or the *chest has serious consequences*. This type of burn will cause *constrictive contraction of the skin* and *produce a tourniquet effect that may impair breathing and/or circulation.*

Mechanism of injury

Identifying the causative agent is of *prime importance* because the nature of the agent has a *direct effect on prognosis and treatment.* The *mechanisms* of *burn injury are flame* and *flash*, *contact*, *scald chemical*, and *electric.*

Flame and flash injuries are the second most common type of burn injury and commonly associated with an inalation injury if the burn has occurred in a closed space. These injuries may occur from house fires (caused by smoking in bed, children playing with matches) or ignited gasoline or propane. Injuries may be combined-partial and full-thickness burns. The amount and duration of the flame will determine the depth of injury.

Contact burns occur from direct contact with a hot substance, such as hot metal, stoves, hot tar, or irons. The area of burn is usually confined to the area where the substance came into contact with the skin.

Scald burns are the most common burn injury, particularly in children. Scald injury may be caused by steam or hot fluids, and may affect a widespread area.

Chemical burns, commonly seen in industry, are caused by strong acids or alkali, such as hydochloric acid and lye. Household chemical burns may occur from accidental exposure to drain cleaners, paint removers, and disinfectants. Serious burns to the eye may occur when a chemical splashes onto the face. Burns to the upper gastrointestinal tract occur when a caustic chemical is ingested.

Electrical burns consist of a small percentage of burn injuries and may be caused by lightning, or by direct to or alternating current. Injury occurs as an electrical current passes directly through the body. Tissue with the highes water content has the least resistance to electrical current

---

<table>
<tr><td>34-4</td><td>

Initial care for major burns

1. Remove victim from source of burn.
2. Douse with water and remove nonadherent, smouldering clothing to stop the burning process.
3. If chemical burn, carefully remove clothing and flush wound with large amounts of water.
4. If electrical burn and victim is still in contact with electrical source, do not touch victim. Remove electrical source with dry non conductive object (rope).
5. Establish patent airway and assess for inhalation injury. Give oxygen if available.
6. Check peripheral pulses to assess circulatory status.
7. Assess and initiate treatment for injuries requiring immediate attention.
8. Remove tight-fitting jewellery or clothing.
9. Cover burn with moist sterile or clean cover.
10. Cover victim with warm dry cover to prevent heat loss.
11. Transport victim to nearest medical facility.

</td></tr>
</table>

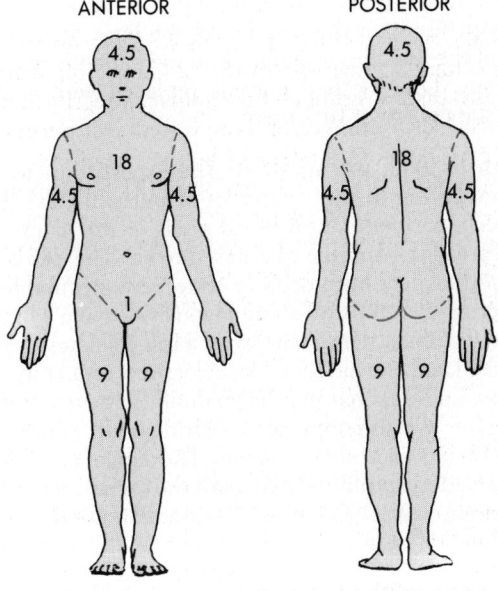

Fig. 34-7 Rule of nones

and consequently, suffers the most damage. Blood, muscles, skin tendons, fat and bones are affected in a decreasing order of resistance. Victims of electrical burns must be checked frequently for signs and symptoms of haemorrhage, intestinal perforation, and cardiac dysrhythmias. The passage of current through the body may cause cardiac arrest at the time of injury.

Pain relief

Pain in extensive burns is best controlled by gentle and minimal handling and by the application of dressings that exclude air from the burned surfaces. The degree of pain is usually inversely proportional to the depth of the burn injury—full-thickness burns cause minimal pain because nerve endings have been destroyed.

In small partial-thickness burns, cool (not cold) compresses on the burn site may provide some relief as long as the victim is kept warm.

The initial care for major burns is summarized in Box 34-4.

Acute Period

The acute period of treatment begins at the end of the emergent period and lasts until the burn wound is healed. The length of this period varies. If the burn is a partial-thickness injury, the acute period extends 10 to 20 days; if the burn is a full-thickness injury over a large percentage of the body requiring surgery for skin grafting, the acute period can last for months.

The nursing care of patients during the acute period of burns is complex. Analysis of date may lead to the identification of numerous nursing diagnoses.

During the *acute period* the *two main principles of management* are: (1) *treatment of the burn wound*, and (2) *avoidance, detection,* and *treatment of complications*. The *most common complications* are *infection* (septicaemia, pneumonia), *renal disease,* and *heart failure*.

Burn treatment methods

Different methods of treating the burned area may be used, depending on the location of the burn, its size and depth, of the facilities available, and the patient's response to therapy. One method may be replaced with another during the course of treatment.

Open or exposure method. The exposure method is used most often in the treatment of burns involving the face, neck, perineum, and broad areas of the trunk. The burned area is cleansed and exposed to air. The exudate of a partial-thickness burn dries in 48 to 72 hours and forms a hard crust then falls off spontaneously, leaving a healed, unscarred surface. The dead skin of a full-thickness burn is dehydrated and converted to black, leathery eschar in 48 to 72 hours. Loose eschar may be gradually removed through the use of hydrotherapy and debridement. uninfected eschar acts as a protective covering. The danger of infection exists as bacteria proliferate beneath the eschar. Spontaneous separation, produced by bacterial action, occurs unless surgical debridemnt is performed first.

Semiopen method. The semiopen wound car method consists of covering the wound with topical antibiotic agents and a thin layer of gauze to help keep the agent in contact with the wound. This method permits the passage of wound exudate through the dressing without the loss of antibiotic cream. The success of semiopen care depends on cleaning the wound once or twice a day. Meticulous semiopen wound care speeds debridement, enhances the development of granulation tissue, and enables earlier grafting.

Closed method. In the closed or occlusive method of burn treatment, the wound are washed and the dressings are changed at least once a day, or in some instances once each shift. Commonly, the dressing consists of gauze impregnated with topical ointments and a gauze wrap. Counter-pressure wrappings (elastic bandages) may be applied. When a dressing is in place, nursing observation includes monitoring for signs of impaired circulation (numbness, pain, and tingling) and for signs of infection (odour on dressings, elevated temperature, and elevated pulse rate).

Application of topical agents. The application of topical agents to the burn wound can help to decrease infection and hasten healing. These agents are effective because damage to blood vessels in the burn area prevents systemic antibiotics from reaching the burn wound. Antibiotics may be given prophylactically or may be withheld until an infection occurs.

Skin grafts. Skin grafts are applied to cover the burn wound and speed healing, to prevent contractures, and to shorten convalescence. Successful grafting reduces the patient's vulnerability to infection and prevents the loss of body heat and water vapour from the open wound. Grafting for cosmetic or functional purposes may be performed during the rehabilitative period. Most skin grafts are applied between the third and twenty-first day after the initial injury, depending on the depth and extent of the burn and the condition of the base.

Grafts are obtained from various sources. An autograft is a graft of skin obtained from the patient's own body. A homograft is a graft of skin obtained from a cadaver 6 to 24 hours after death. A heterograft is a graft of skin obtained from other animals, such as a pig. Synthetic substitutes for skin are currently being investigated.

Homografts may grow or "take", but in a matter of weeks they will be rejected by the body and slough off. The advantage of a temporary graft is to reduce water electrolyte, and protein loss at the burn surface. The covered wound is less painful and allows the patient freedom of movement. Temporary grafts are used until the patient is ready for autogratfts. Often autografting is delayed as a result of complications, such as pneumonia or gastric haemorrhage.

Nursing Care

Burn patients are often frightened and anxious about their injury and the associated treatments. The intensive care unit (ICU) environment can compound these responses.

Burn patients experience both physical and psychological pain. Physical pain is usually focused on specific activities such as wound cleansing and debridement, dressing changes, and physical therapy. The patient may react to physical pain in three ways: (1) by ignoring it, (2) by accepting it, or (3) by overreacting to it. The nurse should not judge whether or not the patient is feeling real pain. the nurse mush instead assess the patient's reaction to pain and intervene appropriately.

Decreasing fear and anxiety

The psychological responses of the patient in the immediate postburn period are in response to a threat to survival. The fear of death is real as the patient senses the acuity of the situation by experiencing pain, disfigurement, isolation, and dependency from being attached to machines and monitors that maintain vital functions. A variety of behaviours may be seen during the acute and emergent phase. Patients' reactions are determined by their personality, their degree of total adjustment to life, and the extent and location of their burns.

The nurse should support and encourage the patient to ease the patient's anxiety. Setting short-term, achievable goals will help to motivate the patient. Providing the family with an explanation of the patient's needs will ease their fears and allow them to encourage the patient.

Facilitating learning

During the period of recovery from a burn injury, the patient and family have enormous learning needs. During the acute period, informational needs are built from the knowledge gained on admission. Explanations of the goals of therapy and expected outcomes much be reinforced frequently because of the stress and overload the patient and family experience.

Preventing hypothermia

As in the emergent period, hypothermia remains a concern. Open burn wounds result in a significant heat loss. The patient's room must be kept at a temperature of 28 to 29 °C with a humidity of 40% to 50%. In addition, heat loss can be minimized by exposing only one burned area at a time during dressing changes.

Preventing infection

Infection control begins at the time the patient is admitted to the hospital and continues until healing is complete. Local and systemic infections (septicaemia) are the most common complications of burns and are the major cause of death, particularly in burns covering more than 25% of the body. Initially autogenous sources are the primary sources if infection because of bacteria that survive in the hair follicles and seat glands beneath the burned tissue. However, the patient is also susceptible to infection from exogenous sources.

The organisms that usually infect burns are *Staphylococcus aureus*, *Pseudomonas aeruginosa*, and the coliform bacilli. In recent years, there has been a high incidence of fungal infections resulting from the use of broad-spectrum antibiotics. *Candida albicans*, which is normally found in the gastrointestinal tract, accounts for the majority of the fungal infections. Cultures of the patient's nose, throat, wound, and unburned skin and also a punch biopsy may be taken on admission and at biweekly intervals to determine the presence of bacteria and their sensitivity to antibiotics.

To prevent the introduction of organisms into the wound, all persons who approach the patient should wear gowns, masks, caps, and gloves. Persons with upper respiratory infections should not be permitted near the patient. Surgical aseptic technique and sterile gloves are used when applying dressings. Care of the severely burned patient in special burn units can contribute to decreased infection because the environment is specifically geared to infection control. If the patient is cared for in a general hospital unit, a private room is essential and all equipment needed by the patient remains in the room. Reverse isolation precautions are initiated if the burn is greater than 25% BSA in an adult or 15% BSA in a child.

Decreasing pain

Psychological pain may be induced or exaggerated because of loneliness. The patient's complaints of pain may be a call for attention that can be met by the presence and touch of the nurse providing care. Anxiety over anticipated procedures that may or may not be painful may cause a progressive increase in the degree of pain experienced. Muscle tension related to fear and apprehension is known to lower the pain threshold. Sleep deprivation, a common occurrence in critical care units, can also make the patient less tolerant of pain. Self-hypnosis or relaxation exercises can be effective in altering the perception of either actual or anticipated discomfort and should be consistently reinforced by the team. (See Chapter 8 for further information about pain and its management.)

Providing nutritional requirements

Metabolism is increased following moderate to severe burns as a result of stress, fluid loss, fever infection, and hypercatabolism. Shivering and the elevated levels of catecholamines, cortisol, and glugagon found shortly after thermal injury increase tissue oxygen consumption and heat production, deplete liver and muscle glycogen stores and fat deposits, and lead to a negative nitrogen balance and weight loss. Protein is broken down, providing amino acids for gluconeogenesis, and amino acids are prevented from incorporating into protein. The diminished rate of protein

---

34-5

Initial treatment of major burns in the emergency room.

1. Establish airway.
2. Initiate fluid therapy by intravenous catheters.
3. Insert indwelling Foley catheter for hourly urine measurement.
4. Insert nasogastric tube to remove stomach contents and prevent gastric distention.
5. Insert central intravenous catheter, if appropriate.
6. Manage pain by intravenous narcotics in small, frequent doses.
7. Provide tetanus prophylaxis.

production prolongs wound healing and increases the patient's susceptibility to infection.

Maintenance of a nutritional support program is critical to survival and is initiated on admission. The goals of the nutritional support program are to establish eating by mouth as soon as possible and to maintain sufficient calorie and protein intake to restore tissue loss. A team approach provides comprehensive input and integrates the efforts of the patient, physician, nurse, pharmacist, dietician, and occupational and physiotherapists.

The protein and caloric needs of the burned patient are highly variable, depending on the extent and depth of injury and the patient's age, sex, preburn nutritional status, and pre-existing diseases. The daily protein requirement is greater than normal as a result of the negative nitrogen balance.

Protein is necessary for tissue repair and healing, not as a source of energy. Therefore, it is important to provide sufficient carbohydrate and fat calories to satisfy energy needs.

Rehabilitation Period

Rehabilitation begins at the time of admission. However, rehabilitation as the third stage of treatment begins when the patient's burn is reduced to less than 20% of BSA and the patient is capable of assuming some self-care activity. The principles of management are to return the patient to a productive place in society and accomplish functional and cosmetic reconstruction. It is important to remember that rehabilitation does not end when the patient is discharged; it may take from 2 to 5 years after discharge for the patient to reach a maximal level of emotional and physical adjustment.

PLASTIC SURGERY

Plastic surgery is concerned with correction or reconstruction of deformities of body structures either present at birth or resulting from disease or trauma. Purposes of the surgery include restoration of function and improvement in appearance.

General Care of the Person Having Plastic Surgery

Preparation for surgery

It is believed that any plastic surgery for an obvious defect is justified if it helps people feel they have a better chance for positive recognition. The plastic surgeon may reshape a nose or repair a deformed hand so that an emotionally stable person will feel more confidence.

Before surgery the surgeon will tell the patient what probably can be done and what changes are possible. It is important to know what the patient has been told so that misunderstandings and misinterpretations can be avoided. Preparation is necessary for the normal appearance of skin grafts and reconstructed tissue immediately after surgery. Postoperative tissue reaction may distort normal contours, suture lines may be reddened, and the colour of the newly transplanted skin may differ somewhat from that of surrounding skin. The appearance of the surgical area changes as the oedema decreases and the suture line becomes less

reddened and indurated. The scar will be less noticeable 6 months after surgery than at 6 days or 6 weeks postoperatively.

The patient who is having plastic surgery may have extensive scarring and deformity and may be exceedingly sensitive to scrutiny. On the other hand, the patient may have little apparent deformity, and it may be difficult to understand why the patient wishes to have surgery. The nurse cannot know what the disfigurement means to the individual and should avoid judgment concerning the necessity of surgery.

Many plastic surgeries are now performed on an outpatient basis. Procedures that require extensive grafting usually require hospitalization.

Maintaining psychological comfort

Plastic surgery raises many of the same concerns of other surgeries. Specific concerns may include the following:
1. Economic
   a. Possible long hospitalization and convalescence for skin grafting
   b. Elective cosmetic surgery may not be performed by the NHS
2. Physical discomfort
3. Physical appearance in postoperative period
4. Final outcome of surgery

These concerns may result in anxiety and mild depression during the first few days after surgery. Empathic communication by the nurse helps the patient identify and deal with concerns.

SKIN GRAFTING

Skin grafting consists of replacing damaged skin with healthy skin to prevent unsightly scars.

Graft Sources

Skin for grafting may be obtained from various sources. The most suitable form is the *autograft,* because it does not provoke an immune response with rejection of the graft. *Homografts* (which are temporary) may be necessary if the patient's condition is poor and if large areas must be covered, as with burns.

Types of Grafts

Plastic surgery may be performed by means of *free grafting,* which consists of cutting tissue from one part of the body and moving it directly to another part. It may also be done by leaving one end of the graft attached to the body to provide a blood supply for the graft until blood vessels form at the new place of attachment (*flap graft*).

The surgeon selects skin for grafting that is similar in texture and thickness to that which has been lost, and studies the normal lines of the skin and its elasticity to avoid noticeable scars. Scar tissue contracts with time, and in normal circumstances this is good because it produces a complete closure of the line of injury. However, in some cases scar tissue may contract in such a way that surrounding tissues are pulled out of normal contour, and distortion may result.

Free grafts

Free grafts are the most commonly used skin grafts. There are several types of free grafts, each with its advantages and limitations. Split-thickness grafts consist of epidermis and varying thicknesses of the dermis. Full-thickness grafts include the entire dermis and epidermis(Fig 34-1). The most widely used type is the intermediate or thick split-thickness graft. This can be cut into large pieces with a dermatome set to ensure a uniform thickness of the graft, and these can then be cut into smaller pieces to match the area to be grafted.

Meshed grafts are either thin or intermediate split-thickness grafts that have been placed through a perforating machine that creates a mesh. Meshed grafts are elastic and can be used to cover larger areas than the original size. They also conform more easily to irregular surfaces and can be placed over less clean bases than standard split-thickness grafts. Cosmetic appearance is poor. Meshed grafts are used frequently to cover large burned areas.

In order to survive, full-thickness grafts must develop their own blood supply (which takes 2 weeks). Regeneration of skin at the donor site is not possible because the underlying tissue has been removed. The donor site heals by *secondary* intention (Chapter 14) with scar formation.

Flap grafts

Flap grafts are used to cover larger defects than can be covered by free grafts. Flap grafts are made by cutting along three sides of a flap (two long and one short side). There are basically two major types of flap grafts. The *transposed* graft is slid over to a nearby skin area to be covered and is sutured in place. The *tube pedicle* graft is formed by suturing the long sides of the graft together to form a tube and then suturing the end to another area of the body. An intermediary site may be used, such as the forearm, in a two-step procedure, to permit moving the tube to a farther site on the body. After the graft has taken, the original site is freed and the graft is sutured to the recipient site.

Island flaps are narrow strips of neurovascular tissue from which the skin has been removed. The flap is transferred to a distant site through a tunnel made *under* the skin. The only scars that remain are at the donor and recipient sites.

Free flap grafts

Development of microsurgical techniques has permitted the use of free flaps. A large amount of tissue can be moved because blood flow is reestablished at the new site by anastomosing the donor blood vessel with a recipient site blood vessel. Some free flaps contain functional nerves that can be reattached to permit sensation at the recipient site. Surgery often takes from 4 to 12 hours. Significant peripheral disease and diabetes mellitus are contraindications for surgery.

Care of the Person with a Skin Graft

Four conditions are necessary for a graft to survive.
1. Adequate vascularization of the recipient site
2. Constant contact with the underlying tissue
3. Immobilization
4. Freedom from infection

Anything that comes between the undersurface of the graft and the recipient area, such as a discharge caused by infection, excess serous fluid, or blood, will float the graft away from close contact and may cause it to die. To prevent floating, some surgeons insert drains at strategic spots along the edges of the graft, or a small catheter is inserted on the edge of the graft under the recipient skin and attached to suction to remove the fluid.

The area is inspected frequently to see if the skin is adhering to the underlying tissue. If fluid collects under the skin graft, it is removed by aspiration with a sterile needle and syringe, or the fluid is rolled to the wound edge with a sterile applicator.

A wide variety of materials are used as dressings. The choice depends on the kind of graft and the surgeon's preference. Often the graft is covered with a piece of coarse mesh gauze anchored to the adjacent skin edges with an elastic bandage to give firm, gentle pressure and to immobilize the area. The first dressing may be covered with a compress of sterile normal saline solution. Because the compress is moist, it fits the contour of the wound better. Continuous pressure is necessary to keep the graft adherent to the recipient bed, but pressure should not be so firm as to cause death of the graft.

Inner dressings on the recipient site are usually changed by the surgeon 1 to 2 days after surgery, and it is usually possible to know then whether the result of the operation is satisfactory.

Before patients with skin grafts are discharged, they need to know how to care for the recipient and donor sites at home until healing has occurred (Box 34-6).

Care of the Patient Undergoing Microvascular Surgery (Free Flaps)

Patients are instructed to refrain from smoking for 1 week before microvascular surgery because of the profound vasoconstrictive effect of nicotine.[54] If trauma has been experienced before surgery, anticoagulant therapy is given to prevent microthrombi in the flap. Following surgery, the patient may be transferred to the intensive care unit for continuous flap monitoring.

The major complication is necrosis of the transposed tissue, resulting from decreased circulation from arterial or venous thrombosis at the flap site. *Arterial* thrombosis may result in complete flap failure within hours after onset; it is

---

Patient Teaching 34-6

The patient with a skin graft

Keep surface of healed graft moistened daily with a skin lotion for 6 to 12 months. (Grafted skin does not sweat; it dries and cracks easily.)
Protect grafted skin from direct sunlight with a sunscreen lotion for at least 6 months.
Wear a strong elastic stocking for 4 to 6 months with grafts on lower extremities.
Report changes in the graft (haematoma, fluid collection) to doctor.

characterized by pallor or coolness of the flap, and no bleeding when the flap is stuck with a needle. *Venous thrombosis* is less critical and occurs more slowly. It is characterized by a warm, mottled flap that oozes dark blood (from continued arterial blood flow); arterial occlusion will eventually occur.[54]

Circulation of the flap may be monitored by a *laser Doppler* that measures the average blood flow from a probe at the flap site. If the postoperative reading falls to below 50% of the preoperative baseline, the surgeon is notified.[16] A second, more precise method of monitoring blood flow is with a photoplethysmographic (PPG) disc. The disc is applied to the flap surface and measures reflected light from pulsatile changes in tissue blood flow.[54] Changes are reflected in waveforms on a monitor.

If the legs are not involved in the surgery, ambulation is started after 24 hours. Involved extremities are elevated to prevent venous engorgement. The patient may be given nothing by mouth for 48 hours in case further surgery for flap ischaemia is necessary.

SCOSMETIC SURGERY

Removal of Skin Markings

Disfiguring marks on the skin may be removed by abrasive action (dermabrasion), by changing the colour through medical dermatattooing, or by laser facial resurfacing.

Either local or general anaesthesia is used for *dermabrasion*. The skin is abraded with a diamond fraise. There is postoperative swelling, discomfort, crusting, and erythema, which may persist for several weeks. The procedure may be done in stages. A hydrogel dressing is applied after surgery. At home, the patient removes the dressing every 12 hours and compresses the surgical area for 15 to 30 minutes with cloths soaked in lukewarm tap water.[34] A new hydrogel dressing is then applied. New skin regenerates in 8 to 10 days.

Medical dermatattooing is performed on an ambulatory basis; no anaesthesia is used, although a sedative may be prescribed to be taken 1 hour before surgery. The procedure is done in several stages; pigment is impregnated into the skin with a tattooing needle. The skin is left exposed to air to dry and crust. An ice bag may be applied to relieve postoperative discomfort. N.B. Not all cosmetic surgery is offered within the NHS.

Laser Surface Resurfacing

Done with a CO_2 laser, this technique may be used to remove skin markings or wrinkles and premalignant lesions.[51] The procedure is done with the patient under general anaesthesia. The CO_2 laser beam destroys bacteria in addition to tissue, therefore risk of infection is decreased. Nerve endings are also destroyed, leading to minimal postoperative discomfort. Following surgery, antibiotic ointment is applied to the surgical area and covered with petroleum-based gauze and dry dressings. After 3 days the dressing is removed and the patient applies frequent warm moist compresses as instructed, to soften and remove skin crusts. Sunscreen must be used for at least 6 months after healing.[51] Types of laser therapy are now used to remove an unwanted tattoo.

SUMMARY

1. Skin disorders that produce marked visual disfigurement may result in alterations in body image and self-esteem.

2. Bacterial skin infections include folliculitis (infections of the hair follicle), furuncles (deep folliculitis), carbuncles (cluster of furuncles), or cellulitis (diffuse infection of skin and subcutaneous tissue); treatment includes warm soaks or hot moist dressings, and topical or systemic antibiotics.

3. Viral skin inflammations include herpes simplex, herpes zoster, and warts; acyclovir is given for herpes simplex in immunocompromised patients and for herpes zoster.

4. Fungal skin inflammations include candidiasis and the dermatophytoses (tinea capitis, corporis, cruris, and pedis); treatment includes topical or oral antifungal drugs.

5. Parasitic infestations include those by lice or scabies mite; treatment includes a topical pediculocide/scabicide.

6. Dermatitis may result from contact with irritants, as an atopic (hypersensitivity) reaction, from stasis of circulation in the legs, or from unknown cause (dandruff). Dressings moistened with aluminium acetate solution and topical steroids may be used for uninfected weeping lesions, and antibiotics may be used for infected lesions.

7. The most common papulosquamous disorder is psoriasis, a chronic condition resulting from rapid cell mitosis. Exacerbations of psoriasis may be treated with occlusive wraps over topical steroid therapy; crude tar therapy, alone or in combination with ultraviolet light; or PUVA therapy.

8. Nonmalignant skin lesions are primarily keratoses (corns, calluses, seborrhoeic keratosis, actinic keratosis) that are characterized by overgrowth and thickening of the epithelium; actinic keratoses result from solar irradiation and may become squamous cell carcinomas.

9. Premalignant lesions include leukoplakia (white or red patches), which may develop into invasive squamous cell carcinoma, and pigmented moles, which may develop into melanoma. Moles that change appearance in colour, size, loss of hair, or bleeding should be reported to the doctor.

10. Squamous cell carcinoma, which may metastasize, and basal cell carcinoma, which rarely metastasizes, may be removed by surgical excision and curettage with electrodesiccation, cryosurgery, or irradiation.

11. Malignant melanomas have a high incidence of metastasis and mortality; they are treated by radical excision, chemotherapy, and immunotherapy.

12. The severity of alarm injury depends on the age of the victim, body part involved, burning agent, size and depth of the burn wound, and the victim's medical history.

13. The initial systemic responce to a burn is the shift of fluid from the intravascular to the interstitial space, creating hypovolemia. After 48 to 72 hours the fluid shifts from the interststial to the intravascular space and hypervolemia occurs.

14. Free grafts (split-thickness, full-thickness) are sections of epidermis and dermis that are taken from a donor area and transplanted to a distant area. Flap grafts include subcutaneous tissue, and one end remains attached to the donor site. Free flap grafts contain skin, subcutaneous tissue, and a major blood vessel, which are transplanted to a distant site with anastomosis of the blood vessel with a recipient vessel.

15. Care of the person with a graft includes (1) applying firm dressings, to maintain graft contact with the underlying tissue; (2) preventing collection of fluid under the graft, to protect against separation of the graft; (3) protecting the graft site from excess pressure and motion, to promote vascularization and prevent separation; and (4) using aseptic technique, to prevent infection.

STUDY QUESTIONS

- Why are counselling and teaching the major nursing strategies for persons with skin disorders?
- Which skin disorders have pruritus as a symptom? What approaches help modify pruritus?
- Mrs. B. tells you that she is thinking about buying a new over-the-counter drug which, although expensive, is being advertised as a cure for psoriasis. Which of the following health teaching approaches would be *most* effective? Explain:
  a. Tell Mrs. B not to waste her money because psoriasis cannot be cured.
  b. Explore her knowledge of psoriasis and experiences she has had with previous therapies.
  c. Suggest she check first with her doctor before buying the drug.
- How would you explain to a family member the pysiological changes following burn injury?
- Explain in your own words the differences among the various types of skin grafts. Why is the postoperative care different from free flap grafts than for other types of grafts?

REFERENCES AND SELECTED READINGS

1. American Cancer Society: *Cancer facts and figures 1991*, Atlanta, 1991, The Society.
2.* Berliner H: Aging skin, pt 1, *Am J Nurs* 86:1138-1141, 1986.
3.* Berliner H: Aging skin, pt 2, *Am J Nurs* 86:1259-1261, 1986.
4.* Bodey GP: Topical and systemic antifungal agents, *Med Clin North Am* 72:637-659, 1988.
5. Buxton PK: ABC of dermatology: eczema and inflammatory dermatoses, *Br Med J* 295:1112-1114, 1987.
6.* Cohen K: Free-flap surgery: nurses make it work, *RN* 51(3):26-29, 1988.
7.* Crawford E et al: Mohs' chemosurgery: day surgery for cutaneous malignancies, *AORN J* 43:464-468, 1986.
8.* Cuzzell JZ: Clues: itching and burning in skin folds, *Am J Nurs* 19(1):23-24, 1990.
9.* Cuzzell JZ: Clues: recurrent, punched-out lesions, *Am J Nurs* 90(5):21-22, 1990.
10.* Cuzzell JZ: Clues: pain, burning, and itching, *Am J Nurs* 90(7):15-16, 1990.
11.* Dolsky RL, Newman J, Fetzek JR: Liposuction: history, techniques, and complications, *Dermatol Clin* 5:313-334, 1987.
12.* Dunn ML, Cockerline EB, Rice MR: Treatment options for psoriasis, *Am J Nurs* 88:1082-1087, 1988.
13.* Epstein E: Common skin disorders, ed 3, Oradell, NJ, 1988, Medical Economics Books.
14.* Feder HM, Renfro L, Schmidt DD: Common questions about herpes simplex, *Hosp Pract* 24(1A):50-62, 1989.
15.* Goodman T: Grafts and flaps in plastic surgery, *AORN J* 48:650-663, 1988.
16.* Goodman T, White S: Microvascular reconstruction: nursing management, *AORN J* 48:666-676, 1988.
17.* Greany D, Goldsmith HS: Cutaneous melanoma: diagnosis and surgical intervention, *AORN J* 42:43-49, 1985.
18.* Gurevich I: Counseling the patient with herpes, *RN* 53(2):22-28, 1990.
19.* Habif TP: *Clinical dermatology: a color guide to diagnosis and treatment*, ed 2, St Louis, 1990, Mosby–Year Book.
20.* Harber LC, Whitman GB: Photosensitivity: classification, *Dermatol Clin* 4:167-170, 1986.
21.* Hartwig PA: Lasers in dermatology, *Nurs Clin North Am* 25(3):657-666, 1990.
22.* Hetland JR: Scabies: managing an outbreak, *Geriatr Nurs* 8:319-321, 1987.
23.* Hood LM: Scabies: are your patients at risk? *Geriatr Nurs* 8:312-315, 1987.
24.* Kaplan AP et al: Allergic skin disorders, *JAMA* 258:2900-2909, 1987.
25.* Kleinsmith D, Perricone NV: Common skin problems in the elderly, *Dermatol Clin* 4:485-499, 1986.
26.* Klotz RW: Herpetic whitlow: an occupational hazard, *JAANA* 58(1):8-12, 1990.
27. Kopf AW: Prevention and early detection of skin cancer/melanoma, *Cancer* 62(8):1791-1795, 1988.
28.* Lawler PE: Be sunsensible: steps toward safety in the sun, *Oncol Nurs Forum* 16(3):424-427, 1989.
29.* Lawler PE, Schreiber S: Cutaneous malignant melanoma: nursing's role in prevention and early detection, *Oncol Nurs Forum* 16(3):345-352, 1989.
30.* LeFort SM: Herpes zoster and postherpetic neuralgia: the need for early intervention in the elderly, *Nurs Pract* 14(3):30-41, 1989.
31.* Loeser JD: Herpes zoster and postherpetic neuralgia, *Pain* 25:149-164, 1986.
32.* Lombardo BL et al: Group support for derm patients, *Am J Nurs* 88:1088-1090, 1988.
33.* Lynn MM, Holdcroft C: Treatment for fungal skin infections: an update, *Nurse Pract* 14(8):64-71, 1989.
34.* McKinnon CC, Fulton JE: Facial dermabrasion, *AORN J* 51:739-750, 1990.
35.* Moosny J: What's wrong with this patient? . . . scabies, *RN* 52(5):61-63, 1989.
36.* Moschella SL, Hurley HA: *Dermatology*, ed 3, Philadelphia, 1991, WB Saunders.
37.* Nichol NH: Atopic dermatitis: the (wet) wrap up, *Am J Nurs* 87:1560-1563, 1987.
38.* Novotny J: Adolescents, acne, and the side-effects of Accutane, *Pediatr Nurs* 15:247-248, 1989.
39.* Parks BR, Smith D: Treatment of head lice and scabies infestations in children, *Pediatr Nurs* 15:522-524, 1989.
40. Pathak MA: Sunscreens: topical and systemic approaches for prevention of acute and chronic sun-induced skin reactions, *Dermatol Clin* 4:321-334, 1986.
40a.* Phillips TJ, Dover JS: Recent advances in dermatology, *New Eng J Med* 326(3):167-177, 1992.
41.* Prigel DL: How to spot melanoma, *Nursing 87* 17(6):60-62, 1987.
42.* Quan M et al: Management of acne vulgaris, *Am Fam Physician* 38:207-218, 1988.
43.* Reese JL: Nursing interventions for wound healing in plastic and reconstructive surgery, *Nurs Clin North Am* 25(1):223-233, 1990.
44.* Reeves JR: Head lice and scabies in children, *Pediatr Infect Dis* 6:598-602, 1987.
45.* Rosenbaum M: Pruritus of unknown origin, *Hosp Pract* 23(10A):19-22, 1988.
46.* Roy DJ: Caring for self-esteem of the cosmetic patient, *Plast Surg Nurs* 6:138-141, 1986.
47.* Sauer GC: *Manual of skin diseases*, ed 6, Philadelphia, 1991, JB Lippincott.
48.* Schaefer DG, Wolf JE: Common dermatological disorders, *Clin Plast Surg* 14:201-208, 1987.
49.* Schroeder SA et al: *Current medical diagnosis and treatment*, Norwalk, Conn, 1991, Appleton & Lange.
50.* Sheahan SL, Seabolt JP: Management of common parasitic infections encountered in primary care, *Nurse Pract* 12(8):19-33, 1987.
51.* Spadoni D, Cain CL: Facial resurfacing: using the carbon dioxide laser, *AORN J* 50:1007-1013, 1989.

*Recommended for student reading.

52.* Stahl S, Hamilton S, Spira M: Surgical treatment of acne scars, *Clin Plast Surg* 14:261-276, 1987.

53.* Stern C: Melanoma, the most lethal skin cancer, *RN* 50(7):12-14, 1987.

54.* Swain D, Shell DH: Microvascular tissue transfer: perioperative nursing considerations, *AORN J* 49:1032-104 3, 1989.

55. Toback AC, Anders JE: Phototoxicity from systemic agents, *Dermatol Clin* 4:223-229, 1986.

56.* Way LW: Current surgical diagnoses and treatment, ed 9, Norwalk, Conn, 1991, Appleton & Lange.

57.* Wyngaarden JB, Smith LH: Textbook of medicine, ed 18, Philadelphia, 1988, WB Saunders.

FURTHER READING

Buxton PK: *ABC of Dermatology,* impression 5, London, 1991, British Medical Association.

du Vivier A: *Atlas of Clinical Dermatology,* Edinburgh, 1986, Churchill Livingstone.

Marrs R: An individual approach to ease frustration. Support for people with eczema, *Professional Nurse* 5(10):522-528, 1990.

Osborne P: Out in the mid-day sun? Nurses' perceptions of the dangers of sun exposure, *The Professional Nurse* 4(10):496-500, 1989.

Stone LA, Lindfield EM and Robertson S: *A Colour Atlas of Nursing Procedures in Skin Disorders,* London, 1989, Wolfe Medical Publications Limited.